TEXTBOOK OF PATHOLOGY

TEXTBOOK OF PATHOLOGY

Rajeswari Kathiah, MD, DNB, MNAMS, DipRCPath, FIME

Head, Department of Pathology
All India Institute of Medical Sciences (AIIMS)
Madurai, Tamil Nadu, India

Gayathri Devi Thanigaimani, MD, DRCOG

Professor, Department of Pathology
Panimalar Medical College Hospital & Research Institute
Chennai, Tamil Nadu, India

Indhu Kannan, MD, DNB, MNAMS, DipRCPath

Consultant Pathologist
Meenakshi Mission Hospital
Madurai, Tamil Nadu, India

ELSEVIER

ELSEVIER

RELX India Pvt. Ltd.
Registered Office: 818, 8th Floor, Indraprakash Building, 21, Barakhamba Road, New Delhi 110 001
Corporate Office: 14th Floor, Building No. 10B, DLF Cyber City, Phase II, Gurgaon-122 002, Haryana, India

Textbook of Pathology, Second Edition, Rajeswari Kathiah, Gayathri Devi Thanigaimani, Indhu Kannan

ISBN: 978-81-312-6983-1
eISBN: 978-81-312-6985-5

Content Strategist: Chandan Kumar
Content Project Manager: Goldy Bhatnagar
Sr Production Executive: Dhan Singh Rana
Sr Graphic Designer: Milind Majgaonkar

Typeset by GW Tech India

Printed in India by Sanat Printers

Preface to the Second Edition

The field of medical education is ever-evolving, and the need for continuous improvement is undeniable. In 2019, the Medical Council of India (MCI) introduced a competency-based curriculum for medical graduates, revolutionizing medical education in India. This new curriculum is designed to be more learner- and patient-centric and outcome- and context-oriented.

Pathology, as a discipline, has witnessed remarkable advancements, especially in areas such as immunopathology and molecular pathology. Additionally, the integration of digital and spatial pathology is transforming diagnostic processes and treatment protocols.

The second edition of our textbook strives to reflect these advancements and align with the new educational framework. We have meticulously structured the book to be practical and user-friendly. Each chapter begins with a list of critical competencies, directly linked to the content that follows. We have incorporated "must-read" topics, scenario-based self-assessment questions, and sections for self-directed learning to cater to inquisitive minds.

New to this edition, we have added mind maps for complex topics, facilitating better retention and recollection. These visual aids are designed to help learners grasp intricate concepts more effectively. To further align with the new assessment methods, we have included scenario-based MCQs with answers at the end of every chapter. Additionally, we have enriched the content with many more pictures to enhance understanding.

Understanding the pressures of competitive exams that students face at the end of their MBBS course, we have tailored the content to support exam preparation and success.

Reflecting on the words of Dr Stanley L Robbins from the first edition of the Textbook of Pathology (1957):

"The pathologist is interested not only in the recognition of structural alterations but also in their significance, i.e., the effects of these changes on cellular and tissue function and ultimately the effects on the patient. It is not a discipline isolated from the living patient but rather a basic approach to a better understanding of disease and therefore a foundation of sound clinical medicine."

We present this quote to highlight the crucial role of the pathologist in the patient care team. Our hope is that this book not only answers the 'why' and 'how' of disease processes but also ignites a passion for pathology, making your learning journey both meaningful and enjoyable.

Rajeswari Kathiah
Gayathri Devi Thanigaimani
Indhu Kannan

Preface to the First Edition

Change is inevitable and medical education is not an exemption. While the traditional curriculum has been in practice for decades, in 2019, the Medical Council of India (MCI) has rolled out a competency-based curriculum for medical graduates, marking a major landmark for medical education in India. The new curriculum attempts to make medical education in India more learner- and patient-centric, gender-sensitive, and outcome- and context-oriented.

Vast strides have also been made in the field of Pathology, embracing rapidly growing branches like immunopathology and molecular pathology. Further innovations in digital and spatial pathology are continuing to be made to adopt the developments in science and technology that can help improve its process.

Any textbook that attempts to provide an overview of Pathology today must incorporate the learner-patient centric competencies needed for success, and the emerging techniques and procedures driving the future of the field. The authors here have endeavoured to do just that.

We have designed the book to have a practical, easy-to-follow structure. The critical competencies have been enlisted at the beginning of every chapter and mapped to the content inside. The "must read" topics, scenario-based self-assessment questions to aid learning and topics for self-directed learning for the inquisitive minds have been included for each chapter. We have centred the content to meet the needs of the learner and have also made them simple and interesting to ensure that the process of learning is enjoyable.

We, the authors have borne in mind the various competitive exams students need to undertake at the end of their MBBS course for progress in their career while preparing the content of the book and attempted to make justice to that as well.

In the first edition of the *Textbook of Pathology (1957)*, Dr Stanley L Robbins, the founding author of perhaps the best known of all pathology textbooks, stated:

"The pathologist is interested not only in the recognition of structural alterations, but also in their significance, i.e, the effects of these changes on cellular and tissue function and ultimately the effect of these changes on the patient. It is not a discipline isolated from the living patient, but rather a basic approach to a better understanding of disease and therefore a foundation of sound clinical medicine."

We leave you with this quote to emphasise the role of the pathologist in the patient care team. Our hope is that this book inspires you to ask 'why' and 'how' and helps you unravel the mysteries behind the various disease processes thereby making you fall in love with this subject.

Rajeswari Kathiah
Gayathri Devi Thanigaimani
Indhu Kannan

Acknowledgements

Dear Readers,
Creating a textbook is a collective effort, and this second edition of the Textbook of Pathology is no exception.

I owe a tremendous amount of gratitude to my dear father, **Mr Kathiah**, whose unwavering belief in my success motivated me to write this textbook, and my mother, **Mrs Sundari Kathiah**, whose love and blessings saw me through this journey. I could not have completed this work without the continual support of my dear soulmate, **Mr Veerasingam**, and my adorable daughters, **Harini** and **Shalini**. Special thanks also to my dear mother-in-law, **Ms Muthulakshmi**, my sweet brother, **Mr Saravanan**, and my dear sister, **Ms Vidyavathy**, for their unconditional love and support throughout my career.

I am deeply indebted to the support offered by my HODs of my previous institution, Professor **Dr Rajalakshmi** and Professor **Dr Meenakshisundaram**, who greatly encouraged and motivated me in writing this book.

Gratitude is also due to my ever-enthusiastic students of AIIMS, Madurai for continuing to inspire me to learn and teach.

Many persons associated with our publisher, Elsevier, deserve our special thanks. Their understanding of our needs, prompt responses, and charming attitudes helped us significantly in reducing stress and simplifying our lives. I would like to extend special mention to the RELX team, with special thanks to Arvind Koul (Head - Content Strategy, Education), Chandan Kumar (Content Strategist), and Goldy Bhatnagar (Content Project Manager) for their exceptional contributions.

I am profoundly grateful to my dear friends who support and stand by me in all my ventures. Your unwavering encouragement has been a pillar of strength throughout this journey.

Special thanks to the contributors for accepting to contribute and completing the task on time. I am also thankful to my dear departmental colleagues and the entire team at **AIIMS, Madurai**, whose immense support made this work possible.

Finally, I would like to acknowledge with gratitude my co-authors, **Dr Indhu** and **Dr Gayathri**, for their tireless work, commitment, and collaboration. I take great pride in working alongside these intelligent professionals and will remain humbled by their dedication.

I must also acknowledge the role of my mentor, **Prof Dr Rajendiran**, whose infectious enthusiasm made me fall in love with this wonderful subject. His guidance and passion have been truly inspiring.

There are many others who may have been left out unintentionally—my special thanks and apologies to all of them.

Rajeswari Kathiah

Dear Readers,
Thank you for choosing our book in your pursuit of pathology. At this juncture, I must express my heartfelt gratitude to many individuals who have been instrumental in my journey. While the list is extensive and difficult to fully enumerate here, I wish to highlight a few significant contributors. Rest assured, those not mentioned by name due to time and space constraints have also played vital roles in my development as a doctor, teacher, and now author.

First and foremost, I extend my deepest thanks to my coauthors, **Dr Rajeswari** and **Dr Indhu**. Their belief in my capabilities and willingness to collaborate has been fundamental to bringing this book to fruition. Our partnership, which began as a casual acquaintance, has blossomed into a labor of passion and commitment. I also appreciate the team at Elsevier for offering me my initial opportunity to become an author.

My family's unwavering support has been the cornerstone of this achievement. My husband, **Dr D Balaji**, has always provided me with complete freedom and encouragement in all my endeavors. My children, **Srividya** and **Varsha**, have graciously sacrificed "mother time" to allow me the space to complete this book. My mother, **Dr A Sivathalam**, has been a constant source of encouragement, while my brother, **Dr T Karthikeyan**, has persistently motivated me to reach greater heights. I also fondly remember my late father, **Mr KP Thanigaimani**, whose faith in my abilities has always driven me to excel.

I am deeply grateful to my professors, **Dr Hemalatha Ganapathy** and **Dr V Rajalakshmi**, who have imparted not only knowledge but also moral values that have shaped my professional journey. The management of **Panimalar Medical College** has been immensely supportive, providing a platform for me to achieve significant milestones. My dear undergraduate students have served as my brand ambassadors, and their enthusiasm has been both inspiring and rewarding.

I also wish to thank my friends from both undergraduate and postgraduate years, especially **Dr R Rajamahendran**, who sparked my passion for teaching. My colleagues and the college administration have made my professional life both beautiful and enjoyable, for which I am profoundly grateful.

In conclusion, this book is a testament to the collective efforts of many wonderful individuals. While I cannot name everyone here, please know that your contributions have been invaluable. This journey from being a doctor to becoming an author has been enriched by your support and encouragement. Thank you all for being an integral part of this journey.

Gayathri Devi Thanigaimani

Dear Readers,
I am deeply indebted to my mentor and my dear friend, **Dr Rajeswari Kathiah**. This book would be immeasurably poor or worse, non-existent without her vision, guidance, and commitment. I am proud of this opportunity to collaborate with her and see firsthand what a stellar professional she is. I am also happy to have worked with **Dr Gayathri** and will cherish this time for ever.

I would like to express my sincere gratitude to **Meenakshi Mission Hospital**, my esteemed institute, for providing me with a supportive and stimulating environment that has fostered my growth and development. The resources, guidance, and opportunities offered by the institute have been invaluable to my progress, and I am deeply thankful for the experience and knowledge gained during my time here. Thank you, Meenakshi Mission Hospital, for helping me unlock my potential and shaping me into the person I am today.

My gratitude also extends to the publisher, Elsevier, for endorsing our work, and for their exceptionally helpful management of this assignment.

Finally, I wish to express my eternal gratitude for the love and support I receive from my friends, family, and extended family, in particular, my husband **Dr Karthikeyan**, my little angel **Riya**, my parents, **Mr and Mrs Kannan**, my dear sister and family and the enduring blessings from **Dr VS Subramanian**, my father in law. This would have proved impossible without them.

Indhu Kannan

Contributors

Dr Rajeswari Kathiah, MD, DNB, MNAMS, DipRCPath, FIME
Head, Department of Pathology
All India Institute of Medical Sciences (AIIMS)
Madurai, Tamil Nadu, India

Dr Gayathri Devi Thanigaimani, MD, DRCOG
Professor, Department of Pathology
Panimalar Medical College Hospital & Research Institute
Chennai, Tamil Nadu, India

Dr Indhu Kannan, MD, DNB, MNAMS, DipRCPath
Consultant Pathologist
Meenakshi Mission Hospital
Madurai, Tamil Nadu, India

Dr V Rajalakshmi, MD
Professor & Head of Pathology
Panimalar Medical College Hospital & Research Institute
Poonamallee, Chennai, Tamil Nadu, India

Dr K Meenakshisundaram, MD
Professor & Head, Department of Pathology
ESIC Medical College & PGIMSR
KK Nagar, Chennai, Tamil Nadu, India

Dr Leena Dennis Joseph, MD
Professor of Pathology
Sri Ramachandra Institute of Higher Education & Research
Porur, Chennai, Tamil Nadu, India

Dr V Eswari, MD
Professor & Head of Pathology
Meenakshi Medical College & Hospital
Kancheepuram, Tamil Nadu, India

Dr S Shanmugapriya, DCP, DNB, PDCC (Nephropath)
Professor of Pathology
ESIC Medical College & PGIMSR
Rajaji Nagar, Bangalore, Karnataka, India

Dr M Lavanya, MD
Professor of Pathology
Sri Venkateshwaraa Medical College Hospital & RC
Ariyur, Puducherry, India

Dr A Sathish Selvakumar, MD
Associate Professor of Pathology
ESIC Medical College & Hospital
Bihta, Patna, Bihar, India

Dr G Anushuya, MD
Associate Professor of Pathology
ESIC Medical College & PGIMSR
KK Nagar, Chennai, Tamil Nadu, India

Dr A Sivaramakrishnan, MD (TM)
Associate Professor of Transfusion Medicine
ESIC Medical College & PGIMSR
KK Nagar, Chennai, Tamil Nadu, India

Dr Vimala Chelladurai, MD
Laboratory Director
Premier Health Center
Chennai, Tamil Nadu, India

Dr Ramya Krishna, D, MD, DNB
Senior resident of Pathology
ESIC Medical College & PGIMSR
KK Nagar, Chennai, Tamil Nadu, India

Reviewers for the Second Edition

Dr Dinisha Einstien, MD
Associate Professor of Pathology
Panimalar Medical College Hospital & Research Institute
Poonamallee, Chennai, Tamil Nadu, India

Dr Prathiba Arumugam, MD
Professor of Pathology
Panimalar Medical College Hospital & Research Institute
Poonamallee, Chennai, Tamil Nadu, India

Dr M Ranjani, MD
Assistant Professor of Pathology
ESIC Medical College & PGIMSR
KK Nagar, Chennai, Tamil Nadu, India

Dr Norton Stephen, MD, DNB
Assistant Professor of Pathology
All India Institute of Medical Sciences (AIIMS)
Madurai, Tamil Nadu, India

Dr Sarumathy Ganesan, MD
Associate Professor of Pathology
Panimalar Medical College Hospital & Research Institute
Poonamallee, Chennai, Tamil Nadu, India

Dr Valli Priyaa, MD, PDF (Nephro)
Assistant Professor of Pathology
All India Institute of Medical Sciences (AIIMS)
Madurai, Tamil Nadu, India

Dr VS Karthikeyan, DNB, DMRD, EDIR
Consultant Radiologist
Aarthi Scans & Labs
Madurai, Tamil Nadu, India

Contents

Competency Map: Pathology

Competency Code	Competency	Core (Y/N)	Chapter No.	Page No.
PA 2.1	Demonstrate knowledge of the causes, mechanisms, types and effects of cell injury and their clinical significance.	Y	2	26
PA 2.2	Describe the etiology of cell injury. Distinguish between reversible-irreversible injury: mechanisms; morphology of cell injury.	Y	2	27, 30
PA 2.3	Intracellular accumulation of fats, proteins, carbohydrates, pigments.	Y	2	45
PA 2.4	Describe and discuss Cell death- types, mechanisms, necrosis, apoptosis (basic as contrasted with necrosis), autolysis.	Y	2	32, 37, 43
PA 2.5	Describe and discuss pathologic calcifications, gangrene.	Y	2	34, 48
PA 2.6	Describe and discuss cellular adaptations: atrophy, hypertrophy, hyperplasia, metaplasia, dysplasia.	Y	2	22
PA 2.7	Describe and discuss the mechanisms of cellular aging and apoptosis.	N	2	37, 50
PA 4.1	Define and describe the general features of acute and chronic inflammation including stimuli, vascular and cellular events.	Y	3	57
PA 4.2	Enumerate and describe the mediators of acute inflammation.	Y	3	66
PA 4.3	Define and describe chronic inflammation including causes, types, nonspecific and granulomatous, and enumerate examples of each.	Y	3	74
PA 5.1	Define and describe the process of repair and regeneration including wound healing and its types.	Y	3	80
PA 6.1	Define and describe oedema and its types, pathogenesis and clinical correlations.	Y	4	100
PA 6.2	Define and describe hyperaemia, congestion and haemorrhage.	Y	4	97, 99
PA 6.3	Define and describe shock and its pathogenesis and stages.	Y	4	116
PA 6.4	Define and describe normal haemostasis and the aetiopathogenesis and consequences of thrombosis.	Y	4	103, 106
PA 6.5	Define and describe embolism and its causes and common types.	Y	4	111
PA 6.6	Define and describe ischaemia–infarction, its types, aetiology, morphological changes and clinical effects.	Y	4	114
PA 11.1	Describe the pathogenesis and features of common cytogenetic abnormalities and mutations in childhood.	N	5	125
PA 11.3	Describe the pathogenesis of common storage disorders in infancy and childhood.	N	5	131
PA 9.1	Describe the principles and mechanisms involved in immunity.	Y	6	157

Competency Code	Competency	Core (Y/N)	Chapter No.	Page No.
PA 9.2	Describe the mechanism of hypersensitivity reactions.	Y	6	170
PA 9.3	Describe the HLA system and the immune principles in transplant and mechanism of transplant rejection.	Y	6	165, 205
PA 9.4	Define autoimmunity. Enumerate autoimmune disorders.	Y	6	178
PA 9.5	Define and describe the pathogenesis of systemic lupus erythematosus.	Y	6	178
PA 9.6	Define and describe the pathogenesis and pathology of HIV and AIDS.	Y	6	197
PA 9.7	Define and describe the pathogenesis of other common autoimmune diseases.	N	6	178
PA 3.1	Describe the pathogenesis and pathology of amyloidosis.	Y	6	210
PA 7.1	Define and classify neoplasia. Describe the characteristics of neoplasia including gross, microscopy, biology, behaviour and spread. Differentiate benign from malignant neoplasms.	Y	7	222
PA 7.2	Describe the molecular basis of cancer.	Y	7	233
PA 7.3	Enumerate carcinogens and describe the process of carcinogenesis.	Y	7	254
PA 7.4	Describe the effects of tumour on the host including paraneoplastic syndrome.	Y	7	261
PA 7.5	Describe immunology and the immune response to cancer.	N	7	248
PA 10.1	Define and describe the pathogenesis and pathology of malaria.	Y	8	299
PA 10.2	Define and describe the pathogenesis and pathology of cysticercosis.	Y	8	304
PA 10.3	Define and describe the pathogenesis and pathology of leprosy.	Y	8	285
PA 10.4	Define and describe the pathogenesis and pathology of common bacterial, viral, protozoal and helminthic diseases.	N	8	276, 282, 286, 291, 292, 293, 294, 301, 302, 304, 306, 307
PA 12.1	Enumerate and describe the pathogenesis of disorders caused by air pollution, tobacco and alcohol.	Y	9	315, 319, 321
PA 12.2	Describe the pathogenesis of disorders caused by protein–calorie malnutrition and starvation.	Y	9	332
PA 12.3	Describe the pathogenesis of obesity and its consequences.	Y	9	339
PA 11.2	Describe the pathogenesis and pathology of tumour and tumour-like conditions in infancy and childhood.	N	10	360
PA 8.1	Describe the diagnostic role of cytology and its application in clinical care.	Y	11	370
PA 8.2	Describe the basis of exfoliative cytology including the technique and stains used.	Y	11	372
PA 23.1	Describe abnormal urinary findings in disease states and identify and describe common urinary abnormalities in a clinical specimen.	Y	11	380

Competency Code	Competency	Core (Y/N)	Chapter No.	Page No.
PA 23.2	Describe abnormal findings in body fluids in various disease states.	Y	11	386
PA 23.3	Describe and interpret the abnormalities in a panel containing semen analysis, thyroid function tests, renal function tests or liver function tests.	Y	11	391
PA 35.3	Identify the aetiology of meningitis based on given cerebrospinal fluid (CSF) parameters.	Y	11	389
PA 25.6	Interpret liver function and viral hepatitis serology panels. Distinguish obstructive from nonobstructive jaundice based on clinical features and liver function tests.	Y	11	393
PA 27.1	Distinguish arteriosclerosis from atherosclerosis. Describe the pathogenesis and pathology of various causes and types of arteriosclerosis.	Y	13	428, 429
PA 27.2	Describe the aetiology, dynamics, pathology types and complications of aneurysms including aortic aneurysms.	Y	13	436
PA 27.3	Describe the aetiology, types, stages pathophysiology, pathology and complications of heart failure.	Y	14	462
PA 27.4	Describe the aetiology, pathophysiology, pathology, gross and microscopic features, criteria and complications of rheumatic fever.	Y	14	489
PA 27.5	Describe the epidemiology, risk factors, aetiology, pathophysiology, pathology, presentations, gross and microscopic features, diagnostic tests and complications of ischaemic heart disease.	Y	14	474
PA 27.6	Describe the aetiology, pathophysiology, pathology, gross and microscopic features, diagnosis and complications of infective endocarditis.	Y	14	491
PA 27.7	Describe the aetiology, pathophysiology, pathology, gross and microscopic features, diagnosis and complications of pericarditis and pericardial effusion.	Y	14	498
PA 27.9	Classify and describe the aetiology, types, pathophysiology, pathology, gross and microscopic features, diagnosis and complications of cardiomyopathies.	N	14	493
PA 27.10	Describe the aetiology, pathophysiology, pathology features and complications of syphilis on the cardiovascular system.	N	14	485
PA 13.1	Describe haematopoiesis and extramedullary haematopoiesis.	Y	15	505, 507
PA 17.2	Enumerate the indications, and describe the findings in bone marrow aspiration and biopsy.	N	15	508
PA 13.3	Define and classify anaemia.	Y	15	511
PA 13.4	Enumerate and describe the investigation of anaemia.	Y	15	543
PA 14.1	Describe iron metabolism.	Y	15	514
PA 14.2	Describe the aetiology, investigations and differential diagnosis of microcytic hypochromic anaemia.	Y	15	514
PA 15.1	Describe the metabolism of vitamin B12 and the aetiology and pathogenesis of vitamin B12 deficiency.	Y	15	517

Competency Code	Competency	Core (Y/N)	Chapter No.	Page No.
PA 15.2	Describe laboratory investigations of macrocytic anaemia.	Y	15	517
PA 15.4	Enumerate the differences and describe the aetiology and distinguishing features of megaloblastic and nonmegaloblastic macrocytic anaemias.	N	15	517
PA 16.1	Define and classify haemolytic anaemia.	Y	15	525
PA 16.2	Describe the pathogenesis and clinical features and haematological indices of haemolytic anaemia.	Y	15	525
PA 16.3	Describe the pathogenesis, features, haematological indices and peripheral blood picture of sickle cell anaemia and thalassaemia.	Y	15	532, 535
PA 16.4	Describe the aetiology, pathogenesis, haematological indices and peripheral blood picture of acquired haemolytic anaemia.	Y	15	538, 540, 542
PA 16.5	Describe the peripheral blood picture in different haemolytic anaemias.	Y	15	525
PA 17.1	Enumerate the aetiology, pathogenesis and findings in aplastic anaemia.	N	15	522
PA 18.1	Enumerate and describe the causes of leucocytosis, leucopenia, lymphocytosis and leukaemoid reactions.	Y	16	554, 556
PA 18.2	Describe the aetiology, genetics, pathogenesis, classification, features and haematological features of acute and chronic leukaemias.	Y	16	563, 579, 587
PA 19.1	Enumerate the causes and describe the differentiating features of lymphadenopathy.	Y	16	559
PA 19.4	Describe and discuss the pathogenesis, pathology and the differentiating features of Hodgkin and non-Hodgkin lymphomas.	Y	16	565
PA 19.6	Enumerate and differentiate the causes of splenomegaly.	Y	16	596
PA 21.1	Describe normal haemostasis.	Y	17	608
PA 21.2	Classify and describe the aetiology, pathogenesis and pathology of vascular and platelet disorders including immune thrombocytopenic purpura and haemophilias.	Y	17	610, 612, 618, 619
PA 21.3	Differentiate platelet from clotting disorders based on the clinical and haematological features.	Y	17	623
PA 21.4	Define and describe disseminated intravascular coagulation, its laboratory findings and diagnosis.	Y	17	620
PA 21.5	Define and describe disseminated intravascular coagulation, its laboratory findings and diagnosis of vitamin K deficiency.	Y	17	622
PA 22.1	Classify and describe blood group systems (ABO and RH).	Y	18	632
PA 22.2	Enumerate the indications, describe the principles and enumerate and demonstrate the steps of compatibility testing.	Y	18	637
PA 22.4	Enumerate blood components and describe their clinical uses.	Y	18	639
PA 22.5	Enumerate and describe infections transmitted by blood transfusion.	Y	18	647

Competency Code	Competency	Core (Y/N)	Chapter No.	Page No.
PA 22.6	Describe transfusion reactions and enumerate the steps in the investigation of a transfusion reaction.	Y	18	641
PA 22.7	Enumerate the indications and describe the principles and procedures of autologous transfusion.	Y	18	647
PA 26.1	Define and describe the aetiology, types, pathogenesis, stages, morphology and complications of pneumonia.	Y	19	685
PA 26.2	Describe the aetiology, gross and microscopic appearance, and complications of lung abscess.	Y	19	693
PA 26.3	Define and describe the aetiology, types, pathogenesis, stages, morphology, complications and evaluation of obstructive airway disease (OAD) and bronchiectasis.	Y	19	660, 667
PA 26.4	Define and describe the aetiology, types, pathogenesis, stages, morphology, microscopic appearance and complications of tuberculosis.	Y	19, 10	679, 285
PA 26.5	Define and describe the aetiology, types, exposure, environmental influence, pathogenesis, stages, morphology, microscopic appearance and complications of occupational lung diseases.	Y	19	670, 675
PA 26.6	Define and describe the aetiology, types, exposure, genetics, environmental influence, pathogenesis, stages, morphology, microscopic appearance, metastases and complications of tumours of the lung and pleura.	Y	19	694, 703
PA 26.7	Define and describe the aetiology, types, exposure, genetics, environmental influence, pathogenesis, morphology, microscopic appearance and complications of mesothelioma.	N	19	703
PA 24.1	Describe the aetiology, pathogenesis, pathology and clinical features of oral cancers.	N	20	710
PA 24.2	Describe the aetiology, pathogenesis, pathology, microbiology, clinical and microscopic features of peptic ulcer disease.	Y	21	739
PA 24.4	Describe the aetiology, pathogenesis and pathological features of carcinoma of the stomach.	Y	21	743
PA 24.5	Describe the aetiology, pathogenesis and pathological features of tuberculosis of the intestine.	N	21	756
PA 24.6	Describe the aetiology, pathogenesis pathological and distinguishing features of inflammatory bowel disease.	Y	21	757
PA 24.7	Describe the aetiology, pathogenesis pathological and distinguishing features of carcinoma of the colon.	Y	21	766
PA 25.1	Describe bilirubin metabolism, enumerate the aetiology and pathogenesis of jaundice and distinguish between direct and indirect hyperbilirubinaemias.	Y	22	805
PA 25.2	Describe the pathophysiology and pathological changes seen in hepatic failure and their clinical manifestations, complications and consequences.	Y	22	782

Competency Code	Competency	Core (Y/N)	Chapter No.	Page No.
PA 25.3	Describe the aetiology and pathogenesis of viral and toxic hepatitis. Distinguish the causes of hepatitis based on the clinical and laboratory features. Describe the pathology, complications and consequences of hepatitis.	Y	22	786
PA 25.4	Describe the pathophysiology, pathology and progression of alcoholic liver disease including cirrhosis.	Y	22	781, 783, 797
PA 25.5	Describe the aetiology, pathogenesis and complications of portal hypertension.	Y	22	784
PA 32.6	Describe the aetiology, pathogenesis, morphology, laboratory findings, morphological features, complications and metastases of pancreatic cancer.	N	23	830
PA 28.1	Describe the normal histology of the kidney.	Y	24	836
PA 28.2	Define, classify and distinguish the clinical syndromes and describe the aetiology, pathogenesis, pathology, morphology, clinical, laboratory and urinary findings, and complications of renal failure.	Y	24	839
PA 28.3	Define and describe the aetiology, precipitating factors, pathogenesis, pathology, laboratory and urinary findings, progression and complications of acute renal failure.	Y	24	839
PA 28.4	Define and describe the aetiology, precipitating factors, pathogenesis, pathology, laboratory urinary findings, progression and complications of chronic renal failure.	Y	24	840
PA 28.5	Define and classify glomerular diseases. Enumerate and describe the aetiology, pathogenesis, mechanisms of glomerular injury, pathology, distinguishing features and clinical manifestations of glomerulonephritis.	Y	24	841
PA 28.6	Define and classify glomerular diseases. Enumerate and describe the aetiology, pathogenesis, mechanisms of glomerular injury, pathology, distinguishing features and clinical manifestations of glomerulonephritis of IgA nephropathy.	Y	24	848
PA 28.7	Enumerate and describe the findings in glomerular manifestations of systemic disease.	Y	24	859
PA 28.8	Enumerate and classify diseases affecting the tubular interstitium.	Y	24	865
PA 28.9	Define and describe the aetiology, pathogenesis, pathology, laboratory and urinary findings, progression and complications of acute tubular necrosis.	Y	24	863
PA 28.10	Describe the aetiology, pathogenesis, pathology, laboratory findings, distinguishing features, progression and complications of acute and chronic pyelonephritis and reflux nephropathy.	Y	24	865
PA 28.11	Define classify and describe the aetiology, pathogenesis, pathology, laboratory and urinary findings, distinguishing features, progression and complications of vascular diseases of the kidney.	Y	24	870
PA 28.12	Define classify and describe the genetics, inheritance, aetiology, pathogenesis, pathology, laboratory and urinary findings, distinguishing features, progression and complications of cystic diseases of the kidney.	Y	24	874

Competency Code	Competency	Core (Y/N)	Chapter No.	Page No.
PA 28.13	Define classify and describe the aetiology, pathogenesis, pathology, laboratory and urinary findings, distinguishing features, progression and complications of renal stone disease and obstructive uropathy.	Y	24	877
PA 28.14	Classify and describe the aetiology, genetics, pathogenesis, pathology, presenting features, progression and spread of renal tumours.	Y	24	879
PA 28.15	Describe the aetiology, genetics, pathogenesis, pathology, presenting features and progression of thrombotic angiopathies.	N	24	872
PA 29.1	Classify testicular tumours and describe the pathogenesis, pathology, presenting and distinguishing features, diagnostic tests, progression and spread of testicular tumours.	Y	25	910
PA 29.2	Describe the pathogenesis, pathology, presenting and distinguishing features, diagnostic tests, progression and spread of carcinoma of the penis.	Y	25	906
PA 29.3	Describe the pathogenesis, pathology, hormonal dependency, presenting and distinguishing features, urological findings and diagnostic tests of benign prostatic hyperplasia.	Y	25	918
PA 29.4	Describe the pathogenesis, pathology, hormonal dependency, presenting and distinguishing features, diagnostic tests, progression and spread of carcinoma of the prostate.	Y	25	919
PA 29.5	Describe the aetiology, pathogenesis, pathology and progression of prostatitis.	N	25	917
PA 28.16	Describe the aetiology, genetics, pathogenesis, pathology, presenting features and progression of urothelial tumours.	N	25	898
PA 30.1	Describe the epidemiology, pathogenesis, aetiology, pathology, screening, diagnosis and progression of carcinoma of the cervix.	Y	26	935
PA 30.2	Describe the pathogenesis, aetiology, pathology, diagnosis, progression and spread of carcinoma of the endometrium.	Y	26	943
PA 30.3	Describe the pathogenesis, aetiology, pathology, diagnosis, progression and spread of leiomyomas and leiomyosarcomas.	Y	26	945, 947
PA 30.4	Classify and describe the aetiology, pathogenesis, pathology, morphology, clinical course, spread and complications of ovarian tumours.	Y	26	949
PA 30.5	Describe the aetiology, pathogenesis, pathology, morphology, clinical course, spread and complications of gestational trophoblastic neoplasms.	Y	26	960
PA 30.6	Describe the aetiology and morphological features of cervicitis.	N	26	934
PA 30.7	Describe the aetiology, hormonal dependence, features and morphology of endometriosis.	N	26	939
PA 30.8	Describe the aetiology and morphological features of adenomyosis.	N	26	941
PA 30.9	Describe the aetiology, hormonal dependence and morphology of endometrial hyperplasia.	N	26	942

Competency Code	Competency	Core (Y/N)	Chapter No.	Page No.
PA 31.1	Classify and describe the types, aetiology, pathogenesis, pathology and hormonal dependency of benign breast disease.	Y	27	969, 975, 979
PA 31.2	Classify and describe the epidemiology, pathogenesis, classification, morphology, prognostic factors, hormonal dependency, staging and spread of carcinoma of the breast.	Y	27	982
PA 31.4	Enumerate and describe the aetiology, hormonal dependency and pathogenesis of gynaecomastia.	N	27	981
PA 32.1	Enumerate, classify and describe the aetiology, pathogenesis, pathology and iodine dependency of thyroid swellings.	Y	28	996, 1003
PA 32.2	Describe the aetiology, cause, iodine dependency, pathogenesis, manifestations, laboratory and imaging features and course of thyrotoxicosis.	Y	28	1001
PA 32.3	Describe the aetiology, pathogenesis, manifestations, laboratory and imaging features and course of thyrotoxicosis/ hypothyroidism.	Y	28	996
PA 32.4	Classify and describe the epidemiology, aetiology, pathogenesis, pathology, clinical and laboratory features, complications and progression of diabetes mellitus.	Y	28	1017
PA 32.5	Describe the aetiology, genetics, pathogenesis, manifestations and laboratory and morphological features of hyperparathyroidism.	N	28	1013
PA 32.7	Describe the aetiology, pathogenesis, manifestations, laboratory and morphological features and complications of adrenal insufficiency.	N	28	1033
PA 32.8	Describe the aetiology, pathogenesis, manifestations, laboratory and morphological features and complications of Cushing syndrome.	N	28	1028
PA 32.9	Describe the aetiology, pathogenesis, manifestations and laboratory and morphological features of adrenal neoplasms.	N	28	1034, 1035
PA 34.1	Describe the risk factors, pathogenesis, pathology and natural history of squamous cell carcinoma of the skin.	Y	29	1062
PA 34.2	Describe the risk factors, pathogenesis, pathology and natural history of basal cell carcinoma of the skin.	Y	29	1064
PA 34.3	Describe the distinguishing features between a naevus and melanoma. Describe the aetiology, pathogenesis, risk factors, morphology clinical features and metastases of melanoma.	N	29	1057
PA 33.1	Classify and describe the aetiology, pathogenesis, manifestations, radiologic and morphologic features and complications of osteomyelitis.	Y	30	1087
PA 33.2	Classify and describe the aetiology, pathogenesis, manifestations, radiologic and morphologic features and complications and metastasis of bone tumours.	Y	30	1090
PA 33.3	Classify and describe the aetiology, pathogenesis, manifestations, radiologic and morphologic features and complications and metastasis of soft tissue tumours.	Y	30	1107

Competency Code	Competency	Core (Y/N)	Chapter No.	Page No.
PA 33.4	Classify and describe the aetiology, pathogenesis, manifestations, radiologic and morphologic features and complications of Paget disease of the bone.	N	30	1084
PA 33.5	Classify and describe the aetiology, immunology, pathogenesis, manifestations, radiologic and laboratory features, diagnostic criteria and complications of rheumatoid arthritis.	N	30	1103
PA 35.1	Describe the aetiology, types and pathogenesis, differentiating factors, CSF findings in meningitis.	Y	31	1129
PA 35.2	Classify and describe the aetiology, genetics, pathogenesis, pathology, presentation sequelae and complications of CNS tumours.	Y	31	1141
PA 36.1	Describe the aetiology, genetics, pathogenesis, pathology, presentation, sequelae and complications of retinoblastoma.	N	31	1154

Cell as a Unit of Health and Disease

1

Gayathri Devi Thanigaimani

CHAPTER OUTLINE

INTRODUCTION

The word pathology stands for **the *study of suffering*** ('pathos' means suffering and 'logy' means study) and it refers to study of diseases. Pathology is broadly divided into general pathology or cellular pathology, haematology and systemic pathology. General pathology is the study of pathology of the cell, the various insults that occur to the cell and the response of the body to the insults at cellular level. Haematology refers to the study of diseases of blood and systemic pathology refers to the study of diseases of the various systems of the body.

Before entering the world of pathology, understanding some terminologies are essential. Each pathological condition is caused by certain agents which are referred to as ***aetiology*** and the factors that increase the likelihood of getting affected are called ***risk factors.*** The mechanism by which a particular aetiological condition causes disease in the human body is called ***pathogenesis,*** whereas the anatomical and histological changes that occur because of the disease are called ***morphological changes.***

Understanding a disease or a disorder is like **solving a puzzle**, the pieces of which are the subjects of your entire course of medicine. The beauty of the puzzle, or rather, understanding of the disease process lies in fitting the centre piece, which is the pathogenesis and morphological changes caused by it.

Various aspects of pathology
Aetiology – What is the cause?
Pathogenesis – Evolution of disease
Morphology – Structural changes
Functional consequences

The word ***'cellular pathology'*** was coined by Rudolph Virchow to symbolize that all diseases originate at the cellular level. So, in essence, modern pathology refers to the study of cellular pathology, and to understand cell pathology a basic understanding of the normal cell structure and function is required. In this chapter, we discuss a few aspects of cell biology that form the basis for understanding cellular abnormalities discussed in the subsequent chapters.

NORMAL CELL STRUCTURE

The animal cell is made up of many structures that have specific roles in the functioning and well-being of the cell. The cell membrane encloses the cytoplasm, in which many double membrane–bound organelles are found, such as **nucleus, mitochondria, endoplasmic reticulum**

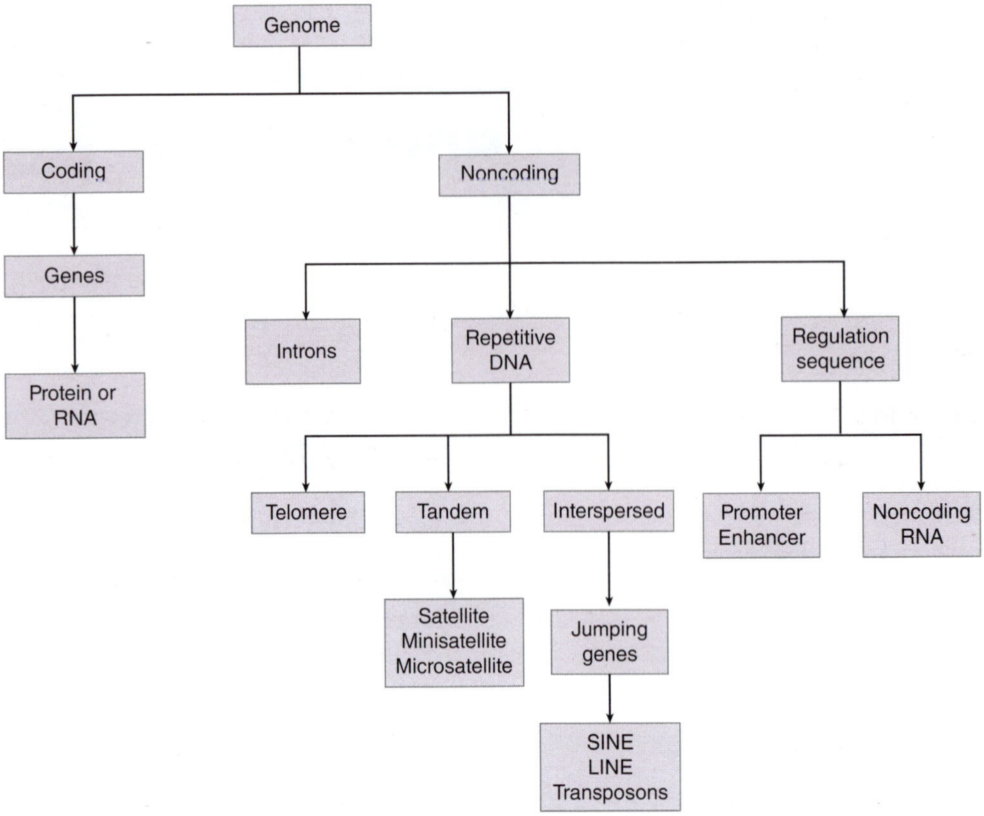

Fig. 1.1 Classification of genes in genome. Genes in the genome are classified into coding genes, that code for proteins and noncoding genes that do not code for proteins.

(ER), Golgi apparatus. The nucleus is the main control centre of the cell because it contains the DNA, which is the key factor for production of proteins that act as building blocks of the organelles. The genetic matter contained in the DNA also controls the functioning of cell, and any defect in the DNA is the root cause of many disorders and neoplastic transformations. The functions of the various organelles and their role in the housekeeping of the cell are discussed later in this chapter.

THE GENOME

The field of biomedical science developed the technique of sequencing the human genome in 2001, which revolutionized our understanding of health and disease. Since then, we have had a remarkable increase in the data archive about our genome, which has inspired scientists to discover new therapies.

The human genome consists of about 3.2 billion base pairs. These are divided into **protein-coding genes or exons** that form 1.5% of the genome and **noncoding genes** that form the remaining 98.5% (Fig. 1.1). The exons code for proteins such as enzymes, structural proteins and signalling molecules that maintain the cell structure (Fig. 1.2). The noncoding part of the genome was initially considered as 'junk DNA' with no significant purpose. But further studies revealed that 80% of the noncoding DNA is

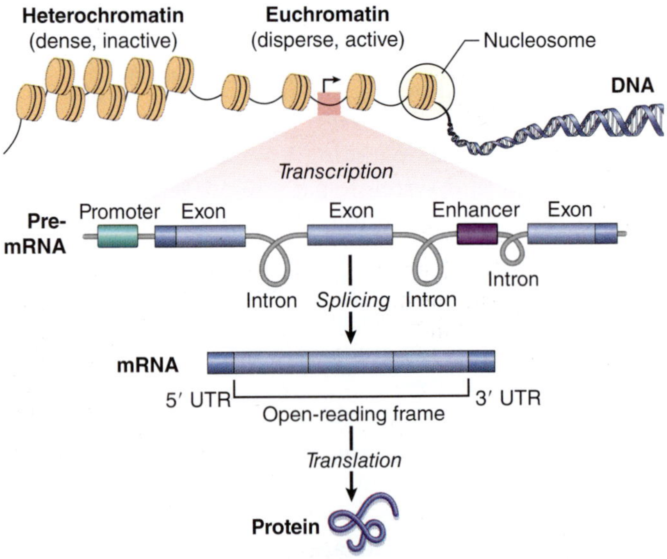

Fig. 1.2 Organization of nuclear DNA and steps in protein formation. The nuclear genetic material is organized into dispersed, transcriptionally active euchromatin or densely packed, transcriptionally inactive heterochromatin. After transcription, the intronic sequences are subsequently spliced out of the pre-mRNA to produce the mRNA that is translated into protein.

involved in regulation of gene expression. For example, the noncoding DNA has certain sequences that act as on and off switches that determine when and where the genes are to be expressed for protein production. Thus, while exons produce the building blocks, the noncoding DNAs provide the blueprint and oversee the construction process. This variation in blueprint is the basis of variation among different species. The noncoding DNAs are classified into the following:

- ***Promoter and enhancer regions*** that bind to transcription factors.
- Binding sites for factors that organize ***higher order chromatin structure.***
- ***Noncoding regulatory RNAs*** that do not form protein but regulate gene expression.
- ***Jumping genes (transposons) which are mobile genetic elements that comprise DNA sequences that have the capacity to move from one chromosomal site to another.*** These vary in number and position even in closely related species.
- ***Introns*** are noncoding regions, interspersed within genes, that are transcribed into mRNA but removed later by RNA splicing.
- Special structural regions such as ***telomeres*** (chromosomal ends) and *centromeres* (chromosomal tethers).

The presence of different traits among individuals of a species is because of the presence of **alleles** for many genes. Alleles are variants of genes, and humans being diploid, inherit one allele from each parent. This creates genetic variations among individuals, and this is referred to as **polymorphism.** It has been identified that polymorphisms that are associated with diseases are more commonly located in noncoding regions than in coding regions.

Recent genomic studies have also revealed that humans share 99.5% of their DNA sequences, and intraspecies variation of genome lies only in 0.5% of the DNA. This very small portion of the DNA is responsible for differences in appearance, character, susceptibility to diseases and response to environmental agents. The following are the two common forms of DNA variation in the human genome:

- **Single nucleotide polymorphism (SNP)** (Fig. 1.3): SNPs denote variations at a single nucleotide position. These may be present in
  - Coding regions: About 1% of SNPs are located here and produce differences in the structure of proteins.
  - Regulatory regions: These alter the gene expression.
  - Neutral SNPs: These have no effect on gene function, but when co-inherited with a disease-causing gene, these can be used as markers to identify the causative gene. This is called *linkage equilibrium.*
- **Copy number variation (CNV)** (Fig. 1.4): They are variations in the number of copies of a particular DNA sequence in the genome of an individual. Their role in disease susceptibility is yet to be established.

FACTORS REGULATING GENE EXPRESSION

Epigenetics (Fig. 1.5)

All terminally differentiated cells have the same genetic composition but differ in their structure and function. This is explained by epigenetics, which induces *silencing*

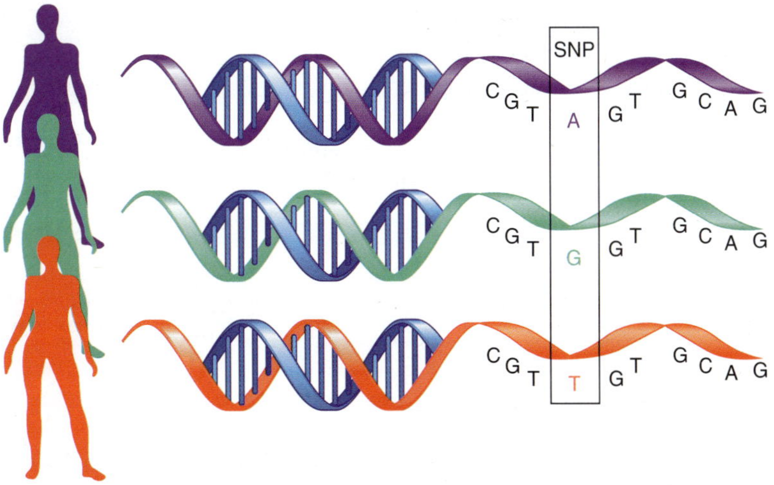

Fig. 1.3 Single nucleotide polymorphisms (SNPs) represent variation in one nucleotide.

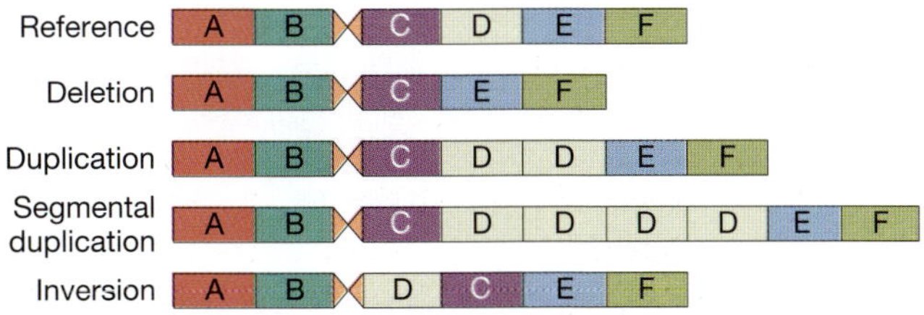

Fig. 1.4 Copy number variation (CNV) – D is a segment in the DNA of the parent. It may get deleted or duplicated or inverted producing variations in their number in the offspring.

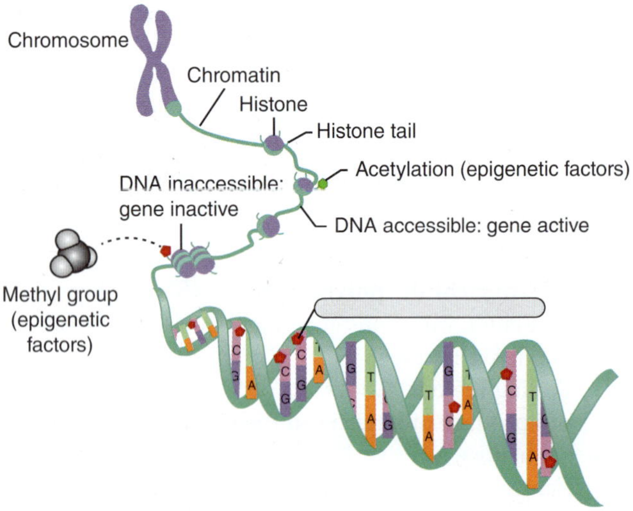

Fig. 1.5 Epigenetics – genes bound to epigenetic factors are silenced while others are active.

of unwanted genes and permits expression of genes required for the functioning of that cell. **Epigenetics is defined as heritable changes in gene expression that are not caused by alterations in the DNA sequence**, i.e. a change in the phenotype and not in the genotype. The nuclear chromatin in the cells exists in two forms – dense transcriptionally inactive *heterochromatin* and sparse transcriptionally active *euchromatin.* Gene expression is controlled by the movement of segments of DNA between the two forms. This is done by modification in histone by *histone acetylation, methylation and phosphorylation, and DNA methylation.*

Evidence now show that epigenetics plays an important role in the causation of cancer and the pathogenesis of diseases. Therefore, scientists are extremely interested in epigenetics because unlike genetic changes, **epigenetic changes are amenable to therapy.** This has given hope for the development of newer therapeutic agents for the treatment of cancer and certain other diseases.

MicroRNA and Long Noncoding RNA

These belong to the family of RNAs that are transcribed by genes but do not undergo translation to form proteins.

- **MicroRNA** (miRNA) (Fig. 1.6)
  MicroRNA are RNA segments of 22-nucleotide length in average. These cause **post-transcriptional silencing of mRNA** and thereby regulate gene expression. This is done by binding to target mRNA and modulating their

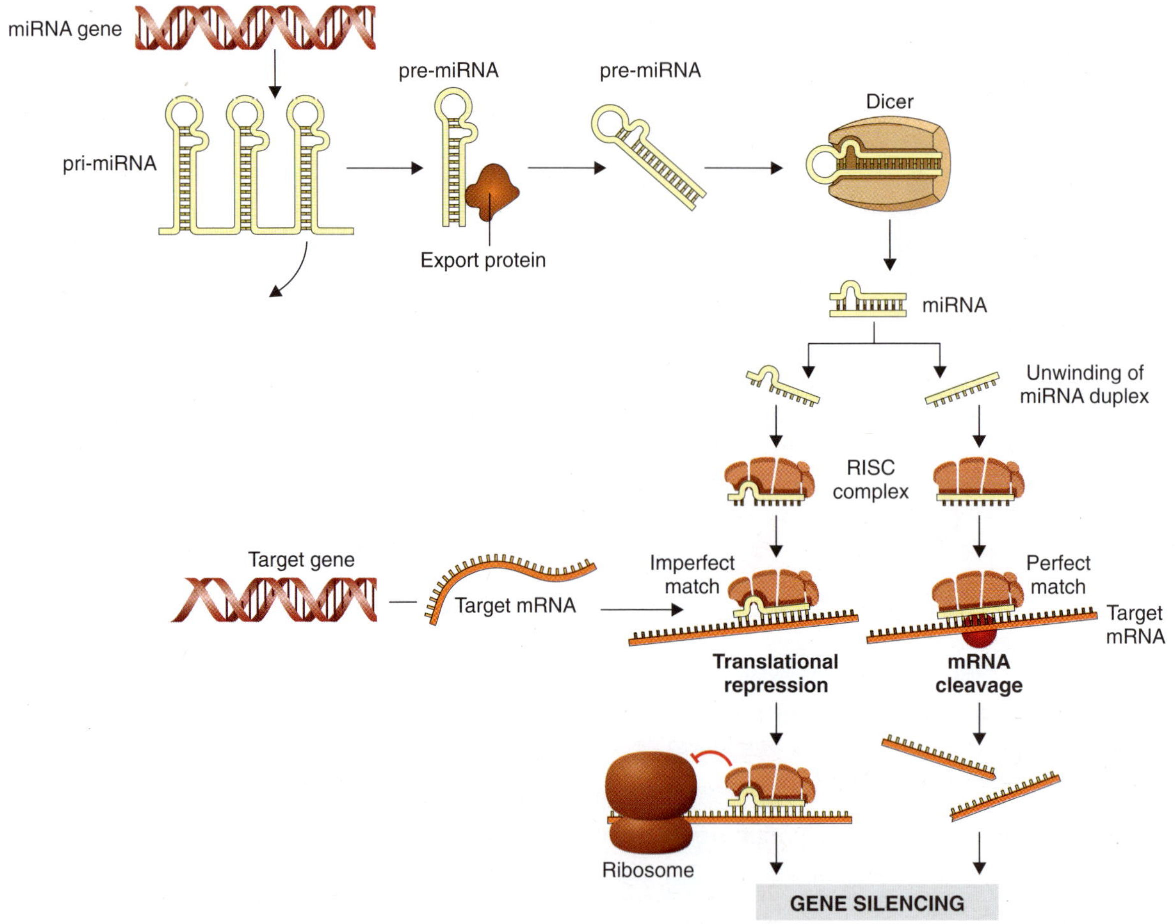

Fig. 1.6 Generation and function of MicroRNA. The miRNA genes are transcribed to produce pre-miRNA that when reaches the cytoplasm is trimmed by the Dicer enzyme to generate mature double-stranded miRNAs. The miRNA is then incorporated into the multiprotein RNA-induced silencing complex (RISC). Base pairing between the single-stranded miRNA and its target mRNA in RISC causes post-transcriptional silencing of target RNA.

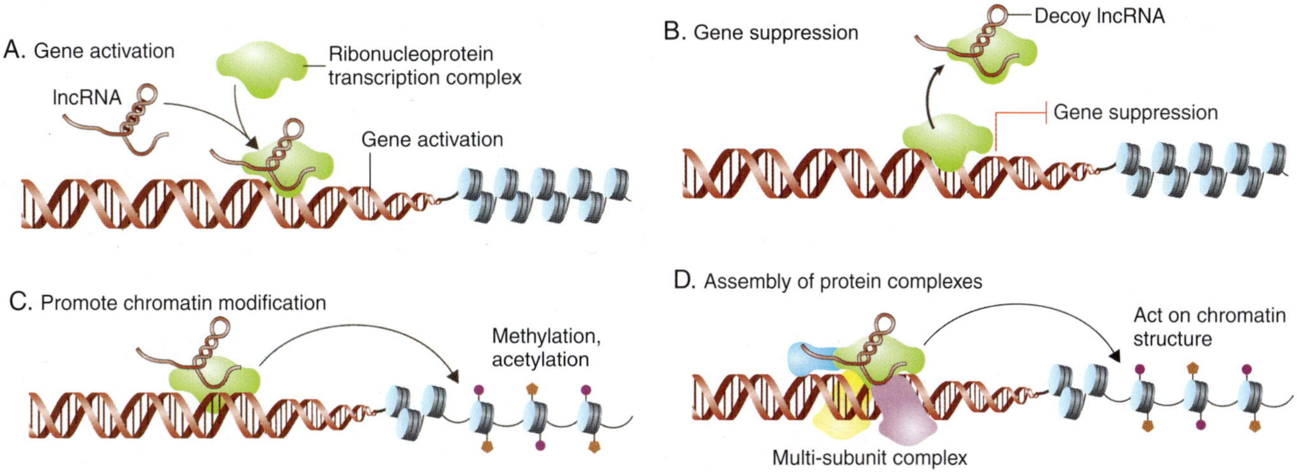

Fig. 1.7 Functions of long noncoding RNA. (A) lncRNAs can facilitate transcription factor binding and thus promote gene activation. (B) Or, lncRNAs can pre-emptively bind transcription factors and thus prevent gene transcription. (C) They can modify the chromatin by binding to acetylases or methylases. (D) In other instances, lncRNAs may act as scaffolding and influence the general chromatin architecture.

translation into corresponding proteins. This mechanism of gene regulation has been identified to play an important role, both in normal development and in pathogenesis of cancer.

Small interfering RNAs (siRNAs) are short sequences of RNA of similar function as miRNA, that are experimentally introduced into cells. Such synthetic siRNAs are used in research to study gene function and are also being investigated as possible therapeutic agents to silence pathogenic genes.

- **Long noncoding RNA (lncRNA)** (Fig. 1.7)
  lncRNAs are noncoding RNAs of length more than 200 nucleotides; these are much more in number in the human genome than miRNAs. These regulate gene expression in many ways and have now been found to play an *important role in carcinogenesis*. These have been found to have their footprint in almost all the hallmark pathways of carcinogenesis, such as activation of oncogenic pathways (e.g. lncRNA ANRIL), tumour suppressor gene function (e.g. lncRNA GAS5), increasing the ability of tumour cells to invade and cause metastasis (lncRNA HOTAIR). Another known function of lncRNA is repression of the X chromosome by XIST causing physiologic X chromosome inactivation. The role of lncRNA in other diseases is also being investigated.

FUNDAMENTAL HOUSEKEEPING MECHANISMS OF CELLS

All cells must perform many housekeeping functions to stay viable. This includes protection from the environment, communication, nutrient acquisition, movement, renewal of senescent molecules, energy generation and molecular catabolism. These functions are allocated to different intracellular organelles (Fig. 1.8) to ensure that injurious degradative enzymes are kept away from the other components of the cell and to provide unique intracellular environment required for each function (Table 1.1).

PLASMA MEMBRANE: PROTECTION AND NUTRITION ACQUISITION

Plasma membranes are fluid bilayers of amphipathic phospholipids, composed of hydrophilic head groups to interact with aqueous environment and hydrophobic lipid tails to interact with each other that form a barrier to passive diffusion of large or charged molecules (Fig. 1.9A). The bilayer consists of different phospholipids, which are distributed asymmetrically to suit their specific function. Phosphatidylserine is predominantly found in inner leaflet (flips to extracellular face during apoptosis – programmed cell death to give 'eat me' signals to phagocytes), glycolipids and sphingomyelins are usually found in extracellular face (helps in cell–cell and cell–matrix interactions), whereas phosphatidylinositol is found on both leaflets.

The next important component of plasma membrane is the proteins that are associated with the lipid bilayer by one of the four mechanisms – as transmembrane proteins; in association with components of lipid bilayer on cytosolic side; by insertion into the membrane using glycosylphosphatidylinositol (GPI) as anchors on the extracellular face; as noncovalent association with true transmembrane proteins (Fig. 1.9B). The functions of these proteins include (1) ion and metabolite transportation; (2) uptake of macromolecules; and (3) cell–ligand, cell–matrix and cell–cell interactions. Some proteins function independently, whereas most aggregate together to form large complexes either in rough ER or in situ.

The external face of the lipid bilayer also contains carbohydrates that are studded on it as oligosaccharides and

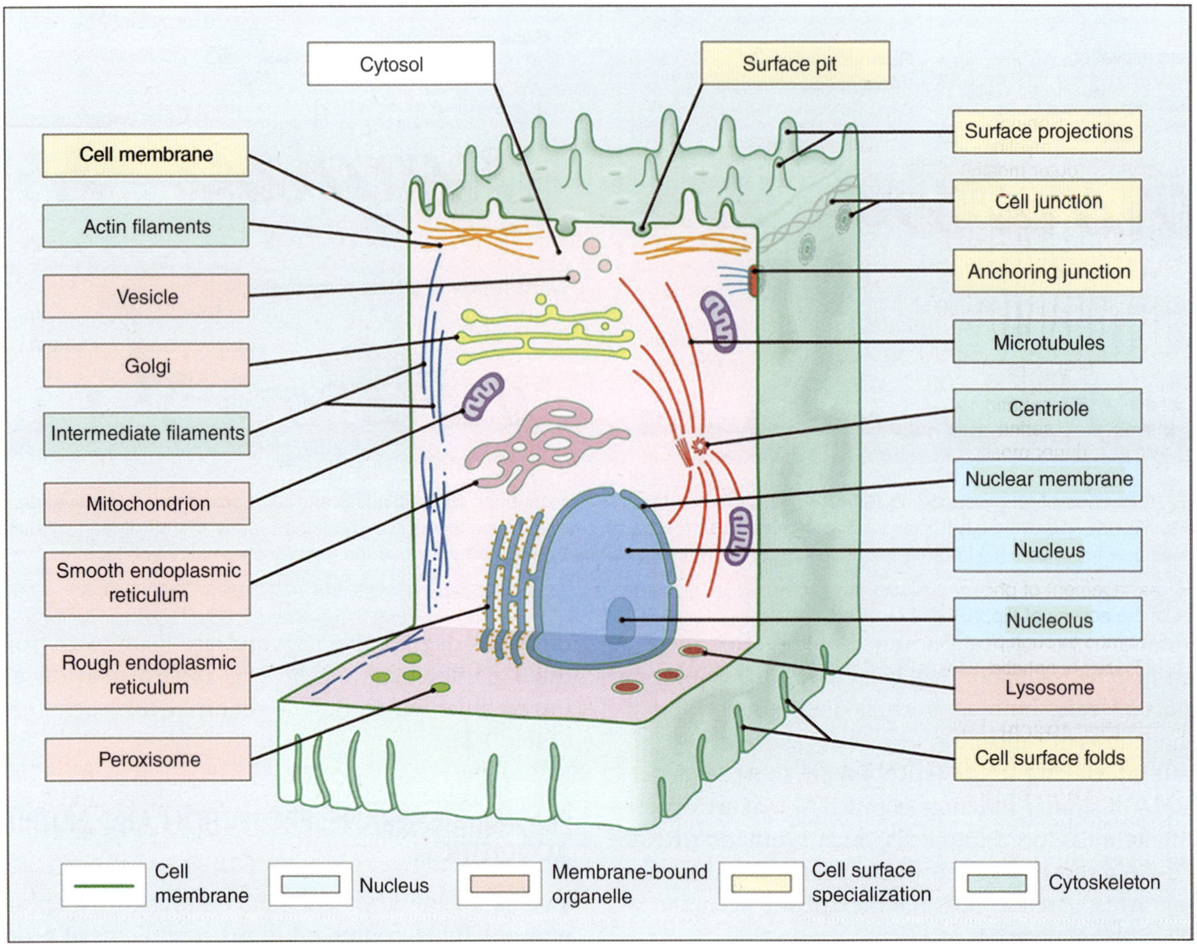

Fig. 1.8 Basic subcellular constituents of cells. (*Source:* From James S. Lowe, Peter G. Anderson and Susan I. Anderson. The Cell. Stevens & Lowe's Human Histology. 5th edition. 2020. Elsevier.)

Table 1.1 Functions of Intracellular Organelles

Category	Organelle	Function
Protein synthesis	Rough endoplasmic reticulum	Proteins for cell membrane and beyond
	Smooth endoplasmic reticulum	Cytosolic proteins
	Golgi apparatus	Assembling of proteins
Catabolism	Lysosomes	Digestion of macromolecules
	Proteasomes	Digestion of proteins into peptides
	Peroxisomes	Breakdown of fatty acids and producing hydrogen peroxide
Movement within cell	Endosomes	Movement of internalized material and newly synthesized material
	Cytoskeleton	Organelles and proteins
Movement of cell in environment	Cytoskeleton	Maintaining cell shape and polarity
Energy production	Mitochondria	Oxidative phosphorylation, synthesis of metabolic intermediates and sensors of cell damage

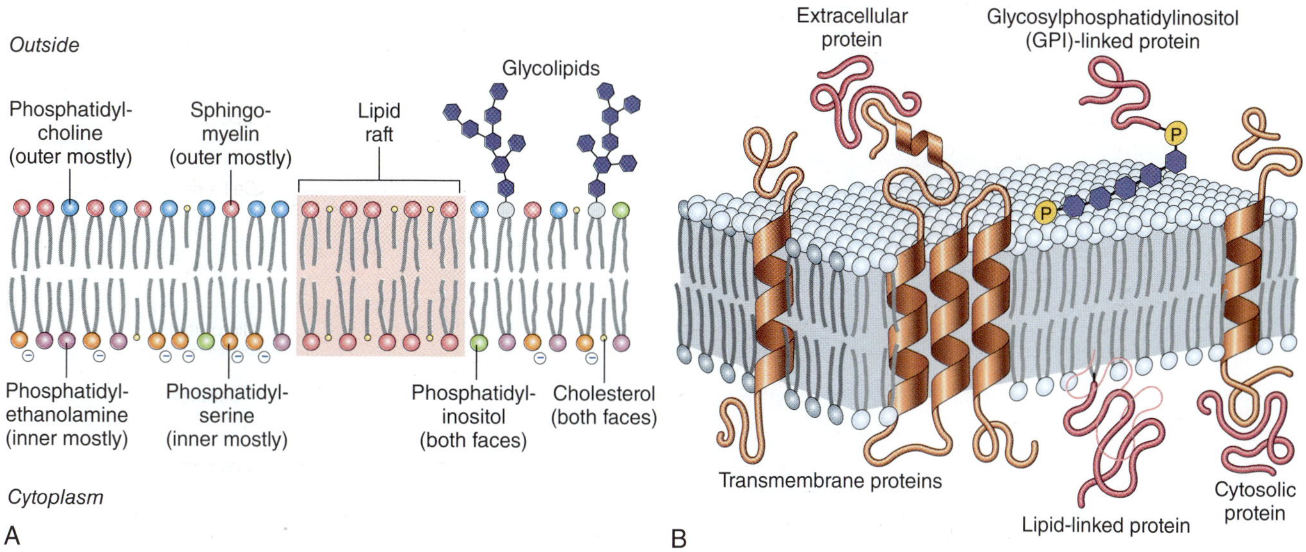

Fig. 1.9 Arrangement of phospholipids and proteins in plasma membrane. (A) The phospholipid distribution within the membrane is asymmetric because of the activity of flippases. (B) Membrane-associated proteins may traverse the membrane, or be attached in the cytosolic face with the plasma membrane through post-translational modifications or addition of palmitic acid or get attached at the extracytoplasmic face with the membrane via glycosylphosphatidylinositol (GPI) linkages. (*Source:* From Robbins & Cotran Pathologic Basis of Disease, 10th edition. 2021. Elsevier.)

polysaccharides attached to glycolipids, glycoproteins and proteoglycans. These form glycocalyx, which is important for barrier function of the plasma membrane and in cell–cell and cell–matrix interactions.

The movement of substances across the plasma membrane occurs through various mechanisms (Fig. 1.10). The important ones are as follows:

- **Passive diffusion:** The molecules crossing the membrane by passive diffusion include nonpolar molecules such as O_2 and CO_2, hydrophobic molecules such as steroid hormones and polar molecules less than 75 Da in mass such as water and ethanol. Plasma membrane is impermeable to polar molecules more than 75 Da in mass and to ions.
- **Channel proteins and carriers:** These help in movement of polar molecules up to 1000 Da in mass, and ions. Channel proteins move solutes on the basis of *size and charge,* and the movement is only passive (higher to lower concentration). The carriers are highly specific to particular solutes, but movement can be either passive or active (lower to higher concentration), and the energy for the active movement is provided by ATPase. These channels play an important role in regulating the water content of the cell by maintaining an appropriate osmotic gradient and in regulating intracellular and intraorganellar pH.
- **Receptor-mediated and fluid phase uptake:** The movement of fluids and macromolecules in the cell takes place by the processes of *endocytosis* (from outside to inside the cell), *exocytosis* (from inside to outside the cell) or *transcytosis* (across the cell from apical to basolateral side of cell). The process of endocytosis may occur by two mechanisms:
  (1) **Potocytosis and caveolae-mediated endocytosis,** which transports small molecules, such as vitamins, by forming invaginations of the plasma membrane, and is important for transmembrane signalling and/or cellular adhesion through receptors and integrins.
  (2) **Pinocytosis and receptor-mediated endocytosis,** which involves uptake of bigger molecules, such as LDL and transferrin, after binding to specific cell-surface receptors.

CYTOSKELETON AND CELL–CELL INTERACTIONS (FIG. 1.11)

Cytoskeleton is an intracellular scaffolding of protein, which helps the cell to maintain its shape and polarity, organize intracellular organelles and to move about.

Structure of Cytoskeleton

It is composed of three types of proteins:

- **Actin microfilaments** (5- to 9-nm diameter fibrils): These form double-stranded helices with a defined polarity. In muscles, these help in contraction by their interaction with myosin, and in nonmuscle cells, these help in controlling the cell shape and movement.
- **Intermediate filaments** (10-nm diameter fibrils): These are large proteins that impart tensile strength to the cells. These are heterogenous and have tissue-specific characteristics.
  - Lamin A, B and C: nuclear lamina of all cells
  - Vimentin: mesenchymal cells
  - Desmin: muscle cells
  - Neurofilaments: axons of neurons
  - Glial fibrillary acidic protein: glial cells around neurons
  - Cytokeratins: epithelial cells; they are subdivided into type I (acidic) and type II (neutral/basic)

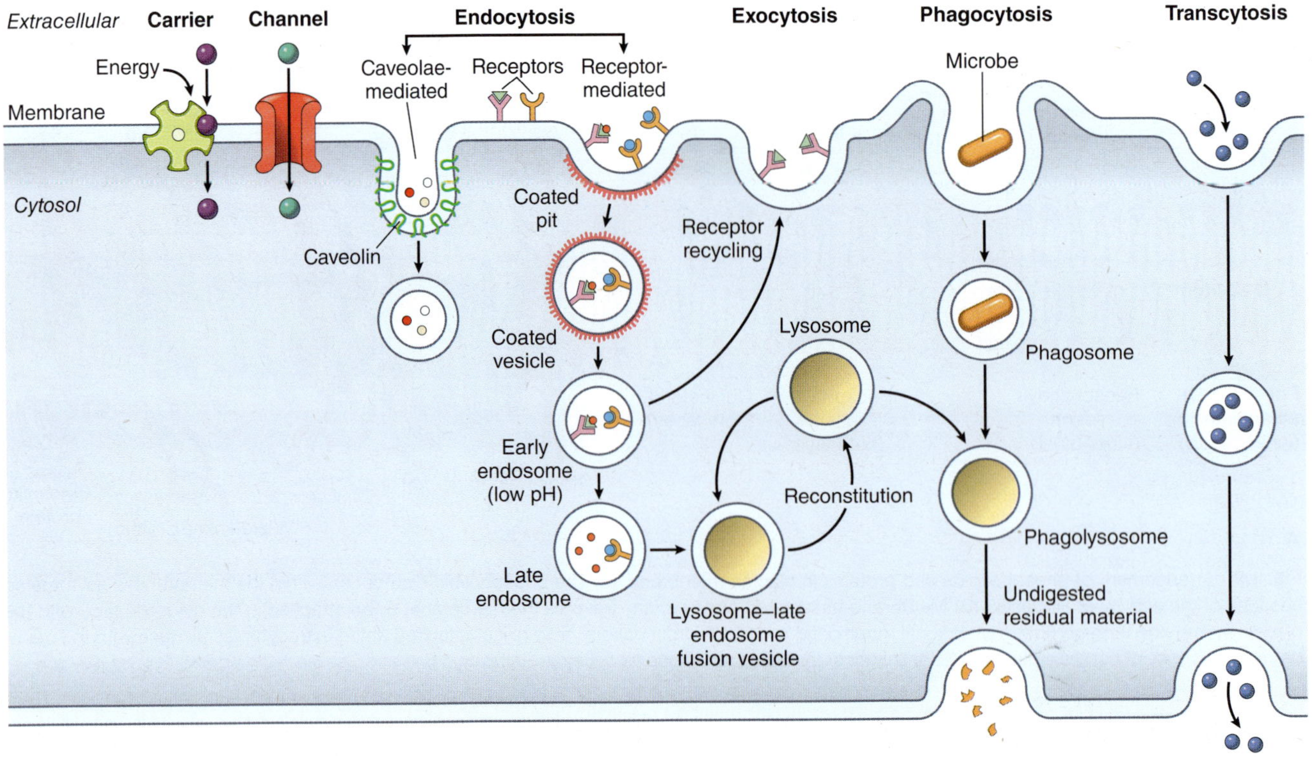

Fig. 1.10 Movement of small molecules and larger structures across membranes. Small, charged solutes can move through channels or carriers. Channels are used when movement is along gradient, whereas carriers are required to move against a concentration gradient. Receptor-mediated and fluid-phase uptake of material (endocytosis) may be by potocytosis or pinocytosis. Phagocytosis involves intake of large particles – typically by specialized phagocytes. Transcytosis involves the transcellular endocytotic transport of a molecule, whereas exocytosis is for the discharge of cellular contents to the extracellular space.

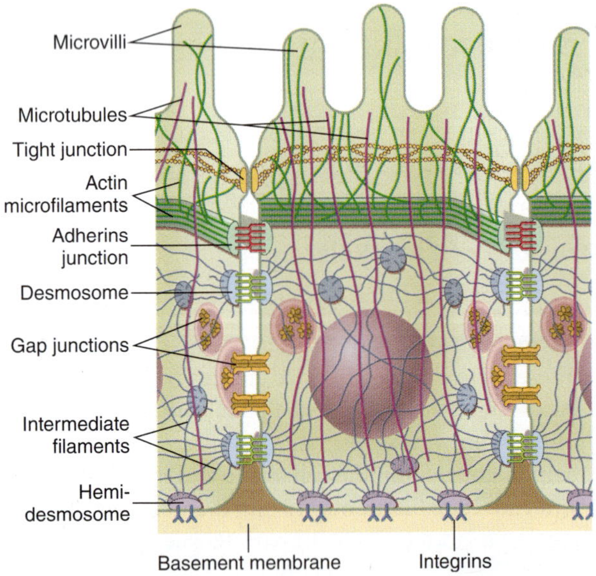

Fig. 1.11 Cytoskeletal elements and cell–cell interactions. Interepithelial adhesion involves proteins forming tight junctions and desmosomes; adhesion to the extracellular matrix involves cellular integrins and hemidesmosomes.

- **Microtubules** (25-nm diameter fibrils): These are dimers of α- and β-tubulin arrayed with specific polarity. Within the cell, these serve as cables for the movement of motor proteins – *kinesins* and *dyneins*. These are also important components of cilia in ciliary epithelium and flagella of sperms.

CELL–CELL INTERACTIONS

The interaction and communication between cells are mediated by forming cell junctions. The three basic types of cell junctions are as follows:

- **Occluding junctions or tight junctions:** These create a continuous barrier by *sealing adjacent cells* together. These are composed of proteins such as occludin, claudin, zonulin and catenin, and help to regulate movement of substances across the cells and maintain polarity. But these junctions are *dynamic* and can dissociate to facilitate inflammatory cell migration or epithelial proliferation.
- **Anchoring junctions or desmosomes:** These *mechanically attach cells* and their cytoskeletons to other cells or to the extracellular matrix (ECM). The major components of desmosomes are glycoproteins called *cadherins*. There are three types of desmosomes made of different type of cadherins as shown in Table 1.2.
- **Communicating junctions or gap junctions:** These microtubules are responsible for transmitting chemical and electrical signals from one cell to another. These are made of transmembrane proteins called connexions that form pores for passage of ions, nucleotides, sugars, amino acids, vitamins and other small molecules. These are critical for *cell–cell communication* such as in cardiac myocytes where rapid transmission of impulses helps the myocardium to contract in a highly coordinated manner to produce a heartbeat.

Table 1.2 Types of Desmosomes

Type	Function	Constituents	Purpose
Spot desmosomes	Small focus of adhesion between cells	Desmogleins, desmocollins	Help to communicate extracellular forces over multiple cells
Hemidesmosomes	Adhesion of cell to ECM	Integrins Focal adhesion complexes	Functional link Generate intracellular signals when there is external shear stress
Belt desmosomes	Broad band of adhesion between cells	E-cadherins	Influence cell shape and motility

ENDOPLASMIC RETICULUM AND GOLGI APPARATUS: BIOSYNTHESIS

The synthesis and degradation of proteins and enzymes in the cell are tightly balanced. ER consists of interconnected branching tubules with a single lumen that has composition similar to the extracellular environment. The membrane may show presence of ribosomes. ER is divided into ***smooth ER that does not have ribosomes and rough ER that has ribosomes attached to its membrane*** (Fig. 1.12). The smooth ER produces proteins for cytosolic release, whereas rough ER produces proteins for other organelles, plasma membrane or releasing to the exterior.

The smooth ER is not very prominent in many cells except those cells that secrete and store steroids (such as liver and adrenals) and muscles where the calcium inside the smooth ER is released into the cytoplasm to enable contraction of the muscles. Because of this specialized function of smooth ER in muscles, here it is called **sarcoplasmic reticulum**. In other cells, release of calcium into the cytoplasm may cause the activation of various enzymes that may even in some circumstances lead to apoptosis.

The ribosomes attached to rough ER translate mRNA and extrude the proteins into the ER lumen or integrate it into the ER membrane. The ***chaperones*** in the ER modify these proteins into N-linked oligosaccharides. This is called *protein folding* and is essential for the normal functioning of the proteins. When this folding does not occur because of defect in the protein or production of excess protein beyond the folding capacity of the ER, the *misfolded proteins* accumulate in the ER leading to *ER stress response* (or unfolded protein response) that may trigger apoptosis.

From the rough ER, the proteins are taken up by the *Golgi apparatus*, an organelle made up of stacked cisternae. The proteins and lipids undergo *glycosylation* in the Golgi apparatus, and this is important in directing the proteins and lipids to their destination. For example, proteins that have mannose phosphate receptor added to them will be directed to lysosomes. Apart from this, the Golgi apparatus helps to recycle proteins and form secretory vesicles to release secretions of the cell extracellularly, such as in goblet cells, bronchial epithelium and plasma cells.

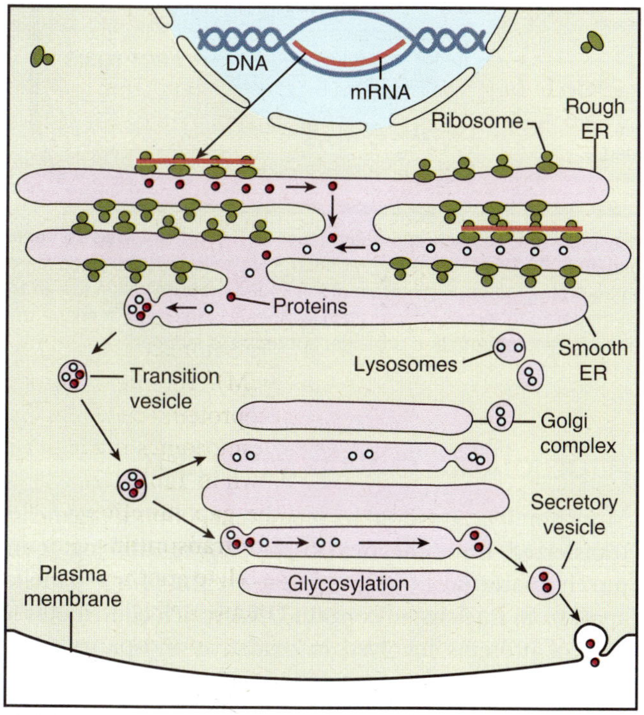

Fig. 1.12 Role of mitochondria and Golgi apparatus. The mRNA from the nucleus is translated into proteins by the ribosomes in the ER which are taken to Golgi apparatus for glycosylation and direction to their destination.

LYSOSOMES AND PROTEASOMES: WASTE DISPOSAL

Lysosomes and proteasomes are the organelles responsible for waste disposal in the cell (Fig. 1.13).

- **Lysosomes** are membrane-bound organelles that contain many enzymes such as proteases, nucleases, lipases, glycosidases, phosphatases and sulphatases that function at a pH less than 5. These enzymes are synthesized in rough ER, glycosylated to mannose-6-phosphate in Golgi apparatus and thereby transported specifically into lysosomes. The macromolecules for digestion reach the lysosomes by three pathways:
  1. *Extracellular material* entering the cell by fluid-phase pinocytosis or receptor-mediated endocytosis

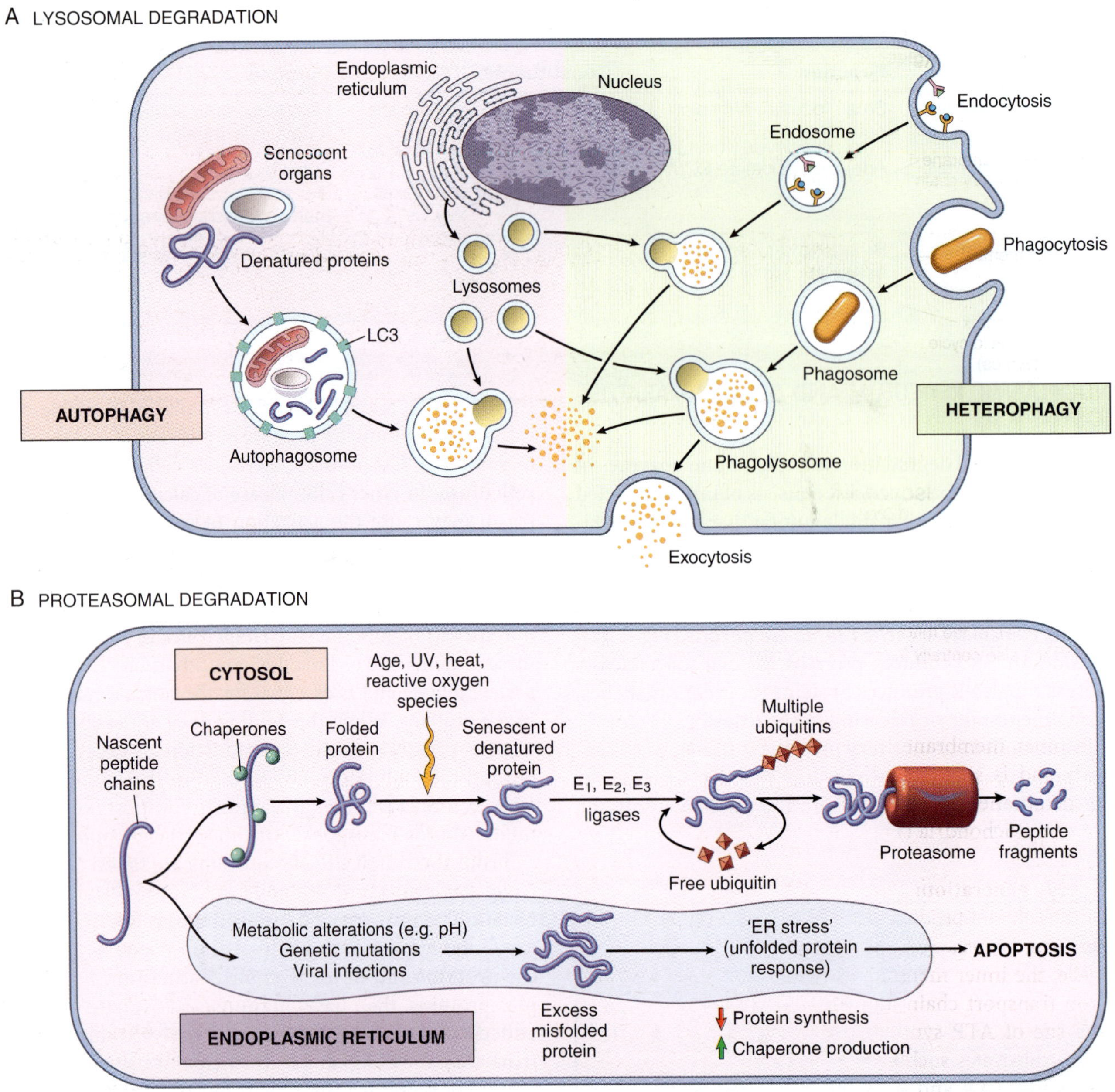

Fig. 1.13 Intracellular catabolism. (A) Lysosomal degradation. Heterophagy (right side) depicts the degradation of their internalized contents, whereas autophagy (left side) depicts the degradation of intracellular organelles. (B) Proteasome degradation. Cytosolic proteins because of various reasons are tagged by multiple ubiquitin molecules for degradation by proteasomes. High levels of misfolded proteins within the endoplasmic reticulum (ER) trigger a protective unfolded protein response which may lead to reduction in protein synthesis or increase in chaperone proteins that can facilitate protein refolding. If this is inadequate to handle the excess of unfolded proteins, apoptosis is induced.

2. *Senescent organelles* and denatured intracellular proteins form an autophagosome and fuse with lysosome for catabolism by a process called autophagy
3. *Microorganisms* that are phagocytosed form a phagosome that fuses with lysosome to form phagolysosome

- **Proteasomes** degrade proteins into small fragments that are later broken down into amino acids and recycled. This mainly includes denatured and misfolded proteins that are bound to ubiquitin.

MITOCHONDRIA: CELLULAR METABOLISM

Mitochondria are double membrane–bound organelles transferred from the ova to the zygote, making them **purely maternal** in origin. These are the only organelle, apart from nucleus, to **contain DNA** which contributes to 20% of proteins involved in oxidative phosphorylation. Owing to the two modes of transcription of mitochondrial proteins (mitochondrial DNA and nuclear DNA), inheritance of mitochondrial disorders may be autosomal, X-linked or maternal. A mitochondrion is composed

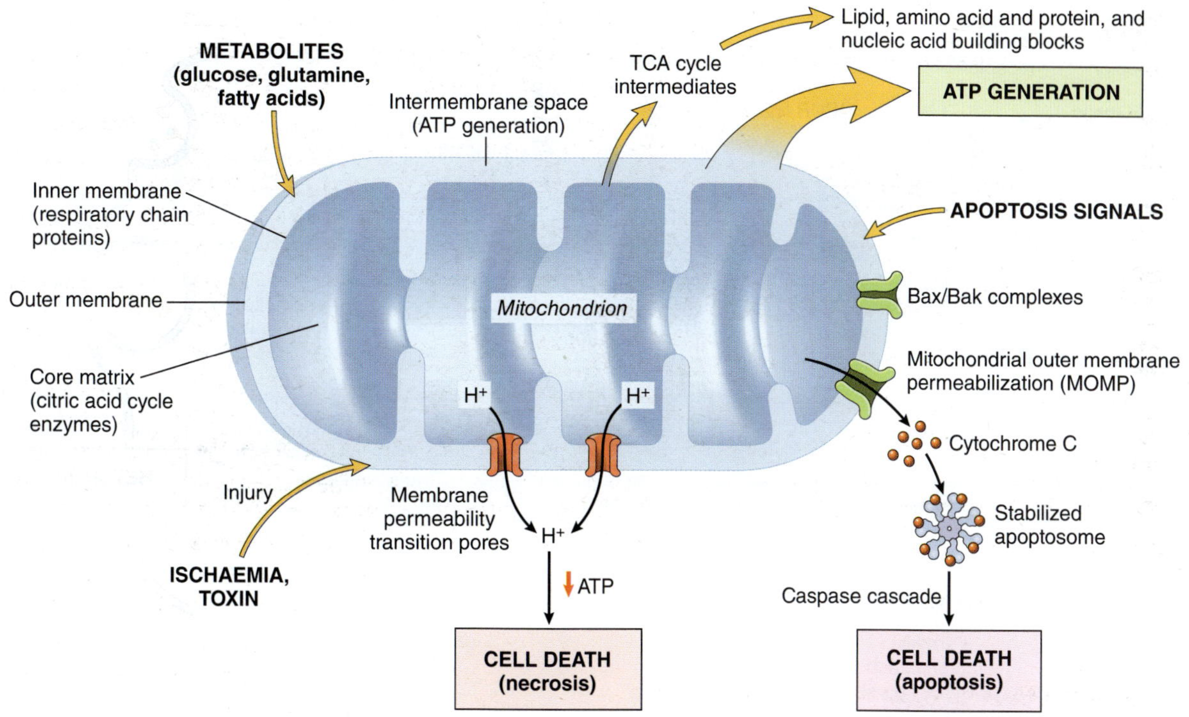

Fig. 1.14 Roles of the mitochondria. Apart from ATP synthesis, mitochondria also act as source of molecules for syntheses of lipids and proteins and are also centrally involved in cell life-and-death decisions.

of an inner membrane that encloses the mitochondrial matrix and is surrounded by an outer membrane with intermembrane space in between. The three major functions of mitochondria (Fig. 1.14) are as follows:

- **Energy generation:** Mitochondria are the powerhouse of the cell and produce ATP by oxidative phosphorylation. The matrix contains enzymes of tricarboxylic acid cycle, the inner membranes bear the enzymes of electron transport chain and the intermembrane space is the site of ATP synthesis. Mitochondrial matrix oxidizes substrates such as glucose, amino acids and fatty acids into CO_2 and drives the hydrogen ion pump to transfer H^+ that was formed in the matrix to the intermembrane space. This creates an *H^+ gradient across the inner membrane* that facilitates the flow of H^+ back into the matrix and, in the process, produces ATP.

  Apart from ATP, the mitochondria can also produce heat energy by using the inner membrane protein *thermogenin*. The by-products produced in this process are the oxygen free radicals. Increase in this radical generation during hypoxia, toxic injury and mitochondrial ageing may lead to *intracellular oxidative stress*.
- **Intermediate metabolism:** The mitochondria provide building blocks for proteins and lipids by shunting some of the intermediates to the synthetic pathway from ATP synthesis. This is called ***Warburg effect,*** and is seen in rapidly growing cells such as benign and malignant tumour cells. It favours cellular growth over cellular maintenance when it receives signals from certain exogenous factors such as growth factors, change in nutrient and oxygen supplies, and cellular signalling pathways.
- **Cell death:** Mitochondria play a major role in both forms of cell death – necrosis and apoptosis.

  Necrosis: External cellular injury may damage the mitochondria by dissipating the proton potential across the inner membrane, which in turn causes failure of ATP synthesis and cell death.

  Apoptosis: This is the programmed cell death that is triggered by extrinsic signals or intrinsic pathways. Mitochondria play a central role in the intrinsic pathway of apoptosis when they become leaky. Important enzymes such as cytochrome C leak into the cytosol and initiate the process. These mechanisms are explained in detail in Chapter 2.

GROWTH FACTORS AND RECEPTORS

Growth factors are substances that stimulate the activity of genes required for cell growth and cell division, by binding to specific receptors in the cell (Fig. 1.15). The functions of growth factors include the following:

1. Stimulate cell proliferation in steady state and injury by
   - Promoting entry of cells into the cell cycle
   - Relieving blocks on cell cycle progression
   - Preventing apoptosis
   - Enhancing biosynthesis of cellular components required for a mother cell to give rise to two daughter cells

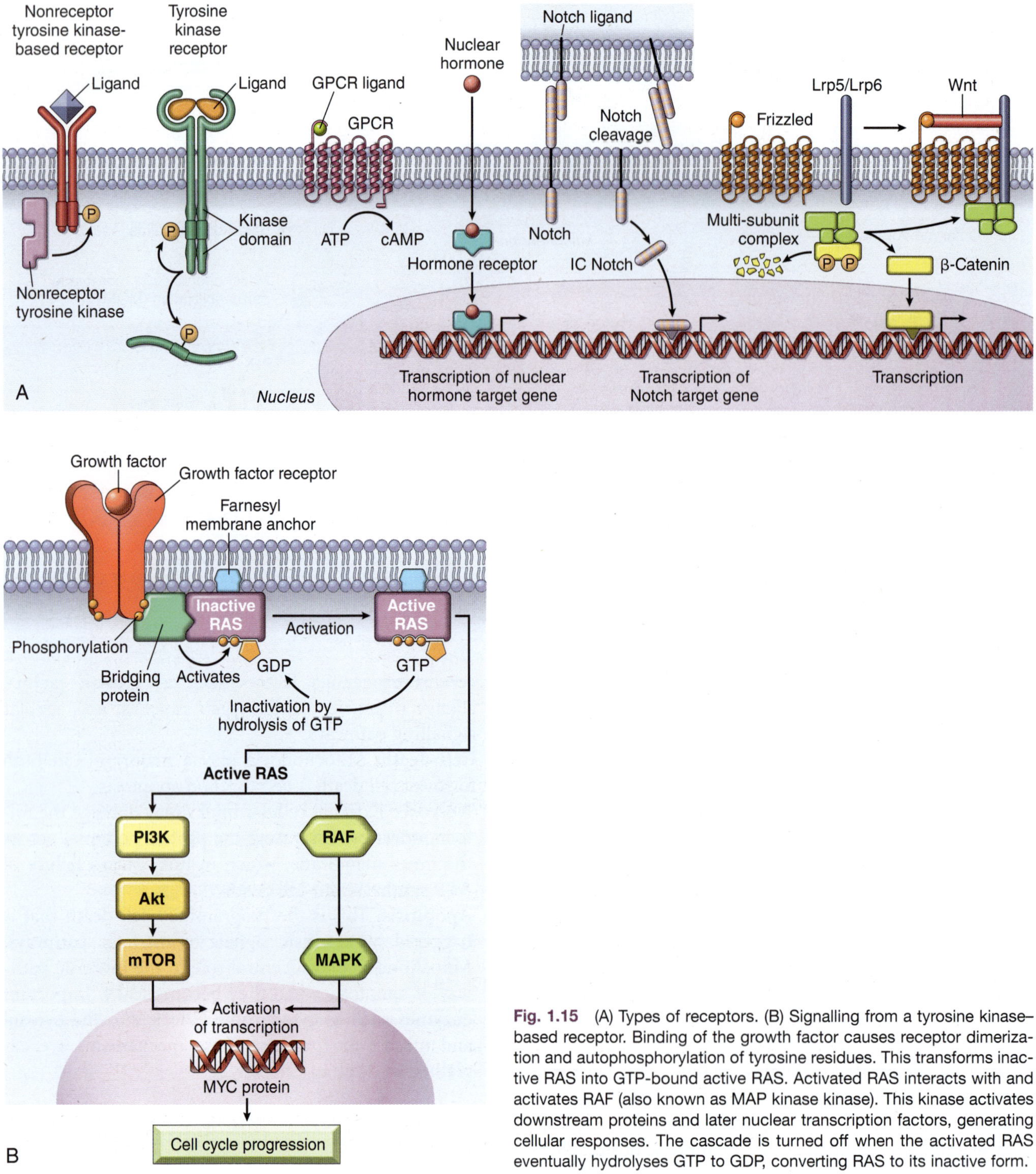

Fig. 1.15 (A) Types of receptors. (B) Signalling from a tyrosine kinase–based receptor. Binding of the growth factor causes receptor dimerization and autophosphorylation of tyrosine residues. This transforms inactive RAS into GTP-bound active RAS. Activated RAS interacts with and activates RAF (also known as MAP kinase kinase). This kinase activates downstream proteins and later nuclear transcription factors, generating cellular responses. The cascade is turned off when the activated RAS eventually hydrolyses GTP to GDP, converting RAS to its inactive form.

2. Control cell migration
3. Drive cell differentiation

These growth factor genes are also referred to as proto-oncogenes. Their uncontrolled activity or constitutive activation converts them into oncogenes causing tumour formation and neoplastic transformation. Some important growth factors are described in Table 1.3.

SIGNALLING PATHWAYS (FIG. 1.16)

Intercellular signalling is very important for communication among cells in multicellular organisms. It is essential for organization of cells, growth, and response to threats and stimuli. Disruptions in these signals may lead to cancer, shock or even cell death. The signals received by

Table 1.3 Important Growth Factors and Their Role

Growth Factor	Produced by	Target Cells	Clinical Relevance
Epidermal growth factor (EGF) and transforming growth factor-α (TGF-α)	Macrophages and some types of epithelial cells	Hepatocytes, fibroblasts and many epithelial cells	EGFR1 mutations/amplification are seen in cancers of lung, head and neck, breast and brain The ERBB2 receptor (also known as HER2) is overexpressed in a subset of breast cancers, and molecular antagonists to them are used in treatment
Hepatocyte growth factor (HGF; also known as scatter factor)	• Fibroblasts • Most mesenchymal cells • Endothelium • Nonhepatocyte liver cells	• Hepatocytes • Biliary, pulmonary, renal, mammary epithelial cells • Epidermal cells	• Morphogen in embryonic development • Promotes cell migration • Enhances hepatocyte survival • Overexpressed or mutated in renal and thyroid papillary carcinomas, and inhibitors to its receptors may be of value for cancer therapy
Platelet-derived growth factor (PDGF)	• Stored in platelet granules and is released on platelet activation • Macrophages, endothelium, smooth muscle cells	• Fibroblast, endothelial and smooth muscle cell proliferation and chemotaxis • Matrix synthesis	Recruitment of the cells into areas of inflammation and tissue injury
Vascular endothelial growth factors (VEGFs) include VEGF-A, -B, -C and -D and **placental growth factor (PGF)**	Endothelium	VEGF-A angiogenesis VEGF-B and PGF vasculogenesis (embryonic vessel development) VEGF-C and -D lymphangiogenesis (angiogenesis and lymphatic development)	Antibodies against VEGF are approved for treatment of renal and colon cancers, ophthalmic diseases including 'wet' age-related macular degeneration, retinopathy of prematurity, and diabetic macular oedema Increased levels of VEGF receptors in pregnant women may cause preeclampsia by removing free VEGF required for maintaining normal endothelium
Transforming growth factor-β (TGF-β) TGF-β1 has widespread distribution, and is referred to as TGF-β	Platelets, endothelium and mononuclear inflammatory cells	Binds to receptors that activate SMADs downstream They often have opposing effects on different tissues and so called pleiotropic	• Scar formation by increasing collagen production and reducing degradation • Fibrosis in lung, liver and kidneys in the setting of chronic inflammation • Terminate inflammatory responses

the cell stimulate specific responses in different cells and are modes of relaying information. Some examples of types of signals are as follows:

- Danger signals, as in the case of damaged or infected cells that trigger neighbouring cells to respond to these signals and help eliminating them.
- Contact with neighbouring cells: These signals help in movement of ions and second messenger molecules between neighbouring cells through adhesion molecules and/or gap junctions.
- Contact with ECM: These help in attachment of leucocytes to other cells during inflammation with the help of integrins.
- Secreted molecules: The important secreted molecules include growth factors, cytokines and hormones.

Extracellular cell–cell signalling pathways may be of different types such as

- **Autocrine:** The molecule acts on the same cell that secretes it.

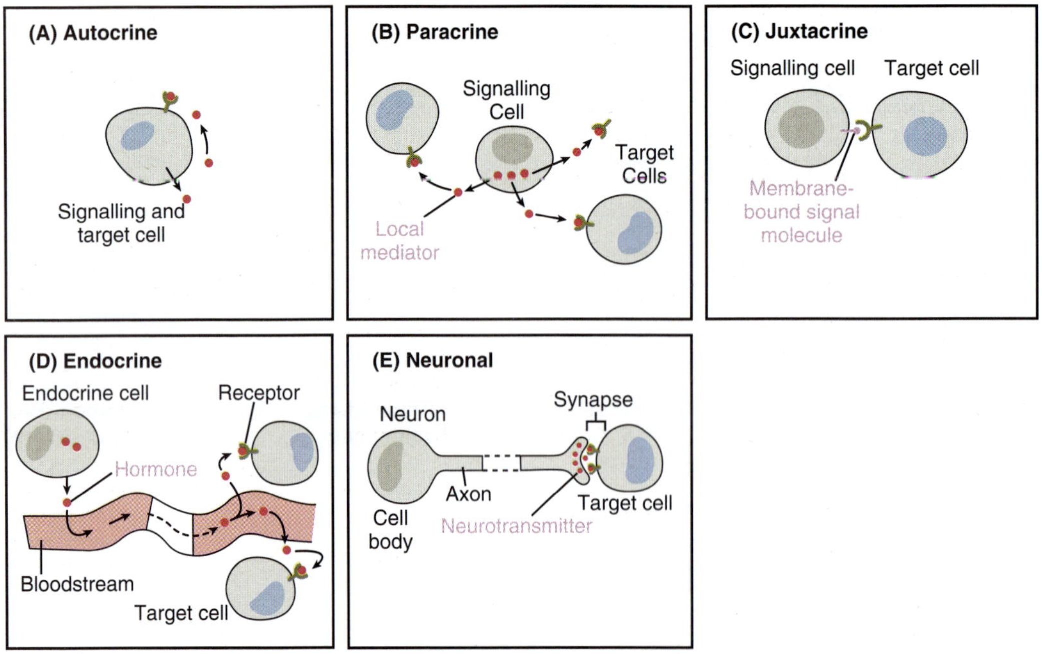

Fig. 1.16 Signalling pathways (refer text).

- **Paracrine:** The molecule acts on the cells in the vicinity in which it is secreted and gets degraded or trapped in ECM quickly. Juxtacrine is a type of paracrine where the molecule is attached to the surface of the secreting cell and activates cells that encounter the secreting cell.
- **Endocrine:** The secreted molecule is carried by blood and acts on distant target organs.
- **Synaptic:** Stimulus is transmitted from neurons to target cells at synaptic junctions, where they are received by specific receptors. The molecules that bind to the receptors are called ligands, and binding of the ligand to the receptor triggers a chain of intracellular events. This ligand–receptor binding is very specific. On the basis of their location, cellular receptors are classified into the following:
- **Cell surface receptors** (transmembrane proteins) that may open ion channels or activate an associated GTP-binding regulatory protein or an associated enzyme, or trigger a proteolytic event.
- **Intracellular receptors** that are activated by lipid-soluble molecules such as vitamin D and steroid hormones.

SIGNAL TRANSDUCTION PATHWAYS

The binding of a ligand to the receptor induces receptor cross-linking, which in turn modifies the intracellular domain of the receptor. This triggers a series of biochemical changes in the cells that lead to signal transduction to the nucleus, where it causes changes in gene expression. The cellular receptors are classified on the basis of the signalling mechanisms and intracellular biochemical pathways they activate (Fig. 1.17).

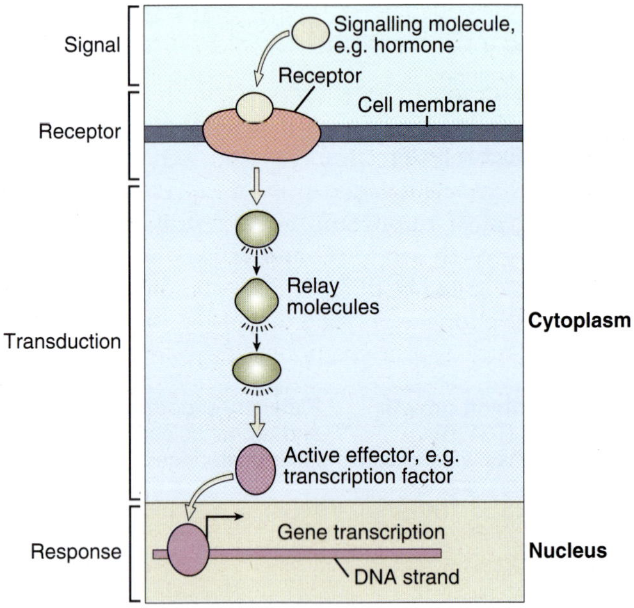

Fig. 1.17 Mechanism of signal transduction.

- **Receptors with kinase activity:** These receptors phosphorylate proteins (such as tyrosine, serine/threonine) through the protein kinase activity. They also have associated phosphatases that reverse the phosphorylation, thus controlling the signalling. These receptors may either have intrinsic tyrosine kinase activity or be associated with intracellular nonreceptor tyrosine kinase enzyme.

- **G protein–coupled receptors**: Interestingly, these receptors traverse the cell membrane seven times and hence called *seven-transmembrane receptors*. When the ligand binds to the receptor, the G protein bound to the receptor is activated through the exchange of GDP for GTP. This generates cyclic AMP (cAMP) and inositol 1,4,5-triphosphate (IP3), of which the latter releases calcium from ER.
- **Nuclear receptors**: Lipid-soluble ligands such as hormones diffuse into cells, activating intracellular nuclear receptors which can either activate or repress gene transcription.
- Other classes of receptors include **Notch receptors** and **frizzled receptors**. The frizzled receptors influence cell development through Wnt signalling pathway.

The process of ligand binding to receptor and receptor activation can trigger various responses in the cells, which include the following:

1. Enzyme activation (or inactivation)
2. Nuclear (or cytoplasmic) localization of transcription factors
3. Transcription factor activation (or inactivation)
4. Actin polymerization (or depolymerization)
5. Protein degradation (or stabilization)
6. Activation of feedback inhibitory (or stimulatory) loops

The activation of receptors and signal transduction pathways alters gene transcription by its effect on transcription factors. These transcription factors may translocate to the nucleus and activate or supress gene expression. **The most important transcription factors that promote growth are MYC and JUN, whereas growth arrest is mediated by p53.** The DNA-binding domains of the transcription factors bind them to specific regions on the genes such as gene promoters and gene enhancers. It is now found that these transcription factors must possess protein–protein interaction domains to control RNA synthesis.

ROLE OF EXTRACELLULAR MATRIX

ECM is a wide array of proteins that lie outside the cell in the interstitium. These help in maintaining the architecture of tissues, and their interaction with cells is critical for development and healing. The remodelling of ECM is a continuous process, and it influences various processes such as repair, fibrosis and tumour metastasis. Their key functions include the following:

- Mechanical support for cell anchorage and maintenance of cell polarity, such as in epithelium
- Control of cell proliferation by controlling growth factor availability
- Scaffolding for tissue renewal and regeneration following tissue injury, such as in cirrhosis
- Establishment of tissue microenvironments, such as in the case of basement membrane of glomeruli that helps in regulating the filtration process

ECM occurs in two basic forms – interstitial matrix and basement membrane (Table 1.4).

Table 1.4 Two Forms of Extracellular Matrix

Interstitial Matrix	Basement Membrane
• It is present between the cells • It is produced by mesenchymal cells • It is a three-dimensional, relatively amorphous gel • It includes fibrillar and nonfibrillar collagens, fibronectin, elastin, proteoglycans and hyaluronate	• It is organized into a membrane on which the epithelium and endothelium rest • It is formed by epithelium and underlying mesenchymal cells • It is a flat lamellar chicken wire mesh • It includes amorphous nonfibrillar type IV collagen and laminin

COMPONENTS OF EXTRACELLULAR MATRIX

ECM is composed of three groups of proteins – the fibrous structural proteins, the hydrated gels and adhesive proteins (Fig. 1.18).

1. **Fibrous structural proteins:** These provide tensile strength and elastic recoil to tissue. They include collagen and elastin.
   Collagens are composed of three separate polypeptide chains braided into a triple helix. These are divided into **fibrillary collagens** (types I, II, III and V) and **nonfibrillary collagens** (type IV, VII and IX). The fibrillary collagens are the major components of the connective tissue of bone, cartilage, tendon, blood vessels, skin and scars. *Lysyl oxidase*, in the presence of *vitamin C*, creates lateral cross-links in these collagens and provides them tensile strength. Hence, vitamin C deficiency causes skeletal deformities in children, bleeding from weak blood vessel walls and poor healing. Nonfibrillary collagens form basement membrane (type IV) or anchor squamous epithelium to the underlying basement membrane (type VII).
   Elastin is responsible for the recoil of tissues after physical deformation. These are found in cardiac valves, large blood vessels, uterus, skin and ligaments. Elastic fibres are made up of central core of elastin surrounded by a meshwork of fibrillin.
2. **Water-hydrated gels:** These include proteoglycans and hyaluronan that provide compressive resistance and lubrication.
   Proteoglycans are present in joint cartilage and provide resistance to compressive forces and lubrication

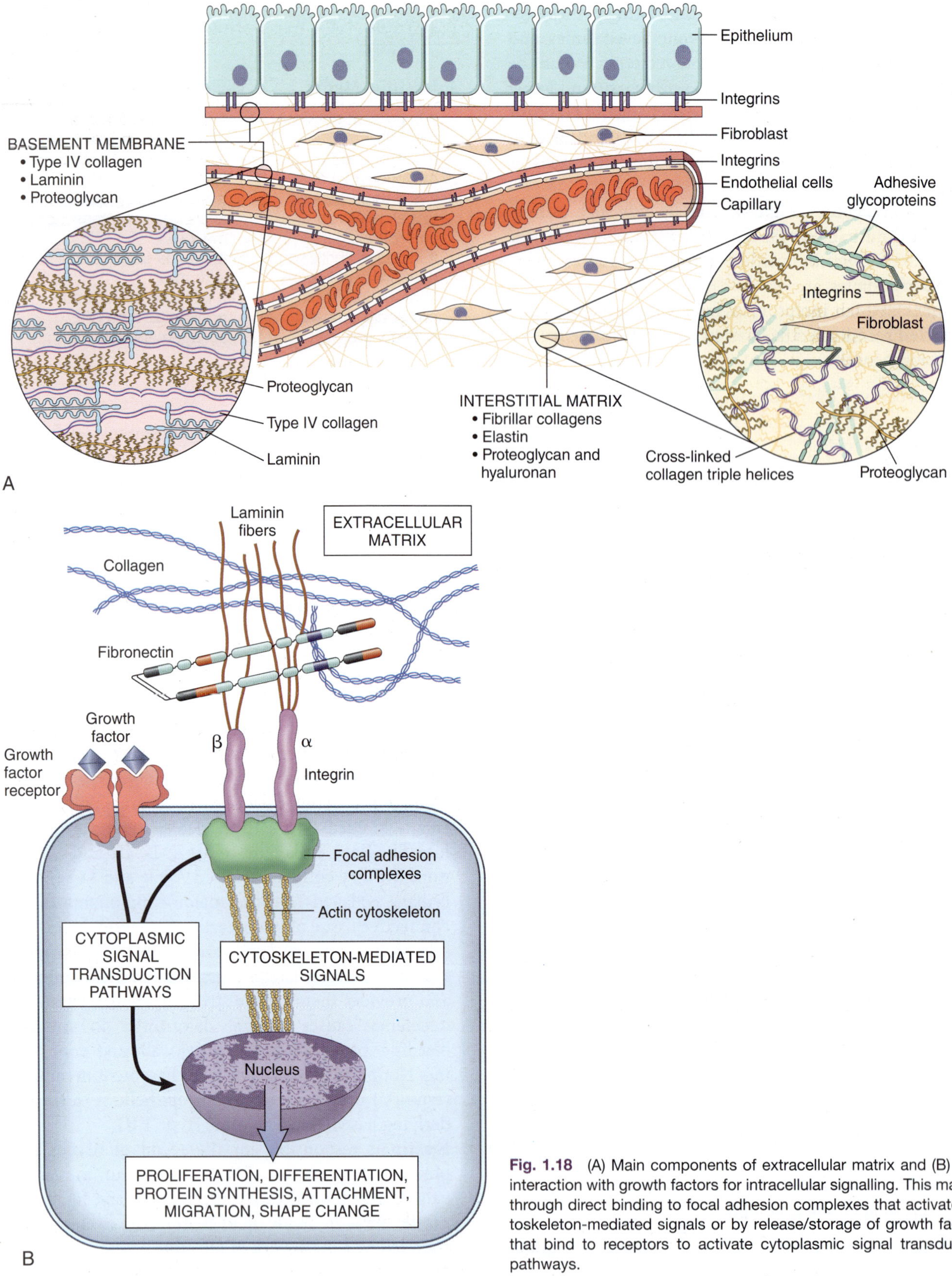

Fig. 1.18 (A) Main components of extracellular matrix and (B) their interaction with growth factors for intracellular signalling. This may be through direct binding to focal adhesion complexes that activate cytoskeleton-mediated signals or by release/storage of growth factors that bind to receptors to activate cytoplasmic signal transduction pathways.

to the adjacent bone. These are composed of *glycosaminoglycans* such as keratin sulphate and chondroitin sulphate attached to hyaluronic acid polymer called **hyaluronan** with the help of proteins. These osmotically absorb water and form gelatin-like compressible gel. These also act as storehouse of growth factors and help in cell proliferation, migration and adhesion.

3. **Adhesive glycoproteins** bind ECM elements to one another and to cells. The important adhesive proteins include *fibronectin* and *laminin*. The receptors of these molecules are called **cell adhesion molecules** (CAMs), which include integrins, immunoglobulins, cadherins and selectins, with the most among them being integrins.
   Fibronectin is a large heterodimer produced by fibroblasts, monocytes and endothelium. It is present in tissues and plasma and plays an important role in wound healing by forming a scaffold for ECM deposition and aiding angiogenesis and re-epithelialization.
   Laminin is the most abundant glycoprotein in basement membrane. It connects cells to underlying ECM components such as type IV collagen and heparan sulphate. It also helps in cell proliferation, differentiation and motility.
   Integrins are a large family of transmembrane glycoproteins that link the intracellular cytoskeleton of cells to ECM components. These play an important role in migration of leucocytes in inflammation and aggregation of platelets in haemostasis. Binding of cells through the integrin receptors can also activate signals for cell locomotion, proliferation and differentiation.

CELL CYCLE

Cell cycle is the sequence of events by which every organism undergoes cellular proliferation (Fig. 1.19). This is critical for growth and development, maintenance of homeostasis, replacement of dead cells and repair of damaged tissue. It involves synthesis of DNA and other cellular constituents followed by their proportionate distribution to two daughter cells. The nonmultiplying cells are said to be in G0 state (resting state). The following are the four important stages of cell cycle:

- **G1 or presynthetic growth phase**
- **S or DNA synthesis phase**
- **G2 or premitotic growth phase**
- **M or mitotic phase**

Cells in G0 state or cells that have completed M phase may enter the cell cycle, on the basis of the nature of cell and presence of growth signals. The cell cycle is controlled by activators, inhibitors and cell cycle checkpoints.

Cell cycle activators include *cyclins* and their associated enzymes *cyclin-dependent kinase* (CDK). Cyclins bind to specific CDKs and activate them, which in turn phosphorylates protein substrates and progresses the cell cycle to the next stage. When the CDK activity is completed, it gets degraded spontaneously, creating a rise and fall in its activity. The four important cyclins of cell cycle are cyclins D, E, A and B and they are produced in this order. Cyclin D is the first to appear and activates cell cycle by binding to CDK4 and later to CDK6.

Cell cycle inhibitors are the factors that inhibit the action of CDK–cyclin complex called *cyclin-dependent*

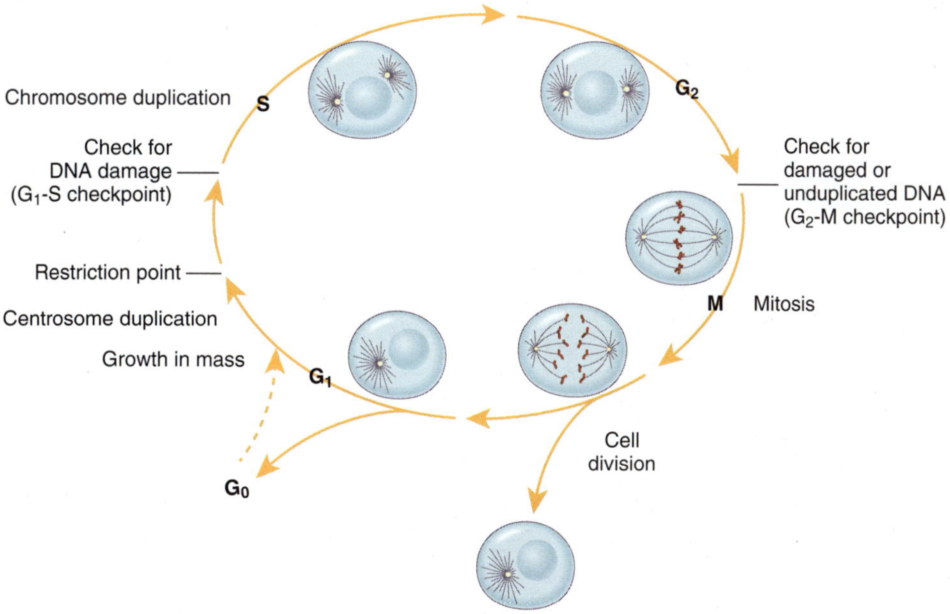

Fig. 1.19 Cell cycle landmarks. This figure depicts the four stages of cell cycle and the two major checkpoints, G1-S and G2-M.

kinase inhibitors (CDKIs). These are divided into two families – CDKIs that inhibit all cyclins (p21, p27 and p57) and CDKIs that inhibit only CDK4 and CDK6 (p15, p16, p18 and p19).

Cell cycle checkpoints are inbuilt surveillance mechanisms within the cell cycle to prevent proliferation of cells with defective DNA. There are two checkpoints:

- **Checkpoint 1 at G1-S transition** that checks the quality of DNA in the cell entering cell cycle and adequacy of growth factors.
- **Checkpoint 2 at G2-M transition** to check the quality of the newly synthesized DNA to be given to daughter cells.

These checkpoints are manned by tumour suppressor genes. Failure of these checkpoints may lead to uncontrolled proliferation of cells or proliferation of cells with defective DNA leading to malignant transformation.

STEM CELLS

Stem cells are specialized cells that are capable of differentiating into various differentiated cells. These play a major role in development of embryo and in replacement of damaged cells in adults so that the tissue population is maintained. There is a delicate balance between dying mature cells and replicating stem cells that helps to maintain tissue homeostasis. The two important properties of stem cells are as follows:

- Ability of stem cells to maintain their numbers called **self-renewal.**
- **Asymmetric division**, in which a stem cell always divides into one daughter cell that becomes differentiated into mature cell and another daughter cell that retains self-renewal property as stem cell (Fig. 1.20).

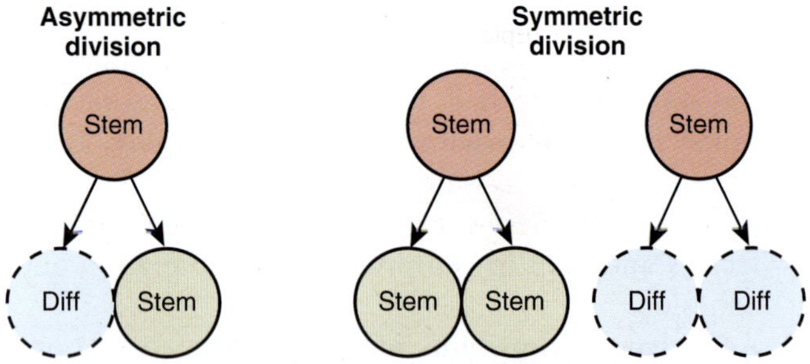

Fig. 1.20 Division of stem cells.

Stem cells belong to two categories:

- **Embryonic stem (ES) cells:** These are found in the blastocyst stage of the embryo in the inner cell mass. These are the ***most undifferentiated cells*** and *totipotent* with the capacity to form any cell in the body, belonging to any of the three germ cell layers (Fig. 1.21).
- **Adult stem cells (also called tissue stem cells):** These are undifferentiated cells found in special ***stem cell niches*** located within differentiated cells. These are usually quiescent but can be stimulated to produce differentiated cells. However, these are not totipotent and can produce only cells native to the tissue in which the stem cells are located (Fig. 1.22). The common stem cell niches are given in Table 1.5.

Among the adult stem cells, ***haematopoietic stem cells*** are one of the most active and well-studied stem cells. These are found in the bone marrow and capable of producing all lineage of blood cells. They are used in bone marrow transplant in leukaemia patients and patients with defective stem cells. The other stem cell

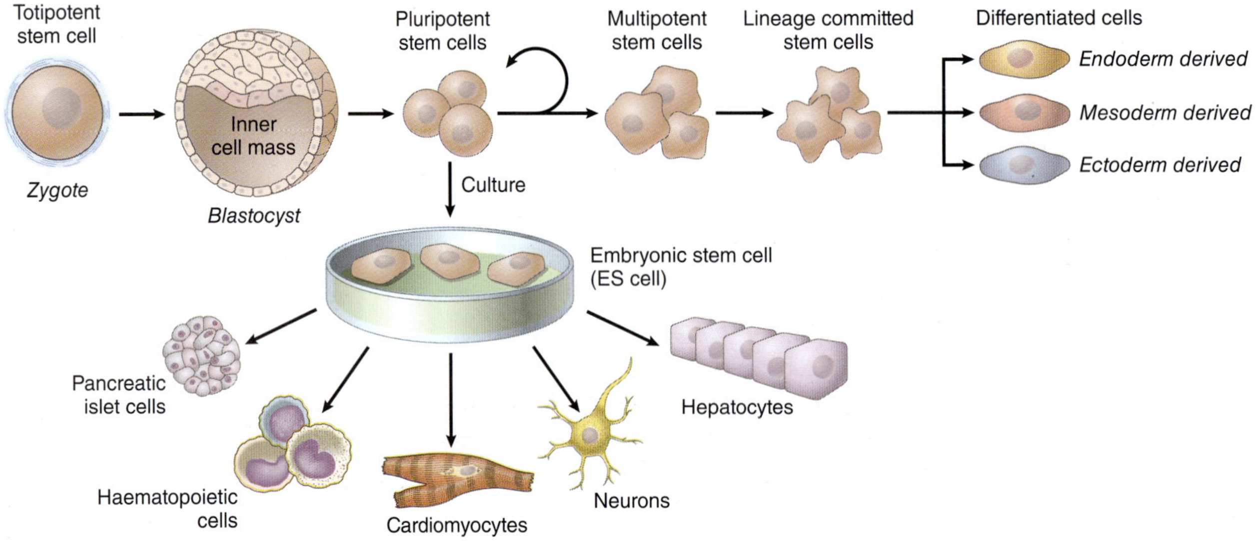

Fig. 1.21 Embryonal stem cells. The zygote divides to form blastocysts, and the inner cell mass of the blastocyst generates the embryo. The pluripotent cells of the inner cell mass, known as embryonic stem (ES) cells, can be induced to differentiate into cells of multiple lineages. ES cells can be cultured in vitro and induced to give rise to cells of all three lineages.

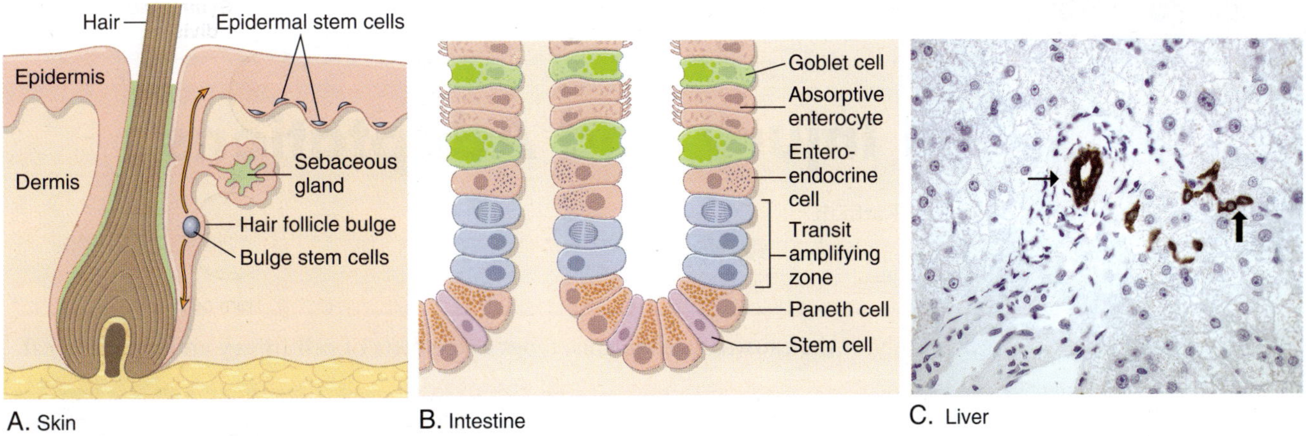

Fig. 1.22 Location of stem cell niches. (A) Skin stem cells are located in the bulge area of the hair follicle, in sebaceous glands, and in the lower layer of the epidermis. (B) Small intestine stem cells are located near the base of the crypt, above Paneth cells. (C) Liver stem cells (oval cells) are located in the canals of Hering (thick arrow), structures that connect bile ductules (thin arrow) to parenchymal hepatocytes. Bile duct cells and canals of Hering are stained here with an immunohistochemical stain for cytokeratin 7.

Table 1.5 Location of Stem Cell Niches

Brain	Subventricular zone and dentate gyrus
Skin	Bulge region of the hair follicle
Cornea	Limbus
Small intestine	Base of crypt
Liver	Oval cells in canals of Hering

found in bone marrow is the ***mesenchymal stem cell*** that can form stromal cells such as cartilage, bone, fat and muscle, and is useful during tissue regeneration to provide a scaffolding.

Regenerative medicine is a new developing branch in medicine, which is based on the ability to isolate, expand and transplant stem cells in humans. Although the transplanted stem cells are capable of regenerating damaged tissues, these possess HLA genes that elicit immunogenic rejection in the transplant recipient. This has motivated scientists to develop techniques in which the differentiated cells obtained from the patient are converted into stem cells called ***induced pluripotent stem cells*** (iPS) and introduced back into the patient. This would help to overcome the problem of immunogenic rejection.

SELF-ASSESSMENT

Self-Assessment Questions

1. Explain the methods of post-translational silencing of mRNA.
2. What are the stages of the cell cycle and the factors that control the cell cycle?
3. Explain the properties and types of stem cells.
4. Explain the structure and functions of mitochondria.
5. Where are lysosomal enzymes produced and how do they reach the lysosomes?
6. Name the cell receptors and mechanism of signal transduction.
7. What are the pathways of cell signalling?

Topics for Self-Directed Learning

1. Role of epigenetics in cancer and its treatment.
2. Various pathways of growth signal transduction in cells and the disorders associated with their defects.
3. Disorders of collagen synthesis and associated syndromes.
4. Evolving technologies in stem cell transplant.

2 Cell Injury and Adaptations

Rajeswari Kathiah

PA 2.1 Demonstrate knowledge about the causes, mechanisms, types and effects of **cell injury** and their clinical significance.

PA 2.2 Describe the aetiology of cell injury. Distinguish between **reversible and irreversible injuries**: mechanisms and morphology.

PA 2.3 Discuss **intracellular accumulation** of fats, proteins, carbohydrates and pigments.

PA 2.4 Describe and discuss cell death: **types, mechanisms, necrosis, apoptosis** (basic as contrasted with necrosis) and **autolysis.**

PA 2.5 Describe and discuss **pathological calcifications** and **gangrene.**

PA 2.6 Describe and discuss cellular adaptations: **atrophy, hypertrophy, hyperplasia, metaplasia** and **dysplasia.**

PA 2.7 Describe and discuss the mechanisms of **cellular ageing and apoptosis.**

CHAPTER OUTLINE

OVERVIEW OF CELLULAR RESPONSES TO STRESS

Cells actively maintain the composition of their immediate environment and intracellular milieu within a narrow range of physiological parameters, thereby staying in a steady state called ***homeostasis.*** They are complex, interconnected systems and even single, local injuries can result in multiple secondary and tertiary effects.

The cells of our body are constantly exposed to a wide variety of stress factors that are listed later in the chapter. Although the cells are designed to handle the impaction because of stress, they succumb beyond a certain limit. In simple terms, cell injury disturbs cellular homeostasis. Cells have a limited reserve of responses to injury, depending on the cell type and the nature of the injury. These responses can be categorized as adaptation, degeneration or death.

Injury to tissues and organs begins at the cellular level. **Rudolf Virchow**, known as the father of cellular pathology, based his study of diseased cells on the observation of structural changes. However, Virchow also stated that biochemical changes in the cell, which preceded the appearance of morphological alterations, gave a more complete explanation of the functional disturbances in diseased cells and, in some cases, were the only detectable changes. Thus, a pathologist must always correlate lesions with their biochemical basis and keep in mind that a cell may be damaged functionally, yet it may have no apparent morphological alterations.

When exposed to physiological stresses or pathological stimuli, cells undergo ***adaptation*** to achieve a new steady state that would help them survive in the new environment. If the stress is severe, the cells become ***reversibly injured***, a point from which they could come back to their native state on regression of the noxious stimuli. If the stress is too severe, then the cells are ***irreversibly injured*** and eventually ***cell death*** occurs.

Cellular responses to injury are not an 'all-or-none' phenomenon. Response to a given stimulus depends on the type, status and genetic makeup of the injured cell, apart from the nature, intensity and focus of the stimulus. Adaptation, reversible injury and cell death may be **stages of progressive deterioration** following exposure to a dangerous stimulus (Flowchart 2.1).

Cell death is more often because of pathological causes; however, physiological causes like embryogenesis may cause cell death also. Variety of causes like ischaemia, infections, toxins and chemicals can give rise to **cell death**, which is the end result of progressive cell injury and is one of the most crucial events in the pathogenesis of disease in any tissue or organ.

Cells can also be injured by one of the following ways, more commonly, when they counteract stress:

- Metabolic derangements and sublethal, chronic injury may be associated with ***intracellular accumulations*** of a variety of substances such as proteins, lipids and carbohydrates.
- ***Pathological calcification*** occurs when calcium gets deposited at sites of cell death or, in normal tissues, because of high levels of serum calcium.
- ***Cellular ageing*** is a normal process and is accompanied by a variety of characteristic morphological and functional changes in the cells.

In this chapter, we discuss the spectrum of cellular injuries and the two patterns of cell death – necrosis and apoptosis – along with sublethal injuries in the form of intracellular accumulation, pathological calcification and cellular ageing.

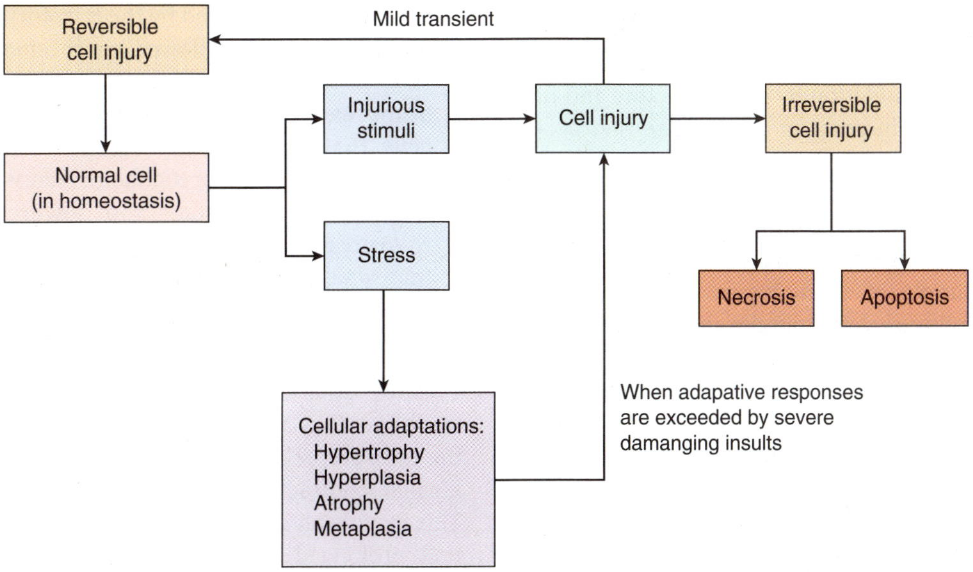

Flowchart 2.1 Schematic representation of stages of cellular responses to stress and injury. (*Source:* From Robbins & Cotran Pathologic Basis of Disease, 10th edition. 2021. Elsevier.)

CELLULAR ADAPTATIONS PA 2.6

Adaptations are reversible changes in the size, number, metabolic activity, morphology or functions of cells in response to environmental stress. A cell may adapt to a stimulus or a sublethal injury positively with increased efficiency and productivity or undergo degeneration with reduced functional capacity. The response to injury can be reversible with eventual restoration of normal or near-normal cellular structure and function or irreversible with progression from degeneration to death of the cell.

Adaptations can be because of physiological or pathological causes and are of four types:

- Hypertrophy
- Hyperplasia
- Atrophy
- Metaplasia

HYPERTROPHY

Increase in the size of cells leading to an increase in the size of the affected organ is referred to as hypertrophy. Thus, the affected organ has larger cells and no new cells.

Tissues composed of ***labile*** (rapidly proliferating cells) and ***stable*** (quiescent cells with the capacity to proliferate whenever needed) ***cells*** respond to stress by undergoing both hyperplasia and hypertrophy. Tissues composed of ***permanent cells*** (nondividing cells) adapt to stress only by hypertrophy because these cells are incapable of proliferation. These include the striated muscles of the heart and skeletal muscles, which are terminally divided cells and have a very limited capacity to divide further and hence respond to stress only by hypertrophy. In many organs, both hypertrophy and hyperplasia coexist and contribute to an increase in the size of the organs.

Hypertrophy can be **physiological or pathological**. Physiological hypertrophy is the result of increased functional demand or stimulation by growth factors and hormones. The massive increase in uterine size that occurs during pregnancy is mainly because of hypertrophy, stimulated by hormones acting on smooth muscles. This leads to increased synthesis of smooth muscle proteins and thus increase in cell and organ size.

Another example of physiological hypertrophy includes the enlarging skeletal muscles in body builders in response to increased demand.

Thus, the most common stimulus for muscle hypertrophy is ***increased workload***. In addition, as an example of pathological hypertrophy in the heart, chronic haemodynamic overload because of hypertension or valvular disease causes increased workload and acts as the stimulus for cardiac hypertrophy. This increase in cell size results in an increase in the strength and work capacity of muscles.

Apart from muscles, adipocytes may also expand in size by depositing more lipids within their cytoplasmic vesicles. Thus, in human adults, the increase in body fat tissue occurs mostly by an increase in the size of adipocytes, not by an increase in the number of adipocytes.

Mechanisms of Hypertrophy

In hypertrophy, the increase in the size of the cells is because of an increase in the synthesis of additional structural proteins. Cardiac hypertrophy is the prototypical example of pathological hypertrophy.

Three steps involved in the pathogenesis of cardiac hypertrophy are as follows:

1. ***Mechanical sensors*** initiated by increased workload, growth factors like TGF-β, insulin-like growth factor-1 (IGF-1) and vasoactive agents coordinate and set off the response.
2. The signals that are generated in the cell membrane activate many signalling pathways, most importantly phosphoinositide 3-kinase (PI3K)/AKT pathway and G-protein-coupled receptor-mediated pathways.
3. This results in the activation of a set of transcription factors like GATA4, nuclear factor of activated T cells (NFAT) and myocyte enhancer factor 2 (MEF2), which work together to increase the synthesis of muscle proteins that cause muscular hypertrophy.

An understanding of these mechanisms has provided insights into the basis of hypertrophy and has helped in the development of target drugs that inhibit the key signalling pathways explained earlier.

Other mechanisms causing hypertrophy include the following:

1. **Switch of contractile proteins from adult to fetal or neonatal forms:** For example, the α isoform of myosin heavy chain is replaced by the β isoform, which has the tendency to cause slower, more energetic and economic contraction.
2. **Some early embryonic genes are re-expressed in cells that undergo hypertrophy:** For example, the gene for atrial natriuretic factor that is expressed only in the embryonic stage and downregulated later is re-expressed in cardiac hypertrophy. This factor promotes salt excretion by the kidneys and leads to a reduction in blood volume, pressure and haemodynamic overload.

Irrespective of the cause and mechanism, when hypertrophy reaches a limit beyond which it cannot withstand the pressure, regressive cellular changes like loss of myofibrillar contractile elements and myocyte death occur. This may result in organ failure, thus highlighting the fact that prolonged and excessive adaptation to stress can progress to significant cell injury and organ failure if the stress is not withdrawn (Fig. 2.1).

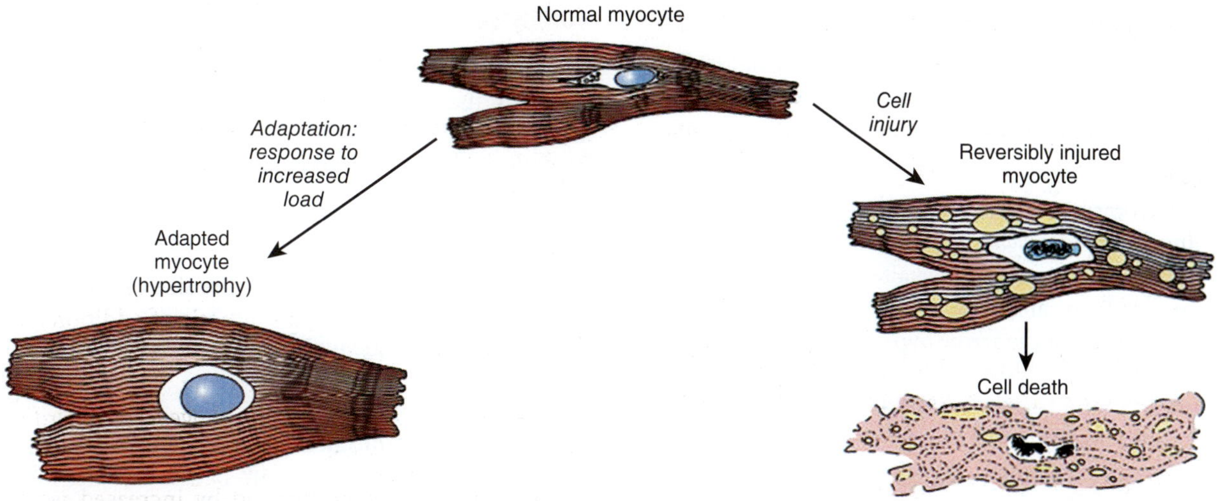

Fig. 2.1 Diagrammatic representation of a normal myocyte, adapted, reversibly injured, and a myocyte that has undergone cell death.

Table 2.1 Examples of Pathological Hypertrophy and Hyperplasia

Organ/Tissue	Condition	Comment
Myocardiums	Right ventricular hypertrophy	Response to pulmonary valve stenosis, pulmonary hypertension or ventricular septal defect
	Left ventricular hypertrophy	Response to aortic valve stenosis or systemic hypertension
Arterial smooth muscle	Hypertrophy of arterial walls	Occurs in hypertension
Capillary vessels	Proliferative retinopathy	Complication of diabetes mellitus
Bone marrow	Erythrocyte precursor hyperplasia	Response to increased erythropoietin production (e.g. because of hypoxia)
Cytotoxic T lymphocytes	Hyperplastic expansion of T-cell populations	Involved in cell-mediated immune responses
Breast	Juvenile hypertrophy (females)	Exaggerated pubertal enlargement
	Gynaecomastia (males)	Owing to high oestrogen levels (e.g. in cirrhosis, iatrogenic, endocrine tumours)
Prostate	Epithelial and connective tissue hyperplasia	Relative excess of androgens stimulates androgen-sensitive central zone
Thyroid	Follicular epithelial hyperplasia	Most commonly because of a thyroid-stimulating antibody (Graves disease)
Adrenal cortex	Cortical hyperplasia	Response to increased ACTH production (e.g. from a pituitary tumour or, inappropriately, from a lung carcinoma)
Myointimal cells	Myointimal cell hyperplasia in atheromatous plaques	Myointimal cells in plaques proliferate in response to platelet-derived growth factor

ACTH, adrenocorticotropic hormone.
(*Source:* From Jonathan Bury, Underwood's Pathology: a Clinical Approach, Elsevier 2019.)

HYPERPLASIA

Increase in the number of cells leading to an increase in the size of the organ as a response to stress is referred to as **hyperplasia**. Only cells capable of dividing further (stable and labile cells), as explained earlier, can adapt to hyperplasia. Hence, tissues composed of ***labile*** (rapidly proliferating cells) and ***stable*** (quiescent cells with the capacity to proliferate in response to the needs) ***cells*** that are capable of dividing further may respond to stress by undergoing both hyperplasia and hypertrophy. Same stimulus can trigger both hyperplasia and hypertrophy and hence these two processes most often coexist. It can be stressed here that the permanent cells cannot undergo hyperplasia. Hyperplasia can be physiological or pathological (Table 2.1).

Physiological Hyperplasia

Hyperplasia occurs when there is a need to increase the functional capacity of hormone-sensitive organs or to compensate for the damage or loss of cells in an organ.

Examples:

1. Development of the breast at puberty under the influence of *oestrogen*
2. Regeneration of the liver after partial hepatectomy under the influence of a variety of *cytokines*
3. Compensatory marrow hyperplasia following blood loss or haemolysis under the influence of *erythropoietin* (this marrow hyperplasia can increase the production of blood cells by as much as eightfold to its usual production capacity)

Pathological Hyperplasia

Pathological hyperplasia is the result of ***excessive or inappropriate actions of growth factors or hormones*** on end organs.

Examples:

1. *Endometrial hyperplasia* because of excessive stimulation by oestrogen
2. *Benign prostatic hyperplasia* because of excessive stimulation by androgen

Mechanism of Hyperplasia (Fig. 2.2)

Hyperplasia is either because of ***proliferation of mature cells*** driven by growth factors and cytokines or because of ***formation of new cells from stem cells.***

Though abnormal, ***hyperplasia is a controlled process*** that regresses completely once the stimulus is removed. But these rapidly proliferating cells could harbour mutations that could result in malignancies. Thus, hyperplasia is a ***precursor lesion for cancerous growth***. For example, endometrial hyperplasia is a risk factor for endometrial carcinoma. Hence, identification, follow-up and treatment of pathological hyperplasia are essential for prevention of cancerous growth.

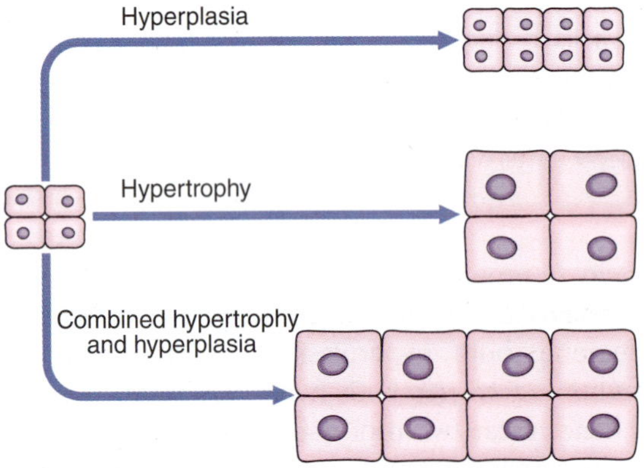

Fig. 2.2 Schematic representation of hyperplasia and hypertrophy. (*Source:* From Jonathan Bury. Disorders of growth, differentiation and morphogenesis. Underwood's Pathology. 7th edition. 2019.)

ATROPHY (FIG. 2.3)

Decrease in the size of an organ or tissue because of decrease in the size and number of the cells is referred to as **atrophy**. Atrophy can be ***physiological or pathological***. Pathological atrophy can be ***local or generalized***.

Examples of physiological atrophy:

- Regression of the notochord during embryogenesis
- Involution of the thyroglossal duct during embryogenesis
- Shrinkage of the uterus following pregnancy
- Atrophy of the endometrium, vaginal epithelium and breast following menopause

Examples of pathological atrophy:

Pathological atrophy occurs because of the following causes:

- **Decreased workload:** Disuse atrophy of skeletal muscles following immobilization of limbs is a classic example. The decrease in skeletal muscle cell size in the beginning is reversible; however, it becomes irreversible with extended duration. Furthermore, the clinical picture may get complicated with additional changes like increased bone resorption and osteoporosis.
- **Loss of nerve supply:** Denervation atrophy of skeletal muscles occurs when the nerves supplying them are damaged.
- **Diminished blood supply:** Ischaemic atrophy of the brain in the old age occurs because of atherosclerosis and reduced blood supply (Figs 2.3 and 2.4).
- **Diminished nutrition:** Atrophy seen in protein–energy malnutrition is because of depletion of skeletal muscle proteins for energy needs after the exhaustion of fat stores. In cancer cachexia, excessive production of TNF results in loss of appetite and lipid stores, leading to muscle atrophy.
- **Loss of hormonal influence:** Atrophy of the endometrium, vaginal epithelium and breast occurs after menopause.

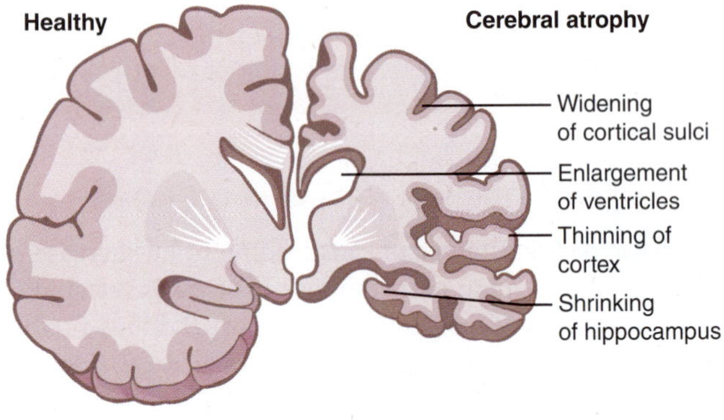

Fig. 2.3 Diagrammatic representation of normal and atrophic brain.

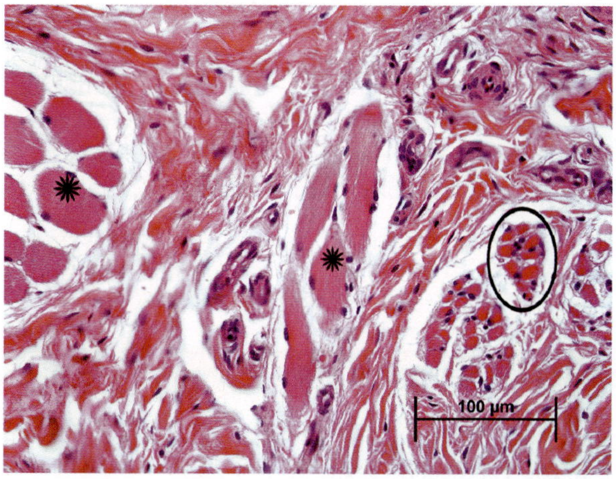

Fig. 2.4 Atrophy because of loss of cellular mass. Skeletal muscle from tongue that atrophied secondary to impairment of the regional blood supply. Affected muscle bundles (circled) are reduced in size, as are individual myofibres. Normal fibres are indicated by an asterisk. (*Source:* From Matthew A. Wallig and Evan B. Janovitz. Morphologic Manifestations of Toxic Cell Injury. Haschek and Rousseaux's Handbook of Toxicologic Pathology. 3rd Edition. 2013. Elsevier.)

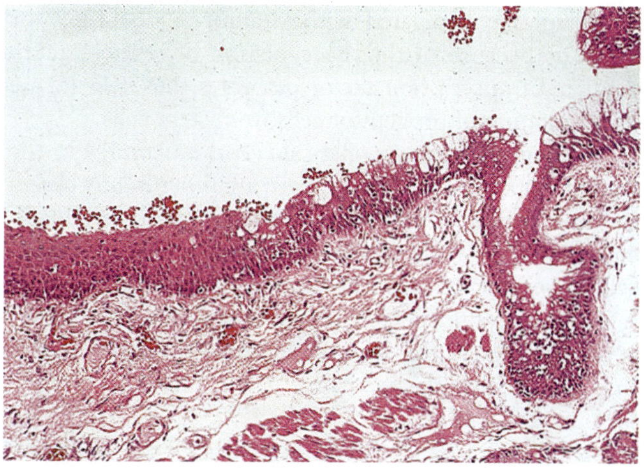

Fig. 2.5 Microscopy of squamous metaplasia of respiratory epithelium in smokers. (*Source:* From Jonathan Bury. Disorders of growth, differentiation and morphogenesis. Underwood's Pathology. 7th edition. 2019.)

- **Pressure atrophy:** Compression of tissues over an extended time can cause atrophy. A common example is pressure atrophy of surrounding tissues caused by an enlarging neoplasm.

Mechanisms of Atrophy

Irrespective of the cause, morphology of cells in atrophy is identical in all the conditions. During the initial stages of atrophy, to bring down the metabolic needs of the cell for survival, *the size of the cell and the number of organelles are reduced.* Atrophic cells contain fewer mitochondria, myofilaments and rough endoplasmic reticulum (ER). Reduction in the cell size is because of *reduced protein synthesis and increased protein degradation.* Reduced metabolic activity is the cause of reduced protein synthesis, and activation of the ubiquitin–proteasome pathway is the cause for increased protein degradation. Thus, early in the process, atrophic cells have ***reduced function*** and as the stress continues or becomes excessive, ***cell death*** by apoptosis occurs.

In many cases, atrophy is accompanied by autophagy, which is explained in the later sections.

Although the terms 'hypoplasia' and 'atrophy' are often used interchangeably, the former is better reserved to indicate the failure in attainment of the normal size or shape of an organ as a consequence of a developmental failure. Although hypoplasia is closely related to atrophy in terms of its pathogenesis, it is a failure in morphogenesis. An example of hypoplasia is the failure in development of the legs in adult patients with neurological deficit in the lower limbs or severe spina bifida.

METAPLASIA

Metaplasia is an adaptive response in which *one type of differentiated cells is replaced by another type of differentiated cells. Both epithelial and mesenchymal cells undergo metaplasia.* In simple terms, metaplasia occurs when one cell type is stressed by the altered environment and hence is replaced by some other tough cell types that can withstand the stress. The most common epithelial metaplasia is columnar to squamous, because squamous epithelium is the toughest epithelium.

Examples of squamous metaplasia:

- Squamous metaplasia of columnar epithelium in the respiratory tract of smokers (Fig. 2.5)
- Squamous metaplasia of columnar epithelium in the excretory ducts of salivary glands and pancreas because of obstruction by stones
- Squamous metaplasia of endocervical epithelium in response to infections and irritation

Squamous to columnar metaplasia: Though not common like squamous metaplasia, the incidence of columnar metaplasia is on the rise and has gained clinical significance. Most importantly, squamous to columnar metaplasia at the lower end of the oesophagus because of acid reflux is referred to as ***Barrett oesophagus.*** This condition is a *forerunner of adenocarcinoma* at the lower end of the oesophagus if untreated for a long time and hence needs early diagnosis and intervention.

Connective tissue metaplasia: This adaptive change refers to the formation of cartilage, bone and adipose tissue in sites that do not normally contain these elements, for example, ***myositis ossificans*** in which bone is formed in muscles following intramuscular haemorrhage.

Mechanisms of Metaplasia

This reversible change is not because of the change in the phenotype of differentiated cells but is because of ***reprogramming of stem cells*** in normal tissues or of undifferentiated mesenchymal cells in connective tissue. This transformation is driven by *cytokines, growth factors and extracellular matrix components* that push the precursor cells to differentiate along the new pathway.

Metaplasia associated with vitamin A deficiency or excess is because of the dysregulation of retinoic acid–regulated transcription factor pathways that help in the differentiation of progenitor cells from stem cells.

Although metaplasia offers ***survival advantage*** to the cells under stress, metaplastic cells are ***functionally defective*** and hence, in some instances, metaplasia is considered undesirable. For example, the metaplastic squamous cells in contrast to the ciliated columnar cells of the respiratory tract cannot secrete mucus and do not have ciliary action to protect the surface. In addition, if the factors that trigger metaplastic change persist, malignant transformation can set in.

Metaplastic change, often viewed as a premalignant condition, requires immediate intervention, either surgical or medical, else it leads to malignant transformation.

OVERVIEW OF CELL INJURY AND CELL DEATH

Cells are injured when the stress is too much for the cells to adapt. Cellular injury may progress through a few stages before ending in cell death.

Reversible cell injury: When the injury is less intense, the functional and morphological damages are reversible on removal of the stimuli.

The hallmark morphological feature of reversible injury is ***cellular swelling*** because of changes in the ion concentration and influx of water into the cell. This is mainly because of loss of function of Na^+,K^+-ATPase pump on the cell membrane, which requires ATP for its function. The mitochondrial dysfunction that occurs during cell injury reduces the oxidative phosphorylation leading to *depletion of ATP*, thereby affecting the function of that pump. The process is discussed in detail later.

Irreversible cell injury: When the injurious stimulus is strong and/or excessive and/or continuous for a cell to tolerate, the cell undergoes irreversible damage. It would reach a point of no return, invariably followed by cell death.

There are two principal types of cell death – ***apoptosis and necrosis***. These two forms of cell death differ in mechanisms, morphology and their role in health and disease.

- **Apoptosis:** This form of cell death is ***highly regulated***, in which the cell kills itself when its DNA or protein is damaged beyond a point of repair. Apoptosis is characterized by dissolution of the nucleus, fragmentation of the cell without loss of membrane integrity and rapid removal of cellular debris by macrophages without inflammation. It can be because of ***physiological or pathological*** causes.
- **Necrosis:** This form of cell death is ***unregulated*** and results in loss of cellular membrane integrity and disturbances in intracellular ion homeostasis. Leakage of cellular contents elicits a brisk inflammatory reaction because the cellular membrane is damaged. Necrosis is ***always pathological*** and is a common mode of cell death that follows ischaemia, infections, trauma and toxin exposures.

All the above-mentioned forms of cell injury and cell death are discussed in detail in the subsequent sections.

CAUSES OF CELL INJURY PA 2.1

Causes of cell injury can be grouped into the following categories (Flowchart 2.2):

1. **Hypoxia:** Hypoxia is an extremely important cause of cell injury and cell death that may be because of ischaemia, cardiorespiratory failure, severe anaemia, carbon monoxide poisoning or severe blood loss. The exact mechanism of hypoxia triggering cell death is by shutting down oxidative phosphorylation and bringing down the energy level of cells.
2. **Physical agents:** Mechanical trauma, extremes of temperature, radiation, electric shock and sudden changes in atmospheric pressure can cause injury to cells.
3. **Chemical agents, drugs and toxins:** Many drugs, high concentrations of sodium and glucose, hyperbaric oxygen and trace amounts of poisons like arsenic, cyanide, pesticides, insecticides and air pollutants can induce cell death.
4. **Infectious agents:** All types of microorganisms, including viruses, bacteria, fungi, rickettsiae and protozoa, can cause mild injury and death of cells.

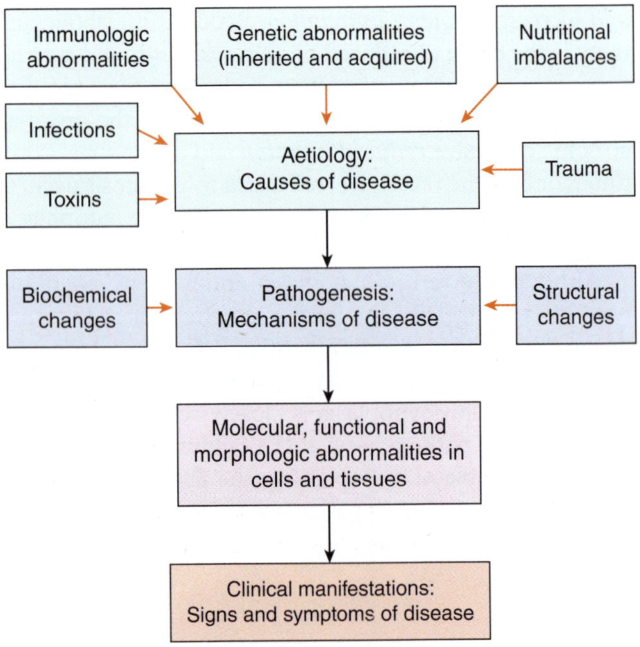

Flowchart 2.2 Causes of cell injury, and cell injury as a cause of diseases.

5. **Immune reactions:** Immune reactions against external agents like microbes and responses against self-antigens in autoimmune diseases can cause cell death.
6. **Genetic diseases:** Genetic diseases ranging from chromosomal disorders (e.g. Down syndrome) to single gene disorders (inborn errors of metabolism) can cause injury to cells and death.
7. **Nutritional imbalances:** Both nutritional deficiency and excess can cause cell injury. Cells may get injured in states of protein deficiency, vitamin deficiencies and also obesity because of multiple mechanisms.
8. **Workload imbalance:** Cells that cannot meet an increased demand may undergo degeneration or death.

MECHANISMS OF CELL INJURY PA 2.2

The way in which a cell responds to an injury depends on many factors like the nature, duration and severity of the injury and the type, state and adaptability of the cell. Nutritional status, hormonal status and metabolic needs of cells also influence the outcome. Similarly, genetic polymorphisms play a major role in the differences in the responses to injury between the individual cells. Cell injury is the result of different biochemical mechanisms affecting many essential cellular components.

All causes of cell injury activate one or more of four final common biochemical mechanisms leading to cell injury. These fundamental biochemical mechanisms of cell injury are the following: **(1) ATP depletion, (2) permeabilization of cell membranes, (3) disruption of biochemical pathways and (4) damage to DNA.**

The above-mentioned four mechanisms are split into **the following seven events of cell injury** (Fig. 2.6):

- ATP depletion
- Mitochondrial damage
- Disturbances of calcium homeostasis
- Oxidative stress
- Defects in membrane permeability
- Damage to DNA
- Damage to proteins

ATP DEPLETION

ATP in a cell is synthesized by oxidative phosphorylation and glycolytic pathway. Decline in cellular ATP is the fundamental cause of cell death. Important causes of ATP depletion are lack of oxygen and nutrients, damage to mitochondria and the effects of some toxins like cyanide. Cellular actions like membrane transport, lipogenesis, protein synthesis and phospholipid turnover are affected when ATP decreases. When it reaches 5%–10% of cellular levels, it severely affects the viability of the cell.

The downstream effects of ATP loss are as follows (Flowchart 2.3):

A. The activity of plasma membrane ***Na^+,K^+-ATPase (sodium pump) is severely reduced,*** resulting in failure of active transport of sodium and potassium. The results are increased intracellular sodium and reduced potassium levels, which culminate in the accumulation of intracellular water, dilation of ER and **cellular swelling**.
B. ***Switching of energy metabolism:*** As already stated, ATP can be generated by two pathways. Hypoxia not only halts the oxidative phosphorylation but also augments anaerobic glycolysis through the production of adenosine monophosphate to generate ATP from breakdown of glycogen. This results in depletion of glycogen and accumulation of lactic acid. The resultant ***intracellular acidosis*** decreases the activity of many enzymes whose functions are dependent on an ideal and stable pH.
C. Damage to calcium pump results in ***influx of calcium,*** leading to many deleterious effects on the cell.
D. Loss of ATP ***affects the protein synthetic machinery*** marked by detachment of the ribosomes, bringing down protein synthesis in the cells.

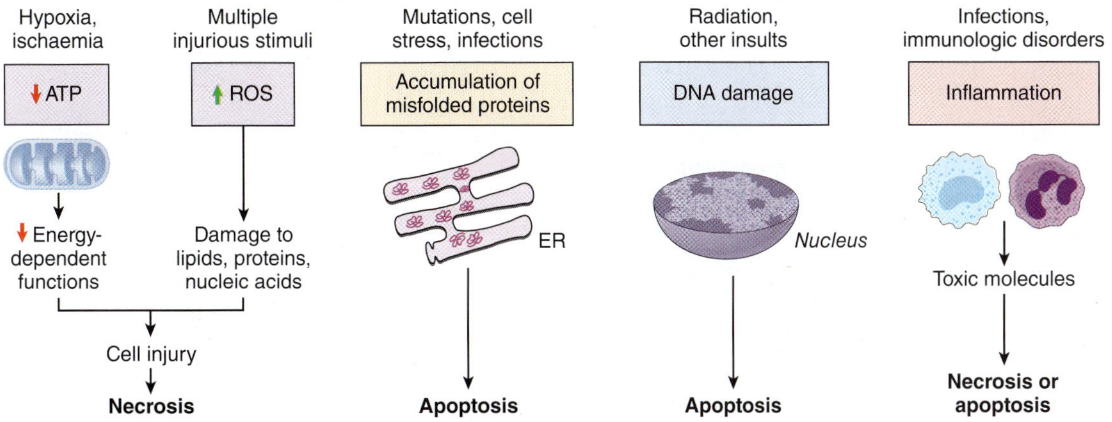

Fig. 2.6 The major biochemical mechanisms and sites of damage in cell injury. Note that the causes and mechanisms of cell death by necrosis and apoptosis are shown as being independent, but there may be overlap. (Based on Vinay Kumar, Abul K. Abbas, and Jon C. Aster. Cell Injury, Cell Death, and Adaptations. Robbins Basic Pathology, 10th edition, Elsevier, 2021.)

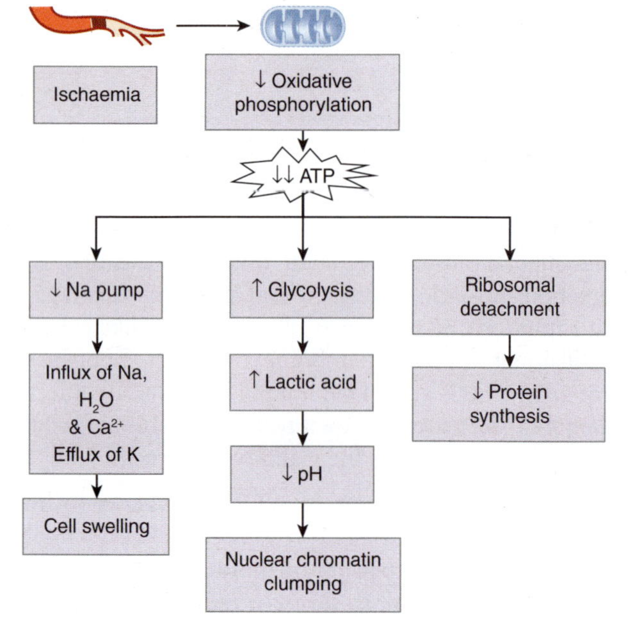

Flowchart 2.3 Sequences of events because of hypoxia and decreased ATP in cell injury.

E. Hypoxia also triggers accumulation of ***misfolded proteins,*** which may also lead to cell death.
F. ***Membranes of the organelles get disrupted,*** resulting in cell death by necrosis.

MITOCHONDRIAL DAMAGE

Uninterrupted functioning of mitochondria with ATP generation is a must for vitality of every cell. But this highly essential cellular organelle is extremely sensitive and can be damaged by hypoxia, increased levels of cytosolic calcium, reactive oxygen species (ROS), toxins or a wide variety of injurious agents.

Three major downstream effects of mitochondrial damage are as follows:

1. Damage to the mitochondria results in the formation of ***mitochondrial permeability transition (MPT) pore,*** a high-conductance channel, in the mitochondrial membrane. Mitochondrial membrane potential is lost because of opening of this channel, resulting in the failure of oxidative phosphorylation and reduction in ATP levels. Cyclophilin D is an important mitochondrial protein and also one of the structural components of MPT pore. The immunosuppressive drug cyclosporine, which is believed to prevent ischaemic injury, acts by inhibiting many cyclophilins including cyclophilin D. This is a classic example of targeted therapy for cell injury.
2. ***ROS*** are generated because of abnormal oxidative phosphorylation.
3. Increased permeability of the outer membrane leaks out proteins like *cytochrome c which may activate caspases and trigger apoptosis* (explained later), leading to cell death.

DISTURBANCES OF CALCIUM HOMEOSTASIS (FIG. 2.7)

Intracellular concentration of calcium is kept at very low concentrations by sequestering it within mitochondria and ER, because calcium is an important mediator of cell injury. Hypoxia and toxins increase the level of cytosolic calcium by mobilizing from intracellular stores and also from outside the cell membrane. The effects of altered cytosolic calcium levels are as follows:

A. **Opening of MPT pore** leads to ATP depletion because of accumulation of calcium within the mitochondria.
B. **Increased cytosolic calcium** activates many destructive enzymes like phospholipases, proteases, endonucleases and ATPases, causing membrane damage, cytoskeletal breakdown, nuclear fragmentation and ATP depletion, respectively.
C. Increased cytosolic calcium also results in **apoptosis** by activation of caspases and by augmenting mitochondrial permeability.

ACCUMULATION OF OXYGEN-DERIVED FREE RADICALS: OXIDATIVE STRESS

Free radical–mediated damage is a major mechanism of cell injury and the basis of many conditions like chemical injury, radiation injury, cellular ageing, ischaemia–reperfusion injury and oxidative burst within phagocytes.

Free Radicals

Free radicals are chemical species that have ***single unpaired electron*** in the outer orbit around the atomic nucleus. Unpaired electrons are *highly reactive and react with proteins, lipids, carbohydrates and nucleic acids.* Some of these reactions become autocatalytic in which the molecules

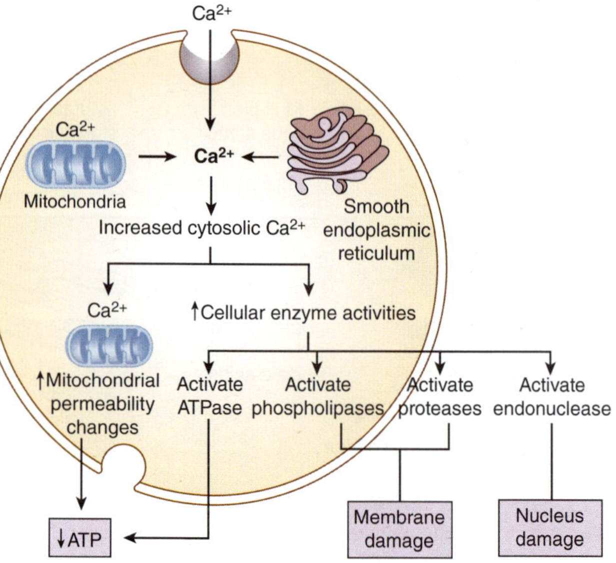

Fig. 2.7 Sequences of increased cytosolic calcium cell injury.

themselves are converted into free radicals following their reaction with free radicals. As one would anticipate, this leads to propagation of the damage.

Free Radicals in Health and Disease ROS are a form of oxygen-derived free radicals that are produced during normal cellular mitochondrial respiration and also generated by phagocytes during their defence against invading microorganisms. In normal circumstances, these are eliminated by the antioxidant reserve of the body. Therefore, in a healthy individual, free radicals are produced at a steady state, without causing cellular damage because of the detoxifying effects of antioxidants. When produced appropriately and in correct quantity, free radicals constitute a part of many physiological actions. But when there is an increased production of free radicals or reduced levels of antioxidants, it results in ***oxidative stress.*** Oxidative stress is the basis of many diseases including cell injury, ageing, cancers and Alzheimer disease.

Production of Free Radicals Free radicals are generated within the cells in the following conditions:

1. ***Redox reactions*** that happen during cellular respiration generate superoxide anion, hydrogen peroxide and hydroxyl ions.
2. Free radicals are generated within the cells during absorption of radiant energy like ***ultraviolet light and X-rays***.
3. During ***inflammation***, rapid bursts of ROS are generated from neutrophils with the action of NADPH oxidase. Xanthine oxidase of cells also generates superoxide free radicals.
4. Certain chemicals and drugs produce free radicals following ***metabolic conversion***, for example, CCL3 from CCL4.
5. Free radicals are also produced during ***Fenton reaction*** (Fig. 2.8), in which transition metals like iron and copper donate or accept free electrons.
6. ***Nitric oxide*** produced by endothelial cells, macrophages and neurons is a free radical and can get transformed to highly reactive ***peroxynitrite*** (ONOO), NO_2 and NO_3^-.

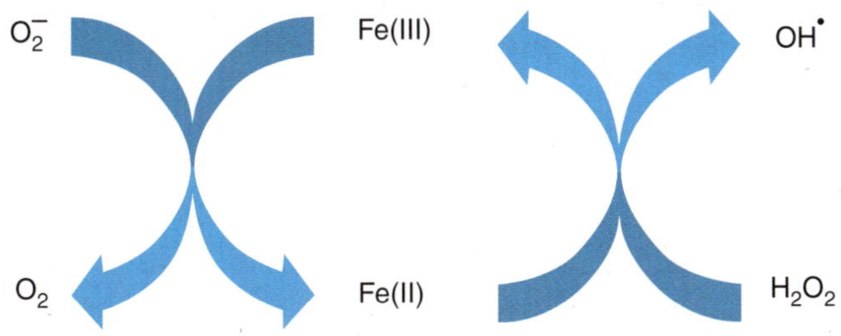

Fig. 2.8 Fenton reaction. (*Source:* Emerging Nanotechnologies in Food Science: Rosa Busquets, Fig. 5.2, Elsevier Inc., 2017.)

Table 2.2 Common Antioxidants Acting as Scavengers of Free Radicals

Enzymes	Vitamins	Proteins
Catalase	Vitamin A	Transferrin
Superoxide dismutase	Vitamin C	Ferritin
Glutathione peroxidase	Vitamin E	Lactoferrin
		Ceruloplasmin
Break down H_2O_2 and O_2	Block or scavenge free radicals	Act by binding to iron or copper and reducing their reactivity

Scavenging of Free Radicals (Table 2.2) Free radicals are ***unstable*** and decay spontaneously. Cells have antioxidants in the form of enzymes, vitamins and proteins. Antioxidants may block the formation of free radicals or inactivate them after their formation. Excess of free radicals is pathological (Fig. 2.9).

Pathological Actions of Free Radicals Three effects of free radicals relevant to cell injury are as follows:

1. ***Lipid peroxidation of membranes:*** This process damages membranes of both cells and organelles.
2. Oxidation of amino acids and ***cross-linking of proteins:*** This leads to loss of enzyme activity, disruption of structural proteins and stimulation of proteosomal degradation of folded and misfolded proteins. This, in turn, induces cellular stress and evokes misfolded protein response.
3. Damage to DNA: ***Double-strand breaks and cross-linking of DNA strands*** with adduct formation occurs that plays a key role in cellular ageing and carcinogenesis.

Hence, it is understood that maintaining a steady state of free radicals and antioxidants is essential for vitality and normal functioning of cells.

DEFECTS IN MEMBRANE PERMEABILITY

Membrane damage which starts as loss of membrane permeability and progresses to frank membrane damage is a constant feature of irreversible injury except in apoptosis. Even the slightest damage, in the form of loss of selective membrane permeability, affects viability and function of a cell. Damage of cell membrane and organelle (subcellular) membrane has serious consequences.

Mechanisms of Membrane Damage

- ***Direct damage*** by toxins, chemicals, complements and physical agents

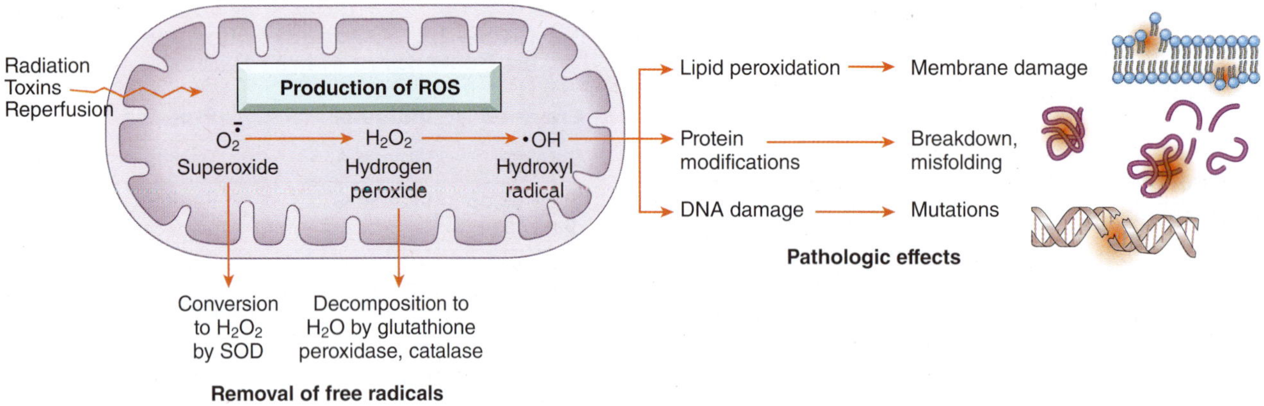

Fig. 2.9 Formation, removal and pathological effects of free radicals in cell injury.

- ***Lipid peroxidation*** of membrane lipids by free radicals
- ***Reduced phospholipid synthesis*** because of defective mitochondrial function and decline in the cellular levels of ATP
- ***Digestion of membrane phospholipids*** by phospholipases, which are activated by increased cytosolic calcium
- ***Damage to cytoskeletal proteins*** by activation of proteases by the increased intracytosolic calcium levels (this results in cellular swelling and indirectly damages the plasma membrane)

Consequences of Membrane Damage (Fig. 2.10)

1. **Plasma membrane damage:** This leads to loss of cellular content, ATP, metabolites, and fluid and osmotic balance.
2. **Mitochondrial membrane damage:** This has deleterious effects on the viability of a cell, as discussed earlier. Mitochondrial membrane damage leads to opening of MPT pore, resulting in decline of ATP production and also setting the stage for apoptosis by releasing pro-apoptotic molecules.

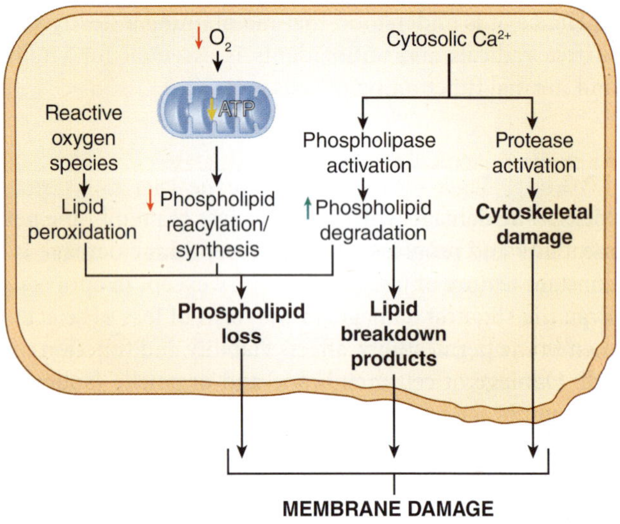

Fig. 2.10 Mechanisms and consequences of membrane damage.

3. **Lysosomal membrane damage:** Lysosomes contain RNases, DNases, proteases and phosphatases, so damage to their membranes results in leakage of these digestive enzymes into the cytoplasm. Here they may be activated by the intracellular acidic pH, resulting in the enzymatic digestion of constituents of cell and death by necrosis.

DAMAGE TO DNA

Irrespective of the DNA repair machinery of a cell, if the injury is too severe to be repaired, DNA gets damaged, leading to apoptosis.

DAMAGE TO PROTEINS

Free radical or inherited mutation-induced defective proteins trigger ***misfolded protein response,*** resulting in cell death by apoptosis.

It is well understood from the preceding discussions that the events of cell injury happen in a sequence. Locating the exact point at which the cell progresses from a reversibly injured state to an irreversibly injured state is essential from the therapeutic point of view, but identifying this switch is not plausible. The features that define morphological irreversibility are as follows:

1. **Inability to reverse mitochondrial dysfunction**
2. **Profound disturbances in cell membrane**

The morphological features of reversible and irreversible cell injuries are discussed in the next section.

MORPHOLOGICAL CHANGES IN CELL INJURY (TABLE 2.3) PA 2.2

Cell injury causes morphological changes in the cell in both reversible and irreversible stages. It can be stressed here that biochemical and ultrastructural changes precede the light microscopic and gross changes in the affected areas. Hence, understanding the biochemical changes and correlating them with morphological changes are very essential for clinicopathological correlation.

Table 2.3 Differences in the Ultrastructural Features of Reversible and Irreversible Injuries

Organelle	Reversible Injury	Irreversible Injury
Cell membranes	Blebs Cellular swelling Myelin figures	Disruption
Mitochondria[a]	Amorphous density	Large flocculent densities Swollen with vacuoles
Cytoskeleton	Aggregation	Disruption
Rough endoplasmic reticulum and ribosomes	Swelling Dispersed ribosomes	Lysis Dispersed ribosomes
Lysosomes	Autophagy occurs	Swollen and ruptured
Nucleus[a]	Clumping of chromatin	Pyknosis Karyolysis Karyorrhexis

[a] Significant changes in an irreversible injury.

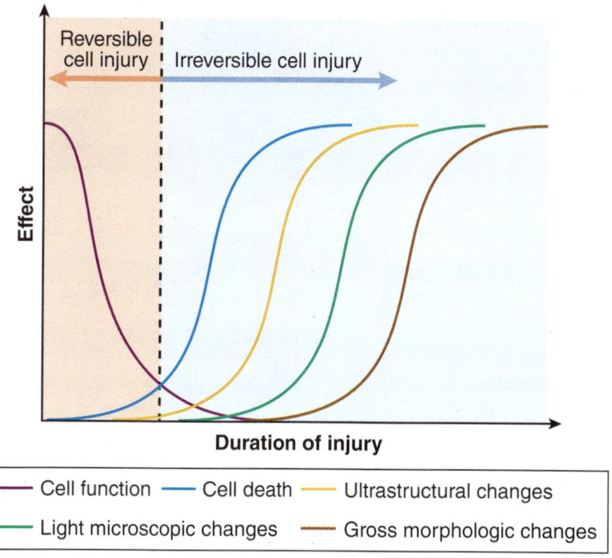

Fig. 2.11 Sequential development of biochemical and morphological changes in cell injury. The relationship among cellular function, cell death and the morphological changes of cell injury. Note that cells may rapidly become nonfunctional after the onset of injury, although they are still viable, with potentially reversible damage; with a longer duration of injury, irreversible injury and cell death may result. Note also that cell death typically precedes ultrastructural, light microscopic and grossly visible morphological changes. (From Anthony Chang et al., Robbins Basic Pathology, Elsevier 2018.)

The sequence of events that follow cell injury is as follows:

- **Decline in cellular function**
- **Biochemical alterations**
- **Ultrastructural changes**
- **Light microscopic changes**
- **Gross morphological changes**

The rapid event that follows cell injury is the decline in cellular function, which may return to its original level if the stimulus is removed. With persistent or intense stimuli, the cell yields to an irreversibly injured state with biochemical and morphological changes.

Early morphological changes can be seen only by electron microscopy, whereas light microscopic changes take time to appear and gross changes become visible to the naked eyes also with further passage of time.

The sequence of changes that occur in myocardial cells in myocardial infarction is discussed in greater detail in Chapter 14.

Fig. 2.11 highlights the order of events in cell injury.

MORPHOLOGICAL CHANGES IN REVERSIBLE CELL INJURY

It is crucial to differentiate an irreversibly injured cell from a reversibly injured cell because the latter can reverse back to its healthy state. Although the morphological changes observed in reversible and irreversible injuries may at times overlap, a few salient differences between them prove useful (Fig. 2.12).

The two salient features of reversible injury that are seen under the light microscope are ***cellular swelling*** and ***fatty change.*** As discussed earlier, cellular swelling is because of the failure of energy-dependent ion pumps in the plasma membrane. Fatty changes are seen in cells that are involved in the process and the cells that are dependent on fat metabolism like hepatocytes and myocardial cells when they are stressed. The ultrastructural differences between reversible and irreversible injuries are given in Table 2.3. The electron microscopic features of reversible and irreversible cell injuries are shown in Fig. 2.13.

Morphology

Hydropic degeneration: 'Hydropic degeneration' and 'cloudy swelling' are the terms used for the microscopic appearance of acute cell swelling. The influx of water in hydropic degeneration dilutes the cytosol, separates its organelles and distends the cell, giving the affected cell a swollen, pale and vacuolated appearance. In renal proximal tubules, swollen epithelial cells impinge on the tubular lumen (Fig. 2.14). In the liver, swollen hepatocytes and endothelial cells compress hepatic sinusoids (Fig. 2.14).

The clear cytoplasmic vacuoles in the affected cells are mainly water-distended mitochondria or cisternae of the Golgi complex or ER. Therefore, these vacuoles are not

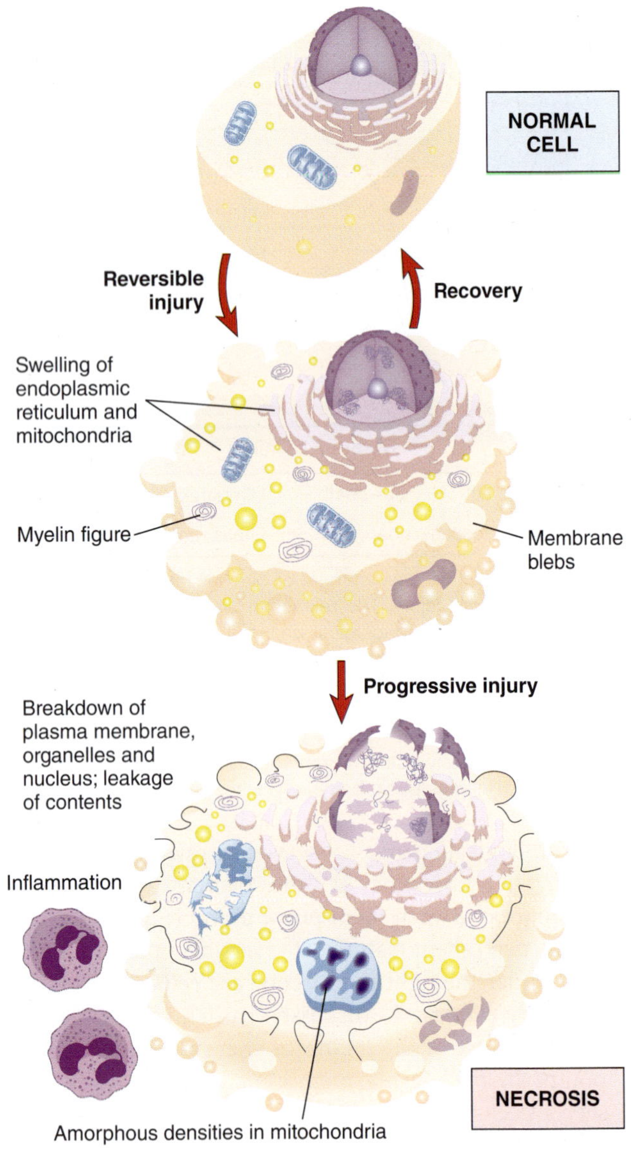

Fig. 2.12 Morphological changes in reversible versus irreversible cell injury. (*Source:* Vinay Kumar, Abul K. Abbas, and Jon C. Aster. Cell Injury, Cell Death, and Adaptations. Robbins Basic Pathology, 10th edition, Elsevier, 2021.)

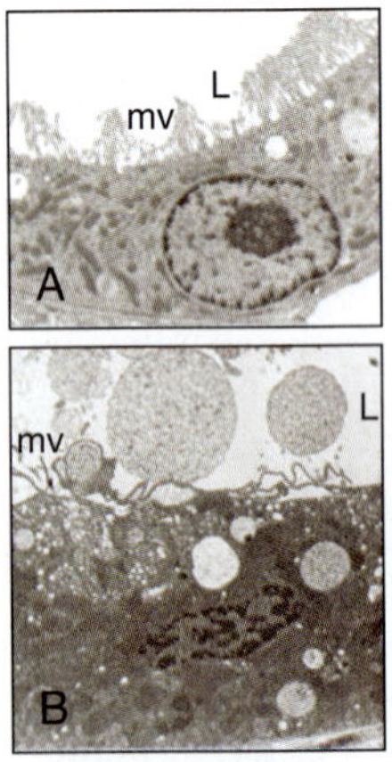

(A) Electron micrograph of a normal epithelial cell of the proximal kidney tubule. Note abundunt microvilli (mv) lining the luminal surface (L).

(B) Epithelial cell of the proximal tubule showing early cell injury resulting from reperfusion following ischemia. The microvilli are lost; blebs have formed. Mitochondria would have been swollen during ischaemia; with reperfusion, they rapidly undergo condensation and become electron-dense.

Fig. 2.13 Electron microscopic features of reversible and irreversible injuries (necrosis) in a kidney.

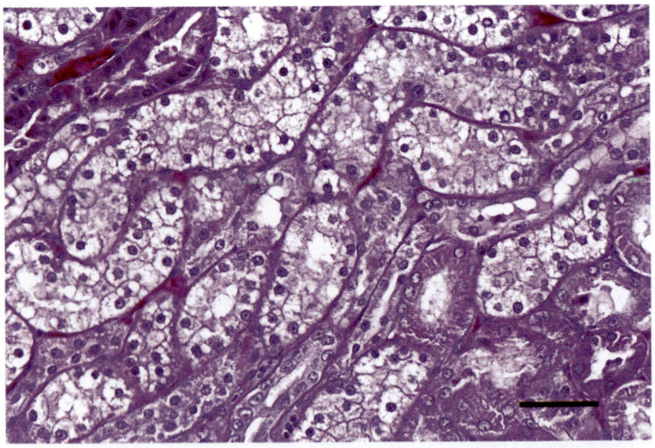

Fig. 2.14 Hydropic change in renal tubular epithelial cells, microscopy. Note the prominent proximal convoluted tubular cell cytoplasmic vacuolation. (*Source:* From Kanwar Nasir M. Khan, Gordon C. Hard, Carl L. Alden. Haschek and Rousseaux's Handbook of Toxicologic Pathology. 2013. Elsevier.)

stained by histochemical techniques used to detect fat or glycogen, the two other causes of cytoplasmic vacuolation. Ballooning degeneration is an extreme variant of hydropic degeneration that is typically seen in keratinocytes of stratified squamous epithelium of the skin.

The ultrastructural features of reversible injury are as follows:

Plasma membrane changes: Blebbing, blunting and loss of microvilli
Mitochondrial alterations: Swelling and formation of small amorphous densities
ER: Dilation with detachment of ribosomes
Cytoplasm: Myelin figures
Nuclear alterations: Disaggregation of granular and fibrillar elements

Morphological changes seen in apoptosis and necrosis are shown in Fig. 2.15.

NECROSIS **PA 2.4**

Necrosis refers to the spectrum of morphological changes that follow cell death in living tissues, largely resulting from ***denaturation*** of intracellular proteins or from the progressive degradative action of **enzymes** on an irreversibly injured cell. The hallmark of necrosis is ***loss of integrity of cell membranes.*** The enzymes that digest the necrotic cell are derived from the lysosomes of the dying cells or from the lysosomes of the leucocytes that are recruited as a part of the inflammatory process. Owing to the loss of membrane integrity, necrotic cells leak their contents to the exterior, thus triggering an inflammatory response. In addition, the membrane disintegration leads to ***leakage of cellular enzymes*** that become detectable in the blood as early as within 2 hours of cell death. Thus, estimation of serum levels of these enzymes can help in detecting tissue-specific cellular injury. Common examples of intracellular enzymes whose levels are elevated in

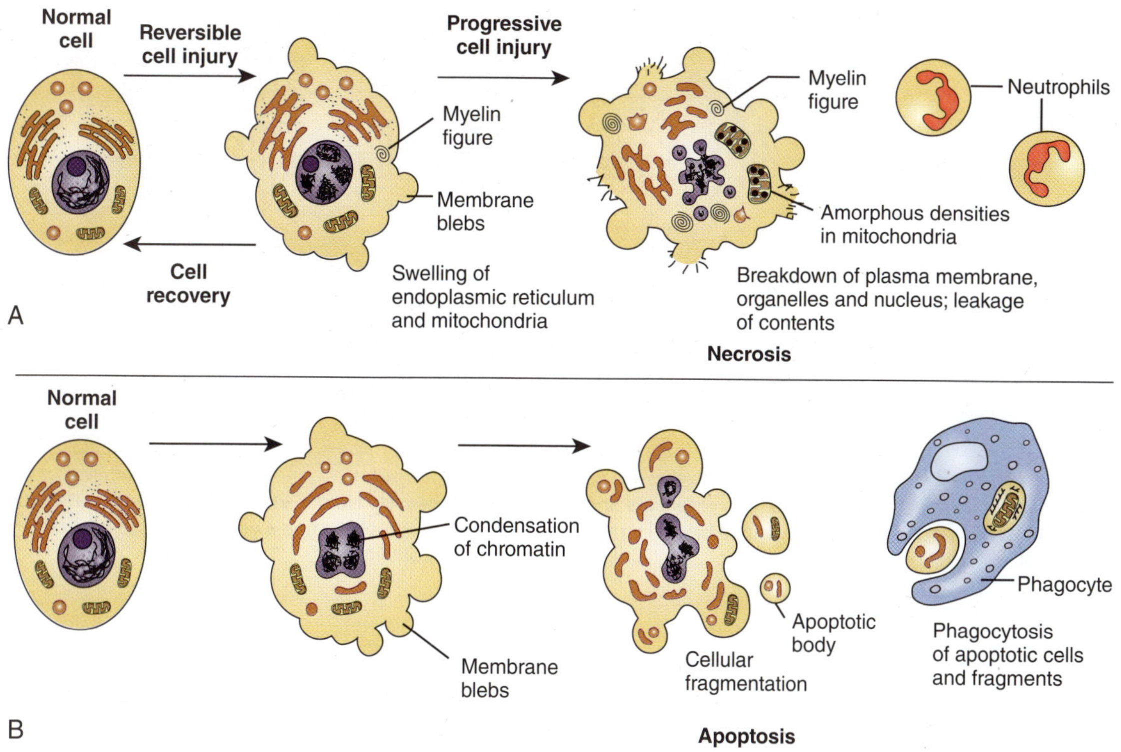

Fig. 2.15 Morphological changes in reversible injury, progressive injury and apoptosis.

necrosis of their parent cell and the associated diseases are listed in Table 2.4.

Morphological Features of Necrosis

Digestion of the contents of the cell and the host response may take many hours to become detectable. As explained earlier, ultrastructural changes precede light microscopic changes, which are followed by gross morphological changes.

Electron microscopy shows the following features:

- ***Plasma membrane:*** Disruption
- ***Membrane of organelles:*** Disruption
- ***Mitochondria:*** Dilation and large amorphous densities
- ***Cytoplasm:*** Myelin figures, amorphous debris, aggregated fluffy material
- ***Nucleus:*** May show one of the following features because of breakdown of DNA:
    - Karyolysis: Dissolution of nucleus and fading of basophilia
    - Pyknosis: Nuclear shrinkage and increased basophilia
    - Karyorrhexis: Fragmentation of pyknotic nuclei

    The above-mentioned changes are followed by complete disappearance of nuclei.

Light microscopic features of necrosis (Fig. 2.16) are as follows:

- ***Increased eosinophilia*** of cytoplasm occurs because of loss of cytoplasmic RNA and denaturation of cytoplasmic proteins.
- ***Glassy homogeneous*** appearance of cells is seen because of loss of glycogen.
- ***Moth-eaten*** appearance of cytoplasm is present because of vacuoles formed after digestion of organelles.

Table 2.4 Common Enzyme Markers of Cell Death

Enzyme	Diseases Associated with Elevation of Enzyme Levels
Aspartate aminotransferase (AST, SGOT)	Viral hepatitis Alcoholic liver disease Acute myocardial infarction
Alanine aminotransferase (ALT, SGPT)	Viral hepatitis Alcoholic liver disease
Creatine kinase-MB (CK-MB)	Acute myocardial infarction Myocarditis Skeletal muscle injury
Lactate dehydrogenase (LDH)	Acute myocardial infarction Myocarditis Skeletal muscle injury
Cardiac troponin (CTn)	Acute myocardial infarction
Lipase	Acute pancreatitis
Amylase	Acute pancreatitis Sialadenitis

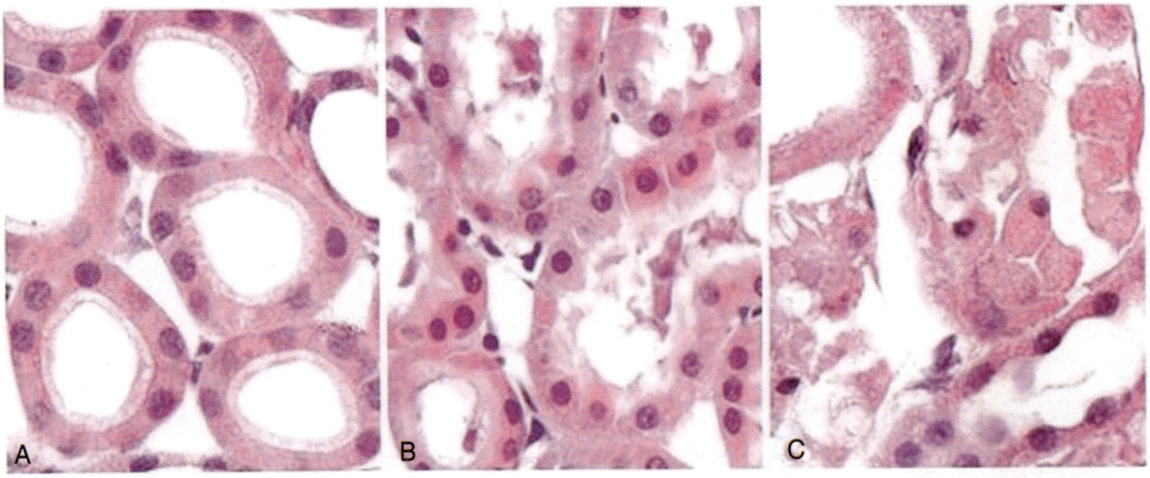

Fig. 2.16 Light microscopic features of normal cell, reversible and irreversible injuries. (A) Normal kidney tubules with viable epithelial cells. (B) Early (reversible) ischaemic injury showing surface blebs, increased eosinophilia of cytoplasm and swelling of occasional cells. (C) Necrotic (irreversible) injury of epithelial cells, with fragmentation, nuclear loss and leakage of contents.

- ***Myelin figures*** (large whorled masses of phospholipids) derived from cell membrane replace dead cells.
- If the myelin figures are not phagocytosed and cleared, these undergo further degradation to fatty acids and ***calcify***.

Gross morphology of necrosis varies according to the pattern of necrosis described in the next section.

MORPHOLOGICAL PATTERNS OF NECROSIS

Necrosis of cells in tissues has several patterns which are morphologically different. These patterns provide clues to the underlying diseases, so identifying them is important.

1. **Coagulative necrosis** (Fig. 2.17)
   Ischaemia may lead to coagulative necrosis in all organs except the brain. The mechanism of degradation is ***protein denaturation***. In this process, enzymes along with structural proteins undergo denaturation and hence proteolysis of dead cells is blocked. Eventually, dead cells remain as eosinophilic anucleate cells for days to weeks before they get cleared by infiltrating leucocytes. The affected tissues have firm consistency. A focal area of coagulative necrosis is called an ***infarct***. Examples of coagulative necrosis are myocardial infarction, viral hepatitis and splenic infarction (Fig. 2.18).
2. **Liquefactive necrosis**
   This pattern of necrosis usually follows ***bacterial infection*** affecting any organ (abscess formation) and ***hypoxia in the brain*** (Fig. 2.19). The mechanism of degradation is ***enzymatic digestion*** of dead cells by enzymes of infiltrating leucocytes. The affected tissue gets transformed to a liquefied viscous mass with pus formation.
3. **Gangrenous necrosis** PA 2.5
   Gangrene of tissues may be of the following two types:
   Dry gangrene is a clinical term used commonly to describe limbs that have lost their blood supply and

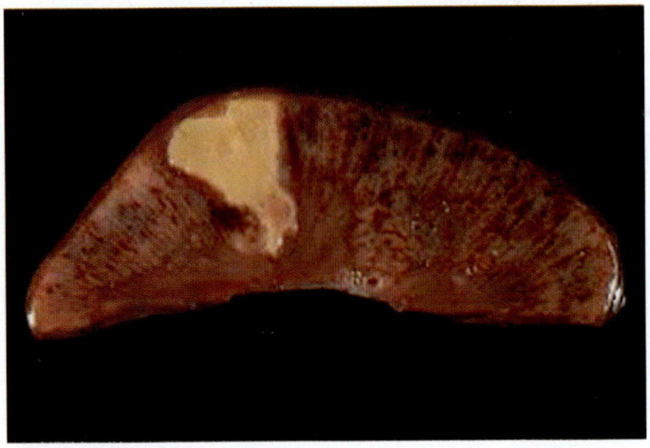

Fig. 2.17 Coagulative necrosis: gross morphology of wedge-shaped infarct of spleen.

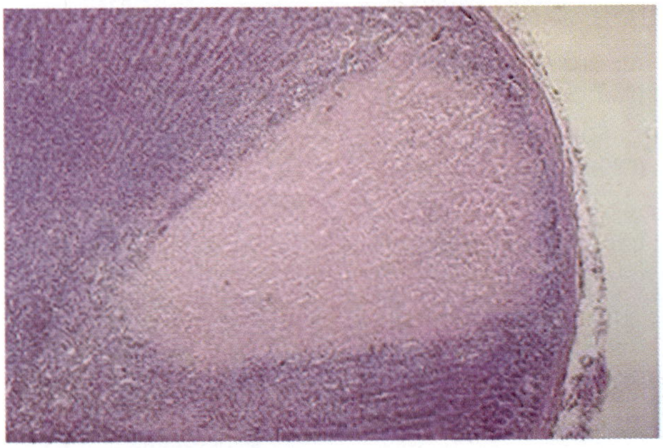

Fig. 2.18 Microscopy of splenic infarct. Note the pale homogeneous areas corresponding to necrosis.

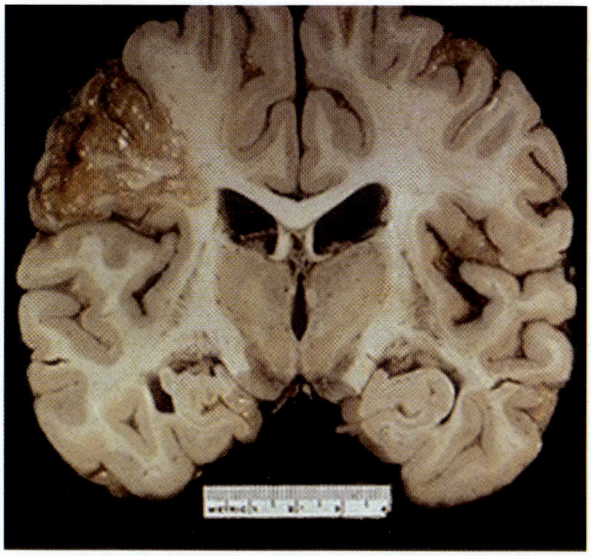

Fig. 2.19 Gross morphology of liquefactive necrosis of brain. Note that the cerebral infarction at the upper left in this image, in the distribution of the middle cerebral artery, demonstrates liquefactive necrosis. Eventually, the removal of the dead tissue leaves behind a cavity.

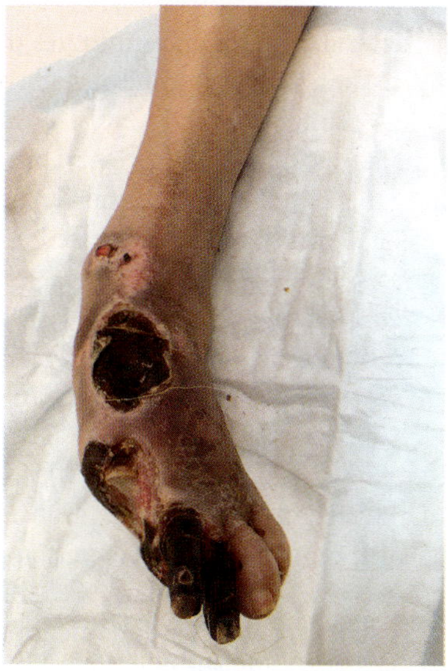

Fig. 2.20 Gross morphology of dry gangrene. Left foot dry gangrene. The patient with extensive left foot dry gangrene that developed after failure to heal at first ray amputation. (*Source:* From Rebecca Scully and Samir Kaushik Shah. Gangrene of the Foot. In Current Surgical Therapy. 13th edition. 2020. Elsevier.)

have undergone ***coagulative necrosis.*** It develops in ischaemic tissue, where the blood supply is inadequate to keep the tissue viable. Gangrene is not a disease in itself but a symptom of other diseases. Dry gangrene occurs mostly because of peripheral artery disease but can also be because of acute limb ischaemia. As a result, individuals with arteriosclerosis, those with high cholesterol, those with diabetes and smokers commonly have dry gangrene. Bacterial infection of dry gangrene is less likely because the limited oxygen in the ischaemic limb restricts putrefaction and bacteria fail to survive. The affected area is dry, shrunken and dark reddish-black (Fig. 2.20). The **line of separation** usually brings about complete detachment, with eventual falling off the gangrenous tissue if not removed surgically, a process referred to as *autoamputation*. Over time, occasionally, dry gangrene may develop into wet gangrene if an infection supervenes.

Wet gangrene is a type of necrosis superimposed with bacterial infections resulting in ***liquefactive necrosis*** as a result of enzymatic action from infiltrating leucocytes. It is more common in moist tissues such as the gut, mouth, cervix and vulva. It usually develops rapidly because of blockage of venous (mainly) or arterial blood flow. The affected part is saturated with stagnant blood, which promotes the rapid growth of bacteria. The toxic products formed by bacteria may often get absorbed, causing systemic manifestation of sepsis and finally death. The affected area is oedematous, soft, putrid, rotten and dark (Fig. 2.21). Owing to

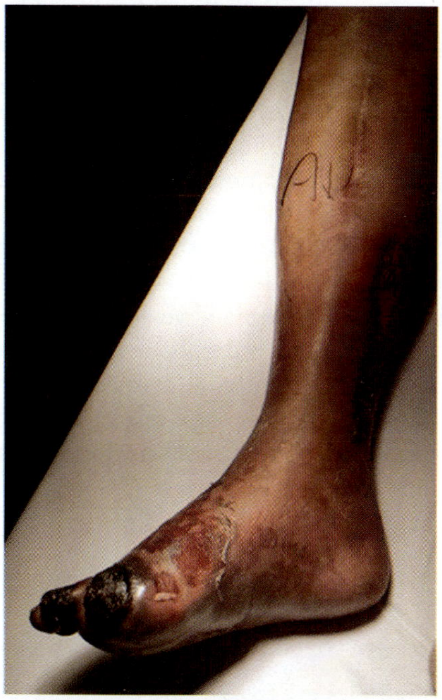

Fig. 2.21 Clinical picture of wet gangrene of the lower limb. Note the oedematous and erythematous tissue proximal to the necrotic tissue. (*Source:* https://thoracickey.com/wet-gangrene/.)

the high mortality associated with wet gangrene, it is treated as a surgical emergency.

Gas gangrene is a type of wet gangrene caused by a bacterial infection that produces gas within the affected tissues. It is most commonly caused by *Clostridium* species, particularly *C. perfringens*. Infection spreads rapidly because the gas produced by the bacteria expands and infiltrates the adjacent healthy tissues. Gas gangrene usually causes necrosis, gas production and sepsis. Progression to toxaemia and shock is often very rapid. Owing to its ability to quickly spread to the surrounding tissues, gas gangrene should be treated as a medical emergency.

4. **Caseous necrosis** (Fig. 2.22)
   This pattern of necrosis is seen with ***tuberculous infections***. It is referred to as caseous (meaning cheese-like), which appears as a friable white area of necrosis when seen with the naked eyes. Microscopic examination of the necrotic area displays an amorphous collection of fragmented or lysed cells and granular debris bordered by inflammatory cells. Often, but not always, such areas of caseous necrosis are surrounded by epithelioid cells forming **granulomas**.
5. **Fat necrosis**
   'Fat necrosis' is a clinical term but is not a specific pattern of necrosis. This type of necrosis is characterized by focal areas of fat destruction that usually follow release of lipase from the pancreas in the background of ***acute pancreatitis***. The fatty acids released because of the action of lipases on the fat combine with calcium to form grossly visible chalky white areas of fat saponification (Fig. 2.23). Microscopy reveals the presence of foci of outlines of necrotic fat cells along with areas of calcification and inflammatory cell infiltration.
6. **Fibrinoid necrosis**
   This special form of necrosis is seen in ***immune reactions*** involving deposition of antigen–antibody complexes along the blood vessel walls. The characteristic bright pink amorphous appearance of the necrotic region is because of the escape of fibrin from the lumen into the vessel wall (Fig. 2.24). Common causes of fibrinoid necrosis are systemic lupus erythematosus, polyarteritis nodosa, malignant hypertension, etc.

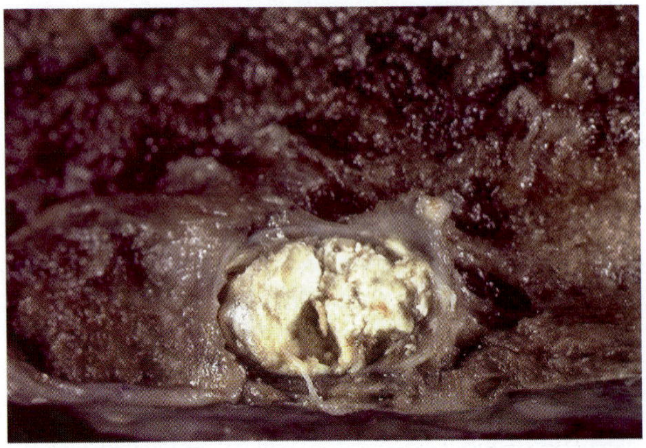

Fig. 2.22 Gross morphology of caseous necrosis, pleura. Note the cheesy appearance of the necrotic area.

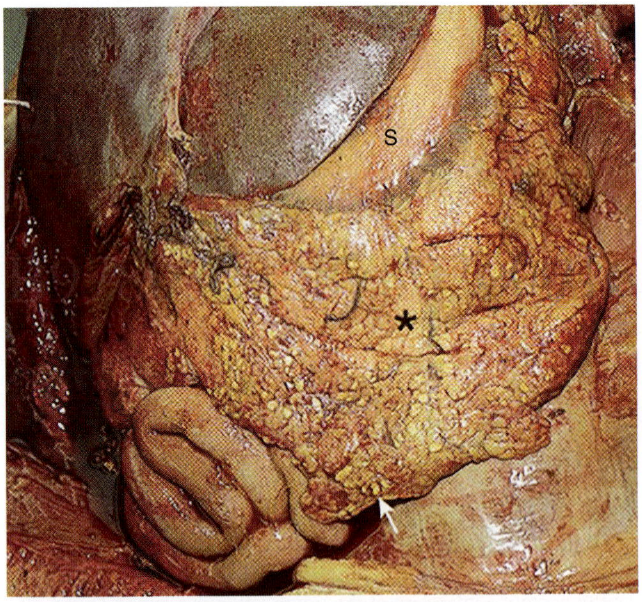

Fig. 2.23 Gross microscopy of fat necrosis of omentum. The chalky white areas in the omentum represent calcium combined with free fatty acids (saponification) that were released on digestion of intracellular lipids by lipase released from the injured pancreas. (*Source:* Autopsy Pathology: A Manual and Atlas, 2nd ed.: Richard L. Davis, Philip C. Ursell, Walter E. Finkbeiner Fig. 15-29, Elsevier Inc., 2009.)

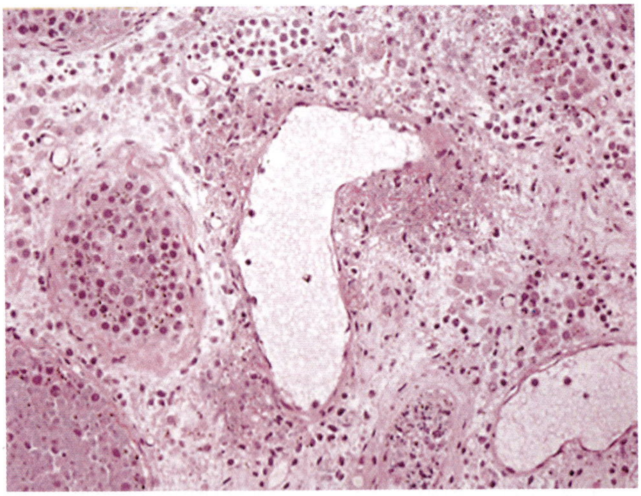

Fig. 2.24 Microscopy of fibrinoid necrosis. Note the bright pink-coloured areas of fibrinoid necrosis. (*Source:* Uropathology, Second Edition: Ming Zhou, George J. Netto, Jonathan I. Epstein, Fig. 195.4, Elsevier Inc., 2023.)

In general, irrespective of the cause and pattern of necrosis, the necrotic cells are cleared by the enzymatic digestion and phagocytosis of the remaining debris by the infiltrating leucocytes. In situations in which the clearance is not done, these act as a nidus for calcium deposition and get calcified, which is the basis for dystrophic calcification (explained later).

ISCHAEMIA–REPERFUSION INJURY

In the preceding sections, we have discussed that the effects of hypoxia and ischaemia are because of blockage of oxidative phosphorylation and the reduction in the levels of cellular ATP and that a cell is initially reversibly injured before it gets irreversibly injured. Although restoration of blood flow reverts the changes if the cell is reversibly injured, it is a *double-edged sword,* because it can also exacerbate damages and augment cell death. This process, known as **ischaemia–reperfusion injury**, also called reperfusion injury or reoxygenation injury, is the tissue damage caused when blood supply returns to the tissue after a brief period of ischaemia. It is important to identify this entity, because this exacerbates the cell damage that occurred during infarction after initiating therapy to restore blood circulation.

Mechanisms of reperfusion injury (Flowchart 2.4) are as follows:

- Reperfusion of ischaemic tissues is often associated with **microvascular injury**, mainly because of increased permeability of capillaries and arterioles that leads to an increase in diffusion and fluid filtration across the tissues.
- Damage to the cell membrane may, in turn, cause the release of more **free radicals.** Such reactive species may also act indirectly in redox signalling to turn on apoptosis.
- Ischaemic tissue has decreased function of free radical scavengers because of cell injury. Once blood flow is reestablished, oxygen species contained in the blood damage the ischaemic tissue because the scavengers that normally deactivate them are not functional now.
- The restored blood flow reintroduces oxygen within cells that damages cellular proteins, DNA and the plasma membrane.
- The **inflammatory response** triggered by the imbalance between ROS and nitric oxide is partially responsible for the damage caused by reperfusion injury.
- Activation of complement system occurs.
- Exacerbation of ***altered calcium homeostasis*** is seen in the injured cells.

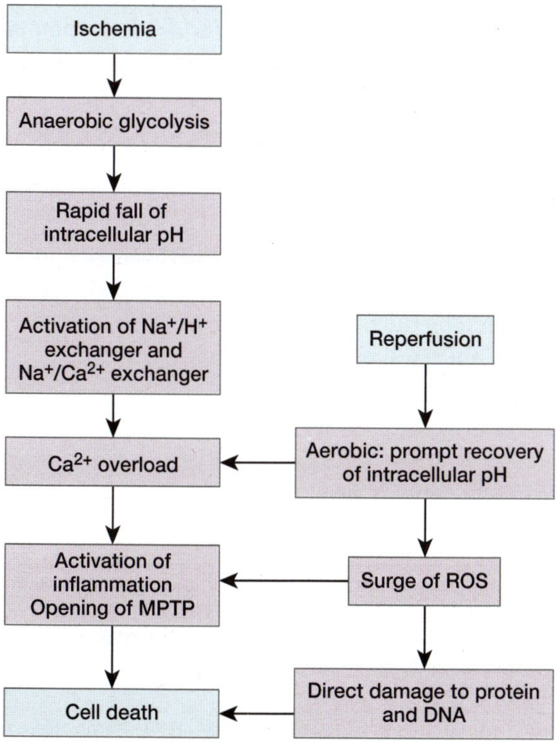

Flowchart 2.4 Mechanisms of reperfusion injury.

It is understood that the mechanisms of reperfusion injury are quite complex, and each factor can complement other. Hence, it is apparent that a combination of molecular and cellular approaches, targeting multiple pathological processes, needs to be adopted to limit the extent of reperfusion injury and to increase the regenerative capacity of ischaemic tissues.

APOPTOSIS — PA 2.4, PA 2.7

Apoptosis is a unique, tightly ***regulated pathway of cell death*** in which cells destined to die activate intrinsic enzymes that degrade the constituents of the cell. It is genetically regulated, so it is also called ***programmed cell death***. Unlike necrosis which is always pathological, apoptosis can be triggered by both physiological and pathological causes.

The history of apoptosis dates back to 1842, when the German scientist Carl Vogt first described its principles. For many years, neither 'apoptosis' nor 'programmed cell death' was a cited term. Two discoveries that brought cell death from obscurity to a major field of research are the following: (1) identification of components of the cell death control and effector mechanisms; and (2) linkage of abnormalities in cell death to human disease, in particular cancer. Only in 1972 was the process recognized by the distinctive morphological features of the membrane-bound fragments. In Greek, apoptosis means the ***'falling off'*** of leaves from a tree. It is named so because of the similarity between the formation of membrane-bound apoptotic bodies and the falling of leaves from trees. The unique feature of apoptosis is that the ***whole process happens rapidly without eliciting inflammation***.

CAUSES OF APOPTOSIS

Unlike necrosis that is always pathological, apoptosis can be because of physiological or pathological causes.

Apoptosis in Physiological Conditions

In the following situations, apoptosis serves as a process to remove the cells that are no longer required:

- The sculpting of an embryo during ***embryogenesis***

- Involution of hormone-dependent tissues on ***withdrawal of hormones*** – endometrial breakdown in menstrual cycle, atrophy of ovaries and endometrium in the postmenopausal period
- ***To maintain constant cell population of labile cells,*** which proliferate continuously like haematopoietic cells and surface epithelial cells of the gastrointestinal tract
- ***Removal of self-reactive lymphocytes*** during the process of immunological tolerance (explained in detail in Chapter 6)
- ***Removal of inflammatory cells*** after they have served their purpose in the battle against microorganisms or foreign agents

Apoptosis in Pathological Situations

The following are the examples of apoptosis in pathological conditions, acting to remove the dead cells:

- ***Damage to DNA*** (when the cellular DNA is irreversibly damaged because of radiation, drugs and hypoxia, apoptosis is triggered by the injured cell to eliminate itself)
- ***Misfolded protein response*** (intracellular protein accumulation can happen because of inherited mutations or because of free radicals; the abnormal protein accumulated in ER causes ER stress that triggers apoptotic cell death)
- Cytotoxic T-cell-mediated cell death following ***viral infections***
- Cytotoxic T-cell-mediated cell death in ***tumours and transplant rejection reactions***
- ***Atrophy of parenchymal organs following duct obstruction*** in the salivary glands and pancreas

MECHANISMS OF APOPTOSIS

Apoptosis results from the activation of a set of enzymes called ***caspases*** – so named because these are cysteine proteases that cleave proteins after aspartic acid residues. Caspases ***exist in their inactive forms*** and must undergo enzymatic cleavage to become an active enzyme. The activation of caspases depends on the *balance between proapoptotic and antiapoptotic proteins. The presence of cleaved active caspases is a biochemical marker for apoptosis.* The whole process of apoptosis is divided into two phases:

I) Initiation phase
II) Execution phase

There are two different types of caspase activation, induced by different conditions that ultimately converge on a common pathway of execution.

A brief insight into the proteins involved in apoptosis (Table 2.5) is as follows:

There are more than 20 proteins in this category that may work for, or against, apoptosis.

Growth factors and other signals that aid in the survival promote the production of antiapoptotic proteins. When cells lose their survival signals, when their DNA is damaged or when ER stress signals are delivered, the sensor category proteins sense the damage and are activated. These, in turn, recruit the proapoptotic proteins and set the stage for apoptosis.

1. **Antiapoptotic proteins:** These function to prevent apoptosis when uninhibited.
2. **Proapoptotic proteins:** When released, these trigger apoptosis.
3. **Sensors:** These proteins sense the cellular damage or stress and maintain the balance between pro- and antiapoptotic proteins.

Phases and Pathways of Apoptosis (Fig. 2.25)

- There are two phases of apoptosis – ***initiation phase and execution phase.*** These two phases are followed by removal or clearance of the apoptotic bodies.
- There are two different pathways of the initiation phase – ***the mitochondrial pathway and the death receptor pathway.*** Both the pathways are functional under different conditions, involve different molecules and serve distinct roles in health and disease but can intersect. These two distinct pathways converge on caspase activation.

Initiation Phase of Apoptosis

a. **The intrinsic or mitochondrial pathway of apoptosis**
   This pathway is the major pathway of apoptosis and is triggered by the following factors:
   - Withdrawal of growth factors

Table 2.5 Examples and Functions of Proteins Involved in Apoptosis

Feature	Antiapoptotic	Proapoptotic	Sensors
Function	These reside in the outer mitochondrial membrane, making it impermeable and thereby preventing leakage of cytochrome c	Following activation, they form a channel to facilitate the leakage of cytochrome c from the intermembranous space of mitochondria into the cytoplasm	Act as umpires by maintaining balance between pro- and antiapoptotic proteins
Examples	BCL2, BCL-XL, MCL1	BAX, BAK	BAD, BIM, BID, Puma, Noxa

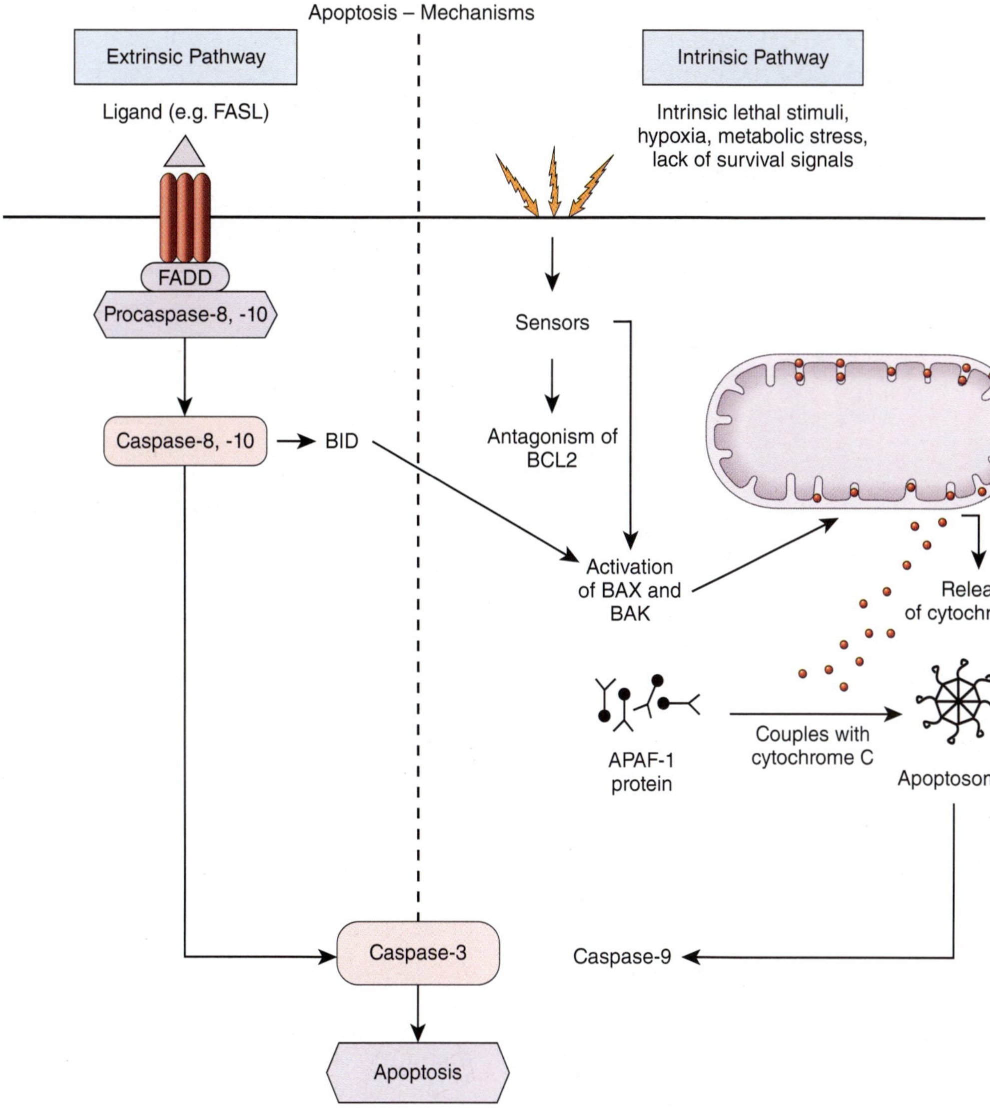

Fig. 2.25 Mechanisms of apoptosis – extrinsic and intrinsic pathways. (*Source:* From Scott A. Oakes, Robbins & Cotran Pathologic Basis of Disease, Elsevier 2021.)

- Withdrawal of hormones on the cell
- Radiation-induced DNA damage
- Toxin-induced DNA damage
- Accumulation of misfolded protein (ER stress)

Cellular stress caused by the aforementioned factors is sensed by the sensor group of proteins that activate the proapoptotic proteins, BAX and BAK, which work together to increase the permeability of the outer membrane of the mitochondria. This step is soon followed by release of mitochondrial proteins, most importantly ***cytochrome c,*** from the mitochondrial intermembrane space into the cytosol. Simultaneously, the functions of ***antiapoptotic proteins are blocked*** and their production is reduced under the influence of the sensors. The release of cytochrome c into the cytoplasm coupled with the decline in the levels and functions of antiapoptotic proteins initiates the process of apoptosis. The released cytochrome c binds to a protein called apoptosis activating factor-1 (***APAF-1***), and forms an apoptosome complex. This complex binds to and activates ***caspase-9*** (the initiator caspase of mitochondrial pathway), which then continues to activate other inactive caspase-9, causing the development of an autoamplification process. At the same time, the other proteins that are released into the cytoplasm along with cytochrome c bind and neutralize the physiological inhibitors of apoptosis in the cell, called inhibitors of apoptotic proteins (IAPs).

b. **The extrinsic or death receptor–initiated pathway of apoptosis** (Fig. 2.26)

This pathway of apoptosis is triggered when the ***death receptors*** on the plasma membrane of cells get engaged. The most common death receptors are ***type 1 TNF receptor***, and their related protein is called ***FAS*** (CD95). The ligand for Fas is Fas ligand (FasL). FasL is expressed on T cells when they react against self-antigens (to

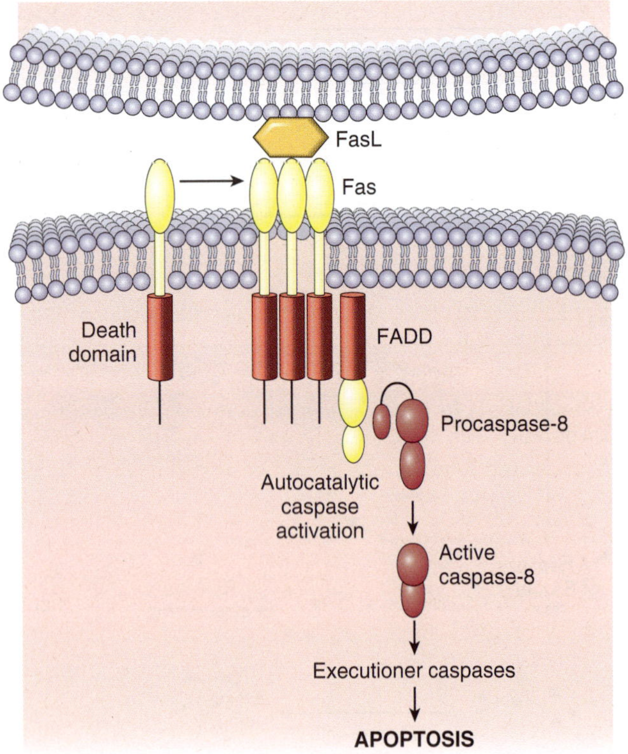

Fig. 2.26 The extrinsic (death receptor–initiated) pathway of apoptosis, illustrated by the events following Fas engagement. FADD, Fas-associated death domain; FasL, Fas ligand. (*Source:* Robbins and Cotran Pathologic Basic of Disease, 10th edition, Elsevier, 2021.)

eliminate self-reactive clones during tolerance development, explained in Chapter 6) and on cytotoxic T lymphocytes to remove virus-infected cells and tumour cells. During activation, when FasL binds to Fas, three or more molecules of Fas bind together and form a binding site for an adaptor protein called Fas-associated death domain (***FADD***) on the cytoplasmic side. FADD after binding activates ***procaspase-8 or procaspase-10*** (in humans) to form caspase-8 or caspase-10, respectively. The activated caspase-8 and caspase-10 continue to activate other procaspase-8 and procaspase-10 – *autoamplification*.

Execution Phase of Apoptosis Irrespective of the pathway, the initiation phases converge on an execution phase. In this phase, a cascade of caspase activation mediates the final phase of apoptosis. The mitochondrial pathway results in the activation of initiator ***caspase-9*** and the death receptor pathway in the activation of initiator ***caspase-8 or caspase-10.*** These caspases activate executioner caspases – ***caspase-3 and caspase-6,*** which further activate ***DNAse enzyme*** and cause enzymatic cleavage of DNA. Caspases also cause **nuclear fragmentation** by degrading the nuclear matrix. ***Blebs on the membrane*** of the affected cells and the apoptotic cell are broken down into smaller fragments called ***apoptotic bodies***, which can be readily engulfed by phagocytes.

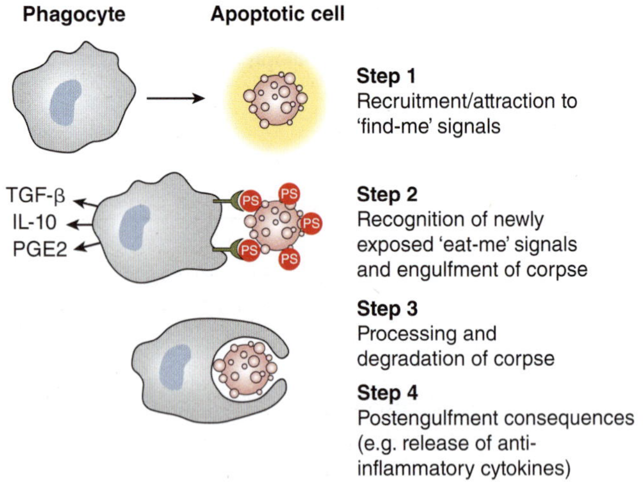

Fig. 2.27 Clearance of apoptotic bodies. (*Source:* Robbins and Cotran Pathologic Basic of Disease, 10th edition, Elsevier, 2021.)

Clearance of Dead Cells The execution phase ends with the formation of apoptotic bodies, followed by the clearance of these fragments.

Apoptotic bodies are rapidly identified, engulfed and cleared by phagocytes before they undergo necrosis. The following factors deliver the 'find me' and 'eat me' signals and help in the identification of apoptotic bodies by phagocytes:

a. ***Flipping of phosphatidylserine*** from the inner aspect of the plasma membrane to the outer aspect that serves as a signal for phagocytes. This is highlighted by staining with annexin V.
b. Apoptotic bodies may be coated with ***thrombospondin***, a glycoprotein released by a number of cells including fibroblasts that serve as a potent chemoattractant for the macrophages.
c. Apoptotic bodies may also be coated with immunoglobulins and complement proteins, especially C1q, which act as ***opsonins*** (described in Chapter 6) and enhance phagocytosis.
d. Dying cells secrete certain soluble factors that attract phagocytes.

The complete process of apoptosis occurs rapidly, and the dead cells get cleared within minutes, leaving no evidence behind (Fig. 2.27).

MORPHOLOGICAL CHANGES IN APOPTOSIS

The following cellular changes induced by apoptosis are best seen by electron microscopy:

- ***Cellular shrinkage:*** The cells shrink with condensation of cytoplasm because of tight packing of organelles.
- ***Chromatin condensation:*** This is the most characteristic feature of apoptosis. The chromatin aggregates peripherally under the nuclear membrane.

- ***Cytoplasmic blebs and apoptotic bodies:*** Apoptotic cells form blebs on the surface, which on detachment become apoptotic bodies.
- ***Phagocytosis of apoptotic bodies:*** Clearance of the apoptotic cells by phagocytes marks the end of the whole process.

The process of apoptosis happens rapidly; hence, it is not easy to detect in tissues. The ***complete absence of inflammation*** makes it even more difficult to identify in tissue sections. By light microscopy and haematoxylin and eosin staining, apoptotic cells appear as rounded masses with deep eosinophilic cytoplasm and fragmented chromatin (Fig. 2.28).

During karyorrhexis, endonuclease activation leaves short DNA fragments which are regularly spaced in size. These give a characteristic '***laddered***' appearance on agar gel electrophoresis. Tests for DNA laddering differentiate apoptosis from necrosis.

DISORDERS ASSOCIATED WITH DYSREGULATED APOPTOSIS

Apoptosis, in excess or deficiency, can lead to diseases.

Examples of conditions because of increased apoptosis and excessive cell death:

- Neurodegenerative diseases like Alzheimer, Huntington and Parkinson diseases
- Ischaemic injury
- Stroke
- Death of virus-infected cells
- Death of tumour cells

Examples of diseases because of defective apoptosis and increased cell survival:

- Cancers associated with TP53 mutation are associated with defective apoptosis and prolonged survival of transformed cells (described in Chapter 7).

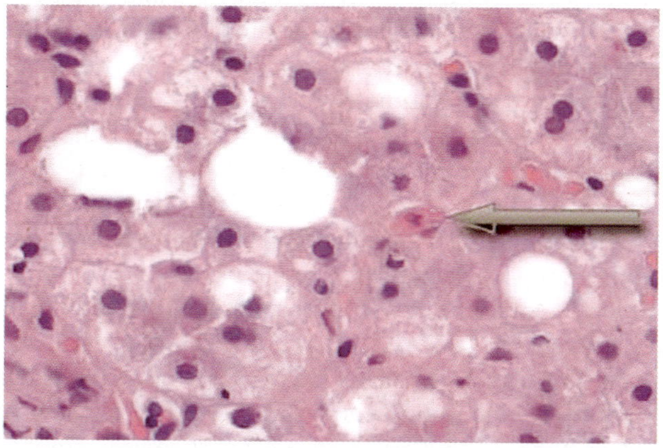

Fig. 2.28 Apoptotic hepatocyte seen in tissue sections, light microscopy, haematoxylin and eosin stain. The arrow points to the apoptotic cell. Note the bright eosinophilic colour of the cytoplasm and the cellular shrinkage.

- Defective apoptosis resulting in failure of clearance of self-reactive lymphocytes is the cause for many autoimmune disorders (described in Chapter 6).

Protein Misfolding

The link between protein misfolding and apoptosis needs special mention. The role of ***chaperones*** in the folding of freshly synthesized proteins, ubiquitination of misfolded polypeptides and targeting of such polypeptides for proteolysis in proteasomes is discussed in Chapter 1. Pathological stimuli that interfere with ER function can disrupt ER homeostasis, impose stress on it and subsequently cause accumulation of unfolded or misfolded proteins in ER. To handle such accumulation of unfolded or misfolded proteins and to restore normal ER functions, the cells have evolved highly specific signalling pathways collectively called the '***unfolded protein response***' (UPR).

UPR activates signalling pathways that accelerates the production of chaperones, enhances proteosomal degradation of abnormal proteins and slows down protein translation to reduce the load of misfolded proteins in the cell. However, if the overload of unfolded or misfolded proteins in ER is not resolved, the prolonged UPR induces ***ER stress***–associated programmed cell death, apoptosis, to remove the stressed cells (Fig. 2.29). This ER stress is now recognized as the basis of many conditions like Alzheimer disease, Huntington disease, cystic fibrosis and type 2 diabetes and has also been implicated in the normal ageing process.

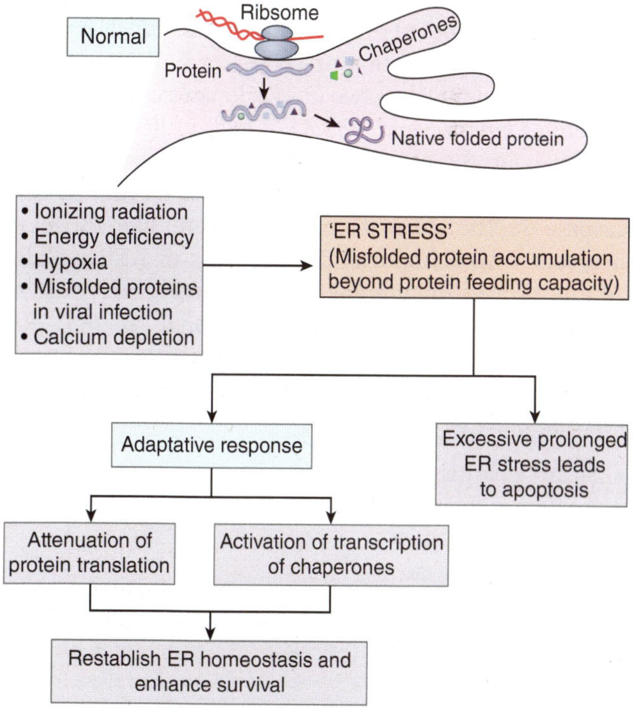

Fig. 2.29 The unfolded protein response and endoplasmic reticulum (ER) stress. (*Source:* Robbins and Cotran Pathologic Basic of Disease, 10th edition, Elsevier, 2021.)

Table 2.6 Differences Between Necrosis and Apoptosis

Feature	Necrosis	Apoptosis
Cell size	Increased	Decreased
Number of cells	Many	Single or many
Plasma membrane	Disrupted	Intact
Nuclear changes	Pyknosis Karyorrhexis Karyolysis	Fragmentation of nuclear DNA into nucleosome-sized fragments
Cellular contents	Leak out of the cell	Intact
Inflammation	Present	Absent
Cause	Always pathological	Physiological or pathological

DIFFERENCES BETWEEN NECROSIS AND APOPTOSIS (TABLE 2.6)

Necroptosis

Necroptosis is a unique form of cell death with ***hybrid features of necrosis and apoptosis*** and is now recognized as an important death pathway in both physiological and pathological conditions. This resembles necrosis morphologically and biochemically but resembles apoptosis also by being ***genetically programmed.*** It is also called ***programmed necrosis.*** Although it is genetically programmed, it does not involve caspases and hence is referred to as ***'caspase-independent programmed cell death'.*** Necroptosis is triggered by ligation of TNFR1 or FAS receptors by their ligands. It involves two unique kinases called *receptor-associated kinase-1 and -3 (RAK-1 and -3).* The binding of ligand to its receptor on the surface of cell membrane forms a multiprotein complex composed of RIP-1,3 and caspase-8. The downstream events are like those of necrosis – mitochondrial damage, loss of ATP, cellular and lysosomal membrane damage and generation of ROS. Hence, *morphological features of a cell that dies because of necroptosis resemble those of necrosis.*

Clinical examples with necroptosis as the mode of cell death are as follows:

- Steatohepatitis
- Acute pancreatitis
- Reperfusion injury
- Parkinson disease
- Cytomegalovirus infection

Pyroptosis

Pyroptosis is a highly inflammatory form of lytic programmed cell death that occurs most frequently on infection with intracellular pathogens and is likely to form part of the antimicrobial response. The process of pyroptosis promotes the rapid clearance of various bacterial, viral, fungal and protozoal infections by removing intracellular replication niches and enhancing the host's defensive responses.

Recognition of pathogen-associated molecular patterns (PAMPs) and damage-associated molecular patterns (DAMPs) (explained in Chapter 6) activates the formation of multiprotein complex inflammasomes, which then activates caspases to initiate pyroptosis. By mechanism, pyroptosis is activated by inflammatory caspases, including caspase-1 (mainly)/4/5 in humans. Caspase-3 activation can take place in both apoptosis and pyroptosis, in an alternative pathway that connects apoptosis and pyroptosis that has been discovered recently.

The inflammasome pathway may be canonical or noncanonical, with the former using caspase-1-activating inflammasomes and the latter using other caspases. The effector of pyroptosis that ultimately leads to cell death by membrane rupture is gasdermin D (GSDMD).

Pyroptosis, as a form of programmed cell death, has many morphological differences as compared with apoptosis. Although both pyroptosis and apoptosis undergo chromatin condensation, in apoptosis, the nucleus breaks into multiple chromatin bodies, whereas in pyroptosis, the nucleus remains intact. In cells that undergo pyroptosis, gasdermin pores are formed on the plasma membrane, resulting in water influx. Cells that undergo pyroptosis exhibit membrane blebbing and produce protrusions known as pyroptotic bodies.

Necroptosis works in a caspase-independent fashion, so it is proposed that both pyroptosis and necroptosis may act as defence systems against pathogens when apoptotic pathways are blocked.

Ferroptosis

Ferroptosis, also called oxytosis, is a recently recognized iron-dependent cell death that is different from other cell death forms, including apoptosis and necrosis. It is regulated by a set of genes and its mechanism involves three primary metabolisms involving thiol, lipid and iron, leading to an iron-dependent generation of lipid peroxidation. Cells affected by ferroptosis show a variety of metabolic changes and, ultimately, cell death.

Iron is an essential part of driving intracellular lipid peroxidation and ferroptosis. Ferroptosis can be prevented by using iron chelators (e.g. deferoxamine), whereas supplying exogenous iron (e.g. ferric ammonium citrate) supports ferroptosis. The imbalance between iron import, storage and export may affect the susceptibility of cells to ferroptosis.

Although many proteins have been shown to regulate ferroptosis, glutathione peroxidase 4 (GPX4) is the central enzyme of this pathway. GPX4 effectively inhibits ferroptosis by reducing and thus limiting lipid peroxides and generation of ROS. This process needs the substrate glutathione (GSH), which is provided by the enzyme xCT

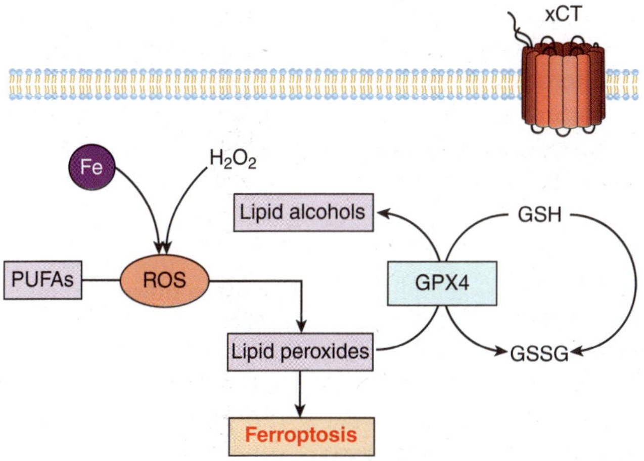

Fig. 2.30 Simplified ferroptotic cascade. Free iron accumulation is an initiator of ferroptosis. GPX4 normally inhibits ferroptosis by limiting lipid peroxides generated by ROS. This process requires the substrate GSH, which is provided by the enzyme xCT, which imports cysteine for GSH synthesis. GPX4, glutathione peroxidase 4; GSH, glutathione; ROS, reactive oxygen species.

via an intermediate step. xCT is the cysteine/glutamate antiporter, which imports cysteine for GSH synthesis (Fig. 2.30).

Ferroptotic cell death is accompanied by a sequence of variations in cell morphology, metabolism and protein expression that helps to discriminate this form of cell death from others. At the cellular and subcellular levels, cells undergoing ferroptotic cell death acquire a characteristic rounded shape before cell death similar to necrotic cells, but there is no cytoplasmic and organelle swelling, or plasma membrane rupture. The nuclei in ferroptotic cells retain their structural integrity, without condensation, chromatin margination, plasma membrane blebbing or formation of apoptotic bodies, which are characteristically seen in apoptosis. The only distinctive morphological feature seen in ferroptosis is mitochondria appearing smaller than normal with increased membrane density.

Ferroptosis has been implicated in several types of cancer. Such forms of cancers have been hypothesized to be highly sensitive to ferroptosis induction. An upregulation of iron levels has also been seen to induce ferroptosis in certain types of cancer, such as breast cancer.

AUTOLYSIS PA 2.4

Autolysis is the digestion of a cell by its own hydrolytic enzymes from lysosomes. This process is also called self-digestion. Autolysis is uncommon in living organisms and usually occurs in necrotic tissue because enzymes act on components of the cell that would not normally serve as substrates for the enzymes. These enzymes are released due to halting of active processes in the cell that provide substrates in healthy, living tissue. Although autolysis resembles the active process of digestion of nutrients by live cells, the dead cells are not actively digesting themselves as is often thought and autolysis in itself is not an active process. Failure of cellular respiration and subsequent failure of oxidative phosphorylation is the trigger of the autolytic process. The reduced availability and subsequent absence of high-energy molecules that are essential to maintain the integrity of the cell and maintain homeostasis causes significant changes in the biochemical operation of the cell.

Failure of delivery of molecular oxygen to cells results in a metabolic shift to anaerobic glycolysis. Glycolysis has a lower yield of ATP than oxidative phosphorylation and generates acidic by-products that decrease the pH of the cell. This acidic environment enables many of the enzymatic processes involved in autolysis.

Limited synthesis of ATP impairs many cellular transport mechanisms that use it, as discussed in the previous sections. The downstream events like water retention, ionic changes and acidification of the cell damage membrane-bound intracellular structures including the lysosome and peroxisome.

Lysosomes are membrane-bound organelles that typically contain a broad spectrum of enzymes capable of hydrolytic digestion of polysaccharides, proteins, nucleic acids, lipids, phosphoric acid esters and sulphates. This process requires compartmentalization and segregation of enzymes and substrates via a single intracellular membrane that prevents unwanted destruction of other intracellular components. Under normal conditions, the molecular machinery of the cell is further protected from lysosomal enzyme digestion by regulation of cytosolic pH. The activity of lysosomal hydrolases is optimal at a moderately acidic pH of 5, which is significantly more acidic than the more basic average pH of 7.2 in the surrounding cytosol. As the products of glycolysis accumulate, pH of the cell decreases which leads to blunting of this protective effect. In addition, lysosomal membranes damaged by water retention in the cell release lysosomal enzymes into the cytosol. These lysosomal enzymes are likely to be active because of the decreased cytosolic pH and are thus free to use cellular components as substrates.

Peroxisomes are responsible for the breakdown of lipids, particularly long-chain fatty acids. In the absence of an active electron transport chain and related cellular processes, there is no metabolic partner for the reducing equivalents in the breakdown of lipids. In autolysis, peroxisomes provide catabolic potential for fatty acids and ROS, which are released into the cytosol because the peroxisomal membrane is damaged by water retention and enzymatic digestion.

Autolysis results in an acidic, anaerobic, nutrient-rich environment that nurtures the activity of invasive and opportunistic microorganisms in a process known as putrefaction. Autolysis and putrefaction are the main processes responsible for the decomposition of remains of dead organisms.

Autolysis is also seen in tissues excised for biopsy which are not fixed immediately in appropriate fixatives. Autolysis in living individuals is accompanied by an inflammatory response, whereas in post-mortem changes, there is a complete absence of inflammatory response. Autolysis during post-mortem changes is rapid in organs like the pancreas and gastric mucosa because they are rich in hydrolytic enzymes; intermediate in organs like the heart, liver and kidney; and slow in fibrous tissue. Analysing the background changes associated with autolysis would help in distinguishing post-mortem changes from ante-mortem changes.

Morphologically, autolysed cells and tissues are identified by their homogeneous, eosinophilic cytoplasm and lack of cellular details. The release of catabolically active enzymes from the subcellular locations of lysosomes initiates an irreversible process that culminates in the complete reduction of dead organisms.

In wound healing, autolytic debridement can be beneficial, in which the body breaks down and liquifies dead tissue so that it can be washed or carried away.

AUTOPHAGY

In Greek, *auto* means self and *phagy* means eating, so autophagy means 'cell eating'. Autophagy is a naturally regulated process in which a ***cell eats its own components.*** The primary organelle involved in autophagy is the **lysosome**. The discovery of autophagy-related genes (Atgs) in yeast in the 1990s allowed researchers to deduce the mechanisms of autophagy, which eventually led to the Nobel Prize in Physiology or Medicine being awarded to Japanese researcher Yoshinori Ohsumi in 2016.

Autophagy is divided into three types on the basis of the mechanism of material delivery to the lysosomes:

1. **Macroautophagy:** This is the ***major form of autophagy***. In this type, portions of cytosol to be degraded are isolated and delivered enclosed within a double-membrane-bound autophagic vacuole – ***autophagosome.***
2. **Microautophagy:** Lysosomal membrane invaginates inwards and delivers the contents.
3. **Chaperone mediated:** Direct translocation occurs across the lysosomal membrane by chaperone proteins.

PROCESS OF AUTOPHAGY

The process of autophagy can be broken down into multiple steps. The formation of autophagosome is the most crucial step in the process of autophagy and is regulated by more than a dozen proteins that act in a coordinated and sequential manner (Fig. 2.31). The steps involved in autophagy are as follows:

1. ***Initiation:*** Formation of the isolation membrane or phagophore by ER
2. ***Elongation:*** Extension of the autophagosomal membrane to surround and capture its target
3. ***Maturation*** of autophagosome
4. ***Fusion*** of autophagosome with lysosome to form autophagolysosome
5. ***Release of lysosomal enzymes*** into the autophagolysosome
6. ***Degradation*** of the engulfed material
7. ***Recycling*** of metabolites

Genetics of autophagy:

More than 10 genes related to autophagy have been identified and are called ***Atgs***.

The nucleation, elongation and closure of the autophagosomal membrane require the function of *light chain 3 (LC3) – a microtubule-associated protein.*

LC3 is the marker of the autophagy process.

Autophagy in Health and Disease

Autophagy is the mechanism for turnover of organelles like ER, mitochondria and lysosomes. In disease, autophagy is seen as an adaptive response to stress, promoting survival of the cells, but in other cases, it appears to promote cell

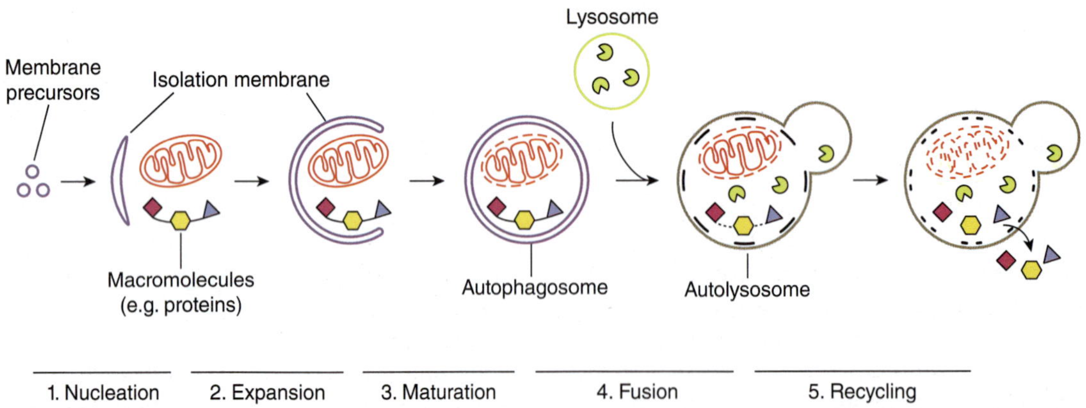

Fig. 2.31 Autophagy delivers cytoplasmic material to the lysosomal compartment for degradation. (1) Membrane donors including Atg9 vesicles nucleate an isolation membrane. (2) The isolation membrane expands and engulfs cytoplasmic cargo material including organelles and macromolecules. (3) The isolation membrane matures into a closed double-membrane autophagosome. (4) The outer autophagosomal membrane fuses with a lysosome (or the vacuole in yeast), leading to the degradation of the inner membrane and the cargo. (5) Components are recycled back into the cytoplasm.

death and morbidity. In extreme cases of starvation, the breakdown of cellular components promotes cellular survival by maintaining cellular energy levels. Dysregulation of autophagy occurs in many disease states including cancers, inflammatory bowel diseases, neurodegenerative diseases and infectious diseases like mycobacterial infections, *Shigella* infection and HSV infection.

INTRACELLULAR ACCUMULATIONS PA 2.3

Intracellular accumulation of abnormal amounts of a variety of substances is one of the major *manifestations of metabolic derangements in cells.* The substance may be a product of the same cell or another cell. It may accumulate within the cytoplasm, within the organelles or within the nucleus. Intracellular accumulation may be because of inherited or acquired causes. In acquired conditions, the accumulation is reversible, at least in the initial stages. In inherited conditions like storage disorders, the accumulation is progressive and might lead to cell death.

The four major mechanisms for intracellular accumulation are as follows (Fig. 2.32):

- ***Defective packaging and transport*** may result in inadequate removal of a substance, for example, fatty changes in the liver.
- ***Inherited deficiency of enzymes*** may result in failure of degradation of the substrate, resulting in its accumulation, for example, storage disorders.
- ***Defects in protein folding*** of substances may result in their accumulation, for example, α_1-antitrypsin deficiency.
- ***Accumulation of abnormal exogenous substance occurs***, for which the cell does not possess any enzyme system to degrade or transport, for example, accumulation of silica.

INTRACELLULAR ACCUMULATION OF LIPIDS

Triglycerides, cholesterol/cholesterol esters and phospholipids can accumulate inside a cell in many conditions. Phospholipid accumulation in the form of myelin figures is seen in necrotic cells.

1. **Triglyceride accumulation – steatosis**
   Steatosis refers to abnormal accumulation of triglycerides within the parenchymal cells of the liver, kidney, heart and muscle. The liver is commonly affected, because it is the major organ involved in fat metabolism. Steatosis of the liver is also called ***fatty liver*** (Fig. 2.33). Common causes include toxins, obesity, diabetes mellitus, protein–energy malnutrition and anoxia. In developed countries, the common causes are alcohol abuse, diabetes and obesity. Fatty liver is discussed in detail in Chapter 22. Tigroid heart is a form of fatty degeneration in which, on post-mortem examination, the heart shows alternate streaks of yellow (fat) and red (normal muscular tissue) colour.

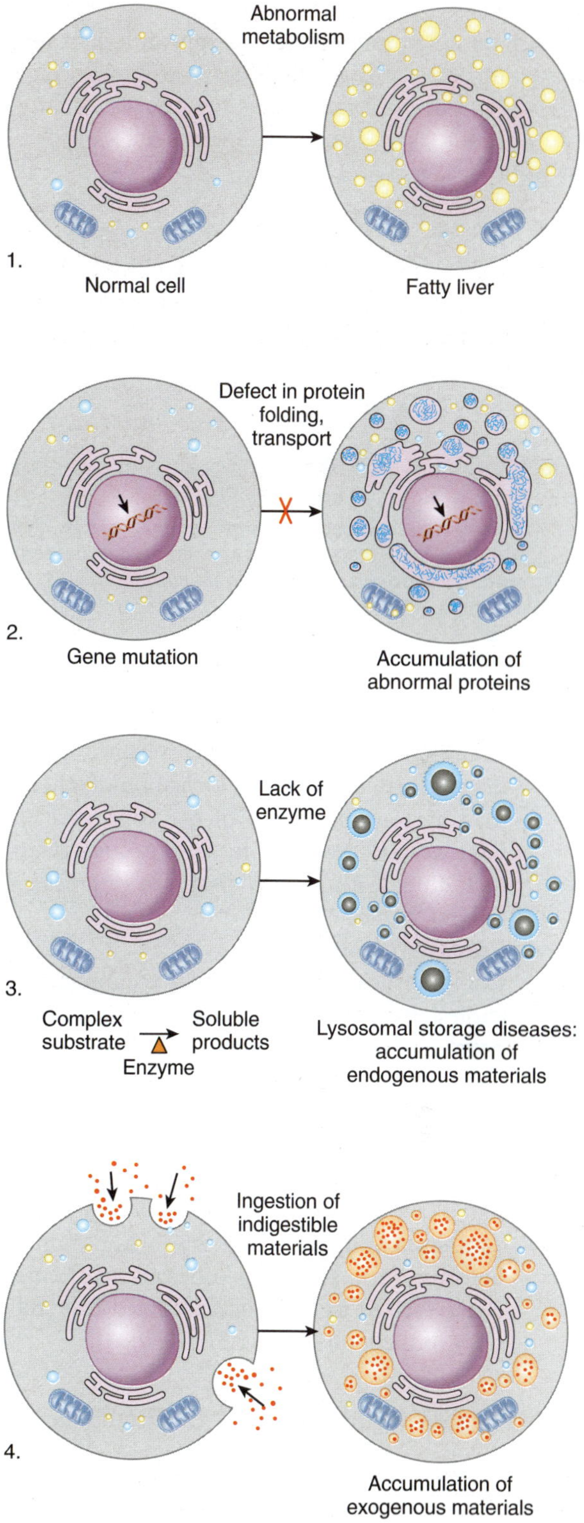

Fig. 2.32 Mechanisms of intracellular accumulations. (*Source:* Robbins and Cotran Pathologic Basic of Disease, 10th edition, Elsevier, 2021.)

2. **Cholesterol and cholesterol esters**
   Accumulation of cholesterol and its esters is always pathological and is seen in the following conditions:
   A. **Atherosclerosis**
   Atheroma is characterized by the presence of foam cells and is the hallmark feature of atherosclerosis. Foam cells are nothing but lipid-laden

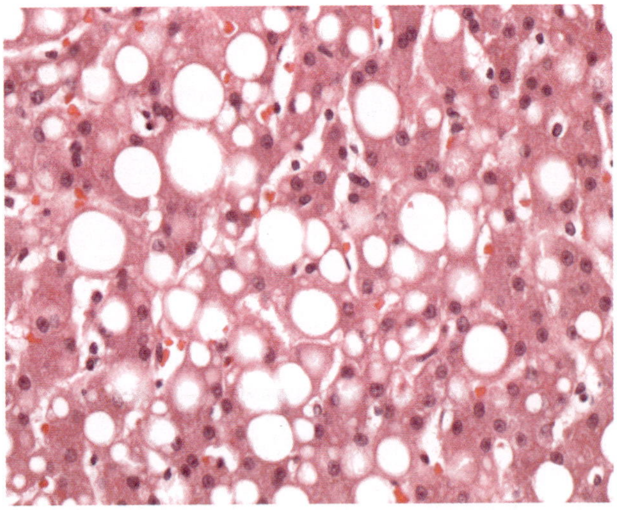

Fig. 2.33 Fatty liver, microscopy. High-power detail of fatty change of the liver. In most cells, the well-preserved nucleus is squeezed into the displaced rim of cytoplasm about the fat vacuole. (*Source:* From Fatty Liver Disease. In MacSween's Pathology of the Liver. 7th edition. 2018. Elsevier.)

smooth muscle cells and macrophages. Aggregation of foam cells and the formation of atheroma may narrow the lumen of the aorta and other large vessels, resulting in serious consequences including death. This is discussed in greater detail in Chapter 13.

B. **Cholesterolosis**
Cholesterolosis refers to focal accumulation of cholesterol-laden macrophages in the lamina propria of the gall bladder.

C. **Xanthomas**
The presence of clusters of foam cells in the subepithelial connective tissue of the skin and tendons produces tumorous masses in acquired and hereditary hyperlipidaemic states and is called xanthoma (Figs 2.34 and 2.35). Xanthoma tuberosum (also known as tuberous xanthoma) is characterized by xanthomas located over tuberosity of the joints (Figs 2.32 and 2.33).

INTRACELLULAR ACCUMULATION OF PROTEINS

Normal or abnormal proteins can accumulate inside a cell, causing cell injury. Intracellular accumulation of protein may be seen as eosinophilic droplets, vacuoles or aggregates.

The following are the conditions associated with intracellular accumulation of proteins:

1. **Russel bodies:** Intracellular accumulation of immunoglobulins is seen in conditions associated with plasma cell proliferation. The immunoglobulins accumulate inside ER and are seen as large, homogeneous and eosinophilic inclusions.

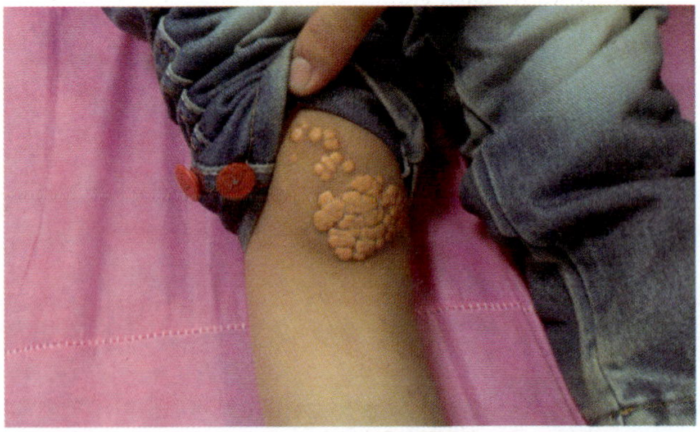

Fig. 2.34 Clinical picture of multiple xanthoma tuberosum.

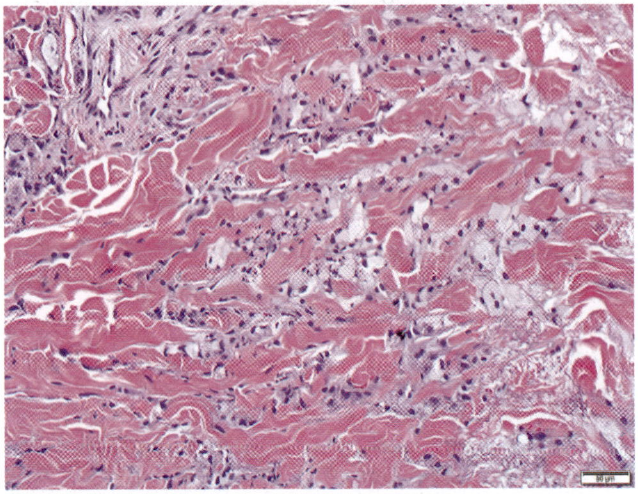

Fig. 2.35 Microscopy of xanthoma. There is admixture of dermal foamy histiocytes with neutrophils and extravascular lipid.

2. **Resorption droplets in proximal renal tubular epithelial cells:** In conditions causing heavy proteinuria, increased reabsorption of proteins occurs in the proximal tubules and can be seen as pink hyaline droplets within the cytoplasm of proximal tubular epithelial cells.
3. **Defective intracellular transport and secretion of critical proteins:** In α_1-antitrypsin deficiency, the inherited defects in protein folding result in misfolded protein response, causing ER stress and cell death.
4. **Accumulation of cytoskeletal proteins:** There are many types of cytoskeletal proteins such as:
   - Microtubules
   - Thin actin filaments
   - Thick myosin filaments
   - Intermediate filaments
   The intermediate filaments provide a flexible intracellular support to the cellular components and are of the following five types:
     - Keratin filaments – in epithelial cells
     - Vimentin filaments – in connective tissue cells
     - Desmin filaments – in muscle cells
     - Neurofilament – in neurons
     - Glial filaments – in astrocytes

In some disease states, these intermediate filaments may accumulate inside the cells. For example, keratin intermediates accumulate within hepatocytes to form ***alcoholic hyaline bodies*** in alcoholic liver disease and neurofilaments accumulate within neurons to form neurofibrillary ***tangles*** in Alzheimer disease.

5. **Aggregation of abnormal proteins:** Proteinopathies or protein aggregation diseases are a group of disorders that are characterized by the accumulation of abnormal or misfolded proteins within the cells (discussed in Chapter 6).

INTRACELLULAR ACCUMULATION OF GLYCOGEN

Glycogen is the storage form of glucose and is stored in cytoplasm of normal cells. In patients with defective glucose or glycogen metabolism, glycogen accumulates excessively within the cells.

In ***diabetes mellitus***, glycogen accumulates within renal tubular epithelial cells, hepatocytes, cardiac myocytes and β cells of the islets of Langerhans. In ***glycogen storage disorders***, because of inherited deficiency of enzymes involved in the synthesis or breakdown of glycogen, it accumulates inside the cells, causing injury to the cells. Glycogen accumulated within cells is microscopically seen as clear vacuoles in routine staining, because it is lost during formalin fixation. It is best demonstrated with alcohol fixation, followed by staining with ***periodic acid–Schiff (PAS) or Best carmine***. Glycogen is ***sensitive to digestion by diastase*** and hence treatment with diastase along with PAS staining proves the intracellular content as glycogen (tissue with a positive PAS-stained vacuole shows negative stain when the tissue is treated with diastase before staining).

INTRACELLULAR ACCUMULATION OF PIGMENTS (TABLE 2.7)

Pigments are coloured substances that may be endogenous or exogenous in origin. These accumulate within cells and may or may not be associated with diseases.

1. **Endogenous pigments**
   a. **Lipofuscin** (Fig. 2.36)
   Also called ***lipochrome or wear and tear pigment***, ***lipochrome*** is composed of lipids and phospholipids complexed with proteins. It is derived by lipid peroxidation of polyunsaturated lipids of the subcellular membranes. Therefore, the presence of lipofuscin indicates free radical–mediated injury. These cells ***undergo slow and regressive changes***. The organs with extensive lipofuscin deposition may have a brown colour; this is referred to as ***brown atrophy.*** Under a bright-field microscope, lipofuscin appears as *yellow-brown granular pigments* in the perinuclear region. Lipofuscin is commonly noted in hepatocytes and cardiac myocytes of ageing patients and patients suffering from protein–energy malnutrition and starvation.
   b. **Haemosiderin** (Fig. 2.37)
   Haemosiderin is a major storage form of iron and when it accumulates excessively within cells, it causes tissue damage and death. Iron metabolism and haemosiderin are explained in detail in Chapter 15. Iron is stored as ferritin in most cells and as haemosiderin in cells of the haematopoietic system under normal circumstances. But when there is a local or systemic excess, the excess haemosiderin may get deposited

Table 2.7 Common Examples for Endogenous and Exogenous Pigments

Endogenous Pigments	Exogenous Pigments
Lipofuscin	Carbon
Melanin	Tattoo
Haemosiderin	
Homogentisic acid	
Bilirubin	

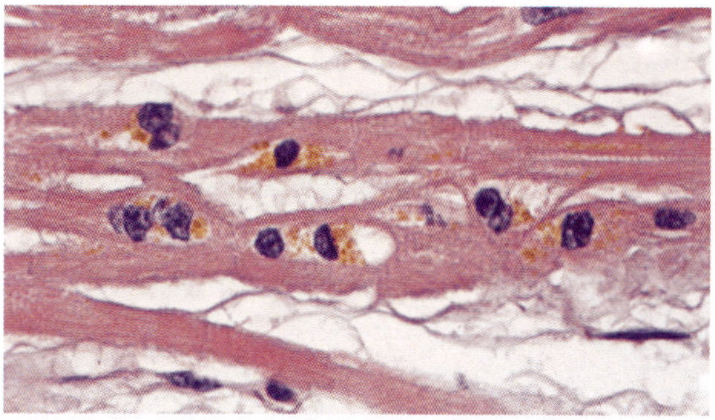

Fig. 2.36 Microscopy of lipofuscin in cardiac myocytes. Note the yellow-brown appearance of the granules. (*Source:* From Radu et al. Histological and immunohistochemical changes of the myocardium in dilated cardiomyopathy. Rom J Morphol Embryol. 2012;53(2): 269-75.)

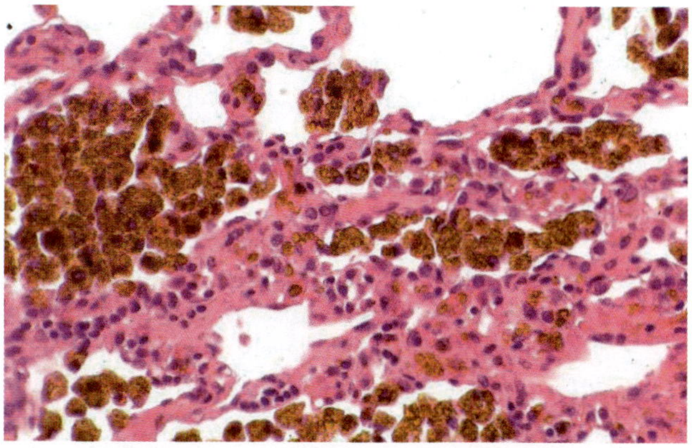

Fig. 2.37 Microscopy of haemosiderosis, lung. Haemosiderin-laden macrophages are seen over the septa and in the alveolar spaces.

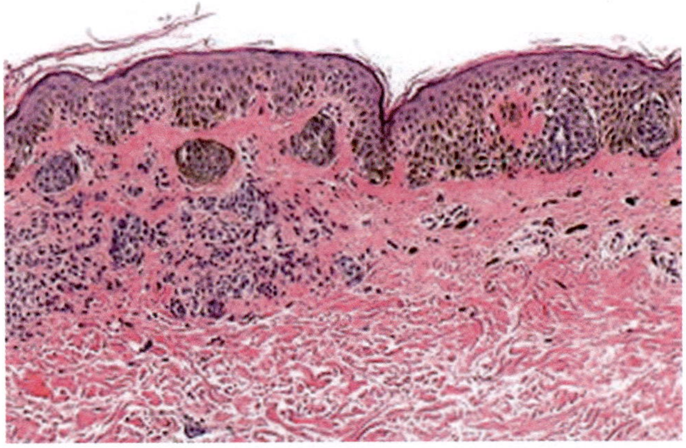

Fig. 2.38 Microscopy of junctional nevus with melanin pigment.

in cells and appear as *golden-brown granular or crystalline inclusions.* In systemic overloaded states, haemosiderin accumulates in multiple organs – a disease state referred to as ***haemosiderosis.***

c. **Melanin** (Fig. 2.38)
Melanin is the pigment present in melanocytes. Excess melanin may be seen in conditions associated with melanocyte proliferation like nevus and malignant melanoma. Melanin appears as *brown-black pigment* in sections and can be highlighted with ***Masson Fontana stain*** and immunohistochemically with ***Melan A, S100 and HMB45.***

d. **Homogentisic acid**
Homogentisic acid is a black pigment that deposits in the skin, connective tissue and cartilage in an inherited disease called ***alkaptonuria.*** The pigmentation is known as ***ochronosis.***

e. **Bilirubin**
Bilirubin is a pigment present in the bile. It is derived from porphyrin ring of the haem moiety of haemoglobin. The normal level of bilirubin in blood is less than 1 mg/dL. Excess of bilirubin is referred to as ***hyperbilirubinaemia*** and the clinical condition is called ***jaundice.*** Metabolism of bilirubin and pathogenesis of jaundice is explained in Chapter 22. Bilirubin, when in excess, deposits in the liver, skin, sclera and many other tissues. High levels of unconjugated bilirubin can cause ***kernicterus***, a toxic brain injury seen in infants.

2. **Exogenous pigments**

a. **Carbon** (Fig. 2.39)
The commonest exogenous pigment accumulated in cells is carbon, which is present in the alveoli of most urban dwellers because of air pollution. Prolonged exposure to high levels of carbon results in ***anthracosis***, a lung disease that is characterized by the accumulation of carbon, *progressing to a fibrosing lung disease or emphysema.*

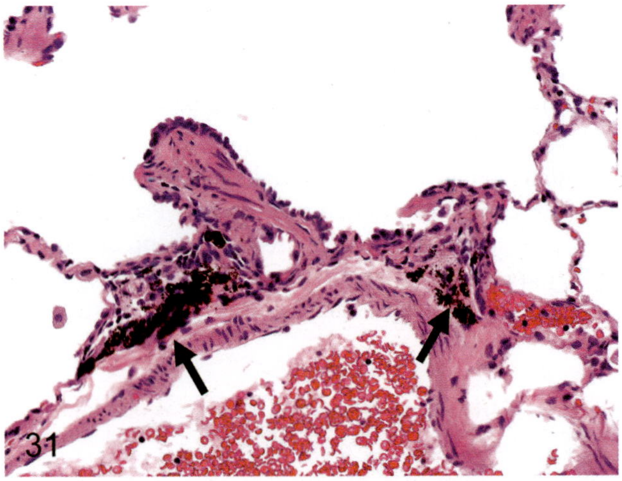

Fig. 2.39 Anthracotic pigment in lung, microscopy.

b. **Tattoo**
Tattooing is a form of localized exogenous pigmentation of the skin. The injected pigments are phagocytosed by the dermal macrophages and remain there forever.

PATHOLOGICAL CALCIFICATION PA 2.5

Pathological calcification is the abnormal deposition of calcium salts along with iron, magnesium and other mineral salts in the tissues.

There are two types of pathological calcification:

- ***Metastatic calcification:*** Calcium deposition in normal tissues because of hypercalcaemia
- ***Dystrophic calcification:*** Calcium deposition in dead and degenerated tissues

DYSTROPHIC CALCIFICATION

Dystrophic calcification occurs in ***dead and degenerating tissues*** and is often a cause of organ dysfunction. All types of necrosis can have areas of dystrophic calcification. In some instances, the calcification can be so extensive that it may convert the affected site into a hard stone. ***Serum calcium is often normal*** in these patients. *Common examples of dystrophic calcification are as follows:*

- Caseous necrosis in tuberculous lesions
- Liquefactive necrosis in chronic abscess
- Fat necrosis following pancreatitis
- Dead parasites like *Schistosoma*
- Atheromas of advanced atherosclerosis
- Valvular heart disease
- Heart valves of aged persons
- Thrombi, especially in veins

Dystrophic calcification is a simple indication of chronic cell injury but is often a cause of organ dysfunction.

METASTATIC CALCIFICATION

Metastatic calcification is a type of pathological calcification that occurs in normal tissues because of ***elevated serum levels of calcium.***

There are five principal causes of metastatic calcification:

1. Increased synthesis of parathyroid hormone (PTH) with resultant bone resorption, for example, hyperparathyroidism
2. Ectopic PTH-related protein secretion by malignant tumours
3. Bone resorption – multiple myeloma, breast cancer with diffuse skeletal secondaries, Paget disease, immobilization
4. Vitamin D–related diseases – sarcoidosis
5. Renal failure causing phosphate retention and secondary hyperparathyroidism

Although metastatic calcification can affect any tissue, the following are the commonly affected sites:

- Interstitial tissues of the gastric mucosa
- Renal interstitium (Fig. 2.40)
- Pulmonary interstitium
- Systemic arteries
- Pulmonary veins

All the above-mentioned tissues secrete acid, have an ***internal alkaline compartment*** and favour calcium deposition.

With smaller deposits, they do not cause any harm, but with massive deposits, they can compromise the function of the tissues.

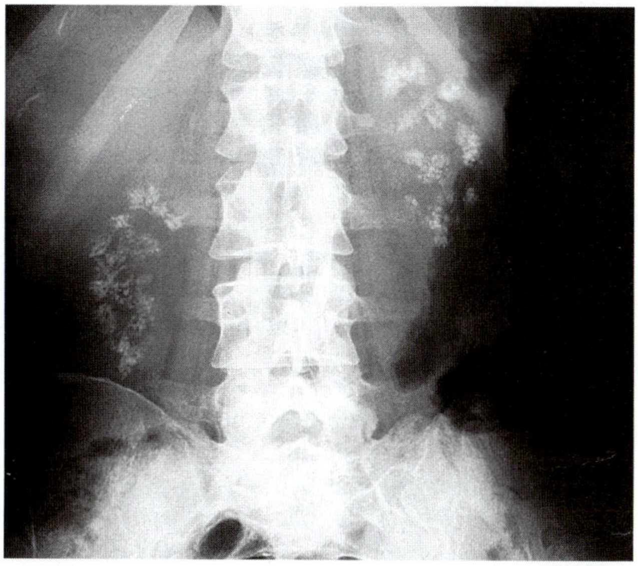

Fig. 2.40 Metastatic calcification, nephrocalcinosis. Plain radiograph showing bilateral metastatic medullary nephrocalcinosis in a patient with distal renal tubular acidosis. (*Source:* From Wei Chen, Rebeca D. Monk and David A. Bushinsky. Nephrolithiasis and Nephrocalcinosis. In Comprehensive Clinical Nephrology. 2019. Elsevier.)

Morphology

Morphologically, both types of calcification look similar. Grossly calcified areas appear as chalky ***white streaks or as large multinodular deposits*** in cases with massive deposits (Fig. 2.41). The affected tissues are gritty to cut.

Microscopically, calcium appears as an *amorphous, basophilic, granular material that may be intracellular or extracellular* (Fig. 2.42). In chronic extensive deposits, heterotopic bone formation may be present. In certain tumours like papillary thyroid carcinoma (PTC) or serous carcinoma of the ovary, dystrophic calcification appears as concentric lamellated structures called ***psammoma bodies*** (Fig. 2.43). These are believed to be formed subsequent to the necrosis of the tip of papillae

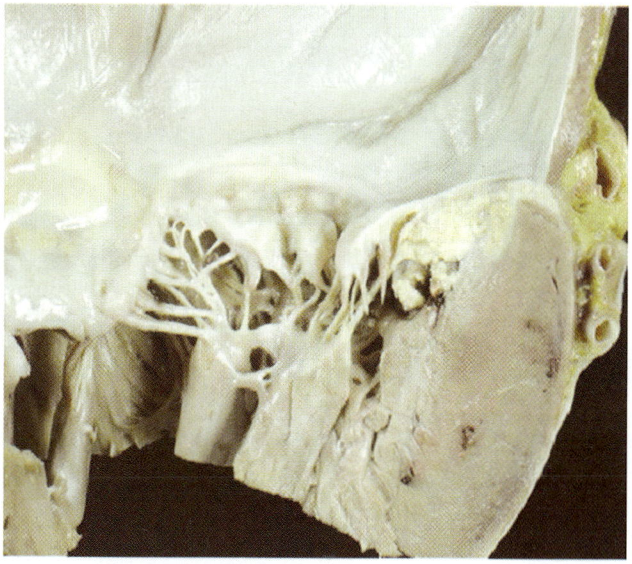

Fig. 2.41 Dystrophic calcification of TB node, gross. A case of severe dystrophic calcification of the three cusps of the aortic valve (on the left) and of the annulus of the mitral valve (on the right), accounting for aortic stenosis and mitral incompetence, respectively.

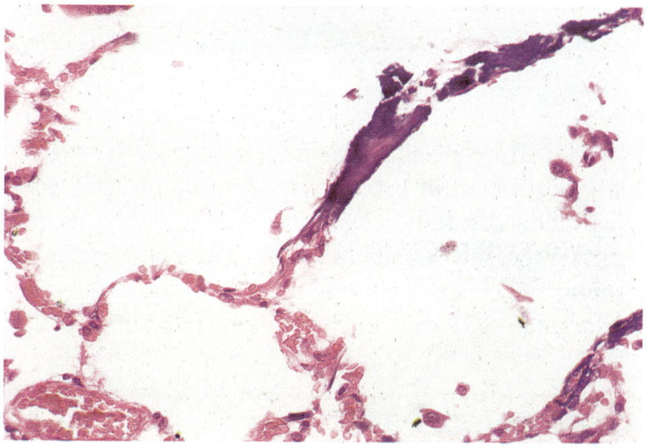

Fig. 2.42 Dystrophic calcification of alveolar walls in a case of hypercalcaemia, microscopy. (*Source:* From Stephen R. Morley. Disorders of metabolism and homeostasis. Underwood's Pathology. 2019. Elsevier.)

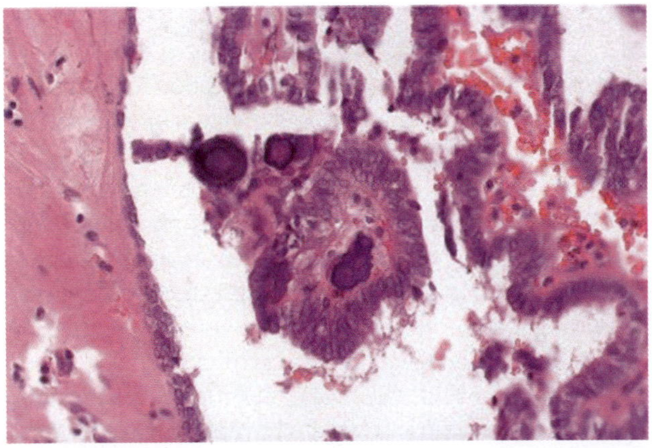

Fig. 2.43 Psammoma bodies: these represent a characteristic feature seen as round, calcified concretions with concentric laminations. Psammoma bodies represent necrotic tumour cell(s) that forms the nidus for deposition of calcium salts. (*Source:* From Bruce M. Wenig. Neoplasms of the Thyroid Gland. In Atlas of Head and Neck Pathology. 3rd edition. 2016. Elsevier.)

Table 2.8 Important Special Stains Relevant to Cell Injury

Substance	Special Stain[a]
Glycogen	Periodic acid–Schiff (PAS) + diastase sensitivity
Fat	Sudan black Oil red O
Haemosiderin	Perl's Prussian blue
Melanin	Masson Fontana
Calcium	Von Kossa Alizarin red
Plasma cells	Pyronin
Copper	Rhodamine Orcein
Apoptotic cells	Annexin V
α_1-Antitrypsin	PAS

[a]Routine stain for tissue sections: haematoxylin and eosin.

in PTC. The concentric calcification because of progressive acquisition of outer layers gives a lamellated configuration. These are commonly seen in PTC. Calcium can be specially stained using *Von Kossa or Alizarin red stains.* Other special stains used in histopathology as relevant to cell injury and proteins are listed in Table 2.8.

CELLULAR AGEING — PA 2.7

Human beings desire to stay immortal and young. Ageing is certainly an unwelcome yet unavoidable phase of life. It is universal, not just for humans but also for every living thing including plants. Ageing begins at birth, and cellular ageing is the cause of ageing in individuals. The theories and research studies on this process date back to 99 BCE. In a most recent advancement in 2019, scientists in London extended the life span of fruit flies by combining doses of lithium, trametinib and rapamycin.

Ageing refers to the ***progressive loss of functional capacity,*** which is a characteristic of senescence, and results in death. Apart from cosmetic reasons, ageing has many health issues because advancing age is a risk factor for many diseases like cancer. Cellular ageing is the result of a progressive decline in cellular function and viability caused by genetic abnormalities and because of the accumulation of cellular and molecular damage following exposure to exogenous influences.

Ageing is not a passive process but is a well-regulated active process. Many researchers have proved that ageing is ***influenced by both genes and environmental factors.*** The major mechanisms of cellular ageing are as follows:

1. DNA damage
2. Cellular replicative senescence
3. Abnormal protein homeostasis
4. Deregulated nutrient sensing

1. **DNA damage**
   Nuclear and mitochondrial DNA sustains damage by many exogenous (physical, chemical and microbiological) and endogenous (ROS) factors. DNA repair enzymes aid in the repair of these damages, but with ageing, the damages outnumber repairs and start accumulating. In diseases because of defective DNA repair, like Bloom syndrome and ataxia telangiectasia, premature ageing occurs. DNA damage is an important cause for cellular ageing.
2. **Cellular replicative senescence**
   Ageing is associated with progressive replicative senescence. Cells have a limited capacity for replication; after a fixed number of cell divisions, they go into a nonreplicative state called cellular senescence.
   There are two mechanisms as the basis for cellular senescence:
   a. **Shortening of telomeres** (Fig. 2.44)
      Telomeres are short, repetitive sequences of DNA that are present at the ends of the chromosomes. Their function is to ensure that in each cell division, the replication is complete and the ends of the chromosomes are not fused or damaged. The telomeres shorten with each cell division. When telomeres become critically short, they can no longer protect the ends of the chromosomes and the cells eventually possess broken DNA which triggers cell-cycle arrest.
      Telomerase is an enzyme that prevents telomere shortening by adding nucleotides to the ends of chromosomes. Germ cells and stem cells (lower levels than germ cells) possess telomerase activity and hence multiply rapidly. Somatic cells do not

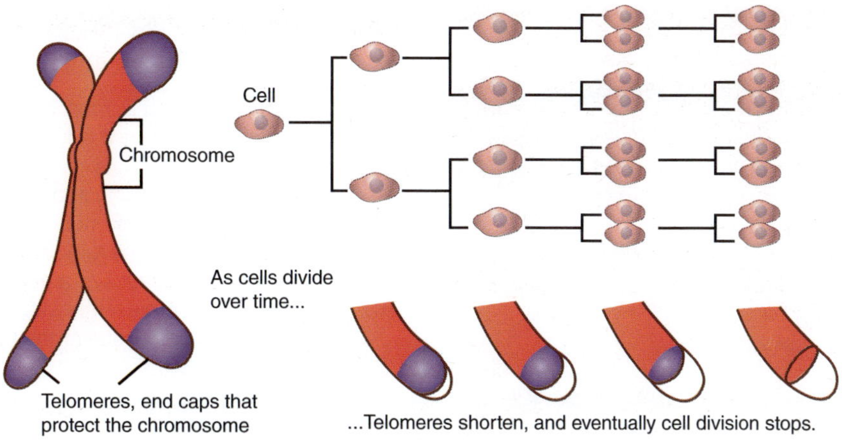

Fig. 2.44 Telomere shortening with cell division.

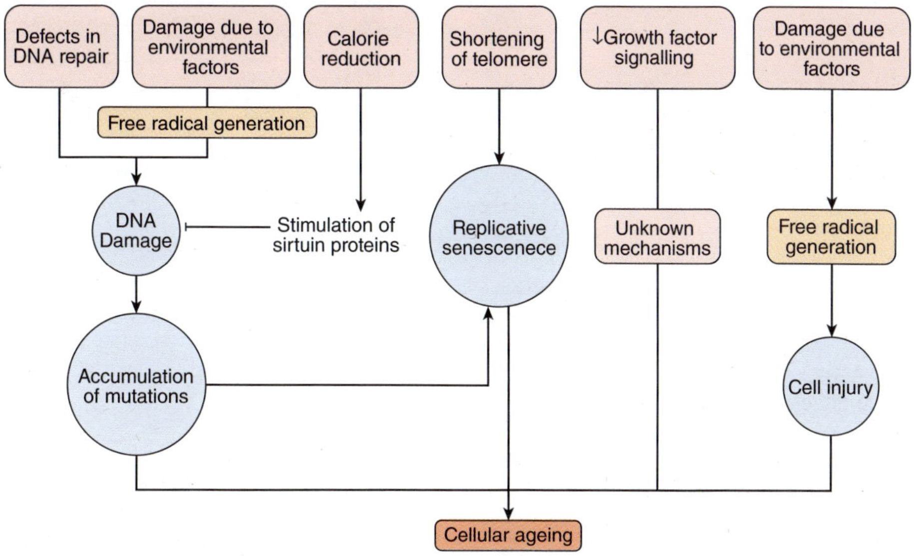

Flowchart 2.5 Mechanisms of cellular ageing. (*Source:* From Vinay Kumar, Abul Abbas, Jon Aster. Robbins & Cotran Pathologic Basis of Disease, 10th edition. Elsevier. 2020.)

have telomerase activity. One of the mechanisms of immortality in neoplastic cells is the reactivation of telomerase enzyme resulting in indefinite proliferation. Telomere shortening is associated with other diseases with premature cell loss, like aplastic anaemia (discussed in Chapter 15).

b. **Tumour suppressor gene activation**
Activation of tumour suppressor genes such as *p16* and *INK4a*, coded by CDKN2A, is associated with cellular ageing. *The function of these proteins is to cause cell-cycle arrest.* Hence, these proteins push the cells out of the cell cycle and along the senescence pathway.

3. **Abnormal protein homeostasis**
Protein homeostasis involves two mechanisms:
   a. Correct folding of proteins mediated by chaperones
   b. Removal of misfolded proteins mediated by ubiquitin–proteasome and autophagy–lysosome systems

   With ageing, both the mechanisms are deranged. Defective protein homeostasis affects cell survival, replication and function. In addition, misfolded proteins cause ER stress and trigger apoptosis.

4. **Deregulated nutrient sensing**
Two mechanisms are involved in sensing the disturbed nutrition, which happens with ageing:
   a. **Attenuation of IGF-1 signalling**
   IGF-1 that promotes anabolic state and aids in cell growth and proliferation gets attenuated.
   b. **Loss of function of sirtuins**
   Sirtuins are a family of NAD-dependent protein deacetylases. These proteins help cells to adapt to environmental stress, food deprivation and DNA damage. These act by many mechanisms including inhibition of apoptosis and inhibition of damage because of free radicals and stimulation of protein folding. Loss of sirtuins is associated with cellular ageing (Flowchart 2.5). ***Calorie restriction increases longevity mainly by augmenting the IGF-1 signalling and the functions of sirtuins.***

SELF-ASSESSMENT

Scenario-Based MCQs

1. A patient is admitted to the emergency room following a car accident. He has multiple injuries and is in shock. Which of the following best describes the primary mechanism of cell injury in this patient?
   A. Hypoxic injury because of reduced blood flow
   B. Chemical injury from medications
   C. Infectious injury from bacteria
   D. Immune-mediated injury
2. A 60-year-old woman with a long history of smoking presents with chronic obstructive pulmonary disease (COPD). Which type of cell injury is most likely predominant in her lung tissues?
   A. Apoptotic injury
   B. Necrotic injury
   C. Free radical–induced injury
   D. Hypoxic injury
3. A patient with a history of alcohol abuse presents with liver dysfunction. Laboratory tests show elevated liver enzymes. The liver injury in this patient is primarily because of:
   A. Reversible cell injury
   B. Irreversible cell injury
   C. Infectious injury
   D. Hypoxic injury
4. A man is rescued from a house fire and treated for carbon monoxide poisoning. His cells are likely experiencing:
   A. Reversible injury because of chemical exposure
   B. Irreversible injury because of hypoxia
   C. Necrosis because of direct thermal damage
   D. Apoptosis because of inflammatory response
5. A patient with diabetes mellitus type 2 shows accumulation of glycogen in liver cells. This is an example of:
   A. Intracellular accumulation of carbohydrates
   B. Intracellular accumulation of proteins
   C. Intracellular accumulation of lipids
   D. Intracellular accumulation of pigments
6. During an autopsy, a pathologist notes abundant lipofuscin pigment in the liver and heart cells of an elderly individual. This finding is indicative of:
   A. Accumulation because of cell injury
   B. Normal ageing process
   C. Pathological pigment accumulation
   D. Infectious process
7. A biopsy from a patient with myocardial infarction shows cells with swollen mitochondria and ruptured membranes. This type of cell death is most consistent with:
   A. Apoptosis
   B. Necrosis
   C. Autophagy
   D. Pyroptosis
8. A patient with HIV/AIDS shows lymphocyte death primarily through a mechanism that involves DNA fragmentation and cell shrinkage. This process is best described as:
   A. Necrosis
   B. Apoptosis
   C. Autolysis
   D. Pyroptosis
9. A patient with chronic renal failure develops metastatic calcification. Which of the following best describes this condition?
   A. Calcification occurring in damaged tissues
   B. Calcification because of high serum calcium levels
   C. Calcification within a tumour
   D. Calcification because of a genetic disorder
10. A diabetic patient presents with a nonhealing foot ulcer showing blackened tissue at the toes. This is most likely:
    A. Wet gangrene
    B. Dry gangrene
    C. Gas gangrene
    D. Caseous necrosis
11. A patient with severe hypertension shows left ventricular hypertrophy. This change in the heart muscle is an example of:
    A. Hyperplasia
    B. Hypertrophy
    C. Metaplasia
    D. Dysplasia
12. A heavy smoker develops squamous metaplasia in the bronchial epithelium. This is an example of:
    A. Adaptive hyperplasia
    B. Reactive hypertrophy
    C. Pathological metaplasia
    D. Physiological dysplasia
13. In an elderly patient, a biopsy shows decreased cell turnover and increased cellular debris. This is indicative of:
    A. Cellular ageing
    B. Chronic inflammation
    C. Infectious process
    D. Neoplastic transformation
14. A patient undergoing chemotherapy shows increased cell death with DNA fragmentation and cell shrinkage. This type of cell death is mainly because of:
    A. Necrosis
    B. Apoptosis
    C. Autolysis
    D. Pyroptosis
15. An individual with long-term exposure to UV radiation shows skin cells with damaged DNA undergoing cell death. The most likely mechanism is:
    A. Necrosis because of direct damage
    B. Apoptosis because of DNA damage
    C. Autophagy because of metabolic stress
    D. Pyroptosis because of inflammation
16. A factory worker is exposed to high levels of lead over several years. This type of cell injury is predominantly:
    A. Hypoxic injury
    B. Chemical injury
    C. Physical injury
    D. Infectious injury
17. A patient with severe anaemia shows signs of tissue hypoxia. This condition is an example of cell injury primarily because of:
    A. Chemical toxicity
    B. Physical trauma
    C. Lack of oxygen
    D. Inflammatory response

18. An individual who ingests a large dose of acetaminophen experiences liver damage. The liver cells are likely undergoing:
    A. Reversible injury
    B. Irreversible injury
    C. Necrosis
    D. Apoptosis
19. A patient recovers from transient ischaemia following a brief episode of cardiac arrhythmia. The cell injury in this case was most likely:
    A. Irreversible necrosis
    B. Reversible hypoxic injury
    C. Chronic inflammation
    D. Apoptotic cell death
20. A patient with chronic alcoholism shows hepatocytes with fatty changes. This is an example of:
    A. Carbohydrate accumulation
    B. Protein accumulation
    C. Lipid accumulation
    D. Pigment accumulation
21. A biopsy from a patient with stroke shows brain cells with eosinophilic cytoplasm and nuclear pyknosis. This is indicative of:
    A. Necrosis
    B. Apoptosis
    C. Autophagy
    D. Senescence
22. A patient with tuberculosis shows caseous necrosis in the lung tissue. This form of cell death is characterized by:
    A. Inflammatory cell death
    B. Coagulative necrosis
    C. Liquefactive necrosis
    D. Fat necrosis
23. An individual with atherosclerosis shows calcification in the arterial walls. This is an example of:
    A. Dystrophic calcification
    B. Metastatic calcification
    C. Physiological calcification
    D. Calcific myonecrosis
24. A patient with chronic asthma shows bronchial wall thickening and increased smooth muscle. This is an example of:
    A. Atrophy
    B. Hypertrophy
    C. Hyperplasia
    D. Dysplasia
25. A patient with Barrett oesophagus, a condition because of chronic acid reflux, exhibits:
    A. Squamous metaplasia
    B. Columnar metaplasia
    C. Fibrous dysplasia
    D. Hypertrophic hyperplasia

Answers

1. (A); 2. (C); 3. (B); 4. (A); 5. (A); 6. (B); 7. (B); 8. (B); 9. (B); 10. (B); 11. (B); 12. (C); 13. (A); 14. (B); 15. (B); 16. (B); 17. (C); 18. (B); 19. (B); 20. (C); 21. (B); 22. (B); 23. (A); 24. (C); 25. (B)

Scenario-Based Questions

1. A factory worker exposed to benzene for several years is diagnosed with bone marrow failure. Discuss the pathophysiological mechanisms of chemical-induced cell injury in this context.
2. A patient experiences a transient ischaemic attack but recovers fully within a few hours. Analyse the cellular changes associated with reversible injury in this case and contrast them with irreversible cell injury.
3. An autopsy of a chronic alcoholic reveals significant fatty changes in the liver. Explain the mechanisms leading to intracellular accumulation of lipids and its consequences in liver cells.
4. A patient suffering from myocardial infarction shows extensive cardiac muscle cell death. Compare and contrast necrosis and apoptosis in the context of myocardial infarction.
5. A patient with chronic renal failure develops extensive vascular calcifications. Discuss the pathogenesis of metastatic calcification and its clinical implications.
6. A hypertensive patient shows left ventricular hypertrophy. Describe the cellular adaptation mechanisms in response to increased workload, focusing on hypertrophy and hyperplasia.
7. An elderly patient with Alzheimer disease shows various signs of cellular ageing. Discuss the mechanisms and implications of cellular ageing in the context of neurodegenerative diseases.
8. A patient is diagnosed with amyloidosis. Discuss the pathogenesis of intracellular protein accumulation and its effects on cell function.
9. A patient with bacterial meningitis shows areas of necrosis in brain tissue. Elaborate on the mechanisms and morphological characteristics of necrosis in infectious diseases.
10. A patient with chronic bronchitis exhibits bronchial epithelial changes. Discuss the types of cellular adaptations that occur in response to prolonged inflammation.
11. A patient undergoing chemotherapy for leukaemia shows high rates of tumour cell apoptosis. Explain the role of apoptosis in cancer therapy and its significance in treatment response.
12. A mountaineer develops acute mountain sickness at high altitude. Analyse the cellular effects of hypoxia and the body's adaptive response.
13. A diabetic patient with a foot ulcer develops dry gangrene. Discuss the pathophysiology of gangrene development in the context of diabetes.
14. A patient receiving radiation therapy for cancer treatment shows signs of radiation-induced cell injury. Describe the cellular response to ionizing radiation and its therapeutic and adverse effects.
15. An elderly patient shows increased lipofuscin accumulation in the heart and liver tissues. Discuss the mechanisms and significance of pigment accumulation in ageing.

Self-Assessment Questions

1. Mechanisms of hypertrophy and metaplasia.
2. Morphological changes in reversible and irreversible injuries.
3. Biochemical mechanisms of cell injury.
4. Different types of necrosis with examples.
5. Mechanism of reperfusion injury.
6. Free radicals in health and disease.
7. Mechanisms of apoptosis.
8. Differences between apoptosis and necrosis.
9. Types of intracellular accumulations and their consequences.
10. Types, pathogenesis and morphology of pathological calcification.
11. Process of cellular ageing.

Topics for Self-Directed Learning

1. Properties of the principal free radicals involved in cell injury.
2. The unfolded protein response and the ER stress.
3. Diseases caused by misfolding of proteins.
4. Comparison and contrast between necroptosis and pyroptosis.
5. Pigments in health and disease.
6. Hyaline change in cells.
7. Porphyrin as an intracellular pigment.
8. The relationship between calories, sirtuins and ageing.

Inflammation, Healing and Repair

3

Gayathri Devi Thanigaimani

PA 4.1 Define and describe the general features of acute and chronic inflammation including stimuli and **vascular and cellular events.**

PA 4.2 Enumerate and describe the **mediators** of acute inflammation.

PA 4.3 Define and describe **chronic inflammation** including causes, types, nonspecific and granulomatous, and enumerate examples of each.

PA 5.1 Define and describe the process of repair and regeneration including **wound healing** and its types.

CHAPTER OUTLINE

OVERVIEW OF INFLAMMATION

Inflammation is the response of a host to eliminate a foreign agent from the body. It occurs in vascularized tissues, whenever there is an infection or damage, by cells and mediators of the host defence system. It is a protective mechanism of the body to remove the injury-causing agents and the tissues damaged by the agent. It is absolutely essential for eliminating infections and for the healing process to occur, but there may be collateral damage to the host tissue when it occurs excessively.

Steps involved in inflammation (Fig. 3.1):

- Recognition of the offending agent
- Recruitment of the host defence components to the site of injury
- Removal of the offending agent
- Response termination
- Repair of damage

Components of inflammation:

- Leucocytes
- Chemical mediators, which are soluble factors produced by cells or derived from plasma proteins
- Antibodies
- Blood vessels that serve to transport the aforementioned factors to the site of inflammation

Beneficial versus harmful effects of inflammation:
Although inflammation helps our body by eliminating the injurious agent, when the response is exaggerated or is misdirected against the body components or does not get terminated after elimination of the inciting agent, it may lead to harmful effects on the host. It has also been implicated in the pathogenesis of some primary metabolic, degenerative and genetic

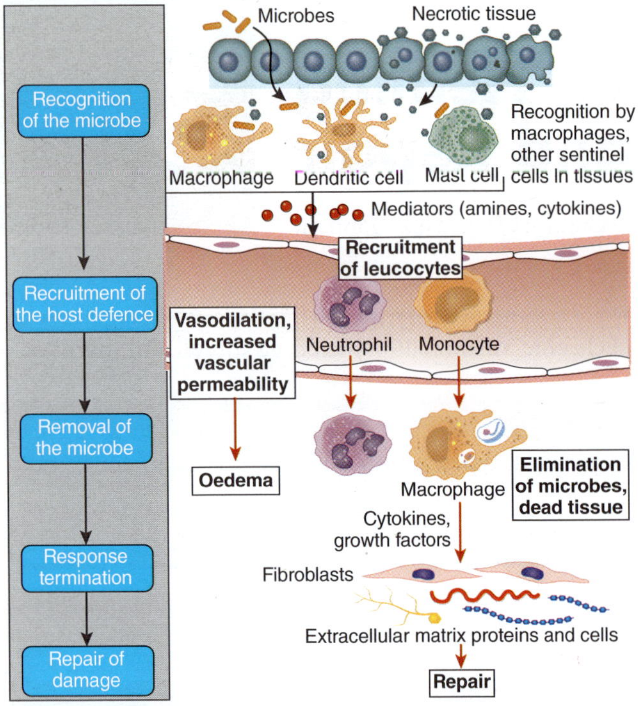

Fig. 3.1 Steps involved in inflammation. (*Source:* From Vinay Kumar, Abul K. Abbas and Jon C. Aster. Inflammation and Repair. In Robbins Basic Pathology 10th edition. 2018. Elsevier.)

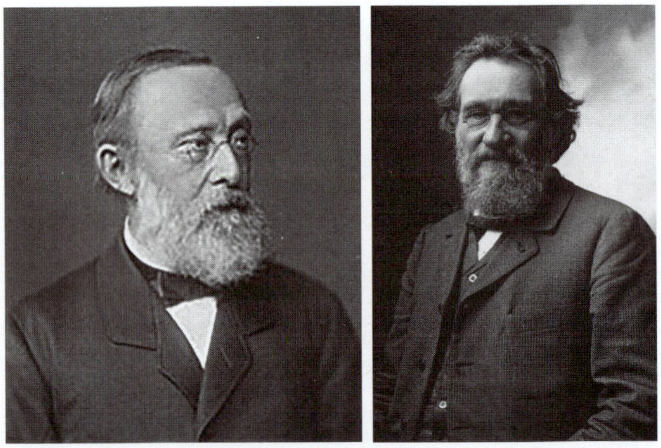

Fig. 3.2 Rudolph Virchow (left) and Elle Metchnikoff (right). (*Source:* Image of Rudolph Virchow and Elie Metchnikoff.)

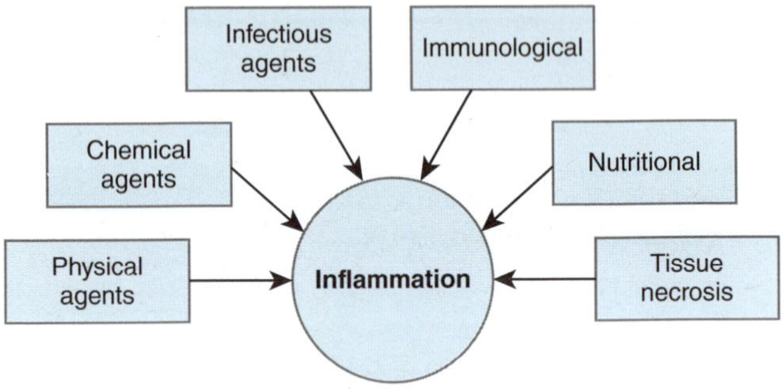

Flowchart 3.1 Causes of inflammation.

disorders. Hence, inflammation may be referred as a 'silent killer'.

Local versus systemic effects of inflammation:
The local response of the tissue at the site of inflammation is universally seen in all types of inflammation, but in some scenarios, there may be a systemic response of the body. This may be because of the mediators that mediate fever, leucocytosis, etc., or may be because of a widely disseminated infection called *sepsis*. Sometimes the systemic response may be exaggerated enough to lead to severe consequences such as in *systemic inflammatory response syndrome*.

HISTORICAL HIGHLIGHTS (FIG. 3.2)

Knowledge about the signs of inflammation dates back to 3000 BCE when *Celsus* first described the four cardinal signs of inflammation – ***rubor*** (redness), ***tumour*** (swelling), ***calor*** (heat) and ***dolor*** (pain). *Rudolf Virchow* in the nineteenth century described the fifth cardinal sign of inflammation ***functio laesa*** or loss of function. The revolutionary conclusion that inflammation was not a disease but rather a response of the body was given by the Scottish surgeon *John Hunter* in 1793. In the 1880s, the process of phagocytosis was discovered by the Russian biologist *Elie Metchnikoff*, and he identified that inflammation was the body's effort to bring phagocytic cells to the injured area to remove the offending bacteria. Furthermore, the role of chemical substances, which are now termed mediators of inflammation, was conceptualized by *Sir Thomas Lewis*.

CAUSES OF INFLAMMATION (FLOWCHART 3.1)

- **Infections** are the most common cause of inflammation. Bacterial, viral, fungal and parasitic infections can cause inflammation directly or by producing toxins. These may cause local or systemic, mild or fatal, and acute or chronic inflammation. However, the outcome depends not only on the causative agent but also on the response of the host.
- **Tissue necrosis**, irrespective of the cause, releases certain chemicals that trigger inflammation. In fact, the presence of inflammation has been noted as one of the features that differentiates necrosis from apoptosis as a mode of cell death.
- **Foreign bodies** that enter the body may damage the tissue or be a source of inflammation.
- **Endogenous substances**, sometimes, may be inert or toxic and when deposited in the tissue may trigger an inflammatory response. Examples of such endogenous bodies include urate crystals as in gout, cholesterol crystals as in atherosclerosis and lipids as in metabolic syndrome.
- **Immune reactions,** also called hypersensitivity reactions, include a group of reactions caused by an exaggerated host response to an external microbe or a misdirected response against the body's own antigen. These cause significant damage to the body, resulting in allergies and

Table 3.1 Features of Acute and Chronic Inflammation

	Acute Inflammation	Chronic Inflammation
Onset	Fast: minutes or hours	Slow: days
Duration of inflammation	Short: several hours to few days	Long: months to years
Cellular infiltrate	Mainly neutrophils	Monocytes/macrophages and lymphocytes
Tissue injury, fibrosis	Usually mild and self-limited	Often severe and progressive
Local and systemic signs	Prominent	Less
Granulation tissue	Absent	Present
Scarring	May be present	Present
Main type of host defence	Innate immunity	Adaptive immunity
Complete resolution	May occur	Always associated with tissue destruction and repair
Main mediators	Vasoactive amines, arachidonic acid metabolites, cytokines and complement mediators	Cytokines produced by macrophages

autoimmune diseases. The antigen is endogenous and cannot be eliminated, so it leads to long-standing chronic destruction of the tissues.

ACUTE VERSUS CHRONIC INFLAMMATION

Acute inflammation is the immediate reaction of the body to an infectious agent or tissue destruction. But when there is a persisting stimulus, the inflammation persists for many days to months and leads to permanent tissue loss and is called chronic inflammation. The differences between them are summarized in Table 3.1.

ACUTE INFLAMMATION PA 4.1

The three major components of acute inflammation are as follows:

- Dilation of small blood vessels causing increased blood flow
- Increased permeability of blood vessels causing leakage of cells and proteins
- Movement of leucocytes from the circulation to the site of inflammation and removal of the offending agent

The inflammatory cells, apart from removing the microbe by phagocytosis, also produce various chemical substances called mediators that lead to many of the effects of inflammation in the local area and systemically. The response in acute inflammation can be subdivided into vascular events and cellular events, with the former preceding the latter. Let us review them in detail.

VASCULAR EVENTS (FIG. 3.3)

Vascular events of acute inflammation include changes in the vascular calibre and vessel wall permeability to cause movement of plasma proteins and inflammatory cells to the site of infection. This increase in vascular permeability is called exudation, and the protein-rich fluid that escapes from the vessel into the interstitial space is called exudate. It also contains inflammatory cells and implies an inflammatory process in the vicinity. The vascular events in order of occurrence are as follows:

- *Transient vasoconstriction* occurs because of neurogenic mechanism, if inflammation has been initiated by a vascular injury.
- *Vasodilation*, mediated by histamine, increases blood flow to the area by opening up new capillary beds leading to erythema (rubor) and warmth (calor).
- *Increased vascular permeability* leads to movement of protein-rich exudate to the extravascular space.
- *Stasis and engorgement* occur because of the increase in viscosity of blood, caused by the fluid movement to extravascular space.
- *Localization of neutrophils* along the vessel wall endothelium occurs to facilitate their movement across the vessel wall into the interstitium.

Increased Vascular Permeability (Fig. 3.4)

This is a very important event in inflammation and so it is essential to study the various mechanisms that lead to this event. It often involves the postcapillary venules and is called the *hallmark of acute inflammation*. The mechanisms that lead to increased permeability may be immediate or delayed, depending on the time taken for the injury or change to occur, and may be transient or prolonged, depending on the time taken for the change to revert or heal. The various mechanisms involved in this process are explained in Table 3.2.

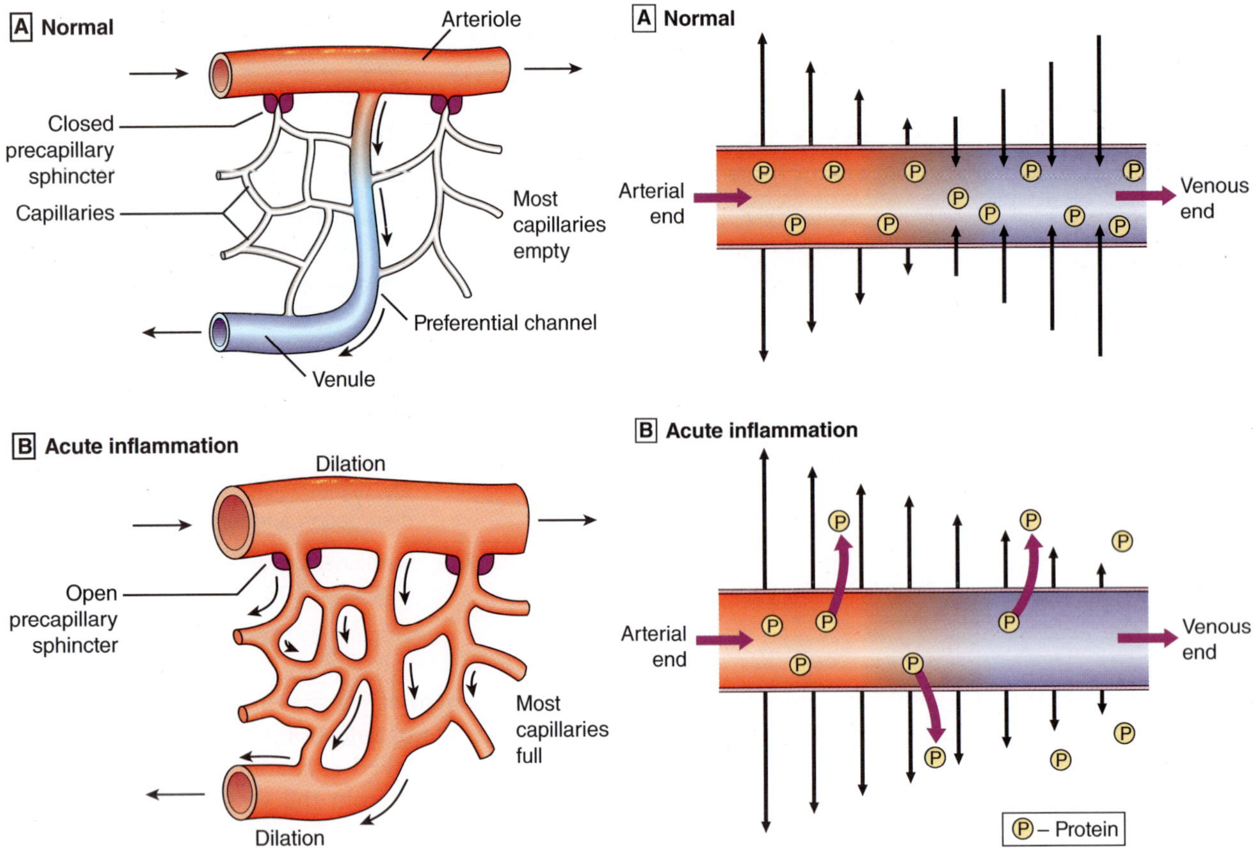

Fig. 3.3 Vascular events in acute inflammation: vasodilation (A) and increased vascular permeability (B). (*Source:* From Timothy J. Stephenson. Inflammation. In Underwood's Pathology. 7th edition. 2019. Elsevier.)

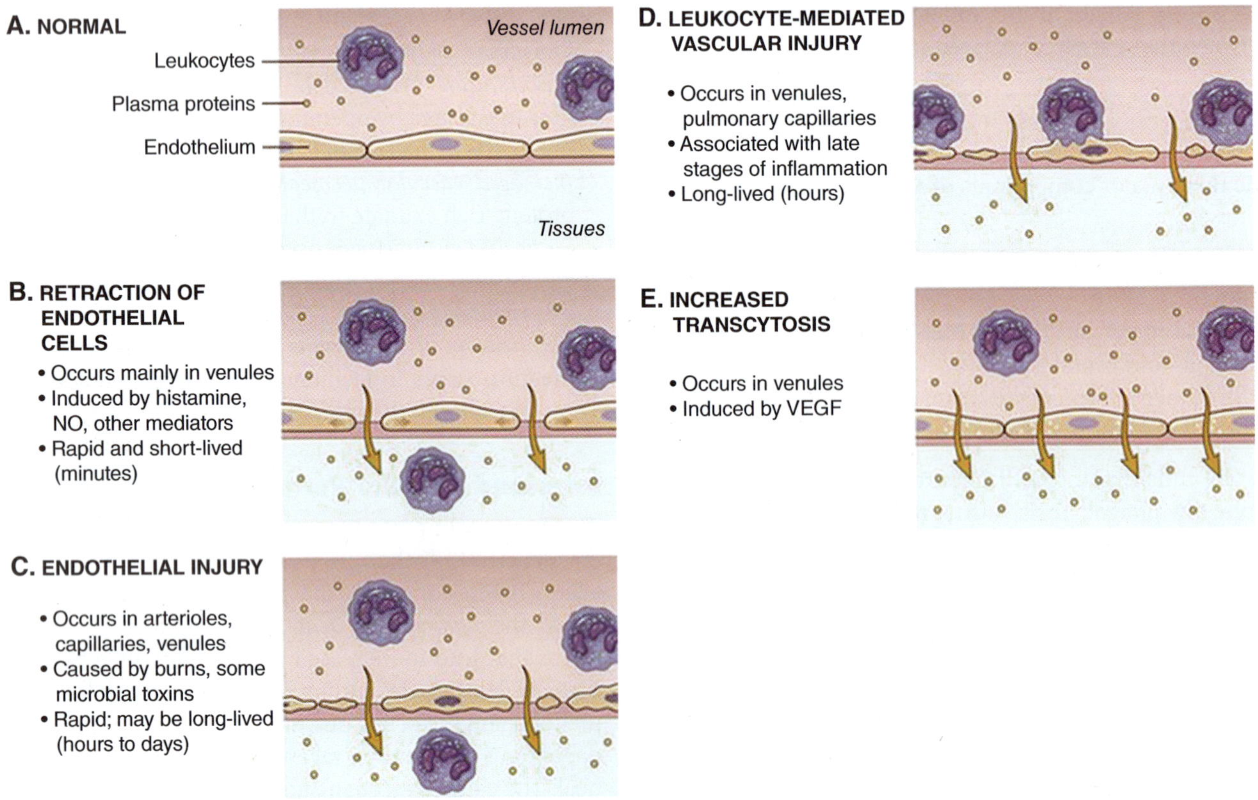

Fig. 3.4 Mechanisms of increased vascular permeability. (*Source:* Robbins 7th edition, Fig. 2.3.)

Table 3.2 Mechanisms of Increased Vascular Permeability

Mechanism	Pathogenesis	Mediator	Type of Response	Example
Contraction of endothelial cells	Increase in interendothelial cell space	Histamine, bradykinin, leukotriene	Immediate transient response	Burns
Retraction of endothelial cells	Reorganization of cytoskeleton	Cytokines, especially IL-1 and TNF	Delayed prolonged response	Late-appearing sunburn
Direct damage of endothelium	Destruction of endothelial cell	Toxins/microbes in circulation	Immediate prolonged response	Snake venom
Cell-mediated damage of endothelium	Destruction of endothelium	Neutrophils that adhere to it	Delayed prolonged response	Late phase of thermal burns
Transcytosis	Movement of fluids and proteins through the endothelial cell	VEGF		Role in inflammation uncertain

IL-1, interleukin-1; TNF, tumour necrosis factor; VEGF, vascular endothelial growth factor.

Response of the Lymphatic System

The lymphatics around the area of inflammation proliferate to help remove the accumulated extravascular oedematous fluid, and take in a lot of inflammatory cells and debris during this process to clean the vicinity. This may lead to secondary inflammation of the lymphatics and the draining lymph nodes, which undergo reactive hyperplasia of the lymphoid follicles. *Lymphangitis* refers to the inflammation of the lymphatic vessels, which may be seen as reddish streaks in the skin adjoining the area of inflammation, and *lymphadenitis* refers to the reactive inflammation of the draining lymph nodes, both of which may cause pain and tenderness. Further discussion about lymph node pathologies is given in Chapter 16.

CELLULAR EVENTS

Movement of leucocytes, especially phagocytic cells, into the interstitium and tissue is very important for removal of the infectious agent and necrotic tissue and for the healing process. On the contrary, these inflammatory cells apart from helping to fight the infection may also cause collateral damage to the surrounding tissues. The entire process is controlled by various chemical mediators, and the ones specific for this movement are the chemokines. The steps are as follows (Fig. 3.5):

1. Within the lumen – margination, rolling and adhesion to the vascular endothelium
2. Migration across the endothelium and vessel wall
3. Outside the lumen – movement in the tissues towards the microbe by chemotaxis
4. Phagocytosis and destruction of the infectious agent

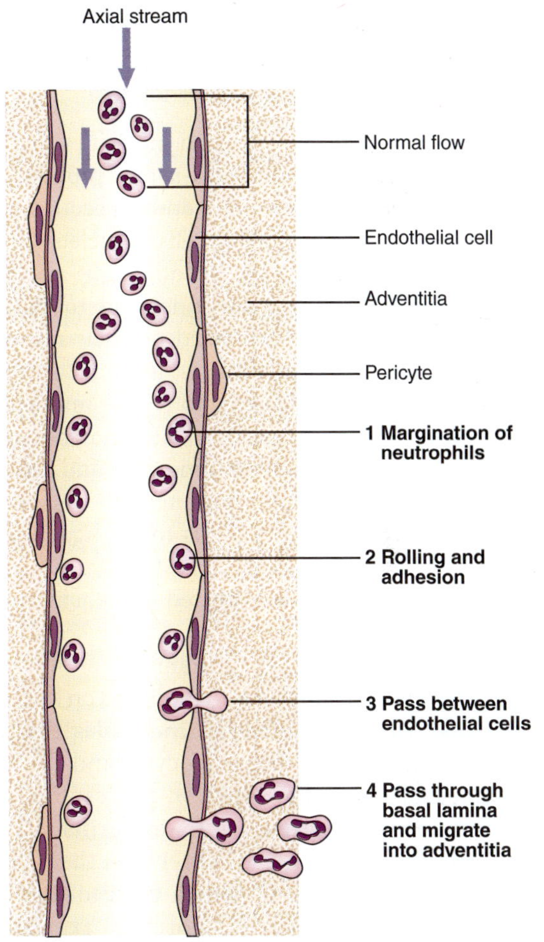

Fig. 3.5 Margination, rolling, adhesion and transmigration. (*Source:* From Timothy J. Stephenson. Inflammation. In Underwood's Pathology 7th edition. 2019. Elsevier.)

Intravascular Events

White blood cells (WBCs) have the tendency, even in normal flowing blood, to occupy a slightly peripheral position than red blood cells (RBCs), which occupy the central axis. Furthermore, during the vascular events, stasis triggers further movement of more leucocytes nearer to the endothelium and this is called **margination**. These cells attach transiently and detach to slow down their flow. This is called **rolling**. In the next step, these cells adhere firmly to the endothelium and stop moving.

Table 3.3 Functions of Adhesion Molecules in Intravascular Cellular Events

Adhesion Molecule	Site	Ligand	Function
E selectin	Endothelium	Sialyl-Lewis ligand (WBC)	Rolling and adhesion
P selectin	Platelets and endothelium	Sialyl-Lewis ligand (WBC)	Rolling
L selectin	WBC	Glycoprotein on endothelium	Rolling
B1 integrin	WBC	VCAM 1	Adhesion
B2 integrin	WBC	ICAM 1	Adhesion and transmigration
Ig PECAM	Endothelium and WBC		Most important for diapedesis

PECAM, platelet endothelial cell adhesion molecule; WBC, white blood cell.

This is called **adhesion**. These processes of rolling and adhesion are mediated by certain adhesion molecules that are expressed on WBCs, platelets and endothelial cells under the influence of cytokines (Table 3.3). The major adhesion molecules are described as follows:

- **Selectins:** These are the adhesion molecules that form low-affinity bonds to facilitate the rolling process. There are three types of selectins, E, P and L selectins, which are expressed on endothelial cells, platelets (also in Weibel–Palade bodies of the endothelium) and leucocytes, respectively. These selectins bind to sialylated oligosaccharide ligands expressed on their responsive cell. Injury to tissue potentiates local macrophages, mast cells and endothelial cells to release interleukin-1 (IL-1), tumour necrosis factor (TNF) and chemokines that act on the selectin-containing cells and redistributes them to the surface for binding to the ligand.
  - **L selectin** on leucocytes binds to the ligand on the endothelium.
  - **E selectin** on cytokine-activated endothelium binds to the ligand on leucocytes.
  - **P selectin** on cytokine-, histamine- or thrombin-activated endothelium binds to the ligand on leucocytes.
- **Integrins:** These are adhesion molecules that form strong bonds between the leucocytes and the endothelium, facilitating the adhesion process. There are two families of integrins, the **β_1 integrins** (VLA-4), which bind to the ligand VCAM-1, and the **β_2 integrins** (LFA-1 and MAC-1), which bind to the ligand ICAM-1. These integrins are normally expressed in low-affinity state on leucocytes, and their ligands on the endothelium are not exposed. Infection- or injury-associated release of IL-1, TNF and chemokines accentuates the expression of the ligands on the endothelium, while transforming the low-affinity integrins into high-affinity ones. This leads to firm adhesion of the leucocytes on the endothelium by reorganizing their cytoskeleton and spreading out on the endothelium.

Migration of Leucocyte Across the Endothelium

Following adhesion to the endothelial surface, the leucocytes migrate outside the vessel wall by moving through the interendothelial space and then piercing through its basement membrane. This process is called **transmigration or diapedesis** (Fig. 3.6). This process is mediated by chemokines by facilitating the expression of the unique adhesion molecule platelet endothelial cell adhesion molecule-1 (PECAM-1), also called CD31. PECAM-1 belongs to the immunoglobulin family and is normally found in the intercellular space of the endothelium. Collagenases secreted by the leucocytes then help in piercing the basement membrane. Once these are outside the vessel, they are guided by the chemokines to reach the target tissue.

Overall, the movement of the leucocytes is greatly influenced by the chemokines and the adhesion molecules activated by them. Deficiency of these adhesion molecules may lead to defective leucocyte migration and an increased risk of infection. It is discussed in detail in Chapter 6.

Chemotaxis (Fig. 3.7)

The migration of leucocytes in tissue along a chemical gradient from the area of a lower concentration to that of a higher concentration of the chemoattractant is called chemotaxis. Chemoattractants may be exogenous or endogenous. The common chemoattractants are given in Table 3.4.

The mechanism of movement is explained in Flowchart 3.2.

The type of inflammatory cells in the infiltrate varies at different points of time. Neutrophils are the first cells to respond and predominate in the initial 6–24 hours. This is because of their large numbers, higher sensitivity to chemokines and firmer attachment to the selectins on the endothelial surface. But they last for only 24–48 hours, after which they undergo apoptosis. The next cells to predominate in the inflammatory site from 24 to 48 hours are the monocytes, because they survive longer and are capable of

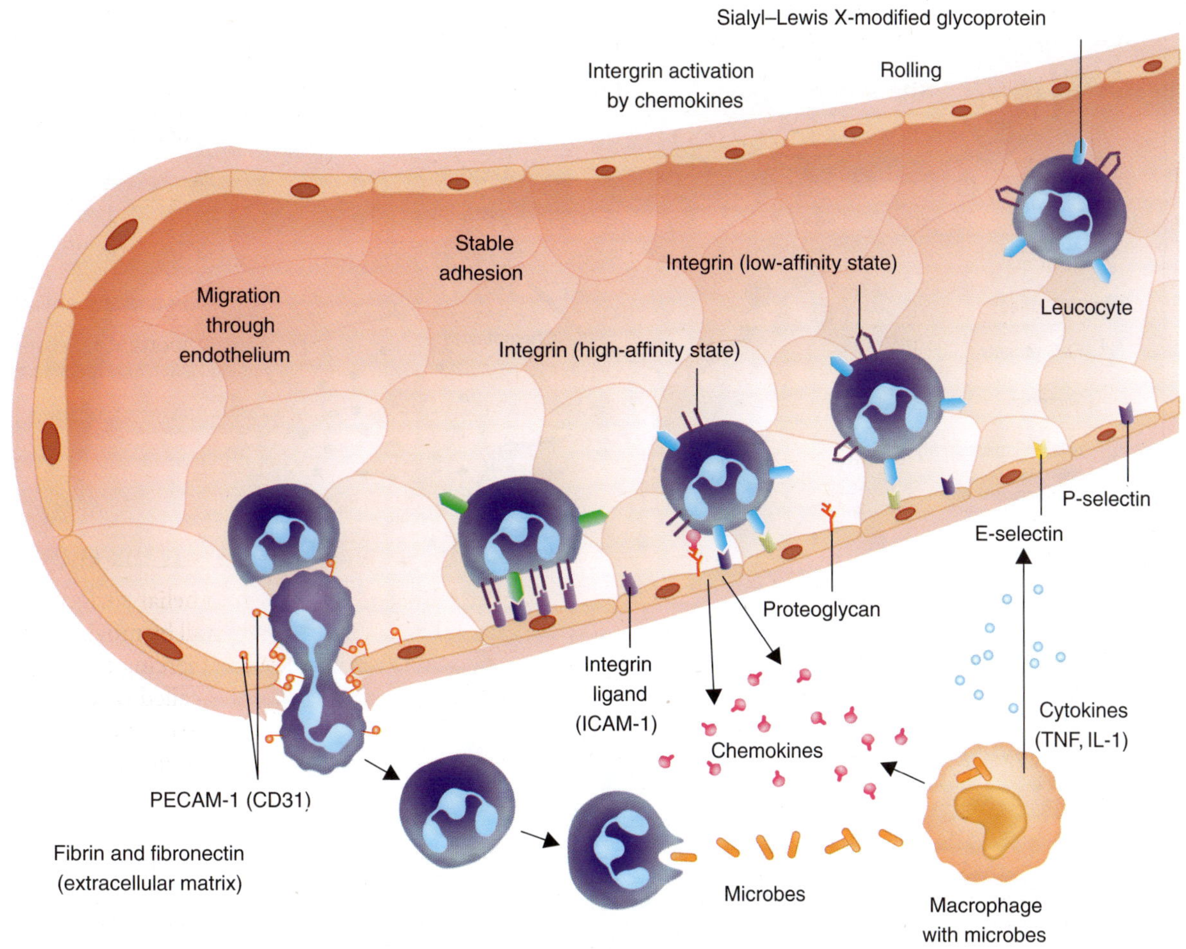

Fig. 3.6 Role of adhesion molecules in leucocyte migration in blood vessels. (*Source:* From Vinay Kumar, Abul K. Abbas and Jon C. Aster. Inflammation and Repair. In Robbins Basic Pathology 10th edition. 2018. Elsevier.)

proliferation in the tissues. There are few exceptions for the aforementioned mechanism:

- Neutrophils predominate for many days in *Pseudomonas* infection.
- Lymphocytes predominate in viral infection.
- Eosinophils predominate in allergic reactions.
- Activated lymphocytes, macrophages and plasma cells predominate in some hypersensitivity reactions.

Phagocytosis

Once the neutrophils reach their site of action, their protective role begins, which is executed in the following three steps:

1) Recognition of the microbe
2) Engulfment of the microbe
3) Killing and degradation of the microbe

Following identification of the microbe, the neutrophil undergoes structural changes with an increase in cytosolic calcium and activation of enzymes (protein kinase C and phospholipase A2), which are collectively called **leucocyte activation**. The migrated neutrophils and the resident macrophages are the major phagocytes, but these differ slightly in their functions (Table 3.5). These work together and help in elimination of the microbe by phagocytosis and killing.

Recognition of microbes: Both leucocytes and macrophages recognize the microbe with the help of receptors present on their surface. The three major receptors are as follows (Fig. 3.8):

- **Mannose receptors** recognize bacterial glycoproteins and glycolipids with the help of terminal mannose and fucose residues that are different from the terminal sialic acid or *N*-acetylgalactosamine present on mammalian glycoproteins and glycolipids.
- **Scavenger receptors** on macrophages bind to bacteria and also to oxidized low-density lipoprotein (LDL) in circulation that are not taken up by the normal hepatic LDL receptors.
- **Opsonization receptors** are high-affinity receptors that recognize and bind to opsonins that coat the microbes. The common opsonins that coat the microbes are IgG immunoglobulin and C3b complement component. The process of opsonins coating the microbe to help the phagocyte identify the target is called opsonization.

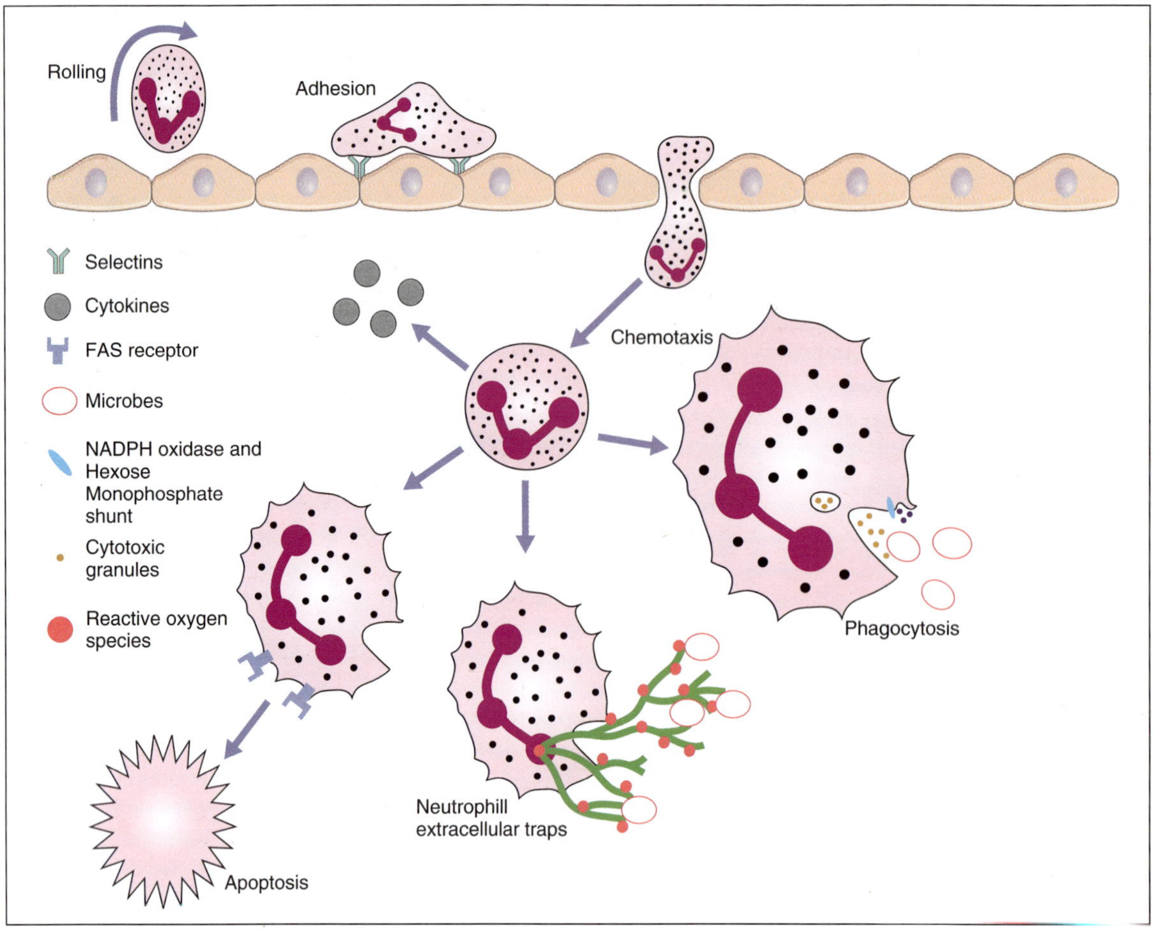

Fig. 3.7 Role of neutrophils after exiting vessels.

Table 3.4 Common Chemoattractants

Exogenous	Endogenous
• Bacterial products • Peptides with *N*-formylmethionine terminal amino acid • Some lipids	• Cytokines, mainly the chemokine group (e.g. IL-8) • Complement products, mainly C5a • Arachidonic acid metabolites, mainly leukotriene B_4

IL-8, interleukin-8.

Engulfment (Fig. 3.9): After the microbe binds to the leucocyte, the leucocyte puts forward pseudopodia on either side that fuse and form a phagosome by pinching off a portion of the cell membrane. This may require cytoskeletal changes and actin polymerization, which are influenced by chemokines that control chemotaxis. The lysosome that is present inside the cell fuses with the phagosome to form the phagolysosome, which is where killing of the microbe takes place.

Killing and degradation

The important factors that help in killing the engulfed bacteria are located in the lysosome and comprise the reactive oxygen species, reactive nitrogen species and lysosomal enzymes (Fig. 3.10). For an easier understanding, the entire reaction can be broken down into the following parts:

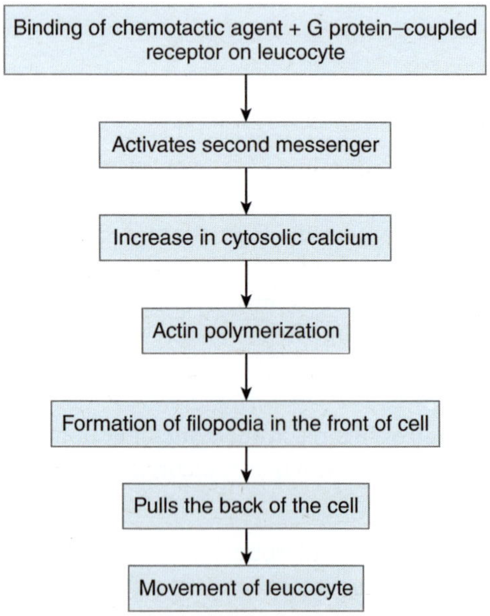

Flowchart 3.2 Mechanism of movement of inflammatory cells.

- **Respiratory burst and formation of superoxide:** The enzyme NADPH oxidase, also called phagocytic

Table 3.5 Differences Between Neutrophils and Macrophages

	Neutrophils	Macrophages
Origin	HSCs in bone marrow	HSCs in bone marrow (in inflammatory reactions) Many tissue-resident macrophages originate from stem cells in yolk sac or fetal liver (early in development)
Life span in tissues	Several days	Inflammatory macrophages: Days or weeks Tissue-resident macrophages: Years
Responses to activating stimuli	Rapid, short-lived, mostly degranulation and enzymatic activity	More prolonged, slower, often dependent on new gene transcription
Reactive oxygen species	Rapidly induced by assembly of phagocyte oxidase (respiratory burst)	Less prominent
Nitric oxide	Low levels or none	Induced following transcriptional activation of iNOS
Degranulation	Major response; induced by cytoskeletal rearrangement	Not prominent
Cytokine production	Low levels or none	Major functional activity; requires transcriptional activation of cytokine genes
NET formation	Rapidly induced, by extrusion of nuclear contents	No
Secretion of lysosomal enzymes	Prominent	Less

HSC, haematopoietic stem cell; iNOS, inducible nitric oxide synthase; NET, neutrophil extracellular trap.
(*Source:* From Vinay Kumar, Abul K. Abbas and Jon C. Aster. Inflammation and Repair. In Robbins Basic Pathology 10th edition. 2018. Elsevier.)

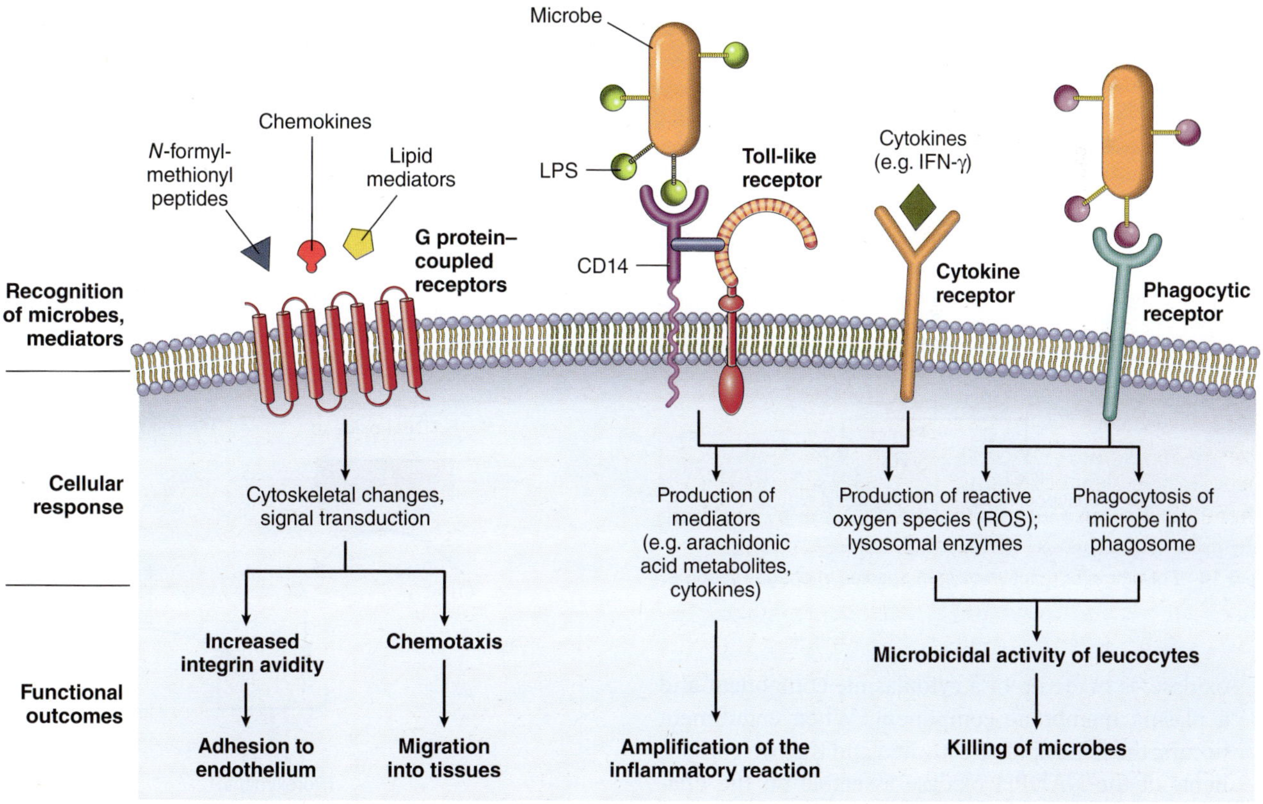

Fig. 3.8 Different types of leucocyte receptors and their stimuli for activation. (*Source:* From Vinay Kumar, Abul K. Abbas and Jon C. Aster. Inflammation and Repair. In Robbins Basic Pathology 10th edition. 2018. Elsevier.)

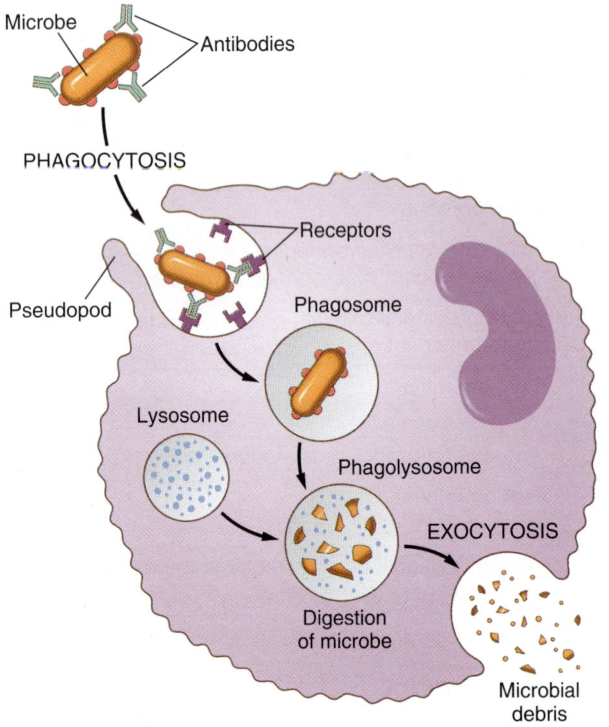

Fig. 3.9 Engulfment and phagolysosome formation. (*Source:* From John E. Hall and Michael E. Hall. Resistance of the Body to Infection: I. Leukocytes, Granulocytes, the Monocyte-Macrophage System, and Inflammation. Guyton and Hall Textbook of Medical Physiology. 14th edition. 2021. Elsevier.)

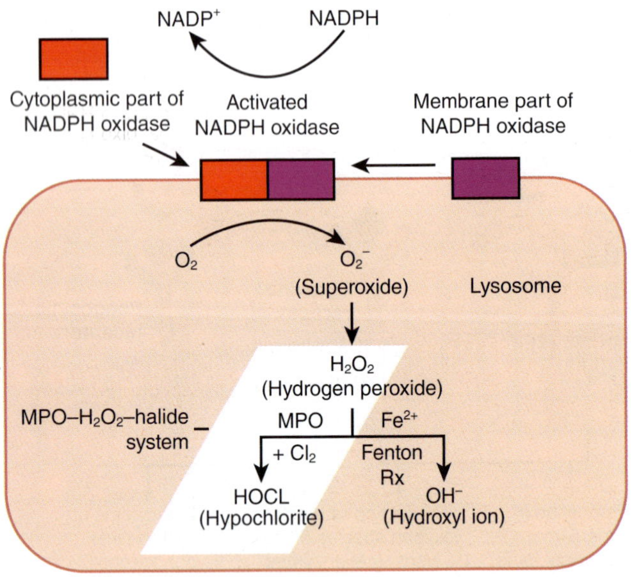

Fig. 3.10 Formation of reactive oxygen species in phagolysosome.

oxidase, is made up of a cytoplasmic component and a plasma membrane component. When engulfment occurs, the neutrophil is activated and the two components of the NADPH oxidase assemble on the phagolysosome membrane and convert O_2 into O_2^- superoxide. This is called respiratory burst; this process occurs only inside the phagolysosome so that the rest of the cell is not damaged.

- **Spontaneous dismutation:** The superoxide thus formed undergoes spontaneous dismutation and gets converted into hydrogen peroxide (H_2O_2; in some places such as the brain, this process is executed by superoxide dismutase). But H_2O_2 is not very efficient and is hence transformed into other compounds.
- **Fenton's reaction:** Some of the H_2O_2 molecules take part in Fenton's reaction in the presence of ferrous ion to form hydroxyl OH^- radical, which is a powerful microbicidal agent.
- **MPO–H_2O_2–halide system:** This is the most powerful antimicrobial system in the neutrophils. *Myeloperoxidase* (MPO) is an enzyme present in the azurophilic granules of the neutrophils. This enzyme in the presence of the halogen chlorine converts H_2O_2 into *hypochlorite,* which destroys the microbes by halogenation or oxidation of proteins and lipids.
- **Formation of reactive nitrogen species** (Fig. 3.11): The inducible nitric oxide synthase (iNOS) enzyme present on the phagolysosome membrane converts the amino acid arginine to nitric oxide (NO) when the neutrophil is activated. Furthermore, NO combines with the superoxide formed during respiratory burst to form peroxynitrite $ONOO^-$, which also has bactericidal properties.
- **Release of lysosomal enzymes:** Monocytes and neutrophils contain lysosomal granules that are discharged into the phagolysosome and help in killing the engulfed microbe. The major enzymes include acid proteases, neutral proteases, defensins, cathelicidins, lysozyme, lactoferrin and major basic protein (found in eosinophils and are cytotoxic to parasites).

Deleterious effect of this stage of phagocytosis is often seen in the tissue surrounding the inflammatory action site because of extracellular release of the reactive oxygen

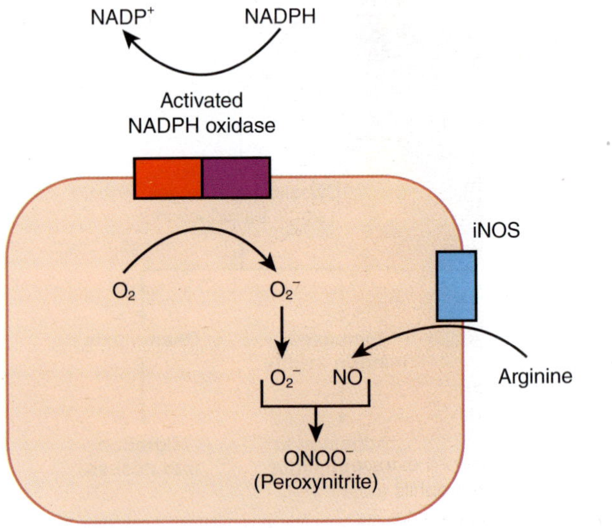

Fig. 3.11 Formation of reactive nitrogen species.

species, nitrogen species and lysosomal enzymes. Hence, as discussed in detail in Chapter 2, our body has many protective mechanisms to counter and prevent the harmful effects of these free radicals. These include:

- *Antioxidant enzymes* such as superoxide dismutase (removes O_2^-), catalase (removes H_2O_2), glutathione peroxidase (removes H_2O_2 and OH^-) and peroxiredoxins (removes HNO_3^-)
- *Serum proteins* such as ceruloplasmin and non-iron-bound transferrin (reduce the availability of metal ions for Fenton's reaction)
- Circulating *antiproteases* such as α_1-antitrypsin and α_2-macroglobulin (inactivate neutrophil proteases)

Neutrophil Extracellular Traps (NETs)

NETs are extracellular meshwork of nuclear chromatin formed by the neutrophil to kill a larger number of microbial agents by trapping them in the mesh and exposing them to a high concentration of microbicidal agents. The neutrophils exhibit this behaviour when they are triggered by infectious pathogens or chemical mediators such as cytokines (interferons and chemokines), complement factors or endogenous danger signals. Formation of NETs called **NETosis** (Fig. 3.12) is beneficial for removal of the pathogen, but when the process is unchecked, it may cause tissue damage and precipitate thrombotic events. NET is composed of *neutrophilic DNA* that gets decondensed and mixed with neutrophilic granular contents such as α-defensins, neutrophil elastase and MPO that have microbicidal properties. The process of NETs leads to the death of neutrophils because of loss of nuclear chromatin and hence it is also called 'beneficial suicide' (Fig. 3.13).

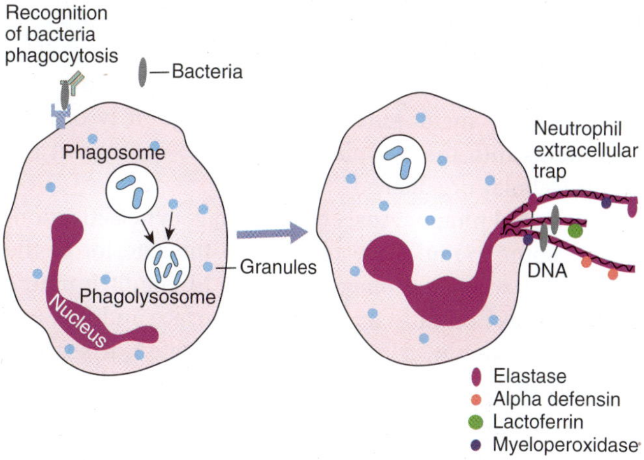

Fig. 3.12 Schematic representation of the NETosis process.

Role of Leucocytes in Tissue Injury

The leucocytes in the process of killing the microbes unintentionally cause damage to the surrounding tissues. This may occur by various mechanisms:

- *Collateral damage* to the surrounding tissues, especially in chronic infections such as tuberculosis
- An *exaggerated response* to certain antigens as in the case of allergy
- *Cross-reactivity* of certain antibodies against host antigens as in autoimmune disorders

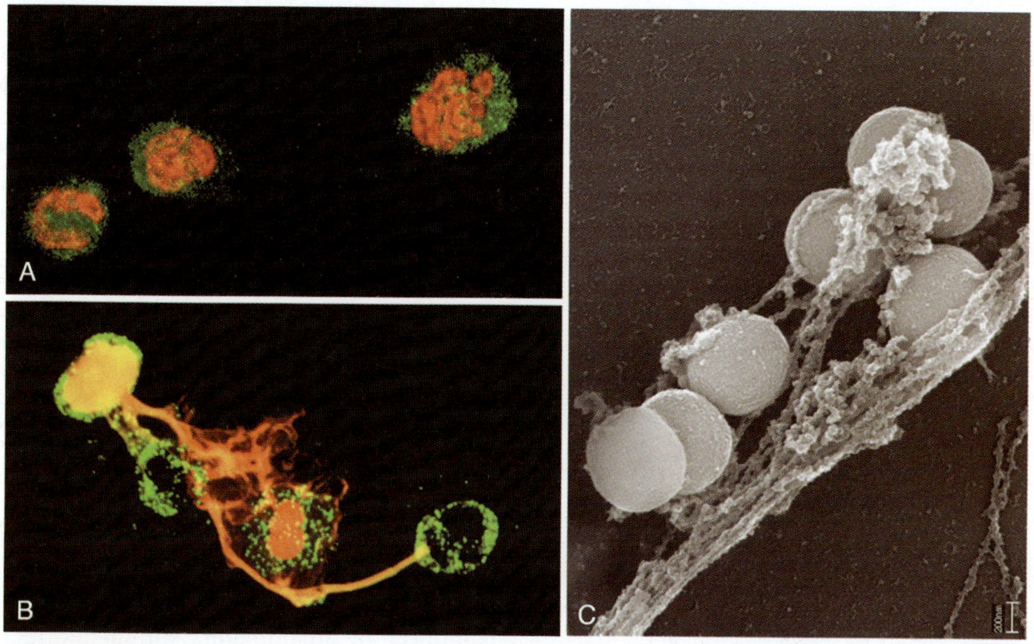

Fig. 3.13 Neutrophil extracellular traps. (A) Healthy neutrophils with nuclei stained red and cytoplasm stained green. (B) Release of nuclear material from neutrophils (note that two have lost their nuclei), forming extracellular traps. (C) Electron micrograph of bacteria (staphylococci) trapped in NETs. (*Source:* From Vinay Kumar, Abul K. Abbas and Jon C. Aster. Inflammation and Repair. In Robbins Basic Pathology 10th edition. 2018. Elsevier.)

- *Damage of the phagolysosome membrane* by the materials ingested in the phagosome such as urate crystals (the crystals may cause physical damage to the phagolysosome membrane, causing leakage of lysosomal contents into the cytoplasm leading to damage of the intracellular organelles)
- **Frustrated phagocytosis** during phagocytic activation, only some granules are released to the exterior of the cell. But when the phagocyte tries to engulf immune complexes bound to an immobile surface and it is unable to ingest it, it gets strongly activated; it secretes plenty of lysosomal contents outside the cell, damaging the tissue in the vicinity.

MEDIATORS OF ACUTE INFLAMMATION PA 4.2

Substances produced by the body to initiate and orchestrate an inflammatory response are called mediators. They control the entire process till the termination of the response. The most important mediators of acute inflammation are vasoactive amines, arachidonic acid (AA) metabolites, cytokines (including chemokines) and complement products (Flowchart 3.3). These are mainly produced by macrophages, dendritic cells and mast cells, but platelets, neutrophils, endothelial cells and most epithelia also contribute to this process. To minimize damage to host tissues, these mediators are released only when they are stimulated; these have a short half-life and are removed quickly from the circulation. But as long as the inflammation is present, these undergo self-amplification by stimulating the synthesis and release of other mediators.

The mediators may be broadly classified into cell-derived mediators and plasma mediators. The cellular mediators originate from the cells involved in the inflammatory process and are released at the site of action by the cell. The mediators may be preformed and present in the lysosomes of the cell or may be synthesized by the cell on activation. On the contrary, plasma mediators are synthesized by the liver and are present in the circulation in an inactive form. They are activated by cleavage and they exhibit their properties only after activation.

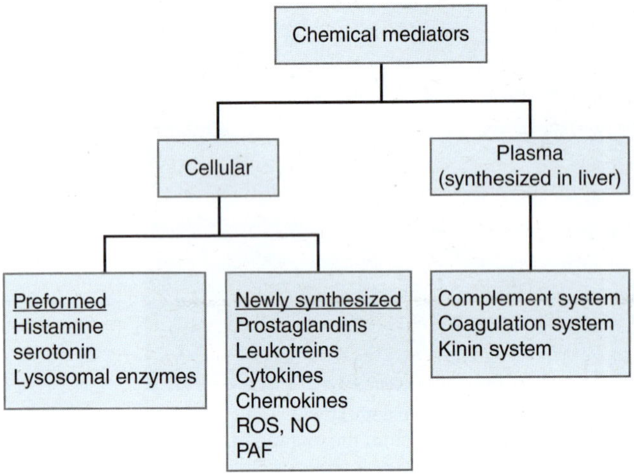

Flowchart 3.3 Classification of chemical mediators.

In the next section, we review the important mediators and their role in inflammation.

Preformed Mediators

Vasoactive Amines Vasoactive amines are the first mediators to be released in inflammation, and these have a significant effect on the blood vessels. They include histamine and serotonin.

Histamine

- Histamine is produced by circulating mast cells (richest source), basophils and platelets.
- Mast cell degranulation may occur because of physical injury such as trauma, because of allergic reaction when antibodies bind to mast cells or because of complement product C3a, C5a action.
- Its actions are exerted on H_1 receptors located in the endothelium of arterioles, capillaries and venules.
- It is the main mediator of the immediate transient phase of increased vascular permeability in the postcapillary venules during acute inflammation.
- It causes vasodilatation, especially of the arterioles.

Serotonin

- Serotonin is present in platelets (dense body granules) and neuroendocrine cells of the gastrointestinal tract (GIT).
- It acts as a neurotransmitter in GIT.
- It has a vasoconstrictor effect on vessels, the role of which in inflammation is not yet ascertained.

Newly Synthesized Cellular Mediators

ARACHIDONIC ACID METABOLITES

These include the lipid mediators, prostaglandin (PG) family and leukotrienes (LTs), which are together called eicosanoids. AA is a 20-carbon polyunsaturated fatty acid that is found within the cell membrane of phospholipids. It may be derived from dietary sources or from the linoleic acid, an essential fatty acid. Increase in cytoplasmic calcium levels activates the enzyme phospholipase A2, which releases AA from the cell membrane and enables it to be acted upon by the two enzymes cyclooxygenases and lipoxygenases.

Cyclooxygenase Pathway AA is acted upon by the enzymes COX-1 and COX-2 to form PGs by the mast cells, macrophages, endothelial cells and many other cell types. COX-1 is constitutively present in many tissues and plays a major role in regulating homeostasis such as mucosal protection in the stomach and maintenance of fluid and electrolyte balance in the kidney. On the contrary, COX-2 is induced by inflammatory stimuli and takes part in inflammation, with not much of a role in normal tissue. There are five important mediators in this family as shown in Flowchart 3.4.

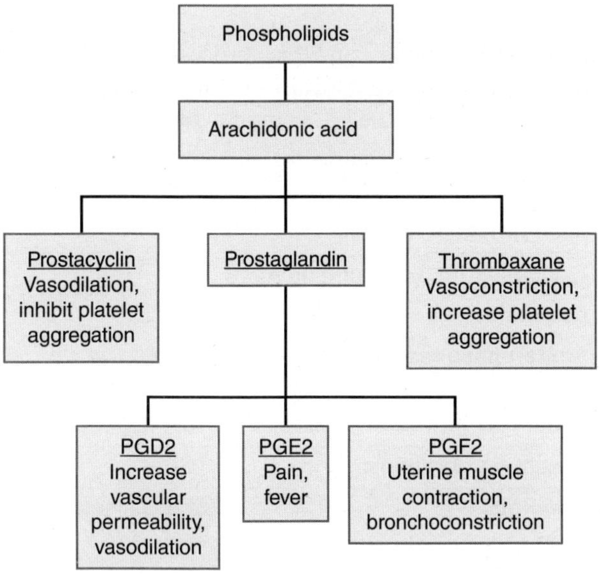

Flowchart 3.4 Cyclooxygenase pathway of arachidonic acid.

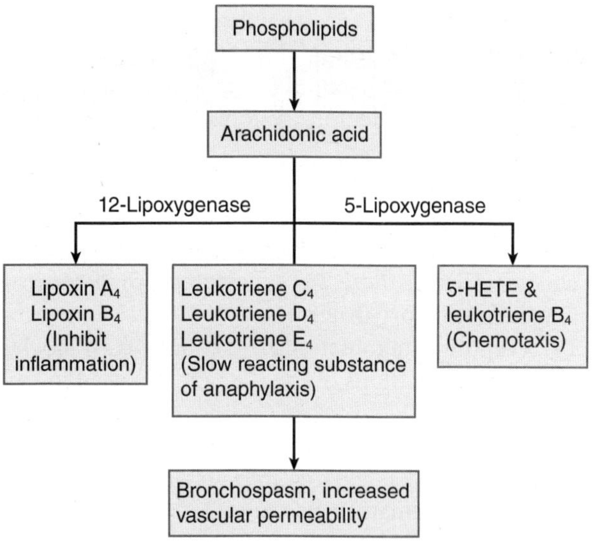

Flowchart 3.5 Lipoxygenase pathway of arachidonic acid.

Prostacyclin (PGI_2)

- Synthesized in the endothelium by the enzyme prostacyclin synthase
- Vasodilator and inhibits platelet aggregation
- Increases vascular permeability and chemotactic effect of other mediators

Thromboxane (TXA_2)

- It is synthesized in platelets by the enzyme thromboxane synthase, which is absent in endothelium.
- It is a vasoconstrictor and increases platelet aggregation.
- Thrombosis of cerebral and coronary vessels may occur if there is an imbalance in prostacyclin and thromboxane synthesis.

Prostaglandin

- PGD_2, PGE_2 and $PGF_2\alpha$ are important PGs, with PGD_2 being the most important one.
- PGD_2 is a chemoattractant for neutrophils.
- PGD_2 and PGE_2 cause vasodilation and an increase in vascular permeability of postcapillary venules.
- $PGF_{2\alpha}$ causes the contraction of uterine and bronchial smooth muscles.
- PGE_2 is responsible for pain and fever during an inflammatory reaction.

Lipoxygenase Pathway This pathway results in the formation of LTs and lipoxins (LXs) (Flowchart 3.5).

LTs: These are formed by lipoxygenase synthase in mast cells and leucocytes. The major LTs are LTB_4, LTC_4, LTD_4 and LTE_4.

- LTB_4 is a powerful chemotactic agent for neutrophils.
- LTC_4, LTD_4 and LTE_4 are important mediators of asthma and are called slow-reacting substance of anaphylaxis (SRS-A). These cause more severe bronchospasm and increased vascular permeability than histamine, but they cause vasoconstriction (histamine is a vasodilator).

LXs: LXA_4 and LXB_4 are produced by platelets, using the intermediate formed by neutrophils. Hence, these require neutrophils and platelets for their synthesis. These mediators are formed at the end of the inflammatory process and help in halting the inflammatory process. By nature, these are anti-inflammatory and inhibit neutrophil chemotaxis.

Transcellular Biosynthesis of Eicosanoids Transcellular biosynthesis is a newly identified mechanism that explains the production of eicosanoids by cells not containing the cyclooxygenase and lipoxygenase enzymes. This requires a donor cell that synthesizes and releases a component of the biosynthetic cascade and an accessory cell that takes up that intermediate and processes it into the final biologically active product using secondary enzymes such as PG isomerases, LTA_4 hydrolases or LTC_4 synthases.

Inhibitors of Eicosanoid Synthesis

- **Cyclooxygenase inhibitors:** There are nonselective inhibitors such as aspirin and nonsteroidal anti-inflammatory drugs (NSAIDs) that inhibit COX-1 and COX-2 or selective COX-2 inhibitors that inhibit COX-2, 200- to 300-fold compared with COX-1. The selective inhibitors were thought to be superior because they suppressed inflammation-associated PG synthesis without primarily affecting homeostasis-associated PGs. But these did not prove very useful, because COX-2 was found to contribute to homeostasis also. Most importantly, these drugs suppressed vasodilator PGI_2 (produced by endothelium) without inhibiting COX-1-associated thromboxane synthesis (in platelets), leading to an unopposed platelet aggregation and vasoconstriction by thromboxane. This increased the risk of cerebral and coronary thrombosis, which led to withdrawal of the drug.

- **Lipoxygenase inhibitors:** Drugs that inhibit LT production such as zileuton are found to be useful in the treatment of asthma.
- **Corticosteroids** inhibit COX 2, phospholipase A2, proinflammatory cytokines such as IL-1 and TNF, and iNOS, the function of which is discussed later in this chapter. Hence, these are considered broad-spectrum anti-inflammatory drugs.
- **LT receptor antagonists** such as montelukast block LT receptors and actions of the LTs, and are used in treating asthma.
- **Fish oil in diet:** Fish oil provides substrates that are more preferably converted into anti-inflammatory lipids than inflammatory eicosanoids.

CYTOKINES

These are proteins produced by many cells that act primarily on immune and inflammatory cells, thereby controlling their role in the process. Some cytokines have unique roles and are listed in Table 3.6.

Let us now review the functions of important cytokines.

Interleukin-1 and Tumour Necrosis Factor IL-1 and TNF are produced in the body in response to inflammatory stimuli such as microbes, foreign bodies, immune complexes or injury. IL-1 is produced by macrophages, dendritic cells and few epithelial/endothelial cells, whereas TNF is produced by macrophages, mast cells and T lymphocytes. These together play an important role in local and systemic effects of inflammation (Fig. 3.14):

- **Endothelial activation:** Upregulation of adhesion molecules and ligands, switching of the endothelium into a

Table 3.6 Common Functions of Cytokines

Proinflammatory cytokines	IL-1, TNF, IFN-γ, chemokines, IL-12
Anti-inflammatory cytokines	TGF-β, IL-10, IL-13, IL-4
Macrophage activation	IFN-γ
Systemic effects of inflammation	IL-1, TNF
Cachexia	TNF, IL-1
Acute-phase response protein production	IL-6, IL-1
Major role in wound healing	TGF-β,
Maximum fibrogenic	TGF-β,
Chemotaxis	Chemokines, IL-17 (neutrophils)

IFN-γ, interferon-γ; IL, interleukin; TGF-β, transforming growth factor-β; TNF, tumour necrosis factor.

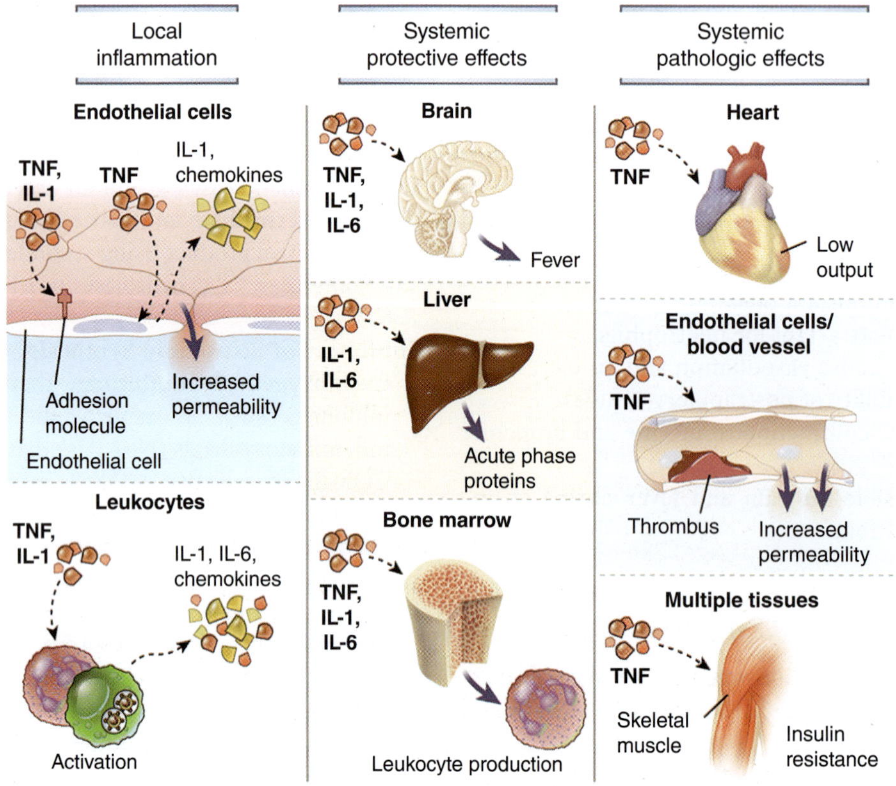

Fig. 3.14 Local and systemic actions of cytokines. (*Source:* From Abul K. Abbas, Andrew H. Lichtman and Shiv Pillai. Innate Immunity. Cellular and Molecular Immunology. 9th edition. 2018. Elsevier.)

procoagulant state from an anticoagulant state and promoting release of other cytokines and other mediators from the endothelium

- **WBC activation:** Increases responsiveness of neutrophils to stimuli, increases microbicidal potential of macrophages and IL-1 also stimulates T Helper 17 cell response
- **Systemic effects of inflammation:** Cause systemic acute-phase responses such as fever, sepsis, leucocytosis, anorexia and fatigue with TNF playing a specific role in causing cachexia by inducing catabolism; in addition, production of acute-phase proteins such as C-reactive protein (CRP) influenced by IL-6 and IL-1
- **Cardiac effects:** Reduce cardiac contractile function leading to reduction in cardiac output
- **Increases insulin resistance** in peripheral tissues

Knowledge about the functions of cytokines has prompted us to try TNF antagonists in the treatment of inflammatory disorders such as rheumatoid arthritis. They have also been tested in the treatment of coronavirus, with promising results. Such patients were found to have an increased risk of mycobacterial infection because of reduced macrophage function.

Chemokines Chemokines are small proteins whose major role is chemotaxis. On the basis of their function, these are classified into homeostatic chemokines, which help in the organization of T and B lymphocytes in their anatomic distribution, and inflammatory cytokines, which play an important role in chemotaxis during inflammation. The two important cytokines that need special mention are CXCR4 and CCR5, which are essential for the attachment of HIV on CD4-positive cells.

On the basis of the cysteine residue arrangement, chemokines may be classified as given in Table 3.7.

NITRIC OXIDE

It is produced by neurons, macrophages and endothelial cells from the amino acid, L-arginine, by the action of the enzyme nitric oxide synthase (NOS). NOS may be one of the following subtypes: nNOS (found in neurons), eNOS (found in endothelium) and iNOS (induced by IL-1, TNF, interferon-γ [IFN-γ] and bacterial endotoxins). Its functions are as follows:

- Neurotransmitter in neurons
- Vasodilation, inhibition of platelet adhesion, aggregation and degranulation, inhibition of WBC adhesion and recruitment in the endothelium
- Microbicidal in inflammatory cells

PLATELET-ACTIVATING FACTOR

It is produced from phospholipids in platelets, mast cells, basophils, macrophages, neutrophils and endothelial cells. Platelet-activating factor causes platelet aggregation, vasoconstriction and bronchoconstriction. However, at low concentration, it has a different effect on the blood vessel, which includes vasodilation and increased vascular permeability.

Plasma-Derived Mediators

Complement System It is a system of about 20 proteins produced by the liver that help in host defence and inflammatory reactions in the body. Their activation leads to release of various cleavage products that serve different roles in inflammation. Once the complement system is activated by the cleavage of C3, it leads to a cascade of activation of enzymes resulting in amplification of the complement activation process (Fig. 3.15). Hence, C3 activation is the critical step in the complement activation and C3 convertase may be formed by any one of the following three pathways:

- **Classical pathway:** Triggered by IgG and IgM antibody that is bound to an antigen
- **Alternative pathway:** Triggered by IgA but can be activated by microbes or cobra venom directly without any antibody
- **Lectin pathway:** Triggered by mannose-binding lectin on the microbe

C3 convertase formed in the classical and alternate pathway is different (C3bBb in the alternative pathway or C4bC2b in the classical and lectin pathways). Irrespective of its composition, it breaks down C3 and releases C3a. The remaining C3b on the cell acts as C5 convertase to cleave C5 into C5a and C5b. C5a is released and C5b

Table 3.7 Classification of Chemokines

Type of Chemokine	CXC Chemokines (αCK)	C-C Chemokines (βCK)	C Chemokines (γCK)	CXC3 Chemokines
Chemotactic on	Neutrophils – mainly induced by microbial products	All WBCs, with not much effect on neutrophils	Lymphocytes	Monocytes and T cells
Examples	IL-8	MCP-1 (monocytes) RANTES Eotaxin (eosinophils)	Lymphotactin	Fractalkaline

IL-8, interleukin-8; MCP-1, monocyte chemoattractant protein 1; WBC, white blood cell.

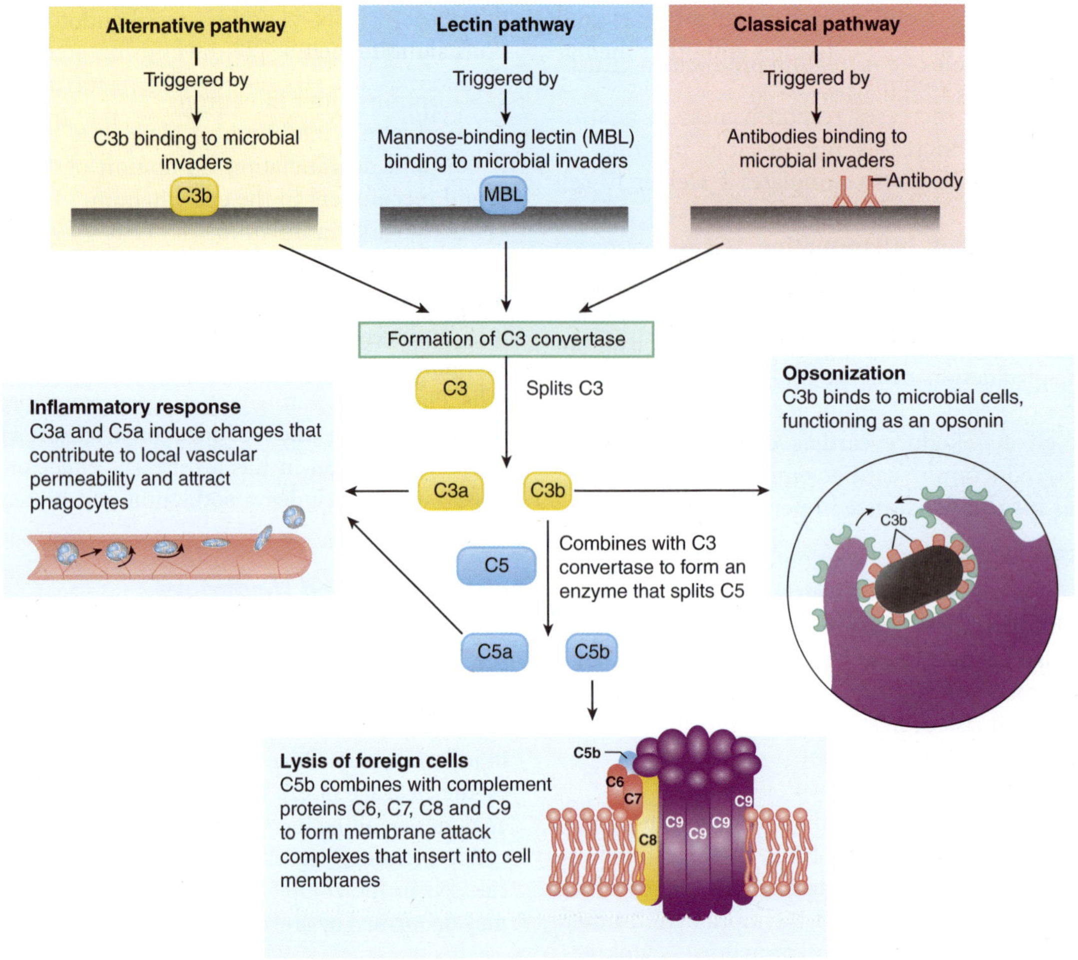

Fig. 3.15 Complement cascade.

combines with the downstream complement components to form the membrane attack complex C5b-9.

The important functions of the complement system components are moderating chemotaxis and anaphylaxis in inflammation, opsonization of microbes for phagocytosis and killing of cells and capsulated microbes such as *Neisseria*. The components for each of these functions are given in Table 3.8.

The complement system also has many regulators in the body to prevent excessive activation and damage of tissues. Damage in autoimmune diseases occurs because of overwhelming of this system beyond its capacity. The main regulators are as follows:

- C1 inhibitor inhibits C1, which is the first protein that activates C3. Deficiency of this inhibitor leads to hereditary angio-oedema.
- CD55 and CD59 bound to the plasma membrane of cells. CD55 (decay-accelerating factor) prevents C3 convertase formation, whereas CD59 (membrane inhibitor of reactive lysis) prevents membrane attack complex formation. Deficiency of these proteins causes paroxysmal nocturnal haemoglobinuria. The disorders associated with complement inhibitor deficiencies are discussed in Chapter 6.

Table 3.8 Functions of Complement Components

Complement Component	Function
C3a, C5a	Anaphylatoxins – release histamine from mast cells and cause vasodilation and increased vascular permeability
C5a	Chemotactic for neutrophil Activates lipoxygenase pathway of AA
C3b	Opsonin that coats microbes and cells for phagocytosis
C5b-9 Membrane attack complex	Causes cell lysis by increasing cell membrane permeability Kills bacteria with thin cell wall such as *Neisseria*

AA, arachidonic acid.

Coagulation System The process of coagulation and inflammation is interlinked at various points and may potentiate the effect of each other. Inflammation activates the endothelium, which turns it into procoagulant state from anticoagulant state, and the protease-activated receptors (PARs), which are activated by thrombin and are found on platelets and leucocytes (discussed in detail in Chapter 4). But the role of coagulation products in initiating inflammation is still not ascertained.

Kinin System Kininogens are the precursor of kinins, which are produced by the action of kallikreins. The most important kinin produced by this mechanism is *bradykinin,* which causes dilation and increased permeability of blood vessels, smooth muscle contraction and pain on injection into the skin. It has a short half-life because of rapid inactivation by the enzyme kininase. It plays a role in anaphylaxis.

Thus, the various cellular and plasma mediators play their role in a very well-orchestrated symphony to eliminate the infectious organism and protect the body (Flowchart 3.6). Although some may have opposite roles, their purpose is to control the infectious agent and to reduce collateral damage to the surrounding tissues.

TERMINATION OF ACUTE INFLAMMATION

The process of termination of an episode of acute inflammation is very much essential to avoid damage to the host tissue. The beneficial effects of inflammation turn into deleterious effects if these are not terminated at the right moment. This occurs usually on removal of the inciting agent because of various control mechanisms which include the following:

- Presence of stimuli is required for the release of mediators that occurs only in bursts.
- Mediators are broken down very quickly and have a short half-life.
- Neutrophils, the key cells of acute inflammation, have a short life span and are removed by apoptosis.
- The AA metabolite pathway changes from LT production to LX production.
- Elimination of inciting agents stimulates production of anti-inflammatory cytokines such as transforming growth factor-β (TGF-β) and IL-10.
- Neural impulses reduce production of TNF by macrophages.

MORPHOLOGICAL PATTERNS OF ACUTE INFLAMMATION

Acute inflammation is associated with dilated blood vessels and the presence of fluid and leucocytes (exudate) in the extravascular space. The identification of pattern of inflammation may help in identifying the aetiology. The patterns of acute inflammation include the following:

Serous inflammation

This is commonly seen in body cavities and is characterized by the presence of clear fluid in these spaces and also in cavities created by tissue destruction. The fluid is a plasma derivative or secreted by mesothelial cells and is sterile with low leucocyte content. Examples include pleural effusion, pericardial effusion, ascites (these may also occur in noninflammatory conditions in which the fluid is called transudate; refer Chapter 4 for further details) and burn blisters (Fig. 3.16).

Fibrinous inflammation

Exudate is a protein-rich fluid seen in acute inflammation. When there is an increase in permeability, fibrin along with other smaller proteins leaks into the extravascular space, especially the body cavities. The leaked fibrin forms a meshwork of threads or an amorphous coagulum in these spaces that may be dissolved by fibrinolysis and removed by macrophages. Failure to degrade the fibrin may lead to ingrowth of blood vessels and scarring. This organization of fibrous tissue in pleural or pericardial space may lead to obliteration of the space with long-term consequences (Fig. 3.17).

Purulent (suppurative) inflammation

Neutrophils, necrotic cell debris and oedematous fluid together constitute pus, which is produced in purulent inflammation. The most common cause of this type of inflammation is pyogenic bacteria staphylococci, which cause liquefactive necrosis in tissues leading to pus formation. This localized collection of pus in tissues, organs or confined space is called *abscess,* which is surrounded by neutrophils. This may later get encircled by vascular dilation and fibroblastic proliferation, as in chronic inflammation (Fig. 3.18). With repair, the abscess gets walled off by connective tissue.

Ulcers (Fig. 3.19)

Sloughing off of the necrotic tissue on the surface of the organ or tissue leads to a defect in the continuity of the tissue and is called an ulcer. Ulcers may be seen on the skin and mucosa of the mouth, GIT or genitourinary tract. Common causes include ischaemia of the skin and subcutaneous tissues of lower extremities and peptic ulcers. The type of inflammatory cells depends on the type of inflammation: neutrophils in acute and mononuclear cells (lymphocytes, macrophages and plasma cells) in chronic inflammation.

OUTCOMES OF ACUTE INFLAMMATION

The outcome of an acute inflammation depends on the nature of injury, severity, the tissue affected and the host's ability to respond to the injury. The outcome is usually one of the following:

- **Complete resolution:** When the injury is limited and the amount of tissue destruction is minimal, regeneration of damaged cells helps in complete resolution. The inflamed region returns back to the normal preinjured histology and function.
- **Healing with scarring or fibrosis:** When there is a significant amount of tissue destruction because of inflammation, the tissue involved cannot regenerate.

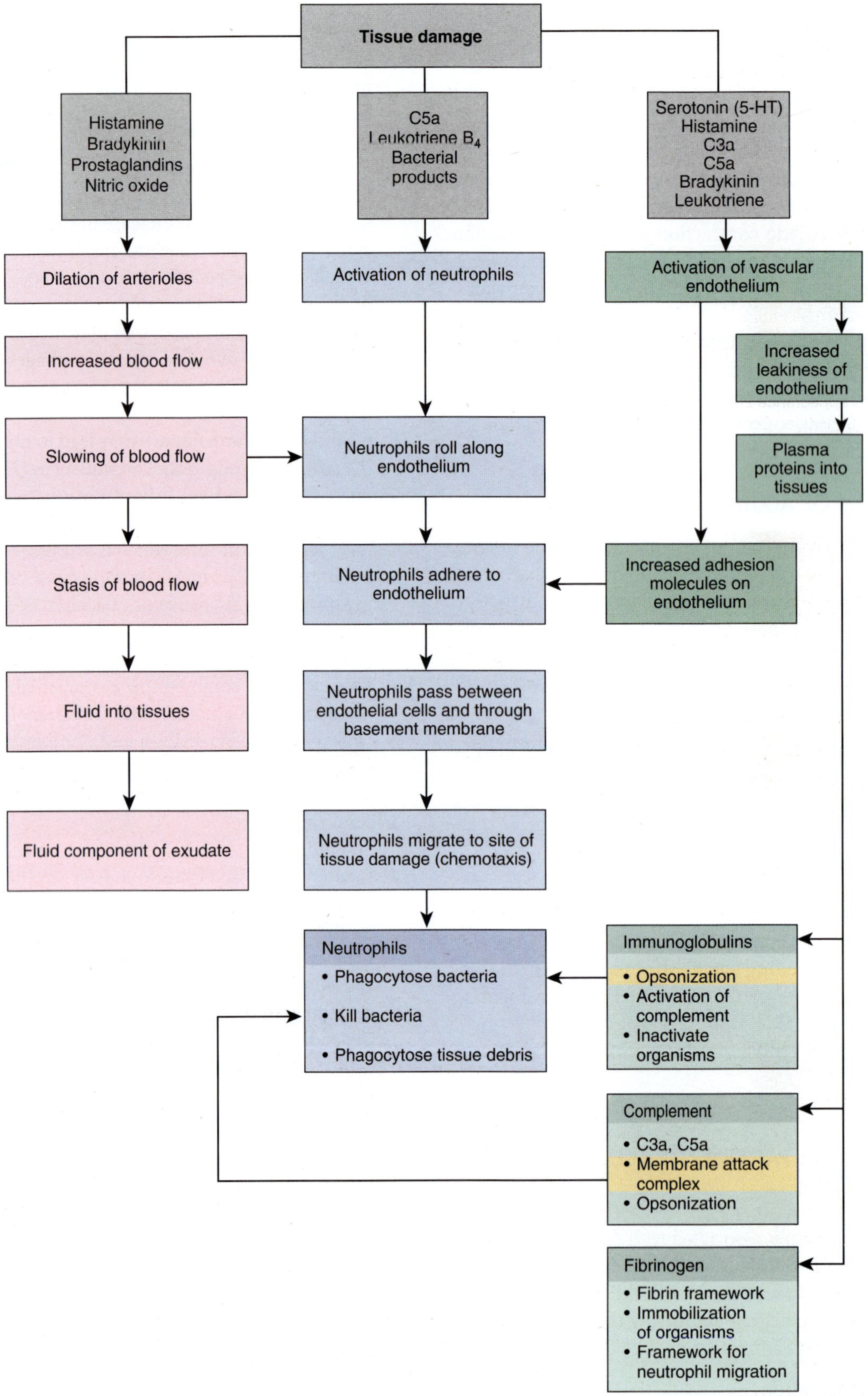

Flowchart 3.6 Role of mediators in the acute inflammatory process – a bird's eye view. (*Source:* From Geraldine O'Dowd, Sarah Bell and Sylvia Wright. Acute inflammation, healing and repair. Wheater's Pathology: A Text, Atlas, and Review of Histopathology. 6th edition. 2020. Elsevier.)

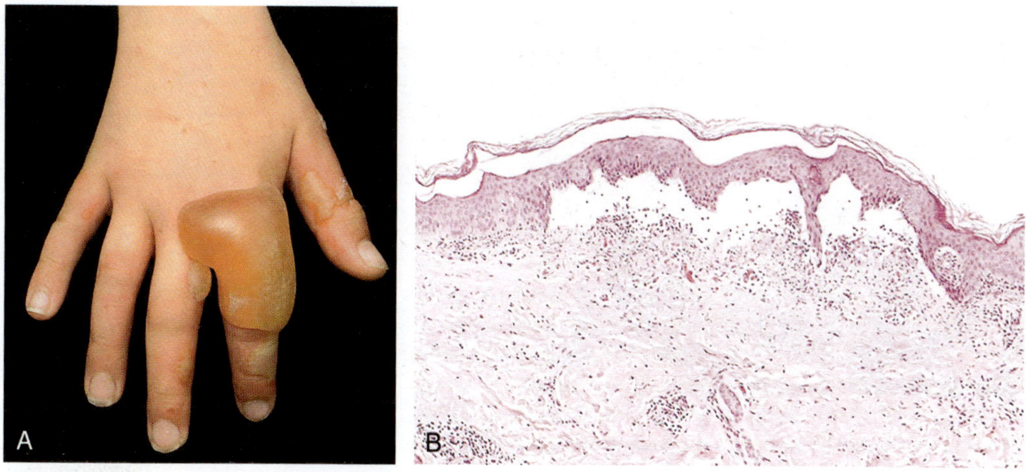

Fig. 3.16 Gross appearance and microscopy of serous inflammation – burn blister. (*Source:* From Mirren Ramniklal Mandalia, Richard Chalmers and Frederick B. Schreuder. Contact with fig tree sap: An unusual cause of burn injury. 2007. Burns; 34:5. 719-721.)

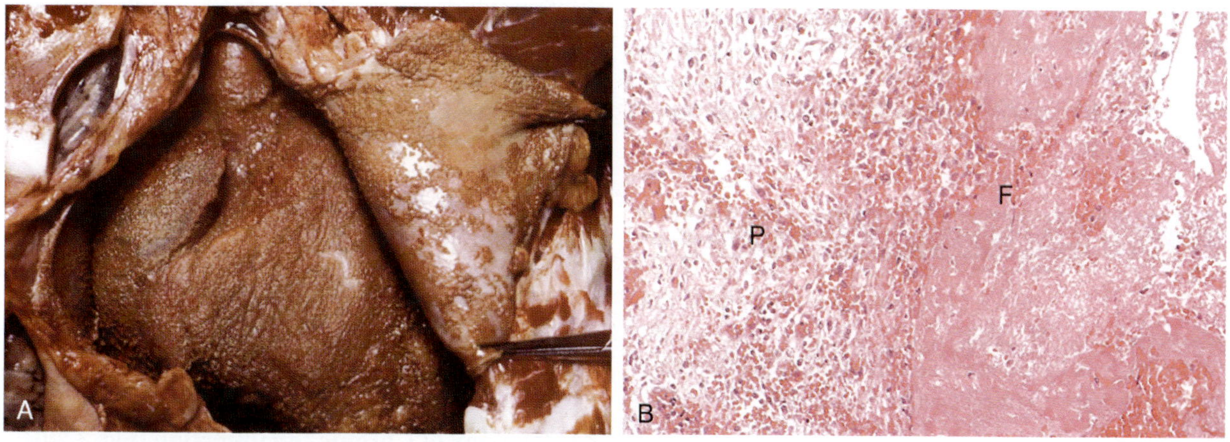

Fig. 3.17 Fibrinous pericarditis, gross. (A) Deposits of fibrin on the pericardium. Microscopy (B) shows a pink meshwork of fibrin exudate (F) overlying the pericardial surface (P). (*Source:* From Vinay Kumar, Abul K. Abbas and Jon C. Aster. Inflammation and Repair. In Robbins Basic Pathology 10th edition. 2018. Elsevier.)

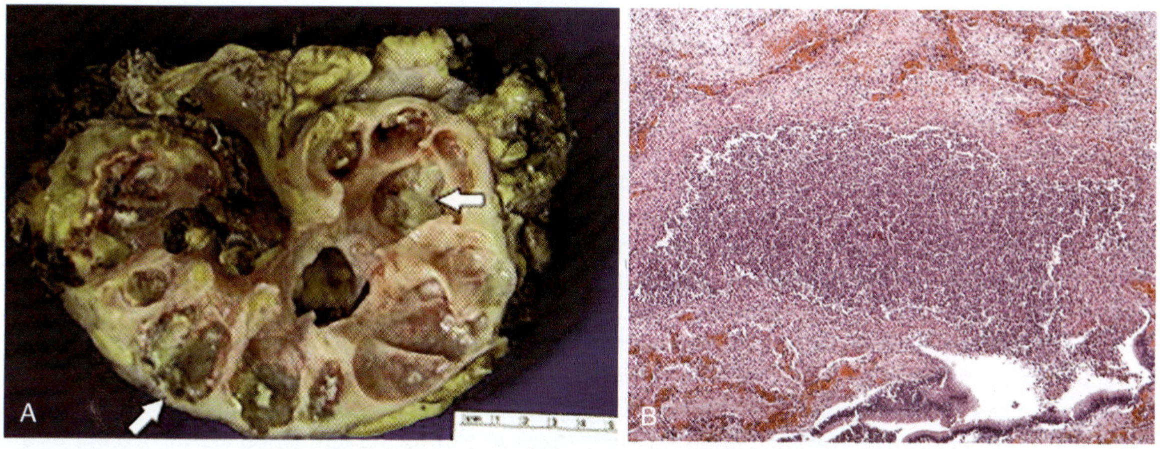

Fig. 3.18 Gross appearance of (A) multiple abscesses (arrows) in the kidney in a case of xanthogranulomatous pyelonephritis. Microscopy (B) shows an abscess wall containing neutrophils and cellular debris and is surrounded by congested blood vessels. (*Source:* (A) From I. Stoica, F. O'Kelly, M.B. McDermott and F.M.J. Quinn. Xanthogranulomatous pyelonephritis in a paediatric cohort (1963–2016): Outcomes from a large single-center series. Journal of Pediatric Urology. 2018. 14; 169.e1-169.e7. (B) From Xanthogranulomatous Pyelonephritis. In Ming Zhou, George J. Netto and Jonathan I. Epstein. High-Yield Uropathology. 2012. Saunders.)

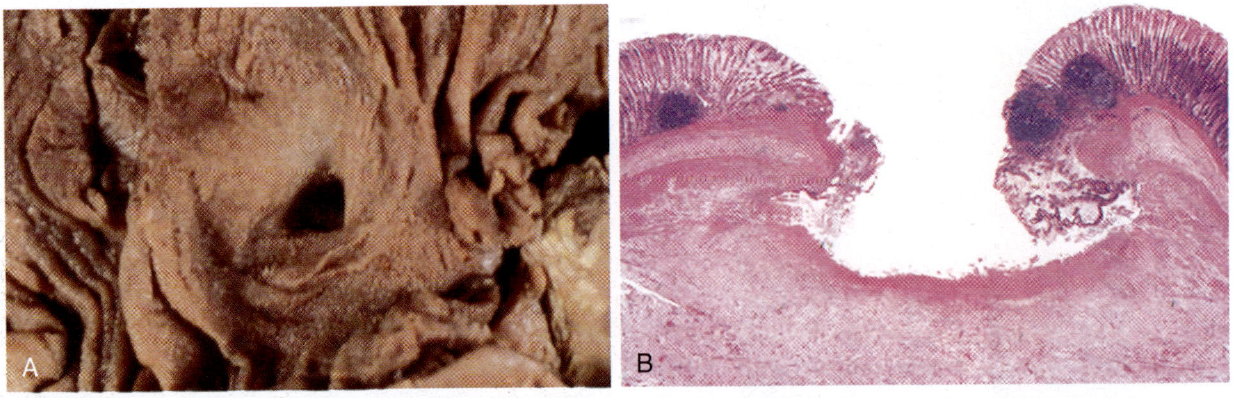

Fig. 3.19 The gross appearance of an ulcer. (A) A chronic duodenal ulcer. (B) Low-power cross-section view of a duodenal ulcer crater with an acute inflammatory exudate in the base. (*Source:* From Vinay Kumar, Abul Abbas, Jon Aster. Robbins & Cotran Pathologic Basis of Disease. 10th Edition. Elsevier. 2020.)

In serous cavities, there is an excess fibrin leakage into the cavity that gets organized and there is an overgrowth of connective tissue leading to scarring.

- **Evolution into chronic inflammation** (discussed later): When the injurious stimuli persist or the healing process is interrupted, acute inflammation progresses to chronic inflammation.

CHRONIC INFLAMMATION PA 4.3

Inflammation that lasts for a long duration of about weeks or months along with tissue injury and repair occurring simultaneously is called chronic inflammation. It may be a sequela of acute inflammation or may arise de nova.

AETIOLOGY OF CHRONIC INFLAMMATION

Background aetiological conditions for chronic inflammation are as follows:

- **Infection** with microorganisms that are persistent for a long duration and difficult to eradicate leads to a delayed type of hypersensitivity reaction. Examples include mycobacteria; some viral, fungal and parasitic infections; and acute bacterial infections of the lung that evolve into chronic lung abscess.
- **Hypersensitivity diseases:** These are a group of disorders that cause inflammatory response in the body because of excessive or inappropriate activation of the immune system. These include inadvertent activation of the immune system against the body's own antigen (autoimmune diseases), excessive unprecedented immune response against microbes in the intestine (inflammatory bowel disease) or an exaggerated immune response against common environmental allergens (allergic response). In all these conditions, the immune reaction occurs in an unwanted scenario, so there is damage to the host tissue. The conditions mostly exhibit a combination of acute and chronic inflammation leading to fibrosis in later stages.
- Sustained exposure to endogenous or exogenous potentially **toxic agents:** Exposure to silica, asbestos and other kinds of exogenous toxic agents may trigger chronic inflammation because of their nondegradable nature, which makes them remain in the body for a prolonged period of time. Similarly, endogenously produced cholesterol and lipids may trigger a chronic inflammation in the vessel wall because of their deposition in these abnormal loci, and lead to conditions such as atherosclerosis.
- Chronic inflammation has been implicated in the pathogenesis of certain other disorders such as Alzheimer disease, metabolic syndrome and the associated type 2 diabetes, and also in certain cancers.

Morphology of Chronic Inflammation (Fig. 3.20)

The presence of *granulation tissue* is the hallmark of chronic inflammation. The tissue appears pink and granular on gross examination. Microscopically, it is composed of the following:

- Mononuclear inflammatory cells such as macrophages, lymphocytes and plasma cells
- Tissue destruction, because of the continued presence of the inciting agent or the inflammatory cells
- Evidence of healing demonstrated by the presence of angiogenesis and fibrosis that represent connective tissue replacement in place of the damaged tissues

CELLS AND MEDIATORS OF CHRONIC INFLAMMATION

The tissue destruction and simultaneous healing that occurs in chronic inflammation are carried out by a cocktail of cells, such as macrophages, lymphocytes and plasma cells with a minor contribution from eosinophils, mast cells, neutrophils and their associated mediators. However, the cells that dominate the picture in chronic inflammation

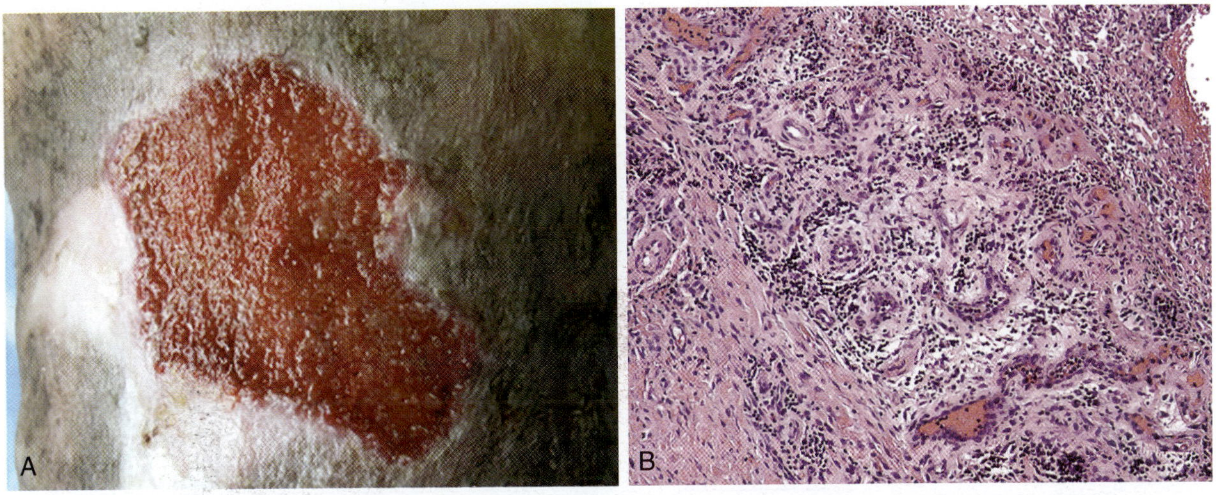

Fig. 3.20 Gross of healthy granulation tissue at the base of a skin ulcer (A). Microscopic appearance of granulation tissue showing blood vessels, fibroblasts and chronic inflammatory cells (B). (*Source:* From Anais Malpica. Nonneoplastic Diseases of the Vagina. Gynecologic Pathology: A Volume in Foundations in Diagnostic Pathology Series. 2nd edition. 2021. Elsevier; From Katherine L. Baquerizo Nole and Robert S. Kirsner. Leg ulcers. Dermatological Signs of Systemic Disease. 5th edition. 2017. Elsevier.)

are the macrophages, followed by lymphocytes. Let us review the role of these cells in chronic inflammation.

Role of Macrophages

Let us first study the origin and function of this cell before we venture into its role in inflammation.

Origin of macrophages: Macrophages originate from the progenitor cells found in the embryonic yolk sac in the early fetal life, followed by the fetal liver in later stages and then from the haematopoietic stem cells of the bone marrow after birth. They may be found in circulation or in tissues and are given different names in different locations. The major difference between the circulating macrophages called monocytes and the tissue macrophages is their life span. The former has a short life span of 1 day, whereas tissue macrophages live for many months to years. Although the monocytes are formed only in the bone marrow, the resident macrophages of the various organs repopulate themselves by local proliferation rather than depending on the bone marrow. The various names given to resident macrophages of the tissues are given in Fig. 3.21, and these together form the reticuloendothelial system.

Pathways of macrophage activation: The monocytes in circulation are recruited to the site of inflammation within

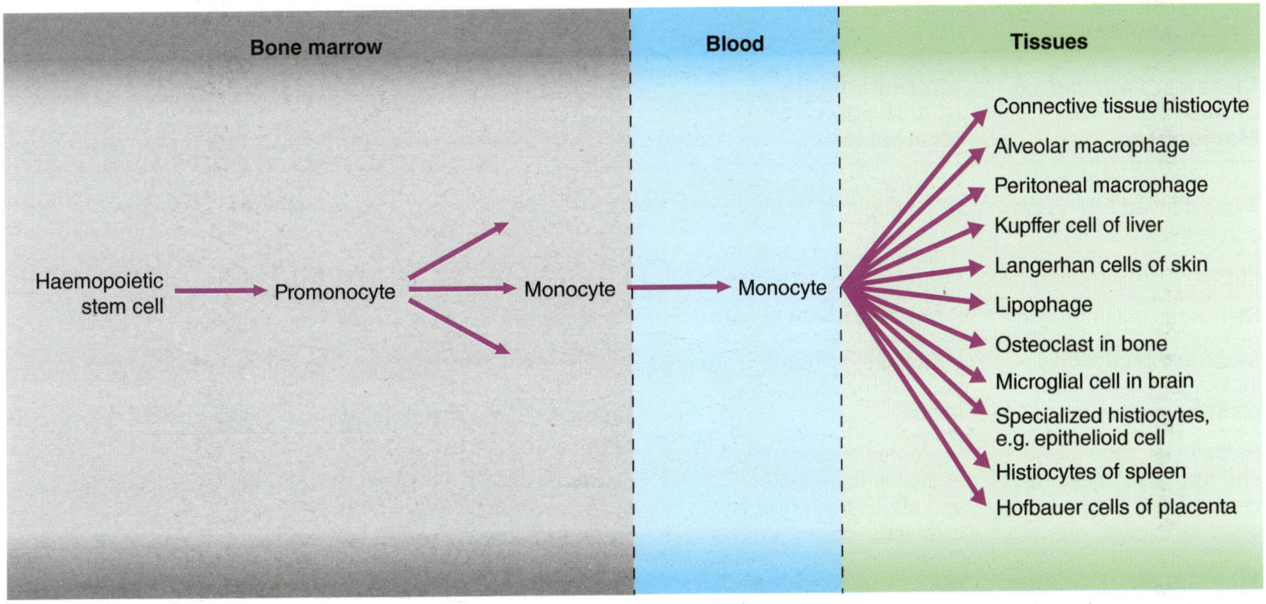

Fig. 3.21 The mononuclear macrophage system. (*Source:* From Timothy J. Stephenson. Inflammation. In Underwood's Pathology 7th edition. 2019. Elsevier.)

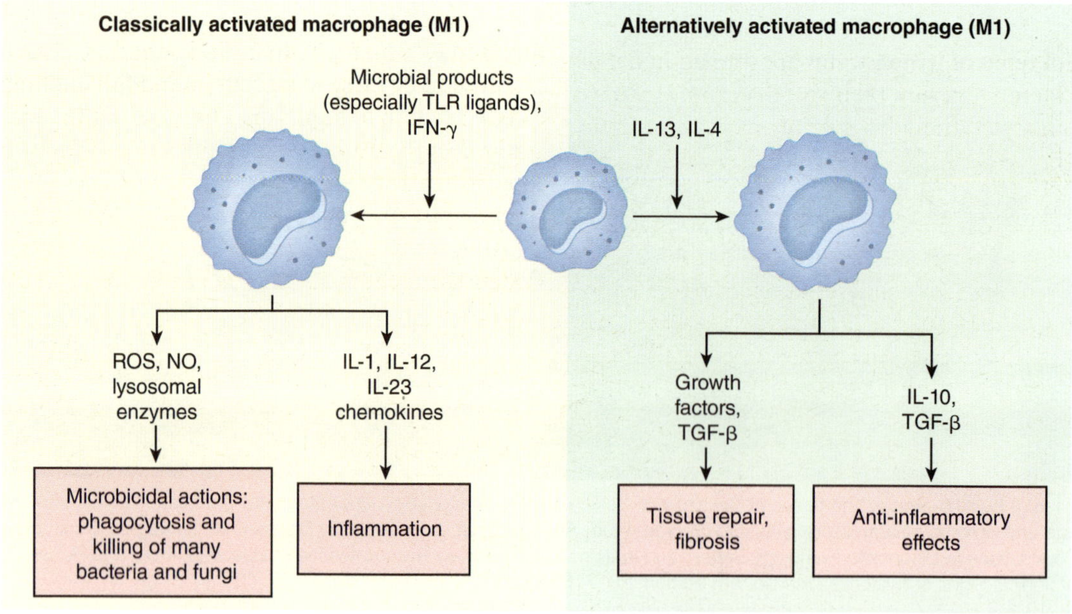

Fig. 3.22 Two types of macrophage activation. (*Source:* From Robbins & Cotran Pathologic Basis of Disease, 10th edition. Elsevier. 2018.)

48 hours by the same mechanism of margination, rolling, adhesion, transmigration and chemotaxis, all mediated by the same adhesion molecules and chemical mediators as the neutrophils. On reaching the tissues, the monocytes get transformed into macrophages. These macrophages may undergo two types of activation that determine their role in inflammation. The differences between these two, M1 and M2 macrophages, are explained in Fig. 3.22 and Table 3.9.

Macrophage in inflammation: Although macrophages help in elimination of the infectious agent, they are the major cells causing tissue damage in chronic inflammation (Fig. 3.23). Their functions are as follows:

- Phagocytosis and riddance of microbes and necrotic tissue
- Tissue repair by fibrosis and scar formation
- Synthesis and secretion of mediators such as cytokines and AA metabolites
- Antigen presentation to T cells
- Respond to activation signals from helper T cells and help in microbe killing

Table 3.9 Pathways of Macrophage Activation

Classical Pathway of Activation – M1 Macrophage	Alternate Pathway of Activation – M2 Macrophage
Activated by microbes, T-cell-derived IFN-γ and crystals such as urate	Activated by T-cell-derived IL-13 and IL-4
Forms M1 macrophage	Forms M2 macrophage
Stimulates inflammation	Stimulates tissue repair
Mediators produced include ROS, NO and proinflammatory cytokines	Mediators include TGF-β, IL-10 and certain growth factors
Helps in microbe killing and may also cause tissue damage	Promotes angiogenesis, activates fibroblasts and stimulates collagen synthesis

IFN-γ, interferon-γ; IL, interleukin; NO, nitric oxide; ROS, reactive oxygen species; TGF-β, transforming growth factor-β.

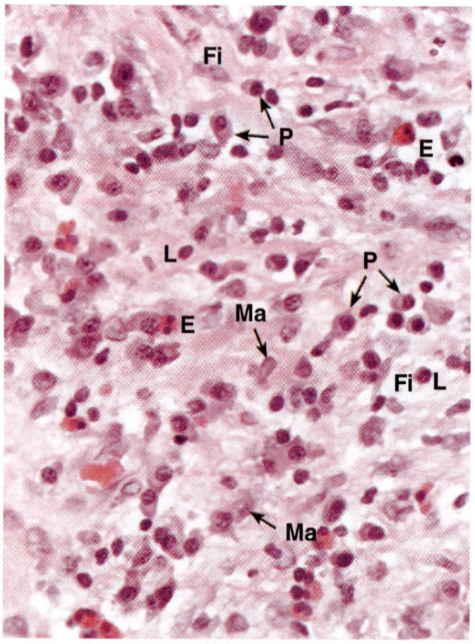

Fig. 3.23 Cells of chronic inflammation. E, eosinophil; Fi, fibroblast; L, lymphocyte; Ma, macrophage; P, plasma cell. (*Source:* From Geraldine O'Dowd, Sarah Bell and Sylvia Wright. Chronic inflammation. In Wheater's Pathology: A Text, Atlas, and Review of Histopathology. 6th edition. Elsevier 2020.)

Role of Lymphocytes

The nature and types of lymphocytes are studied in detail in Chapter 6. Here, we review their role in chronic inflammation. Lymphocytes, though a part of adaptive immune response of the body, may be present in sites of chronic inflammation and when this occurs, the damage caused is exacerbated by the lymphocytes. This is typically seen in autoimmune and hypersensitivity diseases. The migration of lymphocytes to the site of inflammation is mediated by the same adhesion molecules and cytokines as the neutrophils and once they reach the target tissues, they are stimulated by mediators secreted by macrophages such as TNF, IL-1 and chemokines.

T lymphocytes: $CD4^+$ helper T cells help in elimination of the microbe. The macrophages present antigens to these cells and the T cells, in turn, secrete mediators that activate macrophages. This vicious cycle may perpetuate tissue damage in chronic inflammation. The three subsets of these cells perform different functions as given in Table 3.10.

B lymphocytes: The presence of plasma cells and activated B cells at the site of chronic inflammation has been noted along with production of antibodies against the microbes or host antigens; however, their role in chronic inflammation is uncertain.

In some chronic inflammatory conditions, lymphocytes, plasma cells and antigen-presenting cells may aggregate to form **tertiary lymphoid organs** as seen in the synovium of patients with rheumatoid arthritis and in thyroid in Hashimoto thyroiditis. This process is called **lymphoid organogenesis.**

Role of Eosinophils, Mast Cells and Neutrophils

Eosinophils: Eosinophils play a key role in allergic reactions, IgE-mediated reactions and parasitic infections. The specific mediator that attracts eosinophils is eotaxin, a chemokine, and the factor that activates it is IL-5. Eosinophils produce a major basic protein that is capable of parasitic killing and lysis of mammalian cells.

Mast cells: Mast cells or tissue basophils contain a rich plethora of mediators and take part in acute and chronic inflammatory reactions. They have Fc receptors for IgE antibodies using which these antibodies bind on them. Activation of these mast cell–bound IgE antibodies in allergic reaction to foods, insect venom, drugs, etc., leads to their degranulation, and the allergic response which may sometimes have catastrophic consequences.

Neutrophils: Neutrophils, the key cells of acute inflammation, may also be present in chronic inflammation when the inciting agent is persistent or as a response to mediators released by macrophages. Their presence in chronic inflammation is called acute on chronic inflammation and is seen in conditions like osteomyelitis of bone and smoking-related lung injury.

Table 3.10 Role of T Lymphocytes in Chronic Inflammation

Helper T cell	Mediator Secreted	Role
Helper 1	IFN-γ	Activates macrophage by the classical pathway
Helper 2	IL-4, IL-13 IL-5	Activates macrophages by an alternate pathway Recruits and activates eosinophils
Helper 17	IL-17	Recruitment of neutrophils

IFN-γ, interferon-γ; IL, interleukin.

GRANULOMATOUS INFLAMMATION

A variant of chronic inflammation that shows the presence of activated macrophages and scattered T lymphocytes occasionally with central necrosis is called granulomatous inflammation. In an attempt to eliminate the offending agent, the strongly activated lymphocytes may injure the host tissue by activating the macrophages. These activated macrophages resemble epithelial cells because of the newly acquired abundant cytoplasm and are hence called **epithelioid cells,** *which are the hallmark cells of granulomatous inflammation.* These epithelioid cells occasionally fuse to form large cells with many nuclei called **multinucleate giant cells** (Fig. 3.24).

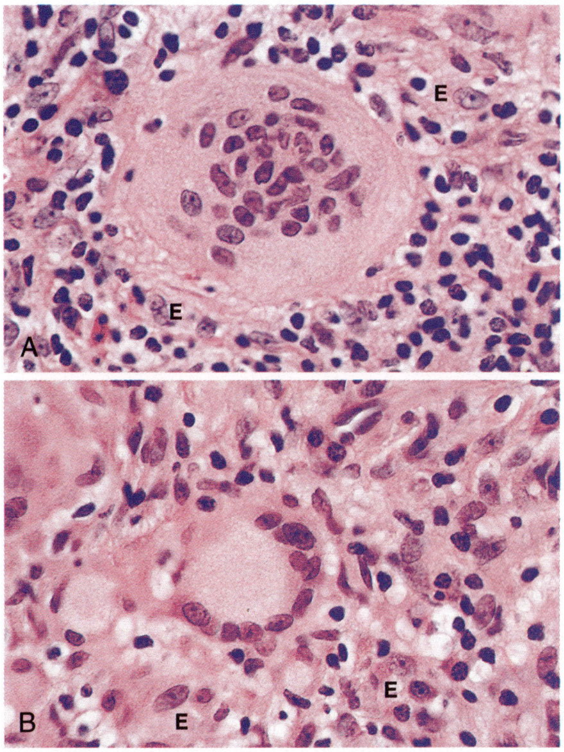

Fig. 3.24 Microscopic appearance of foreign body giant cell (A) and Langhans giant cell (B). E, epithelioid cell. (*Source:* From Geraldine O'Dowd, Sarah Bell and Sylvia Wright. Chronic inflammation. In Wheater's Pathology: A Text, Atlas, and Review of Histopathology. 6th edition. Elsevier 2020.)

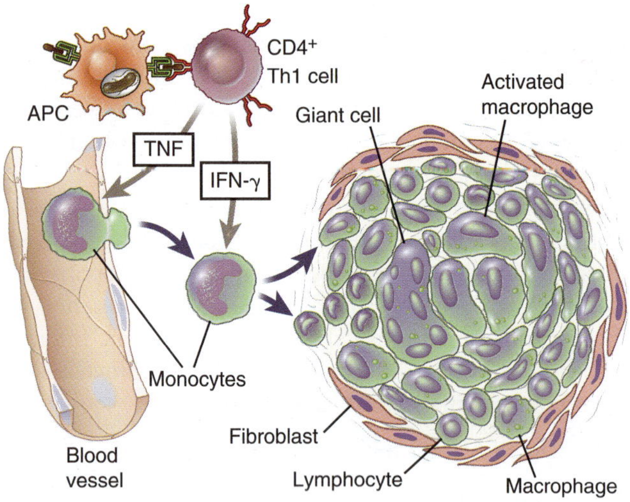

Fig. 3.25 Mechanism of granuloma formation. Activated T cells produce cytokines that recruit macrophages (tumour necrosis factor [TNF], interleukin-17 [IL-17], chemokines) and others that activate macrophages (interferon-γ [IFN-γ]). Activated macrophages, in turn, stimulate T cells by presenting antigens and via cytokines such as IL-12. Prolonged reactions involving T cells and macrophages may result in granuloma formation. (*Source:* From Abul K. Abbas, Andrew H. Lichtman and Shiv Pillai. Hypersensitivity Disorders. In Cellular and Molecular Immunology. 2022. Elsevier.)

The two types of granulomas and their pathogenesis are as follows (Fig. 3.25):

- **Nonimmune granulomas:** These are formed without activation of T-cell immune response. Foreign bodies such as talc, sutures and large fibres are usually the inciting agents. They can be identified at the centre of the granuloma as refractile bodies when viewed under polarized light.
- **Immune granulomas** are formed because of a prolonged T-cell-mediated immune response. These are formed when the macrophage is unable to remove the offending agent or when the microbe is persistent as in tuberculosis or when the antigen is a host antigen. T Helper 1 cell produces IFN-γ, which activates the macrophage, and the macrophage, in turn, produces IL-2 to activate the T cells.

Tuberculosis is considered as the prototype of granulomas, and the granuloma in this condition is called *tubercle*. In countries such as India where tuberculosis is widely prevalent, any granuloma should be considered to be of tuberculous origin unless proven otherwise. Various causes of the granulomas are listed in Table 3.11.

Furthermore, some conditions are associated with unique types of granulomas and need special mention:

- Cat scratch disease – stellate-shaped granuloma
- Syphilis – gumma
- *Plasmodium falciparum* infection – Durck granuloma
- Among the inflammatory bowel diseases, granulomas shown only in Crohn disease both in the lesion and in the draining lymph nodes
- Churg–Strauss syndrome – eosinophilic granuloma

Table 3.11 Causes of Granuloma

Immunological	Nonimmunological
Lymphocyte associated E.g.: 1. Tuberculosis 2. Leprosy 3. Sarcoidosis 4. Cat scratch disease 5. Blastomycosis 6. Histoplasmosis 7. Hodgkin lymphoma	No association with lymphocytes Formed by indigestible material E.g.: 1. Silicosis 2. Foreign Body granuloma
Caseating Granuloma	**Noncaseating Granuloma**
1. Tuberculosis 2. Histoplasmosis 3. Syphilis 4. Coccidiomycosis	1. Tuberculosis 2. Sarcoidosis 3. Hodgkin lymphoma 4. Leprosy

Morphology

Epithelioid cells are plump, elongated cells with abundant pink granular cytoplasm, indistinct cell borders and a slipper-shaped nucleus with central constriction. Granulomas are seen as a collection of such epithelioid cells with lymphocytic rimming around the collection. Later on, they may develop a collar of fibroblasts and connective tissue. In most cases, multinucleated giant cells, containing abundant cytoplasm and many nuclei, formed by the fusion of these epithelioid cells called **Langhans giant cells** may be seen (Fig. 3.26). Apart from these findings, in mycobacteria-associated granulomas, there may be a central area of **caseation necrosis** formed because of hypoxia and free radical injury. It appears as cheesy material in gross and as amorphous, structureless, eosinophilic, granular debris under the microscope. Not all cases of granulomas show caseation necrosis, and it is also possible for tuberculosis to form granuloma without necrosis. Healing of granulomas is achieved by replacement with fibrosis.

SYSTEMIC EFFECTS OF INFLAMMATION (FIG. 3.27)

Although inflammation may occur in localized areas, the cytokine mediators may cause systemic effects in the individual. Systemic effects are invariably encountered in most bacterial and viral infections. These systemic effects are together called **acute-phase response** and are mediated mainly by TNF, IL-1, IL-6 and type 1 interferons. The components of acute-phase response are as follows:

- **Fever:** It is the increase in body temperature by 1–4°C, which is commonly seen in infection-associated

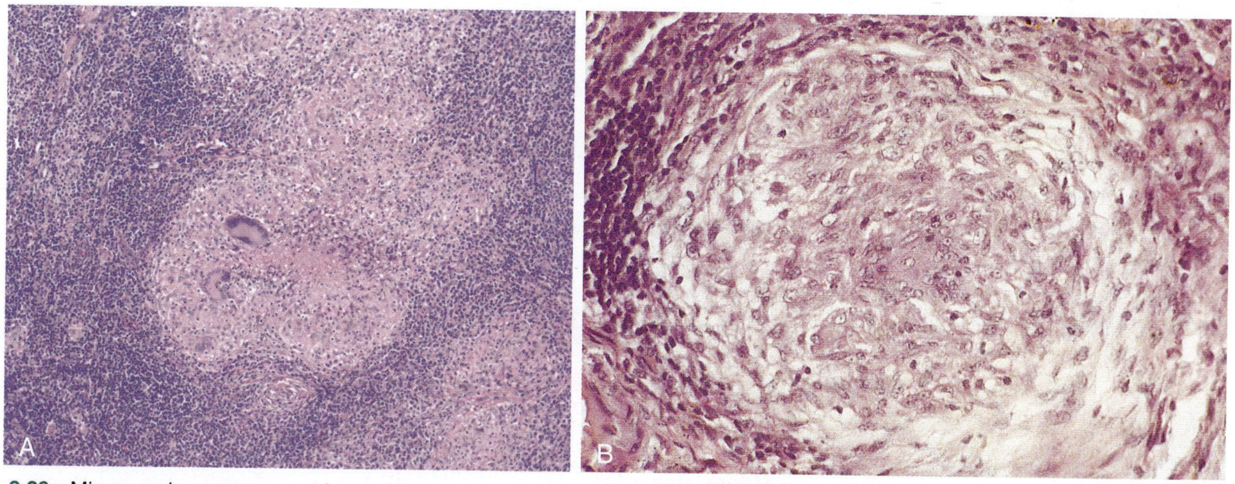

Fig. 3.26 Microscopic appearance of granuloma in tuberculosis with Langhans giant cells (A), with high-power view showing epithelioid cells (B). (*Source:* From Carlos Barrionuevo-Cornejo and Daniela Dueñas-Hancco. Lymphadenopathies in human immunodeficiency virus infection. Seminars in Diagnostic Pathology. 2018. 35; 84-91.)

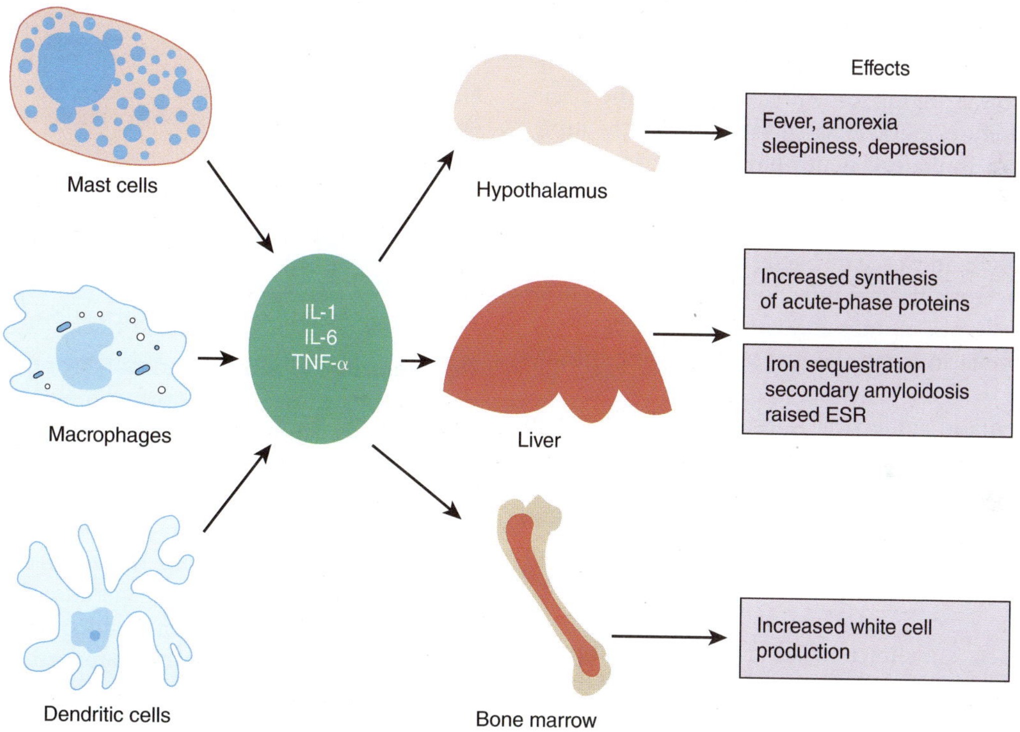

Fig. 3.27 Systemic effects of inflammation.

inflammation. The factors that act on the temperature-regulating centre in the hypothalamus and cause this increase in temperature are called pyrogens. They may be exogenous in origin such as bacterial products (exogenous pyrogens) or endogenous in origin such as IL-1 and TNF (endogenous pyrogens). The pyrogens stimulate prostaglandin PGE_2 production from AA in the vascular cells of the hypothalamus, which stimulates the production of neurotransmitters that reset the temperature set point at a higher level. It is hypothesized that the fever is a protective mechanism to enhance lymphocyte responses. The PG synthesis inhibitors such as NSAIDs and aspirin help reduce fever.

- **Acute-phase proteins** are plasma proteins, produced by the liver, in greater quantities in inflammatory conditions. The most important acute-phase reactants are *CRP, fibrinogen, serum amyloid A (SAA) protein and hepcidin*. The mediators that stimulate their synthesis by the hepatocytes are the cytokines IL-6 (for CRP and fibrinogen) and IL-1 or TNF (for SAA). Effects of these proteins are as follows:
  - These act as opsonins by binding to microbe cell wall and fix complement.

  - These help in removing necrotic cells by binding to the chromatin.
  - These increase erythrocyte sedimentation rate (ESR) by enhancing rouleaux formation as the fibrin makes the RBCs sticky.
  - Secondary amyloidosis occurs because of prolonged production and deposition of these proteins in tissues, especially SAA.
  - CRP levels serve as a marker of myocardial infarction risk in patients with coronary artery disease.
  - Anaemia seen in chronic inflammatory conditions is because of raised levels of hepcidin, which reduces iron absorption from the intestine and release of iron from iron stores.
- **Leucocytosis** is the increase in leucocyte count above normal values, occasionally reaching values of 40,000–100,000 cells/mL. These are common findings in acute bacterial infections. The markedly elevated values are called **leukaemoid reaction** and are discussed in detail in Chapter 6 on WBCs. Initially, there is an accelerated release of cells by IL-1 and TNF into the blood from the bone marrow, bringing some precursors into the circulation. Therefore, it is associated with a rise in the number of more immature neutrophils in the blood, referred to as a left shift. The common changes in WBCs are as follows:
  - Neutrophilia in pyogenic bacterial infection
  - Lymphocytosis in viral infections, such as infectious mononucleosis, mumps and German measles
  - Eosinophilia in some allergies and parasitic infestations
  - Leucopenia in some viral infections, rickettsiae and certain protozoal infections
- **Clinical features** such as increased pulse and blood pressure, reduced sweating to minimize heat loss through the skin, rigors (shivering), chills (search for warmth), anorexia, somnolence and malaise occur because of the effect of cytokines on brain cells.
- **Septic shock** is a clinical triad of disseminated intravascular coagulation, hypotensive shock and metabolic disturbances including insulin resistance and hyperglycaemia. It is because of high levels of IL-1 and TNF produced by the body in disseminated infections such as bacterial sepsis. This is explained in detail in Chapter 4.

HEALING AND REPAIR PA 5.1

An organism's ability to survive largely depends on its capability to handle injurious stimuli and recover from the damages caused by those stimuli. The recovery from an injury by regaining the tissue architecture and function is called healing or repair.

The process of healing starts with the resolution of inflammation and reestablishment of normal homeostasis.

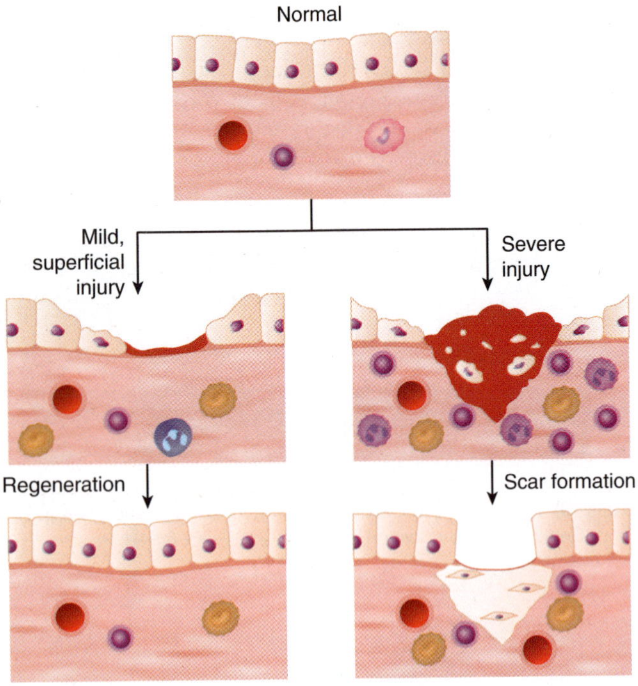

Fig. 3.28 Methods of tissue repair. (*Source:* From Robbins & Cotran Pathologic Basis of Disease, 10th edition. Elsevier. 2018.)

OVERVIEW OF HEALING AND REPAIR

Repair of a damaged tissue can occur by two methods, namely regeneration and scar formation (Fig. 3.28).

Regeneration: Healing that occurs by replacement of the damaged structures to the normal preinjury state is called regeneration. This commonly occurs in the skin and mucosa of intestines that are made of rapidly dividing cells in parenchymal organs such as the liver. When an injury occurs, there is proliferation of the undamaged cells with an additional support from the stem cells. Hence, the main processes involved in regeneration are cell proliferation and tissue regeneration, which are dependent on growth factors, integrity of the supporting framework of extracellular matrix (ECM) and presence of stem cells that can form mature cells.

Scar formation: Healing by deposition of connective tissue results in scar formation, and this enables the tissue to perform its function up to a certain extent. It occurs when the supporting structure is damaged or when the tissue is not capable of regenerating itself. When this excess collagen deposition occurs in organs such as the lung, liver or kidney, it is called *fibrosis*, whereas the collagen deposition in areas of exudate collection is called *organization*.

However, in most areas of inflammation, both types of repair are present to some degree. The mechanisms of cell proliferation, tissue regeneration and connective tissue deposition that occur in the repair process are discussed next.

CELL PROLIFERATION AND TISSUE REGENERATION

The ability of a tissue to undergo repair depends on the capacity of the component cells to proliferate. Hence, on the basis of their intrinsic proliferative capacity, tissues are classified into labile, stable and permanent tissues (Fig. 3.29) and this is given in Table 3.12.

Regeneration of tissues is both by proliferation of mature cells and by formation of mature cells from stem cells. These processes require growth factors and ECM support. The cells around the area of injury, especially the macrophages, secrete these growth factors which then get concentrated by binding to ECM. ECM also produces integrins that help in proliferation by providing growth signals to the surrounding cells. However, **presence of the connective tissue structural framework is necessary for the regeneration to occur**. Damage of the framework leads to incomplete regeneration and scarring.

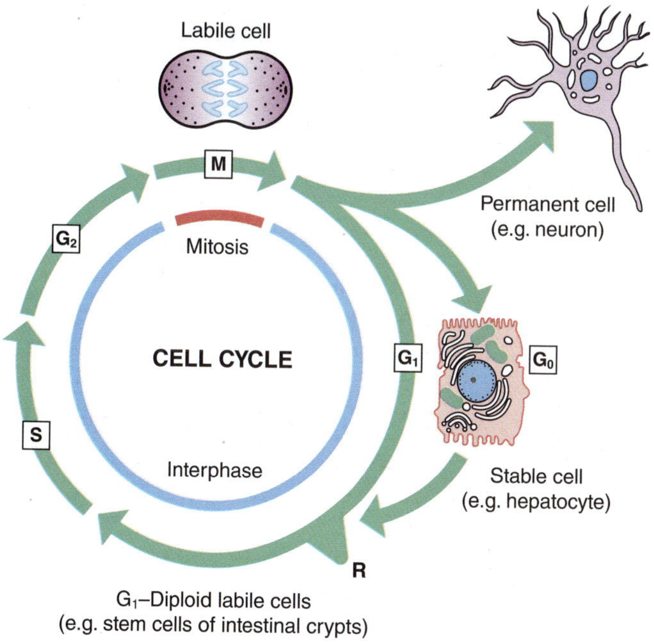

Fig. 3.29 Types of tissue.

Liver Regeneration (Fig. 3.30)

The liver is the only organ in our body that, akin to the tail of the lizard, is capable of regeneration to a great extent. It is seen to occur following partial resection in cases of tumour and in cases of liver donors. The two mechanisms involved in the process include proliferation of reminiscent hepatocytes and production of mature cells from progenitor cells.

About 90% of liver regeneration is achieved by remaining hepatocyte proliferation, which is promoted by the combined actions of cytokines and polypeptide growth factors. The stages of this process are depicted in Flowchart 3.7.

In contrast, regeneration of the liver in cases of chronic liver injury, where viable hepatocytes are scanty, is from progenitor cells. The major contribution is by the **oval cells located in the canals of Herring**, but the factors that control this process are yet to be identified.

Repair by Connective Tissue Deposition

When the aforementioned cell/tissue proliferation is unable to repair the damaged tissue completely because of damage in the framework, or when permanent tissue is damaged, the process of healing is completed by connective tissue deposition, resulting in a scar. The sequence of events in scar formation are given in Flowchart 3.8.

The most important cell in scar formation is the **macrophage**. The *classically activated M1 macrophage* of inflammation is replaced by the *alternatively activated M2 macrophage* during the healing process by unknown mechanisms. These cells help in the following processes:

- Clear the microbes and necrotic tissue
- Provide growth factors for cell proliferation
- Secrete cytokines and other growth factors that stimulate fibroblast proliferation and scar formation

Table 3.12 Types of Tissue

Type of Tissue	Nature	Examples
Labile	Continuously dividing cells that replace lost tissues (occurs by adult cell proliferation and stem cell pool division)	• Haematopoietic cells of bone marrow • Stratified squamous epithelia of the skin, oral cavity, vagina and cervix • The cuboidal epithelia of the ducts draining exocrine organs • The columnar epithelium of the gastrointestinal tract, uterus and fallopian tubes • Transitional epithelium of the urinary tract
Stable	Though silent in normal state, it divides actively when there is an injury (has a limited capacity except liver)	• Parenchyma of liver, kidney and pancreas – endothelial cells, fibroblasts and smooth muscle cells that are essential for wound healing
Permanent	Terminally differentiated cells that do not proliferate (so repair is by scarring)	• Neurons • Cardiac muscle cells • Skeletal muscle

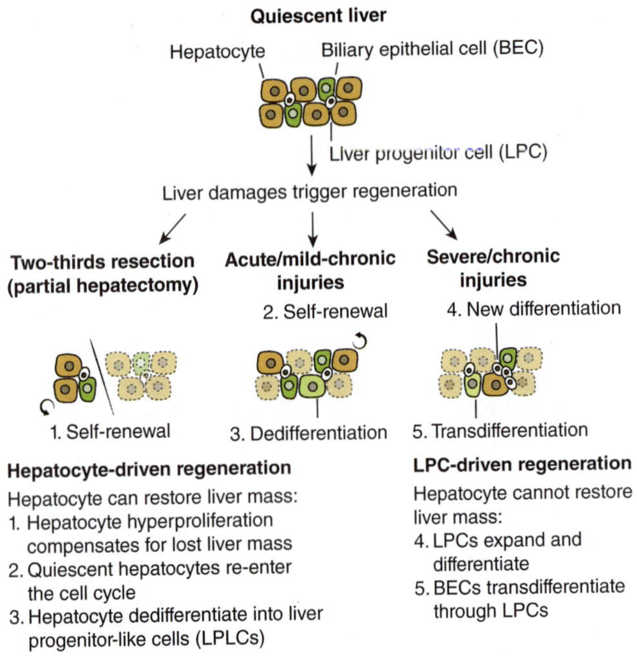

Fig. 3.30 Causes and mechanisms of liver regeneration. (*Source:* From Filippo Macchi, Kirsten C. Sadler, Trends in Genetics, Elsevier 2020.)

Priming phase
Kupffer cells produce IL-6 that make hepatocytes respond to growth signals.

↓

Growth factor phase
- Proliferation of hepatocytes occurs as a response to HGF and TGF-α produced by many cells. This process requires activation of multiple growth genes and inactivation of growth supressor proteins.
- Proliferation of nonparenchymal cells such as Kupffer cells and stellate cells occurs after hepatocyte proliferation.

↓

Termination phase
Hepatocytes stop proliferating and return to G0 phase due to action of TGF-β.

Flowchart 3.7 Stages of liver regeneration.

Steps in Scar Formation

ANGIOGENESIS (FIG. 3.31)

Angiogenesis is the process of new blood vessel formation from existing vessels. The knowledge about the mechanism and the influencing factors has helped in developing treatment modalities that increase or inhibit angiogenesis. The sequence of events is shown in Flowchart 3.9.

The key mediators and growth factors involved in the process of angiogenesis are given in Table 3.13.

Formation of Granulation Tissue Granulation tissue represents the pink fleshy tissue that is formed during the process of healing. It is composed of fibroblasts, loose connective tissue, interspersed new sprouting vessels and chronic inflammatory cells. Depending on the size of deficit to be filled, the granulation tissue is formed to fill the gap of the healing wound. The rich vascularity may make it bleed on touch.

Angiogenesis
Formation of new blood vessels to supply nutrients to the repairing tissue, mediated by VEGF, which also increases vascular permeability and causes oedema.

↓

Formation of granulation tissue
Pink soft granular tissue composed of fibroblasts, thin-walled new leaky vessels, lymphocytes and macrophages is formed in 3 to 5 days. Amount of granulation tissue depends on size of wound and severity of inflammation.

↓

Deposition of connective tissue
Migration and proliferation of fibroblasts with deposition of ECM produced by them.

↓

Scar remodelling
Connective tissue deposition is balanced with degradation to reduce the size of scar just enough to give the maximum strength possible.

Flowchart 3.8 Steps in scar formation.

Deposition of Connective Tissue This process results in the conversion of a pink vascular granulation tissue into a pale avascular collagen-rich scar. This occurs in three steps:

(1) Migration of fibroblasts to the site of injury
(2) Proliferation of fibroblasts
(3) Synthesis and deposition of ECM proteins by these cells

The main factor in this process is **TGF-β**, followed by fibroblast growth factor (**FGF**) and **platelet-derived growth factor (PDGF)** produced mainly by the M2 macrophages in the granulation tissue and other cells such as mast cells and lymphocytes. The functions of TGF-β in the wound are as follows:

- Suppression of inflammation by inhibiting lymphocytes
- Migration and proliferation of fibroblasts
- Increased synthesis of collagen and fibronectin
- Reduced degradation of ECM by inhibiting matrix metalloproteases (MMPs)

Thus, it contributes to scar formation and fibrosis in chronic inflammatory diseases of organs such as the liver, kidney and lung.

Scar Remodelling The balance between ECM protein synthesis and degradation decides the final strength of the scar formed. ECM that is formed and deposited is

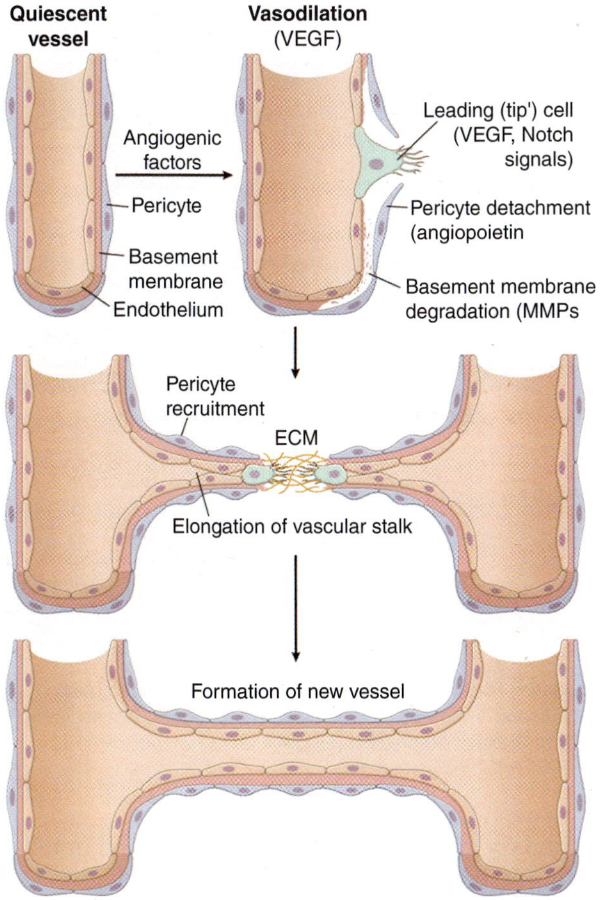

Fig. 3.31 Steps in angiogenesis. (*Source:* From Woo Cheal Cho, George Jour and Phyu P. Aung. Role of angiogenesis in melanoma progression: Update on key angiogenic mechanisms and other associated components. Seminars in Cancer Biology. 2019. 59; 175-186.)

Vasodilation (caused by NO and VEGF)
↓
Vessel sprout formation (by separation of pericytes and breakdown of basement membrane)
↓
Migration of endothelial cells in the direction of injured tissue
↓
Endothelial cell proliferation occurs behind the leading tip cell that is moving forward
↓
Conversion of the stack of proliferated endothelium into capillary tubes
↓
Recruitment of pericytes to envelop the capillary tubes
↓
Endothelial proliferation stops
↓
Basement membrane is deposited

Flowchart 3.9 Sequence of events in angiogenesis.

Table 3.13 Mediators of Angiogenesis

Mediator	Effect
VEGF	Endothelial migration and proliferation Formation of lumen in the capillary tube
FGF	Endothelial proliferation Macrophage and fibroblast migration Epithelial migration in skin wounds
Angiopoietin 1 and 2	Recruitment of pericytes Structural maturation of vessels
PDGF	Recruitment of smooth muscle cells
TGF-β	Suppresses endothelial proliferation
ECM proteins	Sprouting of vessels
Matrix metalloproteinase	Vessel remodelling

ECM, extracellular matrix; FGF, fibroblast growth factor; PDGF, platelet-derived growth factor; TGF-β, transforming growth factor-β; VEGF, vascular endothelial growth factor.

degraded by a group of enzymes called *MMPs*, which include the following:

- Interstitial collagenases – degrade fibrillar collagen
- Gelatinases – degrade amorphous collagen and fibronectin
- Stromelysins – degrade proteoglycans, laminin, fibronectin and amorphous collagen

The activity of these MMPs is strictly controlled by two mechanisms:

- Activation of these MMPs occurs only at the site of injury by proteases such as plasmin.
- Inactivation of these enzymes occurs by tissue inhibitors of matrix metalloproteases (TIMPs) produced by the mesenchymal cells.

Thus, the healing process in our body is performed by a multitude of cells and factors which perform their functions in a coordinated manner to produce a healthy scar with the least loss of function possible.

FACTORS AFFECTING TISSUE REPAIR/WOUND HEALING

Tissue repair may be affected by various extrinsic and intrinsic factors. An understanding of these factors may help reduce the influence of these factors in delaying wound healing. The factors that delay wound healing can be divided into those acting at the site of injury and systemic factors that affect the overall healing tendency of the person.

Local Factors

- Foreign body (sutures, dirt, glass or even bone spicules may hinder the healing process)
- Mechanical factors (movement, torsion, local pressure)
- Infection (causes persistent inflammation)
- Ionizing radiation
- Location of wound (across joints, in the skin, over bones where immobilization becomes difficult)
- Size (surgical wounds have cleaner margins and heal faster than large wounds; extensive wounds have some degree of loss of function)
- Blood supply (areas with poor blood supply, areas with reduced venous drainage and areas with pressure that affect blood flow such as bed sores)
- Type of tissue involved (injuries in organs with labile cells tend to heal by regeneration, whereas those made of permanent cells tend to undergo fibrosis and form scars)

Systemic Factors

1. Hormones (glucocorticoids reduce inflammation and affect collagen synthesis by reducing TGF-β production)
2. Reduced circulating blood volume (hypovolaemia)
3. Metabolic status (diabetes mellitus)
4. Age (wound healing is slower in the old age)
5. Nutritional deficiency (protein, vitamin C, copper and zinc deficiency)

HEALING OF SKIN WOUNDS

Healing of skin wound is an example of combined healing and regeneration of epithelium with deposition of connective tissue. On the basis of the size of the wound, healing may be by first or second intention (Fig. 3.32).

Healing by First Intention/Primary Union

This occurs when the injury has disrupted only the epithelial layer with loss of a relatively less number of epithelial cells and minimal disruption of the basement membrane. The main mechanism is *epithelial regeneration*. The repair consists of inflammation, proliferation of epithelial and other cells and maturation of the connective tissue scar. The best example of healing by first intention is a surgically cut skin wound approximated by sutures (Fig. 3.33).

The steps in wound healing by primary intention are given in Table 3.14.

Healing by Second Intention/Secondary Union

Wounds with a significant loss of tissue because of the larger size of wound, abscess formation, ulceration and parenchymal organs with hypoxic tissue necrosis heal by a combination of *regeneration and scar formation* (Fig. 3.33). This is called healing by second intention.

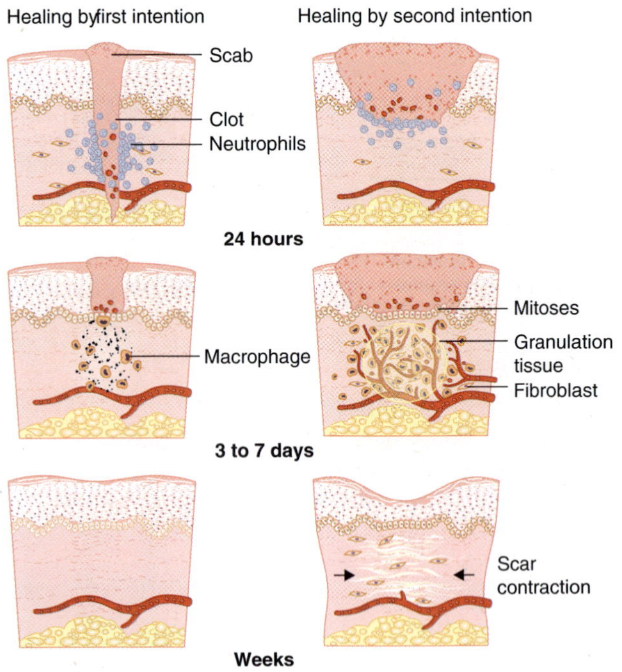

Fig. 3.32 Pictorial representation of stages of wound healing – first and second intentions. (*Source:* From Robbins & Cotran Pathologic Basis of Disease, 10th edition. Elsevier. 2018.)

Secondary union differs from primary union in the following features:

- There is more necrotic tissue and a larger fibrin clot formed has to be removed, resulting in a more intense inflammatory response and an associated injury to the tissues in the vicinity.
- A larger volume of granulation tissue is formed to bridge the gap, resulting in a bigger scar.
- The other steps in wound healing are similar such as epithelial proliferation to normal thickness, deposition of collagen type 3, replacement by collagen type 1 and formation of avascular scar with a permanent loss of dermal appendages in the scar area.
- The unique step in secondary union is **scar contraction** seen in large surface wounds, the purpose of which is to reduce the size of the scar and to approximate the edges of the wound to the maximum amount possible. This is achieved by special cells called *myofibroblasts* found along the edges of the wound, which resemble smooth muscle cells in their contractile ability. With the help of these cells, the wound size is reduced to 5%–10% the original wound size in 6 weeks.

Wound Strength

At the end of 1 week, the wound strength is 10%. But this improves because of the increased rate of collagen deposition versus collagen degradation in the initial 2 months, which is the crucial time of wound healing. Finally, 70%–80% of wound strength is gained at the end of 3 months and this does not improve any further with

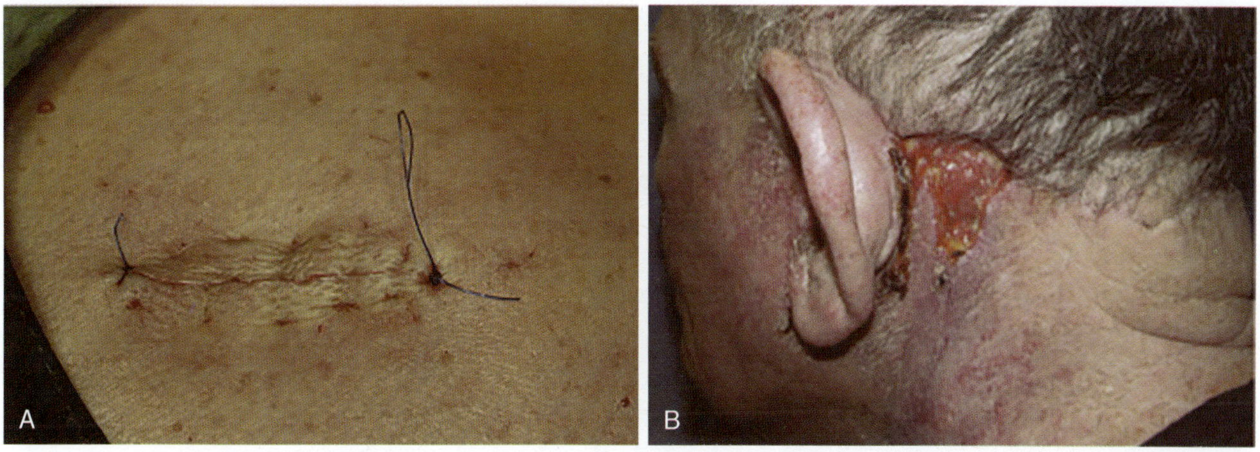

Fig. 3.33 Wound closure without tissue loss (A). Healing by second intention; wound without approximation of skin edges (B). (*Source:* From I. Justan. New type of skin suture–fully buried running mattress suture. Journal of Plastic, Reconstructive & Aesthetic Surgery. 2009; 63:e338-e339; From Abhishek Soni, Ravi Narula, Anil Kumar, Monika Parmar, Manish Sahore and Mohinder Chandel. Comparing Cyanoacrylate Tissue Adhesive and Conventional Subcuticular Skin Sutures for Maxillofacial Incisions—A Prospective Randomized Trial Considering Closure Time, Wound Morbidity, and Cosmetic Outcome. Journal of Oral and Maxillofacial Surgery, 2013: 71: 2152.e1-2152.e8.)

Table 3.14 Steps of Wound Healing by First Intention

Time	Events
Day 0	Blood clot stops bleeding; contains RBCs, fibrin, fibronectin and complement proteins; acts as scaffold for migrating cells Blood clot dehydrates at the surface and causes scab formation
Day 1	Neutrophils in margins of the wound release enzymes to clear debris Epithelial changes – basal cells of epidermis show mitotic activity
Day 2	Continuous thin epithelial layer formed by migrating proliferating epithelium that also deposits the basement membrane
Day 3	Macrophages replace neutrophils Granulation tissue fills the incision space Epithelial thickness approaches normal epidermal thickness
Day 5	Surface epidermis attains normal thickness Granulation tissue fills the wound Fibroblasts are abundant and produce plenty of ECM and collagen fibrils
10–14 days	Accumulation of collagen and fibroblast proliferation Granulation tissue blanches and scar formation occurs WBC, oedema and blood vessels – disappear
1 month	Scar is acellular, and dermal appendages are lost along the incision line Collagen 3 is replaced by collagen 1 by the action of the enzyme collagenase

ECM, extracellular matrix; RBC, red blood cell; WBC, white blood cell.

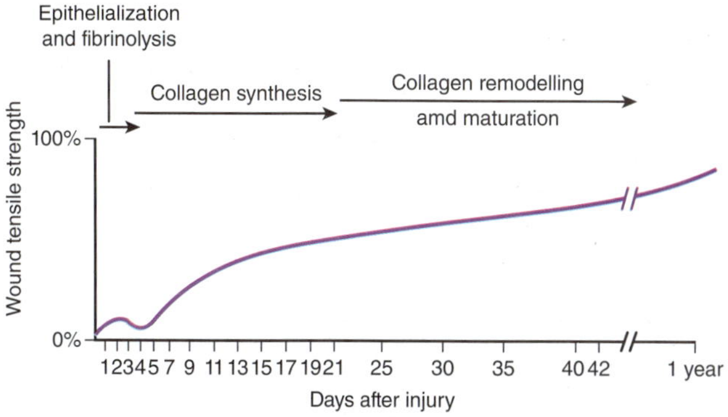

Fig. 3.34 Graph on recovery of wound strength. (*Source:* From Michael G. Franz, David L. Steed and Martin C. Robson. Optimizing Healing of the Acute Wound by Minimizing Complications. Current Problems in Surgery. 2007; 44: 691-763.)

time. A scar can never regain the complete tensile strength as that of normal tissue (Fig. 3.34).

FIBROSIS IN PARENCHYMAL ORGANS

Abnormal excessive deposition of collagen during chronic inflammation in internal organs is called fibrosis. It is similar to scar formation in surface tissues. Fibrosis commonly occurs because of chronic infections and autoimmune disorders, because of loss of significant tissue. It may lead to complete organ failure. The main mediator in this process is the fibrogenic cytokine **TGF-β**, whose production is stimulated by cell death and the production of reactive oxygen species. The origin of collagen is from myofibroblasts in the lung and kidney and stellate cells in liver cirrhosis.

The common systemic disorders associated with parenchymal fibrosis are liver cirrhosis, systemic sclerosis (scleroderma), fibrosing diseases of the lung (idiopathic pulmonary fibrosis, pneumoconiosis, drug,

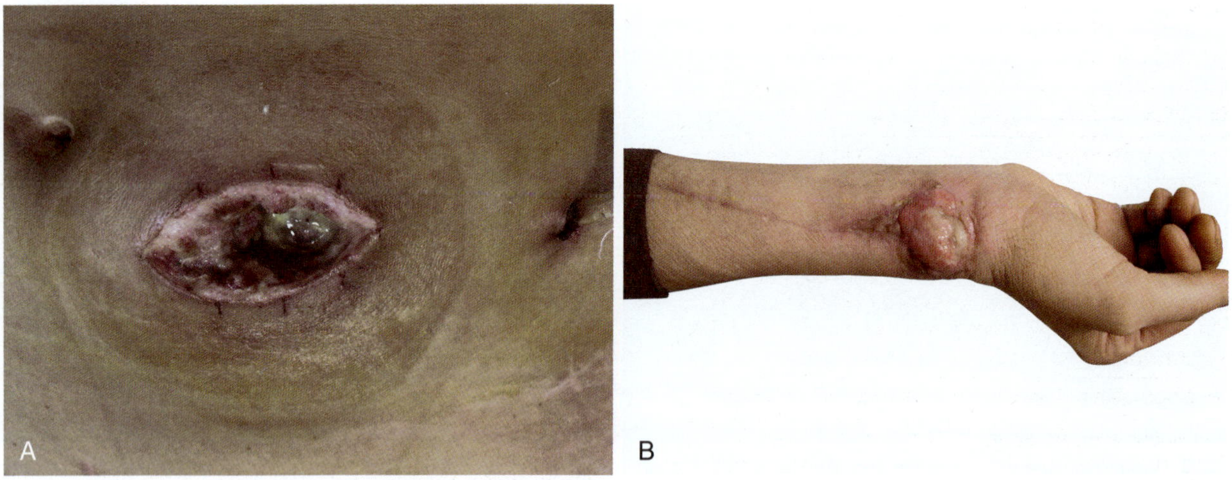

Fig. 3.35 Clinical image of ileostomy scar dehiscence following infection (A). Proud flesh (B). (*Source:* From Elodie Bonin, Valérie Bridoux, Rachid Chati, Sabrina Kermiche, Julien Coget, Jean Jacques Tuech and Horace Roman. Diverting stoma-related complications following colorectal endometriosis surgery: a 163-patient cohort. European Journal of Obstetrics & Gynecology and Reproductive Biology. 2019; 232: 46-53.)

radiation-induced pulmonary fibrosis), end-stage kidney disease and constrictive pericarditis. We shall discuss these conditions in the corresponding systemic chapters.

ABNORMALITIES IN WOUND HEALING

Wound healing is not perfect in all cases. There may be variations because of the following reasons:

- **Delayed wound healing**
  The healing process may not happen in some cases as per the time frame expected because of various reasons such as contamination of the wound site with foreign bodies, compromised blood supply, systemic metabolic disorders such as uncontrolled diabetes mellitus and vitamin C deficiency. Vitamin C is an important factor required for the synthesis of collagen fibres and their cross-linking.
- **Deficient scar formation**
  Occasionally, scars that are formed are not strong enough because of deficiency of granulation tissue formation or quantitative/qualitative defect in collagen deposition. When this occurs in abdominal scars, the abdomen may gape open when there is an increase in intra-abdominal pressure as in vomiting, coughing and constipation. This is called *scar dehiscence,* and it may be superficial or full-thickness dehiscence (Fig. 3.35A). The same defects in surface wounds result in the formation of *ulcers*. The common sites are the lower extremities, and the common reasons for the ulcers are compromised blood supply because of atherosclerosis and loss of sensation as in diabetic peripheral neuropathy.
- **Excessive repair components**
  - An increased amount of granulation tissue formation results in the projection of a mound of pink fleshy granulation tissue above the level of the epithelium. This is called **proud flesh,** and it prevents healing by blocking the re-epithelialization process (Fig. 3.35B).

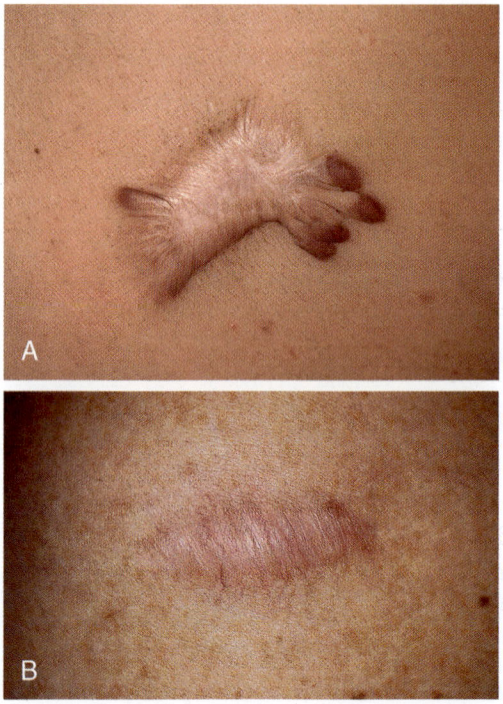

Fig. 3.36 Clinical picture of keloid with claw-like extensions beyond scar margin (A) and hypertrophic scar (B) that is restricted within scar margin. (*Source:* From Jean L. Bolognia & Julie V. Schaffer & Lorenzo Cerroni. Dermatology: 2-Volume Set, 4th Edition. 2020.)

  - An increased amount of collagen synthesis may result in the formation of **hypertrophic scar** and **keloid** (Fig. 3.36). The differences between the two are given in Table 3.15.
  - An increased number of fibroblasts in a wound because of excessive proliferation may result in much firmer and denser tumour masses called **desmoids** or **aggressive fibromatosis**. These are considered low-grade borderline – between benign and malignant – tumours.

Table 3.15 Comparison Between Hypertrophic Scar and Keloid

Hypertrophic scar	Keloid
Formed in thermal or trauma wounds in which the deep dermis is damaged	Formed in people who have inherent tendency to form keloids, especially Afro-Americans
The scar is raised because of excess collagen deposition but is confined to the scar margins	The scar is increased in size beyond the original wound margins and does not regress
Develops within 4 weeks	Develops after 3 months
May occur in scars at any location	Common in scars located over the sternum, earlobe, face and neck

- **Reduced scar contraction**
  The purpose of contraction of scar is to reduce the size of the wound. When the wound is on a hard surface such as bone, the granulation tissue is adherent on the bone and scar contraction does not take place. This results in a large size of wounds.
- **Contractures** (Fig. 3.37)
  Scar contraction is an important step in normal wound healing by second intention. But when it occurs excessively, it results in a deformity and restriction of movement of joints, when the scar is present over a joint. The common sites of contractures are the palms, soles and anterior thorax.

FRACTURE HEALING

The healing of bone fractures is slightly different compared with healing in other tissues. There are two types of healing depending on the method of bone formation – healing by primary union and healing by secondary union.

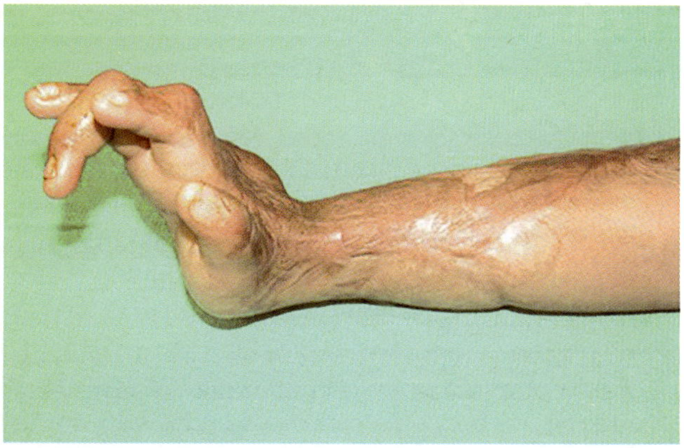

Fig. 3.37 Clinical picture of scar contractures following burns. (*Source:* From Matthew Brown and Kevin C. Chung. Postburn Contractures of the Hand. Hand Clinics, 2017: 33: 317-331.)

Primary Union

Healing by first intention or primary union is an **intramembranous type of ossification** in which bone formation occurs without an intermediary cartilage formation. This occurs when there is complete immobilization of the fracture site achieved by internal fixation. An osteoclast-led cutting cone grows along the long axis of the bone, bridging the fracture site. This osteoclastic invasion is followed by marching osteoblasts that deposit osteoid and form bone directly. In X-ray, this is witnessed as disappearance of fracture line with no evidence of callus.

Secondary Union

Healing by second intention or secondary union is an **enchondral type of ossification** in which bone is formed by replacement of cartilaginous anlage. This type of healing occurs when there is motion at the fracture site during the healing process, such as in cast treatment. This type of healing occurs in five stages. Different parts of the callus may be in different stages at any given point of time. The five stages of fracture healing by secondary intention are as follows (Fig. 3.38):

1. **Haematoma formation:** Fracture causes disruption of not only the bone but also the associated marrow, periosteum, surrounding muscle and blood vessels. This results in the formation of a haematoma made up of platelets, RBCs and WBCs and necrotic debris. The haematoma contains a significant amount of TNF-α, IL-6 and IL-8.

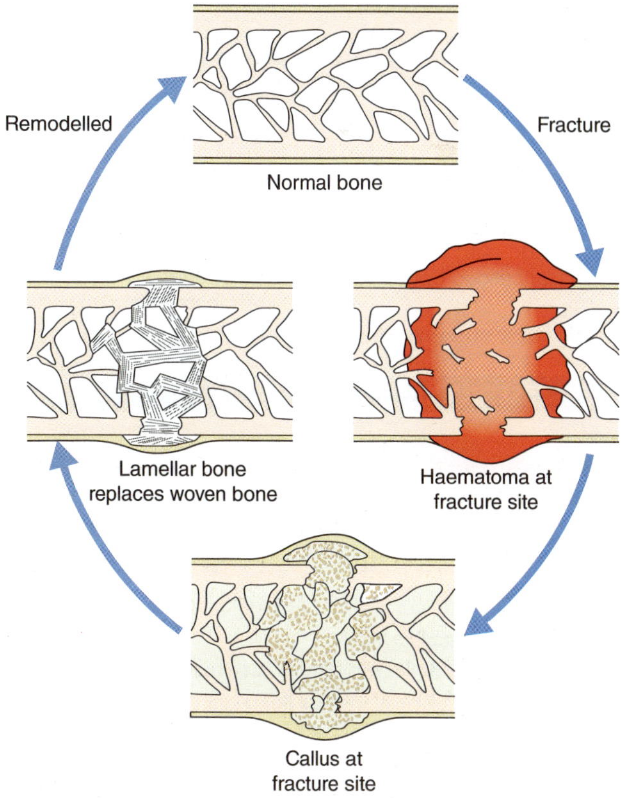

Fig. 3.38 Stages of fracture healing.

This haematoma is essential for the process of healing, and its disruption leads to delayed healing.

2. **Inflammation:** This stage starts within 8 hours of injury. The local hypoxia caused by the injury causes necrosis of surrounding tissues, which, in turn, triggers an inflammatory response. Neutrophils start appearing within 3 hours and are followed by macrophages and lymphocytes that remove the necrotic tissue and stimulate the healing to progress.
3. **Soft callus formation:** This stage starts at around 3 weeks in humans and is initiated by the transformation of progenitor cells into chondrocytes and osteoblasts. These cells replace the fibrous tissue and haematoma with cartilage and osteoid. Type I and II collagen deposition occurs in the matrix during this stage. This stage is seen on the X-ray as fluffy appearance between the fracture ends which are still not united.
4. **Hard callus formation:** The cartilage begins to get calcified with terminal differentiation of chondrocytes. This occurs after many weeks of fracture. The osteoblast and osteoclast population predominates because of death of chondrocytes and the woven bone is deposited. The X-ray shows calcification of fracture callus.
5. **Remodelling:** The formation of bone akin to the normal bone is attempted in this phase. The osteoclasts remove the disorganized woven bone, whereas the osteoblasts lay down the organized lamellar bone. This is mainly mediated by binding of RANKL to RANK, a receptor on the surface of osteoclasts.

Factors influencing fracture healing are as follows:

Factors favouring union	Factors hindering union
• Good blood supply • Good reduction and fixation • Hormones – growth hormone, parathormone, thyroxine • Good nutrition • Cancellous bone	• Compound fracture • Poor blood circulation • Infection • Distraction • Segmental fractures • Osteoporosis • Soft-tissue interposition • Inadequate immobilization

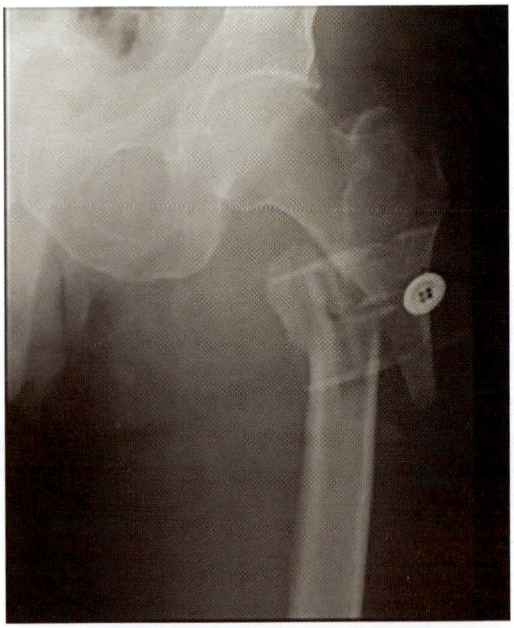

Fig. 3.39 X-ray showing nonunion of the femur. (*Source:* From Paul J. Harwood and David O. Ferguson. An update on fracture healing and non-union. Orthopaedics and Trauma, 2015; 29: 228-242.)

Complications of Fracture Healing

1. **Delayed union:** It occurs when the time taken for the healing to progress is much longer than expected.
2. **Nonunion** (Fig. 3.39): It occurs when the fracture ends fail to unite. This may be atrophic or hypertrophic nonunion. Atrophic nonunion occurs when there is a deficiency in callus formation because of malnutrition, smoking and medications such as steroids. Hypertrophic nonunion occurs when there is exuberant callus formation because of lack of adequate stability at the fracture site.

SELF-ASSESSMENT

Multiple Choice Questions

1. A boy came to outpatient department with trauma to his knee joint. The inflamed joint will show the following except
   A. Swelling
   B. Warmth
   C. Pain
   D. Bluish discolouration
2. A patient presents with acute appendicitis. The most important cell in this pathology is
   A. Neutrophil
   B. Lymphocyte
   C. Eosinophil
   D. Monocyte
3. A 56 year old smoker developed atheroma in his coronary artery. The atheroma is composed of foam cells which are macrophages that have engulfed oxidized LDL. The receptors on the macrophage that helped in this process is
   A. Mannose receptor
   B. Scavenger receptor
   C. Toll like receptor
   D. NOD like receptor
4. A 60 year old female wants to reduce skin changes related to aging. The body's mechanism of reducing aging process by neutralizing the effects of free radicals is mediated by many agents including
   A. Proteases

B. Iron bound transferrin
C. Ceruloplasmin
D. Oxidising agents

5. In patients with Good Pasteur syndrome where antibodies are formed against basement membrane antigens, the leukocyte damages the membrane due to
A. Phagocytosis
B. Frustrated Phagocytosis
C. NETosis
D. Cross reactivity of antigens

6. A 25 year old term pregnant female presents with uterine contractions. The prostaglandin involved in this process is
A. PGI 2
B. PGD2
C. PGE2
D. PGF 2α

7. A 55 year old male went to a pharmacy requesting for pain relief medication and was unethically given COX 2 selective inhibitors. He is at a risk of developing
A. Asthma
B. Cerebral thrombosis
C. Rashes
D. Fever

8. A patient presenting with acute anaphylactic reaction was given steroids as an emergency measure. The function of steroids includes
A. COX 2 inhibition
B. Phospholipase inhibition
C. Cytokine inhibition
D. All the above

9. A 65 year old male with colon carcinoma lost his appetite and looked cachectic. The mediator primarily responsible for this is
A. IL 1
B. TNF
C. IL-6
D. IFN γ

10. A 36 year old male developed HIV infection following unprotected intercourse with a HIV positive female. The chemokine that helped the HIV virus entry into CD 4 cell is
A. CXCR-4 chemokine
B. CC chemokine
C. CXC chemokine
D. C chemokine

11. A 6 year old girl presented with sudden abdominal pain, swelling of her face and breathing difficulty. She gave past history of similar episodes and was diagnosed with hereditary angioedema. The cause of this disorder is
A. Deficiency of C3 convertase
B. Deficiency of C1 inhibitor
C. Deficiency of CD55
D. Deficiency of CD59

12. A 55 year old patient had recurrent episodes of pleural inflammation which led to obliteration of pleural space and adhesion of visceral and parietal pleura. The type of inflammation seen in this patient is
A. Serous inflammation
B. Purulent inflammation
C. Fibrinous inflammation
D. Granulomatous inflammation

13. A 46 year old patient presented with an ulcer, the base of which was covered by a reddish friable tissue called granulation tissue which is composed of all except
A. Fibroblasts
B. Blood vessels
C. Mononuclear inflammatory cells
D. Epithelioid cells

14. A brain biopsy showed many cells of which the macrophages are represented by
A. Astrocytes
B. Microglia
C. Kupfer cells
D. Langerhan cells

15. A 45 year old female underwent thyroidectomy surgery and the thyroid tissue showed lymphoid aggregates. This is due to
A. Reactive lymphadenitis
B. Malignant transformation
C. Lymphoid organogenesis
D. Lymphoma

16. A 27 year old male developed tuberculosis and his lymph node biopsy showed granuloma formation. The important mediator produced by lymphocytes that activates macrophages to form granuloma is
A. IFN γ
B. IL 1
C. IL10
D. TGF β

17. A patient presented to emergency ward with acute abdominal pain and fever. The investigation commonly used as a marker of acute inflammation is
A. Blood hemoglobin
B. Blood CRP levels
C. Blood glucose levels
D. Se Urea levels

18. A 12 year old child presented with an acute allergic response to insect bite. His blood counts may show an increase in
A. Lymphocyte
B. Neutrophil
C. Eosinophil
D. Basophil

19. A 16 year old girl developed deformity of her joint due to healing of a joint trauma with a scar that developed across the joint. This is due to
A. Angiogenesis
B. Scar remodelling
C. Scar contraction
D. Scar weakening

20. A patient who underwent an abdominal surgery would like to know when his surgery scar will regain its full strength to the pre operative status.
A. 1 month
B. 2 months
C. 3 months
D. Never

Answers

1. (D); 2. (A); 3. (B); 4. (C); 5. (B); 6. (D); 7. (B); 8. (D); 9. (D); 10. (A); 11. (B); 12. (C); 13. (D); 14. (B); 15. (C); 16. (A); 17. (B); 18. (C); 19. (C); 20. (D)

Self-Assessment Questions

1. When we prick our finger with a needle, initially there is not much blood oozing out, but a few seconds later, there is an increase in the amount of blood oozing out. How can we explain this phenomenon?
2. A patient reports to an orthopaedic doctor for joint pain. What are the signs the doctor looks for to check inflammation and what is the reason for those signs of inflammation?
3. A patient presents with bacterial pneumonia and fever. What are the mediators involved in the fever process? What are the acute-phase proteins that may be elevated in the patient's blood?
4. A patient inadvertently put on selective COX inhibitors develops cerebral thrombosis. What is the possible mechanism?
5. A patient with a history of recurrent pneumothorax is treated by inducing inflammation to make the parietal pleura to adhere to the visceral pleura and obliterate the pleural space. What type of inflammation is this inducing?
6. A patient with a long-standing ulcer of the foot has red fleshy tissue covering. What is the tissue called and what is the expected microscopic finding of the tissue?
7. A patient with tuberculosis presents with enlarged lymph nodes. What is the type of inflammation seen in the lymph node?
8. How does healing by second intention differ from healing by first intention?
9. A patient who had undergone a major laparotomy surgery postoperatively develops acute pneumonia with severe cough. He presents 1 week after surgery with a burst abdomen (opening up all layers of abdominal sutures). How will you explain this?
10. A patient had a fall and broke his radial bone for which internal fixation is done. What is the type of fracture healing you expect?

Answers

1. Initial vasoconstriction, followed by vasodilation.
2. Calor and rubor – because of vasodilation; dolor and tumour – because of increased vascular permeability.
3. Fever – IL-1, TNF, PGE_2; acute-phase proteins – CRP, fibrinogen, SAA protein and hepcidin.
4. These drugs suppress vasodilator PGI_2 (produced by endothelium) without inhibiting COX-1-associated thromboxane synthesis (in platelets), leading to unopposed platelet aggregation and vasoconstriction by thromboxane. This increases the risk of cerebral and coronary thrombosis.
5. Fibrinous inflammation.
6. Granulation tissue is composed of fibroblasts, proliferating blood vessels and mononuclear inflammatory cells, lymphocytes and macrophages.
7. Granulomatous inflammation.
8. An increased amount of granulation tissue and scar contraction by myofibroblasts.
9. Scar dehiscence because of increased intra-abdominal pressure caused by chronic cough.
10. Primary union.

Topics for Self-Directed Learning

1. Interaction between complement, coagulation and kinin systems.
2. Other pathways in AA metabolism.
3. Role of steroids in inflammation.
4. Types of giant cells and associated conditions.
5. Mechanism of granuloma formation.
6. Mechanism of healing in specific organs such as the liver, brain and kidney.
7. Management of complications of wound healing.
8. Desmoid tumour.

MIND MAPS

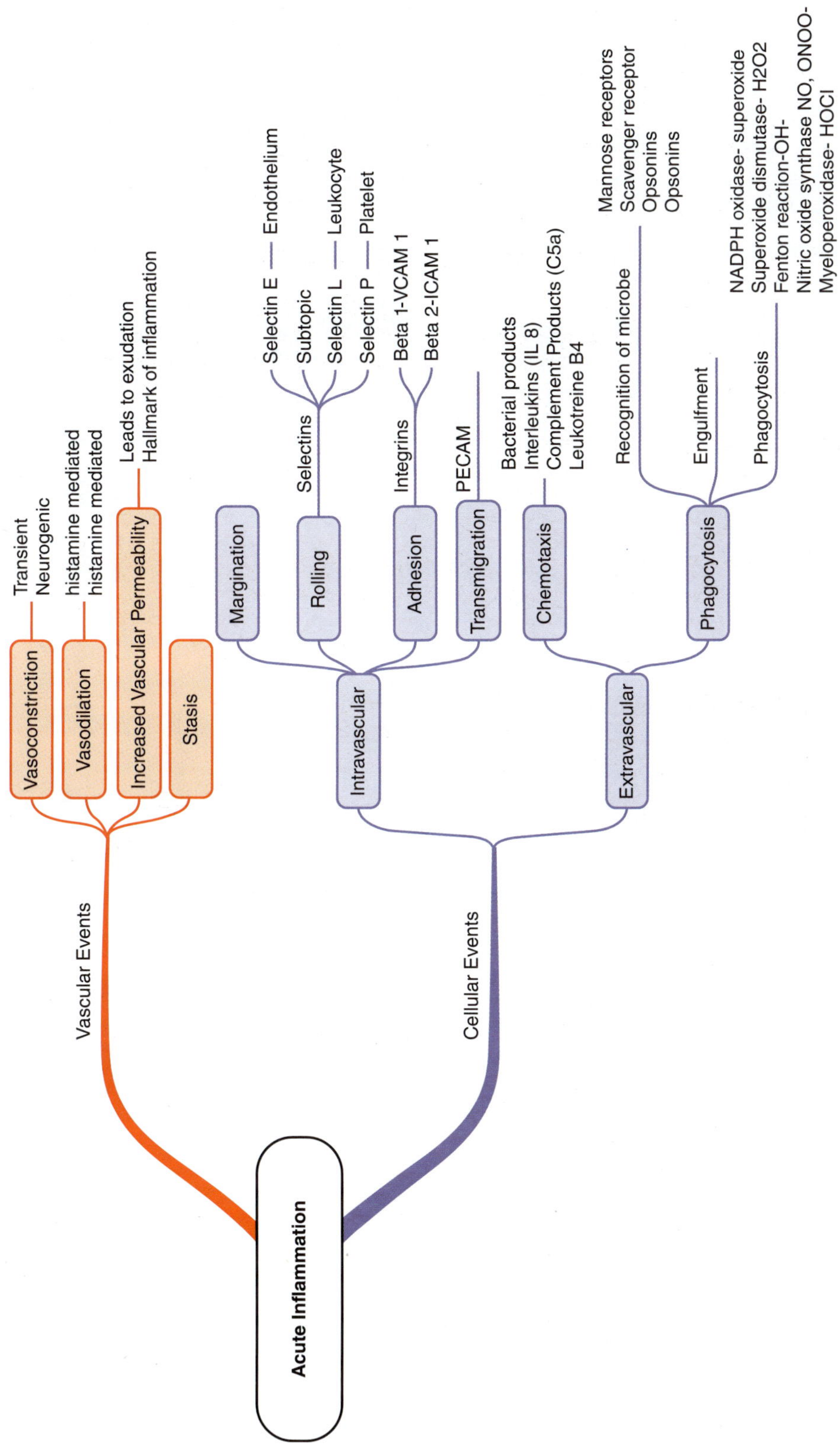
Acute Inflammation
Vascular Events
Vasoconstriction
Transient
Neurogenic
Vasodilation
histamine mediated
histamine mediated
Increased Vascular Permeability
Leads to exudation
Hallmark of inflammation
Stasis
Cellular Events
Intravascular
Margination
Rolling
Selectins
Selectin E — Endothelium
Subtopic
Selectin L — Leukocyte
Selectin P — Platelet
Adhesion
Integrins
Beta 1-VCAM 1
Beta 2-ICAM 1
Transmigration
PECAM
Extravascular
Chemotaxis
Bacterial products
Interleukins (IL 8)
Complement Products (C5a)
Leukotreine B4
Phagocytosis
Recognition of microbe
Mannose receptors
Scavenger receptor
Opsonins
Opsonins
Engulfment
Phagocytosis
NADPH oxidase- superoxide
Superoxide dismutase- H2O2
Fenton reaction-OH-
Nitric oxide synthase NO, ONOO-
Myeloperoxidase- HOCl

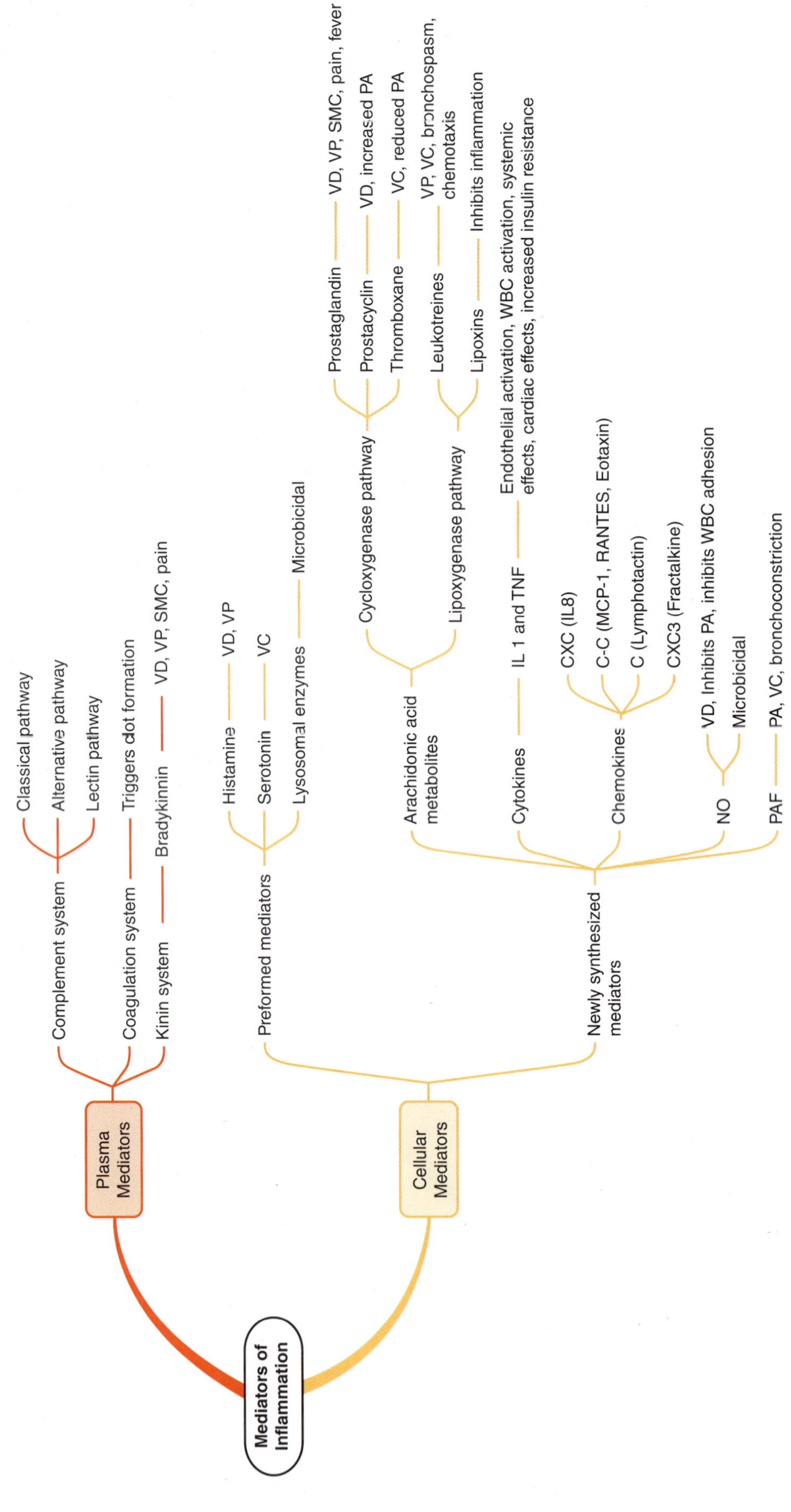
Mediators of Inflammation
Plasma Mediators
Complement system
Classical pathway
Alternative pathway
Lectin pathway
Coagulation system
Triggers clot formation
Kinin system
Bradykinnin
VD, VP, SMC, pain
Cellular Mediators
Preformed mediators
Histamine
VD, VP
Serotonin
VC
Lysosomal enzymes
Microbicidal
Newly synthesized mediators
Arachidonic acid metabolites
Cycloxygenase pathway
Prostaglandin
VD, VP, SMC, pain, fever
Prostacyclin
VD, increased PA
Thromboxane
VC, reduced PA
Lipoxygenase pathway
Leukotreines
VP, VC, bronchospasm, chemotaxis
Lipoxins
Inhibits inflammation
Cytokines
IL 1 and TNF
Endothelial activation, WBC activation, systemic effects, cardiac effects, increased insulin resistance
Chemokines
CXC (IL8)
C-C (MCP-1, RANTES, Eotaxin)
C (Lymphotactin)
CXC3 (Fractalkine)
NO
VD, Inhibits PA, inhibits WBC adhesion
Microbicidal
PAF
PA, VC, bronchoconstriction

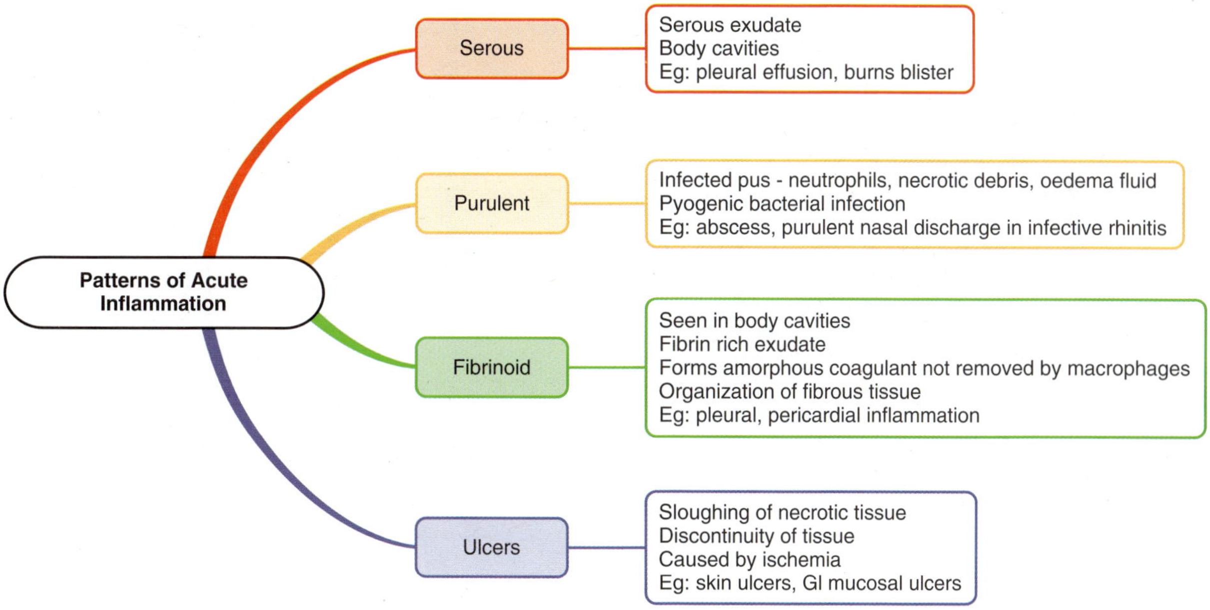
Patterns of Acute Inflammation
Serous
Serous exudate
Body cavities
Eg: pleural effusion, burns blister
Purulent
Infected pus - neutrophils, necrotic debris, oedema fluid
Pyogenic bacterial infection
Eg: abscess, purulent nasal discharge in infective rhinitis
Fibrinoid
Seen in body cavities
Fibrin rich exudate
Forms amorphous coagulant not removed by macrophages
Organization of fibrous tissue
Eg: pleural, pericardial inflammation
Ulcers
Sloughing of necrotic tissue
Discontinuity of tissue
Caused by ischemia
Eg: skin ulcers, GI mucosal ulcers

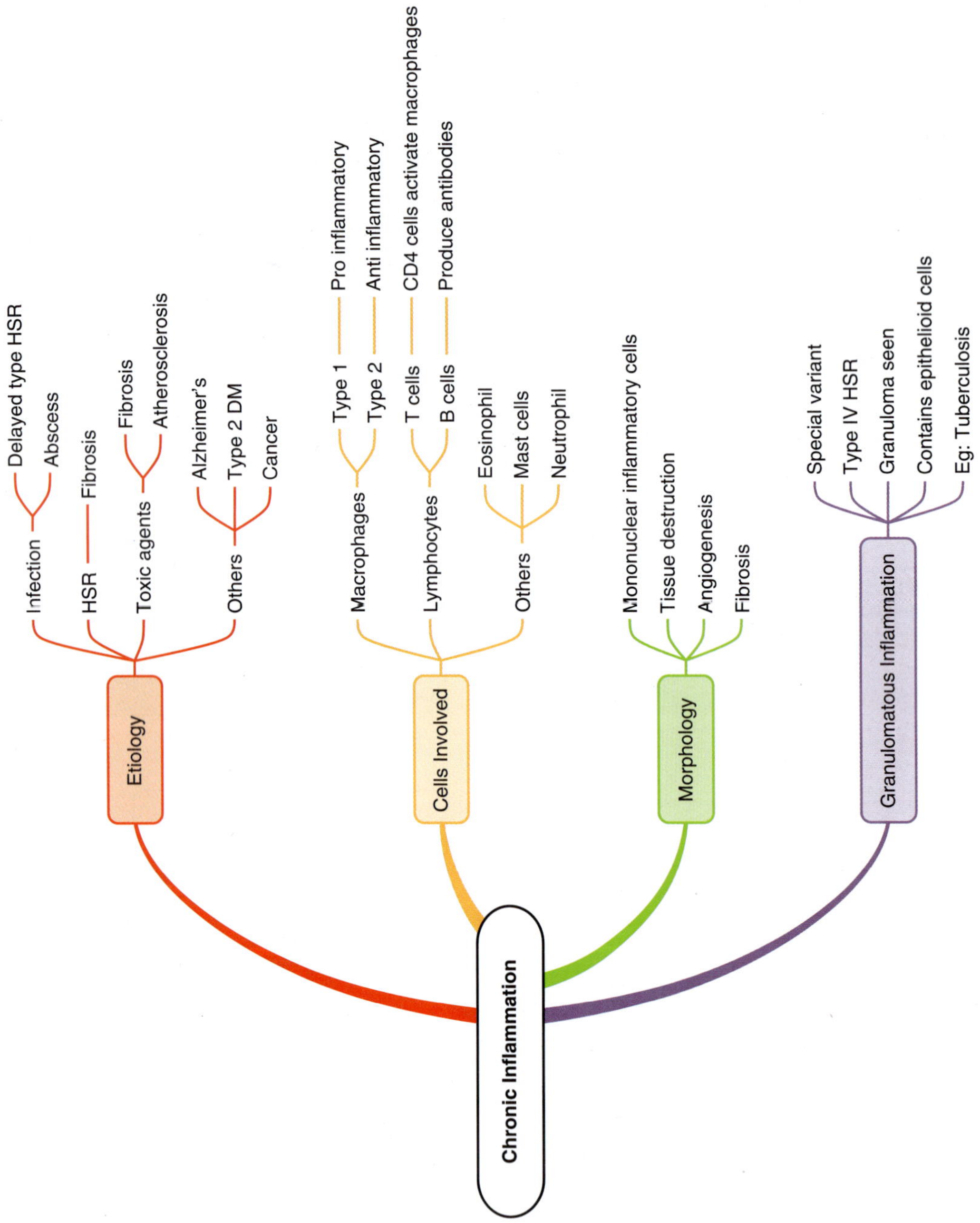
Chronic Inflammation
Etiology
Infection
Delayed type HSR
Abscess
HSR
Fibrosis
Toxic agents
Fibrosis
Atherosclerosis
Others
Alzheimer's
Type 2 DM
Cancer
Cells Involved
Macrophages
Type 1
Pro inflammatory
Type 2
Anti inflammatory
Lymphocytes
T cells
CD4 cells activate macrophages
B cells
Produce antibodies
Others
Eosinophil
Mast cells
Neutrophil
Morphology
Mononuclear inflammatory cells
Tissue destruction
Angiogenesis
Fibrosis
Granulomatous Inflammation
Special variant
Type IV HSR
Granuloma seen
Contains epitheloid cells
Eg: Tuberculosis

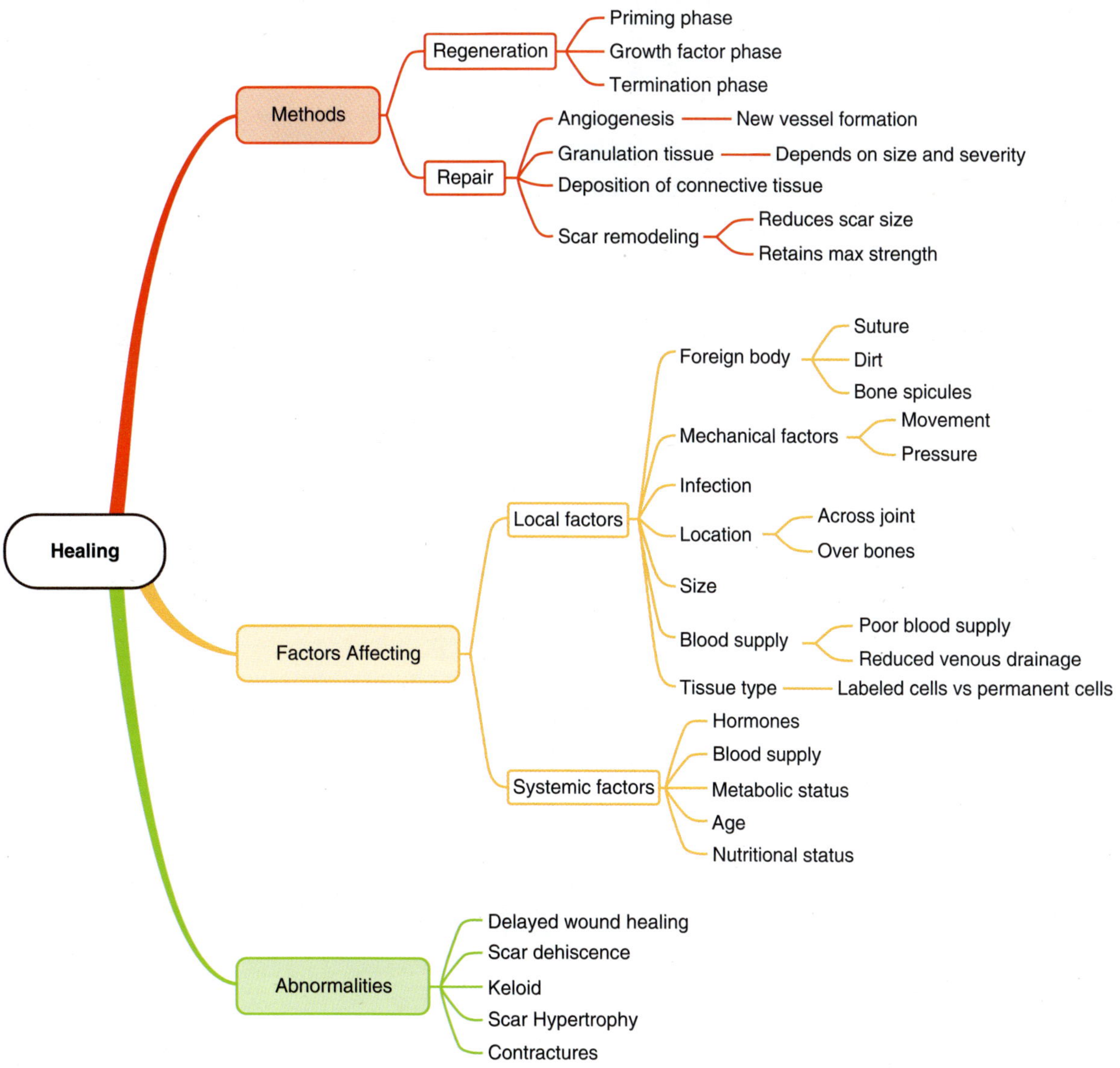
Healing
Methods
Regeneration
Priming phase
Growth factor phase
Termination phase
Repair
Angiogenesis
New vessel formation
Granulation tissue
Depends on size and severity
Deposition of connective tissue
Scar remodeling
Reduces scar size
Retains max strength
Factors Affecting
Local factors
Foreign body
Suture
Dirt
Bone spicules
Mechanical factors
Movement
Pressure
Infection
Location
Across joint
Over bones
Size
Blood supply
Poor blood supply
Reduced venous drainage
Tissue type
Labeled cells vs permanent cells
Systemic factors
Hormones
Blood supply
Metabolic status
Age
Nutritional status
Abnormalities
Delayed wound healing
Scar dehiscence
Keloid
Scar Hypertrophy
Contractures

4 Haemodynamic Disorders

Leena Dennis Joseph

PA 6.1 Define and describe **oedema** and its types, pathogenesis and clinical correlations.

PA 6.2 Define and describe **hyperaemia, congestion and haemorrhage.**

PA 6.3 Define and describe **shock** and its pathogenesis and stages.

PA 6.4 Define and describe normal **haemostasis** and the aetiopathogenesis and consequences of **thrombosis.**

PA 6.5 Define and describe **embolism** and its causes and common types.

PA 6.6 Define and describe **ischaemia–infarction,** its types, aetiology, morphological changes and clinical effects.

CHAPTER OUTLINE

INTRODUCTION

Haemodynamics plays a vital role in human health and circulation of blood, which is crucial for the delivery of oxygen and nutrients and also for the removal of waste generated by metabolism. Under normal circumstances, the fluid is retained within the blood vessels; because of the proteins in the plasma, very little fluid leaks out into the interstitial spaces.

Many pathological conditions can alter this fluid balance by mechanisms such as endothelial injury or dysfunction, increased hydrostatic pressure or decreased proteins in the blood.

Most of the diseases of blood vessels and the cardiovascular system depend on these haemodynamic mechanisms. Haemostasis is the process of blood clotting that prevents excess blood loss through the formation of clot. However, when this occurs within a moving circulation, it is called thrombosis, which may further move away from its site of origin and embolize, leading to haemodynamic disturbances. Thromboembolism contributes to the three major causes of death in developed countries – myocardial infarction, pulmonary embolism and cerebrovascular accident (stroke).

Similarly, inadequate haemostasis can lead to haemorrhage and excess fluid loss, which can compromise the blood flow and result in hypoperfusion and even shock. With this introduction, we discuss the main entities that contribute to the major haemodynamic disturbances in the body.

HYPERAEMIA AND CONGESTION PA 6.2

'Hyperaemia' and 'congestion' are the terms used for localized increase in the volume of blood within dilated vessels in a tissue/organ (Table 4.1).

Hyperaemia is an **active process** in which arteriolar dilatation leads to increased blood flow to a tissue/organ, whereas the impaired venous drainage is a **passive process** and is called venous congestion (Fig. 4.1). If the condition develops rapidly, it is called **acute**; if it is of prolonged duration and has gradual response, it is called **chronic.**

HYPERAEMIA

Hyperaemia is an active process in which arteriolar dilatation leads to increased blood flow to a tissue or organ.

Causes of hyperaemia can be physiological or pathological.

Physiological causes: It may be in response to an increased functional demand; examples are heart and skeletal muscles during exercise.

Table 4.1 Differences Between Hyperaemia and Congestion

	Hyperaemia	Congestion
Process	Active	Passive
Mechanism	Increase in blood supply to the tissue and arteriolar dilatation	Accumulation of venous blood in an organ
Oedema	Absent	Present
Colour	Red	Blue
Oxygenation	Oxygenated blood	Deoxygenated blood
Causes	a. Physiological as in exercise b. Hormonal c. Fever d. Inflammation	Because of generalized congestion as in left ventricular failure, mitral stenosis, constrictive pericarditis
Hypoxia	No	Can cause hypoxia

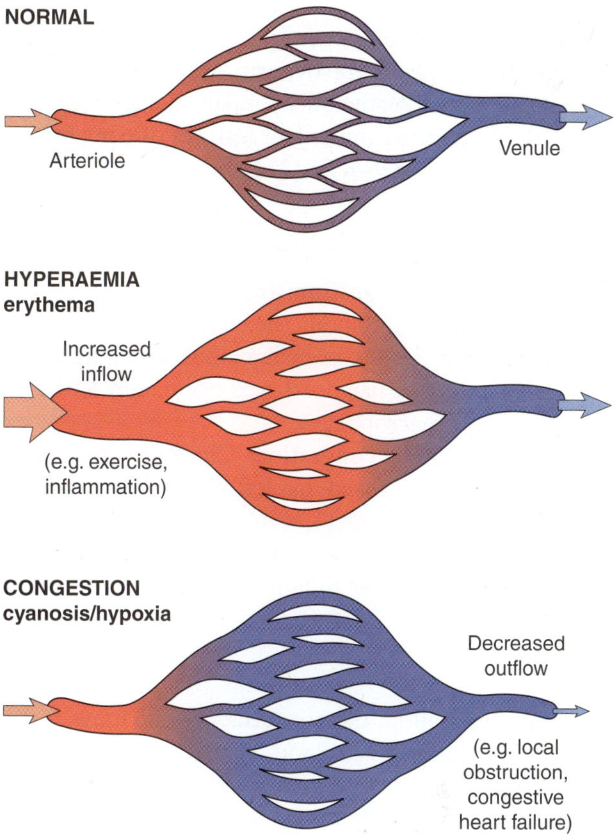

Fig. 4.1 Hyperaemia and congestion.

Pathological causes: It is seen in inflammation and is responsible for the heat (calor) and redness (rubor) of the tissue/organ.

CONGESTION

Congestion is a passive process, resulting from impaired outflow of venous blood from a tissue. Passive congestion may be **systemic**, when it involves multiple organs simultaneously as in congestive cardiac failure, or it may be **localized**, because of venous obstruction as in congestion of the leg veins in deep vein thrombosis (DVT) leading to oedema of the lower extremities. It can also be because of compression of the veins, as seen with external factors, tumours, pregnancy, etc.

Acute congestion develops during shock, or in sudden right-sided heart failure, and occurs in the lung and liver. **Chronic passive** congestion develops slowly over the course of weeks or months, as the outflow of blood from the affected part is slowly reduced or when partial obstruction to the outflow of blood persists.

Morphology

Congested tissues have an abnormal blue-red colour (cyanosis) because of stasis of red blood cells (RBCs) and accumulation of deoxygenated haemoglobin.

Long-standing congestion leads to inadequate tissue perfusion and persistent hypoxia, which can lead to parenchymal cell death and secondary tissue fibrosis.

Here we describe the salient features of congestion in the lung, liver, spleen and kidney.

PULMONARY VENOUS CONGESTION

Acute pulmonary congestion: The alveolar capillaries are dilated and filled with blood. The congestion, which is of a short duration, results in oedematous widening of the alveolar septa. Small haemorrhages occur, and RBCs are engulfed by the macrophages.

Chronic pulmonary congestion: Chronic venous congestion is usually caused by **left-sided heart failure,** which may be secondary to acute myocardial infarction, cardiomyopathies, hypertensive or valvular heart diseases. This leads to a rise in pulmonary venous pressure.

Morphology

In acute congestion, the cut surface of the lungs feels wet and typically oozes blood. In chronic congestion, the lungs are heavy and firm in consistency. The cut surface is dark or rusty brown (brown induration).

In chronic pulmonary congestion, a large number of macrophages containing haemosiderin accumulate in the alveoli. These cells are called **heart failure cells**. There is also the presence of **transudate** in the alveoli. The alveoli are filled with smooth to slightly floccular pink material, a characteristic of pulmonary oedema. **Capillaries** in the alveolar wall are congested with many RBCs (Fig. 4.2).

In cases of a longer duration, the lungs may also become fibrotic, because collagen is laid down in the alveolar walls. Hard brown lungs are called **brown induration**.

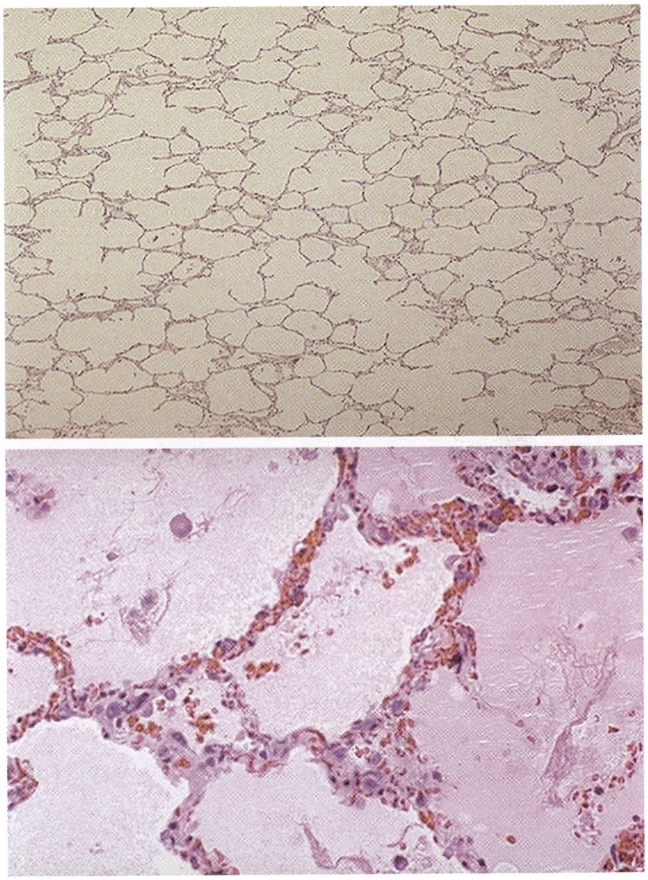

Fig. 4.2 Normal lungs (above) and lungs in chronic venous congestion (below), microscopy. High power, the alveoli in this lung are filled with a smooth to slightly floccular pink material, a characteristic of pulmonary oedema. Note also that the capillaries in the alveolar walls are congested with many red blood cells. (*Source:* https://webpath.med.utah.edu/LUNGHTML/LUNG004.html.)

HEPATIC VENOUS CONGESTION

Acute hepatic congestion: In short-duration congestion, the central vein and sinusoids are distended with blood and there may be even necrosis of centrally located hepatocytes. The periportal hepatocytes that are better oxygenated because of their proximity to the hepatic arterioles may develop fatty change.

Chronic hepatic congestion: Long-standing chronic **right-sided heart failure** increases venous pressure, resulting in chronic venous congestion of the liver. Rare causes include constrictive pericarditis, tricuspid stenosis and obstruction of the inferior vena cava and hepatic vein.

Morphology

The liver increases in size and weight and the capsule appears tense. The cut surface shows **a nutmeg appearance** because of alternate dark and light areas (Fig. 4.3).

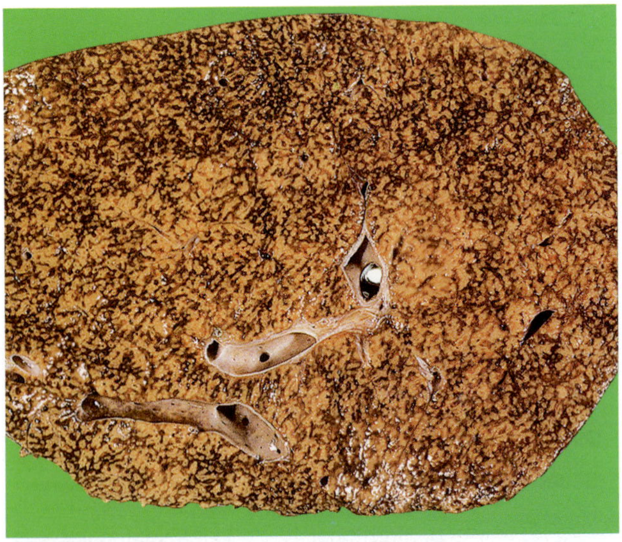

Fig. 4.3 Chronic venous congestion of liver, gross. The variegated light and dark colours reflect fat accumulating in zone 1/2 hepatocytes and central acinar congestion/hepatocellular atrophy. This appearance is compared with the cut surface of a nutmeg ('nutmeg' liver). (*Source:* From S. Kim Suvarna. Cardiovascular system. Underwood's Pathology. 2019. Elsevier.)

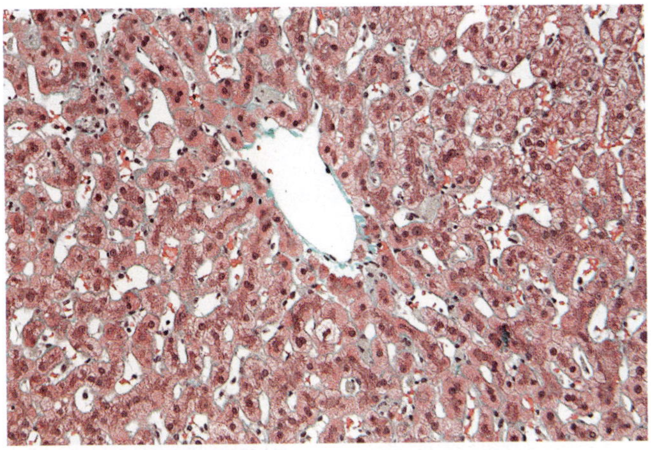

Fig. 4.4 Chronic venous congestion of liver, microscopy. Trichrome stain. Note the presence of perisinusoidal fibrosis and centrilobular (zone III) sinusoidal dilation. (*Source:* https://en.wikipedia.org/wiki/Congestive_hepatopathy.)

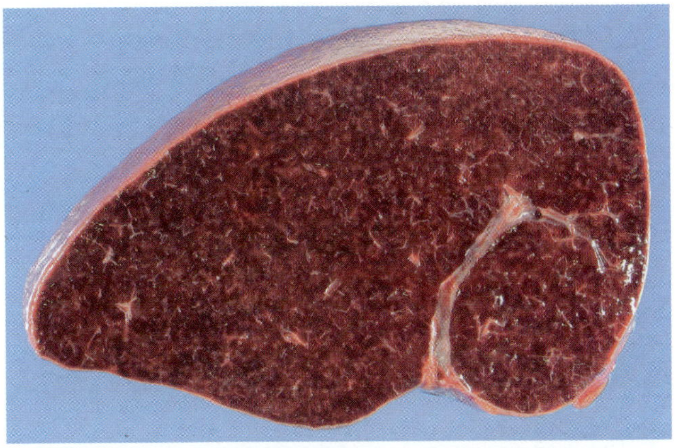

Fig. 4.5 Chronic venous congestion of spleen, gross. A notable feature is the firmness of the unfixed spleen on cut section, feeling almost as firm as liver. In this example, the fibrous trabeculae are also prominent. (*Source:* From Andrew J. Connolly, Walter E. Finkbeiner, Philip C. Ursell and Richard L. Davis. Atlas of Gross Autopsy Pathology. Autopsy Pathology: A Manual and Atlas. 3rd Edition. 2016. Elsevier.)

The congested centrilobular regions are dark red to brown in colour. Congestion is most prominent around the central veins within the hepatic lobules. The periportal hepatocytes, which are better oxygenated regions, appear pale because of fatty change.

Microscopic examination shows **centrilobular hepatocyte necrosis**, haemorrhage and haemosiderin-laden macrophages. Thickening of central veins and fibrosis is seen in prolonged venous congestion. Periportal regions show **fatty change** (Fig. 4.4).

CHRONIC VENOUS CONGESTION OF SPLEEN

Congestive splenomegaly most often occurs in **portal hypertension** because of cirrhosis and right-sided cardiac failure with cor pulmonale. Decreased portal venous drainage leads to congestive splenomegaly.

The increased portal venous pressure causes dilatation of sinusoids, with slowing of blood flow from the cords to the sinusoids. This prolongs the exposure of blood cells to the macrophages, resulting in excessive trapping and destruction leading to hypersplenism. Perivascular haemorrhages result in organization.

Morphology

The spleen is moderately enlarged and can weigh up to 1000 g. It is firm in consistency. It is deeply congested, tense and cyanotic, and the cut surface is grey-tan in colour (Fig. 4.5).

The red pulp is enlarged because of congestion and marked sinusoidal dilatation. **Capillarization** of sinusoids may occur, in which sinusoids are converted into capillaries. There is hyperplasia of reticuloendothelial cells in the red pulp of the spleen and fibrous thickening of the capsule and trabeculae.

Small haemorrhages in the pulp cause foci of scarring, which measure 1–2 mm in diameter and are called **Gamna–Gandy bodies or nodules or siderofibrotic nodules**. The coarse collagen bundles in the scar are encrusted with iron and calcium. A few macrophages containing haemosiderin are present among the collagen bundles.

CHRONIC VENOUS CONGESTION OF KIDNEY

Morphology

The kidneys are slightly enlarged and the medulla is congested.

The changes are mild, and the tubules may show degenerative changes such as cloudy swelling and fatty change.

HAEMORRHAGE PA 6.2

Haemorrhage or bleeding occurs because of rupture of blood vessels, leading to the passage of blood into nonvascular spaces, or exterior of the body, into the hollow organs or body cavities. It is derived from the Greek word '*hem*' for blood and '*orrhage*', which means to burst. Haemorrhage occurs when the integrity of blood vessels is compromised. This can happen because of direct trauma, which disrupts the vessel wall, or through diseases that weaken vessel walls, such as aneurysms or vasculitis. In coagulopathies, even minor vascular injuries can lead to significant bleeding because of impaired clotting. The body's response to acute blood loss includes vasoconstriction to reduce blood flow to the injured area, increased heart rate and cardiac output to maintain circulation, and the mobilization of clotting factors to stop bleeding.

Table 4.2 Causes of Haemorrhage

- Trauma
- Surgical procedures
- Rupture of an aneurysm
- Vitamin C deficiency
- Thrombocytopenia
- Deficiency of coagulation factors
- Tumours and infections
- Atherosclerosis
- Vasculitis
- Hypertension

The common causes of haemorrhage are listed in Table 4.2.

CLINICAL SIGNIFICANCE

On the basis of the size of the haemorrhage, the lesions are classified into the following (Fig. 4.6):

Petechiae: This term is derived from the Italian word for freckle. These are minute 1- to 2-mm diameter haemorrhages into the skin, mucous membranes or serosal surfaces. These could be because of low platelet count, defective platelet function or loss of vascular wall support as in vitamin C deficiency.

These represent rupture of capillaries or arterioles and occur in conjunction with coagulopathies or vasculitis.

A unique type of pinpoint haemorrhages is Janeway lesions, which are seen under the nails in bacterial endocarditis.

Purpura: These are slightly larger haemorrhages (3–5 mm in size). These could be because of trauma or vascular inflammation or increased vascular fragility. Purpura in Greek means *purple*.

Ecchymosis: These are larger 1- to 2-cm lesions, also called bruises. These change colour as the lesion progresses, from red-blue colour of haemoglobin to blue-green colour of bilirubin to golden brown colour of haemosiderin.

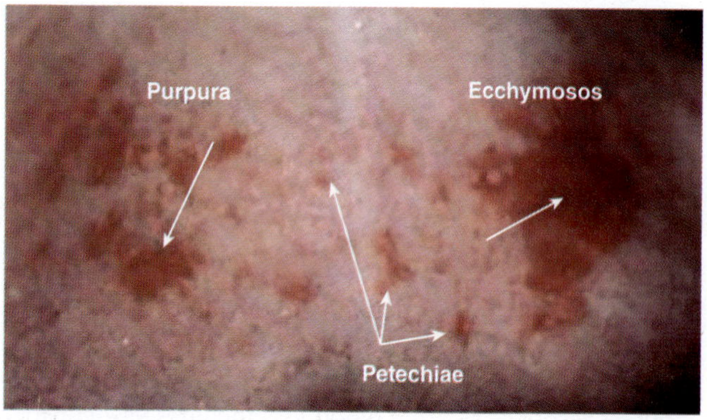

Fig. 4.6 Clinical pictures of petechiae, purpura and ecchymosis. Note the difference in their sizes. (*Source:* https://www.rdhmag.com/career-profession/personal-wellness/article/16405016/petechiae-ecchymoses-or-purpura#&gid=1&pid=2.)

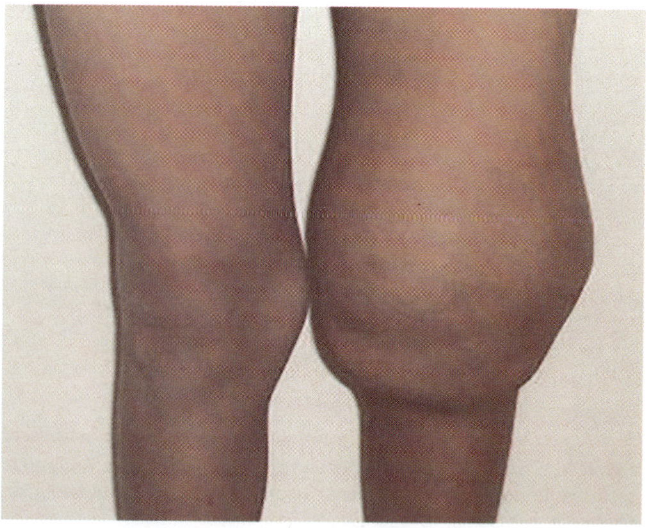

Fig. 4.7 Clinical picture of haemarthrosis. (*Source:* https://link.springer.com/article/10.1007/s00270-012-0480-3.)

Haemarthrosis (Fig. 4.7)**, haemopericardium and haemothorax:** These are haemorrhages that occur in the joint space, pericardium and pleural space, respectively.

Occasional loss of up to 20% of blood volume usually causes no disability. However, even a small bleed into a closed space like the cranial cavity can cause a rise in the intracranial pressure and lead to death.

If a large volume of blood is lost from the body, hypovolaemic shock develops. Repeated minor haemorrhages that cause slow leakage of blood eventually cause iron-deficiency anaemia.

OEDEMA AND EFFUSIONS — PA 6.1

Oedema is defined as an **abnormal and excessive accumulation of free fluid in the interstitial tissue spaces and serous cavities**. The term 'oedema' is derived from the Greek word '*Oidema*', which means swelling.

Normally, around 60% of the body weight is water, of which one-third is present as **extracellular fluid** and two-third as **intracellular fluid.**

The extracellular fluid compartment is present either intravascularly or in the interstitial space. When fluid accumulates in the interstitial space, it is called oedema. Oedema may be localized when it is limited to an organ or limb, e.g. in lymphatic oedema or in allergic oedema.

When oedema is generalized and diffuse, it is called **anasarca or dropsy** (Fig. 4.8) and it is usually detected in the subcutaneous tissues, e.g. renal oedema, cardiac oedema or nutritional oedema.

However, when the fluid accumulates in body cavities, these have specific names:

Abdominal cavity: **Ascites** (Fig. 4.9)
Pleural cavity: **Pleural effusion**

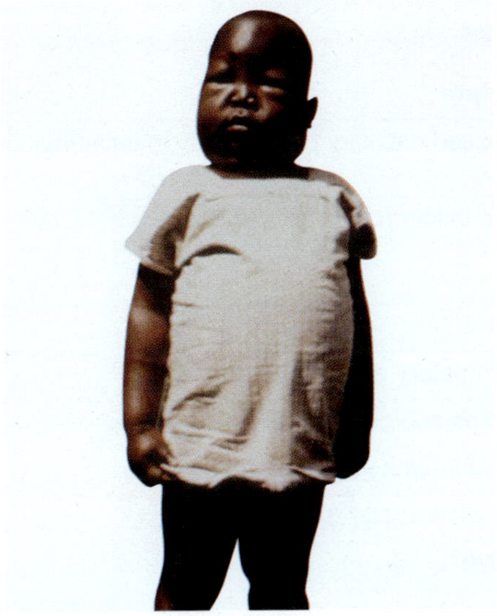

Fig. 4.8 Clinical picture of anasarca. (*Source:* https://en.wikipedia.org/wiki/Anasarca.)

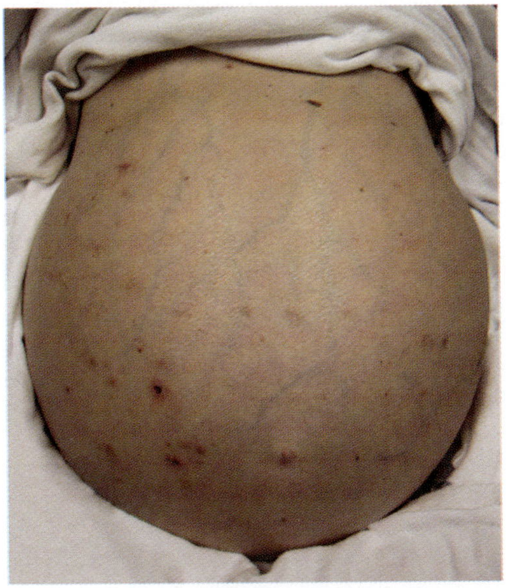

Fig. 4.9 Clinical picture of ascites. Note the prominence of superficial veins. (*Source:* https://en.wikipedia.org/wiki/Ascites.)

Pericardial cavity: **Hydropericardium/pericardial effusion**
Thoracic cavity: **Hydrothorax**

Depending on the fluid composition, the oedematous fluid may be a **transudate or an exudate** (Table 4.3).

A transudate is an ultrafiltrate of the plasma, which occurs because of alterations in the hydrostatic pressure or oncotic pressure (noninflammatory oedema). An exudate is secondary to increased capillary permeability (inflammatory oedema).

PATHOGENESIS

Oedema is caused by mechanisms that interfere with the normal fluid balance of plasma, interstitial fluid and lymph flow (Table 4.4). The normal movement of fluid between the vascular and extravascular (interstitial) spaces is affected by five main factors (Fig. 4.10):

- Elevated capillary hydrostatic pressure
- Reduced plasma osmotic pressure (oncotic pressure)
- Lymphatic obstruction
- Sodium and water retention
- Increased vascular permeability

The pathophysiology of oedema involves an imbalance in the Starling forces that govern fluid exchange across capillary walls. In heart failure, increased hydrostatic pressure because of congested venous circulation leads to fluid transudation into interstitial spaces. In renal disease, reduced albumin synthesis or loss (as in nephrotic syndrome) lowers plasma oncotic pressure, causing fluid leakage. Liver cirrhosis impairs albumin synthesis and can lead to portal hypertension, both contributing to oedema formation.

Elevated Capillary Hydrostatic Pressure

The hydrostatic pressure of the capillaries is the force that drives the fluid from the capillaries to the interstitial space. A rise in the hydrostatic pressure at the venular end of the capillary results in minimal or no reabsorption of fluid, resulting in oedema. Increase in hydrostatic pressure is mainly caused by disorders that impair venous return.

Examples of oedema, depending on this mechanism, are as follows:

- *Oedema of cardiac diseases*, as seen in congestive cardiac failure and constrictive pericarditis (*cardiac oedema)*
- *Ascites in liver diseases*, as seen in cirrhosis (the liver is nodular and fibrotic, with consequent portal hypertension)
- *DVT*, with subsequent obstruction, leading to oedema in the lower extremities
- *Gravid uterus* causing pressure and oedema of the legs
- *Varicose veins* and associated oedema

Reduced Plasma Oncotic Pressure

The plasma oncotic pressure is the pressure exerted by the total amount of plasma proteins, which tend to draw fluid into the vessels. A fall in the total plasma protein levels (hypoproteinaemia of less than 5 g/dL) results in a lower oncotic pressure, which cannot counter the effect of hydrostatic pressure of blood and results in oedema. Albumin is the main plasma protein that exerts osmotic pressure, around four times more than globulin.

Examples of oedema, depending on this mechanism, are as follows:

- *Oedema of renal disease*, as seen in nephrotic syndrome, acute glomerulonephritis
- *Ascites of liver diseases*, in which albumin production is decreased

Table 4.3 Differences Between Transudate and Exudates

Features	Transudate	Exudate
Causes	Increased hydrostatic pressure or decreased oncotic pressure	Increased capillary permeability in inflammation
Pathological states	Congestive heart failure Hypoproteinaemia Nephrotic syndrome	Acute inflammation
Endothelial permeability	Normal	Altered
Fluid nature	Ultrafiltrate of plasma	Inflammatory extravascular fluid
Composition	Water and dissolved electrolytes	Proteins and cellular debris
Colour	Straw-coloured	Yellowish-white opaque appearance
pH	Alkaline (>7.3)	Less alkaline (<7.3)
Specific gravity	<1.012	>1.020
Protein content	Low (<3 g/dL)	High
Glucose content	Same as that of blood	Low in infection
Ratio of LDH levels in fluid and serum	Low (<0.6)	High (>0.6)
Light microscopy	Inflammatory cells are absent	Neutrophils in acute inflammation Macrophages and lymphocytes in chronic inflammation

LDH, low-density lipoprotein.

Table 4.4 Pathophysiological Categories of Oedema

Mechanism	Causes
Elevated hydrostatic pressure	***Impaired venous return*** • Congestive heart failure • Constrictive pericarditis • Ascites because of liver cirrhosis • Venous obstruction/compression because of tumours, thrombosis and lower extremity inactivity ***Arteriolar dilatation*** • Heat • Neurohormonal dysregulation
Reduced plasma oncotic pressure	Protein-losing glomerulopathies Malnutrition Liver cirrhosis Protein-losing gastroenteropathy
Lymphatic obstruction	Inflammatory Neoplastic Postirradiation Postsurgical
Sodium retention	Excessive salt intake with renal insufficiency Increased tubular reabsorption of sodium • Renal hypoperfusion • Increased renin–angiotensin–aldosterone secretion
Inflammation	Acute inflammation Chronic inflammation

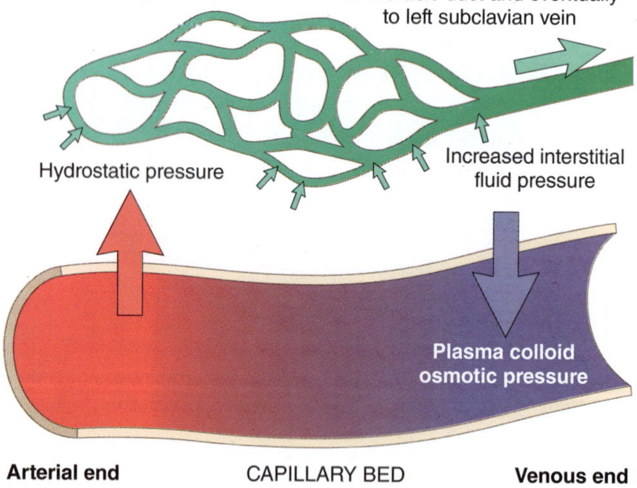

Fig. 4.10 Hydrostatic, oncotic pressure and lymphatic flow in health. (*Source:* From Vinay Kumar, Abul K. Abbas and Jon C. Aster. Hemodynamic Disorders, Thromboembolic Disease, and Shock. In Robbins & Cotran Pathologic Basis of Disease. 10th edition. 2021. Elsevier.)

- *Protein-losing enteropathies*
- *Protein malnutrition*
- *Malabsorption syndrome*

Lymphatic Obstruction

In the normal course, the interstitial fluid that escapes is cleared by the lymphatic system. If there is an obstruction in the lymphatic drainage, it can result in oedema.

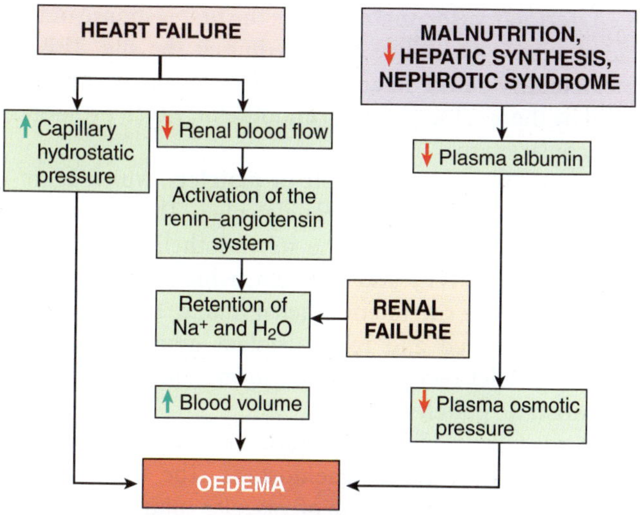

Fig. 4.11 Mechanisms of oedema in heart failure, renal failure, malnutrition, liver failure and nephrotic syndrome. (*Source:* From Robbins & Cotran Pathologic Basis of Disease, 10th edition. 2021. Elsevier.)

Examples of oedema, depending on this mechanism, are as follows (Fig. 4.11):

- Occlusion of the lymphatics by inflammation and fibrosis, by *Wuchereria bancrofti* as in filariasis, leads to chronic lymphoedema of the scrotum in male patients and elephantiasis in both sexes.
- Removal of the axillary lymph nodes in mastectomy for carcinoma of the breast can lead to lymphoedema of the affected arm.
- Infiltration and obstruction of the superficial lymphatics in breast cancer can cause oedema of the overlying skin (*peau d'orange*).
- External pressure on the lymphatics can also produce lymphoedema.
- Occlusion of the lymphatic channels by malignant cells can also result in lymphatic oedema.

Sodium and Water Retention

The majority of sodium is reabsorbed by the proximal convoluted tubules of the kidney under the influence of either intrinsic renal mechanisms or extrarenal mechanisms, whereas water balance is controlled by antidiuretic hormone (ADH).

INFLAMMATION

Oedema in inflammation is discussed in Chapter 3, 'Pathological basis of inflammation'.

MORPHOLOGY OF OEDEMA

Subcutaneous tissue: Oedema can be diffuse or conspicuous in regions with high hydrostatic pressure. The localization may be dependent on gravity, as seen in the legs, when a person is ambulatory, or in the sacrum, as seen when a person is bedridden **(dependent oedema)**.

Finger pressure over the oedematous tissue may result in displacement of the interstitial fluid, leaving a depression and this is called **pitting oedema**.

Because of increase in hyaluronic acid and chondroitin sulphate, patients develop pretibial **nonpitting oedema** in myxoedema and retrobulbar oedema in Graves disease (exophthalmos).

Periorbital oedema is the classical localization of oedema in renal dysfunction, as the oedematous fluid tends to collect in areas of loose connective tissues.

Pulmonary oedema: Lungs are two or three times their normal weight, and the cut surface brings forth frothy, blood-tinged fluid.

Brain oedema can be localized or generalized. The swollen brain exhibits narrowed sulci and distended gyri, which are compressed by the skull.

Effusions: These may involve body cavities as seen in hydrothorax, hydropericardium or ascites. The fluid may be a transudate or an exudate; it may even be chylous, as seen in lymphatic obstruction.

Microscopy

Oedema is easily recognized as clearing and separation of the extracellular matrix (ECM) and cell swelling.

Clinical Features

Looking out for *subcutaneous oedema* may help in ruling out a cardiac or renal disease.

Treating oedema is important because it impairs wound healing and clearance of infections.

Pulmonary oedema can present as dyspnoea as a result of impedance in oxygen diffusion and also at times may get complicated with bacterial infection.

Ascitic fluid can also get infected with bacteria, leading to a serious and sometimes fatal infection.

Brain oedema is life threatening; when severe, the brain may herniate through the foramen magnum or the brainstem vascular supply may get compressed. This may cause death of the patient.

HAEMOSTASIS PA 6.4

Normal haemostasis is a series of regulated processes that finally lead to the formation of a blood clot that limits bleeding from an injured vessel. The pathological counterpart of this mechanism is thrombosis, which is the formation of a blood clot within an uninjured intact blood vessel.

Normal haemostasis is a process involving **endothelium, platelets and clotting factors** that occurs at the site of vascular injury and culminates in the formation of a blood clot, reducing the extent of bleeding.

Haemostasis is achieved through the steps given next (Fig. 4.12).

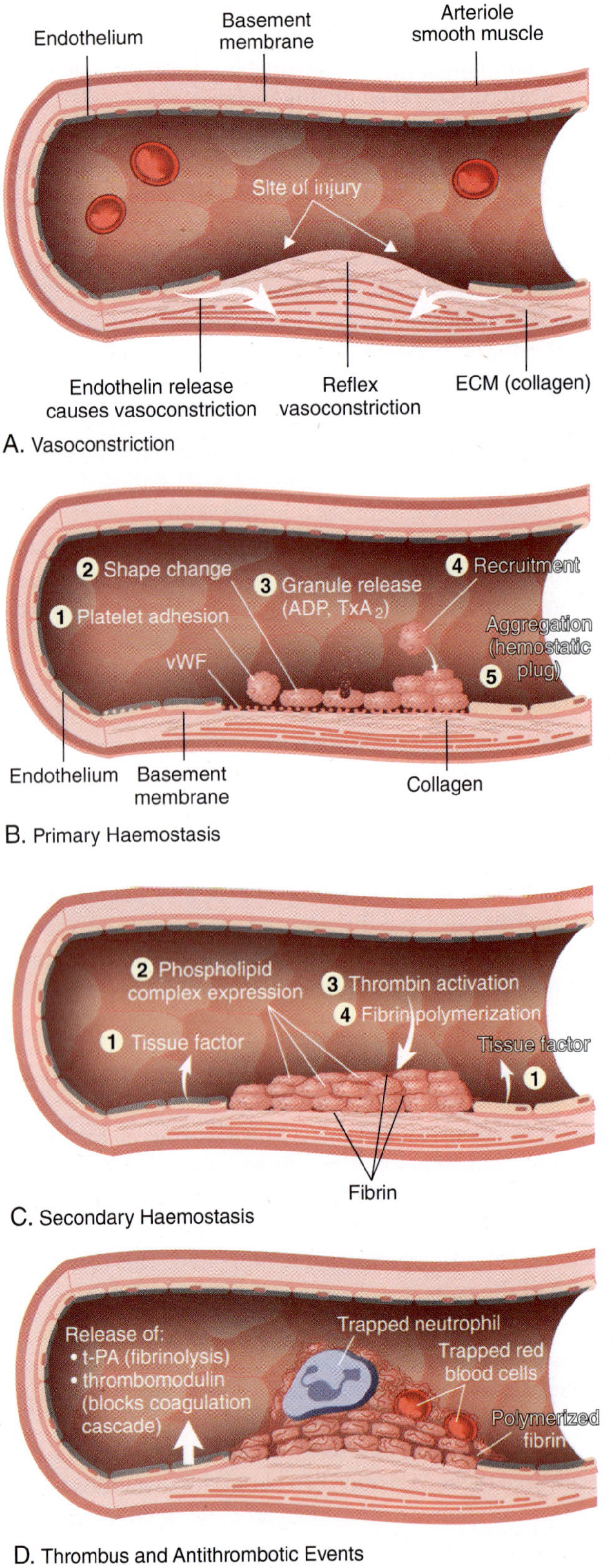

Fig. 4.12 Events in haemostasis – vasoconstriction, primary haemostatic plug formation, secondary haemostatic plug formation, thrombus and antithrombotic events. (*Source:* From Robbins & Cotran Pathologic Basis of Disease, 10th edition. 2021. Elsevier.)

Arteriolar vasoconstriction is the first response of the blood vessels to reduce the bleeding at the site. This is mediated by reflex neurogenic mechanisms and facilitated by the local secretion of endothelin, which promotes vasoconstriction.

This is followed by the **role of platelets,** which aggregate to form the primary platelet plug. This is brought about by the exposure of the subendothelial von Willebrand factor (vWF) and collagen, which cause platelet adhesion to the site of endothelial injury. These platelets become activated and release potent granules, causing further platelet recruitment and formation of a **primary haemostatic platelet plug.**

This is followed by the formation of a secondary platelet plug and secondary haemostasis. The tissue factor, which is released at the site of vascular injury, binds and activates factor VII, which leads to the formation of thrombin. Thrombin cleaves the circulating fibrinogen into insoluble fibrin, creating a fibrin meshwork and forming a secondary plug. This process is called **secondary haemostasis.**

The aggregated platelets and fibrin undergo contraction to form a solid permanent plug, which prevents further bleeding from the site of injury. This clot formation is kept in check by the counter-regulatory mechanisms such as tissue plasminogen activator, which is produced by the endothelial cells.

ROLE OF ENDOTHELIUM IN NORMAL HAEMOSTASIS

Endothelial cells have both prothrombotic and antithrombotic properties. The balance between the two properties determines whether a thrombus is formed or not (Fig. 4.13).

The antithrombotic properties are based on the fact that they have antiplatelet, anticoagulant and fibrinolytic effects.

The **antiplatelet effect** is mediated by the fact that an intact endothelium prevents platelet adhesion and also produces inhibitors of platelet aggregation, such as prostacyclin (PGI_2), nitric oxide (NO) and adenosine diphosphatase, which degrade adenosine diphosphate.

The **anticoagulant effect** of the endothelium is mediated by the presence of heparin-like molecules, thrombomodulin and tissue pathway inhibitor.

The **fibrinolytic effects** are mediated by the presence of tissue plasminogen activator (t-PA), which degrades the thrombus as soon as it forms.

The **prothrombotic properties** of the endothelium are brought forth by the three basic features of the endothelium, which include platelet effects, procoagulant effects and antifibrinolytic effects.

The injured endothelium exposes the subendothelial connective tissue which allows adhesion of platelets. vWF is also a cofactor that helps in platelet binding.

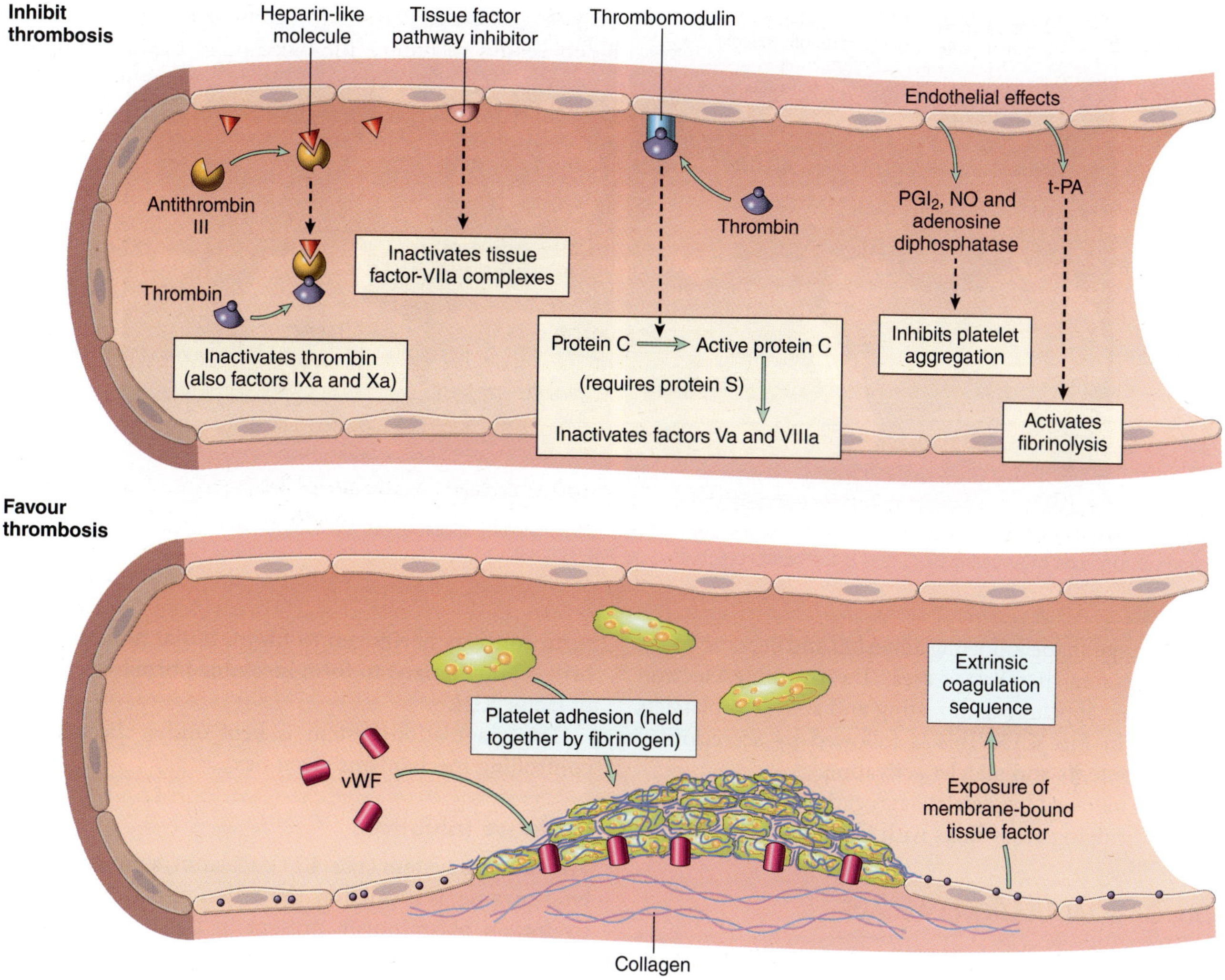

Fig. 4.13 Role of endothelium in haemostasis and thrombosis.

The endothelial cells secrete tissue factor, which activates the extrinsic coagulation pathway and promotes clot formation.

Endothelial cells also secrete inhibitors of plasminogen activators, which reduce fibrinolysis and tend to favour thrombosis.

ROLE OF PLATELETS IN NORMAL HAEMOSTASIS

Platelets play a critical role in haemostasis by the formation of a primary platelet plug to seal the vascular defect and by providing a surface for the clotting factors to act. These anucleate cell fragments are produced by megakaryocytes in the bone marrow. The platelets function via glycoprotein surface receptors, contractile cytoskeleton and two types of granules – the α-granules and the dense granules. These undergo a sequence of reactions that culminate in the formation of a platelet plug via platelet adhesion, activation and aggregation (Fig. 4.14).

Platelet adhesion is mediated by interactions with vWF, which acts as a bridge between the platelet surface receptor glycoprotein Ib (GpIb) and exposed collagen.

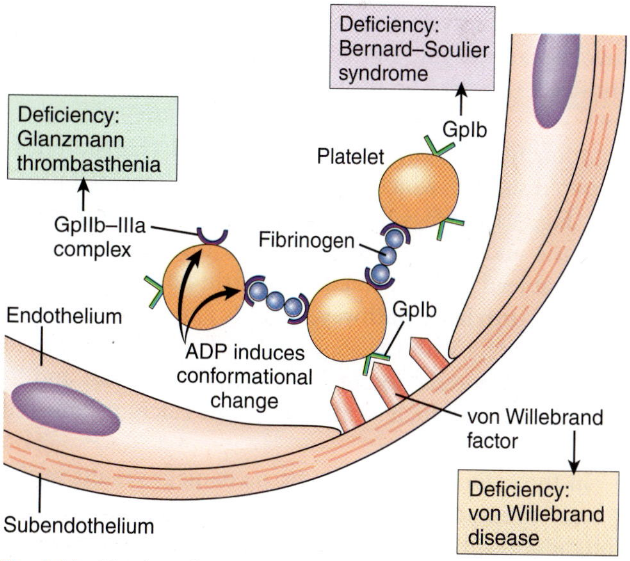

Fig. 4.14 Platelet adhesion and aggregation. von Willebrand factor functions as an adhesion bridge between subendothelial collagen and the glycoprotein Ib (GpIb) platelet receptor. Aggregation is accomplished by fibrinogen bridging GpIIb–IIIa receptors on different platelets. ADP, adenosine diphosphate. (*Source:* From Robbins & Cotran Pathologic Basis of Disease, 10th edition. 2021. Elsevier.)

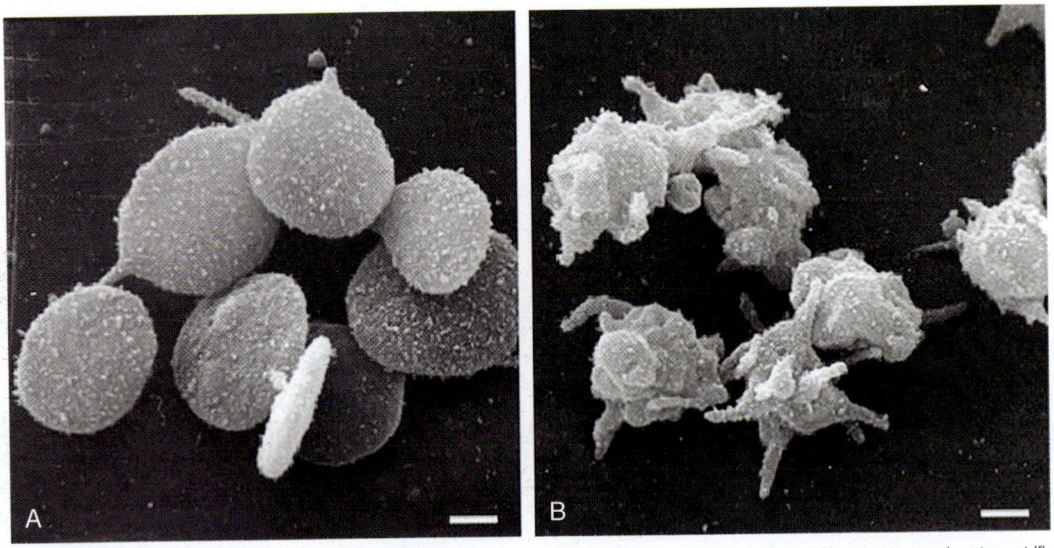

Fig. 4.15 Scanning electron microscopic pictures of resting and activated platelets. (*Source:* https://www.researchgate.net/figure/Scanning-electron-micrographs-of-A-resting-37-C-and-B-temperature-activated-20_fig7_6923881.)

These change shape following adhesion and become spiky, thus increasing the surface area. The scanning electron microscopic appearance of resting and activated platelets is shown in Fig. 4.15. This is followed by secretion of granule contents and platelet activation.

This is followed by platelet aggregation, which is facilitated by bridging cross-links with fibrinogen.

ROLE OF COAGULATION CASCADE

The coagulation cascade is a series of amplifying enzymatic reactions that lead to deposition of an insoluble fibrin clot. It is a sequence of events in which the clotting factors are activated and passed on to the next stage, where they activate the next factor. Each reaction step involves an enzyme (an activated coagulation factor), a substrate (inactive proenzyme form of a coagulation factor) and a cofactor (a reaction accelerator). All these components are assembled on a negatively charged phospholipid surface, which is provided by the activated platelets. Fig. 4.16 shows the schematic representation of the intrinsic and extrinsic pathways and the common pathway that lead to the formation of fibrin polymers.

In the **intrinsic pathway**, there is activation of factor XII on contact with the abnormal surface, which leads to a sequential interaction of factors XI, IX and VIII and finally factor X, which work along with calcium ions and platelet factor 3.

In the **extrinsic pathway**, tissue damage results in the release of tissue factor or thromboplastin. Tissue factor on interaction with factor VII activates factor X.

The **common pathway** begins where both intrinsic and extrinsic pathways converge to activate factor X, which forms a complex with factor Va and platelet factor 3 in the presence of calcium ions. This complex activates prothrombin (factor II) to thrombin (factor IIa), which, in turn, converts fibrinogen to fibrin. Initial monomeric fibrin is polymerized to form insoluble fibrin by activation of factor XIII.

The coagulation system is kept under check by the controlling mechanisms given next.

Protease Inhibitors

Fibrinolytic system (Fig. 4.17): Plasmin, a potent fibrinolytic enzyme, is formed by the action of plasminogen activator on plasminogen present in the normal plasma. Two types of plasminogen activators are identified:

- t-PA, which is derived from endothelial cells and leucocytes
- Urokinase-like plasminogen activator, which is present in the plasma

THROMBOSIS PA 6.4

Thrombosis is defined as the process of formation of a solid mass in the circulating blood from the constituents of flowing blood. The solid mass formed is called a thrombus, and it consists of an aggregate of coagulated blood containing platelets, fibrin and entrapped cellular elements of blood.

AETIOPATHOGENESIS

There are three primary abnormalities which can contribute to a thrombus formation, and these constitute the Virchow triad (Fig. 4.18). These include the following three components:

- **Injury to the endothelium**
- **Stasis or turbulent flow (changes in the blood flow)**
- **Hypercoagulability of blood**

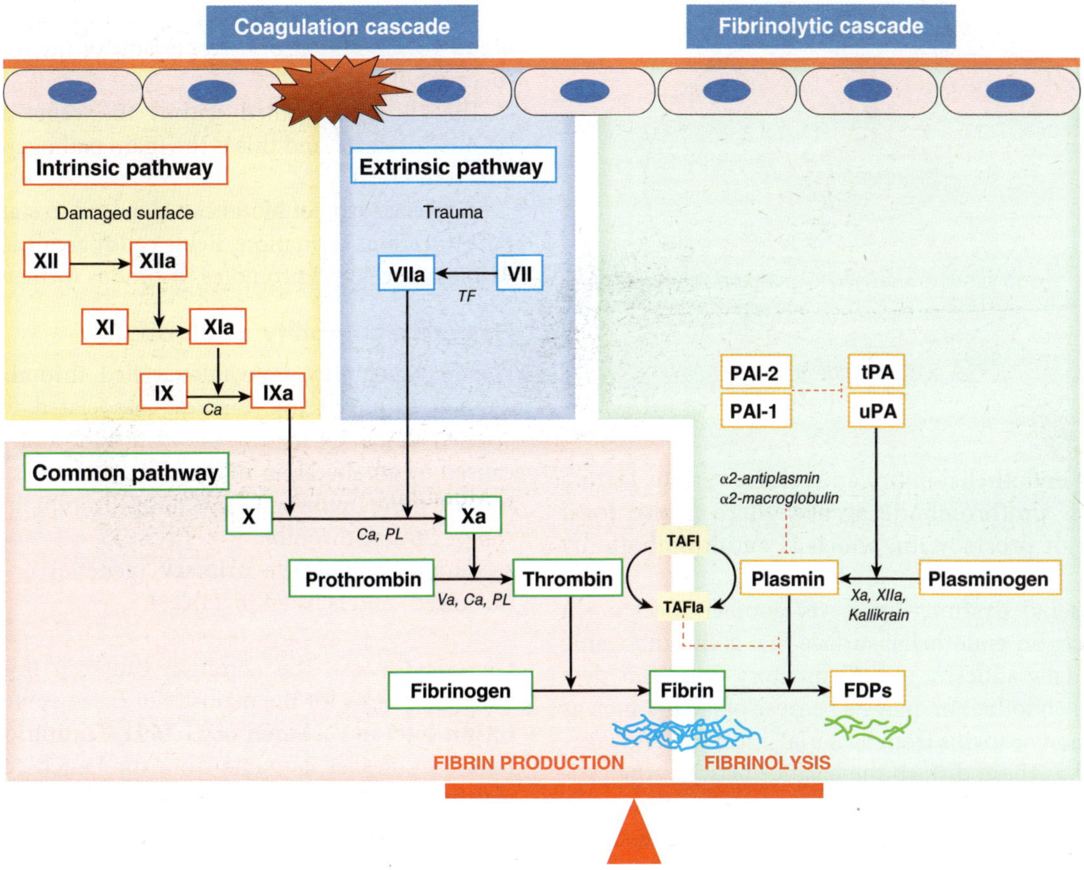

Fig. 4.16 Coagulation and fibrinolytic systems.

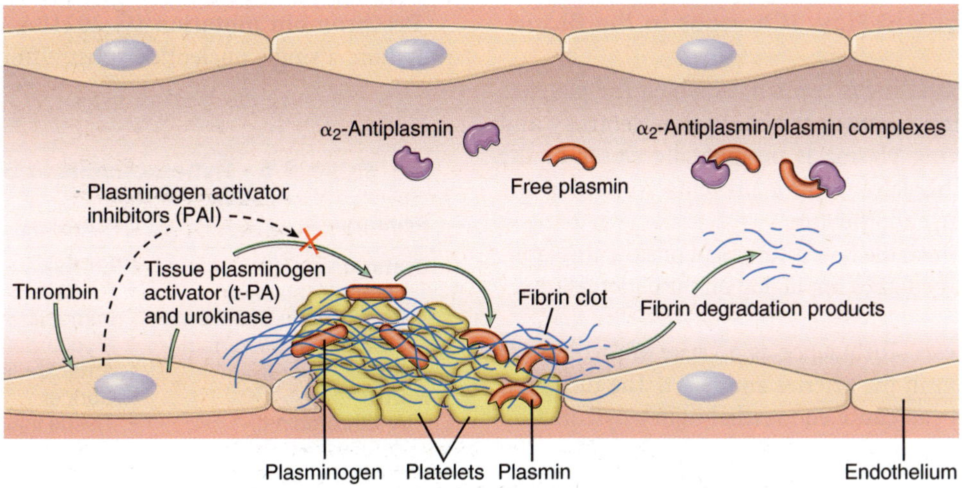

Fig. 4.17 Role of fibrinolytic system in haemostasis and thrombosis.

Injury to the Endothelium

Endothelial injury may be either physical damage or endothelial dysfunction. The physical damage to the endothelium leads to thrombosis in the heart or in the arterial circulation. Normal vascular flow prevents platelet adhesion to the endothelium. However, in the context of an endothelial injury, the platelets adhere to the damaged endothelium and build up to form a thrombus.

A thrombus can form within the **chambers of the heart**, as seen in myocardial infarction, with damage to the myocardium and the endothelium. Thrombi that can form on the cardiac valves are called **vegetations**. These vegetations are seen in infective endocarditis as well as other forms of endocarditis, such as Libman–Sacks endocarditis and nonbacterial thrombotic endocarditis.

These thrombi can also be formed in the blood vessels, as seen in atherosclerotic plaques or in various forms of vasculitis.

The **damage to the endothelium** exposes the highly thrombogenic subendothelial ECM. Platelets adhere to

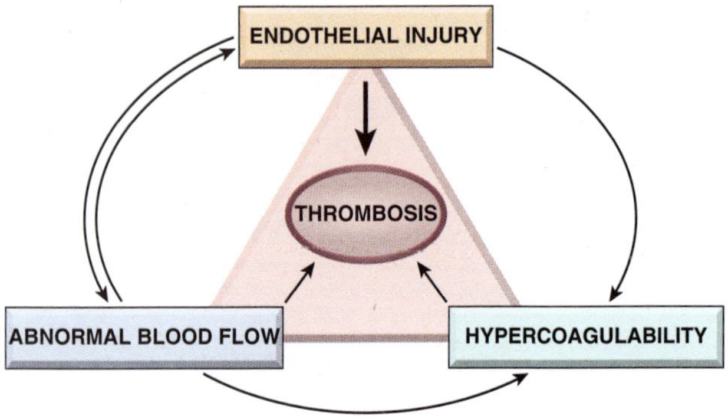

Fig. 4.18 Virchow triad.

the site of endothelial injury and release various factors that act as prothrombotic agents. There is also local depletion of prostacyclin, which is antithrombotic by nature.

Endothelial dysfunction is yet another mechanism that induces an endothelial surface that is thrombogenic or abnormally adhesive to inflammatory cells. This dysfunctional endothelium may be because of factors such as hypertension or toxins from bacterial infections and cigarette smoke. These disturb the balance between the prothrombotic and antithrombotic properties of the endothelium, tilting it towards the prothrombotic state. There is also a reduction in the antithrombotic factors, such as thrombomodulin, PGI_2 and t-PA.

Stasis or Turbulent Flow (Changes in the Blood Flow)

The normal blood flow is laminar, in which the platelets and cellular components of the blood flow centrally and the slower moving plasma is peripherally closer to the endothelium. This laminar flow prevents contact of the platelets with the endothelium.

In a state in which the flow is turbulent or slow, this laminar flow is disturbed, thus impinging on the endothelium.

Aetiopathogenesis Turbulence as a cause of thrombosis is more common in the arteries and heart. The turbulent stream of blood can cause endothelial injury/dysfunction and **increase the prothrombotic properties**. This disturbed flow also brings about a greater contact of platelets with the endothelium. In situations of stasis, there is also a lack of movement of blood, thus causing a lack of clearance of activated clotting factors. The stasis of blood in potential dilated spaces also prevents the inflow of clot inhibiting factors.

In clinical situations of myocardial infarction, arrhythmias or atrial fibrillation, there are increased chances of a thrombus forming within the dilated cardiac chambers (mural thrombus).

Dilated cardiomyopathy is yet another scenario in which stasis in the dilated chambers of the heart can cause thrombosis.

Thrombosis can also occur within atherosclerotic blood vessels and also in aneurysms of the blood vessels (because of stasis).

The thrombi formed within the veins are mainly because of stasis, and this is the main pathogenetic mechanism in DVT.

Hyperviscosity of blood can also lead to stasis and initiate thrombus formation. Sickle cell anaemia also leads to vascular stasis and promotes thrombus formation.

Hypercoagulability of Blood

Hypercoagulability state (also called thrombophilia) is defined as a systemic disorder associated with an increased tendency for the blood to clot and is basically caused by an alteration in coagulation factors. These factors are more important for venous thrombi than for arterial or cardiac thrombi.

Aetiology could be primary (genetic) or secondary (acquired) and is listed in Table 4.5.

Genetic Causes The common cause in this category, which accounts for the majority of cases, is **factor V mutation (factor V Leiden or G 1691A mutation)**. Leiden mutation derives its name from the Dutch city where it was first described. It is commonly seen in patients with DVT. The mutation alters the amino acid residue in factor V and renders it resistant to proteolysis by protein C. This leads to loss of an important antithrombotic counter-regulatory mechanism.

Prothrombin mutation (G 20210A variant): In this mutation, a single nucleotide substitution (G to A) in the

Table 4.5 Hypercoagulable States

Primary	Secondary
Common	**High risk**
• Factor V mutation	• Prolonged state of immobilization
• Prothrombin mutation	• Myocardial infarction
• Elevated levels of factor VIII, IX, XI or II	• Atrial fibrillation
Rare	• Cancer
• Antithrombin III deficiency	• Tissue injury
• Protein C deficiency	• Fracture
• Protein S deficiency	• Surgery
Very rare	• Burns
• Fibrinolysis defects	• Prosthetic heart valves
• Homozygous homocystinuria	• DIC
	• Antiphospholipid antibody syndrome
	Low risk
	• Cardiomyopathy
	• Hyperoestrogenic states
	• Nephrotic syndrome
	• Oral contraceptive pills
	• Smoking
	• Sickle cell anaemia

DIC, disseminated intravascular coagulation.

3′-untranslated region of the prothrombin gene is a fairly common allele. This variant results in increased prothrombin transcription and is associated with a nearly threefold increased risk of venous thrombosis.

Less common hypercoagulable causes include **antithrombin C deficiency, protein C deficiency or protein S deficiency**. Patients with these deficiencies are usually adolescents or young adults and often present with venous thrombosis and recurrent thromboembolism.

Very rare causes of genetic hypercoagulable states include **defects in fibrinolysis** and also **homozygous homocystinuria**. Elevated homocysteine levels contribute to arterial and venous thrombosis and also play an important role in atherosclerosis. The prothrombotic effects of homocysteine may be attributed to the thioester linkages formed between homocysteine metabolites and a variety of proteins, including fibrinogen. An inherited deficiency of cystathione-β-synthase leads to a marked elevation in homocysteine levels.

These genetic factors are very important to recognize because heterozygous individuals are at an increased risk of venous thrombosis with risk factors such as pregnancy, prolonged bed rest or prolonged immobilization. These may be the cause of significant morbidity in younger patients (younger than 50 years).

Secondary or Acquired Causes Among the secondary (acquired) causes of hypercoagulable states, the most important factors are prolonged bed rest or immobilization, myocardial infarction, atrial fibrillation, tissue injury, cancer, prosthetic cardiac valves, disseminated intravascular coagulation (DIC), heparin-induced thrombocytopenia (HIT) and antiphospholipid antibody (APLA) syndrome, to name a few.

In most of these situations, stasis or vascular injury promotes thrombosis. The hypercoagulable state seen with oral contraceptive usage and pregnancy may be related to the increased hepatic synthesis of coagulation factors and reduced synthesis of antithrombin III.

In certain cancers, the tumour products act as procoagulant factors and predispose to thrombosis. With advanced age, there is an increased tendency for the formation of thrombosis, which depends on the increased platelet aggregation and decreased synthesis of prostacyclin from the endothelium.

Heparin-Induced Thrombocytopenia Syndrome Among the acquired causes, HIT syndrome needs a special mention because it is seen in approximately 5% of patients who are treated with unfractionated heparin (for therapeutic anticoagulation). These patients develop autoantibodies that bind complexes of heparin and platelet membrane protein (platelet factor 4). These antibodies also bind similar complexes present on the endothelial surfaces. This adhesion results in platelet activation, aggregation and consumption of platelets as well as endothelial injury. The consumption of these platelets leads to thrombocytopenia. Newer low-molecular-weight fractionated heparin produces fewer autoantibodies. This entity is discussed in detail in Chapter 17.

Antiphospholipid Antibody Syndrome This is a condition in which there are detectable circulating antibodies that bind to phospholipids. The proteins that are mainly targeted by these antibodies include β_2 glycoprotein I, a plasma protein that associates with the surface of the endothelial cells and trophoblasts, and prothrombin.

These antibodies bind to these proteins and induce a hypercoagulable state in vivo. The exact mechanism is not known. In vitro, the antibodies interfere with the phospholipids and thus inhibit coagulation. These antibodies also cause a false-positive reaction during the serological testing for syphilis. This is because the antigen in the standard assay for syphilis is embedded in cardiolipin.

APLA syndrome can be divided into primary and secondary forms. When seen in patients with a known autoimmune disease, it is called secondary APLA, also known as **lupus anticoagulant**. A classical example is reported in patients with systemic lupus erythematosus.

In primary APLA syndrome, the patients present with a hypercoagulable state, without having any known autoimmune disease. In rare cases, it may manifest after exposure to certain drugs or infections.

These patients are treated with anticoagulation and immunosuppression.

MORPHOLOGY OF THROMBI

On the basis of their site of origin, thrombi can be classified into arterial or cardiac thrombi and venous thrombi.

Arterial or cardiac thrombi arise at the sites of endothelial injury or turbulence. These arterial thrombi arise at a point and propagate in a retrograde manner towards the direction of the heart. These propagating thrombi are loosely attached to the vessel wall and so have a tendency to embolize.

Thrombi occurring in the heart chambers or aortic lumen are called **mural thrombi** (Fig. 4.19). These can form when there is abnormal myocardial contraction, as observed with arrhythmias, dilated cardiomyopathy or myocardial infarction. Atherosclerotic lesions in the aorta and aortic aneurysms can also lead to thrombus formation. Arterial thrombi are usually occlusive.

Venous thrombi (phlebothrombosis) are usually secondary to stasis. They tend to extend in the direction of blood flow. Venous thrombi are also occlusive; they can propagate towards the heart and can be seen as a long cast within the vessel lumen that can embolize and cause obstruction. These are formed in a slow-moving setting, so venous thrombi predominantly contain red cells and hence appear red. The lower extremity veins are the most common sites for a venous thrombosis, but these can also be seen in the upper extremities, periprostatic plexus, etc.

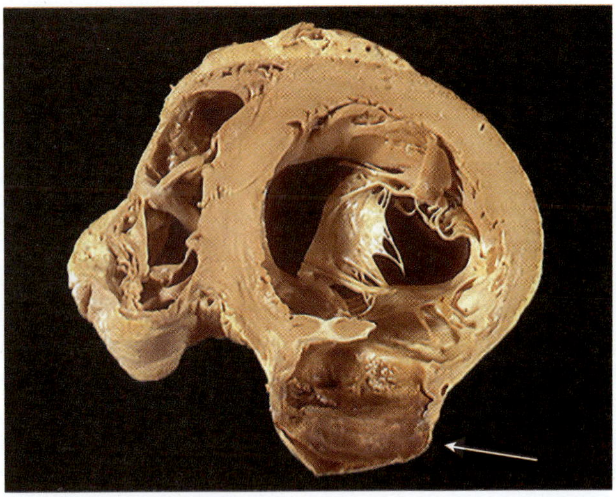

Fig. 4.19 Mural thrombi, gross. A cross-section through the heart reveals a ventricular aneurysm with a very thin wall at the arrow. Note the presence of a mural thrombus within the aneurysm. (*Source:* https://webpath.med.utah.edu/CVHTML/CV143.html.)

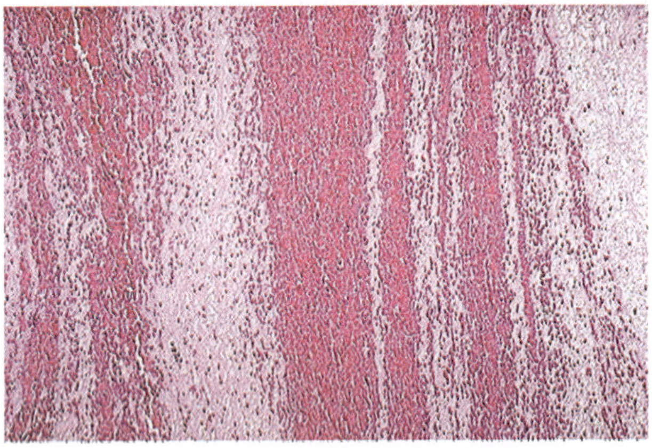

Fig. 4.20 Lines of Zahn. Note the alternating pale pink bands of platelets with fibrin and red bands of RBCs in thrombus. RBC, red blood cell.

The thrombi usually have visible laminations called **lines of Zahn** (Fig. 4.20). Venous thrombi can also be seen grossly under the microscope. These are pale platelet and fibrin layers alternating with dark red cell-rich layers. These layers are seen only in flowing blood, hence are used to differentiate from antemortem thrombosis.

Another confusing aspect is with **postmortem clots**. These however are gelatinous and have a red dependent portion and a yellow upper portion resembling 'chicken fat'. Furthermore, postmortem clots are not attached to the vessel wall, as against red thrombi that are firmly attached to the wall and have grey strands of fibrin.

Thrombi developing on cardiac valves are called **vegetations**. When blood-borne infective organisms cause thrombi to form on the valves, it is called infective endocarditis. Sterile vegetations are called nonbacterial thrombotic endocarditis, and the vegetations seen in systemic lupus erythematosus are called Libman–Sacks endocarditis. These appear verrucose on gross examination and are also sterile.

FATE OF THROMBUS

Thrombi evolve through the following four processes:

- **Propagation:** A thrombus enlarges in size with the addition of more platelets and fibrin, thus progresses in size, making it more vulnerable to vascular occlusion or embolization.
- **Embolization:** The thrombus may get dislodged from its site of origin and embolize by getting transported to a distant place.
- **Dissolution:** The fresh thrombus may at times get dissolved by the activation of the fibrinolytic factors and thus lead to the shrinkage in the size of the thrombus. The older thrombi are resistant to fibrinolytic effect. Hence, dissolution is more a feature of fresh thrombus.
- **Organization and recanalization** (Fig. 4.21): Older thrombi become recanalized by the ingrowth of endothelial cells and fibroblasts. Later, capillary channels may form through the thrombus, creating new lumina, thus establishing connectivity. There are also chances that the organized thrombus can get incorporated into the vessel walls.

CLINICAL FEATURES

The most important feature of thrombi is their potential to cause obstruction of arteries and veins. Thrombi also have a greater tendency to embolize.

Venous Thrombosis (Phlebothrombosis)

Most of the venous thrombi occur in the superficial or deep veins of the leg. **Superficial venous** thrombi are usually seen in the saphenous venous system, commonly in a setting of varicose veins. The local effects include pain and congestion of the affected leg. The **deep vein thrombi** arise from the large leg veins at or above the knee joint, such as popliteal, femoral and iliac veins. These are more serious in nature, because they have greater chances of embolization.

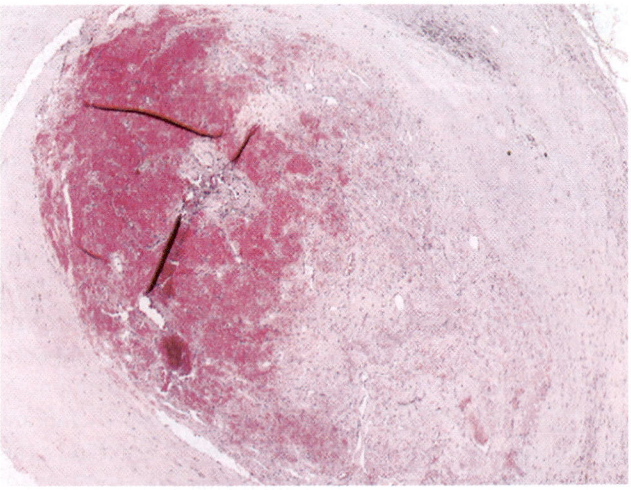

Fig. 4.21 Organization of thrombus. Note the stenosis of the vessel. (*Source:* https://medicine.tamu.edu/class-files/histopathology/Histopathology%20Study%20Guide/Hemodynamic/Organized%20Thrombus.htm.)

Deep vein thrombi are associated with hypercoagulable states, heart failure, bed rest and immobilization.

Arterial and Cardiac Thromboses

Atherosclerosis can predispose to arterial thrombi because of its association with endothelial injury and the abnormal blood flow. Myocardial infarction can predispose to cardiac mural thrombi by producing stasis in the noncontractile cardiac muscle. Both cardiac and mural thrombi can embolize and cause ischaemic damage and infarction in the organs where they are lodged, be it the brain, kidneys, spleen or any other organ.

EMBOLISM PA 6.5

An embolus is a detached intravascular solid, liquid or gaseous mass that is carried by the blood from its point of origin to a distant site where it can cause tissue dysfunction or infarction.

TYPES OF EMBOLI

Emboli can be classified on the basis of the following:

A. ***Physical nature of the emboli***
Solid: For example, thromboemboli, atheromatous material, tumour emboli, tissue fragments, bacterial clumps or foreign body material
Liquid: Fat, bone marrow and amniotic fluid
Gaseous: Air and other gases

B. ***Whether infected or not***
Bland: When the embolus is sterile
Septic: When the embolus is infected

C. ***Depending on the source of the emboli***
Endogenous: When it is from within the body
Exogenous: When it is introduced from outside

D. ***On the basis of their origin***
Thromboembolism: A vast majority of emboli are dislodged thrombi; hence, they are called thromboemboli. These may cause pulmonary embolism or systemic embolism.

Pulmonary Embolism

Pulmonary emboli mostly originate from the deep venous thromboses and are the most common form of thromboembolic disease. The common veins of origin are the popliteal, femoral or iliac veins and rarely pelvic veins or vena cava.

Risk factors: The major risk factor is postsurgery or after prolonged immobilization. The risk becomes more with other conditions such as advanced age, obesity and pregnancy.

Fragmented thrombi from DVT are carried through progressively large veins and the right side of the heart before entering the pulmonary circulation. The **consequences** of pulmonary thrombosis depend on the size of both the embolus and the vessels.

Fate of Pulmonary Embolism Small pulmonary emboli may travel to the smaller branches of pulmonary arteries and may resolve spontaneously. Most of them are clinically silent, with no consequences. These may become organized in the vessel walls with the passage of time.

When the emboli obstruct 60% or more of the pulmonary circulation, it is called **massive pulmonary embolism**. If an embolus lodges at the bifurcation of the main pulmonary artery, it is called a **saddle embolus** (Fig. 4.22). It produces an acute and massive obstruction to the blood flowing to the lungs, thus resulting in acute ventricular failure, which may present with a massive shock.

Multiple recurrent pulmonary emboli may fuse to form a single large mass.

Consequences Most of the small pulmonary emboli do not produce infarcts. However, in a compromised patient with congestive heart failure or chronic lung disease, they may present with a **pulmonary infarction.**

It is a red infarct in the lung, because of its dual blood supply, where the bronchial artery supplies the compromised zone. The area of the infarct is pyramidal in shape, with the base towards the pleural surface. Later when healing starts, granulation tissue starts growing in from the edges of the infarct, with consequent fibrous scar.

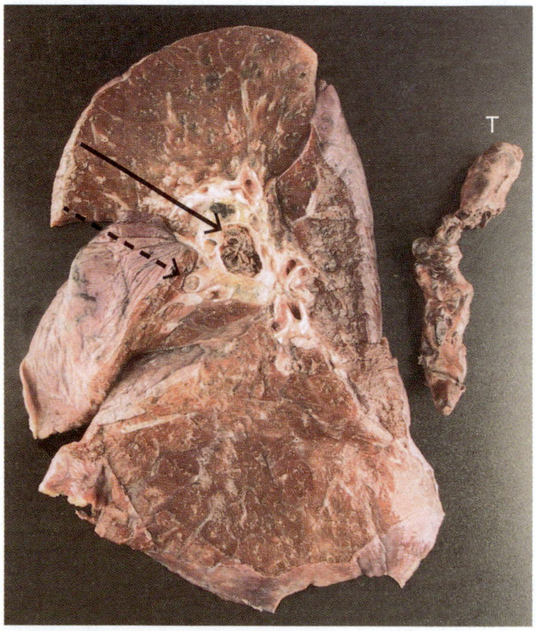

Fig. 4.22 Pulmonary thrombus, gross. This is referred to as 'saddle embolus', which bridges across the pulmonary artery as it divides into right and left main pulmonary arteries. The thrombus often has the outlines of the vein in which it formed. (*Source:* Raj Dasgupta, David G. Hicks, R. Michelle Koolaee, et al.: Pathology Case Reports: Beyond the Pearls, Fig. 27.1, Elsevier Inc., 2022.)

Obstruction of the medium-sized pulmonary arteries can result in **pulmonary haemorrhage**, when there is a rupture of the blood vessels after the obstruction by emboli.

Multiple recurrent pulmonary emboli can cause mechanical blockage of the arterial bed, which results in pulmonary hypertension and subsequent right ventricular failure.

In some rare cases, the embolus can pass through an interatrial or interventricular defect and gain access to the systemic circulation and this is called **paradoxical embolus.**

Clinical Presentation Cough, stabbing pleuritic pain, shortness of breath and occasional haemoptysis may be the presenting features. A person with one episode of pulmonary embolism is at risk for a recurrent episode.

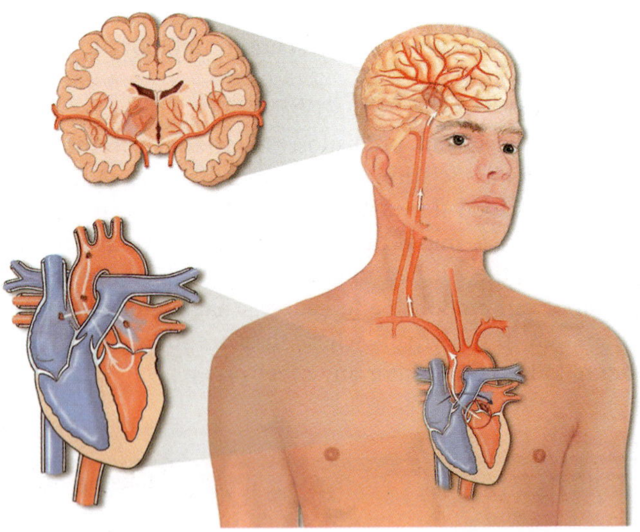

Fig. 4.23 Pathway of paradoxical embolism.

Systemic Thromboembolism

Systemic thromboembolism is defined as the embolism in which emboli occlude the systemic arterial circulation. These emboli usually produce infarcts in the region supplied by the involved vessels. The consequence of embolization depends on the calibre of the occluded vessel, collateral supply and vulnerability of the affected tissue to anoxia.

Cardiac Causes The most common source of systemic thromboembolism is from **intracardiac mural thrombi**, which are seen secondary to a myocardial infarction, or from a thrombus formed in the dilated left atrium following a stenosed mitral valve secondary to a rheumatic heart disease. In these settings, an atrial fibrillation can dislodge the thrombus. The cardiac mural thrombi contribute to 85% of the arterial emboli. Dilated cardiomyopathy is another setting in which a thrombus can form within the dilated chambers of the heart, which can later embolize. Bacterial endocarditis and other valvular vegetations can also lead to septic infarcts.

Causes in Blood Vessels Thrombi on ulcerated atherosclerotic plaques can also embolize, as can thrombi from aneurysms.

The thrombi from the venous circulation can pass through a septal defect and enter the systemic circulation, causing systemic thromboembolism, the paradoxical emboli (Fig. 4.23).

Consequences The arterial emboli can travel to various organs, as against the venous emboli, which usually lodge in the pulmonary vascular bed. These may get lodged at sites of luminal narrowing as seen at the bifurcation of blood vessels or in vessel constrictions or in areas of atherosclerotic plaques.

When an embolus gets lodged, it propagates locally and finally causes infarction of the affected tissues. In certain situations, these can undergo fragmentation and lysis. On the basis of the site of occlusion, the organ undergoes ischaemia and coagulative necrosis.

The most common site for the embolus to lodge is the **lower extremity**, as seen in approximately 75% of cases. These emboli can lead to gangrene of the extremities.

Brain is another site where the thrombi may lodge at the cerebral artery and cause ischaemic necrosis of the brain (liquefactive necrosis). The middle cerebral artery is the most common site of arrest of arterial thrombi in branches of the carotid artery.

Emboli in the mesenteric vessels of the **intestine** can cause infarction of the bowel. **Renal** artery emboli can cause small peripheral infarcts in the kidneys. The spleen and upper extremities are less commonly affected.

The fragmented vegetations of bacterial endocarditis can cause **mycotic aneurysms** or lead to a **pyaemic abscess.**

Treatment of pulmonary embolism, the most common form of thromboembolic disease, typically involves anticoagulation to prevent further clot formation. In cases of large or life-threatening emboli, thrombolytic therapy may be used to dissolve the clot. For prevention, risk factor modification, including anticoagulation in high-risk scenarios like major surgery, is crucial.

Fat Embolism

Fat embolism is the presence of emboli comprising fat microglobules in the circulation.

Aetiology

- **Fracture of long bones and severe skeletal injuries** (with long bone fractures, bone marrow fragments enter the circulation and lodge in small blood vessels of the lung, skin, kidneys, brain and other organs, producing ischaemia and haemorrhage)
- Extensive trauma to fat-laden tissue
- Burns

- Rarely orthopaedic procedures
- During vigorous cardiopulmonary resuscitation

Clinical Features Patients may develop potentially fatal **fat embolism syndrome**, which is characterized by pulmonary distress, cutaneous petechial haemorrhages and various neurological manifestations.

Pulmonary manifestations: A patient may develop dyspnoea and tachypnoea because of the presence of fat microglobules in pulmonary capillaries.

Haematological manifestations: A patient may develop thrombocytopenia and anaemia. Thrombocytopenia is because of adherence of platelets to fat microglobules. Hence, a patient may develop petechial haemorrhages over the chest and upper extremities. Anaemia may result from red cell aggregation to the fat globules or even haemolysis.

Neurological manifestations: Numerous petechial haemorrhages in the brain parenchyma manifest as irritability, restlessness, delirium, loss of consciousness and cerebral oedema, and, in some cases, may even cause herniation within a week with a fatal outcome.

Fat embolism syndrome may be because of both mechanical obstruction and biochemical injury. The fat microemboli along with red cells and platelets aggregate together and cause mechanical obstruction. Biochemical injury is produced by the free fatty acids that are released from the fat globules. These free fatty acids cause local toxic injury to the endothelium, with resultant platelet aggregation and granulocyte recruitment. Release of injurious free radicals and chemical mediators potentiates the biochemical injury.

Laboratory Diagnosis

Bronchoalveolar lavage: It is performed to demonstrate fat in the alveolar macrophages, which are highlighted by fat stains such as Sudan III, Sudan IV, Sudan Black, osmic acid and oil red O. The fat microglobules are engulfed by the alveolar macrophages.

Histopathology (Fig. 4.24): In autopsy specimens, frozen section examination reveals the presence of fat globules in the pulmonary arterioles and alveoli. The routine processing dissolves the fat and thus fat is seen as colourless vacuoles by haematoxylin–eosin staining.

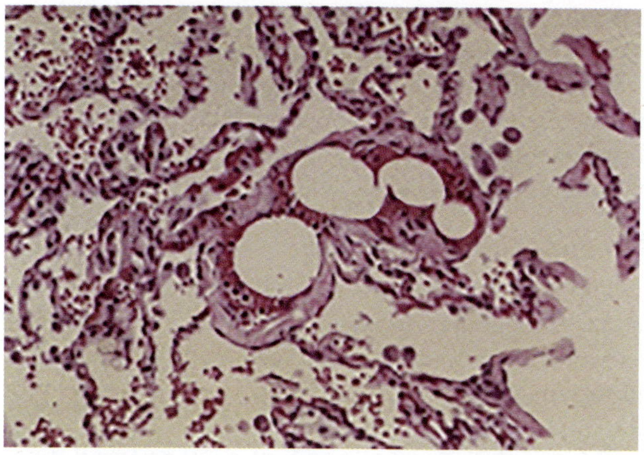

Fig. 4.24 Fat embolism, microscopy. Bone marrow embolus in the pulmonary circulation. The cellular elements on the left side of the embolus are haematopoietic cells, and the cleared vacuoles represent marrow fat. (*Source:* Anthony W. Alfrey: Rapid Review Pathology, 6th ed. Fig. 5.9, Elsevier Inc., 2024.)

Air Embolism

Air embolism occurs when air is introduced into the venous or arterial circulation.

Causes

- Trauma: Air enters the circulation through any penetrating wound or injury, as seen in a wound over the neck or a chest wall injury.
- During surgical procedures: Air may be introduced during invasive procedures such as laparoscopic procedures and thoracocentesis, into the coronary artery during bypass surgeries, into the cerebral circulation during neurosurgeries in a sitting position or in haemodialysis.
- Abortions: Air can also be introduced into the vessels during an abortion by a faulty technique.

Aetiopathogenesis More than 100 mL of air is needed to be introduced into the vessels for it to manifest clinically as air embolism. These air bubbles tend to coalesce and cause physical obstruction in the circulation.

Decompression Sickness This is a special form of air embolism seen in deep-sea divers, scuba divers and underwater construction workers who are exposed to rapid changes in atmospheric pressure. When air is breathed at high atmospheric pressure, as seen in deep-sea diving, a large amount of inert gases, such as **nitrogen or helium**, is dissolved in the blood, body fluids and tissues. When the individual ascends suddenly from high atmospheric pressure to normal atmospheric pressure, these gases bubble out in the circulation and cause physical obstruction and injury.

The physical obstruction manifests as **bends and chokes** because of small vessel obstruction. This causes reduced blood supply to the skeletal muscle and supporting tissues, in and about the joints, causing muscular and joint pain called bends.

The obstruction to the pulmonary blood vessels causes oedema, haemorrhage and respiratory distress manifesting as chokes.

If there is ischaemia to the blood vessels of the brain, it can lead to even coma and death.

Chronic decompression sickness: This is also called **Caisson disease** (named after pressurized underwater vessels used during bridge construction), in which workers in the pressurized vessels may develop acute and chronic forms of decompression sickness. This can also lead to avascular necrosis of the bone. The bones commonly involved are the head of the femur, tibia and humerus.

Treatment of acute decompression sickness involves placing the individual in a high-pressure chamber, which forces the gas bubbles back into the solution, and then decompressing gradually.

Amniotic Fluid Embolism

Amniotic fluid embolism is a very severe complication of labour and develops when amniotic fluid along with fetal cells and debris enters the maternal circulation. This usually occurs through ruptured blood vessels or a tear in the placental membranes.

This may be seen as a complication of maternal delivery, usually at the end of labour and the immediate postpartum period. From the venous circulation, amniotic fluid emboli enter the right side of the heart and finally rest in the pulmonary circulation. It may precipitate the mechanism of highly fatal DIC.

Morphology

The amniotic fluid emboli are composed of squamous cells that are shed from the fetal skin, lanugo hair, fat from vernix caseosa and mucin derived from the fetal respiratory or gastrointestinal tract. There is also pulmonary oedema and diffuse alveolar damage or acute respiratory distress syndrome (ARDS) (Fig. 4.25).

This condition usually presents in the immediate postpartum period, and the patient usually presents with severe dyspnoea, cyanosis and neurological impairment ranging from headache to seizures. There can also be bleeding as a manifestation of DIC. The patient may also develop shock and coma, and even die.

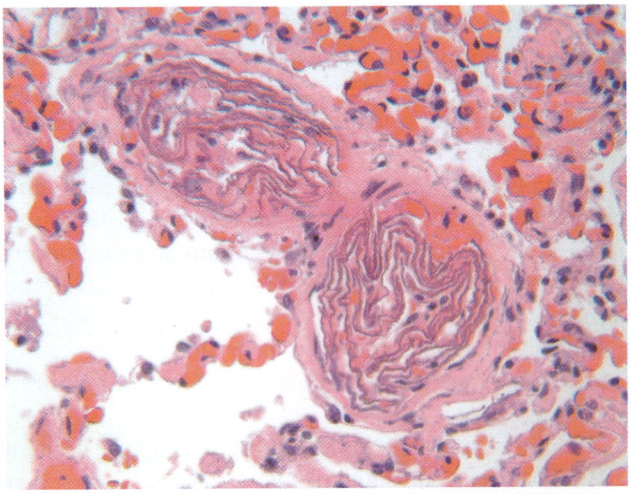

Fig. 4.25 Amniotic fluid embolism, microscopy. Note that the two small pulmonary arterioles are packed with laminated swirls of fetal squamous cells. There is marked oedema and congestion. (*Source:* From The Lungs in Obstetric and Gynecologic Diseases. Stephen E. Lapinsky and Catherine Nelson-Piercy. The Lungs in Obstetric and Gynecologic Diseases. Murray & Nadel's Textbook of Respiratory Medicine. 7th edition. Elsevier.)

INFARCTION PA 6.6

An infarct is a localized area of ischaemic necrosis that is caused by occlusion of either the arterial blood supply or the venous drainage.

Most of the infarcts are areas of coagulative necrosis because of sudden occlusion of the arterial blood supply and resultant ischaemia. Cellular outlines are maintained, but structural details are lost in this type of necrosis.

CLINICAL EXAMPLES OF INFARCTS

- Myocardial infarction – heart
- Pulmonary infarction – lungs
- Cerebral infarction – brain
- Intestinal infarction – bowel/intestine
- Gangrene – extremities

CAUSES OF INFARCTS

Most of the infarcts are caused by the following:

- **Arterial causes:** Occlusion of the lumen leads to most of the infarcts, which could be because of either a thrombus or an embolus. There could be a vasospasm in the vessel wall, or a haemorrhage into the atheromatous plaque, which can also lead to complete occlusion and narrowing, with subsequent infarction. External compression by a tumour can also lead to infarction.
- **Venous causes:** The occlusion of the veins can be because of a thrombus or an embolus, or it could be because of external compression, as seen in strangulated hernia.

FACTORS THAT DETERMINE THE OUTCOME OF AN INFARCT

The outcome may be minimal effect or death of the tissue, on the basis of the following factors:

1. **Nature of the blood supply**
   Dual blood supply: Organs or tissues with a double blood supply, such as the liver, lung, hand and forearm, are less likely to develop infarction.
   End arterial blood supply: Organs that have end arteries with no collaterals are more prone to undergo infarction.
2. **Rate of occlusion**
   Slow occlusion is less likely to produce infarction than rapid occlusion. This may be because it provides more time to develop collateral circulation pathways.
3. **Vulnerability of the tissues to hypoxia**
   Certain tissues such as neurons and cardiac myocytes are more vulnerable to ischaemic damage as compared with skeletal muscles. Neurons can undergo necrosis even if blood supply is occluded for 3–4 minutes. However, cardiac myocytes can withstand ischaemia for up to 20–30 minutes.

4. **Oxygen content of the blood:** The damage is faster in patients with anaemia or cyanosis than in a person with normal oxygenation of blood.

CLASSIFICATION OF INFARCTS

A. **On the basis of colour**

Pale infarct: If an infarct is white or pale in colour, it is called a pale infarct. These infarcts usually occur in arterial occlusion of solid organs, especially when there is an end arterial blood supply, as seen in the heart, spleen and kidney. It is also seen in tissues with increased density.

Red infarct: When the infarct is red and haemorrhagic, it is called a red infarct. This usually occurs because of venous occlusion in organs with loose textured tissues, such as the lungs. It is also seen in organs with a dual blood supply, such as the lungs and small intestine.

Red infarct is also seen in previously congested tissues and also when the blood flow is reestablished to a site of previous arterial occlusion. It is also seen with torsion ovary or torsion testis, when the twisting of the pedicle of the organs causes occlusion of the thin-walled veins, leading to blockage of the venous drainage.

B. **Presence or absence of infection**

Septic infarct: When the infarct is infected, it is called a septic infarct. This can happen in two situations – one, when a fragment from vegetation of bacterial endocarditis blocks an artery and causes infarction and the bacteria present in the embolus get seeded in the infarcted area. The other condition is when the patient develops bacteraemia, and there is secondary bacterial seeding of the infarct.

Bland infarct: When the infarct is free of infection, it is called a bland infarct.

C. **According to the age of the infarct**

Recent or fresh infarct

Old or healed infarct

PATHOGENESIS OF INFARCT

Localized hyperaemia: This is the first event because of local hypoxia that occurs after obstruction to the blood supply.

Within a few hours, there is oedema over the affected part along with haemorrhage. There are few cellular changes such as cloudy swelling and degeneration that occur before necrosis and are seen within 12–48 hours. There is proteolysis of the dead tissue along with RBC lysis.

This is followed by acute inflammatory infiltrate. Blood pigments, secondary to lysis of RBCs, are deposited in the area of infarct. The infarct now becomes pale grey because of loss of RBCs. Finally, healing sets in with the formation of granulation tissue.

Reperfusion injury can occur after the restoration of blood flow to ischaemic tissues. Although reperfusion is essential to salvage viable tissue, it can paradoxically cause additional cellular damage because of oxidative stress and inflammation. This phenomenon is particularly significant in myocardial infarction and stroke, in which timely restoration of blood flow is critical to minimize tissue damage.

Morphology

Pale infarcts: Grossly, these are usually wedge-shaped, in which the occluded vessel is at the apex and the base is at the periphery or the surface of the organ (Fig. 4.26). These are usually seen in solid organs such as the heart, kidney and spleen and also in dry gangrene of the extremities. The colour evolves from poorly defined and

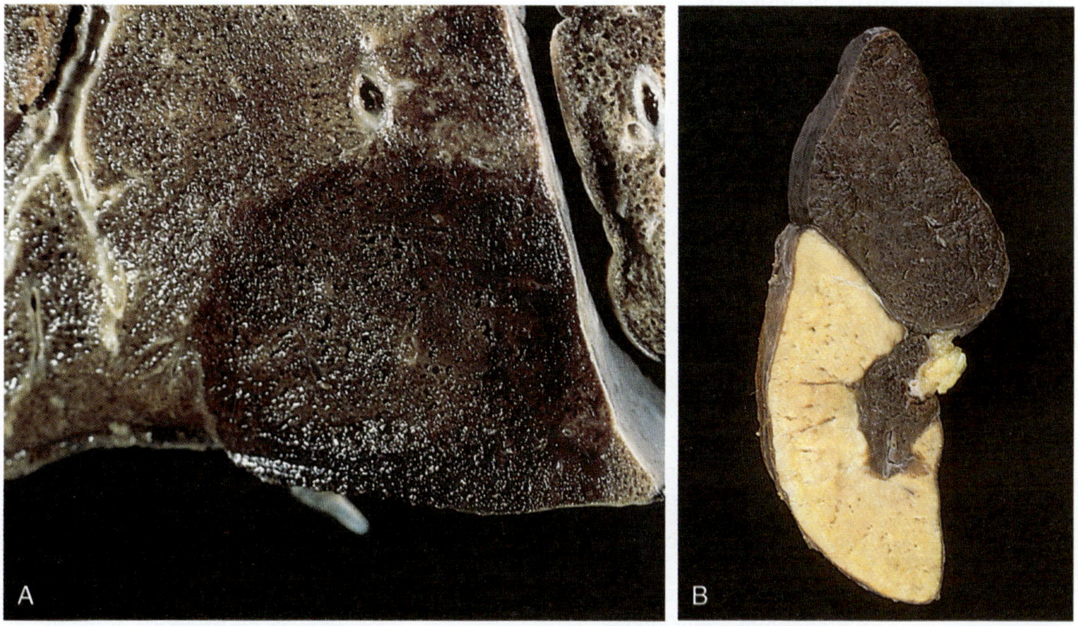

Fig. 4.26 Red and white infarcts, gross. (A) Haemorrhagic, roughly wedge-shaped pulmonary red infarct. (B) Sharply demarcated white infarct in the spleen. (*Source:* From Ischaemia, infarction and shock. In Simon S. Cross. Underwood's Pathology, 7th edition. 2019. Elsevier.)

haemorrhagic red when fresh to the sharply defined pale colour later.

Red infarcts: These infarcts are seen as sharply circumscribed areas of necrosis that are firm in consistency and dark red to purple in colour. These are seen in organs with a double blood supply such as the liver and lungs and also in organs with extensive collateral circulation, such as the small intestine.

Under a microscope, both pale and red infarcts show areas of ischaemic coagulative necrosis. Acute inflammatory cells are seen in the area within a few hours and reach their peak within 1–2 days. Changes of frank necrosis appear after 4–10 hours.

The healing process starts at the margins, and the dead cells are eaten up by the macrophages by the process of phagocytosis. Parenchymal regeneration takes place where there are stable or labile cells; in areas where there are permanent cells, the area gets filled up with granulation tissue.

SHOCK PA 6.3

Shock is a result of inadequate tissue perfusion, leading to cellular dysfunction and organ failure. The word 'shock' is derived from the Dutch word 'Schokken', meaning jolt or jerk.

Failure of the circulatory system because of a decreased cardiac output or reduced effective circulatory blood volume leads to systemic hypotension, with consequent tissue hypoperfusion, hypoxia and cell injury. The injury being reversible initially becomes irreversible later on and leads to organ failure and death.

CLASSIFICATION

There are three major categories of shock, on the basis of the aetiology (Table 4.6):

- Hypovolaemic shock
- Cardiogenic shock
- Septic shock

There are few other types of shock also:

Neurogenic shock: Less commonly, when shock results from loss of vascular tone because of spinal cord injury or improper technique of anaesthesia, it is called neurogenic shock.

Anaphylactic shock: This results from systemic vasodilation and increased vascular permeability that is triggered by an immunoglobulin E–mediated hypersensitivity reaction.

Here, we describe hypovolaemic, cardiogenic and septic shock in detail.

Hypovolaemic Shock

This type of shock occurs because of **low cardiac output**, which could be because of the following:

- Loss of blood, as in haemorrhage
- Loss of plasma, as seen in severe burns
- Loss of body fluids, as seen in severe vomiting or diarrhoea

Loss of fluid leads to a decreased circulating blood volume, low cardiac output, hypotension and a state of shock.

Cardiogenic Shock

Cardiogenic shock is a type of shock that results from failure of the heart to pump blood (**myocardial pump failure**). This is seen in the following conditions:

- Myocardial infarction
- Myocarditis
- Papillary muscle rupture and cardiac rupture
- Cardiac tamponade
- Pulmonary embolism
- Ventricular arrhythmias

In the above-mentioned conditions, direct myocardial damage or a mechanical abnormality of the heart leads to a low-cardiac-output state, resulting in a reduced cardiac output and blood pressure. In a cardiac tamponade, there is extrinsic compression of the heart, which leads to a

Table 4.6 Types of Shock with Clinical Examples and Principal Mechanisms

Type of Shock	Clinical Examples	Principal Mechanisms
Cardiogenic	Myocardial infarction Ventricular rupture Arrhythmia Cardiac tamponade Pulmonary embolism	Failure of myocardial pump resulting from intrinsic myocardial damage, extrinsic compression or obstruction to outflow
Hypovolaemic	Fluid loss (e.g. haemorrhage, vomiting, diarrhoea, burns or trauma)	Inadequate blood or plasma volume
Shock associated with systemic inflammation	Overwhelming microbial infections (bacterial and fungal) Superantigens (e.g. toxic shock syndrome) Trauma, burns, pancreatitis	Activation of cytokine cascades; peripheral vasodilation and pooling of blood; endothelial activation/injury; leucocyte-induced damage, disseminated intravascular coagulation

(*Source:* From Vinay Kumar, Abul Abbas, Jon Aster. Robbins & Cotran Pathologic Basis of Disease. 10th Edition. Elsevier. 2020.)

decreased cardiac output. In pulmonary embolism, there can be an outflow obstruction, leading to a decreased output. The decreased cardiac output leads to decreased tissue perfusion and resulting shock.

Septic Shock

This type of shock is because of severe sepsis that results in hypotension by causing vasodilation and peripheral pooling of blood. It is associated with dysfunction of multiple organs. It is also called **endotoxic shock**.

Septic shock is commonly caused by gram-positive or gram-negative bacteria, but fungus, protozoa or even rickettsiae can also lead to septic shock. The common gram-positive organisms are *Staphylococcus aureus*, enterococci, *Streptococcus pneumoniae* and some gram-negative bacteria. This type of shock is associated with systemic inflammation, and the triggers may include superantigens, as seen in toxic shock syndrome.

There is an overwhelming response of the immune system, with activation of cytokine cascades, peripheral vasodilation and pooling of blood. There is also endothelial activation or injury, leucocyte-induced damage and DIC.

The inflammatory mediators thus produced cause arterial dilatation, vascular leakage and venous blood pooling. These result in tissue hypoperfusion, leading to a cellular hypoxia and consequent organ failure.

Pathogenesis of Septic Shock (Fig. 4.27) Various microorganisms have microbial constituents that can trigger the process. Various players of inflammation, such as neutrophils, macrophages, dendritic cells and endothelial cells, and soluble products of the innate immune system, such as the complement, are activated by these microorganisms and their products.

Factors that play a major role in the pathophysiology of septic shock include the following:

- Inflammatory and counter-inflammatory responses
- Endothelial activation and injury
- Induction of a procoagulant state
- Metabolic abnormalities
- Organ dysfunction

Inflammatory and counter-inflammatory responses

Proinflammatory response is triggered through activation of receptors on cells of the innate immune system.

- The components of the microbial cell wall get engaged with the receptors that are present on the surface of these cells, such as Toll-like receptors. This engagement leads to release of chemical mediators of inflammation, such as TNF, IL-1 and IFN-γ.
- Markers of acute inflammation, such as C-reactive protein and procalcitonin, are also elevated.
- It also leads to the production of reactive oxygen species and lipid mediators that activate the

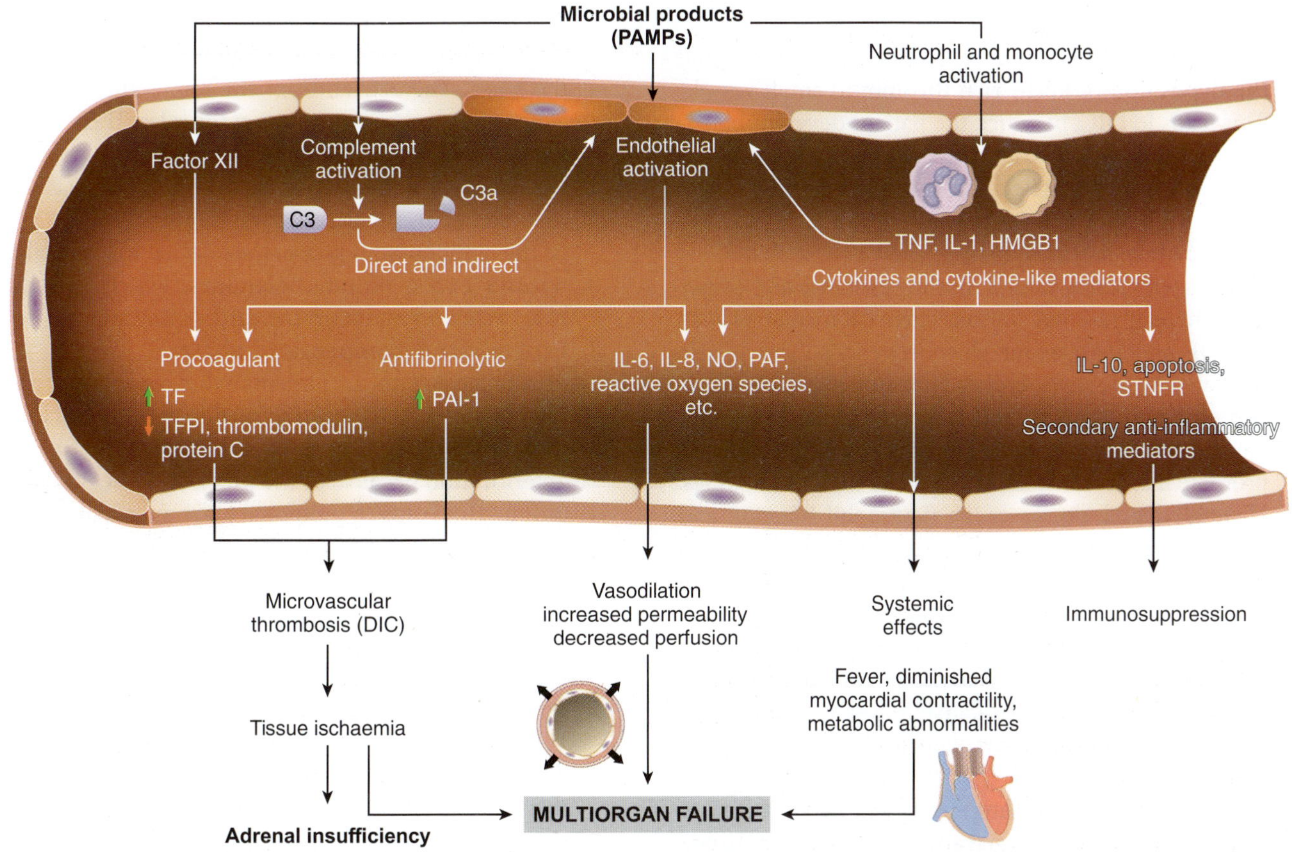

Fig. 4.27 Major pathogenic pathways in septic shock. (*Source:* From Robbins & Cotran Pathologic Basis of Disease, 10th edition. 2021. Elsevier.)

endothelial cells to upregulate the expression of adhesion molecules. This leads to production of more cytokines and chemokines.

- There is also the activation of complement cascade, leading to the production of anaphylatoxins (C3a, C5a), chemotactic fragments and opsonins.
- There is also an activation of the coagulation pathway through factor XII and also through endothelial activation.

There is also activation of the counter-regulatory immunosuppressive mechanism.

Endothelial activation and injury

This may be mediated by either microbial constituents or proinflammatory state. The cytokines lead to loosening of the endothelial cells and leakage of protein-rich fluid with subsequent oedema, which further impairs tissue perfusion.

Endothelial activation also upregulates the production of NO and other vasoactive inflammatory mediators such as complement components that further worsen systemic hypotension.

Induction of a procoagulant state

The ensuing microbial infection with its endotoxins can lead to the activation of factor XII. There can also be an increase in proinflammatory cytokines such as IL-6 and production of tissue factor. In a microbial infection, there is also reduction in the endothelial anticoagulant factors such as tissue factor pathway inhibitor, thrombomodulin and protein C. The state of sepsis also reduces fibrinolysis by increasing the plasminogen activator inhibitor 1 expression.

All these lead to systemic activation of thrombin and the deposition of fibrin-rich thrombi in small vessels. This leads to DIC, in which the patient develops bleeding manifestations because of consumption of coagulation factors and platelets. DIC is discussed in greater detail in Chapter 17.

Metabolic abnormalities

Patients with sepsis exhibit insulin resistance and consequent hyperglycaemia. Various chemical mediators such as TNF and IL-1 favour gluconeogenesis. This is also mediated by the stress-induced hormones such as glucagon, growth hormones and glucocorticoids. The proinflammatory mediators also suppress insulin release and promote insulin resistance in the liver and other tissues. Hyperglycaemia decreases the neutrophil function and suppresses bactericidal activity. Sepsis may be associated with an adrenal insufficiency and subsequent decrease in glucocorticoid deficiency. This may result from decreased functioning of the intact glands or adrenal necrosis resulting from DIC (called Waterhouse–Friderichsen syndrome). The reduced oxidative phosphorylation and switchover to anaerobic glycolysis lead to lactic acidosis.

Organ dysfunction

Systemic hypotension, thrombosis and oedema lead to decreased delivery of oxygen and nutrients to the tissues. All these cause further organ damage, which can ultimately lead to adult respiratory distress syndrome.

STAGES OF SHOCK

Shock is a progressive disorder that goes through the following three phases:

1. Nonprogressive (compensated/reversible) phase
2. Progressive decompensated phase
3. Irreversible phase

1. **Nonprogressive (compensated/reversible) phase**

   In this phase, the body attempts to maintain adequate cerebral and coronary blood supply by redistribution of blood so that the **vital organs are adequately perfused** and oxygenated. This is facilitated by the activation of various **neurohormonal mechanisms** that cause widespread vasoconstriction of the peripheries and attempts by the kidney to conserve the fluid. If adequate treatment is provided, the homeostasis is maintained and it is reversible.

   The vasoconstriction is mediated by the neural and humoral factors (e.g. baroreceptors, chemoreceptors and renin–angiotensin system). It is a response to hypotension and tissue hypoxia and is mainly seen in the vessels of the skin and abdominal viscera. It increases the peripheral resistance, heart rate (tachycardia) and blood pressure. Clinically, cutaneous vasoconstriction is responsible for the cool and pale skin seen in initial stages of shock.

   The **kidneys** also play a major role in restoring the fluid imbalance and improving the venous return to the heart. The activation of the renin–angiotensin–aldosterone mechanism is one of the roles. There is also release of ADH because of decreased effective circulating volume. The glomerular filtration rate (GFR) is also reduced because of arteriolar vasoconstriction.

   In the compensated phase, the adrenal medulla also releases excess of catecholamines, which increase heart rate and maintain the cardiac output.

2. **Progressive decompensated phase**

   This stage occurs in patients who have other risk factors such as a preexisting cardiovascular and lung disease. The persistence of shock leads to further deterioration because of the preexisting health condition. This leads to pulmonary hypoperfusion with resultant pulmonary oedema and tachypnoea.

   At this stage, there is switch to anaerobic glycolysis, which results in metabolic lactic acidosis. Clinically, at this stage, the patient develops confusion and worsening of the renal function.

3. **Irreversible decompensated shock**

   When the shock is so severe that no recovery takes place in spite of compensatory mechanisms and therapy, it is called irreversible decompensated shock.

This stage is characterized by progressive damage to the vessel wall, which becomes unresponsive to the vasoconstrictors and leads to **progressive vasodilation**. This leads to peripheral pooling of blood and further deterioration in the effective circulating volume. There is also **increased vascular permeability**, which further compromises the effective circulatory volume.

Progressive fall in blood pressure and reduced blood flow to the myocardium cause coronary insufficiency and myocardial ischaemia, resulting in further depression of cardiac function, reduced cardiac output and decreased blood flow. Further pulmonary hypoperfusion causes respiratory distress because of pulmonary oedema, tachypnoea and ARDS. There is also ischaemic damage to the other vital organs such as the heart, kidneys and brain. The damaged tissues release prothrombotic factors and activate the coagulation cascade, thus promoting thrombosis. The thrombi further impair the blood flow, leading to worsening of the tissue damage. Clinically, the patient presents with features of coma, worsened heart function and progressive renal failure.

Morphology

All the above-mentioned changes in the organs are secondary to hypoxic injury, and salient changes can be noted in the adrenals, kidneys, lungs, brain, heart and gastrointestinal tract.

Changes in Kidneys

Hypoxia causes acute tubular necrosis, which is a major consequence of shock.

Gross: Kidneys are enlarged, swollen and congested, and the cortex appears pale. Cut surface shows pooling of blood in the outer regions of the medulla.

Microscopy

Proximal tubules are dilated with focal necrosis of tubular epithelial cells. There may be pigmented casts within the lumina, caused mainly by haemoglobin or myoglobin.

Interstitium shows oedema, and there is the presence of mononuclear cells in the interstitium and within tubules.

Changes in Adrenals

The adrenals show lipid depletion in the cortical cells, with focal haemorrhage in cases of severe shock. Massive haemorrhagic necrosis of the entire adrenal gland is found in Waterhouse–Friderichsen syndrome, which is associated with severe meningococcal septicaemia.

Changes in Lungs

The lungs are generally not affected in hypovolaemic shock because of their dual blood supply. But in septic shock, the changes are very prominent and are called shock lungs.

Grossly, the lungs are heavy and wet.

Microscopy shows features of ARDS. The changes include congestion, interstitial and alveolar oedema, interstitial lymphocytic infiltrate, alveolar hyaline membrane, and thickening and fibrosis of the alveolar septa.

Changes in Heart

The heart is more vulnerable to the effect of hypoxia and shows haemorrhages and necrosis, consequent to ischaemia, more so in the subepicardial and subendocardial regions.

Haemorrhagic Gastroenteropathy

Hypoperfusion of the alimentary tract results in mucosal and mural infarction called haemorrhagic gastroenteropathy.

Grossly, the lesions are multifocal and widely distributed throughout the bowel. The lesions are superficial ulcers and reddish purple in colour. The adjacent bowel mucosa is oedematous and haemorrhagic.

Microscopically, the involved surface of the bowel shows dilated and congested vessels and haemorrhagic necrosis of the mucosa.

CLINICAL FEATURES

The classical features are low blood pressure, subnormal temperature, feeble and irregular pulse, and shallow respiration.

Hypovolaemic and Cardiogenic Shock

Patients with hypovolaemic and cardiogenic shock present with altered sensorium, cyanosis, oliguria, weak rapid pulse, tachypnoea, and cool, clammy extremities. Patients with hypovolaemic shock may survive with appropriate management.

Septic Shock

The skin initially may be warm and flushed because of peripheral vasodilation. Patients with septic shock or cardiogenic shock associated with massive myocardial infarction usually have a high mortality rate.

Whatever the type of shock, the primary threat to life is the underlying initiating event, such as a myocardial infarction, severe haemorrhage or a bacterial infection. The cardiac, cerebral and pulmonary events further aggravate the morbidity. The renal damage ensues with progressive oliguria, acidosis and electrolyte imbalance.

Prognosis varies with the origin of shock and its duration. Hypovolaemic shock can be treated effectively, particularly in young patients. However, the prognosis is not all that good with septic or cardiogenic shock.

SELF-ASSESSMENT

Multiple Choice Questions

1. A 45-year-old woman presents with lower extremity swelling. She has a history of congestive heart failure. The swelling is most likely because of
   A. Hypercoagulability
   B. Reduced plasma oncotic pressure
   C. Elevated capillary hydrostatic pressure
   D. Lymphatic obstruction
2. A patient presents with sudden onset of shortness of breath. A CT scan reveals a pulmonary embolism. The embolism most likely originated from
   A. Coronary arteries
   B. Deep veins of the leg
   C. Carotid arteries
   D. Pulmonary veins
3. A 60-year-old man with a history of hypertension presents with haematuria. Imaging shows left renal vein thrombosis. This condition is an example of
   A. Arterial thrombosis
   B. Venous thrombosis
   C. Microangiopathic haemolytic anaemia
   D. Disseminated intravascular coagulation
4. A patient in the ICU develops sudden hypotension, tachycardia and cool extremities after significant blood loss. This is indicative of
   A. Septic shock
   B. Cardiogenic shock
   C. Hypovolaemic shock
   D. Neurogenic shock
5. A 70-year-old man with a history of smoking presents with acute chest pain and ECG changes indicative of a myocardial infarction. This is an example of infarction because of
   A. Venous occlusion
   B. Arterial occlusion
   C. Vasospasm
   D. Haemorrhage
6. A patient presents with a swollen, painful leg. Doppler ultrasound reveals deep vein thrombosis. The immediate risk associated with this condition is
   A. Cellulitis
   B. Pulmonary embolism
   C. Chronic venous insufficiency
   D. Varicose veins
7. During surgery, a patient experiences an accidental air embolism. This type of embolism is characterized by
   A. Solid mass in circulation
   B. Liquid mass in circulation
   C. Gaseous mass in circulation
   D. Bacterial mass in circulation
8. A patient with liver cirrhosis presents with abdominal distension and shifting dullness on percussion. This is indicative of
   A. Ascites because of hypoproteinaemia
   B. Gastrointestinal bleeding
   C. Hepatic encephalopathy
   D. Cholelithiasis
9. A young woman in labour develops sudden respiratory distress and seizures. This is most likely
   A. Pulmonary embolism
   B. Amniotic fluid embolism
   C. Myocardial infarction
   D. Eclampsia
10. A patient with a prosthetic heart valve presents with signs of stroke. The most likely cause is
    A. Haemorrhagic stroke
    B. Ischaemic stroke because of thromboembolism
    C. Vasospasm
    D. Hypertensive encephalopathy
11. A 55-year-old man presents with chest pain and is diagnosed with a pulmonary embolism. A risk factor for this condition is
    A. Hyperlipidaemia
    B. Hypertension
    C. Prolonged immobility
    D. Diabetes mellitus
12. A patient with a history of atrial fibrillation develops sudden onset of right-sided weakness. The most likely diagnosis is
    A. Haemorrhagic stroke
    B. Ischaemic stroke
    C. Transient ischaemic attack
    D. Peripheral neuropathy
13. A 30-year-old woman with systemic lupus erythematosus presents with recurrent miscarriages. Laboratory tests reveal prolonged PTT. She is likely suffering from
    A. Haemophilia A
    B. von Willebrand disease
    C. Antiphospholipid antibody syndrome
    D. Disseminated intravascular coagulation
14. A patient with chronic kidney disease presents with generalized oedema. This is most likely because of
    A. Decreased plasma oncotic pressure
    B. Increased hydrostatic pressure
    C. Sodium and water retention
    D. Lymphatic obstruction
15. A patient is diagnosed with myocardial infarction and subsequently develops cardiogenic shock. This is an example of shock because of
    A. Myocardial pump failure
    B. Vasodilation and peripheral pooling of blood
    C. Hypovolaemia
    D. Anaphylactic reaction
16. In a patient with septic shock, the underlying mechanism is most likely
    A. Vasodilation and peripheral pooling of blood
    B. Myocardial pump failure
    C. Severe blood loss
    D. Spinal cord injury
17. A 40-year-old obese woman undergoing surgery is at an increased risk for which of the following postoperative complications?
    A. Arterial thrombosis
    B. Venous thromboembolism
    C. Haemorrhagic stroke
    D. Myocardial infarction
18. A 65-year-old man with atrial fibrillation who forgot to take his anticoagulant medication is at an increased risk for
    A. Haemorrhagic stroke
    B. Deep vein thrombosis
    C. Ischaemic stroke
    D. Pulmonary embolism

19. A young adult presents with painful swelling in the leg after a long flight. Doppler ultrasound confirms deep vein thrombosis. What is the most probable underlying mechanism?
    A. Venous stasis
    B. Arterial vasospasm
    C. Hypercoagulability
    D. Endothelial injury
20. A patient with a known history of deep vein thrombosis suddenly develops chest pain and shortness of breath. The most likely diagnosis is
    A. Acute myocardial infarction
    B. Pulmonary embolism
    C. Pneumonia
    D. Acute asthma attack

Answers

1. (C); 2. (B); 3. (B); 4. (C); 5. (B); 6. (B); 7. (C); 8. (A); 9. (B); 10. (B); 11. (C); 12. (B); 13. (C); 14. (C); 15. (A); 16. (A); 17. (B); 18. (C); 19. (A); 20. (B)

Self-Assessment Questions

1. A 65-year-old man with a history of hypertension and myocardial infarction presents with bilateral ankle swelling and shortness of breath. Describe the underlying pathophysiological mechanisms contributing to his oedema.
2. A patient with chronic kidney disease is experiencing persistent oedema. Explain how renal dysfunction can lead to the development of oedema in this patient.
3. During an autopsy, a pathologist notes that one organ is bright red and another is dark and cyanotic. Discuss the differences between hyperaemia and congestion that could account for these findings.
4. A patient with a history of chronic heart failure presents with hepatomegaly and a 'nutmeg' appearance of the liver on imaging. Explain the pathogenesis and morphological changes seen in chronic venous congestion of the liver in this context.
5. In a case of pleural effusion, laboratory analysis shows a low protein content in the pleural fluid. Discuss the differences between transudate and exudate, and what this finding suggests about the underlying pathology.
6. A patient develops a deep vein thrombosis after a long-haul flight. Describe the aetiopathogenesis, morphology and potential consequences of this thrombosis.
7. Compare and contrast the pathophysiological mechanisms and potential outcomes of pulmonary and systemic thromboembolism.
8. After a traumatic fracture, a patient develops respiratory distress and petechial haemorrhages. Outline the definition, etiological factors, clinical features and laboratory investigations that would help confirm a diagnosis of fat embolism in this case.
9. A patient presents with a myocardial infarction. Discuss the causes, pathogenesis, types and morphological changes associated with infarcts in this context.
10. A patient in the ICU develops septic shock following a bacterial infection. Describe the causes, pathogenesis, stages and clinical features of septic shock in this scenario.

Topics for Self-Directed Learning

1. Iatrogenic lymphatic obstruction as a cause of oedema.
2. Role of endothelium in health and disease.
3. Role of thrombin in health and disease.
4. Link between inflammation and thrombosis.
5. Genetic causes and the types of mutations in primary hypercoagulable states.
6. Management for different types of air embolism.
7. Role of cytokines in shock.
8. Role of Toll-like receptors in septic shock.

MIND MAPS

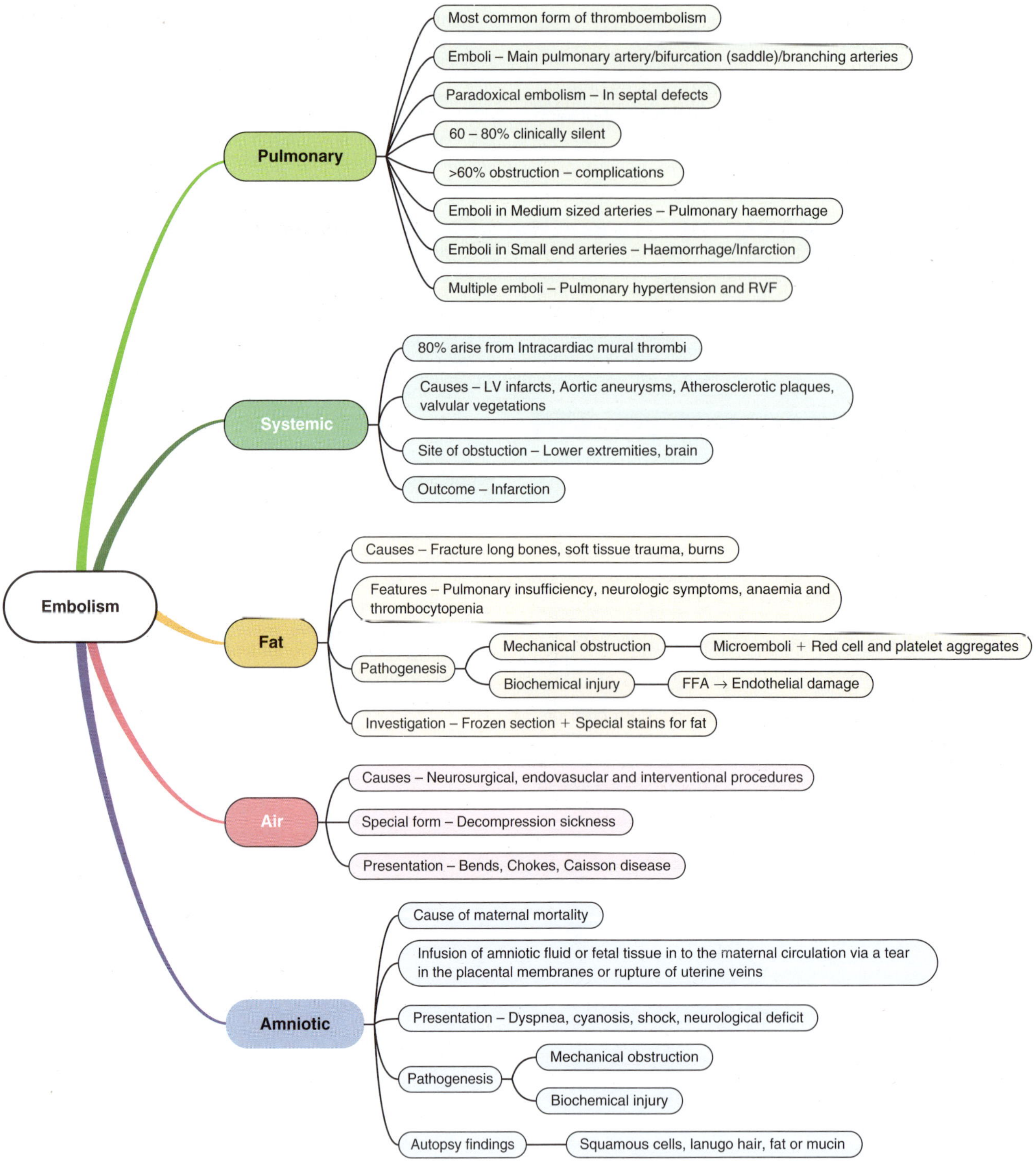
Embolism
Pulmonary
Most common form of thromboembolism
Emboli – Main pulmonary artery/bifurcation (saddle)/branching arteries
Paradoxical embolism – In septal defects
60 – 80% clinically silent
>60% obstruction – complications
Emboli in Medium sized arteries – Pulmonary haemorrhage
Emboli in Small end arteries – Haemorrhage/Infarction
Multiple emboli – Pulmonary hypertension and RVF
Systemic
80% arise from Intracardiac mural thrombi
Causes – LV infarcts, Aortic aneurysms, Atherosclerotic plaques, valvular vegetations
Site of obstuction – Lower extremities, brain
Outcome – Infarction
Fat
Causes – Fracture long bones, soft tissue trauma, burns
Features – Pulmonary insufficiency, neurologic symptoms, anaemia and thrombocytopenia
Pathogenesis
Mechanical obstruction
Microemboli + Red cell and platelet aggregates
Biochemical injury
FFA → Endothelial damage
Investigation – Frozen section + Special stains for fat
Air
Causes – Neurosurgical, endovasuclar and interventional procedures
Special form – Decompression sickness
Presentation – Bends, Chokes, Caisson disease
Amniotic
Cause of maternal mortality
Infusion of amniotic fluid or fetal tissue in to the maternal circulation via a tear in the placental membranes or rupture of uterine veins
Presentation – Dyspnea, cyanosis, shock, neurological deficit
Pathogenesis
Mechanical obstruction
Biochemical injury
Autopsy findings
Squamous cells, lanugo hair, fat or mucin

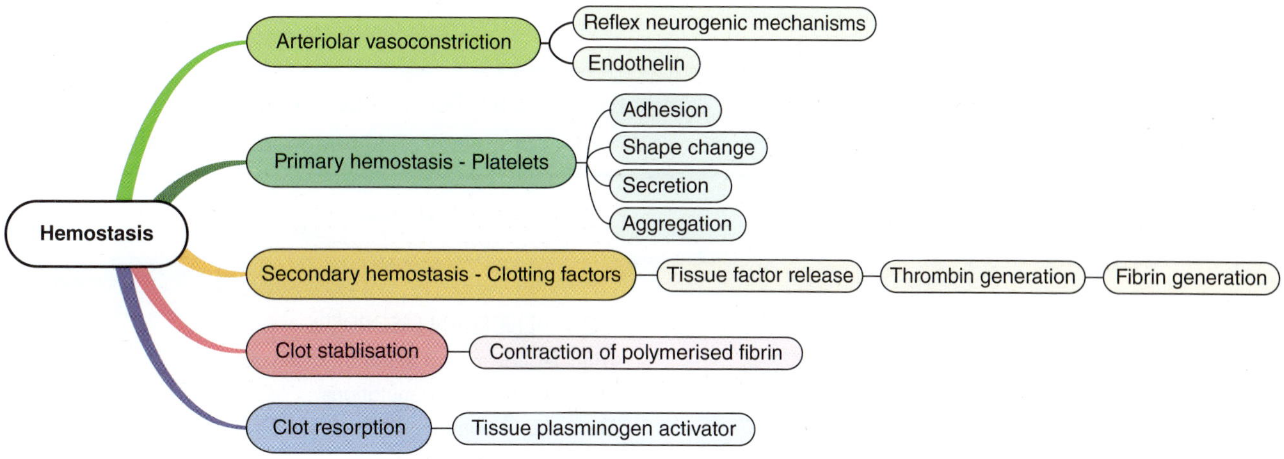
Hemostasis
Arteriolar vasoconstriction
Reflex neurogenic mechanisms
Endothelin
Primary hemostasis - Platelets
Adhesion
Shape change
Secretion
Aggregation
Secondary hemostasis - Clotting factors
Tissue factor release
Thrombin generation
Fibrin generation
Clot stablisation
Contraction of polymerised fibrin
Clot resorption
Tissue plasminogen activator

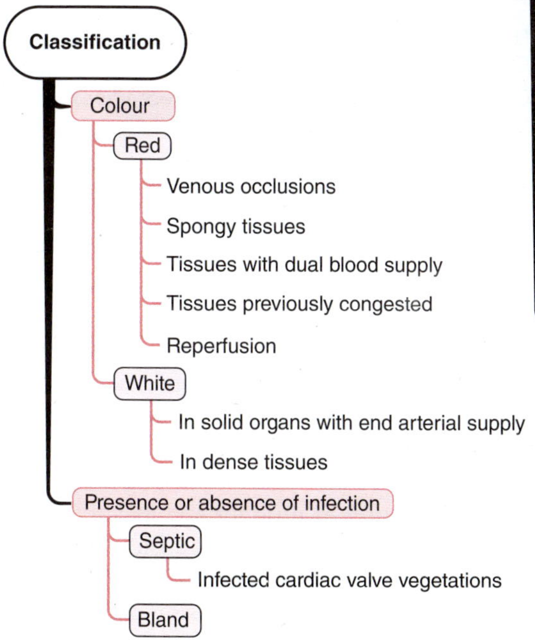
Classification
Colour
Red
Venous occlusions
Spongy tissues
Tissues with dual blood supply
Tissues previously congested
Reperfusion
White
In solid organs with end arterial supply
In dense tissues
Presence or absence of infection
Septic
Infected cardiac valve vegetations
Bland

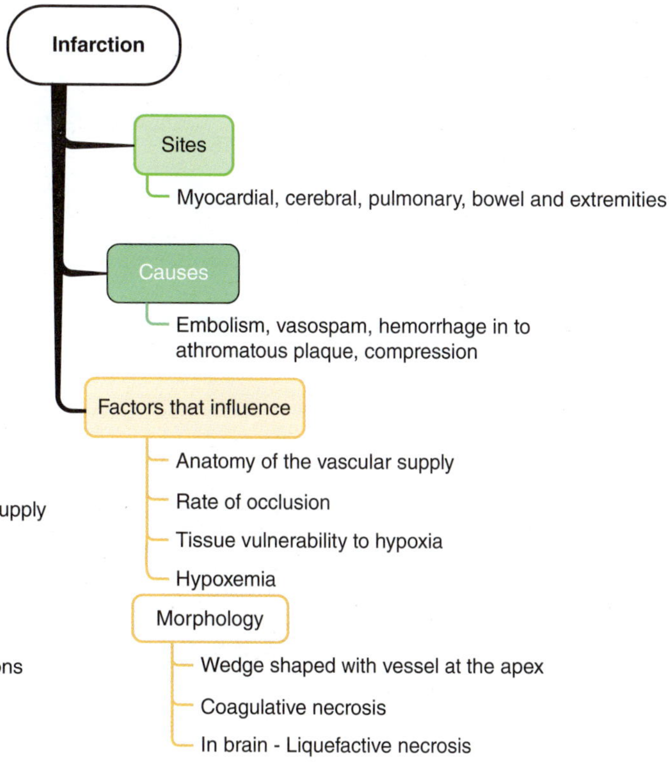
Infarction
Sites
Myocardial, cerebral, pulmonary, bowel and extremities
Causes
Embolism, vasospam, hemorrhage in to athromatous plaque, compression
Factors that influence
Anatomy of the vascular supply
Rate of occlusion
Tissue vulnerability to hypoxia
Hypoxemia
Morphology
Wedge shaped with vessel at the apex
Coagulative necrosis
In brain - Liquefactive necrosis

5 Genetic Disorders

M Lavanya

PA 11.1 Describe the pathogenesis and features of common cytogenetic abnormalities and mutations in childhood.
PA 11.3 Describe the pathogenesis of common storage disorders in infancy and childhood.

CHAPTER OUTLINE

INTRODUCTION

GENES AND HUMAN DISEASES

The Human Genome project in 2003 drafted the entire human genome. A human genome consists of about 3.2 billion DNA base pairs, arranged in 23 pairs of chromosomes as triplet sequence called genes. **Genes are the functional unit of hereditary**. Any abnormality in the gene or chromosome may give rise to genetic disorders.

Genetic diseases can be broadly classified as follows (Table 5.1):

- **Disorders because of single gene mutation**
  a. Mendelian disorders
  b. Disorders with non-Mendelian inheritance
- **Chromosomal disorders**
- **Complex multigenic disorders**

Disorders because of single gene mutation

These diseases are caused by **mutation in a single gene** with large effects and usually follow the classical Mendelian pattern of inheritance (also known as **Mendelian disorders**), with some exceptions. These are generally rare and are more common in a selective population.

Examples: Haemophilia A, commonly seen in the males of the royal families of England; sickle cell anaemia, common in areas endemic to malaria

Chromosomal disorders

These diseases are caused by **changes in the chromosome structure or number** and may involve the autosomes or sex chromosomes. These are uncommon diseases with a high penetrance. (**Penetrance** is the likelihood of disease expression in a person with a mutated gene.)

Examples: Down syndrome (trisomy 21), Klinefelter syndrome (47XXY)

Complex multigenic disorders

These diseases are more common in occurrence and have a low penetrance. These are caused by the **interaction of multiple genes, polymorphisms and environmental factors**. Polymorphism refers to the variations in a gene within a population. Some variant genes

Table 5.1 Classification of Genetic Disorders

1. **Disorders with single gene mutation**
   a. **Mendelian disorders**
      i. Autosomal inheritance
         1. Autosomal dominant
         2. Autosomal recessive
      ii. Sex-linked inheritance
         1. X-linked dominant
         2. X-linked recessive
   b. **Disorders with non-Mendelian inheritance**
      i. Trinucleotide-repeat mutation
      ii. Mitochondrial gene mutation
      iii. Genomic imprinting
      iv. Gonadal mosaicism
2. **Chromosomal disorders**
   a. Changes in chromosomal structure
   b. Changes in chromosome number (cytogenetic disorder)
      i. Involving autosomes
      ii. Involving sex chromosomes
3. **Complex multigenic disorders**

(polymorphism) are associated with a small increase in the risk of developing the disease. Several such variant genes are needed for the occurrence of a disease, so it is termed multigenic or polygenic. Environmental factors also play an important role in the pathogenesis of these diseases, hence termed multifactorial.

Examples: Atherosclerosis, diabetes mellitus, hypertension

MUTATIONS

A mutation is defined as a **permanent change** in the genetic material. Mutations can occur in germ cells or somatic cells. Germ cell mutations are transmitted to the progeny and give rise to inherited diseases. Somatic cell mutations are acquired mutations and are not transmitted or inherited but may give rise to neoplasia.

Mutations can **occur spontaneously or can be acquired**. Acquired mutations develop on exposure to some chemical or physical agents called **mutagen or carcinogen**. Examples of carcinogens are alkylating agents, azo dyes and radiation exposure.

Types of Gene Mutation and Its Effects

1. **Point mutation:** These mutations are characterized by changes in a single nucleotide base in the DNA sequence and can occur in the coding or noncoding region of DNA.

   Types of point mutation:

   a. **Missense mutation:** Here, the point mutation changes the genetic code by substituting one amino acid for another. It is of two types:

      Conservative missense mutation: The substituted amino acid has a similar biochemical property as that of the original.

      Nonconservative missense mutation: The substituted amino acid is biochemically different and alters the protein function.

      Example: Sickle cell anaemia – point mutation in the β-globin chain (sixth position) substitutes the amino acid valine for glutamic acid. This alters the biochemical properties of haemoglobin and results in sickle-shaped red blood cells (RBCs).

   b. **Nonsense mutation:** The point mutation results in the formation of a stop codon.

      Example: β-thalassaemia – here, the mutation causes premature termination of β-globin gene translation. As a result, there is reduced formation of β-globin chain, causing severe anaemia.

   c. **Silent mutation:** Here, the altered codon codes for the same amino acid and hence the mutation has no effect.

2. **Deletions and insertions:** One or more nucleotides are added or removed from the coding sequence. The DNA sequence is read as a trinucleotide code. If the number of nucleotides inserted or deleted is not in multiples of 3, then the entire reading frame of the DNA strand downstream gets changed or shifted. This is called **frameshift mutation** and results in the addition of many improper amino acids to the protein.
3. **Trinucleotide repeats (TNRs):** These mutations are characterized by the amplification of a sequence of trinucleotides. An example is fragile X syndrome – there are 250–4000 tandem repeats in contrast to a normal average of 29 repeats of the trinucleotide CGG within the gene called familial mental retardation 1 (FMR1) gene.

MENDELIAN DISORDERS PA 11.1

INHERITANCE PATTERNS

The laws of inheritance were postulated by Gregor Mendel (1822–1884) from his studies on garden pea. Genetic disorders because of a single gene defect (monogenic disorders) classically follow the Mendelian law of inheritance with few exceptions.

Classification of Mendelian Disorders

Autosomal inheritance

Autosomal dominant (AD)

Autosomal recessive (AR)

Sex-linked inheritance

X-linked recessive

X-linked dominant

Note: Mutations in the Y chromosome affect the spermatogenesis and cause infertility in the affected male. Hence, no Y-linked inheritance disorders are known.

Table 5.2 List of Mendelian Disorders

System/Inheritance	Autosomal Dominant	Autosomal Recessive	X-linked Recessive
Nervous	Huntington disease Neurofibromatosis Myotonic dystrophy	Friedreich ataxia Spinal muscular atrophy	Fragile X syndrome
Haematology	Hereditary Spherocytosis von Willebrand disease	Sickle cell anaemia Thalassaemia	Haemophilia A and B Glucose-6-phosphate dehydrogenase deficiency
Musculoskeletal	Marfan syndrome Ehlers–Danlos syndrome (some variants) Osteogenesis imperfecta Achondroplasia	Ehlers–Danlos syndrome (some variants)	Duchenne muscular dystrophy
Metabolic	Familial hypercholesterolaemia Acute intermittent porphyria	Cystic fibrosis Phenylketonuria Galactosaemia Homocystinuria Lysosomal storage diseases Glycogen storage diseases α_1-Antitrypsin deficiency Wilson disease Haemochromatosis Alkaptonuria	Diabetes insipidus Lesch–Nyhan syndrome
Renal	Autosomal dominant polycystic kidney disease	Autosomal recessive polycystic kidney disease	
Gastrointestinal	Familial polyposis coli		
Immunity			Chronic granulomatous disease Agammaglobulinaemia Wiskott–Aldrich syndrome

The list of Mendelian disorders is given in Table 5.2. The characteristic features of each group of disorders are described briefly.

Autosomal Inheritance

Autosomal Dominant Disorders

- AD disorders are genetic disorders that require only one defective allele to manifest in an individual.
- The gene involved is located in the autosomal chromosome. Hence, **males and females are equally affected.**
- The disease manifests in the heterozygous and homozygous states.
- The age of onset is delayed.
- **Pedigree chart** (family tree) (Fig. 5.1)
  - One of the parents is usually affected.
  - When the affected person marries a normal person, the offspring has a 50% chance of inheriting the disease.
  - All the generations will have some affected persons.
  - When both parents are normal, the child may get an AD disorder because of a new mutation, and in such cases, there is no risk for the siblings.
- **Variations in penetrance and expression are seen.**
  Penetrance is given as a percentage; 75% penetrance means that only 75% of the individuals with inherited mutation will express the disease. The remaining 25% are phenotypically normal.

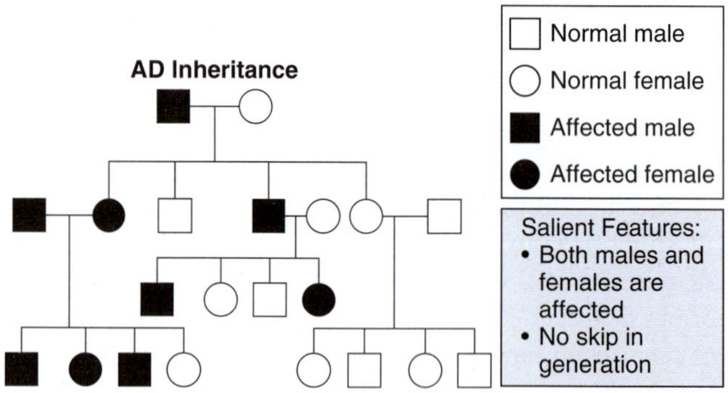

Fig. 5.1 Pedigree chart of autosomal dominant disorders.

Expression is the phenotypic manifestation of the mutation. Some mutations can have one or more phenotypic expressions.

Example: Neurofibromatosis type I (NFI) can manifest as multiple brown-coloured macules (*café au lait* spots), Lisch nodules in the iris, freckles in the axilla and groin, neurofibromas of the skin, gliomas of the optic nerve and skeletal deformities. Individuals

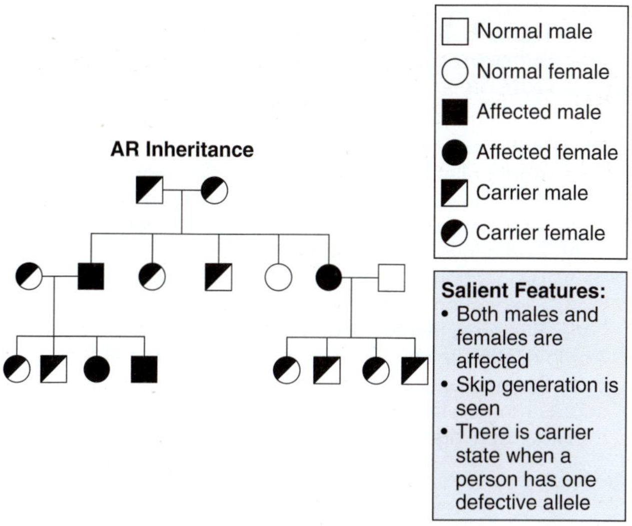

Fig. 5.2 Pedigree chart of autosomal recessive disorders.

inheriting the NFI gene can vary in their expression from one to all the characteristics of the disease.

- The mutant gene usually encodes for a structural protein or regulatory protein.

Autosomal Recessive Disorders

- AR disorders are genetic disorders that require both the alleles to be defective to manifest in an individual.
- Most metabolic diseases show AR inheritance.
- The disease can manifest only in the homozygous state. It is characterized by complete penetrance and full expression.
- The onset of symptoms occurs early in life.
- Parents are usually normal (heterozygotes). Skip in generation is seen (Fig. 5.2).
- A person who carries one defective allele but does not manifest the disorder because of the other normal allele is called a carrier.
- The siblings of an affected person have 25% (one in four) chance of inheriting the disease.
- These are more common in consanguineous marriages.
- If the affected person marries a normal individual, none of the offspring are affected.

Sex-Linked Inheritance

- Females have two X chromosomes; hence, the X-linked traits can be dominant or recessive.
- Males having one X chromosome are **hemizygous**, and they express the trait regardless of whether it is dominant or recessive.

X-Linked Recessive Disorders (Fig. 5.3)

- These are disorders in which the defective allele on the X chromosome manifests only in the absence of a normal counterpart.
- Males are commonly affected. In men, the Y chromosome does not carry the same genes and hence they are affected when they have one defective allele on the X chromosome.

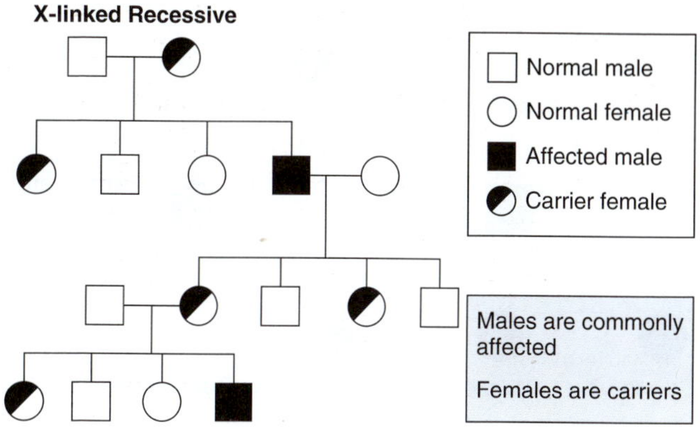

Fig. 5.3 Pedigree chart of X-linked recessive disorders.

- On the contrary, in women, both the X chromosomes need to have defective alleles to manifest the disorder, which is very rare.
- The affected male does not transmit the disease to his sons but transmits the defective X chromosome to all his daughters who now have one defective X chromosome and become carriers (Fig. 5.3).
- The carrier females do not manifest the disease but have 50% (one in two) chance of transmitting the disease to her sons and 50% chance of her daughters being carriers.
- Very rarely, because of random inactivation of the normal X chromosome (Lyon hypothesis), these disorders may manifest in a heterozygous (carrier) female.
- In addition, when a carrier female marries an affected male, their daughter may be homozygous for the defective X chromosome and manifest it.

X-Linked Dominant Inheritance

- In X-linked dominant inheritance, the disease is expressed when a defective allele is present on one X chromosome irrespective of the allele on the other chromosome.
- Females are affected twice more than males.
- The affected female transmits the disease to half of her children (50% chance in both males and females).
- The affected male transmits the disease to all his daughters, but none of his sons are affected (Fig. 5.4).
- **Examples:** These include vitamin D–resistant (familial hypophosphataemic) rickets and ornithine transcarbamylase deficiency.

AUTOSOMAL DISORDERS WITH DEFECTS IN STRUCTURAL PROTEINS

Marfan syndrome and Ehlers–Danlos syndrome (EDS) are common connective tissue disorders with AD inheritance.

MARFAN SYNDROME

Marfan syndrome is an inherited connective tissue disorder affecting multiorgan systems. The principal changes

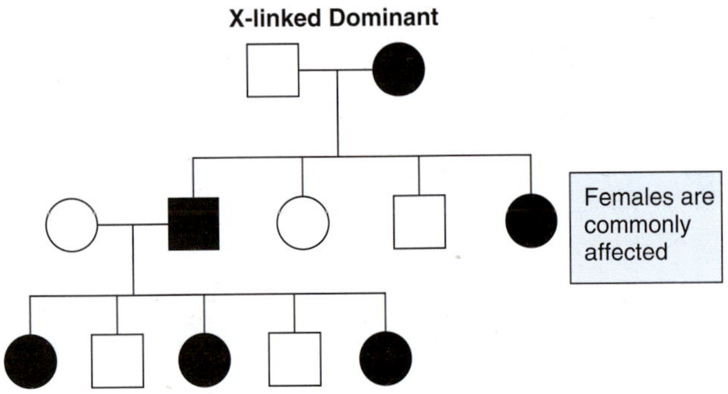

Fig. 5.4 Pedigree chart of X-linked dominant inheritance.

are seen in the **skeleton, cardiovascular system, skin and eyes**.

Incidence	:	One in 5000
Inheritance	:	Autosomal dominant
Genetic defect	:	Missense mutation in FBN1 gene on chromosome 15q21.1
Protein defect	:	**Fibrillin-1**, an extracellular glycoprotein

Pathogenesis

Fibrillin is an extracellular glycoprotein that forms microfibrils and also provides the scaffold for elastin deposition. The microfibrils are present widely in the connective tissue, with an increased concentration being present in the **aorta, heart, ligaments and ciliary zonules of eyes.** Hence, these organs are mainly affected if fibrillin is abnormal.

Mutations in fibrillin-1 gene can result in the following:

1. **Loss of structural support:** Abnormal fibrillin-1 protein weakens the connective tissue framework and gives rise to the characteristic features.
2. **Excessive activation of transforming growth factor-β (TGF-β):** TGF-β is a multifunctional cytokine that regulates cell proliferation and a variety of inflammatory reactions. Normally, microfibrils sequester TGF-β and loss of microfibrils leads to excessive activation of TGF-β, which causes the following:
   a. Cardiovascular changes because of the prevention of vascular smooth muscle development
   b. Loss of extracellular matrix (ECM) because of the activation of metalloproteases

Morphology

Skeletal system
- Patients are abnormally tall with long extremities.
- The fingers are long and tapering (arachnodactyly/spider fingers).
- The skull is long (dolichocephalic) with prominent frontal eminence.
- Chest: Pectus excavatum (concave sternum) or pectus carinatum (pigeon chest) may be present.
- Spine: Kyphosis, scoliosis and disc prolapse are seen.
- Tendons and ligaments are lax, leading to hyperextensibility of the joints (double jointed).

Cardiovascular system
- Aortic root dilation and mitral valve prolapse are the common lesions.
- The aortic root dilation is because of cystic medial necrosis of the vessel wall. Progressive dilation can lead to aortic incompetence and aortic dissection (a life-threatening complication).

Eyes
- Subluxation or dislocation of the lens
- Severe myopia

Table 5.3 Clinical Diagnosis of Marfan Syndrome on the Basis of Revised Ghent Criteria

Diagnostic scenarios

I. Aortic dilation/aneurysm with dislocation of lens
II. Aortic involvement with FBN1 mutation
III. Aortic involvement and systemic involvement
IV. Aortic involvement and family history
V. Dislocation of lens and FBN1 mutation
VI. Dislocation of lens and family history
VII. Systemic involvement and family history

Aortic dilation/aneurysm is considered a cardinal feature. The rest of the morphological changes are given scores ranging from 1 to 3, and the total score ≥7 is considered a significant systemic involvement.

Clinical Features

The lesions described are characteristic of Marfan syndrome. However, because of varied expressivity, the clinical diagnosis of Marfan syndrome relies on a set of defined clinical criteria named **'revised Ghent criteria'** (Table 5.3). These criteria are based on the family history, clinical features and mutation of the fibrillin gene.

Treatment

Patients with Marfan syndrome usually die early by 30–40 years of age.

Administration of antihypertensive drugs (β-blockers) and replacement of the aorta and valves with prosthetic grafts have greatly increased the life expectancy of patients with Marfan syndrome.

EHLERS–DANLOS SYNDROME

EDS is a group of inherited connective tissue disorders characterized by remarkable **hyperextensibility of the skin, joint hypermobility and tissue fragility**. There are 13 clinical types of EDS according to the 2017 international classification (Table 5.4).

Table 5.4 Clinical Classification of EDS (2017 International Classification)

EDS Clinical Types	Inheritance	Mutations	Protein	Clinical Features	Complications
1. Classical EDS	AD	COL5A1, COL5A2	Type V collagen	Hyperextensibility of skin Joint hypermobility	Extreme fragility, delayed wound healing
2. Classical-like EDS	AR	TNXP	Tenascin XB	Hyperextensibility of skin	
3. Cardiac-valvular	AR	COL1A2	Type I collagen	Severe progressive cardiac-valvular problems (aortic valve, mitral valve)	Valvular diseases
4. Vascular EDS	AD	COL3A1	Type III collagen	Translucent skin and prominent blood vessels	Rupture of blood vessels and hollow viscera
5. Hypermobile EDS	AD	Unknown	Unknown	Generalized joint hypermobility	Dislocations
6. Arthrochalasia EDS	AD	COL1A1, COL1A2	Type I collagen	Congenital hip dislocation Joint hypermobility	Dislocations
7. Dermatosparaxis EDS	AR	ADAMTS2	ADAMTS−2	Extreme skin fragility with skin tears	Bladder rupture, diaphragmatic rupture
8. Kyphoscoliotic EDS	AR	PLOD1 FKBP14	LH1, FKBP22	Congenital muscle hypotonia, early onset kyphoscoliosis	Rupture of blood vessels
9. Brittle cornea syndrome	AR	ZNF469 PRDM5	ZNF469 PRDM5	Thin cornea, blue sclera, keratoconus	Eyeball rupture
10. Spondylodysplastic EDS	AR	B4GALT7 B3GALT6	β4GalT7 β3GalT6	Short stature, hypotonia	
11. Musculocontractural EDS	AR	CHST14 DSE	D4ST 1 DSE	Muscle contractures, craniofacial features	Recurrent dislocations
12. Myopathic EDS	AD/AR	COL12A1	Type 12 collagen	Muscle hypotonia, joint contractures	
13. Periodontal EDS	AD	C1R, C1S	C1r, C1s	Periodontal disease, precocious tooth loss	

AD, autosomal dominant; AR, autosomal recessive; EDS, Ehlers–Danlos syndrome.

Prevalence : One in 5000
Protein defect : Fibrillar collagen
Genetic defect : EDS is caused by mutations in genes that encode collagen and enzymes that modify the collagen
Inheritance : Autosomal dominant, Autosomal recessive

Pathogenesis

Mutations in the genes that encode structural collagen or its modifiers cause significant weakness and loss of tensile strength in supporting structures throughout the body. The changes are prominently seen in the **skin, joints, arteries and hollow viscera.**

Clinical Features (Fig. 5.5)

The characteristic clinical features are hyperextensibility of the skin and hypermobility of the joints. These can be elicited clinically by stretching the skin, bending the thumb to touch the forearm and hyperextension of the knee joint.

Complications

The dreaded life-threatening complications in these cases are rupture of blood vessels and hollow viscera such as the intestines and bladder.

Diagnosis

Diagnosis is made by characteristic clinical features and molecular studies.

AUTOSOMAL DISORDERS WITH DEFECTIVE RECEPTOR PROTEINS

FAMILIAL HYPERCHOLESTEROLAEMIA

Familial hypercholesterolaemia is the most commonly occurring inherited disorder. It is characterized by high level

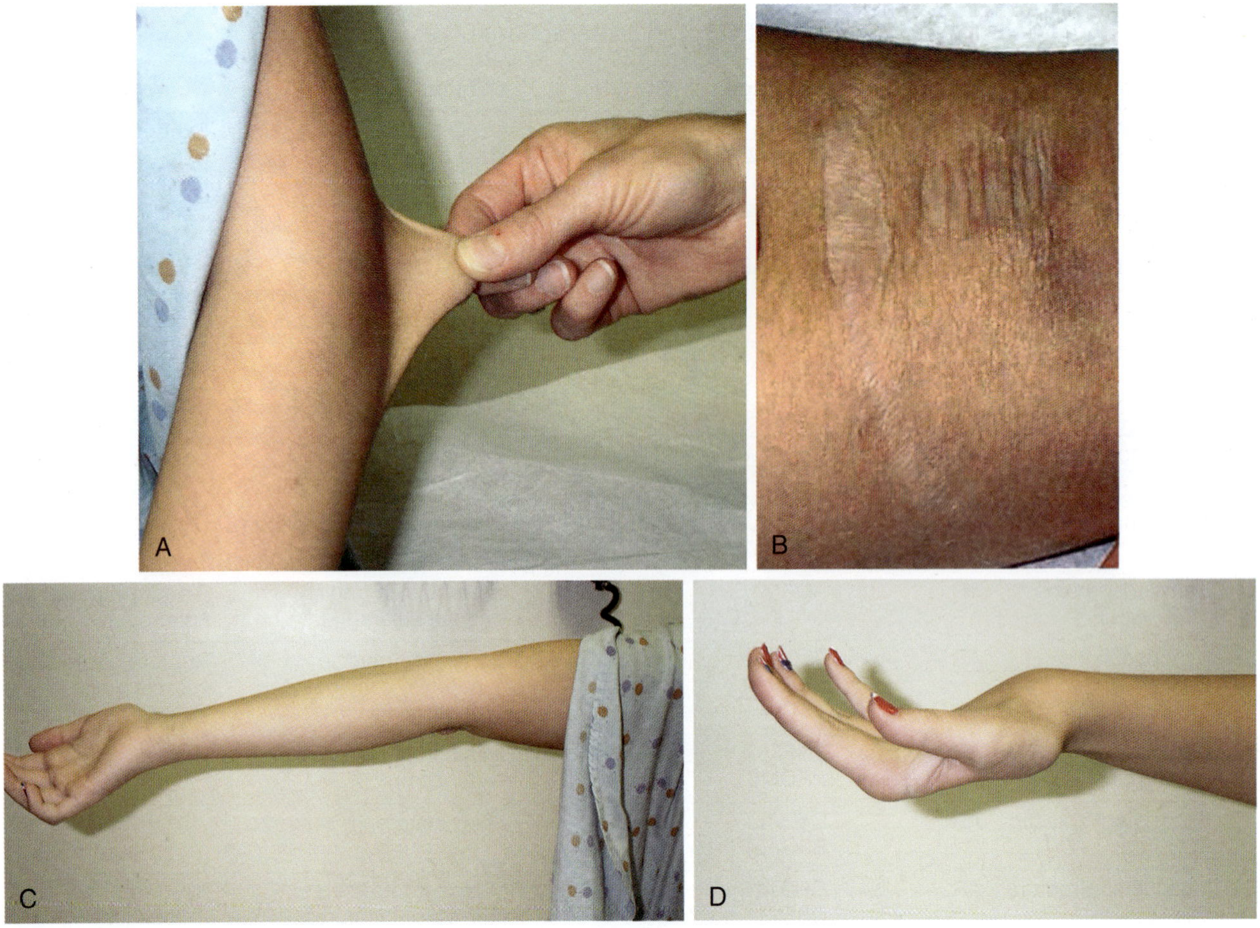

Fig. 5.5 Ehlers–Danlos syndrome classical type. (A) Note the marked hyperextensibility of the skin over this child's arm. (B) These widened atrophic scars have the thin papery texture that is characteristic of Ehlers–Danlos syndrome. (C and D) Hyperextensibility of the joints of the elbow and fingers is also seen. (*Source:* From Ehlers-Danlos Syndromes. Elsevier Point of Care. 2022. Elsevier.)

of low density lipoprotein (LDL) in blood and cholesterol deposits in arteries, tendon and skin. The defect is in the receptor protein of LDL namely LDL receptor (LDLR).

Prevalence	:	One in 500; most common inherited disorder
Protein defect	:	LDL receptor
Genetic defect	:	LDLR gene on chromosome 19
Inheritance	:	Autosomal dominant Homozygotes have more severe disease than heterozygotes

Pathogenesis (Fig. 5.6)

LDL is the carrier of cholesterol esters in circulation. Cholesterol esters bind to LDL receptors, located on the surface of liver cells, and the LDL–LDLR complex is internalized. The endosomal vacuole so formed fuses with the lysosome and the complex is broken down and the cholesterol present is used or converted to storage forms. A defect in LDL receptor causes high circulating levels of LDL (rich in cholesterol esters) that are taken up by tissue macrophages that accumulate to form plaques (atherosclerotic plaque in blood vessels) or nodules of lipid-laden macrophages (xanthomas of the skin and tendon).

More than 900 mutations are identified, which are classified into 5 groups (Table 5.5).

Clinical Features

Persons with familial hypercholesterolaemia have high levels of blood cholesterol from birth. The levels vary in the heterozygous and homozygous states.

Normal cholesterol level	:	<200 mg/dL
Familial hypercholesterolaemia		
Heterozygous	:	<350 mg/dL
Homozygous	:	600–1200 mg/dL

Persons with familial hypercholesterolaemia develop premature atherosclerosis and xanthomas of the tendons and skin. These patients develop symptoms of coronary artery disease by 40 years of age and usually die of myocardial infarction.

Treatment

Treatment with statins significantly reduces the level of blood cholesterol and thereby reduces the morbidity and mortality because of coronary artery disease.

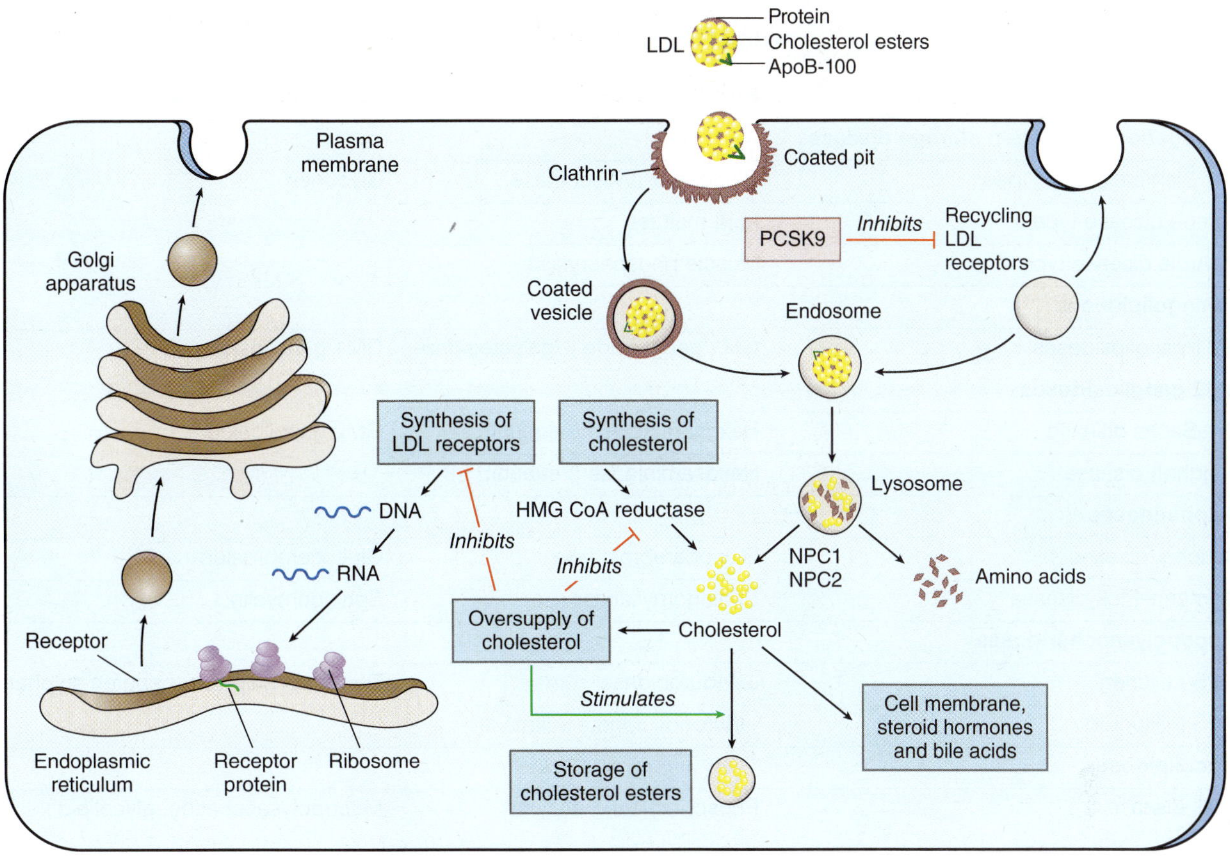

Fig. 5.6 Pathogenesis of familial hypercholesterolaemia.

Table 5.5 Classification of Familial Hypercholesterolaemia

Class	Genetic Defect	Result	Type of Defect
I	Translation of mRNA in the endoplasmic reticulum	No LDL receptors are formed	Quantitative
II	Post-translational modification in the Golgi apparatus	LDL receptors are formed but are functionally defective	Qualitative
III	Transport to the cell surface	No LDL receptors on the cell membrane	Quantitative
IV	Clustering of LDL receptors at clathrin-coated pit	LDL receptors on the surface do not bind LDL	Qualitative
V	Recycling of LDL receptors	LDL receptors do not dissociate from LDL in lysosomes	Quantitative

LDL, low-density lipoprotein.

AUTOSOMAL DISORDERS WITH ENZYME DEFECTS PA 11.3

LYSOSOMAL STORAGE DISEASES

Lysosomes are cytoplasmic membrane-bound vesicles containing various hydrolytic enzymes. These enzymes are active only at acidic pH and hence called acid hydrolases. The function of lysosomes is to break down complex macromolecules into small diffusible molecules.

Lysosomal storage diseases (LSDs) result from mutation in the genes coding for the **lysosomal acid hydrolases**. This results in deficiency of the enzyme and accumulation of the undigested macromolecule within the lysosome. The distended lysosomes lead to poor cell function, cell injury and cell death.

LSDs are classified into subgroups on the basis of the accumulated substrates (Table 5.6). More than 50 LSDs are known, and the list is expanding. Only the important diseases are discussed here.

Table 5.6 List of Important Lysosomal Storage Diseases

Lysosomal Storage Diseases	Enzyme Deficiency	Substrate Accumulated
Glycogenosis/glycogen storage diseases		
von Gierke disease type I	Glucose-6-phosphatase	Glycogen
Pompe disease type II	Acid maltase	
McArdle disease type V	Muscle phosphorylase	
Sphingolipidoses		
GM1 gangliosidoses	GM1 ganglioside β-galactosidase	GM1 ganglioside
GM2 gangliosidoses		
Tay–Sachs disease	Hexosaminidase α subunit	GM2 ganglioside
Sandhoff disease	Hexosaminidase β subunit	
Sulphatidoses		
Gaucher disease	Glucocerebrosidase	Glucocerebroside
Niemann–Pick disease	Sphingomyelinase	Sphingomyelin
Mucopolysaccharidoses		
MPS I (Hurler)	α-l-Iduronidase	Dermatan sulphate, heparan sulphate
MPS II (Hunter)	l-Iduronosulphate sulfatase	
Mucolipidoses		
I-cell disease	Phosphorylating enzyme	Mucopolysaccharide, glycolipid

Sphingolipidoses

Sphingolipidoses are LSDs characterized by the accumulation of lipids derived from breakdown of the cell membrane. **Cerebrosides, gangliosides, sphingomyelin and sulphatides** are sphingolipid components of the cell membrane. These are broken down into sphingosine and fatty acid by a complex metabolic pathway involving various lysosomal acid hydrolases. Deficiency of these enzymes results in the accumulation of the macromolecule **sphingolipid** (Fig. 5.7).

Tay–Sachs Disease (GM2 gangliosidoses)

Tay–Sachs disease is characterized by **GM2 ganglioside** accumulation because of enzyme deficiency.

Mutation	:	HEXA gene on chromosome 15
Enzyme deficient	:	Hexosaminidase A
Substrate accumulated	:	GM2 ganglioside
Inheritance	:	Autosomal recessive
Occurrence	:	It is more prevalent in Ashkenazi Jews; carrier rate is 1 in 30 in Jews and 1 in 100,000 in the non-Jewish population
Organ affected	:	Brain

Pathogenesis Because of deficiency of **hexosaminidase A enzyme**, its substrate GM2 ganglioside (the complex lipid) gets accumulated in the lysosomes of all cells but more prominently in the neurons of the brain and ganglion cells of the retina. This results in a progressive destruction of the neurons and proliferation of microglia.

Morphology (Fig. 5.8)

Brain

Macroscopy: The brain shows marked atrophy.

Microscopy: Neurons are **ballooned** with cytoplasmic vacuoles. These vacuoles represent the lysosomes distended with GM2 ganglioside (complex lipid). In retina, ganglion cells are distended with similar inclusions.

Special stains: Fat stains (oil red O and Sudan black) are positive in the vacuoles.

Electron microscopy: The neurons show numerous cytoplasmic membranous bodies (lysosomes with a whorled configuration of membranes – onion skin appearance).

Clinical Features Infants are normal at birth and present with progressive mental and motor deterioration at about 6 months of age. Examination of the eye reveals the characteristic **cherry-red spot in the macula**. The child reaches a vegetative state by 1–2 years of age and usually dies between 2 and 3 years of age.

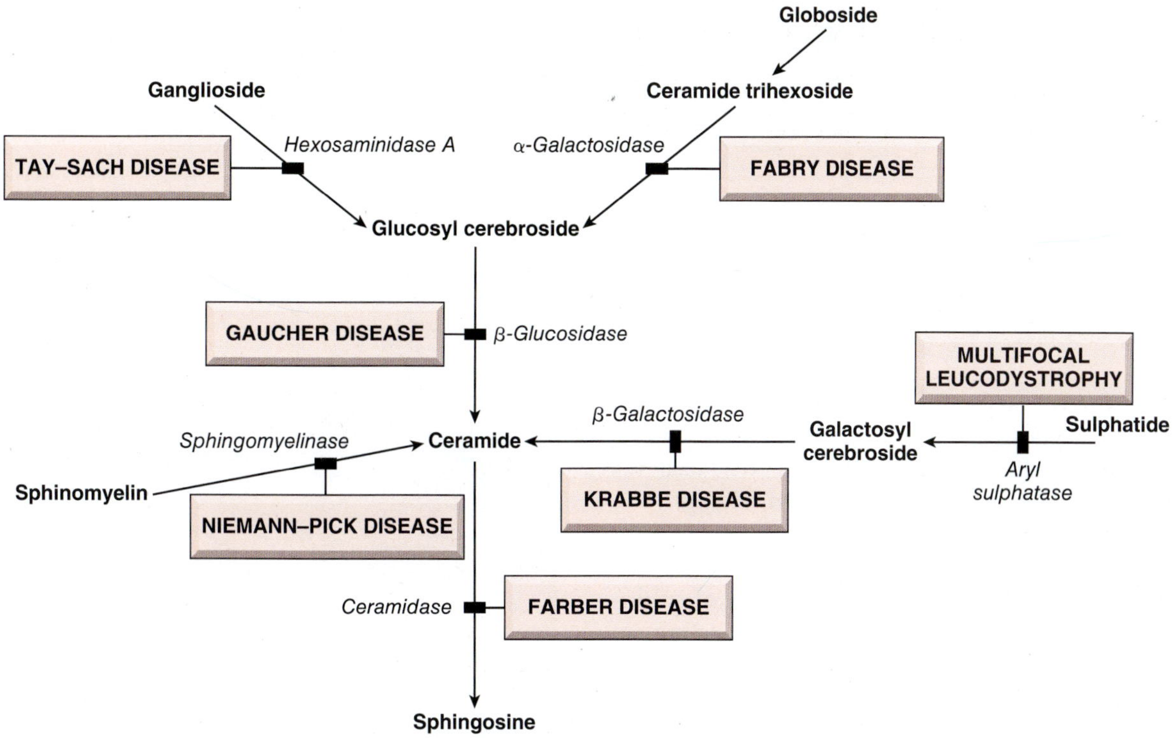

Fig. 5.7 Pathogenesis of sphingolipidoses.

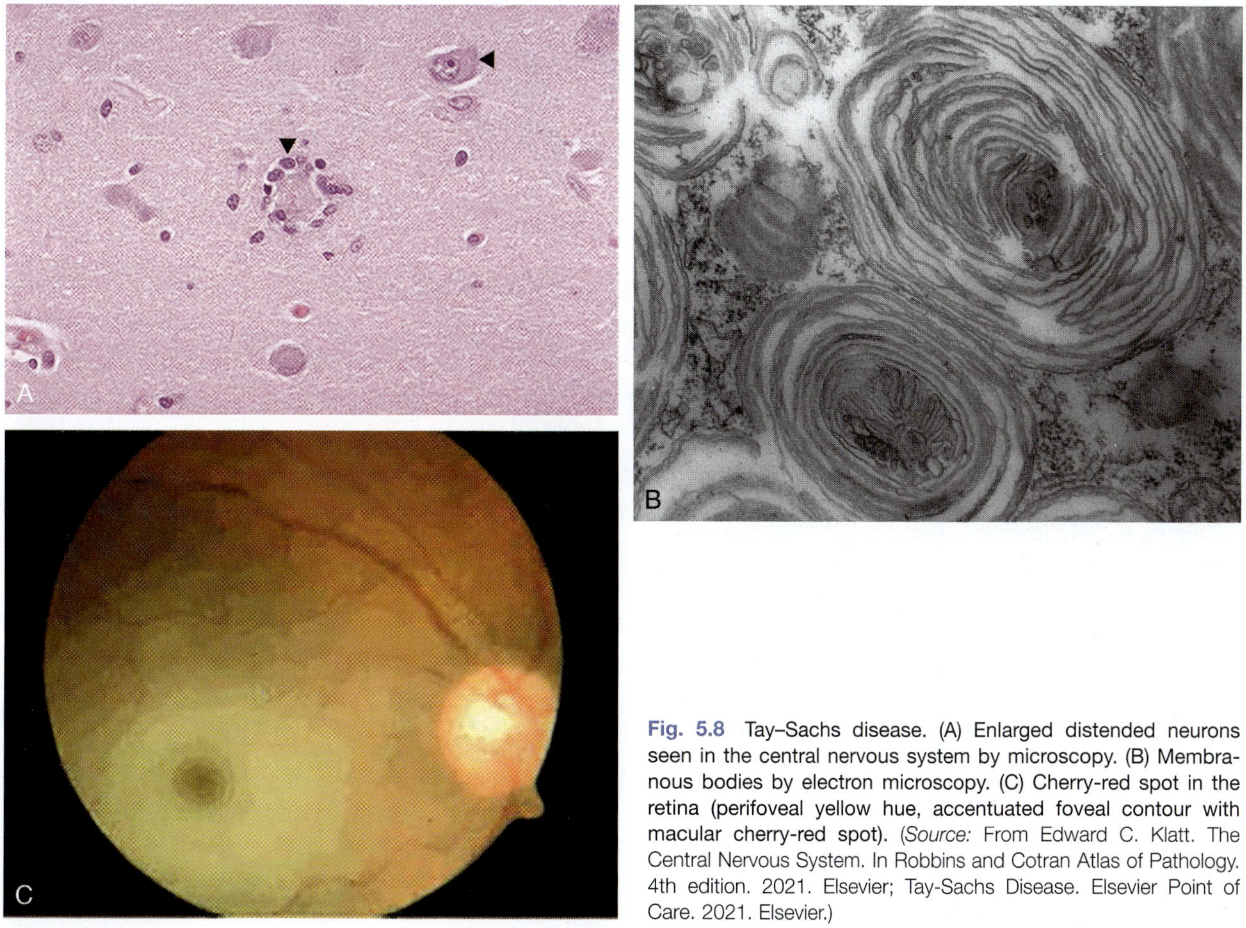

Fig. 5.8 Tay–Sachs disease. (A) Enlarged distended neurons seen in the central nervous system by microscopy. (B) Membranous bodies by electron microscopy. (C) Cherry-red spot in the retina (perifoveal yellow hue, accentuated foveal contour with macular cherry-red spot). (*Source:* From Edward C. Klatt. The Central Nervous System. In Robbins and Cotran Atlas of Pathology. 4th edition. 2021. Elsevier; Tay-Sachs Disease. Elsevier Point of Care. 2021. Elsevier.)

Table 5.7 Types of Niemann–Pick disease

Type	Gene mutation	Pathology	Clinical feature
Type A	SMAD 1	Deficiency of sphingomyelinase	Organomegaly, severe neurological involvement Death within 3 years
Type B	SMAD 1	Deficiency of sphingomyelinase	Organomegaly Survive to adulthood
Type C	NPC 1, NPC 2	Defect in lipid transport protein	Hydrops fetalis, stillbirth, neonatal hepatitis, progressive neurological deterioration

Diagnosis Enzyme assay and DNA analysis are performed for antenatal diagnosis and detection of the carrier state.

Possibility of chaperone therapy is under trial (as mutations in HEXA gene affect the protein folding).

Niemann–Pick Disease

Niemann–Pick disease is caused by **deficiency of sphingomyelinase**, leading to lysosomal accumulation of sphingomyelin in various organs. It is classified into three types on the basis of gene mutation and clinical presentation: Type A, Type B and Type C (refer Table 5.7).

Mutation	:	SMPD 1 gene in Type A and Type B NPC 1 or NPC 2 gene in Type C
Enzyme deficient	:	Sphingomyelinase
Substrate accumulated	:	Sphingomyelin
Inheritance	:	Autosomal recessive
Occurrence	:	More prevalent in Ashkenazi Jews
Organs affected	:	Brain (myelin sheath), spleen and liver

Pathogenesis Membrane lipid (sphingomyelin) is broken down by the enzyme (acid sphingomyelinase) to ceramide. Defect in the enzyme (SMAD 1 mutation) leads to the accumulation of sphingomyelin, and an abnormality in lipid transport proteins (NPC 1 and 2 mutations) causes cholesterol and glycolipids to accumulate in the lysosomes.

Morphology (Fig. 5.9)

The characteristic feature is **foam cells** – large macrophages with numerous small vacuoles in the cytoplasm. The vacuoles represent the lysosomes distended with sphingomyelin and cholesterol. The foam cells are widely distributed in all organs. It is marked in the spleen, liver and lymph nodes, causing organomegaly.
Brain: Atrophy with vacuolization and ballooning of neurons can be seen.
Eyes: Cherry-red spot in the retina is present.
Special stains: Fat stains are positive in the vacuoles.
Electron microscopy: It reveals distended lysosomes with whorls of a lamellar structure called **zebra bodies**.

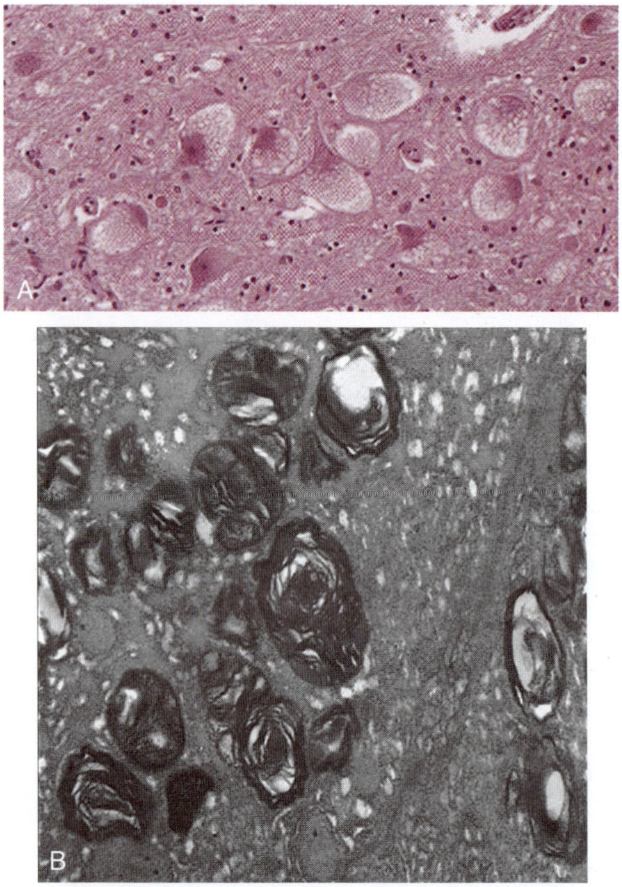

Fig. 5.9 Niemann–Pick disease. (A) Foam cells by microscopy – ballooned neurons in the oculomotor nucleus. (B) Zebra bodies by electron microscopy. (*Source:* From David Ellison, Seth Love, Leila Chimelli, Brian N. Harding, James S. Lowe, Harry V. Vinters, Sebastian Brandner and William H. Yong. Lysosomal and peroxisomal disorders. Neuropathology. 3rd edition. 2013. Elsevier.)

Clinical Features Type A disease presents at early infancy with hepatosplenomegaly and progressive mental retardation. The child usually dies before 1–2 years of age. In Type B disease, the child survives to adulthood with organomegaly, but without central nervous system (CNS) involvement. Progressive neurological disease without organomegaly is characteristic of Type C disease.

Diagnosis Biochemical assay is performed for sphingomyelinase activity in the liver or bone marrow biopsy.

DNA analysis is performed for SMAD 1 and NPC 1 and NPC 2 mutations.

Gaucher Disease

Gaucher disease is the *most common LSD*. It is characterized by glucosylceramide (**glucocerebroside**) accumulation in lysosomes of macrophages.

Mutation	:	Mutations in β-glucosidase gene on chromosome 1 (1q21)
Enzyme deficient	:	Glucocerebrosidase
Substrate accumulated	:	Glucocerebroside
Inheritance	:	Autosomal recessive
Occurrence	:	Most common among LSD in general (1 in 50,000) and more prevalent in Ashkenazi Jews
Organs affected	:	Spleen, liver and brain

Pathogenesis Glucocerebrosides are derived from the catabolism of membranes from senescent leucocytes and RBCs. Deficiency of glucocerebrosidase results in the accumulation of glucoceramide in the macrophages and brain.

Morphology (Fig. 5.10)

The characteristic feature is the presence of **Gaucher cell** (distended macrophages) all over the body. Gaucher cell are large cells (90 microns in diameter) with eccentrically placed nuclei and abundant fibrillary cytoplasm. The cytoplasm resembles **crumpled tissue paper**. These cells are formed from tissue-specific macrophages (splenic macrophages in the spleen, Kupffer cells in the liver, alveolar macrophages in the lungs), except in the brain where they are formed from periadventitial cells in the Virchow–Robin space.
Special stain: Periodic acid–Schiff (PAS) stain is strongly positive.
Electron microscopy: It reveals elongated and distended lysosomes in the cytoplasm.

Clinical Features Three clinical subtypes have been described:

- Type I or chronic non-neuronopathic form
- Type II or acute neuronopathic form
- Type III or intermediate form

Type I disease is the most common form and is characterized by glucocerebroside accumulation in all organs except the brain. The spleen and skeletal muscles are prominently involved. Life expectancy of these patients is only slightly reduced.

Type II disease presents in infancy with severe neurological involvement. There is no detectable level of enzyme activity in the tissues. Patients die at an early age.

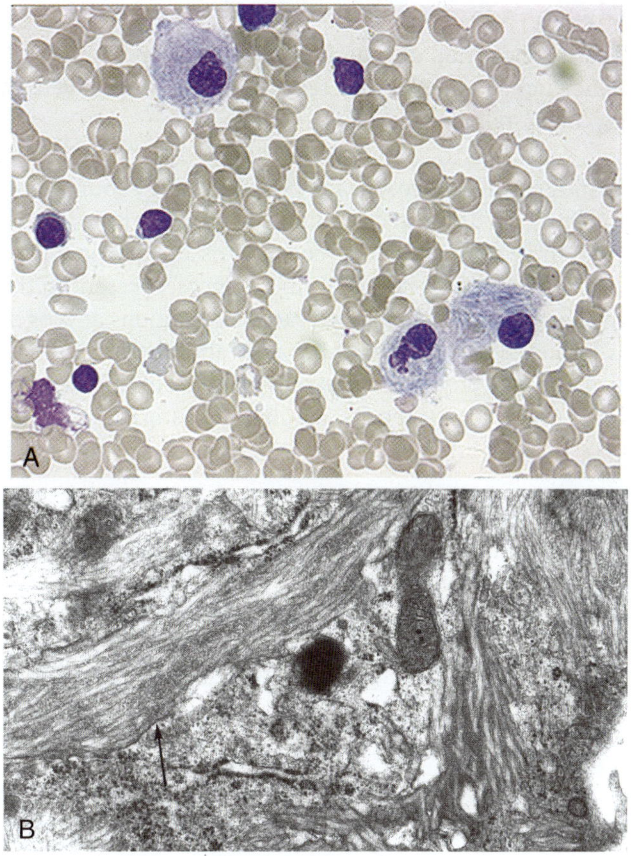

Fig. 5.10 Gaucher disease. (A) Gaucher cell in bone marrow aspirate. (B) Gaucher inclusions by electron microscopy – membrane-bound twisted inclusions of glucosylceramide and phospholipids (arrow). (*Source:* From Gregory A. Grabowski, T. Andrew Burrow, Nancy D. Leslie and Carlos E. Prada. Lysosomal Storage Diseases. Nathan and Oski's Hematology and Oncology of Infancy and Childhood. 8th edition. 2015. Elsevier; Stephan vom Dahl and Eugen Mengel. Lysosomal storage diseases as differential diagnosis of hepatosplenomegaly. Best Practice & Research: Clinical Gastroenterology. 2010. 24; 619-628.)

Type III disease is intermediate between type I and type II diseases. These patients have systemic involvement initially and then develop progressive neurological deterioration in adolescence.

The clinical finding common in all types is massive splenomegaly.

Diagnosis Biochemical enzyme assay (glucocerebrosidase levels) and genetic studies (glucocerebrosidase gene mutation) in peripheral blood leucocytes or in cultured skin fibroblast are performed. Bone marrow biopsy reveals the presence of Gaucher cells.

Prenatal diagnosis can be made on amniotic fluid and chorionic villi biopsy.

Treatment Treatment with recombinant enzymes is highly effective but is expensive.

Allogenic haematopoietic stem cell transplantation (HSCT) can offer cure.

Glycogen Storage Diseases (Glycogenosis)

These are a group of inherited disorders that result from deficiency of one of the several enzymes involved in glycogen metabolism.

Pathogenesis Glucose is the primary energy source, and the body needs a constant supply of glucose. It is derived from three sources: diet, glycogenolysis and gluconeogenesis. Glycogen is a storage form of glucose, present in the liver and muscles. In hypoglycaemic conditions, glycogen is broken down to glucose for utilization by tissues. The deficiency of any of the enzymes involved in the metabolism of glycogen results in glycogen storage diseases (GSDs) (Fig. 5.11).

Clinical Features GSDs can be classified into three major subgroups on the basis of clinical presentation and organ involvement (Table 5.8):

1. **Hepatic form** (GSD types 0, I, III, VI, IX) is characterized by hepatomegaly and low blood glucose levels.
2. **Myopathic form** (GSD types V, VII) is characterized by muscle weakness.
3. Others
   a. Hepatic and myopathic forms (GSD types III, IV) involve both the liver and the muscle.
   b. GSD type II (Pompe disease) involves all organs, but involvement of the heart is predominant.

Severity of the disease can vary from severe, which is fatal in infancy, to mild with a normal life span.

Morphology (Fig. 5.12)
Liver biopsy shows glycogen deposits (empty vacuoles) in the cytoplasm of hepatocytes and steatosis. These findings may be accompanied by fibrosis or cirrhosis. There is an increased risk of development of hepatocellular carcinoma.

Special stain: PAS is positive for glycogen in hepatocytes.

Diagnosis Traditionally, diagnosis is made by liver or muscle biopsy findings and enzyme assay. Nowadays, biopsies are no longer required for diagnosis.

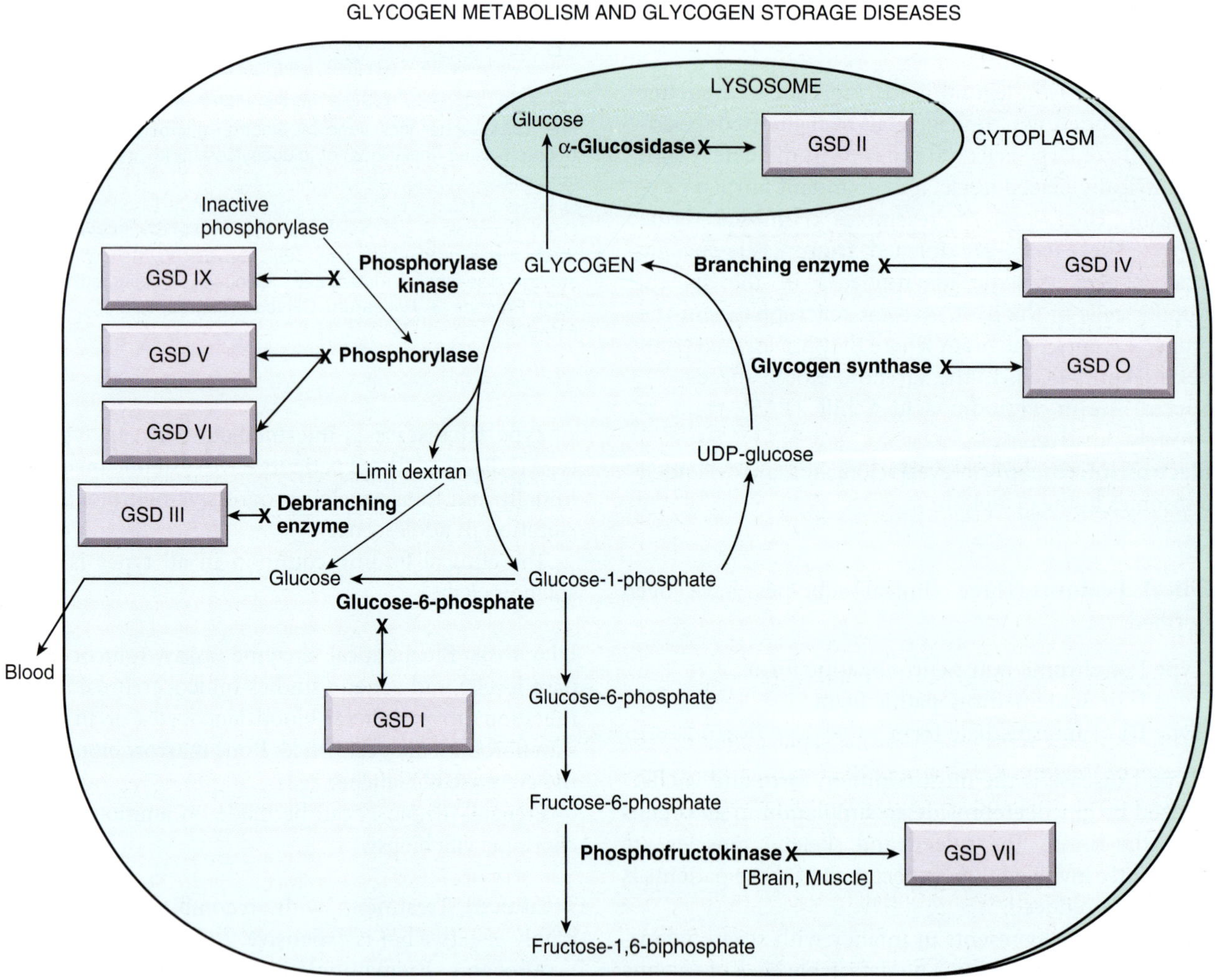

Fig. 5.11 Pathogenesis of glycogen storage diseases.

Table 5.8 Glycogen Storage Disease Types

GSD Type	Enzyme Deficiency	Gene Mutation	Inheritance	Clinical Presentation
Type 0	Glycogen synthase	GYS2	AR	Hypoglycaemia, diabetes
Type I (von Gierke disease)	Glucose-6-phosphatase	G6PC	AR	Hepatomegaly, renomegaly
Type II (Pompe disease)	α-1,4-Glucosidase	GAA	AR, X-linked dominant	Cardiomegaly, muscle hypotonia
Type III (Cori disease)	Glycogen debranching enzyme	AGL	AR	Hepatomegaly, muscular involvement
Type IV (Andersen disease)	Glycogen branching enzyme	GBE	AR	Hepatomegaly, muscular involvement
Type V (McArdle disease)	Muscle phosphorylase	PYGM	AR	Muscle involvement (painful cramps following exercise)
Type VI (Hers disease)	Liver phosphorylase	PYGL	AR	Hepatomegaly
Type VII (Tarui disease)	Muscle phosphofructokinase	PFKM	AR	Muscle involvement
Type IX	Phosphorylase kinase	PHKA2, PHKB	AR, X-linked recessive	Hepatomegaly
Type XI (Fanconi–Bickel syndrome)	GLUT 2 transporter	SLC2A2	AR	Hepatomegaly

AR, autosomal recessive; GSD, glycogen storage disease.

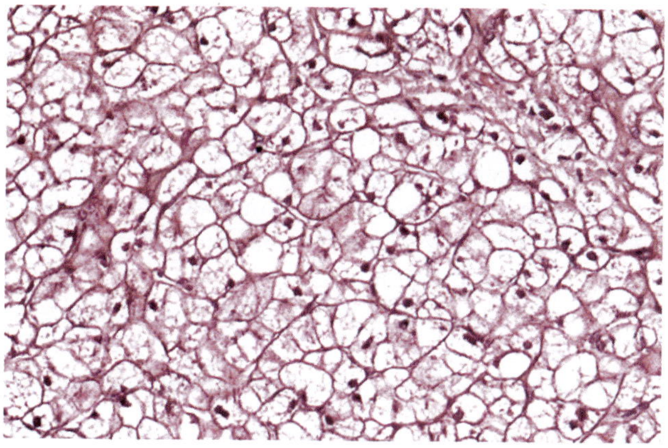

Fig. 5.12 Glycogen storage diseases. Liver cells show cytoplasmic empty vacuoles. (*Source:* From Jay H. Lefkowitch. Childhood Liver Disease and Metabolic Disorders. Scheuer's Liver Biopsy Interpretation. 10th edition. Elsevier.)

DNA mutation analysis is the gold standard for diagnosis and can also be used for prenatal diagnosis.

Treatment Diet therapy and enzyme replacement are the mainstay of treatment. The aim of the treatment is to prevent hypoglycaemia and metabolic complications.

Mucopolysaccharidoses

Mucopolysaccharidoses (MPSs) are a group of inherited disorders resulting from deficiency of enzymes involved in the degradation of mucopolysaccharides (glycosaminoglycans).

Pathogenesis Mucopolysaccharides are complex carbohydrates linked to proteins. Examples include dermatan sulphate, heparin sulphate and chondroitin sulphate. These are abundantly present in the connective tissue. Deficiency of any of the enzymes involved in their degradation results in mucopolysaccharide accumulation within lysosomes in various tissues. There are several types that have AR mode of transmission, except Hunter (type II) disease (Table 5.9).

Morphology

The accumulated mucopolysaccharides are seen in macrophages, endothelial cells, intimal smooth muscle cells and fibroblast throughout the body, causing organomegaly (spleen, liver, bone marrow, lymph nodes and heart). These cells appear to have clear cytoplasm under the microscope and are called the **balloon cells.**

Special stain: PAS stains the mucopolysaccharides accumulated in the cytoplasm.

Electron microscopy shows numerous minute vacuoles (distended lysosomes). In neurons, **lamellated zebra bodies** are seen.

Clinical Features In general, all the types are characterized by coarse facial features, clouding of the cornea, joint stiffness and mental retardation. In Hurler syndrome, children are normal at birth but develop hepatosplenomegaly

Table 5.9 Types of Mucopolysaccharidoses

Type	Enzyme Deficiency	Inheritance
Type I (Hurler)	α-Iduronidase	AR
Type II (Hunter)	Iduronate sulphatase	XR
Type III (Sanflippo)	Heparan sulphatase α-*N*-Acetylglucosaminidase Acetyl-CoA α-Glucosamine acetyl transferase *N*-Acetylglucosamine-6-sulphatase	AR
Type IV (Morquio)	Galactosamine-6-sulphate sulphatase β-Galactosidase	AR
Type VI (Maroteaux–Lamy)	*N*-Acetylgalactamine-4-sulphatase	AR
Type VII (Sly)	β-Glucuronidase	AR
Type IX (Natowicz)	Hyaluronidase I	AR

AR, autosomal recessive; XR, X linked recessive.

by 6–24 months of age. They progressively develop stunted growth, coarse facial features and skeletal deformities and usually die by 6–10 years of age because of cardiovascular complications. Hunter syndrome (type II MPS) has X-linked recessive inheritance with a mild clinical course and the absence of corneal clouding.

Diagnosis Characteristic clinical features include increased urinary excretion of mucopolysaccharides and enzyme assays. Neonatal screening can be performed with urine test. Prenatal diagnosis is made through enzyme assay and DNA analysis.

Treatment Enzyme replacement therapy and treatment of specific symptoms are performed through a multidisciplinary approach.

HSCT has been partially successful. Following HSCT, glycosaminoglycan accumulation in various tissues is reduced except in the brain.

NON-MENDELIAN DISORDERS

Non-Mendelian disorders are **single gene disorders that do not follow the classical Mendelian laws of inheritance.** These are classified as follows:

- TNR mutation diseases
- Mutations in mitochondrial genes
- Genomic imprinting
- Gonadal mosaicism

TRINUCLEOTIDE-REPEAT MUTATION DISEASES

Trinucleotide repeat (TNR) mutation occurs when the number of repetitive sequence of trinucleotides present in a gene is more than normal. TNR mutations are the major cause of neurological and neuromuscular diseases (Table 5.10).

The general features of TNR mutations are as follows:

- They cause highly unstable DNA.
- The number of repeats in the diseased gene continues to increase with each inheritance.
- There is a generation that has premutation before the successive development of full mutation, in which the number of repeats is above normal but not high enough to cause clinical symptoms.
- The repeats may occur in coding or noncoding regions of the genome.
- They alter function of the gene product or the gene expression.

Table 5.10 Trinucleotide-Repeat Mutation Diseases

Disease	Repeats	Gene	Chromosome Locus	Abnormal Protein Product
TNR expansions in noncoding regions				
Fragile X syndrome	CGG	FMR1	Xq27.3	FMR1 protein
Friedreich ataxia	GAA	FXN	9q21.2	Frataxin
Myotonic dystrophy	CTG	DMPK	19q13.3	Myotonic dystrophy protein kinase
TNR expansions in coding regions				
Huntington disease	CAG	HTT	4p16.3	Huntington
Spinocerebellar ataxia	CAG	ATXN1	6p23	Ataxin 1
Spinobulbar muscular atrophy	CAG	AR	Xq12	Androgen receptor

AR, autosomal recessive; FMR1, familial mental retardation 1; TNR, trinucleotide repeat.

Fragile X Syndrome

Fragile X syndrome is the **second most common inherited cause of mental retardation** (the most common cause is Down syndrome). The term 'fragile X' refers to the appearance of fragile or unstable sites in the X chromosome when cultured in folate-deficient media. These sites are observed as break, constrictions or loss of staining in the X chromosome. The fragile site associated with fragile X syndrome is called FRAXA (Fig. 5.13).

Incidence	:	One in 1550 for males One in 8000 for females
Karyotyping	:	Constrictions/discontinuity in staining in the X chromosome
Molecular pathogenesis		
Gene involved	:	FMR1 (familial mental retardation 1) gene at chromosome Xq27.3
Protein product	:	FMRP (familial mental retardation protein)
Mutation	:	Trinucleotide (**CGG**) repeat mutation in the promoter region of FMR1 gene

TNR mutation is said to occur when the number of repeats is more than the normal. On the basis of the number of repeats, the mutations are classified as premutation and mutation (Table 5.11).

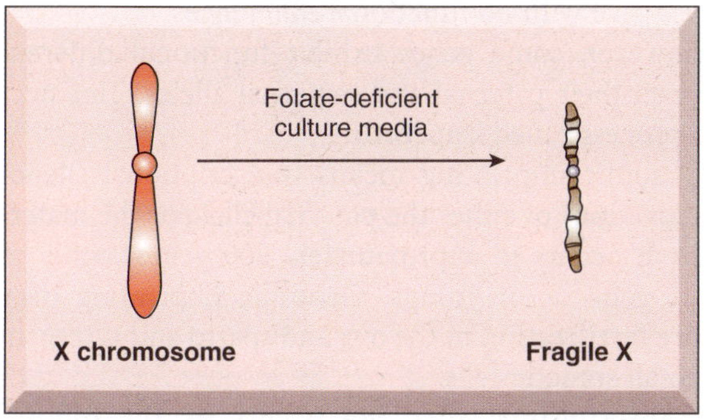

Fig. 5.13 Fragile sites on the chromosome in fragile X syndrome.

Table 5.11 Classification of Mutation in Fragile X Syndrome

Number of Trinucleotide Repeats	Mutation	Diseases
5–50	No mutation	Normal
55–200	Premutation	Fragile X-associated tremor/ataxia Fragile X-associated primary ovarian insufficiency
>200	Full mutation	Fragile X syndrome

Full mutation causes silencing or loss of function of FMR1 gene and thereby marked reduction in the production of FMRP, whereas premutations cause gain of function of FMR1 gene.

Inheritance: X-linked non-Mendelian inheritance

The characteristic features of fragile X inheritance are as follows (Fig. 5.14):

- With each inheritance, the number of TNR increases and the amplification of the repeats from a permutation to a full mutation occurs only during oogenesis and not during spermatogenesis. When TNR is more than 200, it is known as **full mutation**.
- **Carrier males** carry TNR premutation in the X chromosome. They are clinically normal but can transmit the mutation to all daughters. Sons are normal.
- **Carrier females** transmit the mutation to 50% of sons and 50% of daughters after amplifying it during oogenesis.
- Sons who inherit full mutation are affected.
- Daughters inherit full mutation from their mother.
  a. Only 50% are affected because of unfavourable lyonization (the normal X chromosome undergoes inactivation and the mutated X chromosome is active).
  b. The remaining 50% are unaffected because of inactivation of the mutated X chromosome (favourable lyonization).
- **Anticipation:** Severity of clinical symptoms worsens with each successive generation.

Clinical Features

Males are more severely affected than females.

Affected males have the following:

- Mental retardation (intelligence quotient [IQ]: 20–60)
- Facial features: Long face, large mandible, large everted ears
- Macro-orchidism (large testes) at puberty
- Hyperextensible joints

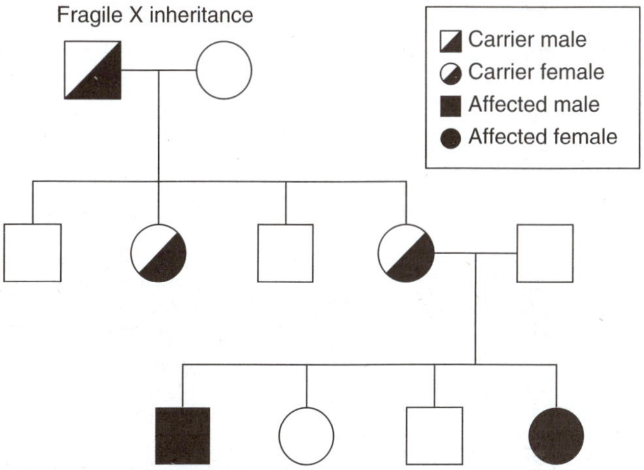

Fig. 5.14 Pedigree chart of fragile X syndrome.

Individuals with premutations accumulate the mRNA in the cell that are toxic to the cell. The individuals may hence develop the following conditions:

- **Fragile X tremor/ataxia:** It includes intentional tremors and cerebellar ataxia. It may progress to parkinsonism.
- **Fragile X-associated primary ovarian syndrome:** It contains a wide spectrum of ovarian disorders.

Diagnosis Diagnosis is made on the basis of clinical features and genetic testing (karyotyping and Southern blot or polymerized chain reaction [PCR]).

MITOCHONDRIAL GENE MUTATIONS

Mitochondria are the only sites for extranuclear genetic material known as mitochondrial DNA (mtDNA). mtDNA contains only 37 genes, out of which 13 genes code for enzymes involved in oxidative phosphorylation of ATP. The rest of the mitochondrial proteins are inherited by nuclear DNA.

The inherited mitochondrial diseases are caused by mutations occurring either in the nuclear DNA or in mtDNA. Mutations in mtDNA are much more common than those in nuclear DNA because of the following:

1. Exposure to reactive oxygen species released during mitochondrial oxidative phosphorylation
2. Lack of DNA repair mechanisms

The special features of diseases because of mutations in mtDNA are as follows:

- **Maternal inheritance:** The mother transmits the disease to all her offspring. But the affected father does not transmit the disease. This is because during fertilization, the zygote inherits mtDNA only from the ova (Fig. 5.15).
- **Heteroplasmy:** Numerous copies of mtDNA are present in a cell. Mutations may affect some but not all copies of mtDNA. Hence, deleterious/mild mutations may coexist with normal mtDNA within the same cell or an individual as a whole. The disease manifests when the number of mutated mtDNAs reaches a minimum threshold level.

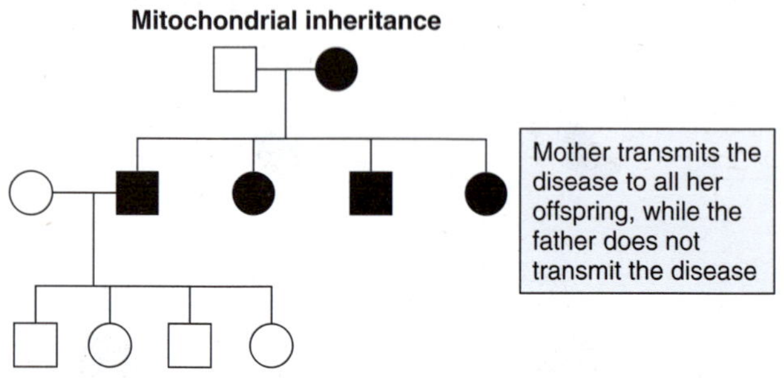

Fig. 5.15 Pedigree chart of disorders because of mitochondrial inheritance.

- **Variable expressivity:** During each cell division, the cytoplasm containing the mutant and normal mitochondria is randomly distributed to daughter cells. Hence, the proportion of mutant mtDNA and normal mtDNA in individual cells varies greatly. This results in a varied clinical expression of the disease.

Pathogenesis

The main function of mitochondria is ATP production by oxidative phosphorylation. Mitochondrial diseases are a group of inherited diseases characterized by a **defect in oxidative phosphorylation** that affects the organs most dependent on oxidative phosphorylation such as the brain, skeletal muscles, heart, kidney and liver. These present as a multisystem disease with predominant neuromuscular involvement.

Clinical Features

Leber hereditary optic neuropathy is a prototype of this disorder. Its characteristic features are as follows:

- Visual impairment, which progresses to bilateral loss of vision
- Cardiac conduction defects
- Neurological deficits

GENOMIC IMPRINTING

Most autosomal genes are expressed as two alleles: one maternal and the other paternal. Both the alleles are said to be active with no functional differences.

However, some genes exhibit functional differences between their paternal and maternal alleles. This occurs by a process called **imprinting.**

Genomic imprinting means transcriptional silencing (inactivation) of either the paternal allele or the maternal allele. It occurs in approximately 200 genes, either as a single gene or in groups. Genomic imprinting **occurs before fertilization** in the ova and sperm and is transmitted to all somatic cells.

Transcriptional silencing occurs by the following two mechanisms:

- DNA methylation of CG nucleotides
- Histone H4 deacetylation and methylation

Genomic imprinting is of two types:

- Maternal imprinting: Silencing of the maternal allele
- Paternal imprinting: Silencing of the paternal allele

Genomic imprinting is best studied with two unrelated genetic syndromes, Prader–Willi syndrome and Angelman syndrome, which were later found to have similar genetic abnormality.

Pathogenesis (Fig. 5.16)

Band 11.2 in the long arm of chromosome 15 harbours the gene for both Prader–Willi syndrome (PWG) and Angelman

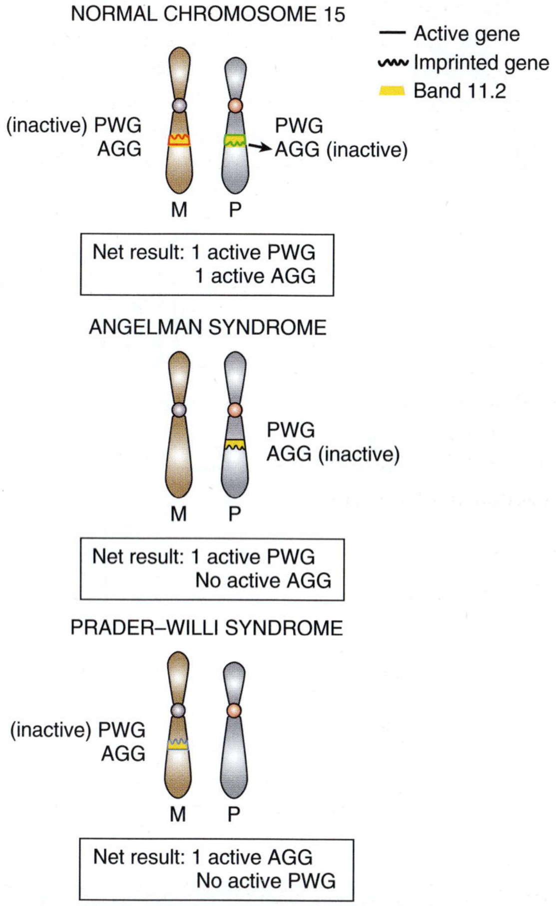

Fig. 5.16 Pathogenesis of Prader–Willi syndrome and Angelman syndrome.

syndrome (AGG). Normally, there is imprinting (inactivation) of PWG gene in the maternal chromosome and imprinting of AGG gene in the paternal chromosome. This results in chromosome 15 carrying an active AGG gene in the maternal chromosome and an active PWG gene in the paternal chromosome in all individuals.

Deletion of the band region (q11.2) on maternal chromosome 15 causes loss of the active AGG gene, resulting in Angelman syndrome. The same deletion if it occurs in the paternal chromosome causes loss of active PWG and results in Prader–Willi syndrome (Table 5.12).

Deletion is the most common cause (70%) of these syndromes. The other causes are as follows:

1. Uniparental disomy: 20%–25%
2. Defective imprinting: 1%–4%

Uniparental disomy: This is a condition in which both the chromosomes of a homologous pair are inherited from one parent. In patients with Prader–Willi syndrome without karyotypic abnormality, both chromosomes 15 are maternally derived. These individuals do not have functionally active paternal allele and manifest the disease.

Defective imprinting: In this condition, the functionally active allele carries the imprint. In Prader–Willi syndrome, the paternal allele carries the maternal imprint, whereas in Angelman syndrome, the maternal allele carries the paternal imprint.

Molecular Pathogenesis

In **Angelman syndrome**, the gene involved is **UBE3A** gene that encodes for ubiquitin ligase. It catalyses the transfer of activated ubiquitin to the target protein. Selective imprinting of the paternal allele of this gene occurs in specific regions of the brain. Hence, deletion of the functionally active maternal allele causes mental retardation. In other tissues, both the alleles are active.

In **Prader–Willi syndrome**, there is loss of function of '**SNORP family of genes**'. This group of genes is imprinted in the maternal allele. These genes encode for small nucleolar RNA that causes the modification of ribosomal RNA.

Clinical Features

The clinical features in these syndromes are different. This served as the basis for identification of this type of inheritance. The question why a mutation at a particular site gave two different types of presentation in affected

Table 5.12 Comparison of Prader–Willi syndrome and Angelman syndrome

Features	Prader–Willi Syndrome	Angelman Syndrome
Karyotypic abnormality	Deletion of band q12 in the long arm of chromosome 15 (paternal) Del (15) (q11.2q13)	Deletion of band q12 in the long arm of chromosome 15 (maternal) Del (15) (q11.2)
Gene/genes involved	Group of genes: SNORP family of genes (PWG)	Single gene: UBE3A gene (AGG)
Molecular pathogenesis	Maternal allele (PWG): Genomic imprinting **Paternal allele (PWG): Deletion**	Paternal allele (AGG): Genomic imprinting **Maternal allele** (AGG): **Deletion**
Clinical features	Mental retardation Short stature, small hands and feet Hypotonia Profound hyperphagia Obesity Hypogonadism	Mental retardation Ataxic gait Seizures Inappropriate laughter – *happy puppets*

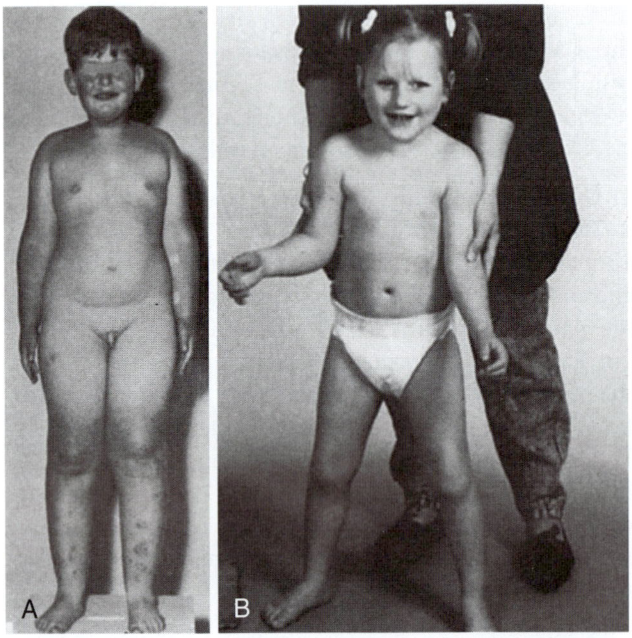

Fig. 5.17 Clinical picture of Prader–Willi syndrome (A) and Angelman syndrome (B). (*Source:* From Bruce M. Carlson. Cleavage and Implantation. Human Embryology and Developmental Biology. 6th edition. 2019. Elsevier.)

individuals led to the identification of genomic imprinting (Fig. 5.17).

Diagnosis

Karyotyping is performed in patients with typical clinical features.

Molecular diagnosis by fluorescence in situ hybridization (FISH) or array comparative genomic hybridization (CGH) is performed to detect deletions in band q11.2 on chromosome 15, and DNA methylation studies are conducted to detect uniparental disomy.

GONADAL MOSAICISM

Gonadal mosaicism typically presents as an AD disease in multiple offspring from phenotypically normal parents. This is against the rules for AD inheritance (one of the parents should be affected).

Pathogenesis: This condition is because of mutations that occur during early embryonic development only in few of the cells that are destined to form future gonads. This results in mosaicism of gonads as these are composed of two types of germ cells: normal germ cells giving rise to normal gametes and mutated germ cells giving rise to gametes that carry the mutation. When the offspring is formed by normal gametes, the offspring is normal, whereas the offspring formed with gametes carrying mutations has the disorder. The mutations initially occurred in only germ cells of the parent, so the somatic cells of the parent are normal and the parent is not affected (Fig. 5.18).

Diagnosis: Karyotyping shows mutation only in germ cells, not in somatic cells.

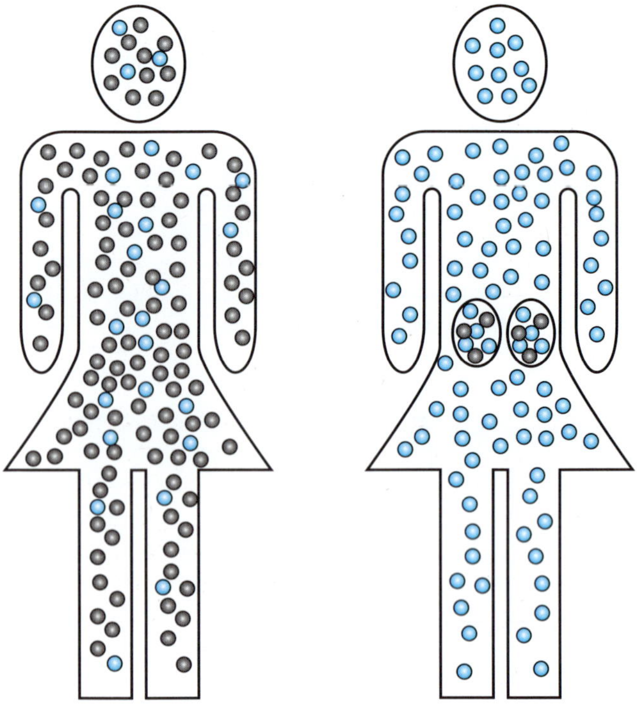

Fig. 5.18 Constitutional mosaicism (the entire body is composed of normal and abnormal cells) versus gonadal mosaicism (only the gonads are composed of normal and abnormal cells).

COMPLEX MULTIGENIC DISORDERS/ MULTIFACTORIAL DISORDERS

Multifactorial disorders result from a **complex interplay between multiple genes and environmental factors** to produce a disease. These diseases are often clustered in families and do not follow the Mendelian laws of inheritance (Table 5.13).

PATHOGENESIS

Multifactorial disorders are complex multigenic disorders that occur when **several polymorphisms are coinherited.** Normally, more than one-fourth of the human genes have polymorphic alleles. This heterogeneity leads to a

Table 5.13 Common Diseases that Follow Multifactorial Inheritance

Adults	Children
Diabetes mellitus type 2	Cleft lip/cleft palate
Hypertension	Pyloric stenosis
Atherosclerosis	Hirschsprung disease
Psoriasis	Congenital heart disease
Ankylosing spondylitis	Anencephaly, meningomyelocoele
Gout	Congenital talipes equinovarus

wide variation in susceptibility of individuals to certain diseases. These are further complicated by interaction with environmental factors.

Inheritance of these diseases is studied by population genetics. These studies have found the following:

- The number of involved genes for any disease is not known.
- Each polymorphism varies in significance. For example, in diabetes mellitus type 1, 20–30 genes are implicated, of which 6–7 are important.
- Some polymorphisms are common to multiple diseases of the same type, e.g. inflammatory arthritis.
- Expression of symptoms is proportional to the number of mutated genes.
- Risk in first-degree relatives is the same (5%–10%).
- Environmental influence modifies the phenotypic expression of complex traits. For example, in diabetes mellitus type 2, the individuals first manifest the disease after weight gain (obesity).

Complex multigenic disorders are usually suspected when these diseases have a wide range of severity. However, these should be differentiated from single mutant gene diseases in having reduced penetrance and variable expressivity.

CHROMOSOMAL DISORDERS

Cytogenetics is the study of chromosomes. Any abnormality detected in the number or structure of chromosomes is known as chromosomal/cytogenetic disorders. These are classified as follows:

1. **Cytogenetic disorders involving autosomes**
   a. With numerical aberration – trisomy 21 (Down syndrome)
   b. With structural aberration – chromosome 22q11.2
2. **Cytogenetic disorders involving sex chromosomes**
   a. Klinefelter syndrome (47XXY)
   b. Turner syndrome (45X0)

The chromosomes are studied using cytogenetic techniques: conventional – karyotyping; and molecular – FISH and DNA microarray.

NORMAL KARYOTYPING

Karyotyping is the first cytogenetic technique developed for chromosomal analysis. A normal human cell has 46 chromosomes: 22 pairs of autosomes and 2 sex chromosomes – XX in females and XY in males.

Principle: Chromosomes are best studied during the **metaphase** stage in mitosis, when the chromosomes are condensed and appear as two chromatids connected at the centromere. Hence, for karyotyping, cell division is arrested at the metaphase stage. The chromosomes are then harvested, stained and analysed (Fig. 5.19).

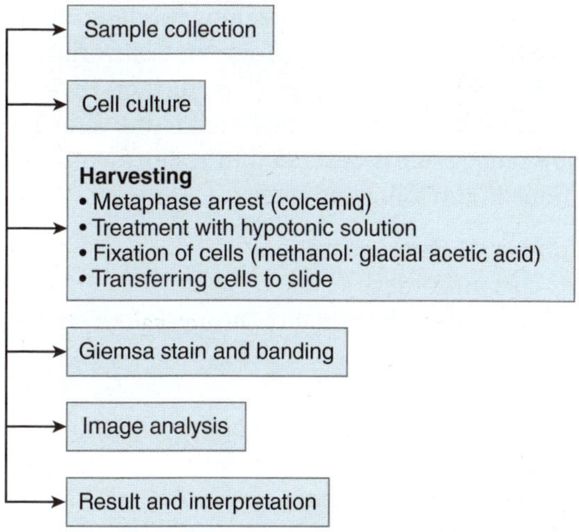

Fig. 5.19 Steps in karyotyping.

Sample Collection

Karyotyping can be performed on any mitotically active cell. The commonly used cells are peripheral blood lymphocytes.

Sources of cells for karyotyping are as follows:

Routine karyotyping – **lymphocytes from peripheral blood, fibroblast from skin biopsy**
Prenatal diagnosis – amniocytes from amniotic fluid, chorionic cells from chorionic villi sampling
Preimplantation diagnosis – blastomere cells from embryo
Leukaemia diagnosis – bone marrow leucocytes
Tumour genetics – tumour cells

Procedure

Proliferating cells in the culture are arrested at the metaphase stage by the use of colcemid (mitotic spindle inhibitor). The cells are treated with hypotonic solution (for swelling of cells and separation of chromosomes) and fixed. The chromosomes are then collected on a slide, stained with Giemsa stain and photographed. A computer-based image analysis is performed for arranging the chromosomes on the basis of their length and position of the centromere. Staining causes the appearance of light- and dark-stained regions on the chromosome, which are used for banding. Banding divides each arm of the chromosome into regions, bands and sub-bands. This helps in identification and detection of the exact location of structural aberrations in the chromosome.

Types of Chromosomal Banding

G-banding (Giemsa stain)
Q-banding (quinacrine stain)
C-banding (stains the centromere)
NOR banding (nucleolar organizing regions)
R-banding (reverse banding)

Cytogenetics Nomenclature

The short arm of the chromosome is designated as 'p' (petit) and the long arm as 'q' (the next alphabet). Each arm is further divided into regions bordered by prominent bands and numbered from the centromere in the ascending order. Each region is further divided into bands and sub-bands and numbered in the same manner. Karyotyping result is described in a shorthand system of notations in the following order:

1. Number of chromosomes
2. Sex chromosomes
3. Chromosomal abnormality (numerical or structural)

Example

1. 47XY, +21
   47: Number of chromosomes
   XY: Sex chromosomes (male)
   +21: Addition of extra chromosome 21
2. 46XX, (del) 22q11.2
   46: Number of chromosomes
   XY: Sex chromosomes
   Abnormality (deletion) in chromosome 22, long arm, region 1, band 1, sub-band 2

Cytogenetic Terminology

Some of the common terminologies used in cytogenetics for chromosome number are as follows:

Haploid	:	Single set of chromosomes (n)
Diploid	:	Two sets of chromosomes (2n)
Euploid	:	Normal chromosomal component

The terminologies used in genetic diseases because of abnormality in the number or structure of chromosomes are given in the next sections.

Numerical Abnormalities of Chromosomes

Polyploid	:	Abnormal number of the haploid set of chromosomes (3n, 4n). Triploidy: 3n Tetraploidy: 4n
Aneuploid	:	Chromosomal number is not a multiple of the haploid set (2n − 1, 2n + 1, 2n ± 2). Causes are nondisjunction and anaphase lag.
Trisomy	:	Addition of an extra chromosome to the diploid set of chromosomes (2n + 1).
Monosomy	:	Loss of one chromosome from the diploid set (2n − 1).
Mosaicism	:	Individuals having two or more populations of cells with different chromosomal numbers (e.g. 46XX/47XX + 21, 45X/47XXY).
		Failure of chromosomes to separate during mitosis or meiosis.
Meiotic nondisjunction	:	It results in two different types of gametes – one containing an extra chromosome and the other is deficient for a chromosome. Fertilization of these gametes by normal gametes results in zygotes having aneuploidy (2n + 1 and 2n − 1, respectively).
Mitotic nondisjunction	:	It results in daughter cells having one extra chromosome and one less chromosome. During early development, this can result in two populations of cells with different chromosomal number within the same individual (somatic mosaic).
Anaphase lag	:	One chromosome in meiosis or one chromatid in mitosis lags behind and is left out of the cell nucleus. This results in one normal gamete/cell and one with one chromosome less.

Structural Abnormalities of Chromosomes (Fig. 5.20)

Deletion: Loss of a segment of chromosome.
Insertion: Addition of a segment of chromosome.
Ring chromosome: Chromosomal breaks occur at both the ends of the chromosome, followed by fusion of the ends, resulting in a ring structure.
Inversion: It occurs when two breaks occur in a chromosome, followed by reincorporation of the inverted segment.
Translocation: This comprises a transfer of a segment of one chromosome to another. It is of two types: balanced and unbalanced (Fig. 5.21).
Balanced translocation: It occurs by translocation of chromosomal segments with no loss of genetic material.
Unbalanced translocation: Translocation is associated with loss of genetic material.
Robertsonian translocation (Fig. 5.22): Translocation between two acrocentric chromosomes results in the formation of a very large chromosome containing both long arms and a small product, which is usually lost.
Isochromosome (Fig. 5.23): It is the chromosome having two long arms or two short arms. It occurs when one of the arms is lost and the remaining arm gets duplicated.

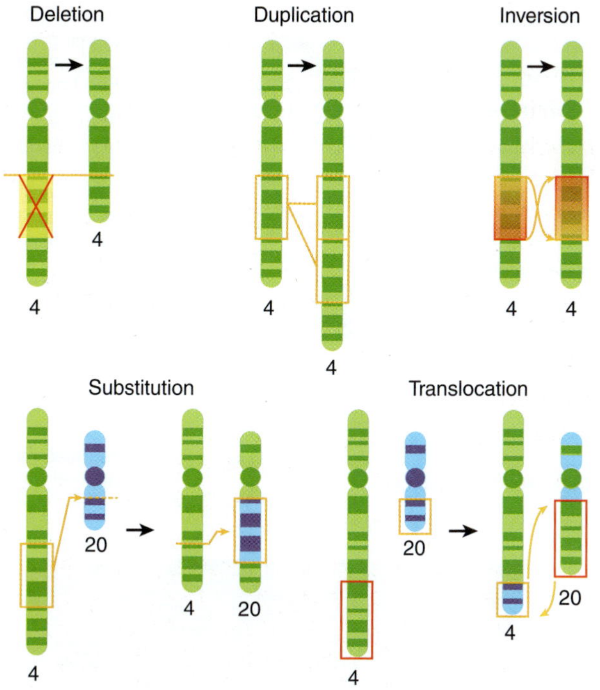

Fig. 5.20 Structural abnormalities of chromosomes.

AUTOSOMAL DISORDERS

Trisomy 21 (Down syndrome)

Down syndrome is the most common chromosomal disorder characterized by the presence of extra chromosome 21 in the human genome. It is the **most common cause of mental retardation**.

Karyotype: It is **47XX,** +21.
Incidence: This is 1 in 800. The chance of having a child with Down syndrome increases with maternal age.

Pathogenesis (Fig. 5.24) The causes for trisomy 21 are as follows:

1. **Meiotic nondisjunction – 95%**
2. **Robertsonian translocation – 4%**
3. **Mosaicism – 1%**

Meiotic nondisjunction means failure of homologous chromosomes to separate, resulting in gametes having one extra chromosome and one less chromosome (Fig. 5.24). Fertilization of such gamete having two chromosomes 21 with a normal gamete results in trisomy 21. According to genetic studies, the extra chromosome 21 has a maternal origin.
Robertsonian translocation involves transfer of segments between two acrocentric chromosomes (e.g. chromosome 21 and chromosome 14) resulting in the formation of a very large chromosome with long arms of both chromosomes. The tiny short arms are usually lost. This translocation is seen in 1 in 1000 apparently normal individuals. When these individuals produce a progeny, the fertilized ovum has two normal chromosomes 21 but the translocated segment on chromosome 14 acts as a third chromosome and results in Down syndrome. Karyotyping shows normal chromosomal numbers with the translocated segment of chromosome 21. These cases are inherited in families.
Down syndrome **mosaics** have a mixture of cells with 46 and 47 chromosomes. It occurs when mitotic nondisjunction of chromosome 21 occurs during early embryogenesis. These children have only mild symptoms.

Molecular pathogenesis According to the ***gene dosage hypothesis***, the clinical features of Down syndrome result from the overexpression of certain 'disease-causing genes' in a trisomic state. These genes are involved in mitochondrial energy pathway, CNS development and folate metabolism. The exact mechanism is still not known.

Clinical features The characteristic clinical features are as follows (Fig. 5.25):

- Mental retardation (IQ: 25%–50%)
- Facial features: Flat facies, slanting palpebral fissure, depressed nasal bridge, prominent epicanthal folds and low-set ears
- Hypotonia of muscles
- Congenital heart disease seen in 40% of cases; the most common cause of death in early childhood
- Intestinal stenosis
- Presence of a single horizontal palmar crease (simian crease)
- Excess gap between the first and second toes (saddle gap)

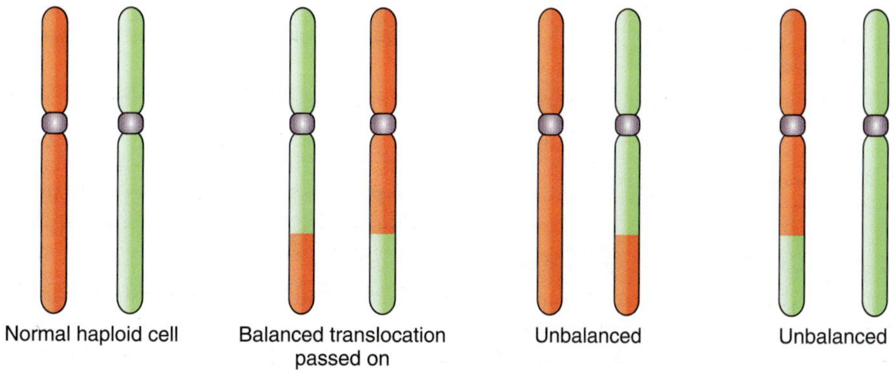

Fig. 5.21 Balanced and unbalanced translocation.

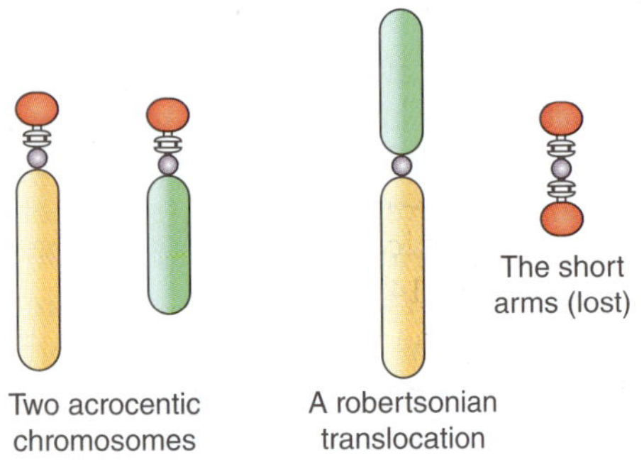

Fig. 5.22 Robertsonian translocation of chromosomes.

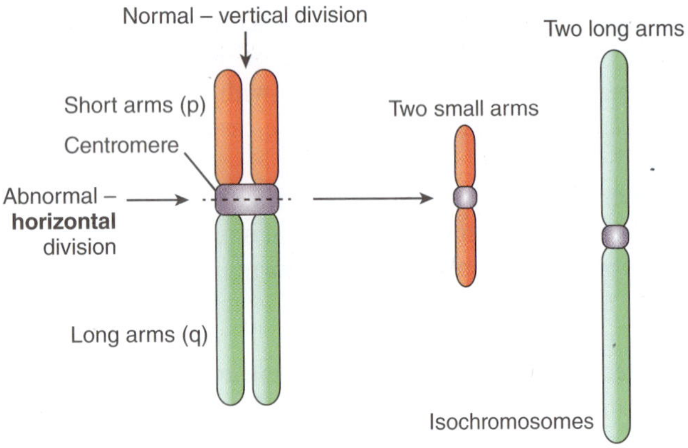

Fig. 5.23 Isochromosome.

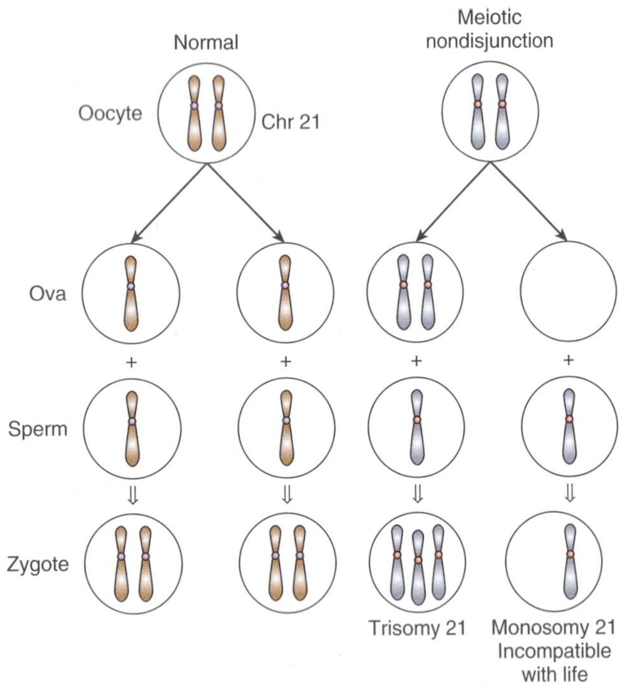

Fig. 5.24 Pathogenesis of Down syndrome.

- Increased risk of developing the following diseases:
  a. Acute leukaemia in those older than 20 years (the most common form is acute myeloid leukaemia)
  b. Neurodegenerative disease such as Alzheimer disease in those older than 40 years

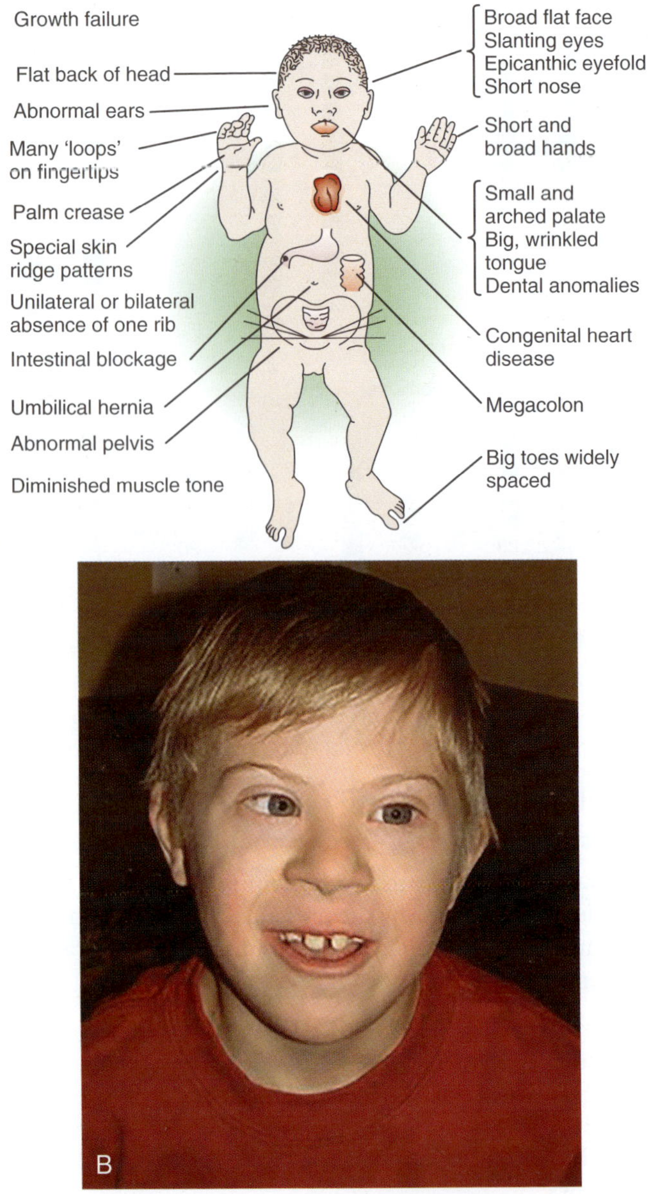

Fig. 5.25 Features of Down syndrome (A) and the clinical picture of a child with Down syndrome showing epicanthal folds, midface hypoplasia, microcephaly, strabismus and irregularly spaced dentition. (*Source:* From Melissa A. Davidson. Primary Care for Children and Adolescents with Down Syndrome. Pediatric Clinics of North America, 2008; 55:1099-1111.)

The improvised medical care has increased the life expectancy of individuals with Down syndrome to 47 years.

Diagnosis Diagnosis is made at birth by identifying characteristic clinical features or prenatally by using various screening and diagnostic tests.

Prenatal screening test for Down syndrome includes certain biochemical tests on maternal blood and ultrasonography.

Prenatal diagnostic tests for Down syndrome can be invasive or noninvasive.

Invasive: Karyotyping of fetal cells from amniocentesis/chorionic villus sampling is performed.

Table 5.14 Pathology and Clinical Features of Edwards and Patau Syndromes

Trisomy	Edwards Syndrome	Patau Syndrome
Karyotype	47XX, +18 47XY, +18	47XX, +13 47XY, +13
Pathology	Presence of one extra chromosome 18	Presence of one extra chromosome 13
Pathogenesis	Meiotic nondisjunction Mosaicism Robertsonian translocation	Meiotic nondisjunction Mosaicism Robertsonian translocation
Risk factor	Advanced maternal age	Advanced maternal age
Clinical features	Mental retardation Prominent occiput Small jaw (micrognathia) Low-set ears Umbilical hernia Overriding of digits Rocker bottom feet Congenital heart defects Horseshoe kidney	Mental retardation Microcephaly Microphthalmia Cleft lip and palate Polydactyly Rocker bottom feet Congenital heart defects Horseshoe kidney
Life expectancy	<1 year	<1 year

Noninvasive: Fetal-derived free DNA in the maternal blood is studied for the overexpression of chromosome 21 genes (next-generation sequencing).

Other Trisomies Trisomies involving other autosomal chromosomes are usually associated with multiple congenital anomalies, and the affected babies usually die within 1 year of life. Edwards syndrome (trisomy 18) and Patau syndrome (trisomy 13) are briefly described in Table 5.14.

Chromosome 22q11.2 Deletion Syndrome

Chromosome 22q11.2 syndrome is caused by deletion of a small fragment in the long arm of chromosome 22 at a specific locus. The clinical presentation of this syndrome varies greatly and involves multiple organ systems. Hence, it has been known in the past as various distinct entities:

- DiGeorge syndrome
- Velocardiofacial syndrome
- CATCH 22 syndrome
- Conotruncal anomaly face syndrome

All the above-mentioned entities are now grouped together on the basis of their common chromosomal abnormality as 22q11.2 deletion syndrome.

Incidence : One in 4000
Karyotype : 46XX, (del) 22q11.2

Pathogenesis: The clinical heterogeneity of this syndrome reflects as variation in the position and size of the deleted fragment. The deleted fragment in chromosome 22 contains about 30–40 genes. TBX1 (T-box transcription factor) is one of these genes that acts on PAX9 gene that controls the development of the palate, parathyroid and thymus. Deletion of TBX1 gene results in abnormality of all these organs.

Clinical Features The characteristic clinical features are as follows:

- Congenital heart defects
- Abnormalities of the palate
- Facial dysmorphism
- Developmental delay
- T-cell immunodeficiency
- Hypocalcaemia
- Increased risk of developing psychotic illness – schizophrenia

Diagnosis: Diagnosis is based on clinical features and confirmed with detection of the deletion by FISH.

SEX CHROMOSOMAL DISORDERS

Cytogenetic disorders involving sex chromosomes are more common than autosomal disorders. Their general features are as follows:

- These are difficult to diagnose at birth.
- These are recognized at the time of puberty because of problems related to sexual development and fertility.
- The more the number of X chromosomes, the greater is the severity of mental retardation.

Special Features of Sex Chromosomes

Before discussing the sex chromosomal disorders, let us consider the special features of sex chromosomes:

1. Lyonization or inactivation of all but one X chromosome
2. Less amount of genetic material in the Y chromosome

Lyon Hypothesis Males carry one X chromosome but have the same amount of gene product as females (XX). This discrepancy was explained by Lyon hypothesis. It states:

- In cells having two or more X chromosomes, there is **spontaneous inactivation of all but one X chromosome.**
- The inactivated X chromosome presents as condensed heterochromatin. This is readily visualized in the cells as a dark-staining small mass attached to the nuclear membrane and is called **Barr body or chromatin body** (Table 5.15; Fig. 5.26).
- Either the paternal X chromosome or the maternal X chromosome is inactivated randomly in the blastomere stage.
- The inactivation is **permanent** and transmitted to its progeny cells. Hence, normal females are in reality mosaics with two populations of cells: one with inactivation of the paternal X chromosome and another with inactivation of the maternal X chromosome.
- Some genes escape inactivation and are expressed by both X chromosomes.
- Both X chromosomes are active during oogenesis.

Table 5.15 Number of Barr Bodies Per Cell According to the Karyotype

Karyotype	Number of X Chromosome	Number of Barr Bodies
46XY	1	0
46XX	2	1
45X	1	0
47XXY	2	1
48XXXY	3	2
48XXXX	4	3

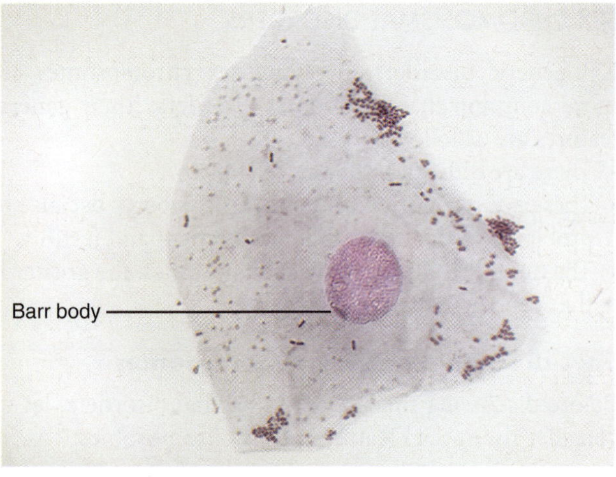

Fig. 5.26 Barr body in squamous cell. (*Source:* https://en.wikipedia.org/wiki/Barr_body.)

Molecular Basis of X Inactivation The **XIST gene** present on the X chromosome codes for a noncoding RNA, and this noncoding RNA coats the X chromosome to make it inactive. In an active X chromosome, the XIST allele is switched off.

Y chromosome The Y chromosome is necessary for male organ development. Irrespective of the number of X chromosomes, the presence of a single Y chromosome determines the male sex. The important genes in Y chromosomes are as follows:

- SRY gene (sex-determining region Y gene) dictates testicular development.
- MSY or male-specific Y region contains 75 genes involved in spermatogenesis.

The two most common sex chromosomal disorders **(Klinefelter syndrome and Turner syndrome)** are described here. The differences between the common chromosomal syndromes are given in Table 5.16.

Klinefelter Syndrome

Individuals with Klinefelter syndrome are phenotypic males having one Y chromosome and two or more X chromosomes.

Klinefelter syndrome is one of **the most common causes of male hypogonadism and infertility**.

Incidence: One in 660 live male births

Karyotype: Two types of karyotypic abnormality seen:

1. Classical pattern (90%): 47XXY, 48XXXY, 49XXXXY
2. Mosaic pattern: 46XY/47XXY, 47XXY/48XXXY

Pathogenesis The cause of Klinefelter syndrome in a classical pattern is **meiotic nondisjunction** during gametogenesis.

According to Lyon hypothesis, individuals with extra X chromosomes should be normal because all but one X chromosome are inactivated. But the abnormal phenotype in these patients is explained by the following:

- There may be overexpression of some genes that escape inactivation.
- The androgen receptor (AR) gene on the X chromosome has a variable CAG repeat region. Short CAG repeats in AR gene code for more sensitive receptors, whereas long repeats code for less sensitive receptors. Usually, the X chromosome having AR genes with shorter CAG repeats is inactivated and this exacerbates the hypogonadism.

Clinical Features (Fig. 5.27) **Klinefelter syndrome is diagnosed** after puberty, usually because of lack of development of secondary sexual characters or during investigation for infertility. The clinical features are as follows:

- Male hypogonadism – causes reduced spermatogenesis and male infertility

Table 5.16 Differences Between Chromosomal Syndromes

	Down syndrome	Klinefelter syndrome	Turner syndrome
Definition	Cytogenetic disorder affecting autosomes	Cytogenetic disorder affecting sex chromosomes	Cytogenetic disorder affecting sex chromosomes
Cause	Trisomy of chromosome 21	Trisomy of sex chromosome	Monosomy of sex chromosome
Classical karyotype	46XX, +21 46XY, +21	47XXY	45X0
Incidence	One in 700 live births	One in 600 live male births	One in 2000 live female births
Pathogenesis	Meiotic nondisjunction • Extra chromosome is of maternal origin	Meiotic nondisjunction • Extra chromosome is of maternal origin	Meiotic nondisjunction • Lost X chromosome is of paternal origin
Phenotypic sex	Male or female	Male	Female
Characteristic clinical feature	Mental retardation	Failure of secondary sexual development, infertility	Failure of secondary sexual development, primary amenorrhoea, infertility
Other features	Characteristic facies Simian crease Cardiovascular abnormalities	Tall stature Small atrophic testes Small penis Loss of beard Gynaecomastia	Small stature Webbed neck Atrophic (streak) ovaries Infantile genitalia Poor breast development
Increased risk	Acute leukaemia Alzheimer disease	Diabetes mellitus Osteoporosis	Gonadoblastoma (with additional Y component)
Diagnosis	Prenatal/at birth	At puberty	At puberty
Barr body	Females: 1 Males: 0	1	0

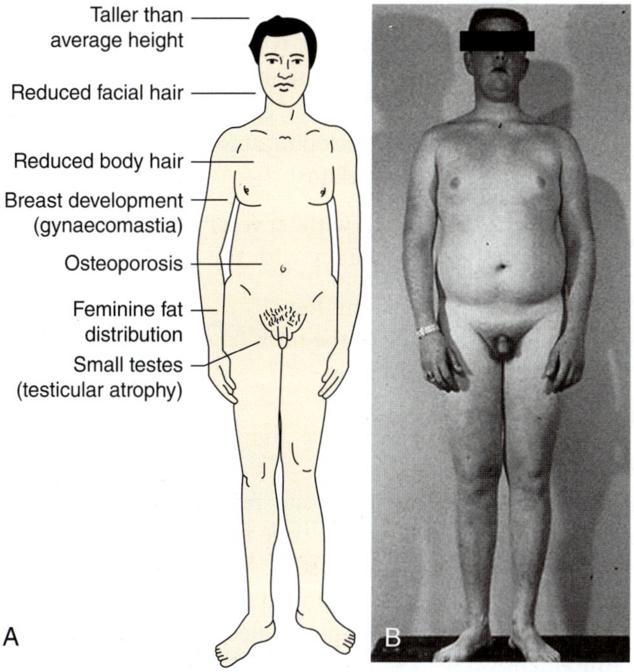

Fig. 5.27 (A) Features of Klinefelter syndrome. (B) Clinical image – on the left side is a man with classical 47XXY Klinefelter syndrome, presenting with androgen deficiency of prepubertal onset with eunuchoidal body proportions, small penis, sparse chest and pubic hair, poor muscle development, prepubertal fat distribution and very small testes. (*Source:* From Alvin M. Matsumoto and Bradley D. Anawalt. Testicular Disorders. Williams Textbook of Endocrinology. 14th edition. 2020. Elsevier.)

- Distinctive body habitus
  Tall stature
  Abnormally long legs
  Small atrophic testes
  Small penis
- Lack of secondary male characteristics – deep voice, beard and male distribution of pubic hair
- Gynaecomastia – a 20-fold more risk of developing breast carcinoma in those with gynaecomastia
- Mitral valve prolapse in 50% of cases
- Mean IQ lower than normal
- Increased incidence of type 2 diabetes and metabolic syndrome
- Increased incidence of osteoporosis and bone fractures

Laboratory Findings

Plasma follicle-stimulating hormone (FSH) levels: Constantly elevated
Plasma testosterone levels: Reduced
Plasma oestradiol levels: Increased

Morphology of Testicular Biopsy

Gross: Bilateral testes are atrophic.
Microscopy: The seminiferous tubules are atrophic. These appear hyalinized with loss of germ cells. Sometimes, the

tubules appear primitive (filled with cords of cell with no lumen or no evidence of spermatogenesis).
Leydig cell hyperplasia is seen in the interstitium.

Treatment Treatment with testosterone causes virilization but does not restore fertility.

Turner Syndrome

Individuals with Turner syndrome are **phenotypic females with monosomy of the X chromosome**. It is the most common sex chromosomal abnormality in females.

Incidence: One in 2500 live female births
Karyotype: There are three types of karyotypic abnormalities:

1. Classical Turner syndrome (57%): 45X
2. Partial monosomy of the X chromosome (14%): 46X,i (Xq), 46X,r (X), 46XX,del (Xp), 46XX,del (Xq)
3. Mosaic type (29%): 45X/46XX, 45X/46XY, 45X/47XXX

Pathogenesis (Fig. 5.28) In classical Turner syndrome, complete monosomy of the X chromosome occurs because of **meiotic nondisjunction** during gametogenesis.

Partial monosomy of the X chromosome may occur because of structural aberrations such as:

- Isochromosome of the long arm of the X chromosome following loss of the short arm
- Ring chromosome, following deletion of portions of both long arms and short arms
- Deletion of portions of the long arm or short arm

Patients with mosaic Turner syndrome have variable proportion of cells with 45X karyotype. Phenotypic abnormalities are severe in those with a high proportion of 45X cells, whereas presentation is almost normal in those with a lower proportion of 45X cells.

With the use of more sensitive cytogenetic techniques, many patients with Turner syndrome have been found to be mosaics (75%). Studies have shown that 99% of the conceptus with 45X karyotype abort spontaneously. Loss of one X chromosome is lethal. Hence, many scientists question the existence of patients with classical Turner syndrome and believe all of them to be mosaics.

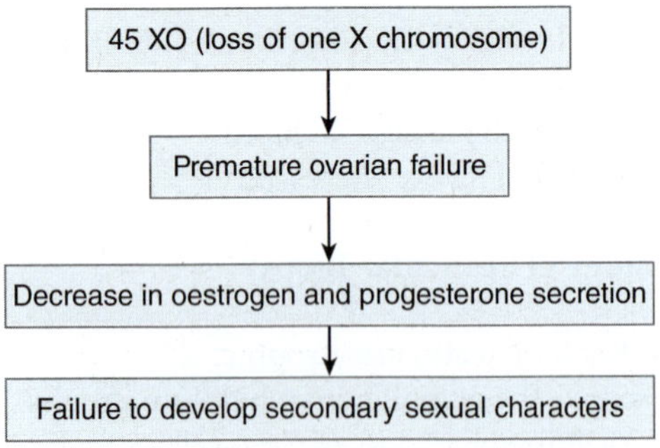

Fig. 5.28 Pathogenesis of Turner syndrome.

In females, both X chromosomes are active during oogenesis and are needed for the development of ovaries. In Turner syndrome, the loss of one X chromosome leads to **premature ovarian failure** (complete loss of oocytes by 2 years of age). Ovarian failure, in turn, decreases the hormone production (oestrogen and progesterone) and results in the failure of secondary sexual development.

Molecular Pathogenesis One of the important genes associated with Turner syndrome phenotype is **short stature homeobox (SHOX) gene at Xp22.33.** This gene is active in both X chromosomes in females and has an active homologue in the Y chromosome. Thus, loss of one copy of SHOX gene results in short stature and skeletal abnormalities.

Clinical Features (Fig. 5.29) The clinical features of Turner syndrome vary markedly. Most commonly, these present at adolescence or early adulthood with primary amenorrhoea. Turner syndrome is **the most important cause of primary amenorrhoea.**

The other clinical features are as follows:

- Short stature (<150 cm)
- Low posterior hairline
- Webbing of the neck
- Broad chest with widely placed nipples (poor breast development)
- Cubitus valgus
- Congenital heart disease: Coarctation of the aorta and bicuspid aortic valve
- Reproductive system: Delayed puberty with infantile genitalia and streak ovaries (there is a **higher risk of developing gonadoblastoma** in patients with a Y component [e.g. 45X/46XY])
- An increased risk of developing autoimmune thyroiditis, obesity and diabetes mellitus

Sometimes, patients with severely affected Turner syndrome present in infancy with the following:

- Oedema of the hand and foot
- Swelling of the nape of the neck (cystic hygroma)
- Congenital heart disease

Treatment Growth hormone therapy is performed for short stature.

Oestrogen and progesterone replacement therapy is performed around 12 years of age for the development of secondary sexual characteristics. The hormone replacement therapy has to be continued till menopause.

Excision of gonads is performed in patients with Y component.

MOLECULAR GENETIC DIAGNOSIS

Molecular genetic diagnosis is one of the most dynamic and transforming fields in laboratory medicine. It was

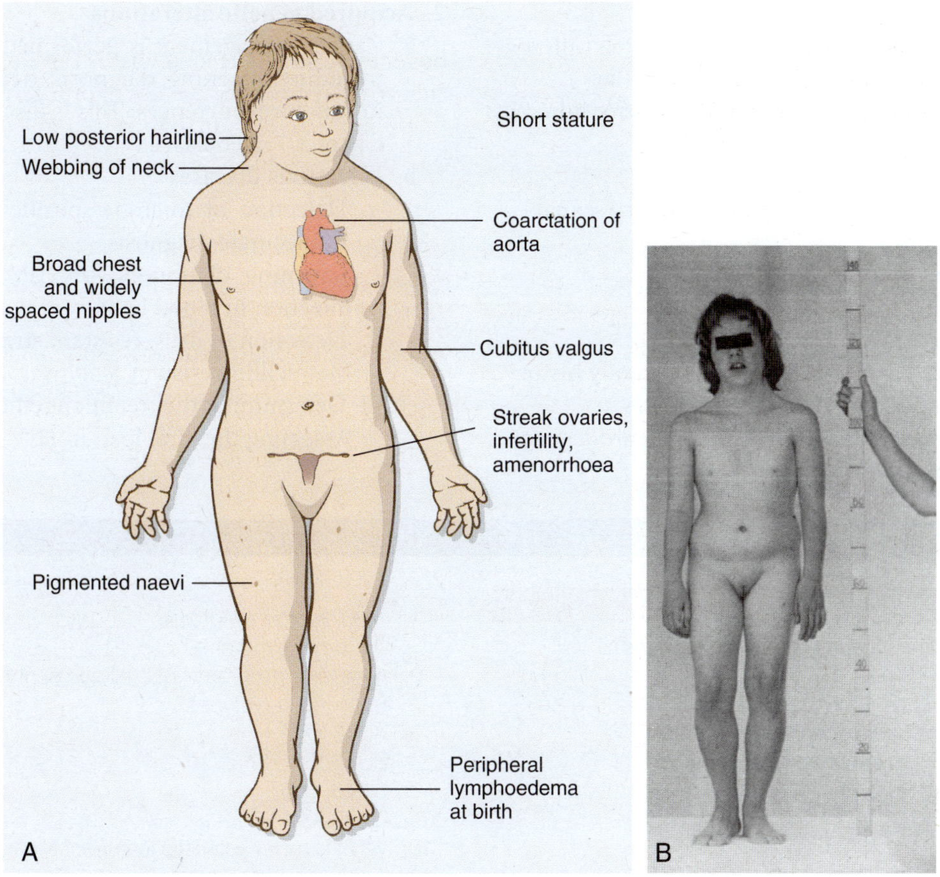

Fig. 5.29 (A) Features of Turner syndrome. (B) Turner syndrome in a girl aged 14 years 10 months with the typical form of the syndrome of gonadal dysgenesis (Turner syndrome – 45X). She was short and sexually infantile, except for the appearance of sparse pubic hair, and had a short webbed neck, shield-like chest with widely separated nipples, bilateral metacarpal signs, puffiness over the dorsum of the fingers, cubitus valgus, increased number of pigmented nevi, characteristic facies and low-set ears. (*Source:* From Dennis M. Styne. Physiology and Disorders of Puberty. Williams Textbook of Endocrinology. 14th edition. 2020. Elsevier; Vinay Kumar, Abul K. Abbas and Jon C. Aster. Genetic and Pediatric Diseases. Robbins Basic Pathology. 10th edition. 2021.)

used in the past for the diagnosis of inherited genetic disorders. In the present era, the field has rapidly developed and revolutionized the health care system with application in the field of oncology and infectious diseases.

A disease manifests because of changes taking place at the genetic level. These changes in DNA are transcribed to RNA and then translated to protein molecules. Molecular diagnosis means studying the molecular markers (DNA, RNA, protein) for changes associated with the disease condition. Studying the genetic material (DNA, RNA) and its interactions is called ***genomics,*** whereas studying the protein product is called ***proteomics.***

APPLICATIONS OF MOLECULAR DIAGNOSTIC TECHNIQUES

1. **Inherited genetic alterations**

   Inherited genetic diseases are often diagnosed by cytogenetic studies: conventional karyotyping and molecular diagnostic techniques. These may be performed at any age.

Age-wise indications for diagnosing inherited genetic diseases include the following:

Prenatal period

Prenatal testing should be performed for fetuses that are at an increased risk of inheriting a genetic disease:

- Advanced maternal age
- Fetal anomalies on ultrasound scan
- Parents with known balanced chromosomal rearrangement
- Family history of genetic diseases: Cystic fibrosis, spinomuscular atrophy
- Bad obstetric history: Abortion/stillbirth/sudden infant death syndrome

Fetal DNA for prenatal testing can be obtained by noninvasive or invasive techniques.

Noninvasive	:	Maternal blood is collected to obtain cell-free DNA of fetal origin
Invasive	:	Amniocentesis: 11–14 weeks Chorionic villus biopsy: 15–17 weeks Umbilical cord blood: 16–20 weeks

Neonatal/infancy
- Multiple congenital anomalies
- Mental retardation/development delay
- Suspicion of Down syndrome or other syndromes
- Suspicion of metabolic syndrome

Young adults
- Failure of development of secondary sexual characters
- Primary amenorrhoea
- Infertility

Older adults
- Inherited cancer syndromes – a family history of colon cancer, breast cancer, etc.
- Risk assessment for developing neurodegenerative disorders

2. **Acquired genetic alterations**
   a. Cancer management is performed at various levels including screening, diagnosis, treatment and monitoring for recurrences. This is discussed in detail in Chapter 7: Neoplasia.
   b. **Infectious diseases**
      i. Detection of microbe-specific genetic material for accurate diagnosis
         Screening of donors for HIV and hepatitis B infection in blood bank
      ii. Detection of drug-resistant strains of microbes
         Methicillin-resistant *Staphylococcus aureus*
      iii. Determining the treatment efficacy
         Assessing the viral load in HIV infection

SELF-ASSESSMENT

Multiple Choice Questions

1. What is the primary cause of Down syndrome?
   A. Deletion mutation
   B. Nondisjunction of chromosome 21
   C. Point mutation in a specific gene
   D. Translocation involving chromosome 21
2. In Marfan syndrome, which gene is typically mutated?
   A. BRCA1
   B. FBN1
   C. HEXA
   D. SRY
3. Which of the following is an example of an autosomal recessive disorder?
   A. Marfan syndrome
   B. Neurofibromatosis type I
   C. Tay–Sachs disease
   D. Familial hypercholesterolaemia
4. Turner syndrome is characterized by which karyotype?
   A. 47,XXY
   B. 45,X
   C. 47,XXX
   D. 46,XY
5. What is the primary effect of mutations in the LDLR gene?
   A. Sickle cell anaemia
   B. Cystic fibrosis
   C. Familial hypercholesterolaemia
   D. Haemophilia
6. Which disorder is associated with a CGG trinucleotide repeat expansion?
   A. Huntington disease
   B. Fragile X syndrome
   C. Down syndrome
   D. Klinefelter syndrome
7. Gaucher disease results from a deficiency in which enzyme?
   A. Hexosaminidase A
   B. Glucocerebrosidase
   C. Sphingomyelinase
   D. β-Glucosidase
8. Which condition is associated with a chromosomal deletion at 22q11.2?
   A. Down syndrome
   B. Klinefelter syndrome
   C. DiGeorge syndrome
   D. Turner syndrome
9. Klinefelter syndrome typically presents with which of the following karyotypes?
   A. 47,XXY
   B. 45,X
   C. 46,XY
   D. 47,XXX
10. What is a characteristic feature of Niemann–Pick disease?
    A. Hypotonia
    B. Spherocytosis
    C. Foam cells
    D. Macro-orchidism
11. Which of the following is a feature of autosomal dominant inheritance?
    A. Both parents must be carriers.
    B. The disease manifests only in the homozygous state.
    C. One affected parent can pass the disorder to the offspring with a 50% probability.
    D. The disease is more common in males.
12. In Tay–Sachs disease, accumulation of which substance is observed?
    A. Amyloid protein
    B. GM2 ganglioside
    C. Glucocerebroside
    D. Fibrillin-1
13. Which disorder is characterized by the presence of café au lait spots?
    A. Neurofibromatosis type I
    B. Marfan syndrome
    C. Ehlers–Danlos syndrome
    D. Gaucher disease
14. Which is a common symptom of Ehlers–Danlos syndrome?
    A. Joint hypermobility
    B. Aortic root dilation
    C. Cherry-red spot in the macula
    D. Sickle-shaped red blood cells
15. What is the primary defect in fragile X syndrome?
    A. A deletion mutation on the X chromosome
    B. Overexpression of the FMR1 gene
    C. Trinucleotide repeat expansion in the FMR1 gene
    D. Mutation in the SHOX gene

16. Which genetic disorder is associated with a 'cherry-red spot' in the eye?
    A. Tay–Sachs disease
    B. Marfan syndrome
    C. Niemann–Pick disease
    D. Gaucher disease
17. Lysosomal storage diseases are primarily caused by what type of genetic alteration?
    A. Deletions in structural genes
    B. Mutations in genes coding for lysosomal acid hydrolases
    C. Overexpression of metabolic pathway genes
    D. Translocations involving metabolic genes
18. Which of the following is a feature of X-linked recessive disorders?
    A. Females are more commonly affected than males.
    B. Affected males transmit the disorder to their sons.
    C. Male carriers are asymptomatic.
    D. Males are commonly affected, and females are usually carriers.
19. In genomic imprinting, transcriptional silencing occurs because of
    A. DNA methylation and histone modification
    B. Overexpression of certain genes
    C. Gene duplication
    D. Nonsense mutations
20. Which disorder involves a defect in oxidative phosphorylation?
    A. Cystic fibrosis
    B. Leber hereditary optic neuropathy
    C. Sickle cell anaemia
    D. Haemophilia A

Answers

1. (B); 2. (B); 3. (C); 4. (B); 5. (C); 6. (B); 7. (B); 8. (C); 9. (A); 10. (C); 11. (C); 12. (B); 13. (A); 14. (A); 15. (C); 16. (A); 17. (B); 18. (D); 19. (A); 20. (B)

Scenario-Based Questions

1. A 15-year-old male patient came to the ophthalmology outpatient department (OPD) with diminished vision. The boy was tall with long fingers. On auscultation, the boy had a crisp mid-systolic click. On ophthalmic examination, the boy had superotemporal subluxation of the lens. The boy's father had died 5 years back with sudden chest pain. What is the diagnosis and the probable genetic mutation the boy is having?
2. A 10-year-old girl was brought to the hospital with complaints of shoulder dislocation. On examination, her other joints were hypermobile and her skin was hyperextensible. Her mother also gave history that the child got bruised easily following insignificant injuries and commented that the child's father and her paternal aunt had hypermobile joints. What is the probable diagnosis and defective gene product in this condition?
3. A 4-year-old male child presented with vomiting and progressive deterioration of psychomotor function. On examination, he had hepatosplenomegaly and cherry-red spot was observed in the retina. Liver biopsy showed the presence of vacuolated hepatocytes. Under the electron microscope, the vacuoles appeared to be engorged lysosomes containing zebra bodies. What is the diagnosis? How will you confirm it?
4. A 6-year-old girl was admitted to the hospital with complaints of abdominal distension with pain (on/off) since 2 months. On examination, there was hepatosplenomegaly. Her complete blood cell count revealed pancytopenia. Bone marrow biopsy showed macrophages with fibrillary cytoplasm resembling a wrinkled tissue paper and was positive for periodic acid–Schiff stain. What is the diagnosis? Describe its pathogenesis.
5. A healthy 23-year-old primigravida at 8 weeks of pregnancy presented with complaints of abdominal pain and vaginal spotting. On examination, she had minimal vaginal bleeding and was admitted for observation and advised bed rest. The next day, she had spontaneous abortion. What is the most common cause of miscarriage in the first trimester?
6. A 33-year-old primigravida who did not attend routine antenatal check-up delivered a baby boy by normal vaginal delivery at the hospital. The paediatrician noted that the baby had upslanting palpebral fissure, depressed nasal bridge, single palmar crease and a wide gap between the first and second toes. What is the probable diagnosis? Describe the clinical features and complications of this condition.
7. A 23-year-old woman came to the hospital with complaints of primary amenorrhoea. She had a short stature, webbing of the neck, broad chest with poorly developed breast and infantile genitalia. What is the diagnosis? Describe its cytogenetic abnormality.
8. A couple, who had been married for 3 years, came to the clinic for infertility workup. The male partner was 7 feet tall and thin built with long legs. On examination, he had gynaecomastia and small testes. Which karyotypic abnormality can cause this presentation?
9. At a genetic counselling centre, the counsellor elicited history that 4 adult males and 2 females in a family of 12 over 3 generations were having intellectual disability, which was more severe in males than in females. On examination, the males were healthy and had enlarged testes. What is the diagnosis? Explain the inheritance pattern.

Answers

1. Marfan syndrome.
2. Ehlers–Danlos syndrome.
3. Niemann–Pick disease.
4. Gaucher disease.
5. Chromosomal aberration.
6. Down syndrome.
7. Turner syndrome.
8. Klinefelter syndrome.
9. Fragile X syndrome.

Topics for Self-Directed Learning

1. Differences between heredity and familial diseases.
2. How to construct and analyse the pedigree chart for genetic diseases.
3. Holandric genes and inheritance.
4. Role of electron microscopy in the diagnosis of lysosomal storage diseases.
5. Differences between inborn errors of metabolism and lysosomal storage diseases.
6. Hermaphroditism and pseudohermaphroditism.
7. Role of genetic polymorphism in health and disease.

MIND MAPS

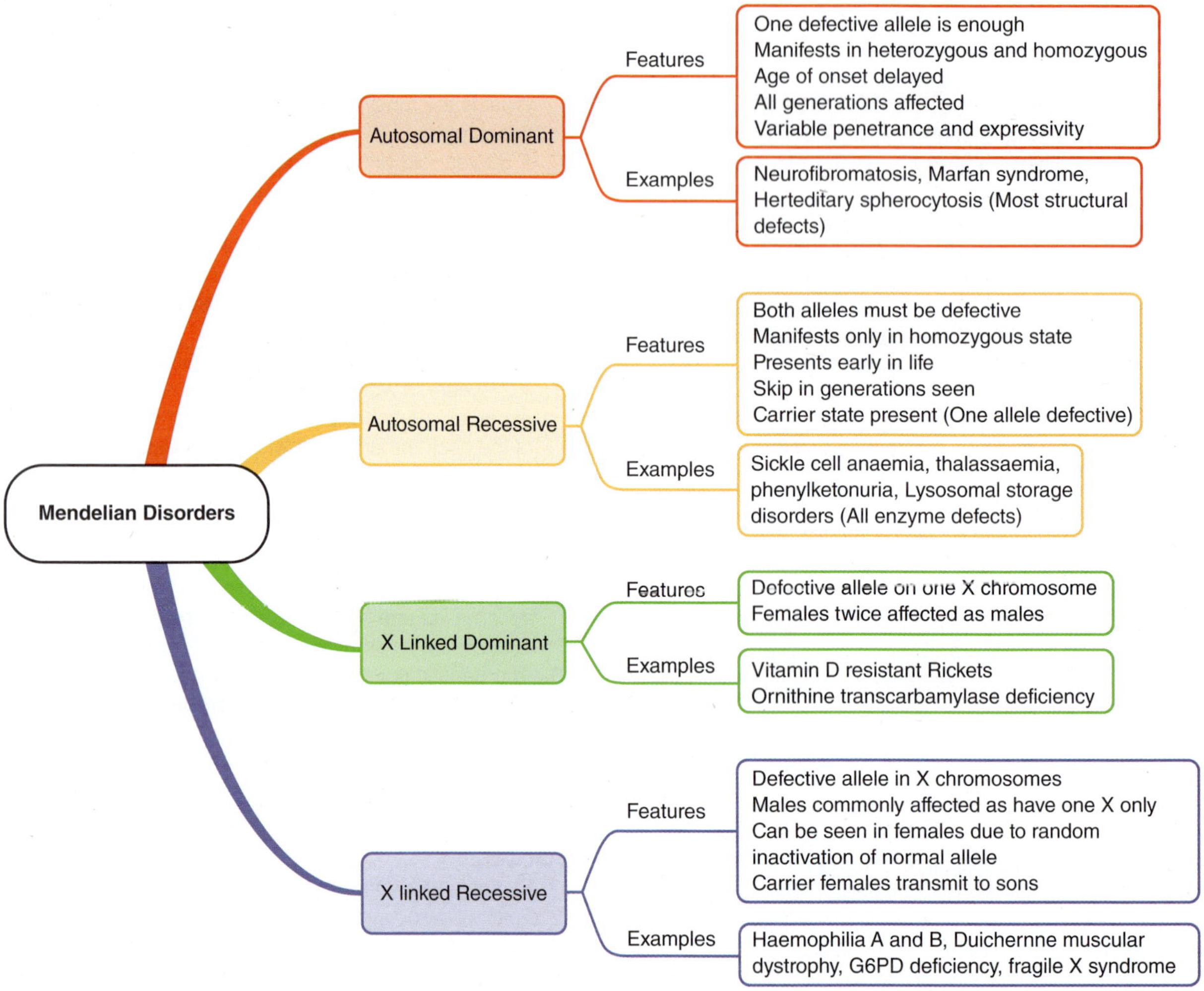
Mendelian Disorders
Autosomal Dominant
Features
One defective allele is enough
Manifests in heterozygous and homozygous
Age of onset delayed
All generations affected
Variable penetrance and expressivity
Examples
Neurofibromatosis, Marfan syndrome, Herteditary spherocytosis (Most structural defects)
Autosomal Recessive
Features
Both alleles must be defective
Manifests only in homozygous state
Presents early in life
Skip in generations seen
Carrier state present (One allele defective)
Examples
Sickle cell anaemia, thalassaemia, phenylketonuria, Lysosomal storage disorders (All enzyme defects)
X Linked Dominant
Features
Defective allele on one X chromosome
Females twice affected as males
Examples
Vitamin D resistant Rickets
Ornithine transcarbamylase deficiency
X linked Recessive
Features
Defective allele in X chromosomes
Males commonly affected as have one X only
Can be seen in females due to random inactivation of normal allele
Carrier females transmit to sons
Examples
Haemophilia A and B, Duichernne muscular dystrophy, G6PD deficiency, fragile X syndrome

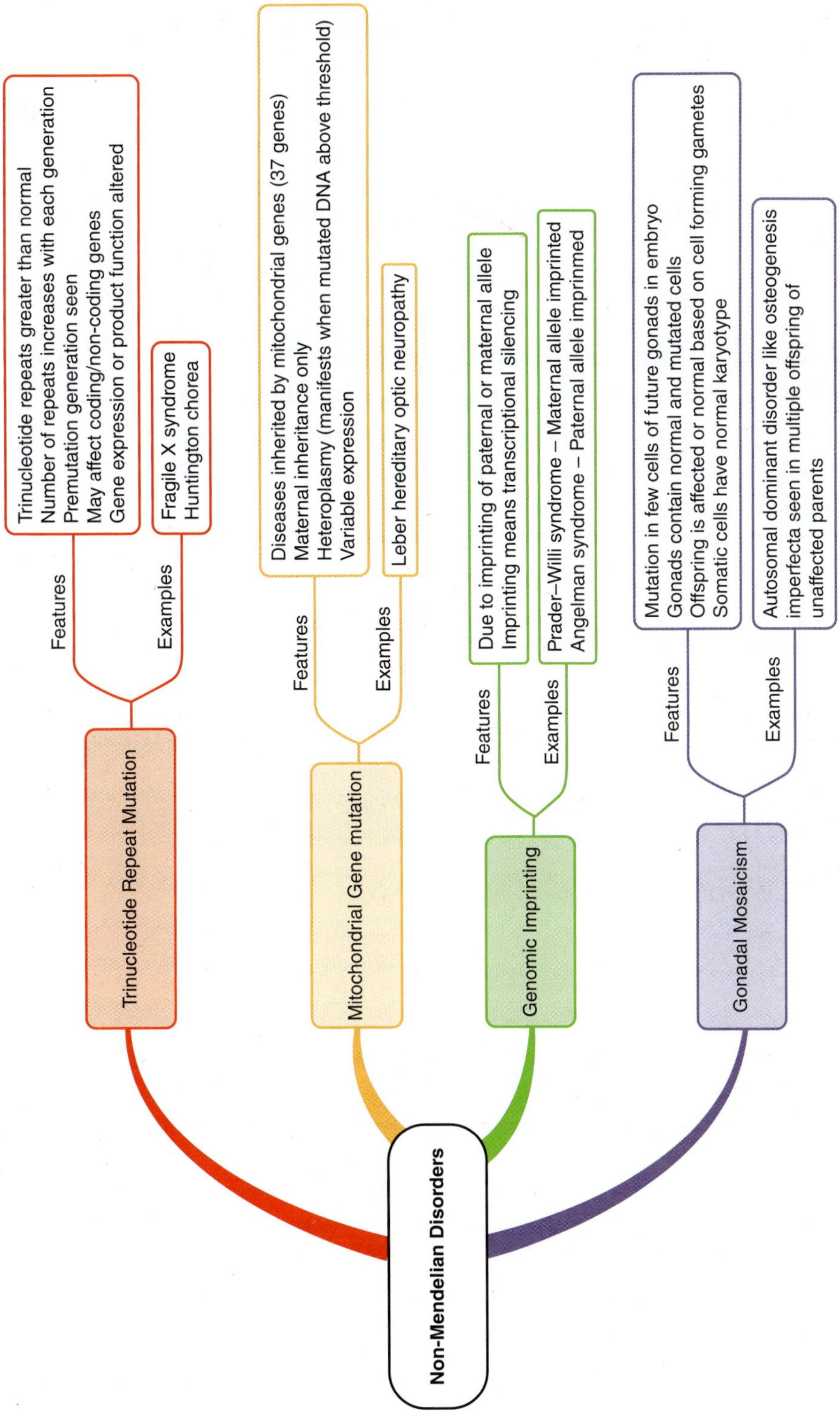
Non-Mendelian Disorders
Trinucleotide Repeat Mutation
Features
Trinucleotide repeats greater than normal
Number of repeats increases with each generation
Premutation generation seen
May affect coding/non-coding genes
Gene expression or product function altered
Examples
Fragile X syndrome
Huntington chorea
Mitochondrial Gene mutation
Features
Diseases inherited by mitochondrial genes (37 genes)
Maternal inheritance only
Heteroplasmy (manifests when mutated DNA above threshold)
Variable expression
Examples
Leber hereditary optic neuropathy
Genomic Imprinting
Features
Due to imprinting of paternal or maternal allele
Imprinting means transcriptional silencing
Examples
Prader–Willi syndrome – Maternal allele imprinted
Angelman syndrome – Paternal allele imprinmed
Gonadal Mosaicism
Features
Mutation in few cells of future gonads in embryo
Gonads contain normal and mutated cells
Offspring is affected or normal based on cell forming gametes
Somatic cells have normal karyotype
Examples
Autosomal dominant disorder like osteogenesis imperfecta seen in multiple offspring of unaffected parents

6 Immune Disorders

Rajeswari Kathiah

PA 9.1 Describe the **principles and mechanisms involved in immunity.**

PA 9.2 Describe the mechanism of **hypersensitivity reactions.**

PA 9.3 Describe the HLA system and the immune principles in transplant and mechanism of **transplant rejection.**

PA 9.4 Define autoimmunity. Enumerate **autoimmune disorders.**

PA 9.5 Define and describe the pathogenesis of **systemic lupus erythematosus.**

PA 9.6 Define and describe the pathogenesis and pathology of **HIV** and **AIDS.**

PA 9.7 Define and describe the pathogenesis of other **common autoimmune diseases.**

PA 3.1 Describe the pathogenesis and pathology of **amyloidosis.**

CHAPTER OUTLINE

THE IMMUNE SYSTEM

The **immune system** is a host defence system comprising many biological structures and processes that protects us from diseases and is essential for survival. At the same time, the immune system by itself is capable of causing tissue injury and diseases. *Immunology* is the study of all aspects of the immune system.

Disorders of the immune system can lead to autoimmune diseases, inflammatory diseases and cancer. Immunodeficiency occurs when the immune system is less active than normal, resulting in recurring and serious life-threatening infections. In humans, immunodeficiency may be the result of a genetic disease such as severe combined immunodeficiency (SCID) or an acquired condition such as human immunodeficiency virus (HIV)/acquired immunodeficiency syndrome (AIDS) or because of the use of immunosuppressive drugs. In contrast, autoimmunity is the result of hyperactive immune system attacking normal tissues as if they were foreign organisms. Common autoimmune diseases include Hashimoto thyroiditis, rheumatoid arthritis, type 1 diabetes mellitus and systemic lupus erythematosus (SLE). Hypersensitivity reactions (HSRs) are the result of overactivity of the immune system in response to a variety of endogenous and exogenous antigens.

This chapter deals with disorders of the immune system along with amyloidosis, which is characterized by the deposition of abnormal proteins and suppression of immunity. To better understand the immune system and its related disorders, the next section describes the normal functioning and maturation of the immune system.

THE NORMAL IMMUNE RESPONSE PA 9.1

INTRODUCTION

An **immune response** is a reaction that occurs in humans or in any other organism for the purpose of defending against foreign agents. These agents include a wide variety of different microorganisms including bacteria, viruses, parasites and fungi that could cause serious disorders to the health of the host if not cleared from the body.

There are two distinct aspects of the immune response, the innate and the adaptive, which work together to protect us against pathogens (Fig. 6.1).

The innate immunity – the body's first response to a pathogen – is known to be a nonspecific and quick response to any pathogen. Components of the innate immune response include physical barriers like the skin and mucous membranes; immune cells such as neutrophils, macrophages and monocytes; and many other soluble factors including cytokines, surfactant and complement.

On the other hand, **the adaptive immunity** is the body's immune response that is targeted against specific antigens and thus it takes longer to activate the components involved. The adaptive immune system includes cells such as dendritic cells, T cells and B cells as well as antibodies, which directly interact with the antigens, thereby mounting a strong response against the pathogens.

Layered Immune Response

The immune system offers protection against the pathogens with multiple layers of defence of increasing specificity. In simple terms, physical barriers like the surface epithelia prevent entry of pathogens, but if a pathogen breaches such barriers, the other components of the innate immune system that include the neutrophils and macrophages mount an immediate but nonspecific response. If pathogens successfully escape the innate response, the second layer of protection, the adaptive immune system, which is activated by the innate immune system, attacks with a much stronger and pathogen-specific response. The immune system also comprises specific cells to recognize or rather remember pathogens previously encountered, allowing it to respond faster and more effectively when the same pathogen is encountered again.

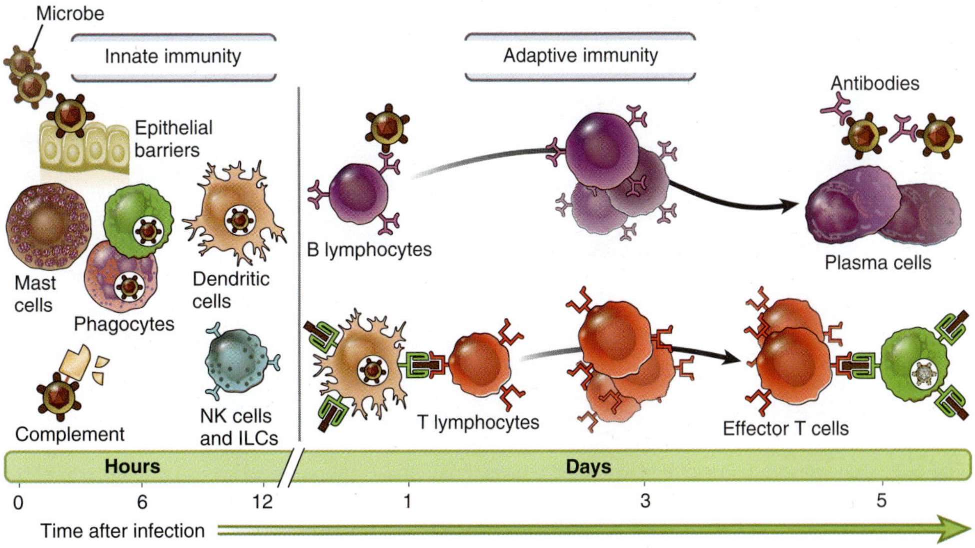

Fig. 6.1 Principal mechanisms of innate and adaptive immune response. *(Source:* https://basicmedicalkey.com/introduction-to-the-immune-system-nomenclature-general-properties-and-components/.)

Thus, during development, exposure to pathogens confers **active immunity**, which is a specific response to a target antigen and takes from few days to weeks to develop but lasts longer, sometimes lifelong, and immunological memory helps to recognize the pathogen in later life. A classic example of **natural active immunity** includes chickenpox infection, following which the adaptive immune response offers lifelong immunity. **Artificial active immunity** can be induced by vaccination that contains a live attenuated or inactivated form of the pathogen.

Active immunity involves the exposure of the pathogen, whereas **passive immunity** refers to the process of providing ready-made antibodies to the individual. Neonates have little or no exposure to microbes and are especially vulnerable to infection, but several layers of passive protection are offered by the mother. During pregnancy, immunoglobulin G (IgG) is transferred from the mother to her fetus directly through the placenta, providing the newborns with high levels of antibodies of the same specificity as their mother at the time of birth. Breast milk also contains antibodies that are transferred from the mothers to the gut of the infants to offer protection against pathogens until the newborns can synthesize their own antibodies. This is referred to as **natural passive immunity**, as the fetus and the newborn do not actually have any memory cells or antibodies but can only borrow them. This passive immunity is for the short term, lasting from a few days to months following which the immunity matures and gains antigenic experience. Artificially, immunoglobulins generated in disease-exposed individuals can be collected, pooled and injected into susceptible persons. Human hepatitis B immunoglobulin and human rabies immunoglobulin are examples of **artificial passive immunity**.

TISSUES OF THE IMMUNE SYSTEM

The immune system consists of the following organs (Fig. 6.2):

Generative or primary or central lymphoid organs: The site where lymphocytes mature and become competent

The central lymphoid organs are the thymus where the T lymphocytes mature and the bone marrow where all blood cells and B lymphocytes mature. These organs are discussed in detail in Chapter 16, and the process of maturation is discussed later under the 'Immunological tolerance' section.

Peripheral or secondary lymphoid organs: The site where adaptive immune responses against pathogens are initiated

Lymph nodes, spleen, organized mucosal and cutaneous lymphoid tissues, antigen-presenting cells (APCs) and lymphocytes constitute peripheral lymphoid organs.

Lymph nodes and spleen are discussed in Chapter 16.

The cutaneous and mucosal lymphoid systems are located under the epithelia of the skin or mucosa. The mucosa-associated lymphoid tissue (MALT) is a diffuse system of small concentrations of lymphoid tissue found in various submucosal sites of the body.

The components of MALT are categorized into the following:

- Gut-associated lymphoid tissue (**GALT**; Peyer patches are a component of GALT found in the lining of the small intestine)
- Bronchus-associated lymphoid tissue (**BALT**)
- Nasal-associated lymphoid tissue (**NALT**)
- Conjunctiva-associated lymphoid tissue (**CALT**)
- Larynx-associated lymphoid tissue (**LALT**)

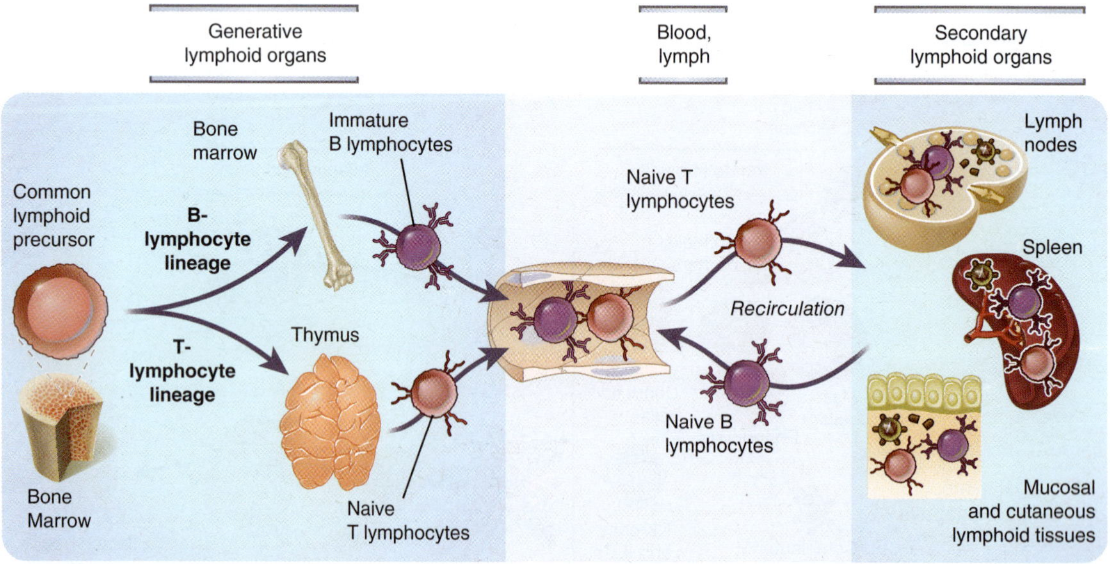

Fig. 6.2 Generative and peripheral lymphoid organs. From Abul K. Abbas, Andrew H. Lichtman and Shiv Pillai. Cells and Tissues of the Immune System. Cellular and Molecular Immunology. 9th edition. 2018.

- Skin-associated lymphoid tissue (**SALT**)
- Vulvovaginal-associated lymphoid tissue (**VALT**)
- Testis-associated lymphoid tissue (**TALT**)

These lymphocytes react with the antigens when there is a breach in the epithelium. Pharyngeal tonsils and Peyer patches of the small intestine are anatomically defined mucosal lymphoid tissues. More than half of the body's lymphocytes are present in the mucosal tissues, and most of them are memory cells. The segregation of B and T cells in lymph nodes and spleen is discussed in Chapter 16.

Lymphocyte Recirculation

Lymphocyte recirculation refers to the continuous transport of large numbers of naive lymphocytes between blood and lymphoid organs. Naive B and T lymphocytes after completing their maturation in the bone marrow and thymus, respectively, circulate in blood for about 30 minutes before lodging into the lymphoid and nonlymphoid organs. Even in these locations, they do not reside permanently but re-enter the blood vessels and lymphatic system to perform their duties in providing immune response to our body. Human body contains as many as 5×10^{11} lymphocytes that travel through blood every day. Naive T and B lymphocytes enter the lymph nodes or organized lymphoid tissues by selectively adhering to and transmigrating through the high endothelial venules.

INNATE IMMUNITY

Innate immunity is also called native immunity. It is always present, ready to defend against organisms and eradicate damaged cells. It is a network of components that are listed later. The role of each component is discussed next.

Components of innate immunity can be divided into five groups, with their members as follows:

Components of Innate Immunity

1. **Surface barriers and their secretions**
2. **Pattern recognition receptors**
   A. Toll-like receptors (TLRs)
   B. Nod-like receptors (NLRs)
   C. Other receptors
3. **Cellular components**
   A. Phagocytes
   B. Dendritic cells
   C. Granulocytes
   D. Innate lymphoid cells (ILCs)
4. **Complement system**
5. **Others**
   A. Mannose-binding protein
   B. C-reactive protein
   C. Surfactant

Surface Barriers and Their Secretions

The epithelia of the skin, gastrointestinal (GI) tract, genitourinary tract and respiratory tract act as mechanical barriers to the entry of pathogens from the external environment. Apart from being physical barriers, these also secrete antimicrobial molecules like *defensins,* which act as chemical barriers and have commensal flora that act as biological barriers. Apart from these, enzymes such as lysozyme and phospholipase A2 found in saliva, tears and breast milk also have antibacterial properties. Vaginal secretions become slightly acidic after menarche and serve as a chemical barrier, whereas semen contains defensins and zinc to kill pathogens. In the stomach, gastric acid serves as a powerful chemical defence against ingested pathogens.

Pattern Recognition Receptors (Fig. 6.3)

Cells of the innate immune system are capable of recognizing molecular structures on the surface of the microbial pathogens with the help of pattern recognition receptors (PRRs). These receptors are germline-encoded host sensors that detect molecules typical for the pathogens. These are proteins expressed mainly by the cells of the innate immune system such as macrophages, monocytes, dendritic cells, neutrophils and epithelial cells to identify the following two categories of molecules:

A. **Pathogen-associated molecular patterns (PAMPs)** – associated with microbial pathogens
B. **Damage-associated molecular patterns (DAMPs)** – associated with components of the host's cells that are released during cell injury or death

PRRs are located in all the cellular compartments where microbes may be present – plasma membrane receptors detect extracellular pathogens, endosomal receptors detect ingested pathogens and cytosolic receptors detect pathogens in the cytoplasm.

Toll-Like Receptors Toll-like receptors (TLRs) are the best known PRRs that are located in the plasma membrane and endosomal vesicles. They were first discovered in *Drosophila.* Till date, 10 functional members of the TLR family have been described in humans and each recognizes a different set of microbial molecules. All these receptors signal by a common pathway that converges in the activation of two sets of receptors:

i. NF-κB
ii. Interferon regulatory factors (IRFs)

The net result of activation of these two pathways is the secretion of cytokines and stimulation of the other host defence mechanisms that are essential for innate and adaptive immunity. It can be understood that

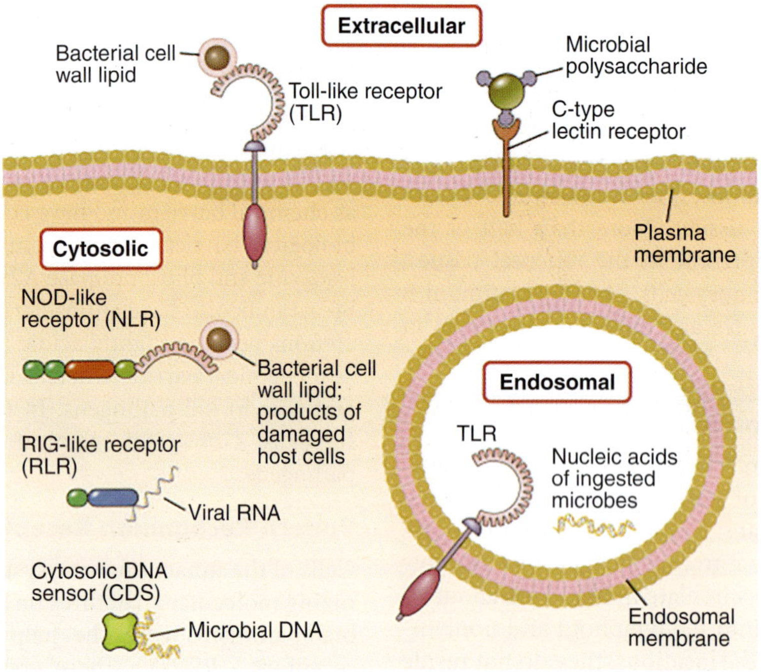

Fig. 6.3 Cellular receptors for microbes, products of damaged cells and foreign agents. (*Source:* https://www.google.com/url?sa=i&url=https%3A%2F%2Fbasicmedicalkey.com%2Finnate-immunity-the-early-defense-against-infections%2F&psig=AOvVaw1E0YCI4ILoNWoq8OlaVihn&ust=1605799155995000&source=images&cd=vfe&ved=0CAIQjRxqFwoTCljCx5uyjO0CFQAAAAAdAAAAABAD.)

germline loss-of-function mutation of TLRs, though rare, is associated with life-threatening immunodeficiency syndromes. The types of TLRs and their specificity are given in Table 6.1.

Table 6.1 Types of TLR and the Pathogen Binding to It

Type of TLR	Pathogen Binding to It
TLR 1	Bacteria
TLR 2	Gram-positive bacteria, fungi
TLR 3	DsRNA virus
TLR 4	Gram-negative bacteria
TLR 5	*Toxoplasma gondii*
TLR 6	Mycoplasma
TLR 7	Single-stranded RNA virus
TLR 8	Single-stranded RNA virus
TLR 9	DNA virus
TLR 10	Unknown
TLR 11, 12	*T. gondii*
TLR 13	Bacteria and virus

TLR, Toll-like receptor.

Nod-Like Receptors and the Inflammasome Nod-like receptors (NLRs) are PRRs located in the cytoplasm that have the potential to recognize a wide range of substances including products released from injured and dead cells, loss of intracellular potassium ions and some microbial products. Many of this type of receptors signal via a cytosolic multiprotein complex called the *inflammasome*. **Inflammasome complex** acts by activating an enzyme *caspase-1* that cleaves IL-1 and IL-18 from their precursor molecules. As discussed in Chapter 3, IL-1 is a proinflammatory cytokine that mediates inflammation through recruitment of phagocytes and induction of fever.

'Autoinflammatory syndrome' is a group of diseases characterized by periodic fever syndromes because of gain-of-function mutations in NLRs and related proteins and loss-of-function mutations in regulators of the inflammasome. NLRs are involved in the inflammation associated with many diseases such as:

- Atherosclerosis
- Type 2 diabetes mellitus
- Gout

Other Receptors The other receptors that are involved in the innate immune response and their spectrum of activity are as follows:

C-type lectin receptors (CLRs) – detect fungal glycans
RIG-like receptors (RLRs) – detect viral nucleic acid
Mannose receptors – detect microbial sugars

Hence, it is stressed here that all the subsequent reactions of innate and adaptive immunity are dependent on the function of these receptors.

Cellular Components

Cellular components of innate immunity include phagocytes, dendritic cells, granulocytes and innate lymphocytes.

Phagocytes Monocytes and neutrophils are phagocytes in the circulation and can rapidly be recruited to the sites of infection. Tissue monocytes are called macrophages and are professional phagocytes. The process of phagocytosis is described in detail in Chapter 3. Macrophages and dendritic cells have prominent roles in adaptive immunity also, so their functions are explained in detail in the subsequent sections.

Dendritic Cells Dendritic cells are phagocytes in the tissues in which they are located, mainly in the skin, nose, lungs, stomach and intestines, and remain in contact with the external environment. These cells have been termed dendritic because of their resemblance to neuronal dendrites and spine-like projections, but later it was confirmed that these dendritic cells are in no way related to the nervous system. Dendritic cells serve as a link between the body tissues and the innate and adaptive immune systems. These may be classified as *interdigitating dendritic cells* of the mucosa and *follicular dendritic cells* (FDCs) of the lymph nodes. The former is the most important APC to T cells, one of the key cell players of the adaptive immune system.

Granulocytes This category of cells includes those cells that have granules in their cytoplasm, **neutrophils, mast cells, basophils and eosinophils**. The role played by mast cells, basophils and eosinophils is discussed in detail in Chapter 3.

Innate Lymphoid Cells Innate lymphoid cells (ILCs) are derivatives of the common lymphoid progenitors. These cells are defined by the absence of antigen-specific B-cell receptor (BCR) or T-cell receptors (TCRs) because of the absence of recombination activating gene, described later. ILCs express neither myeloid nor dendritic cell markers.

Natural Killer Cells Natural killer (NK) cell is a member of the ILC family and a lymphocyte that plays important roles in innate and adaptive immunity. NK cells make up approximately 5%–10% of peripheral blood lymphocytes and express **CD16** (a receptor for IgG Fc tails). This provides NK cells the ability to attack IgG-coated target cells, a phenomenon referred to as antibody-dependent cellular cytotoxicity (**ADCC**) (Fig. 6.4).

NK cells do not directly attack invading microbes. The function of NK cells is to detect and destroy severely injured and abnormal cells such as virus-infected and tumour cells.

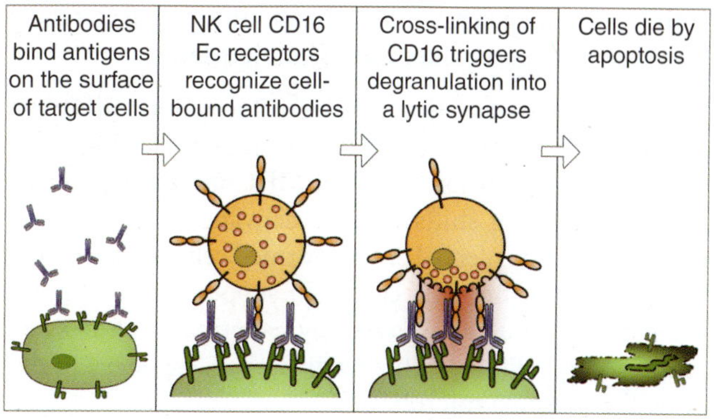

Fig. 6.4 ADCC of NK cells. ADCC, antibody-dependent cellular cytotoxicity; NK, natural killer. (*Source:* https://www.google.com/url?sa=i&url=https%3A%2F%2Fen.wikipedia.org%2Fwiki%2FAntibody-dependent_cellular_cytotoxicity&psig=AOvVaw0SHSxtWMddkOS7TLtPSFXI&ust=1605804824295000&source=images&cd=vfe&ved=0CAIQjRxqFwoTCKjHv6fHjO0CFQAAAAAdAAAAABAK.)

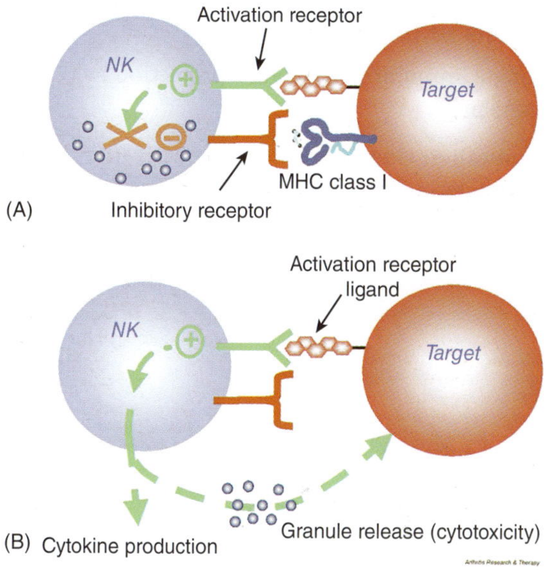

Fig. 6.5 Activating and inhibiting receptors of NK cells. NK, natural killer. (*Source:* https://www.google.com/url?sa=i&url=https%3A%2F%2Farthritis-research.biomedcentral.com%2Farticles%2F10.1186%2Far1034%2Ffigures%2F1&psig=AOvVaw1Orxsp0JaHjutRaej8K33R&ust=1605804721955000&source=images&cd=vfe&ved=0CAIQjRxqFwoTCIjp6fbGjO0CFQAAAAAdAAAAABAN.)

NK cells act by the signals delivered by activating and inhibitory receptors present on target cells (Fig. 6.5).

- **Activating receptors** are a group of receptors that are involved in recognizing the surface molecules induced by a variety of stress such as infections and DNA damage. Hence, these receptors enable NK cells to recognize and attack damaged and infected cells.
- **Inhibitory receptors** recognize self-class I major histocompatibility complex (MHC) molecules, which are expressed on all healthy cells and prevent NK cells from attacking normal cells. They recognize target cells by a mechanism known as *'missing self'* in which

they recognize virus-infected and tumour cells by their failure to express class I MHC molecules.

Viral infection and neoplastic transformation induce the expression of ligands for activating receptors while suppressing the expression of class I MHC molecules. Hence, when the balance shifts towards activation, NK cells get engaged and the infected or transformed cells are destroyed.

Apart from this, NK cells also support early defence against intracellular pathogens by secreting cytokines like interferon-γ (**IFN-γ**), which activate macrophages to destroy the ingested microbes.

Regulation of NK cell activity by cytokines:

- IL-2 and IL-15 stimulate the proliferation of NK cells.
- IL-12 activates the destruction of target cells and stimulates secretion of IFN-γ.

Role played by the complement system is discussed in detail in Chapter 3.

Reactions of Innate Immunity

The innate immune system offers protection by two major mechanisms:

Inflammation: Complement system activation and cytokine mediate inflammation, and the process is discussed in detail in Chapter 3.

Antiviral defence: *Type 1 interferon* produced in response to viral antigens acts on infected and uninfected cells and inhibits viral replication, which is referred to as antiviral state.

Apart from the aforementioned mechanisms, innate immunity generates danger signals that stimulate adaptive immune response. Unlike adaptive immunity, innate immunity does not have immunological memory or antigen specificity.

ADAPTIVE IMMUNITY

The adaptive immune system consists of lymphocytes and their products, most importantly, the antibodies. Lymphocytes of adaptive immunity are equipped with highly diverse receptors to detect a wide range of antigens.

Adaptive immunity is of the following two types (Fig. 6.6):

1. **Humoral immunity** – by **B lymphocytes** and their antibodies, which act against extracellular microbes and their toxins
2. **Cell-mediated immunity** – by **T lymphocytes**, which act against extra- and intracellular microbes

Cells of the adaptive immune system

T and B lymphocytes, the two pillars of adaptive immune response, have significant heterogeneity and are specialized

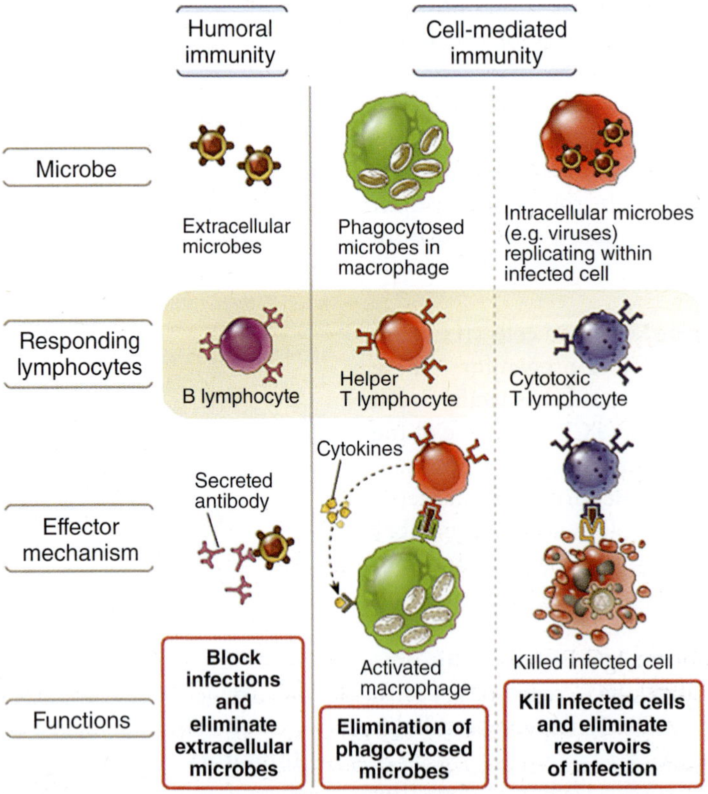

Fig. 6.6 Types of adaptive immunity. In humoral immunity, B lymphocytes secrete antibodies that eliminate extracellular microbes. In cell-mediated immunity, some T lymphocytes secrete soluble proteins called cytokines that recruit and activate phagocytes to destroy ingested microbes and other T lymphocytes kill infected cells. (*Source:* https://basicmedicalkey.com/introduction-to-the-immune-system-nomenclature-general-properties-and-components/.)

in molecular properties and functions. The human body has about 2 trillion lymphocytes, constituting 20%–40% of white blood cells (WBCs), and their total mass is about the same as that of the brain or liver. The peripheral blood contains 2% of circulating lymphocytes, and the remaining lymphocytes reside within the tissues and lymphatic system. Owing to their migrating nature, lymphocytes are capable of immune surveillance throughout the body and home into any site of infection. Mature lymphocytes that have not met any specific antigen are referred to as *naive* (immunologically inexperienced) lymphocytes. Subsequently, when the lymphocytes are activated by antigens and other signals, they differentiate into effector cells, which necessitate actions to eliminate microbes, and memory cells, which live in a state of heightened awareness and are able to mount an immune response against the microbes when they return. In lymphoid organs, different classes of lymphocytes are segregated anatomically in such a way that they interact with each other only when required to do so by encountering with antigens and other stimuli.

Let us discuss the diversity of T and B lymphocytes before describing the process of lymphocyte differentiation into effector and memory cells.

Lymphocyte Diversity As already mentioned, our body has lymphocytes with specificity for a wide range of antigens even before they are exposed to the antigens. Later, when we are exposed to a particular antigen, the lymphocyte that has receptor specific to that antigen undergoes activation and proliferation. This concept is referred to as **clonal selection** (Fig. 6.7).

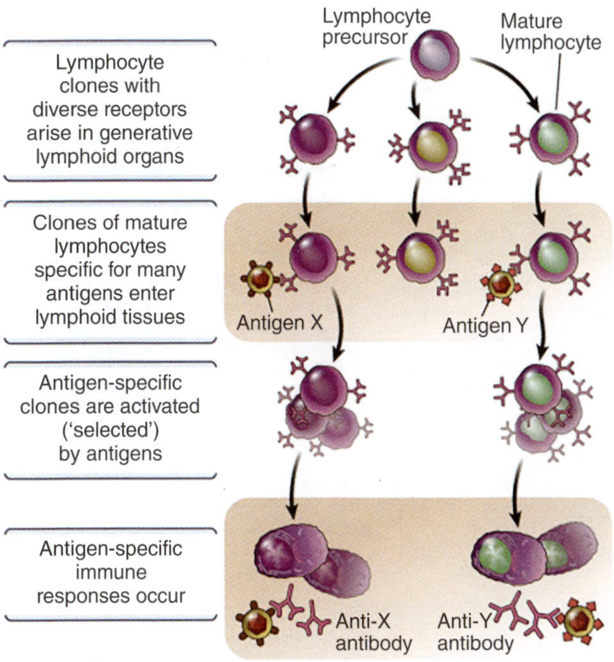

Fig. 6.7 Clonal selection of lymphocytes. The diagram shows only B lymphocytes giving rise to antibody-secreting cells, but the same principle applies to T lymphocytes. The antigens shown are surface molecules of microbes, but clonal selection is true for all extracellular and intracellular antigens. (*Source:* https://basicmedicalkey.com/introduction-to-the-immune-system-nomenclature-general-properties-and-components/.)

The theory states that in a preexisting group of lymphocytes, a specific antigen activates only its counter-specific cell, which then induces that particular cell to multiply, producing identical clones for antibody production. Such activation occurs in secondary lymphoid organs such as spleen and lymph nodes. Lymphocytes of the same specificity constitute a clone, and all the members of the same clone express identical antigen receptors that are different from the receptors expressed in other clones. There are around 10^{12} lymphocytes in immunocompetent individuals, and approximately 10^7–10^9 clones express receptors specific for different antigens. It is estimated that the number of cells specific for any 1 antigen is fewer than 1 in 100,000 lymphocytes. Phases of humoral immune responses are shown in Fig. 6.8.

Antigen Receptor Diversity It is an amazing fact that the immune system is capable of producing an expansive range of receptors, far more than could be individually encoded in the genome, which is referred to as antigen receptor diversity. Antigen receptor diversity is generated by *somatic recombination of the genes* that code for antigen receptors. Genes for antigen receptors are present in the germline of all the cells of the body, including lymphocyte progenitors. The genes for these receptors consist of spatially separated portions that cannot be expressed as mRNAs. These gene segments are assembled by recombination, and the DNA sequence variation is introduced at the sites where the gene segments are joined at the time of maturation of lymphocytes. This results in the formation of many different genes that can be transcribed and translated into antigen receptors, with diverse amino acid sequences, especially in the regions of the receptors that recognize and bind antigen. The enzymes involved in the recombination of these gene segments are the product of the recombination activating genes – **RAG-1** and **RAG-2**.

It should be stressed here that germline antigen receptor genes are present in all cells of the body but only T and B lymphocytes possess *recombined antigen receptor genes* – the TCR in T cells and immunoglobulins in B cells. Thus, in normal individuals, TCR antigen is polyclonal and monoclonal TCR populations are hallmarks of malignancy, as well as a few nonmalignant conditions like HIV infection, Epstein–Barr virus (EBV) infections, autoimmunity or immunodeficiency. In the present era, PCR, southern blotting and flow cytometry have emerged as detection methods to discriminate these polyclonal and monoclonal populations using TCR PCR fragments or TCR antibodies.

T Lymphocytes T lymphocytes arise from haematopoietic stem cells (HSCs) and develop in the thymus. The peripheral blood contains a greater proportion of mature

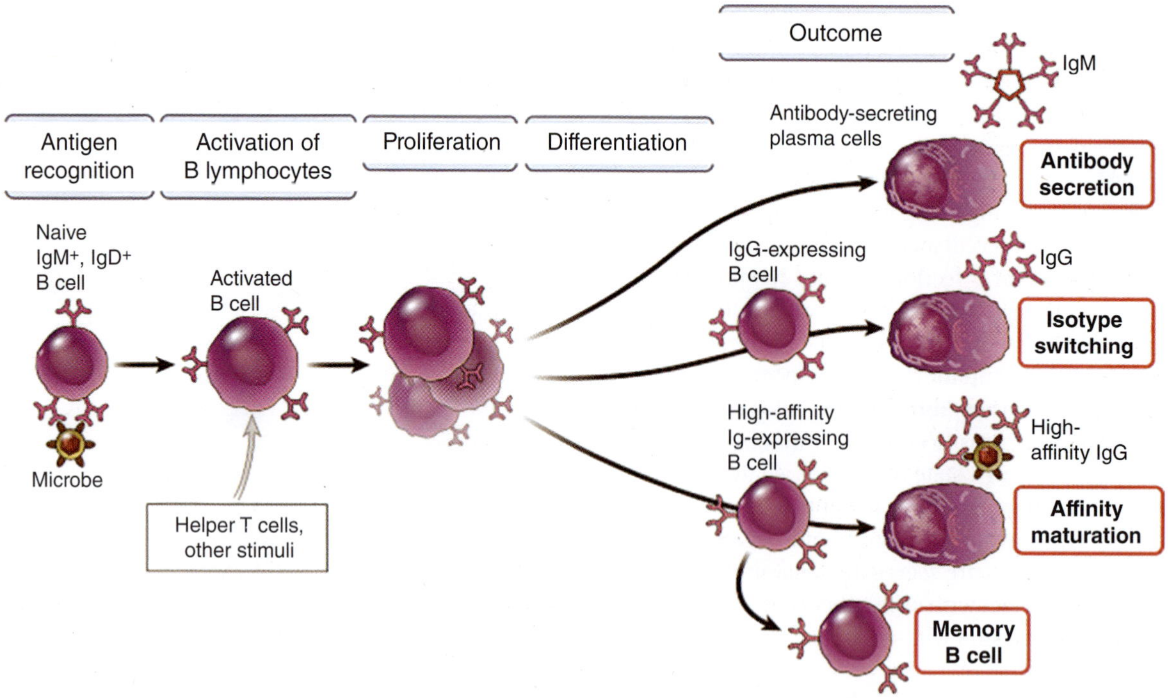

Fig. 6.8 Phases of humoral immune responses. Naive B lymphocytes recognize antigens; under the influence of helper T cells and other stimuli (not shown), the B cells are activated to proliferate, giving rise to clonal expansion, and to differentiate into antibody-secreting plasma cells. Some of the activated B cells undergo heavy-chain isotype switching and affinity maturation, and some become long-lived memory cells. (*Source:* https://www.google.com/url?sa=i&url=https%3A%2F%2Fbasicmedicalkey.com%2Fhumoral-immune-responses-activation-of-b-lymphocytes-and-production-of-antibodies%2F&psig=AOvVaw1BfCjEozazzOcAE79TelOO&ust=1605805307182000&source=images&cd=vfe&ved=0CAIQjRxqFwoTCLD_qlvJjO0CFQAAAAAdAAAAABAm.)

T cells that constitute 60%–70% of total lymphocytes. In peripheral lymphoid organs, these reside in the T-cell zones.

Groups of specific, differentiated T cells have important roles in controlling and shaping the immune responses by providing a variety of immune-related functions. The three major categories of T cells involved in distinct functions are as follows:

- **Helper T cells** function majorly to stimulate B cells to produce antibodies and to activate other cells of the immune response to destroy the pathogens. They have many subsets and have been discussed later.
- **Cytotoxic T cells** are involved in the destruction of infected cells.
- **Regulatory T cells** are crucial for immunological memory, for shutting down T-cell immunity at the end of an immune reaction and, most importantly, to suppress autoreactive T cells that have escaped tolerance mechanisms (explained later).
- **Memory T cells** provide the immune system with 'memory' against previously encountered microbes.

T-Cell Receptor Complex (Fig. 6.9) Every T cell identifies a specific cell-bound antigen by means of an antigen-specific TCR. TCR is composed of a disulphide-linked heterodimer made up of α- and β-polypeptide chains, each having a variable antigen-binding region and a constant region. Almost 95% of the T cells have this configuration

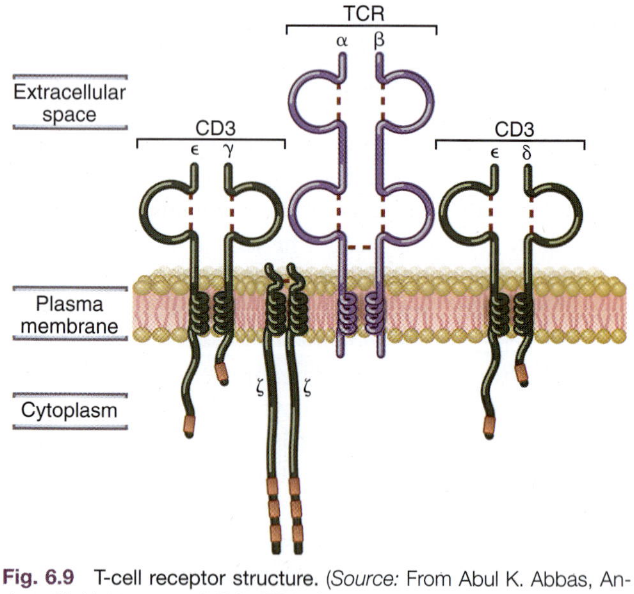

Fig. 6.9 T-cell receptor structure. (*Source:* From Abul K. Abbas, Andrew H. Lichtman and Shiv Pillai. Cellular and Molecular Immunology, Edition 10. Elsevier. 2021.

and are referred to as αβ TCR. Such **αβ TCR** recognizes peptide antigens only when they are presented by MHC molecules on the surface of APCs. This phenomenon is called **MHC restriction,** and this ensures that T cells recognize only cell-associated antigens.

Every TCR is covalently bound to the CD3 complex, which is made up of six polypeptide chains and the ζ chain dimer. These are identical in all the T cells and hence are markers for T-cell lineage and are involved in the transduction of signals into the T cells that are stimulated by binding of antigen to the TCR. **TCR, CD3 and ζ form the TCR complex**.

A minor fraction of T cells express another type of TCR composed of γ and δ chains. This type of **γδ TCR** identifies peptides, lipids and tiny molecules without the need for antigen presentation by MHC molecules. Hence, these aggregate at epithelial surfaces like the skin and mucosa of the GI and urogenital tracts, suggesting their sentinel role against the pathogens that try to enter through the epithelia. Another minor fraction of T cells coexpress the markers of NK cells and are called **NK-T cells**.

CD4, CD8, CD28 and integrins are additional surface markers expressed by T cells. CD4 and CD8 are coreceptors in T-cell activation and are mutually exclusive in subsets of αβ T cells. These initiate signals that are necessary for T-cell activation. Around 60% of mature T cells are $CD4^+$ and 30% are $CD8^+$. Integrins are adhesion molecules that enhance the attachment of T cells with APCs.

The series of changes that take place in APCs and T cells is explained later.

B Lymphocytes B lymphocytes develop from HSCs in the bone marrow and are the only cells in the body that are capable of producing antibodies. Mature B lymphocytes comprise 10%–20% of lymphocytes in peripheral blood and peripheral lymphoid tissues.

B-Cell Receptor Complex (Fig. 6.10) B cells recognize antigens with the help of BCR complex. Membrane-bound surface immunoglobulins of the types **IgM and IgD** present on naive B cells are the antigen-binding component of B cells. In addition to these surface immunoglobulins, B-cell antigen receptor complex contains **Igα** (CD79a) and **Igβ** (CD79b), which are essential for signal transduction following antigen binding to the surface IgM/IgD. These are similar to CD3 and ζ chain dimer of T cells. Apart from these, B cells also express complement receptor 2, also called **CR2 or CD21,** which identifies complement products released during innate immune responses, and **CD40,** which receives activating signals from helper T cells.

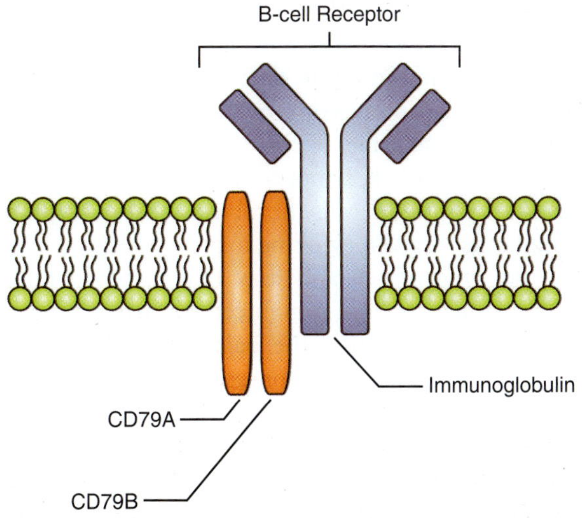

Fig. 6.10 B-cell receptor structure. (*Source:* https://www.google.com/url?sa=i&url=https%3A%2F%2Fen.wikipedia.org%2Fwiki%2FB-cell_receptor&psig=AOvVaw36qQH2XjsJNeUMxXydAbgy&ust=1605865360427000&source=images&cd=vfe&ved=0CAIQjRxqFwoTCJjlwuWoju0CFQAAAAAdAAAAABAJ.)

After antigen binding and stimulation, B cells mature into plasma cells to produce antibodies and memory cells. Every single plasma cell can produce hundreds to thousands of antibodies per second, which is an example of the astonishing power of the immune response to handle pathogens.

Dendritic Cells Dendritic cells are the most professional and important APCs that initiate responses against protein antigens, and, as mentioned earlier, these cells have a role in innate immunity also. Dendritic cells are located under the epithelia and express many receptors like TLRs and lectins for capturing and responding to microbes and are recruited to the T-cell zones of lymphoid organs where they present antigens to T cells. All these features make dendritic cells the most competent APCs in adaptive immune response.

Immature dendritic cells located within the epidermis are called **Langerhans cells;** another type of dendritic cells located in the germinal centres of the lymphoid follicles in the spleen and lymph nodes is called FDCs. FDCs present antigens to B cells in the germinal centre.

Macrophages Macrophages are derivatives of HSCs and are a part of the mononuclear phagocyte system. The cells are discussed in detail along with their role in inflammation in Chapter 3 and only the functions of macrophages relevant to adaptive immune response are discussed here.

1. Macrophages, being phagocytes, play a significant role in innate immunity, the first line of defence.
2. Macrophages are efficient APCs that detect, phagocytose, process and present the antigens as peptide fragments to T cells.
3. Macrophages phagocytose and destroy target antigens opsonized by IgG or C3b and play a role in the effector phase of humoral immune response.
4. Macrophages activated by T cells gain intensified ability to destroy and eliminate the phagocytosed antigens in some forms of cell-mediated immunity.

Thus, macrophages play major roles in all forms of immunity.

Major Histocompatibility Complex PA 9.3

MHC is a large locus on the DNA containing a set of closely linked *polymorphic genes* that code for cell surface proteins that are crucial for the adaptive immune system. The complex is also called **human leucocyte antigen (HLA) complex**. The complex has been termed MHC because it was discovered during the study of tissue compatibility for transplantation. It was later proved that tissue rejection because of MHC incompatibility is an experimental artefact masking the actual function of MHC molecules, which is binding antigens derived from self-proteins/pathogens and the antigen presentation on the cell surface for recognition by the appropriate T cells. MHC molecules mediate interactions of leucocytes with other leucocytes and other cells of the immune system. In addition, MHC determines the compatibility of donors for organ transplant and one's susceptibility to autoimmune diseases.

The combination of HLA alleles in every individual is called **HLA haplotype**. Every one of us inherits one set of HLA from each parent and hence every HLA locus expresses two different molecules. Owing to the polymorphism associated with HLA genes, infinite combinations of molecules exist in the population and HLA profile of most individuals do not match. This is the basis for transplant rejection reactions between individuals as the donors MHC molecules are recognized as foreign and immune response is mounted. Immunosuppressive agents, as a part of treatment before transplantation, are given to suppress the response by HLA.

In humans, the MHC region is located on chromosome 6. The MHC gene family is divided into three subgroups: class I MHC, class II MHC and class III MHC. These genes are highly polymorphic and among all those genes present in MHC region, there are two types of genes coding for the proteins class I MHC molecules and class II MHC molecules that are directly involved in the antigen presentation. The genetic organization of the HLA complex and the structure of HLA molecules is shown in Fig. 6.11.

On the basis of their structure, distribution and function, MHC proteins are classified into two major classes.

Class I MHC Class I MHC molecules are expressed on all nucleated cells and platelets, i.e. in all cells except red blood cells. These present **intracellular antigens** to cytotoxic T cells following which the cytotoxic T lymphocytes trigger the target cells to undergo apoptotic cell death. Thus, class I MHC molecules mediate cellular immunity, a primary means to handle intracellular pathogens such as viruses, some bacteria and rickettsia.

A class I MHC molecule is a heterodimer consisting of a polymorphic α or heavy chain bound covalently to a smaller nonpolymorphic protein called **β_2-microglobulin.** The α chains of class I MHC molecules are encoded by three genes – HLA-A, HLA-B and HLA-C – which lie close to each other in the MHC locus. The extracellular portion of α chain is divided into three domains – **α_1, α_2 and α_3**. The α_1 and α_2 domains form a cleft or groove that is the site of peptide binding. The polymorphic amino acid residues line the lateral sides and base of the peptide-binding groove, which is the basis for binding of different class I alleles with different peptides.

Class I MHC molecules present peptides derived from proteins such as viral and tumour antigens. $CD8^+$ T lymphocytes recognize and receive peptides only when presented by class I MHC molecules. This phenomenon is called **class I MHC restriction** (Fig. 6.12).

Class II MHC Class II MHC molecules are expressed on the surface of cells involved in the immune response, i.e. APCs, B lymphocytes, dendritic cells, etc.; class II MHC molecules are encoded in a locus called HLA-D, which has three subregions: HLA-DP, HLA-DQ and HLA-DR.

Class II MHC molecule is also a heterodimer composed of noncovalently associated α and β chains that are polymorphic. The extracellular domains of α and β chains have two domains referred to as **$\alpha_1\alpha_2$** and **$\beta_1\beta_2$**, respectively. The peptide-binding cleft faces outward and is formed by the association between $\alpha_1\beta_1$ domains that are polymorphic. Polymorphism of class II MHC molecules is associated with distinctive binding of antigenic peptides.

Class II MHC molecules present processed antigens derived from **extracellular microbes** and soluble proteins to $CD4^+$ helper T cells. $CD4^+$ T lymphocytes recognize and receive peptides only when presented by class II MHC molecules. This phenomenon is called **class II MHC restriction.**

MHC molecules play the two crucial roles in mediating T-cell-mediated immune responses:

1. Immune response can be mounted only if an individual inherits the genes for those MHC molecules that bind to the peptides derived from the antigens.
2. MHC molecules segregate the cytoplasmic and internalized antigens and ensure that the appropriate immune response is mounted.

The role of HLA in autoimmune diseases is discussed later.

Role of Cytokines in Immune Response

Cytokines include chemokines, interferons, interleukins, lymphokines and tumour necrosis factors (TNFs) but generally not hormones or growth factors. These are produced by a broad range of cells that include immune cells like macrophages, B lymphocytes, T lymphocytes, and cells like endothelial cells, fibroblasts and many types of stromal cells. A given cytokine may be produced by more than one type of cell and may have a broad range of actions. Cytokines act through cell surface receptors and function by modulating the balance between humoral and cell-based immune responses, as well as by regulating the maturation, growth and responsiveness of particular cell population. Some cytokines enhance or inhibit the action of other cytokines in complex ways. Cytokines are important in health and disease, specifically in host immune responses, trauma, sepsis, cancer and reproduction.

Interactions between cells involved in immune response are essential, and such interactions are mediated by cytokines called interleukins. Cytokines may have

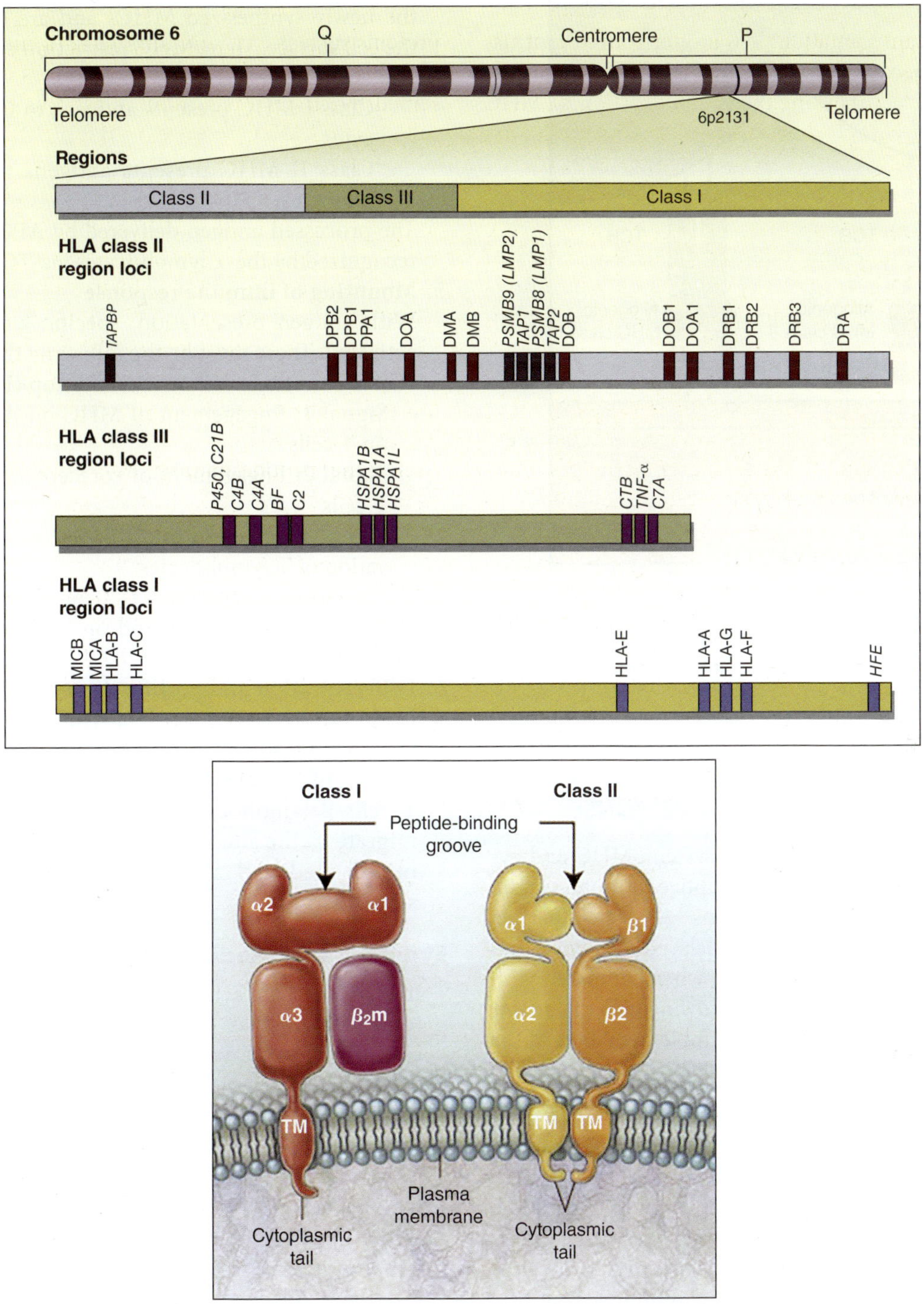

Fig. 6.11 Genetic organization of the HLA complex and structure of HLA molecules. HLA, human leucocyte antigen. (*Source:* From Emeline Masson Frenet and Andromachi Scaradavou. Human Leukocyte Antigens. In Transfusion Medicine and Hemostasis. 3rd edition. 2019. Elsevier.)

autocrine (act on the cells that produce them), paracrine (act on the neighbouring cells) or endocrine (act on cells at a distance) actions.

Cytokines are messenger molecules of the immune system and are involved in different types of immune responses as follows:

- Cytokines of innate immune response – TNF, IL-1, IL-12, type 1 interferons and chemokines (these are produced by macrophages, dendritic cells and NK cells)
- Cytokines of adaptive immune response – IL-2, IL-4, IL-5, IL-17, IFN-γ, TGF-β and IL-10.
- Colony-stimulating factors (these stimulate haematopoiesis, GM-CSF and IL-7)

Cytokines have many therapeutic applications. Some cytokines have been developed into protein therapeutics using recombinant DNA technology, and many cytokine antagonists are used in the treatment of various inflammatory diseases in the present era of medicine.

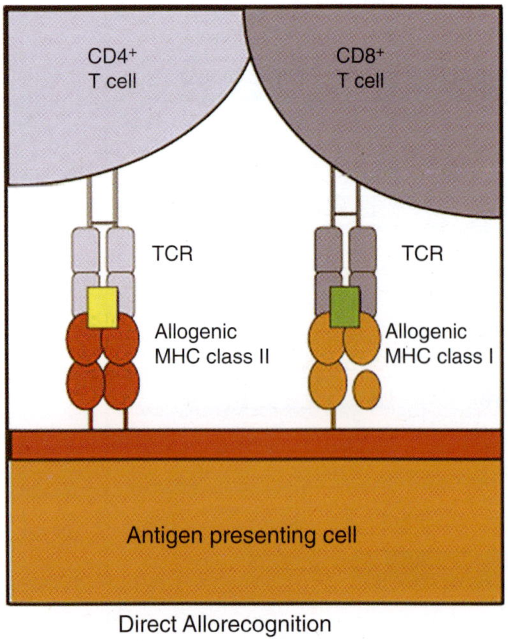

Fig. 6.12 MHC restriction. MHC, major histocompatibility complex. (*Source:* https://www.google.com/url?sa=i&url= https%3A%2F%2Fwww.sciencedirect.com%2Fscience%2Farticle%2Fpii%2FS0161589007006220&psig=AOvVaw1v_uvy0K7ZFrNgjFlD4slM&ust=1605865832058000&source=images&cd=vfe&ved=0CAIQjRxqFwoTCJjDucqqju0CFQAAAAAdAAAAABAD.)

OVERVIEW OF ADAPTIVE IMMUNE RESPONSE

Having discussed the immune cell system, MHC and cytokines, we now review how the adaptive immune system functions in eliminating pathogens. As stated earlier, adaptive immune response is a delayed response and takes days to even weeks to develop when compared with innate immune response. The following are the major events in sequence involved in the implementation of the adaptive immune response:

1. **Recognition of antigens**
   The first and the most important event in the immune response is initiated by APCs (dendritic cells, macrophages, etc.), which detect the entry of antigens with the help of their receptors and carry them to the draining lymph nodes. B lymphocytes also detect the antigens with the help of their surface immunoglobulins.
2. **Phagocytosis and processing of antigens by APCs**
   After detecting the antigens, they are internalized and processed within APCs. Cytoplasmic proteins are degraded by proteasomes, and the peptides are transported into the endoplasmic reticulum. Internalized proteins are proteolytically digested in endosomes or lysosomes.
3. **Production of MHCs by APCs**
   Appropriate MHCs according to the nature of the proteins are freshly synthesized simultaneously in APCs when the antigens are processed.
4. **Presentation of antigens by APCs to T lymphocytes**
   Processed peptides bind to the antigen-binding cleft of the newly synthesized MHCs and are transported to the cell surface. Here, MHC restriction comes into play as stated earlier.
   - Class I MHC presents antigens to $CD4^+$ lymphocytes.
   - Class II MHC presents antigens to $CD8^+$ lymphocytes.

   The processed antigen delivered by APCs via MHC is recognized by the T lymphocytes via TCR.
5. **Mounting of immune response**
   With antigen presentation, specific lymphocytes are activated. There must be the following three signals for effective immune response to develop (Fig. 6.13):
   Signal 1: Engagement of MHC on APCs and TCR on T cells
   Signal 2: Engagement of coreceptors on APCs and T cells
   Signal 3: Secretion of cytokines by APCs and activation of T lymphocytes
   Coreceptors CD28 and CD80 or CD86 are present on the surface of T cells and on the surface of APCs, respectively.
6. **Differentiation and proliferation of effector cells**
   In this step, the appropriate lymphocyte population is activated, followed by proliferation and differentiation of effector cells (helper T cells/cytotoxic T cells/B lymphocytes/NK cells/macrophages) that migrate to the site of injury. The sequence of events in cell-mediated and humoral immunity is listed separately.

Events in Cell-Mediated Immunity

- If $CD8^+$ cells are activated, they differentiate into cytotoxic lymphocytes that destroy the target cells and eliminate the reservoirs.
- $CD4^+$ T cells secrete IL-2 and also express IL-2 receptors to self-stimulate themselves and proliferate (autocrine effect).
- When the antigens are presented by macrophages or B lymphocytes, $CD4^+$ cells by using their CD40 ligand (CD40L) and cytokines activate the macrophages and B lymphocytes expressing CD40 receptor. Thus, the activated macrophages and B cells are able to eliminate the bacteria.
- The helper T-cell family has many members; each of them is driven by a certain set of cytokines and carries out different functions as shown in Table 6.2.

Events in Humoral Immunity

After activation, B cells proliferate and differentiate into plasma cells and secrete antibodies. B-cell responses can be T-cell dependent or T-cell independent on the basis of the nature of the antigens. Protein antigens elicit T-cell-dependent response that is quite complex yet sophisticated, whereas polysaccharide and lipid antigens elicit T-cell-independent responses that are simple.

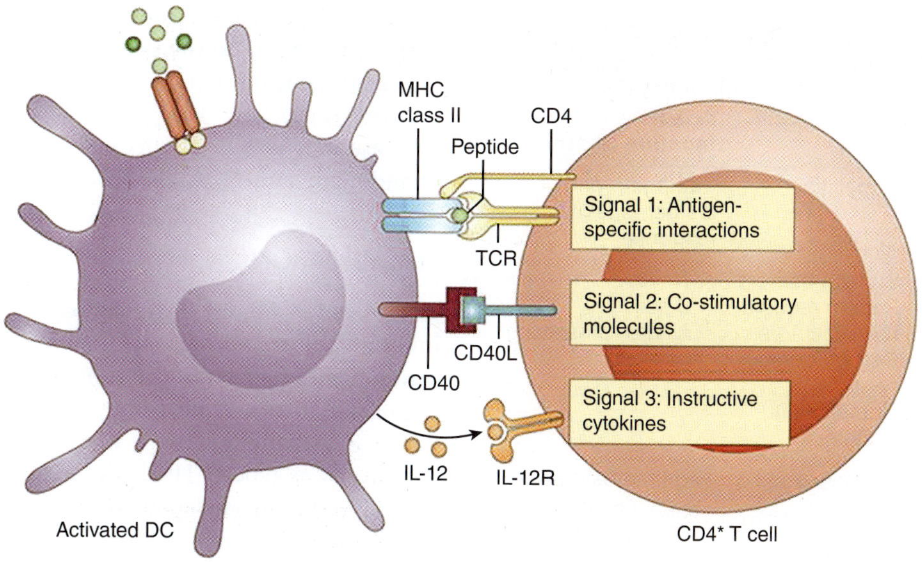

Fig. 6.13 Cellular signals in immune response. (*Source:* From Macmillan Publishers Ltd: Nature Reviews Immunology, 14, 719–730.)

Table 6.2 Helper T-Cell Subsets, Cytokines Associated with them and their Functions

Helper T-Cell Subset	Cytokines Produced	Cytokines That Induce the Subset	Functions	Role in Disease
Th1	IFN-γ	IFN-γ IL-12	Key defence against intracellular pathogens and tumours	Autoimmune diseases Type IV hypersensitivity reactions
Th2	IL-4 IL-5 IL-13	IL-4	Defence against extracellular pathogens Stimulate B cells to differentiate and secrete antibodies Defence against helminthic parasites	Allergic reactions Type I hypersensitivity reactions
Th17	IL-17 IL-22	TGF-β IL-6 IL-1 IL-23	Defence against gut pathogens and at mucosal barriers Recruitment of neutrophils and monocytes	Autoimmune diseases Chronic inflammatory diseases

IFN-γ, interferon-γ.

In T-cell-dependent responses, helper T cells are activated by the three signals mentioned earlier and express CD40L along with secretion of cytokines. This leads to activation of B cells, followed by two reactions:

- **Isotype switching:** Naive B cells produce IgM and IgD. In isotype switching induced by IFN-γ and IL-4, B cells are activated to produce antibodies of different classes or isotypes.
- **Affinity maturation:** Production of antibodies with increased affinities for the antigen improves the quality of the immune response.

The actions of antibody are as follows:

- Neutralization of the microbes occurs by binding of antibodies.
- Opsonization of microbes is followed by phagocytosis and degradation.
- Antibodies help in complement activation and destruction.
- IgA is a mucosal antibody that neutralizes the microbes in the mucosa.
- IgE acts against helminths.
- Transplacental transport of IgG offers protection to the newborns.

With all the aforementioned steps, an effective immune response is mounted following which the antigen is eliminated, leading to a decline in the immune response. The memory cells survive for a long time and take care of immunogenic memory.

Table 6.3 Innate Versus Adaptive Immune Systems

Feature	Innate Immune System	Adaptive Immune System
Specificity	Nonspecific	Pathogen- and antigen-specific response
Components	• Surface barriers • Pattern recognition receptors • Cellular components • Complement system	• T cells • B cells • Antigen-presenting cells
Timing of response following exposure	Immediate and maximal	Lag time between exposure and maximal response
Receptors used	100 different receptors to recognize 1000 molecular patterns	Only two receptors (TCR and immunoglobulins) each with millions of variations to recognize millions of antigens
Immunological memory	No immunological memory	Immunological memory is characteristically seen

TCR, T-cell receptor.

INNATE VERSUS ADAPTIVE IMMUNITY

The differences between innate and adaptive immune systems are listed in Table 6.3.

With a detailed description of a normal immune response, we now turn our discussion to the disorders of the immune system.

HYPERSENSITIVITY REACTIONS PA 9.2

INTRODUCTION

Hypersensitivity refers to undesirable reactions produced by the immune system and includes allergies and autoimmunity. It is referred to as an excessive or harmful reaction of the immune system to the antigens, and these reactions are generally damaging, uncomfortable and occasionally fatal. These reactions require presensitization of the host.

These reactions can be triggered by the following:

- Microbial or environmental antigens like pollen, drugs and foods may trigger autoimmune reactions.
- Self-antigens, which are capable of producing an immune response, may cause autoimmune reactions.

These can be because of the failure in regulating the balance between the effector mechanisms of immune responses and their control mechanisms. The mechanism is similar to the general defence against pathogenic organisms and may be uncontrolled, excessive or misdirected.

These may also occur because of inheritance of HLA and many non-HLA-like susceptibility genes.

CLASSIFICATION

The Gell and Coombs classification, which is based on the immunological mechanism that mediates the disease, distinguishes four types of immune responses that result in tissue damage. A fifth type has been recently added, which is actually a subtype of type 2, and hence many consider it as type II HSR. The five types, their mechanisms, mediators, histopathological lesions and common diseases are listed in Table 6.4.

IMMEDIATE (TYPE I) HYPERSENSITIVITY

Type I hypersensitivity (or **immediate hypersensitivity**) is a rapidly developing allergic reaction provoked by exposure to a specific type of antigen referred to as an allergen by ingestion, inhalation, direct contact or injection in a previously sensitized genetically predisposed individual. These reactions are referred to as allergy and may occur as a local reaction or systemic disorder (anaphylaxis). Local reactions are diverse, and the manifestations depend on the portal of allergen entry. Systemic reactions often follow injection of an antigen as that happens with bee sting but can also be precipitated by ingestion of antigens and may be fatal if not noticed and managed immediately.

Pathogenesis

Type I hypersensitivity can be further classified into **immediate-** and **late-phase** reactions. The immediate HSR occurs minutes after exposure and includes release of vasoactive amines and lipid mediators that leads to vasodilation, vascular leakage, muscle spasm and glandular secretions. The late-phase reaction occurs 2–24 hours after exposure and may last for many days. It includes the release of cytokines and infiltration of tissues with eosinophils, basophils, monocytes and T cells and is characterized by tissue destruction in the form of mucosal epithelial damage.

The following are the criteria to be met for the development of type I HSR:

- Individual – genetically predisposed
- Exposure – second and subsequent (with first exposure, no clinical manifestation)
- Antigen – polyvalent (able to bind to more than one antibody at a time)
- Antibody – should be present over mast cells (sensitized mast cells)

Table 6.4 Types, Mechanisms, Mediators, Lesions and Common Clinical Examples

Type, Other Names	Principal Mediators	Mechanisms	Histopathological Changes	Clinical Examples
I Immediate Allergy Anaphylactic	IgE	Production of IgE antibody → immediate release of vasoactive amines and other mediators from mast cells; later recruitment of inflammatory cells	Vascular dilation, oedema, smooth muscle contraction, mucus production, tissue injury, inflammation	Atopy Anaphylaxis Asthma
II Cytotoxic Antibody dependent	IgM IgG Complement	Production of IgG, IgM → binds to antigen on target cell or tissue → phagocytosis or lysis of target cell by activated complement or Fc receptors; recruitment of leucocytes	Phagocytosis and lysis of cells; inflammation; in some diseases, functional derangements without cell or tissue injury	Autoimmune haemolytic anaemia Rheumatic heart disease
III Immune complex	IgG Complement Neutrophils	Deposition of antigen–antibody complexes → complement activation → recruitment of leucocytes by complement products and Fc receptors → release of enzymes and other toxic molecules	Inflammation, necrotizing vasculitis (fibrinoid necrosis)	Systemic lupus erythematosus Rheumatoid arthritis Serum sickness
IV Delayed Cell-mediated Antibody independent	T lymphocytes	Activated T lymphocytes → (1) release of cytokines, inflammation and macrophage activation; (2) T-cell-mediated cytotoxicity	Perivascular cellular infiltrates; oedema; granuloma formation; cell destruction	Contact dermatitis Mantoux test Chronic transplant rejection
V Inhibitory	IgG	IgG class antibodies directed towards cell surface antigens have an inhibiting effect without destruction of the target	Lymphocytic infiltrate without tissue injury	Graves disease Myasthenia gravis

IgG, immunoglobulin G.

Immediate Reaction The master regulator of immediate HSR is the **Th2** subtype of helper T cells that stimulate the production of IgE antibodies.

1. In this reaction, the first step is the antigen capture and presentation by APCs to naive $CD4^+$ helper T cells. As a response to this, IL-4 is secreted at the site, driving the helper T cell differentiation towards Th2. As explained in the previous sections, the cytokines of Th2 response such as IL-4, IL-5 and IL-13 are secreted. Functions of these cytokines are described later.
2. B cells are stimulated by CD4 T cells + Th2 cells to produce IgE antibodies specific to that polyvalent antigen.
3. During this sensitization process, IgE antibodies get bound to Fc receptors on the surface of tissue mast cells and basophils. Mast cells and basophils coated by IgE antibodies are hence 'sensitized'.
4. Subsequent exposure to the same allergen cross-links the bound IgE on sensitized cells, resulting in anaphylactic degranulation. This results in the immediate and explosive release of pharmacologically active preformed mediators from storage granules, which are responsible for the immediate reaction and early clinical manifestations.
5. Arachidonic acid helps in the concurrent synthesis of inflammatory lipid mediators that are responsible for the late-phase reaction and tissue damage.
   The principal effects of these products are vasodilation and smooth muscle contraction. The important preformed and freshly synthesized mediators involved and their specific actions in type I hypersensitivity are discussed here.

Late-Phase Reaction In the late phase of type I HSR (Fig. 6.14), leucocytes are recruited to the sites of the reaction and are responsible for the amplification and sustained nature of the inflammatory response even without any additional exposure to the triggering antigen. The predominant inflammatory cell responsible for the tissue damage and clinical symptoms is eosinophil.

Mediators and Factors

All the mediators and their functions are described in Chapter 3 and their functions relevant to immediate hypersensitivity are discussed here.

- **Histamine:** This mediator acts on histamine receptors 1 and 2 and causes increased vasopermeability and

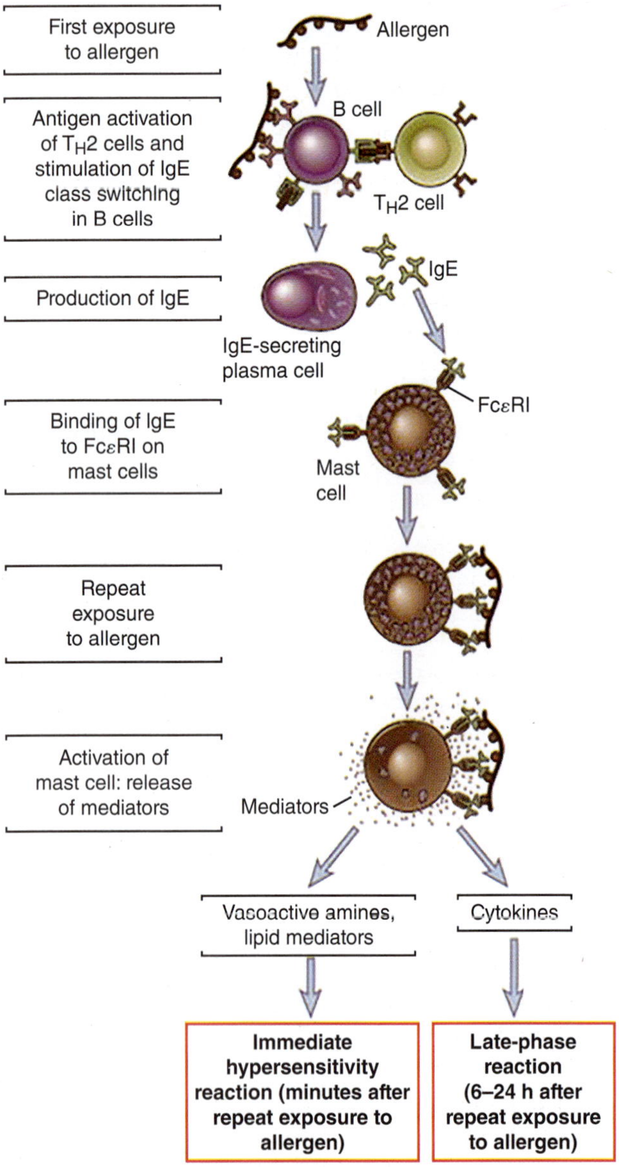

Fig. 6.14 Sequence of events in type I hypersensitivity.

vasodilation, enhanced mucus production, contraction of smooth muscles of the airway and GI tract, pruritus, cutaneous vasodilation and increased gastric acid secretion.

- **Tryptase:** Tryptase is a major protease released by mast cells that cleaves and activates C3 and C5 apart from playing a role in airway remodelling. It is a good marker of mast cell activation. Other protease enzymes such as acid hydrolases also help in these actions.
- **Chemotactic factors:** Eotaxin, an eosinophilic chemotactic factor of anaphylaxis, causes eosinophil chemotaxis and an inflammatory factor of anaphylaxis results in neutrophil chemotaxis. Eosinophils release *major basic protein* and, together with the activity of neutrophils, can cause significant tissue damage in the later phases of allergic reactions.
- **Proteoglycans:** Heparin seems to be important in storing the proteases already formed and may play a role in the production of α-tryptase.

Newly Formed Mediators

1. **Arachidonic acid metabolites**
   a. **Leukotrienes – produced via the lipoxygenase pathway**
      - **Leukotriene B4** stimulates neutrophil chemotaxis and activation and augmentation of vascular permeability.
      - **Leukotrienes C4 and D4** are potent bronchoconstrictors and increase vascular permeability and cause arteriolar constriction.
      - **Leukotriene E4** enhances bronchial responsiveness and increases vascular permeability.
      - **Leukotrienes C4, D4 and E4** comprise what was previously known as the slow-reacting substance of anaphylaxis.

   b. **Cyclooxygenase products**
      - **Prostaglandin D2** is produced mainly by mast cells and acts as a bronchoconstrictor, peripheral vasodilator, coronary and pulmonary artery vasoconstrictor, platelet aggregation inhibitor, neutrophil chemoattractant and enhancer of histamine release from basophils.
      - **Prostaglandin F2α** acts as a bronchoconstrictor, coronary vasoconstrictor, peripheral vasodilator and platelet aggregation inhibitor.
      - **Thromboxane A2** causes platelet aggregation and bronchoconstriction.
2. **Platelet-activating factor (PAF):** It acts as a platelet aggregator and is also a very potent mediator in allergic reactions. It increases vascular permeability and causes chemotaxis and degranulation of eosinophils and neutrophils as well as bronchoconstriction.
3. **Adenosine:** This is a bronchoconstrictor that also potentiates IgE-induced mast cell release of mediators.
4. **Bradykinin:** Kininogenase released from the mast cell can act on plasma kininogens to produce bradykinin. An additional (or alternative) route of kinin generation, involving activation of the contact system via factor XII by mast cell–released heparin, has been described. Bradykinin increases vasopermeability, vasodilation, hypotension, smooth muscle contraction, pain and activation of arachidonic acid metabolites. However, its role in IgE-mediated allergic reactions has not been clearly demonstrated.
5. **Cytokines:** These play a major role in mediating late-phase reactions.
   - **IL-4:** It stimulates and maintains Th2 cell proliferation and switches B cells to IgE synthesis.
   - **IL-5:** It is a key factor in the maturation, chemotaxis, activation and survival of eosinophils. IL-5 also primes basophils for histamine and leukotriene release.
   - **IL-6:** It promotes mucus production.
   - **IL-13:** It has several of the same effects as IL-4.
   - **TNF-α:** TNF acts as a proinflammatory cytokine that activates neutrophils and eosinophils and increases monocyte chemotaxis.

All the aforementioned mediators are responsible for the manifestations of immediate HSRs along with causing inflammatory changes contributing to epithelial cell damage.

Clinical Manifestations

Allergic reactions can occur as immediate reactions, late-phase reactions or chronic allergic inflammation. The clinical consequences of type I HSR largely depend on the route and severity of antigen exposure.

Systemic exposure: This is because of a large dose of antigen that can cause catastrophic and systemic release of vasoactive, bronchoactive and inflammatory mediators that manifests as anaphylactic shock.

Local exposure: Local exposure to antigen usually causes a localized release of vasoactive, bronchoactive and inflammatory mediators that can manifest differently depending on the exposed organ:

- *Epidermal exposure:* Urticaria
- *Inhalation:* Allergic rhinitis
- *Ingestion:* Diarrhoea

The collective biological activities of the aforementioned mediators can cause variable clinical responses depending on the organ systems affected, as follows:

- **Urticaria/angio-oedema:** Release of these mediators in the superficial layers of the skin can cause pruritic wheals with surrounding erythema. If deeper layers of the dermis and subcutaneous tissues are involved, angio-oedema results. Angio-oedema is swelling of the affected area; it tends to be painful rather than pruritic.
- **Allergic rhinitis:** In the upper respiratory tract, sneezing, itching, nasal congestion, rhinorrhoea and itchy or watery eyes are the common presentation.
- **Allergic asthma:** In the lower respiratory tract, these mediators can cause bronchoconstriction, mucus production and inflammation of the airways, resulting in chest tightness, shortness of breath and wheezing.
- **Anaphylaxis:** There are two forms of anaphylaxis:
  Systemic anaphylaxis: In some individuals, a severe reaction occurs within minutes of development of type I hypersensitivity, leading to symptoms such as acute asthma, laryngeal oedema, diarrhoea, urticaria and shock. Classic examples are penicillin allergy and bee sting allergy.
  Local anaphylaxis (atopy): Ten per cent of the population has 'atopy' and is easily sensitized to allergens that cause a localized reaction when inhaled or ingested, producing symptoms. Classic examples are food allergies and hay fever due to ragweed pollen allergy.

Continuous or repeated exposure to an allergen (e.g. a cat-allergic patient who owns a cat) can result in chronic allergic inflammation. This results in structural and functional changes to the affected tissue. Furthermore, a repeated allergen challenge can result in increased levels of antigen-specific IgE, which ultimately can cause further release of IL-4 and IL-13, thus increasing the propensity for Th2 cell/IgE–mediated responses.

TYPE (ANTIBODY-MEDIATED) II HYPERSENSITIVITY (FIG. 6.15)

Antibody-mediated type II HSR is an antibody-mediated process in which IgG and IgM antibodies directed against antigens on cells or extracellular matrix result in cell lysis and tissue damage or loss of function within 2–24 hours. The antibodies may be against endogenous antigens (autoantibodies) or exogenous antigens. The mechanisms by which the antibodies cause tissue damage are as follows:

- Opsonization and phagocytosis
- Complement activation and direct injury
- Complement activation and inflammation
- Antibody-dependent cellular cytotoxicity (ADCC)

1. **Opsonization and phagocytosis**
   Phagocytosis is the major mechanism by which cells coated with antibodies are destroyed. Cells opsonized by IgG antibodies are recognized by phagocyte Fc receptors, which are specific for the Fc portions of some IgG subclasses. In addition, when IgG or IgM antibodies are deposited on the cell surfaces, they may activate the complement system by the classical pathway. This generates by-products like C3b and C4b, which are also powerful opsonins. These opsonize the target cells following which phagocytosis and clearance occur.
2. **Complement activation and direct injury**
   The cross-linked antibodies normally activate the classical pathway of the complement cascade that results in the generation of the 'membrane attack complex' that disrupts membrane integrity of the target cells by 'drilling holes' through the lipid bilayer, causing osmotic lysis of the cells.
3. **Complement activation and inflammation**
   When antibodies target host cells, the complement activation, apart from direct injury and opsonization, can also induce potent inflammation. Release of C5a and other chemotactic agents recruits inflammatory cells and release of anaphylatoxins such as C5a and C3a as by-products of complement activation promotes vascular permeability. When the leucocytes are activated by engagement of their C3b and Fc receptors, substances like lysosomal enzymes and reactive oxygen species are released which are toxic to the tissues.
4. **Antibody-mediated cell-mediated cytotoxicity**
   Cells coated with IgG antibodies can also be destroyed by NK cells, which bind to the target via their receptors for the Fc fragment of IgG. The NK cells cause lysis of the coated cells even without phagocytosing the opsonized material. This activation of NK cells by antibodies leading to cell destruction is referred to as 'ADCC'.

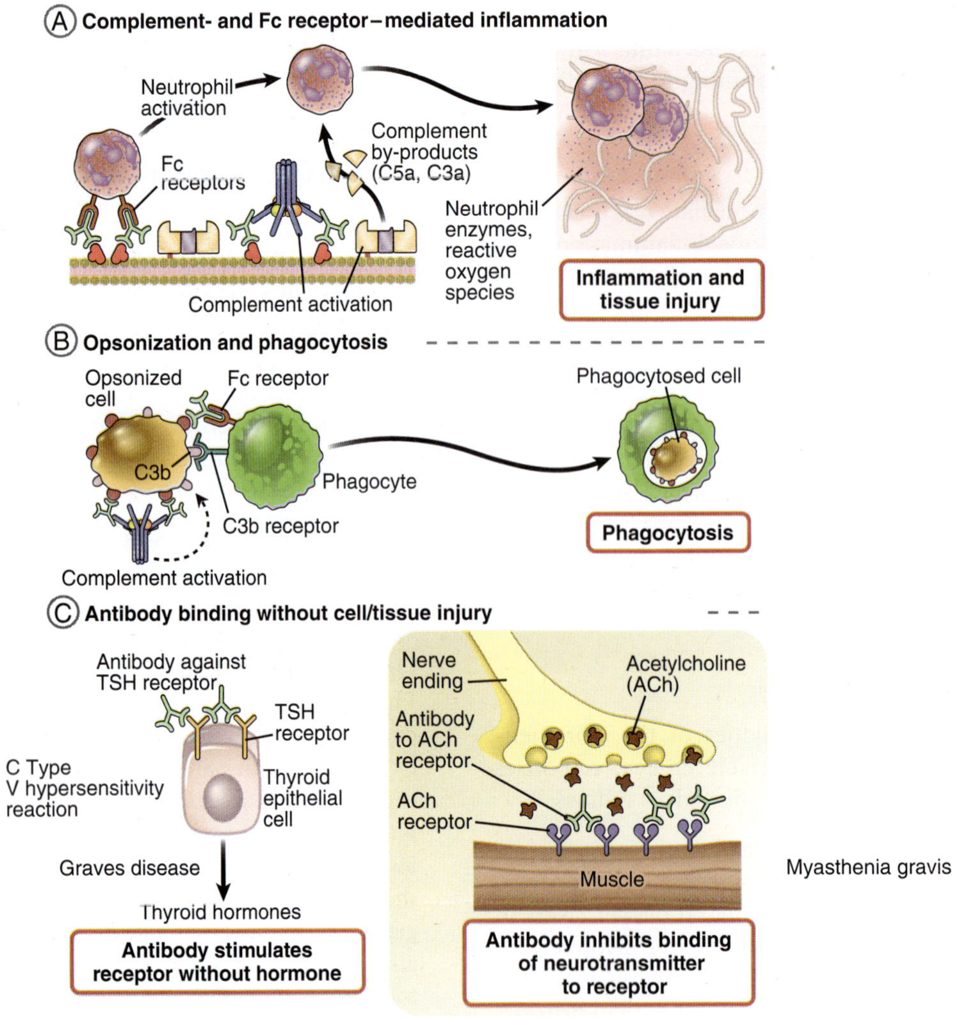

Fig. 6.15 Mechanisms of antibody-mediated hypersensitivity. (*Source:* From Abul K. Abbas, Andrew H. Lichtman and Shiv Pillai. Hypersensitivity: Disorders Caused by Immune Responses. In Basic Immunology: Functions and Disorders of the Immune System. 6th edition. Elsevier. 2020.)

5. **Antibody-mediated cellular dysfunction**
Binding of antibodies can also disrupt the normal functioning of the bound protein without causing injury or destruction. In myasthenia gravis, the binding of the antibodies to the acetylcholine receptors blocks the receptor and prevents activation of the receptor by acetylcholine, leading to muscle weakness. Similarly, in Graves disease, the binding of antibodies to the thyroid receptors blocks the receptor but in addition stimulates the receptor, leading to hypersecretion of thyroid hormone. This HSR is described in detail later.

Clinical Consequences

The clinical consequences of type II hypersensitivity largely depend on the host tissue involved or the target protein and the manner in which antibodies cause damage (Table 6.5).

1. **Rhesus incompatibility**
After sensitization in the first pregnancy or blood transfusion, when an Rh –ve mother conceives with an Rh +ve fetus, small numbers of fetal erythrocytes that pass across the placenta stimulate a memory response that causes destruction of fetal erythrocytes by the IgG antibodies. This disorder is discussed in detail in Chapter 10.
2. **Mismatch transfusion reactions**
Natural antibodies to major blood group antigens (A, B) bind to erythrocytes in the transfused blood carrying the target antigens that results in massive haemolysis. This disorder is discussed in detail in Chapter 18.
3. **Cell destruction because of autoantigens**
Antibodies to a variety of self-antigens such as those on the basement membranes of the lungs and kidneys (Goodpasture syndrome) and erythrocytes (autoimmune haemolytic anaemia) can result in damaging reactions.
4. **Drug-induced haemolytic anaemia**
Drugs such as penicillin, cephalosporin and streptomycin act as hapten and can be absorbed nonspecifically by the surface proteins on erythrocytes and cause IgG-mediated damage to red cells.

Table 6.5 Examples of Type II Hypersensitivity Reactions and the Target Antigen in Each Disease

Disease	Target Antigen
Autoimmune haemolytic anaemia	Red cell membrane proteins
Autoimmune thrombocytopenic purpura	Platelet membrane proteins
Goodpasture syndrome	Noncollagenous protein BM of glomeruli and lung alveoli
Acute rheumatic fever	Streptococcal cell wall antigen Antibody cross-reacts with myocardial antigen
Pemphigus vulgaris	Proteins present in the interepidermal junctions
ANCA-positive vasculitis	Neutrophil granule proteins
Insulin-resistant diabetes	Insulin receptor
Pernicious anaemia	Intrinsic factor of gastric parietal cells

BM, basement membrane.

TYPE III (IMMUNE COMPLEX–MEDIATED) HYPERSENSITIVITY (FIG. 6.16)

Type III hypersensitivity is caused by the generation of immune complexes or antibody–antigen complexes in circulation, which induce injurious inflammation following deposition in host tissue. The antigens that are part of the complexes can be exogenous or endogenous. In type III reactions, the antibody–antigen complex is preformed and circulates prior to deposition, whereas in type II reactions, antibody directly binds to antigens that are fixed components of the injured tissue. Type II and III HSRs against self-antigens are the basis of autoimmune disorders. Immune complex deposition in the tissues results in systemic autoimmune disorders, but many such deposits prefer to attack the kidneys and small blood vessels and hence present with restricted manifestations. Hence, immune complex disease can be systemic or localized.

Systemic Immune Complex Disease

The pathogenesis of systemic immune complex disease has three phases:

1. **Formation of immune complexes**
   Endogenous antigens that frequently cause complex formation with antibodies are host DNA. Exogenous antigens may be pharmacologically administered agents or from a microbial source. These complexes accumulate when normal phagocytosis and clearance in the spleen and liver become defective or when the complexes are too small to be recognized by macrophages. In either case, the antibody binds to the antigen, resulting in a macromolecular immune complex that subsequently precipitates out of plasma and deposits in host tissues.
2. **Deposition of immune complexes**
   In the second phase, the immune complexes formed are deposited. Preferred sites of deposition tend to be the small blood vessels of the kidney, joints and skin.

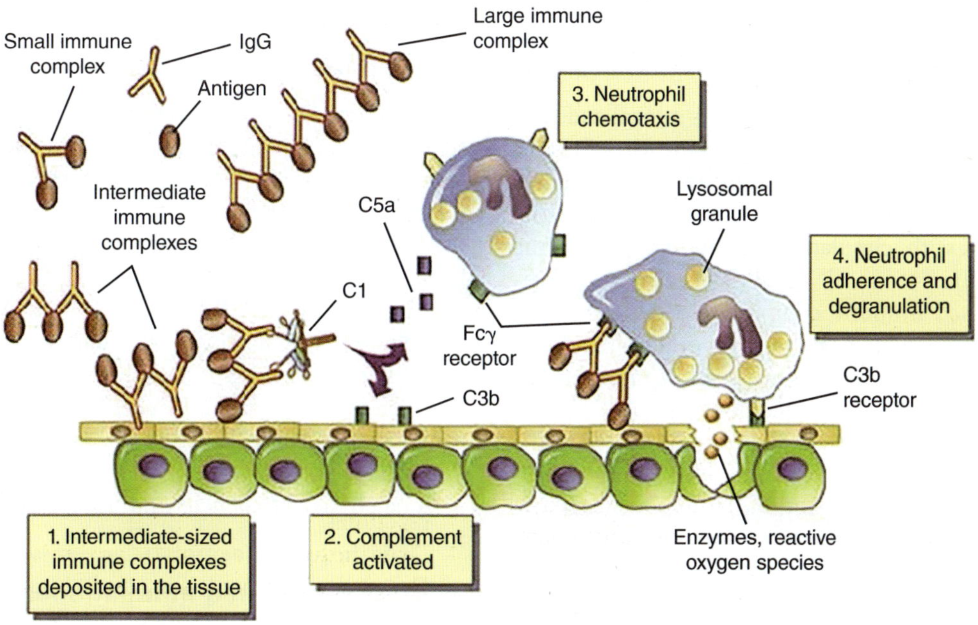

Fig. 6.16 Sequence of events in type III hypersensitivity reaction. (*Source:* From Abul Abbas Andrew Lichtman Shiv Pillai. Cellular and Molecular Immunology. 9th Edition. 2016. Elsevier.)

The glomerulus is one of the most preferred sites of complex deposition because plasma is stringently filtered by the glomerular basement membrane. Factors like the size of the complex and the proportion of antigens to antibodies influence the deposition. Medium-sized complexes and the ones with excess antigen are the most dangerous.

3. **Inflammation and tissue damage**
   - After deposition, complexes activate the classical pathway of the complement cascade, resulting in the release of C3a and C5a that recruit neutrophils and macrophages. In addition, the Fc region of antibodies within the complex can directly recruit neutrophils and macrophages.
   - The neutrophils that are recruited release a number of substances like prostaglandins, lysosomal enzymes and free oxygen radicals around the complexes, causing damage to the tissues at the site of immune complex deposition. These may also activate platelets to cause aggregation, thrombus formation and blockage of blood vessels, leading to ischaemic cell death.

   This phase may present as fever, proteinuria, joint pain, urticaria, vasculitis, etc. Complement proteins may be detected at the site of injury, which can lead to reduced serum levels of C3 protein that are sometimes used as a marker to monitor the disease.

As the circulating immune complexes generally deposit within the vasculature, the primary histopathological sequelae of type III HSRs is **necrotizing vasculitis**, dominated by an acute inflammatory picture that ends in fibrinoid necrosis. The immune complexes can be seen by electron microscopy as electron-dense deposits and by immunofluorescence microscopy as granular lumpy deposits of immunoglobulin and complement along the glomerular basement membrane.

Two reactions are prototypical examples for type III hypersensitivity (Table 6.6), which deserve mention here:

Arthus reaction: The Arthus reaction is a localized area of tissue necrosis characterized by in situ formation of antigen–antibody complexes generally after the intradermal injection of an antigen. This is seen in a previously sensitized host with circulating antibodies against the antigen. It manifests as local vasculitis because of deposition of IgG-based immune complexes in dermal blood vessels. Arthus reactions have been reported after vaccination and can occur after tetanus toxoid–containing or diphtheria toxoid–containing vaccines.

Acute serum sickness: In this condition, the immune system reacts to antiserum from other individuals or species that contain proteins or antibodies used to treat certain diseases. Nowadays, this is rare because of discontinuation of the usage of antiserum from other species. It presents with a triad of symptoms like fever, rashes and joint pain, all of which are attributed to inflammation mediated by immune deposition. This is often seen in

Table 6.6 Examples of Type III Hypersensitivity

Disease	Target Antigen	Major Clinical Manifestations
Arthus reaction	Antigens from many tissues	Cutancous vasculitis
Systemic lupus erythematosus	Nuclear antigens	Skin lesions Arthritis Nephritis
Polyarteritis nodosa	Hepatitis B virus surface antigen	Systemic vasculitis
Reactive arthritis	Several bacterial antigens	Acute arthritis
Serum sickness	Various antigens	Arthritis Nephritis Vasculitis
Poststreptococcal glomerulonephritis	Streptococcal cell wall antigens	Nephritis
Rheumatoid arthritis	Antibody (IgG and IgM) complexes	Arthritis
Farmer lung	Inhaled antigens (often mould or hay dust)	Alveolar inflammation

IgG, immunoglobulin G.

diseases such as SLE, which is associated with persistent antibody responses to autoantigens. Membranous glomerulonephritis and several vasculitis types occur because of the same cause, but the inciting antigens remain unknown.

TYPE IV (DELAYED-TYPE OR CELL-MEDIATED) HYPERSENSITIVITY (FIG. 6.17; TABLE 6.7)

The cell-mediated or delayed-type or type IV hypersensitivity is caused by inflammation resulting from cytokines produced by $CD4^+$ T cells and cell lysis by $CD8^+$ T cells. Certain environmental and self-antigens induce $CD4^+$-mediated chronic inflammatory diseases, including autoimmune diseases, whereas viral infections induce the production of $CD8^+$ T cells.

Delayed hypersensitivity is a major mechanism of defence against various intracellular pathogens, including mycobacteria and fungi. Hence, in patients with AIDS or other immunosuppressive states associated with loss of $CD4^+$ cells, the host response against intracellular pathogens such as *Mycobacterium tuberculosis* is markedly impaired.

$CD4^+$ Cell-Mediated Inflammation

Whenever an antigen is administered into the skin of a previously immunized individual, a detectable cutaneous

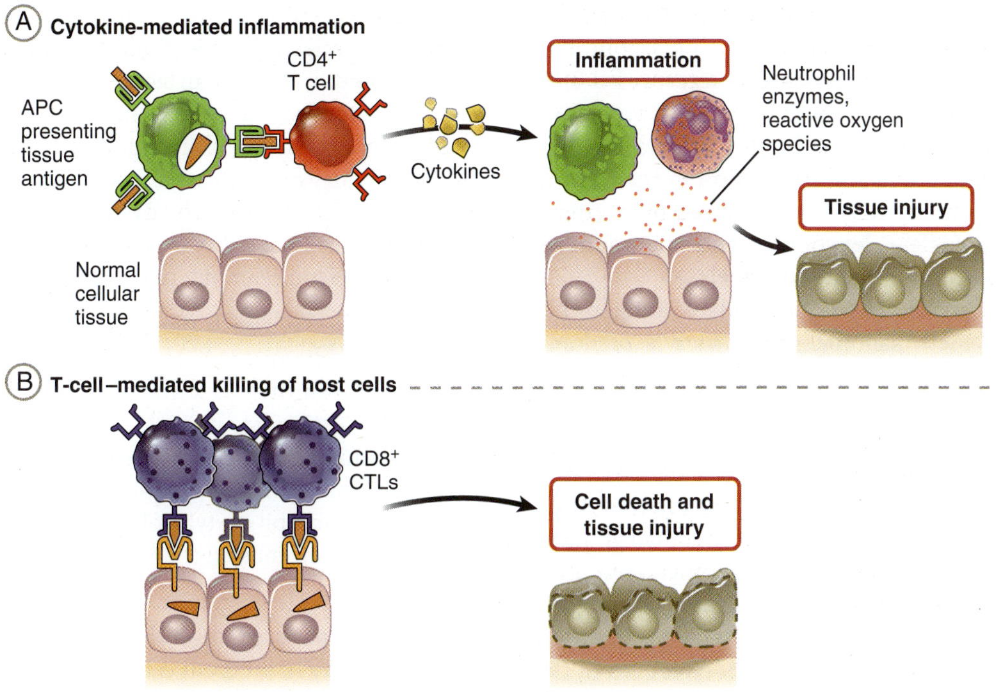

Fig. 6.17 $CD4^+$ T-cell-mediated tissue injury – type IV hypersensitivity. (*Source:* From Abul K. Abbas, Andrew H. Lichtman and Shiv Pillai. Hypersensitivity: Disorders Caused by Immune Responses. In Basic Immunology: Functions and Disorders of the Immune System. 6th edition. Elsevier. 2020.)

reaction develops within 24–48 hours. Owing to this time lag, this is called delayed-type reaction. Th1 and Th17 cells produce inflammation in specific organs. The inflammatory reaction associated with Th1 cells is dominated by activated macrophages and that associated with Th17 cells by a greater neutrophil component. The stages in the development of the reaction are as follows:

Table 6.7 Examples of Type IV Hypersensitivity Reaction

Disease	Target Antigen	Features
Type 1 diabetes mellitus	Pancreatic β-cell proteins	Insulitis β-Cell damage
Allergic contact dermatitis	Environmental chemicals (e.g. urushiol) Metals (e.g. nickel) Topical medication	Epidermal necrosis Inflammation Skin rash Blisters
Granulomas	Various, depending on the underlying disease	Walled-off lesions containing epithelioid cells and other cells
Hashimoto thyroiditis	Thyroglobulin antigen	Follicular thyroiditis Hypothyroidism
Inflammatory bowel disease	Self-antigens	Cytokine release Recruitment of macrophages because of hyperactivation of T cells and other immune cells Inflammation

1. **Activation of $CD4^+$ T cells**
   The antigens presented by the dendritic cells (APCs) to $CD4^+$ T cells induce the secretion of IL-12 that stimulates the proliferation of T cells in an autocrine manner. Differentiation towards Th1 or Th17 is dependent on the cytokines produced by APCs. If IL-12 is produced, differentiation towards Th1 is stimulated, whereas production of IL-1, IL-6 and IL-23 favours differentiation towards Th17 cells.
2. **Responses of Th1 cells**
   On exposure to an antigen, Th1 cells release cytokines like IFN-γ, the predominant mediator of type IV HSR, which activates macrophages by the classical pathway. The following changes are induced by IFN-γ:
   - There occurs a marked increase in the ability of macrophages to phagocytose and kill microorganisms.
   - Class II MHC molecules are expressed at a higher amount for antigen presentation.
   - Macrophages secrete TNF, IL-1 and chemokines, which promote inflammation.
   - There occurs augmented production of IL-12, which helps in amplifying the Th1 response.

Activated Th17 secrete cytokines like IL-17, IL-22 and chemokines. They recruit neutrophils and monocytes to the reaction site and augment the ongoing inflammation.

Clinical Examples of $CD4^+$ T Cells Causing Inflammatory Reactions The prototypical example of delayed-type hypersensitivity (DTH) is the *tuberculin reaction* or *the*

Mantoux test. The Mantoux test involves the intradermal administration of purified *M. tuberculosis* protein derivative and the body's response is interpreted after 48–72 hours. Patients who have been previously exposed to the bacteria will develop a delayed HSR manifested by reddening and induration in the dermis, which is histopathologically characterized by accumulation of mononuclear leucocytes and macrophages causing cuffing around the blood vessels.

With some persistent and nondegradable antigens like tubercle bacilli, the inflammatory infiltrate is predominantly macrophages for 2–3 weeks. With the persistence of the antigens, macrophages often undergo morphological alterations, obtain more cytoplasm and transform into *epithelioid cells.* An aggregate of epithelioid cells surrounded by a collar of lymphocytes is referred to as **granuloma.** This pattern of inflammation, called granulomatous inflammation, is associated with increased levels of $CD4^+$ and Th1 cells. It can also be caused by indigestible foreign bodies, which activate macrophages without eliciting an adaptive immune response. Examples of this reaction include the following:

- Contact dermatitis caused because of contact with urushiol, the antigen of ivy or poison oak, which manifests as itchy, vesicular dermatitis
- Some of the drug reactions
- Rheumatoid arthritis
- Multiple sclerosis
- Inflammatory bowel disease

$CD8^+$ T-Cell-Mediated Cytotoxicity

In this type of T-cell-mediated reaction, $CD8^+$ CTLs kill antigen-expressing target cells with the help of enzymes and perforins. After recognition of target cells, $CD8^+$ CTLs secrete these enzymes that enter the target cells by endocytosis. Perforin facilitates the release of the granzymes, the proteases that cleave and activate caspases, which induce apoptosis of the target cells. These granzymes are present as complexes. Activated CTLs also express Fas ligand (FasL), which is similar to TNF, that binds to Fas expressed on target cells and triggers apoptosis. Following viral infections and exposure to some contact-sensitizing agents, IFN-γ is released. $CD8^+$ T-cell-mediated cytotoxicity is associated with graft rejection and response against viruses.

Other diseases because of $CD8^+$ cytotoxicity are erythema multiforme (mild form), Stevens–Johnson syndrome and toxic epidermal necrolysis (severe form).

TYPE V (STIMULATORY) HYPERSENSITIVITY

Type V stimulatory HSR is not considered as a separate entity, because many believe that it belongs to type II HSR. The term 'stimulatory', though, used is not a perfect term for this type of hypersensitivity because the antibodies in this category not only are stimulatory but may also be inhibitory. When IgG class antibodies directed towards cell surface antigens have a stimulating effect on their target, they bind to the cell surface receptors and either prevent the intended ligand binding with the receptor or mimic the effects of the ligand. The antibodies do not cause cell injury or death as in type II hypersensitivity and instead cause **stimulation or dysfunction**, so this is considered as a separate entity by some experts.

The two classic examples under this type are as follows:

- **Graves disease**, which presents with hyperthyroidism and thyrotoxicosis, is because of the presence of antibodies against thyroid-stimulating hormone (TSH) receptor that stimulate it.
- **Myasthenia gravis**, which presents with muscle weakness and paralysis, is because of the presence of antibodies that inhibit acetylcholine binding with its receptor at the neuromuscular junction and downmodulates the receptors.

We have discussed the roles played by each type of hypersensitivity in different categories of diseases ranging from allergy to multisystem disorders like SLE. It should be stressed here that most diseases have more than one type of HSR as the underlying mechanism, although one type dominates.

AUTOIMMUNE DISORDERS PA 9.4, PA 9.5, PA 9.7

Autoimmunity is the presence of antibodies and T lymphocytes directed against normal components of a person. These components are called autoantigens or self-antigens and typically consist of proteins (or proteins complexed to nucleic acids). The antibodies and T lymphocytes that recognize autoantigens are called '**autoantibodies**'. The mere presence of autoantibodies is not indicative of an autoimmune disorder because these may be seen in normal individuals also. In addition, antibodies may be produced following damage to tissues to enhance the clearance process.

Hence, three requirements should be met before a disorder is categorized as truly caused by autoimmunity:

- Presence of an immune reaction specific for some self-antigen
- Evidence that such a reaction is not secondary to tissue damage but is of primary pathogenic significance
- Absence of another well-defined cause of the disease

Autoimmune diseases have varied clinical manifestations and can be broadly classified into two categories:

1. **Organ-specific** autoimmune diseases, in which immune responses are against a single organ or tissue, e.g. pemphigus vulgaris
2. **Systemic** autoimmune diseases, in which the immune reactions are against a wide range of antigens, e.g. SLE

Autoimmunity is because of the loss of self-tolerance and hence we discuss the immunological tolerance mechanisms before we discuss the individual autoimmune diseases.

IMMUNOLOGICAL TOLERANCE (FIG. 6.18)

Immune system not only educates its cell population to mount an effective immune response but also trains them effectively not to do so with its self-antigens through a process called immunological tolerance. Immunological tolerance is a state of immune unresponsiveness specific to a particular antigen or a set of antigens induced by previous exposure to that antigen or a set of antigens. In short, lack of responsiveness to one's own antigens is called self-tolerance, which is the basis for an individual's ability to live in harmony with his or her immune system without developing autoimmunity. Tolerance is an active process and, in fact, a learning experience for T cells. Failure of immunological tolerance is fundamental for autoimmune disorders. Immunological tolerance is said to occur mechanistically at two levels: central and peripheral.

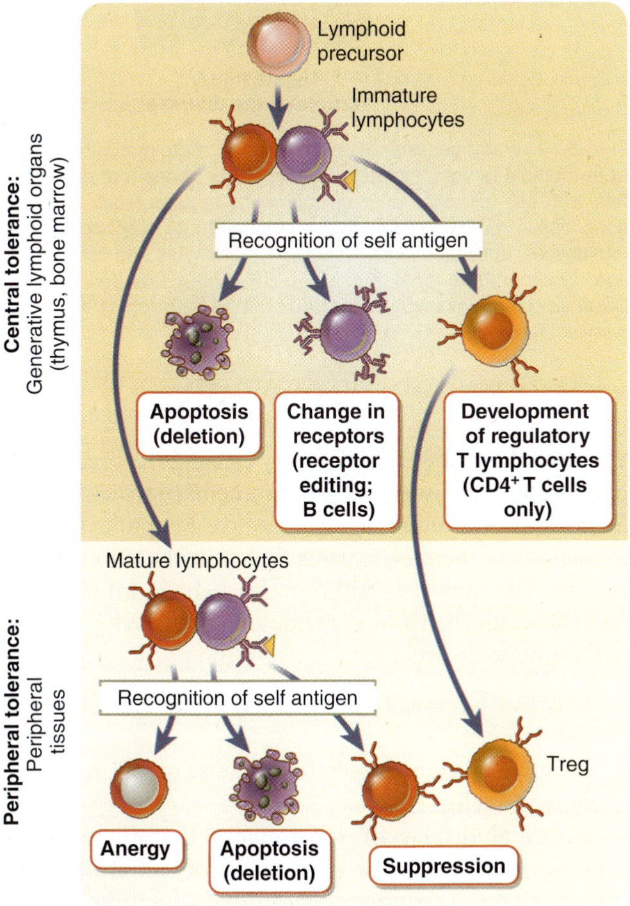

Fig. 6.18 Mechanisms of immunological tolerance. (*Source:* From Abul K. Abbas, Andrew H. Lichtman and Shiv Pillai. Immunologic Tolerance and Autoimmunity. In Cellular and Molecular Immunology. 9th edition. Elsevier 2018.)

Central Tolerance

During the process of central tolerance, the immature T and B cells are taught and tested for their reaction towards self-antigens and the ones that try to mount immune response are picked up and selectively deleted.

T Cells For T cells, central tolerance happens at the level of thymus, and for B cells, it happens at the level of bone marrow.

The chief mechanism of T-cell tolerance is the deletion of autoreactive T cells in the thymus so that the individual is rendered self-tolerant. Immature T cells migrate from the bone marrow to the thymus, where they encounter peptides derived from endogenous proteins bound to MHC molecules on thymic epithelial cells.

Positive selection, also called thymic education, ensures that only clones with TCRs and moderate affinity for self-MHC are allowed to develop. **Negative selection** by means of apoptosis occurs when T cells have extremely high affinity for the MHC–self-peptide complexes. The remaining cells leave the thymus to function in the periphery as mature, functional $CD4^+$ or $CD8^+$ T cells. A protein called **AIRE** (autoimmune regulator) induces the expression of some peripheral tissue–restricted self-antigens in the thymus and is crucial for deletion of immature T cells specific for these antigens.

B Cells During their development in the bone marrow, B lymphocytes reactivate the machinery of antigen receptor gene rearrangement and start expressing new antigen receptors that are not specific for self-antigens. This process is referred to as **receptor editing**. B cells that have not undergone receptor editing undergo apoptotic cell death.

It should be stressed here that central tolerance is not a foolproof mechanism and is error prone in which a significant proportion of self-reactive clones escape the training process and enter the peripheral blood. If not controlled peripherally, such self-reactive clones have the ability to cause tissue injury.

Peripheral Tolerance There are four major mechanisms that act in the periphery to identify and handle self-reactive T and B cells:

- **Clonal anergy**
  Lymphocytes that try to mount an immune response against self-antigens in the periphery are rendered inactive by a process called 'clonal anergy'. As we have discussed in the previous sections, T cells require first two signals for the further events to occur, which include the interaction of TCR on T cells with MHC molecules on APCs and the engagement of costimulatory molecules. Resting dendritic cells in normal tissues do not express adequate levels of

costimulatory molecules. When these cells present self-antigens to self-reactive T cells, the second signal is not generated and such self-reactive T cells are made anergic. Two inhibitory receptors that act like costimulatory molecules but in an opposite manner help in this process. These are CTLA4 and PD-1 that send inhibitory signals to T cells when they encounter self-antigens. B cells are also affected by anergy because they do not receive activation signals from inactivated self-reactive T cells.

- **Deletion by apoptosis**
  When T cells recognize self-antigens, they may receive signals for apoptosis by the unopposed expression of proapoptotic protein **Bim** or by **FasL** expression, which is a death receptor that activates the extrinsic pathway of apoptosis. The mechanisms are discussed in detail in Chapter 2. The role played by Fas-mediated apoptosis is clear from the cases in which 'autoimmune lymphoproliferative syndrome (ALPS)', an autoimmune disorder, develops because of the absence of Fas or FasL.
- **Suppression by regulatory T cells**
  Regulatory T cells are a subpopulation of T cells that function to downregulate the immune response after the elimination of the pathogen and also prevent T cells from reacting against self-antigens, fetus and commensal microbes. The major class of regulatory T cells expresses **CD25** (α chain of the IL-2 receptor) and **FOXP3**, both of which are essential for the development and maintenance of regulatory T cells. Mutations in FOXP3 result in the development of an autoimmune disorder called immune dysregulation, polyendocrinopathy, enteropathy, X-linked (IPEX), and mutation in IL-2 or IL-2 receptor is associated with the development of type 1 diabetes, multiple sclerosis and a rare multiorgan autoimmune disease.
- **Antigen sequestration in immune-privileged sites**
  Some antigens like those of the **testis, eye and brain** are anatomically placed in hidden locations (immune-privileged sites) where they are barred from communicating with the blood and lymph. Owing to this, the cells of the immune system do not come across such antigens during their training period and are ignored by the immune system. Nothing worrisome happens as long as they remain hidden. Any trauma or infection that causes the release of these cryptic antigens triggers the immune system, which assumes them as foreign and mounts a prolonged immune response. This is the basis of post-traumatic orchitis and uveitis.

PRINCIPLES AND FEATURES OF AUTOIMMUNE DISEASES (FIG. 6.19)

Autoimmunity is the result of interplay between inheritance of susceptibility genes and environmental factors.

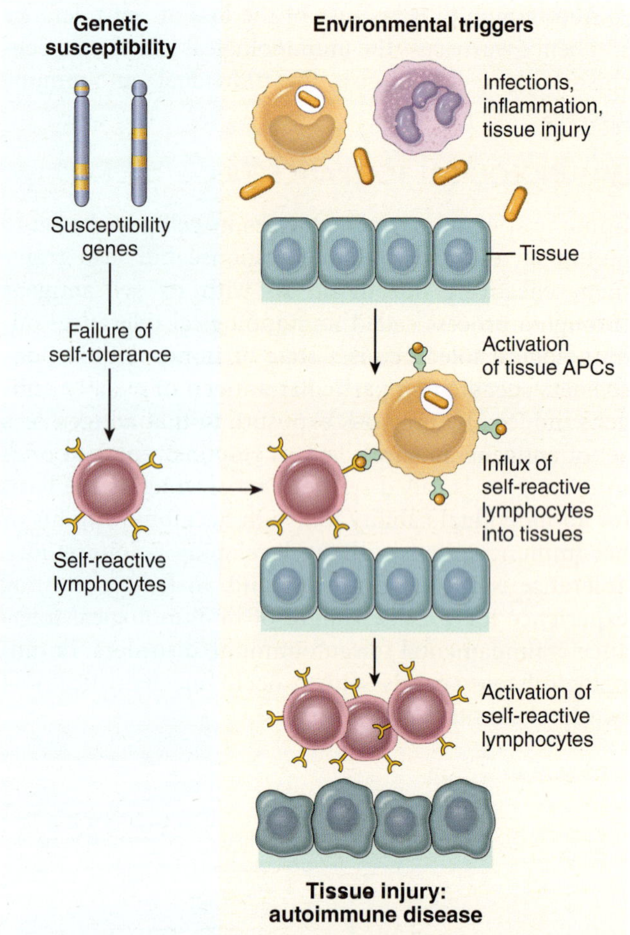

Fig. 6.19 Pathogenesis of autoimmunity. Autoimmunity results from multiple factors, including susceptibility genes that may interfere with self-tolerance and environmental triggers (such as infections, tissue injury and inflammation) that promote lymphocyte entry into tissues, activation of self-reactive lymphocytes and tissue damage. (*Source:* From Vinay Kumar, Abul K. Abbas and Jon C. Aster. Diseases of the Immune System. Robbins Basic Pathology. 10th edition. Elsevier 2018.)

Susceptibility genes contribute by causing the breakdown of self-tolerance, whereas environmental factors like infections act by activating self-reactive lymphocytes. The following are the mechanisms that contribute to autoimmunity, although it is still not clear which among these postulated mechanisms contribute to the development of autoimmune disorders:

- Defective tolerance as explained under immunological tolerance
- Defective immune regulation because of failure of regulatory T cells
- Abnormal display of self-antigens that includes increased expression or persistence of self-antigens or formation of neoantigens because of structural changes induced by the injuries
- Inflammation triggered by microbes or cell injury that leads to the activation of adaptive immune response

Role of Susceptibility Genes

It is clearly understood that most autoimmune disorders are complex multigenic and multifactorial disorders. The genes that contribute to autoimmune disorders belong to both HLA and non-HLA categories. Tables 6.8 and 6.9 contain the list of HLA genes and non-HLA genes, respectively, and their associated autoimmune disorders.

Role of Environmental Factors

The environmental factor that plays a major role in the development of autoimmune disorders in susceptible individuals is infections, followed by ultraviolet (UV) radiation and smoking. The following are the mechanisms by which infections trigger immune reactions in autoimmune diseases:

- Infections upregulate the expression of costimulators over APCs, which are normally downregulated for self-antigens (Fig. 6.20).
- Molecular mimicry: Microbes may express antigens that have similar amino acid sequences of self-antigens. Hence, immune responses against the microbes may be misdirected towards self-antigens, resulting in tissue damage.
- By inducing polyclonal B-cell activation, microbes can stimulate the production of autoantibodies.
- The tissue injury caused by microbial infections can structurally modify self-antigens and convert them to neoantigens, which get targeted by immune cells because they are sensed as non-self-antigens.
- The cytokines whose production is stimulated by microbes activate and recruit self-reactive lymphocytes to the sites of self-antigens.

UV radiation acts by causing cell death and leads to the exposure of nuclear antigens that triggers the self-reactive lymphocytes to mount an immune response. Smoking acts by modifying the self-antigens.

Table 6.8 Association of HLA Genes and Autoimmune Disorders

Disease	HLA Allele
Rheumatoid arthritis	DRB1 DRB1
Type 1 diabetes	DRB1*0301-DQA1*0501 DQB1*0201 haplotype DRB1*0401-DQA1*0301 DQB1*0302 haplotype DRB1*0301/0401 haplotype heterozygotes
Multiple sclerosis	DRB1*1501
Systemic lupus erythematosus	DRB1*0301 DRB1*1501
Ankylosing spondylitis	B*27
Coeliac disease	DQA1*0501-DQB1*0201

HLA, human leucocyte antigen.

Table 6.9 Association of non-HLA Genes and Autoimmune Disorders

Gene	Associated Disease
PTPN22	Rheumatoid arthritis Inflammatory bowel disease
IL23R	Inflammatory bowel disease Psoriasis Ankylosing spondylitis
CTLA4	Rheumatoid arthritis
IL2RA	Multiple sclerosis
NOD2	Inflammatory bowel disease
ATG16	Inflammatory bowel disease

HLA, human leucocyte antigen.

General Features of Autoimmune Disorders

The common features shared by autoimmune disorders are the following:

- Autoimmune disorders are chronic with relapses and remissions.
- The damage caused is often progressive.
- The clinical manifestations are based on the nature of the underlying immune response.

With this background, we proceed with the discussion of specific autoimmune diseases. Table 6.10 lists both systemic and organ-specific autoimmune disorders. The systemic diseases are more inclined to involve blood vessels and connective tissues and therefore they are often called *collagen vascular diseases* or connective tissue diseases. We focus here on selected systemic autoimmune diseases as organ-specific disorders are discussed in relevant chapters.

SYSTEMIC LUPUS ERYTHEMATOSUS

SLE is an autoimmune disease characterized by the presence of autoantibodies against nuclear and cytoplasmic antigens, multisystem inflammation, protean clinical manifestations and a relapsing and remitting course. It has a prevalence of as high as 1 in 2500 in certain populations, affecting women with a frequency of 1:700. The female-to-male ratio is 9:1 during the reproductive age group of 17–55 years, whereas it is only 2:1 for disease developing during childhood or after the age of 65 years. The higher incidence of SLE in females could be attributed to the elevated hydroxylation of oestrogen, the abnormally decreased levels of androgens and differences seen in gonadotropin-releasing hormone (GnRH) levels.

Aetiology

Genetic and environmental factors play major roles in the failure of immunological tolerance, which is the fundamental defect in the pathogenesis of SLE.

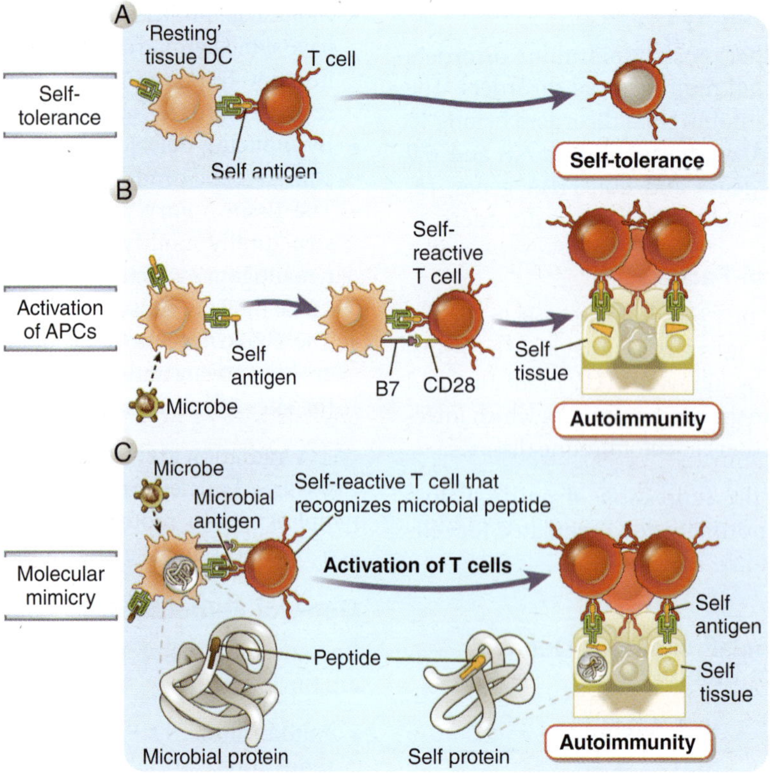

Fig. 6.20 Role of infections in autoimmunity. (*Source:* From Abul K. Abbas, Andrew H. Lichtman and Shiv Pillai. Immunologic Tolerance and Autoimmunity. In Cellular and Molecular Immunology. 9th edition. Elsevier 2018.)

Table 6.10 Autoimmune Diseases

Systemic	Organ Specific
Diseases Mediated by Antibodies	
Systemic lupus erythematosus	Autoimmune haemolytic anaemia Autoimmune thrombocytopenia Myasthenia gravis Graves disease Pernicious anaemia Goodpasture syndrome
Diseases Mediated by T Cells	
Rheumatoid arthritis Systemic sclerosis Sjögren syndrome	Type 1 diabetes mellitus Multiple sclerosis
Diseases Postulated to be Autoimmune	
Polyarteritis nodosa Inflammatory myopathies	Inflammatory bowel diseases Primary biliary cirrhosis Autoimmune hepatitis

Genetic Factors Genetic factors play a clear-cut role in SLE, with a sibling risk ratio 8- to 29-fold higher than that in the general population and a 10-fold increase in disease concordance in identical twins. There is also a 24%–56% concordance rate in monozygotic twins compared with a 2%–5% risk in dizygotic twins.

The current understanding of SLE points towards a large number of genes being involved in a multifactorial-type inheritance pattern in most patients.

- Genome-wide association studies have identified more than 60 risk loci for SLE susceptibility across populations. Most of the loci with a strong association with SLE are involved with the immune system.
- Genes previously associated with other autoimmune diseases have been identified to be associated with SLE such as diabetes-associated *PTPN2* and rheumatoid arthritis–associated *STAT4.*
- Genetic studies also reveal the presence of disruptions in lymphocyte signalling, clearance of complement and immune complexes, interferon response, apoptosis and DNA methylation.
- Several genes associated with T-cell function and signalling, including *PTPN22, TNFSF4, PDCD1, IL10, BCL6, IL16 and STAT4,* have been associated with SLE.
- Some patients demonstrate inherited deficiencies of complement components, such as C2, C4 or C1q, leading to defective removal of circulating immune complexes by the mononuclear phagocyte system. This favours tissue deposition of the immune complexes.
- The deficiency of C1q results in defective phagocytic clearance of apoptotic cells that may elicit an immune response.
- Most of these loci encode proteins involved in lymphocyte signalling that may play a role in lupus pathogenesis.

Epigenetic Factors Epigenetics refers to inherited changes in gene expression caused by mechanisms like DNA methylation and post-translational modifications of histones other than DNA base sequence changes. Extensive genetic studies offer insights into the epigenetics of SLE – hypomethylation of genes involved in osmotic lysis, apoptosis, inflammation and cytokine pathways has been associated with SLE.

MHC genes regulate production of particular autoantibodies like HLA-DQ locus and the production of anti-double-stranded DNA, anti-Sm and antiphospholipid antibodies (APLAs). Epigenetic mechanisms may represent the missing link between genetic and environmental risk factors.

Immunological Factors Failure of self-tolerance in B cells results from defective elimination of self-reactive B cells. $CD4^+$ helper T cells specific for nucleosomal antigens also escape tolerance and contribute to the production of high-affinity pathogenic autoantibodies. Increased production of B-cell-activating factor (BAFF) cytokine increases the life span of B cells.

Circulating type I interferons produced by dendritic cells play a role in lymphocyte activation in SLE where self-nucleic acids mimic their microbial counterparts. These cytokines may activate dendritic cells and B cells to promote Th1 responses, all of which may stimulate the production of pathogenic autoantibodies.

Environmental Factors Triggers of SLE include UV light, demethylating drugs and viruses or endogenous viral-like elements. Sunlight is the most obvious environmental factor that may exacerbate SLE. UV light may modulate the immune response, for example, by stimulating keratinocytes to produce IL-1, a cytokine known to promote inflammation. EBV may reside in and interact with B cells and promote interferon-α (IFN-α) production by plasmacytoid dendritic cells that increase the production of antibodies. It is well established that around 100 drugs induce autoantibodies in a significant number of patients who may or may not be symptomatic.

Genetic predisposition may play a role in the case of certain drugs, particularly those agents that are metabolized by acetylation such as procainamide and hydralazine, with the disease more likely to develop in patients who are slow acetylators. These drugs may alter gene expression in $CD4^+$ T cells by inhibiting DNA methylation and inducing overexpression.

Pathogenesis

Many experimental models have postulated the sequence of events in SLE:

1. UV radiation exposure and other environmental culprits lead to apoptosis of cells.
2. A large volume of nuclear antigens is generated because of inadequate clearance of nuclei.
3. Defective immunological tolerance is the result of abnormalities in B and T cells.
4. Such lymphocytes are stimulated by the self-antigens.
5. Production of autoantibodies occurs against the antigens.
6. Antigen–antibody complexes bind to Fc receptors on B and dendritic cells and are processed.
7. The processed nuclear antigens are presented to the T cells.
8. B cells are stimulated by T cells via CD40L to produce autoantibodies.
9. T-cell activation leads to the production of cytokines.
10. Repeated cycles of antigen release and immune activation lead to the production of high-affinity autoantibodies.

Mechanisms of Tissue Injury in SLE

Most lesions in SLE are because of the presence of autoantibodies.

- Immune complex deposition (type III HSR) leads to complement activation and deposition of complement and immunoglobulins in the glomeruli and blood vessels.
- Antiphospholipid syndrome can result in arterial or venous thromboses or present as pregnancy-related complication. The antibodies are produced against the target β_2-glycoprotein 1 and are found to have a greater association with thrombosis. When these features are associated with SLE, it is called secondary APLA syndrome, whereas in the absence of SLE, it is called primary APLA syndrome.
- Autoantibodies specific for red blood cells, WBCs and platelets opsonize these cells and promote their phagocytosis and lysis. Antinuclear antibodies (ANAs) cannot penetrate an intact cell, so the formation of immune complex is possible only if the cell nuclei are exposed. In tissues, nuclei of damaged cells react with ANAs, lose their chromatin pattern and become homogeneous to produce the so-called **lupus erythematosus (LE) bodies** or **haematoxylin bodies**. The LE cell is a neutrophil or macrophage that has engulfed the denatured nucleus of an injured cell. It may be seen in peripheral blood and pericardial and pleural effusions, but with the emergence of more specific and sophisticated tests, demonstration of LE cell is no longer used for the diagnosis of SLE.

Morphology

All the clinical features of SLE are caused by the deposition of immune complexes at various sites, and the most characteristic lesions are noted in blood vessels, kidneys, connective tissue and skin.

Blood Vessels Capillaries, small arteries and arterioles may demonstrate **acute necrotizing vasculitis** with characteristic **fibrinoid necrosis**. With time, the vessels undergo fibrous thickening with narrowing.

Renal The kidney is the most commonly involved visceral organ. Renal involvement in SLE is called

lupus nephritis. Although only approximately 50% of patients with SLE develop clinically evident renal disease, biopsy studies demonstrate some degree of renal involvement in most patients if examined by electron microscopy or immunofluorescence. Therefore, for the sake of prognosis, it is important to correctly classify the extent of renal involvement. Glomerular disease usually develops within the first few years of SLE onset and is often asymptomatic. The present system of SLE classification categorizes glomerular lesions of SLE into six groups or classes. There may be overlap within these classes and in due course lesions progress from one class to another. Class I is the least common type, class IV is the most common type and class VI is associated with the worst prognosis.

Acute or chronic renal failure may cause symptoms related to uraemia, proteinuria and fluid overload. Acute nephritic disease may manifest as hypertension and haematuria. Nephrotic syndrome may cause oedema, weight gain or hyperlipidaemia.

Class I

It is an uncommon renal lesion in lupus nephritis and is defined as **minimal mesangial lupus nephritis**. It is characterized by the accumulation of immune complex in the mesangium identified by immunofluorescence or electron microscopy, without concomitant light microscopic alterations.

Class II

It is defined as **mesangial proliferative lupus nephritis** characterized by any degree of mesangial hypercellularity (defined as three or more cells per mesangium) in association with mesangial immune deposits. These lesions may be associated with isolated small immune deposits involving the peripheral capillary walls.

Class III

It is defined as **focal lupus nephritis** involving less than 50% of all glomeruli. The glomeruli that are affected usually show segmental (affecting only a portion of the glomerulus) or global (involving the entire glomerulus) endocapillary proliferative lesions or inactive glomerular scars. These may or may not be associated with capillary wall necrosis and crescents and subendothelial deposits. In assessing the extent of the lesions, glomeruli with both active and sclerotic lesions are taken into account. Focal or diffuse mesangial alterations (including mesangial proliferation or mesangial immune deposits) may accompany the focal glomerular lesions.

Class IV

It is the most common and also the most severe form of lupus nephritis and is defined as **diffuse lupus nephritis** involving 50% or more glomeruli in the biopsy. In the affected glomeruli, it may be segmental or global and hence further subclassified into class IV segmental (IV-S) or class IV global (IV-G). The affected glomeruli show proliferation of endothelial, mesangial and epithelial cells with or without crescent formation. Extensive subendothelial immune complex deposits may give rise to the characteristic circumferential thickening of the capillary wall leading to the '**wire loop**' lesions when seen under a light microscope. The subdivision for segmental and global lesions is based on evidence suggesting that diffuse segmental lupus nephritis may have an outcome that is different from that of diffuse global lupus nephritis. Fibrinoid necrosis is usually associated with endocapillary hypercellularity and may therefore be a more severe expression of the same pathogenetic mechanism. Patients with this class of lupus nephritis present with haematuria, proteinuria and hypertension with or without renal failure.

Class V

Class V is defined as **membranous lupus nephritis** characterized by diffuse thickening of the capillary walls because of the deposition of immune complexes in the subepithelial zone. A high degree of mesangial hypercellularity may be seen and scattered subendothelial immune deposits may be identified by electron microscopy or immunofluorescence. The lesions are commonly associated with an increased production of basement membrane–like material. Patients with this class of lupus nephritis present with nephrotic syndrome.

Class VI

This lesion is defined as advanced sclerosing lupus nephritis and is characterized by global glomerulosclerosis in 90% or more of the cases and in which there is clinical or pathological evidence that the sclerosis is attributable to lupus nephritis. There is no evidence of ongoing active glomerular disease. Class VI may represent the advanced stage of other chronic stages.

Dermatological Cutaneous manifestations of SLE include malar rash, photosensitivity and discoid lupus. **Malar rash** (Fig. 6.21) is characterized by erythema over the cheeks and nasal bridge that is occasionally painful or pruritic. Butterfly appearance on the face because of malar rash is histologically characterized by vacuolar degeneration of the basal layer of the epidermis, dermal oedema and perivascular inflammation.

Photosensitivity in SLE may be either acute or chronic after sun exposure, with expected duration of approximately 2 days in classical cases with an appearance of rash.

Discoid lupus is a chronic lupus rash that is plaque-like in character, with follicular plugging and scarring often developing in sun-exposed areas. It may be a part of systemic lupus or may represent discoid lupus without organ involvement as a separate diagnostic entity.

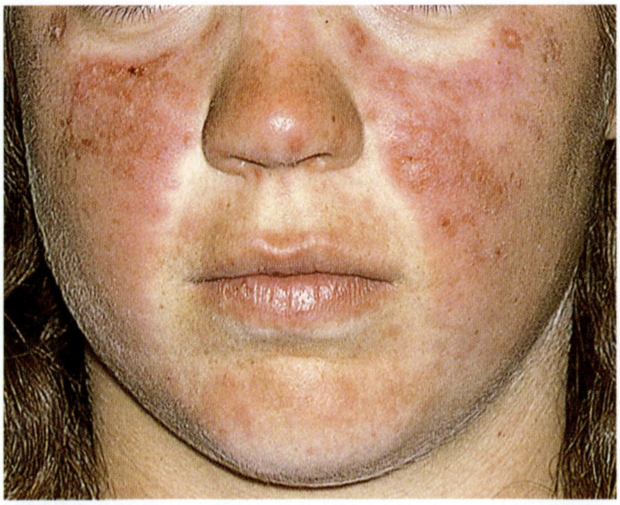

Fig. 6.21 Malar rash in SLE, clinical picture – cutaneous disease. Acute cutaneous LE (SLE). The classical butterfly rash occurs in 10%–50% of patients with acute LE. LE, lupus erythematosus; SLE, systemic lupus erythematosus. (*Source:* From James G.H. Dinulos. Connective Tissue Diseases. Habif's Clinical Dermatology. 7th edition. Elsevier 2021.)

Discoid lesions can develop in up to 25% of patients with SLE; a small case series suggested that the presence of such lesions may indicate a milder disease or less renal involvement. In another review, it was reported that patients with discoid lesions rarely progressed to SLE. However, there is a 5% risk of discoid lupus disease developing into the systemic condition.

Musculoskeletal Arthralgia, myalgia and frank arthritis involving the small joints of the hands, wrists and knees causing joint pains are the initial manifestations. In contrast to rheumatoid arthritis, SLE arthritis or arthralgia may be asymmetrical, with pain that is disproportionate to the swelling. Characteristic hand deformities are swan neck deformities that result from recurrent synovitis and inflammation of the joint capsule, tendons and ligaments. However, an important point to note is that the joint involvement in SLE is usually **nonerosive**.

Another important consideration is the increased prevalence of avascular necrosis (AVN) in about 44% of the SLE population in the first year of therapy with high-dose corticosteroids.

Neurological Seizures related to SLE may be generalized or partial and may precipitate status epilepticus because of damage of neurons by immune complex deposition. Psychosis may manifest as paranoia or hallucinations.

Transverse myelitis with spastic paraparesis and sensory loss at a given level is a rare but severe complication of SLE or APLA syndrome. Stroke and transient ischaemic attack (TIA) may be related to APLA or SLE vasculitis. Migraine headaches may be linked to antiphospholipid syndrome.

Pulmonary Multiple pulmonary complications, including pleurisy, pleural effusion, pneumonitis, pulmonary hypertension and interstitial lung disease, may occur and their risk increases with the use of long-term steroids. Pleuritis, a formal diagnostic criterion for SLE, induces chest pain and pleural effusion that is exudative, with an elevated lactate dehydrogenase level. Pleurisy with pleuritic chest pain with or without pleural effusions is the most common feature of acute pulmonary involvement in SLE. Most seriously, haemoptysis may herald diffuse alveolar haemorrhage, a rare, acute, life-threatening pulmonary complication of SLE.

Cardiac Pericarditis is the most common cardiac feature of SLE that is often relieved when the patient leans forward. Myocarditis may occur in SLE with heart failure symptoms. Coronary vasculitis manifesting as angina or infarction is rarely reported. Pulmonary hypertension may present with indolent chest pain or dyspnoea. Valvular abnormalities, primarily of the mitral and aortic valves, manifest as diffuse leaflet thickening and become dysfunctional on using steroids. It takes the form of single or multiple 1- to 3-mm warty deposits on any heart valve, distinctively on either surface of the leaflets. Libman–Sacks endocarditis is noninfectious but may manifest as symptoms similar to those of infective endocarditis in patients with SLE or antiphospholipid syndrome. More commonly, accelerated ischaemic coronary artery disease (CAD) is associated with SLE and may present indolently as atypical anginal pain. Risk factors for atherosclerosis, including hypertension, obesity and hyperlipidaemia, are more common in patients with SLE than in the population at large. In addition, immune complexes and APLAs may cause endothelial damage and promote atherosclerosis.

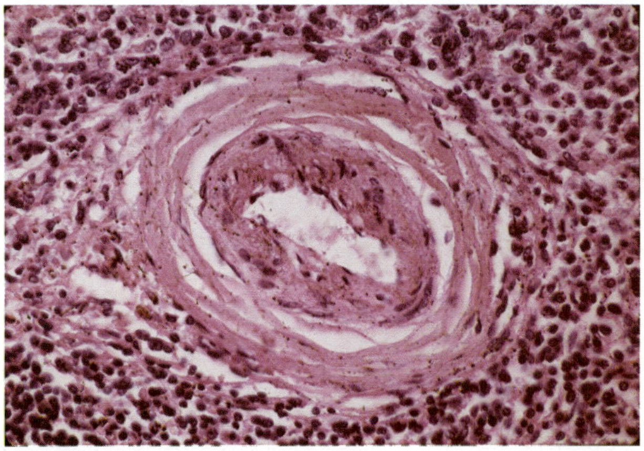

Fig. 6.22 Spleen in SLE, microscopy – small artery with concentric collagen formation around a vessel. This is also termed ***onion skinning.*** SLE, systemic lupus erythematosus. (*Source:* From Attilio Orazi, Sonam Prakash. Differential Diagnosis in Surgical Pathology. Elsevier 2015.)

Spleen (Fig. 6.22) Splenomegaly is a common finding, with capsular thickening and follicular hyperplasia being common features. Other than these, concentric intimal and smooth muscle cell hyperplasia of the central penicilliary arteries results in the characteristic *'onion skin lesions'*.

Signs and Symptoms of SLE

SLE is a chronic inflammatory multisystem disease that can affect almost any organ system, although it mainly involves the skin, joints, kidneys, blood cells and nervous system. Its presentation and course are highly variable, ranging from indolent to fulminant.

The classical presentation of the triad – fever, joint pain and rash – in a woman of childbearing age should prompt investigation to confirm or rule out the diagnosis of SLE. In patients with suggestive clinical findings, a family history of autoimmune disease should raise further suspicion of SLE.

The common clinical presentations are listed in Table 6.11, and the system-wise manifestations are discussed along with morphology.

Diagnosis of SLE

As SLE is a multisystem disorder with extremely variable presentation, the diagnosis is based on the combination of clinical, laboratory and morphological findings.

Familiarity with the diagnostic criteria helps clinicians to recognize SLE and to subclassify this complex disease on the basis of the pattern of target organ manifestations.

Table 6.11 Clinical and Pathological Manifestations of SLE

Clinical Manifestation	Prevalence (%)
Haematological	100
Fatigue	80–100
Arthritis, arthralgia and myalgia	80–90
Skin	85
Fever	55–85
Weight loss	60
Renal	50–70
Neuropsychiatric	25–35
Pleuritis	45
Pericarditis	25
Gastrointestinal	20
Raynaud phenomenon	15–40
Ocular	5–15
Peripheral neuropathy	15

SLE, systemic lupus erythematosus.

Hence, the American College of Rheumatology (ACR) has established a complex set of criteria for the clinical assessment of this disorder that was initially proposed in 1997 and was later updated in 2012 by the Systemic Lupus International Collaborating Clinics (Table 6.12). A patient is classified as having SLE if four of the clinical and immunological criteria are present at any time (not necessarily concurrently), including at least one clinical and one immunological criteria. ACR and the European League Against Rheumatism (EULAR) also have published new criteria for the classification of SLE in 2019.

Autoantibodies in SLE (Table 6.13)

The hallmark feature of SLE is the production of autoantibodies against nuclear and cytoplasmic components of the cell and some cell surface antigens of blood cells that form the basis of the pathogenicity, clinical features and diagnosis of this condition. Serological evidence of the presence of specific antibodies is essential for confirming the diagnosis. Broadly, the autoantibodies fall under two categories – ANAs and other autoantibodies.

ANAs: These are directed against nuclear antigens and can be grouped into the following four types:

- Antibodies to DNA
- Antibodies to histones
- Antibodies to nonhistone proteins bound to RNA
- Antibodies to nucleolar antigens

Indirect immunofluorescence, which can identify antibodies that bind to a variety of nuclear antigens, including DNA, RNA and proteins (collectively called generic ANAs), is widely used. The pattern of nuclear fluorescence suggests the type of antibody present in the patient's serum. This does not specify the cause because a combination of patterns is a frequent finding. **Antibodies to double-stranded DNA and the Smith (Sm) antigen are virtually diagnostic of SLE.**

In addition to ANAs, patients with lupus have a host of other autoantibodies such as:

- **APLAs** are present in 40% of cases that are formed against epitopes of plasma proteins that are exposed when the proteins are in complex with phospholipids. Such proteins are prothrombin, annexin V, β_2-glycoprotein 1 and proteins C and S. Antibodies against the phospholipid–β_2-glycoprotein complex also bind to cardiolipin antigen and hence may give a false-positive test result for syphilis. Some of these antibodies interfere with in vitro clotting tests and are hence called lupus anticoagulant.
- Some antibodies in SLE are directed against red cells, platelets and lymphocytes.

Course and Management of SLE

The course of SLE is highly variable and unpredictable. Even without treatment, some patients have an indolent course with mild manifestations for decades. Most patients, even with proper treatment, have a relapsing and remitting course.

Table 6.12 Revised Criteria for the Classification of SLE

Criterion	Definition
Clinical and Laboratory Criteria	
Acute cutaneous lupus	Malar rash (fixed erythema, flat or raised, over the malar eminences), photosensitivity
Chronic cutaneous lupus	Discoid rash: erythematous raised patches with adherent keratotic scaling and follicular plugging
Nonscarring alopecia	Diffuse thinning or hair fragility in the absence of other causes
Oral or nasal ulcers	Oral or nasopharyngeal ulceration, usually painless
Joint disease	Nonerosive synovitis involving two or more peripheral joints, characterized by tenderness, swelling or effusion
Serositis	Pleuritis (pleuritic pain or rub or evidence of pleural effusion), pericarditis
Renal disorder	Persistent proteinuria >0.5 g/24 h, or red cell casts
Neurological disorder	Seizures, psychosis, myelitis or neuropathy in the absence of offending drugs or other known causes
Haemolytic anaemia	reticulocytosis, low haptoglobin, elevated indirect bilirubin, elevated LDH AND positive Coomb's test
Leucopenia or lymphopenia	Leucopenia: <4.0 × 10^9 cells/L (4000 cells/mm^3) total on two or more occasions, *or* Lymphopenia: <1.5 × 10^9 cells/L (1500 cells/mm^3) on two or more occasions
Thrombocytopenia	Thrombocytopenia: <100 × 10^9 cells/L (100 × 10^3 cells/mm^3) in the absence of offending drugs and other conditions
Immunological Criteria	
Antinuclear antibody (ANA)	Abnormal titre of ANA by immunofluorescence
Anti-dsDNA antibody	Abnormal titre
Anti-Sm antibody	Presence of antibody to Sm nuclear antigen
Antiphospholipid antibody	Positive finding of antiphospholipid antibodies on the basis of the following: (1) An abnormal serum level of IgG or IgM anticardiolipin antibodies (2) A positive test for lupus anticoagulant using a standard test (3) A false-positive serological test for syphilis known to be positive for at least 6 months and by negative *Treponema pallidum* immobilization or fluorescent treponemal antibody absorption test
Low complement	Low C3, C4 or CH50
Direct Coombs test	Assay for anti–red cell antibody in the absence of clinically evident haemolytic anaemia

SLE, systemic lupus erythematosus.

The flare-ups are managed with corticosteroids or immunosuppressive drugs. With the currently available drugs, the outcome has improved with better survival rates. The most common causes of death are renal failure, intermittent infections and CAD. Patients may also develop complications because of long-term immunosuppression.

RHEUMATOID ARTHRITIS

Rheumatoid arthritis is an autoimmune disorder with multisystem involvement, primarily affecting the joints. The disease most often begins between the ages of 30 and 50 years and three-fourths of the affected patients are women. It manifests as joint pain worst in the mornings, stiffness, swelling and decreased movement of the joints. Small joints in the hands and feet are most commonly affected along with other organs, such as the eyes, skin or lungs. Beneath the skin in elbows, etc., firm lumps, called rheumatoid nodules, are found.

To stress the systemic autoimmune nature of the disease, the disease is mentioned here and is discussed in detail in Chapter 30.

SJÖGREN SYNDROME

Sjögren syndrome is an autoimmune disease that affects the exocrine glands. The primary symptoms are dry mouth (xerostomia) and dry eyes (keratoconjunctivitis sicca) because of functional impairment of the glands. The disease may be an isolated condition or associated with other autoimmune diseases like rheumatoid arthritis, SLE or scleroderma. The former is called the primary Sjögren syndrome or sicca syndrome and the latter is the secondary form of Sjögren syndrome. Other symptoms

Table 6.13 Autoantibodies Detected in Autoimmune Diseases

Autoimmune Disease	Type of Autoantibody
SLE	Anti-dsDNA Anti-U1-RNP Anti-Smith antigen Antiphospholipid Generic ANAs
Systemic sclerosis	Anti-DNA topoisomerase 1 Anticentromere proteins Anti-RNA polymerase III
Sjögren syndrome	Anti-Ro/SS-A Anti-La/SS-B
Autoimmune myositis	Anti-histidyl aminoacyl-tRNA synthetase, Jo1 Anti-Mi-2 nuclear antigen Anti-MDA5 Anti-TIF1γ nuclear protein
Rheumatoid arthritis	Anti–cyclic citrullinated peptides (CCP) Rheumatoid factor

ANA, antinuclear antibody; SLE, systemic lupus erythematosus.

include dry skin, vaginal dryness, chronic cough, numbness of the limbs, muscle pain, joint pains and thyroid problems. Those affected are also at an increased risk (5%) of lymphoma. The disorder most often affects women, with the female to male ratio being 9:1, and the median age of onset is around 50–60 years.

Pathogenesis (Fig. 6.23)

Although the exact cause is unknown, it is believed to involve a combination of genetic and environmental triggers such as exposure to viruses like human T-lymphotropic virus (HTLV), HIV, hepatitis C virus (HCV), EBV and cytomegalovirus (CMV) or bacteria. These trigger such attacks in susceptible individuals and cause cell damage, followed by apoptosis of these glandular cells. This leads to the exposure of the antigens that are recognized by the self-reactive T cells because of failure of immunological tolerance in these individuals. These viruses may also induce the disease by 'molecular mimicry' when these have similar amino acid sequence and the antibodies produced against them cross-react with the self-antigens.

Sjögren syndrome is a systemic chronic inflammatory disorder characterized by lymphocytic infiltrate composed of $CD4^+$ T cells, B cells, plasma cells and fibrosis in the exocrine organs, predominantly the lacrimal and salivary glands. However, it may also affect the respiratory, GI and urogenital linings. Affected individuals may have a family history of this disease and they express certain MHC genes like HLA-DR 52, HLA-DR3, HLA-B8 and HLA-DQ2, HLA-DQA1 and HLA-DQB1 in the HLA regions, which may be the reason for their susceptibility. Here, T-cell and B-cell activation is implicated by the release of cytokines. The dendritic cells especially produce BAFF, which further releases ANAs like anti-SS-A and anti-SS-B antibodies.

The ANAs against ribonucleoproteins are detected in 90% of such patients by the immunofluorescence techniques. Hence, these are used as serological markers but are not characteristic of Sjögren syndrome because these may also be seen in cases of SLE. The net result is inflammation, tissue damage and, eventually, fibrosis. SS-A antibodies indicate early disease onset, longer disease duration and extraglandular manifestations such as cutaneous vasculitis and nephritis.

Morphology (Fig. 6.24)

Microscopy reveals characteristic lymphocytic sialadenitis with intense lymphocytic infiltration to the extent of formation of lymphoid follicles with germinal centres. The lining epithelial cells of the ducts may show hyperplasia, leading to obstruction. In due course, the acini undergo changes like atrophy, hyalinization and fibrosis and are later replaced with fat. The lack of tears leads to dryness of the corneal epithelium, eventually leading to inflammation, erosion and ulceration. The oral mucosa may atrophy, with inflammatory fissuring and ulceration. Dryness and crusting of the nose may lead to ulcerations and even perforation of the nasal septum.

Clinical Features (Fig. 6.25)

Symptoms are because of inflammatory destruction of the exocrine glands. The eyes become dry, itchy, painful and present as keratoconjunctivitis sicca with blurring of vision and a scratchy sensation of sand and gravel in the eyes. In the salivary glands, xerostomia is seen with cracks and fissures of the oral structures, especially in the tongue and buccal mucosa. It can lead to secondary conditions like altered taste, inflamed papillae, high susceptibility to dental caries and candidiasis.

Extraglandular manifestations include synovitis, diffuse pulmonary fibrosis and peripheral neuropathy associated with high titres of antibodies specific for SS-A. Even though defects of tubular function including renal tubular acidosis, uricosuria, phosphaturia and histologically prominent tubulointerstitial nephritis may occur, glomerular disease is uncommon in Sjögren syndrome.

Lip biopsy is essential for the diagnosis of Sjögren syndrome. The lymph nodes of patients with Sjögren syndrome are often hyperplastic, with the most intense lymphocytic response seen in the focal points of salivary and lacrimal glands filled with a mixture of polyclonal T and B cells. In about 5% of patients, the emergence of a dominant B-cell clone is usually indicative of the development of a marginal zone lymphoma, an incidence that is 40-fold higher than that in the normal population.

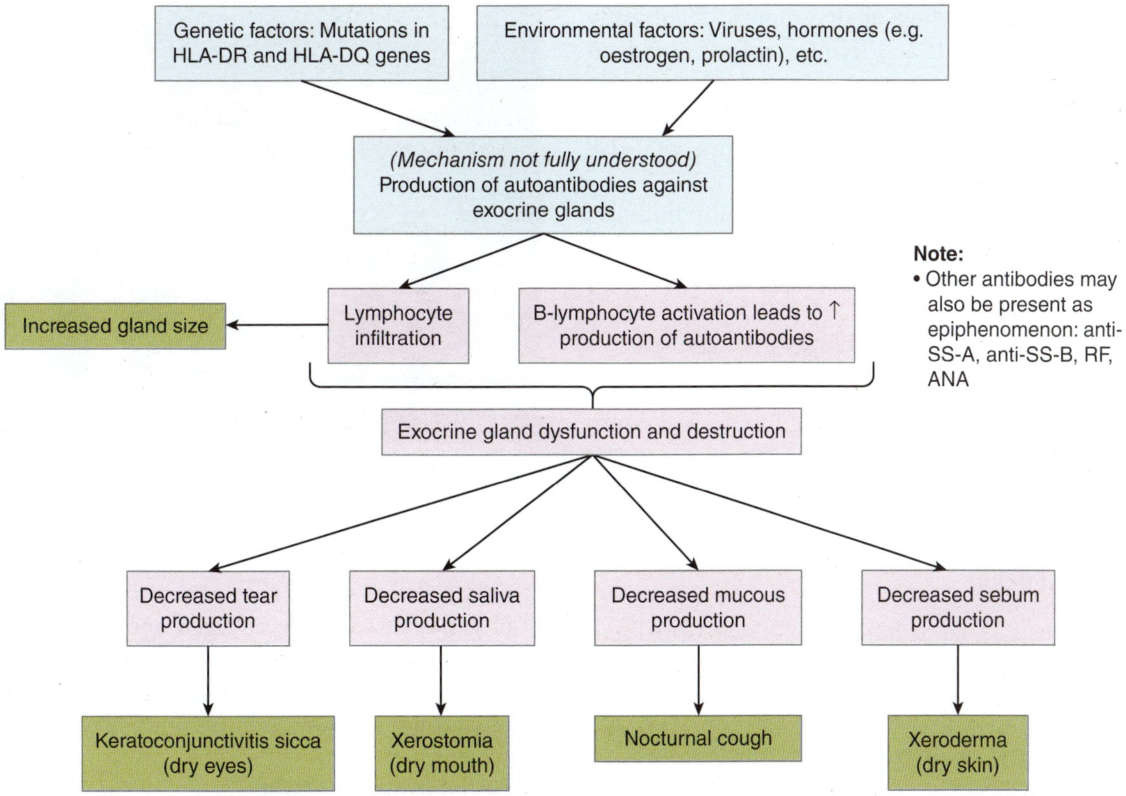

Fig. 6.23 Pathogenesis and clinical findings of Sjögren syndrome. (*Source:* https://www.google.com/url?sa=i&url=https%3A%2F%2Fcalgaryguide.ucalgary.ca%2F1496%2F&psig=AOvVaw3HJJR3GPSj8yfUFZebguJa&ust=1605969845427000&source=images&cd=vfe&ved=0CAIQjRxqFwoTCMiGn4euke0CFQAAAAAdAAAAABAP.)

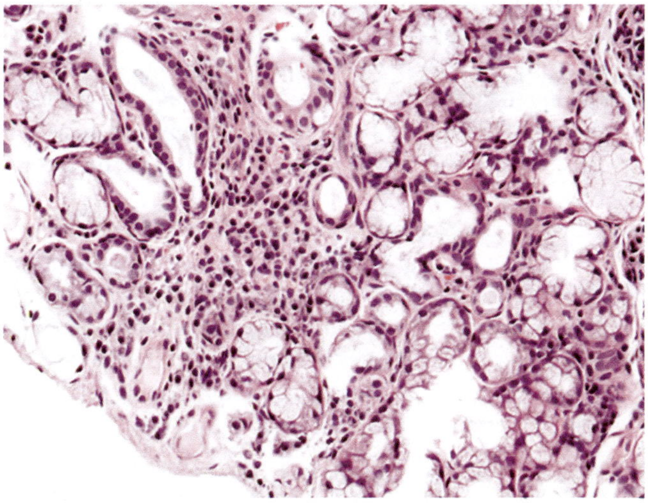

Fig. 6.24 Microscopy of salivary gland in Sjögren syndrome – focal lymphoid infiltration in the minor salivary gland associated with Sjögren syndrome. Lip biopsy. (*Source:* https://en.wikipedia.org/wiki/Sj%C3%B6gren_syndrome#/media/File:Sjogren's_syndrome_(2).jpg.)

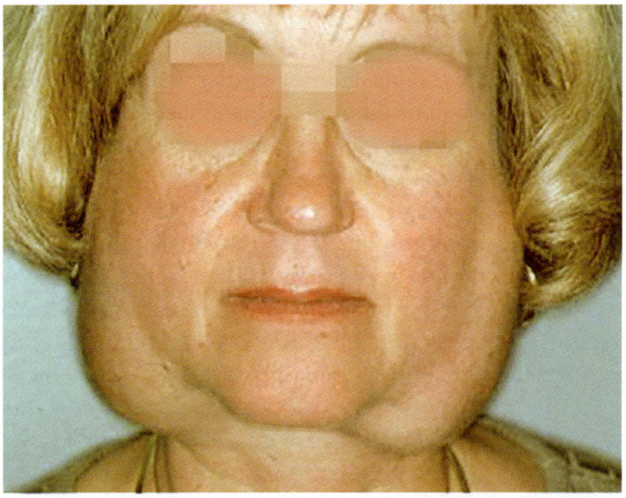

Fig. 6.25 Clinical picture of Sjögren syndrome. Note the marked bilateral parotid enlargement. (*Source:* https://emedicine.medscape.com/article/332125-overview.)

Diagnosis of Sjögren Syndrome

According to the American–European Consensus Group (AECG) classification system, the diagnosis of primary Sjögren syndrome requires **at least four of the criteria given next**; in addition, either criterion 5 or criterion 6 must be included. Sjögren syndrome can be diagnosed in patients who have no sicca symptoms or even without performing a biopsy if three of the four objective criteria are fulfilled. The criteria are as follows:

1. Ocular symptoms – dry eyes for more than 3 months, foreign body sensation and use of tear substitutes more than three times daily

2. Oral symptoms – feeling of dry mouth, recurrently swollen salivary glands and frequent use of liquids to aid swallowing
3. Ocular signs – Schirmer test performed without anaesthesia (<5 mm in 5 minutes) and positive vital dye staining results
4. Oral signs – abnormal salivary scintigraphy findings, abnormal parotid sialography findings and abnormal sialometry findings (unstimulated salivary flow <1.5 mL in 15 minutes)
5. Positive minor salivary gland biopsy findings
6. Positive anti-SSA or anti-SSB antibody results

Secondary Sjögren syndrome is diagnosed when symptoms of oral or ocular dryness exist in the presence of a connective tissue disease or other autoimmune disease along with criterion 3, 4 or 5.

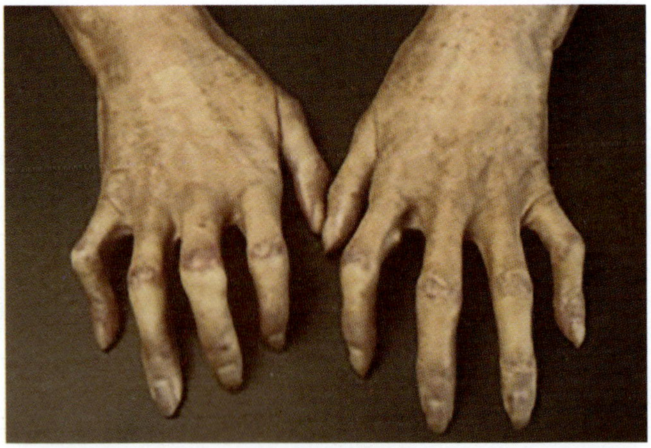
Fig. 6.26 Sclerodactyly in limited cutaneous disease. (*Source:* From Joanne Szczygiel Cunha. Scleroderma (Systemic Sclerosis). Ferri's Clinical Advisor 2021. Elsevier 2021.)

SYSTEMIC SCLEROSIS

Systemic sclerosis is an autoimmune disease predominantly affecting the skin along with some visceral organs and is characterized by intense inflammatory infiltrate, widespread damage to blood vessels and diffuse fibrosis. The disease was previously called *scleroderma* because of the predominant cutaneous manifestations but is presently referred to as systemic sclerosis because of its involvement in multiple systems. On the basis of the disease distribution and manifestations, it is divided into the following types:

1. **Diffuse scleroderma** starts as a widespread skin involvement with early progression to involve multiple organs. Death in cases with visceral involvement generally follows renal failure, cardiac failure, intestinal malabsorption or pulmonary insufficiency.
2. **Limited scleroderma** has limited skin involvement and late systemic involvement.
3. **CREST syndrome** involves limited scleroderma along with other features like **c**alcinosis, **R**aynaud phenomenon, o**e**sophageal dysmotility, **s**clerodactyly (Fig. 6.26) and **t**elangiectasia. Patients may have gastro-oesophageal reflux disease (GERD) but predominantly develop skin tightening over the face and distal to the elbows and knees. This type is also characterized by slow progression because the disease is limited more to the skin but may get complicated by pulmonary hypertension.

Systemic sclerosis is about four times more common among women than among men. It is most common among people aged 50–60 years and is rare in children.

Pathogenesis

There are three major processes involved in the pathogenesis of systemic sclerosis – autoimmune responses, vascular damage and fibrosis.

- **Autoimmunity:** Autoimmune response is generated by the production of $CD4^+$ cells, which release cytokines like TGF-β and IL-13 that stimulate fibroblasts and inflammatory cells. They also stimulate transcription of genes that encode collagen and other extracellular matrix proteins (e.g. fibronectin) in fibroblasts. Other cytokines recruit leucocytes and propagate the chronic inflammation. Humoral immunity may also be seen in the form of ANAs that may cause fibrosis, but the mechanism is not clear.
- **Vascular damage:** Vascular damage in systemic sclerosis predominantly affects the microvasculature. Damage to the endothelium, followed by platelet aggregation, leads to release of platelets and endothelial-derived growth factors (e.g. PDGF, TGF-β) that trigger perivascular fibrosis and collagen accumulation. Vascular smooth muscle cells also show an increased expression of adrenergic receptors leading to constriction. Intimal proliferation is evident in the digital arteries of patients with systemic sclerosis. All these lead to widespread narrowing of the microvasculature, causing ischaemic injury and scarring.
- **Fibrosis:** The accumulation of alternatively activated macrophages, actions of fibrogenic cytokines produced by infiltrating leucocytes, an intrinsic abnormality of fibroblasts that causes them to produce excessive amounts of collagen, hyperresponsiveness of fibroblasts to these cytokines and scarring that follows ischaemic damage caused by the vascular lesions – all contribute to the process of fibrosis.

Genetic predisposition such as polymorphisms in *COL1A2* and $TGF\text{-}\beta_1$ may influence severity and development of the disease and has a familial predisposition. CMV and parvovirus B19 are sometimes claimed to be the epitope of this disease.

Morphology (Fig. 6.27)

In systemic sclerosis, although any organ may be involved, prominent changes are seen in the skin, GI tract, kidney, musculoskeletal system, blood vessels, lungs, heart and peripheral nerves.

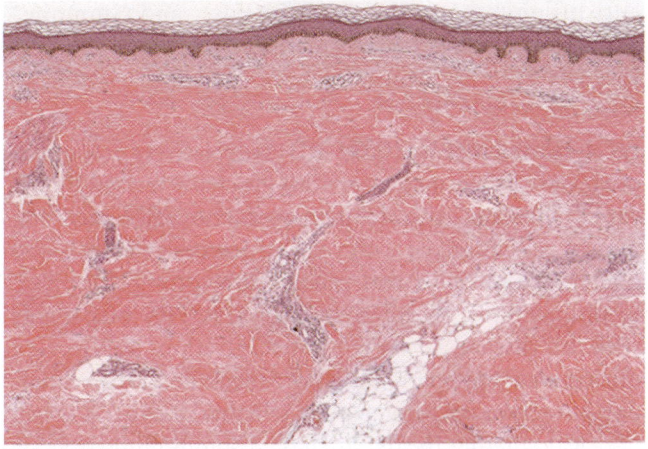

Fig. 6.27 Microscopic image of systemic sclerosis. Note the atrophy of dermal appendages because of fibrosis. (*Source:* https://www.google.com/url?sa=i&url=http%3A%2F%2Fwww.pathologyoutlines.com%2Ftopic%2Fskinnontumorscleroderma.html&psig=AOvVaw1Qc2u09hkR2b6Jdm6RdjxW&ust=1605950044401000&source=images&cd=vfe&ved=0CAIQjRxqFwoTCPjY96TkkO0CFQAAAAAdAAAAABAD.)

Skin **Diffuse sclerotic atrophy** involves the fingers and distal regions of the upper extremities and extends proximally to involve the upper arms, shoulders, neck and face in diffuse type of scleroderma. Microscopically, oedema, perivascular infiltrates containing $CD4^+$ Th2 cells, swelling and degeneration of collagen fibres (which appear eosinophilic), loss of rete ridges and atrophy of dermal appendages because of fibrosis can be observed. Focal and sometimes diffuse subcutaneous calcifications may develop, especially in patients with CREST syndrome. Loss of blood supply may lead to cutaneous ulcerations and atrophic changes in the terminal phalanges sometimes requiring amputation. In advanced stages, the face becomes a drawn mask and the fingers take on a tapered, claw-like appearance, with limitation of motion in the joints.

Digestive Tract The most common manifestation in the oesophagus is reflux oesophagitis, which may be complicated by oesophageal stricturing or benign narrowing of the oesophagus with progressive atrophy and collagenous replacement of muscularis, leading to dysphagia and chest pain. It may worsen because of progressive fibrosis. If this is left untreated, acid from the stomach may enter the oesophagus, causing oesophagitis and GERD.

The duodenum is frequently dilated and may be slow to empty, and the grossly dilated, atonic organ may produce a sump effect. Part of the colon may be pseudo-obstructed because of fibrosis or may present as ischaemic colitis. Scleroderma may also be associated with gastric antral vascular ectasia (GAVE) or *watermelon stomach,* in which atypical blood vessels found radially arranged around the pylorus of the stomach may cause upper GI bleeding and iron-deficiency anaemia in patients.

Kidneys The most important clinical complication of scleroderma involving the kidney is *scleroderma renal crisis,* which is seen in two-thirds of the patients. It is considered as a poor prognostic factor. Symptoms of scleroderma renal crisis are malignant hypertension with evidence of acute organ damage, hyperreninaemia, azotaemia and microangiopathic haemolytic anaemia. Apart from this, the high blood pressure, haematuria and proteinuria may also be indicative of renal crisis. Glomerular changes are not generally noticed.

Approximately 7%–9% of all patients with diffuse cutaneous scleroderma develop renal crisis at some point in the course of their disease, but it is more common in those with rapid skin involvement and those with antibodies against RNA polymerase (60%).

In hypertensive patients, vascular alterations like concentric intimal thickening because of deposition of mucinous or finely collagenous material are more pronounced. They are often associated with fibrinoid necrosis involving the arterioles along with thrombosis and infarction.

Musculoskeletal The first joint symptoms that patients with scleroderma have are nonspecific joint pain because of hypertrophy and hyperplasia of synovial tissues that can lead to arthritis or cause discomfort and restricted joint mobility because of calcinosis. Inflammatory myositis similar to polymyositis may develop, but joint destruction is not prominent in scleroderma.

Lungs Lung function impairment is almost universally seen in patients with diffuse scleroderma on pulmonary function testing. Some patients may develop pulmonary hypertension secondary to pulmonary dysfunction, which may be progressive, and lead to right-sided heart failure. The earliest manifestation of this may be a decreased diffusion capacity on pulmonary function testing. Pulmonary and interstitial fibrosis is a common manifestation.

Other pulmonary complications in more advanced disease include aspiration pneumonia, pulmonary haemorrhage and pneumothorax.

Clinical Features

Distinctive features of systemic sclerosis are the striking cutaneous changes, notably skin thickening. Oesophageal motility is impaired, and the lower oesophageal sphincter is incompetent, leading to dysphagia in around half of these patients. Gastro-oesophageal reflux and secondary strictures may also develop. The intestinal muscularis mucosa degenerates, leading to pseudodiverticula in the colon and ileum. Abdominal pain, intestinal obstruction or malabsorption syndrome with weight loss and anaemia reflect involvement of the small intestine. Interstitial and peribronchial fibrosis may cause respiratory difficulties because of pulmonary fibrosis, which may lead to right-sided cardiac dysfunction. Myocardial fibrosis may cause either arrhythmias or cardiac failure. Intimal hyperplasia of small arteries causes Raynaud phenomenon with episodic vasoconstriction. In long-standing involvement of the lungs, pulmonary hypertension may develop. Intimal hyperplasia of interlobular and arcuate arteries may occur in the kidneys, causing renal ischaemia and hypertension with mild proteinuria in 30% of patients. All of these lead to malignant hypertension with slow progression to renal failure.

Diagnosis

Diagnosis of systemic sclerosis requires appropriate clinical symptoms and signs, presence of autoantibodies, specifically anticentromere and anti-scl70/anti-topoisomerase antibodies, and, occasionally, biopsy. Patients with these antibodies are more likely to have underlying pulmonary fibrosis and peripheral vascular disease. Ninety per cent of patients have a detectable ANA. Anticentromere antibody is more common in the limited form (80%–90%) and is associated with CREST syndrome in many cases than in the diffuse form (10%). In general, patients with limited disease live longer than those with systemic sclerosis with diffuse visceral involvement at the outset. Anti-scl70 is more common and more specific in the diffuse form (30%–40%) and in African American patients (who are more susceptible to the systemic form).

Pulmonary disease has become the major cause of death in systemic sclerosis because renal crisis responds to treatment.

INFLAMMATORY MYOPATHIES

The inflammatory myopathies are a group of diseases with no known cause and are characterized by chronic muscle inflammation accompanied by muscle weakness. These can be primary or associated with other autoimmune diseases. The three main types of chronic, or persistent, inflammatory myopathies are polymyositis, dermatomyositis and inclusion body myositis (IBM). This group of disorders is discussed in detail in Chapter 30.

MIXED CONNECTIVE TISSUE DISEASE

Mixed connective tissue disease (MCTD) is a rare autoimmune disorder that is characterized by features commonly seen in three different connective tissue disorders: SLE, scleroderma and polymyositis. It is most commonly seen in women younger than 30 years. Signs and symptoms vary but may include Raynaud phenomenon; heart, lung and skin abnormalities; rheumatoid arthritis–like symptoms; kidney disease; muscle weakness; hypomotility of the oesophagus; anaemia; lymphadenopathy; and certain neurological symptoms. Hence, it cannot be seen as a separate entity but is a combination of the three diseases. In some cases, it may progress to full-blown SLE or scleroderma and may lead to complications such as pulmonary hypertension, renal disease and interstitial lung disease. Medications such as corticosteroids, nonsteroidal anti-inflammatory drugs (NSAIDs) and immune-suppressing drugs help to manage symptoms.

IgG4-RELATED DISEASE

IgG4-related disease (**IgG4-RD**) is a relatively new group of chronic inflammatory conditions characterized by tissue infiltration with lymphocytes and IgG4-secreting plasma cells admixed with varying degrees of fibrosis and obliterative phlebitis that usually show prompt response to oral steroids. In approximately 51%–70% of patients with this disease, *serum* IgG4 concentrations are elevated during an acute phase that may contribute to the pathology but the exact pathogenesis remains unclear. It is still not clear whether the disease has an autoimmune basis or not, but B cells seem to play a key role in the pathogenesis.

This condition was initially noticed in cases of autoimmune pancreatitis when lesions were developed in other organs; now, it has been shown to involve many other organs like the biliary tree, salivary glands, periorbital tissues, kidneys, lungs, lymph nodes, meninges, aorta, breast, prostate, thyroid, pericardium and skin. It commonly affects middle- and old-aged people.

It is a relapsing–remitting disease associated with a tendency to develop mass-forming, tissue-destructive lesions at multiple sites. The lesions show characteristic histopathological appearance of inflammation and the deposition of connective tissue at the affected anatomical sites that can lead to organ dysfunction, organ failure or even death if not treated. These include Mikulicz syndrome (enlargement and fibrosis of salivary and lacrimal glands), Riedel thyroiditis, idiopathic retroperitoneal fibrosis, autoimmune pancreatitis and inflammatory pseudotumours of the orbit, lungs and kidneys.

Early detection is important to avoid organ damage and potentially serious complications, and the disease can be treated with rituximab, an anti-B-cell reagent.

IMMUNODEFICIENCY DISORDERS

OVERVIEW

Immunodeficiency is a state in which the immune system's ability to fight infectious disease and cancer is compromised or entirely absent. It can be primary or secondary. Primary immunodeficiency syndromes are because of inherited causes, but most cases of immunodeficiency are acquired or secondary because of extrinsic factors that affect the patient's immune system. A person who has an immunodeficiency of any kind is said to be **immunocompromised**. An immunocompromised person may be particularly vulnerable to opportunistic infections, in addition to normal infections that could affect any individual. Immunodeficiency also decreases cancer immunosurveillance, in which the immune system scans the cells of the body and kills the transformed ones (explained in detail in Chapter 7).

We discuss the well-defined primary immunodeficiencies and AIDS, the most fatal example of secondary immunodeficiency.

PRIMARY IMMUNODEFICIENCY (FIG. 6.28)

Primary immunodeficiency can be because of defects in innate or adaptive immunity. In a minority of cases, primary immunodeficiency may be associated with inherited systemic diseases.

Defects in Innate Immunity (Table 6.14)

Inherited defects in early innate immune response affect leucocyte function or the complement system.

Defects in Leucocyte Function

1. **Leucocyte adhesion defects (LADs)**
   LADs are characterized by defective adhesion because of the absence of adhesion proteins required for the binding of leucocytes with the endothelium, which is crucial for the leucocytes to escape from blood to the sites of antigen for effective phagocytosis. It is understood that however effective the phagocytic functions of WBCs are, if the adhesion is defective, phagocytosis is not possible. There are two types of LADs – leucocyte adhesion deficiency type 1 (LAD1) and leucocyte adhesion deficiency type 2 (LAD2).
   LAD1 is characterized by a defect in the synthesis of the β_2 chain shared by the integrins LFA-1 and Mac-1. **LAD2** is characterized by deficiency of the enzyme fucosyltransferase resulting in the absence of sialyl-Lewis X, the fucose-containing ligand for E- and P-selectins. Patients with LAD1 and LAD2 are prone to bacterial infections, which are recurrent and frequently life-threatening.
2. **Defects of phagolysosome function**
   - **Chédiak–Higashi syndrome** is a classic example of defective phagolysosome function, which is an autosomal recessive disease characterized by defective fusion of phagosomes and lysosomes leading to impaired phagocyte function and susceptibility to infections. The gene that is mutated is the *LYST* gene, which normally codes for a protein that is involved in lysosomal trafficking. The abnormalities seen are neutropenia, defective degranulation and delayed or ineffective microbial degradation. Owing

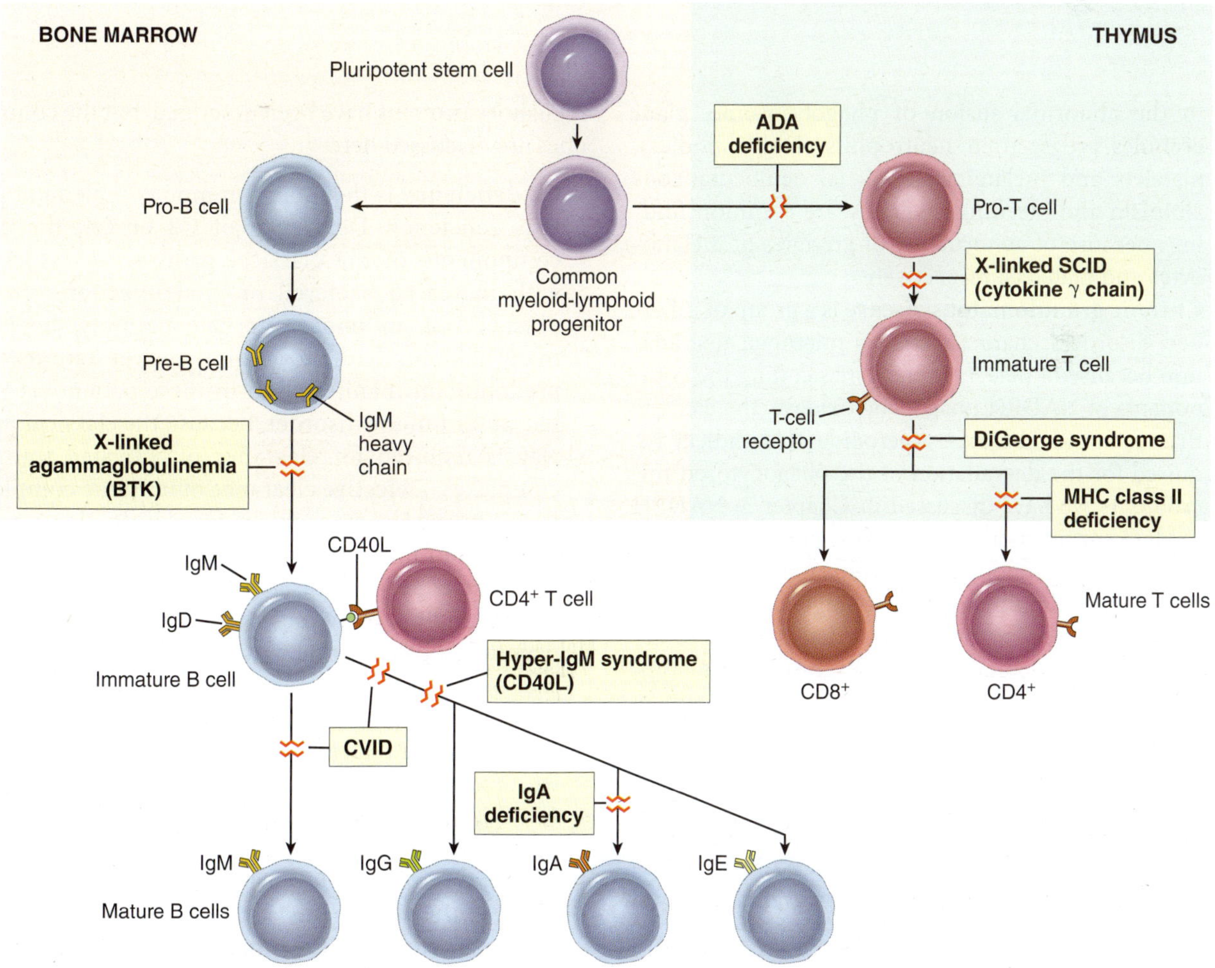

Fig. 6.28 Primary immunodeficiency diseases. (*Source:* From Vinay Kumar, Abul K. Abbas, and Jon C. Aster. Diseases of the Immune System. Robbins Basic Pathology. 10th Edition. 2018. Elsevier.)

Table 6.14 Defects in Innate Immunity

Disease	Abnormality
Defects in Leucocyte Function	
Leucocyte adhesion deficiency 1	Defective leucocyte adhesion because of mutations in β chain of CD11/CD18 integrins
Leucocyte adhesion deficiency 2	Defective leucocyte adhesion because of mutations in fucosyltransferase required for synthesis of sialylated oligosaccharide, which are the receptors for selectins
Chédiak–Higashi syndrome	Decreased leucocyte functions because of mutations affecting proteins involved in lysosomal membrane trafficking
Chronic granulomatous disease • X-linked	Decreased oxidative burst • Phagocyte oxidase (membrane component)
• Autosomal recessive	• Phagocyte oxidase (cytoplasmic component)
Myeloperoxidase deficiency	Decreased microbial killing because of defective MPO–H_2O_2 system
Defects in the Complement System	
C2, C4 deficiency	Defective classical pathway activation results in reduced resistance to infection and reduced clearance of immune complexes
C3 deficiency	Defects in all complement functions
Deficiency of complement regulatory proteins	Excessive complement activation Clinical syndromes include angio-oedema, paroxysmal nocturnal haemoglobinuria

to the abnormal fusion of phagolysosome, giant granules are seen in neutrophils (Dohle bodies), platelets and melanocytes. Partial oculocutaneous albinism and bleeding tendency are common findings because of abnormality of granules of melanocytes and platelets, respectively.

- **Chronic granulomatous disease** is a group of inherited disorders characterized by microbial degradation because of defects in the genes coding the components of NADPH phagocytic oxidase, the enzyme that acts and liberates superoxide free radical required for the degradation of the phagocytosed microbe. As we have discussed in Chapter 3, NADPH oxidase enzyme is a complex made of membrane and cytoplasmic components that come together with the phagocytic stimuli and act as a single unit. X-linked defect of chronic granulomatous disease leads to deficiency of membrane-bound components (gp-91phox) and the autosomal recessive defect leads to the deficiency of cytoplasmic components (p47phox and p67phox) of the enzyme complex. The disease is microscopically characterized by macrophage-rich chronic inflammatory reaction that tries to control the infection as neutrophils fail to do so. Such collections of activated macrophages form granulomas and hence the disease derived its name.

Defects in Complement System Deficiencies of every component of the complement system including the regulatory proteins have been described, but the common ones are discussed here.

- **C2 deficiency** is the most common complement protein deficiency. Deficiency of C2 or C4, the early components of the classical pathway, is associated with increased bacterial or viral infections. In the presence of an intact alternate pathway, however, many patients have no clinical manifestations. The predominant manifestation in these patients is SLE-like autoimmune disorder, because the classical pathway is required for clearance of activated immune complexes. Defective clearance of immune complexes is the proposed mechanism for the development of such autoimmune disorders.
- **C3 deficiency** is associated with recurrent and life-threatening pyogenic infections, because C3 is a component of both classical and alternate pathways. There is also an increased incidence of immune complex diseases like glomerulonephritis.
- **Properdin and factor D deficiencies** are associated with recurrent pyogenic infections but are rare.
- **C5, C6, C7, C8 and C9 deficiencies** are associated with increased susceptibility to recurrent gonococcal and meningococcal infections, because these complement proteins are components of the membrane attack complex required to lyse the thin walls of *Neisseria*.
- **Mannose-binding lectin defect** is associated with an increased susceptibility to infections.

- **C1 inhibitor (C1INH) deficiency** is associated with hereditary angio-oedema, because this regulator protein is involved in the inhibition of factor XII and kallikrein system apart from C1. The uninhibited kallikrein leads to overproduction of bradykinin, which is a potent vasodilator and causes life-threatening oedema of the skin, larynx and GI tract.
- **CD55-, CD59- and C8-binding protein deficiency:** CD55-, CD59- and C8-binding proteins are regulators of complement and their deficiency is associated with the development of paroxysmal nocturnal haemoglobinuria (PNH), a form of haemolytic anaemia (discussed in Chapter 15).

Defects in Adaptive Immunity

Adaptive immunity defects are further classified into B-cell defects/T-cell defects or both. The defects can be abnormalities of lymphocyte maturation or activation.

1. **SCID**

   SCID is a group of genetically heterogeneous diseases that have in common combined defects in both cell-mediated and humoral immune responses. The primary defect lies at the level of T cells, and this secondarily affects the B cells, resulting in the severe and combined clinical picture. Children born with this defect develop oral thrush because of candidiasis, extensive diaper rash, with extreme susceptibility to a wide range of pathogens, and failure to thrive. Graft-versus-host disease (GVHD) may also develop because of transplacental transfer of maternal T cells to the fetus. Without HSC transplantation, death of the child occurs before 1 year. There are two forms of SCID – X-linked and autosomal–recessive.

   X-linked SCID: This is the most common form of SCID because of mutation of the common γ chain (γc) subunit of cytokine receptors. This is a component of the receptors for a wide range of cytokines that include IL-2, IL-4, IL-7, IL-9, IL-11, IL-15 and IL-21. Signals from these receptors, especially IL-7, are crucial for the survival and proliferation of T-cell precursors. Absence of such signals leads to significant defect in the development of lymphocytes.

   Autosomal–recessive SCID is commonly because of deficiency of the enzyme *adenosine deaminase (ADA),* which leads to the accumulation of the substrate deoxyadenosine and its derivative deoxy-ATP that are toxic to the immature lymphocytes. Several other less common causes of SCID such as mutations of RAG genes, JAK3 and many other signalling molecules have been described.

   The net result in all the forms of SCID is reduced numbers of T cells with functionally defective B cells (although their quantity is normal). The thymus is small and devoid of lymphoid cells, with other lymphoid tissues being hypoplastic.

   HSC transplantation is the main modality of treatment, but gene therapy has been successfully tried in X-linked SCID. ADA deficiency can be treated with enzyme replacement therapy.
2. **X-linked agammaglobulinaemia (Bruton agammaglobulinaemia)**

   X-linked agammaglobulinaemia, also called Bruton agammaglobulinaemia, is a common form of primary immunodeficiency characterized by the inability of the B-cell precursors to develop into mature B cells because of deficiency of the Bruton tyrosine kinase (BTK) enzyme, the gene for which is located at Xq21.22. The function of this enzyme is essential for the development of BCR complex over B cells and also for proliferation and survival of B cells. In Bruton agammaglobulinaemia, maturation of B cells is arrested and proliferation is inhibited because of the deficiency of BTK enzyme.

   As the disease is X linked, it is seen almost exclusively in males, with few exceptions. The disease manifests with recurrent bacterial infections usually 6 months after birth when the maternal immunoglobulins are depleted. The causative organisms are always capsulated bacteria, such as *Haemophilus influenzae*, *Streptococcus pneumoniae* or *Staphylococcus aureus,* and viruses such as enteroviruses, which are normally neutralized and cleared by opsonizing antibodies and phagocytosis. Owing to the deficiency of mucosal IgA seen in Bruton disease, intestinal pathogens like *Giardia lamblia* cause recurrent illness.

   The disease is characterized by the following features:
   - Normal numbers of pre-B cells
   - Absent or reduced B cells in blood
   - B-cell regions of lymphoid organs being hypoplastic
   - Reduced serum levels of all classes of immunoglobulins
   - Normal T-cell counts, T-cell regions and T-cell responses

   In addition, a significant number of these patients develop autoimmune disorders like arthritis because of breakdown of self-tolerance and chronic infections in the face of immunodeficiency. Patients are treated with immunoglobulin replacement therapy and may reach adulthood.
3. **DiGeorge syndrome**

   DiGeorge syndrome, also called thymic hypoplasia, is because of the failure of thymus development and hence results in T-cell deficiency. The thymus is a derivative of *third and fourth pharyngeal pouches* along with parathyroids, some of the C cells of the thyroid and the ultimobranchial body. In the majority of cases, DiGeorge syndrome is because of deletion of gene at chromosome **22q11**. One such gene is **TBX1**, which is essential for the branchial arch and great vessel development.

   The disease has the following characteristic features:
   - Recurrent fungal and viral infections because of loss of T-cell-mediated immunity

- Reduced numbers of T cells in the blood
- T-cell regions of the lymphoid organs that are hypoplastic
- Normal numbers of B cells but with defective function
- Tetany because of the absence of parathyroids
- Congenital defects of the heart and great vessels because of the absence of ultimobranchial body
- Abnormal appearance of the face, eyes and ears

4. **Hyper-IgM syndrome**
Hyper-IgM syndrome is because of defect in the activation of B cells. Let us review three events in the activation of B cells, dendritic cells and macrophages that happen normally before discussing the pathogenesis and the features of the disease.
   - B cells are activated by antigen-activated T cells by CD40–CD40L interaction between B cells and T cells.
   - CD40 is also expressed by dendritic cells and macrophages, and their interaction with $CD4^+$ cells is crucial for their activities.
   - The function of activation-induced cytidine deaminase (**AID**), a DNA editing enzyme, is essential for class switching and affinity maturation (explained earlier).

   In hyper-IgM syndrome, there is either absence of CD40L on $CD4^+$ T cells or deficiency of AID enzyme because of loss-of-function mutations.
   The characteristic features of this disease are the following:
   - Elevated levels of IgM antibodies
   - Reduced levels of IgG, IgA and IgE antibodies
   - Normal numbers of B and T cells
   - Ineffective macrophages and dendritic cells
   - Impaired cell-mediated and humoral immunity
   - Patients presenting with recurrent pyogenic infections
   - Development of autoimmune haemolytic anaemia, thrombocytopenia and neutropenia because of aberrant activity of IgM
   - Infiltration of plasma cells in the mucosa of the GI tract
5. **Common variable immunodeficiency (CVID)**
CVID is a relatively common disease that may be inherited or sporadic. This disease occurs because of inability of the B cells to differentiate into plasma cells, which may be because of intrinsic B-cell defects or $CD4^+$ T-cell defects. Many cases are associated with the loss-of-function mutation of either the gene that codes for BAFF, a cytokine receptor that plays a key role in the differentiation and survival of B cells, or the gene that codes for inducible costimulator (ICOS), which is involved in T-cell activation and T- and B-cell interactions.
The characteristic features of the disease are the following:
   - Hypogammaglobulinaemia involving all classes of antibody
   - Normal or near-normal numbers of B cells in blood
   - Hyperplastic B-cell regions in lymphoid organs because of proliferation of B cells but showing defective maturation in response to an antigen
   - Recurrent pyogenic and enteroviral infections
   - Increased incidence of autoimmune diseases
   - Increased incidence of lymphoid malignancies
6. **IgA deficiency**
Isolated IgA deficiency is a common immunodeficiency in most populations across the world with an incidence of 1 in 600 persons in the United States, although it is less common in Africans and Asians. In most cases, the exact cause is unknown, whereas, in some cases, the disease is because of defective BAFF, the receptor for B-cell-activating cytokine.
The characteristic features of the disease are the following:
   - Extremely low levels of serum and secretory IgA
   - Normal serum levels of other classes of immunoglobulins
   - Defective mucosal immunity
   - Recurrent respiratory, GI and urogenital tract infections
   - Increased incidence of allergic and autoimmune diseases
   - Severe anaphylactic reaction following transfusion of blood containing normal IgA
7. **X-linked lymphoproliferative disease**
X-linked lymphoproliferative disease is characterized by the selective inability to eliminate EBV, leading to a severe form of infectious mononucleosis and B-cell lymphomas. In the majority of cases, the disorder is because of mutations in the gene that codes for serum amyloid P-component (SAP). SAP is an adapter protein that is involved in the activation of NK, T and B cells. It is also essential for the development of follicular helper T cells and hence the disease is characterized by absent or poorly formed germinal centres and failure to form high-affinity antibodies. For reasons still not known, there is no increased incidence of other viral infections.

Immunodeficiencies Associated with Systemic Diseases

1. **Ataxia-telangiectasia**
Ataxia-telangiectasia is an autosomal recessive disorder because of mutation of the gene located on the chromosome 11 that codes for the protein ATM. ATM is involved in stabilizing the DNA, sensing DNA damage and orchestrating the apoptosis of the cells with damaged DNA and DNA recombination events like immunoglobulin isotype switching. The role played by ATM in prevention of tumour development is discussed in Chapter 7. Defective DNA repair and accumulation of damaged DNA occur in the absence of ATM.

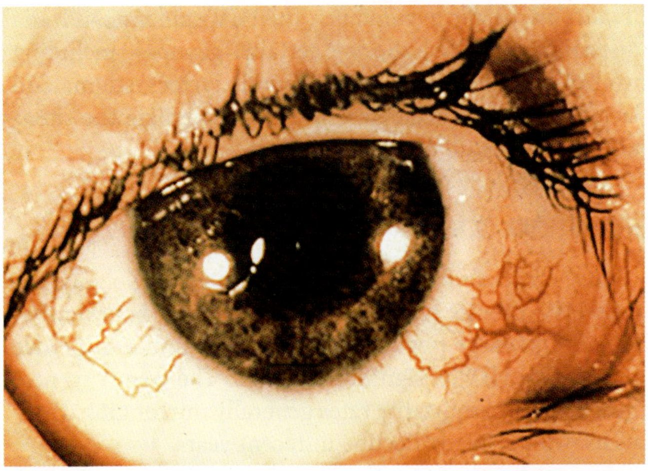

Fig. 6.29 Ataxia-telangiectasia. Characteristic telangiectasias in the bulbar conjunctiva usually develop in those aged between 3 months and 6 years. (*Source:* From Rajiv Varma and Shelley D. Williams. Neurology. Zitelli and Davis' Atlas of Pediatric Physical Diagnosis. 7th edition. Elsevier 2018.)

The disease is characterized by the following features:

- Ataxia (abnormal gait)
- Telangiectasias (vascular malformations) (Fig. 6.29)
- Neurological deficits
- Immunodeficiency – mostly humoral (deficiency of IgA and IgG2) but may also be combined
- Frequent infections
- Higher incidence of autoimmune diseases
- Increased incidence of tumours with advancing age

2. **Wiskott–Aldrich syndrome**
Wiskott–Aldrich syndrome is an X-linked disorder because of mutation in the gene located at Xp11.23 that codes for Wiskott–Aldrich syndrome protein, WASP. WASP plays a role in linking antigen receptors with cytoskeletal proteins and is involved in cytoskeleton-dependent responses like signal transduction and cell migration. The exact function of WASP relevant to lymphocytes and platelets is still not clear. HSC offers cure.
The characteristic features of the disease are the following:
   - Recurrent infections because of defects in cellular immunity
   - Thrombocytopenia
   - Eczema
   - Ineffective humoral response
   - Low serum IgM and normal IgG levels
   - Elevated serum IgA and IgE levels
   - Higher incidence of lymphomas

SECONDARY IMMUNODEFICIENCY

Secondary immune deficiencies or acquired deficiencies, as a group, are more frequent than primary immune deficiencies and are caused by severe malnutrition, chronic diseases such as uncontrolled diabetes, immunosuppressive medications, chemotherapy and certain malignancies such as leukaemia. Immunodeficient state is common in people having defective lymphocytic maturation, inadequate immunoglobulin synthesis or depleted lymphocytes because of certain infections or drugs. The mechanisms of the common causes of secondary immunodeficiency are listed in Table 6.15.

Table 6.15 Causes of Secondary Immunodeficiency

Disease	Mechanism
HIV infection	Loss of $CD4^+$ helper T cells
Chemotherapy	Bone marrow suppression
Radiotherapy	Bone marrow suppression
Leukaemias	Suppression of normal haematopoietic elements
Metastatic deposits in bone marrow	Suppression of normal haematopoietic elements
Malnutrition	Inhibition of lymphocyte maturation and function
Drugs	Lymphocyte depletion
Infections	Lymphocyte depletion
Splenectomy	Reduced phagocytosis
Diabetes	Multifactorial

HIV, human immunodeficiency virus.

ACQUIRED IMMUNODEFICIENCY SYNDROME PA 9.6

AIDS, caused by the retrovirus, HIV, a lentivirus that can be transmitted between individuals, is the most common secondary immunodeficiency disease. It is characterized by profound immunosuppression that leads to opportunistic infections, secondary neoplasms and neurological manifestations.

GLOBAL OVERVIEW

Prevalence: As of the latest reports, more than 38 million people worldwide live with HIV/AIDS, with Sub-Saharan Africa bearing the brunt of the epidemic. A notable prevalence is also observed in various regions, including Eastern Europe, Central Asia and parts of Latin America.
New infections: Annually, about 1.5 million new HIV infections are reported globally. The rate of new infections has shown a declining trend in many regions because of improved awareness and preventive strategies, although some areas still report rising numbers.

Mortality: Globally, HIV/AIDS-related deaths have significantly decreased from their peak in the early 2000s, largely because of the widespread availability of effective ART. However, mortality rates remain high in regions with limited access to these lifesaving treatments.

TRENDS OVER TIME

Historical perspective: HIV/AIDS first emerged as a global health issue in the early 1980s. Initially identified among specific high-risk groups, it quickly became evident that the virus could affect anyone. Over the decades, the pandemic has evolved, with varying patterns observed in different parts of the world.
Recent trends: The past few years have seen a global decrease in new HIV infections and AIDS-related deaths, largely attributable to the widespread availability of effective ART and improved access to HIV testing and prevention services.

TRANSMISSION MODES

Sexual transmission: The primary mode of HIV transmission globally is through unprotected sexual intercourse. The virus can be transmitted in both heterosexual and homosexual encounters, with the specifics of transmission dynamics varying by region and population.
Parenteral transmission: HIV can also be transmitted through exposure to infected blood, notably among intravenous drug users sharing needles. The transmission through blood transfusions has drastically reduced in regions where blood screening is rigorously practiced.
Mother-to-child transmission (MTCT): HIV can be transmitted from an infected mother to her child during pregnancy, childbirth or breastfeeding. However, the implementation of ART during pregnancy and delivery, and to the newborn, has significantly reduced the rates of MTCT.

EPIDEMIOLOGY IN INDIA

Prevalence in India: India has an estimated 2.1 million people living with HIV, making it one of the largest HIV-positive populations in the world. The prevalence rate is around 0.22%, which is lower than that in many other countries but still significant because of the large population base.
Regional variations: The epidemic in India shows substantial regional variation, with the highest prevalence rates found in the southern and northeastern states. States like Andhra Pradesh, Karnataka, Maharashtra and Manipur have reported higher rates compared with the national average.
Transmission patterns: In India, heterosexual transmission accounts for the majority of new HIV infections. However, there are significant transmission rates among key populations, including sex workers, men who have sex with men and intravenous drug users.

Impact on specific populations: The HIV epidemic in India disproportionately affects certain groups, including women and children. Socioeconomic factors, stigma and lack of access to healthcare further exacerbate the situation for these vulnerable populations.

STATISTICAL COMPARISONS

Global versus Indian data: When compared globally, India's HIV prevalence rate is relatively low. However, because of its large population, the total number of people living with HIV is significantly high. The trends in new infections and mortality rates generally mirror global patterns, with a steady decline in recent years.
Temporal trends: Over the past decade, India has seen a decline in both new HIV infections and AIDS-related deaths. This is attributed to increased awareness, better access to ART and preventive measures.

ECONOMIC AND SOCIAL IMPACT

Healthcare burden: The HIV epidemic imposes a substantial burden on healthcare systems, both in India and globally. The cost of treatment and care, coupled with the loss of productivity because of illness, has significant economic implications.
Social implications: HIV/AIDS carries a heavy social stigma, which can lead to discrimination and marginalization of affected individuals. This stigma not only impacts the health and well-being of people living with HIV but also hampers effective response and prevention efforts.

HIV

HIV is a nontransforming human retrovirus belonging to the Lentivirus family. Two genetically different but related forms of HIV, called HIV-1 and HIV-2, have been isolated from patients with AIDS. HIV-1 is the most common type associated with AIDS in the United States, Europe and Central Africa, whereas HIV-2 causes a similar illness principally in West Africa and India. Specific tests for HIV-1 and HIV-2 are available, and blood collected for transfusion is routinely screened for both HIV-1 and HIV-2 seropositivity.

HIV is a spherical (80–110 nm), enveloped virus (Fig. 6.30). The envelope is made up of a lipid part derived from the host cell membrane and a protein part with two components – glycoprotein 120 (**gp120**), which are projected as knob-like spikes on the surface, and glycoprotein 41 (**gp41**), which forms the anchoring transmembrane pedicles. It also has an icosahedral nucleocapsid with a protein core. The inner core contains the following:

- The major capsid protein p24
- Nucleocapsid protein p7/p9
- Viral enzymes – integrase, reverse transcriptase and protease
- Two copies of viral genomic RNA

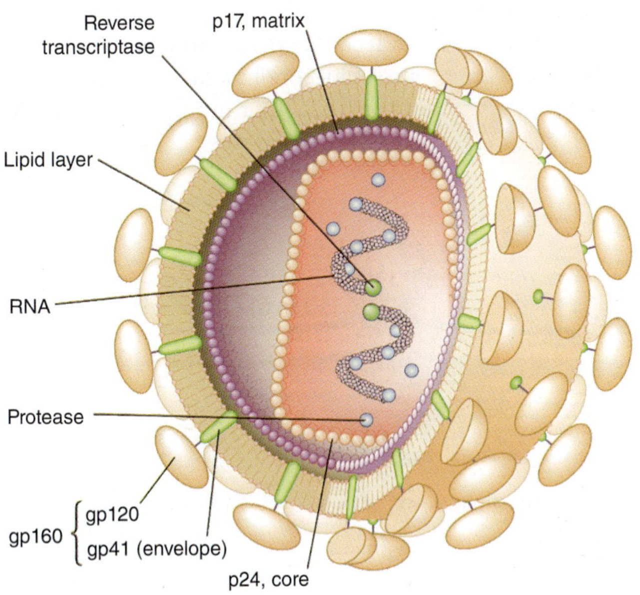

Fig. 6.30 Structure of HIV virion. Two molecules of single-stranded RNA are shown within the nucleus. The reverse transcriptase polymerase converts viral RNA into DNA (a characteristic of retroviruses). The protease includes integrase (p32 and p10). The p24 (core protein) levels can be used to monitor HIV disease. p17 is the matrix protein; gp120 is the outer envelope glycoprotein that binds to cell surface CD4 molecules; and gp41, a transmembrane protein, influences infectivity and cell fusion capacity. HIV, human immunodeficiency virus. (*Source:* From Janet D. Wilson and Jane Anderson. Sexually transmitted infections and human immunodeficiency virus. Kumar and Clark's Clinical Medicine. 10th edition. Elsevier. 2021.

HIV contains some structural and nonstructural genes:

1. **Structural genes:** Structural genes code for various components of the virus.
   - The **gag** gene codes for the core and shell of the virus where p7 constitutes the nucleocapsid and p24 and p15 constitute the core antigens.
   - The **pol** gene codes for viral enzymes such as reverse transcriptase, protease and integrase.
   - The **env** gene codes for the envelope glycoprotein (gp160), which is cleaved into two parts – gp120, which is the main receptor of HIV that binds to CD4 molecules on host cells and initiates infection, and gp41, the protein that promotes fusion.
2. **Nonstructural genes:** Nonstructural genes regulate viral replication and play a key role in the pathogenesis of HIV. HIV contains several other accessory genes, including tat, rev, vif, nef, vpr and vpu.
   For example, tat is a transcriptional activation gene that is essential for HIV-1 replication. nef (negative factor gene) downregulates CD4 receptor expression on the cell surface of infected T cells, thereby enhancing release of virions and infectivity of other cells, and vif (viral infectivity factor gene) influences the infectivity of viral particles.

Antigenic variation and diversity: HIV shows extensive antigenic diversity because of high rates of mutation that is believed to be because of the error-prone nature of reverse transcriptase enzyme and the mutation-prone env gene against which antibodies are produced, making development of vaccine against HIV extremely difficult.

Life Cycle of HIV

Receptor Attachment and Replication of Virus (Fig. 6.31)

HIV infects cells through the CD4 molecule by using it as a receptor and various chemokine receptors as coreceptors. The requirement for CD4 binding explains the selective tropism of the virus for $CD4^+$ T cells and other $CD4^+$ cells like monocytes/macrophages and dendritic cells. Chemokine receptors, particularly CCR5 and CXCR4, serve as coreceptors for HIV.

There are two types of HIV on the basis of their use of the coreceptors:

1. **R5 strains** use CCR5 and preferentially infect cells of the monocyte/macrophage lineage, hence referred to as **M-tropic**. These strains are dominant in acute infection.
2. **X4 strains** use CXCR4 and are **T-tropic**, preferentially infecting T cells. These strains are dominant in the chronic phase of infection.

The HIV envelope contains two noncovalently associated glycoproteins, surface gp120 and the transmembrane protein gp41. The initial step in infection is the binding of the gp120 envelope glycoprotein to CD4, which leads to a conformational change that produces a new recognition site on gp120 for the coreceptors CCR5 or CXCR4.

- DC-SIGN, a dendritic cell–specific lectin receptor present in the skin and mucosal surfaces, can also bind to HIV-1 that facilitates the transport of HIV by dendritic cells to lymphoid organs where HIV replicates further in T cells.

The events that follow receptor and coreceptor attachment are as follows:

- **Fusion:** Fusion of HIV to host cell takes place by gp41, the fusion protein after the $CD4^+$–gp120 attachment. However, HIV can infect only activated T cells and memory T cells, whereas naive T cells remain resistant to infection.
- **Penetration and uncoating:** After fusion, HIV nucleocapsid enters the host cell cytoplasm, followed by uncoating and release of two copies of ssRNA and viral enzymes.
- **Reverse transcription:** Viral reverse transcriptase mediates transcription of its ssRNA into ssDNA so that DNA–RNA hybrid is formed. RNA is degraded by viral endonuclease, and ssDNA replicates to form dsDNA, which then forms proteins by transcription.

The nucleoprotein complex thus formed comprises linear dsDNA, gag matrix protein, accessory vpr protein and viral integrase. This is called preintegration complex, which is transported into the host cell nucleus.

- **Integration:** The viral dsDNA gets integrated into the host cell chromosome with the help of viral integrase to

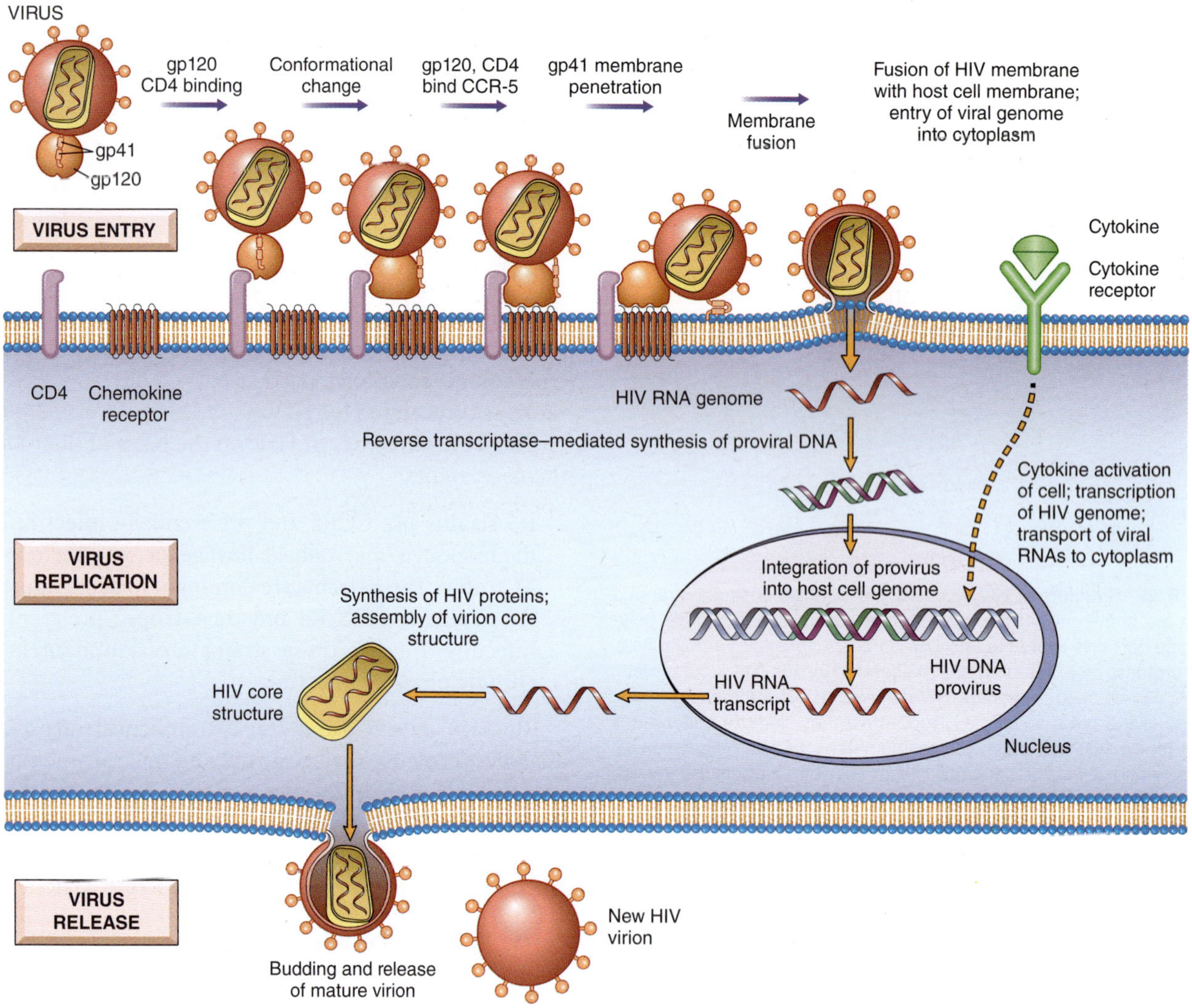

Fig. 6.31 The life cycle of HIV showing the steps from viral entry to production of infectious virions. HIV, human immunodeficiency virus. (*Source:* From Vinay Kumar, Abul K. Abbas and Jon C. Aster. Diseases of the Immune System. Robbins Basic Pathology. 10th edition. Elsevier 2018.)

form the provirus, which may remain latent for several months to years.

- **Latency:** HIV is different in that it is able to replicate even in the latent state and is infectious to other neighbouring cells, killing the infected cells because of extensive viral budding.

Completion of the life cycle of the virus occurs only after cell activation of $CD4^+$ cells, which most often leads to cell lysis. Even with potent antiviral therapy, the memory $CD4^+$ T cells affected by then remain latent in the lymph nodes for months to years.

Pathogenesis (Fig. 6.32) HIV predominantly affects two important systems of the human body:

1. Immune system
2. Central nervous system

HIV Infection of the Immune System Binding of NF-κB to sequences within the promoter regions of genes is required to activate the transcription of HIV proviral DNA for increasing the virion production, virion release and cell lysis. Hence, conditions that upregulate NF-κB help in the survival and proliferation of the virus in the host. These conditions include the following:

- Antigens or cytokines that upregulate transcription factors like NF-κB, which stimulate transcription of genes encoding cytokines such as IL-2 and its receptor, which in resting T cells is held inactive in the cytoplasm.
- TNF and other cytokines produced during physiological activation of macrophages also stimulate NF-κB activity.
- HIV-infected people are at an increased risk for recurrent exposure to other infections, which also lead to increased lymphocyte activation and production of proinflammatory cytokines.

HIV affects the T and non–T cells, resulting in profound immune suppression.

Mechanism of T-Cell Depletion HIV exerts its effect on the memory and activated T cells and lyses around 2 billion CD4 T cells (cytopathic effect of the virus), but it cannot

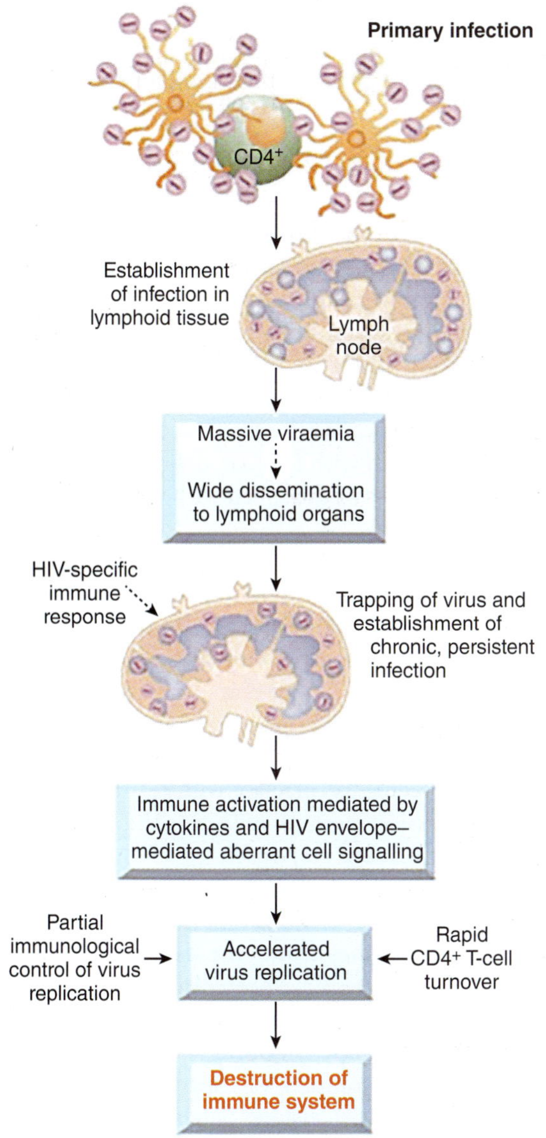

Fig. 6.32 Pathogenesis of HIV infection. HIV, human immunodeficiency virus. (*Source:* Illustrated by Katie Ris. From Anthony S Fauci. HIV and AIDS: 20 years of science. Nature. 2003: 9;839–843.

infect the naive T cells. This is because the naive T cells contain an enzyme APOBEC3G that causes cytosine-to-uracil DNA mutations that prevent further replication. But in the activated T cells, this gene is degraded by proteases regulated by the vif gene.

When $CD4^+$ cells are lost in the beginning, up to a point, the immune system replaces this loss and hence the number of cells may appear normal or even falsely higher for a certain period of time. In addition to direct cytopathic effect by viral budding, interference of protein synthesis and various other mechanisms mentioned later contribute to loss of T cells:

- Apoptosis-induced cell death by chronic activation of infected cells
- Progressive destruction of lymphoid architecture and cellular composition
- Pyroptosis of infected cells by activation of inflammasome pathway
- Qualitative defects in T cells and loss of Th1 response
- Direct infection of thymic progenitor cells
- Improper production of cytokines required for activation of T cells
- Fusion of infected and uninfected cells with the formation of syncytia (giant cells), which can occur because gp120 expressed on infected cells binds to CD4 molecules on uninfected T cells, followed by cell fusion and cell death

Infection of Non-T Cells In addition, HIV affects the macrophages, dendritic cells, B cells and neural cells.

Macrophages: HIV mainly infects the terminally differentiated macrophages, which may not replicate further, with the help of vpr gene that induces the formation of preintegration complex. Some may bud virions from the intracellular vacuoles and act as reservoirs of infection, especially in the later stages when CD4 levels are low. This is possible because macrophages are comparatively resistant to their cytopathic effects. Such infected monocytes show decreased chemotaxis, reduced cytokine production, impaired microbial resistance, etc.

Dendritic cells: Mucosal dendritic cells through a lectin receptor bind to HIV and carry the virus to the lymph nodes to present it to the CD4 cells. The viral particles bind to the processes of the FDCs. FDCs have receptors for the Fc portion of immunoglobulins and hence they trap HIV virions coated with anti-HIV antibodies. The antibody-coated virions localized to FDCs retain the ability to infect $CD4^+$ T cells as they traverse the intricate meshwork formed by the dendritic processes of the FDCs.

B cells: HIV-specific activation of B cells is induced by the ongoing HIV replication leading to B-cell hyperplasia in lymph nodes, plasma cell increase in the bone marrow and hypergammaglobulinaemia. But a state of decreased B-cell responses to specific immunogens and non-HIV pathogens prevails because of improper T-cell activation and intrinsic B cells. Apart from these, B cells are affected by infection with EBV and CMV, overexpression of gp41 and increased cytokine production.

HIV Infection of the Central Nervous System Macrophages from the lymph nodes affect the microglia in the brain. As neurons are not infected by HIV, the extent of neuropathological changes is often less than that might be expected from the extreme clinical manifestation. Neurological deficit is caused indirectly by viral products and by cytokines like IL-1, TNF and IL-6 along with nitric oxide (induced by fusion protein) and certain molecules that are secreted.

Course of HIV Infection Following mucosal infection, the clinical picture of HIV infection is divided into three major phases:

1. Acute retroviral syndrome
2. Middle chronic phase
3. AIDS

1. **Acute HIV disease or acute retroviral syndrome**
   During entry of HIV, the mucosal lymphoid tissues are the primary target and are associated with death of a large number of mucosal T cells that form the major compartment of T cells in the body. This occurs because of the damaged epithelium and failure of mucosal barriers. Then the virus spills over into bloodstream to cause primary viraemia, affecting all helper T cells, dendritic cells and macrophages (or acute mononucleosis-like syndrome), and this coincides with an initial flu-like illness that occurs in many patients (50%–75%) 3–6 weeks after the primary infection and resolves in the next 2–4 weeks. There is a significant drop in the numbers of circulating CD4 T cells to around 10^9 cells at this stage.
2. **Middle chronic phase or phase of clinical latency**
   The next clinical phase can be asymptomatic or may have persistent generalized lymphadenopathy (PGL) or develop symptoms because of minor opportunistic infections.
   Asymptomatic stage
   Adequate humoral (neutralizing antibodies) and cell-mediated immune (CD8 T cells) response develops within 1 month in most of the patients. As a result, viraemia drops down and CD4 T-cell count becomes normal, marking initial containment of the virus. It is important to note that this is a state of clinical latency but not of microbiological latency. The immune response cannot clear the HIV infection completely as HIV-infected cells persist in the lymph nodes, and there is a high level of ongoing viral replication. However, once the latency is broken, the disease progresses rapidly and death usually occurs within 2 years if left untreated. The HIV–RNA levels are used to find the disease progression, and this equilibrium between the viral load and the host response marks the *viral set point*.
   PGL
   As a result of HIV replication in lymph nodes, 25%–30% of asymptomatic but infected people develop lymphadenopathy more than 1 cm in size at one or more noncontiguous sites that persist for at least 3 months. PGL must be distinguished from other causes of lymphadenopathies such as lymphoma.
3. **AIDS**
   After a variable period of clinical latency, the CD4 T-cell level starts falling. On the basis of the count, it is classified into three categories: $CD4^+$ cells greater than or equal to 500 cells/μL, 200–499 cells/μL, and fewer than 200 cells/μL. Eventually patients develop constitutional symptoms such as unexplained diarrhoea lasting for more than 1 month, weight loss of more than 10% of body weight, fatigue, malaise and night sweats.
   Gradually, the patient moves towards the advanced end stage of HIV infection called AIDS, often within 7–10 years in the absence of any treatment. It is characterized by a rapid fall in CD4 T-cell count (usually <200 cells/μL), and the host defence drops as the number of infected cells and the viral burden increase.
   HIV escapes the host response by various means such as destruction of the $CD4^+$ T cells that are critical for effective immunity, antigenic variation and downmodulation of class I MHC molecules on infected cells so that viral antigens are not recognized by $CD8^+$ CTLs.
   A coreceptor switch idea was proposed in which the virus relying solely on CCR5 to enter its target cells starts relying on either CXCR4 or both CCR5 and CXCR4, which causes further infection.
   Patients infected with HIV are divided into two categories, on the basis of the speed with which they progress to AIDS:
   - **Rapid progressors:** These patients progress to AIDS within 2–3 years.
   - **Long-term nonprogressors:** These patients remain asymptomatic with stable $CD4^+$ and low viral load even after 10 years (*elite controllers* – those with undetectable plasma virus). The inheritance of particular HLA alleles to maintain high T-cell levels seems to correlate with resistance to disease progression, perhaps reflecting the ability to mount antiviral T-cell responses.

Clinical Features The clinical manifestations range from acute to severe illness, and the features of acute and chronic middle phases have been discussed in the previous sections. Here, we discuss the common signs and symptoms of the final phase, AIDS. It should be stressed here that the symptom complex varies greatly with geographical distribution. A typical adult patient with AIDS presents with fever, weight loss, diarrhoea, generalized lymphadenopathy, multiple opportunistic infections, neurological disease and, in many cases, secondary neoplasms. At present, the various combinations of antiviral therapy have reduced the overall risk of disease progression.

A list of AIDS-defining opportunistic infections and tumours in patients with HIV is given in Table 6.16.

Clinical features of AIDS are discussed under three headings – opportunistic infections, tumours and CNS involvement.

Opportunistic Infections

Opportunistic infections such as oral candidiasis (thrush), vaginal candidiasis and herpes zoster set in secondary to profound immune suppression and may be associated with extensive mycobacterial tuberculosis or some neoplasms. Depending on the CD4 T-cell count, various infections occur.

Many of these infections represent reactivation of latent infections, which are normally kept in check by our immune system but are not completely eradicated,

Table 6.16 AIDS-Defining Opportunistic Infections and Tumours in Patients Infected with HIV

1. Infections	
Protozoal and helminthic infections	*Cryptosporidium* or *Cystoisospora* (enteritis) *Pneumocystis* (pneumonia or disseminated infection) *Toxoplasma* (pneumonia or CNS infection)
Fungal infections	*Candida* (oesophageal, tracheal or pulmonary) *Cryptococcus* (CNS infection) *Coccidioides* (disseminated) *Histoplasma* (disseminated)
Bacterial infections	*Mycobacterium* ('atypical', e.g. *Mycobacterium avium-intracellulare*, disseminated or extrapulmonary; *Mycobacterium tuberculosis*, pulmonary or extrapulmonary) *Nocardia* (pneumonia, meningitis, disseminated) *Salmonella* infections, disseminated
Viral infections	Cytomegalovirus (pulmonary, intestinal, retinitis or CNS infections) Herpes simplex virus (localized or disseminated infection) Varicella-zoster virus (localized or disseminated infection) Progressive multifocal leucoencephalopathy
2. Neoplasms	Kaposi sarcoma Primary lymphoma of brain Invasive cancer of the uterine cervix

AIDS, acquired immunodeficiency syndrome; CNS, central nervous system; HIV, human immunodeficiency virus.

because the infectious agents have evolved to coexist with the hosts or remain latent. About 60%–70% of deaths in patients with HIV can be contributed to these opportunistic infections, which includes the following:

Candidiasis: Candidiasis is caused by *Candida,* affecting the skin, nails and mucous membranes of the bronchi, mouth, oesophagus and vagina, and its appearance indicates transformation in otherwise asymptomatic people.
CMV infection: CMV mainly infects patients with very low titre of CD4 count and can infect multiple parts of the body, causing pneumonia, gastroenteritis or mucosal ulcerations, encephalitis and sight-threatening retinitis or chorioretinitis.
Mycobacterium infection: Atypical tuberculosis caused by atypical mycobacteria, *M. tuberculosis,* can either remain localized in the lungs or get disseminated to the larynx, lymph nodes, etc., and is more common in those with very low $CD4^+$ count. *Mycobacterium avium* **complex (MAC)** or *Mycobacterium kansasii* is a major contributor of pulmonary and extrapulmonary infections in patients with AIDS. The scary part of increased mycobacterial infections in patients with AIDS is the rising incidence of resistance to antitubercular drugs.
JC virus infection: JC virus is a human papova-like virus that causes **progressive multifocal leucoencephalopathy** which is fatal. Symptoms may include loss of muscle control, paralysis, blindness, speech problems and an altered mental state.
Salmonella infection: Septicaemia induced by *Salmonella* seen in patients with AIDS is a severe form of infection in which the bacteria exceed the immune system's ability to control them. Diarrhoea is the predominant symptom which may also be caused by other enteric bacteria like *Shigella* and *Cryptosporidium.*
Infection by other organisms: *Coccidioides immitis* is most commonly acquired by inhaling the spores, which can lead to pneumonia that is sometimes called desert fever, San Joaquin Valley fever or valley fever. Similarly, *Pneumocystis jirovecii* may cause pneumonia in around 15% of untreated patients along with *Cryptococcus, Toxoplasma gondii, Histoplasma capsulatum,* CMV, etc. *Cryptococcus* can also spread to the brain, causing cryptococcal meningitis. It can also infect the skin, bones or urinary tract. *T. gondii* causes encephalitis and is responsible for 50% of all HIV-related mass lesions in CNS. *Persistent diarrhoea,* which is commonly seen in untreated patients with advanced AIDS, is often caused by infections with protozoans such as *Cryptosporidium, Isospora belli* or microsporidia. These patients present with chronic, profuse, watery diarrhoea. Herpes simplex virus in patients with AIDS can also cause bronchitis, pneumonia and oesophagitis.

Tumours

In total, 25%–40% of HIV-infected patients may present with associated malignancies. This group includes the three AIDS-defining malignancies: high-grade B-cell non-Hodgkin lymphoma (NHL), Kaposi sarcoma (KS) and invasive cervical cancer.

KS: This vascular neoplasm is caused by a virus called Kaposi sarcoma herpesvirus (KSHV) or human herpesvirus 8 (HHV-8) and is the most common of all the tumours in HIV-infected patients. HIV is the major cofactor without which KSHV cannot progress to forming KS lesions. KS appears as firm pink or purple spots on the skin that can be raised or flat. It can be life-threatening and more aggressive in HIV cases than the classical KS seen in non-HIV-infected patients, because it is widespread and affects multiple organs.
Lymphomas: Immune suppression rather than HIV itself is implicated in the pathogenesis of an increased incidence of lymphomas and other non-AIDS-defining malignancies, including Hodgkin lymphoma, which is seen

at a 10-fold higher rate in patients with AIDS than in the normal population. Possible explanations are as follows:

- **T-cell immunodeficiency.**
  As explained by the mechanisms of T-cell depletion under pathogenesis above.
- **Unchecked proliferation of B cells:** Aggressive B-cell lymphoma infected by EBV-like oncogenic viruses develops, because T cells that generally restrain the proliferation of B cells are deficient. Patients with AIDS have high levels of cytokines IL-6, which are growth factors for B cells and activate them. In the absence of T-cell immunity, these activated EBV-infected clones proliferate and eventually acquire additional somatic mutations, leading to their outgrowth as full-blown EBV-positive B-cell lymphomas, which may extend to extranodal sites such as CNS, gut, lungs and eyes.
- **Germinal centre B-cell hyperplasia** (Fig. 6.33): Profound germinal centre B-cell hyperplasia may occur, diversifying immunoglobulin genes of B cells via lesions introduced into their DNA by the enzyme activation-induced cytidine deaminase (AID). This may extend to cause mutations in oncogenes implicated in B-cell lymphomagenesis. Mutations in oncogenes such as MYC and BCL6 lead to the development of Burkitt lymphoma and diffuse large B-cell lymphoma. Thus, the striking germinal centre B-cell hyperplasia that occurs early in HIV infection may contribute to lymphomagenesis by simply increasing the number of B cells that are 'at risk' for acquiring potential lymphoma-initiating events.

Cervical cancer is an AIDS-defining illness, because women living with HIV are commonly associated with squamous cell carcinoma of the cervix. Human papillomavirus (HPV) is more likely to cause preinvasive lesions of the cervix, squamous intraepithelial lesion (SIL), which can quickly progress to invasive cancer if left untreated. Women living with HIV infection are more likely to develop invasive cervical cancer and cervical dysplasia. This high risk of cervical cancer in patients with AIDS is attributed to the diminished immune surveillance.

CNS Involvement

Approximately half of the patients infected with HIV present with CNS manifestations, whereas around 90% of HIV-infected patients demonstrate some form of CNS involvement at autopsy. Complications of the nervous system can occur in more than 40% of patients with HIV infection. CNS is predominantly affected by lymphomas, and opportunistic infections as discussed in the earlier sections. CNS infections in HIV-positive persons contribute to 15%–25% of AIDS-related deaths. Two major causes of CNS opportunistic infections are tuberculous meningitis (TBM) and cryptococcal meningitis. Apart from these infections, aseptic meningitis and acute demyelinating polyneuropathy (AIDP) can be the presenting symptoms of acute HIV infection. Vacuolar myelopathy, peripheral neuropathy and progressive encephalopathy may also be associated.

Morphology

All the other lesions seen in AIDS are discussed in their respective chapters and here we discuss the morphology of lymph nodes in HIV infection.

Enlarged lymph nodes in the initial phases of HIV infection reveal marked hyperplasia of B-cell follicles. The follicles are enlarged, prominent and often serpiginous. The mantle zones that surround the follicles are often attenuated, and the germinal centres impinge on interfollicular T-cell zones. This stage represents the polyclonal B-cell activation that is seen in HIV-infected persons. As the disease advances, the phase of B-cell proliferation subsides and gives way to severe

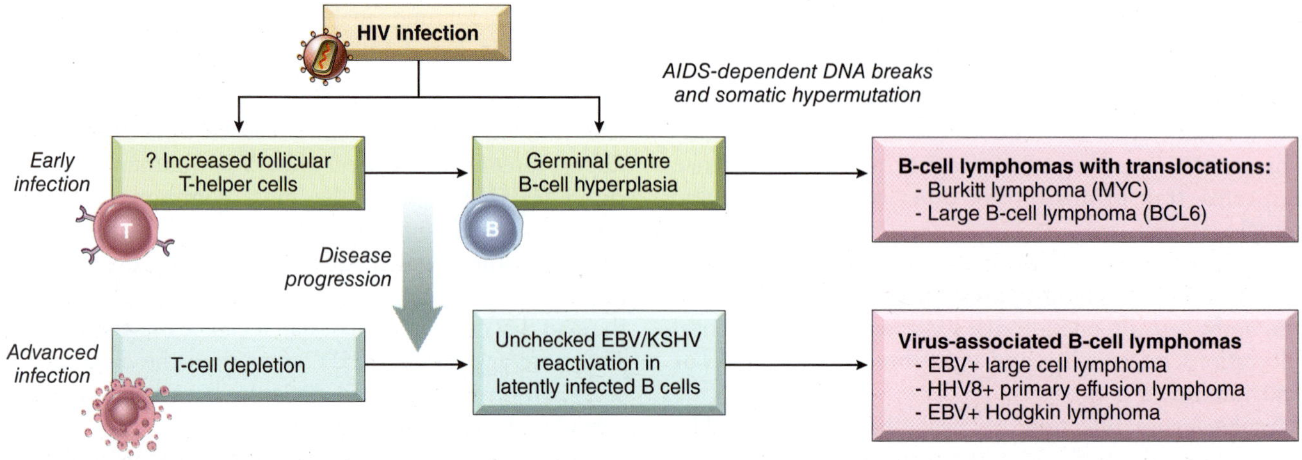

Fig. 6.33 A model for the pathogenesis of B-cell lymphomas in HIV infection. HIV infection results in several changes that may cooperate to produce B-cell lymphomas. An increase in T follicular helper cells early in the course of the disease is postulated, but its basis is unknown. HIV, human immunodeficiency virus. (*Source:* From Vinay Kumar, Abul K. Abbas and Jon C. Aster. Diseases of the Immune System. Robbins Basic Pathology. 10th edition. Elsevier 2018.)

lymphoid involution. The lymph nodes are depleted of lymphocytes, and the germinal centres may even become hyalinized. Such tiny, atrophic, '**burnt-out**' lymph nodes may have numerous opportunistic pathogens within the macrophages. Owing to severe immunosuppression, inflammatory responses to infections, both in the nodes and at the extranodal sites, may be sparse, absent or atypical. For example, mycobacteria may not evoke granuloma formation, because $CD4^+$ cells are deficient. Similar burnt-out changes are seen in the spleen and thymus.

Antiretroviral Drug Therapy

Antiretroviral medications prevent HIV from multiplying, thus protecting the cells that the virus would otherwise target. With the advent of highly active antiretroviral therapy (HAART), the incidence of lymphoma along with various opportunistic infections could be controlled and hence the mortality rate has fallen substantially in HIV-infected populations.

More than 25 antiretroviral drugs from 6 distinct drug classes have been developed for the management of HIV infection. When a combination of at least three effective drugs that target the enzymes or glycoproteins are used in a motivated, compliant patient, HIV replication can be reduced to below the level of detection and also be maintained for long periods. The rationale behind using three drugs is that even when a drug-resistant virus breaks through, there are several second- and third-line options to combat the virus. Once the virus is suppressed, the progressive loss of $CD4^+$ T cells is halted and gradually over a period of time, the peripheral blood $CD4^+$ T-cell count increases and often returns to normal levels.

A fraction of patients with HIV infection with advanced stage on antiretroviral therapy (ART) may develop a paradoxical deterioration of their clinical condition as their immune system recovers. This is referred to as *'immune reconstitution syndrome (IRIS)'*, which is associated with increasing $CD4^+$ T-cell count and decreasing viral load and is thought to be because of poorly controlled host response to the high burden of antigen from persistent microbes.

TRANSPLANT REJECTION REACTIONS PA 9.3

INTRODUCTION

Transplantation is the act of transferring cells, tissues or organs from one site to another, more commonly performed between different individuals. The failure of an organ system can be corrected with transplantation of a functioning organ (e.g. kidney, liver, heart or lung) from a donor. However, the immune system remains the most frightening barrier to offer transplantation as a routine treatment. As we have discussed in the earlier sections, the immune system has elaborate and effective mechanisms developed to handle and destroy foreign agents. The same mechanisms are involved in the rejection of transplanted organs, which are recognized as foreign by the recipient's immune system.

Understanding these mechanisms is essential, because it helps in identifying the clinical features of rejection and hence in making an early diagnosis and delivering appropriate management. Understanding these mechanisms is also crucial to develop strategies to minimize rejection and to develop new drugs and treatments that blunt or overcome the effects of the immune system on transplanted organs, thereby ensuring the success of transplantation.

TYPES OF GRAFT

The degree of immune response to a graft depends mainly on the degree of genetic disparity between the grafted organ and the host. The major antigenic differences between a donor and a recipient that result in rejection of transplants are because of the differences in HLA alleles between the donor and the recipient. HLA genes are highly polymorphic, so there are always some differences between all the individuals, except identical twins. Understanding the types of graft is essential before discussing the essence of transplant rejection.

- **Xenografts** are grafts between members of different species. They have the most disparity and elicit the maximal immune response and undergo rapid rejection.
- **Allografts** are grafts between members of the same species that differ genetically. This is the most common form of transplantation. The extent to which allografts undergo rejection depends on the degree of histocompatibility between the donor and the recipient.
- **Isografts**, which are grafts between genetically identical individuals (e.g. monozygotic twins), do not undergo rejection because of histocompatibility.
- **Autografts** are grafts from one part of the body to another of the same individual (e.g. skin grafts). They do not elicit rejection.

The extent and type of response also vary with the type of the transplanted tissue or organ. Organs such as the eyes and brain are immunologically privileged; these have minimal or no immune system cells and can tolerate even mismatched grafts. This is the reason behind the success rate of corneal transplant. Skin grafts are not initially vascularized and so do not manifest rejection until they establish blood supply. Heart, kidneys and liver are highly vascular organs, and transplantation of these organs leads to a vigorous cell-mediated response in the host.

METHODS TO IMPROVE AND PROLONG GRAFT SURVIVAL

The two most important methods to improve graft survival are as follows:

1. **HLA compatibility testing and matching**
   The value of HLA matching between the donor and the recipient is not uniform for all types of transplantation and varies with different solid organ transplants. In kidney transplants, there is substantial benefit if all the polymorphic HLA alleles are matched. However, HLA matching is usually not performed for transplants of the liver, heart and lungs because other considerations such as anatomic compatibility, severity of the underlying illness and the need to minimize the time of organ storage override the potential benefits of HLA matching.
2. **Use of immunosuppressants**
   Except for identical twins, immunosuppressive therapy is a must in all donor–recipient combinations. Immunosuppressive drugs currently used include steroids to reduce inflammation, mycophenolate mofetil to inhibit lymphocyte proliferation and tacrolimus to inhibit T-cell responses. Additional methods that are used to treat rejection include T-cell- and B-cell-depleting antibodies and pooled intravenous IgG and plasmapheresis. Another recently developed strategy is the administration of proteins that bind to B7 costimulators that block signal 2 generation in immune response.
   Although immunosuppression prolongs graft survival, it comes with its own price, which is an increased susceptibility to opportunistic infections. The most frequent infectious complications are reactivation of polyoma virus, development of EBV-induced lymphomas, HPV-induced squamous cell carcinomas and KS. All these lesions are probably because of reactivation of latent viral infections, precipitated by diminished host defences.
   To overcome the high risks associated with the use of immunosuppressants, strategies are being tested to induce donor-specific tolerance in graft recipients.

MECHANISMS OF ALLOGRAFT REJECTION

Rejection is a process in which the T lymphocytes and antibodies produced against the antigens of the graft react and destroy the tissue grafts. Although other cells are also involved, the **T cells are central in the graft rejection** reaction. The rejection reaction consists of two phases: the sensitization phase and the effector phase.

Sensitization phase

In this phase, the $CD4^+$ and $CD8^+$ T cells, using their TCR complex, recognize the alloantigens expressed on the cells of the foreign graft. These are presented by APCs via their MHC through the generation of three signals of the immune response as discussed in previous sections.

At least two distinct, but not necessarily mutually exclusive, pathways of allograft rejection exist: the direct and the indirect pathways. Each pathway leads to the generation of different sets of allospecific T-cell clones and results in graft rejection.

The graft antigens are either presented directly to recipient T cells by graft APCs or the graft antigens are picked up by host APCs, processed like any other foreign antigen and presented to the host T cells. These are called the direct and indirect pathways of recognition of alloantigens, respectively.

Both the pathways lead to the activation of $CD8^+$ T cells, which develop into CTLs, and $CD4^+$ T cells, which become cytokine-producing effector cells, mainly Th1 cells. The direct pathway is the most important for CTL-mediated acute transplant rejection, and the indirect pathway plays a greater role in chronic transplant rejection.

The frequency with which T cells recognize the foreign antigens in a graft is much higher than the frequency of T cells recognizing other pathogens. Hence, it is understood that immune responses to allografts are stronger than responses to microbes. Such strong reactions can destroy grafts rapidly and hence powerful immunosuppressive agents are required to control them. B lymphocytes also recognize antigens (as they always do) in the graft, including HLA and other antigens that differ between the donor and the recipient.

Effector phase

Graft rejection is classified into **hyperacute, acute and chronic**, on the basis of their clinical and pathological features. This historical classification was initially proposed by clinicians on the basis of rejection of kidney allografts and has stood the test of time. Each type of rejection is mediated by a specific kind of immune response.

PATTERNS OF GRAFT REJECTION

Hyperacute graft rejection (Fig. 6.34)

Hyperacute rejection is mediated by humoral immunity, with preformed antibodies specific for the antigens present on graft endothelial cells resulting in the rejection of the transplanted organs within minutes to hours. The preformed antibodies may be natural IgM antibodies specific for blood group antigens or may be antibodies specific for allogeneic MHC molecules that were stimulated by prior exposure to allogeneic cells because of blood transfusions, pregnancy (especially with multiparity) or transplantation of another organ. As soon as the graft is transplanted and blood flow is restored, the antibodies bind to antigens on the graft vascular endothelium and activate the complement system. This leads to rapid endothelial injury, thrombosis, vascular occlusion and ischaemic necrosis of the graft. Hyperacute rejection is fortunately rare nowadays, as every donor–recipient pair is matched for blood type and also potential recipients are tested for antibodies against the cells of the prospective donor with a cross-match test.

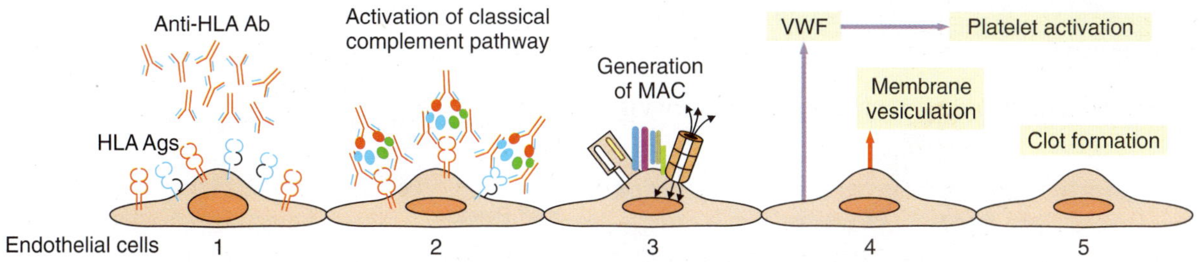

Fig. 6.34 Sequence of events in hyperacute rejection. (*Source:* https://revistanefrologia.com/en-immune-response-histology-humoral-rejection-articulo-S2013251416300712#imagen-6.)

Acute graft rejection

Acute rejection can be mediated by T cells or antibodies that are activated by alloantigens in the graft. It occurs within days or weeks after transplantation and is the chief cause of early graft failure. It also may appear immediately or much later after transplantation, when the immunosuppression is tapered or terminated. On the basis of the role of T cells or antibodies, acute rejection is divided into two types, although both patterns are present in most rejecting grafts.

Acute cellular rejection (Fig. 6.35) is mediated by $CD8^+$ CTLs or $CD4^+$ T lymphocytes. $CD8^+$ CTLs may directly destroy graft cells or $CD4^+$ cells may secrete cytokines and induce inflammation, damaging the graft. T cells may also react against graft vessels, leading to vascular damage.

Acute antibody-mediated (or humoral) rejection is mediated by antibodies and targets vascular endothelium. Antibodies bind to vascular endothelium and activate complement via the classical pathway. The resultant inflammation induces endothelial damage and results in graft failure.

Chronic rejection (Fig. 6.36)

Chronic rejection is a form of graft damage mediated by cell-mediated immunity that occurs over months or years, leading to progressive loss of graft function. It manifests as interstitial fibrosis and gradual narrowing of graft blood vessels, and this is termed *graft arteriosclerosis.* The activated T cells react against graft alloantigens and secrete cytokines, which stimulate the proliferation and functions of fibroblasts and vascular smooth muscle cells in the graft. In a small fraction of cases, alloantibodies also contribute to chronic rejection.

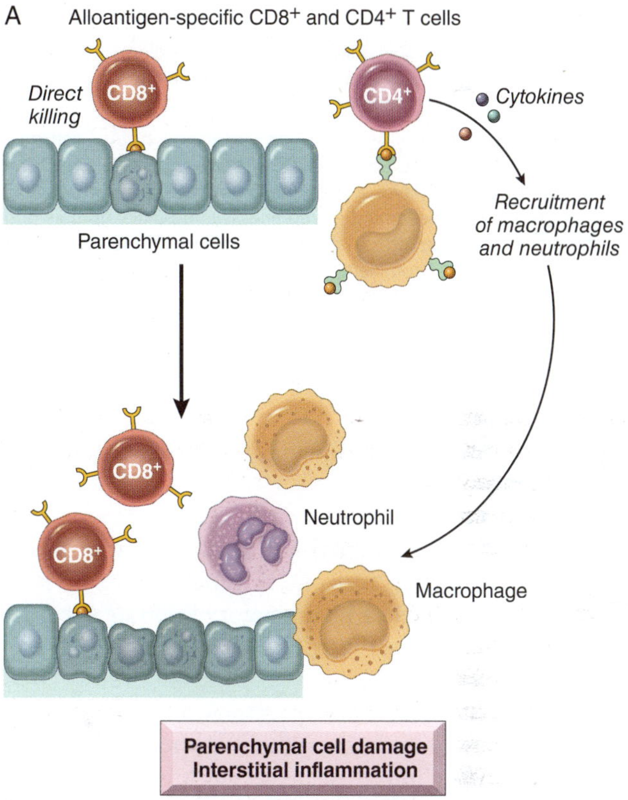

Fig. 6.35 Pathogenesis of acute cellular rejection. (A) Destruction of graft cells by T cells. Acute T-cell-mediated rejection involves direct killing of graft cells by $CD8^+$ CTLs and inflammation caused by cytokines produced by CD4 T cells. (B) Acute cellular rejection of a kidney graft, manifested by inflammatory cells in the interstitium and between epithelial cells of the tubules (tubulitis). Collapsed tubules are outlined by wavy basement membranes. (C) Rejection vasculitis in a kidney graft. An arteriole is shown with inflammatory cells attacking and undermining the endothelium (endotheliitis) *(arrow)*. (*Source:* From Robbins & Cotran Pathologic Basis of Disease, 10th edition. 2021. Elsevier.)

MORPHOLOGY OF GRAFT REJECTION

Here, we discuss the morphological features of rejection in kidney allografts, but similar histopathological changes are seen in other organ transplants.

Hyperacute rejection

In hyperacute rejection, the affected grafted kidney rapidly becomes cyanotic and mottled, and passes few drops of bloody urine. Almost all the arterioles and arteries exhibit acute **fibrinoid necrosis** of their walls and thrombotic occlusion of their lumen. Neutrophils rapidly accumulate within the arterioles, glomeruli and peritubular capillaries. As these reactions get intensified, the glomerular capillaries also undergo thrombotic occlusion, leading to necrosis of the renal cortex.

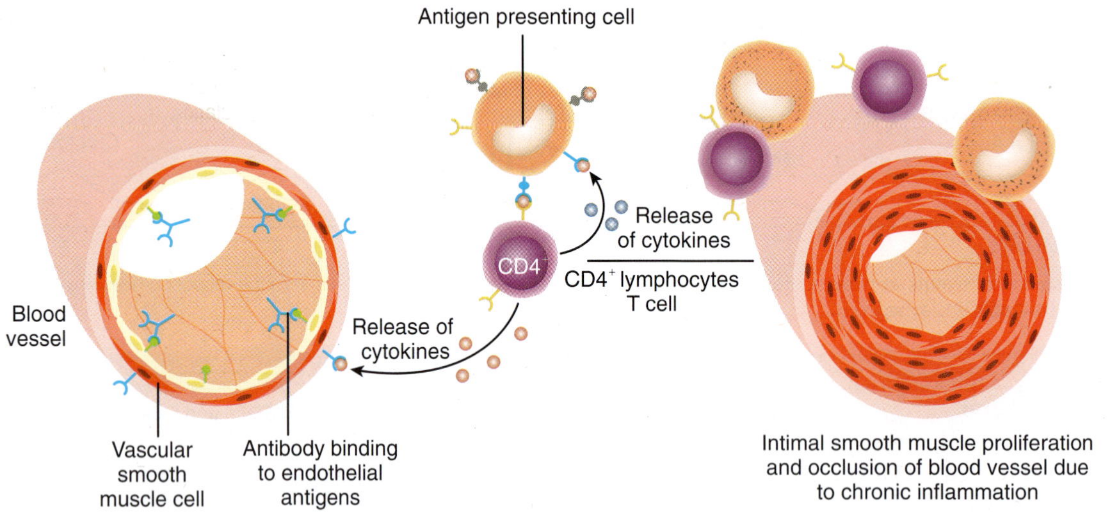

Fig. 6.36 Pathogenesis of chronic cellular rejection. (A) Graft arteriosclerosis caused by T-cell cytokines and antibody deposition. (B) Graft arteriosclerosis in a cardiac transplant. (C) Transplant glomerulopathy, the characteristic manifestation of chronic antibody-mediated rejection in the kidney. The glomerulus shows inflammatory cells within the capillary loops (glomerulitis), accumulation of mesangial matrix and duplication of the capillary basement membrane. (D) Interstitial fibrosis and tubular atrophy, resulting from arteriosclerosis of arteries and arterioles in a chronically rejecting kidney allograft. In this trichrome stain, the blue area *(asterisk)* shows fibrosis, contrasted with the normal kidney *(top right)*. An artery with prominent arteriosclerosis is shown *(bottom right)*. (*Source:* From Vinay Kumar, Abul K. Abbas and Jon C. Aster. Diseases of the Immune System. Robbins & Cotran Pathologic Basis of Disease. 10th Edition. Elsevier. 2021.)

Acute rejection

Acute cellular rejection may produce two different patterns of injury.

1. In the *tubulointerstitial pattern*, there is extensive interstitial and tubular inflammation associated with focal tubular injury. The mononuclear inflammatory infiltrate is composed of activated $CD4^+$ and $CD8^+$ T lymphocytes.
2. The *vascular pattern* shows inflammation of vessels with or without necrosis of vessel walls. The affected vessels display swollen endothelial cells with lymphocytic infiltrate in the space between the endothelium and the vessel wall, a finding referred to as **endotheliitis or intimal arteritis.**

Acute humoral rejection is characterized by damage to glomeruli and small blood vessels. Glomerular inflammation and peritubular capillaritis are predominant features because of the deposition of complement products, generated as a result of activation of the complement system by the antibody-dependent classical pathway. Small vessels may also show focal thrombosis (Fig. 6.37).

Chronic rejection (Fig. 6.38)

Chronic rejection displays vascular changes predominantly, with intimal thickening and vascular occlusion. Kidney grafts with chronic rejection display glomerulopathy, with *duplication of the basement membrane*, secondary to chronic endothelial injury and peritubular capillaritis characterized by multilayering of peritubular capillary basement membranes. Interstitial fibrosis and tubular atrophy with loss of renal parenchyma may be seen because of the vascular lesions. Interestingly, interstitial mononuclear cell infiltrates are typically sparse.

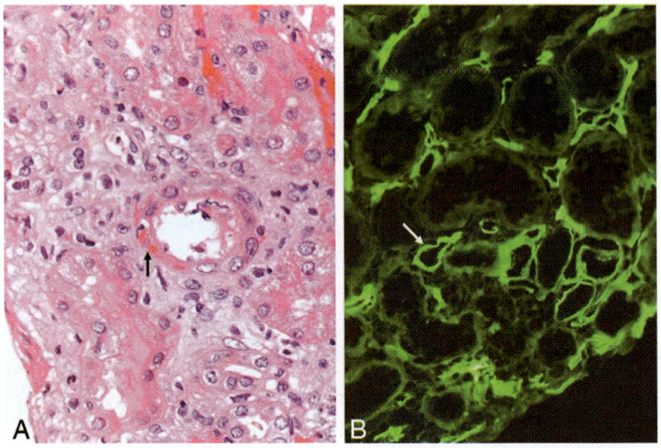

Fig. 6.37 Morphology of acute humoral rejection. (A) Acute humoral rejection. Transmural arteritis (fibrinoid necrosis of the vascular wall) (H&E). (B) C4d deposits in the peritubular capillaries (immunofluorescence). H&E, haematoxylin–eosin. (*Source:* https://revistanefrologia.com/en-immune-response-histology-humoral-rejection-articulo-S2013251416300712#imagen-7.)

CLINICAL IMPLICATIONS

Hyperacute rejection has to be identified immediately as the affected kidneys are nonfunctional and have to be removed at the earliest. The current immunosuppressive therapy is

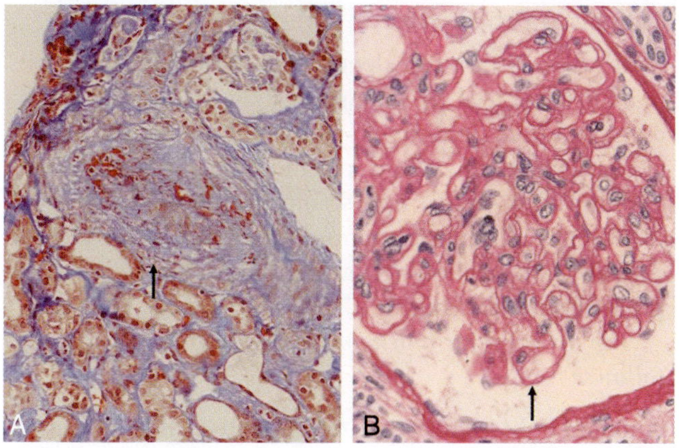

Fig. 6.38 (A) Transplant vasculopathy. Myointimal proliferation with vascular occlusion (Masson trichrome). (B) Transplant glomerulopathy. Disseminated duplication of the glomerular basement membrane (PAS). (*Source:* https://revistanefrologia.com/en-immune-response-histology-humoral-rejection-articulo-S2013251416300712#imagen-8.)

designed mainly to prevent and reduce acute rejection by preventing the activation of alloreactive T cells. The early recognition of cellular rejection is very important because, in the absence of accompanying humoral rejection, most patients respond well to immunosuppressive therapy.

Although treatment to prevent or curtail acute rejection has steadily improved, leading to better 1-year survival of transplants, chronic rejection is refractory to most currently used therapies and is becoming the principal cause of graft failure.

HAEMATOPOIETIC STEM CELL TRANSPLANTATION

HSC transplantation is offered as cure for many stem cell disorders like aplastic anaemia, immunodeficiency syndromes, sickle cell anaemia and PNH. Somatic cell gene therapy, in which HSCs obtained from affected patients are genetically reengineered and transplanted back, is under evaluation for use in some primary immunodeficiency states. Milestone achievement in HSC transplantation is the harvesting of stem cells from peripheral blood unlike in olden days when marrow aspiration was performed for the harvesting. This is performed with the use of cytokines to mobilize them from the marrow and to improve the yield. Umbilical cord blood, which is a rich source of stem cells, is also used for harvesting. The two major complications commonly associated with HSC transplantation that differentiate it from other solid organ transplantation are as follows:

- **Immunodeficiency**
- **GVHD**

Immunodeficiency

Immunodeficiency is a common complication that is associated with HSC transplantation. The reasons are as follows:

1. Iatrogenic (in all the cases of HSC transplantation, an immunodeficient state is induced in the host with the help of chemotherapy and radiation to clear the immune cells; this is performed to create space for the transplanted cells to engraft and establish themselves without getting rejected)
2. The underlying disease, e.g. aplastic anaemia
3. Prior treatment
4. Delay in the repopulation of the host's immune system
5. Development of GVHD with injury to the immune system

Identification of the immunodeficient state of the patient is essential because the host becomes a prey for a wide range of simple pathogens and even commensals. CMV infection is worth mentioning here, because it is very common in such patients and is because of the activation of previously acquired silent infection. This is discussed in detail in Chapter 8.

Graft-Versus-Host Disease

The difference between conventional transplant rejection reaction and GVHD is that in a conventional transplant rejection reaction, the immune system of the host rejects the graft, whereas in GVHD, the immune cells present in the graft reject the host.

The three principal features of GVHD are as follows:

- The graft contains immunocompetent cells – lymphocytes.
- The host is immunologically crippled.
- The graft is not rejected by the host.

The reason why GVHD is commonly seen as a complication of HSC transplantation is the immunodeficient state seen in the recipient of HSC transplantation and the presence of immunocompetent donor lymphocytes in the transplant. The immunocompetent cells present in the donor inoculum recognize the host's HLA antigens as foreign and mount an immune response. Depending on the timing of the clinical presentation, GVHD is divided into two forms: acute and chronic. $CD8^+$ CTLs and sensitized donor T cells are the cause of the disease. In both the forms, the most commonly affected organs are the skin, liver and GI tract.

1. **Acute GVHD**
   Acute GVHD occurs within days to weeks and can last up to 100 days. The clinical manifestations include generalized rash and desquamation, cholestatic jaundice because of destruction of small bile ducts and bloody diarrhoea because of mucosal ulceration.
2. **Chronic GVHD**
   Chronic GVHD may follow acute GVHD or can be precipitated slowly at any point of time after transplantation. Clinical manifestations include extensive cutaneous injury with damage to dermal appendages and fibrosis. Involvement of the liver and GI tract manifests as cholestatic jaundice and oesophageal strictures.

It is clear that the donor lymphocytes are the cause of GVHD, and their selective depletion before transplantation is associated with no risk of GVHD. Of course, this blessing comes with its own curse because of the fact that lymphocytes are needed for the engraftment, inhibition of EBV-infected clones and suppression of leukaemia cells. Hence, the depletion of lymphocytes is associated with the reemergence of leukaemia, development of lymphomas and also graft failure.

AMYLOIDOSIS PA 3.1

Amyloidosis is not a single disease entity but a group of disorders caused by extracellular deposition of insoluble abnormal amyloid fibrils that alter the normal function of tissues.

Rudolph Virchow, in 1854, introduced and popularized the term 'amyloid', meaning 'starch-like', to denote a macroscopic tissue abnormality that exhibited a positive iodine staining reaction. Subsequent light microscopic studies with polarizing optics demonstrated the inherent birefringence of amyloid deposits, a property that increased intensely after staining with Congo red stain. In 1959, electron microscopic examination of ultrathin sections of amyloidotic tissues demonstrated the presence of fibrils of indeterminate length and invariably 80–100 Å in width. Using the criteria of congophilia and fibrillar morphology, a wide range of biochemically distinct forms of amyloid have been identified.

Amyloid deposits are primarily extracellular, but reports exist of fibrillary structures within macrophages and plasma cells. It is deposited in various tissues and organs of the body in various disease processes. Although its presence can be suspected with clinical examination, morphological identification of this substance is essential for the diagnosis. With continuous accumulation, such amyloid deposits in tissues may cause pressure atrophy and organ failure in due course of the disease.

PROPERTIES OF AMYLOID PROTEINS

It should again be emphasized here that amyloid is not a single chemical entity. Till date, 36 proteins have been identified as being amyloidogenic in humans. Although all amyloid proteins have morphological similarity, there are three major and many minor biochemical forms deposited in tissues because of varied pathogenic mechanisms.

Physical Properties of Amyloid

Irrespective of the clinical form and chemical nature, all amyloid proteins have similar physical properties, the reason being their morphological similarity.

Electron microscopic features: Continuous nonbranching fibrils are present with a diameter of approximately 7.5–10 nm.

X-ray crystallography and infrared spectroscopic features: Characteristic β-pleated sheet conformation of amyloid proteins is the reason behind their congophilic nature and characteristic birefringence.

Chemical Properties of Amyloid

Nearly 90%–95% of the deposits consist of amyloid fibrils that are produced by the aggregation of misfolded proteins, and the remaining 5%–10% of the deposits consist of components such as glycosaminoglycans (GAGs), apolipoprotein E (apoE) and serum amyloid P-component (SAP). Such proteins arise from proteins expressed by the cells at the deposition site or precipitate systemically after production at a local site.

The three major biochemical forms of amyloid are as follows:

Amyloid light-chain protein (AL protein) is composed of complete immunoglobulin light chains or the amino terminal fragments of light chains or both. This type of amyloid protein is the product of neoplastic proliferation of plasma cells; in a majority of AL amyloids, λ chains are found.

Amyloid-associated protein (AA protein) found in the fibrils is because of the proteolysis of a larger precursor called serum amyloid-associated (SAA) protein that is synthesized in the liver and circulates in the blood. The production of SAA protein by the liver is increased in inflammatory states as part of the acute-phase response. Hence, this form of amyloidosis is associated with chronic inflammation and is called secondary amyloidosis or reactive amyloidosis.

β-Amyloid (Aβ) protein forms the core of cerebral plaques found in Alzheimer disease as well as the amyloid deposited in walls of cerebral blood vessels in individuals with Alzheimer disease. The Aβ protein is derived by proteolysis of amyloid precursor protein. This form of amyloid is discussed in Chapter 31.

CLASSIFICATION SYSTEMS

Historical classification of amyloidosis was clinically based, whereas modern classification systems are biochemically and clinicopathologically based.

Older classification systems: Until 1970s, the idea of a single amyloid substance predominated. Many descriptive classification systems were proposed on the basis of the organ distribution of amyloid deposition and clinical findings. Most such classification systems included primary and secondary amyloidosis. Some systems also included myeloma-associated, familial and localized amyloidosis. Such classification systems that are based on aetiology provide little information and are no longer used and recommended.

Modern classification of amyloidosis: This system classifies amyloidosis on the basis of the chemical composition of the amyloid protein, i.e. the type of amyloid fibril. Amyloidosis is referred to with a capital A (for amyloid), followed by short form for the fibril protein. Names such as AA describe the protein but not necessarily the clinical phenotype. Great importance is now given to appropriate and timely typing and classification of each type of amyloid-related disease to focus on treatment and to plan appropriate monitoring. A given amyloid fibril may be associated with amyloid deposition in a wide range of clinical settings, so a more practical approach to the classification of amyloidosis is a combined biochemical–clinical classification and is given in Table 6.17.

PATHOGENESIS (FIG. 6.39)

Amyloidosis is the result of deposition of abnormally folded proteins, which, being insoluble, tend to aggregate. Normally, such misfolded proteins are degraded extracellularly by macrophages or intracellularly in proteasomes

Table 6.17 Classification of Amyloidosis

Type	Clinically Related Precursor Protein	Major Clinical Settings
Systemic	Immunoglobulin light chains	Plasma cell dyscrasias
	Transthyretin	Familial amyloidosis Senile cardiac amyloidosis
	AA amyloidosis	Inflammation-associated amyloidosis Familial Mediterranean amyloidosis
	β_2-Microglobulin	Dialysis associated amyloidosis
	Immunoglobulin heavy chains	Systemic amyloidosis
Localized	Calcitonin	Medullary thyroid carcinoma
	Amylin	Insulinoma Type 2 diabetes
	Atrial natriuretic factor	Isolated atrial amyloidosis
	β-Precursor protein	Alzheimer disease Down syndrome
	Prion protein	Prion diseases
	Lactoferrin	Familial corneal amyloidosis
	Prolactin	Pituitary amyloidosis
	Keratin	Cutaneous amyloidosis
	Medin	Aortic amyloidosis in the elderly people

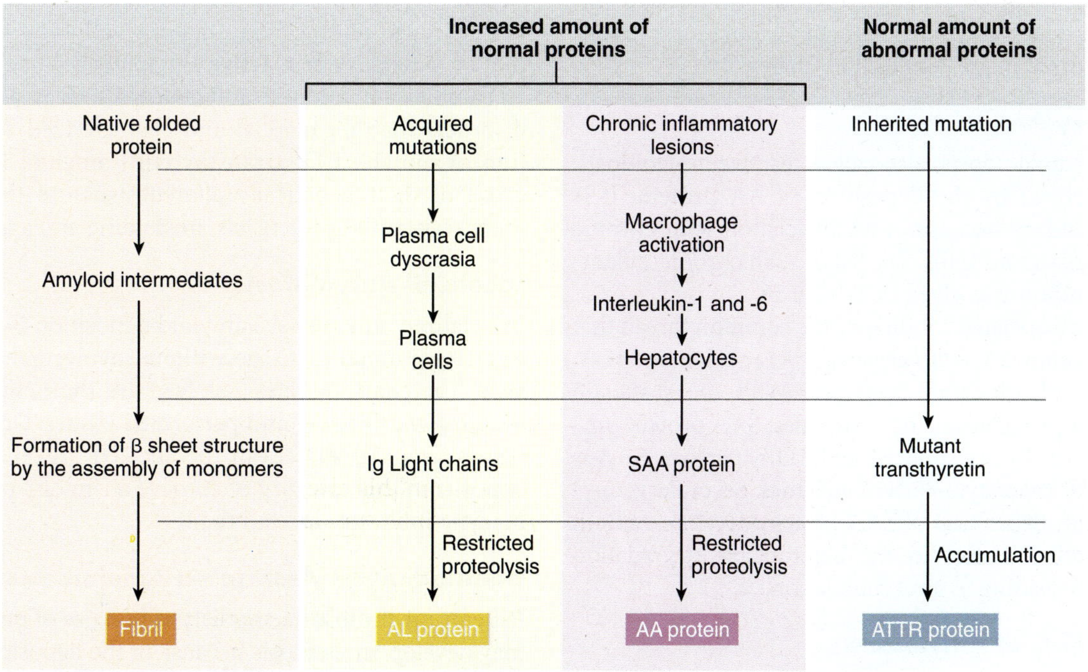

Fig. 6.39 Pathogenesis of amyloidosis – the proposed mechanisms underlying deposition of the major forms of amyloid fibrils. (*Source:* From Vinay Kumar, Abul Abbas, Jon Aster. Robbins & Cotran Pathologic Basis of Disease, 10th edition. Elsevier. 2020.)

as discussed in Chapter 1. In amyloidosis, failure of such degradative mechanisms leads to the accumulation of the misfolded proteins. The proteins that get deposited in amyloidosis are broadly divided into two categories:

1. Increased production of normal proteins with an inherent tendency to fold improperly
2. Mutant proteins with a tendency to misfold and aggregate

On the clinical basis, systemic amyloidosis is subclassified into primary and secondary amyloidosis.

Primary Amyloidosis

Amyloidosis associated with plasma cell dyscrasias.

This is the most common form of amyloidosis and is characterized by systemic distribution. The amyloid fibril that gets deposited in this category is AL type, which is immunoglobulin light chains produced by the defective plasma cell. In up to 15% of patients with multiple myeloma (discussed in Chapter 16), systemic amyloidosis is associated. The excess light chains synthesized by the neoplastic plasma cells may be kappa or lambda. Such free light chains are present in serum and urine and get deposited in tissues as amyloid. Specific amino acid sequence of the light chains determines their amyloidogenic potential.

Most patients with primary amyloidosis may not have any form of overt plasma cell dyscrasia or any other underlying disease and such cases are categorized as primary amyloidosis. But all cases have an excess of monoclonal immunoglobulins or light chains in their serum and urine and mostly exhibit increase in marrow plasma cells, which may be the source of excess light chains. Hence, this confirms that all the cases of primary amyloidosis have silent plasma cell dyscrasia or monoclonal gammapathy, which has a tendency to produce antibodies without forming mass lesions and is discussed in greater detail in Chapter 16.

Secondary Amyloidosis

Secondary amyloidosis, also called reactive amyloidosis, is characterized by the deposition of AA protein. It is called secondary because of its association with chronic inflammatory conditions. The list of such chronic inflammatory conditions is given in Table 6.18.

Table 6.18 Conditions Associated with Secondary or Reactive Amyloidosis

Rheumatoid arthritis
Ankylosing spondylitis
Inflammatory bowel disease
Tuberculosis
Leprosy
Bronchiectasis
Chronic osteomyelitis
Renal cell carcinoma
Hodgkin lymphoma
GI tract malignancies
Lung cancer
Urogenital carcinoma
Heroin drug abuse
Narcotic abuse

GI, gastrointestinal.

In all the associated conditions, the common thread that runs is inflammation with elevated levels of IL-6 and IL-1, which are inflammatory cytokines. With the sustained elevation of proinflammatory cytokines, SAA protein production by the liver is induced. In healthy persons, SAA is degraded by monocyte-derived enzymes. Secondary amyloidosis with deposition of SAA protein develops only in persons with a defect in the macrophage degradation mechanism, leading to its accumulation.

Heredofamilial Amyloidosis

This category of amyloidosis is rare and occurs in limited geographic regions. The most common type in this group is familial Mediterranean fever, which is an 'autoinflammatory syndrome' associated with overproduction of the proinflammatory cytokine, IL-1, as a response to inflammatory stimuli. The gene that is mutated in this disease codes for a protein called *pyrin,* which is responsible for the overproduction of IL-1. The disease is clinically characterized by recurrent attacks of fever and polyserositis and is common in Armenians, Sephardic Jews and Arabians. The type of amyloid fibril that gets deposited is AA, because of the inflammatory aetiology similar to that of secondary or reactive amyloidosis.

Familial amyloidotic polyneuropathies is a group of disorders that are familial and characterized by deposition of mutant TTR (transthyretin) amyloid fibrils because of their genetically altered structure that makes them resistant to proteolysis, misfolding and aggregation.

Localized Amyloidosis

In localized amyloidosis, amyloid deposition is restricted to a single organ or tissue without involvement of other sites. The common sites involved are the lungs, larynx, skin, tongue, bladder and periorbital tissues. Grossly, it is seen as nodular masses in the affected organs. Amyloid deposits in this category often have a rim of lymphoplasmacytic infiltrates around them.

Haemodialysis-Associated Amyloidosis

Patients on chronic haemodialysis because of renal failure may develop amyloidosis because of the deposition of β_2-microglobulin. The level of this protein is elevated in such patients because of the failure of its removal by the dialysis membrane. β_2-Microglobulin gets deposited in sites like joints, muscle, tendons and ligaments and may present with carpal tunnel syndrome. This form of amyloidosis is now reduced in incidence with the advent of new dialysis filters that remove β_2-microglobulin effectively.

Amyloid of Ageing

Apart from many other risks, ageing is also complicated with the development of amyloidosis in individuals because of unknown mechanisms. The amyloid protein that gets deposited in this category is normal TTR, transthyretin, and the common organ affected is the heart; hence, the term 'senile cardiac amyloidosis' was used earlier. Patients may present with restrictive cardiomyopathy or arrhythmias or remain asymptomatic and diagnosed incidentally.

Endocrine Amyloid

Some endocrine tumours, such as medullary thyroid carcinoma, phaeochromocytoma and pancreatic islet tumour, may have microscopic deposits of amyloid. Amyloid deposition is also noted in the islets of Langerhans in type 2 diabetes. In these cases, the amyloid fibrils are derived from polypeptide hormones or special proteins like islet amyloid polypeptide.

MORPHOLOGY

Amyloid deposition in tissues and organs may take any form, with no consistent pattern of involvement. Some common features are described here. The deposition of amyloid in heredofamilial conditions is varied, and the common organs affected by primary and secondary amyloidosis in decreasing order of frequency are as follows:

Primary amyloidosis: Heart, GI tract, respiratory tract, peripheral nerves, skin and tongue

Secondary amyloidosis: Kidneys, liver, spleen, lymph nodes, adrenals and thyroid

Amyloid deposits are not seen grossly; however, when there is a huge accumulation of amyloid, the organ is commonly enlarged with waxy firm consistency. Histologically, the amyloid deposition is always extracellular and begins between cells, often closely adjacent to the basement membranes. As the amyloid accumulates progressively, it encroaches on the cells and destroys them. Perivascular and vascular deposits are common in amyloidosis because of plasma cell proliferation.

The histopathological diagnosis of amyloid is based almost entirely on its staining characteristics. With the routine haematoxylin–eosin (H&E) stain, amyloid appears bright pink in colour. The most common stain used is the dye Congo red, which under ordinary light imparts a pink or red colour to amyloid deposits. With polarizing microscopy, the Congo red–stained amyloid shows the so-called apple-green birefringence. This exclusive reaction is shared by all forms of amyloid and is caused by the cross-β-pleated configuration of amyloid fibrils. Confirmation can be obtained by electron microscopy. Immunohistochemistry can differentiate the different chemical forms of amyloid.

The morphological forms by which amyloidosis affects organs is variable.

Kidney: Renal amyloidosis (Fig. 6.40) is the most common and also the most serious form of amyloidosis. Grossly, the kidneys may be of normal size and colour but in advanced stages, these may be shrunken because of ischaemia caused by vascular compromise induced by the deposition of amyloid within the vessel walls. Microscopically, amyloid is deposited primarily in the glomeruli, but the interstitial peritubular tissue and

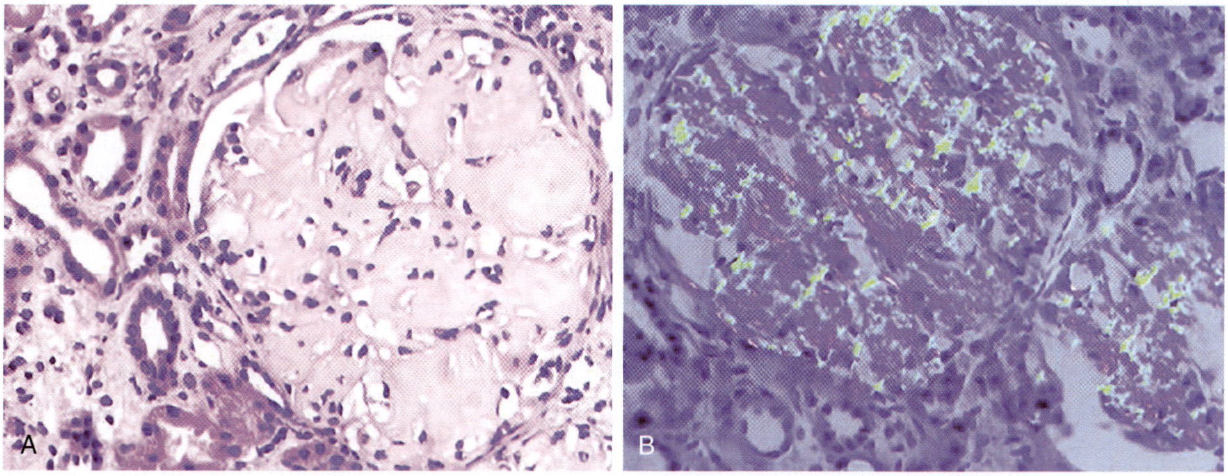

Fig. 6.40 Morphology of renal amyloidosis – H&E and polarized Congo red. It shows glomeruli with an expansion of the mesangial matrix by amorphous, pale eosinophilic, (A) Acellular material and orange–red staining of eosinophilic material with apple-green birefringence on (B) polarization microscopy. H&E, haematoxylin–eosin. (*Source:* https://www.google.com/url?sa=i&url=https%3A%2F%2Fwww.researchgate.net%2Ffigure%2FH-E-100x-and-500x-magnification-and-Congo-red-staining-Polarized-Congo-red-Showing_fig1_309335512&psig=AOvVaw3FUUAp4wJnG73rKU6IpXqF&ust=1605940937446000&source=images&cd=vfe&ved=0CAIQjRxqFwoTCKC0jq7CkO0CFQAAAAAdAAAAABAD.)

blood vessels are also affected. The glomerular deposits first appear as subtle enlargement of the mesangial matrix, accompanied by uneven widening of the basement membranes of the glomerular capillaries. In due course, such deposits cause capillary narrowing and distortion of the glomerular vascular tuft. With progression of the disease, the capillary lumens are obliterated, and the obsolescent glomerulus is flooded by confluent masses or interlacing broad ribbons of amyloid.

Spleen: Amyloidosis of the spleen may be grossly unremarkable or may cause moderate to marked splenomegaly. For unknown reasons, one of the following two patterns of deposition is seen:

- **Sago spleen:** The deposits are largely limited to the splenic follicles, producing tapioca-like granules on gross examination.
- **Lardaceous spleen:** The amyloid involves the walls of the splenic sinuses and connective tissue framework in the red pulp. Fusion of the early deposits gives rise to large map-like areas of amyloidosis.

Liver: Amyloid deposits in the liver may be grossly unremarkable or may cause moderate to marked hepatomegaly. The deposit appears first in the space of Disse and then progressively encroaches on hepatic parenchymal cells and sinusoids. In due course, pressure atrophy and loss of hepatocytes occur, leading to total replacement of large areas of liver parenchyma. Blood vessels are frequently involved. Even with extensive involvement, liver function is generally preserved.

Heart: The heart may be affected in any form of systemic amyloidosis and is the major organ affected in senile systemic amyloidosis. It may appear grossly unremarkable or may be enlarged and firm. Amyloid deposition begins as focal subendocardial accumulation and within the myocardium between the muscle fibres. Progression of the disease eventually causes pressure atrophy of the myocardial fibres. The conduction system may be damaged with subendocardial amyloid deposits, which is the reason for the electrocardiographic abnormalities noted in some patients.

Other organs

- 'Tumour-forming amyloid of the tongue' is the term used for nodular deposits in the tongue that may cause macroglossia.
- A unique form of amyloid is found in the plaques as well as blood vessels of brains in patients with Alzheimer disease.
- Amyloidosis of peripheral and autonomic nerves is a feature of several familial amyloidotic neuropathies.
- As mentioned earlier, depositions of amyloid in patients on long-term haemodialysis are most prominent in the carpal ligament of the wrist, resulting in compression of the median nerve (carpal tunnel syndrome).

CLINICAL FEATURES

The clinical presentation of amyloidosis is varied and ranges from asymptomatic to life-threatening features. The symptoms depend primarily on the site of amyloid accumulation. Kidneys and heart are the most commonly involved organs. Renal amyloidosis can cause nephrotic syndrome with or without uraemia. Renal failure is a common cause of death in systemic amyloidosis.

Cardiac amyloidosis may cause both systolic and diastolic heart failure, conduction disturbances and arrhythmias, restrictive cardiomyopathy or constrictive pericarditis. AA amyloidosis usually spares the heart.

Amyloidosis of CNS usually presents with sensory and autonomic neuropathies. Sensory neuropathy is of symmetrical pattern and progresses in a distal-to-proximal manner. Autonomic neuropathy can present as orthostatic hypotension but may manifest more gradually with nonspecific GI symptoms like constipation, nausea or early satiety.

Amyloidosis of the tongue may be massive and cause obstructive sleep apnoea, speech disturbances and swallowing difficulties. Amyloid deposition in the throat may cause hoarseness. GI tract involvement may manifest as malabsorption with sprue-like appearance.

Vascular amyloidosis leads to vascular fragility, which may cause spontaneous or post-traumatic bleeding. A rare manifestation is amyloid purpura, with a susceptibility to bleeding with bruising around the eyes, termed 'raccoon eyes'. This is caused by amyloid deposition in the blood vessels and a reduced activity of thrombin and factor X, two clotting proteins that lose their function after binding with amyloid.

Amyloid deposition in the synovial space results in enlarged shoulders, which is seen as 'shoulder pad sign'. Amyloid proteins may be deposited inside the knees, hands, wrists, elbow, hip and ankle, causing joint pain.

Uncommonly, a collection of amyloids can grow large enough to be called an 'amyloidoma', a macroscopic lump of amyloid that can cause mass effect on soft tissues or bone.

INVESTIGATIONS

Histopathological demonstration of amyloid deposits in tissues is essential for the diagnosis of amyloidosis. The most common sites sampled are the kidneys (when renal symptoms are present) or rectal or gingival mucosa in systemic amyloidosis. Abdominal fat pad aspiration and Congo red staining can be used in suspected cases of systemic amyloidosis. In suspected cases of primary amyloidosis, urine and serum protein immunoelectrophoresis should be performed. Bone marrow examination should be performed to check for the presence of multiple myeloma or monoclonal plasmacytosis in such patients. A rapid and specific test for amyloidosis is scintigraphy with radiolabelled serum amyloid P component that also provides information regarding the extent of amyloidosis to follow-up patients on treatment.

TREATMENT AND PROGNOSIS

The management of primary and reactive amyloidosis is treating the underlying illness. In general, the prognosis of reactive amyloidosis is relatively better than that of primary amyloidosis, which has a poor prognosis. New treatment strategies aimed at correcting protein misfolding and inhibiting fibrillogenesis are under development.

SELF-ASSESSMENT

Scenario-Based MCQs

1. A 35-year-old woman with recurrent infections and high levels of IgM is diagnosed with a primary immunodeficiency. This condition most likely involves a defect in:
   A. T lymphocytes
   B. B lymphocytes
   C. Macrophages
   D. Neutrophils
2. During spring, a patient experiences severe allergic reactions characterized by sneezing and watery eyes when exposed to pollen. This reaction is typically mediated by:
   A. Cell-mediated cytotoxicity
   B. Immune complex–mediated tissue injury
   C. IgE-mediated mast cell degranulation
   D. Delayed-type hypersensitivity
3. A patient who has undergone a kidney transplant develops graft rejection 1 week after surgery. This rejection is most likely mediated by:
   A. Antibody-mediated destruction of graft
   B. T-cell-mediated cytotoxicity
   C. Complement activation
   D. Neutrophil infiltration
4. A patient presents with joint pain and a skin rash. Laboratory tests reveal the presence of autoantibodies. This condition exemplifies:
   A. A response to foreign antigens
   B. A failure of the immune system to recognize self-antigens
   C. A hypersensitivity reaction to drugs
   D. Immune tolerance to self-antigens
5. A 30-year-old female with a butterfly rash, joint pain and renal dysfunction is diagnosed with a chronic autoimmune disease. The most likely diagnosis is:
   A. Rheumatoid arthritis
   B. Systemic lupus erythematosus
   C. Scleroderma
   D. Dermatomyositis
6. An HIV-positive patient develops severe immunodeficiency and opportunistic infections. This progression is characteristic of:
   A. Early HIV infection
   B. Chronic HIV infection
   C. AIDS
   D. Post-HIV syndrome
7. A 40-year-old man with dry mouth, dry eyes and arthritis is suspected of having an autoimmune disorder affecting exocrine glands. The probable diagnosis is:
   A. Systemic lupus erythematosus
   B. Rheumatoid arthritis
   C. Sjögren syndrome
   D. Multiple sclerosis
8. A patient with chronic joint inflammation, morning stiffness and symmetric arthritis is most likely suffering from:
   A. Osteoarthritis
   B. Rheumatoid arthritis
   C. Psoriatic arthritis
   D. Gouty arthritis
9. A patient with a long-standing history of rheumatoid arthritis shows nodular deposits in organs on imaging. These deposits are likely composed of:
   A. Amyloid fibrils
   B. Granulomatous tissue
   C. Fibrinoid material
   D. Neutrophil extracellular traps
10. A patient with a history of multiple allergies develops a rapid, severe reaction to a bee sting, characterized by difficulty breathing and hypotension. This reaction is typical of:
    A. Type I hypersensitivity
    B. Type II hypersensitivity
    C. Type III hypersensitivity
    D. Type IV hypersensitivity
11. A patient with a heart transplant develops a fever, dyspnoea and cough 3 months post-transplant. A biopsy shows lymphocytic infiltration and myocyte damage. This is indicative of:
    A. Acute cellular rejection
    B. Antibody-mediated rejection
    C. Chronic rejection
    D. Hyperacute rejection
12. In a patient with systemic lupus erythematosus, the presence of which antibody is most indicative of renal involvement?
    A. Anti-Smith antibody
    B. Anti-dsDNA antibody
    C. Antiphospholipid antibody
    D. Anti-Ro/SSA antibody
13. A 25-year-old male presents with back pain and stiffness that improves with exercise. X-ray reveals sacroiliitis. This presentation is suggestive of:
    A. Osteoarthritis
    B. Ankylosing spondylitis
    C. Rheumatoid arthritis
    D. Psoriatic arthritis
14. A patient with HIV shows a CD4+ T cell count of 200 cells/μL. This finding is critical for the diagnosis of:
    A. Early HIV infection
    B. Chronic HIV infection
    C. MHC
    D. Post-HIV syndrome
15. A patient develops a severe haemolytic reaction after receiving a blood transfusion because of a mismatch. This type of reaction is categorized as:
    A. Type I hypersensitivity
    B. Type II hypersensitivity
    C. Type III hypersensitivity
    D. Type IV hypersensitivity
16. A young woman with no significant medical history develops a low platelet count, kidney dysfunction and a positive antinuclear antibody (ANA) test. The most likely diagnosis is:
    A. Haemolytic anaemia
    B. Idiopathic thrombocytopenic purpura
    C. Systemic lupus erythematosus
    D. Acute lymphocytic leukaemia

17. A patient presents with a chronic cough and hilar lymphadenopathy. Biopsy shows noncaseating granulomas. This presentation is most suggestive of:
    A. Sarcoidosis
    B. Tuberculosis
    C. Systemic lupus erythematosus
    D. Rheumatoid arthritis
18. A 50-year-old female with recurrent urinary tract infections and glomerulonephritis is found to have low levels of C3 complement. This finding is most indicative of:
    A. Classical pathway activation
    B. Alternative pathway activation
    C. Lectin pathway activation
    D. Complement inhibitor deficiency
19. A patient diagnosed with Graves disease presents with hyperthyroidism. The pathogenesis of this disease primarily involves:
    A. Cell-mediated destruction of thyroid follicles
    B. Antibody-mediated stimulation of thyroid hormone synthesis
    C. Deposition of immune complexes in the thyroid gland
    D. T-cell-mediated inhibition of thyroid hormone synthesis
20. A patient with systemic sclerosis shows skin thickening and Raynaud phenomenon. The underlying pathogenesis of this disease is characterized by:
    A. Vasculitis and granuloma formation
    B. Fibrosis and autoantibody production
    C. Complement activation and immune complex deposition
    D. T-cell-mediated cytotoxicity
21. During a hypersensitivity pneumonitis investigation, a patient's lung biopsy reveals lymphocytic infiltration and granuloma formation. These findings are consistent with a reaction primarily mediated by:
    A. IgE antibodies
    B. IgG antibodies
    C. T lymphocytes
    D. Neutrophils
22. A child with a severe combined immunodeficiency (SCID) is prone to frequent infections because of a lack of functional:
    A. B and T lymphocytes
    B. Macrophages and dendritic cells
    C. Neutrophils and eosinophils
    D. Natural killer cells and monocytes
23. In a patient with myasthenia gravis, the primary pathophysiological mechanism is:
    A. Destruction of acetylcholine receptors by cytotoxic T cells
    B. Formation of antibodies against acetylcholine receptors
    C. Deposition of immune complexes at neuromuscular junctions
    D. Direct viral damage to motor neurons
24. A patient with coeliac disease shows damage to intestinal villi. This pathology is primarily because of an immune response against:
    A. Gluten
    B. Lactose
    C. Casein
    D. Fructose
25. In a case of Hashimoto thyroiditis, the thyroid gland is primarily affected by:
    A. Antibody-mediated stimulation
    B. T-cell-mediated destruction
    C. Deposition of immune complexes
    D. Complement activation
26. A patient with a kidney transplant develops a fever and tenderness over the graft site 2 days post-transplant. This scenario most likely indicates:
    A. Acute cellular rejection
    B. Antibody-mediated rejection
    C. Chronic rejection
    D. Hyperacute rejection
27. An individual with Goodpasture syndrome develops rapidly progressive glomerulonephritis and lung haemorrhage. The pathogenesis of this condition involves autoantibodies targeting:
    A. Basement membrane collagen
    B. Epithelial cell antigens
    C. Endothelial cell antigens
    D. Myeloperoxidase
28. A patient with SLE presents with neurological symptoms. Brain MRI shows white matter changes. These symptoms are most likely related to:
    A. Vasculitis
    B. Lupus nephritis
    C. Antiphospholipid antibody syndrome
    D. Direct central nervous system involvement
29. A patient experiences severe asthma attacks when exposed to cat dander. This type of hypersensitivity reaction is primarily mediated by:
    A. IgE antibodies and mast cells
    B. T lymphocytes
    C. Immune complex deposition
    D. Autoantibodies
30. In a patient who received a liver transplant, the development of jaundice and elevated liver enzymes 2 months post-transplantation suggests:
    A. Acute cellular rejection
    B. Chronic rejection
    C. Graft-versus-host disease
    D. Hyperacute rejection

Answers

1. (B); 2. (C); 3. (B); 4. (B); 5. (B); 6. (C); 7. (C); 8. (B); 9. (A); 10. (A); 11. (B); 12. (B); 13. (C); 14. (B); 15. (C); 16. (A); 17. (A); 18. (B); 19. (B); 20. (B); 21. (C); 22. (A); 23. (B); 24. (A); 25. (B); 26. (D); 27. (A); 28. (A); 29. (A); 30. (B).

Scenario-Based Questions

1. A patient with recurrent bacterial infections has a laboratory test revealing low immunoglobulin levels. Discuss the possible types of primary immunodeficiencies this patient might have and their pathophysiology.
2. Describe the mechanism of action and potential therapeutic uses of monoclonal antibodies in autoimmune diseases, using a specific disease as an example.
3. A child is diagnosed with severe combined immunodeficiency (SCID). Explain the genetic basis and immunological deficiencies associated with SCID.
4. Discuss the role of helper T cells in orchestrating the immune response, emphasizing their interaction with other immune cells.
5. Explain how immune tolerance is maintained in the body and the mechanisms by which this tolerance can be broken, leading to autoimmunity.
6. A patient with systemic lupus erythematosus (SLE) presents with a range of symptoms. Describe the pathogenesis of SLE and its systemic effects.
7. Illustrate the process of antigen processing and presentation, highlighting its significance in initiating an immune response.
8. A patient undergoing chemotherapy develops neutropenia. Discuss the consequences of neutropenia on the immune system and potential strategies to manage this condition.
9. Describe the different types of hypersensitivity reactions with examples, focusing on their underlying immunological mechanisms.
10. A patient receives a kidney transplant and later shows signs of transplant rejection. Discuss the different types of transplant rejection and their immunological basis.
11. Explain the concept of immunological memory and its importance in vaccine development, using a specific vaccine as an example.
12. Discuss the role of cytokines in the immune response, particularly in the context of inflammatory diseases.
13. A patient with HIV infection progresses to AIDS. Describe the pathogenesis of HIV and how it leads to the clinical manifestations of AIDS.
14. Explain the principle behind immunotherapy for cancer, including a discussion on checkpoint inhibitors.
15. A patient presents with anaphylaxis following a bee sting. Describe the immunological basis of anaphylaxis and its emergency management.
16. Discuss the role of the complement system in immunity, including its activation pathways and role in disease processes.
17. A patient with rheumatoid arthritis shows improvement with TNF inhibitors. Discuss the pathogenesis of rheumatoid arthritis and the role of TNF in its progression.
18. A patient presents with symptoms of allergy. Discuss the diagnostic approaches for allergic diseases, including skin tests and serological assays.
19. Explain the concept of herd immunity and its significance in controlling infectious diseases, particularly in the context of a vaccination programme.
20. A patient with chronic inflammatory disease develops kidney dysfunction and a biopsy reveals amyloid deposits. Discuss the pathogenesis of amyloidosis in the context of chronic inflammation, including the types of proteins involved and the systemic effects of amyloid deposition.
21. A 45-year-old woman presents with persistent dry eyes and dry mouth. She is subsequently diagnosed with Sjögren syndrome. Explain the immunological mechanisms underlying Sjögren syndrome, including the role of autoantibodies and the impact on exocrine glands.
22. In a patient with SLE, a renal biopsy shows lupus nephritis. Describe the immunopathology of lupus nephritis, focusing on the role of autoantibodies, immune complexes and the complement system in damaging the renal glomeruli.

Topics for Self-Directed Learning

1. TLR family and their microbial spectrum.
2. Detection of transplant rejection.
3. Autoinflammatory syndromes.
4. Diseases with IL-17 response.
5. Ten diseases having more than one type of hypersensitivity reaction.
6. Role of CTLA-4 in health and diseases.
7. HLA association in autoimmune diseases.
8. Non-HLA genes associated with autoimmune diseases.
9. Molecular mimicry in diseases.
10. Antiphospholipid antibody syndrome.
11. CREST syndrome.
12. Post-transfusion GVHD.
13. Hereditary angio-oedema.
14. X-linked lymphoproliferative syndrome.
15. Secondary immunodeficiency states and their mechanism other than AIDS.

MIND MAPS

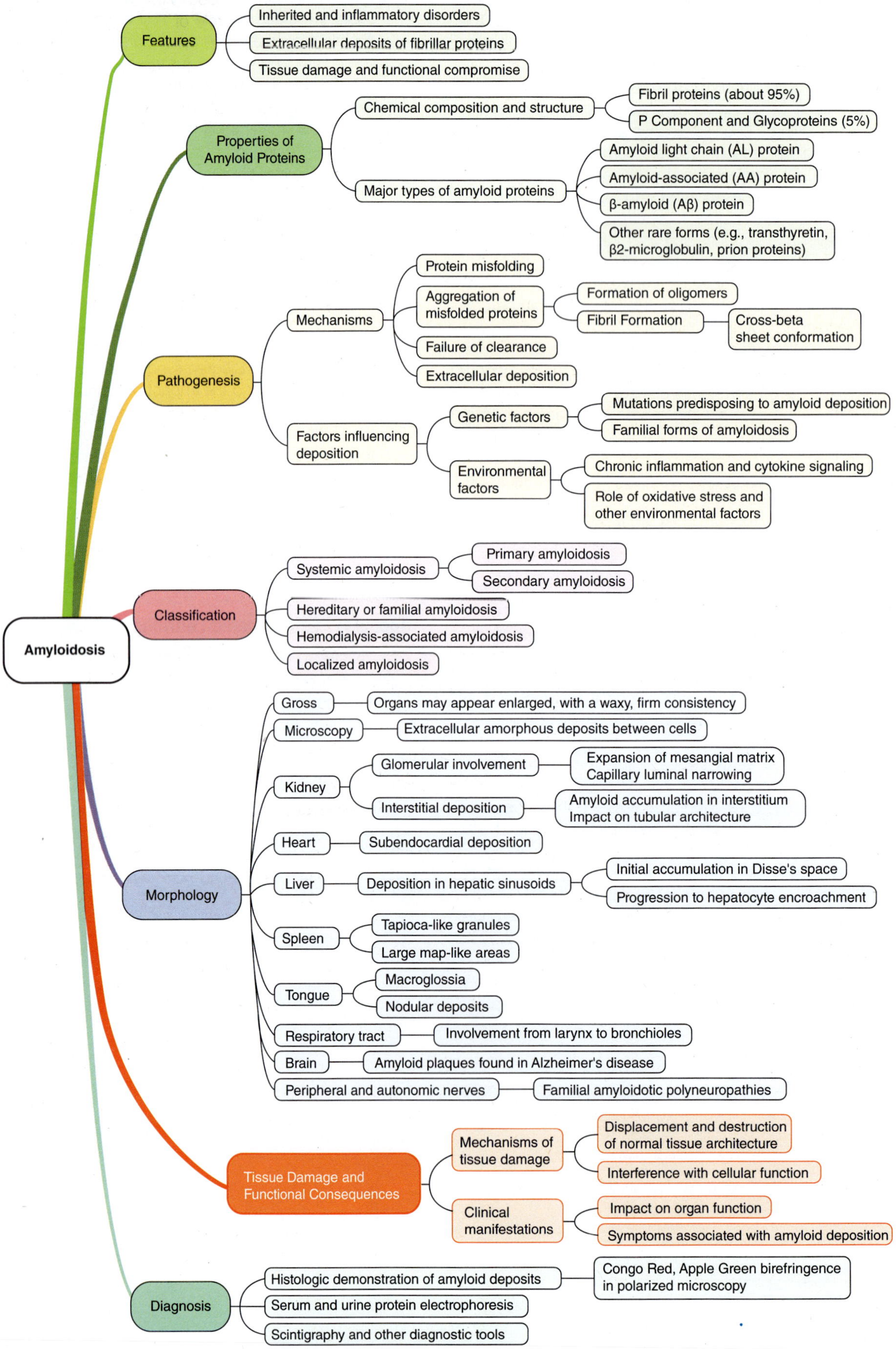
Amyloidosis
Features
Inherited and inflammatory disorders
Extracellular deposits of fibrillar proteins
Tissue damage and functional compromise
Properties of Amyloid Proteins
Chemical composition and structure
Fibril proteins (about 95%)
P Component and Glycoproteins (5%)
Major types of amyloid proteins
Amyloid light chain (AL) protein
Amyloid-associated (AA) protein
β-amyloid (Aβ) protein
Other rare forms (e.g., transthyretin, β2-microglobulin, prion proteins)
Pathogenesis
Mechanisms
Protein misfolding
Aggregation of misfolded proteins
Formation of oligomers
Fibril Formation
Cross-beta sheet conformation
Failure of clearance
Extracellular deposition
Factors influencing deposition
Genetic factors
Mutations predisposing to amyloid deposition
Familial forms of amyloidosis
Environmental factors
Chronic inflammation and cytokine signaling
Role of oxidative stress and other environmental factors
Classification
Systemic amyloidosis
Primary amyloidosis
Secondary amyloidosis
Hereditary or familial amyloidosis
Hemodialysis-associated amyloidosis
Localized amyloidosis
Morphology
Gross
Organs may appear enlarged, with a waxy, firm consistency
Microscopy
Extracellular amorphous deposits between cells
Kidney
Glomerular involvement
Expansion of mesangial matrix Capillary luminal narrowing
Interstitial deposition
Amyloid accumulation in interstitium Impact on tubular architecture
Heart
Subendocardial deposition
Liver
Deposition in hepatic sinusoids
Initial accumulation in Disse's space
Progression to hepatocyte encroachment
Spleen
Tapioca-like granules
Large map-like areas
Tongue
Macroglossia
Nodular deposits
Respiratory tract
Involvement from larynx to bronchioles
Brain
Amyloid plaques found in Alzheimer's disease
Peripheral and autonomic nerves
Familial amyloidotic polyneuropathies
Tissue Damage and Functional Consequences
Mechanisms of tissue damage
Displacement and destruction of normal tissue architecture
Interference with cellular function
Clinical manifestations
Impact on organ function
Symptoms associated with amyloid deposition
Diagnosis
Histologic demonstration of amyloid deposits
Congo Red, Apple Green birefringence in polarized microscopy
Serum and urine protein electrophoresis
Scintigraphy and other diagnostic tools

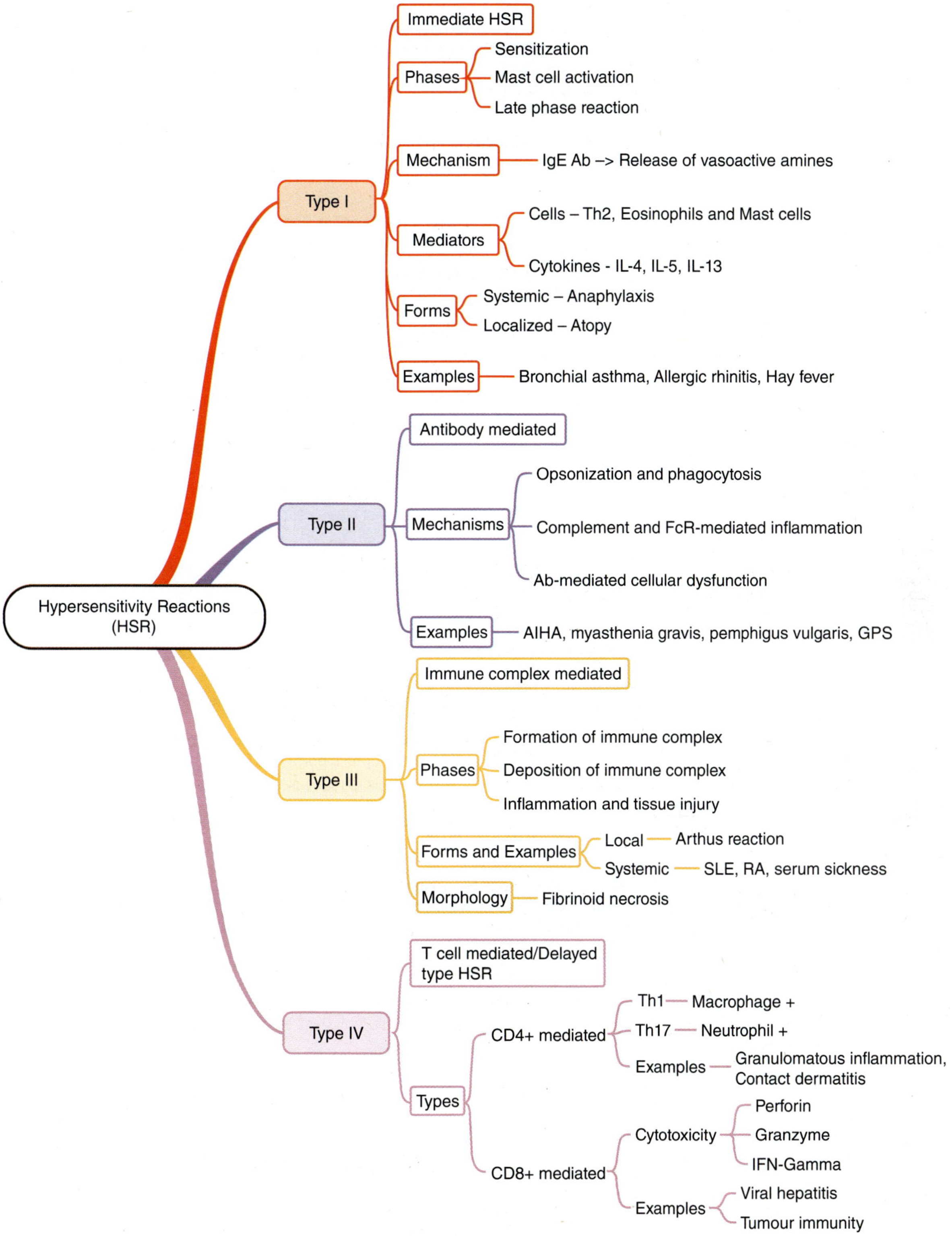
Hypersensitivity Reactions (HSR)
Type I
Immediate HSR
Phases
Sensitization
Mast cell activation
Late phase reaction
Mechanism
IgE Ab –> Release of vasoactive amines
Mediators
Cells – Th2, Eosinophils and Mast cells
Cytokines - IL-4, IL-5, IL-13
Forms
Systemic – Anaphylaxis
Localized – Atopy
Examples
Bronchial asthma, Allergic rhinitis, Hay fever
Type II
Antibody mediated
Mechanisms
Opsonization and phagocytosis
Complement and FcR-mediated inflammation
Ab-mediated cellular dysfunction
Examples
AIHA, myasthenia gravis, pemphigus vulgaris, GPS
Type III
Immune complex mediated
Phases
Formation of immune complex
Deposition of immune complex
Inflammation and tissue injury
Forms and Examples
Local
Arthus reaction
Systemic
SLE, RA, serum sickness
Morphology
Fibrinoid necrosis
Type IV
T cell mediated/Delayed type HSR
Types
CD4+ mediated
Th1
Macrophage +
Th17
Neutrophil +
Examples
Granulomatous inflammation, Contact dermatitis
CD8+ mediated
Cytotoxicity
Perforin
Granzyme
IFN-Gamma
Examples
Viral hepatitis
Tumour immunity

- **Systemic Lupus Erythematosus (SLE)**
  - **Introduction to SLE**
    - Definition: Autoimmune disease involving multiple organs.
    - Characterized by a wide array of autoantibodies, especially antinuclear antibodies (ANAs).
    - Chronic, remitting, and relapsing illness.
    - Injury caused by immune complexes and binding of antibodies to various cells and tissues.
  - **Epidemiology**
    - Prevalence: Up to 1 in 2500 in certain populations.
    - Predominantly affects women (female-to-male ratio of 9:1 in reproductive age).
    - Higher prevalence in blacks and Hispanics compared to whites.
    - Manifestation: Most common in twenties and thirties, but can occur at any age.
  - **Autoantibodies in SLE**
    - Hallmark: Production of autoantibodies, particularly ANAs.
    - Pathogenicity: Formation of immune complexes or direct attack on target cells.
    - Examples: Antibodies to double-stranded DNA and Smith (Sm) antigen.
    - Diagnostic value: Helps in diagnosis and management of SLE.
  - **Diagnostic Tests**
    - ANA Detection:
      - Methods: Indirect immunofluorescence, ELISAs.
      - Patterns: Homogeneous, rim, speckled, nucleolar, centromeric.
    - Other Autoantibodies: Against blood cells, phospholipid-protein complexes.
  - **Pathogenesis**
    - Genetic Factors: Contributions from MHC and non-MHC genes.
    - Immunologic Factors: Defective self-tolerance in B and T cells, activation of CD4+ helper T cells, role of type I interferons.
    - Environmental Factors: UV light exposure, sex hormones, drugs.
  - **Mechanisms of Tissue Injury**
    - Immune Complex Deposition: Type III hypersensitivity reaction.
    - Antibody-mediated Cytopenias: Examples include immune thrombocytopenic purpura (ITP).
    - Antiphospholipid Antibody Syndrome: Thrombotic complications.
    - Neuropsychiatric Manifestations: Antibodies crossing blood–brain barrier.
  - **Morphology**
    - Organ Involvement: Skin, kidneys, blood vessels, joints, CNS, serosal membranes, heart, lungs, spleen, lymph nodes.
    - Key Lesions: Necrotizing vasculitis, glomerulonephritis, skin rashes, joint synovitis, Libman-Sacks endocarditis.
  - **Clinical Features**
    - Variable Presentation: Fever, rash, joint pain, chest pain, photosensitivity, renal involvement, haematologic abnormalities.
    - Course: Relapsing and remitting, acute or indolent.
    - Complications: Renal failure, infections, coronary artery disease.
  - **Subtypes of Lupus**
    - Chronic Discoid Lupus Erythematosus.
    - Subacute Cutaneous Lupus Erythematosus.
    - Drug-Induced Lupus Erythematosus.
  - **Treatment and Prognosis**
    - Treatment: Corticosteroids, immunosuppressive drugs.
    - Prognosis: Improved survival rates, common causes of death include renal failure and infections.

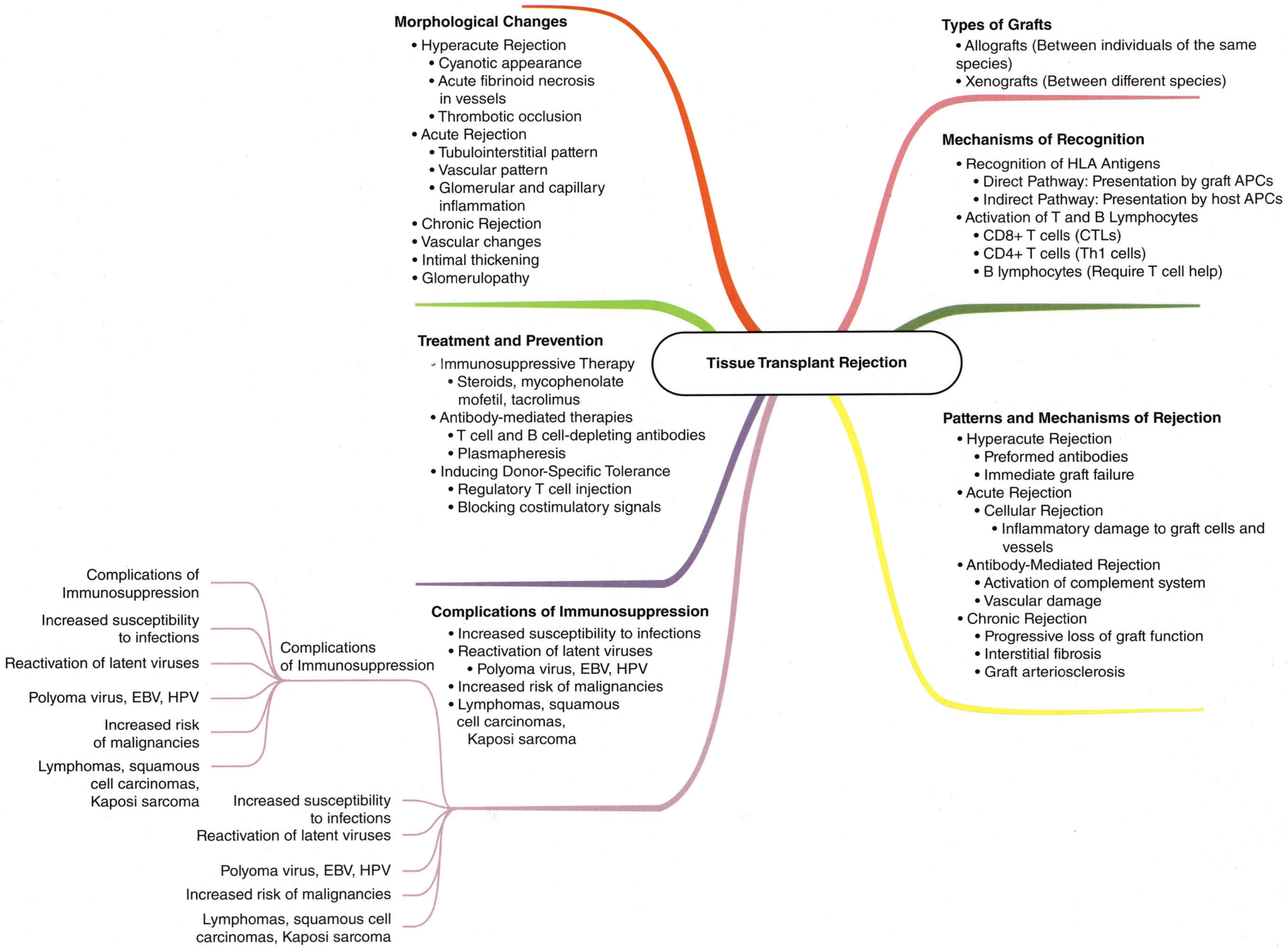
Tissue Transplant Rejection
Morphological Changes
• Hyperacute Rejection
• Cyanotic appearance
• Acute fibrinoid necrosis in vessels
• Thrombotic occlusion
• Acute Rejection
• Tubulointerstitial pattern
• Vascular pattern
• Glomerular and capillary inflammation
• Chronic Rejection
• Vascular changes
• Intimal thickening
• Glomerulopathy
Types of Grafts
• Allografts (Between individuals of the same species)
• Xenografts (Between different species)
Mechanisms of Recognition
• Recognition of HLA Antigens
• Direct Pathway: Presentation by graft APCs
• Indirect Pathway: Presentation by host APCs
• Activation of T and B Lymphocytes
• CD8+ T cells (CTLs)
• CD4+ T cells (Th1 cells)
• B lymphocytes (Require T cell help)
Treatment and Prevention
• Immunosuppressive Therapy
• Steroids, mycophenolate mofetil, tacrolimus
• Antibody-mediated therapies
• T cell and B cell-depleting antibodies
• Plasmapheresis
• Inducing Donor-Specific Tolerance
• Regulatory T cell injection
• Blocking costimulatory signals
Patterns and Mechanisms of Rejection
• Hyperacute Rejection
• Preformed antibodies
• Immediate graft failure
• Acute Rejection
• Cellular Rejection
• Inflammatory damage to graft cells and vessels
• Antibody-Mediated Rejection
• Activation of complement system
• Vascular damage
• Chronic Rejection
• Progressive loss of graft function
• Interstitial fibrosis
• Graft arteriosclerosis
Complications of Immunosuppression
• Increased susceptibility to infections
• Reactivation of latent viruses
• Polyoma virus, EBV, HPV
• Increased risk of malignancies
• Lymphomas, squamous cell carcinomas, Kaposi sarcoma
Complications of Immunosuppression
Complications of Immunosuppression
Increased susceptibility to infections
Reactivation of latent viruses
Polyoma virus, EBV, HPV
Increased risk of malignancies
Lymphomas, squamous cell carcinomas, Kaposi sarcoma
Increased susceptibility to infections
Reactivation of latent viruses
Polyoma virus, EBV, HPV
Increased risk of malignancies
Lymphomas, squamous cell carcinomas, Kaposi sarcoma

7 Neoplasia

Rajeswari Kathiah

PA 7.1 Define and classify neoplasia. Describe the characteristics of neoplasia including gross, microscopy, biology, behaviour and spread. **Differentiate benign from malignant neoplasms.**

PA 7.2 Describe the **molecular basis of cancer.**

PA 7.3 Enumerate **carcinogens** and describe the process of **carcinogenesis.**

PA 7.4 Describe the effects of tumour on the host including **paraneoplastic syndrome.**

PA 7.5 Describe immunology and the **immune response to cancer.**

CHAPTER OUTLINE

OVERVIEW PA 7.1

Cancer is one of the leading causes of death across the globe. It is also one of the leading causes of morbidity among people of all ages. The desire of mankind to conquer this dreaded disease is still unquenchable. In this chapter, we describe the nomenclature, tumour biology, molecular basis, morphological features and diagnostic methodologies of neoplasms.

NOMENCLATURE (TABLE 7.1)

The term 'neoplasm' refers to the tumour mass itself. The process that results in a neoplasm is called neoplasia. ***'Tumour'*** is synonymous with neoplasm. ***'Oncology'*** is the study of neoplasms. In the words of British oncologist Willis, *'A neoplasm is an abnormal mass of tissue, the growth of which exceeds and is uncoordinated with that of the normal tissues and persists in the same excessive manner after cessation of the stimuli which evoked the change'.*

Table 7.1 Nomenclature of Tumours

Cell of Origin – Histogenesis	Benign Tumours	Malignant Tumours
Tumours of Epithelial Origin		
Squamous cell	Squamous papilloma	Squamous cell carcinoma
Glandular cell	Adenoma	Adenocarcinoma
	Papilloma	Papillary carcinoma
	Cystadenoma	Cystadenocarcinoma
Basal cell		Basal cell carcinoma
Transitional cell	Transitional cell papilloma	Transitional cell carcinoma
Renal cell	Renal tubular adenoma	Renal cell carcinoma
Liver cell	Hepatic adenoma	Hepatocellular carcinoma
Germ cell		Seminoma Nonseminomatous germ cell tumours
Placental cell	Hydatidiform mole	Choriocarcinoma
Melanocytes	Nevus	Malignant melanoma
Tumours of Mesenchymal Origin		
Stroma and its derivatives	Lipoma	Liposarcoma
	Fibroma	Fibrosarcoma
	Chondroma	Chondrosarcoma
	Osteoma	Osteosarcoma
Tumours of Muscle Origin		
Skeletal muscle	Rhabdomyoma	Rhabdomyosarcoma
Smooth muscle	Leiomyoma	Leiomyosarcoma
Tumours of Haematopoietic Origin		
Haematopoietic cells		Leukaemias Myeloma
Lymphoid tissue		Lymphomas
Tumours of Blood Vessels and their Surface Coverings		
Blood vessels	Haemangioma	Angiosarcoma
Lymphatics	Lymphangioma	Lymphangiosarcoma
Mesothelium	Benign fibrous tumour	Mesothelioma
Tumours from More Than One Cell of Origin		
Salivary gland	Pleomorphic adenoma	Malignant mixed tumour
Tumours from More Than One Cell of Origin and More Than One Germ Cell Layer		
Totipotent cells in germ cells or in embryonic rests	Mature teratoma	Immature teratoma

In the molecular era, neoplasm can be defined as *'growth that is triggered by a series of acquired mutations affecting a single cell and its clonal progeny'.*

All tumours have two fundamental components:

1. ***Parenchyma,*** which is made up of neoplastic cells
2. ***Stroma,*** which supports the parenchymal cells and is composed of connective tissue and blood vessels

The classification and biological behaviour of tumours are primarily based on the parenchymal component, but their growth and spread are dependent on the stroma. '**Desmoplasia**' is the term used to describe the abundant stroma produced by neoplastic parenchymal cells (Fig. 7.1). Tumours with scant connective tissue are soft and fleshy, whereas tumours with abundant stroma are hard and scirrhous.

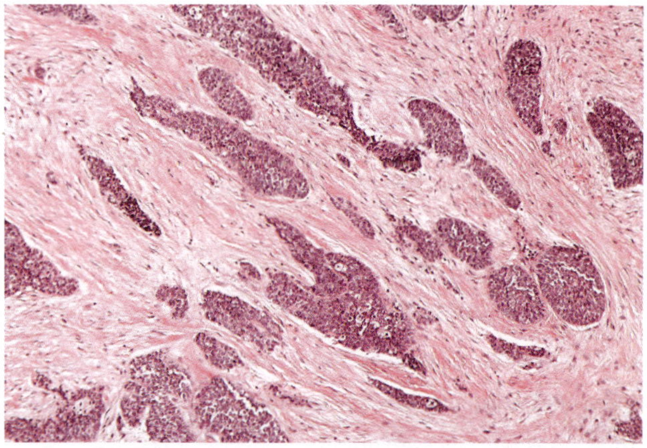

Fig. 7.1 Desmoplasia seen in desmoplastic small round cell tumour. (*Source:* https://www.google.com/url?sa=i&url=https%3A%2F%2Fen.wikipedia.org%2Fwiki%2FDesmoplasia&psig=AOvVaw0EKzqVCc_E1cfBFkWIBqcl &ust=1607155858198000&source=images&cd=vfe&ved=0CAIQjRxqFwoTCLjM-MTws-0CFQAAAAAdAAAAABAD.)

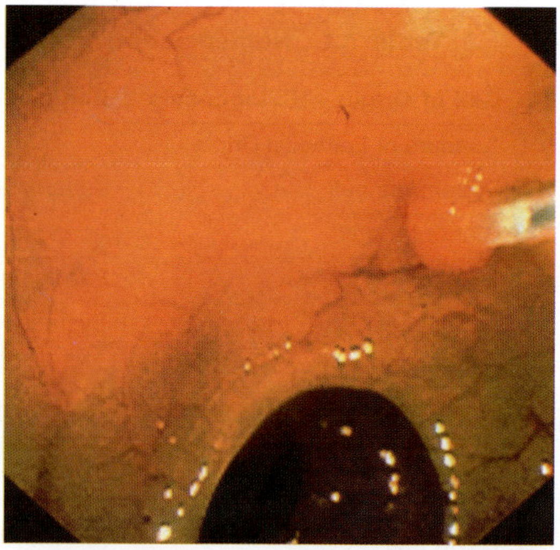

Fig. 7.2 Endoscopic view of hyperplastic polyp. Hyperplastic polyps are typically small (<5 mm) and are about the same colour as the surrounding colonic mucosa.

Benign Tumours

Localized, noninvasive, innocent-looking tumours, which are amenable for surgical removal, comprise the benign category. Although nonaggressive in nature, these tumours can be a cause of significant morbidity and at times death.

Tumours are classified according to their cell of origin, macroscopic architecture or microscopic pattern. Benign tumours are designated by adding the suffix *-oma* to the name of the cell of origin.

Malignant Tumours

Malignant tumours are also referred to as 'cancers', derived from the Latin word for 'crab' because of their invasive behaviour. Malignant tumours can **invade locally and spread to distant** sites. The outcome of malignant tumours is not always unfavourable and is dependent on the tumour type, stage of presentation and grade of the tumour (described later).

Malignant tumours arising from epithelial cells are called ***carcinomas***, those arising from stroma are called ***sarcomas*** and those from blood-forming cells are called leukaemias and lymphomas. Sometimes, the organ or tissue of origin can be identified and added, as in hepatocellular carcinoma (HCC), salivary duct carcinoma, etc.

Other terminologies in naming tumours are as follows:

- Tumours composed of immature cells are called **blastomas** along with the name of organ or cell of origin such as retinoblastoma and neuroblastoma.
- The term '***polyp***' is used for a neoplasm, benign or malignant, that produces a macroscopically visible projection above a mucosal surface and projects into the lumen (Fig. 7.2).
- **Mixed tumours:** A mixed tumour can be benign or malignant and is the result of a divergent differentiation of a single neoplastic clone. For example, a mixed tumour of the salivary gland, which is also called pleomorphic adenoma, arises from a single clone with the capacity to differentiate into epithelial, myoepithelial and stromal cells (Figs 7.3 and 7.4).
- **Teratoma** refers to the tumour composed of immature and mature cells derived from more than one germ layer, at times from all the three germ layers. This tumour is commonly seen in the ovary and testis (Figs 7.5 and 7.6).
- **Hamartoma:** This is a disorganized mass composed of cells belonging to that site.
- **Choristoma:** This refers to the heterotopic rest of cells. An example is pancreatic tissue in submucosa of the gastrointestinal tract.

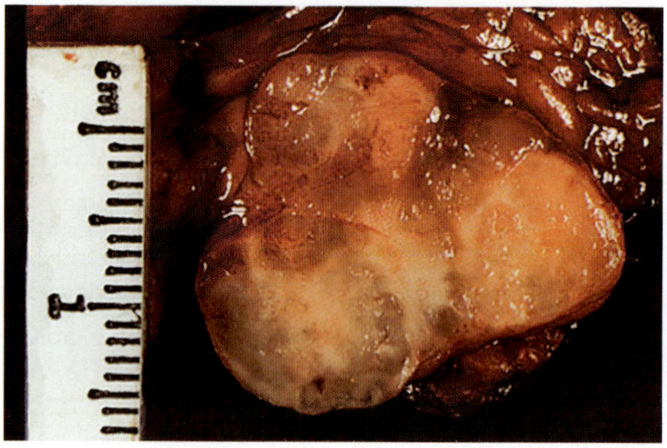

Fig. 7.3 Mixed tumour, gross; note the glistening appearance. (*Source:* Jonathan B. McHugh. Major and Minor Salivary Glands. In Rosai and Ackerman's Surgical Pathology. 11th edition. 2018 Elsevier.)

FEATURES OF MALIGNANT NEOPLASMS

Differentiating a malignant tumour from a benign tumour is extremely important in the diagnostic workup,

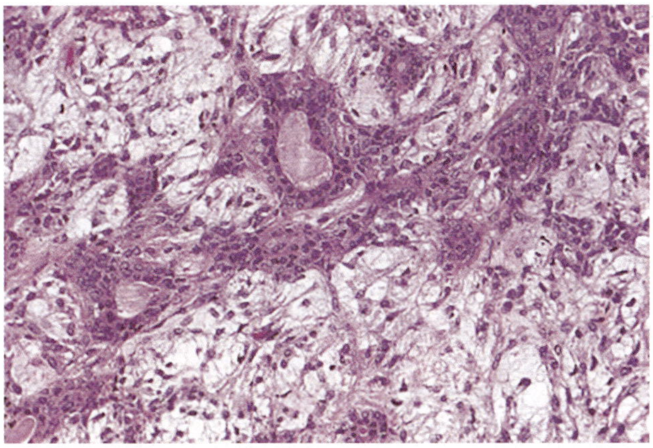

Fig. 7.4 Mixed tumour, microscopy; epithelial and myoepithelial cells are seen in myxoid background. (*Source:* Jonathan B. McHugh. Major and Minor Salivary Glands. In Rosai and Ackerman's Surgical Pathology. 11th edition. 2018 Elsevier.)

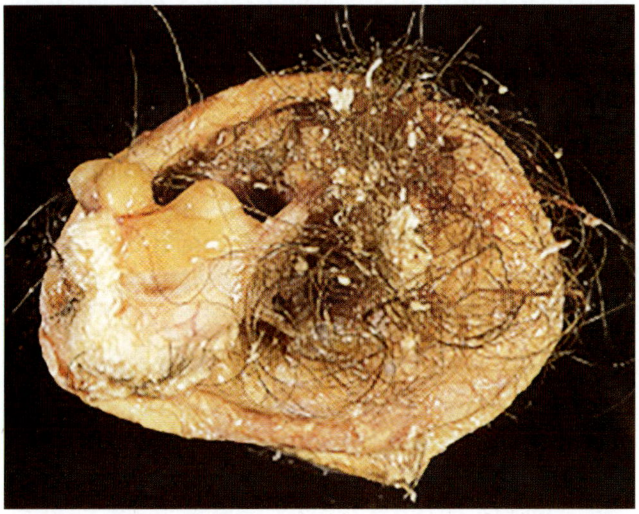

Fig. 7.5 Teratoma of ovary, gross – cyst filled with hair and keratinous debris with one solid nodular area (Rokitansky protuberance). (*Source:* From Mary Segars Dolan, Cherie Hill and Fidel A. Valea. Benign Gynecologic Lesions: Vulva, Vagina, Cervix, Uterus, Oviduct, Ovary, Ultrasound Imaging of Pelvic Structures. Comprehensive Gynecology. 7th edition. 2017. Elsevier.)

and the management of patients with an overdiagnosis is as bad as of those with an underdiagnosis. The differences between benign and malignant tumours are listed in Table 7.2. Characteristics and hallmark features of malignant tumours that would help in differentiating a malignant tumour from a benign tumour are listed in Fig. 7.7. Not all malignant tumours have all the mentioned features. These may occur singly or in combination and should be clearly documented in the histopathology report. These features are not just helpful in differentiating malignant tumours from benign ones but also helpful in grading the tumours and prognosticating them, which is explained in detail later.

- Differentiation and anaplasia
- Pleomorphism

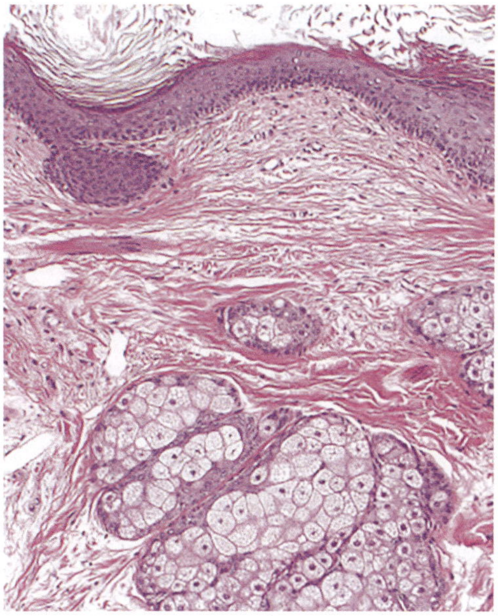

Fig. 7.6 Mature cystic teratoma, microscopy – this cyst is lined by mature epidermis and is subtended by connective tissue containing exuberant dermal appendages (pilosebaceous follicles). (*Source:* From Mary Segars Dolan, Cherie Hill and Fidel A. Valea. Benign Gynecologic Lesions: Vulva, Vagina, Cervix, Uterus, Oviduct, Ovary, Ultrasound Imaging of Pelvic Structures. Comprehensive Gynecology. 7th edition. 2017. Elsevier.)

Table 7.2 Differences Between Benign and Malignant Tumours

Characteristics	Benign Tumours	Malignant Tumours
Differentiation	Well-differentiated appearance Structure similar to that of tissue of origin Little or no anaplasia	Usually some lack of differentiation Structure often atypical Variable degree of anaplasia
Growth rate	Slow progressive expansion Rare mitotic figures Normal-appearing mitotic figures	Slow-to-rapid growth Erratic growth rate Mitotic figures often numerous Mitotic figures sometimes abnormal
Local invasion	No invasion Cohesive and expansile growth Capsule often present	Local invasion Infiltrative growth Usually no capsule
Metastasis	No metastasis	Frequent metastasis (definitive criterion for malignancy)

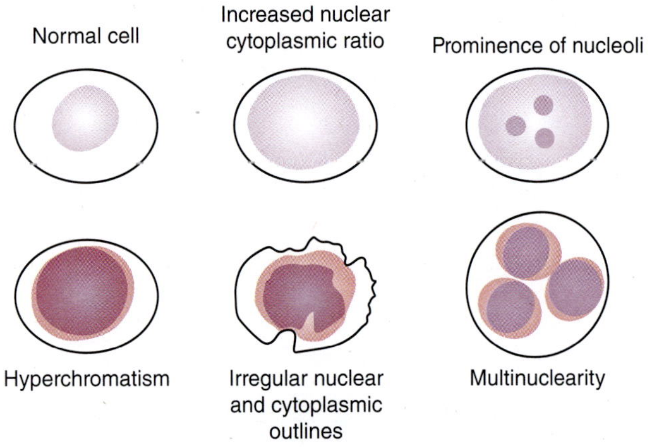

Fig. 7.7 Nuclear features of malignancy.

- Atypical nuclear features
- Atypical mitosis
- Loss of polarity
- Necrosis

  Hallmark features of malignancy are the following:
  - Local invasion
  - Metastasis

Differentiation and anaplasia

The extent to which the neoplastic cells resemble their cell of origin, both physically and physiologically, is called differentiation. Malignant tumours are further classified into mild, moderate and poorly differentiated according to their extent of resemblance to their corresponding normal tissue. Differentiating a well-differentiated malignancy (Fig. 7.8) from benign tumours is not simple, and other factors of malignancy need to be accounted for. Lack of differentiation is called **anaplasia.** Poorly differentiated cells are anaplastic, and anaplasia is the hallmark of malignancy.

Pleomorphism

Differences in size and shape of cells are referred to as pleomorphism. Cells in malignant tumours most often exhibit pleomorphism but not always. Cells within the same tumour may range from small cells to tumour giant cells with nuclear features of malignancy. Although pleomorphism is a feature of malignancy, some benign tumours also exhibit pleomorphism. Hence, this feature should be accounted for along with other features of malignancy (Fig. 7.9).

Atypical nuclear features

The following atypical nuclear features may be present in cells of malignant tumours singly or in combination:

- **Increased nuclear cytoplasmic ratio – may reach up to 1:1**
- **Irregular nuclear shape**
- **Irregularly clumped chromatin**
- **Hyperchromatic nuclei**
- **Abnormally large prominent nucleoli**

Exceptionally, malignant tumours might look bland with innocent-looking nuclei. Hence, careful examination for the presence of other features of malignancy is of immense help in arriving at the diagnosis.

Atypical mitosis

Mitotic figures are only markers for rapid cell growth and are not specific for malignant tumours. They are seen in a variety of normal tissues and in rapidly proliferating benign tumours. **Atypical mitotic figures** in the form of

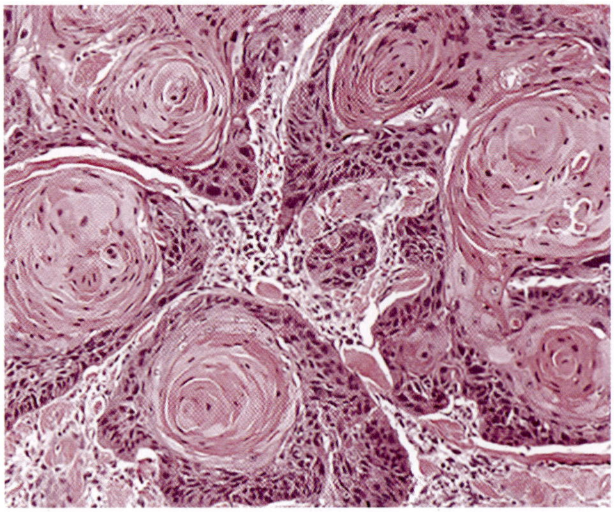

Fig. 7.8 Well-differentiated malignant tumour, microscopy – squamous cell carcinoma with many keratin horns and tumours recapitulating their normal counterparts. (*Source:* From Daniel J. Santa Cruz and Alejandro A. Gru. Tumors of the Skin. Diagnostic Histopathology of Tumors. 5th edition. 2021. Elsevier.)

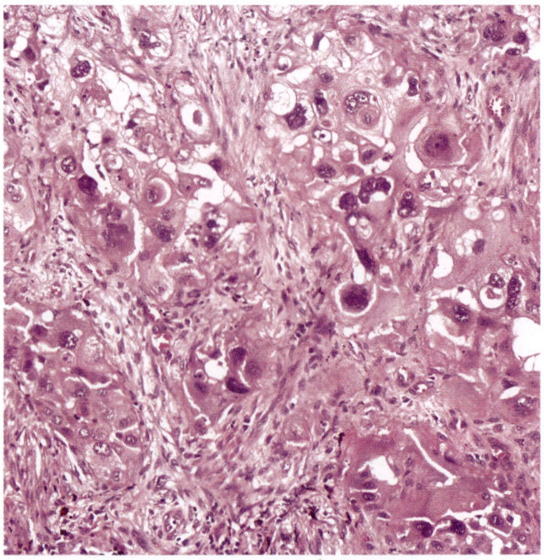

Fig. 7.9 Nonkeratinizing poorly differentiated squamous cell carcinoma. Poorly differentiated squamous cell carcinoma (SCC) shows vague nests of high-grade tumour cells with massive cytologic atypia. Poorly differentiated SCC cells can retain their eosinophilic cytoplasm and may be confused for large cell carcinoma.

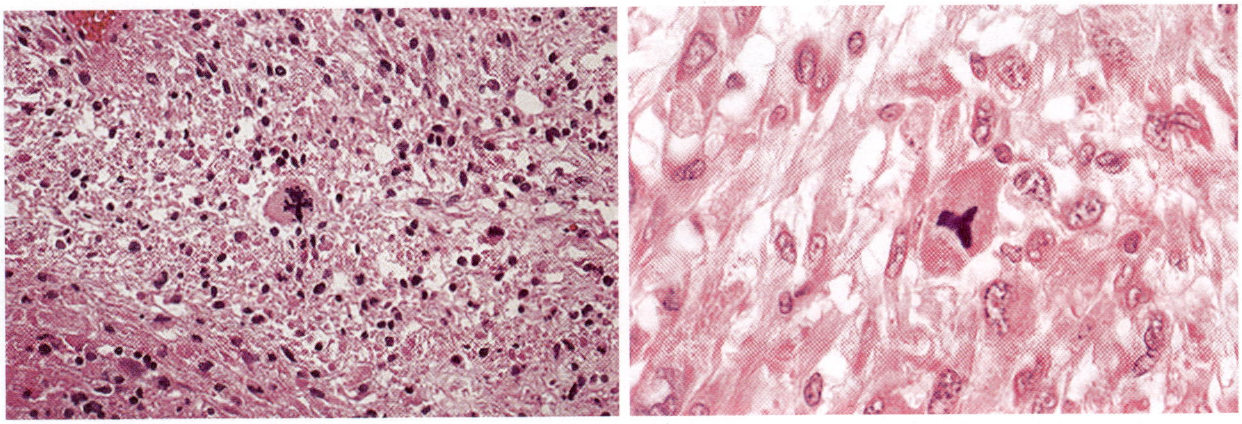

Fig. 7.10 Atypical mitotic figures in a malignant tumour. (*Source:* From Alomari, Ihab; Patel, Pranav M. Takayasu Arteritis. Elsevier 2022.)

tripolar, quadripolar or multipolar spindles (contrasted with the bipolar spindles of normal cells) are indicative of malignancy (Fig. 7.10). Assessing the mitotic activity status of a tumour is extremely helpful in grading many tumours. Mitotic figures can be counted by naked eye examination of the tissue sections, but this method is inaccurate and error prone. There are many markers for assessing the mitotic activity of the tumour population, and a few commonly used methods are as follows:

- Ki-67 labelling
- MIB1 index labelling
- Phosphohistone H3
- S-phase fraction

However, some malignant tumours are mitotically inactive. Hence, low or lack of mitotic activity should not be the sole criterion to rule out malignancy.

Loss of Polarity (Fig. 7.11)

Disturbance in the polarity of cells refers to **loss of alignment of the tumour cells to the basement membrane**, which is particularly evident in epithelial malignancies.

Necrosis

Tumour cells have an enormous need for oxygen and nutrients that are usually provided by new blood vessels. Despite this, rapidly growing malignant tumours frequently encounter hypoxia and nutrient deprivation because of insufficient blood supply. This results in central areas of ischaemic necrosis. Necrosis is included in many grading systems and is also an important diagnostic and prognostic marker for many malignant tumours (Fig. 7.12).

Hallmark Features of Malignancy

Local Invasion Most benign tumours are encapsulated (Fig. 7.13) within a fibrous capsule that creates a plane that makes the tumour discrete, palpable, mobile and easily resectable. In contrast, malignant tumours are poorly demarcated with lack of cleavage plane and are characterized by progressive infiltration, invasion and destruction of the surrounding tissues (Fig. 7.14). Invasiveness makes the resection more difficult.

Carcinoma in situ (CIS) is considered as the preinvasive phase of carcinoma that displays all the cellular features of malignancy except invasion of the basement

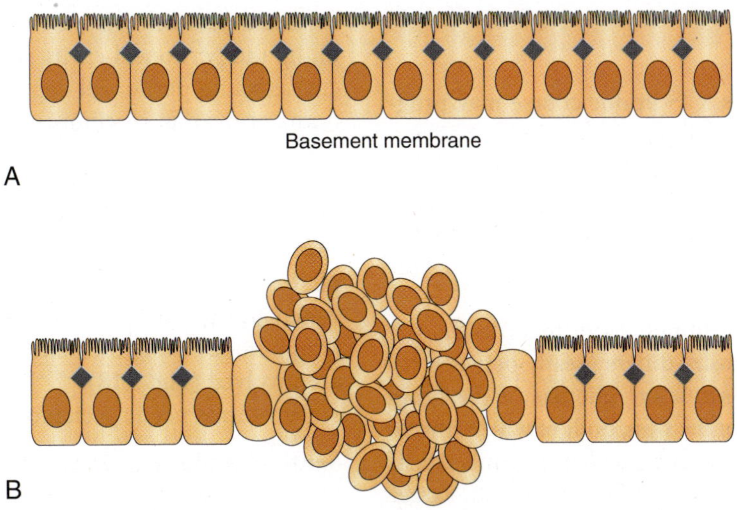

Fig. 7.11 Excessive growth with loss of polarity and tissue disorganization are hallmark features of malignancy.

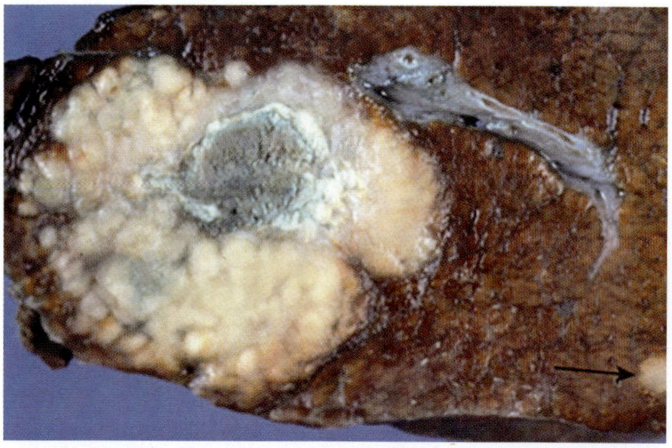

Fig. 7.12 Malignant tumour with necrosis – hepatocellular carcinoma, gross. (*Source:* From Laura W. Lamps. Liver: Tumors and Tumorlike Conditions. In Rosai and Ackerman's Surgical Pathology. 11th edition. Elsevier 2018.)

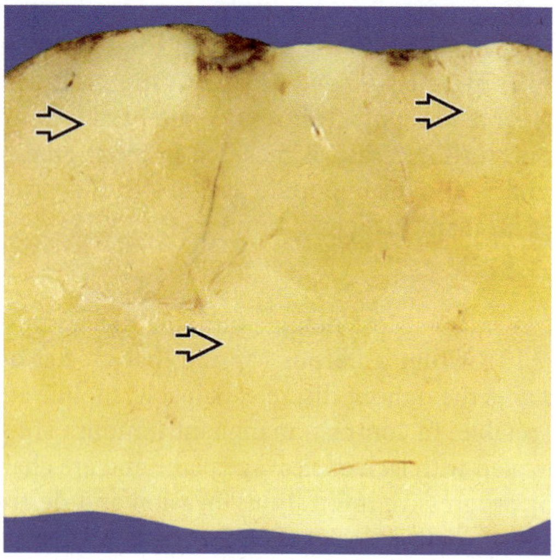

Fig. 7.13 Benign encapsulated tumour, gross; note the circumscription and the presence of delicate capsule surrounding the tumour. (*Source:* https://www.google.com/url?sa=i&url=https%3A%2F%2Fvoices.uchicago.edu%2Fgrosspathology%2Fbone-soft-tissue%2Flipoma%2F&psig=AOvVaw2EeVgrLG4BX4m8TKuJ7bXb&ust=1606482185979000&source=images&cd=vfe&ved=0CAIQjRxqFwoTCIDO89OioO0CFQAAAAAdAAAAABAD.)

membrane and metastasis. CIS in due course may progress to invasive carcinoma.

Metastasis Metastasis is **the most reliable feature of malignancy**. It is defined as the spread of tumour to distant sites that are physically discontinuous with the primary site of tumour.

Although all malignant tumours can metastasize, the rate at which they metastasize differs greatly between tumours. Exceptions to this rule are gliomas of the brain and basal cell carcinoma of the skin, both of which invade early but metastasize rarely. The incidence of metastasis correlates with anaplasia, rapid tumour growth, larger size and aggressive local invasion in most cases.

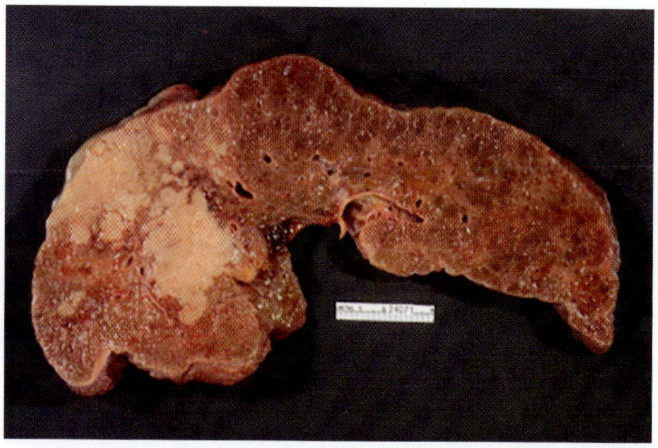

Fig. 7.14 Malignant tumour with invasion, gross – hepatocellular carcinoma. Poorly encapsulated hepatocellular carcinoma consisting of two dominant nodules with multiple smaller satellite nodules, arising in a background of cirrhosis. (*Source:* From Laura W. Lamps. Liver: Tumors and Tumorlike Conditions. In Rosai and Ackerman's Surgical Pathology. 11th edition. Elsevier 2018.)

Differences between benign and malignant neoplasms are shown in Fig. 7.15.

PATHWAYS OF SPREAD OF MALIGNANT TUMOURS

Spread of tumours from primary to distant secondary sites, a characteristic feature of malignant tumours, may occur by one of the following three pathways:

- Direct seeding of body cavities or surfaces
- Lymphatic pathway
- Haematogenous pathway

Direct Seeding of Body Cavities or Surfaces

This type of spread occurs when a malignant tumour penetrates into the body cavity or surface. It most often involves the peritoneal cavity, but pleural, pericardial, subarachnoid and joint spaces may also be involved. Seeding of the peritoneal cavity is a common characteristic feature of ovarian carcinomas, but the peritoneal deposits tend to be noninvasive and do not penetrate the organ. '**Pseudomyxoma peritonei**' is a term used for a gelatinous mass filling the peritoneal cavity seen in association with mucin-secreting peritoneal deposits from appendiceal carcinoma or ovarian carcinomas (Figs 7.16 and 7.17).

Lymphatic Pathway

This is **the most common pathway for initial spread of carcinomas**, but sarcomas may also use this route. Lymphatic vessels supplying the periphery of tumours are invaded by the tumour cells as the first step. Eventually, lymph nodes along the natural routes of these lymphatics are involved (Fig. 7.18).

Few terms need special mention here:

Sentinel node (Fig. 7.19): The first node in the regional lymphatic basin that receives lymph flow from the primary tumour is the sentinel node.

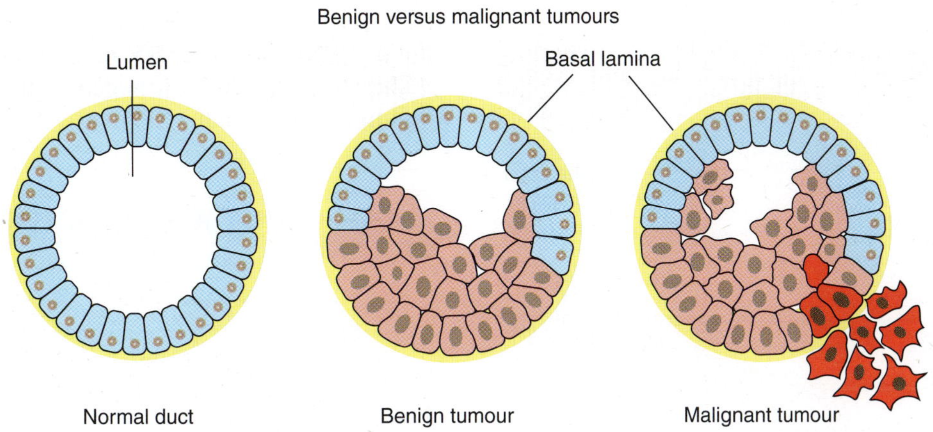

Fig. 7.15 Differences between benign and malignant tumours – schematic diagram.

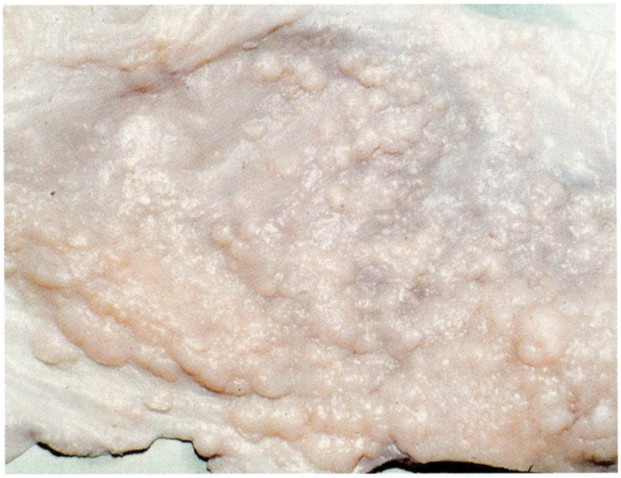

Fig. 7.16 Peritoneal deposits of metastatic carcinoma.

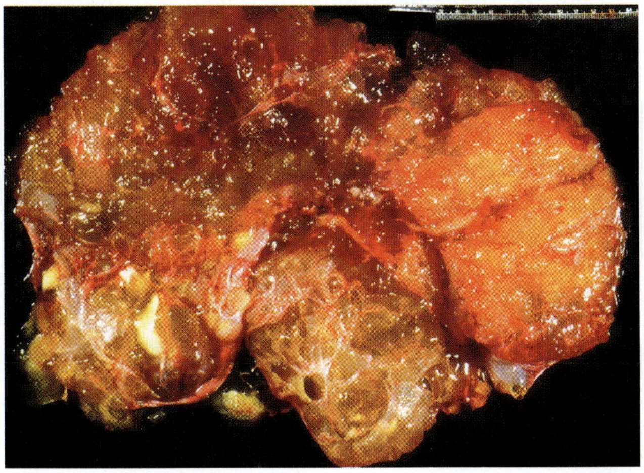

Fig. 7.17 Pseudomyxoma peritonei. A large mass of mucoid tissue with a prominent jelly-like consistency has been evacuated from the abdomen.

Skip metastasis: Owing to venous lymphatic anastomoses or obliteration of lymphatic channels because of inflammation or radiation, locoregional lymph nodes may be bypassed and result in skip metastases of distant nodes.

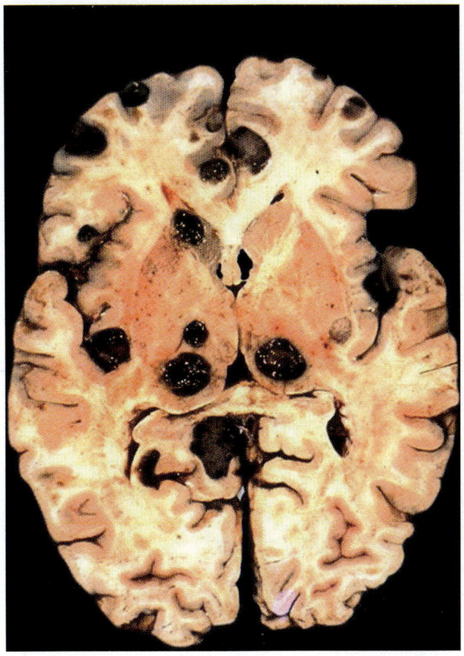

Fig. 7.18 Metastatic melanoma of CNS.

At least in the beginning, locoregional lymph nodes function to prevent the dissemination of the tumour by mounting an immune response against the tumour cells and destroying them. This may cause enlargement of the involved nodes with reactive changes. Hence, it should be stressed here that enlargement of the lymph nodes in the regional lymphatic basin could be because of reactive changes or secondaries and needs careful microscopic examination.

Haematogenous pathway

Sarcomas typically use this pathway for dissemination. Veins are easily penetrated by tumour cells compared with the thick-walled arteries, except in some uncommon conditions. With the invasion of the veins, tumour cells follow the venous flow draining the site of the primary tumour and come to rest in the first capillary bed they

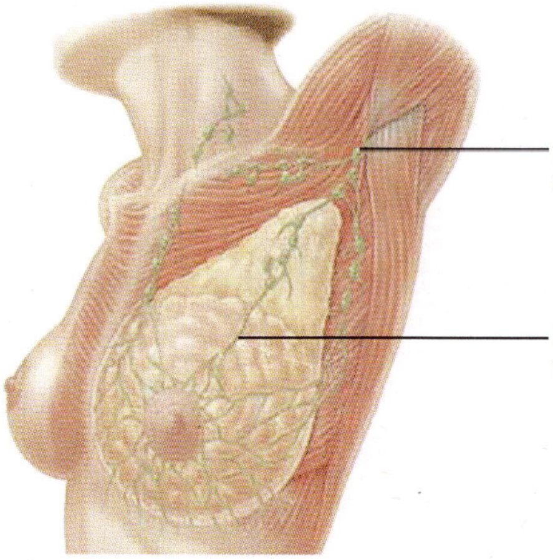

Fig. 7.19 Sentinel node.

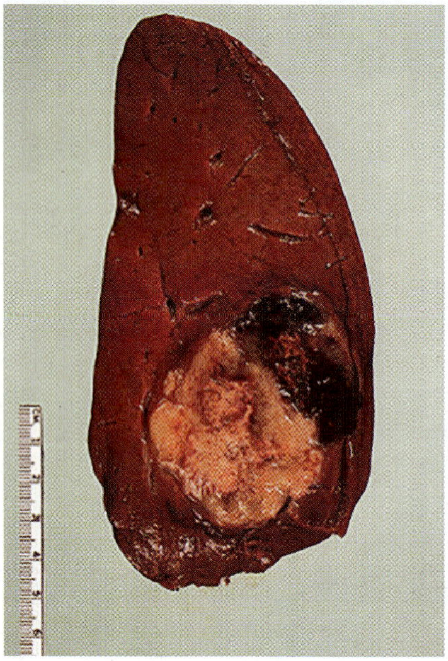

Fig. 7.20 Metastatic melanoma deposits in liver, gross; note the characteristic black colour. (*Source:* From Laura W. Lamps. Liver: Tumors and Tumorlike Conditions. In Rosai and Ackerman's Surgical Pathology. 11th edition. Elsevier 2018.)

come across. The ***liver and the lungs are the most commonly involved sites*** by the haematogenous pathway because caval blood flows to the lungs and the portal blood flows to the liver (Fig. 7.20).

Cancers of the prostate and thyroid may involve the paravertebral plexus and are associated with frequent vertebral metastases. Tumours like renal cell carcinoma and HCC have the tendency to invade and grow inside the veins without widespread dissemination. Careful microscopic examination of tumour areas for the presence of **lymphovascular invasion (LVI)** is extremely essential, because it is important in assessing the prognosis and designing treatment protocol. Apart from these mechanisms, many tumours have their preferred sites of metastasis for unknown reasons.

Examples include bronchogenic carcinomas involving the adrenals and brain.

EPIDEMIOLOGY AND AETIOLOGY OF CANCER

EPIDEMIOLOGY OF CANCERS

Cancer is the second leading cause of death globally and was responsible for an estimated 9.6 million deaths in 2018. Almost one in six deaths overall is because of cancer. About 70% of deaths from cancer occur in low- and middle-income countries because of late-stage presentation, inaccessibility to diagnosis and treatment. Alarmingly, the World Health Organization (WHO) predicts that the number of new cancer cases is expected to rise by approximately 70% over the next 20 years. In 2017, only 26% of low-income countries reported having pathology services available in the public sector in contrast to 90% of high-income countries.

The economic impact of cancer is significant and is increasing. Globally, cancer aetiology and epidemiology have received significant attention from researchers and policy makers. Although there is considerable overlap in common types of cancers worldwide, developing countries tend to have a higher incidence and death rates for viral infection–related cancers such as hepatitis-related liver cancer and human papillomavirus (HPV)–related cervical cancer. Only one in five low- and middle-income countries has the necessary data to drive cancer policy.

With the ongoing demographic and epidemiological transition, cancer is emerging as the major public health concern in India. Cancer is now the leading cause of catastrophic health spending, distress financing, increased expenditure and loss of lives in India. Cancer mortality has doubled from 1990 to 2016. India's cancer incidence is predicted to almost double as a result of demographic changes alone in 2040.

The most common cancers are as follows (Fig. 7.21; Table 7.3):

- Lung – 2.09 million cases
- Breast – 2.09 million cases
- Colorectal – 1.80 million cases
- Prostate – 1.28 million cases
- Skin cancer (nonmelanoma) – 1.04 million cases
- Stomach – 1.03 million cases

The most common causes of cancer deaths are as follows:

- Lung – 1.76 million deaths
- Colorectal – 862,000 deaths
- Stomach – 783,000 deaths
- Liver – 782,000 deaths
- Breast – 627,000 deaths

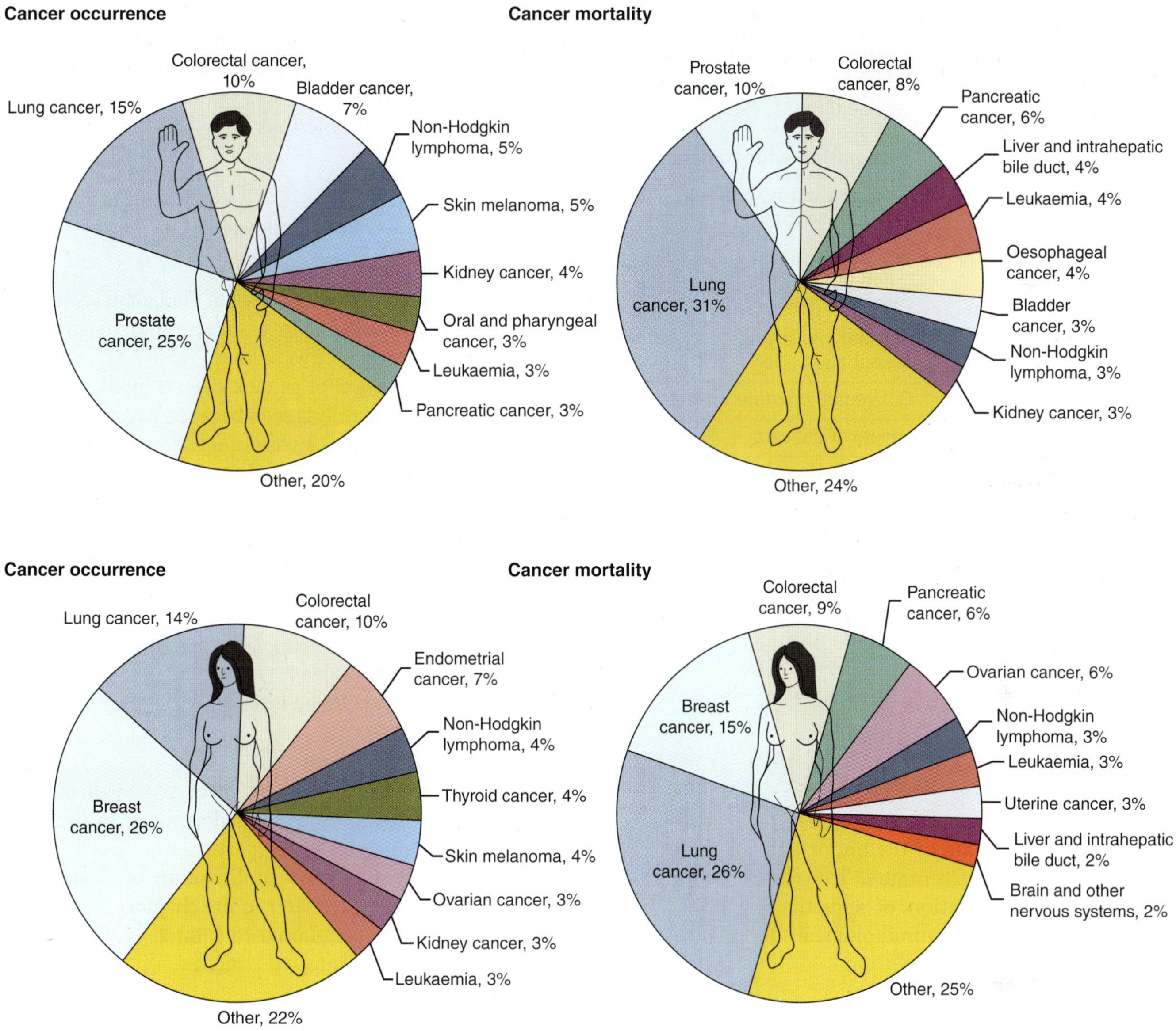

Fig. 7.21 Common cancers by occurrence and mortality in the United States in men and women. (*Source:* Jemal A, Siegel R, Ward E, et al. (2008). "Cancer statistics, 2008". CA Cancer J Clin. 58 (2): 71–96.)

Table 7.3 The Top Five Common Cancers in Indian Men and Women

	Men	Women
1	Lip, oral cavity	Breast
2	Lung	Lip, oral cavity
3	Stomach	Cervix
4	Colorectal	Lung
5	Oesophagus	Stomach

Reference: http://cancerindia.org.in/cancer-statistics/.

AETIOLOGY OF CANCERS

- **Environmental factors**
- **Age**
- **Acquired predisposing conditions**
- **Genetic predisposition**

Environmental Factors (Table 7.4)

Environment is the most dominating factor in the development of cancer and is the major reason for the wide variation in the geographic distribution of tumours. Modifying or avoiding key risk factors can significantly reduce the burden of cancer. The following factors are the common causes of malignancies:

- **Smoking**
- **Infectious agents**

Table 7.4 Common Environmental Carcinogens and Their Associated Cancers

Environmental Factors	Association with Cancers
Smoking	Lung, oral cavity, pharynx, larynx, oesophagus, pancreas, bladder
Infectious agents	Listed under 'Microbial carcinogenesis'
Alcohol	Oropharynx, larynx, oesophagus, liver
Diet	Colorectal, prostate, breast
Obesity	Variety of cancers
Hormonal imbalance	Breast, endometrium
Environmental carcinogens	Listed under the section chemical carcinogens

- **Alcohol**
- **Diet**
- **Obesity**
- **Hormonal imbalance**
- **Environmental carcinogens**

  Important factors are discussed in detail in Chapter 9.

Age

Advancing age is one of the important risk factors for the development of tumours. The reason behind this fact is the accumulation of somatic mutations along with the reduction in immunological surveillance as the age advances.

Acquired Predisposing Conditions

The diseases under this heading can be categorized as follows:

- Chronic inflammatory lesions
- Precursor lesions
- Immunodeficiency states

Each entity is detailed as follows:

a. **Chronic inflammatory states**
The mechanisms of development of malignancies (most commonly carcinomas) in a background of chronic inflammatory lesion are as follows (Table 7.5):
   i. The acquisition of genetic defects by the rapidly proliferating cells is seen because 'a restless soil is a fertile soil' for cancerous development.
   ii. Chronic inflammation increases the pool of stem cells, which are at a higher risk of transformation.
   iii Reactive oxygen species (ROS) produced as a part of immune response further induce genetic damage.
   iv. Metaplastic change induced by chronic inflammation is a forerunner of malignancy. Barret oesophagus is a classical example for this entity (Fig. 7.22).

b. **Precursor lesions** (Table 7.6)
Precursor lesions belong to the three categories shown in Table 7.6.

c. **Immunodeficiency states**
The major mechanism of the development of malignancies (most commonly haematogenous) in the immunocompromised states (particularly T-cell deficiency) is the unchecked proliferation of oncogenic viruses. This is detailed later in the chapter.
Example: Burkitt lymphoma in human immunodeficiency virus (HIV)–infected patients.

Table 7.5 List of the Common Malignancies that Arise from Chronic Inflammatory Background

Inflammatory Lesion	Associated Malignancy	Causative Agent
Asbestosis Silicosis	Mesothelioma Bronchogenic carcinoma	Asbestos fibres Silica particles
Chronic bronchitis	Bronchogenic carcinoma	Smoking Silica Asbestos
Cystitis	Bladder carcinoma	Chronic indwelling catheter
Inflammatory bowel disease	Colorectal carcinoma	
Lichen sclerosus	Vulvar squamous cell carcinoma	
Chronic pancreatitis	Pancreatic carcinoma	Alcohol
Barrett oesophagus	Oesophageal carcinoma	Gastric acids
Sjögren syndrome	MALT lymphoma	
Dermal inflammation	Malignant melanoma	UV light

UV, ultraviolet.

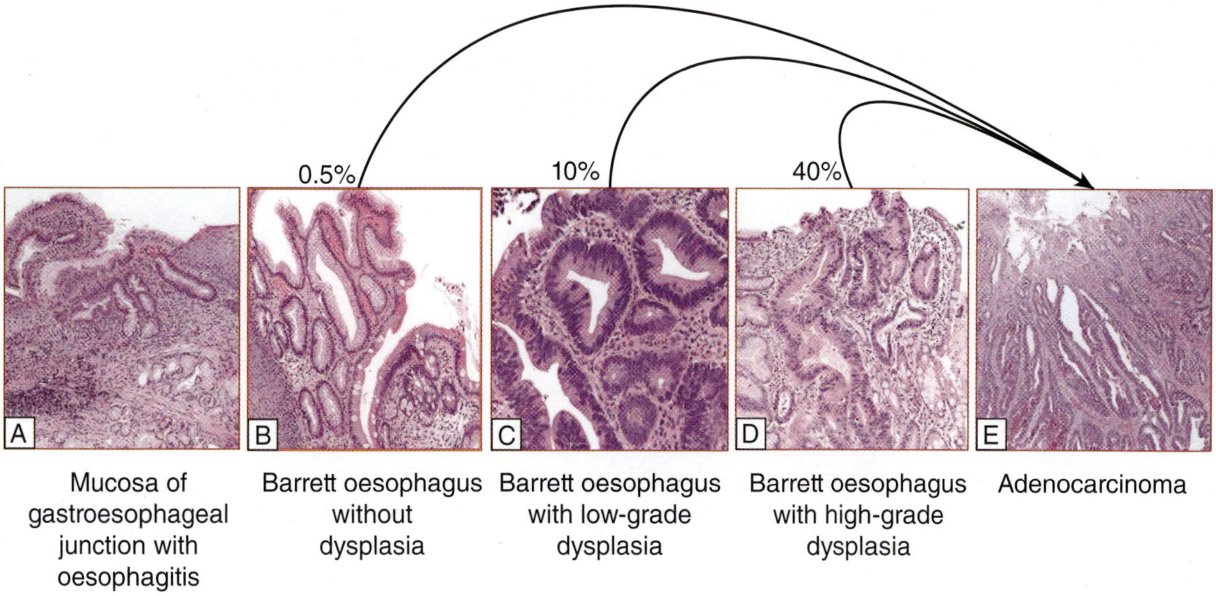

Fig. 7.22 Progression of long-standing Barrett oesophagus to oesophageal adenocarcinoma. (*Source:* https://www.spandidos-publications.com/10.3892/ijo.2012.1481.)

Table 7.6 Precursor Lesions and their Associated Malignancies

Precursor Lesion Category	Examples
Chronic inflammatory background	Barrett oesophagus Squamous metaplasia of bladder in schistosomiasis Colonic metaplasia in atrophic gastritis
Noninflammatory hyperplasia	Endometrial hyperplasia Oral leucoplakia
Benign neoplasms	Villous adenoma of the large intestine

Inherited predisposition to cancer

Genetic predisposition plays an important role in many cancers. More important is the **complex interaction between the genetic predisposition and the environmental factors.** Genetic factors can also influence the outcome of environmentally induced tumours. Apart from mutations, genetic polymorphisms of the enzymes involved in the conversion of procarcinogens to carcinogens influence the susceptibility to develop cancers. This is explained in a greater detail in the subsequent sections.

MOLECULAR BASIS OF MALIGNANCIES PA 7.2

Genetic change is the fundamental step for malignant transformation.

The following are the facts regarding genetic changes associated with malignancies:

1. **Nonlethal mutation** is the basis of carcinogenesis.
2. Genetic changes are **heritable** and are passed on to daughter cells. Hence, all the cells in a tumour are derivatives of the single transformed cell – **monoclonality**.
3. The common cancer-causing mutations involve the following genes:
   a. **Proto-oncogenes**
   b. Tumour suppressor genes
   c. **Genes involved in apoptosis**
   d. **Genes involved in DNA repair**
4. Cancer develops through **stepwise accumulation of complementary mutations** (Fig. 7.23). The process starts with ***initiating mutations,*** followed by acquisition of several ***driver mutations,*** which is succeeded by ***passenger mutations*** affecting the genes that maintain genomic integrity. Tumour progression is characterized by acquisition of **additional mutations**.
5. In addition to genetic changes, ***epigenetic alterations*** contribute to the characteristics of malignant cells. This may take the form of ***DNA methylation or histone modifications***. Unlike genetic mutations, epigenetic changes are reversible with drugs and hence are the areas of great interest for research.

MOLECULAR HALLMARKS OF MALIGNANCIES (FIG. 7.24)

The following are the fundamental molecular changes in cells that are considered as molecular hallmarks of malignancy:

1. Self-sufficiency in growth signals – mutation of proto-oncogenes

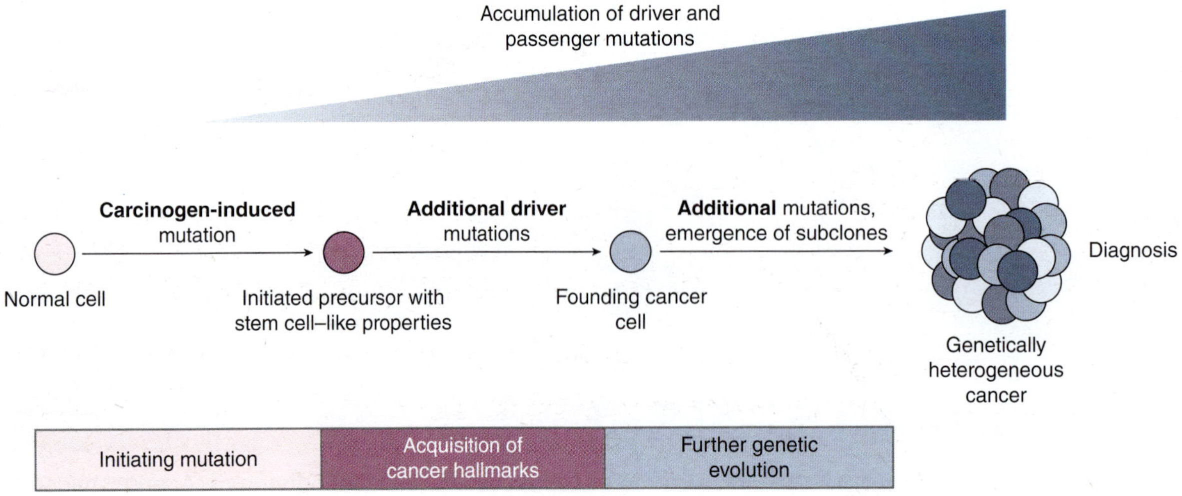

Fig. 7.23 Stepwise accumulation of mutations in chemical carcinogenesis. (*Source:* From Vinay Kumar, Abul K. Abbas and Jon C. Aster. Neoplasia. Robbins Basic Pathology. 10th edition. Elsevier 2018.)

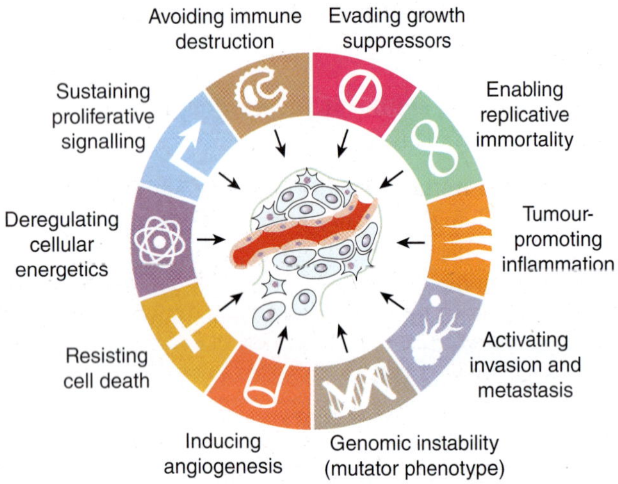

Fig. 7.24 Molecular hallmarks of cancer – eight cancer hallmarks and two enabling factors (genomic instability and tumour-promoting inflammation). Most cancer cells acquire these properties during their development, typically because of mutations in critical genes. (*Source:* From Vinay Kumar, Abul K. Abbas and Jon C. Aster. Neoplasia. Robbins Basic Pathology. 10th edition. Elsevier 2018.)

2. Insensitivity to growth inhibitory signals – mutation of tumour suppressor genes
3. Abnormal cellular metabolism – Warburg effect
4. Evasion of apoptosis
5. Limitless replication
6. Sustained angiogenesis
7. Local invasion
8. Distant metastasis
9. Evasion of host immune response

Apart from these molecular changes, ***genomic instability and cancer-promoting inflammation*** are considered enabling characteristics because these favour cellular transformation and tumour progression.

Each event is described next.

SELF-SUFFICIENCY IN GROWTH SIGNALS: MUTATION OF PROTO-ONCOGENES

Protein products of proto-oncogenes are essential for the normal cellular function. Understanding the steps involved in normal growth factor signalling pathways (Fig. 7.25) helps us in understanding the growth factor signalling pathways in cancer (Fig. 7.26). The role of proto-oncogenes is reviewed as given next.

Proto-oncogenes code for the following set of growth-promoting factors:

a. Growth factors (ligand or primary messenger)
b. Receptor for growth factors
c. Signal transduction proteins

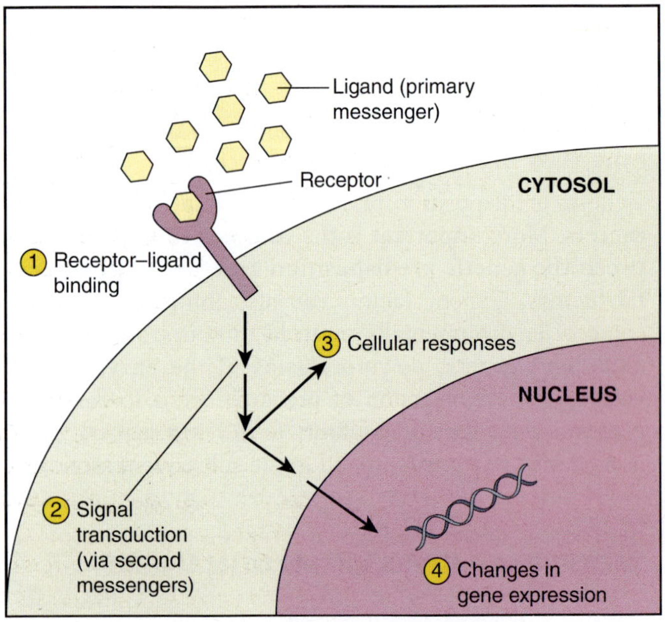

Fig. 7.25 Steps involved in normal growth factor signalling pathways. (*Source:* https://www.slideshare.net/bijitadutta123/signalling-mechanism-in-cell-growth.)

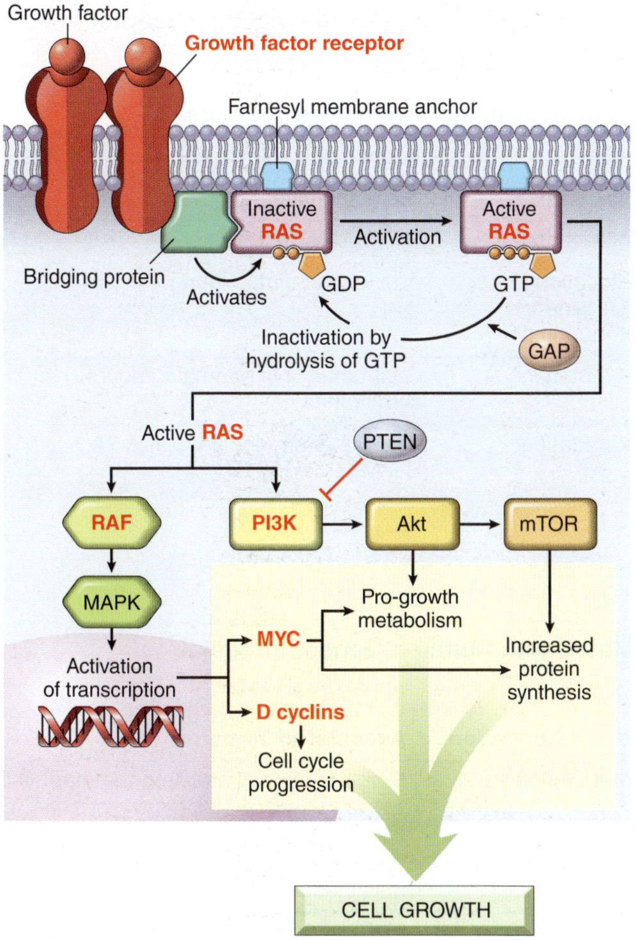

Fig. 7.26 Growth factor signalling pathways in cancer. (*Source:* From Vinay Kumar, Abul K. Abbas and Jon C. Aster. Neoplasia. Robbins Basic Pathology. 10th edition. Elsevier 2018.)

d. Nuclear transcription factors
e. Cell-cycle proteins and regulators

Mutated proto-oncogenes are called **oncogenes**. The proteins coded by oncogenes are called **oncoproteins**, and they function to promote the growth of tumour cells. Most of the oncogenes code for components of the cellular signalling system to promote growth of tumour cells. Oncogenes are categorized and described next.

Growth Factors

Growth factors are small polypeptides, elaborated by many cells, that normally act on another cell to promote its proliferation. These are produced only when there is a stimulus for a cell to proliferate. When proto-oncogenes get transformed to oncogenes, these become autonomous and the growth factors are produced even in the absence of a stimulus (Table 7.7). Furthermore, a cancer cell may produce the growth factor it requires for its stimulation by itself.

Receptors for Growth Factors

Growth factors need the presence of growth factor–specific cell surface receptors for their actions. These receptors are

Table 7.7 Common Examples of Tumours Associated with Mutations in Growth Factor Genes

Growth Factors	Proto-Oncogene	Mode of Activation	Associated Tumours
PDGF-β	PDGFB	Overexpression	Astrocytoma
TGF-α	TGFA	Overexpression	Astrocytoma
FGF	HST1FGF3	Overexpression Amplification	Osteosarcoma Bladder carcinoma Breast carcinoma
HGF	HGF	Overexpression	Hepatocellular carcinoma Follicular carcinoma thyroid

FGF, fibroblast growth factor; HGF, hepatocyte growth factor; PDGF-β, platelet-derived growth factor-β; TGF-α, transforming growth factor-α.

transmembrane proteins and have two surfaces: an extracellular portion that has a domain for binding growth factor, and an intracellular cytoplasmic domain that has an enzyme-activating area which triggers cellular proliferation.

When the genes for growth factor receptors get mutated, these become autonomous and stimulate cell proliferation without the binding of growth factors (Table 7.8).

Targeted therapy: Drugs that specifically bind and inhibit these mutated growth factor receptors resulting in tumour growth cessation have been discovered and are in widespread use. This targeted therapy may not be effective in advanced cancers in which the tumour cell population has subclones with resistance to targeted therapy.

Signal Transduction Proteins

The signalling pathways can be receptor tyrosine kinase or nonreceptor tyrosine kinase pathways. Signal transduction proteins are present in the cytoplasm of cells and function to transduce the signals from the growth factor receptors to the nucleus of the cell, stimulating intracellular growth activation pathways. When the genes for signal transduction proteins get mutated, these become autonomous and stimulate cell proliferation without the activation of growth factor receptors (Table 7.9) is shown in Fig. 7.26.

Transcription Factors

The binding of growth factors with their receptors and the consequent activation of signalling pathways result in stimulation of nuclear transcription factors that promote cellular proliferation. When the genes for nuclear transcription factors get mutated, these become autonomous and stimulate cell proliferation without the activation of growth factor receptors and the signal transduction proteins. There

Table 7.8 Common Examples of Tumours Associated with Mutated Growth Factor Receptor Genes

Growth Factors Receptors	Proto-Oncogene	Mode of Activation	Associated Tumours
EGF – receptor family	ERBB1 – EGFR	Mutation	Adenocarcinoma of lung
	ERBB2 – HER	Amplification	Breast carcinoma
PDGF receptor	RET	Point mutation	Gliomas, leukaemias
ALK receptor	ALK	Translocation Fusion gene Point mutation	Adenocarcinoma of lung
Receptor for KIT ligand	KIT	Point mutation	Gastrointestinal stromal tumours, seminomas
Receptor for neurotropic factors	RET	Point mutation	Multiple endocrine neoplasia 2A, B – MEN 2A and B

PDGF, platelet-derived growth factor.

Table 7.9 Common Examples of Tumours Associated with Mutated Genes for Signal Transduction Proteins

Signal Transduction Proteins	Proto-Oncogene	Mode of Activation	Associated Tumours
GTP-Binding Proteins	KRAS	Point mutation	Colon, pancreas and lung tumours
	HRAS	Point mutation	Bladder and kidney tumours
	NRAS	Point mutation	Melanomas and haematological malignancies
RAS signal transduction	BRAF	Point mutation Translocation	Melanoma, leukaemias Colon cancers
Nonreceptor tyrosine kinase	ABL	Translocation Point mutation	Chronic myelogenous leukaemia Acute lymphoblastic leukaemia
JAK/STAT	JAK2	Translocation	Myeloproliferative disorders
NOTCH	NOTCH 1	Point mutation Translocation Gene rearrangement	Leukaemias Lymphomas

are many known transcription factors like MYC, MYB, JUN, FOS and REL, but of all these proteins, **MYC is the most commonly mutated transcription factor in human tumours.**

MYC Proto-Oncogene MYC is a family of regulator genes and proto-oncogenes that code for transcription factors. The MYC family consists of three closely related human genes: c-myc (MYC), l-myc (MYCL) and n-myc (MYCN).

MYC is activated by various mitogenic signals, and the protein products of MYC proto-oncogenes are transcription factors that activate the expression of many pro-growth genes through RAS/MAPK pathways. By modifying the expression of its target genes, MYC stimulation results in many biological effects. MYC promotes the growth of both normal and neoplastic cells.

Few of its major functions are as follows:

- Promotion of cell growth by upregulating cyclins and downregulating cell-cycle inhibitors
- Promotion of protein synthesis by upregulating rRNA genes and their processing
- Downregulation of apoptosis
- MYC upregulation being the basis for metabolic reprogramming and the Warburg effect, which is the fourth hallmark of cancer
- Stem cell self-renewal and reprogramming of somatic cells into pluripotent stem cells

MYC gene is mutated and amplified in many human cancers like Burkitt lymphoma, small-cell carcinoma lung, neuroblastoma and many other cancer types including breast, colorectal, pancreatic, gastric and endometrium (Table 7.10).

Table 7.10 Common Examples of Tumours Associated with Mutated MYC Gene

Transcription Factors	Proto-Oncogene	Mode of Activation	Associated Tumours
MYC	**CMYC**	Translocation	Burkitt lymphoma
	NMYC	Amplification	Neuroblastoma
	LMYC	Amplification	Small-cell carcinoma of lung

Cell-Cycle Proteins and Regulators

The process of growth factor binding with its receptors is followed by activation of signalling pathways and activation of transcription pathways. This ultimately leads to upregulation of cyclins and cyclin-dependent kinases, all of which function to push the cells into the cell cycle and regulate the orderly progression of cells through the various phases of the cell cycle to cause cellular proliferation (Fig. 7.27). When the genes for cyclins and cyclin-dependent kinases get mutated, they become autonomous and stimulate cell proliferation without the involvement of the preceding factors (Table 7.11). A similar unconditional proliferation occurs when cyclin-dependent kinase inhibitors (CDKIs), which prevent the uncontrolled proliferation of cells, are mutated. Gain-of-function mutations in genes for cyclins and cyclin-dependent kinases and loss-of-function mutations in genes for CDKIs result in tumour (Fig. 7.28).

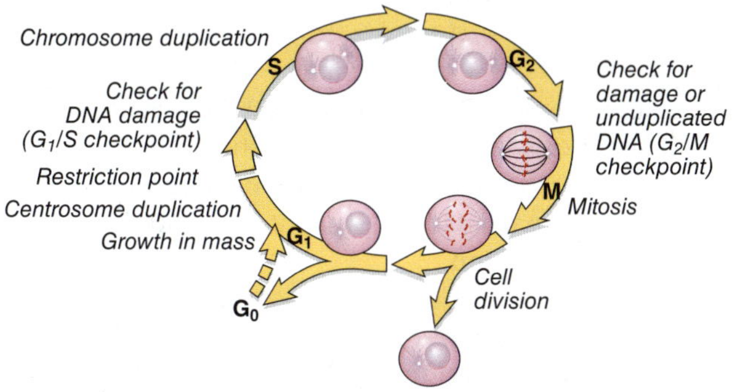

Fig. 7.27 Cell-cycle landmarks. (*Source:* From Vinay Kumar, Abul K. Abbas and Jon C. Aster. The Cell as a Unit of Health and Disease. Robbins Basic Pathology. 10th edition. 2018. Elsevier.)

INSENSITIVITY TO GROWTH INHIBITORY SIGNALS: MUTATION OF TUMOUR SUPPRESSOR GENES (TABLE 7.12)

The products of tumour suppressor genes function by applying brakes in the cell cycle and prevent them from unwanted proliferation. The mechanisms of tumour suppressor genes to prevent cellular proliferation are as follows:

- As cell-cycle checkpoints
- Inducing cell-cycle arrest
- Inducing apoptotic cell death
- Shifting the cells to postmitotic differentiated pool without replication

The two most important tumour suppressor proteins are **RB and p53,** which are called the 'governor of cell proliferation' and the 'guardian of our genome', respectively.

Salient features and functions of some of the above-listed tumour suppressor genes are described next.

Table 7.11 Common Examples of Tumours Associated with Mutated Genes for Cell-Cycle Proteins and Regulators

Cell-Cycle Proteins and Regulators	Proto-Oncogene	Mode of Activation	Associated Tumours
Cyclins	Cyclin D1	Translocation Amplification	Mantle cell lymphoma Breast carcinoma Oesophageal carcinoma Multiple myeloma
Cyclin-dependent kinases (CDK)	CDK4	Amplification	Glioblastoma Melanoma
Cyclin-dependent kinase inhibitors (CDKI)	p16	Inactivation	Melanoma Pancreatic carcinoma Glioblastoma

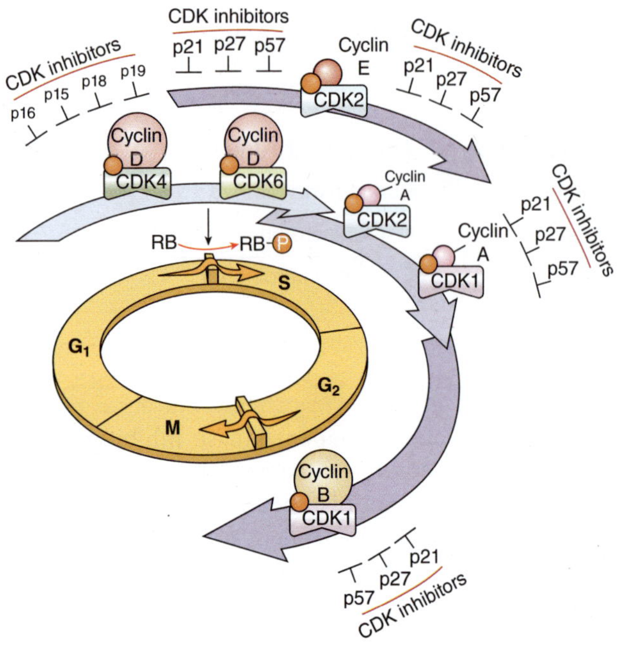

Fig. 7.28 Role of cyclins, CDKs and CDK inhibitors in cell cycle. (*Source:* From Vinay Kumar, Abul K. Abbas and Jon C. Aster. The Cell as a Unit of Health and Disease. Robbins Basic Pathology. 10th edition. 2018. Elsevier.)

TP53, the caretaker of cells

TP53 is a major tumour suppressor gene whose protein product functions to prevent cellular proliferation by various mechanisms (Fig. 7.29). The gene is located on chromosome 17p13.1 and is the most commonly mutated gene in human cancers that is detected in more than 50% of cancers. Loss-of-function mutations of both alleles of TP53 gene are acquired mutations in most cases of tumour development. Persons born with inherited or germline mutation of one of the two alleles of the TP53 gene are said to have **Li–Fraumeni syndrome** and develop tumour when the second allele gets mutated. Individuals with this syndrome are at a multifold risk of developing multiple primary tumours at a younger age. The syndrome complex comprises a variety of tumours like sarcomas, breast cancer, leukaemias, brain tumours and adrenocortical carcinomas.

TP53 codes for its protein product p53, which acts at many levels to prevent cancer development.

- First, with the help of a large network of signals, it senses cellular stresses like damages to DNA, shortened telomeres, hypoxia and excessive pro-growth signals induced by MYC and RAS.
- These signals release p53, which is bound to its inhibitor MDM2, and activate it. The mechanisms that trigger the release of p53 from its inhibitor MDM2 are given next.

Hypoxia and DNA Damage Hypoxia and DNA damage result in the upregulation of two important protein kinases involved in the activation of p53: (1) **ATM** – ataxia–telangiectasia mutated; (2) **ATR** – ataxia–telangiectasia and RAD3 related. These two enzymes release p53 from MDM2 and result in the accumulation of p53.

Activation of Oncoproteins When pro-growth pathways are abnormally activated by oncoproteins like RAS, the expression of **p14/ARF** gets augmented. This releases p53 by degrading of MDM2.

- The outcomes following p53 activation and accumulation in a cell are different in different cells on the basis of the scenario. The events that accompany p53 activation are as follows (Fig. 7.29):
  - **Transient arrest of cell cycle**
  - **DNA repair**
  - **Cellular apoptosis**
  - **Cellular senescence**

Transient Arrest of Cell Cycle The p53-mediated growth inhibitory action is by transcription of CDKN1A gene. This gene induces production of p21, which acts at the late G1 phase and halts the cell cycle by inhibiting CDK4/cyclin D. The purpose of this step is to give enough resting time for the cells to get their damaged DNA repaired. This form of cell-cycle arrest is **temporary and reversible**. Once the damaged DNA is repaired, the cells are permitted to re-enter the cell cycle by the fall of p53 levels in the cells.

DNA Repair This is the **most essential step** because the DNA damage induced by a variety of insults gets repaired under the influence of p53. GADD45 is the p53 responsive stress protein that repairs the damaged DNA.

Cellular Apoptosis Cells with DNA damage that cannot be repaired by the repair mechanisms are made to undergo apoptosis by p53. This is actually a protective mechanism to prevent proliferation of cells with irreparable DNA damage, failing which it could result in neoplastic transformation.

Cellular Senescence Cellular senescence is different from transient cell-cycle arrest and is a state of **permanent arrest**. What exactly decides the fate of a cell as cellular senescence or apoptotic cell death is not yet clear.

Thus, abnormal cells with damaged DNA are blocked from replication and clonal expansion by effectively functioning p53. With all the functions of p53 explained, one can imagine the effects of loss of p53 functions in a cell. If a cell has no reserve of its functioning p53, DNA damages go unrepaired with accumulation of driver mutations in oncogenes and other genes, which ultimately results in the expansion of malignant clone and tumour formation.

The two other important facts about p53 mutations are as follows:

1. Tumours with p53 mutations are relatively **resistant to chemotherapy and radiotherapy,** the two common modalities of treatment of malignant tumours.
2. Cells with mutated p53 acquire a **mutator phenotype** with a tendency to incur additional mutations at a rate higher than that of other cells.

Table 7.12 List Of Common Tumour Suppressor Genes and the Tumours Associated with their Mutation

Gene	Protein	Familial Syndromes	Sporadic Tumours
TP53	p53 protein	Li–Fraumeni syndrome	Most cancers in humans
RB	Retinoblastoma protein	Familial retinoblastoma syndrome	Retinoblastoma Osteosarcoma Cancers of breast, colon and lung
APC	Adenomatous polyposis coli protein	Familial colonic polyps and cancers	Carcinoma of stomach, colon, pancreas and melanoma
NF-1	Neurofibromin	Type 1 neurofibromatosis	Neuroblastoma Juvenile myeloid leukaemia
NF-2	Merlin	Type 2 neurofibromatosis	Schwannoma, meningioma
PTEN	Phosphatase and tensin homologue	Cowden syndrome	Many cancers and lymphomas
BRCA1, BRCA2	Breast cancer-1 and breast cancer-2	Familial breast and ovarian carcinoma Male breast cancer Chronic lymphocytic leukaemia	-
MSH2, MLH1, MSH6	MSH2, MLH1, MSH6	Hereditary nonpolyposis colon carcinoma	Cancer of colon and endometrium
PTCH	Patched	Gorlin syndrome	Basal cell carcinoma, medulloblastoma
WT1	Wilms tumour 1	Familial Wilms tumour	Wilms tumour
MEN1	Menin	MEN-1 syndrome	Pituitary, parathyroid and pancreatic carcinoma
CDH1	E-cadherin	Familial gastric cancer	Gastric carcinoma, lobular carcinoma breast
VHL	von Hippel–Lindau protein	von Hippel–Lindau syndrome	Renal cell carcinoma
SMAD2, SMAD4	SMAD2, SMAD4	Juvenile polyposis	Colonic and pancreatic carcinoma
SDHB, SDHD	Succinate dehydrogenase complex subunits B and D	Familial paraganglioma and pheochromocytoma	Paraganglioma
STK11	Liver kinase B1 (LKB1)/STK11	Peutz–Jeghers syndrome	Diverse cancers
CDKN2A	P16/INK4a and p14/ARF	Familial melanoma	Cancers of pancreas, breast, oesophagus and melanoma

APC, adenomatous polyposis coli.

RB, a Negative Regulator of Cell Cycle (Fig. 7.30)

RB protein is expressed in every cell and is lost or inactivated in most of the human tumours.

Role of RB Gene in Regulation of Cellular Differentiation

RB exists in an active hypophosphorylated state in resting cells and is converted to an inactive hyperphosphorylated state in cells entering the cell cycle. In its active hypophosphorylated state, RB forms a complex with E2F transcription factors, inhibiting the production of cyclins and cyclin-dependent factors required for driving the cells in the cell cycle. When the growth factor signalling pathways are activated, RB gets hyperphosphorylated and goes into an inactive state, leaving E2F in the active state. This enhances the expression of cyclins and cyclin-dependent kinases and drives cells through the G1/S transition. **RB is the key player of the cell cycle,** regulating the balance between the cell-cycle proteins and their inhibitors.

Loss of control over cell cycle is the most important step in the development of malignancies. This happens when the following occur:

- Loss of function of RB
- Loss of inhibitors of cell cycle such as p16/INK4a

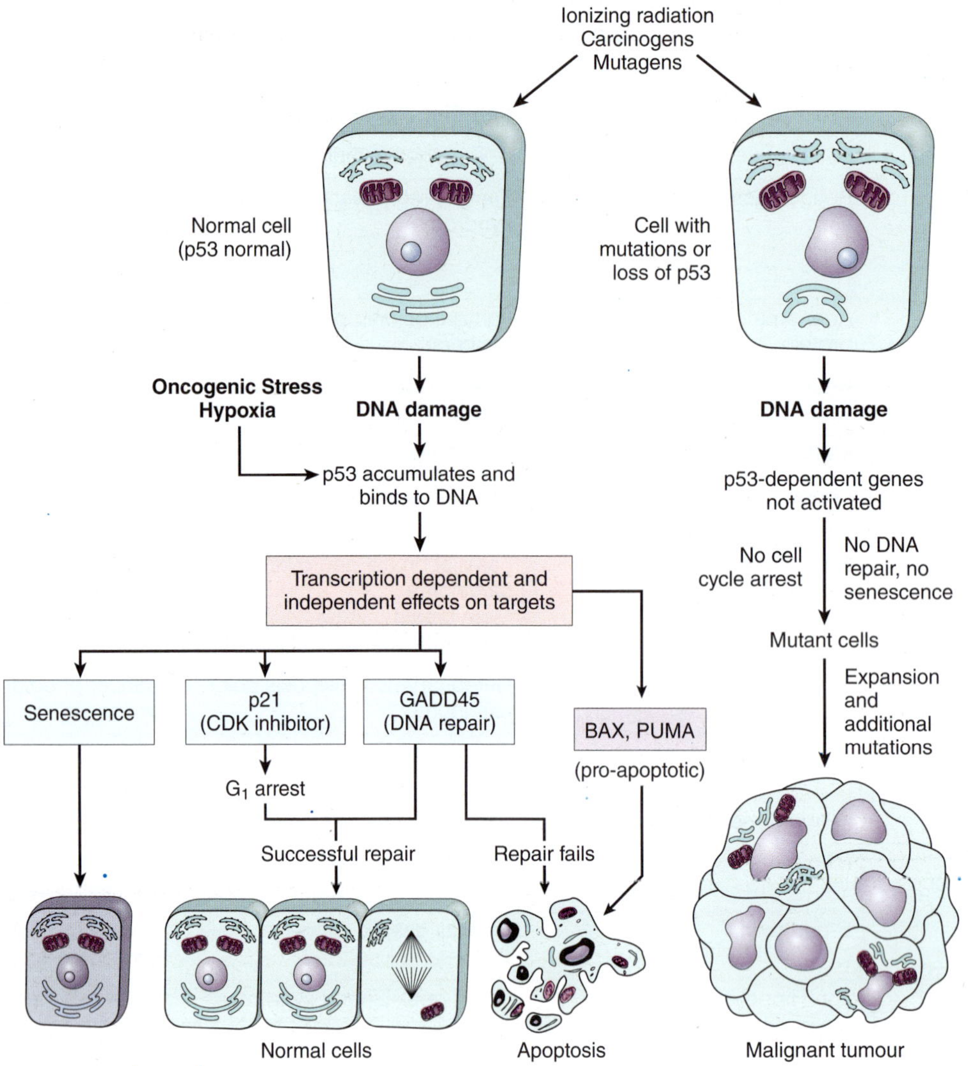

Fig. 7.29 Role of p53 in genomic integrity. (*Source:* From Vinay Kumar, Abul K. Abbas and Jon C. Aster. Neoplasia. Robbins Basic Pathology. 10th edition. Elsevier 2018.)

- Increased levels of cyclin D or CDK4 that cause phosphorylation of RB
- Inactivation of RB protein by the protein products of oncogenic viruses, **E7 protein induced by HPV** being a typical example (E7 protein binds with hypophosphorylated RB protein and prevents it from binding to E2F transcription factor, thus setting the stage for the mutated/cancerous cells to replicate)

APC

Adenomatous polyposis coli (APC) gene is a tumour suppressor gene that suppresses the growth-promoting signalling pathways through its protein product APC protein (Fig. 7.31). It majorly functions as the gatekeeper of colonic neoplasia. Familial adenomatous polyposis (FAP) syndrome is an autosomal dominant syndrome characterized by the development of innumerable adenomatous polyps that are precancerous with a high risk of undergoing malignant transformation before the patient turns 50 years of age. Apart from its role in the development of FAP syndrome, 70%–80% of sporadic cases of colorectal carcinoma are associated with loss-of-function mutation of APC gene, highlighting its guardian nature over colonic epithelial cells.

E-Cadherin

E-cadherin is a protein present on the surface of cells that help to maintain intercellular adhesions. β-Catenin is an intracellular protein that binds to the cytoplasmic tail of E-cadherin. It is a growth-promoting protein that can translocate to the nucleus and induce the production of proteins for cellular proliferation. When the E-cadherin gene, also known as **CDH1**, is mutated with loss of expression of the protein on the surface of cells, β-catenin is unbound and uninhibited and thus stimulates cell proliferation. Loss of expression of E-cadherin is associated with cancers of the breast, colon, pancreas, oesophagus and prostate. Inherited loss of E-cadherin is associated with the development of familial gastric carcinoma. E-cadherin function is also lost when activating mutations affect the β-catenin gene.

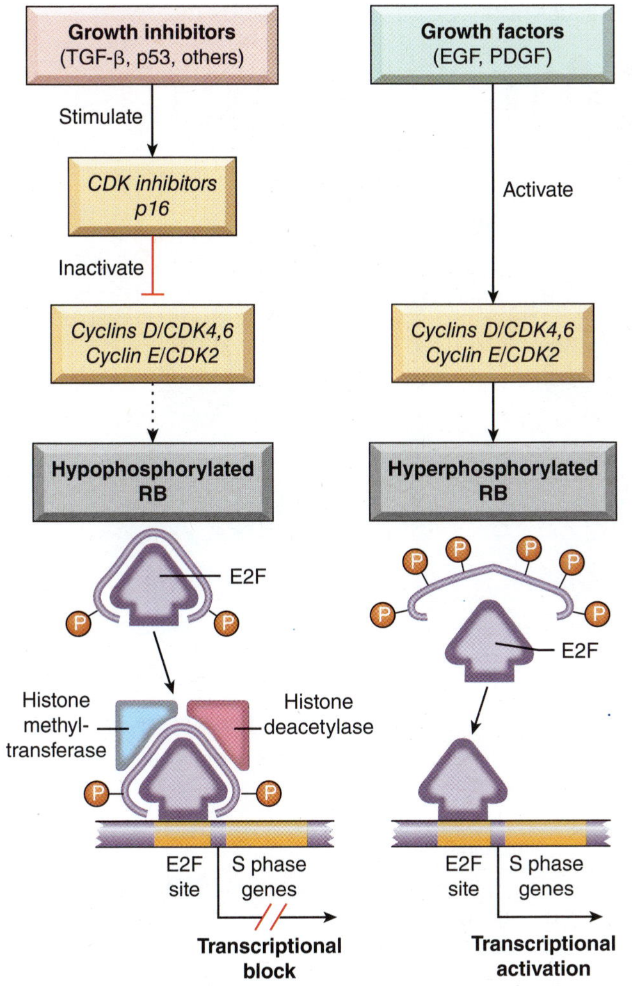

Fig. 7.30 Role of RB in cell-cycle regulation. (*Source:* From Vinay Kumar, Abul K. Abbas and Jon C. Aster. Neoplasia. Robbins Basic Pathology. 10th edition. Elsevier 2018.)

NF1

NF1 gene codes for a protein called **neurofibromin** that applies brake to the RAS signalling pathways. In the absence of neurofibromin because of NF1 gene mutation, RAS pathway is uninhibited, resulting in cellular proliferation and development of tumours. In inherited NF1 mutations, patients develop a syndrome called **neurofibromatosis type 1** characterized by the development of gliomas of the optic nerve and numerous neurofibromas, some of which may develop into malignant peripheral nerve sheath tumours.

NF2

NF2 gene codes for a protein called **neurofibromin 2** or **Merlin**, which belongs to a family of cytoskeletal proteins involved in the transfer of signals including growth inhibitory signals between cells. Inherited NF2 mutation is characterized by the development of bilateral schwannomas of the acoustic nerve, meningiomas and ependymomas.

Other important tumour suppressor genes like **BRCA1** and **BRCA2** are explained in Chapter 27.

ABNORMAL CELLULAR METABOLISM: WARBURG EFFECT

Discovery of the Warburg effect is a breakthrough in cancer research. Otto Warburg was awarded with Nobel Prize in 1931 for discovering the altered metabolic state of cancer cells. His discovery received great attention only over the last 10 years and has emerged as the most active area of cancer research.

Normal cells depend on mitochondrial oxidative phosphorylation for the production of ATP in the presence of oxygen and switch to anaerobic glycolysis only when there is hypoxia.

According to the Warburg effect, ***'cancer cells have a different form of cellular metabolism characterized by very high levels of glucose uptake and accelerated conversion of glucose to lactose via the glycolytic pathway, even in the presence of sufficient oxygen'*** (Fig. 7.32).

The Warburg effect is the fundamental basis of positron emission tomography (**PET**) **scan**, in which patients are injected with ^{18}F-fluorodeoxyglucose, a nonmetabolizable derivative of glucose, which is preferentially taken up by the tumour cells and rapidly dividing cells like those of the bone marrow. Most malignant tumours, especially the fast-growing ones and secondary deposits, are PET positive.

It was unclear for so many years as to why the cancer cells choose the less efficient glycolytic pathway as their metabolic pathway.

The reasons postulated are as follows:

Although the glycolytic pathway is comparatively inefficient in the generation of ATP and generates only 2 ATPs for every molecule of glucose when compared with oxidative phosphorylation that generates 36 ATPs per molecule of glucose, it **generates carbon moieties** that are required for the production of cellular components (DNA, RNA, lipids, proteins, organelles, etc.) for the rapidly dividing tumo ur cells.

This preference for anaerobic glycolysis is not an exclusive feature of tumour cells, because it is also the preferred metabolic pathway for all rapidly dividing normal cells. Hence, the Warburg effect is not cancer specific but specific for any rapidly proliferating cell.

The molecular basis for this metabolic switch is the activation of oncogenes and the growth-promoting signalling pathways that involve the following pathways and proteins:

- **PI3K/AKT signalling**
- **MYC overexpression**
- **Receptor tyrosine kinase activity**

Many tumour suppressors like p53, PTEN and STK11 act to inhibit the metabolic switchover to the Warburg effect.

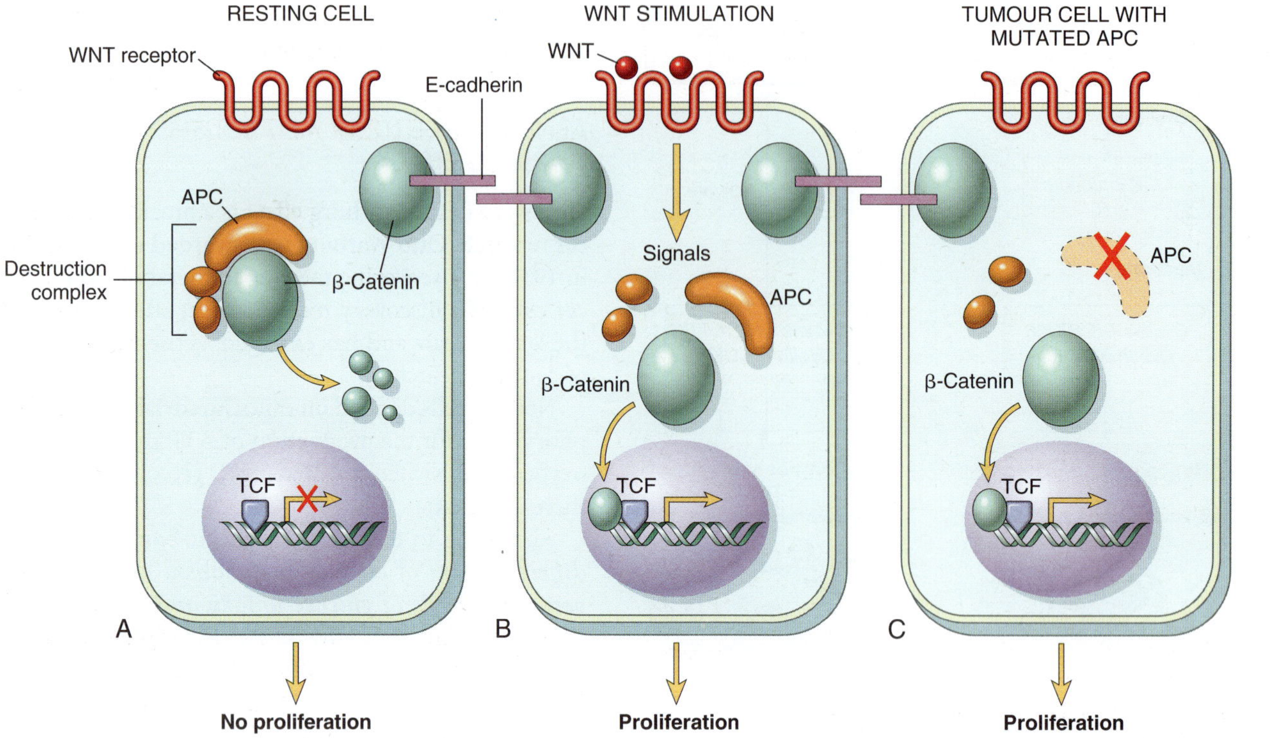

Fig. 7.31 The role of APC in regulating the stability and function of β-catenin and E-cadherin. APC, adenomatous polyposis coli. (*Source:* From Vinay Kumar, Abul K. Abbas and Jon C. Aster. Neoplasia. Robbins Basic Pathology. 10th edition. Elsevier 2018.)

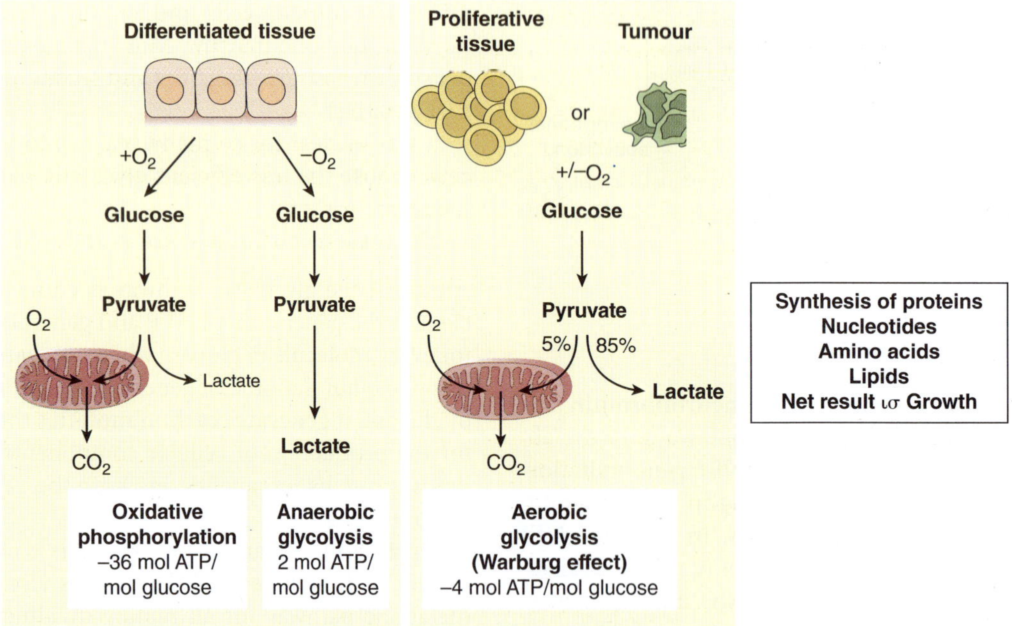

Fig. 7.32 Metabolic pathways of normal versus cancer cells.

EVASION OF APOPTOSIS

Expansion of tumour cell population occurs by three major mechanisms:

- **Activating mutations in proto-oncogenes**
- **Inactivating mutations in tumour suppressor genes**
- **Mutations in genes involved in apoptosis**

Apoptosis is one of the protective mechanisms that functions to eliminate the unwanted cells and prevent the proliferation of transformed cells. It is induced by many triggers including DNA damage.

As described in Chapter 2, apoptosis is activated by two different pathways in the initiation phase that converge on the execution phase. Proteins that regulate apoptosis fall under three categories.

In healthy cells, antiapoptotic proteins dominate and maintain the integrity of the outer membrane of mitochondria. When the intrinsic pathway gets activated by withdrawal of growth factors, DNA damage, radiation or chemicals, the sensors sense the stress and disrupt the integrity of the outer membrane of the mitochondria, releasing the proapoptotic proteins.

Reduced apoptosis or its resistance plays a vital role in carcinogenesis. There are multiple ways a malignant cell can avoid apoptosis. **Generally, the mechanisms of evasion of apoptosis can be divided into the following categories:**

1. **Disruption of balance between proapoptotic and antiapoptotic proteins**
   It is not the absolute quantity of these proteins but rather the ratio of these pro- and antiapoptotic proteins that plays an important role in the regulation of cell death. Over- and underexpression of certain genes have been found to contribute to cancer development by reducing apoptosis in cancer cells.
   Such alterations commonly seen are as follows:
   - Overexpression of BCL2
   - Underexpression of Bax
2. **Defects or mutations in p53**
   As discussed earlier, p53 is a tumour suppressor protein that induces apoptosis in cells with DNA damage. In tumours with TP53 mutation, cells with unrepaired DNA proliferate by escaping apoptosis. Defects in p53 tumour suppressor gene have been linked to more than 50% of human cancers.
3. **Reduced function of caspases**
   As discussed in Chapter 2, caspases play a central role in apoptosis, being the important players in the initiation and execution of apoptosis. Downregulation of caspases is associated with carcinogenesis.
   Examples include loss of expression of caspase-9 in colorectal cancer and caspase-3 in breast cancer.
4. **Impaired signalling through death receptor**
   Death receptors and their ligands are key players in the extrinsic pathway of apoptosis. Many abnormalities in the death signalling pathways that lead to evasion of the extrinsic pathway of apoptosis have been identified. Such abnormalities include (1) downregulation of the receptors and (2) impairment of receptor function. These may lead to the development of malignancies and also resistance to treatment.
5. **Increased expression of IAPs**
   IAPs are a group of structurally and functionally similar proteins that regulate apoptosis. Dysregulated IAP expression has been reported in many cancers (Fig. 7.33). **Survivin**, an IAP, has been reported to be overexpressed in many cancers, especially in non-small-cell lung carcinomas.

LIMITLESS REPLICATION

Every cancer has some cells that possess the capacity to proliferate indefinitely. The mechanisms for this immortality are as follows:

- Escape from senescence
- Escape from mitotic crisis
- Capacity for self-renewal

Escape from Senescence (Fig. 7.34)

Telomeres progressively shorten with increasing cell divisions, even in stem cells. M1 or mortality stage is defined as senescence in which the cell's telomeres are critically short to induce cell-cycle arrest. This M1 phase is also referred to as Hayflick limit. After a fixed number of cell divisions, cells undergo senescence by mechanisms that are still not clearly understood. Levels of p53 and INK4a/p16 get upregulated in cells, attaining the senescent state. Premalignant cells that have obtained a number of oncogenic alterations can bypass M1 and enter an extended life span. Such tumour cells escape senescence through mutations in p53 or other genes involved in RB-dependent G1/S phase of the cell cycle. By escaping from senescence, cells have increased proliferative capacity but this does not confer immortality to the cells. In crisis (referred to as M2 crisis), there is a balance between cell growth and apoptosis and the vast majority of the cell population dies. A rare cell can upregulate telomerase activity and continue to proliferate.

Escape from Mitotic Crisis

As explained in Chapter 2, under cellular ageing, after a fixed number of cell divisions, cells undergo mitotic crisis and death. This is triggered by critically shortened telomeres and exposed ends of the chromosomes. In such situations, cells with intact p53 undergo death by apoptosis. In cells with TP53 mutation, double-strand DNA breaks are followed by dicentric chromosome formation and new double-strand breaks occur. Numerous rounds of this bridge–fusion–breakage cycle lead to massive chromosomal instability and numerous mutations. Such cells usually undergo death. But if telomerase is reactivated, these cells survive, proliferate and form a tumour.

Self-Renewal

At least some cells in all cancers are stem cell–like and these are referred to as cancer stem cells. They may arise by transformation of normal stem cells or through acquired mutations that confer 'stemness' to the cells. Cancer stem cells undergo asymmetric division, i.e. with every cell division, one daughter cell remains as cancer stem cell and maintains the stem cell population.

Thus, cancer cells possess limitless replicative potential and maintain their population through mutations that

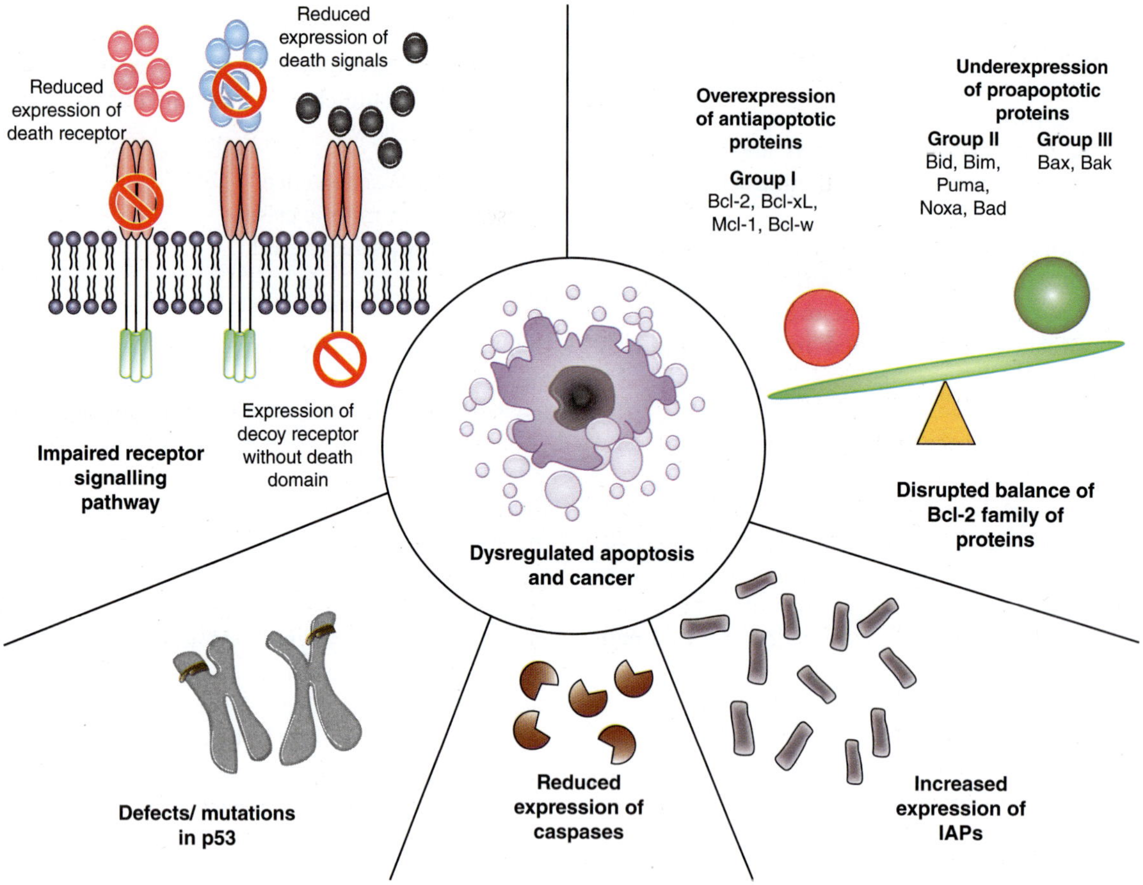

Fig. 7.33 Dysregulated apoptosis in malignancy.

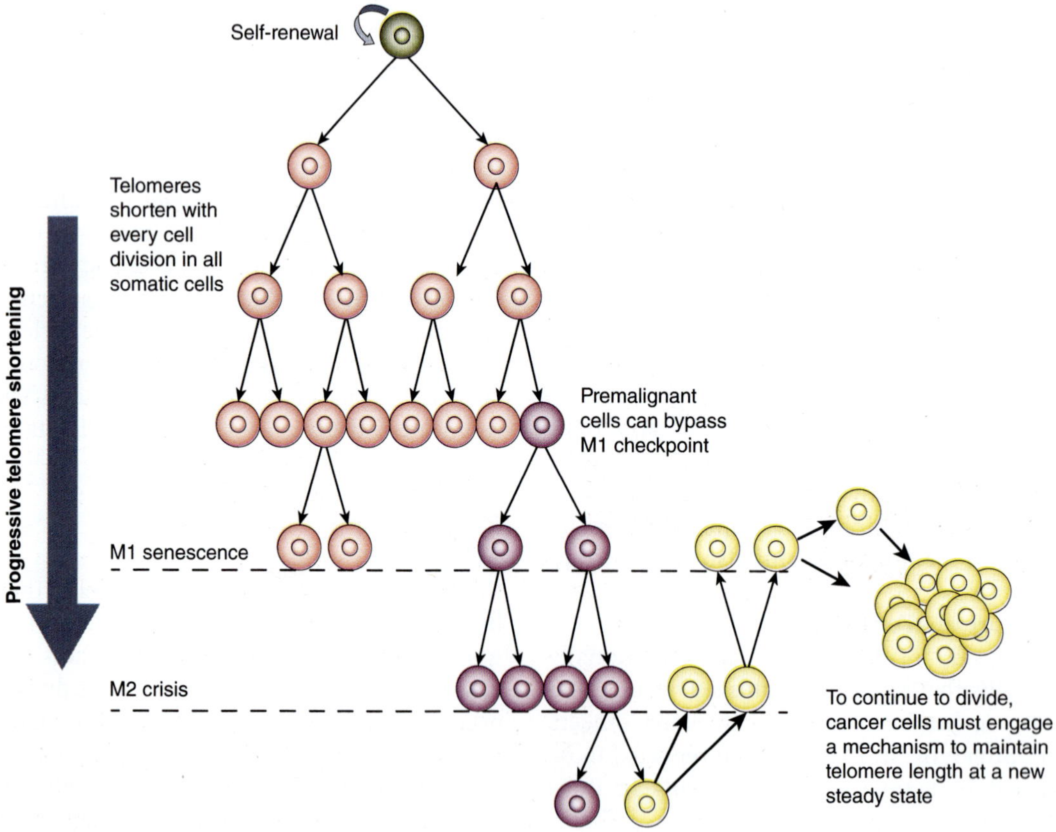

Fig. 7.34 Evasion of M1 senescence and M2 crisis in cancer cells.

inactivate senescence signals, and reactivate telomerase and self-renewal of cancer stem cells.

SUSTAINED ANGIOGENESIS

Angiogenesis is essential for any tumour growth and development. Like normal tissues, tumour cells require delivery of oxygen and nutrients for their survival and growth. Oxygen and nutrients can diffuse through tissues from blood vessels for a maximum of 2 mm. The tumours have a rapidly growing tendency, so they undergo necrosis without adequate blood supply. Hence, to meet the requirements of these expeditiously proliferating cells, neoangiogenesis is stimulated. Neoangiogenesis is a process by which new blood vessels arise from previously existing blood vessels (Fig. 7.35).

Angiogenesis is regulated by the balance between factors promoting and inhibiting it. In tumours with angiogenesis, the balance tips toward factors that induce angiogenesis. After a variable period of vascular quiescence, tumours switch to the angiogenic phase. The angiogenic factors are produced by tumour cells, inflammatory cells like macrophages and stromal cells.

Angiogenesis in tumours is the net result of exaggerated levels of angiogenic factors and depressed levels of antiangiogenic factors.

The molecular basis for the angiogenic switch in tumours is as follows:

- Hypoxia → HIF1α → VEGF and bFGF
- Activating mutations of RAS and MYC → VEGF and bFGF
- Inactivating mutations of p53 → ↓ thrombospondin-1

The effects of angiogenesis on tumours are multiple:

- It supplies the required oxygen and nutrition to the growing tumour cells.
- It helps the removal of waste from the cells.
- The young endothelial cells release factors for the growth of tumour cells.
- These vessels help tumour to metastasize widely.

These new blood vessels supplying the tumours often show **haphazard growth pattern and are dilated and leaky.** This feature offers a clue in angiograms.

Angiogenesis is central to any tumour, so newer drugs that target angiogenesis have been developed but their efficacy is still under study.

LOCAL INVASION

Invasion and metastasis are the two hallmark features of malignancy. Local invasion along with metastasis is the major cause of morbidity and mortality associated with cancers. Although the two processes are different, both have common mechanism for interaction of tumour cells with stroma. The communication between tumour cells and the stroma is not passive but **dynamic and interactive.**

The extracellular matrix (ECM) exists in two different forms:

1. Basement membrane
2. Interstitial connective tissue

Local invasion literally means the invasion of ECM, which is an active process and is divided into four major steps (Fig. 7.36):

- Dissociation of cancer cells from each other
- ECM degradation
- Attachment of tumour cells to ECM components
- Locomotion of tumour cells

DISSOCIATION OF CANCER CELLS FROM EACH OTHER

This is the first step in the process of invasion. Normally, epithelial cells are cemented to each other through intercellular adhesion molecules and ECM. The major intercellular

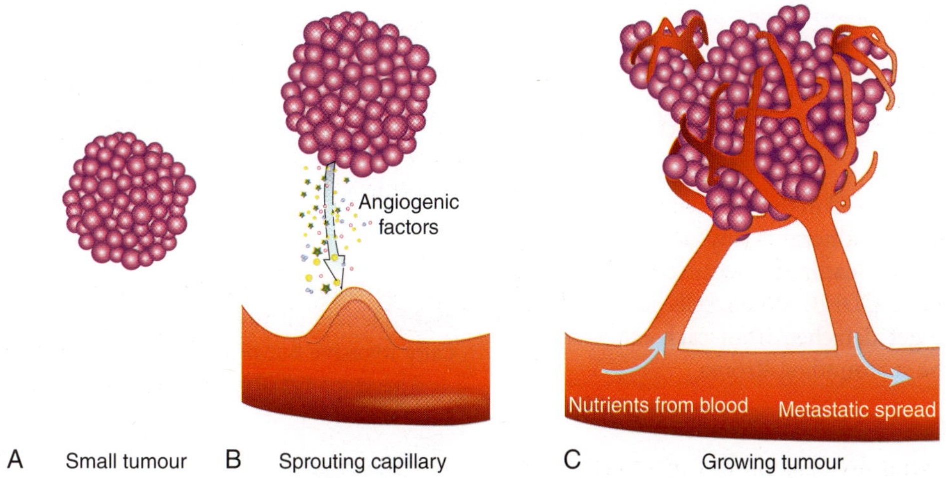

Fig. 7.35 Neovascularization in tumorigenesis.

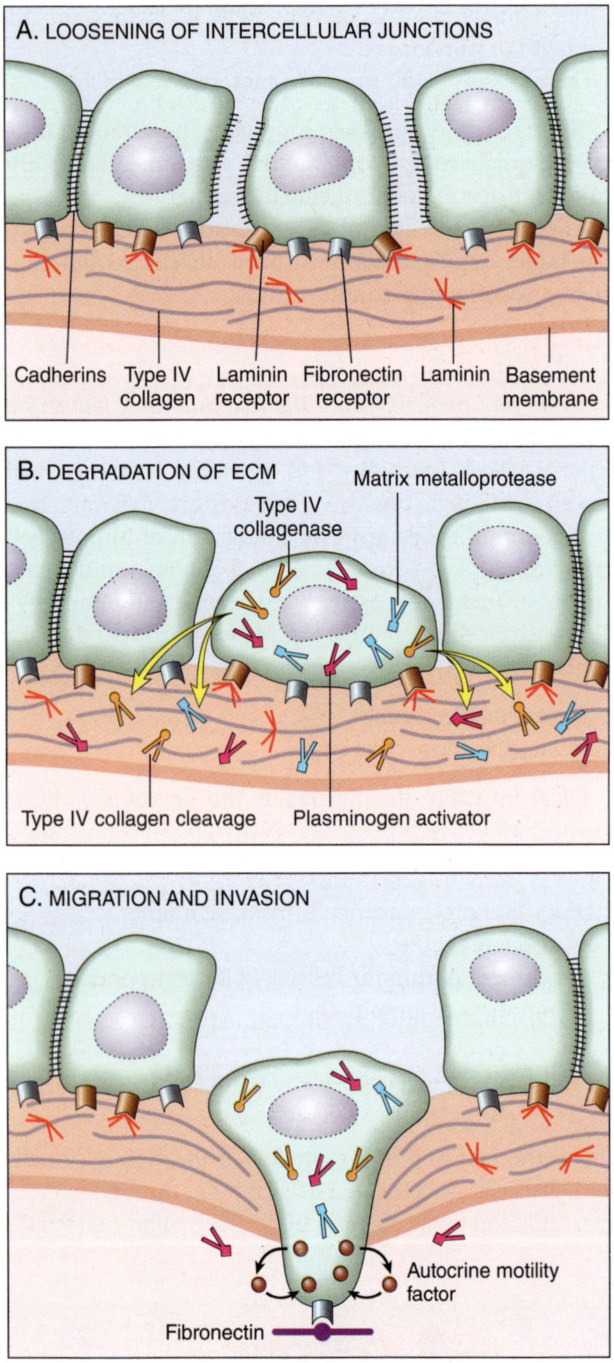

Fig. 7.36 Sequence of events in the invasion of epithelial basement membranes by a tumour. (*Source:* From Vinay Kumar, Abul K. Abbas and Jon C. Aster. Neoplasia. Robbins Basic Pathology. 10th edition. Elsevier 2018.)

adhesion molecule involved in the cell–cell attachment and transfer of signals is E-cadherin. Many cancers are associated with the **loss of E-cadherin** because of inactivating mutation of its gene CDH1. When cells fail to express E-cadherin, these get detached from each other and get ready to invade the surrounding stroma.

Extracellular Matrix Degradation

This occurs following dissociation of cancer cells in the process of local invasion. Matrix degradation requires **matrix metalloproteinases** (MMPs) and many other proteases that are secreted by the tumour cells, stromal cells and infiltrating inflammatory cells.

MMPs serve many functions in cancer development:

I. Remodelling of ECM
II. Release of growth factors for tumour cells from ECM
III. Stimulation of angiogenesis
IV. Chemotactic for tumour cells

In many cancers, expression of MMPs is increased and inhibitors of MMPs tissue inhibitors of metalloproteinases (TIMP) are reduced, leading to invasion.

Attachment of Tumour Cells to ECM Components

After the initial steps of dissociation from adjacent cells and degradation of ECM, cancer cells get attached to ECM components. Tumour cells express proteolytically generated **receptors for matrix components.** Action of MMPs on matrix proteins induces new binding sites on them that bind with the receptors on tumour cells.

Locomotion of Tumour Cells

After their attachment with matrix proteins, tumour cells move through the degraded basement membrane and areas of matrix proteolysis by the process called **'locomotion'**. The mechanism of locomotion is exactly similar to chemotaxis of inflammatory cells seen in inflammation with cytoskeletal remodelling, formation of pseudopods and moving forward.

Factors that help in the forward movement of tumour cells are as follows:

- Cytokines secreted by tumour cells
- Factors released from matrix degradation
- Growth factors released from matrix proteins
- Hepatocyte growth factor secreted by stromal cells

The levels of these factors are elevated in many locally invasive tumours, highlighting their role in the locomotion of tumour cells.

DISTANT METASTASIS

Metastasis is a Greek word meaning **'displacement'.** The development of secondary malignant growth at a distance from the primary site of malignancy is called metastasis. Although the metastatic process is very inefficient, with only 0.01% of circulating tumour cells capable of forming secondary deposits, it is the **primary cause of cancer morbidity and mortality**. It is a dynamic process that involves a series of sequential and interrelated steps. Metastasis follows the same steps as those involved in invasion. Hence, all tumours with distant metastasis are locally invasive but not all invasive tumours metastasize.

The steps involved in the process of metastasis are as follows:

I. The steps for invasion
II. Intravasation into the circulatory and lymphatic systems

III. Evasion of immune attack
IV. Vascular dissemination and homing
V. Invasion and proliferation in distant organs

Each step is detailed as follows:

I. **The steps for invasion** (Fig. 7.37): The four steps involved are described under 'Local invasion'.
II. **Intravasation into the circulatory and lymphatic systems:** Intravasation is the process of entry of tumour cells into the bloodstream and is an essential step in the development of distant metastasis. Tumour cells invade into normal tissue, often towards lymphatics or blood vessels. On reaching the vessel, these cells must degrade the basement membrane and then cross the endothelial barrier to enter the circulation. In the circulation, tumour cells may be destroyed by shear stress or by apoptosis, induced by nonattachment with the matrix or by the immune response. Tumour cells may overcome all these effects by forming clumps with other tumour cells or platelets. These then get successfully lodged in a distant capillary bed, from where they can undergo extravasation to other organs and form secondaries.
III. **Evasion of immune attack:** This is discussed in the subsequent sections.
IV. **Vascular dissemination, extravasation and homing**
Although the anatomic location and vascular drainage of the tumour dictate the sites of secondary deposits through vascular dissemination, many tumours have affinity for specific sites of metastasis (Table 7.13). This situation can be explained in part by the architecture of the circulatory system and the natural routes of blood flow.
Circulating cancer cells often establish new tumours downstream from their originating organ. The lungs, the first organs through which the systemic blood flows first, and the liver, the first organ through which the portal blood flows, are the common sites of metastases. But circulation alone does not explain all cases of preferential spread. Clinical evidence suggests that a homing mechanism is responsible for some unlikely metastatic deposits.
This ***homing phenomenon*** may be related to tumour cell recognition of specific exit sites from the circulation or to awareness of a particularly favourable ***'soil'*** in another tissue. This may happen because of an affinity that exists between receptor proteins on the

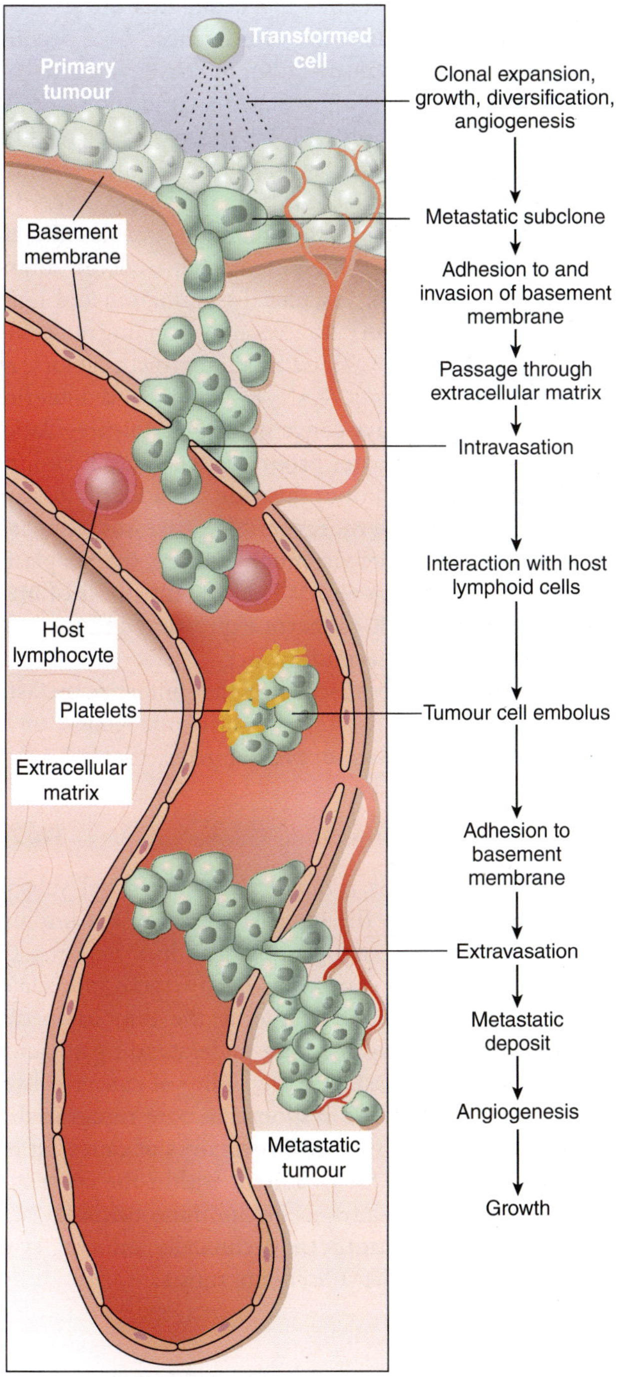

Fig. 7.37 The process of invasion and metastasis. (*Source:* From Vinay Kumar, Abul K. Abbas and Jon C. Aster. Neoplasia. Robbins Basic Pathology. 10th edition. Elsevier 2018.)

Table 7.13 List of Cancers with their Selective Sites of Secondary Deposits

Primary Tumour	Common Sites of Secondary Deposits
Breast	Lung, liver, bones
Colon	Liver, peritoneum, lung
Kidney	Lung, liver, bones
Lung	Adrenals, liver, lung
Prostate	Liver, lung, bones
Pancreas	Liver, lung, peritoneum
Thyroid	Lung, liver, bones
Stomach	Liver, peritoneum, lung

surface of cancer cells and molecules that are abundant in specific tissues.

Examples:

- **CD44** adhesion molecule expressed by normal lymphocytes; when expressed by tumour cells, these selectively home in lymphoid tissues.
- Breast cancer cells may express the chemokine receptor **CXCR4,** which has affinity for cells with CXCL12 expression that results in the movement of the cancer cells from their primary sites of formation.

The lungs, liver, brain and bones are the most common sites for metastases for solid tumours.

The symptoms because of metastases depend on the organs involved.

Examples of metastatic sites and their associated symptoms are as follows:

Lymph node metastases: Lymphadenopathy
Lung secondaries: Cough, haemoptysis and dyspnoea
Liver secondaries: Hepatomegaly, nausea and jaundice
Bone metastases: Bone pain, pathological fracture
Brain metastases: Neurological symptoms like headache, vertigo and seizures

V. **Colonization and proliferation at distant organs**

Once the tumour cells land on their preferred sites of secondary growth, they invade, colonize the tissues and grow further by inducing angiogenesis. Tumour cells secrete growth factors, cytokines and ECM molecules that interact with the resident stromal cells, making the new site a second home for the tumour cells. Most often these grow to only small and clinically insignificant sizes. Tumour cells might remain dormant with micrometastases without progression for several years, as is noted in melanoma, breast and prostatic carcinoma. Molecular mechanisms of homing and colonization are still not completely understood and are areas of intense research.

Molecular Basis of Metastasis

The following are the theories proposed to explain the emergence of metastatic phenotypes:

- **The clonal evolution model:** A subset of tumour cell subclones acquires a pattern of gene expression that is essential for completing the steps of metastasis.
- **Metastatic signature:** Many metastasis-associated gene expression events have been identified that correlate with the development of metastases. Among the genes favouring metastasis are many molecules that arise from the cells of the microenvironment rather than the tumour per se. Tumours with such metastatic signatures develop a tendency to spread during early stages of carcinogenesis.
- **Additional mutations for metastasis:** This model states that the metastatic signature is essential but not sufficient for the development of metastasis and the acquisition of additional mutations is needed to provoke tumour cells to move distantly.
- **Influence of stromal cells, inflammatory cells and angiogenesis:** Metastasis is not only dependent on the properties of tumour cells but also dependent on characteristics of the stroma surrounding the tumour cells, infiltrating inflammatory cells and angiogenesis.

Epithelial-to-Mesenchymal Transition (Fig. 7.38)

There is a growing evidence suggesting that the ability of tumour tissue to metastasize is influenced by a peculiar phenotype modulation in tumour tissue architecture known as epithelial-to-mesenchymal transition (EMT). The essential features of EMT are the loss of intercellular attachments and augmentation of cell motility, resulting in the release of epithelial cells from the parent tissue. The resulting mesenchymal-like phenotype enables the tumour cells with metastatic potential to undergo migration, tumour invasion, vascular dissemination and homing. Many transduction pathways and signalling molecules act to cause this EMT. These include growth factors, receptor tyrosine kinases, RAS, β-catenin and integrins. Most of these pathways converge on the downregulation of E-cadherin, **the master programmer of EMT,** and this is a critical event in tumour invasion. E-cadherin loss and EMT could be **transient, reversible processes**, regulated by the tumour microenvironment. Hence, the neoplastic cells that have undergone EMT during the phase of invasion seem to regain E-cadherin expression and their cohesive quality at the secondary foci.

There are few genes discovered that influence metastasis either by favouring it, 'metastasis oncogenes', or by inhibiting it, 'metastasis suppressor genes' (Table 7.14).

EVASION OF HOST IMMUNE RESPONSE PA 7.5

Immuno-oncology is a rapidly evolving novel subspecialty that deals with the interplay between the immune system and cancer pathogenesis. The link between the immune system and cancer has been widely appreciated over a century, and understanding the tumour-specific immune response improves the understanding of cancer resistance. Not surprisingly, the ability of cancer cells to evade the host immune response is now recognized as one of the most distinguished hallmarks of cancer. It has provided a platform for treatment within the context of immunotherapy. The advances in immuno-oncology have made cancer **immunotherapy** clinically more relevant and is described in the subsequent topics.

Cancer Immunoediting

The immune system, apart from trying to eliminate tumour cells, can also promote tumour progression through chronic inflammation, immune selection of

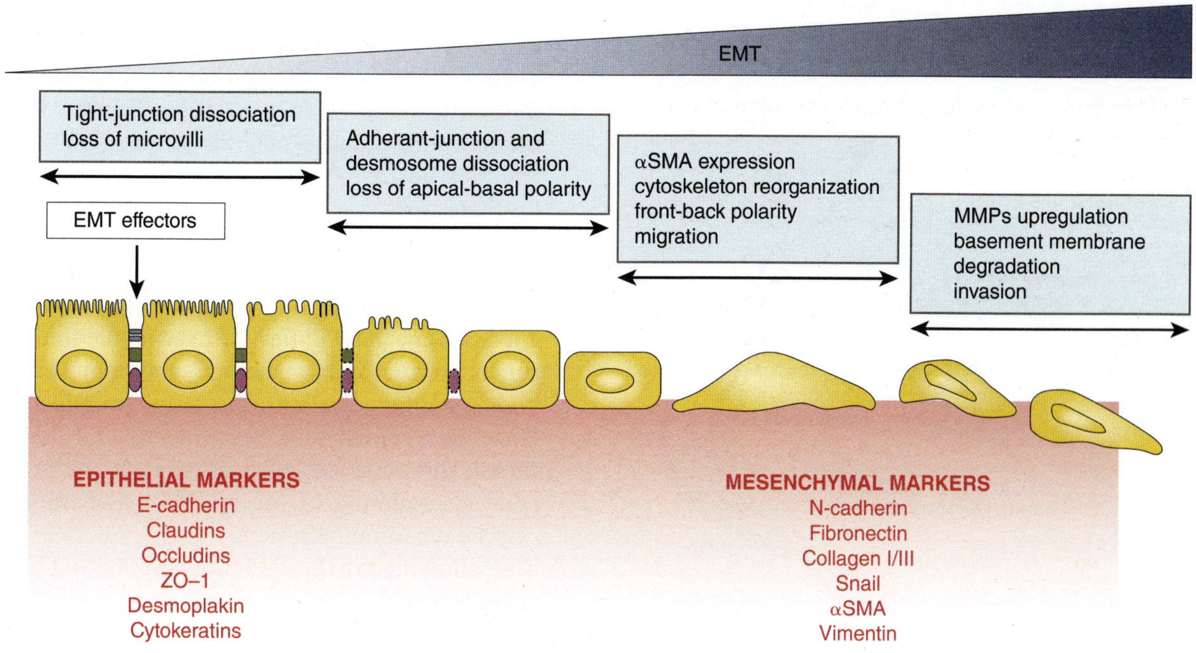

Fig. 7.38 Epithelial-to-mesenchymal transition.

Table 7.14 Genes Favouring and Suppressing Metastasis

Metastasis Oncogenes	Metastasis Suppressor Genes
SNAIL	NM23
TWIST	KAI1
RAGE	KISS1

poorly immunogenic variants and suppression of antitumour immunity. This dual host protective and tumour-promoting action of immunity is referred to as 'cancer immunoediting'.

Tumour antigens, antitumour effector cells, immune surveillance and evasion are discussed as follows:

a. **Tumour antigens** (Table 7.15)
Tumour antigens, produced by tumour cells, are antigenic substances with the ability to trigger immune response in the host. They are classified according to their source and molecular structure.

b. **Antitumour effector cells and mechanisms**
Interaction of immune cells with the developing tumour is complex and includes tumour-specific cells. The immune system may identify the tumour antigens presented on tumour cells and destroy tumour cells by a variety of mechanisms. Although most haematopoietic cells and some tissue cells, under certain circumstances, can eliminate tumour cells, the term 'antitumour effector cells' has generally been used to describe cells specially trained and equipped for tumour cell elimination. Antitumour effector cells include those of the innate immune system (natural killer [NK] cells, macrophages) and the adaptive immune system (cytotoxic T lymphocytes and B lymphocytes) (Fig. 7.39).

Table 7.15 List of Major Classes of Tumour Antigens with Examples

Class of Tumour Antigens	Examples
Products of mutated genes	RAS, p53, BCR-ABL
Oncogenic virus–induced antigens	E6, E7 by human papillomavirus EBNA by Epstein–Barr virus
Overexpressed or aberrantly expressed cellular proteins	Tyrosinase, MART in melanomas overexpressed MAGE, BAGE aberrantly expressed in melanomas
Oncofetal antigens	Carcinoembryonic antigen (CEA) α-Fetoprotein (AFP)
Cluster differentiation antigens	CD20 by mature B-cell lymphomas CD15 and CD30 by Hodgkin lymphoma
Altered surface glycolipids and glycoproteins	CA-125 in ovarian carcinomas and CA-19-9 in pancreatic carcinoma MUC-1 in breast and ovarian carcinomas

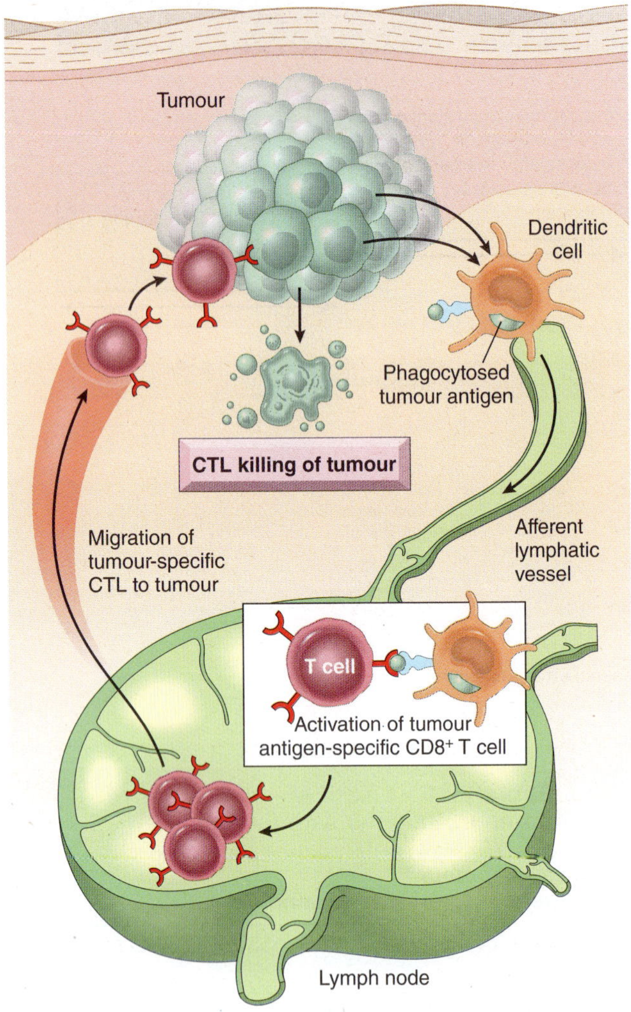

Fig. 7.39 Antitumour immune response by cytotoxic T lymphocytes. (*Source:* From Vinay Kumar, Abul K. Abbas and Jon C. Aster. Neoplasia. Robbins Basic Pathology. 10th edition. Elsevier 2018.)

Two distinct categories of antitumour effector cells have been described:

- Tumour specific
- Tumour nonspecific

Tumour-specific antitumour effector cells and mechanisms

This category includes clonally expanded T lymphocytes expressing a unique T-cell receptor and identifying tumour epitopes with major histocompatibility complex (MHC) molecules. These T lymphocytes, along with the B cells that produce tumour-specific antibodies and dendritic cells that process and present tumour antigens, are responsible for antitumour adaptive immunity.

Tumour nonspecific antitumour effector cells and mechanisms

Effector cells like NK cells, NK-T cells and macrophages that are not MHC restricted come under this category.

It remains unclear as which of these effectors plays a major role in the elimination of tumour targets in vivo. Theoretically, these effector mechanisms lead to tumour rejection, but in reality, this is not a foolproof mechanism, because a majority of the tumours expand and metastasize in the presence of antitumour effector mechanisms.

c. **Immune surveillance**

The link between cancer cells and the immune system was first recognized by *Rudolf Virchow* more than 150 years ago. *Paul Ehrlich* first stated that tumour cells can be recognized as 'foreign' and removed by the body's immune system. The term 'immune surveillance' was coined by *Lewis Thomas and Macfarlane Burnet*. Immune surveillance refers to the process of constant scanning of the body for any transformed cells by the immune system.

The following are the evidences supporting 'immune surveillance':

a. Lymphocytic infiltrates in and around tumours
b. Reactive changes in the lymph nodes at the draining regions of the tumours
c. A high incidence of cancers in immunodeficient people
d. Presence of tumour-specific T cells and antibodies in patients
e. Response of advanced cancers to immunotherapies
f. Experimental results

d. **Immune evasion** (Fig. 7.40)

When the immune system is intact and functional, how do tumour cells escape immune surveillance? The answer to this question is that the tumour cells can release factors to suppress host immunity and are capable of changing their identity so as not to be recognized by the immune system as foreign.

Most cancers occur in people without any immunodeficiency state. This is because of the ability of the tumour cells to evade attack by the immune system through several mechanisms.

Factors that Tumours Exploit to Avoid Immune Responses

- **Outgrowth of antigen-negative variants:** When the tumour progresses, strongly antigenic clones are removed and a selective outgrowth of antigen-negative variants occurs because of immunoediting.
- **Suppressive regulatory T cells:** Immunosuppression in the tumour microenvironment mediated by regulatory T cells and other types of suppressive cells seems to be a major mechanism of tumour immune evasion. Evidence also suggests that transforming growth factor (TGF)-β produced by tumour cells aids in the conversion of helper T cells into suppressive regulatory T cells that play a major role in immune evasion of tumour cells.

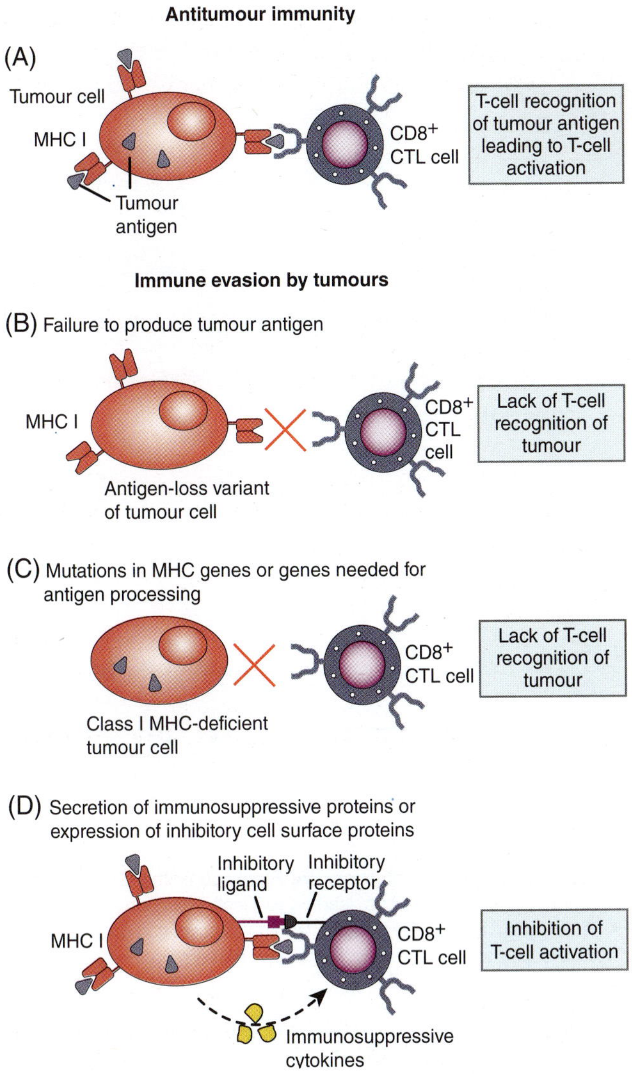

Fig. 7.40 Major mechanisms of immune evasion by tumour cells.

- **Defective antigen presentation:** Tumours escape immune surveillance by downmodulating antigen-processing machinery affecting the MHC I pathway and other tumour antigens. Thus, expression of tumour antigen is downregulated, which would result in the escape of tumour cells from the attack of cytotoxic T lymphocytes.
- **Immunosuppressive mediators:** Immunosuppressive mediators like TGF-β, IL-10 and PGE_2 released by tumour cells inhibit host immune response.
- **Tolerance and immune deviation:** Most tumour cells fail to express costimulatory molecules and can thereby induce anergy or tolerance to immune cells and escape attack by them.
- **Apoptosis:** Many studies have shown that cancer cells remove tumour-specific cytotoxic lymphocytes through apoptosis.
- **Activation of pathways that inhibit T-cell activation**
  It may be recalled that when CTLA4 molecules are expressed on $CD8^+$ lymphocytes, they prevent the signal 2 of immune response by blocking the engagement between the costimulatory molecules (CD28 on T cells and B7 on APCs) by selectively binding to B7 on APCs. Following this event, there is no immune response and the T cells also go into a state of prolonged unresponsiveness called anergy. Tumour cells upregulate the expression of CTLA4 by a variety of mechanisms that are still not completely understood and evade the immune system.
  Apart from this, tumour cells upregulate the expression of PD-L1 and PD-L2, both of which function to activate the programmed death-1 (PD-1) receptor on effector T cells. When upregulated, these cell surface proteins act to induce T-cell inactivation and death.
  On the basis of these two mechanisms, drugs that block CTLA4, PD-L1 or PD-1 receptors are approved and used in the management and treatment of patients with advanced solid tumours and some forms of lymphoma, with promising results. This form of treatment is referred to as 'immunotherapy' (Fig. 7.41) and is discussed later in the chapter.

GENOMIC INSTABILITY

Genetic instability is characteristic of most cancer cells. It is defined as the **increased tendency of genomic alteration during cell division.** Cancer is the result of mutation in multiple genes that control cell division and tumour suppression. The maintenance of genomic stability is essential for cellular integrity to prevent errors that could arise from DNA replication, endogenous genotoxicity and exogenous stress. Genomic integrity is closely monitored by several surveillance mechanisms, DNA damage checkpoints, DNA repair machinery and mitotic checkpoint. A defect in the regulation of these mechanisms frequently results in genomic instability, which pushes the affected cells towards malignant transformation.

Important DNA surveillance mechanisms are as follows:

1. TP53
2. ATM protein
3. Fanconi anaemia complex
4. DNA repair pathways:
   - Nucleotide excision repair (NER)
   - Base excision repair (BER)
   - Mismatch repair (MMR)
   - DNA double-strand break repair (DSBR)

TP53

The role played by TP53 in protecting the genome from genotoxic agents by inducing DNA repair and triggering cell-cycle arrest if the cells are irreversibly damaged has been discussed in great detail in the previous sections.

Ataxia–Telangiectasia-Mutated Protein

ATM is the gene mutated in ataxia–telangiectasia and is essential for recognizing and responding to the damage

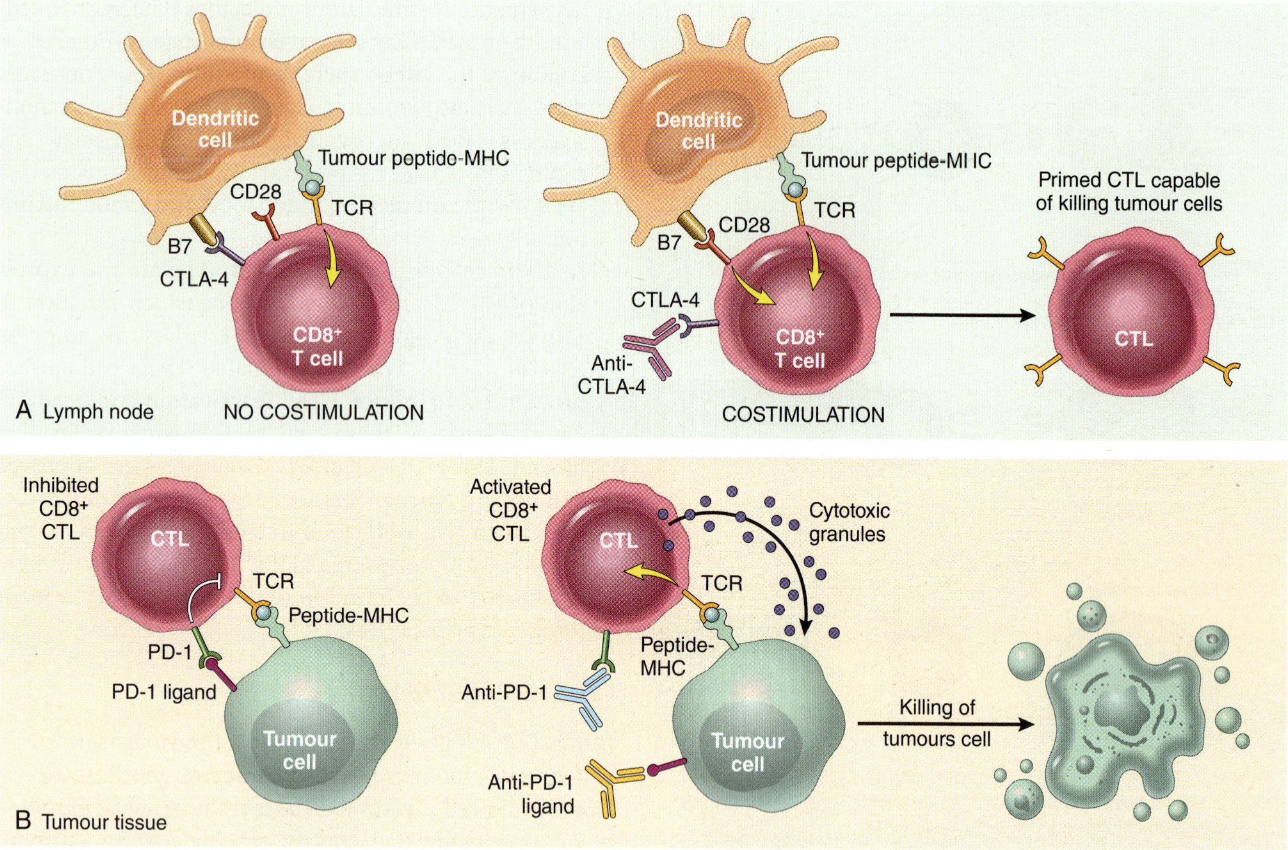

Fig. 7.41 Mechanism of immunotherapy – activation of host antitumour immunity by checkpoint inhibitors. (A) Blockade of the CTLA4 surface molecule with an inhibitor antibody allows cytolytic CD8$^+$ T cells (CTLs) to engage B7 family coreceptors, leading to T-cell activation. (B) Blockade of PD-1 receptor or PD-1 ligand by inhibitory antibodies abrogates inhibitory signals transmitted by PD-1, again leading to activation of CTLs. PD-1, programmed death-1. (*Source:* From Vinay Kumar, Abul K. Abbas and Jon C. Aster. Neoplasia. Robbins Basic Pathology. 10th edition. Elsevier 2018.)

caused to DNA by ionizing radiation. **Bloom syndrome** is characterized by defective ATM protein, and individuals with this syndrome are predisposed to a variety of malignancies.

Fanconi Anaemia Complex

Fanconi anaemia complex is composed of 13 genes all of which function to correct DNA damages. One such protein is BRCA2, which is mutated in some cases of **familial breast cancer** and also in some cases of Fanconi anaemia.

DNA Repair Pathways

Nucleotide Excision Repair Pathway DNA damage induced by ultraviolet (UV) light, exogenous chemicals like aflatoxin B_1 and chemotherapeutic drugs like cisplatin are usually repaired by the NER pathway. This pathway functions through multiple steps:

1. Recognition of the lesion site
2. Incision of the damaged site
3. Synthesis of DNA
4. Ligation of the uncoupled flanks by specific ligase enzymes

Examples of diseases with a defective NER pathway include xeroderma pigmentosum and Cockayne syndrome.

Base Excision Repair The BER pathway is perhaps the most fundamental and ubiquitous DNA repair mechanism in all oxygen-dependent higher organisms. This pathway recognizes, removes and replaces the bases modified by deamination, methylation and oxidation.

The steps involved in the process are as follows:

1. Altered bases are recognized and removed by specific DNA glycosylase enzymes.
2. New bases are synthesized by polymerase delta/epsilon.
3. Ligation of the open ends occurs by ligase enzymes.

Mismatch Repair and Microsatellite Instability (Fig. 7.42) Microsatellite instability (MSI) is a genetic condition that predisposes to mutations that result from impaired DNA MMR. Nonfunctioning MMR is represented by MSI. The function of MMR is to rectify the errors that occur during DNA replication spontaneously. Cells with mutated MMR are unable to correct such errors that occur in their DNA. This would result in the generation of novel microsatellite fragments.

Microsatellites are repeated sequences of DNA made up of repeating units of one to six base pairs. The length of the microsatellites is highly variable from person to person and contributes to DNA 'fingerprint', which

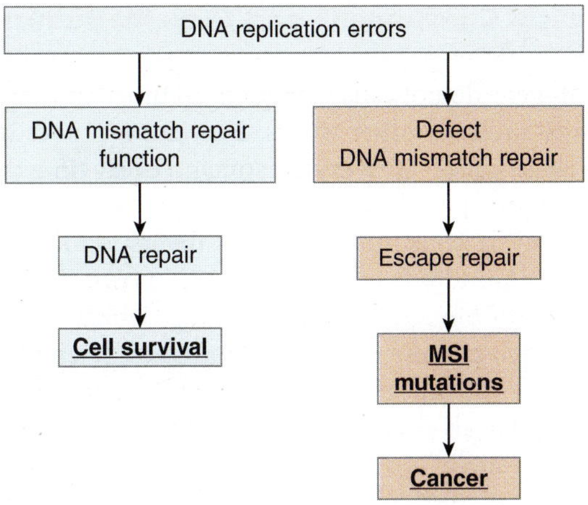

Fig. 7.42 Outcomes in the face of intact mismatch repair pathway and its defect.

imparts each individual with microsatellites of unique length. Microsatellites are also known as **simple sequence repeats** (SSRs).

MMR functions to remove base mismatches formed by exogenous and endogenous agents that induce base deamination, oxidation and methylation. It also plays a major role in repairing the base–base mismatches derived from insertions, deletions and replication errors.

The steps involved in the process are as follows:

1. Recognition of the DNA lesion – MutS and MutL
2. Discrimination of the strand
3. Excision of the lesion by exonucleases
4. Repair of the damage caused by polymerases

The following are the common proteins that function to detect the mismatched bases:

MutS
- MSH1–6
- MLH1
- MLH3

MutL
- PMS1
- PMS2

MSI is associated with cancers of the colon, stomach, endometrium, ovary, hepatobiliary tract, urinary tract, brain and skin.

An example of diseases because of a defective MMR pathway is **Lynch syndrome** – hereditary nonpolyposis colon cancer syndrome.

DNA Double-Strand Break Repair Double-strand DNA breaks are repaired by the DSBR system. There are two major pathways:

Nonhomologous end joining (NHEJ): Broken DNA strands are ligated.
Homologous repair (HRR): Broken homologous DNA sequences are repaired.

An example of diseases because of a defective NHEJ pathway is hereditary breast ovarian cancer syndrome.

An example of diseases because of a defective HRR pathway is syndromes with brain development defects.

Mutator Phenotype

Mutator phenotype refers to **the increase in mutation rate of cancer cells**. This hypothesis was formulated to account for the disparity between the infrequency of spontaneous mutations in normal cells and the large number of mutations observed in human tumours. This hypothesis states that genomic instability is present in precancerous lesions and drives tumour development by increasing the spontaneous mutation rate. The identification of mutations in DNA repair genes in hereditary cancers provides strong support for this hypothesis. This hypothesis relates the genomic instability in precancerous conditions to mutations in caretaker genes, which means that these genes are primarily involved in maintaining genomic stability.

CANCER-ENABLING INFLAMMATION

Nonresolving inflammation is one of the consistent findings of the tumour microenvironment. The connection between inflammation and tumour was first described in the 19th century and is currently accepted as an enabling characteristic of cancer. The evidence for this association is shown by the epidemiology, histopathology and inflammatory profiles of the tumours and is reinforced by the efficacy of anti-inflammatory agents in prophylaxis.

On one side, tumours can induce inflammation, and on the other side, chronic inflammation in the setting of tumour can unleash a greater potential from the tumour. The relationship between cancer and inflammation is well known and an area of intense research in the recent years. Cancers arising from chronic inflammation are discussed in the previous sections, and the mechanisms of cancers enabling inflammation are discussed here.

In patients with advanced cancers, the inflammatory reaction induced can be very extensive, leading to systemic signs of inflammation such as anaemia, cachexia and fatigue. Similarly, many experimental studies have proven that inflammatory cells alter the local tumour microenvironment to enable many hallmarks of cancer. These alterations may be because of interactions between tumour cells and inflammatory cells or through the actions of inflammatory cells on the stromal cells.

The mechanisms underlying this process are as follows:

Release of factors for proliferation
Inflammatory cells and resident stromal cells secrete growth factors like epidermal growth factor (EGF) and proteases that can release growth factors from ECM.
Suppression of growth inhibitors
It is already known that cell–cell and cell–matrix interactions suppress cell growth. Inflammatory cells release

proteases that degrade the adhesion between the cells and the matrix and enable the cells to proliferate.

Increased resistance to cell death

Tumour-associated inflammatory cells prevent **anoikis**, a form of death of cells that occurs when the cells get detached from basement membranes.

Induction of angiogenesis

Release of angiogenic factors like VEGF promotes angiogenesis, helping the tumour cells to sustain growth.

Stimulation of invasion and metastasis

TGF-β released by inflammatory cells induces EMTs. Both TNF and EGF induce mobility of tumour cells, and proteases stimulate invasion.

Evasion of immune response

Factors secreted by the inflammatory cells like TGF-β, IL-2 and Il-13 help the tumour cells to evade the host immune response.

The net effect of the inflammatory system is to positively affect tumour development.

CARCINOGENIC AGENTS AND CARCINOGENESIS PA 7.3

A carcinogen is any substance, chemical, radiation or microbial organism that promotes carcinogenesis. It is discussed under the following headings:

- **Chemical carcinogenesis**
- **Radiation carcinogenesis**
- **Microbial carcinogenesis**

CHEMICAL CARCINOGENESIS

Chemical carcinogens are chemicals that may increase the risk of cancer by altering cellular mechanism or damaging DNA in the cells exposed to them. Although carcinogenicity is generally associated with synthetic chemicals, it is equally likely to occur because of natural and synthetic substances. Carcinogens are not necessarily toxic on immediate exposure; thus, their effects can be more often insidious.

The history of chemical carcinogenesis is punctuated by key epidemiological observations and animal experiments that recognized cancer-causing chemicals. This led to increasingly insightful experiments to establish molecular mechanisms and the awareness about reducing human exposure.

In 1914, Boveri made important observations on chromosomal changes, including aneuploidy. His analysis of mitosis in frog cells and its extrapolation to human cancers is an early example of a basic research finding generating an important hypothesis. The first experimental model of cancer in rabbits exposed to coal tar was performed by Yamagiwa and Ichikawa in Japan and was later confirmed by Pott's epidemiological observation of scrotal cancer in chimney sweepers.

Chemical Carcinogens and Their Mechanisms (Table 7.16)

Carcinogens do not cause cancer at all times and under all circumstances. In other words, a carcinogen does not always cause cancer in every person and every time there is an exposure.

Chemicals constitute the most diverse group of carcinogens. Hundreds of chemicals are known to be carcinogenic to humans. Understanding which chemicals cause which cancers is one of our greatest scientific challenges. All human beings are exposed to trace amounts of many chemicals in day-to-day life. These everyday exposures are usually too small to cause health problems and cancers.

A carcinogen is termed **genotoxic** if it covalently binds to cellular DNA. Chemical carcinogens cause genetic and epigenetic changes in susceptible cells, imparting a selective growth advantage. The affected cells can undergo clonal expansion, become genetically unstable and get transformed to neoplastic cells (Table 7.17).

Table 7.16 List of Major Chemical Carcinogens

Directly Acting Carcinogens	Indirectly Acting Carcinogens
Alkylating agents β-Propiolactone Dimethyl sulphate Diepoxybutane Anticancer drugs like cyclophosphamide, nitrosoureas, chlorambucil	**Aromatic amines, amides and azo dyes** Benzidine β-Naphthylamine Dimethylaminoazobenzene
Acylating agents Dimethylcarbamyl chloride 1-Acetyl-imidazole	**Polycyclic and heterocyclic aromatic hydrocarbons** Benzopyrene Benzanthracene Dibenzanthracene Methylcholanthrene
	Natural and microbial products Aflatoxin B_1 and other mycotoxins Betel nut Griseofulvin Hydrazines Methylxanthines Pyrrolizidine alkaloids Thiourea Tannins
	Miscellaneous Vinyl chloride Nickel Chromium Nitrosamines and amides Insecticides Pesticides

Table 7.17 Cancers associated with various chemicals

Cancer	Chemicals
Lung	Arsenic, asbestos, cadmium, coke oven fumes, chromium, coal gasification, nickel refining, radon, soot, tars, silica
Larynx	Asbestos, isopropyl alcohol, mustard gas
Pharynx	Formaldehyde, mustard gas
Liver	Arsenic, vinyl chloride
Bladder	Aluminium, rubber, leather, benzidine
Skin	Arsenic, coal tar, mineral oils
Nasal cavity and paranasal sinuses	Formaldehyde, isopropyl alcohol, mustard gas, nickel, leather dust, wood dust
Mesothelioma	Asbestos
Soft-tissue sarcoma	Chlorophenols

The first stage of chemical carcinogenesis is tumour **initiation**, which involves exposure of normal cells to chemical carcinogens (Fig. 7.43). All initiators are **highly reactive electrophiles** that can react with electron-rich sites of the cell such as DNA, RNA and proteins. These carcinogens cause **permanent genetic damage** to DNA, providing the initiated cells with an altered responsiveness to their microenvironment and a proliferative advantage when compared with adjacent normal cells.

Cells transformed by initiators pass on the damage to their daughter cells. Initiation is a **rapid and irreversible** process; however, **initiation alone is not enough** for the development of a tumour.

Initiation is followed by **promotion**, resulting in proliferation of the initiated cells to a much greater extent than normal cells, and enhances the probability of additional genetic damage. But promoters are nontumorigenic by themselves, because these do not affect DNA directly and their actions are reversible.

This classical view of two-step chemical carcinogenesis is not only conceptually important but also an oversimplification of our increasing understanding of the complex biological processes that are deregulated in cancer.

Genotoxic carcinogens may be either directly acting or indirectly acting, i.e. requiring metabolic conversion.

Direct-Acting Carcinogens Direct-acting carcinogens **do not need metabolic conversion** to become carcinogenic, but most of them are weak. Some chemotherapeutic drugs come under this category. These drugs are helpful to attain cure in many cancers but later give rise to second tumours in 'cured' people.

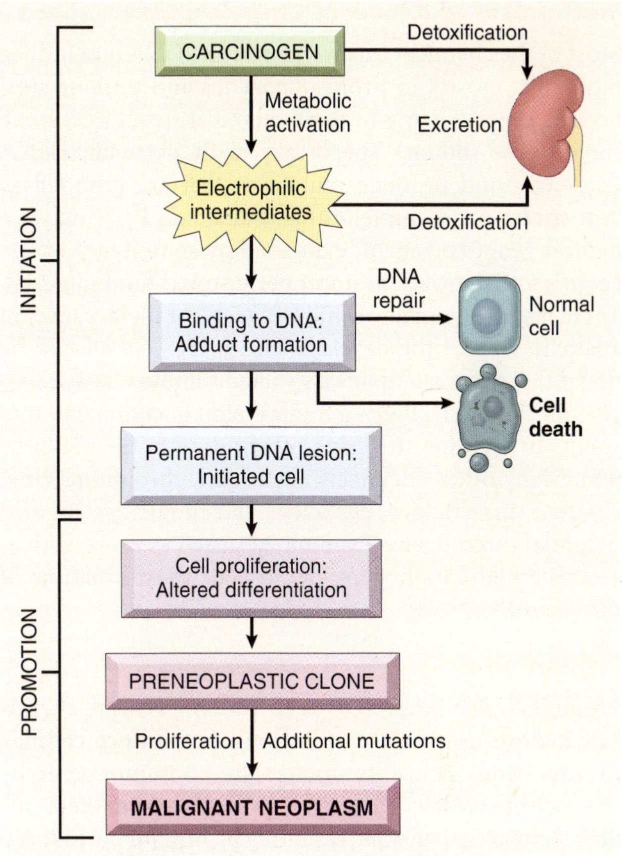

Fig. 7.43 Events in chemical carcinogenesis. (*Source:* From Vinay Kumar, Abul K. Abbas and Jon C. Aster. Neoplasia. Robbins Basic Pathology. 10th edition. Elsevier 2018.)

Indirect-acting Carcinogens Indirect-acting carcinogens **need metabolic conversion** to get transformed to active agents. Some metabolic pathways activate the procarcinogens. Cytochrome P450–dependent mono-oxygenases are involved in the conversion of most of these procarcinogens. The genes that encode these sets of enzymes are polymorphic, so the susceptibility to cancer development is partly related to the particular polymorphic variant that a person inherits.

This can be explained by the enzyme CYP1A1, a product of the P450 gene, which is responsible for the metabolism of polycyclic aromatic hydrocarbon, a toxin found in tobacco smoke. About 10% of the white population has a highly inducible form of CYP1A1, which confers higher susceptibility to lung cancer in association with smoking. If a person inherits the susceptible genotype, he or she has a sevenfold higher risk of developing lung cancer even with light smoking compared with smokers without this susceptible genotype for the enzyme. It should also be emphasized that apart from such genetic susceptibility of metabolic enzymes, environmental factors like age, sex, nutritional status and exposure to other toxins also influence the development of cancer in such individuals.

Mechanism of Action of Chemical Carcinogens

Most of the chemical carcinogens target DNA and induce mutations mostly in proto-oncogenes and tumour suppressor genes. Owing to their chemical structures, some carcinogens interact specifically with particular DNA sequences and produce mutations that are grouped as **'hot spots'.** An example of this is aflatoxin B_1, which is a natural genotoxic agent, expressed by some types of *Aspergillus*, that grows on improperly stored food material. There is a strong relationship between the dietary level of aflatoxin B_1 and the development of HCC. It should be noted that these aflatoxin-associated tumours have a specific mutation in TP53 – a transversion in codon 249 that results in arginine-to-serine substitution in the p53 protein. Many other chemicals like nickel, chromium, vinyl chloride, insecticides, pesticides and fungicides are also potential carcinogens. Even nitrites used as preservatives are potential carcinogens because of the formation of nitrosamines.

Promotion of Chemical Carcinogenesis

Promoters, also referred to as co-carcinogens, are chemicals that **do not induce mutations, but induce cellular proliferation**. Hence, promoters are nontumorigenic by themselves. Initiated cells on exposure to promoters undergo clonal expansion, resulting in tumour formation. During proliferation, certain subclones of the initiated cells suffer additional mutations, which would eventually accumulate all the necessary events for neoplastic transformation. In organs containing stable cells like the liver, the stimulus for proliferation is the initiator chemical itself, which, by causing death of a large number of cells, shifts the resting cells from G0 phase to active phases of the cell cycle. Examples of promoters include hormones such as oestrogen and androgen, drugs such as diethylstilbestrol, chemicals such as phorbol esters and phenol.

Prediction of chemical carcinogenicity is of great importance to human risk assessment.

RADIATION CARCINOGENESIS

The carcinogenic potential of ionizing radiation was recognized soon after Roentgen's discovery of X-rays in 1895. By 1902, the first radiation-induced cancer was reported arising in an ulcerated portion of the skin. Within a few years, a large number of such skin cancers had been observed and the first case of leukaemia was reported in five radiation-exposed workers in 1911. Both Marie Curie and her daughter Irene were thought to have died from complications associated with radiation-induced leukaemia, after working with radioactive isotopes. Many studies have shown an increased cancer risk from radiation exposure – for example, the increased incidence of second malignancies in children treated by radiation for their first malignancy. The detailed long-term studies of atom bomb survivors in Japan have made a major contribution to the assessment of the radiation dose–related risk of developing malignancy. In addition, the possible additive effects of radiation with other carcinogenic agents add another factor to the existing issue.

Radiant energy in the following forms is carcinogenic:

- UV rays from sunlight
- Ionizing radiation
  - Electromagnetic rays
  - Particulate rays

Ultraviolet Radiation

Ultraviolet radiation (UVR) is quite a prominent environmental toxin. It has been implicated in the initiation and progression of photocarcinogenesis, especially in fair-skinned individuals. Exposure to UVR causes several health hazards in humans including skin diseases, immunosuppression, photoageing, cataract and skin cancers. UVR exposure elicits numerous cellular and molecular events that include the production of inflammatory mediators, DNA damage, epigenetic modifications and oxidative damage–mediated activation of signalling pathways. **UVR-initiated signal transduction pathways** are responsible for the tumorigenesis effects.

UVR is associated with the development all types of skin cancers like malignant melanoma, squamous cell carcinoma and basal cell carcinoma. The main source of UVR is the sun, although it can also be obtained from man-made sources like welding torches and tanning beds. The risk of tumour development because of UVR depends on **the type of UV rays, the duration and intensity of the exposure and the quantity and function of the protective melanin in the skin**. For melanoma, it is the intense intermittent exposure, as in sunbathing, that acts as a strong risk factor, whereas for nonmelanoma skin cancers, it is the total cumulative effect that matters.

On the basis of the wavelength, UVR is categorized into three types: **ultraviolet C (UVC: 200–280 nm), ultraviolet B (UVB: 280–320 nm)** and **ultraviolet A (UVA:320–400 nm)**. UVC is highly mutagenic but does not reach the earth's surface because it is completely absorbed by the ozone layer. UVA and UVB wavelengths representing 95% and 5% of the UV spectrum, respectively, reach the earth. UVB is 20-fold less abundant than UVA, but its energy is more efficiently absorbed by cellular molecules, resulting in cellular damages at significantly lower doses than of UVA.

Absorption of UVR by DNA generates the mutagenic cyclobutane **pyrimidine dimers** (CPDs) linking pyrimidine bases in the same DNA strand. These changes are the major cause of skin cancers, because they lead to signature UV mutations. UVR-induced ROS and DNA lesions cause **secondary DNA double-strand breaks**, especially in replicating DNA. Usually, such defects are identified and corrected by the **NER pathway**. It is understood that with excessive sun exposure, the capacity of NER is exceeded and the error-prone nontemplated DNA repair mechanisms take over, allowing the cells with DNA damage to survive, resulting in cancer. This is well illustrated by the high incidence of multiple malignancies in patients with a defective NER pathway, i.e. **xeroderma pigmentosum.**

Ionizing Radiation

Radiation of certain wavelengths called ionizing radiation has enough energy to cause damage to DNA and induce cancer. Ionizing radiation includes electromagnetic rays like **radon, X-rays, gamma rays** and particulate rays like α particles, β articles, protons and neutrons.

Some major contributors are discussed here:

Radon: Radon is the most significant contributor to an individual's background radiation exposure, and the dosage is variable from location to location. Radon gas from natural sources can accumulate in buildings and can also be found in some spring waters and hot springs. Studies show a clear link between lung cancer and high concentrations of radon. It should also be stressed that residential exposure to radon gas has similar cancer risks as passive smoking. Radon is a more potent risk factor for cancer when it is combined with other cancer-causing agents such as smoking and tobacco.

Medical imaging: Medical imaging contributes almost as much radiation dose to people as natural background radiation. Computed tomographic (**CT**) **scans** alone, which account for half the medical imaging doses to individuals, are roughly estimated to be responsible for 0.4% of current cancers in the United States. This stresses the need to minimize radiation exposure, wherever and whenever possible.

Occupational: Some workers are exposed to radiation without being classified as nuclear energy workers like airline crews, mine workers and workers in granite building. They all are at a high risk of cancer development without protective equipment like lead aprons and face masks.

Accidental: The most severe nuclear accident is the Chernobyl nuclear disaster. Such accidents lead not only to death of people but also to acute radiation syndrome and cancer-related morbidity and mortality. The survivors of Hiroshima and Nagasaki atomic bombing reported a high incidence of leukaemias and many solid tumours like cancers of the breast, colon, thyroid and lungs over a prolonged period of time.

The common malignancies that arise with ionizing radiation exposure are as follows:

- **Myeloid leukaemias**
- **Thyroid cancer**
- **Breast cancer**
- **Lung cancer**
- **Salivary gland malignancies**

The organs that are relatively resistant to radiation-induced tumour development are the skin, bone and gastrointestinal tract. However, it should be stressed that any cell can get transformed with sufficient exposure to radiant energy.

MICROBIAL CARCINOGENESIS

Human microbial carcinogens include a diverse group of viruses, bacteria and parasitic worms. These carcinogens may act directly by integrating their genetic material into the host and disrupting their normal cellular functions or indirectly through inflammation or immunosuppression. Microorganism-related cancers are more common in developing countries, and improvements in hygiene and sanitation are associated with the development interventions for cancer prevention. Although the list of microbial carcinogens is long, only a few human oncogenic viruses and *Helicobacter pylori* are discussed here.

Viral Carcinogens (Table 7.18)

Viruses are the causative agents of **10%–15% of human cancers** worldwide. The most common mechanism for viral carcinogenesis is **genomic instability**, causing accumulation of mutations, DNA aberrations and damage. Although each virus has its own specific mechanism for promoting carcinogenesis, the majority of oncogenic DNA viruses encode oncogenes that transform infected cells, most often by targeting **TP53 and RB.**

Oncogenic viruses are classified as oncogenic RNA and DNA viruses.

Oncogenic RNA Viruses

Human T-Cell Leukaemia Virus Type 1 (HTLV-1)

HTLV-1 is **the most potent oncogenic virus** and potentially the most important oncogenic risk factor when

Table 7.18 List of Oncogenic Viruses and their Genome and Associated Cancers

Virus	Genome	Associated Cancers
HTLV-1	RNA virus	Adult T-cell leukaemia
HCV	RNA virus	Hepatocellular carcinoma
KSHV	DNA virus	Kaposi sarcoma Pleural effusion lymphoma
EBV	DNA virus	Burkitt lymphoma Nasopharyngeal carcinoma
HBV	DNA virus	Hepatocellular carcinoma
HPV	DNA virus	Carcinoma cervix Carcinoma penis Anogenital cancers Head and neck cancers
SV40	DNA virus	Mesothelioma Non-Hodgkin lymphoma

EBV, Epstein–Barr virus; HBV, hepatitis B virus; HCV, hepatitis C virus; HPV, human papillomavirus; HTLV-1, human T-cell leukaemia virus type 1.

compared with all other carcinogens, including chemical carcinogens. A unique and aggressive T-cell leukaemia (ATL) was discovered in Japan from which a new retrovirus, HTLV-1, was discovered in the United States and Japan at the same time. Apart from the aggressive leukaemia, HTLV-1 is also the cause of a type of myelopathy/tropical spastic paraparesis.

Like HIV, HTLV-1 spreads by sexual intercourse, transfusion of unscreened blood products and breast-feeding. Leukaemia develops only in 3%–5% of infected people and that too following a long latent period of 40–60 years. Like HIV, this virus has a tropism for $CD4^+$ cells and hence affects **helper T cells** as its major target for infection and neoplastic transformation.

HTLV-1 is an enveloped, dimeric, positive-sense, single-stranded RNA virus and like any other retrovirus its genome encodes the structural proteins and enzymes such as **gag, env and pol**. In addition, it contains a special region referred to as the pX region that encodes regulatory proteins such as **Tax**, HBZ and Rex. A significant number of adult T-cell leukaemias express FOXP3, a marker of regulatory T cells, the function of which is to suppress the immune responses. This is the basis of profound immunosuppression seen in patients with ATL. Unlike other oncogenic viruses, HTLV-1 neither contains an oncogene nor has consistent integration adjacent to a proto-oncogene. However, in leukaemic cells, viral integration has a clonal pattern, confirming that HTLV-1 must have been present at the moment of transformation. Some of the major events in the leukaemogenesis are attributable to the expression of Tax protein expressed by its gene, which is essential for viral replication. Tax is also responsible for the proliferation of the transformed cells, making them susceptible to acquire additional mutations.

The exact mechanisms of HTLV-1 and the process of leukaemogenesis of the virus are still being explored.

Hepatitis C Virus (HCV) Owing to its close association with hepatitis B virus (HBV), HCV is discussed under HBV.

Oncogenic DNA Viruses

Three well-studied oncogenic viruses are as follows:

- HPV
- HBV
- Epstein–Barr virus (EBV)

Several mechanisms that underlie the ability of oncogenic viruses to transform normal cells to malignant cells have been described here.

Human Papillomavirus HPV is a group of viruses with small, double-stranded circular DNA. These viruses have strict tropism for mucosal and cutaneous stratified squamous epithelial cells of the host. A subset of these viruses has been demonstrated to be the causative factor for many human cancers including cervical squamous cell carcinoma, a majority of oropharyngeal cancers and a subset of head and neck squamous cell carcinomas. Cervical cancer is the most common cancer in the developing countries, accounting for 7.5% of all cancer deaths in females.

Table 7.19 Classification of HPV Types According to their Oncogenicity

Category	Common HPV types
High risk	16, 18, 31, 33, 35
Intermediate risk	26, 53, 66
Low risk	6, 11, 40, 42

HPV, human papillomavirus.

The HPV family comprises more than 170 different members. Some types cause benign squamous papillomas, whereas a few special types are the causative factors for malignant tumours. Hence, HPV subtypes are classified into low-, intermediate- and high-risk categories on the basis of their oncogenic potential (Table 7.19).

In the benign lesions, HPV genome is present in the nonintegrated episomal form, whereas in malignant lesions, it is integrated into the host genome. This strongly suggests that the integration of the viral genome into the host genome is essential for malignant transformation. Like HTLV-1, the viral integration site is not constant and is random, but the pattern is clonal. Cells with integrated viral genome express more genomic instability. Such integration also interrupts the viral DNA within the E1/E2 open-reading frame, resulting in the disruption of E2 viral repressor. The E2 gene is responsible for repressing E6 and E7, and its loss leads to the overexpression of the viral oncoproteins **E6 and E7**, the two most essential factors in the carcinogenesis of HPV. Both the proteins complement each other in their actions. The mechanism of action of E6 and E7 proteins is discussed in the next sections (Fig. 7.44).

Actions of the Oncoplayer E6 E6 protein from high-risk HPV types has a high affinity for **p53**, and its major function is to bind and promote degradation of p53, the tumour suppressor protein. It also stimulates the expression of TERT for telomerase reactivation and immortality of the transformed cells.

Actions of the Oncoplayer E7 E7 protein from high-risk HPV types has a high affinity for **RB**, and it acts by binding to RB protein, displacing E2F transcription factor that is normally sequestered by RB. Owing to this effect, cells are driven into the cell cycle, overcoming the G1–S transition. In addition to this, E7 can bind and activate cyclins E and A, causing the cells to proliferate.

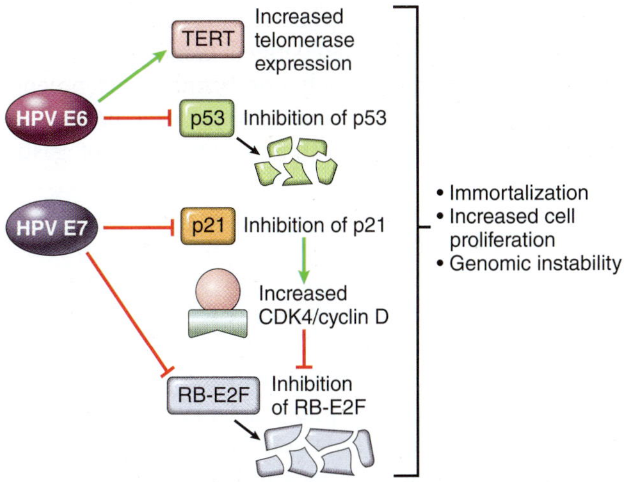

Fig. 7.44 Mechanism of action of E6 and E7 in human papillomavirus (HPV)-induced cancers – transforming effects of HPV E6 and E7 proteins. The net effect of HPV E6 and E7 proteins is to immortalize cells and remove the restraints on cell proliferation. (*Source:* From Vinay Kumar, Abul K. Abbas and Jon C. Aster. Neoplasia. Robbins Basic Pathology. 10th edition. Elsevier 2018.)

All the high-risk HPV types express their oncogenic potential through E6 and E7 proteins, which inactivate the two most important tumour suppressors p53 and RB, activate cyclins and help in the evasion of apoptosis leading to immortality of transformed cells.

Administration of HPV vaccine prevents the development of cervical cancer to a large extent, stressing the oncogenic role played by HPV. Although HPV infection is the major risk factor for the development of cervical cancer, other factors like coexisting microbial infections, cigarette smoking, nutritional deficiencies, hormonal disturbances and immunodeficient states have been implicated in the pathogenesis of cervical cancer.

Epstein–Barr Virus EBV is a herpes virus known to infect the majority of the world population and is associated with many human tumours like **Burkitt lymphoma, B-cell lymphomas in immunocompromised persons, Hodgkin lymphoma subtypes, nasopharyngeal carcinoma,** gastric carcinoma, T-cell lymphoma and NK-cell lymphoma. It is most commonly associated with the development of B-cell lymphomas and nasopharyngeal carcinoma.

In immunocompetent individuals, EBV infection results in polyclonal B-cell activation or a self-limited episode of infectious mononucleosis, whereas in immunodeficient individuals, it takes the virulent form with its ability to evade the weakened immune system.

EBV infects B lymphocytes and oropharyngeal epithelial cells. **CD21** on B lymphocytes is the receptor for EBV through which it gains entry. After the infection, B cells do not die but are latently infected and express virus-induced oncoproteins. EBV-related malignancies are associated with the latent form of infection, and many EBV-encoded latent proteins are known to mediate cellular transformation. These include six nuclear antigens and three latent membrane proteins. One such EBV-encoded protein is LMP-1, which plays a major role in the oncogenesis of EBV. Two nuclear antigens, EBNA-1 and EBNA-2, are also involved equally in the pathogenesis.

The role of LMP1, EBNA and other oncoproteins are described as follows:

1. **LMP-1:** This protein functions as a constitutively active CD40 receptor, stimulating B cells to proliferate autonomously. LMP-1 also suppresses apoptosis by overexpressing BCL-2. This results in the proliferation of latently infected cells.
2. **EBNA:** This oncogene and its products activate many proto-oncogenes including cyclins and stimulate cellular proliferation.
3. **vIL10:** This viral cytokine expressed by cells latently infected by EBV acts by preventing the attack of B cells by monocytes and macrophages.

T-cell immunity against EBV antigens controls and eliminates most of the EBV-infected cells, but a small percentage of cells downregulate the expression of these immunogenic antigens. Such cells persist for a very long period in the host. With acquisition of additional mutations, malignant tumours arise, i.e. acquisition of **MYC oncogene** resulting in the emergence of Burkitt lymphoma (Fig. 7.45) in EBV-infected people. In patients with immune dysregulations, there is sustained B-cell proliferation. In areas with endemic Burkitt lymphoma, the high incidence is attributed to the immune dysregulations induced by the concomitant endemic infections like malaria.

Hepatitis B and C Viruses There is a close association between HBV and HCV infection and the development of **HCC**. An estimated 75% of all HCC cases occur because of chronic infection with HBV or HCV, and the incidence of HCC is on the rise. Areas with endemic hepatitis caused by HBV and HCV have a very high incidence of HCC.

The exact mechanism of tumorigenesis of HBV is not yet clearly understood. HBV DNA gets integrated into the host genome, and there is no consistent pattern of integration. In spite of the integration, HBV does not encode any viral oncoproteins and the oncogenic effects of HBV are actually multifactorial.

The predominant effects are because of **chronic inflammation** induced by the immune response and the resultant liver cell regeneration that follows the death of hepatocytes culminating into genomic instability. In addition, **HBx**, an HBV gene, can activate many transcription factors and signal transduction pathways, stimulating cell proliferation. Apart from this, viral integration with the

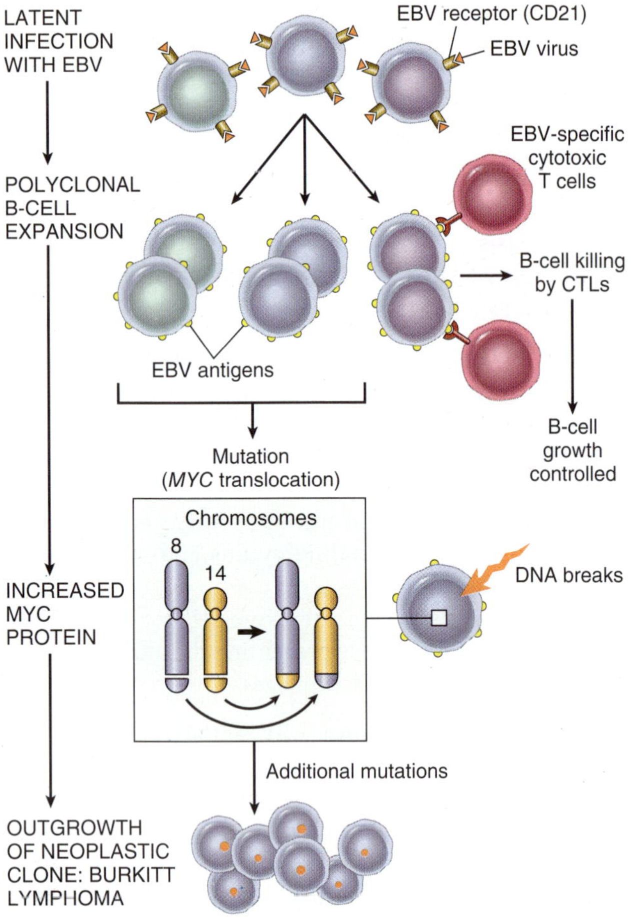

Fig. 7.45 Pathogenesis of EBV-associated Burkitt lymphoma. EBV, Epstein–Barr virus. (*Source:* From Vinay Kumar, Abul K. Abbas and Jon C. Aster. Neoplasia. Robbins Basic Pathology. 10th edition. Elsevier 2018.)

host genome causes structural chromosomal changes that dysregulate oncogenes and tumour suppressor genes.

HCV is also very strongly associated with the development of HCC, but the mechanism of action of HCV is less well understood. Like HBV, HCV acts by inducing **chronic inflammation and rebound regeneration**. Apart from this, HCV core protein may have a direct effect on the development of HCC by stimulating growth-promoting pathways.

Helicobacter Pylori

H. pylori is the first bacterium to be classified as a microbial carcinogen. It was first associated with peptic ulcer but now is strongly linked to the genesis of **gastric adenocarcinomas and gastric lymphomas**. The basis of gastric adenocarcinoma development is the chronic inflammation–induced proliferation of gastric epithelial cells. The bacterium initially causes chronic gastritis, which progresses to gastric atrophy, intestinal metaplasia, dysplasia and invasive malignancy. Among infected individuals, approximately 10% develop severe gastric lesions such as peptic ulcer disease and roughly around 1%–3% progress to gastric carcinoma.

The mechanism of *H. pylori*–associated gastric carcinogenesis has not been well defined. Genotypes of *H. pylori* strains, host genetic polymorphisms, environmental factors like high-salt diet and smoking have been determined to be associated with the occurrence of gastric carcinoma.

H. pylori strains harbouring the Cag gene or producing **CagA** are related to enhanced inflammation and risk of peptic ulcers and carcinoma. CagA acts by penetrating into the gastric epithelial cells where it initiates the events for cellular proliferation.

H. pylori is also associated with the risk of development of gastric B-cell lymphomas, which are often called lymphomas of mucosa-associated lymphoid tissue (MALTomas). Genesis of gastric B-cell lymphomas appears to be different from the development of gastric adenocarcinomas but is still not completely understood. Strain-specific factors of *H. pylori* and polymorphisms of IL-1β and TNF genes are thought to decide the outcome. It is postulated that *H. pylori* infection leads to proliferation of T cells against *H. pylori*, leading to the stimulation of polyclonal B-cell proliferation. Till this stage, B cells are polyclonal and are dependent on T cells for their proliferation and hence the disease is completely reversible with eradication of the bacterium using antibiotics.

With sustained infection and inflammation, acquisition of additional mutations occurs and provides the cells with survival and growth advantage because of constitutive NF-kB activation leading to the development of monoclonal 'MALToma'. At this stage, MALToma can no longer be controlled with antibiotics and would continue to grow further and deeper.

CLINICAL PRESENTATION OF TUMOURS

All tumours, including benign tumours, can cause morbidity and mortality, although malignant tumours are more dangerous. A good understanding of the clinical aspects of tumours is important, because these tumours are the ones that bring the patients for clinical workup. Ultimately, the importance of neoplasms lies in their effects on the patients. The clinical presentation can be because of any of the following reasons:

- **Mass effects**
- **Hormonal effects**
- **Cancer cachexia**

The cause and effects of these are discussed in the next sections.

MASS EFFECT OF TUMOURS

Location of tumours is the most critical determinant of the clinical presentation of all tumours. Tumours may compress adjacent normal structures and lead to their dysfunction. This is commonly seen in intracranial neoplasms, including the benign ones, which compress the brain because of inelasticity of the skull vault. Increased pressure on the brain may lead to symptoms such as confusion, headache, nausea or localized neurological signs.

Other syndromes commonly caused by mass effect are as follows:

- **Spinal cord compression** can be caused by lesions within the spinal canal. More often, a bony metastasis can erode the structural support of vertebrae, resulting in collapse and compression of the spinal cord.
- **Superior vena cava obstruction** can occur when mediastinal lymph nodes or adjacent lung lesions expand and compress the superior vena cava. Obstruction leads to poor return of blood from the head, neck and arms. Patients present with a swollen, flushed upper trunk. Occasionally, it may cause thrombosis of the great blood vessels or venous sinuses of the brain that can be fatal.
- Metastasis to the psoas muscle may occur in cancer cervix, resulting in compression of the lumbar plexus. This can cause neuropathic pain in the associated nerve distributions.

HORMONAL EFFECTS

Endocrine neoplasms may retain the secretory hormonal function of their normal counterparts. This is particularly true of benign neoplasms, for example:

- A thyroid adenoma may secrete thyroxine, resulting in hyperthyroidism.
- An insulinoma of the endocrine pancreas may cause hypoglycaemia by excessive insulin secretion.
- A parathyroid adenoma may produce parathyroid hormone, leading to hypercalcaemia and osteoporosis.

CANCER CACHEXIA

Cachexia is the progressive loss of lean muscle, fat, energy and appetite seen in patients with malignancy. This is partly because of an increased basal metabolic rate. Mechanisms of cachexia are not completely understood, but are thought to be related to production of cytokines by the tumour and the immune system that disturb the homeostasis of the muscle and fat stores. One-third of deaths in patients with cancer is partially attributable to cancer cachexia. There is also evidence of systemic inflammation. There is no effective and specific treatment of cancer cachexia other than cure of the tumour.

Unfortunately, a significant number of cancers remain silent till the late stage when they are picked up by the signs of metastatic disease and most such cancers become rapidly fatal.

PARANEOPLASTIC SYNDROMES (TABLE 7.20) PA 7.4

Paraneoplastic syndromes are a group of rare presentations triggered by a neoplasm that cannot be explained by its anatomic location, compression, infiltration or metastasis. These are defined as clinical syndromes because of **nonmetastatic systemic effects** that accompany malignant tumours. These effects are the result of substances or hormones produced by the tumour that are not normally produced by the parent cell of origin. The symptoms can be endocrine, neuromuscular, musculoskeletal, cardiovascular, haematological, dermatological, bone and soft-tissue changes or miscellaneous changes. Newer theories suggest these syndromes to be an altered immune response to a neoplasm.

In summary, paraneoplastic syndromes are:

- Not related to the local effects or distant spread of tumour
- Not related to production of hormones related to the tumour's cell of origin

Paraneoplastic syndromes may be the first or most prominent presentation of a malignant tumour in a significant number of cases. When a patient without any history of cancer presents with one of the typical paraneoplastic syndromes, a suspicion of cancer should be raised and investigated further. Their clinical importance is because of the fact that these syndromes may produce symptoms similar to those of metastases. These may also cause significant morbidity or mortality.

Hypercalcaemia is the most common paraneoplastic syndrome. Malignancy should be ruled out in patients presenting with symptomatic hypercalcaemia, because malignancy is the most common cause.

Mechanisms of hypercalcaemia are as follows:

- **Osteolysis** induced by the primary bone malignancy (multiple myeloma) or metastatic deposits
- Elaboration of calcaemic humoral substances by extraosseous neoplasms (the most common substance associated with it is parathyroid hormone-related protein [**PTHRP**])

Hypercalcaemia induced by the second mechanism is considered to be paraneoplastic.

Common malignancies associated with paraneoplastic hypercalcaemia are **carcinomas of the breast, kidney, lung and ovary**. The most common lung carcinoma associated with paraneoplastic hypercalcaemia is squamous cell carcinoma. Other than PTHRP, factors like IL-1, TGF-α, TNF and dihydroxyviatmin D are also commonly produced by these paraneoplastic tumours.

Endocrinopathies are common paraneoplastic syndromes. The cancers associated with this manifestation are not of endocrine origin, and their manifestation is because

Table 7.20 Paraneoplastic Syndromes and their Associated Malignancies and Mechanisms

Clinical Syndromes	Common Malignancies Associated	Mechanism
Endocrinopathies		
Cushing syndrome	Small-cell carcinoma of lung Pancreatic neoplasms Neural tumours	ACTH or ACTH-like factors
Hypercalcaemia	Small-cell carcinoma of lung Breast carcinoma Renal cell carcinoma Adult T-cell leukaemia	PTHRP
SIADH	Small-cell carcinoma of lung Intracranial neoplasms	Antidiuretic hormone Atrial natriuretic peptide
Hypoglycaemia	Fibrosarcoma Ovarian malignancy	Insulin or insulin-like factors
Polycythaemia	Renal cell carcinoma Hepatocellular carcinoma Cerebellar haemangioma	Erythropoietin
Dermatological Disorders		
Acanthosis nigricans	Gastric carcinoma Bronchogenic carcinoma Endometrial carcinoma	Epidermal growth factor
Dermatomyositis	Bronchogenic carcinoma Breast carcinoma	Immunological
Neuromuscular disorders		
Myasthenia gravis	Bronchogenic carcinoma Thymic tumours	Immunological
Bone and soft-tissue changes		
Hypertrophic osteoarthropathy and clubbing of digits	Bronchogenic carcinoma	Unknown
Vascular and haematological changes		
DIC	APML Prostatic carcinoma	Procoagulant factors
Venous thrombosis	Prostatic carcinoma Bronchogenic carcinoma	Prothrombotic factors
NBTE	Advanced malignancies	Prothrombotic factors
Red cell aplasia	Thymic tumours	Unknown
Miscellaneous		
Nephrotic syndrome	Many cancers	Tumour antigens, immune complex

ACTH, adrenocorticotropic hormone; APML, acute promyelocytic leukaemia; DIC, disseminated intravascular coagulation; NBTE, nonbacterial thrombotic endocarditis; PTHRP, parathyroid hormone–related protein; SIADH, syndrome of inappropriate antidiuretic hormone secretion.

of ectopic hormone production. Among the various endocrinopathies, **Cushing syndrome** is the most common endocrinopathy. About half of the patients with Cushing syndrome as endocrinopathy have carcinoma of the lung, mostly of small-cell type. The syndrome is because of excessive production of corticotropin for which the precursor molecule is pro-opiomelanocortin. Patients with lung cancer accompanied by Cushing syndrome as paraneoplastic endocrinopathic presentation have elevated serum levels of corticotropin and pro-opiomelanocortin.

Other less common paraneoplastic syndromes are acanthosis nigricans, hypertrophic osteoarthropathy, migratory thrombophlebitis, disseminated intravascular coagulation, neuromyopathic paraneoplastic syndromes, etc.

Owing to their protean manifestations, paraneoplastic syndromes should be managed by a multidisciplinary team.

LABORATORY DIAGNOSIS OF CANCER

Management of cancer starts with cancer diagnosis. Cancer diagnosis includes three stages:

1. Location of the tumour process
2. Evaluation of the tumour extension
3. Determination of the tumour's histological nature

LOCATION OF THE TUMOUR PROCESS

Location of the tumour process requires a thorough clinical examination with adequate anamnesis and laboratory investigations. The complete evaluation for a suspected tumour usually starts with complete history taking and physical examination. There should always be a strong correlation between the clinical diagnosis and the results of diagnostic tests. The approach to laboratory diagnosis of cancer has become more specialized, more complex, more sophisticated and more comprehensive in the recent years. Complementary examinations like imaging techniques, endoscopy, haematological examination and biochemical changes are adjuvant or sometimes irreplaceable in the workup of the location of a tumour.

EVALUATION OF THE TUMOUR EXTENSION AND DETERMINATION OF THE TUMOUR'S HISTOLOGICAL NATURE

Once a diagnosis of cancer has been made, the patient undergoes a series of investigations including imaging modalities like PET scan to determine the characteristics of the tumour tissue and the extent of spread of the tumour in the body.

Once the tumour is suspected and evaluated, a biopsy, which may be a Tru-Cut tissue or a wedge biopsy for histopathological examination, is performed to confirm the diagnosis.

Further evaluation through pathological grading and the TNM system for staging facilitates the establishment of low-error diagnosis and prognosis.

Grading and Staging of Tumours

Grading: Grading of a tumour is based on **its differentiation and other factors like morphological patterns, mitosis and necrosis**. Each tumour has different schemes for grading that categorizes tumours into two to four grades. Although grading is essential for the selection of treatment protocol and assessing prognosis, it does not correlate with biological behaviour of tumours in all cases. In general, higher-grade tumours are more aggressive and carry worse prognosis than lower-grade malignancies. Some of the commonly used grading systems for different tumours are listed in Table 7.21.

Table 7.21 Commonly used Grading Systems for Different Tumours

Grading System	Tumours Graded Using the System
Bloom–Richardson grading system	Breast carcinoma
Gleason grading system	Prostatic carcinoma
Fuhrman grading system	Renal cell carcinoma
FNCLCC grading system	Soft-tissue sarcoma

Staging: Cancer staging is a process of determining the **anatomical extent of the disease**. In addition to classifying a tumour on the basis of its microscopic characteristics, it is essential to classify it on the basis of its extent. The stage generally takes into account the size of a tumour, its invasion into adjacent organs, spread to regional lymph nodes and spread to distant locations.

Cancer staging can be divided into clinical and pathological stages.

Clinical stage is based on all of the available information obtained before removal of the tumour.

Pathological stage adds additional information obtained by microscopic examination by a pathologist after the tumour has been removed surgically.

Clinical and pathological stages often differ because different criteria are used. Pathological staging is usually considered to be more accurate because it allows direct examination of the entire tumour unlike clinical staging that is limited by the fact that the information is obtained by indirect observation of a tumour. However, both staging types often complement each other. Not every tumour is surgically removable or entirely assessable, so pathological staging is not always possible. In addition, in some cases, surgery is preceded by other treatments like neoadjuvant chemotherapy and radiotherapy, which shrink the tumour and induce morphological alterations, so the pathological stage may underestimate the actual stage.

The most widely used system across the globe is the American Joint Committee on Cancer Staging. This system uses a classification system called the TNM system (***T*** for primary tumour, ***N*** for regional node involvement and ***M*** for metastases).

The primary tumour is categorized into T1 to T4 on the basis of the size, and Tis indicates in situ lesion.

Nodal status is categorized into N1 to N3 on the basis of the number of nodes involved, and N0 indicates no nodal involvement. Nx denotes nodes not assessed.

Metastatic status is denoted by M1 or sometimes M2 depending on the presence and number of metastases, and M0 indicates the absence of metastasis. Mx denotes metastasis not assessed.

In the TNM system, clinical and pathological stages are indicated by the prefix alphabets **'c' and 'p' before the stage, respectively.**

This staging system is used for most forms of cancer, except brain tumours, leukaemias and lymphomas.

Laboratory Tests for Tumours

The laboratory tests for tumours are broadly categorized into the following types:

- Morphological tests
- Immunohistochemistry (IHC)
- Flow cytometry
- Circulating tumour cells
- Tumour markers/biomarkers
- Molecular genetics/cytogenetics

Morphological Tests for Tumours

Cytological and histopathological examinations comprise morphological tests. Cytological examination has the benefit of being noninvasive and has less turnaround time for the reports. Samples for cytological examination may be obtained by fine needle aspiration or cytological smears. Cytology has its own limitations in that a 'normal cytology never excludes the possibility of existence of cancer'.

Clinical information is extremely essential for accurate pathological diagnosis but is often overseen by the clinicians. In addition, histopathological examination requires the harvesting of a sufficiently extensive tumour portion to establish the diagnosis. In the case of total surgical removal, the entire specimen is examined macroscopically and microscopically. In other situations, incision biopsies are performed and the samples are subjected to histopathological examination. Although the evaluation of a tumour has gone much beyond morphology, no test can replace the histopathological examination, which should always be given its due importance. Fine needle aspiration cytology (FNAC), cytological smears and frozen section are discussed in Chapter 11.

IHC, flow cytometry and circulating tumour cells are discussed in Chapter 12.

TUMOUR MARKERS

Tumour markers are biomarkers that are found in blood and body fluids that can be elevated by the presence of a tumour. There are many types of tumour markers, each indicative of a particular tumour and can be used in the detection of cancers. These markers are produced directly by the neoplastic cells or by non-neoplastic cells in response to the presence of a neoplasm. These markers can be determined in serum or rarely in urine or other body fluids by immunoassays or enzyme activity. The markers can also be tested using IHC on tissues, but with this method, they cannot be accurately quantified.

Classification (Table 7.22)

Tumour markers can be enzymes, hormones, fragments of proteins, peptides or carbohydrates depending on their chemical nature.

Table 7.22 Classification of Tumour Markers and Their Associated Tumours

Tumour Marker	Associated Tumours
Oncofetal Antigens	
α-Fetoprotein (AFP)	Hepatocellular carcinoma, nonseminomatous germ cell tumours
Carcinoembryonic antigen	Carcinoma of pancreas, colon, lung and stomach
Hormones	
Human chorionic gonadotropin	Choriocarcinoma, nonseminomatous germ cell tumours
Catecholamines	Pheochromocytoma
Calcitonin	Medullary carcinoma thyroid
Ectopic hormones	Refer Table 7.20
Mucins	
CA 15-3	Breast carcinoma
CA 27-29	Breast carcinoma
CA 19-9	Carcinoma of pancreas and colon
CA 125	Surface epithelial tumours of ovary
Enzymes	
Neuron-specific enolase	Neuroblastoma, small-cell carcinoma of lung
Prostatic acid phosphatase	Carcinoma prostate
Placental alkaline phosphatase	Seminoma, dysgerminoma
Tumour-Specific Proteins	
Immunoglobulin	Multiple myeloma
Prostate-specific antigen	Carcinoma of prostate
Fragmented Cell-Free DNA	
TP53, RAS mutants in sputum and serum	Carcinoma lung
TP53, RAS mutants in stool and serum	Carcinoma pancreas
TP53, APC, RAS mutants in stool and serum	Carcinoma colon
Hormone Receptors	
Oestrogen receptor	Breast carcinoma
Progesterone receptor	Breast carcinoma

Uses of Tumour Markers

- **Screening** for common cancers: For example, elevated prostate-specific antigen (PSA) level is a useful evaluation tool to screen prostatic carcinoma.
- **Diagnosis** of specific cancer types: Although tumour markers are not primarily used to diagnose tumours,

they are helpful in certain types of brain tumours where biopsy is not feasible.

- **Confirmation of tumour diagnosis:** Tumour markers are used to verify certain characteristics of tumours like tumour burden and aggressiveness to design the treatment protocol.
- **Monitoring of tumour recurrence after treatment:** For example, elevation of human chorionic gonadotropin in a patient treated for choriocarcinoma suggests recurrence.
- **Staging of tumours:** Some tumour markers are included in the staging workup of tumours. For example, serum levels of α-fetoprotein are measured to assess stage, estimate prognosis and follow response to treatment.
- **Assessment of prognosis:** Many tumour markers are measured to assess the prognosis of the patients.
- **Assess the response to treatment:** Measurement of pre- and post-treatment levels of tumour markers helps in the assessment of tumour response to treatment.

The applied aspects of many tumour markers are discussed under the specific tumours in other chapters. Few commonly used markers are explained here.

One of the most widely used tumour markers is **PSA**, which is the marker for carcinoma of the prostate. Although it has low sensitivity and specificity, like any other tumour marker, its elevated levels in an elderly male definitely raise a strong suspicion regarding carcinoma of the prostate. Markers like PSA, carcinoembryonic antigen (CEA) and α-fetoprotein are not specific for carcinomas and thus cannot be depended on as valuable markers for early detection of cancers. But these can be used to monitor disease activity, especially after excision.

Recent tumour markers are fragmented cell-free circulating DNA molecules that include mutated **APC, TP53 and RAS sequences**. These markers can be detected in stool, serum or sputum according to the associated tumours.

Although not every patient with cancer has a raised level of a tumour marker, the appropriate use of tumour markers provides great opportunities for improving the management of patients with cancer by improving the efficiency of detection and assessing the efficacy of treatment.

MOLECULAR GENETICS/CYTOGENETICS

Molecular techniques are being increasingly used nowadays in the workup of tumours and are discussed in detail in Chapter 12. These techniques are used in the evaluation of tumours with the following applications:

- Diagnosis of malignancy
- Assessing the prognosis
- Therapeutic decision making
- Detecting minimal residual disease
- Diagnosis of hereditary predisposition to malignancy
- Guiding the choice of targeted therapy

MOLECULAR PROFILING OF TUMOURS: PRECISION ONCOLOGY

Molecular profiling of tumours involves the use of various technologies to understand the underlying characteristics of malignant cells.

Molecular studies of individual tumours have gone beyond the analysis of individual genes to entire genome sequencing, assessing epigenetic modifications, quantification of expressed RNAs in a tumour population, simultaneous quantification of proteins and studying cell metabolites.

TARGETED THERAPY (FIG. 7.46)

Implementation of therapies like imatinib and trastuzumab has opened a new era of genomic-driven medicine

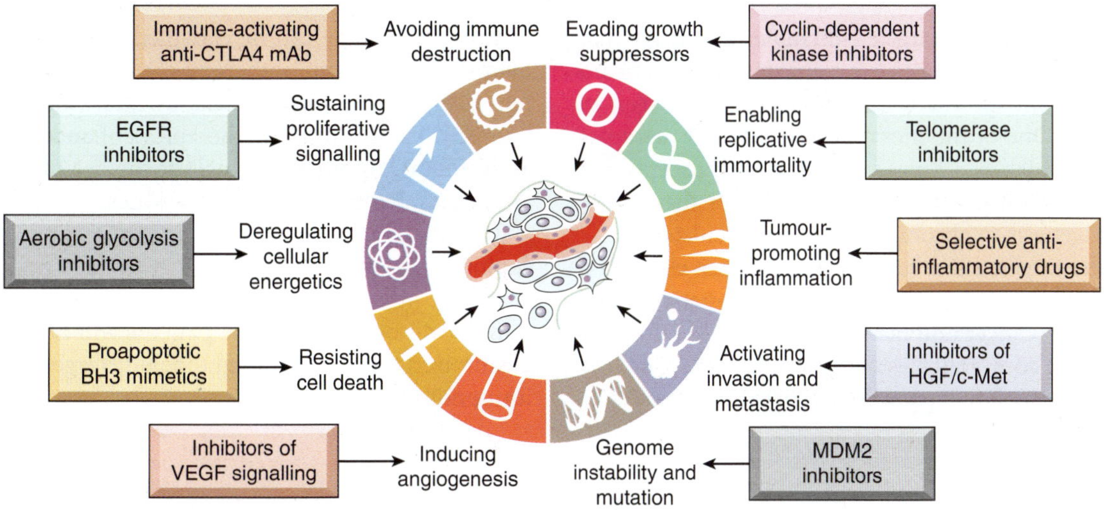

Fig. 7.46 Therapeutic targeting of the hallmarks of cancer – examples. (*Source:* From Vinay Kumar, Abul K. Abbas and Jon C. Aster. Neoplasia. Robbins Basic Pathology. 10th edition. Elsevier 2018.)

in oncology. Imatinib given as a targeted medicine to patients with chronic myeloid leukaemia (CML) prolongs overall survival of the treated patients, which could be matched with that in the general population, and trastuzumab for HER2-expressing breast cancer allows for a 35%–50% reduction in mortality in the adjuvant setting and a 20% reduction in mortality of patients with metastatic disease.

Precision oncology ensures comprehensive molecular profiling of the individual patient's tumour sample that enables to define a draggable target or multiple targets in some cases. This helps the clinician to tailor treatment better than that on the basis of current clinical workup and histopathology report.

The number of tumour-specific molecular aberrations has grown exponentially in the last decade, with significant survival benefits obtained from biomarker matching therapies in many cancer types. This has drastically changed the 'one-size-fits-all' approach of treatment of patients with cancer to focusing on precision medicine on the basis of genomic variants.

The major impact of cancer genome sequencing has been in the following areas of research:

- Identification of new mutations in many cancers
- Description of the complete set of genetic lesions in every tumour
- Exposing the genetic heterogeneity of individual tumours

More efforts are being taken to develop newer, simpler, faster and cost-effective sequencing methods that permit identification of therapeutically targetable genetic abnormalities. Identification of molecular targets and treatment with targeted therapy have completely changed the outlook of cancer treatment and prognosis.

Targeted cancer therapies are expected to be more effective than the conventional chemotherapy and less toxic to normal cells. Many targeted therapies are examples of immunotherapy that uses immune mechanisms for therapeutic goals.

The most successful targeted therapies are drugs that target preferentially a protein or enzyme that carries a genetic mutation specific to cancer cells and not seen in normal cells. One of the most successful target therapies is imatinib, which is a kinase inhibitor with exceptional affinity for the oncofusion protein BCR-Abl that drives the tumorigenesis in chronic myelogenous leukaemia.

There are targeted therapies for lung cancer, colorectal cancer, breast cancer, multiple myeloma, prostatic cancer, head and neck cancer and many others.

Some of the commonly tested molecular targets and the drugs given in such malignancies are listed in Table 7.23.

Table 7.23 List of Commonly Tested Target Molecules in Malignancies and the Drugs Used

Target Molecule	Malignancy	Targeted Therapy
Abl	CML	Imatinib (Gleevec)
Kit	GIST	Imatinib (Gleevec)
PDGFR	GIST	Imatinib (Gleevec)
EGFR	Lung carcinoma	Gefitinib
HER2	Breast carcinoma	Herceptin
VEGF ligand	Colorectal carcinoma	Bevacizamab
FLT3	AML	PKC-412
VEGFR, RAF	RCC, melanoma	BAY 43-9006

CML, chronic myeloid leukaemia.

IMMUNOTHERAPY

Cancer immunotherapy, also called **immuno-oncology**, is the artificial stimulation of the immune system to treat cancer. This form of cancer therapy exploits the fact that cancer cells often have tumour antigens, molecules on their surface that can be detected by the antibodies of the immune system. Although normal antibodies bind to external pathogens, the modified immunotherapy antibodies bind to the tumour antigens, marking and identifying the cancer cells for the immune system to inhibit or kill.

Although targeted therapy uses drugs to attack specific cancer cells, drugs used for immunotherapy do not attack cancer cells directly. Instead, they stimulate the patient's immune system to recognize cancer cells as foreign antigens and mount an immune response, resulting in their destruction.

Immunotherapy can be classified as active, passive or hybrid. Active immunotherapy directs the immune system to target the tumour cells by attacking the tumour antigens. Passive immunotherapies enhance the existing antitumour responses and include the use of monoclonal antibodies, lymphocytes and cytokines.

Results of immunotherapy are promising and being explored much more nowadays. Days are not far when complete molecular profiling of every patient's tumour sample will be done and the patients will be treated with customized therapy that might include targeted drugs and immunomodulators.

SELF-ASSESSMENT

Scenario-Based MCQs

1. A 35-year-old woman presents with a palpable, painless mass in her breast. Biopsy shows cells resembling normal mammary cells, forming duct-like structures. The mass is well demarcated and movable. What is the most likely diagnosis?
   A. Invasive ductal carcinoma
   B. Fibroadenoma
   C. Ductal carcinoma in situ
   D. Lobular carcinoma
2. A pathologist observes a tumour under the microscope characterized by a high degree of cellular differentiation, minimal nuclear atypia and no evidence of invasion into the surrounding tissues. Which feature best classifies this tumour?
   A. Benign
   B. Malignant
   C. Metastatic
   D. Premalignant
3. A patient's lung tumour biopsy shows spindle-shaped cells arranged in a haphazard manner, with numerous mitotic figures and areas of necrosis. The tumour infiltrates the surrounding pulmonary tissue. This description most likely indicates:
   A. Benign neoplasm
   B. Malignant neoplasm
   C. Infectious granuloma
   D. Benign fibrous tissue
4. A 45-year-old man presents with a slow-growing, painless mass on his right forearm. MRI reveals a well-circumscribed mass not invading the surrounding tissues. The most likely characteristic of this mass is:
   A. High metastatic potential
   B. Rapid growth and ulceration
   C. Well-differentiated cells and tissue structure
   D. Poorly defined margins and invasion
5. A biopsy of a skin lesion shows a well-demarcated, noninvasive growth composed of neoplastic cells that resemble the normal epidermal structure. This is indicative of:
   A. Malignant melanoma
   B. Basal cell carcinoma
   C. Squamous cell carcinoma
   D. Keratoacanthoma
6. A liver biopsy reveals a mass with well-differentiated hepatocytes arranged in cords, lacking invasive growth and confined to a distinct region. This description suggests the mass is:
   A. Hepatocellular carcinoma
   B. Hepatic adenoma
   C. Focal nodular hyperplasia
   D. Hepatic metastasis
7. A thyroid nodule biopsy in a 40-year-old woman shows cells with clear cytoplasm and centrally located nuclei, organized into follicles filled with colloid. This pattern is characteristic of:
   A. Papillary carcinoma
   B. Follicular adenoma
   C. Medullary carcinoma
   D. Anaplastic carcinoma
8. A patient presents with a rapidly growing tumour in the colon. Histopathology reveals poorly differentiated cells, high mitotic activity and invasion into the muscularis propria. The most likely diagnosis is:
   A. Adenomatous polyp
   B. Hyperplastic polyp
   C. Colorectal adenocarcinoma
   D. Colorectal lymphoma
9. A research laboratory identifies a mutation in the BRCA1 gene in a family with a high incidence of breast and ovarian cancer. This mutation most likely leads to:
   A. Increased DNA repair efficiency
   B. Enhanced tumour suppressor gene function
   C. Impaired DNA damage response
   D. Activation of oncogenes
10. A biopsy from a patient with lung cancer shows overexpression of the EGFR gene. This finding is significant because it suggests:
    A. A potential target for tyrosine kinase inhibitors
    B. Resistance to radiation therapy
    C. Indication of a benign process
    D. Decreased tumour aggressiveness
11. In a case of colorectal cancer, a patient's tumour shows a mutation in the APC gene. This mutation is primarily associated with:
    A. Inhibition of apoptosis
    B. Increased cell adhesion
    C. Activation of Wnt signalling pathway
    D. Suppression of angiogenesis
12. A 50-year-old patient with chronic myeloid leukaemia (CML) has a confirmed BCR-ABL fusion gene. This genetic alteration is typically associated with:
    A. Increased sensitivity to immunotherapy
    B. High potential for metastasis
    C. Constitutive tyrosine kinase activity
    D. Hormone receptor positivity
13. A tumour analysis reveals a mutation in the PTEN gene. This alteration is likely to result in:
    A. Enhanced DNA repair mechanisms
    B. Decreased PI3K/AKT signalling
    C. Increased cell cycle arrest
    D. Increased PI3K/AKT signalling
14. In a patient with melanoma, the presence of a V600E mutation in the BRAF gene suggests:
    A. Poor prognosis and aggressive behaviour
    B. Increased susceptibility to BRAF inhibitors
    C. Resistance to chemotherapy
    D. Lack of metastatic potential
15. A study on breast cancer cells reveals overexpression of HER2/neu. This finding is clinically relevant because it:
    A. Confers a good prognosis
    B. Indicates sensitivity to trastuzumab
    C. Suggests a hormonal aetiology
    D. Implies a slower rate of tumour growth
16. A 60-year-old man with a history of smoking presents with lung cancer. Which type of carcinogen is most likely responsible for his condition?
    A. Chemical
    B. Viral
    C. Radiation
    D. Hormonal
17. A patient develops liver cancer after years of chronic hepatitis B infection. This is an example of carcinogenesis by:
    A. Chemical agents
    B. Dietary factors
    C. Oncogenic viruses
    D. Physical agents

18. A laboratory study shows that UV radiation causes thymidine dimers in DNA, leading to skin cancer. This is an example of:
    A. Direct-acting carcinogen
    B. Procarcinogen
    C. Promoter
    D. Complete carcinogen
19. In an industrial setting, workers exposed to asbestos develop mesothelioma. Asbestos acts as a(n):
    A. Initiator
    B. Promoter
    C. Complete carcinogen
    D. Indirect carcinogen
20. A study finds that a certain food additive, when metabolized, becomes a carcinogenic compound. This additive is best described as a(n):
    A. Direct-acting carcinogen
    B. Procarcinogen
    C. Cocarcinogen
    D. Initiator
21. A research finds that certain hormonal therapies increase the risk of breast cancer. These therapies act as:
    A. Initiators
    B. Promoters
    C. Complete carcinogens
    D. Indirect carcinogens
22. A population study links a high-fat diet to an increased risk of colon cancer. This dietary factor is acting as a(n):
    A. Direct-acting carcinogen
    B. Promoter
    C. Complete carcinogen
    D. Indirect carcinogen
23. A patient with a genetic predisposition to colorectal cancer has a higher risk when exposed to dietary carcinogens. This is an example of:
    A. Synergism
    B. Additive effect
    C. Antagonism
    D. Independence
24. A 58-year-old woman with lung cancer develops Cushing syndrome. This is most likely because of:
    A. Metastasis to the adrenal glands
    B. Paraneoplastic syndrome
    C. Direct tumour invasion of the pituitary gland
    D. Side effects of chemotherapy
25. A patient with pancreatic cancer experiences migratory thrombophlebitis ('Trousseau syndrome'). This condition is an example of:
    A. Direct tumour effect
    B. Chemotherapy side effect
    C. Paraneoplastic syndrome
    D. Metastasis
26. A man with small-cell lung cancer presents with muscle weakness and hyporeflexia. Laboratory tests show hyponatraemia. This is indicative of:
    A. SIADH
    B. Hypercalcaemia
    C. Lambert–Eaton syndrome
    D. Cachexia
27. A patient with renal cell carcinoma develops high blood calcium levels without bone metastases. This is most likely because of:
    A. Direct bone invasion by the tumour
    B. Paraneoplastic syndrome
    C. Renal failure
    D. Vitamin D deficiency
28. A woman with ovarian cancer experiences ataxia, dysarthria and loss of motor coordination. These symptoms are likely because of:
    A. Metastasis to the brain
    B. Paraneoplastic cerebellar degeneration
    C. Side effects of chemotherapy
    D. Progression of the primary tumour
29. A patient with prostate cancer develops deep vein thrombosis and pulmonary embolism. These complications are most likely related to:
    A. Tumour invasion into blood vessels
    B. Hypercoagulable state because of cancer
    C. Side effects of hormone therapy
    D. Physical inactivity
30. A patient with melanoma shows increased levels of cytotoxic T lymphocytes in the tumour microenvironment. This indicates:
    A. Immune escape by the tumour
    B. Effective immune response against the tumour
    C. Suppression of the immune system
    D. Ineffective antigen presentation
31. A patient with lung cancer is found to have tumours expressing high levels of PD-L1. This finding suggests a potential benefit from:
    A. Chemotherapy
    B. Radiation therapy
    C. Immunotherapy with PD-1/PD-L1 inhibitors
    D. Hormonal therapy
32. In a study, cancer cells are found to downregulate MHC class I molecules. This mechanism primarily helps the tumour to:
    A. Enhance antigen presentation
    B. Promote inflammation
    C. Evade immune detection
    D. Stimulate T-cell activation
33. A patient with breast cancer benefits from a treatment that enhances the activity of NK cells. This therapy primarily aims to:
    A. Promote antibody-dependent cellular cytotoxicity
    B. Induce apoptosis in cancer cells
    C. Block hormone receptors
    D. Inhibit angiogenesis
34. A tumour infiltrate of a patient with colon cancer shows a high proportion of regulatory T cells (Tregs). This finding suggests:
    A. Strong antitumour immunity
    B. Suppression of the immune response
    C. Active inflammation
    D. Effective response to chemotherapy
35. In a clinical trial for a cancer vaccine, the vaccine aims to stimulate:
    A. Tumour angiogenesis
    B. Downregulation of tumour antigens
    C. Immune tolerance to the tumour
    D. Immune response against tumour-specific antigens

Answers

1. (B); 2. (A); 3. (B); 4. (C); 5. (D); 6. (B); 7. (B); 8. (C); 9. (C); 10. (A); 11. (C); 12. (C); 13. (D); 14. (B); 15. (B); 16. (A); 17. (C); 18. (D); 19. (D); 20. (B); 21. (B); 22. (B); 23. (A); 24. (B); 25. (C); 26. (A); 27. (B); 28. (B); 29. (B); 30. (B); 31. (C); 32. (C); 33. (A); 34. (B); 35. (D)

Scenario-Based Questions

1. A 45-year-old patient presents with a slowly growing, painless mass in the neck. Imaging suggests that it is a lipoma. Discuss the pathogenesis of benign tumours, using this scenario as a basis.
2. A patient is diagnosed with non-small-cell lung cancer. Describe the molecular changes often seen in this type of cancer, explaining how they contribute to cancer development and progression.
3. A community living near an industrial plant has an unusually high rate of bladder cancer. Discuss the potential carcinogens involved and their mechanisms of action.
4. A patient with lung cancer develops symptoms of Cushing syndrome. Explain the pathophysiology of paraneoplastic syndromes, using this case as an example.
5. A patient with melanoma shows rapid tumour progression despite an initially effective immune response. Discuss how cancer cells can evade the immune system and potential therapeutic strategies.
6. A patient has two different tumours: a fibroadenoma in the breast and an invasive ductal carcinoma. Compare and contrast these tumours in terms of pathology.
7. A patient with a history of chronic ulcerative colitis is diagnosed with colon cancer. Describe the process of carcinogenesis, including initiation, promotion and progression.
8. A patient with breast cancer tests positive for BRCA1 mutation. Discuss the roles of oncogenes and tumour suppressor genes in cancer, using BRCA1 as an example.
9. A patient is diagnosed with acute lymphoblastic leukaemia. Detail the diagnostic process, treatment options and prognosis, focusing on this specific cancer type.
10. A 55-year-old male smoker with a sedentary lifestyle is diagnosed with pancreatic cancer. Analyse how lifestyle factors might have contributed to his cancer risk.
11. A patient with advanced melanoma receives immunotherapy. Discuss the principles and mechanisms of immunotherapy in cancer treatment.
12. A region with high levels of air pollution sees increased lung cancer rates. Discuss the impact of environmental carcinogens on public health and prevention strategies.
13. A woman undergoes a mammogram that reveals a suspicious lesion. Explain the techniques used in cancer detection and their advantages and limitations.
14. A family has a history of Lynch syndrome. Discuss the role of genetics in cancer predisposition, using this family as an example.
15. A patient with metastatic prostate cancer is offered a trial of a new targeted therapy. Explore the emerging therapies in oncology, focusing on their mechanisms and potential impacts.

Additional Questions

1. Differences between benign and malignant tumours.
2. Pathways of spread of malignant tumours.
3. Environmental carcinogens.
4. Acquired predisposing conditions for malignancy.
5. Molecular hallmarks of malignancy.
6. Common proto-oncogenes and tumour suppressor genes and their associated malignancies.
7. Role of RAS in tumours.
8. Role of MYC in tumours.
9. Role of RB and TP53 in prevention of cancers.
10. Role of angiogenic factors in the development of neoplasms.
11. Role of MMPs in neoplasms.
12. Major classes of tumour antigens.
13. Tumour immunity.
14. DNA repair pathways.
15. Chemical carcinogenesis.
16. Microbial carcinogenesis.
17. Paraneoplastic syndromes.
18. Tumour markers.
19. Grading and staging of tumours.
20. Role of IHC in tumours.

Topics for Self-Directed Learning

1. Chromothripsis.
2. Autophagy in tumour cells.
3. Targeted therapy.
4. Anoikis.
5. MMPs and their inhibitors.
6. MMT genes involved.
7. Dysregulation of cancer-associated genes.
8. Desmoid tumour.
9. Effects of fertilizers and pesticides on human health.
10. Carcinogens found in the current Indian diet.
11. Neoplasms with mutated succinate dehydrogenase complex.
12. Role of stromal elements in metastasis.
13. PD-L1 and PD-L2 expression by tumour cells.
14. Role of IHC in tumours.
15. NextGen sequencing.
16. BRAFomas.
17. DNA microarray.
18. Metabolome.
19. Transcriptome.
20. Plastic as a carcinogen.

MIND MAPS

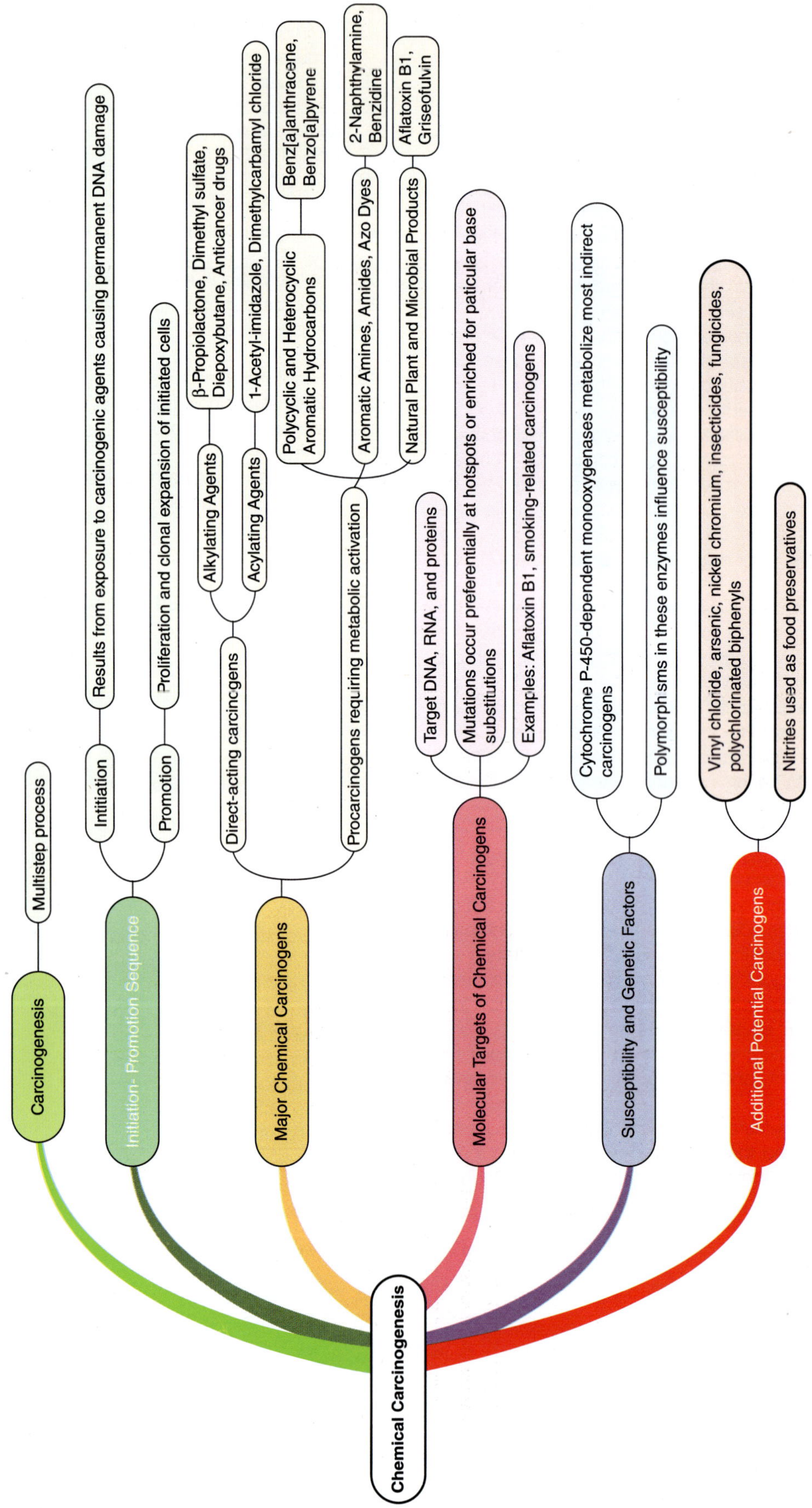

Chemical Carcinogenesis
Carcinogenesis
Multistep process
Initiation- Promotion Sequence
Intitiation
Results from exposure to carcinogenic agents causing permanent DNA damage
Promotion
Proliferation and clonal expansion of initiated cells
Major Chemical Carcinogens
Direct-acting carcinogens
Alkylating Agents
β-Propiolactone, Dimethyl sulfate, Diepoxybutane, Anticancer drugs
Acylating Agents
1-Acetyl-imidazole, Dimethylcarbamyl chloride
Procarcinogens requiring metabolic activation
Polycyclic and Heterocyclic Aromatic Hydrocarbons
Benz[a]anthracene, Benzo[a]pyrene
Aromatic Amines, Amides, Azo Dyes
2-Naphthylamine, Benzidine
Natural Plant and Microbial Products
Aflatoxin B1, Griseofulvin
Molecular Targets of Chemical Carcinogens
Target DNA, RNA, and proteins
Mutations occur preferentially at hotspots or enriched for paticular base substitutions
Examples: Aflatoxin B1, smoking-related carcinogens
Susceptibility and Genetic Factors
Cytochrome P-450-dependent monooxygenases metabolize most indirect carcinogens
Polymorph sms in these enzymes influence susceptibility
Additional Potential Carcinogens
Vinyl chloride, arsenic, nickel chromium, insecticides, fungicides, polychlorinated biphenyls
Nitrites used as food preservatives

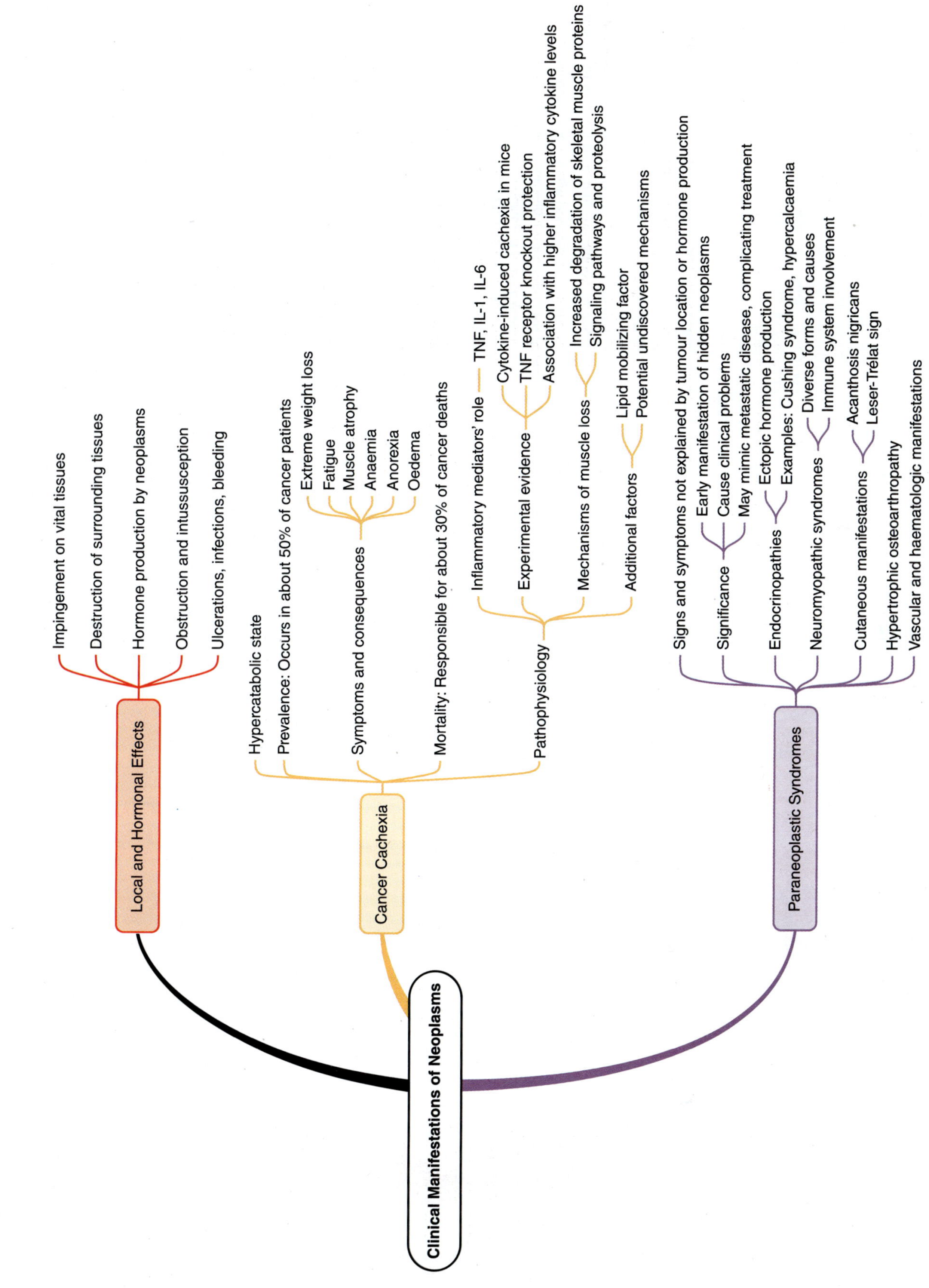
Clinical Manifestations of Neoplasms
Local and Hormonal Effects
Impingement on vital tissues
Destruction of surrounding tissues
Hormone production by neoplasms
Obstruction and intussusception
Ulcerations, infections, bleeding
Cancer Cachexia
Hypercatabolic state
Prevalence: Occurs in about 50% of cancer patients
Symptoms and consequences
Extreme weight loss
Fatigue
Muscle atrophy
Anaemia
Anorexia
Oedema
Mortality: Responsible for about 30% of cancer deaths
Pathophysiology
Inflammatory mediators' role
TNF, IL-1, IL-6
Experimental evidence
Cytokine-induced cachexia in mice
TNF receptor knockout protection
Association with higher inflammatory cytokine levels
Mechanisms of muscle loss
Increased degradation of skeletal muscle proteins
Signaling pathways and proteolysis
Additional factors
Lipid mobilizing factor
Potential undiscovered mechanisms
Paraneoplastic Syndromes
Signs and symptoms not explained by tumour location or hormone production
Significance
Early manifestation of hidden neoplasms
Cause clinical problems
May mimic metastatic disease, complicating treatment
Endocrinopathies
Ectopic hormone production
Examples: Cushing syndrome, hypercalcaemia
Neuromyopathic syndromes
Diverse forms and causes
Immune system involvement
Cutaneous manifestations
Acanthosis nigricans
Leser-Trélat sign
Hypertrophic osteoarthropathy
Vascular and haematologic manifestations

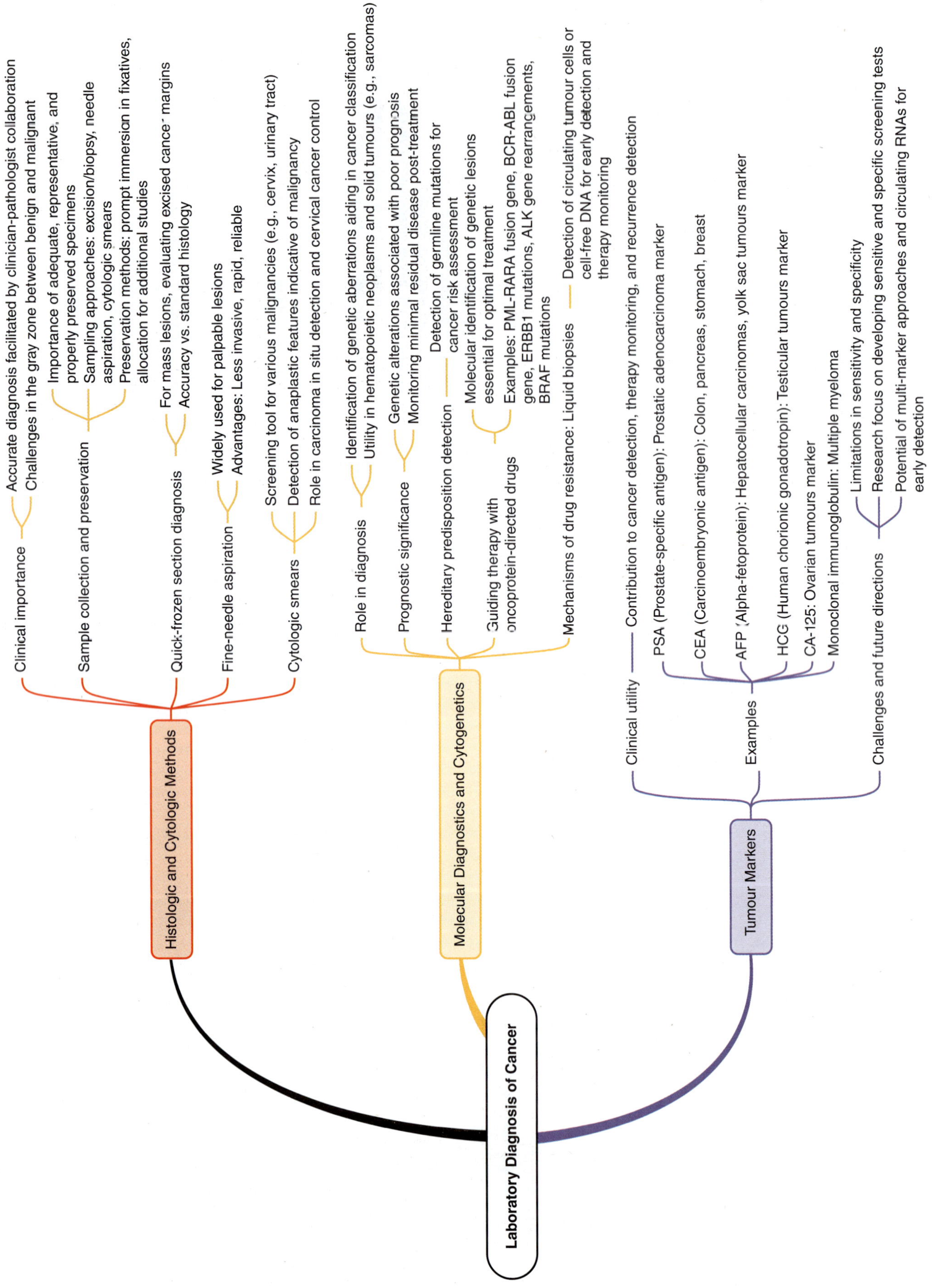
Laboratory Diagnosis of Cancer
Histologic and Cytologic Methods
Clinical importance
Accurate diagnosis facilitated by clinician-pathologist collaboration
Challenges in the gray zone between benign and malignant
Sample collection and preservation
Importance of adequate, representative, and properly preserved specimens
Sampling approaches: excision/biopsy, needle aspiration, cytologic smears
Preservation methods: prompt immersion in fixatives, allocation for additional studies
Quick-frozen section diagnosis
For mass lesions, evaluating excised cancer margins
Accuracy vs. standard histology
Fine-needle aspiration
Widely used for palpable lesions
Advantages: Less invasive, rapid, reliable
Cytologic smears
Screening tool for various malignancies (e.g., cervix, urinary tract)
Detection of anaplastic features indicative of malignancy
Role in carcinoma in situ detection and cervical cancer control
Molecular Diagnostics and Cytogenetics
Role in diagnosis
Identification of genetic aberrations aiding in cancer classification
Utility in hematopoietic neoplasms and solid tumours (e.g., sarcomas)
Prognostic significance
Genetic alterations associated with poor prognosis
Monitoring minimal residual disease post-treatment
Hereditary predisposition detection
Detection of germline mutations for cancer risk assessment
Guiding therapy with oncoprotein-directed drugs
Molecular identification of genetic lesions essential for optimal treatment
Examples: PML-RARA fusion gene, BCR-ABL fusion gene, ERBB1 mutations, ALK gene rearrangements, BRAF mutations
Mechanisms of drug resistance: Liquid biopsies
Detection of circulating tumour cells or cell-free DNA for early detection and therapy monitoring
Tumour Markers
Clinical utility
Contribution to cancer detection, therapy monitoring, and recurrence detection
Examples
PSA (Prostate-specific antigen): Prostatic adenocarcinoma marker
CEA (Carcinoembryonic antigen): Colon, pancreas, stomach, breast
AFP (Alpha-fetoprotein): Hepatocellular carcinomas, yolk sac tumours marker
HCG (Human chorionic gonadotropin): Testicular tumours marker
CA-125: Ovarian tumours marker
Monoclonal immunoglobulin: Multiple myeloma
Challenges and future directions
Limitations in sensitivity and specificity
Research focus on developing sensitive and specific screening tests
Potential of multi-marker approaches and circulating RNAs for early detection

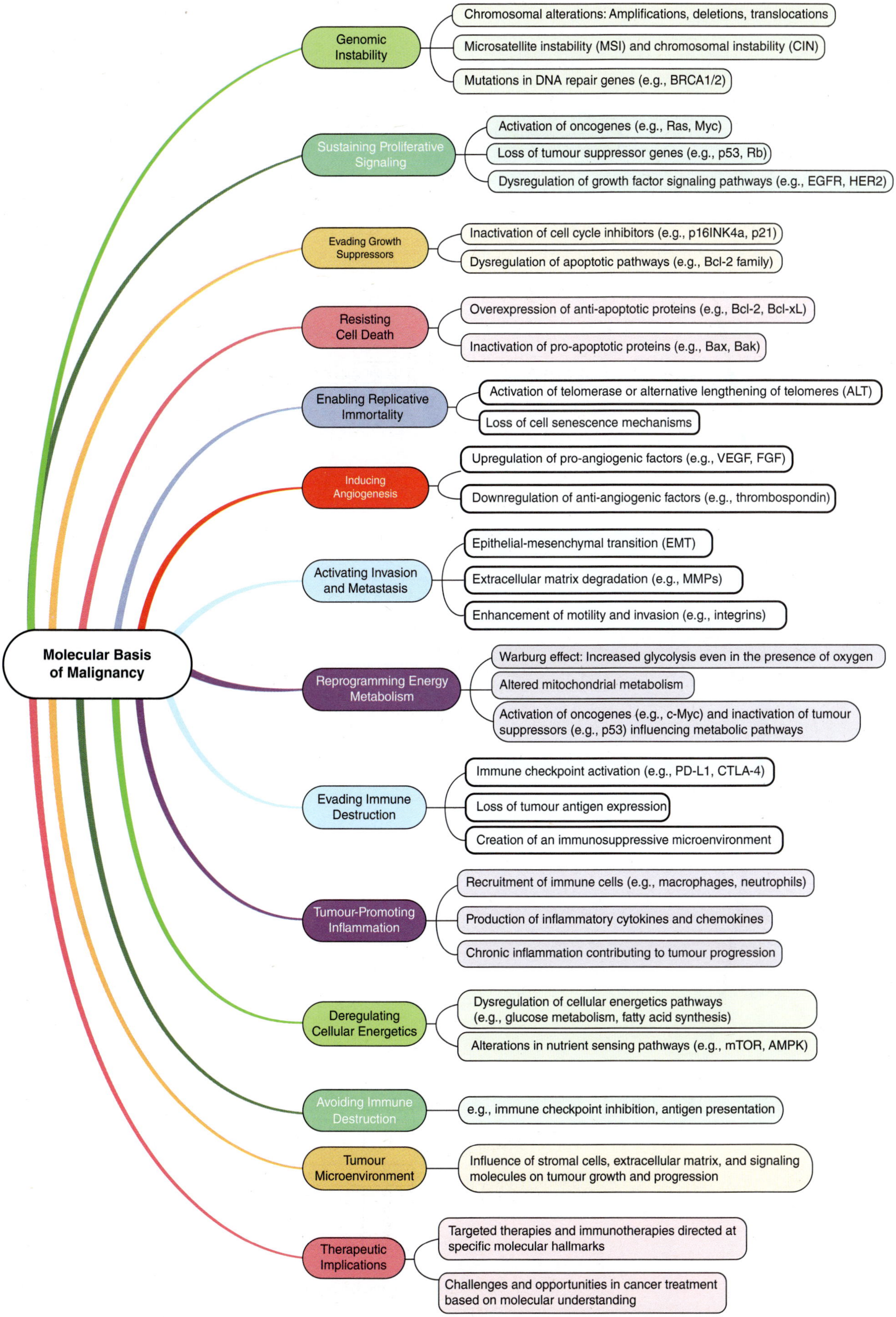
Molecular Basis of Malignancy
Genomic Instability
Chromosomal alterations: Amplifications, deletions, translocations
Microsatellite instability (MSI) and chromosomal instability (CIN)
Mutations in DNA repair genes (e.g., BRCA1/2)
Sustaining Proliferative Signaling
Activation of oncogenes (e.g., Ras, Myc)
Loss of tumour suppressor genes (e.g., p53, Rb)
Dysregulation of growth factor signaling pathways (e.g., EGFR, HER2)
Evading Growth Suppressors
Inactivation of cell cycle inhibitors (e.g., p16INK4a, p21)
Dysregulation of apoptotic pathways (e.g., Bcl-2 family)
Resisting Cell Death
Overexpression of anti-apoptotic proteins (e.g., Bcl-2, Bcl-xL)
Inactivation of pro-apoptotic proteins (e.g., Bax, Bak)
Enabling Replicative Immortality
Activation of telomerase or alternative lengthening of telomeres (ALT)
Loss of cell senescence mechanisms
Inducing Angiogenesis
Upregulation of pro-angiogenic factors (e.g., VEGF, FGF)
Downregulation of anti-angiogenic factors (e.g., thrombospondin)
Activating Invasion and Metastasis
Epithelial-mesenchymal transition (EMT)
Extracellular matrix degradation (e.g., MMPs)
Enhancement of motility and invasion (e.g., integrins)
Reprogramming Energy Metabolism
Warburg effect: Increased glycolysis even in the presence of oxygen
Altered mitochondrial metabolism
Activation of oncogenes (e.g., c-Myc) and inactivation of tumour suppressors (e.g., p53) influencing metabolic pathways
Evading Immune Destruction
Immune checkpoint activation (e.g., PD-L1, CTLA-4)
Loss of tumour antigen expression
Creation of an immunosuppressive microenvironment
Tumour-Promoting Inflammation
Recruitment of immune cells (e.g., macrophages, neutrophils)
Production of inflammatory cytokines and chemokines
Chronic inflammation contributing to tumour progression
Deregulating Cellular Energetics
Dysregulation of cellular energetics pathways (e.g., glucose metabolism, fatty acid synthesis)
Alterations in nutrient sensing pathways (e.g., mTOR, AMPK)
Avoiding Immune Destruction
e.g., immune checkpoint inhibition, antigen presentation
Tumour Microenvironment
Influence of stromal cells, extracellular matrix, and signaling molecules on tumour growth and progression
Therapeutic Implications
Targeted therapies and immunotherapies directed at specific molecular hallmarks
Challenges and opportunities in cancer treatment based on molecular understanding

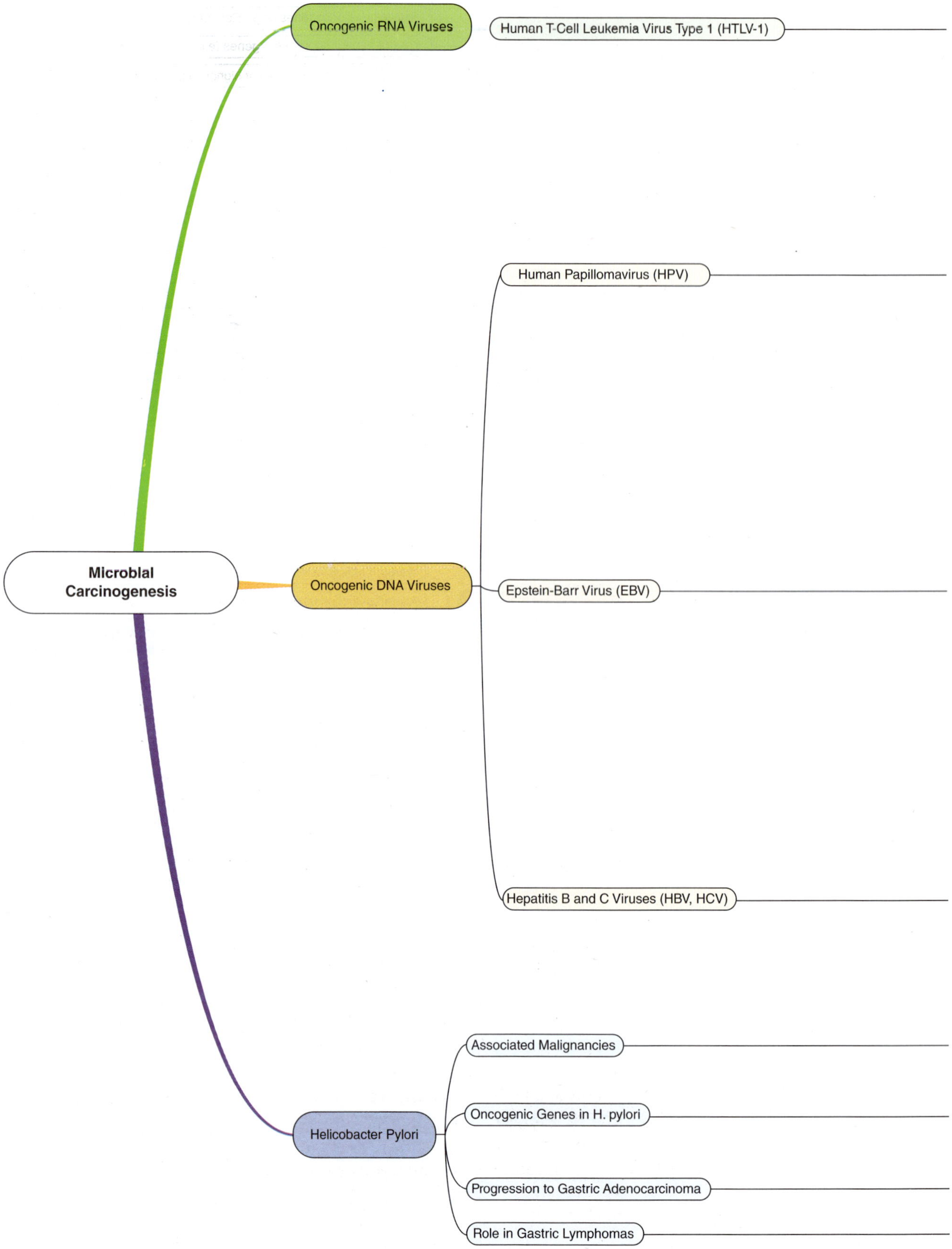
Microblal Carcinogenesis
Oncogenic RNA Viruses
Human T-Cell Leukemia Virus Type 1 (HTLV-1)
Oncogenic DNA Viruses
Human Papillomavirus (HPV)
Epstein-Barr Virus (EBV)
Hepatitis B and C Viruses (HBV, HCV)
Helicobacter Pylori
Associated Malignancies
Oncogenic Genes in H. pylori
Progression to Gastric Adenocarcinoma
Role in Gastric Lymphomas

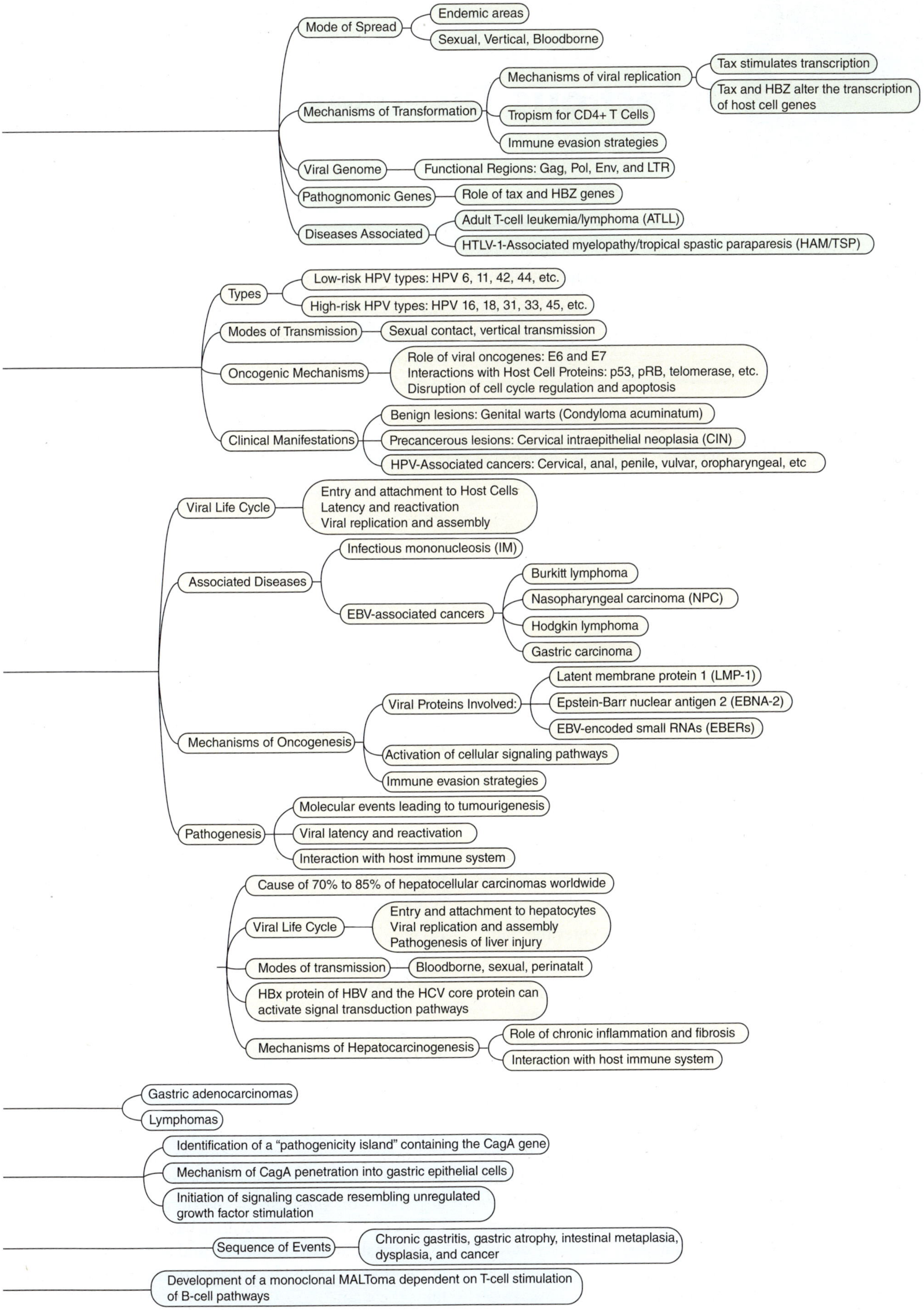
Mode of Spread
Endemic areas
Sexual, Vertical, Bloodborne
Mechanisms of Transformation
Mechanisms of viral replication
Tax stimulates transcription
Tax and HBZ alter the transcription of host cell genes
Tropism for CD4+ T Cells
Immune evasion strategies
Viral Genome
Functional Regions: Gag, Pol, Env, and LTR
Pathognomonic Genes
Role of tax and HBZ genes
Diseases Associated
Adult T-cell leukemia/lymphoma (ATLL)
HTLV-1-Associated myelopathy/tropical spastic paraparesis (HAM/TSP)
Types
Low-risk HPV types: HPV 6, 11, 42, 44, etc.
High-risk HPV types: HPV 16, 18, 31, 33, 45, etc.
Modes of Transmission
Sexual contact, vertical transmission
Oncogenic Mechanisms
Role of viral oncogenes: E6 and E7
Interactions with Host Cell Proteins: p53, pRB, telomerase, etc.
Disruption of cell cycle regulation and apoptosis
Clinical Manifestations
Benign lesions: Genital warts (Condyloma acuminatum)
Precancerous lesions: Cervical intraepithelial neoplasia (CIN)
HPV-Associated cancers: Cervical, anal, penile, vulvar, oropharyngeal, etc
Viral Life Cycle
Entry and attachment to Host Cells
Latency and reactivation
Viral replication and assembly
Associated Diseases
Infectious mononucleosis (IM)
EBV-associated cancers
Burkitt lymphoma
Nasopharyngeal carcinoma (NPC)
Hodgkin lymphoma
Gastric carcinoma
Mechanisms of Oncogenesis
Viral Proteins Involved:
Latent membrane protein 1 (LMP-1)
Epstein-Barr nuclear antigen 2 (EBNA-2)
EBV-encoded small RNAs (EBERs)
Activation of cellular signaling pathways
Immune evasion strategies
Pathogenesis
Molecular events leading to tumourigenesis
Viral latency and reactivation
Interaction with host immune system
Cause of 70% to 85% of hepatocellular carcinomas worldwide
Viral Life Cycle
Entry and attachment to hepatocytes
Viral replication and assembly
Pathogenesis of liver injury
Modes of transmission
Bloodborne, sexual, perinatalt
HBx protein of HBV and the HCV core protein can activate signal transduction pathways
Mechanisms of Hepatocarcinogenesis
Role of chronic inflammation and fibrosis
Interaction with host immune system
Gastric adenocarcinomas
Lymphomas
Identification of a “pathogenicity island” containing the CagA gene
Mechanism of CagA penetration into gastric epithelial cells
Initiation of signaling cascade resembling unregulated growth factor stimulation
Sequence of Events
Chronic gastritis, gastric atrophy, intestinal metaplasia, dysplasia, and cancer
Development of a monoclonal MALToma dependent on T-cell stimulation of B-cell pathways

8 Infectious Diseases

Gayathri Devi Thanigaimani

PA 10.1 Define and describe the pathogenesis and pathology of **malaria.**
PA 10.2 Define and describe the pathogenesis and pathology of **cysticercosis.**
PA 10.3 Define and describe the pathogenesis and pathology of **leprosy.**
PA 10.4 Define and describe the pathogenesis and pathology of **common bacterial, viral, protozoal and helminthic diseases.**

CHAPTER OUTLINE

INTRODUCTION

Infectious diseases refer to the illnesses caused by germs (such as bacteria, viruses and fungi) that enter the body, multiply and cause various manifestations.

- Some infectious diseases are contagious (or communicable), i.e. they spread from one person to another.
- Some infectious diseases are airborne, waterborne, fomite borne or vector borne.
- **Emerging infections** are infections that have increased recently or are threatening to increase in the near future. These infections could probably be the following:
  - Completely new (like SARS, MERS, COVID-19)
  - Reappearing in an area (e.g. dengue in south Florida and certain diseases in Africa)
  - Old infections that have become resistant to antibiotics (e.g. methicillin-resistant *Staphylococcus aureus* [MRSA] and the deadly Gram-negative infections that are cropping up in hospitals)

Zoonotic diseases are infectious diseases of animals that spread to humans by mosquitoes, fleas or ticks or by contact with animals; these diseases include the following:

- Lyme disease (spread by ticks)
- West Nile virus disease (spread by mosquitoes)
- Rabies (spread by bats and other mammals)

COMMON BACTERIAL INFECTIONS

GRAM-POSITIVE BACTERIAL INFECTIONS PA 10.4

Gram-positive bacteria are bacteria that stain positive in Gram staining test. This test is used to classify bacteria into two broad categories – Gram-positive and Gram-negative – on the basis of the permeability of their cell wall to the stain. Gram-positive bacteria take up the crystal violet stain used in the test and appear purple because of the thick peptidoglycan layer in their cell wall that retains the stain.

Gram-positive cocci like *Staphylococcus*, *Streptococcus* and *Enterococcus* are common causes of infection, whereas rod-like *Corynebacterium diphtheriae*, *Listeria*, *Bacillus anthracis* and *Nocardia* are less common. Here, we discuss some of the common diseases caused by Gram-positive organisms.

Staphylococcal Infections

The prototype of staphylococcal genus is *S. aureus*. These are pyogenic Gram-positive cocci present in clusters, as part of the normal flora in the nasal passages, skin and mucous membranes. These cause skin lesions, abscesses, sepsis, pneumonia, osteomyelitis, endocarditis and toxic shock syndrome (TSS). The other important members of this group include coagulase-negative staphylococci – *S. epidermis* (which causes opportunistic infections in catheterized patients, patients with prosthetic valves and drug addicts) and *S. saprophyticus* (which causes urinary tract infections [UTIs] in young women).

Pathogenesis *S. aureus* possesses various virulence factors that help in colonization of the bacteria, which include the following:

- Surface proteins involved in adherence of the bacteria and evasion of host immune response
- Enzymes such as coagulase, DNase, lipase, staphylokinase and the drug resistance–providing β-lactamase to degrade host structures
- Haemolytic toxins and exfoliative toxins
- Proteins that cause antibiotic resistance
- Polysaccharide capsule present in staphylococci infecting prosthetic valves and catheters that helps them attach to artificial materials and resist phagocytosis
- Surface protein A present in some staphylococci, which binds the Fc portion of immunoglobulins, allowing the organism to escape antibody-mediated killing

Superantigens: These are toxins that induce food poisoning and *TSS* (Fig. 8.1). This group of toxins includes TSST-1 and enterotoxin type B, which causes TSS associated with tampon use. These toxins cause polyclonal T-cell proliferation by binding to major histocompatibility complex (MHC) molecules, leading to release of excess of cytokines like tumour necrosis factor (TNF) and IL-1, which triggers a systemic inflammatory response syndrome, characterized by fever, erythematous rash, hypotension, coagulopathy, shock, multiple organ failure and tissue necrosis.

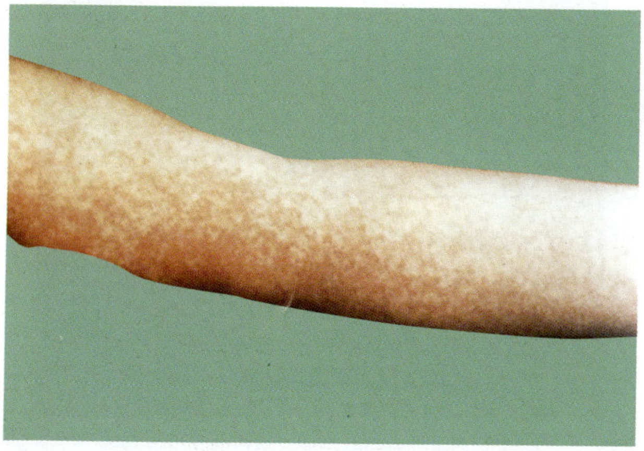

Fig. 8.1 Toxic shock syndrome: erythroderma – morbilliform rash. (*Source:* From Toxic Shock Syndrome. Elsevier Point of Care. 2021.)

MRSA is a group of staphylococci that are resistant to all penicillin and cephalosporin antibiotics. It is mainly found in healthcare facilities, but community-acquired MRSA has become common nowadays.

Morphology

S. aureus causes pyogenic inflammation resulting in local destruction of host tissue. It causes plenty of skin lesions (carbuncle, boils, scalded skin syndrome, impetigo) as well as abscesses, sepsis, osteomyelitis, endocarditis, pneumonia, food poisoning and TSS. It produces golden yellow colony on culture media.

In skin, these infections are centred around the hair follicles except impetigo which is restricted to the superficial epidermis.

- A boil, also called a **furuncle**, is a deep infection of the hair follicle which may form an abscess with suppurative infection of the skin and subcutaneous tissue. The lesions, single or multiple, are commonly seen in moist hairy areas like the axillae, groin and submammary folds.
- **Carbuncle** is a deeper suppurative infection that spreads into the deep subcutaneous fascia and erupts as multiple adjacent skin sinuses.
- **Hidradenitis** develops as a result of inflammation and infection of the apocrine glands of the axilla and groin. It presents as pea- to marble-sized lumps under the skin that can be painful, and they often tend to enlarge and drain pus.

Lung infections occur because of haematogenous spread or as secondary infection during a viral infection. These are characterized by polymorphonuclear infiltrates with tissue destruction.

Scalded skin syndrome (Ritter disease) (Fig. 8.2) is caused by an exfoliative toxin and is common in children with *S. aureus* infection of the skin or nasopharynx. It takes the form of superficial fragile blisters that burst, and histopathology reveals desquamation at the granulosa layer of the epidermis.

Clinical Manifestations

Intravascular	Infective carditis, bacteraemia, septic thrombophlebitis
Respiratory	Otitis media, pneumonia, empyema

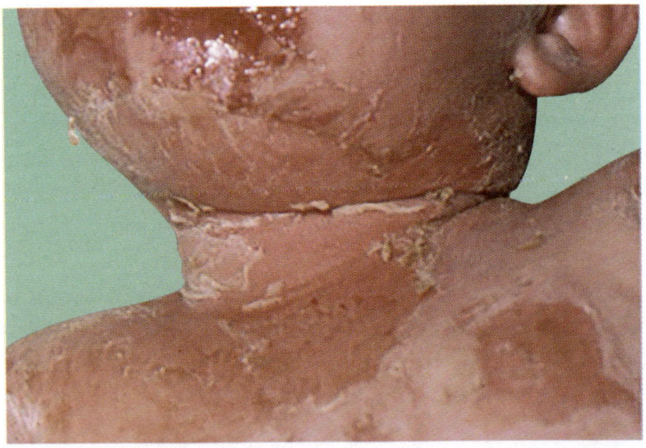

Fig. 8.2 Staphylococcal scalded skin syndrome with extensive erythema and exfoliation. (*Source:* From Maureen Rogers, Rod Phillips and Li-Chuen Wong. Skin disorders. Practical Paediatrics. 7th Edition. Elsevier 2021.)

Skin and soft tissue	Boils, impetigo, abscesses, cellulitis, fasciitis, surgical and traumatic wound infections
Foreign body associated	Catheters and intrauterine devices
Bone related	Osteomyelitis and septic arthritis
Other invasive infections	Meningitis, surgical site infection
Toxin mediated	Staphylococcal TSS, food poisoning, necrotizing pneumonia, bullous impetigo, staphylococcal scalded skin syndrome

Penicillin is the common choice of treatment. Combination therapy with gentamicin may be used to treat serious infections such as endocarditis; in cases of severe bacteraemia, vancomycin is the recommended drug of choice.

Streptococcal Infections

Streptococci are Gram-positive cocci present in pairs or chains. These are responsible for suppurative infections of the skin, oropharynx, lungs and heart valves and other nonsuppurative postinfectious syndromes like rheumatic fever and glomerulonephritis.

- *Group A streptococci* (GAS) cause pharyngitis, tonsillitis, scarlet fever, impetigo, TSS, cellulitis and necrotizing fasciitis.
- *S. agalactiae* (group B) may cause chorioamnionitis in pregnancy and septicaemia and meningitis in newborns by colonizing the female genital tract.
- *S. pneumoniae*, α-haemolytic streptococci, cause meningitis in children and adults and community-acquired pneumonia in older adults.
- *Viridans* group streptococci are part of the normal flora of the mouth and may cause endocarditis.

Pathogenesis The pathogenic factors of streptococci are as follows:

- Streptococci have capsules that resist phagocytosis.
- *S. pyogenes* expresses M protein, a surface protein that prevents bacteria from being phagocytosed, and a complement C5a peptidase that degrades this chemotactic peptide.
- *S. pyogenes* secretes a phage-encoded pyrogenic exotoxin that causes fever and rash in scarlet fever (Fig. 8.3).
- Streptococcal infection induces production of anti-streptococcal M protein antibodies and stimulates T cells. These cross-react with cardiac proteins, leading to poststreptococcal acute rheumatic fever.
- *S. pneumoniae* produces pneumolysin, a toxin that inserts into host cell membranes and lyses cells, greatly increasing tissue damage.
- *S. mutans* produces caries tooth by metabolizing sucrose to lactic acid (which causes demineralization of tooth enamel) and by secreting high-molecular-weight glucans that promote aggregation of bacteria and plaque formation on the teeth.
- Virulent *S. pyogenes* causes a rapidly progressive necrotizing fasciitis and puerperal sepsis.

Morphology and Clinical Manifestations Organs or sites infected by streptococci display the following features:

- Diffuse interstitial neutrophilic infiltrates occur.
- Furuncles, carbuncles and impetigo similar to those caused by staphylococci are present.
- **Erysipelas** is a rapidly spreading erythematous cutaneous swelling that may begin on the face forming a butterfly-shaped swelling or, less frequently, on the body or extremity. The rash has a sharp, serpiginous and well-demarcated border.
- Streptococcal **pharyngitis**, a major predecessor of poststreptococcal glomerulonephritis, manifests as

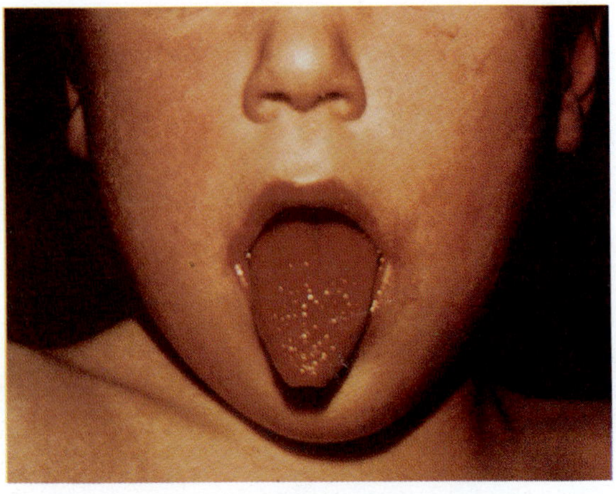

Fig. 8.3 Scarlet fever – characteristic erythematous rash on tongue called strawberry tongue. (*Source:* From Toxic Shock Syndrome. Elsevier Point of Care. 2021.)

oedema, epiglottic swelling and punctate abscesses of the tonsillar crypts, accompanied by cervical lymphadenopathy. When associated with peritonsillar or retropharyngeal abscess, it may cause airway obstruction.
- *S. pneumoniae* is an important cause of **lobar pneumonia**.
- **Scarlet fever** manifests as punctate erythematous rash that is prominent over the trunk and inner aspects of the arms and legs. The face is rarely involved except for a circumoral pallor. Scarlet fever is commonly seen in children between 3 and 15 years of age.

Penicillin remains the treatment of choice for infections because of GAS including pharyngitis and skin and soft-tissue infections. Macrolides (erythromycin, azithromycin) and lincosamides (clindamycin) are commonly used first-line drugs against group A streptococcal infections in patients with β-lactam allergies.

Enterococcal Infections

Enterococci are Gram-positive cocci that grow in chains and belong to Lancefield group D streptococci that do not exhibit any lysis on blood agar. These have two species – *E. faecalis* and *E. faecium*. Enterococci are often resistant to commonly used antibiotics and hence pathogenic. They are a significant cause of endocarditis and UTI. Enterococci are low-virulence bacteria that do not have an antiphagocytic capsule but injure host tissue by producing enzymes.

Diphtheria

Diphtheria is a serious infection caused by the bacterium *C. diphtheriae*, a Gram-positive rod with Chinese letter arrangement that spreads from person to person through respiratory droplets during coughing and sneezing. People can also get infected by touching infected open sores or ulcers.

Diphtheria is fatal in 5%–10% of cases. In children younger than 5 years and adults older than 40 years, the fatality rate may be as high as 20%. But there is a downward trend over the course of the last two decades, even in developing countries, which is shown by 3300 deaths in 2013, compared with 8000 deaths in 1990. Better standards of living, mass immunization, improved diagnosis, prompt treatment and more effective health care have led to this decrease in cases worldwide.

Pathogenesis These bacteria most commonly infect the respiratory system. Once into the respiratory system, these may infect the mucosa of the pharynx, larynx and nose and later cause enlargement of cervical lymph nodes (**bull neck**) (Fig. 8.4). The bacterial toxin damages the respiratory tissue and within 2–3 days, the dead tissue forms a thick, grey coating on the surface of the pharynx or larynx, the '**grey pseudomembrane**' (Fig. 8.5).

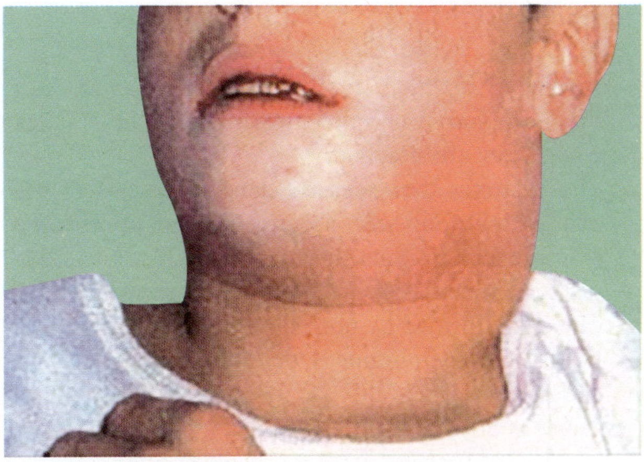

Fig. 8.4 Bull neck appearance in a patient with diphtheria. (*Source:* From Kathryn S. Moffett. Pediatric Infectious Disease. Oral and Maxillofacial Surgery Clinics, 2012; 24: 469-486.)

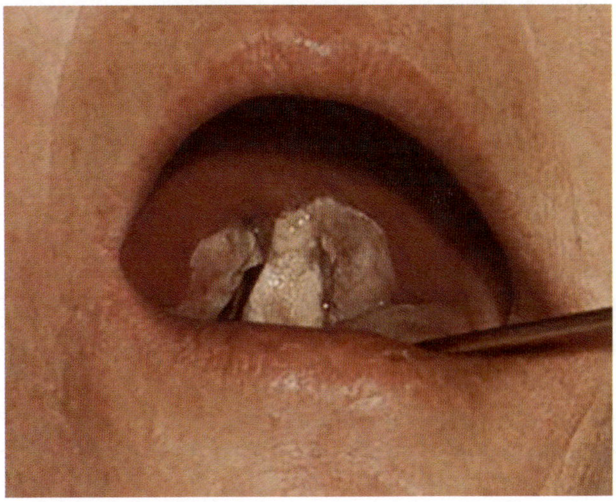

Fig. 8.5 Lesions in the pharynx of a patient with diphtheria with the characteristic 'grey pseudomembrane'. (*Source:* From Kathryn S. Moffett. Pediatric Infectious Disease. Oral and Maxillofacial Surgery Clinics, 2012; 24: 469-486.)

The toxin may also enter the bloodstream and affect the heart, nerve and kidney, leading to myocarditis, polyneuropathy, paralysis or renal failure. The bacteria can also infect the skin, causing open sores or ulcers, but these rarely progress to systemic illness.

Diphtheria toxin is composed of single polypeptide chain with two fragments, fragment A and fragment B, held together by disulphide bonds. Fragment B gains the toxin entry into the host cell and on entering the cell, inside the endosome, the toxin is split into its individual A and B fragments. Fragment A inhibits the synthesis of new proteins in the affected cell by catalysing ADP-ribosylation of elongation factor EF-2 – a protein that is essential in the translation step of protein synthesis. ADP-ribosylation of EF-2 prevents protein synthesis.

Morphology

- Inhaled *C. diphtheriae* proliferate on the mucosa of the nasopharynx, oropharynx, larynx or trachea where they are attached.
- The exotoxin thus released causes necrosis of the epithelium along with a dense **fibrinosuppurative exudate** which sometimes forms a grey to black superficial membrane, called pseudomembrane, because it is formed by nonviable tissue. During resolution, the membrane is digested by enzymes or coughed up.
- There is an intense neutrophilic infiltration in the underlying tissues with marked vascular congestion, interstitial oedema and fibrin exudation which may lead to bleeding and asphyxiation as the membrane sloughs off.
- With the entry of exotoxin into the blood and systemic distribution, there may be fatty changes in the myocardium with isolated myofibre necrosis, polyneuritis with degeneration of the myelin sheaths and axis cylinders (less common), fatty changes and focal necrosis of the liver, kidney and adrenal parenchymal cells.

Investigations and Management **Laboratory diagnosis may be made by the following**

- Demonstration of *C. diphtheriae* by Gram stain of throat swab
- Growth of bacteria in the culture
- **Toxin demonstration** by in vitro tests like Elek's gel precipitation test, detection of tox gene by polymerase chain reaction (PCR) and enzyme-linked immunosorbent assay (ELISA)
- Histological diagnosis of diphtheria by demonstration of groups of bacteria in the pseudomembrane by special stains

Vaccine Quinvaxem is a widely administered pentavalent vaccine which is a combination of five vaccines that protect babies from diphtheria, among other common childhood diseases. Diphtheria vaccine is usually combined at least with tetanus vaccine (Td) and often with pertussis (DTP, DTaP, TdaP, Tdap) vaccine also.

Listeriosis

Listeria monocytogenes is a Gram-positive, rod-shaped, flagellated bacterium that appears as short chains. It is the agent of listeriosis, a serious infection caused by eating food contaminated with this bacterium. Listeriosis has been recognized as an important public health problem in the United States. The disease affects primarily pregnant women, newborns and adults with weakened immune systems.

The bacterium apparently invades via the intestinal mucosa. It attaches to D-galactose receptors on susceptible intestinal cells by means of D-galactose residues on its surface. The bacterium is taken up (also by nonphagocytic cells) by induced phagocytosis, which is mediated by a membrane-associated protein called internalin. Once ingested, the bacterium produces listeriolysin (LLO) and two phospholipases to escape from the phagosome, multiply and invade adjacent cells.

The effective host response is cell-mediated immunity (CMI), involving interferon (IFN) produced by $CD4^+$ (T helper 1) cells and direct lysis of infected cells by $CD8^+$ (Tc) cells. Both these defence mechanisms are based on IFN-γ production and result in the formation of granulomas.

Morphology

- It presents as inflammation with numerous neutrophils. It causes a form of **meningitis** that is similar to that caused by pyogenic bacteria.
- **Focal abscesses** with greyish or yellow nodules, representing necrotic amorphous tissue debris, can occur in any organ, including the lung, liver, spleen and lymph nodes.
- Macrophages appear in large numbers, but granulomas are rare in long-term infections.
- Infants born with *L. monocytogenes* sepsis often have a papular red rash over the extremities and listerial abscesses can be seen in the placenta. A smear of the meconium discloses the Gram-positive bacilli.

Listeriosis is an overt form of the disease, with the mortality rate greater than 25%.

Clinical Manifestations The two main clinical manifestations are **sepsis and meningitis**. Bacteraemia should be treated for 2 weeks and meningitis for 3 weeks, and for brain abscess, at least 6 weeks of treatment is required. Ampicillin generally is the drug of choice; gentamicin is also added frequently for its synergistic effects. The overall mortality rate is 20%–30%. In pregnancy-related cases, around 20% may result in fetal loss or neonatal death, but mothers usually survive.

Nocardiosis

Nocardiosis is caused by slender, aerobic, Gram-positive, acid-fast organisms arranged in branching filaments. They are found in soil and cause opportunistic infections in immunocompromised patients.

The most common form of human nocardial disease is a slowly progressive pneumonia, the common symptoms of which include cough, dyspnoea (shortness of breath), weight loss and fever. It may also spread to the pleura or chest wall. Preexisting pulmonary disease, especially pulmonary alveolar proteinosis, increases the risk of contracting ***Nocardia pneumonia***. Any organ may get affected if a systemic spread takes place.

One of the main pathogenic effects of *Nocardia* species is **encephalitis**. In about 25%–33% of people, *Nocardia* infection takes the form of encephalitis and/or brain abscess formation. *Nocardia* may also cause a variety of cutaneous infections such as actinomycetoma (especially *N. brasiliensis*), lymphocutaneous disease, cellulitis and subcutaneous abscesses. It elicits a suppurative response with central liquefaction and surrounding granulation and fibrosis, but granuloma formation is rare.

Anthrax

Anthrax is caused by rod-shaped, Gram-positive, spore-forming facultative anaerobic bacterium *B. anthracis* that usually grows in chains. It is spread by contact with the bacterial spores, which often appear in infectious animal products. Contact is by breathing in or by consumption of food contaminated with spores or through broken skin. Human-to-human spread is not a feature of these bacilli. People at risk include those working with animals or animal products, travellers, postal workers and military personnel. It is one of the most likely agents to be used in a biological attack.

It is quite common in Africa and central and southern Asia. Globally, at least 2000 cases occur a year, with about 2 cases a year in the United States. Without treatment, the risk of death from cutaneous anthrax is 24%. For intestinal infection, the risk of death is 25%–75%, whereas respiratory anthrax has a mortality rate of 50%–80% even with treatment.

Pathogenesis Lethality of the anthrax disease is because of the bacterium's two principal virulence factors:

- ***Poly-D-glutamic acid capsule***, which protects the bacterium from phagocytosis by host neutrophils
- Tripartite protein toxin, called ***anthrax toxin***, which is a mixture of three protein components: protective antigen (PA), oedema factor (EF) and lethal factor (LF) (PA plus LF produces *lethal toxin* and PA plus EF produces *oedema toxin*; these toxins cause death and tissue swelling [oedema], respectively)

These toxins lead to an overproduction of TNF-α and IL-1β, causing vascular leakage of fluid and cells, ultimately leading to hypovolaemic shock and septic shock.

Morphology

Necrosis and exudative inflammation rich in neutrophils and macrophages are the characteristic features of anthrax.

The ensuing lesions include the following:

- Numerous foci of haemorrhage occur in the mediastinum.
- Haemorrhagic lymphadenitis of hilar and peribronchial lymph nodes occurs.
- Perihilar interstitial pneumonia occurs with infiltration of macrophages and neutrophils.
- Mediastinal lymph nodes are expanded by oedema and macrophages containing phagocytosed apoptotic lymphocytes.
- *B. anthracis* may commonly be seen in the alveolar capillaries and venules and, to a lesser degree, within the alveolar space and draining hilar lymph nodes.

Clinical Manifestations

Skin Cutaneous anthrax (Fig. 8.6) is the most common form (>90% of anthrax cases) and is also known as **hide-porter's disease**. It is the least dangerous form but takes time to achieve complete recovery.

Cutaneous anthrax presents as a painless boil-like skin lesion that eventually forms an ulcer with a black centre (**eschar**). In general, cutaneous infection occurs at the site of spore penetration around 2–5 days after exposure. Nearby lymph nodes may become infected, reddened, swollen and painful. Soon, a scab forms over the lesion and falls off in a few weeks.

Lungs Inhalation anthrax (Fig. 8.7) usually develops within a week or may take up to 2 months after exposure. Affected individuals begin to experience fever, chills and fatigue. These symptoms may be accompanied by cough, shortness of breath, chest pain and nausea or vomiting, making inhalation anthrax difficult to distinguish from influenza and community-acquired pneumonia. This is often described as the prodromal period (1–6 days). This stage reflects infection of the lymph nodes in the chest, a condition called **haemorrhagic mediastinitis**, causing bloody fluid to accumulate in the chest cavity, thereby causing shortness of breath.

The second (**pneumonia**) stage occurs when the infection spreads to the lungs. The patient may then develop

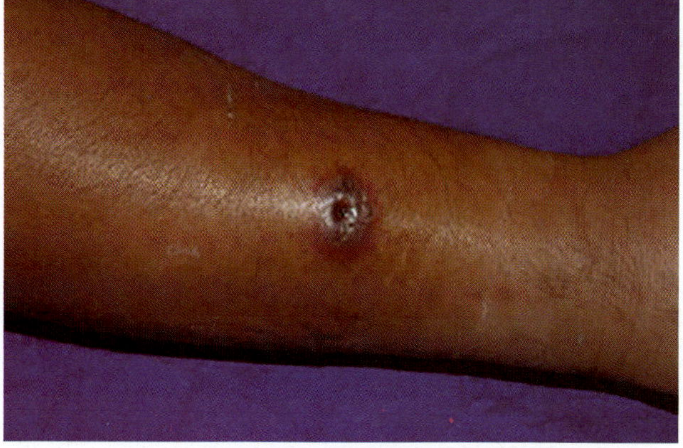

Fig. 8.6 Clinical picture of cutaneous anthrax. (*Source:* From Anthrax. Elsevier point of care. 2022.)

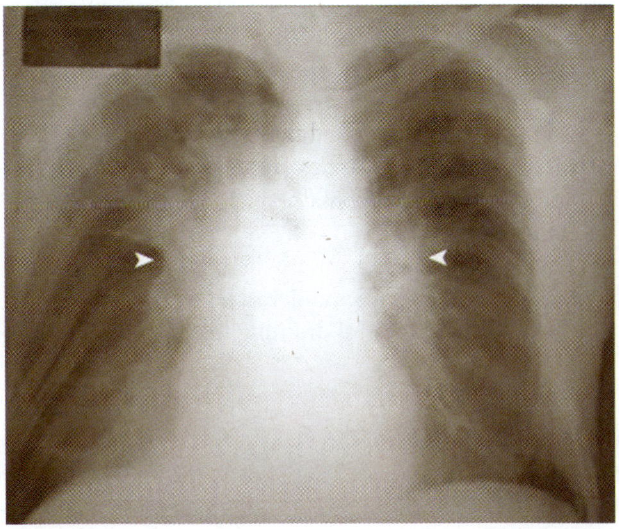

Fig. 8.7 X-ray appearance of inhalation anthrax showing mediastinal widening due to enlarged nodes. (*Source:* From Anthrax. Elsevier point of care. 2022.)

the fulminant phase because of bacteraemia which may cause meningitis. Symptoms include high fever, extreme shortness of breath, shock and rapid death within 48 hours in fatal cases.

Gastrointestinal Gastrointestinal (GI) infection, the rarest form of anthrax, is caused by consuming anthrax-infected meat and is characterized by diarrhoea, potentially with blood, abdominal pain, acute inflammation of the intestinal tract and loss of appetite. GI infections can be treated but usually have fatality rates of 25%–60%.

Investigations and Management Investigations such as Gram staining and growth in culture media are recommended along with rapid diagnostic techniques like PCR, immunofluorescence and microscopy.

There are several options for treating patients with anthrax, including intravenous antibiotics and antitoxins. Patients with severe illness need to be hospitalized and given aggressive treatment, such as continuous fluid infusion and breathing through mechanical ventilators.

GRAM-NEGATIVE BACTERIAL INFECTIONS PA 10.4

Gram-negative bacteria are bacteria that do not retain the crystal violet stain in the Gram staining method used for bacterial classification. These have a cell envelope, which is composed of a thin peptidoglycan cell wall sandwiched between an inner cytoplasmic cell membrane and an outer membrane which protects them from various antibiotics. Gram-negative bacteria range from commensals such as *Escherichia coli* to pathogenic bacteria such as *Pseudomonas aeruginosa*, *Chlamydia trachomatis* and *Yersinia pestis*. Some of the common diseases caused by Gram-negative organisms are discussed here.

Neisserial Infection

Neisseria is one of the Gram-negative diplococci, resembling two coffee beans with their concave surfaces facing each other. These are aerobic bacteria having stringent nutrient requirements and grow best on enriched media such as lysed sheep's blood agar. The common *Neisseria* causing infection in humans are *N. meningitides* and *N. gonorrhoeae* which are elaborated in the following table:

N. meningitides	***N. gonorrhoeae***
It causes a range of diseases embraced by the term invasive meningococcal disease, most commonly cerebrospinal meningitis	Sexually transmitted disease: Gonorrhoea Males: Urethritis Females: Pelvic inflammatory disease, infertility, ectopic pregnancy Neonates: Conjunctivitis, which is preventable by instillation of silver nitrate or antibiotics in the newborn's eyes
It colonizes the oropharynx as a commensal and occasionally enters the blood where the capsule inhibits opsonization and destruction of the bacteria by complement proteins	It primarily causes infection of the anogenital tract or the cervical mucosa
Serogroup A, B, C, Y and W-135 meningococcal infections can be prevented by vaccines	No vaccines are available yet

N. meningitidis has many serotypes; however, five of them cause the majority of cases. Invasive disease mainly occurs when people encounter new strains to which they are not immune, especially in crowded quarters such as military barracks or college dormitories. The complement system provides effective first-line defence and increased rates of serious infection are seen among people who have inherited defects in the complement proteins (C5–C9) which form the membrane attack complex and in patients with paroxysmal nocturnal haemoglobinuria.

N. gonorrhoeae is the second leading cause of sexually transmitted infections (STIs), second only to *C. trachomatis*. It may go unnoticed in women and present later with pelvic inflammatory disease (Fig. 8.8). The virulence of the organism is more evident in patients unable to mount a complement response, just like in meningococcal infection. The spread of infection may lead to arthritis, and in neonates born to infected mothers, it may lead to blindness. However, it is one of the causes of preventable blindness. The highest incidence areas

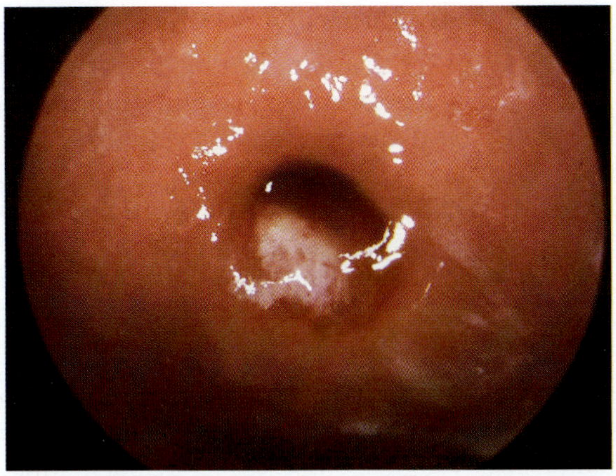

Fig. 8.8 Purulent endocervical exudate seen at cervical os in gonococcal cervicitis. (*Source:* From Jeanne M. Marrazzo and Michael A. Apicella. Neisseria gonorrhoeae (Gonorrhea). Mandell, Douglas, and Bennett's Principles and Practice of Infectious Diseases. 9th edition. Elsevier 2020.)

include Africa and the Western Pacific (including China and Australia) regions.

Pathogenesis *Neisseria* organisms adhere to and invade the nonciliated epithelial cells at the site of entry (nasopharynx, urethra or cervix) mediated by their long pili, which bind to CD46, a protein expressed on all human nucleated cells. OPA proteins (so named because they make bacterial colonies opaque), located in the outer membrane of the bacteria, increase binding to epithelial cells and promote its entry. *Neisseria* use antigenic variation as a strategy to escape the immune response. The endotoxin released by the bacteria increases TNF production and causes further damage to the host.

Pertussis

Also known as *whooping cough*, pertussis is an acute, highly contagious respiratory disease, caused by the Gram-negative bacteria *Bordetella pertussis*. It spreads by droplets and fomites. Secondary bacterial pneumonia is the most common complication seen in children along with neurological complications like seizures and encephalopathy. Pertussis complications in adults include difficulty in sleeping, urinary incontinence, pneumonia and rib fracture. The features are insidious in onset and are characterized by nonspecific cough and mild fever throughout. During the course of infection, patients develop cough with the characteristic whoop due to laryngotracheal bronchitis.

Pathogenesis Pertussis is primarily a toxin-mediated disease which impairs the host defences by inhibiting neutrophils and macrophages and paralyzing the cilia.

- *B. pertussis* colonizes the brush border of the bronchial epithelium and inactivates macrophages using a filamentous haemagglutinin.
- Pertussis toxin is a typical A–B toxin that is composed of five subunits.
- *B. pertussis* also produces a toxic adenylate cyclase that inhibits phagocytosis in neutrophils and causes apoptosis of macrophages.

Pseudomonas Infection

P. aeruginosa is an opportunistic, aerobic, Gram-negative bacillus that is a common cause of hospital-acquired infection. It severely affects people with cystic fibrosis, neutropenia or severe burns leading to sepsis. Many people with cystic fibrosis die of pulmonary failure secondary to chronic infection with *P. aeruginosa*.

Pathogenesis *P. aeruginosa* produces several toxins that contribute to local tissue damage.

- *Exotoxin A*, like diphtheria toxin, inhibits protein synthesis by ADP, leading to the death of host cells.
- It secretes damaging *enzymes* that destroy extracellular matrix (elastase), kills leucocytes (leucocidin) and destroys cell membranes (haemolysins).
- In the lungs of people with cystic fibrosis, *P. aeruginosa* secretes a mucoid exopolysaccharide called *alginate*, which forms a biofilm that protects bacteria from antibodies, complement, phagocytes and antibiotics.
- *Pyocyanin* is a virulence factor which lyses the host cells by oxidative stress.

Morphology

Pseudomonas causes **necrotizing pneumonia** with striking pale necrotic centres and red, haemorrhagic peripheral areas in the terminal airways. On microscopy, in areas of coagulative necrosis, masses of organisms are seen, mostly concentrated in the walls of blood vessels, giving a picture of Gram-negative bacterial **vasculitis.** It is also accompanied by thrombosis and haemorrhage. **Bronchial obstruction** is caused by mucus plugging and, in severe cases, may result in **bronchiectasis** and **pulmonary fibrosis**. In skin burns, *P. aeruginosa* proliferates widely, penetrating deeply into the veins and spreading haematogenously. Well-defined necrotic and haemorrhagic oval skin lesions, called **ecthyma gangrenosum**, often appear. Disseminated intravascular coagulation (DIC) is a frequent complication of *P. aeruginosa*.

Clinical Manifestations *Pseudomonas* is often a cause of hospital-acquired infection. It may lead to antibiotic-resistant pneumonia that is difficult to treat. The sepsis caused by *Pseudomonas* infection of skin burns is a difficult complication for the patient. Apart from these, it also causes corneal keratitis in contact lenses wearers, endocarditis and osteomyelitis in intravenous drug abusers, external otitis (swimmer's ear) in healthy individuals and severe external otitis in people with diabetes.

Plague

Plague, an invasive, frequently fatal disease, is caused by *Y. pestis*, a Gram-negative, facultative, intracellular organism. It is transmitted from rodents to humans by flea bites. Also named Black Death, plague has been responsible for 3 great pandemics that killed an estimated 100 million people.

Pathogenesis *Y. pestis* is primarily a rodent pathogen, with humans being an accidental host. The flea draws viable *Y. pestis* organisms into its intestinal tract when it bites an infected person or rodent. Some *Y. pestis* in the flea are then regurgitated when the flea gets its next blood meal, thus transferring the infection to a new host. On entry into humans, most of the organisms are phagocytosed and killed by the polymorphonuclear leucocytes. A few bacilli are taken up by tissue macrophages which, unable to kill *Y. pestis*, become providers of a protected environment for the organisms to synthesize their virulence factors.

The organism then quickly spreads to the draining lymph nodes, which get swollen, tender and haemorrhagic. This gives rise to the characteristic black **buboes** that are responsible for the name of this disease and later spread to involve the liver, spleen and lungs. Lung involvement in the patient may lead to severe bacterial pneumonia, resulting in discharge of a large number of viable organisms into the air during coughing fits. About 50%–60% of untreated patients will die if remain untreated.

Morphology

The distinctive histological features include the following:

1. Massive proliferation of the organisms
2. Early appearance of protein-rich and polysaccharide-rich effusions with few inflammatory cells
3. Necrosis of tissues and blood vessels with haemorrhage, thrombosis, marked tissue swelling and lymph node enlargement (buboes)
4. Neutrophilic infiltrates that accumulate adjacent to necrotic areas as healing begins

Bubonic Plague	Pneumonic Plague	Septicaemic Plague
There is a small pustule or ulcer in the leg which becomes pulpy and coloured and ruptures through the skin	Severe, confluent, haemorrhagic and necrotizing bronchopneumonia, often with fibrinous pleuritis. The person also has trouble breathing, bloody sputum, chest pain and fever.	All the lymph nodes and organs that are part of the reticuloendothelial system develop foci of necrosis. Fulminant bacteraemia also induces DIC with thrombi. Other symptoms include diarrhoea, extreme weakness, bleeding, shock and gangrene.

Chancroid (Soft Chancre)

Chancroid is an STI that is caused by the bacteria *Haemophilus ducreyi*. It presents with painful sores and ulcers on the skin. The disease is most prevalent in the sub-Saharan African regions along with many European countries. It is commonly observed in men with lower socioeconomic status who have unprotected sex.

Morphology

In males, the primary lesion is usually on the penis; in females, most lesions occur in the vagina or the periurethral area (Fig. 8.9). These lesions are not indurated and originate as pustules at the site of inoculation and progress to ulcerated lesions. The regional lymph nodes become enlarged and tender in about 50% of cases within 1–2 weeks after primary infection and if left untreated, these may form chronic draining ulcers.

Microscopically, it is seen as three layers:

1. Superficial zone of neutrophilic infiltrate, debris and fibrin
2. Granulation tissue with necrotic and thrombotic vessels
3. Dense lymphoplasmacytic inflammatory infiltrate

Granuloma Inguinale

Also called **donovanosis**, it is a sexually transmitted chronic inflammatory disease caused by *Klebsiella granulomatis*, a Gram-negative rod-shaped bacterium. The disease is rare in the United States, although it is endemic in some tropical and developing areas, including India. Small, painless nodules appear after about 10–40 days of contact with the bacteria. Later, the nodules burst, creating open, fleshy and oozing lesions. The infection spreads, mutilating the infected tissue, and will continue to destroy the tissue until treated.

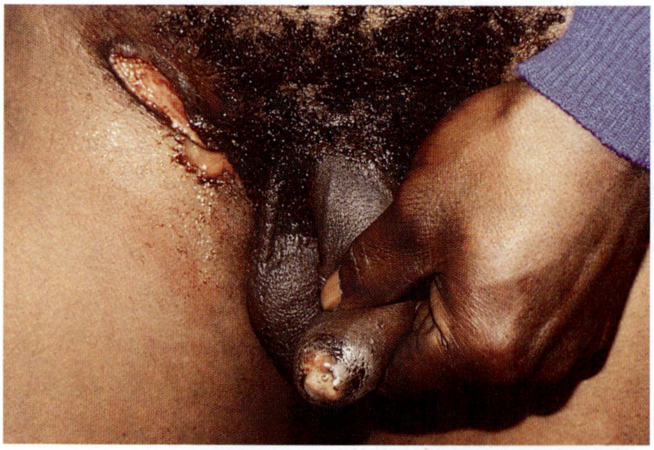

Fig. 8.9 Ulcer (chancroid) found on prepuce. Inguinal lymph nodes are enlarged with erythema of the skin. (*Source:* From Chancroid. Elsevier point of care. 2021.)

Morphology

The lesions appear as raised papules on the mucosal layer of genitalia, mouth and pharynx which may ulcerate and become a **granulomatous mass**. As the lesion enlarges, its borders are raised and indurated and, if untreated, may form **strictures** in the genital regions. On microscopy, there is marked epithelial hyperplasia similar to cancer, along with mononuclear infiltrate and neutrophils beneath the ulcer. On Giemsa staining, characteristic **Donovan bodies** are seen within the macrophages which are nothing but encapsulated coccobacilli.

MYCOBACTERIAL INFECTIONS

Mycobacteria are slender, weakly Gram-positive aerobic rods that grow in straight or branching chains. These have a unique waxy cell wall composed of unusual glycolipids and lipids including mycolic acid that make them acid-fast. There are various types of mycobacterial species:

- *Mycobacterium tuberculosis*, which causes tuberculosis (TB) infection
- *Mycobacterium leprae*, which causes leprosy
- *Mycobacterium ulcerans*, responsible for causing Buruli ulcers
- *Mycobacterium bovis*, which causes TB in cattle
- *Mycobacterium paratuberculosis*, which is associated with Crohn disease
- *Mycobacterium fortuitum* and *M. haemophilum*, which show skin infections with draining abscesses

Tuberculosis **PA 26.4**

TB is a serious chronic pulmonary and systemic disease that is most often caused by *M. tuberculosis*, and transmitted by humans with active infection releasing mycobacteria in their sputum. Oropharyngeal and intestinal TB, contracted by drinking milk contaminated with *M. bovis*, are rare in countries where milk is routinely pasteurized.

Epidemiology A total of 1.3 million people died from TB in 2022. Worldwide, TB is one of the top 10 causes of death and the second leading cause from a single infectious agent (after COVID-19 and ranking above HIV/AIDS). It is preventable and treatable.

Multidrug-resistant (MDR) TB remains a public health crisis and a health security threat. The World Health Organization (WHO) estimates that there were 484,000 new cases with resistance to rifampicin – the most effective first-line drug – of which 78% had MDR TB. Globally, TB incidence is falling at a rate of about 2% per year.

This topic has been dealt with in detail in Chapter 19, 'The Lung'.

Atypical Mycobacterial Infections Atypical mycobacterial infections are caused by certain *mycobacteria* other than those that cause TB and leprosy. Most of these infections are caused by *Mycobacterium avium* complex that includes *M. abscessus*, *M. fortuitum* and *M. kansasii*.

Atypical mycobacterial infections are categorized into the following types:

- Pulmonary disease
- Lymphadenitis
- Skin and soft-tissue disease
- Disseminated disease

Atypical mycobacterial infections are diagnosed on tissue culture. The infections have specific pathological features on skin biopsy.

Treatment of atypical mycobacterial infections depends on the organism that is infecting and the severity of the infection. In most cases, a combination of antibiotics from the sensitive group that include rifampicin, ethambutol, isoniazid, minocycline, ciprofloxacin, clarithromycin, azithromycin and cotrimoxazole is used. Surgical removal of enlarged lymph nodes and aggressive debridement of infected skin lesions are sometimes necessary. In severe cases, skin grafts might be required to repair the surgical wound.

Leprosy **PA 10.3**

Leprosy is an infectious disease caused by a bacillus, *M. leprae*. The disease mainly affects the skin, the peripheral nerves, mucosa of the upper respiratory tract and the eyes. Leprosy is curable with multidrug therapy (MDT). Leprosy is likely transmitted via droplets, from the nose and mouth, during close and frequent contact with untreated cases. According to WHO, leprosy still occurs in more than 120 countries, with more than 200,000 new cases reported every year.

Pathogenesis: *M. leprae* is an intracellular bacillus that is taken up by the macrophages and gets disseminated to various parts of the body through the blood. The ideal temperature for its replication is 32–34°C, which is prevalent in the relatively cooler tissues of the skin and extremities. The average incubation period of the disease is 5 years. Symptoms may occur within 1 year but can also take as long as 20 years or even more to occur. At the sites of proliferation, the bacilli bind to Schwann cells and cause nerve injury such as demyelination and loss of nerve function (specifically loss of axonal conductance). Its virulence factor is its cell wall, which is akin to that of *M. tuberculosis*. The immune response of the body is mainly by CMI, which explains the delayed type of hypersensitivity reaction to dermal injection of bacterial extract lepromin seen in patients.

Clinical classification: Ridley and Jopling classified leprosy clinically into the following types (Fig. 8.10):

- Tuberculoid (TT)
- Borderline tuberculoid (BT)
- Mid-borderline (BB)

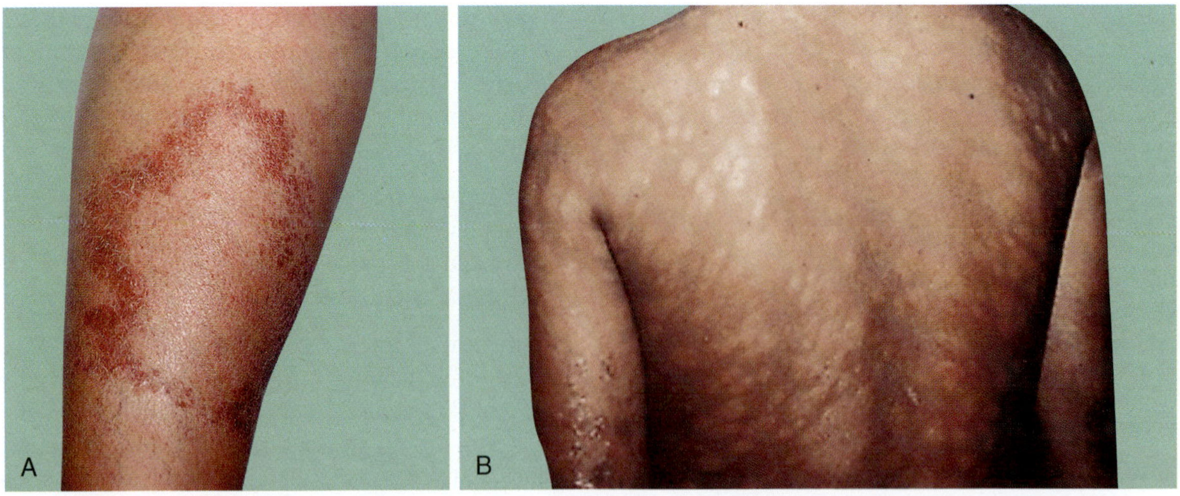

Fig. 8.10 Clinical picture of tuberculoid leprosy with a well-marked peripheral margin and a central zone of healing (A) and lepromatous leprosy showing symmetrical multiple lesions (B). (*Source:* From Joel D. Ernst. Goldman-Cecil Medicine, 2-volume Set. Elsevier. 2020.)

- Borderline lepromatous (BL)
- Lepromatous (LL)

The two ends of the spectrum, tuberculoid leprosy and lepromatous leprosy, have different methods of presentation, pathogenesis and prognosis. This variation is attributed to the difference in the host T lymphocyte response. The differences are given in Table 8.1.

Borderline leprosy is of intermediate severity between tuberculoid leprosy and lepromatous leprosy and is the most common form. Skin lesions appear band-like and resemble tuberculoid leprosy, but the lesions are more numerous and irregular, with large patches which might affect a whole limb. Peripheral nerve involvement with weakness and loss of sensation is often seen. This type is unstable and may become more like lepromatous leprosy or may undergo a reversal reaction, becoming more like the tuberculoid form. It is marked by macrophages with abundant granular, occasionally foamy cytoplasm (*Virchow cells*).

Leprosy may involve nerves without any skin changes. This unusual occurrence is called **pure neural leprosy**.

Leprosy is treated with a combination of antibiotics. MDT is required and drugs like dapsone are used with rifampicin, and clofazimine is added for some disease types. WHO recommends that prophylactic medicine be given to those people who are in close contact with someone who has leprosy. The bacille Calmette–Guérin (BCG) vaccine offers a variable amount of protection against leprosy in addition to its target of TB. The treatment may last for 2–3 years for complete cure.

SPIROCHAETAL INFECTIONS

Spirochaetes are Gram-negative bacteria that are long, helically coiled and corkscrew shaped.

Spirochaetes are distinguished from other bacterial phyla by the location of their flagella, sometimes called axial filaments, which run lengthwise between the bacterial inner and outer membranes in the periplasmic space. Most spirochaetes are free living and anaerobic. Most of the species are pathogenic, e.g. *Treponema pallidum* subspecies, which cause treponematoses such as syphilis and yaws.

Syphilis **PA 10.4**

Syphilis is an STI that is caused by the bacterium *T. pallidum*. It is too slender to be seen by Gram staining, so it is usually visualized by silver stains and immunofluorescence. It can be treated easily using antibiotics and thereby progression of the disease is preventable. Transplacental transmission may occur in the presence of active disease during pregnancy and may result in congenital syphilis. Untreated syphilis may lead to stillbirth, neonatal death, prematurity, low birth weight and lifelong health problems to the infected infant. A total of 67% of women with untreated syphilis will have an adverse outcome of pregnancy, including 26% who will have fetal loss or a stillbirth. Syphilis increases the risk of HIV transmission by two to five times, and coinfection is common (30%–60% in some urban centres). In 2015, Cuba became the first country to eliminate mother-to-child transmission of syphilis. WHO estimates that 7.1 million adults between 15 and 49 years old acquired syphilis globally in 2020.

Clinical Manifestations The clinical manifestation of syphilis depends on the stage of the disease, which is classified as follows (Fig. 8.13):

Primary stage: During the first stage, single or multiple sores or **chancres** appear (Fig. 8.14), where the organism

Table 8.1 Features of Tuberculoid Leprosy Versus Lepromatous Leprosy

Feature	Tuberculoid Leprosy	Lepromatous Leprosy
Common sites	Skin and nerves.	Skin, peripheral nerves, anterior eye chamber, upper airways, testes, hands and feet.
Immune response	$\mathbf{T_H}1$ response associated with production of IL-12 and IFN-γ. IFN-γ causes an effective host response and hence the microbial burden is low. These patients have adequate cell-mediated immunity. The infection becomes localized and tends to heal.	Weak $\mathbf{T_H}1$ response, which produces a weak cell-mediated immunity. These patients have weak cell-mediated immunity. Bacilli multiply and accumulate.
Lepromin test	Lepromin test is positive.	Lepromin test is negative.
Antibody response	No antibodies are formed.	Antibodies are produced which form immune complexes with free antigens and cause vasculitis, glomerulonephritis and erythema nodosum.
Skin lesions	Skin lesions are generally 1–5 in count and are asymmetrical. There is definitive loss of sensation.	Skin lesions appear to be 5 or more in number and are symmetrical. There may or may not be any loss of sensation.
Description	Dry, scaly skin lesions that lack sensation. There is an asymmetric involvement of large peripheral nerves which may lose their sensation and appear swollen. These lesions appear large and as erythematous plaques, with hyperpigmented sharp outer margins fading centrally to a hypopigmented flattened, anaesthetic clear zone of healing.	Symmetric skin thickening and nodules (more severe form of disease). These lesions are small but multiple with erythematous macules and papules, especially on the face, ears, wrists, elbows and knees. The facial lesions may, with progression, coalesce to yield distinctive leonine facies. Lesions in the nose may cause persistent inflammation and discharge bacilli.
Nerve involvement	Nerve involvement by granulomatous inflammation is the main feature of this disease, leading to loss of sensation and muscle atrophy. This may lead to skin ulcers, contractures, paralysis, autoamputation and keratitis with corneal ulcers (if the facial nerve is involved).	Symmetrical involvement of the ulnar and peroneal nerves by minimal inflammation may be seen, leading to loss of sensation and trophic changes in the hands and feet.
Bacillary load	There is a strong host defence mechanism, so bacilli are never found; therefore, it is also called **paucibacillary**.	Owing to the presence of abundant bacteria, it is also referred to as **multibacillary**.
Microscopy	Histology shows the presence of granulomas (Fig. 8.11).	Histology shows lipid-laden macrophages filled with abundant masses of lepra bacilli (globi) (Fig. 8.12). These cells are called lepra cells.

IFN, interferon.

has entered the body. Sores are usually firm, round and painless and can easily go unnoticed. This stage lasts about 3–6 weeks, and healing occurs even without treatment. Spread occurs by haematogenous or lymphatic dissemination.

Secondary stage: During the secondary stage, painless skin rashes and/or mucous membrane lesions are seen in the mouth, vagina or anus. The rash may start during the healing period of the primary lesion or several weeks after the sore has healed. It consists of rough, red or reddish-brown maculopapular, scaly or pustular spots on the palms of the hands and/or the bottoms of the feet. Plaques called ***condylomata lata*** appear in moist regions of the skin such as the anogenital region, inner thighs and axillae. Other symptoms include fever, swollen lymph glands, sore throat, patchy hair loss, headaches, weight loss, muscle aches and fatigue.

Latent stage: The latent stage of syphilis is a period during which there are no visible signs or symptoms of syphilis.

Tertiary stage: Most people with untreated syphilis do not develop tertiary syphilis. However, when it does happen, it can affect many different organ systems. Tertiary syphilis may occur 10–30 years after the primary infection as cardiovascular syphilis, neurosyphilis or benign tertiary syphilis. **Cardiovascular syphilis** may present with syphilitic infection, leading to progressive dilatation of the aortic root, aneurysms and aortic regurgitation, the basic pathogenesis being immune mediated. **Neurosyphilis**

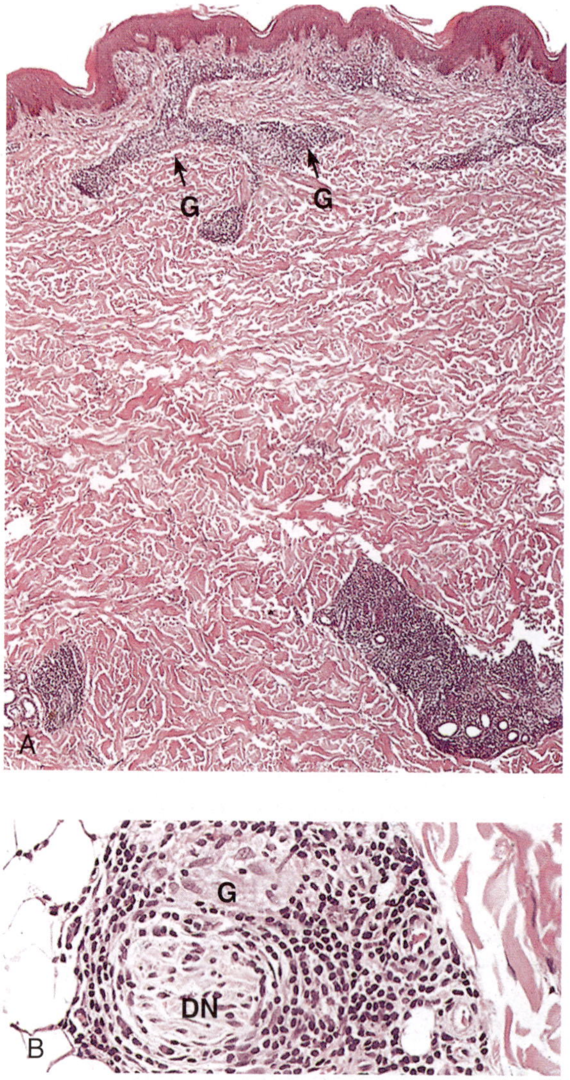

Fig. 8.11 Microscopy of tuberculoid leprosy showing granulomas (G) in the dermis (A) and perineural inflammatory infiltrate (DN, dermal nerve) (B). (*Source:* From Geraldine O'Dowd, Sarah Bell, Sylvia Wright. Wheater's Pathology: A Text, Atlas, and Review of Histopathology. Elsevier. 2019.)

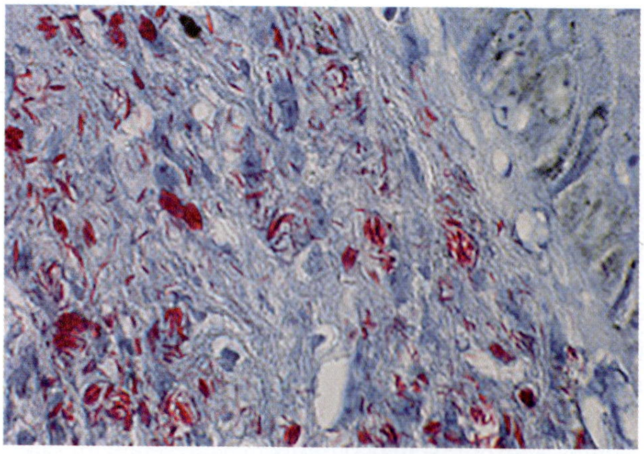

Fig. 8.12 Fite-Faraco stain of lepromatous leprosy showing numerous acid-fast lepra bacilli (red) within lepra cells. (*Source:* From Geraldine O'Dowd, Sarah Bell, Sylvia Wright. Wheater's Pathology: A Text, Atlas, and Review of Histopathology. Elsevier. 2019.)

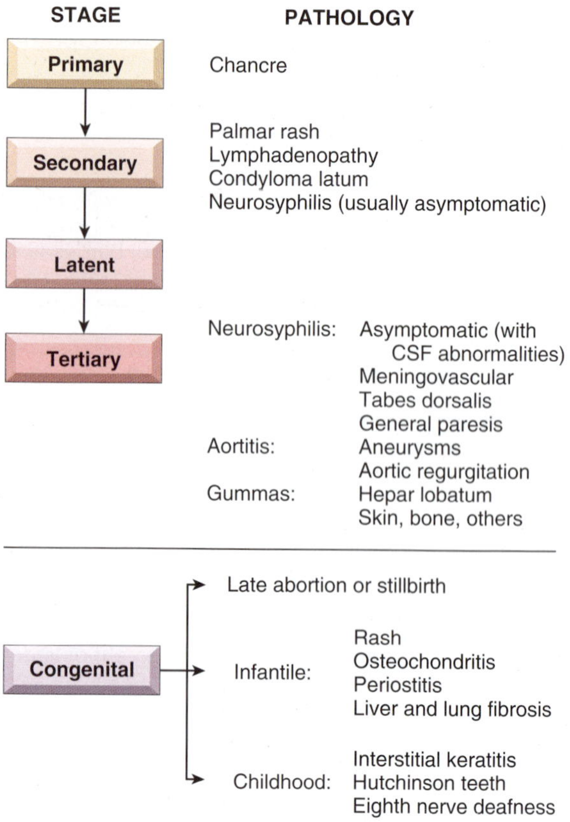

Fig. 8.13 Clinical manifestations of syphilis. (*Source:* From Anthony Chang, Lora Hedrick Ellenson, Jonathan I. Epstein, et al. Robbins Basic Pathology. Elsevier. 2018.)

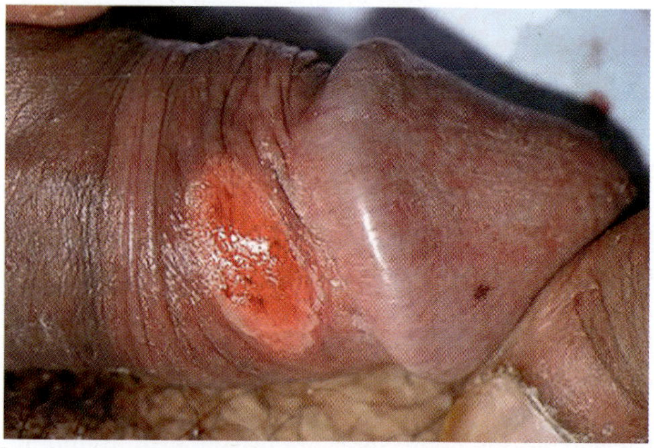

Fig. 8.14 Syphilitic chancre on penile skin. (*Source:* From Syphilis. Elsevier Point of Care. 2022.)

may be symptomatic or asymptomatic. Investigation to identify neurosyphilis is hence required in all syphilitic patients for appropriate diagnosis. The cerebrospinal fluid (CSF) abnormalities (one-third of patients) that help in the diagnosis include increased inflammatory cells, elevated protein levels, decreased glucose levels and the presence of anti-spirochaete antibodies in CSF.

Benign tertiary syphilis presents with **gummas**, which are nodular lesions that may appear on the bones, skin and mucous membrane of the mouth and the upper airway, due to delayed-type hypersensitivity reactions. It causes pain, tenderness, swelling and pathological fractures.

Congenital syphilis: Congenital syphilis is passed on to the child from the mother who acquired the disease prior to or during pregnancy. Symptoms of early (infantile) congenital syphilis include fever, skin problems, low birth weight, nasal discharge and bullous skin rash causing sloughing of the skin. In late (tardive) congenital syphilis, symptoms of the disease do not usually become apparent until 2–5 years of age. In rare cases, the disease may remain latent for years, with symptoms presenting only in adulthood. Penicillin is an effective treatment of syphilis during pregnancy.

Morphology

Primary syphilis: The chancre is an elevated, reddened and firm papule which may get eroded to form a clean shallow ulcer with an adjacent button-like mass. On histology, there is plasma cell infiltration with scattered macrophages and lymphocytes and **proliferative endarteritis**. The regional lymph nodes are enlarged.

Secondary syphilis: Red lesions occur in the mouth or vagina containing the most organisms and are the most infectious.

Tertiary syphilis: It most frequently involves the aorta, central nervous system (CNS), liver, bones and testes. Occlusion of the vasa vasorum results in scarring of the media of the proximal aortic wall, causing loss of elasticity. There may be narrowing of the coronary artery ostia caused by subintimal scarring, leading to an increased chance of myocardial ischaemia. Diffuse thickening of the wall of the ascending aorta by gelatinous intimal plaques separated by creases, furrows and radiating scars gives the '**tree bark' appearance**, a characteristic feature.

Syphilitic gummas: These are white-grey, single or multiple, microscopic lesions of varying sizes ranging from tubercles to large tumour-like masses. The gummas occur in most organs, but particularly in the skin, subcutaneous tissue, bone and joints. The rash of congenital syphilis is more severe than that of adult secondary syphilis. It is a bullous eruption of the palms and soles of the feet associated with epidermal sloughing.

Syphilitic osteochondritis and periostitis may affect any bone, but the lesions of the nose and lower legs are most distinctive. Destruction of the vomer causes the characteristic saddle nose deformity. Periostitis of the tibia leads to excessive new bone growth on the anterior surfaces and anterior bowing or **saber shin**.

In the **liver**, diffuse fibrosis permeates and isolates the hepatic cells into small nests along with the characteristic lymphoplasmacytic infiltrate and vascular changes. Scarring due to gummas may cause a distinctive hepatic lesion known as **hepar lobatum**. On histological examination, the gummas have centres of coagulated, necrotic material and margins composed of palisading macrophages and fibroblasts surrounded by large numbers of mononuclear leucocytes, chiefly plasma cells. Treponemes are scant in gummas and are difficult to demonstrate.

The lungs may be affected by **diffuse interstitial fibrosis**. In the syphilitic stillborn, the lungs appear pale and airless (*pneumonia alba*). The generalized infection may lead to a diffuse interstitial inflammatory reaction in virtually any organ.

The late manifestations of congenital syphilis include a distinctive triad of **interstitial keratitis, Hutchinson teeth** (small incisors shaped like a screwdriver often with notches in the enamel) (Fig. 8.15) and **eighth nerve deafness.** In addition to interstitial keratitis, the ocular changes include choroiditis and abnormal retinal pigmentation. Eighth nerve deafness and optic nerve atrophy develop secondary to meningovascular syphilis.

Laboratory Diagnosis Diagnosis is by demonstration of spirochaete by dark-ground microscopy or by serology, the latter being the mainstay of diagnosis. It includes the following:

- Nontreponemal test: Venereal disease research laboratory (VDRL) and rapid plasma reagin (RPR) measure the antibody to cardiolipin present in both host tissues and *T. pallidum*.
- Treponemal test: Fluorescent treponemal antibody test (FTA-ABS), *T. pallidum* haemagglutination assay (TPHA) and *T. pallidum* immobilization assay (TPI) measure the specific antibodies to *T. pallidum*.

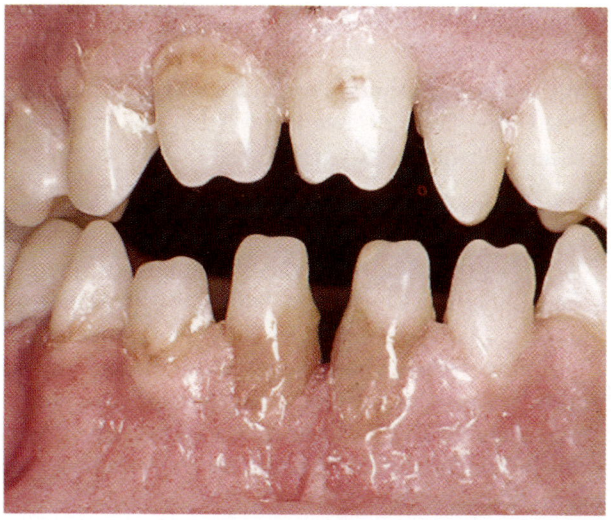

Fig. 8.15 Hutchinson teeth in congenital syphilis (late manifestation). (*Source:* From Syphilis. Elsevier Point of Care. 2022.)

Treatment

Early Infections The first-line treatment is benzathine benzylpenicillin.

Late Infections Large doses of penicillin are preferred because benzathine penetrates poorly into the brain in cases of neurosyphilis. Treatment at this stage solely limits further progression of the disease and has a limited effect on damage which has already occurred.

Lyme Disease

Lyme disease is the most common vector-borne disease in the United States. It is caused by the bacterium *Borrelia burgdorferi* and, rarely, *Borrelia mayonii*. Typical symptoms include fever, headache, fatigue and a characteristic skin rash called erythema migrans. If left untreated, infection can spread to joints (causing chronic arthritis), the heart and the nervous system.

Pathogenesis The pathogens on entry into the vector ticks are localized in their midgut. The influx of blood into the tick's gut during a blood meal causes change in the surface structure of *Borrelia* that facilitates the penetration of the tick's gut by the bacteria and migration via the haemolymph to the salivary gland. From there, the pathogens may be transmitted with the saliva during feeding by the tick. The main pathogenicity is caused by the immune response against the persistent bacteria and the inflammatory reactions produced (by cytokines IL-6 and TNF) by the host cells.

Morphology

A distinctive feature of Lyme disease is arteritis, producing **onion skin–like lesions** like in lupus. In addition, infection can cause extensive erosion of cartilage in large joints. In conditions in which the brain is affected, CSF is hypercellular, due to marked lymphocytic infiltrate, and also contains IgG antibodies.

Clinical Manifestations Clinical features are diverse, but death is rare. Lyme disease involves multiple organ systems and is divided into three stages:

- **Stage 1 (localized infection)**: This phase lasts for 4–12 weeks. The organism multiplies and spreads into the dermis of the skin, at the site of the bite, causing erythema migrans, which has a '*bull's-eye*' appearance.
- **Stage 2 (disseminated infection)**: In this phase, the organism spreads haematogenously throughout the body to cause lymphadenopathy, lymphocytic meningitis, cranial nerve involvement (facial nerve palsy) and cardiovascular system involvement (myocarditis, pericarditis or heart block).
- **Stage 3 (persistent infection)**: It often affects the knee or possibly the hip, other large joints or the temporomandibular joint, causing chronic arthritis. Lyme disease may cause chronic encephalomyelitis that resembles multiple sclerosis.

Management Lyme disease is diagnosed on the basis of symptoms, objective physical findings (such as erythema migrans rash, facial palsy or arthritis), a history of exposure to infected ticks and possibly laboratory tests that include PCR and ELISA.

Antibiotics are the mainstay of treatment. A recombinant vaccine on the basis of the outer surface protein is tried in endemic areas despite the autoimmune changes that may be caused by its usage.

COMMON VIRAL INFECTIONS

The various diseases caused by viruses are grouped into four categories:

- **Acute infection:** An acute viral infection is characterized by rapid onset of disease, a relatively brief period of symptoms and resolution within few days. It is usually accompanied by early production of infectious virions and elimination of infection by the host immune system. The manifestations vary on the basis of the susceptibility of the host to each virus.
  Examples include mumps virus, which has one genetic subtype and infects only once. Influenza virus has many genetic variants and can cause reinfection.
- **Latent infection:** In latent infections, the disease does not present overtly but the host is unable to eliminate the virus. This equilibrium between the host and the parasite may be achieved in various ways. The virus may exist in a truly latent noninfectious occult form, possibly as an integrated genome or an episomal agent, or as an infectious and continuously replicating agent, termed persistent viral infection.
  Infectious agents causing chronic persistent infections escape cell-mediated immune response. The mechanisms are as follows:
  - Generation of cells that escape cell-mediated immune response
  - Downregulation of MHC production in infected cells so that these agents are not recognized and destroyed by T cells
  - Infection of cells of immunoprivileged sites such as the brain

  Examples of latent infection include chronic congenital rubella, cytomegalovirus (CMV) infection, Epstein–Barr virus (EBV) infection, hepatitis B, HIV infection, latent herpes simplex virus (HSV) infection, varicella zoster virus (VZV), adenovirus and some retroviral infections.
- **Chronic infection:** During chronic infection, the immune system is unable to overcome the viral replicatory

mechanisms, resulting in persistent viraemia, e.g. HIV and hepatitis B virus (HBV) infection.
- **Transforming infections:** These viruses transform an infected cell into a benign or a malignant tumour cell by accentuating various survival mechanisms.

The common viral infections under each category are discussed here.

ACUTE VIRAL INFECTIONS

Measles (Rubeola) PA 10.4

The measles virus is a **single-stranded, enveloped RNA virus** of the paramyxovirus family and it causes measles, an infection of the respiratory system. Symptoms include fever, cough, runny nose, red eyes and generalized maculopapular and erythematous rash. The virus is highly contagious and is spread by coughing and sneezing, but it is vaccine preventable.

Pathogenesis The measles virus has two envelope glycoproteins on the viral surface – haemagglutinin (H) and membrane fusion protein (F). These proteins are responsible for host cell binding and invasion. The virus replicates in the respiratory tract and disseminates to many tissues like the skin, conjunctiva, small blood vessels, lymph nodes and CNS.

Although preformed antibodies are useful for passive immunization, cellular immunity appears more important in host defence against measles. In general, CD4 T cells help to control the virus by secretion of cytokines, whereas CD8 T cells directly eliminate cells infected with measles virus.

Morphology

- Epithelial giant cells with viral inclusions and reticuloendothelial (**Warthin–Finkeldey**) giant cells with eosinophilic nucleus and cytoplasmic **Cowdry type A inclusion bodies** may be found in lymphoid tissue with marked follicular hyperplasia and large germinal centres (Fig. 8.16).
- Dilated blood vessels, oedema and perivascular infiltrate of cells manifest as reddish rashes all over the body.
- The characteristic **Koplik spots** (Fig. 8.17) are ulcerated mucosal lesions in the oral cavity near the Stensen ducts associated with inflammation and neovascularization.

Clinical Manifestations Unvaccinated patients at a high risk to develop severe measles include infants younger than 6 months and immunocompromised individuals. Such individuals should receive passive immunization after a recognized exposure.

Complications of measles, including pneumonia, encephalitis, keratitis and haemorrhagic rashes (**black measles**), occur in roughly 1 per 1000–2000 cases. More common, less severe complications include otitis media and croup. Some rare, late complications are subacute sclerosing panencephalitis and measles inclusion body encephalitis.

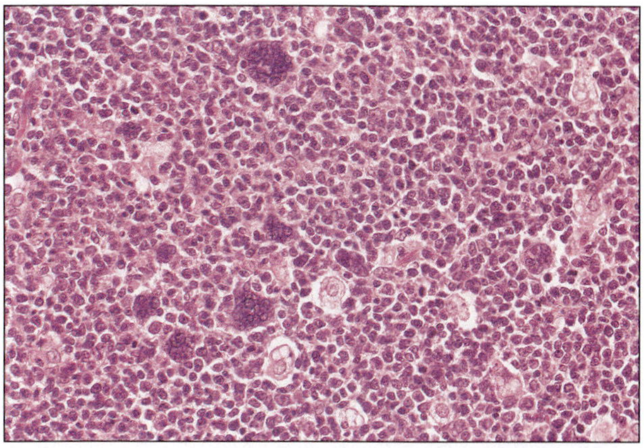

Fig. 8.16 Measles tonsillitis. Reactive follicular epithelial hyperplasia with interfollicular multinucleated Warthin–Finkeldey-type giant cells. (*Source:* From Bruce M. Wenig. Atlas of Head and Neck Pathology. Elsevier. 2016.)

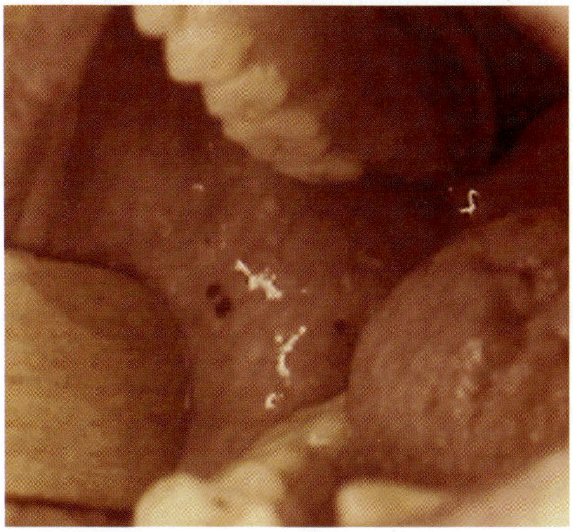

Fig. 8.17 Koplik spots in buccal mucosa. (*Source:* From Rubeola. Elsevier Point of Care. 2022.)

Mumps PA 10.4

Mumps occurs as a result of a **single-stranded RNA virus** and spreads through respiratory secretions, saliva and fomites. The virus has an incubation period of 16–18 days during which the person remains asymptomatic. Initial signs and symptoms often include fever, muscle pain, headache, poor appetite and feeling generally unwell. This is usually followed by painful swelling of one or both parotid salivary glands. About one-third of people have mild or no symptoms. The virus enters the cells of the respiratory tract and replicates and spreads haematogenously with the help of two surface glycoproteins – haemagglutinin (HA) and neuraminidase (NA).

Complications may include the following:

- In **mumps parotitis**, the virus infects the ductal epithelial cells and desquamates the cells, causing classical pain and swelling. The glands are enlarged bilaterally (70% of cases) with dough-like consistency. Microscopy reveals leucocytic infiltration and an oedematous interstitium. The necrotic debris fills the lumen and causes focal damage to the epithelium lining.
- Meningitis and encephalitis are present with demyelination and vascular damage (15%).
- Pancreatitis also releases enzymes which destroy the parenchyma and cause fat necrosis and infiltration with neutrophils (4%).
- There is inflammation of the heart.
- Permanent deafness can occur.
- Testicular inflammation (**mumps orchitis**) with oedema and focal haemorrhage or infarction due to compromised blood supply which uncommonly results in infertility may occur. Women may develop ovarian swelling, but this does not increase the risk of infertility.

Polio PA 10.4

Poliovirus is an unencapsulated **spherical enterovirus.** The main mode of transmission is the faecal–oral route. Poliovirus infects human cells by binding to an immunoglobulin-like receptor, **CD155** (also known as the poliovirus receptor), on the cell surface which facilitates an irreversible conformational change of the viral particle, which is necessary for viral entry. Following attachment to the host cell membrane, the virus may enter the cell by two ways: via the formation of a pore in the plasma membrane through which the RNA is 'injected' into the host cell cytoplasm or via virus uptake by receptor-mediated endocytosis. It replicates in the gut mucosa and spreads through the lymphatics, causing viraemia. Poliovirus uses two mechanisms to evade the immune system: the acidic nature of the stomach and its ability to replicate at a rapid rate.

A smaller proportion of people with poliovirus infection develop serious symptoms due to brainstem involvement (bulbar poliomyelitis), whereas the common type affects the spinal cord and causes paraesthesia (feeling of pins and needles in the legs). Complications include meningitis and paralysis or weakness in the arms or legs or both. Occasionally, paralysis of the respiratory muscles may occur and cause death.

Inactivated polio vaccine (IPV) and oral polio vaccine (OPV) are the two forms of vaccine on the basis of the three serotypes of poliovirus. Polio was eradicated in 2019, and this was made possible because the virus affects only humans, shows limited variations and could be easily neutralized by antibodies generated by immunization.

LATENT VIRAL INFECTIONS

Herpes Simplex Viral Infections PA 10.4

HSV is categorized into two types: herpes simplex virus type 1 (HSV-1) and herpes simplex virus type 2 (HSV-2), which differ serologically but are related genetically and cause similar infections.

HSV-1 is mainly transmitted by oral-to-oral contact and causes not only oral herpes (which can include symptoms known as 'cold sores') but also cutaneous and genital herpes. HSV-2 is an STI that causes genital herpes.

Most of the oral and genital herpes infections are asymptomatic. Symptoms of herpes include painful blisters or ulcers at the site of infection. Herpes infections are most contagious when symptoms are present but can still be transmitted to others in the absence of symptoms. **Infection with HSV-2 increases the risk of acquiring and transmitting HIV infection.**

After its entry and replication in the skin and mucous membranes, the virus is transported along sensory nerves to the nerve cell bodies, where it resides lifelong. It remains latent in most individuals, synthesizing only the latency-associated viral RNA transcripts (LATs) until conditions like decreased immune function, stress and sunlight exposure occur.

Morphology (Fig. 8.18)

Condition	Description
Herpetic gingivostomatitis	Commonly caused by HSV-1 infection Vesicular eruption in the oral mucosa
Herpes labialis	Commonly referred to as cold sores or fever blisters (by ballooning degeneration of epithelial cells)
Herpes genitalis	More common in HSV-2 infection Inflamed papules and vesicles on the outer surface of the genitals
Herpetic whitlow and herpes gladiatorum	It is a painful infection that typically affects the fingers or thumbs
Corneal lesions	Herpes epithelial keratitis – damage caused by the virus Herpes stromal keratitis – damage caused by immunological reaction to the virus
Neonatal infection	From infected mothers to children
Herpesviral encephalitis and herpesviral meningitis	Caused by the transmission of HSV-1 to the brain's temporal lobe or to the brainstem

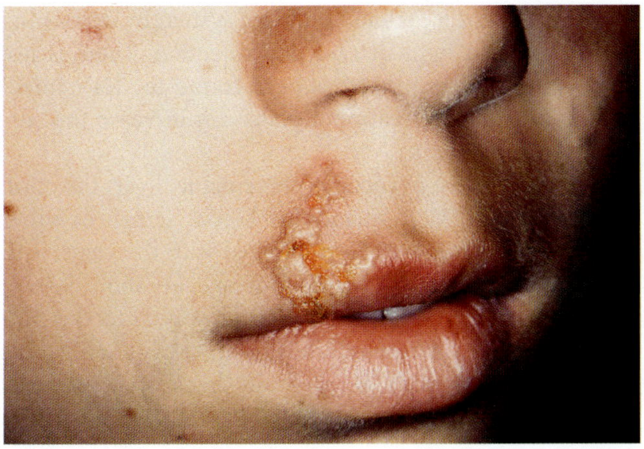

Fig. 8.18 Herpetic labialis. (*Source:* From Philip Buttaravoli, Stephen M. Leffler. Minor Emergencies. Elsevier. 2012.)

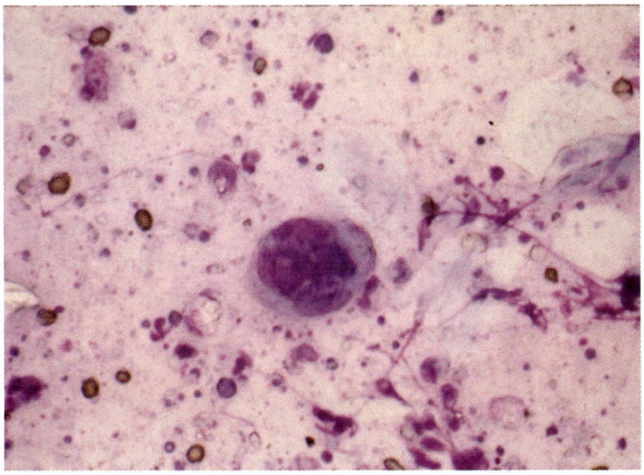

Fig. 8.19 Positive Tzanck preparation showing a multinucleated giant cell typical of a herpesvirus infection. (*Source:* From James G. Marks, Jeffrey J. Miller. Lookingbill and Marks' Principles of Dermatology. Elsevier. 2019.)

One of the less expensive and easy tests performed to distinguish herpetic lesions from varicella lesions is the **Tzanck smear** (Fig. 8.19). It involves scraping the base of a fresh deroofed or ruptured vesicular lesion and examining the material obtained under the microscope by spreading on a glass slide and staining with Giemsa. The presence of characteristic multinucleated giant cells helps in the diagnosis.

Varicella Zoster Virus Infections **PA 10.4**

It is the causative organism of chickenpox (an acute infection [mild in children and severe in adults and immunocompromised hosts]) and shingles (a latent infection [source of morbidity in the older people]).

Primary VZV causes **chickenpox** (varicella), which may result in complications including encephalitis, pneumonia or bronchitis, due to the virus per se or secondary bacterial infection. VZV enters through the respiratory system and even when clinical symptoms of chickenpox have resolved, it remains dormant in the nervous system of the infected person (virus latency) in the trigeminal and dorsal root ganglia. The infection presents as vesicles that fill with pus, rupture and scab before healing. The infection is most contagious 1–2 days before the rashes appear. In about 10%–20% of cases, VZV reactivates later in life, producing a disease known as **shingles or herpes zoster**.

Morphology

Rashes appear after a respiratory discomfort and extend in a centrifugal pattern. The lesions are manifested by multiple vesicles **limited to specific dermatomes**. The vesicles ulcerate in time and form encrusted lesions on the epidermis. Microscopy shows an intraepithelial vesicle with epithelial cells containing inclusion bodies. The vesicle then ruptures over time, heals by regeneration and leaves no scar.

In shingles, the virus affects the sensory nerves of various dermatomes, causing severe pain in the case of the trigeminal nerve. The vesicles cause intense itch and burning sensation and may ulcerate on scratching, leaving exudate and haemorrhage on the skin. If the geniculate nucleus is involved (**Ramsay Hunt syndrome**), it causes facial paralysis.

Cytomegalovirus **PA 10.4**

CMV is a member of a group of herpesviruses which latently infect monocytes and their bone marrow progenitors that may get reactivated when the cellular immunity is depressed. It acts by hiding from and actively suppressing the immune responses shown by our body. In the United States, nearly one in three children is already infected with CMV by the age of 5 years. Over half of adults have been infected with CMV by the age of 40 years.

Spread of Infection People with CMV infection may pass the virus in body fluids such as saliva, urine, blood, tears, semen and breast milk. CMV is spread from an infected person through any of these secretions or tissue transplants.

Morphology

- As the name implies, the cells and the nucleus are enlarged and are pleomorphic.
- There are prominent basophilic inclusions in the nucleus and the cytoplasm. In the nucleus, the inclusion bodies are surrounded by a clear halo separating it from the nuclear membrane (**owl's eye**) (Fig. 8.20).
- The epithelium of various organs like the kidney is affected along with the neurons (brain) and alveolar macrophages (lungs), causing areas of focal necrosis.

Clinical Features

Congenital Up to 40% of babies born to women who are newly infected with CMV during pregnancy become

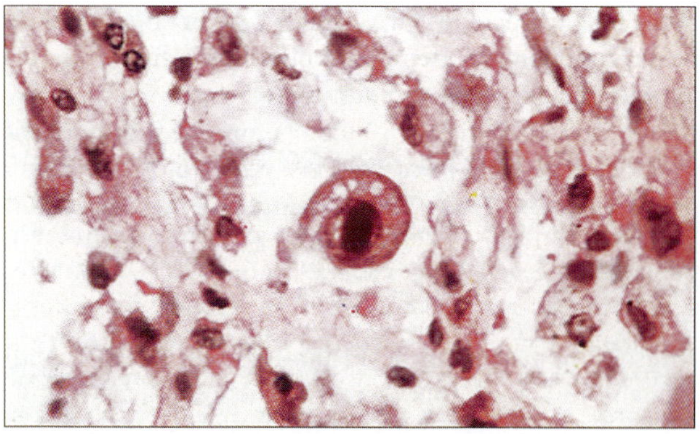

Fig. 8.20 Owl's eye appearance of CMV inclusions in the nucleus. CMV, cytomegalovirus. (*Source:* From Richard V. Goering, Hazel M. Dockrell, Mark Zuckerman, Peter L. Chiodini. Mims' Medical Microbiology and Immunology. Elsevier. 2019.)

infected, whereas a CMV infection prior to pregnancy is less likely to be transmitted to the baby. Newborns with CMV infection are likely to be born premature with low birth weight. Other possible problems include a small brain (microcephaly) or other nervous system disorders that can cause seizures, deafness, mental retardation or death. A fraction of the infected babies may develop serious disability. It develops as the classical cytomegalic inclusion disease.

Immunosuppression Persons who have had an organ or **bone marrow transplant and those with AIDS** can develop serious illness due to reactivation of CMV and much more severe illness if they never had CMV infection in the past and acquire a new infection.

Reactivated CMV infection can affect many parts of the body:

- CMV retinitis affects the eyes and can cause blindness.
- Pneumonia caused by CMV can be life-threatening.
- CMV can affect any part of the GI tract, including the liver and pancreas.
- CMV can infect the brain and other parts of the nervous system, causing symptoms like headache, confusion and leg weakness.

CMV can be easily prevented by practicing proper hygiene, washing hands, avoiding contact with tears and saliva, avoiding sharing of food and glass used by infected persons and also by being careful with the disposal of wastes and usage of contraception methods.

CHRONIC VIRAL INFECTIONS

Persistent or chronic viral infections are characterized as those in which the virus is not cleared but remains in certain specific cells of the infected individuals. Persistent infections may involve stages of both latent and productive infections without rapidly killing or even producing excessive damage to the host cells, e.g. HIV and HBV infection.

- **HIV** weakens a person's immune system by destroying the cells that fight disease and infection. There is not any effective cure that has been found for HIV infection, but proper treatment plans can increase the survival rate by years.
- **Hepatitis B** is a vaccine-preventable liver infection caused by HBV. It spreads by blood, semen or other body fluids from a person infected with the virus. Risk for chronic infection is related to age, i.e. about 90% of infants with hepatitis B develop chronic infection like cirrhosis or liver cancer, whereas only 2%–6% of adults who have hepatitis B as adults become chronically infected.

Both these infections can spread through sexual contact; sharing needles, syringes or other drug injection equipment; or from a mother to her baby at birth. HIV and HBV are discussed in greater detail in Chapter 6 and Chapter 22, respectively.

TRANSFORMING VIRAL INFECTION

Human Papillomavirus — PA 10.4

Human papillomavirus (HPV) is the most common viral infectious agent of the reproductive tract that is common in sexually active people. Skin-to-skin genital contact can transmit the infection. HPV infections usually resolve without any intervention within a few months after acquiring the disease, and about 90% clear within 2 years. However, a small proportion of infections with certain types of precancerous HPV strains (types 16 and 18) can persist and progress to invasive cervical cancer. In 2020, approximately 342,000 women died from cervical cancer; about 90% of these deaths occurred in low- and middle-income countries. There is also evidence linking HPV infection with cancers of the anus, vulva, vagina, penis and oropharynx. This topic is dealt with further in Chapter 7.

Epstein–Barr Virus — PA 10.4

EBV is best known as the cause of **infectious mononucleosis** ('mono' or 'glandular fever'). It is also associated with various nonmalignant, premalignant and malignant lymphoproliferative diseases such as **Burkitt lymphoma**, haemophagocytic lymphohistiocytosis and Hodgkin lymphoma and other diseases like hepatitis, meningoencephalitis and pneumonitis.

The majority of primary EBV infections throughout the world are subclinical. Antibodies to EBV have been demonstrated in all population groups with a worldwide distribution, and approximately 90%–95% of adults are EBV seropositive.

Infectious mononucleosis is a benign lymphoproliferative disorder that predominantly occurs in late adolescents and is characterized by fever, sore throat, generalized lymphadenopathy, splenomegaly and appearance of atypically activated mononucleosis cells.

Pathogenesis EBV spreads through body fluids like saliva. It can infect both B cells and epithelial cells of the oropharynx. The mechanisms for entering these two cells are different.

To enter B cells, viral glycoprotein gp350 binds to its cellular receptor **CD21**. Then, viral glycoprotein gp42 interacts with cellular class II MHC molecules. This triggers fusion of the viral envelope with the cell membrane, allowing EBV to enter the B cell. Human CD35 is an additional attachment factor that can provide a route for entry of EBV into CD21-negative cells, including immature B cells. EBV infection of B cells can either lyse the cell to release virions that can infect other B cells (B-cell neoplasms) or remain latent as an extrachromosomal episome and act as a reservoir of infection.

To enter epithelial cells, viral protein BMRF-2 interacts with cellular β1 integrins. This triggers fusion of the viral envelope with the epithelial cell membrane, allowing EBV to enter the epithelial cell. Once EBV enters the cell, the viral capsid dissolves and the viral genome is transported to the cell nucleus.

EBV is a herpetic lymphotropic microorganism. In the acute phases of the infection, proliferating EBV-infected B cells are controlled primarily by natural killer (NK) T cells, helper $CD4^+$ T cells and cytotoxic suppressor ($CD8^+$) NK T cells. Owing to this T-cell response, the number of EBV-infected cells drops significantly during the next 4–6 weeks. During convalescence, human leucocyte antigen (HLA)-restricted cytotoxic T lymphocytes maintain EBV under control by targeting the latently expressed Epstein–Barr nuclear antigen (EBNA)-3 protein. Reactivation of latent infection results in uncontrolled proliferation of the B cells. It may also lead to the production of autoantibodies that precipitate immune-mediated thrombocytopenia.

Morphology

- **Generalized lymphadenopathy** is a hallmark of infectious mononucleosis; any group of lymph nodes may be involved. However, massive mediastinal and hilar lymph nodes can cause respiratory distress. Mesenteric lymphadenopathy can mimic acute appendicitis. Lymph node enlargement tends to subside over a period of days to weeks.
- **Pharyngitis** characterized by sore throat is the cardinal symptom of infectious mononucleosis. Tonsils are enlarged, can cause obstruction of the airway and are reddened, tender and covered with an exudate in more than 50% of patients.
- The **liver** shows minimal disease with infiltration by lymphocytes and monocytes in the portal area and minor degeneration of the hepatocytes, often manifesting as jaundice and can cause hepatitis.
- **Nervous system manifestations**
  Neurological disorders can occur in association with clinical findings typical of infectious mononucleosis. These include aseptic meningitis, encephalitis, Guillain–Barré syndrome, optic neuritis, cranial nerve palsy, transverse myelitis, acute cerebellar ataxia, dysautonomia, subacute sclerosing panencephalitis, psychosis, Parkinson-like syndrome and CNS lymphoma.
- **Haematological manifestations**
  Peripheral blood shows absolute lymphocytosis, with 5%–80% of the cells being large **atypical lymphocytes** (Fig. 8.21). Occasionally, patients develop transient thrombocytopenic purpura. Other rare complications are haemolytic anaemia, aplastic anaemia, agranulocytosis and agammaglobulinaemia.

Diagnosis of this condition is based on lymphocytosis, positive heterophile antibody reaction **(monospot test)** and rising titre for specific antibodies for EBV.

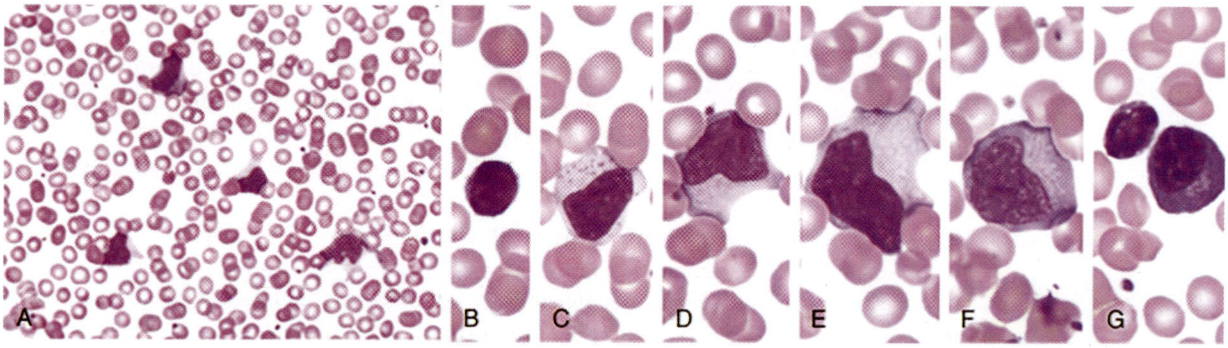

Fig. 8.21 Peripheral smear showing atypical lymphocytes in infectious mononucleosis. Low power (A) shows a moderately high white blood cell count and many reactive lymphocytes. Higher power illustrates small resting lymphocyte (B) for comparison, large granular lymphocyte (C), atypical forms (D–F), also referred to as 'reactive' lymphocytes, and circulating plasma cell (G). (*Source:* From Lauren J. Maskin, Russell J. McCulloh. Ferri's Clinical Advisor 2021. Elsevier. 2021.)

Treatment of EBV infection mainly focuses on symptomatic treatment. Vaccines are still under trial for EBV, but most people become infected with EBV and gain adaptive immunity.

COMMON FUNGAL INFECTIONS

Fungi are eukaryotic organisms and include yeasts (individual cells or in chains) and moulds (multicellular filaments – hyphae). These can be identified in histopathology with the help of special fungal stains like **Gomori's methenamine silver stain** and **periodic acid–Schiff stain**. Fungal infection is common in those taking long-term antibiotics and those who are immunocompromised, and it can present as follows:

- **Cutaneous and superficial mycoses** (dermatomycoses) include infections such as athlete foot and ringworm, in which fungal growth occurs only in the superficial layers of the skin, nails or hair.
- **Subcutaneous mycoses** penetrate below the skin to involve the subcutaneous, connective and bone tissues and may spread through lymphatics.
- **Systemic or deep mycoses** affect internal organs and become widely disseminated throughout the body. This type is often fatal.
- Opportunistic fungal infections are infections by commensals in the body that cause life-threatening infection in immunocompromised hosts.
- **Endemic mycoses** are caused by dimorphic fungi which cause serious systemic infection.

YEAST

Candidiasis

Candidiasis is a fungal infection caused by *Candida* sp., the most common being *Candida albicans. Candida* normally lives on the skin in places such as the mouth, throat, gut and vagina as a normal commensal. It may cause infections if it grows out of control or if it spreads haematogenously. *Candida* species are yeasts, but their buds fail to detach and become elongated to form the **pseudohyphae**.

Pathogenesis Its pathogenicity is governed by the coordinated phenotypic switching between the different phase-specific genes, and each of these variants shows altered colony morphology, antigenicity and virulence. The virulence factors include adhesins and enzymes such as proteases and catalase.

Their ability to form biofilms helps to evade host immune response and antifungals.

But neutrophils and macrophages phagocytose and oxidatively destroy *Candida*, forming the first line of defence. The dendritic cells also potentiate this, especially in HIV-infected patients and those with inherited defects in T_H17 response.

Clinical Manifestations

- **Candidiasis of the skin (cutaneous candidiasis or cutaneous moniliasis):** Superficial skin is a common location for this fungal infection. The lesions appear as well-circumscribed, red and sometimes itchy patches of varying sizes and shapes. They are usually rimmed with small, red-coloured pustules and are commonly found in folds of the skin, i.e. the underarms, under the breasts, the navel, the groin or the folds of the buttocks (e.g. diaper rash) or the webbing between the toes and the fingers. Crusts may form on the scalp, possibly causing hair loss. The infection may spread to the face, fingertips or trunk. Patients with diabetes and burn infections are more prone to superficial infections.

  Diaper rash is a cutaneous infection of the perineum of infants, the region in contact with the wet diapers.
- **Vulvovaginitis or vaginitis:** Pregnant women and women with diabetes are prone to this common fungal infection. It usually presents as a thick white or yellow vaginal discharge (leucorrhoea) with itching and redness of the female genitalia (vagina and vulva).
- **Infection of the glans penis** may be seen in men whose sexual partners have candidal vulvovaginitis and in men with diabetes mellitus.
- **Oral candidiasis (thrush):** This form of candidiasis affects the mouth. It first appears as a creamy white patch or sore on the tongue or mucous membranes of the mouth. When the corners of the mouth are red (inflamed), eroded and cracked because of a *Candida* infection, the condition is called **perleche.**
- *Candida* infection around the nails is called **candidal paronychia.**
- **Systemic candidiasis:** This is the most serious *Candida* infection seen in patients with neutropenia, leukaemia, chemotherapy or transplantation. It affects many parts of the body and is usually caused by an immune deficiency. It may lead to endocarditis, endophthalmitis, meningitis, renal abscesses or rarely osteomyelitis.

Cryptococcosis

Cryptococcus is an encapsulated yeast, an obligate aerobe that grows in both plants and animals. It affects both the immunocompetent and the immunocompromised hosts. It replicates by the process of budding. It is a facultative intracellular pathogen that can use host phagocytes to spread within the body and infect the lungs and brain. It includes two encapsulated yeast species which are described in Table 8.2.

Pathogenesis *Cryptococcus* evades the host defences using its virulence factors as follows:

- The polysaccharide capsule which inhibits phagocytosis
- Enzymes that aid in tissue invasion
- Production of melanin which has antioxidant properties

Table 8.2 Features of *Cryptococcus neoformans* and *C. gattii*

C. neoformans	*C. gattii*
Present in soil and bird droppings; spreads by inhalation	It is associated with certain species of trees and is present in soil
Infects immunocompromised patients with AIDS, leukaemia and lymphoma, transplant patients and patients undergoing steroid therapy	Infects immunologically normal individuals
Causes meningoencephalitis	Large lesions are produced with mass effects and radiological appearance of a neoplasm

Morphology

In healthy individuals, the fungi cause a chronic granulomatous reaction with inflammatory infiltrate and giant cells. When grown as yeast, *C. neoformans* has a prominent capsule which hampers its differentiation from other fungus in Gram-stained smears of purulent exudates. Under the microscope, India ink stain, which does not enter the capsule, is used for identification of the fungi in CSF. The capsule of the organism appears as a clear halo around the cells (Fig. 8.22). In tissues, mucicarmine stain provides specific staining of polysaccharide cell wall in *C. neoformans.*

Clinical Manifestations

- **Pulmonary forms:** In immunocompetent individuals, the infection is asymptomatic. However, in immunosuppressed hosts, chronic pulmonary infections may cause large masses in the lobes of the lungs, segmental pneumonia, pleural effusions and lymph node enlargement.

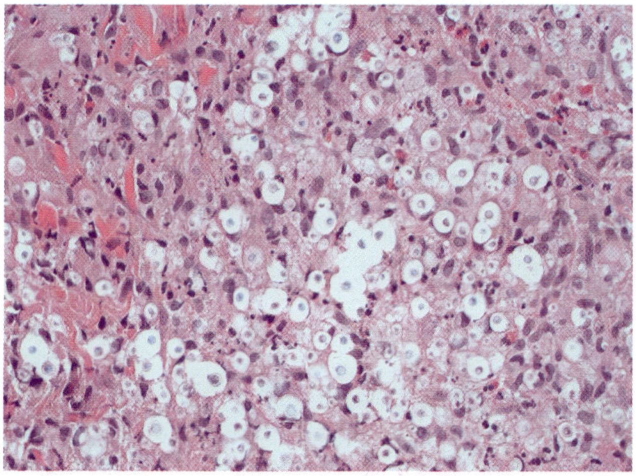

Fig. 8.22 Cryptococcosis. Numerous grey-appearing yeast forms are surrounded by mucinous capsular material. (*Source:* From James W. Patterson. Weedon's Skin Pathology. Elsevier. 2021.)

- **Disseminated forms:** In immunocompromised people, it causes the following:
  - CNS infections, especially of the brain, leading to complications such as hydrocephalus and blindness
  - Cutaneous or skin infections such as papules, plaques and ulcers

Infections of other organs or systems may include chorioretinitis, otitis, myocarditis, endocarditis, gastroduodenitis and hepatitis.

MOULDS

A **mould** is a fungus that grows in the form of multicellular filaments called *hyphae. The* network of these tubular branching hyphae, called a mycelium, is considered a single organism. The hyphae may be septate or aseptate and branching or nonbranching. Here, we describe the two common diseases affecting humans that are caused by moulds – aspergillosis and zygomycosis.

Aspergillosis

Aspergillus fumigatus and *A. flavus* are the most frequently identified ubiquitous organisms capable of living under extensive environmental stress. Most people are thought to inhale thousands of *Aspergillus* spores daily but without effect because of an efficient immune response.

Aspergillosis is thought to affect more than 14 million people worldwide, with allergic bronchopulmonary aspergillosis and chronic pulmonary aspergillosis being considerably more prevalent than invasive aspergillosis.

Pathogenesis Collectively, this group of diseases is referred to as aspergillosis and is broadly broken down into three categories – **allergic, chronic and invasive**.

The fungi enter as droplets and are captured by the alveolar macrophages where they are phagocytosed and killed. In the immunocompromised people, the fungus may cause invasive aspergillosis and also damage the host by provoking the release of many proinflammatory mediators, the most important one being TNF-α. In patients with neutropenia, there may be a rapid and uncontrolled hyphal growth of the invasive fungi, leading to fatal complications. *Aspergillus* produces **aflatoxin**, a carcinogen that leads to liver cancer, discussed in Chapter 7.

Morphology

On microscopy, *Aspergillus* species are reliably demonstrated by silver stains, e.g. Gridley's stain or Gomori's methenamine silver stain. These give the fungal walls a grey-black colour. The hyphae of *Aspergillus* species range in diameter from 2.5 to 4.5 µm. *Aspergillus* hyphae form fruiting bodies and show septate filaments which tend to have **dichotomous branching that is progressive and primarily at acute angles of around 45°** (Fig. 8.23).

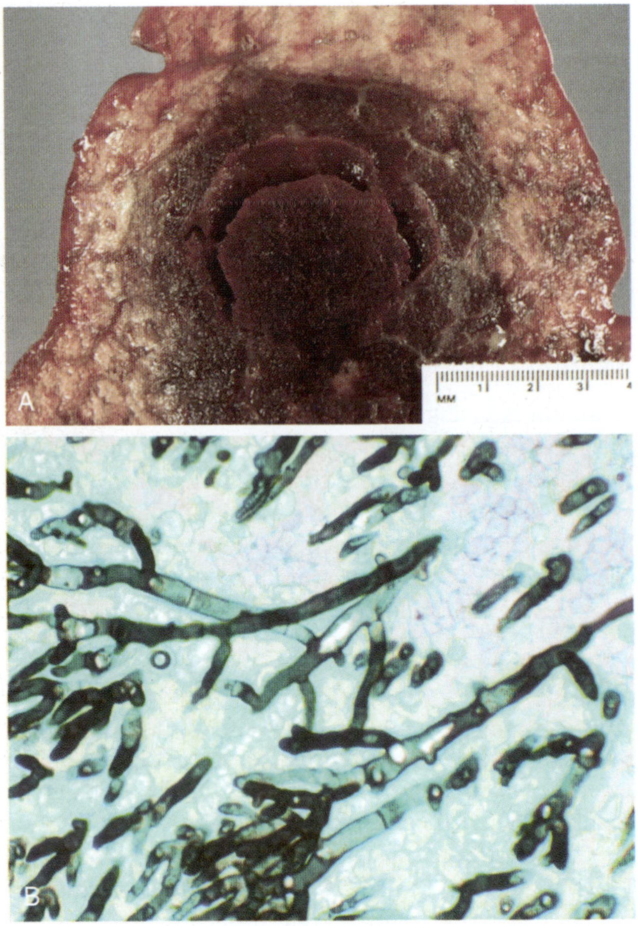

Fig. 8.23 Invasive aspergillosis (gross appearance) of the lung (A). Gomori's methenamine silver stain (B) shows septate hyphae with acute-angle branching. (*Source:* From Anthony Chang, Lora Hedrick Ellenson, Jonathan I. Epstein, et al. Robbins Basic Pathology. Elsevier. 2018.)

Laboratory Investigations On chest X-ray and computed tomography (CT), pulmonary aspergillosis classically manifests as a halo sign and, later, as an air crescent sign. An *Aspergillus* antigen skin test or blood test for *Aspergillus*-specific IgE can be used to screen for allergic bronchopulmonary aspergillosis.

Zygomycosis

The family of fungi mucormycetes, which includes *Mucor*, *Rhizopus*, *Lichtheimia* and *Cunninghamella*, causes the disease **mucormycosis** mainly in immunocompromised individuals and in patients with neutropenia, diabetes mellitus, corticosteroid use, iron overload and breakdown of cutaneous barrier.

Pathogenesis In a normal host, primary defence mechanisms against zygomycosis include sequestration of iron in the serum by specialized iron-binding proteins and phagocytes along with endothelial cells, which regulate vascular tone and permeability. Acting in concert, these mechanisms prevent the establishment of infection in tissue and subsequent endovascular invasion.

In susceptible hosts, normal defence mechanisms break down.

- In diabetic ketoacidosis (DKA), the acidic pH causes the dissociation of free iron from sequestering proteins. This release of free iron allows rapid fungal growth.
- Deficiency in cell number (neutropenia) or functional defects occur.
- Damage of endothelial cells by the fungus allows fungal angioinvasion, thrombosis and thereby tissue necrosis and dissemination of the fungal infection.

Morphology

Microscopically, large, **nonseptate hyphae with 90° angle branching** and nonparallel walls causing tissue necrosis and haemorrhage are seen, the primary sites being nasal sinuses, lungs and the GI tract (Fig. 8.24). In certain conditions, the fungus may spread to the orbits and the brain, giving rise to **rhinocerebral mucormycosis**, where it may cause meningoencephalitis. Lung involvement is rare, but if involved, it causes haemorrhagic pneumonia with vascular thrombi and distal infarctions.

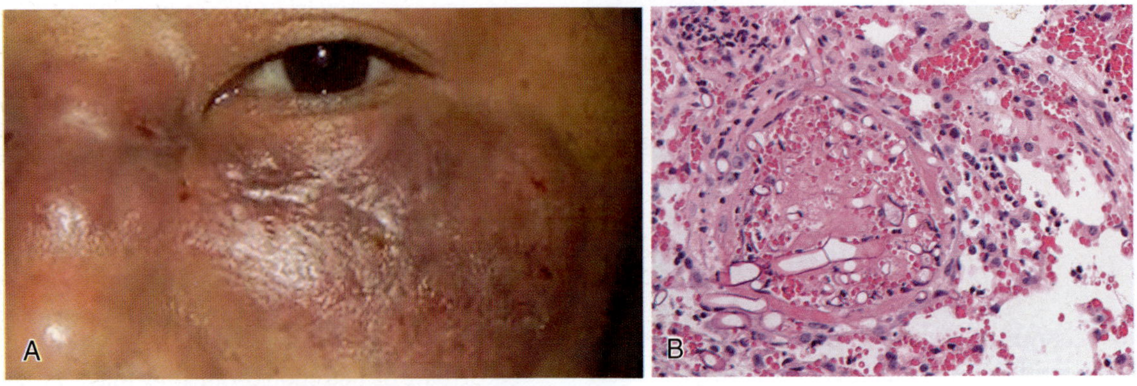

Fig. 8.24 Clinical picture of mucormycosis involving the orbit (A) and microscopy of biopsy tissue showing pauciseptate, broad-based ribbon-like *Mucor* (B). (*Source:* From Dimitrios P. Kontoyiannis. Goldman-Cecil Medicine, 2-volume Set. Elsevier. 2020.)

Mucormycosis can also affect the lungs, skin and GI tract in neonates, or get disseminated in immunocompromised patients.

Investigations and Management The biopsy specimen of the infected tissue is more reliable for detection because the swabs of the tissue or discharge is generally unreliable.

Amphotericin B is the drug of choice, which is administered once the infection is detected and the treatment is continued till the fungus is eradicated from the body. In certain cases, surgical removal of the 'fungal ball' is indicated.

PARASITIC INFECTIONS

Parasitosis, or parasitic infections, is a group of infectious diseases caused or transmitted by parasites. Parasitic infections cause a tremendous burden of disease in both the tropics and the subtropics, as well as in more temperate climates. Of all parasitic diseases, malaria causes the most deaths globally. Malaria kills approximately 660,000 people each year, most of them young children in sub-Saharan Africa. There are three important types of parasitic infections:

- Protozoal infections
- Helminthic infections
- Ectoparasites

The most common protozoal and metazoal infections are discussed in detail here.

PROTOZOAL INFECTIONS

Malaria PA 10.1

Malaria is caused by unicellular protozoans which are intracellular parasites. The protozoan is transmitted to people through the bites of infected **female *Anopheles* mosquitoes**. Children younger than 5 years are the most vulnerable group affected by malaria. WHO estimates that the African region carries a disproportionately high share of the global malaria burden. There are five species – *Plasmodium falciparum* (the cause of **severe cerebral malaria**), *P. vivax, P. ovale, P. knowlesi* and *P. malariae*.

Life Cycle and Pathogenesis (Fig. 8.25) All the species have similar life cycles, although *P. falciparum* contributes to greater virulence. The life cycle involves only humans and mosquitoes, but it passes through several morphologically distinct forms in its development. The infectious stage of *Plasmodium* is the sporozoite, which is found in the salivary glands of female mosquitoes.

In humans

- **Exoerythrocytic stage:** During a blood meal, malaria-infected female *Anopheles* mosquito inoculates sporozoites into the human host. Sporozoites infect liver cells within minutes by binding to the hepatocyte receptor for the serum proteins thrombospondin and properdin. The sporozoites replicate within the hepatocyte and release around 30,000 merozoites (asexual, haploid forms) when the cell ruptures. This stage is asymptomatic. Infections with *P. vivax and P. ovale* are unique in that they form hypnozoites that remain latent in the hepatocytes and cause relapses of malaria later.
- **Erythrocytic stage:** The merozoites released from the liver cells bind to glycophorin molecules on the surface of RBCs and invade them by active membrane penetration. Once they enter RBCs, the merozoites grow within the digestive vacuoles and hydrolyse haemoglobin using various enzymes. The stages within RBC that may be seen on the peripheral smear examination are as follows:
  - *Trophozoite*, the first stage in RBC, is made of a single chromatin mass.
  - *Schizont*, the next stage, has multiple chromatin masses which develop into *merozoites*, which when released infect other RBCs. Paroxysmal fever (due to the release of cytokines like TNF by the host cells) with chills and rigors occurs when merozoites are released into the blood.
  - *Gametocytes* are the sexual erythrocytic stages (gametocytes) which are taken up by the mosquito during its blood meal.

In mosquito

The parasite's multiplication in the mosquito is known as the sporogonic cycle.

In the mosquito's gut, the microgametes penetrate the macrogametes and form zygotes which invade the midgut wall of the mosquito and develop into oocysts. The oocysts grow and release sporozoites, which reach the mosquito's salivary glands. Inoculation of the sporozoites into a new human host perpetuates the malarial life cycle.

***P. falciparum* causes more severe disease than other species, and its greater pathogenicity is because of the following reasons:**

- *P. falciparum* can infect RBCs of any age, whereas other species infect only either the young RBCs or the old RBCs.
- It causes red cells to clump together (**rosette**) and to stick to endothelial cells lining the small blood vessels (**sequestration**), thereby blocking the blood flow and leading to ischaemia. This causes cerebral manifestations and death in children. *P. falciparum* uses proteins like *erythrocyte membrane protein 1* to bind to endothelial cells by using ligands like CD36, VCAM-1, ICAM-1, E-selectin and thrombospondin.
- *GPI-linked proteins*, including merozoite surface antigens, are released from infected red cells and induce the

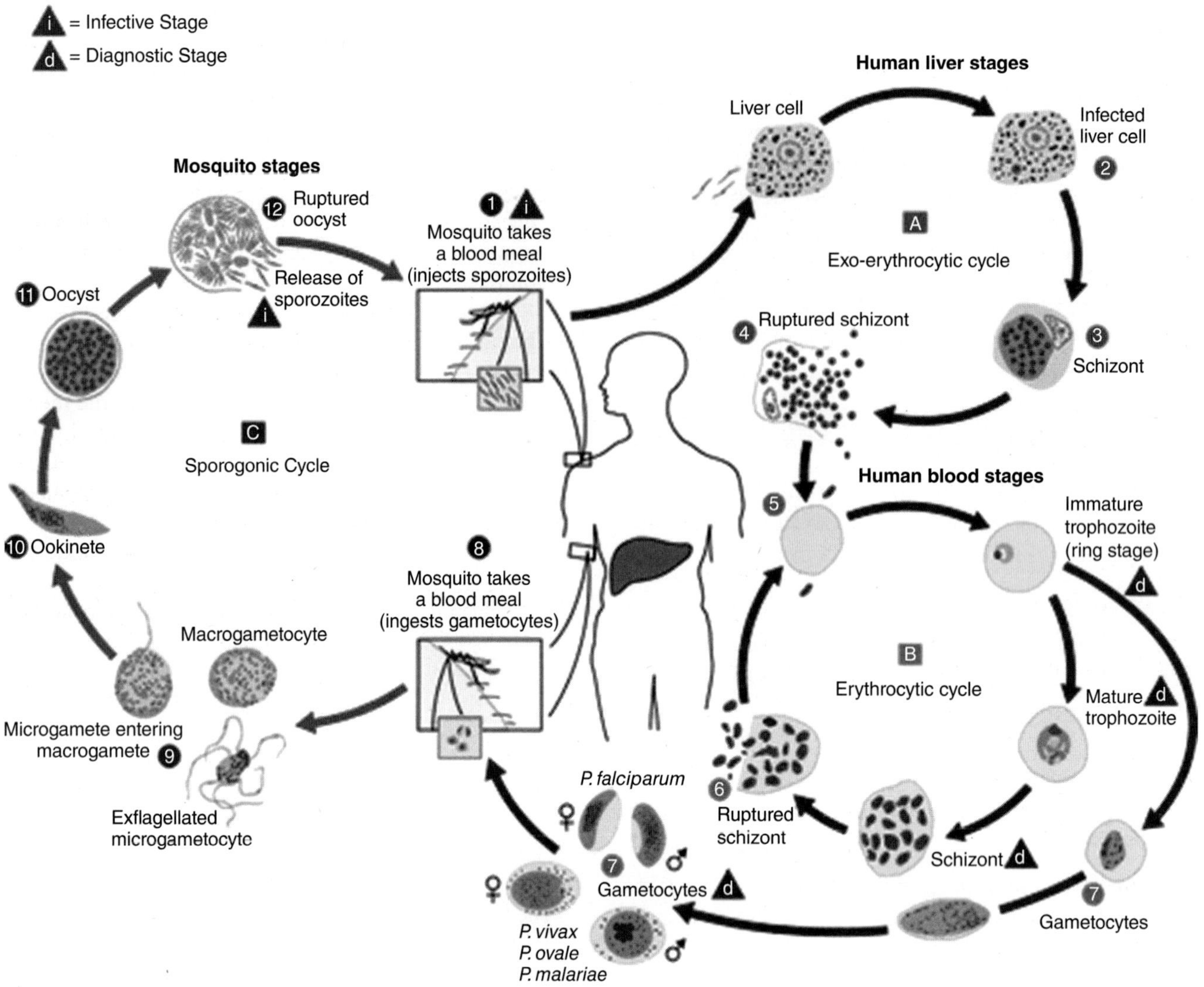

Fig. 8.25 Life cycle of the human malaria parasites. (*Source:* From Rosemary M. Olivero, Elizabeth D. Barnett. Feigin and Cherry's Textbook of Pediatric Infectious Diseases. Elsevier. 2019.)

production of TNF, IFN-γ and IL-1 and other cytokines which suppress the production of red cells, increase fever, stimulate the production of reactive nitrogen species and induce the expression of endothelial receptors.

Host Factors Host resistance to *Plasmodium* can be intrinsic factors such as reduced susceptibility of RBCs or acquired by repeated and prolonged exposure. In endemic areas, protective mutations occur in RBCs, which in the heterozygous form provide selective advantage against malaria. There are four broad classes of mutations:

- Point mutations in globin genes – sickle cell disease (HbS), HbC disease (haemoglobinopathies)
- Globin deficiencies – α and β thalassaemia
- Mutations affecting red cell enzymes – G6PD deficiency
- Mutations causing red cell membrane defects – absence of DARC (Duffy surface blood group), band 3 and spectrin

P. vivax enters red cells by binding to Duffy blood group antigen; most of the West African population is not susceptible, because it does not have the Duffy antigen. Individuals living in endemic areas often gain partial immune-mediated resistance to malaria, evidenced by reduced illness despite infection. But these protozoans have strategies to evade the host immune response *such as* antigenic variation seen in *P. falciparum* to escape the antibody response to PfEMP1.

Morphology

The diagnostic test for malarial infection is the examination of Giemsa-stained peripheral blood smear, which permits the number, density and asexual stages of the parasite to be identified.

P. falciparum infection leads to the following:

- Splenomegaly, due to congestion and hyperplasia of the red pulp. In chronic infection, the spleen undergoes fibrosis and forms a thick capsule and fibrous trabeculae. There are numerous macrophages with engulfed parasitized red cells, and the phagocytes contain granular brown-black birefringent haemozoin pigment, which makes the spleen appear **grey or black**.

- The liver is enlarged and pigmented because of the Kupffer cells being heavily laden with malarial pigment, parasites and cellular debris.
- The kidneys are congested and enlarged, with pigment in glomeruli and haemoglobin casts in the tubules.
- Pigmented phagocytic cells may be present in the bone marrow, lymph nodes, subcutaneous tissue and lungs.
- In **cerebral malaria**, brain vessels are plugged with parasitized red cells. There are ring haemorrhages around the vessels due to vascular stasis and small focal inflammatory reactions (malarial or **Durck granulomata**). With further hypoxia, the neurons get degenerated along with inflammatory infiltrates in the meninges and focal ischaemic softening.
- Nonspecific focal hypoxic lesions in the heart may be caused by progressive anaemia and circulatory stasis in the chronically ill person.

Clinical Features Symptoms of malaria develop as early as 7 days after being bitten by an infectious mosquito to as late as several months or more after exposure. Cerebral malaria is characterized by fever and influenza-like symptoms, including chills, headache, myalgia and malaise; these symptoms occur intermittently. In severe disease, seizures, mental confusion, kidney failure, acute respiratory distress syndrome, coma and death may occur. In the nonimmune people, death is caused by pulmonary oedema or DIC. Suspected or confirmed malaria, especially *P. falciparum* infection, is a medical emergency requiring urgent intervention because clinical deterioration can occur rapidly and unpredictably.

Blackwater fever is a complication seen only in *P. falciparum* infection in which RBCs undergo intravascular haemolysis, releasing haemoglobin directly into the blood. This results in haemoglobinuria, which produces the characteristic black-coloured urine and may occasionally cause acute renal failure. It is also seen in G6PD-deficient patients taking quinine for malarial treatment.

Prevention: Control of mosquitoes and their further breeding is the most important preventive measure that can be undertaken. Insecticide-treated mosquito nets and indoor spraying with residual insecticide are used at present.

Treatment: The best available treatment, particularly for *P. falciparum* malaria, is artemisinin-based combination therapy (ACT). Antimalarial medicines can also be used to prevent malaria. For travellers to the endemic area, malarial chemoprophylaxis is recommended. In endemic regions, sulphadoxine–pyrimethamine can be given to pregnant women and children as a prophylactic measure.

WHO recommends microscopy or malaria rapid diagnostic test (RDT) to be performed in all patients with suspected malaria before treatment is administered. Diagnostic testing improves the overall management of patients with febrile illnesses and may also help to reduce further spread and emergence of drug resistance by reserving antimalarials for those who actually have the disease.

Leishmaniasis **PA 10.4**

Leishmaniasis is caused by an obligate, intracellular and kinetoplast-containing protozoan parasite that is transmitted by the bite of infected **sandflies**. It causes chronic inflammatory disease of the skin, mucous membranes and viscera. There are three main forms of leishmaniasis:

1. **Visceral:** *Leishmania chagasi* (also known as *Leishmania donovani*; causes kala-azar, which is the most serious form of the disease)
2. **Cutaneous:** *Leishmania mexicana*, which is the most common form
3. Mucocutaneous: *Leishmania braziliensis*

The disease is associated with malnutrition, population displacement, poor housing and a weak immune system, especially T-cell dysfunction as in AIDS.

Life cycle and pathogenesis: Life cycle of the sandfly and the steps in leishmaniasis are discussed as follows:

1. The sandflies inject the infective stage, metacyclic **promastigotes**, into the host during blood meals.
2. Metacyclic promastigotes in the puncture wound are phagocytized by the macrophages.
3. Promastigotes transform into amastigotes.
4. Amastigotes multiply in infected cells and affect different tissues, depending on the tissue specificity of the species.
5. Sandflies become infected during blood meals on infected hosts when they ingest macrophages infected with amastigotes.
6. In the midgut of sandflies, parasites differentiate into promastigotes.
7. The promastigotes multiply, differentiate into metacyclic promastigotes and migrate to the proboscis.

Promastigotes produce two abundant surface glycoconjugates, lipophosphoglycan and zinc-dependent proteinase Gp63, which contribute to their virulence.

Resistance and susceptibility to *Leishmania* are mediated through T_H1 and T_H2 responses. $CD4^+$ cells play a major role. *Leishmania* evades host immunity by impairing the development of the T_H1 response and release IFN-γ which with the help of reactive oxygen species kills the parasites within the macrophages.

Morphology

In **cutaneous leishmaniasis** (Fig. 8.26), a well-demarcated skin lesion develops at the site of a sandfly bite, usually within several weeks to months. Multiple lesions may occur after multiple infective bites or with metastatic spread. Their appearance varies. The initial lesion is often a papule that slowly enlarges, ulcerates centrally and develops a raised, erythematous border where intracellular parasites are concentrated. Ulcers are typically painless and cause no systemic symptoms unless secondarily infected. Lesions usually heal spontaneously after several months but may persist for years. The healed lesions leave a depressed, burn-like scar.

Diffuse cutaneous leishmaniasis, a rare syndrome, results in widespread nodular skin lesions resembling those of lepromatous leprosy. It results from cell-mediated anergy to the organism.

Mucosal leishmaniasis starts with a primary cutaneous ulcer. This lesion heals spontaneously; progressive mucosal lesions may not become apparent for months to years. Typically, patients have nasal stuffiness, discharge and pain. Over time, the infection may progress, resulting in gross mutilation of the nose, palate or face.

In **visceral leishmaniasis**, the clinical manifestations usually develop gradually over weeks to months after inoculation of the parasite but can also present acutely. Irregular fever, hepatosplenomegaly, pancytopenia and polyclonal hypergammaglobulinaemia with a reversed albumin to globulin ratio occur. In some patients, there are twice-daily temperature spikes. Emaciation and death occur within months to years in patients with progressive infections. Relapse may occur years after initial infection.

Investigations and Management Tissue specimens - skin sores (cutaneous leishmaniasis) or from the bone marrow (visceral leishmaniasis) - can be examined for the parasite under a microscope, in special cultures and by molecular tests (Fig. 8.27). Blood tests that detect antibody to the parasite can be helpful in cases of visceral leishmaniasis. Molecular tests like PCR are highly sensitive and use minicircle kinetoplast DNA found in the parasite as its identification mark.

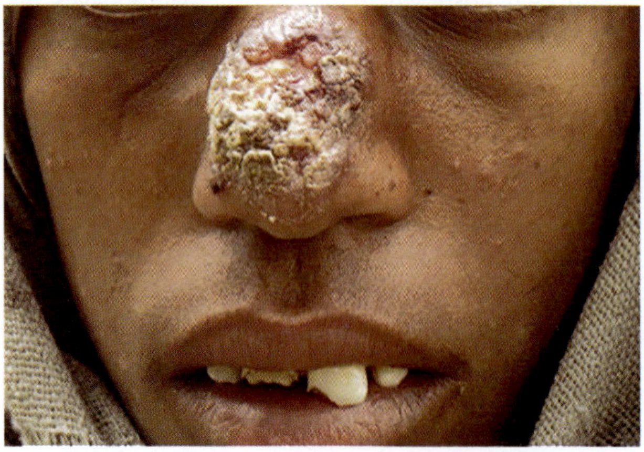

Fig. 8.26 Cutaneous leishmaniasis. (*Source:* From Marleen Boelaert, Shyam Sundar. Manson's Tropical Infectious Diseases. Elsevier. 2014.)

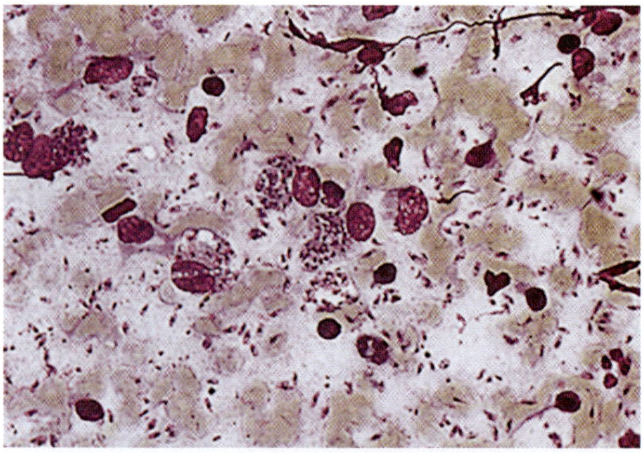

Fig. 8.27 Smear from skin biopsy of a patient with diffuse cutaneous leishmaniasis showing a large number of amastigotes. (*Source:* From Marleen Boelaert, Shyam Sundar. Manson's Tropical Infectious Diseases. Elsevier. 2014.)

METAZOAL INFECTIONS

Lymphatic Filariasis **PA 10.4**

Filariasis is a parasitic disease caused by an infection with nematodes *Wuchereria bancrofti* and *Brugia* species. These nematodes are spread by blood-feeding insects such as **blackflies and mosquitoes.** Filariasis is prevalent throughout the tropics and subtropics of Asia, Africa, the Western Pacific and parts of the Caribbean and South America. The following are its manifestations:

- Asymptomatic microfilaremia
- Recurrent lymphadenitis
- Chronic lymphadenitis with swelling of the dependent limb or scrotum (elephantiasis)
- Tropical pulmonary eosinophilia

Life Cycle and Pathogenesis The adult worm lives in the human lymph vessels, mates and produces millions of microscopic worms, also known as **microfilariae** (Fig. 8.28). Microfilariae circulate in the human blood and get transferred into the mosquito when it bites a person who is infected. They grow and develop inside the mosquito. When the mosquito bites another person, the larval worms pass from the mosquito into the human skin and travel to lodge in the lymph vessels. These larval worms grow into adult worms in a process that takes 6 months or more. An adult worm lives for about 5–7 years.

Symptoms result primarily from inflammatory reactions to the adult worms which damage the human host. Some people may also develop IgE-mediated hypersensitivity reactions to the small larval parasites (microfilariae)

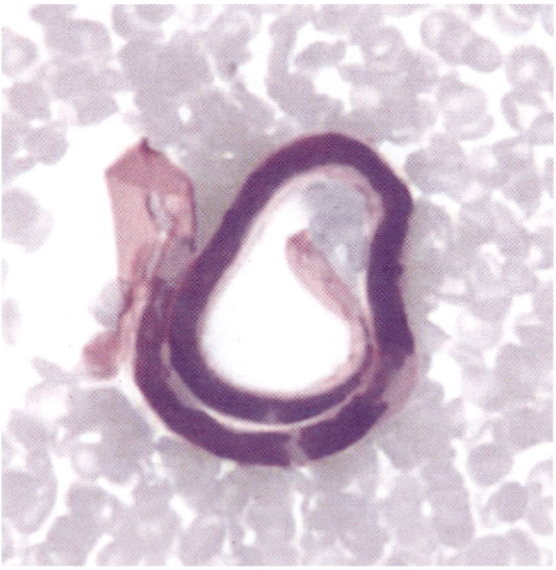

Fig. 8.28 Microfilaria of *Brugia* in the peripheral smear. (*Source:* From Omar Lupi, Christopher Downing, Michael Lee, et al. Mucocutaneous manifestations of helminth infections Nematodes. Journal of the American Academy of Dermatology. Elsevier. 2015.)

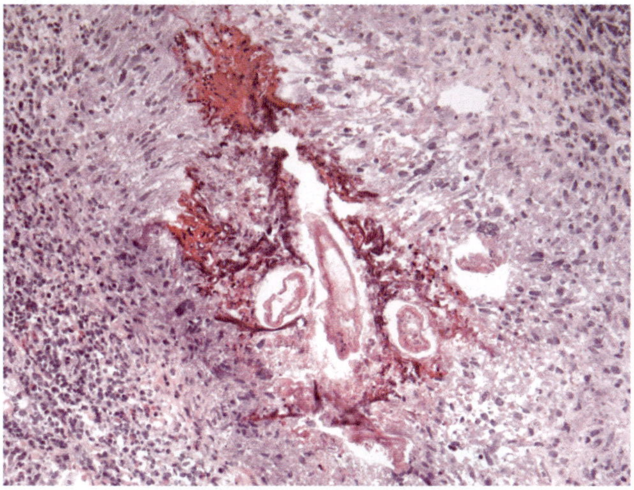

Fig. 8.29 Low power shows an adult worm surrounded by palisading granulomatous inflammation. (*Source:* From Judith A. Ferry. Diagnostic Pathology of Infectious Disease. Elsevier. 2018.)

as in **tropical pulmonary eosinophilia.** IgE and eosinophils are stimulated by IL-4 and IL-5 and secreted as a part of the T_H2-cell response. There is also a granuloma formation seen around the parasites which is part of the T_H1-mediated immune response.

Morphology

In the lymph nodes, the live, dead or calcified worms may be surrounded by (1) mild inflammation, (2) **eosinophilia** with haemorrhage and fibrin deposition and (3) **granuloma** (Fig. 8.29). Those who develop the chronic stages of elephantiasis are usually free from microfilariae (amicrofilaraemic).

Clinical Features The most obvious symptom of lymphatic filariasis is **elephantiasis** – oedema with thickening of the skin and underlying tissues along with persistent lymphoedema, subcutaneous fibrosis and epithelial hyperkeratosis. Elephantiasis results when the parasites lodge in the lymphatic system, obstructing the lymph flow.

Elephantiasis affects mainly the lower extremities, although the ears, mucous membranes and amputation stumps may also be affected. However, different species of filarial worms tend to affect different parts of the body; *W. bancrofti* can affect the legs, arms, vulva, breasts and scrotum (causing hydrocele formation), whereas *Brugia timori* rarely affects the genitals.

Prolonged untreated filariasis may have other complications, which may require surgical intervention, such as:

- Inflammatory: These include lymphangitis, cellulitis, abscess, focal spots, fibromyositis and sterility.
- Obstructive: These include elephantiasis (Fig. 8.30) of limbs and genitalia, chyluria and lymphatic varix of the spermatic cord.
- Allergic: The complications include urticaria, filarial fever and pruritis.

The rare lung involvement by microfilaria may present with eosinophilia and epithelioid granulomas around dead microfilaria (**Meyers–Kouwenaar bodies**).

Laboratory Investigations The diagnosis of filariasis requires examination of a blood smear using a finger-prick test for the presence of the larval round worm *W. bancrofti* or *B. malayi*. The number of parasites (parasitaemia) in the blood is higher during the night, so blood samples are best

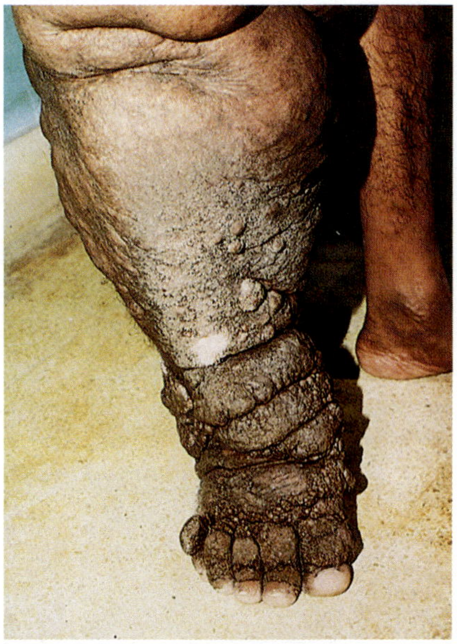

Fig. 8.30 Elephantiasis in filarial infection. (*Source:* From Karen M. Frank, Alexander J. McAdam. Robbins & Cotran Pathologic Basis of Disease. Elsevier. 2021.)

obtained at night. When parasites are not found in the blood, the adult worms may occasionally be found in a lymph node sample from an infected individual.

Onchocerciasis PA 10.4

Onchocerciasis, commonly known as '**river blindness**', is caused by the parasitic worm *Onchocerca volvulus*. It is transmitted to humans through exposure to repeated bites of infected **blackflies** of the genus *Simulium*. These blackflies breed along fast-flowing rivers and streams, causing blindness in people living near rivers, giving the name 'river blindness' to the disease. It is the leading cause of preventable blindness in sub-Saharan Africa. More than 99% of infected people live in African countries.

Clinical Features Onchocerciasis is an **eye and skin** disease. Symptoms are caused by the microfilariae, which move around the human body in the subcutaneous tissue where they mate. This elicits an intense inflammatory response in which the organism is surrounded by mixed infiltrate of inflammatory cells with fibrin and giant cells, producing a characteristic nodule (**onchocercoma**). Infected people may show symptoms such as severe itching.

Skin changes include pigmentation along with chronic itchy dermatitis and scaling that result in a '**leopard skin**' or '**elephant skin**' appearance. There may be thinning of the skin with loss of elasticity, which gives the skin a '**cigarette-paper**' appearance and can contribute to conditions such as '**hanging groin**', which is a sac of atrophic skin containing sclerosed inguinal or femoral lymph nodes. This condition predisposes to hernia.

Infected people may also develop eye lesions which can lead to visual impairment and permanent blindness. It begins as punctate keratitis with small opacities, caused by degenerating microfilariae which evoke an eosinophilic infiltrate. This is followed by sclerosing keratitis (Fig. 8.31) which is sometimes accelerated on the usage of antifilarial drugs – **Mazzotti reaction**.

Laboratory Investigations

- The gold standard test is the skin snip biopsy. The biopsy is performed using a sclerocorneal biopsy punch or by elevating a small cone of the skin (3 mm in diameter) with a needle and shaving 2 mg of tissue off with a scalpel which can be placed under a microscope to view the parasite.
- Nodulectomy of skin nodules can be performed to observe the microfilariae in the specimen.
- Slit lamp eye test can be performed in patients with ocular infections.

The recommended treatment is ivermectin. Ivermectin kills the larvae and prevents them from causing damage, but it does not kill the adult worm. Hence, it should be given every 6 months for the life span of the adult worms (i.e. 10–15 years) or for as long as the infected person has evidence of skin or eye infection. There is a promising treatment using doxycycline that kills the adult worms by killing the *Wolbachia* bacteria on which the adult worms depend to survive.

Cysticercosis PA 10.2

Human cysticercosis is caused by the egg form of *Taenia solium* (also called pork tapeworm), which is transmitted through the oral–faecal route. The pork tapeworm is particularly common in Asia, sub-Saharan Africa and Latin America. It is most prevalent where humans live in close contact with pigs.

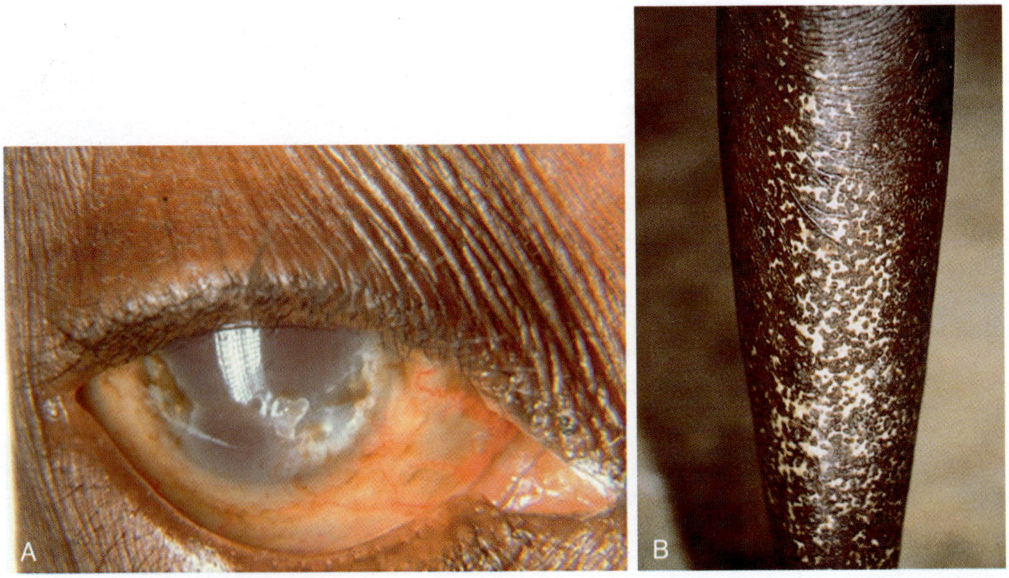

Fig. 8.31 Onchocerciasis, eye manifestation sclerosing keratitis (A) and leopard appearance of skin (B). (*Source:* From Wayne Grayson, Eduardo Calonje. Mckee's Pathology of the Skin. Elsevier. 2020. From Thomas B. Nutman. Hunter's Tropical Medicine and Emerging Infectious Diseases. Elsevier. 2020.)

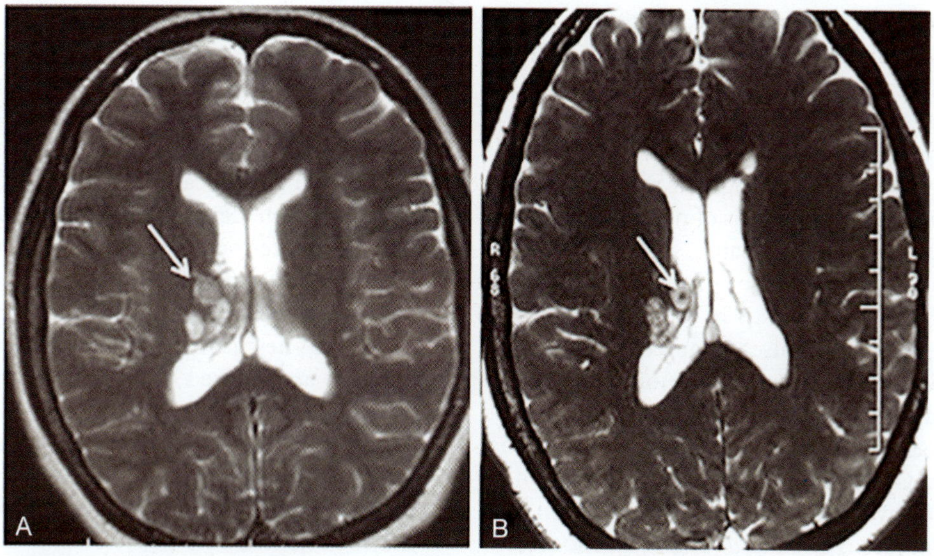

Fig. 8.32 Magnetic resonance image of a person with neurocysticercosis showing many cysts (arrow in A) and a scolex within the cyst (arrow in B) within the brain. (*Source:* From Samir Noujaim, Lawrence Bahoura, Daniel L. Noujaim, Marie Tominna. Neuroradiology. Elsevier. 2019.)

Pathogenesis Infection of humans may be due to ingestion of larvae or eggs by consuming contaminated water or food.

- Ingestion of larval cysts leads to attachment of cysts to the small intestine wall and development into adult tapeworms in about 2 months. This causes mild abdominal symptoms but does not cause cysticercosis.
- Ingestion of eggs leads to its hatching in the intestine to release larvae. The larvae penetrate the gut, enter the bloodstream and invade host tissues, where they encyst and cause cysticercosis. The viable cysts produce *taeniaestatin* and *paramyosin*, which help to evade the immune system and thereby tend to remain asymptomatic. Death of the cyst evokes an inflammatory response in the host, damaging the tissues.

Clinical Features It can affect any organ, but its significant manifestations are seen in the muscles, brain, eyes and skin. The initial host reaction is often avoided through the encystment of the larvae, but degenerating cysts release larval antigens that produce a vigorous host response and cause the clinically apparent syndrome through inflammatory mediators and surrounding oedema.

- **Muscles:** Cysticerci can develop in any voluntary muscle. Invasion of the muscle can cause inflammation of the muscle, with fever and eosinophilia, which starts as muscle swelling and later progresses to atrophy and scarring. In most cases, it is asymptomatic because the cysticerci die and become calcified.
- **Nervous system: Neurocysticercosis** (Fig. 8.32) causes symptoms such as headache and increased intracranial pressure, but the precise location of the cysts, which may be intraparenchymal, attached to the arachnoid or freely floating in the ventricular system, decides the specific symptoms and prognosis. The cysts are ovoid and white to opalescent, mostly grape-sized and contain an invaginated scolex with hooklets that are bathed in clear cyst fluid (Fig. 8.33). The cyst wall is thick and does not evoke host inflammatory response when it is intact. When cysts degenerate, the inflammatory response causes focal scarring and calcifications, which may be distinguished by radiography.
- **Eyes:** In some cases, cysticerci may be found in the eyeball, extraocular muscles and under the conjunctiva (*subconjunctiva*) and may cause visual difficulties.

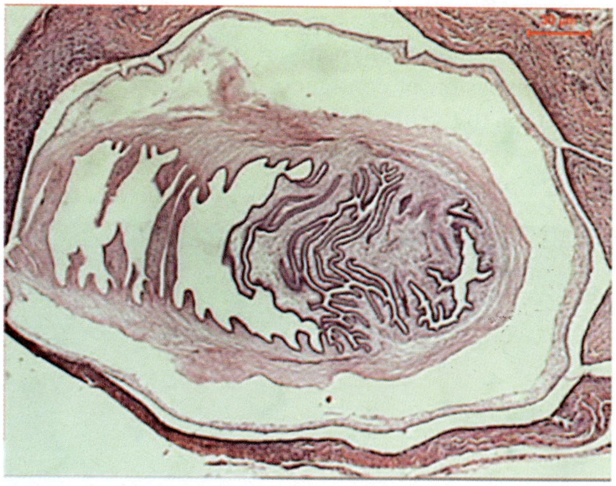

Fig. 8.33 Microscopically, duct-like invaginations, lined by double-layered eosinophilic membrane, are seen in the larval form in a case of oral cysticercosis. (*Source:* From Durgashankar Meena, Mayank Gupta, Vijay Kumar Jain, Rajendra Kumar Arya. Isolated intramuscular cysticercosis: Clinicopathological features, diagnosis and management – A review. Journal of Clinical Orthpaedics and Trauma. Elsevier. 2016. From Ana Carolina Prado Ribeiro, Maria Cecília Luvizotto, Ana Maria Pires Soubhia, Alvimar Lima de Castro. Oral cysticercosis: case report. Oral Surgery, Oral Medicine, Oral Pathology, Oral Radiology, and Endodontology. Elsevier. 2007.)

- **Skin:** *Subcutaneous* cysts are in the form of firm, mobile nodules, occurring mainly on the trunk and extremities. Subcutaneous nodules may be painful.

Laboratory Investigations The diagnosis may be made by aspiration of the cyst. CT or magnetic resonance imaging (MRI) is useful in the diagnosis of neurocysticercosis. Eosinophilia is also a useful indicator.

Hydatid Disease PA 10.4

Echinococcosis is a parasitic disease caused by tapeworms of the *Echinococcus* type. Humans are infected through ingestion of parasite eggs present in the contaminated food, water or soil or after direct contact with animal hosts like dogs. **Cystic echinococcosis**, also known as hydatid disease or hydatidosis, is caused by infection with the species *Echinococcus granulosus* and is the most common type of echinococcosis.

Life Cycle and Pathogenesis After being ingested, the egg develops into a larval oncosphere, which penetrates the intestinal mucosa and enters the portal circulation or lymphatics. Once it reaches the target organ, it forms a rounded, multinucleated mass that becomes cystic and progressively enlarges. Hydatid cysts grow slowly, about 1 mm in diameter per month. The development of morbidity is related to several factors including the number, size, site and stage of cyst development, host reaction and pressure effects of the cyst on adjacent tissues. Erosion of cysts into the biliary or bronchial trees can cause obstruction. Cysts can get infected and form bacterial abscesses. Ruptured cysts may cause severe allergic reactions including anaphylaxis and may lead to seeding of daughter cysts to other organs. Alveolar hydatid disease carries a high mortality without surgery, because of liver failure, invasion of contiguous structures or sometimes metastasis to the brain.

Morphology

The most common organ affected is the liver, followed by lungs. The cysts in echinococcosis are spherical, consisting of one compartment, and are usually filled with a clear fluid – called hydatid fluid. Later, multiple septations can develop. Microscopically, the hydatid cyst or metacestode consists of an outer, opaque, non-nucleated laminated external cuticle and an inner, nucleated, germinal layer that gives rise to brood capsules containing new larvae called protoscolices. These cyst contents are referred to as '**hydatid sand**' (Fig. 8.34). The outer wall may be surrounded by dense granulomatous inflammation composed of a zone of fibroblasts, giant cells and mononuclear and eosinophilic cells from the host inflammatory reaction. Later, these may be replaced by a dense fibrous capsule. Microcalcifications and necrotic cavitation may be present.

Clinical Features The disease often starts without symptoms and may last for years. The symptoms and signs that occur depend on the location and size of cysts. Hydatid disease usually begins in the liver but can spread to other parts of the body, such as the lungs or brain. When the liver is affected, the person may have abdominal pain, hepatomegaly, cholestasis, biliary cirrhosis, portal hypertension and ascites. Lung disease may cause cough, dyspnoea, haemoptysis and pleuritis.

Laboratory Investigations One of the most common ways to diagnose hydatid disease is to look for the presence of asymptomatic cysts. Many asymptomatic cysts can be located using **ultrasound imaging** apart from CT and MRI.

Serological tests like **immunoblot**, **indirect haemagglutination test** (IHA) and **ELISA** are also useful. These

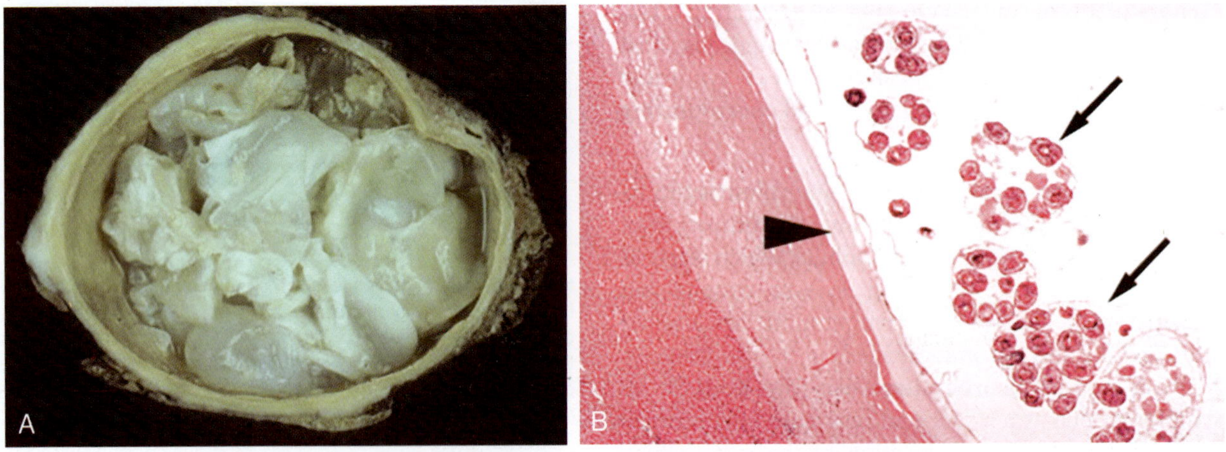

Fig. 8.34 Gross image of hydatid cyst filled with daughter cysts (A) and the cross-section of a hydatid cyst in the liver showing an outer laminated layer (arrowhead) and internal brood capsules (arrows) filled with protoscolices (B). (*Source:* From Bernhard Stamm, Marcela Fejgl, Cornelia Hueber. Satellite cysts and biliary fistulas in hydatid liver disease. A retrospective study of 17 liver resections. Human Pathology. Elsevier. 2008.)

tests are 80%–100% effective with liver cysts, but only 50%–60% effective when cysts are located in other organs.

Strongyloidiasis PA 10.4

Strongyloidiasis is caused by the nematode called *Strongyloides stercoralis*. It is more common in the tropics, subtropics and warm temperate regions.

Life Cycle and Pathogenesis The worms live in the soil and infect humans when larvae penetrate the skin, enter the circulation, travel to the lungs (**Loffler syndrome**) and then travel to the trachea to be swallowed. In the small intestine, the larvae moult twice and become adult female worms which further produce eggs that yield rhabditiform larvae. The rhabditiform larvae can either be passed in the stool or cause autoinfection.

In some people, particularly those with organ transplantation, lymphoma, HIV or immunosuppressive medications, *Strongyloides* can cause a **hyperinfection syndrome** which affects the CNS and can lead to death if untreated. The diagnosis is made by blood and stool tests. Another feature of *Strongyloides* is autoinfection in which these autoinfective larvae penetrate the wall of the ileum or colon or the skin of the perianal region, enter the circulation to reach the lungs and repeat the cycle.

Morphology

Many adult worms, larvae and eggs are found in the crypts of the duodenum and ileum, with eosinophilic infiltrate in the lamina propria (Fig. 8.35). On hyperinfection, the worms penetrate the lymphatics and blood vessels along with mononuclear infiltrate. Adult female worms approximately 2 mm in length may be seen and are found within the crypts. The mucosa may resemble pseudomembranous colitis.

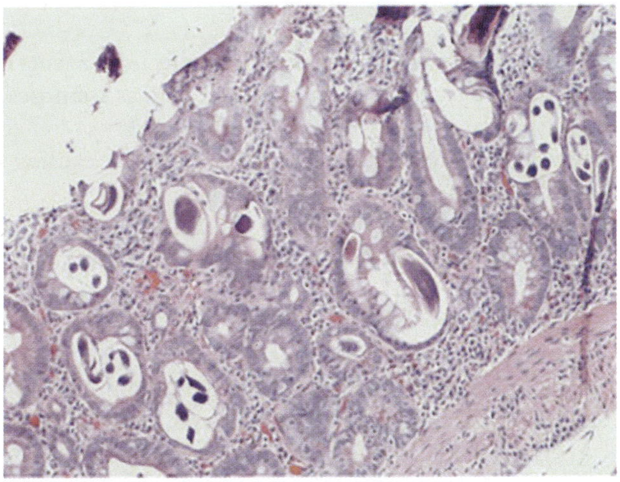

Fig. 8.35 Active inflammation and *Strongyloides* eggs, larvae and adult worms. (*Source:* From Pierre Hindy, Russell Parvin, Kayane Hanna, Frank Gress. Gastrointestinal Endoscopy. Elsevier. 2011.)

Clinical Features Uncomplicated disease: Frequently, infected persons are asymptomatic. In certain cases, mild symptoms may appear, which are listed as follows:

- GI symptoms: Abdominal pain and diarrhoea/constipation
- Pulmonary symptoms (Loffler syndrome): Fever, cough and dyspnoea due to pulmonary infiltrate
- Dermatological manifestations: Urticarial rashes in the buttocks and waist areas as well as larva currens; eosinophilia generally present

Laboratory Investigations The gold standard for diagnosis is demonstrating the organism in stool, sputum or other infected body fluid or tissue.

Treatment includes elimination of the organism by using antihelminthic drugs, *ivermectin* being the most effective.

Schistosomiasis PA 10.4

Schistosomiasis, also known as **snail fever** and **bilharzia**, is a disease caused by parasitic flatworms called schistosomes. The disease is spread by contact with fresh water contaminated with the parasites released from infected **freshwater snails**. High-risk groups include children, farmers, fishermen and people using unclean water.

The common species are the following:

- *Schistosoma mansoni* and *S. japonicum* which affect the liver and the gut, with hepatic cirrhosis being the most common cause of death
- *S. haematobium* causing chronic granulomatous bladder inflammation that may present as haematuria, obstructive uropathy and carcinoma

Life Cycle and Pathogenesis *Schistosoma* eggs are eliminated from humans in faeces or urine. Under appropriate conditions, the eggs hatch and release miracidia, which swim and penetrate specific **snail** intermediate hosts. On release of cercariae from the snail, the infective cercariae swim, penetrate the skin of the human host and shed their forked tails, becoming schistosomulae. The schistosomulae migrate via venous circulation to the lungs, from there to the heart, then develop in the liver and finally exit the liver via the portal vein system when mature. Male and female adult worms copulate and reside in the mesenteric venules, causing inflammation and spreading the infection.

Intestinal schistosomiasis

- Eggs become lodged in the intestinal wall and cause an immune system reaction called a *granulomatous reaction*. This immune response can lead to obstruction of the colon and blood loss and is seen externally as potbelly.
- Eggs can migrate and become lodged in the liver, leading to hepatic fibrosis and portal hypertension.

Morphology

Organism	Morphology
Early *S. mansoni* or *S. japonicum* infections	Gross morphology shows white, pinhead-sized granulomas in the gut and liver Microscopy reveals *Schistosoma* eggs containing miracidium surrounded by granuloma
Late *S. mansoni* or *S. japonicum* infections	Colon: Patches and pseudopolyps Liver: Irregular surface with cut surface showing fibrosis, granulomas but no regenerating nodules Lung: Granulomatous pulmonary arteritis Kidney: Mesangioproliferative, membranous glomerulopathy
S. haematobium	Inflammatory cystitis with granulomas and mucosal erosions Fibrosis of the ureteral wall, leading to obstruction and hydronephrosis Predisposes to squamous cell carcinoma of the bladder

Clinical Features If symptoms do appear, they usually take 4–6 weeks from the time of infection. Severe hepatic fibrosis is a serious manifestation of chronic schistosomiasis. Within 12 hours of infection, tingling sensation or light rash mimicking scabies, commonly referred to as '*swimmer's itch*', may occur because of irritation at the point of entrance. A total of 2–10 weeks later, the patient may develop fever, aches, cough, diarrhoea, chills or gland enlargement.

Laboratory Investigations and Management Diagnosis is by finding eggs of the parasite in a person's urine or stool. It can also be confirmed by finding antibodies against the disease in the blood.

Praziquantel, a prescription medication, is the drug of choice to treat infections caused by all schistosome species.

EMERGING INFECTIOUS DISEASES

Emerging infectious diseases are infections that have recently appeared within a population or those whose incidence or geographic range is rapidly increasing or threatens to increase in the near future. Emerging infections can be caused by the following:

- Previously undetected or unknown infectious agents
- Known agents that have spread to new geographic locations or new populations
- Previously known agents whose role in specific diseases has previously gone unrecognized
- Re-emergence of agents whose incidence of disease had significantly declined in the past but now has reappeared (this class of diseases is known as **re-emerging infectious diseases**)

WHO warned in its 2007 report that infectious diseases are emerging at a rate that has not been seen before. Since the 1970s, about 40 infectious diseases have been discovered, including SARS, MERS, Ebola, chikungunya, avian flu, swine flu, Zika and most recently a new COVID-19 pandemic caused by a new strain of coronavirus.

People now are travelling much more frequently and far greater distances than in the past, are living in more densely populated areas and often are coming into closer contact with wild animals. This increases the potential for emerging infectious diseases to spread rapidly and cause global epidemics.

In addition, there is a potential for diseases to emerge because of deliberate introduction into human, animal or plant populations for terrorist purposes, as discussed in the section 'Agents of bioterrorism'. These diseases include anthrax, smallpox and tularaemia.

FACTORS IN THE EMERGENCE OR RE-EMERGENCE OF INFECTIOUS DISEASES

For an emerging disease to become established, at least two events must occur:

1. The infectious agent must be introduced into a vulnerable population.
2. The agent must have the ability to spread readily from person to person and cause disease and sustain itself within a population.

There are many factors involved in the emergence of new infectious diseases or the re-emergence of 'old' infectious diseases (Table 8.3).

- Some result from natural processes such as the evolution of pathogens over time, but many are a result of **human behaviour** and practices like population growth, migration from rural areas to cities, international air travel, poverty, wars and destructive ecological changes due to economic development and land use.
- Many emerging diseases arise when infectious agents in animals are passed to humans (referred to as **zoonoses**). As the human density increases, the possibility of contact between humans and animals also increases, causing a serious threat.
- **Climate change** is increasingly becoming a concern as a factor in the emergence of infectious diseases. As the earth's climate warms and habitats are altered, diseases can spread into new geographic areas. For example, warming temperatures allow mosquitoes – and the diseases transmitted by them – to expand their range into regions where they previously have not been found.
- **Antimicrobial resistance** occurs because of the acquired resistance of pathogens to antimicrobial medications such as antibiotics. Bacteria, viruses and other microorganisms can change over time and develop

Table 8.3 Factors That Contribute to the Emergence of New Diseases

Factor of Emergence	Example
Microbial adaptation	Genetic drift and shift in influenza A.
Climate change	Diseases transmitted by animal vectors such as mosquitoes (e.g. West Nile fever) are moving further from the tropics as the climate warms.
Economic development	Use of antibiotics to increase meat yield of farmed cows leads to antibiotic resistance.
Changes in human demographics and travel facilitating rapid global spread	SARS-related coronaviruses.
Bioterrorism	Anthrax attacks.
Indiscriminate land use	Dam construction and irrigation systems can encourage malaria and other mosquito-borne diseases.
Use of indiscriminate pesticides	Industrial farming reduces/eliminates biological controls (e.g. dragonflies, amphibians, insectivorous birds, spiders) of known disease vectors (e.g. mosquito, tick, biting midge).
Wildlife trade	This has been linked to zoonotic emergence and spread of new infectious diseases in humans. Crowded and unhygienic wet markets and wildlife farms have been implicated in animal-to-human transmission of emergent viruses, including novel coronaviruses and influenza viruses. Complex issues surrounding the commerce and consumption of bushmeat are also of particular concern.

resistance to the drugs used to treat diseases caused by the pathogens. Examples include MRSA and vancomycin-resistant enterococci.

- **Decline in vaccine coverage:** Even in the presence of safe and effective vaccines, many people choose not to get vaccinated. This has been a particular problem with the measles vaccine. Measles, a highly contagious and serious infection that was eliminated from the United States in 2000 and from the Western Hemisphere in 2016, has returned in certain areas because of an increase in the number of people opting for vaccine exemptions. This has been driven by an anti-vaccine movement that was founded largely on an invalid and discredited study that claimed a link between a vaccine against measles and autism. As a result of the decline in vaccine coverage, measles cases are highest by far this decade, with more than 1000 cases of measles reported in the United States in the first half of 2019.

Agents of Bioterrorism As technologies for genetically modifying organisms have advanced and become more accessible, it has become easier and less expensive to alter the genetic makeup of viruses and bacteria. The potential for misuse of synthetic biology capabilities increases and expands the threat of bioweapons. The tools could be used for the creation of pathogenic microorganisms or the modification of existing microorganisms to make them more dangerous. These agents are categorized into three, on the basis of the degree of threat to human beings (Table 8.4).

The development of vaccines, antimicrobial drugs and the proven eradication of smallpox have created hope and a broader field of research for the infectious diseases to be controlled or even eliminated. However, the current realization that infectious diseases continue to emerge and re-emerge (including the possibility of bioterrorism) underscores the challenges ahead in infectious disease research.

SPECIAL TECHNIQUES FOR DIAGNOSIS OF INFECTIOUS DISEASES

Identification of infectious agents has always been considered a domain of microbiologists. But the role pathologists play is far more significant and important. Isolation of microorganism can help us to identify its presence, but the role of that microorganism in the current pathogenesis cannot be implicated. It is like capturing the murder convict but not able to prove his or her involvement because of lack of evidence. The role of a pathologist now is akin to a public prosecutor who provides the appropriate evidence linking the culprit to the murder scene. Demonstration of tissue destruction and inflammatory response to the microorganism is the only way to differentiate a commensal from an infectious agent and implicate it in the current disease process. Considering this, it is also prudent to be aware that in certain situations such as in TB, the sensitivity and specificity of identifying the organism by histochemical

Table 8.4 Definition of Potential Bioterrorism Agent Categories

Category A	Category B	Category C
Pose the highest risk to national security	Pose the second highest risk to national security	Emerging pathogens that could be engineered for mass dissemination
Can be easily disseminated or transmitted from person to person	Are moderately easy to disseminate	Are easily produced and disseminated
Have high mortality rates with potential to cause public panic and social disruption	Produce moderate morbidity but low mortality	Have the potential for high morbidity and mortality rates and a major health impact
Require special public health preparedness actions	Require enhanced diagnostic capacity and disease surveillance	
Examples include *Bacillus anthracis* (anthrax), variola major (smallpox) and *Yersinia pestis* (plague)	Examples include *Brucella* sp. (brucellosis), *Vibrio cholerae* (cholera) and *Coxiella burnetii* (Q fever)	Examples include hantavirus, Nipah virus and yellow fever

stains may be low. Hence, a combined approach should be followed to conclude the diagnosis.

The role of a pathologist in the diagnosis of infection is as follows:

- Establish morphological diagnosis of infection
- Assess immunocompetence of the host
- Narrow the differential diagnosis of possible pathogens
- Confirm results of microbiological cultures
- Evaluate the relevance of microbiological cultures
- Establish diagnosis unrelated to infection
- Identify concomitant infection in a primary inflammatory or neoplastic disorder
- Identify new pathogens

The techniques to be used by a surgical pathologist include the following:

- Patterns of inflammation
- Histochemical staining
- Immunohistochemical staining
- Molecular diagnosis
- In situ hybridization (ISH)

Patterns of inflammation: The patterns of inflammation, already studied in Chapter 2, give a clue to the type of organism likely to have caused it. The common patterns are enumerated in Table 8.5.

Table 8.5 Patterns of Inflammation and Their Common Causative Organisms

Type of Inflammation	Example
Exudative inflammation	Pyogenic bacteria
Necrotizing inflammation	Gram-negative bacteria, amoebiasis
Granulomatous inflammation	Mycobacteria, fungi
Histiocytic inflammation	*Rhodococcus*, *Legionella*, Whipple disease
Eosinophilic inflammation	Fungi, parasites
Cytopathic changes	Viruses
No response	Host anergy

HISTOCHEMICAL STAINS

Although routine staining with haematoxylin and eosin (H&E) may stain the organisms, special stains make them clearly visible and easily identifiable in tissues and fluids. Moreover, the density of the organisms determines the ability to identify them in the microscopic sections. In case of viruses, the cytopathic changes enable their identification more than the virus per se. The commonly used special stains are given in Table 8.6.

IMMUNOHISTOCHEMICAL STAINS

Recently, many immunostains using antibodies directed against microbial antigens have been identified (Table 8.7). Some are available widely, but many are now available only in referral centres for infectious diseases. These immunostains help to identify the organism with accuracy, but the possibility of cross-reactivity of antibodies between organisms should be borne in mind.

MOLECULAR DIAGNOSIS

Nucleic acid–based tests aim to identify the DNA/RNA of the organism. Nowadays, these tests are of great importance in the diagnosis and management of viral infection.

Most nucleic acid–based tests are designed to identify the presence of a microorganism (called **qualitative testing**) and are more sensitive than all the earlier mentioned tests. However, for certain infections, such as HIV infection and hepatitis C, tests are available to measure the

Table 8.6 Special Stains for Organisms

Organism	Stains Used
Viruses	
Cytomegalovirus	H&E (intranuclear and cytoplasmic inclusions); IHC; PAS and GMS (intracytoplasmic inclusions)
Herpesvirus	H&E (intranuclear inclusions); IHC
Measles virus	H&E (intranuclear inclusions, polykaryons)
Respiratory syncytial virus	H&E (polykaryons); IHC
Parainfluenza virus	H&E (intracytoplasmic inclusions)
Bacteria	
Gram-positive, Gram-negative, *Nocardia*, actinomycetes	Tissue Gram, GMS (all)
Legionella	Silver impregnation
Mycobacteria tuberculosis	Ziehl–Neelsen; PCR
Atypical mycobacteria	Modified Ziehl–Neelsen, PCR
Fungi	
Histoplasma	GMS, PAS
Cryptococcus	H&E, GMS, PAS, mucicarmine; Fontana, IHC
Blastomyces	H&E, GMS, PAS, mucicarmine (weak)
Coccidiomyces	H&E, GMS, PAS
Candida	H&E, GMS, PAS, Gram stain; IHC
Aspergillus	H&E, GMS, PAS, IHC
Parasites	
Protozoa	H&E, PAS, Gram stain (microsporidia); IHC (*Toxoplasma*)
Metazoans	H&E, trichrome stain
Echinococcus	GMS in chitinous wall, modified Ziehl–Neelsen (hooklets)

H&E, haematoxylin and eosin; PCR, polymerase chain reaction.

Table 8.7 Infectious Agents for Which Immunostains Are Available

Fungi	Viruses and Bacteria
Aspergillus (genus only)	Herpesvirus 1 (cross-reacts with herpesvirus 2)
Cryptococcus	Varicella zoster
Histoplasma	Cytomegalovirus
Candida spp.	Respiratory syncytial virus
Coccidioides immitis	Actinomycetes
Pneumocystis jirovecii	Epstein–Barr (Epstein–Barr-encoded RNA)

amount of genetic material that is present (**called quantitative testing**) to determine the severity of the infection. Quantitative tests can also be used to monitor response to treatment and reactivation of infection. These tests also help to check the microorganisms for genes or gene mutations that make the microorganism resistant to a drug and in identification of new strains.

The commonly used methods are ISH and PCR. ISH is widely used in the identification of both HPV and the strain in Pap smears. The presence of high-risk strains in cervical biopsies showing dysplasia guides the management plan. PCR is the most sensitive method available to identify organisms because it can amplify the genetic material and make them easily detectable.

Other tests used to identify microorganisms are as follows:

- Tissue microarray
- Confocal microscopy
- Laser capture microdissection (LCM)
- In situ PCR assay
- Proteomics

These tests are described in detail in Chapter 12, 'Advanced Diagnostic Techniques'.

SELF-ASSESSMENT

Multiple Choice Questions

1. Members of the herpesvirus family have been linked to several human diseases. Which of the following conditions is not caused by viruses from the herpes family?
   A. Cervical intraepithelial neoplasia (CIN) III
   B. Chickenpox
   C. Infectious mononucleosis
   D. Kaposi sarcoma
2. The life cycle of the malarial parasite in humans is made up of a number of stages. Which of the following options describes the correct sequence of events?
   A. Sporozoite injection, merozoite release, ring-stage trophozoite production, growth into schizonts and erythrocytic schizogony
   B. Growth into schizonts, sporozoite injection, erythrocytic schizogony, ring-stage trophozoite production and merozoite release

C. Sporozoite injection, growth into schizonts, merozoite release, ring-stage trophozoite production and erythrocytic schizogony
D. Merozoite release, erythrocytic schizogony, growth into schizonts, ring-stage trophozoite production and sporozoite injection

3. Helminths are eukaryotic parasitic worms that live in and obtain nutrients from their hosts. Which of the following options is not a transmission route for helminths?
A. Faeco-oral transmission
B. Active transmission
C. Primary transmission
D. Bite

4. Which of the following conditions is most likely to be affecting a 15-year-old girl who is otherwise completely healthy and has recently started dating her first boyfriend?
A. Leishmaniasis
B. Infectious mononucleosis
C. Lymphoma
D. Myelofibrosis

5. A 30-year-old man, an intravenous drug user, reports recent onset of weakness and visual problems. On examination, you notice leucoplakia on the tongue and spots of candidiasis on the buccal membranes, making you suspect immunocompromise. Which of the following conditions is most likely to be affecting this patient?
A. Devic disease
B. Charcot–Marie–Tooth disease
C. Tabes dorsalis
D. Progressive multifocal leukoencephalitis

6. A 30-year-old Mexican presents with dysphagia for solid foods, odynophagia, recurrent hiccups and regurgitation. Imaging studies of the upper gastrointestinal tract show accentuated dilation of the oesophagus with irregular motility and a hypertonic gastroesophageal sphincter compatible with achalasia. Serological tests show high titres of IgG antibodies directed against *Trypanosoma cruzi*. Which of the following strategies allows *T. cruzi* to evade intracellular cytolytic activity?
A. Avoidance of phagolysosome fusion
B. Escape from the phagosome
C. Resistance to lysosomal enzyme
D. Avoidance of phagolysosome acidification

7. A 35-year-old man reports symptoms of rhinitis. In a smear taken from his nostrils, the presence of *Staphylococcus epidermidis* is detected. Which of the following measures should be taken?
A. Nasal lavage with saline serum
B. No treatment required
C. Methicillin resistance test
D. Rifampicin treatment of people who have had contact with the patient

8. Indicate the biological effect of M protein as a bacterial virulence factor:
A. Activation of adenylate cyclase
B. Activation of cytokine production
C. Binding
D. Invasion

9. Which organism produces the disease known as melioidosis?
A. *Pseudomonas aeruginosa*
B. *Stenotrophomonas maltophilia*
C. *Burkholderia mallei*
D. *Burkholderia pseudomallei*

10. A rabbit breeder has a large ulcerous lesion on the back of the hand, lymphadenopathy, fever, chills and general malaise. Possible tularaemia is suspected. Which of the following virulence mechanisms is characteristic of the infection-causing microorganism?
A. Production of A–B toxin
B. Production of β-lactamase
C. Intracellular growth
D. Lipooligosaccharide release

11. Which of the following microorganisms is correctly associated with its transmission medium?
A. *Bacillus cereus*: Eggs
B. *Brucella*: Smoked meat
C. *Salmonella*: Shellfish
D. *Listeria monocytogenes*: Ice cream

12. Which of the following parameters is most important in determining whether a virus is transmitted in aerosols?
A. Structure of the shell
B. Structure of the genome
C. Host cell
D. Lytic virus release

13. The herpes simplex virus can counteract the action of protein kinase R and reactivate protein synthesis to resist the action of which of the following cellular factors produced by the infected cell?
A. IFN-α
B. IL-1
C. IL-12
D. TNF-β

14. Which of the following options does the term viral tropism refer to?
A. Attraction of viral particles by specific tissue types in the host
B. Attachment of viral particles to certain transmitting molecules (e.g. blood cells) to promote the infectious spread of the virus
C. Recognition and binding of a virus to a limited number of host cells, infecting some tissues but not others
D. Attraction of viral particles by specific host types

15. Paroxysmal fever, chills and rigor occur when:
A. Hepatocyte ruptures and releases merozoites
B. Latent hypnozoites live in the liver
C. Merozoites enter RBC
D. Merozoites are released into blood by rupture of RBC

16. The genetic mutation that is disastrous for malarial infection is:
A. Sickle cell heterozygote
B. Homozygous sickle cell disease
C. G6PD-deficient female carriers
D. α thalassaemia carrier

17. The most serious manifestation of cysticercosis is because of:
A. Larvae attaching to the gut wall
B. Encystment in muscles
C. Encystment in CNS
D. Malnutrition

18. The pattern of disease in leprosy is determined by:
A. Pathogenicity of infecting bacteria
B. Antibody response of the host
C. Helper T lymphocyte response
D. Toxin produced by *M. leprae*

19. Identify the true statement with respective to lepromatous leprosy:
A. It causes asymmetric skin lesions.
B. Nerves are enclosed by granulomatous inflammation.
C. The host helper 1 response is strong.

D. The skin biopsy shows lepra cells filled with masses of lepra bacilli.

20. The bacterial infection that causes pseudomembrane formation in the nasopharynx and oropharynx is:
    A. *S. pyogenes*
    B. *C. diphtheriae*
    C. *S. aureus*
    D. Tuberculosis
21. The important risk factor for the development of *Neisseria* infection is:
    A. Defect in complement proteins
    B. Young age
    C. Reduced antibody production
    D. Malnutrition
22. The characteristic morphological feature of syphilis seen in all stages of syphilis is:
    A. Granuloma formation
    B. Proliferative endarteritis
    C. Bacterial vasculitis with thrombosis and haemorrhage
    D. Necrotizing inflammatory lesions in skin and GI mucosa
23. Parasites transmitted by blood transfusion include all of the following, EXCEPT:
    A. *Trypanosoma cruzi*
    B. *Leishmania donovani*
    C. *Plasmodium malariae*
    D. *Loa loa*
24. Pseudohyphae are seen in:
    A. *Aspergillus*
    B. *Candida*
    C. Mucormycetes
    D. *Cryptococcus*
25. Cowdry type A intranuclear inclusions are seen in:
    A. Herpes simplex virus infection
    B. Poliovirus infection
    C. Cytomegalovirus infection
    D. Epstein–Barr virus infection

Answers

1. (A); 2. (C); 3. (C); 4. (B); 5. (D); 6. (B); 7. (B); 8. (C); 9. (D); 10. (C); 11. (D); 12. (C); 13. (A); 14. (C); 15. (D); 16. (B); 17. (C); 18. (C); 19. (D); 20. (B); 21. (A); 22. (B); 23. (D); 24. (B); 25. (A)

Scenario-Based Questions

1. An 8-year-old male child presented with evening rise of temperature. His father was treated for cough with expectoration for 6 months. On examination, there were palpable matted cervical lymph nodes. What is the probable diagnosis?
2. A 30-year-old male presents to OPD with rashes on his palms and soles for the past 5 days. He also gives a history of a painless ulcer on his penis a few weeks back which resolved spontaneously. He confesses to having multiple sexual partners. What is the probable diagnosis?
3. A 27-year-old male presents with a reddish patch over the left arm which is gradually increasing in size for the past 5 months. On examination, there is a single erythematous skin lesion on the left arm measuring 5 × 3 cm with decreased sensation. What is the probable diagnosis?
4. A 47-year-old post–renal transplant female presents to the emergency department with complaints of fever, progressive shortness of breath, cough and pleuritic chest pain for the past 2 days. She has productive cough with thick sputum tinged with blood. Sputum examination shows septate hyphae showing dichotomous branching at acute angles highlighted by silver stain. What is the causative organism?
5. A 57-year-old male is brought to the emergency department with headache, nausea and episodic vomiting for the past couple of days with dizziness, confusion and irritability. CSF examination shows organisms with clear halo around the cells with India ink stain. What is the causative organism?
6. A 39-year-old female presents with fever, aches, cough, diarrhoea and chills. She also has light itchy rashes over the legs. She gives a history of swimming in a lake few days back. Urine examination reveals presence of ova. What is the probable diagnosis?
7. A 40-year-old male was admitted with fever, chills and rigor for 3 days. He now has clouding of consciousness and passes dark-coloured urine. What is the probable diagnosis?
8. A 32-year-old female presents to OPD with fever and painful blisters and ulcers around the mouth. On examination, there are multiple vesicular eruption in the oral mucosa. What is the causative organism?
9. A 19-year-old male presents with complaints of fever, sore throat, generalized lymphadenopathy and splenomegaly. Peripheral smear examination shows activated atypical lymphocytes. What is the probable diagnosis?
10. A 20-year-old bone marrow transplant recipient presented with complaints of diarrhoea and abdominal pain. Colonoscopic biopsy showed large cells with prominent basophilic inclusions in the nucleus surrounded by a clear halo. What is the most likely organism?
11. Describe the morphology of a hydatid cyst.
12. What is bioterrorism?

Answers

1. Extrapulmonary tuberculosis.
2. Syphilis.
3. Leprosy.
4. *Aspergillus*.
5. *Cryptococcus*.
6. Schistosomiasis.
7. Cerebral malaria.
8. Herpes simplex virus.
9. Infectious mononucleosis.
10. Cytomegalovirus.

Topics for Self-Directed Learning

1. Infections transmitted by mosquitoes.
2. Infections transmitted by ticks and mites.
3. Organisms that are endemic in India that mandate vaccination of foreigners entering the Indian subcontinent.
4. Vaccines that are required to be taken by Indians for travel to Africa.
5. Trypanosomiasis.
6. Yellow fever.
7. Coronavirus and the pandemic of 2020.
8. Role of haemoglobinopathies in offering protection against malaria.

9 Environmental and Nutritional Disorders

Rajeswari Kathiah, Gayathri Devi Thanigaimani

PA 12.1 Enumerate and describe the pathogenesis of disorders caused by **air pollution, tobacco and alcohol.**
PA 12.2 Describe the pathogenesis of disorders caused by **protein–calorie malnutrition and starvation.**
PA 12.3 Describe the pathogenesis of **obesity** and its consequences.

CHAPTER OUTLINE

INTRODUCTION

Diseases that arise in humans because of exposure to harmful substances in their immediate environment are termed environmental diseases. These diseases can be caused by factors such as smoking, excessive alcohol consumption, and exposure to toxic elements in nature, like the mercury contamination experienced in Minamata Bay. Other sources include radiation from nuclear power plants and the aftermath of atomic bombings. A notable example from India is the Bhopal gas tragedy, which highlights the dangers of chemical exposure and hazardous environments.

On the other hand, diseases resulting from improper dietary habits are known as nutritional diseases. These conditions are more frequently observed in children and the elderly. Malnutrition, which affects approximately one in every seven people globally, is primarily driven by poverty.

In this chapter, we explore the prevalent diseases associated with environmental risks and nutritional imbalances, including both deficiencies and excesses.

ENVIRONMENTAL EFFECTS ON GLOBAL DISEASE BURDEN

The global disease burden, a comprehensive analysis initiated by the World Health Organization (WHO) in 1990, offers a detailed statistical assessment of disease incidence and their causes worldwide. It employs the metric of DALYs (disability-adjusted life years), combining years of life lost because of premature mortality and years lived with disability. The current trends in global health are as follows:

- There has been a marked increase in deaths from HIV/AIDS and related infections, along with a notable rise in fatalities from noncommunicable diseases, especially cancer. Emerging infectious diseases, including fungal infections and the recent COVID-19 pandemic, also pose significant health challenges. India's average life expectancy has impressively risen from 45 years in 1965 to approximately 70 years currently, nearing the life expectancy of developed countries, which ranges from 79 years in the United States to 81 years in the United Kingdom.

- Undernutrition remains the primary global health concern, leading to morbidity and premature deaths. It is responsible for nearly half of the mortality in children under 5 years in developing countries. Conversely, there is an escalating trend of childhood overweight and obesity in low- and middle-income countries, growing 30% faster than in developed nations.
- Cardiovascular diseases, including ischaemic heart disease, stroke, heart failure and peripheral arterial disease, are the foremost causes of global mortality and significantly diminish life quality.
- In developing countries, infectious diseases account for half of the top 10 causes of death. In 2008, around 8.8 million children younger than 5 years died, with half of these deaths occurring in sub-Saharan Africa as a result of pneumonia, diarrhoea, malaria, HIV/AIDS and measles. In addition, neonatal deaths from conditions like sepsis and tetanus in the first month of life constituted 7% of the fatalities, whereas malnutrition, exacerbating infections such as TB and meningitis, contributed to over one-third of all child deaths.

ENVIRONMENTAL POLLUTION

Humans have been causing damage to the environment in different ways. Land, water, air and noise pollution are among the significant ones. This behaviour of mankind has led to adverse effects on the health and safety of the ecosystem in the form of spread of infections, damage to various internal organs, climate change, melting of glaciers, increasing the global water levels, altering the quality of food produce, and many other effects. Xenobiotics are substances found in animals or humans that are foreign to them and are derived from some external source. Most pollutants act as xenobiotics and cause harm to animal and human life (Fig. 9.1). In this chapter, we review the impact of air pollution and metal pollution on the health of humans.

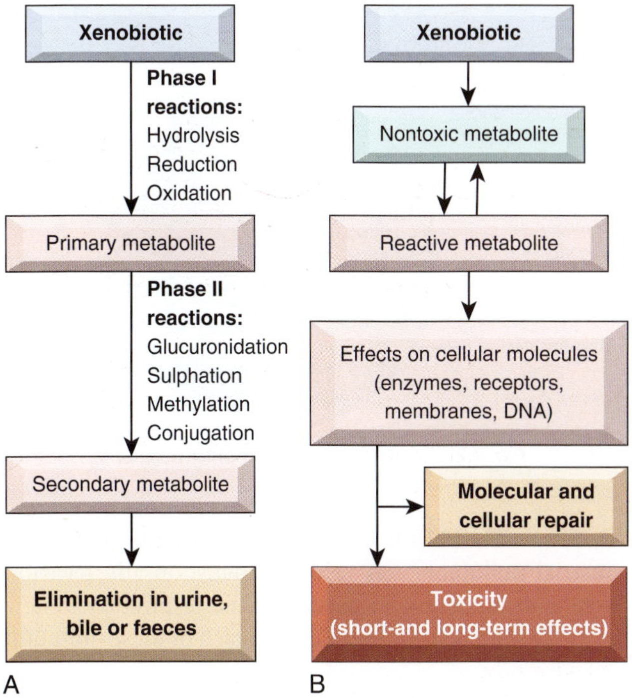

Fig. 9.1 Xenobiotic metabolism. **(A)** Xenobiotics can be metabolized to nontoxic metabolites and eliminated from the body (detoxification). **(B)** Xenobiotic metabolism may also result in the formation of a reactive metabolite that is toxic to cellular components. If repair is not effective, short- and long-term effects develop. (*Source:* Based on Hodgson E: A Textbook of Modern Toxicology, 3rd ed. Hoboken, NJ, Wiley, 2004.)

AIR POLLUTION PA 12.1

Air is an essential element of life. Atmosphere along with lithosphere and hydrosphere forms the biosphere, making life possible on earth. But humans, by the usage of vehicles, air conditioners, refrigerators, etc., have polluted and highly contaminated the air. Hence, organizations across the world are trying to save the environment, and are in the run for purification of air. Apart from the hazardous pollutants in air, microbes and organisms cause various diseases. In developing countries such as India, infectious diseases are the leading cause of illness and death, and these are caused by the transmission of organisms mostly through the air, i.e. airborne diseases.

The Pollutants and Types of Air Pollution (Fig. 9.2)

Over the decades, after the invention of fire around 300,000 years ago, burning has caused release of gases and pollutants into the atmosphere. This phenomenon multifolded when fossil fuels came into use. The pollutants have been changing over time because the substances being burnt also changed over time. The types of air pollutants include primary and secondary air pollutants. Primary pollutants are those that enter the atmosphere directly in the active form and cause harm. Examples are carbon oxides, nitrogen oxides, sulphur oxides, lead, particulate matter (PM) and volatile organic compounds. Secondary air pollutants are those that have undergone change after reaching the atmosphere because of sunlight or any other chemical reaction. Examples are ozone (its chemical reaction is interesting). Air pollution is studied by classifying it as indoor and outdoor air pollution.

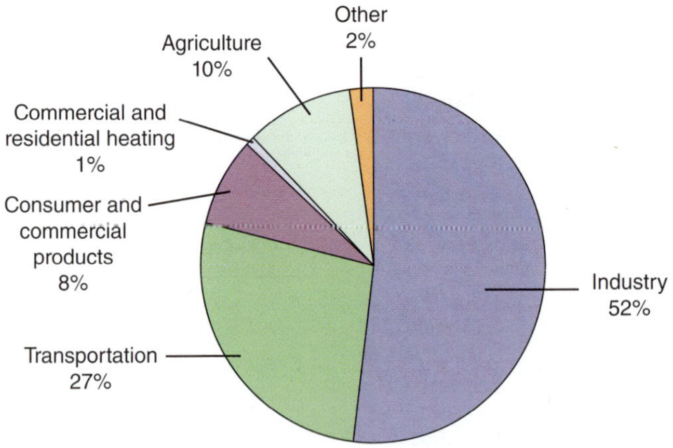

Fig. 9.2 Sources of emissions of air pollutants.

Outdoor Air Pollution Outdoor pollutants such as industrial pollutants and vehicle exhaustion affect various organs in our body, in particular the respiratory system. Now we shall discuss the effects of each of these pollutants on our body.

Ozone is an entity which is present in the stratosphere, and protects us from the harmful UV radiations. But the increased release of chlorofluorocarbons from refrigerators, air conditioners, etc. has caused a huge hole in the ozone layer over the Antarctic region. This has led to the melting of ice, which in turn led to the loss of habitat for animals and also increase in the water level. This comes under the banner of global warming. But the same ozone when present in lower altitude acts as a xenobiotic and causes harm to us. At ground level, ozone is formed by the reaction of nitrogen oxides and volatile organic compounds released from industries and motor vehicle exhausts. On entering our body, ozone forms free radicals which are highly reactive and cause extensive tissue damage. They predominantly cause inflammation of the upper respiratory tract along with reduced lung function and difficulty in breathing. This can predispose to various other conditions and is extremely harmful to people who already have hypersensitivity or COPD. Ozone-related damage shows seasonal variations because it requires sunlight for its formation, and hence it is more prevalent during summer and autumn.

Sulphur dioxide is another air pollutant which can cause harm to humans. It is formed because of combustion of fossil fuels that contain sulphur. This also releases other forms of sulphur such as H_2S, H_2SO_4 and other salts. These can cause direct harm or combine with clouds and cause acid rain which is the main reason for the yellowing of white marble of Taj Mahal, one of the seven wonders of the world. Sulphur also combines with ozone, thus increasing its harmful effects. PM is the major cause of pulmonary inflammation and CVS effects. This pollutant is present in air all around us because of industrialization and transportation. On the basis of size, they can be fatal. The lower the size, the more chances of it crossing the nasal mucosa and reaching the small airways. The fatal size is the ultrafine particles of <10 μm in diameter. When they reach the alveoli, they cause inflammation because of entry of foreign body. The level of suspended particulate matter (SPM) is used as an indicator of air pollution in many places even in India. PM can also come from natural sources such as dust, sand and gravel. These are usually larger in size and much harmless, and are expelled out by sneezing. The other sources are from exhaust from vehicles and industries. They are found in greater concentration in urban areas, affecting the people in big cities.

Carbon has two oxides, carbon monoxide (CO) and carbon dioxide (CO_2). Carbon dioxide causes havoc on the earth by causing global warming along with other greenhouse gases, whereas CO is poisonous to our body. CO is formed mainly because of incomplete oxidation. It can be produced inside houses in a fireplace or from vehicles without maintenance or because of rash driving, making emission checks from vehicles important. Sometimes when CO accumulates in a closed space, it can be fatal because of its higher affinity to haemoglobin than oxygen, producing carboxyhaemoglobin which is a poor carrier of oxygen. CO poisoning is fatal at 60%–70% concentration. Exposed individuals are often rendered unconscious at lower levels because of central nervous system (CNS) depression and are unaware of the impending danger of death. The person must be immediately removed from the exposure and treated.

Morphological Changes due to Pollutants The major system affected by the air pollutants is the respiratory system. The pollutants act primarily by aggravating the underlying respiratory problems such as asthma, COPD and pneumonia, but normal individuals may also suffer the impact. The first response of the body is to eliminate the pollutant either through the air passage or by phagocytosis with macrophages. This may cause inflammation mediated by chemical mediators such as interleukins, prostaglandins and vasoactive amines. Ozone produces reactive oxygen species (ROS) which cause tissue damage. Certain pollutants may get deposited and the macrophage phagocytose them and form nodules such as in silicosis.

Carbon particles also settle down and cause blackening of the airways especially seen in smokers. **CO poisoning** shows different morphology on the basis of its level of poisoning, i.e. it can be either acute or chronic. When the level of carboxyhaemoglobin is 10%–20%, a person will experience headache and nausea. When levels go higher than 20%, exposed individuals experience tachycardia due to tissue hypoxia because carboxyhaemoglobin does not allow oxygen to bind to haemoglobin. Because of the hypoxia, ischaemia develops in CNS. After ischaemia sets in, neurological changes may be irreversible even on treatment. Because of the carboxyhaemoglobin in circulation, the skin and the oral mucosa get a **cherry red colour.**

Indoor Air Pollution The indoor air is comparatively cleaner than outdoor air but can also contain pollutants. Outdoor pollutants can sometimes enter the internal environment but different pollutants may also occur indoors. Although their levels may be low in indoor air, they may be more dangerous because of the closed space and longer duration of exposure. The common sources are as follows:

- Burning of wood in fire places during winter releases various oxides including CO which can cause harm in a closed room.
- Bioaerosols are microorganisms that pose increased risk in closed spaces and include diseases such as viral pneumonia, Legionnaire disease, common cold and the recently prevalent coronavirus.
- Various gas leaks can cause poisoning; examples are radon from the soil, granite or building materials, lead particulates from old paint and also soot particles from fireplace. Radon has been noted to cause lung cancer in uranium miners.
- Other exposure includes exposure in working places, such as formaldehyde, paints and deodorants.
- The sick building syndrome is a health problem attributed to indoor pollutants.

These indoor pollutants can cause asthma attacks just like outdoor pollutants and may aggravate the underlying conditions. Hence, when we find such an exposure, we need to find the source and try to prevent further exposure and not just treat the symptoms. Children, elderly and people with comorbid conditions must be given proper care to prevent such exposures because they are more susceptible to its ill effects.

METALS AS ENVIRONMENTAL POLLUTANTS

The heavy metals often noted to cause harmful effects in humans include cadmium, lead, arsenic and mercury.

Cadmium

Cadmium is a heavy metal which is highly toxic to the body and mainly affects the kidneys and lungs. It produces free radicals, the ROS, and causes injury. Cadmium is being used extensively, such as in batteries, alloys and also in paints, making it a potential occupational hazard but scientists have not found an effective way to recycle it.

Back in 1912, in Japan, there was a mass exposure of cadmium in a village because of irrigation of rice field with cadmium-containing water. This had led to widespread outbreak of a disease called 'itai-itai' that means 'ouch-ouch' disease. The disease mostly affected postmenopausal women and caused osteoporosis, osteomalacia and renal disease. Apart from ingestion and inhalation, it also gains entry through the skin, on exposure to cadmium paints. Cadmium is stored in the kidney and liver. It is detoxified by conversion into the harmless form but when the levels goes beyond 50 ng/mL in blood, it leads to acute toxicity.

Methods of toxicity:

- Cadmium affects proliferation, differentiation and apoptosis by causing DNA damage by formation of free radicals and ROS.
- It also prevents cellular respiration and affects oxidative phosphorylation by binding to mitochondria.
- It decreases the activity of antioxidant enzymes such as superoxide dismutase.

Effects of cadmium on various systems – clinical presentation:

- **Skeletal system**: It causes demineralization. It causes severe pain in joints, spine, and sometimes can even cause deformities. Because of decalcification, the bones are brittle and are susceptible to fracture.
- **Renal system**: It causes proteinuria and renal dysfunction because of renal damage. It can be diagnosed by decrease in the GFR or loss of protein and calcium.
- **Reproductive system**: It disturbs the development of this system in not only humans but also many other mammals. It affects both men and women, decreasing the level of hormones and causing infertility.
- **Cardiovascular system:** Cadmium toxicity acts as a predisposing condition to thrombus formation by disrupting the endothelial cell and its function.
- Recent studies tell that cadmium can also affect the **brain**.
- **Cadmium** is also **carcinogenic**. It may cause lung cancer, prostatic cancer and renal cancer.

Treatment:

First step of any poisoning treatment is cleaning the exposed part and removal from/of the source. If it was ingested, it may be removed from the body by emesis or gastric lavage. This helps in prevention of the cadmium from reaching the blood by reducing absorption. In individuals in whom cadmium has entered the blood and formed bound forms, chelating agents such as EDTA and dimercaprol may be used to eliminate it.

Lead

Lead is a highly poisonous metal which when inhaled or swallowed affects almost every organ and system in the human body. Its prevalence in the human body (adult average of 120 mg) is exceeded only by zinc and iron among the heavy metals. A small amount of lead (1%) is stored in bones; the rest is excreted in urine and faeces within a few weeks of exposure. Continual exposure in excess amounts may result in its bioaccumulation. As of 2019, the global burden of disease attributable to lead exposure has changed. The age-standardized death, measured by population attributable fraction (PAF), due to lead exposure increased from 1.30% in 1990 to 1.56% in 2019. This indicates a gradual increase in the health impact of lead exposure globally. These data contrast with the 2009 WHO report that estimated lead poisoning to account for approximately 0.6% of the global burden of disease. Some countries have lead hot spots, such as battery recycling plants, smelters, refineries, mines, hazardous waste sites and sites where waste is burned in the open. Sometimes even low level of lead which is considered to be safe can cause toxic symptoms; this condition is called subclinical lead poisoning. It causes defects in intellectual capacity, behavioural problems such as hyperactivity and irritability.

Toxicity:

Sources of lead include paint, dust, soil, drinking water and air. Most of the ingested or inhaled lead is absorbed into the bloodstream. The primary cause of its toxicity is its ability to interfere with the functioning of enzymes. It does so by binding to the sulphydryl groups found on many enzymes, or mimicking and displacing other metals which act as cofactors in many enzymatic reactions. Because of its interaction, high levels of calcium and iron provide some protection from lead poisoning whereas low levels cause increased susceptibility.

Effects:

Lead can cause severe damage to the brain, kidneys and ultimately death.

- By mimicking calcium, lead can cross the blood–brain barrier (BBB). It degrades the myelin sheath of neurons, reduces their numbers, interferes with neurotransmission routes and decreases neuronal growth in the human body.
- Lead inhibits porphobilinogen synthase and ferrochelatase, preventing both porphobilinogen formation and the incorporation of iron into protoporphyrin IX, the final step in haem synthesis. This causes ineffective haem synthesis and microcytic anaemia.
- In kidneys, lead causes proximal tubular injury that progresses to tubulointerstitial disease and fibrosis. Lead accumulation in the proximal tubule leads to hyperuricaemia and gout called saturnine gout.
- High-dose exposure to lead causes an increased incidence of hypertension and stroke.
- Lead causes muscle and joint pain. It also inhibits healing of fractures and delays cartilage mineralization.
- Children exposed in early life develop short stature, weight loss and weakness. Sensory, motor, intellectual and psychologic impairments have been noted, including reduced IQ and learning disabilities (Fig. 9.3).

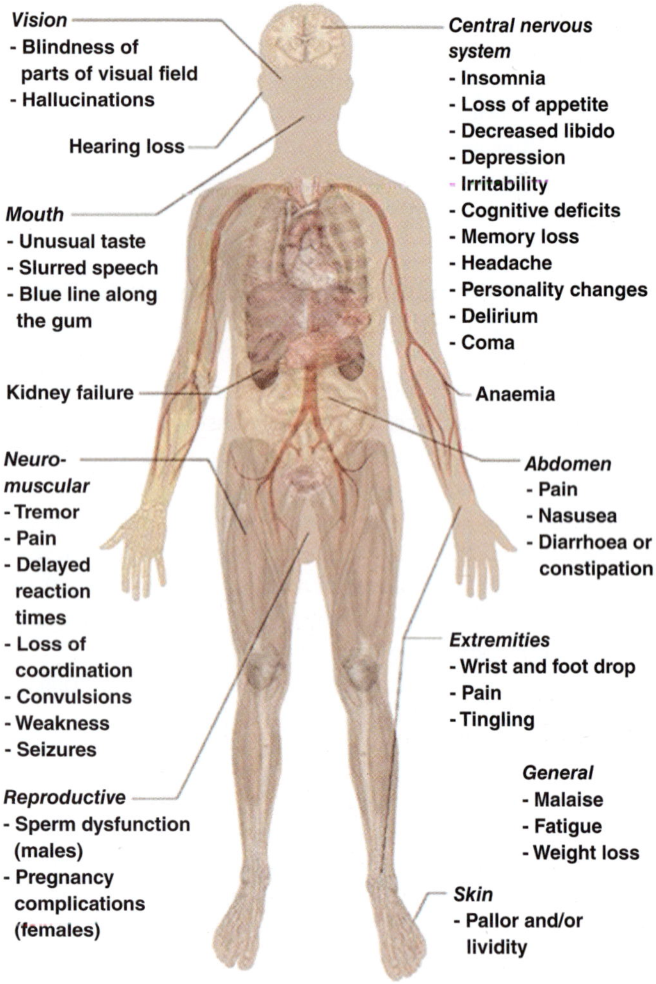

Fig. 9.3 Manifestations of lead poisoning.

Morphology

The major anatomic targets of lead toxicity are the bone marrow and blood, nervous system, gastrointestinal tract and kidneys.

Bone marrow: Ring sideroblasts are seen (RBC precursor with iron-laden macrophages).

- Microcytic hypochromic anaemia (in peripheral smear because of defective haemoglobin synthesis)
- Punctate basophilic stippling of RBCs

CNS: Brain damage can be subtle, producing mild dysfunction, or it can be massive and lethal.

- In children, mild cases show ill-defined subtle changes, but in severe cases, there is marked brain oedema, demyelination of the cerebral and cerebellar white matter, diffuse astrocytic proliferation, psychoses, seizures and coma.
- In adults, the CNS is less often affected, but frequently a peripheral demyelinating neuropathy appears, typically involving the motor nerves of the most commonly used muscles. Thus, the extensor muscles of the wrist and fingers are often the first to be affected (causing wrist drop), followed by paralysis of the peroneal muscles (causing foot drop).

Kidneys: The proximal tubular cells show a characteristic nuclear inclusion made of protein aggregates. It may progress to interstitial renal fibrosis and renal failure.

Mercury

Mercury exists in three forms – metallic/elemental mercury, inorganic mercury (mostly mercury chloride) and organic mercury (mostly methyl mercury). Exposure to mercury can occur through contaminated fish, metallic mercury from dental amalgams, mercury emissions and releases from thermal power generation, artisanal and small-scale gold mining or disposal of mercury-containing products. Metal mercury vapour enters the bloodstream after absorption through the respiratory tract. It then penetrates the BBB and accumulates in brain tissues. When elemental mercury in the brain tissues gets oxidized, it cannot exit the brain through the BBB. Therefore, it remains in the brain tissue for prolonged periods.

Clinical manifestations:

- **Early manifestations** include skin rashes, fatigue, myalgia, headache and sleep disturbances. Gastrointestinal symptoms such as dyspepsia, nausea, vomiting and urinary symptoms such as frequency, incontinence, sensation of incomplete urine voiding may occur. It can also cause paraesthesia of the extremities, gum swelling and red eye.
- **Late manifestations** include **erythrism**, characterized by increased irritability, lack of patience, avoidance of people, excessive shyness and insomnia. Mercury poisoning may also induce flapping tremor, initially occurring as a resting tremor and later may progress to intention tremor, accompanied by a rough and rhythmic movement. At first, the tremor usually involves the hands and later it affects the eyelids, lips, tongue and head. Frequent episodes of coarse jerky movements may be observed. Cognitive impairment, disturbances in memory and attention may develop. Kidney damage ranges from mild albuminuria to renal failure. Acrodynia, contact dermatitis and hyperpigmentation in skin can also be observed.

Arsenic

Exposure to arsenic can occur either through the oral route (mainly water) or inhalation (pesticides and mining activities) which can lead to various health intimidations, manifesting in the gastrointestinal system, skin, nervous system and heart. It was a common murder weapon among the royalties and was fondly referred to as king of poisons. In the 19th century, one-third criminal cases of poisoning involved arsenic and one probable reason for this was its easy availability. In many cases, medical examiners were unable to find if poison was the reason for death because the symptoms were similar to other disorders.

EFFECTS OF TOBACCO PA 12.1

The tobacco epidemic is one of the biggest public health threats the world has ever faced, killing more than 8 million people a year around the world. More than 7 million of those deaths are the result of direct tobacco use, whereas around 1 million deaths are the result of non-smokers being exposed to secondhand smoke.

SMOKING

All forms of tobacco are harmful, and there is no safe level of exposure to tobacco. Cigarette smoking is the most common form of tobacco use worldwide. Other tobacco products include waterpipe tobacco, various smokeless tobacco products, cigars, cigarillos, roll-your-own tobacco, pipe tobacco, bidis and kreteks. Waterpipe tobacco use is damaging to health in similar ways to cigarette tobacco use. However, the health dangers of waterpipe tobacco use are often little understood by users.

Smokeless tobacco use is highly addictive and damaging to health. Smokeless tobacco contains many cancer-causing toxins and its use increases the risk of cancers of the head, neck, throat, oesophagus and oral cavity (including cancer of the mouth, tongue, lip and gums) as well as various dental diseases.

Over 80% of the 1.3 billion tobacco users worldwide live in low- and middle-income countries, where the burden of tobacco-related illness and death is heaviest. Tobacco use contributes to poverty by diverting household expenditure from basic needs such as food and shelter to tobacco.

The economic costs of tobacco use are substantial and include significant health care costs for treating the diseases caused by tobacco use as well as the lost human capital that results from tobacco-attributable morbidity and mortality. In some countries, children from poor households are employed in tobacco farming to boost family income. Tobacco-growing farmers are also exposed to a number of health risks, including the 'green tobacco sickness'.

Tobacco smoke contains around 7500 toxicologically significant chemicals, with more than 70 of them being identified carcinogens (Table 9.1). Some smoke components, such as CO, hydrogen cyanide (HCN) and nitrogen oxides, are gases. Others, such as formaldehyde, acrolein, benzene and certain *N*-nitrosamines, are volatile chemicals contained in the liquid–vapour portion of the smoke aerosol. The radioactive element polonium-210 is also known to occur in tobacco smoke. The chemical composition of smoke depends on puff frequency, intensity, volume and duration at different stages of cigarette consumption. Nicotine, an alkaloid, present in tobacco leaves is responsible for its addictive effect. It binds to nicotinic acetylcholine receptors in the brain and causes increased catecholamine release from sympathetic neurons which apart from giving

Table 9.1 Effects of Selected Tobacco Smoke Constituents

Substance	Effect
Tar	Carcinogenesis
Polycyclic aromatic hydrocarbons	Carcinogenesis
Nicotine	Ganglionic stimulation and depression; tumour promotion
Phenol	Tumour promotion; mucosal irritation
Benzo[a]pyrene	Carcinogenesis
Carbon monoxide	Impaired oxygen transport and utilization
Formaldehyde	Toxicity to cilia; mucosal irritation
Nitrogen oxides	Toxicity to cilia; mucosal irritation
Nitrosamine	Carcinogenesis

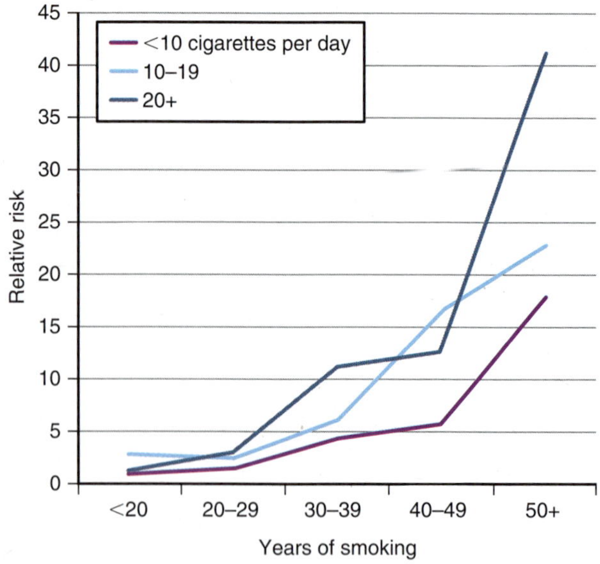

Fig. 9.4 Relative risk of lung cancer in smokers. (*Source:* https://www.ncbi.nlm.nih.gov/pmc/articles/PMC3749017/figure/f2-squmj1303-345-358/?report=objectonly)

a happy feeling causes an increase in heart rate, blood pressure, cardiac output and contractility.

Smoking and Lung Damage

Smoking causes lung diseases by directly damaging the tracheobronchial mucosa leading to irritation and inflammation. It causes COPD which includes emphysema (locally recruited leucocytes produce elastase which injures the lung tissue) and chronic bronchitis (due to inflammation and increased mucus production), which is dealt in detail in Chapter 19.

The risk of developing tobacco-related health hazards is dose dependent and is expressed as pack-years which is calculated by multiplying number of cigarette packs smoked per day with the number of years of smoking. Its effect is cumulative and increases with increase in duration of smoking (Fig. 9.4). However, it is a relief that abstinence from smoking reduces the overall mortality and cardiovascular disease risk within 5 years. Although the lung cancer risk reduces within 5 years, it persists for approximately 30 years.

The nicotine and other carcinogens in smoke are excreted by the body but a part of them acts as indirect carcinogen and gets metabolized by the liver into active carcinogens (Fig. 9.5). The enzyme cytochrome P450 (CYPs), while converting the chemicals into water-soluble form for excretion, also produces electrophilic intermediates. These intermediates form DNA adducts which if not repaired effectively, cause mutations and malignant transformations. The perception of the general public is that not all smokers develop carcinoma. The explanation lies in the fact that different people metabolize the indirect carcinogen into active form at different rates. When the balance between excretion and metabolization tilts in favour of faster metabolism, the risk of malignant transformation is more.

Studies show that thousands of mutations can be produced by carcinogens in tobacco smoke in experimental settings. Moreover, concomitant smoking increases the risk of cancer in people exposed to other carcinogens. There is a 10-fold higher incidence of lung carcinomas in asbestos workers and uranium miners who smoke as compared with those who do not smoke, and the interaction between tobacco and alcohol consumption in the development of oral cancers is well documented.

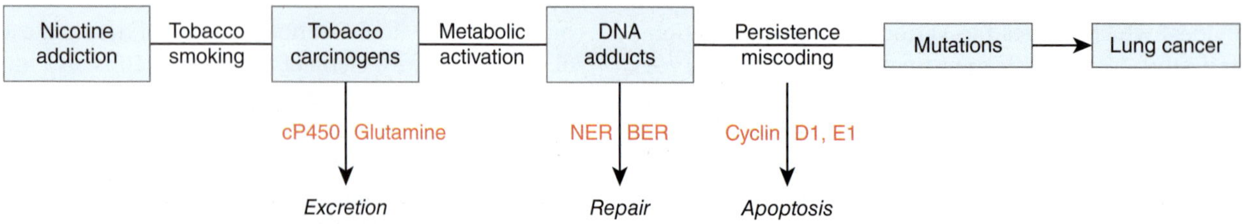

Fig. 9.5 Link between nicotine addiction and lung cancer via tobacco smoke carcinogens and carcinogenesis. cP450, cytochrome P450 enzyme; NER, nucleoside excision repair; BER, base pair excision repair. (*Source:* Adapted from: Hecht SS. Tobacco smoke carcinogens and lung cancer.)

Smoking and Other Organs

1) **Cardiovascular disease:**
   - Smoking causes stroke and coronary heart disease, which are leading causes of death in the United States.
   - Early signs of cardiovascular disease may even be seen in people who smoke less than five cigarettes per day.
   - Smoking damages blood vessels and occludes the lumen causing thrombosis (peripheral vascular disease).
   - Embolus from the thrombus may obstruct the blood flow to the brain and cause intracranial haemorrhage and stroke.
2) **Cancer**: It leads to neoplastic conditions in the bladder, blood (acute myeloid leukaemia), cervix, colon and rectum (colorectal), oesophagus, kidney and ureter, larynx, liver, oropharynx (includes parts of the throat, tongue, soft palate and the tonsils), pancreas, stomach, trachea, bronchus and lung.
3) **Reproductive organs**: As tobacco contains polycyclic hydrocarbons and nitrosamines, smoking both actively and passively by pregnant women may cause stillbirth, low birth weight, preterm delivery and teratogenic effect in fetus. It may lead to reduced fertility in men also.
4) **Musculoskeletal system**: Smoking can affect bone health. Postmenopausal women who smoke are at greater risk of osteoporosis making them prone to fractures than women who have never smoked. Smoking is also a risk factor for rheumatoid arthritis.

Other important manifestations include the following (Fig. 9.6):

- Smoking may affect the teeth, gums and cause tooth loss.
- Smoking can increase chances of cataracts and age-related macular degeneration (AMD).
- Smoking is found to be associated with type 2 diabetes mellitus. The risk of developing diabetes is 30%–40% higher for active smokers compared with nonsmokers.
- Smoking causes general adverse effects on the body, including inflammation and decreased immune function.

Apart from active smoking, exposure to tobacco in environmental air as passive smoking also increases the risk of developing atherosclerosis and myocardial infarction. This risk can be estimated by measuring blood levels of cotinine, a metabolite of nicotine. Although this is on the reducing side, passive smoking poses a significant risk to children and those with respiratory disorders such as asthma.

EFFECTS OF ALCOHOL — PA 12.1

Alcohol is a well-known beverage in many communities consumed for socialization. When consumed in small quantities, it does not affect health, but excess intake may lead to serious social, physical and mental problems. Although illicit drug addiction is more spoken about, alcohol consumption and addiction are far bigger problems. In an average, approximately 50% of adult population in the United States consume alcohol

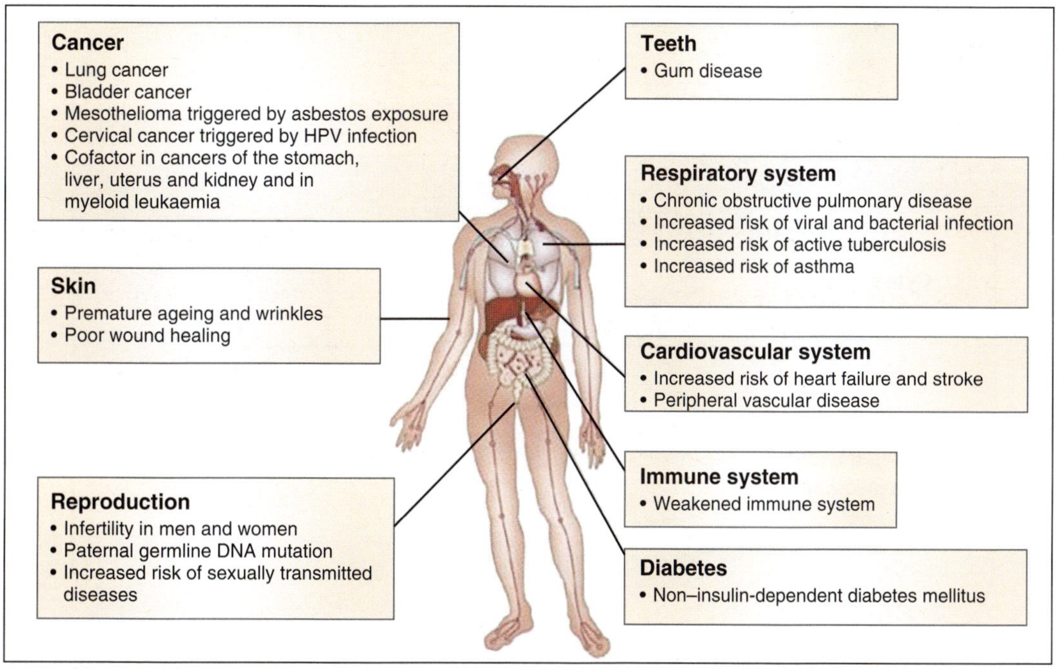

Fig. 9.6 Effects of smoking.

with chronic alcoholism being noted in approximately 12%–20%. Alcohol causes serious morbidity and mortality because of alcohol-related accidents, suicides and homicides, apart from the liver damage and cirrhosis associated with it.

Absorption of ethanol starts in the stomach but most of the absorption is done by the intestine. After absorption, alcohol reaches the bloodstream and is proportionally distributed to tissues and fluids (Fig. 9.7). The proportion of alcohol distributed to a tissue depends on its relative water content, i.e. more the water content of the tissue, more is the absorption of alcohol. Approximately 10% of the blood levels of alcohol are excreted in urine, sweat and breath which produces the odour and lays the basis of breath test for alcohol. The legally permissible limit of alcohol level in blood for driving is 80 mg/dL. This level is reached on the consumption of

- Three standard drinks
- Approximately three bottles of beer
- 450 mL of wine
- 120–150 mL of 80-proof distilled spirits

Following absorption, alcohol is converted into acetaldehyde by

- Alcohol dehydrogenase, which is present in the cytoplasm of hepatocytes and is the major pathway of alcohol metabolism.
- Microsomal ethanol oxidizing system that gets activated at high blood alcohol levels and involves cytochrome P (CYP) liver enzymes. These enzymes, especially CYP2E1, are induced in chronic alcoholics and increase their alcohol tolerance levels and also increase the metabolism of various other drugs, carcinogens and anaesthetics. However, when narcotics or sedatives are taken along with alcohol, alcohol blocks the function of CYP increasing the bioavailability of the drug and potentiating its effect and may lead to grave consequences.
- Catalase which metabolizes less than 5% of ethanol.

Acetaldehyde is then oxidized to acetate by aldehyde dehydrogenase. The toxic metabolites produced during the metabolism of alcohol include the following:

I. Acetaldehyde: It is a direct product produced during alcohol metabolism and is toxic to the body. Its production depends on the level of alcohol dehydrogenase in the body and its duration of action depends on the level of aldehyde dehydrogenase in the body. Individuals who have the inactive allele of aldehyde dehydrogenase will not be able to tolerate alcohol and hence suffer from severe nausea, tachycardia, flushing and hyperventilation.

II. Increased NADH/NAD ratio: Alcohol metabolism by alcohol dehydrogenase converts NAD to NADH, thereby reducing the availability of NAD for its function in the liver. This affects fatty acid oxidation and removal of lactate, leading to fat accumulation in liver (fatty liver) and lactic acidosis as discussed in Chapter 22.

III. ROS: Alcohol metabolism in liver may produce free radicals that cause lipid peroxidation of hepatocyte cell membrane.

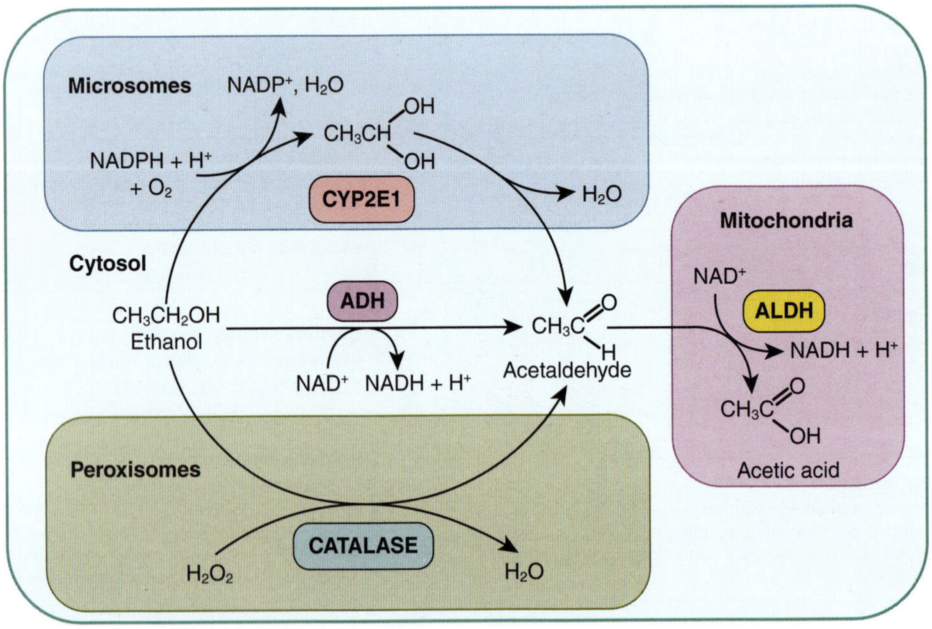

Fig. 9.7 Metabolism of ethanol: Oxidation of ethanol to acetaldehyde by three different routes and the generation of acetic acid. ALD, alcohol dehydrogenase; ALDH, aldehyde dehydrogenase.

THE ADVERSE OUTCOMES OF ETHANOL CONSUMPTION

The effects of alcohol can be acute that are immediate or chronic that are long term due to chronic alcoholism.

Acute alcoholism: It affects the CNS, gastrointestinal system and the liver. These effects may be reversed on discontinuation.

CNS: Initially depresses subcortical structures and later stimulates these structures, causing disordered cortical, motor and intellectual functions. At very high levels, it may suppress the medullary centres, including the respiratory centre causing respiratory depression.

Gastrointestinal system: Gastritis, ulcers, Mallory–Weiss tear and Boerhaave syndrome.

Liver: Acute fatty change.

Chronic alcoholism: Chronic alcoholism may affect any organ of the body apart from the liver and stomach.

Liver: Alcoholic hepatitis and cirrhosis may develop and lead to portal hypertension. Cirrhosis also increases the risk of hepatocellular carcinoma.

Stomach: Severe gastritis, ulceration and perforation may occur. Oesophageal varices and related complications may develop because of portal hypertension.

Pancreas: It may cause acute and chronic pancreatitis.

Heart: Alcoholic cardiomyopathy, which is a type of dilated cardiomyopathy, may occur. Hypertension may develop in alcoholics and risk of atherosclerosis is increased because of their effect on HDL (levels are decreased).

Nutritional deficiency: Thiamine deficiency may lead to peripheral neuropathies and the *Wernicke–Korsakoff syndrome*. Alcoholism may also lead to malnutrition and multiple vitamin deficiencies.

Teratogenic effect: Increased consumption of alcohol during pregnancy results in fetal alcohol syndrome.

Although alcohol has many adverse effects, when consumed in moderate levels, it has beneficial effects such as increase in HDL levels, reduced platelet aggregation and lower fibrinogen levels. However, this cardioprotective effect may be because of the other variable factors seen in people who have a controlled moderate alcohol consumption such as relaxed lifestyle and less stress.

INJURY BY PHYSICAL AGENTS

Injury can be defined as harm caused to a person physically or mentally. It can also be referred to as a discontinuity in tissue or living body. Injuries by physical agents have different forms. They include:

- Mechanical injuries
- Thermal injuries
- Electrical injuries
- Radiation injuries
- Injury due to noise

MECHANICAL INJURY

These are the injuries inflicted by force with or without weapons. These defects are categorized in detail under forensic medicine. The pathology includes abrasions, contusions, lacerations, stab wounds, etc. It can be occupational when one inflicts injury while using the machinery or it can be an assault when it is inflicted upon by another individual. Sometimes it can also be due to carelessness because even accidents can cause bruising. Forensic medicine is a separate medical speciality that deals with wound inspection and investigations, to ascertain the cause of death.

THERMAL INJURY

These are injuries caused when body is exposed to temperature beyond its level of tolerance. It can be caused by extreme heat or extreme cold. The normal body temperature is 37°C (98.6°F). When the body temperature rises, the condition is called hyperthermia. This can be caused by overheat or burns. When the temperature falls, it is called hypothermia. This is caused by extreme low temperatures. Thermal injuries have been seen throughout history, attributed to both human mistakes and at times natural events like forest fire and snowstorms.

Thermal Burns

Thermal injury may be caused by burns, scalds or inhalation of smoke. Every year, nearly 3500 people die because of fire and smoke-related injuries. But because of improved treatment protocols, prevention of wound infection and appropriate care, there is an improvement in survival rates of the burn victims.

The effects of the injury depend on depth of the burns, percentage of body surface involved, extent of smoke inhalation and efficiency/promptness of treatment. Burns are classified into three categories on the basis of depth of involvement for efficient management and prognosis.

The complications associated with burns include the following:

- Burn site infection: The most common organism causing infection is *Pseudomonas aeruginosa* and others include common hospital-acquired bacteria, such as methicillin-resistant *Staphylococcus aureus*, and fungi, especially *Candida* species. The presence of more than 10^5 organisms in the surrounding unburned tissue is considered as invasive infection. Toxins released by these organisms may also lead to septic shock and acute respiratory distress syndrome (ARDS).
- Sepsis and organ failure have drastically reduced because of efficient wound debridement, management and treatment.
- Airway and lung injury due to smoke inhalation may occur due to the presence of various toxic gases in the smoke. They may directly injure the mucosa and cause inflammation or diffuse into the lungs and cause pneumonitis.

Hyperthermia Hyperthermia is increase in body temperature **greater than 37.5–38.3°C (99.5–100.9°F).** It may be caused by extreme heat during summer or by burns. The main effects of hyperthermia are as follows:

- Dehydration: The body starts to lose water and it can cause various problems because water is a major component of the body.
- Heat cramps occur because of loss of electrolytes in sweat when the body tries to lower its temperature by using the sweat mechanism. Cramping of muscles is the hallmark of heat cramps often seen in those performing vigorous exercise.
- Heat exhaustion is the most common effect of hyperthermia. It is the sudden collapse of the individual because of cardiovascular shock caused by dehydration-related hypovolaemia. Rehydration may help the person to re-establish the balance.
- Heat stroke is the end stage when the thermoregulatory mechanisms fail and the core body temperature raises leading to multiorgan failure.

Hypothermia Hypothermia occurs when the temperature falls below **35°C to 32.2°C (95°F to 89.9°F).** It is usually seen in countries that experience extreme cold temperature during winter. When the temperature falls up to 90°F, the patient loses consciousness. Conditions such as high humidity, wet clothing and alcohol-induced peripheral vasoconstriction seen at high blood oxygen levels may aggravate the speed of temperature drop. The effects of hypothermia may be direct due to crystallization of intracellular and extracellular water and indirect due to the circulatory changes caused by low temperature.

ELECTRICAL INJURY

Electricity has been considered one of the greatest discoveries. It is seen in lightning, homes, workplaces, etc. But because our body is a good conductor of electricity, we can get injuries when current passes through our body. When electricity passes through our body, various organs react differently. It also depends on the voltage because low voltage just gives a jerk and very high voltages may cause death. The two common effects of electrical shock are burns and ventricular fibrillation due to disruption in the conduction of impulses in the heart. The voltage at home is from 120 to 220 V and when it passes through the body for quite some time, it can cause burns at the entry and exit points. However, it is an alternating current and causes tetanic muscle spasm. This leads to irreversible clutching of the live wire, extending the duration of contact and hence, worsening the outcome owing to ventricular fibrillation. Very high voltages may also cause spasm of the respiratory muscles causing asphyxia and paralysis of medullary centre of respiration. Lightening can cause extensive burns and death because its intensity ranges from 1 million to 100 million volts.

RADIATION INJURY

Radiation is the emission or transmission of energy in the form of waves or particles through space or through a material medium. There are various types of radiations which include:

- Electromagnetic radiation – radio waves, microwaves, infrared, visible light, ultraviolet, X-rays and gamma (γ) radiation
- Particle radiation – alpha (α) radiation, beta (β) radiation and neutron radiation (particles of nonzero rest energy)
- Acoustic radiation – ultrasound, sound and seismic waves (dependent on some physical transmission medium)
- Gravitational radiation – radiation that takes the form of gravitational waves, or ripples in the curvature of spacetime

Radiation and radioactive substances are used in medicine for diagnosis (X-ray, CT scan), treatment (cancer radiation therapy) and research. All modern communication systems use different forms of electromagnetic radiation where variations in the intensity of the radiation are used to represent changes in the sound, pictures or other information being transmitted. In the field of science, radiation plays a key role in techniques such as radiocarbon dating in which researchers use radioactive atoms to determine the age of materials that were once part of a living organism.

Radiation can be categorized into ionizing or nonionizing depending on the energy of the radiated particles. Ionizing radiation carries more than 10 eV, which has the ability to release tightly bound electrons from an atom and convert them into ions. Such released electrons can do the same to the surrounding atoms triggering a cascade reaction which is damaging to the tissues. Alpha radiation–, beta radiation– or gamma radiation–emitting radioactive substances are the major source of ionizing radiation. Although it includes the commonly used X-rays and gamma rays, the significant damage causing ones are alpha rays and beta rays.

The nonionizing energies of the lower ultraviolet spectrum cannot ionize atoms, but can disrupt the interatomic bonds which form molecules. Sunburn is caused by long-wavelength ultraviolet rays from the sun, which are energetic enough to damage skin cell DNA. Longer electromagnetic waves like visible light, infrared and microwaves, cannot break chemical bonds but cause vibrations perceived as heat. Radio waves, with even longer wavelengths, are generally considered harmless as they do not have sufficient energy to heat tissues or alter cells.

These rays are both boon and bane to mankind because they are useful in various fields but they also lead to producing adverse short- and long-term effects such as fibrosis, mutagenesis, carcinogenesis and teratogenesis.

Measuring radiation: Different units of measure are used, depending on what aspect of radiation is being measured and this is given in the following table:

Unit	Purpose
Curie	Amount of radiation emitted by radioisotope
Gray	Amount of radiation absorbed by tissue per unit mass
Sievert	Equivalent dose that produces same biological effect on tissue; given by absorbed dose multiplied by biological effectiveness of the radiation

To determine a person's biological risk, numbers are assigned to each type of ionizing radiation (alpha and beta particles, gamma rays and X-rays) depending on the ability of that type of radiation to transfer energy to the cells of the body. This number is known as the quality factor (Q). The dose-dependent effect on specific organs is given in Table 9.2.

Factors Affecting the Biological Effects of Radiation

Apart from the characteristics of the radiation, the factors that determine the extent of injury are as follows:

- **Type of radiation:** Various types of radiation differ in penetrability, which is determined by the energy lost per unit distance travelled (kiloelectron volts per micrometre). This value is high for alpha particles, lower for beta particles and even less for gamma rays and X-rays. Thus, alpha particles penetrate a short distance but induce heavy damage, whereas gamma rays travel longer distance but produce much lesser damage.
- **Intensity and frequency of exposure:** A single large exposure produces much more damage than fractionated doses given with recovery intervals between the doses. The intervals give time for cells to repair the damages before the next exposure, reducing the cumulative effect.
- **Field size:** Even smaller doses can produce significant damage when given to a large area of our body. The newer methods in radiation therapy, hence, have changed to higher doses delivered directly to the tumour tissue alone with proper shielding of surrounding tissue, thereby reducing the field size.
- **Nature of cell:** Rapidly dividing cells are more affected than nondividing or stable cells because the DNA of dividing cells is a vulnerable target to the ionizing radiation (Fig. 9.8). In normal cells, DNA damage causes p53 activation and repair or apoptosis as detailed in Chapter 7: Neoplasia. When damage exceeds the capacity of p53 gene or if the gene is ineffective, the damage occurs especially to cells in G2 phase during exposure. Hence, rapidly dividing cells such as gonads, skin, lymphoid tissue, bone marrow and gastrointestinal mucosa are the most affected, whereas muscle and nerve are the least affected.
- **Availability of oxygen:** Molecular oxygen is known to have the ability to potentiate the effect of radiation by generating free radicals. The amount of molecular oxygen rather than the rate of oxygen utilization by the cells is an important factor for increasing the sensitivity of cells to radiation. Hypoxic areas such as centre of large tumours are, hence, insensitive to radiation therapy.
- **Vascular damage:** Damage to the blood vessel endothelium leads to narrowing of blood vessels and ischaemic changes to the tissues. This leads to impaired

Table 9.2 Estimated Threshold Doses for Acute Radiation Effects on Specific Organs

Health Effect	Organ	Dose (Sv)
Temporary sterility	Testis	0.15
Depression of haematopoiesis	Bone marrow	0.50
Reversible skin effects (e.g. erythema)	Skin	1–2
Permanent sterility	Ovaries	2.5–6
Temporary hair loss	Skin	3–5
Permanent sterility	Testis	3.5
Cataract	Lens of eye	5

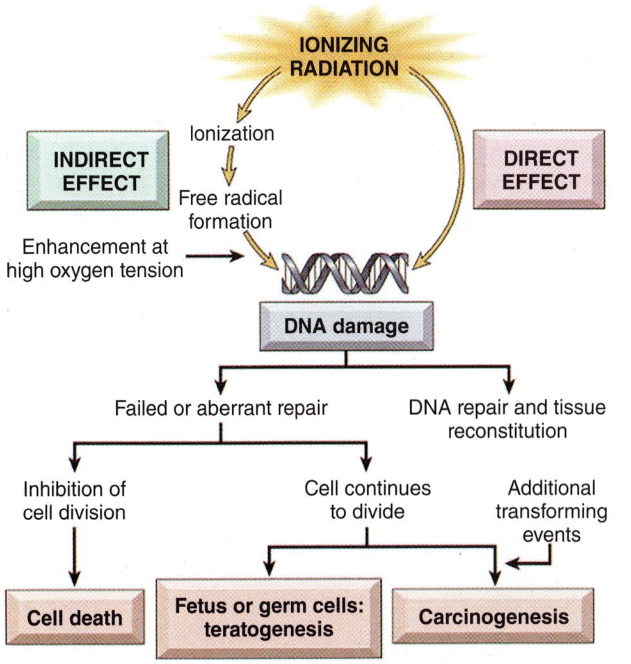

Fig. 9.8 Effects of ionizing radiation on DNA and its consequences. The effects on DNA can be direct, or most importantly, indirect, through free radical formation.

healing and fibrosis. Moreover, release of proinflammatory mediators enhances the damage to blood vessels and tissues. This effect may manifest as late effects in tissue such as brain, kidney, liver, muscle in the form of cell death, atrophic changes and fibrosis.

Morphology

Cellular changes: The cytoplasm shows swelling, distortion of mitochondria and disintegration of endoplasmic reticulum. Plasma membrane may appear disrupted. The nucleus shows swelling, chromatin clumping and condensation. Overall, the cells show marked nuclear and cellular pleomorphism, giant nucleus and mitotic figures making it extremely difficult to differentiate residual tumour from radiotherapy-induced cell changes microscopically.

Chromosomal changes: Structural changes such as DNA breaks, deletions, translocations and fragmentations may occur.

Vascular changes: Immediate changes are minimal with only vascular dilation but with time endothelial swelling and vacuolation may develop later on proceeding to necrosis and dissolution of vessel wall or subintimal fibrosis. The vessel may also get occluded with thrombus or rupture. All these lead to ischaemic changes in tissue supplied by the vessel (Fig. 9.9).

Biological Effects of Radiation

The biological effects of radiation may show two patterns of damage – the stochastic effect and deterministic effect. The stochastic effect of radiation shows a linear pattern of dose-related damage. The damage of the tissue starts from the initial exposure and there is no safe threshold limit for exposure. In contrast, deterministic effect shows damage to tissue only when the dose exceeds the safe threshold limit but beyond this limit the damage is markedly exaggerated irrespective of the exposure dose, i.e. it does not show a linear relationship with the dose. The graph helps to understand the pattern. DNA damage and carcinogenesis show the stochastic effect, whereas damage to tissue such as bone marrow and radiation sickness shows deterministic effect.

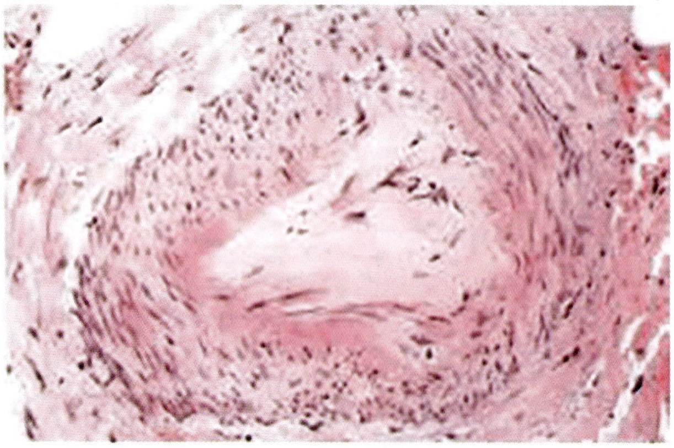

Fig. 9.9 Radiation-induced chronic vascular injury with subintimal fibrosis occluding the lumen. (*Source:* American Registry of Pathology © 1990.)

Early radiation effects: When a high dose of radiation is subjected over a short time span, individuals experience certain acute changes. Some of which are explained as follows:

1) **Total body irradiation:** These are divided into four phases:
   1. The prodromal period (48 hours) – symptoms include anorexia, nausea, vomiting and diarrhoea.
   2. The latent period (from 48 hours to 2–3 weeks) is asymptomatic.
   3. The manifest phase (6–8 weeks after exposure) refers to the time period when variable symptoms appear on the basis of radiation dose.
   4. The recovery period – if the patient survives, recovery occurs from 6 weeks to several months after exposure.
2) **Radiation sickness:** The symptoms can be mild, such as loss of appetite, apathy and mild fatigue, or evident only on laboratory tests with mild lymphopenia.
3) **Haematopoietic and lymphoid systems:** These systems are highly susceptible to any form of radiation. Severe lymphopenia with shrinkage of spleen and lymph nodes is a common feature and the extent of repair depends on the dose of radiation.

   The haematopoietic precursors in the bone marrow are very sensitive and radiation-induced damage may lead to marrow aplasia, and with severe radiation, it may even cause permanent aplastic anaemia. The fall in blood counts parallels the lifespan of the cells and recovery depends on the bone marrow precursor potential to replenish the lost cells. Neutropenia starts within days, thrombocytopenia occurs at the end of 1 week and red cell count decreases in 2–3 weeks. The recovery of neutrophil count and platelet count may require 2–3 months, whereas that of the red cells takes longer.
4) **Acute regional effects:** Skin erythema, gastrointestinal oedema and ulceration are some regional effects seen.

Delayed radiation effects:

1) **Fibrosis**: Fibrosis is the loss of normal tissue components and replacement by matrix and disorganized collagen fibrils. This often results in the loss of organ function and frequent tissue contractions and scarring. Radiation fibrosis syndrome (RFS) is a progressive fibrotic tissue sclerosis with various clinical symptoms in the irradiation field. It is usually a late complication of radiation therapy and may occur weeks or even years after treatment. Genetic factors

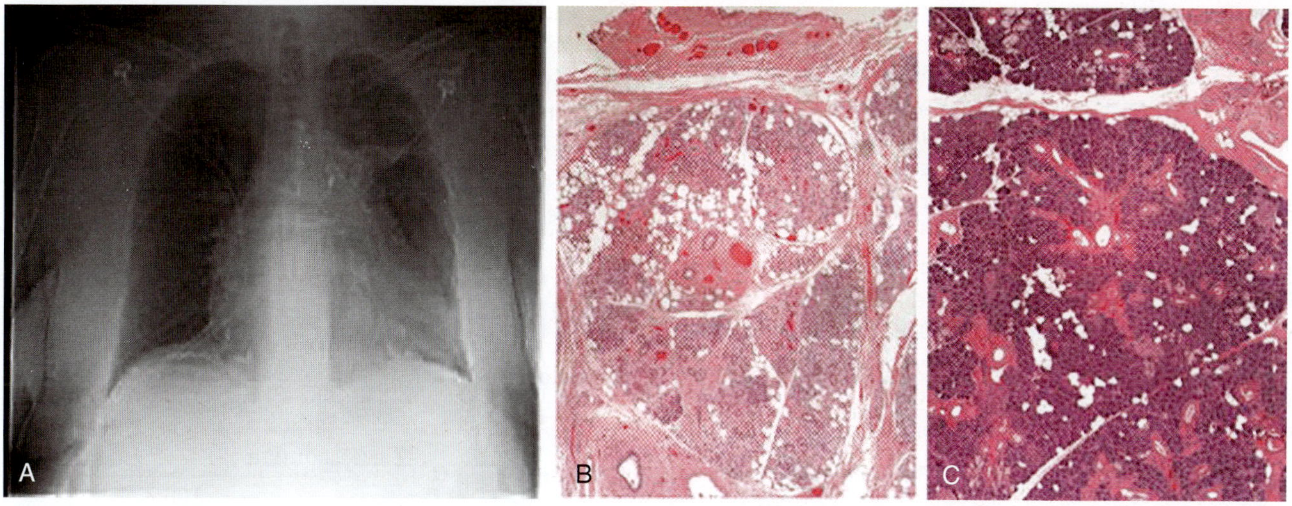

Fig. 9.10 Radiation-induced fibrosis. X-ray shows radiation-induced fibrotic lung injury **(A)** and fibrosis seen in salivary gland **(B)** in contrast with normal salivary gland **(C)**.

seem to play a role in continuation of detrimental effects even after the initial stimulus is removed. It may affect the soft tissue, neural tissue, musculoskeletal and cardiopulmonary systems. Commonly affected organs are lungs and salivary glands in head and neck irradiation, and colorectal and pelvic areas following treatment of cancer of cervix, prostate or rectum (Fig. 9.10).

2) **DNA damage**: Radiation can produce a variety of alterations in the DNA material, such as exchange of bases, destruction of sugars, cross-links and formation of dimers and breaks in between them, but the most serious of them are the double-stranded breaks (DSBs). These ionizing radiations cause DSBs at a rate of 35 DSBs per cell per gray. These DSBs are repaired by homologous recombination or nonhomologous end joining (NHEJ), the latter being more common. But these repair mechanisms may remove portion of the epigenetic markers of the DNA, which regulate the gene expression and also cause mutations. Hence, if these cells escape the cell cycle check points and proliferate, it may lead to cancer. Furthermore, these cells may produce cytokines and growth factors, thus affecting the normal unirradiated cells around them which is called **radiation-induced bystander effect** which are nontarget effects of radiation.

3) **Cancer risks**: Cancer is the most important concern following radiation exposure. Tissues with a high rate of cell proliferation share higher risk of tumour induction. The exposure to carcinogenic agents can be majorly from areas with high radon source; iatrogenic following X-rays, CT scans or radiotherapy; occupational such as in nuclear energy plants; and occasionally by accidental exposure such as during the Chernobyl disaster and partial meltdowns at the Fukushima I Nuclear Power Plant in Japan. Cancer becomes evident only after a long period of latency following the first exposure which causes damage. Leukaemia first appears 2–5 years after exposure, whereas solid tumours appear after at least 10 years or several decades later. The tumours reported to be associated with radiation include multiple myeloma, and cancers of the breast, colon, thyroid, ovary, lung, urinary bladder, stomach, CNS (other than brain) and oesophagus.
Prolonged exposure to ultraviolet radiation from the sun can lead to melanoma and other skin malignancies. **Chronic radiation keratosis** is a precancerous keratotic skin lesion that may arise on the skin many years after exposure to ionizing radiation. In individuals with reduced DNA repair mechanism such as in BLOOM syndrome and xeroderma pigmentosum, the inability to correct intrinsic mutations caused by the radiation exposure greatly increases the risk of developing cancer. Also in others, reduced DNA repair capacity with age and exposure to higher doses of radiation increases the risk of cancer. The carcinogenic effect of radiation is discussed in detail in Chapter 7.

4) **Teratogenic effect**: The classical triad of effects of radiation on the embryo, which is highly radiosensitive, is growth retardation, embryonic/fetal/neonatal death and congenital malformation. At each stage of growth, each organ shows greater vulnerability. During the first 2 weeks of conception, the effect of radiation may lead to miscarriage of the embryo. Following this period and up to 8 weeks, the fetus is vulnerable to congenital malformations. Exposure after organogenesis may cause mental retardation and organ-specific effects.

INJURY DUE TO NOISE

Noise pollution has been on the rise in the current world. When it increases beyond a level, sound causes ear damage and sometimes deafness also. Listening to loud noises for a long period of time can cause temporary or permanent damage to hearing. The injury can manifest as tinnitus, hyperacusis, otalgia and vertigo (because cochlea of inner ear plays an important role in maintaining balance). Small noises can cause headache, dizziness also. Normal hearing range is between 20 and 20,000 Hz. Occupational exposure to loud noises from heavy machinery, attending loud music concerts frequently, and exposure to gun fires and explosions by the army, navy and air force can cause severe noise-related problems.

NUTRITIONAL DISEASES

SOURCES AND NUTRITIONAL IMPORTANCE OF NUTRIENTS

Nutrients are organic or inorganic substances essential for our body to maintain the basic functions. There are six major classes of nutrients – carbohydrates, lipids, proteins, vitamins, minerals and water. Carbohydrates, lipids and proteins are regarded as macronutrients. Vitamins and minerals are regarded as micronutrients. Water does not yield energy but it is required in large amounts. Vitamins can be water soluble or fat soluble. Minerals on the basis of their dietary requirements can be classified as major elements or macrominerals and trace elements or microminerals. We will focus our discussion on the common macro- and micronutrients in the subsequent sections.

Carbohydrates

Carbohydrates are the principal source of energy to our body. They are present in food in three major forms as follows:

1. Starch: It is a complex carbohydrate and an important source of calories. It is present in vegetables (tubers and roots), grains, etc.
2. Sugars: These are the simplest form of carbohydrate. They can be sucrose (table sugar), fructose (fruit sugar) and lactose (milk sugar).
3. Cellulose: This form of carbohydrate is not digested and does not provide any energy.

Glycaemic Index Glycaemic index (GI) is an important parameter related to foods containing carbohydrate. It is a system in which carbohydrate-containing foods are numbered from 0 to 100, according to the amount of blood sugar elevation following their consumption. It is calculated by the following formula:

$$\text{Glycaemic index (GI)} = \frac{\text{Glucose response to test food}}{\text{Glucose response to standard food}} \times 100$$

The quantity of food is standardized to 50 g. The response is taken as plasma glucose level taken 3 hours after consuming food.

On the basis of GI values, food is divided into three categories: Low GI (1–55), e.g. fruits and pulses; medium GI (56–69), e.g. sweet corn and banana; high GI (70–100), e.g. rice and potato.

Glycaemic Load Glycaemic load (GL) is a numerical value that shows the change in blood glucose levels caused by the food. It is calculated by the following formula:

$$\text{Glycaemic load (GL)} = \frac{\text{Carbohydrate content (g)} \times \text{Glycaemic index}}{100}$$

The carbohydrate content is the total amount of carbohydrate present in the meal.

Carbohydrate-rich foods are divided into three categories on the basis of GL values: Low GL (1–10), medium GL (11–19) and high GL (more than 20).

Dietary Fibres The term dietary fibres refer to the total amount of nondigestible substances present in the foods of plant origin.

They are of two types:

1. **Soluble fibre** that forms gel-like material when dissolved in water. These fibres are useful in lowering blood cholesterol and glucose levels.
2. **Insoluble fibre** that is insoluble in water. These fibres help in movement of food through the alimentary canal and increase the bulk of stool. They are used in patients suffering from constipation.

Total dietary fibre can be divided into nonstarch polysaccharides and lignin. Nonstarch polysaccharides can be further divided into noncellulosic polysaccharides and cellulose. Noncellulosic polysaccharides include hemicelluloses, pectin and other polysaccharides (Flowchart 9.1).

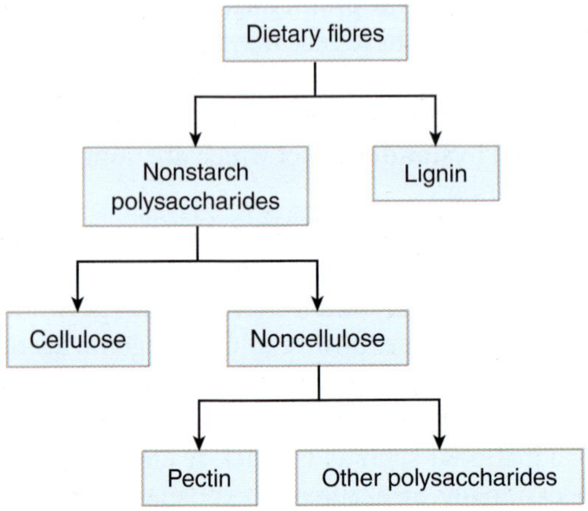

Flowchart 9.1 Types of dietary fibres.

Function Food rich in fibre contribute to weight-reducing diets because of their role in creating satiety and lowering cholesterol. They have also been useful in patients suffering from constipation and decreases the risk of colonic cancer by enhancing bowel motility. They also lower blood glucose levels which helps patients with diabetes to maintain good glycaemic control.

Proteins Proteins are essential components in the diet and are made up of amino acids. Amino acids are classified into two main classes based on their nutritional requirement – essential and nonessential amino acids. Essential amino acids cannot be synthesized in our body and have to be supplemented through diet. They include methionine, threonine, tryptophan, valine, isoleucine, leucine, phenylalanine and lysine. Nonessential amino acids can be synthesized in the body. They include glycine, alanine, serine, tyrosine, cysteine, glutamic acid, aspartic acid, asparagine, glutamine and proline. Arginine and histidine can be partly synthesized and are called semi-essential amino acids.

Limiting Amino Acids and Supplementary Effect Essential amino acids, which are found to be major limiting amino acids, are lysine and threonine found in cereals (wheat and rice), cysteine and methionine found in legumes and tryptophan in maize. Thus, combination of cereals with legumes can be followed to receive all the essential amino acids. This is called the supplementary effect.

Biological Value of Protein Biological value (BV) of protein is the ratio between the amount of protein retained in the body from the absorbed protein.

$$\text{Biological valve (BV)} = \frac{\text{Retained protein}}{\text{Absorbed protein}} \times 100$$

Sources of Protein Sources of protein include animal sources such as meat, dairy products, fish, and plant sources such as legumes, cereals and pulses.

Functions Proteins are required for growth, repair and maintenance of our body. They provide energy, immunity and maintain the osmotic pressure. Apart from this, they also produce numerous substances (muscular proteins, fibrous proteins, membrane proteins, globular proteins, etc.) with varying functions which are discussed in the respective chapters.

Minerals

Minerals are inorganic micronutrients. The daily requirement of macrominerals is more than 100 mg and they include calcium, phosphorus, magnesium, sodium, potassium, sulphur and chloride. The daily requirement of microminerals is less than 100 mg and they include iron, copper, zinc, selenium, molybdenum and iodine. Table 9.3 describes the source, functions and the deficiency states of common minerals.

ROLE OF ANTIOXIDANTS IN HEALTH AND DISEASE

Antioxidants are compounds that inhibit oxidation, which produces free radicals leading to a chain reaction that damages the cells of various organs. Antioxidants perform a variety of functions and act as free radical scavenger, hydrogen donor, electron donor, peroxide decomposer, singlet oxygen quencher, enzyme inhibitor, synergist and metal-chelating agents. Antioxidants such as thiols or ascorbic acid (vitamin C) terminate these chain reactions. To balance the oxidative stress, plants and animals have a complex systems of overlapping antioxidants, such as glutathione and enzymes (e.g. catalase and superoxide dismutase [SOD]), produced internally, which is complemented by dietary antioxidants such as vitamin C and vitamin E.

Antioxidants are further classified as endogenous antioxidants, produced by the body and exogenous antioxidants provided through food supplements. They can also be classified on the basis of the method of synthesis – natural and artificial. Apart from this, on the basis of their action, they are classified into two types – enzymatic and nonenzymatic, which is shown in Fig. 9.11.

1) **Enzymatic antioxidants**: Enzymatic antioxidants work by breaking down and removing the free radicals. The antioxidant enzymes convert free radicals to hydrogen peroxide (H_2O_2) and then to water, in a multistep process in the presence of cofactors such as copper, zinc, manganese and iron. These include primary enzymes – amino acids with primary structure (e.g. catalase), and secondary enzymes – amino acids in helical or beta-pleated forms (e.g. G6PD).
2) **Nonenzymatic antioxidants**: Nonenzymatic antioxidants primarily intercept and terminate the free radical chain reactions. Few examples of the nonenzymatic antioxidants are vitamin C, vitamin E, plant polyphenol, carotenoids and glutathione.
   a) **Flavonoids**: These are the most common group of polyphenolic compounds in the human diet and are found ubiquitously in plants. They boost cellular immune response and also have antioxidant properties. They contribute to vision, brain and urinary tract health. Flavonoids have negligible direct antioxidant activity in the body, but the increase in antioxidant capacity of blood seen after consumption of flavonoid-rich foods is because of production of uric acid from flavonoid depolymerization and excretion.
   b) **Vitamins and minerals**: These micronutrients are essential for the proper functioning of various metabolic cycles in our body. Vitamins C and E, which are ubiquitous among raw plant foods, are confirmed as dietary antioxidants; whereas vitamin A

Table 9.3 Minerals and Their Sources, Function and Deficiency States

Mineral	Source	Function	Deficiency
Calcium	Dairy products mainly milk, green leafy vegetables fish	Part of hydroxyapatite in bones and teeth, muscle contraction, nerve impulse conduction, component of coagulation pathway and activation of enzymes such as adenylyl cyclase and nitric oxide synthase	Carpopedal spasms; Chvostek and Trousseau signs are positive; osteopenia and osteoporosis
Phosphorus	Milk, meat, cereals and nuts	Part of hydroxyapatite in bones and teeth, activation of enzymes, energy storage in the form of high-energy phosphates	Rare
Magnesium	Dark chocolates, avocado and nuts	Activation of enzymes such as hexokinase and pyruvate kinase	Hyperexcitability, cardiac arrhythmia
Sodium	Salt, canned and processed food	Maintenance of membrane potential, active transport of substances and fluid balance	Rare Dehydration, hypotension and tremors
Potassium	Fruits and vegetables	Maintenance of membrane potential and fluid balance	Muscle weakness and cardiac arrhythmia
Chloride	Salt and vegetables	Fluid balance	Rare
Iron	Meat, green leafy vegetables and jaggery	Cofactor of enzyme, oxygen transport	Microcytic anaemia
Copper	Meat, green leafy vegetables, nuts and legumes	Cofactor of enzymes such as superoxide dismutase and cytochrome C oxidase	Menkes disease, microcytic anaemia, weakening of blood vessels and hypopigmentation
Zinc	Meat, seafood, legumes and nuts	Cofactor of enzymes such as superoxide dismutase, DNA and RNA polymerase and reverse transcriptase	Acrodermatitis enteropathica, alopecia, growth and mental impairment and defective wound healing
Selenium	Meat and seafood	Component of selenoprotein, antioxidant	Keshan disease
Iodine	Iodized salt and sea foods	Thyroid hormone production	Goitre, fatigue and weight gain
Fluorine	Water, tea, grape juice, wine and resins	Protection of enamel	Dental caries and toothache
Manganese	Nuts, fruits and vegetables	Cofactor of enzymes such as manganese superoxide dismutase, arginase and pyruvate carboxylase	Rare, impaired growth

becomes an antioxidant following metabolism of provitamin A beta-carotene and cryptoxanthin.

- **Vitamin A (retinol)**, also synthesized by the body from beta-carotene and found in dark green, yellow and orange vegetables and fruits, offers protection from solar radiation damage. Carrots, squash, broccoli, sweet potatoes, tomatoes (which gain their colour from the compound lycopene) are good sources of vitamin A.
- **Vitamin C (ascorbic acid)** is a water-soluble compound that fulfils several roles in human beings. Ascorbic acid is required for the conversion of the procollagen to collagen by oxidizing proline residues to hydroxyproline. In other cells, it is maintained in its reduced form by reaction with glutathione, which can be catalysed by protein disulphide isomerase and glutaredoxins. Ascorbic acid is a redox catalyst which can reduce, and thereby neutralize, ROS such as hydrogen peroxide. Sources include citrus fruits (e.g. oranges and sweet lime), green peppers, broccoli, green leafy vegetables, black currants, strawberries, blueberries, tomatoes, lemons, etc.
- **Vitamin E**, including tocotrienol and tocopherol, is a fat-soluble vitamin that protects lipids. Sources include wheat germ nuts, seeds, whole grains, green leafy vegetables, kiwifruit, vegetable oil and fish liver oil. Alpha-tocopherol is the main form in which vitamin E is consumed. Recent studies showed that some tocotrienol isomers have significant antioxidant properties.
- **Minerals such as selenium, zinc, magnesium, manganese and iodide** play a key role as antioxidants. The acute effects of zinc are produced by two

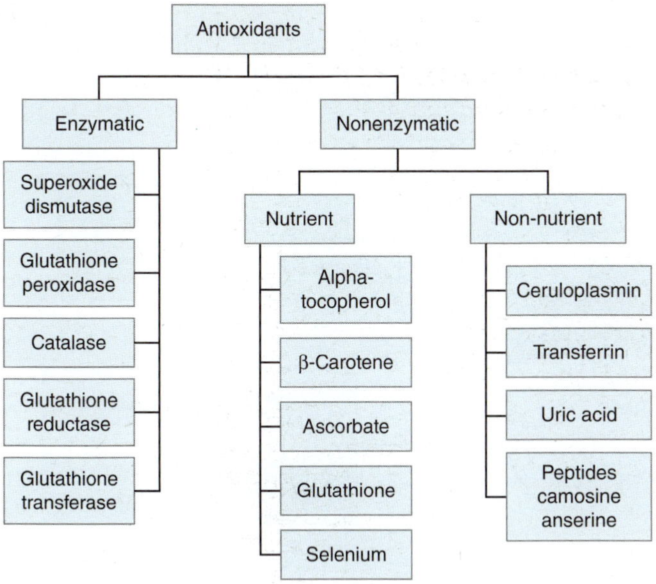

Fig. 9.11 Antioxidants.

mechanisms: Protection of protein sulphydryls and reduction of hydroxyl radical formation from H_2O_2 through the antagonism of redox-active transition metals, such as iron and copper. It chelates transition metals and prevents them from catalysing the production of free radicals in the cell.

c) **Organophosphorus compounds:** Glutathione has antioxidant properties because the thiol group in its cysteine moiety is a reducing agent and can be reversibly oxidized and reduced. In cells, glutathione is maintained in the reduced form by the enzyme glutathione reductase which in turn reduces other metabolites and enzyme systems, such as ascorbate in the glutathione–ascorbate cycle, glutathione peroxidases and glutaredoxins, thus eliminating oxidants.

d) **Carotenoids:** The beneficial properties of members of the carotenoid family such as alpha-carotene, beta-carotene, gamma-carotene, lycopene, lutein, zeaxanthin, beta-cryptoxanthin, astaxanthin carotenoids in prevention of various diseases, such as tumour formation, cardiovascular diseases and vision disturbances, have been documented. This is because of their roles as antioxidants, activation of certain gene expression associated with cell-to-cell communication, provitamin A activity, modulation of lipoxygenase activity and immune response.
   - **Beta-carotene**, which is referred to as a provitamin of vitamin A (retinol), is required for the fulfilment of visual functions. Beta-carotene protects the skin from harmful effects of UV light by preventing the formation of ROS and has anti-inflammatory properties. It counteracts the oxidative damage of cellular lipids, proteins and DNA caused by sunlight and prevents the formation of erythema, premature ageing of the skin, development of photodermatitis and skin cancer.
   - **Lycopene**, synthesized by many plants and microorganisms, is an antioxidant that cannot be synthesized by animals and humans. Lycopene is reported to have a higher antioxidant capacity than other carotenoids, and in particular lycopene has been proven to reduce the risk of prostate cancer.

e) **Uric acids:** Uric acid, the antioxidant with the highest concentration in human blood, is produced from xanthine by the enzyme xanthine oxidase, and is an intermediate product of purine metabolism. Antioxidant activities of uric acid are complex because it does not react with some oxidants, such as superoxide, but does act against peroxynitrite, peroxides and hypochlorous acid.

Free radicals are produced in the body because of exposure to radiation, some environmental pollutants and as by-products of normal metabolism and cause damage to the cells.

The '**antioxidant hypothesis**' postulated in 1987, linked the high content of antioxidants present in plant foods with their health benefits through a direct effect on the reduction of oxidative stress. However, clinical trials supplementing healthy people with antioxidants gave contrasting results, with some intervention studies showing a protective effect, whereas in others no evidence of benefits or even an increase in mortality was described. Many antioxidants that penetrate the body through ingestion, inhalation or skin can be harmful. These substances can generate free radicals that could accumulate. This accumulation can cause damage and even death because of the biological consequences. For example, in the skin, there is a defence antioxidant against UV radiation which is formed by melanin and antioxidant enzymes. This defence prevents swelling, wrinkling and skin cancer. The benefit of antioxidant uptake has been demonstrated in certain conditions such as diabetes, asthma, haemodialysis, thalassaemia, rheumatoid arthritis, systemic attack, postmenopause, schizophrenia, depression and leukaemia (Fig. 9.12).

ROS, generated during excessive oxidative stress, are responsible for the pathophysiology of various cardiovascular disorders including atherosclerosis, cardiac hypertrophy, cardiomyopathy, heart failure, ventricular remodelling, ischaemia/reperfusion injury and myocardial infarction. Cellular 'redox homeostasis' generally maintains the healthy physiology in cardiac myocytes and endothelial cells. However, during excessive oxidative stress, the body's endogenous system fails to maintain normal physiology necessitating an antioxidant supplementation, which could scavenge the free radicals and other toxic radicals. Several antioxidants such as beta-carotene, lycopene, quercetin, resveratrol, vitamin C and vitamin E have shown preventive and therapeutic benefits in different forms of cardiovascular diseases.

The brain is one of the most energy-consuming organs and is entirely dependent on aerobic metabolism. This

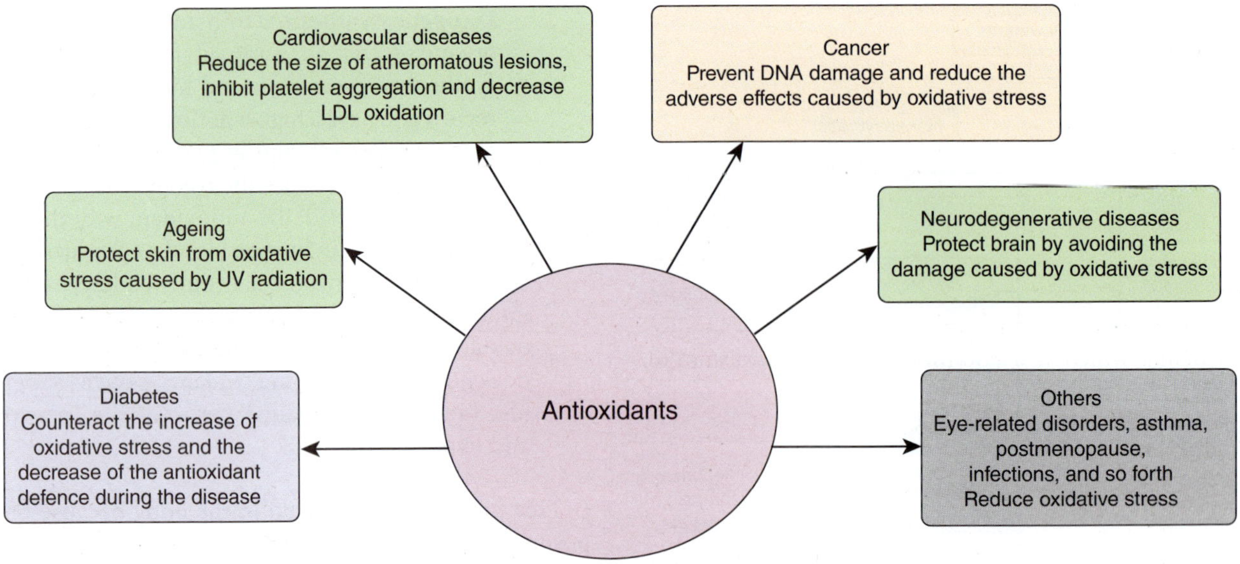

Fig. 9.12 Role of antioxidants in health.

organ uses glutamate as its neurotransmitter and stores high concentrations of iron, making it a superproducer of free radicals. Fortunately, to help detoxify ROS, powerful antioxidant enzymes exist within neurons just like other cells. The three main categories of antioxidant enzymes are catalases, SOD and glutathione peroxidases. These endogenous antioxidants along with the supplementary products are essential to prevent neurodegenerative disorders such as dementia and Alzheimer.

In anticancer therapy, antioxidants play a major role. Active oxygen and its various by-products may be involved in carcinogenesis through two possible mechanisms: Induction of gene mutations that result from cell injury, and the effects on signal transduction and transcription factors. Although these antioxidants offer defence against the effects of free radicals on cells, they may act as a double-edged sword and produce toxic effects at high concentration by overactivating the Nrf2 protein that regulates the antioxidant properties.

DISORDERS OF NUTRITION

Nutritional diseases can be classified into two types: Malnutrition and obesity depending on the availability of nutrients in humans. Even excess of nutrients can be harmful because what is seen in obesity is associated with many clinical consequences and is discussed in detail in the later part of this chapter.

A normal diet normally contains:

1) Adequate energy in the form carbohydrates, fats and proteins
2) Sufficient amino acids and fatty acids which are essential for making proteins and lipids
3) Recommended dietary allowance of vitamins and minerals to aid metabolism

Malnutrition can be due to inadequate intake or inefficient digestion or absorption. Malnutrition leads to loss of fat and muscle mass, weight loss, lethargy and generalized weakness.

Causes of Malnutrition

Following are the common causes of malnutrition:

- Poverty: Poor people suffer from nutritional deficiencies, and in poor countries, crop failures, livestock death, war, political upheaval, etc. lead to malnutrition. Poverty has been the leading cause of malnutrition.
- Infections: Protein–energy malnutrition (PEM) increases the susceptibility to infections and vice versa, forming a vicious cycle.
- Chronic alcoholism: Alcoholics generally have deficiencies of vitamins B1, B6, B9, A, etc., which can be because of poor intake, defective utilization, increased needs or increased rate of loss. The failure to recognize the deficiency can lead to irreversible brain damage (Wernicke encephalopathy and Korsakoff psychosis).
- Inadequate food intake: This is a cause of malnutrition, especially in infants, adolescents and pregnant women.
- Eating disorders: Anorexia nervosa, bulimia, etc. affect individuals who are concerned with body image and weight and lead to malnutrition in the long run.

PROTEIN–ENERGY MALNUTRITION PA 12.2

PEM is a serious disorder that preferentially affects children. Approximately 43% of children in developing countries are stunted and 50% of child deaths are related to malnutrition. PEM also occurs in older and debilitating patients in nursing homes and hospitals. Mini Nutritional Assessment (MNA) is the tool used to measure the nutritional status of older people. Weight loss of more than 5%

associated with PEM showed increased risk of mortality by almost fivefold in them.

Malnutrition is determined according to the following parameters:

a) Body mass index (BMI) (weight in kilograms per height in metre square) has a normal range of 18.5–25 kg/m^2. Therefore, BMI less than 16 is considered as malnutrition. A child whose weight falls less than 80% of normal is also considered as a child with malnutrition. However, many a times, weight may be masked by generalized oedema, which is a common feature of kwashiorkor, explained later.
b) Evaluation of fat stores (thickness of skinfolds).
c) Muscle mass (reduced midarm circumference).
d) Levels of serum proteins.

Marasmus and kwashiorkor: PEM is a form of malnutrition that is defined as a range of conditions arising from coincident lack of dietary protein and/or energy (calories) in varying proportions. The condition can be classified as mild, moderate and severe degrees. The two ends of the spectrum are marasmus and kwashiorkor. They both differ with respect to the alterations of the two regulated protein compartments in the body.

1) Somatic component: Proteins in skeletal proteins (more affected in marasmus).
2) Visceral component: Protein stores in the visceral organs, primarily the liver (more affected in kwashiorkor).

Marasmus: A child is considered to be suffering from marasmus when weight falls to less than 60% of normal for sex, weight, height and age. Such a child suffers from growth retardation, loss of muscle and depletion of somatic protein components. The depletion of proteins is an adaptive mechanism to provide the body with amino acids and energy. As the leptin production drops down, it stimulates the hypothalamic–pituitary–adrenal axis to increase the cortisol production which induces lipolysis. With loss of muscles, the extremities are emaciated, and so by comparison, the head appears too large for the body. Other manifestations of marasmus are because of anaemia, vitamin deficiencies and immune deficiency.

Kwashiorkor: Kwashiorkor is commonly seen in African children who have been weaned too early and subsequently fed poor diet. It is also seen in patients suffering from chronic diarrhoea and those with chronic protein loss such as in cases of protein-losing enteropathies, nephrotic syndrome or extensive burns.

The differences between marasmus and kwashiorkor are given in Table 9.4.

Table 9.4 Differences Between Marasmus and Kwashiorkor

Marasmus	Kwashiorkor
Infants are commonly affected	Children till 3 years of age are affected
Both calorie and protein deficiencies	Predominantly proteins are deficient
Somatic protein component gets depleted	Visceral protein component, more precious and critical for survival gets depleted
Serum albumin levels are normal or slightly decreased	Severe hypoalbuminaemia is a common feature
No generalized oedema	There is generalized or dependent oedema which masks the loss in weight
Severe muscle wasting	Muscle wasting is mild or absent
Subcutaneous fat is metabolized and used as fuel	Subcutaneous fat is preserved

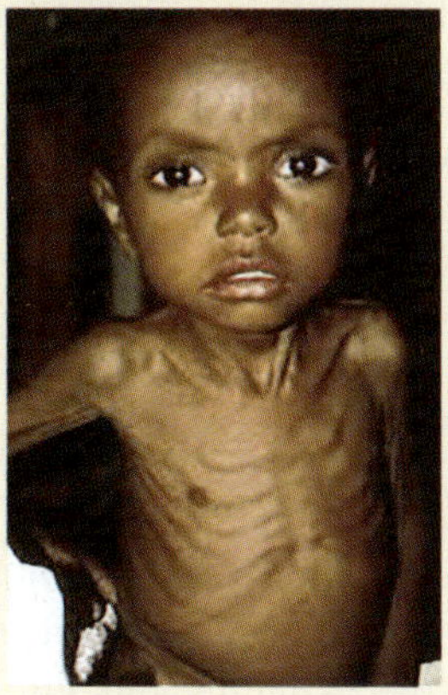

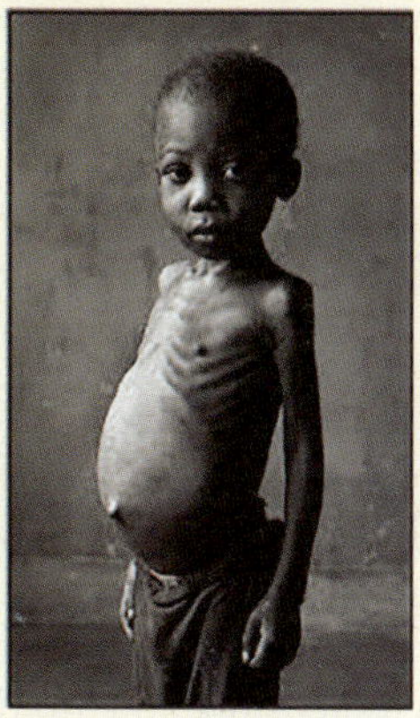

Morphology

Main anatomic changes seen in PEM are growth failure, peripheral oedema in kwashiorkor and loss of body fat and atrophy of muscles in marasmus.

Liver is enlarged and fatty in kwashiorkor. Small bowel shows a decrease in the mitotic index in crypts of glands along with mucosal atrophy and loss of microvilli. The enzyme production is disturbed, often manifested as disaccharidase deficiency because of which the affected patients will not be able to respond to milk-based diets.

Bone marrow becomes hypoplastic, both in case of marasmus and kwashiorkor. The peripheral blood reveals mild anaemia, which is multifactorial in origin such as iron, folate and protein deficiencies or because of the myelosuppressive effects of infection.

Brain appears atrophic with reduction in the number of neurons and impaired myelination of white matter in children who are born to malnourished mothers and in those suffering from PEM in the first few years of life.

The extent of growth failure and the severity of hypoproteinaemia, hypoalbuminaemia and electrolyte imbalances in persons with PEM are predictors of prognosis. Another important complication of malnutrition is micronutrient deficiencies. Vitamin deficiencies are also commonly associated with all forms of malnutrition, with deficiencies in the fat-soluble vitamins being more common.

ANOREXIA NERVOSA AND BULIMIA

Anorexia nervosa and bulimia are eating disorders leading to malnutrition.

Anorexia Nervosa

Anorexia nervosa is a potentially life-threatening eating disorder characterized by the inability to maintain a minimal normal weight, an excessive fear of weight gain, relentless dietary habits that prevent weight gain, and a disturbance in the way in which body weight and shape are perceived. This disorder most commonly affects teens, women and individuals who are keen to maintain body weight such as actors and athletes. There are two main forms of anorexia discussed as follows:

- Restricting type, in which severe limitation of food intake is the primary means to weight loss
- Binge-eating/purging type, in which there are bouts of food intake that are compensated by self-induced vomiting, diuretic or laxative abuse and/or excessive exercise

Peculiar patterns of eating such as breaking food into small pieces, hiding foods or eating food in a specific order may be observed. There is generalized loss of muscle which causes fatigue and loss of cardiac muscle that leads to hypotension and bradycardia. Vitamin and mineral deficiency may also occur. Affected persons are more prone to fractures owing to the development of osteoporosis. Endocrine abnormalities are present and amenorrhea is commonly seen in affected women. Behaviourally, the patient may demonstrate a blunted affect and display psychomotor retardation, especially in the later stages of the disease. Serious complication of anorexia is development of cardiac arrhythmia and hypokalaemia-associated sudden death.

Bulimia

Bulimia is a psychiatric condition characterized by recurrent episodes of binge eating (eating more than the average person in a 2-hour period, accompanied by a sense of loss of control), repetitive inappropriate compensatory behaviours to avoid weight gain. Such eating episodes occur at least once a week for a period of 3 months.

Bulimia is often confused with anorexia nervosa, especially the binge-eating type, because of overlapping of features between them. The main differentiating factor is the body weight. People with anorexia are generally underweight, whereas bulimic patients are normal or overweight. People with bulimia can develop anorexia later in life.

Patients with bulimia may commonly present with gastrointestinal symptoms such as pharyngeal irritation, abdominal pain, haematemesis (from oesophageal irritation; rarely, from actual tears, which may be fatal), difficulty swallowing, bloating, flatulence, constipation and gastroesophageal reflux disease (GERD) apart from the symptoms of malnutrition.

Patients affected by both the disorders are treated with cognitive behavioural therapy, psychotherapy and nutritional rehabilitation counselling along with the nutritional support.

VITAMIN DEFICIENCY

Vitamin deficiency refers to long-term lack of a vitamin. Vitamins are organic molecules that are needed in minor quantities for the proper functioning of the body. Because most of the vitamins cannot be produced by our body in sufficient quantities, they need to be obtained through the diet. Regular intake of recommended dietary allowance of all the 13 vitamins is important for health. Among all the vitamins, A, D, E and K are fat soluble, whereas all the rest are water-soluble vitamins. It is essential to differentiate fat-soluble vitamins from water-soluble vitamins because fat-soluble vitamins require fat for their absorption and hence their absorption is affected in fat malabsorption states. They are also stored in our body and hence can lead to hypervitaminosis that refers to symptoms caused by vitamin level in excess of the normal blood levels. On the contrary, for water-soluble vitamins, manifestations of deficiency occur quickly but toxicity is rare because they can be easily eliminated by our body in urine. Some vitamins can be synthesized endogenously such as vitamin D from precursor steroids, with the help of sunlight, vitamin K and biotin from intestinal microflora and niacin from tryptophan.

Vitamin deficiency can be primary (due to defective intake) or secondary (due to defective absorption, transport, storage or metabolic conversion). In the following sections, vitamins A, D, C, E and K are discussed in detail because of their wide-ranging activities and the morphologic changes of deficient states.

Vitamin A

Vitamin A is the name given to a group of closely related compounds that include retinol, retinal, and retinoic acid, which have similar biological activities. The generic term retinoids encompass vitamin A in its varied forms that include both natural and synthetic chemicals that are structurally related to vitamin A, but may not necessarily have vitamin A–like biological activity. Retinoids are derived from carotenoids, which originated in archaebacteria towards the beginning of evolutionary time. Chemical structures of carotenoids and retinoids are very similar. Retinol, retinal and retinoic acid are the vitamers of vitamin A.

Vitamin A is a fat-soluble vitamin. Dietary availability is mainly in the form of preformed vitamin A (beta-carotene) from plant sources (e.g. yellow and leafy green vegetables such as carrots, squash and spinach) or as provitamin A (retinyl esters) from animal sources (e.g. liver, fish, eggs, milk and butter). Retinol is the most active retinoid and generally bound to proteins or converted into retinyl esters for transport and storage. The two main transporters of vitamin A are chylomicrons and retinol-binding protein (RBP) and they are mainly stored in the Ito cells of the liver.

The dietary vitamin A is absorbed and converted into retinol in the enterocytes. They are then esterified to form retinyl esters which bind to chylomicrons and enter blood through lymph. Liver takes them up through apolipoprotein E and acts as a reserve organ. From the liver, these are distributed to all cells in need of the vitamin. Once taken up by the peripheral tissues, retinol may be stored as retinol ester or oxidized to form retinoic acid (as shown in Fig. 9.13), which has important effects on epithelial differentiation and growth.

In the eyes, retinol is oxidized to retinal which binds with opsin to form rhodopsin (visual pigment) (Fig. 9.13). In the rest of the cells, retinol is converted into retinoic acid because of its high affinity towards retinoic acid receptor (RAR) and retinoic X receptor (RXR) present in the DNA. The binding of the ligand to the receptor leads to gene activation which eventually leads to transcription and later translation to form specific proteins.

Functions of vitamin A include maintenance of normal vision; regulation of cell growth and differentiation, especially in mucus-secreting epithelium; regulation of lipid metabolism; and host resistance to infection. The effects of vitamin A on infections are because of immune-stimulating effects by still poorly understood mechanisms. Vitamin A is also used in the treatment of acne, premature ageing of skin and acute promyelocytic leukaemia.

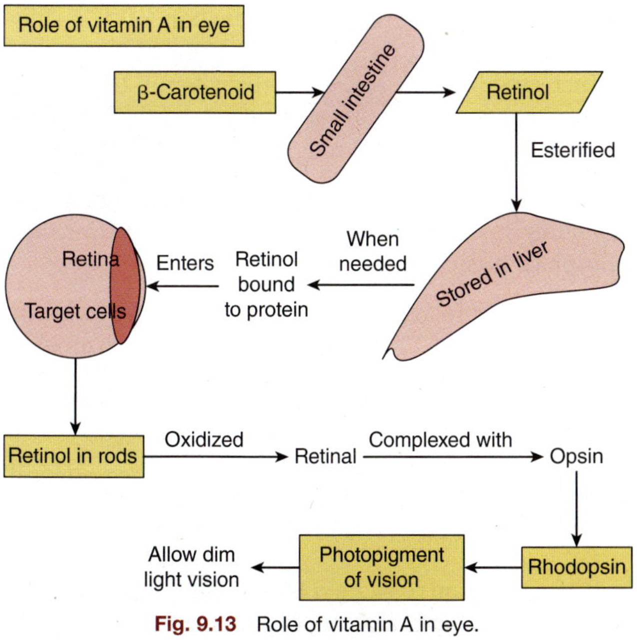

Fig. 9.13 Role of vitamin A in eye.

Deficiency of vitamin A leads to the following conditions:

- Impaired vision – night blindness
- Epithelial metaplasia and keratinization – in eyes, xerophthalmia (xerosis conjunctivae, Bitot spot, keratomalacia and blindness)
- Squamous metaplasia of epithelial lining of respiratory tract (loss of mucociliary epithelium – predisposition to infection) and urinary tract (predisposition to kidney stones)
- Vitamin A deficiency causes immune deficiency which increases the risk of infection which in turn reduces bioavailability of retinol and leads to a vicious cycle (Fig. 9.14)

Toxicity Excessive accumulation of vitamin A (topical application or consumption of vitamin A) leads to toxicity. Toxicity can be acute or chronic. Acute toxicity is due to intake of a large amount of vitamin A over a short period of time and the symptoms include headache, dizziness, vomiting, stupor and blurred vision. Such symptoms may cause clinical picture like that of brain tumour and hence is termed as 'pseudotumour cerebri'. Chronic toxicity is due to intake of vitamin A over a longer duration and the symptoms include weight loss, anorexia, vomiting, nausea, bone pain and high risk for fracture. Synthetic retinoids are contraindicated in pregnancy because these can lead to teratogenicity.

Vitamin D

Vitamin D is a fat-soluble vitamin and its deficiency has been escalating as a common problem worldwide. Production of this vitamin mainly depends on exposure to sunlight and, therefore, it is called sunshine vitamin. Functions of vitamin D include maintenance of adequate levels of ionized calcium and phosphate levels in plasma, bone mineralization and neuromuscular transmission.

Metabolism of Vitamin D The most important source of vitamin D in humans (approximately 90% of the required vitamin D) is its endogenous synthesis from the precursor, 7-dehydrocholesterol, in a photochemical reaction that requires solar or artificial UV light in the range of 290–315 nm (UVB radiation). This reaction leads to the synthesis of cholecalciferol, known as vitamin D3. The term vitamin D is used to refer to vitamin D3. Endogenous production of vitamin D is not uniform among people, and individuals with dark skin generally have a

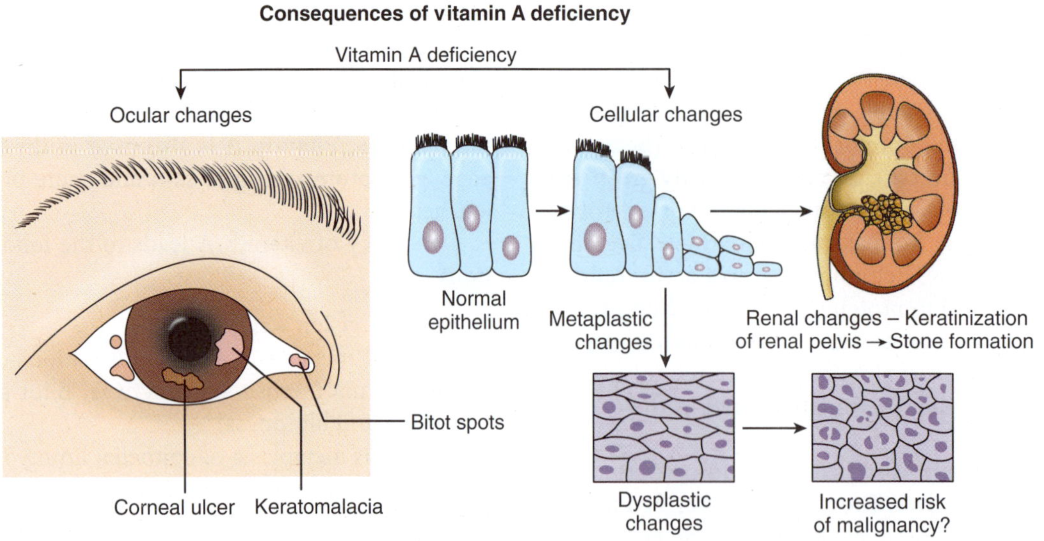

Fig. 9.14 Vitamin A deficiency, its major consequences in the eye and in the production of keratinizing metaplasia of specialized epithelial surfaces, and its possible role in epithelial metaplasia. Not depicted are night blindness and immune deficiency.

lower level of vitamin D production because of melanin pigmentation. Dietary sources of vitamin D include deep sea fish, fish oil, plants and grains.

The main events in vitamin D metabolism are summarized as follows:

1. Vitamin D is synthesized photochemically from 7-dehydrocholesterol in the skin and partly absorbed from foods and supplements in the gut.
2. Vitamin D from both the sources binds to plasma α1-globulin (vitamin D–binding protein [DBP]) and gets transported into the liver.
3. In the liver, it is converted into 25-hydroxycholecalciferol [25-(OH)-D], by the action of 25-hydroxylases, including CYP27A1 and other CYPs.
4. Following this, it is then converted into 1,25-dihydroxyvitamin D [1α,25$(OH)_2$D3], the most active form of vitamin D, by the enzyme 1α-hydroxylase in the kidney.
5. Active vitamin D3 may then bind to vitamin D receptors which interact with vitamin D response elements (VDRE) and cause transcription of DNA to produce the required effect.

Functions of Vitamin D Vitamin D, like retinoids and steroid hormones, binds to high-affinity nuclear receptor. Such receptors are located in most cells of the body. Plasma levels of calcium and phosphorus are regulated through the receptors located in small intestine, bones and kidneys. Apart from this, vitamin D appears to also act through mechanisms that do not involve transcription of target genes, such as the opening of calcium channels through activation of protein kinase C (PKC) by binding to membrane-associated vitamin D receptors. In addition to these functions, vitamin D has immunomodulatory and antiproliferative effects.

Mineralization of Bone Vitamin D plays a major role in the mineralization of osteoid matrix and epiphyseal cartilage in both long and flat bones. Osteoblasts that are stimulated by vitamin D, synthesize osteocalcin which is a calcium-binding protein involved in the deposition of calcium during bone development. Development of flat bones and long bones is discussed in Chapter 30.

Regulation of Vitamin D Three mechanisms regulate the production of 1,25-dihydroxyvitamin D in the kidney (Fig. 9.15):

1. Secretion of parathyroid hormone (PTH): It is secreted in response to hypocalcaemia, and augments the conversion of 25-(OH)-D into 1,25-dihydroxyvitamin D by upregulating the expression of 1α-hydroxylase.
2. Hypophosphataemia: This upregulates 1α-hydroxylase expression, increasing the production of 1,25-dihydroxyvitamin D.
3. Increased levels of 1,25-dihydroxyvitamin D: It downregulates its own synthesis through inhibition of 1α-hydroxylase activity, through a feedback mechanism.

Vitamin D has different effects on different organs and is mainly involved in the maintenance of calcium and phosphate homeostasis.

- In intestine: Increases calcium absorption by activating transcription of TRPV6 (calcium epithelial channels)
- In kidneys: Increases calcium reabsorption by activating transcription of TRPV5 (calcium epithelial channels)
- In bone: Stimulates osteoblasts to synthesize osteocalcin which is involved in the deposition of calcium during development of bone

The interaction of vitamin D with parathormone in the regulation of blood calcium:

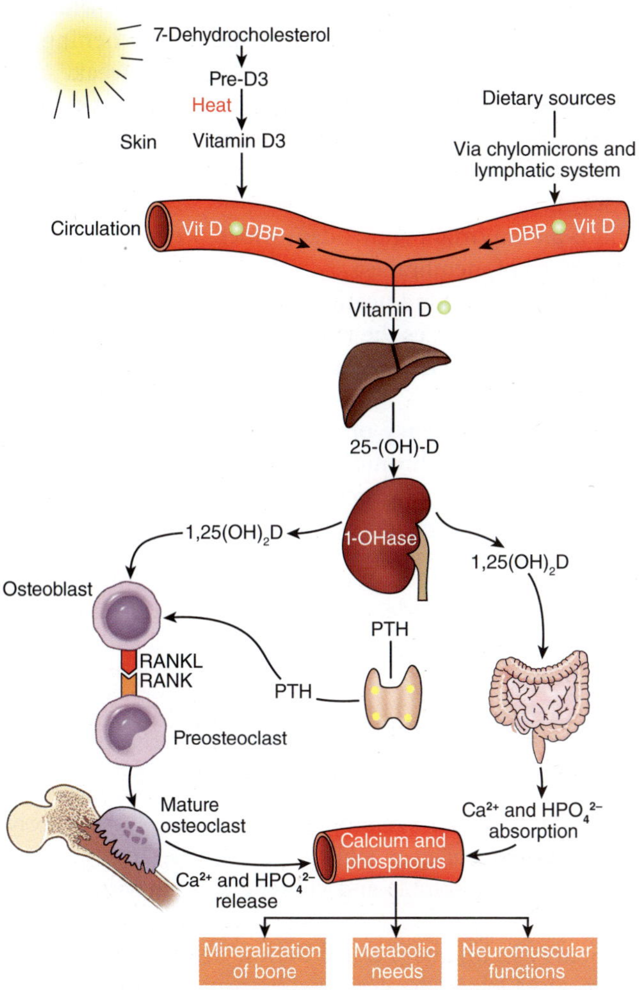

Fig. 9.15 Vitamin D metabolism. Vitamin D is produced from 7-dehydrocholesterol in the skin or is ingested in the diet. It is converted in the liver into 25-(OH)-D and in the kidney into 1,25-dihydroxyvitamin D ($1,25(OH)_2D$), the active form of the vitamin. $1,25(OH)_2D$ stimulates the expression of RANKL, an important regulator of osteoclast maturation and function, on osteoblasts and enhances the intestinal absorption of calcium and phosphorus. DBP, vitamin D–binding protein (α1-globulin).

In individuals with vitamin D deficiency, serum calcium levels fall and reflexly PTH production is elevated, leading to the following consequences (Fig. 9.16):

1. Activation of renal 1α-hydroxylase resulting in the increase of active vitamin D and calcium absorption.
2. Increased resorption of calcium from bone by osteoclasts.
3. Reduced excretion of calcium by kidneys.
4. Increased excretion of phosphate by kidneys.

With all the above-mentioned events, serum calcium levels may be restored but the problem of hypophosphataemia coupled with bone resorption leads to defective mineralization of bone.

Deficiency Vitamin D deficiency may be caused by limited exposure to sunlight (northern latitude inhabitants,

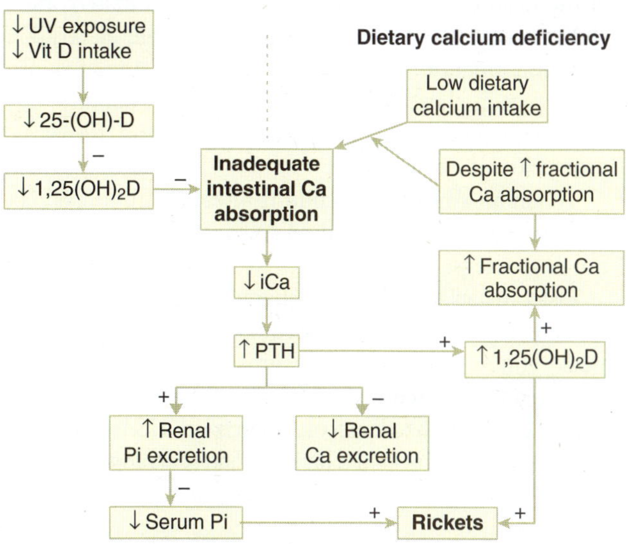

Fig. 9.16 Vitamin D deficiency. Illustration of pathogenesis of vitamin D deficiency and dietary calcium deficiency rickets. +, stimulatory effect; −, suppressive effect; Ca, calcium; iCa, ionized calcium; Pi, inorganic phosphate; PTH, parathyroid hormone; Vit D, vitamin D.

completely veiled women), renal disorders, phosphate depletion and malabsorption disorders.

Deficiency of vitamin D leads to rickets (children), osteomalacia (adults) and hypocalcaemic tetany (due to reduced ionized calcium levels in plasma which is required for normal neural excitation and muscle relaxation).

Morphology

Deficiency of vitamin D leads to excess unmineralized matrix in both rickets and osteomalacia.

Following sequence of events has been observed in patients with rickets:

- Inadequate calcification and failure of cartilage cells to mature leads to overgrowth of epiphyseal cartilage
- Persistence of irregular masses of cartilage that project into the marrow cavity
- Osteoid matrix deposition in inadequately mineralized cartilage
- Enlargement and lateral expansion of osteochondral junction
- Abnormal overgrowth of capillaries and fibroblasts, weakening the poorly formed bone
- Microfractures and stresses on the disorganized zones
- Skeletal deformation due to loss of structural rigidity

Features of rickets include the following which depend on the severity of the process, duration of the disease and extent of damage.

When the affected child is a nonambulatory infant, the head and chest are the major sites of stress. The child so presents with frontal bossing and squared appearance of the head due to excess of unmineralized matrix, rachitic rosary due to overgrowth of cartilage at costochondral junction, craniotabes due to softening of skull bone, pigeon chest deformity due to inward bending of ribs (with weakened metaphyseal ends) and forward protrusion of sternum.

When an ambulatory child is affected, spine, pelvis and tibia are affected leading to lumbar lordosis and bowing of legs.

Osteomalacia in adults is characterized by excess of persistent osteoid due to inadequate mineralization and weak bones. Fractures, be it gross or microfractures, mostly affect vertebral bodies and femoral neck. The excess unmineralized osteoid matrix in H&E staining appears as pink, thickened layer of matrix arranged about the more basophilic normally mineralized trabeculae.

Vitamin D insufficiency which is more common in elderly increases the risk of bone loss and hip fracture.

Vitamin D toxicity is not seen with excessive exposure to sunlight, whereas excessive intake of oral doses of vitamin D is associated with toxicity. It causes metastatic calcification (due to hypercalcaemia), bone pain, loss of appetite, thirst and weakness.

Vitamin C

As discussed earlier, vitamin C is a water-soluble vitamin. Vitamin C is also regarded as antiscorbutic vitamin because it protects against scurvy. Scurvy was described as early as the time of ancient Egypt. It was a limiting factor in long-distance sea travel, often killing huge number of people. During the Age of Sail, it was assumed that at least half of the sailors die of scurvy on a major trip. James Lind is fondly remembered as the man who helped to conquer this killer disease. His experiment on board a naval ship in **1747** showed that oranges and lemons were a cure for scurvy. Until 1932, ascorbic acid was not identified and synthesized. Humans and other primates are not capable of synthesizing ascorbic acid (the active form of vitamin C) and require a constant supply through diet.

Source Sources of vitamin C include citrus fruits, berries, milk, liver, fish and is abundant in a variety of fruits and vegetables.

Metabolism Absorption occurs through sodium-dependent vitamin C transporters (SVCTs) present in intestine. Apart from the intestine, SVCTs are found in the cells of renal tubules, liver, brain, skeletal muscle and many other organs.

Functions Ascorbic acid has many important functions that are listed as follows:

- It acts as a coenzyme for hydroxylases. One of the most important examples for this is hydroxylation of procollagen by propyl and lysyl hydroxylases, which is essential for the cross-linking and strengthening of collagen. Hence, in its absence, collagen is weak.
- Synthesis of norepinephrine requires hydroxylation of dopamine, a step that requires vitamin C.
- It enhances iron absorption by maintaining the ferrous form.
- It is an important antioxidant which prevents oxidative damage of membranes.
- It promotes wound healing.
- Vitamin C reduces the risk of cataract.
- Vitamin C also has immunomodulatory effects.

Deficiency Deficiency of vitamin C is common among older individuals, chronic alcoholics, persons with mental disability and people who live alone.

Manifestations of scurvy include:

- Sore gums and loose teeth are noticed.
- Bone disease: Inadequate osteoid formation is a hallmark of scurvy. Generalized osteopenia and cortical thinning are also seen.
- Haemorrhage and healing defects are common.
- Nonspecific symptoms such as fatigue, irritability and depression are common manifestations.

Majority of the symptoms are because of the poorly hydroxylated collagen which lacks tensile strength and becomes more soluble and vulnerable to enzymatic degradation.

Scurvy in infants is called Barlow disease, the classical form of which is characterized by bruises, broken bones and sores that will not heal. Fortunately, it is rarely seen nowadays.

Vitamin C toxicity is rare, as expected with a water-soluble vitamin.

Vitamin E

Vitamin E or tocopherol is composed of four tocopherols (α, β, γ and δ) and four tocotrienols (α, β, γ and δ) present in food. All eight forms have antioxidant property but cannot be interconverted. Alpha-tocopherol is the only form of vitamin E that can cause deficiency symptoms.

Sources Alpha-tocopherol is found in certain vegetable oils (sunflower, safflower, soya bean, cottonseed, palm, and wheat germ and olive oil), whole grains, nuts and green leafy vegetables.

Metabolism Vitamin E is absorbed in the small intestine and incorporated into chylomicrons, by which it is carried into circulation. The hepatocytes take up these alpha-tocopherols and combine them with VLDL. The VLDL-bound vitamin is transported to other organs. Most of the tocopherols are stored in adipose tissue and the rest are excreted in faeces.

Functions

- Vitamin E acts as an important antioxidant. It scavenges peroxyl radicals and terminates the oxidation of polyunsaturated fatty acids.
- Vitamin E inhibits protein kinase C leading to inhibition of platelet aggregation, reduced proliferation of monocytes, macrophages, neutrophils and vascular smooth muscle cells.
- Vitamin E may directly bind to the enzymes involved in signal transduction and can change the activity of these signal transduction enzymes.

Deficiency Deficiency of vitamin E in humans is very rare. It can cause oxidative damage of tissues, neurological abnormalities such as peripheral neuropathy, ataxia and haemolytic anaemia.

Vitamin K

Vitamin K is a fat-soluble vitamin and exists in two bioactive forms (vitamin K1 and vitamin K2) and one synthetic form (vitamin K3). Vitamin K1 or phylloquinone is a plant product and is active in animals. It is responsible for the production of coagulation factors. Vitamin K2 (menaquinone) is synthesized by the gut bacteria which converts vitamin K1 into vitamin K2. The synthetic type is vitamin K3 (menadione) which interferes with glutathione and causes toxicity. Therefore, it is not useful in the treatment of vitamin K deficiency.

Sources Sources of vitamin K include leafy vegetables, broccoli, cabbage, lettuce and certain plant oils.

Functions

- Vitamin K is essential for the synthesis of coagulation proteins. Gamma-carboxylation of the coagulation factors (factors II, VII, IX, and X) helps them to bind with calcium ions. Therefore, it plays an important role in coagulation pathway. This is explained in detail in Chapter 16.
- Osteocalcin and matrix gamma-carboxyglutamate protein are K-dependent proteins found in bone.

Deficiency

- Vitamin K deficiency impairs the coagulation process leading to bleeding and bruising.

Mechanism

- Vitamin K1 is the major dietary form of vitamin K. It is absorbed in the jejunum and ileum and incorporated into chylomicrons. They then enter into liver and other peripheral tissues. Vitamin K is mainly excreted through faeces.
- Vitamin K cycle: Vitamin K is reduced by vitamin K epoxide reductase (VKOR) to vitamin K hydroquinone. Vitamin K hydroquinone is then converted by vitamin K–dependent carboxylase to vitamin K epoxide. Vitamin K epoxide is reconverted to vitamin K by VKOR. Mutations in the enzymes can result in bleeding disorders or resistance to anticoagulation.

Toxicity

There are no known toxicities associated with vitamin K1 or vitamin K2. Vitamin K3 is toxic, it increases the uptake of oxygen by liver, leading to rise in lipid peroxidation. This causes marked damage and death of hepatocytes and manifests with signs of jaundice, hyperbilirubinaemia and haemolytic anaemia.

The major functions and deficiency states of common vitamins are listed.

The functions, causes of deficiency and the symptoms of trace element deficiency are given in Table 9.5.

OBESITY

PA 12.3

Obesity is a disease of chronic calorie imbalance in which the intake of calories exceeds their consumption by body leading to abnormal or excessive fat accumulation. Although similar, the term overweight is practically defined as an excess of body weight for height. Normal, healthy men have a body fat percentage of 15%–20%, whereas normal, healthy women have a body fat percentage of approximately 25%–30%. However, because differences in weight among individuals are only partly the result of variations in body fat, the body weight, though easily obtained, remains a limited index of obesity.

BMI, also known as the Quetelet index, is used commonly to define obesity. In general, BMI correlates closely with the degree of body fat in most settings; however, this correlation is weaker at low BMIs. BMI is the most commonly used screening tool to estimate overweight and obesity. It is calculated by dividing weight in kilograms by square of height in metres. Individuals with BMI of 30 or higher are considered as obese.

Other indices used to estimate the degree and distribution of obesity include the four standard skin thicknesses (i.e. subscapular, triceps, biceps and suprailiac) and various anthropometric measures, of which waist and hip circumferences are the most important. Skinfold measurements are the least accurate means to assess obesity. waist-to-hip ratio (WHR) is used to assess excess abdominal fat. It plays an important role because fat accumulated in the trunk and abdominal cavity poses a higher risk than subcutaneous tissue accumulation in gluteal and lower extremities.

The present standard techniques for measuring visceral fat volume are abdominal computed tomography (CT) scanning (at L4–L5) and magnetic resonance imaging (MRI) techniques.

Obesity has become a significant worldwide issue, reaching epidemic levels in both developed countries like the United States and developing nations such as India. Around 50% of adults in these regions are obese, and

Table 9.5 Selected Trace Elements and Their Deficiency Syndromes

Element	Function	Basis of Deficiency	Clinical Features
Zinc	Component of enzymes, principally oxidases	Inadequate supplementation in artificial diets Interference with absorption by other dietary constituents Inborn error of metabolism	Rash around eyes, mouth, nose and anus called acrodermatitis enteropathica Anorexia and diarrhoea Growth retardation in children Depressed mental function Depressed wound healing and immune response Impaired night vision Infertility
Iron	Essential component of haemoglobin as well as several iron-containing metalloenzymes	Inadequate diet Chronic blood loss	Hypochromic microcytic anaemia (Chapter 15)
Iodine	Component of thyroid hormone	Inadequate supply in food and water	Goitre and hypothyroidism (Chapter 28)
Copper	Component of cytochrome C oxidase, dopamine β-hydroxylase, tyrosinase, lysyl oxidase and unknown enzymes involved in cross-linking collagen	Inadequate supplementation in artificial diet Interference with absorption	Muscle weakness Neurologic defects Abnormal collagen cross-linking
Fluoride	Mechanism unknown	Inadequate supply in soil and water Inadequate supplementation	Dental caries
Selenium	Component of glutathione peroxidase Antioxidant with vitamin E	Inadequate amounts in soil and water	Myopathy Cardiomyopathy (Keshan disease)

alarmingly, children and adolescents are increasingly affected too. The primary causes of this trend are identified as the consumption of high-calorie diets, intake of refined food products, and a predominantly sedentary lifestyle. These factors together contribute to the escalating obesity rates observed globally.

Classification of Obesity

Although many classifications and definitions for degrees of obesity are accepted, the most widely accepted classifications are those from the World Health Organization (WHO), based on BMI. WHO designations include the following:

- **Grade 1** overweight (commonly called overweight): BMI of 25–29.9 kg/m^2
- **Grade 2** overweight (commonly called obesity): BMI of 30–39.9 kg/m^2
- **Grade 3** overweight (commonly called severe or morbid obesity): BMI of 40 kg/m^2 or higher

Pathogenesis

In simple terms, obesity is a disorder of energy homeostasis. Obesity is a multifactorial disease in which genetic, environmental and psychological factors interact and influence the energy balance. Of these, the major mechanism is the neurohumoral pathway which regulates the energy intake and expenditure. The master regulator of this pathway is the hypothalamus. When it receives signals from the periphery that the stores are adequate, catabolic circuits are triggered and when the signals convey that the stores are inadequate, anabolic circuits are triggered. The downstream events of activation of anabolic circuits are increase in food intake and reduction of energy expenditure, whereas activation of catabolic circuits leads to reduced food intake and increased energy expenditure.

Neurohumoral mechanisms operate with three components – afferent signals, efferent signals and central processing system.

Afferent signals can be long-term signals (leptin and insulin) which regulate the body weight or short-term signals (adiponectin, ghrelin and peptide YY-PYY) which regulate hunger and satiety. These signals stimulate neurons of the arcuate nucleus in the hypothalamus. These first-order neurons in the arcuate nucleus are mainly of two types. They are pro-opiomelanocortin/cocaine and amphetamine-regulated transcripts (POMC/CART) and neuropeptide Y/agouti-related peptide (AgRP/NPY). POMC/CART neurons enhance the production of MSH which acts on its receptor present on second-order neurons. This in turn leads to production of hormones that enhance weight reduction. Similarly, when AgRP/NPY neurons are stimulated, NYY is produced which acts on Y1/5 receptors. This results in production of orexigenic factors which enhance uptake of food, eventually leading to weight gain (Figs 9.17 and 9.18).

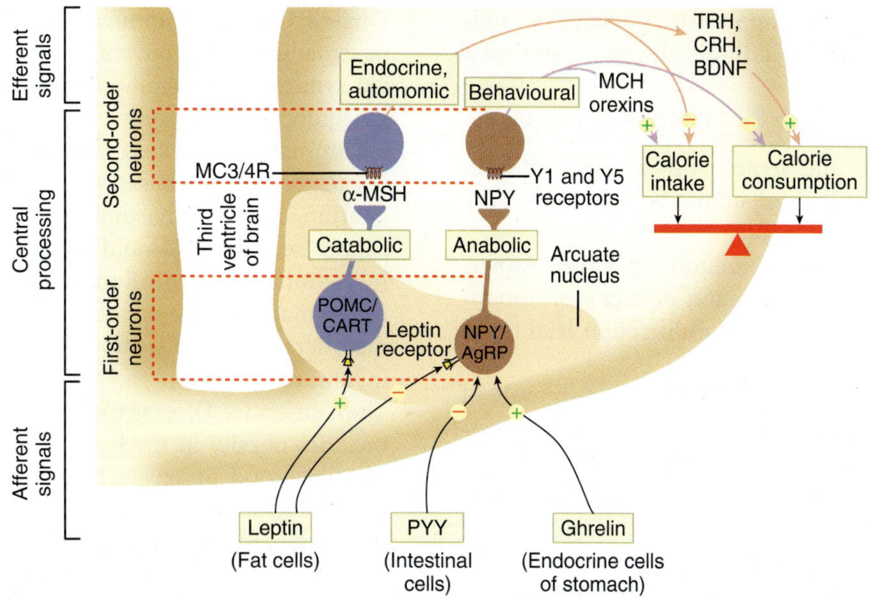

Fig. 9.17 Neurohumoral circuits in the hypothalamus regulating energy balance. Shown are POMC/CART anorexigenic neurons and NPY/AgRP orexigenic neurons in the arcuate nucleus of the hypothalamus and their pathways. BDNF, brain-derived neurotrophic factor; CRH, corticotropin-releasing hormone; TRH, thyroid-releasing hormone; MCH, melanin-concentrating hormone; PYY, peptide YY.

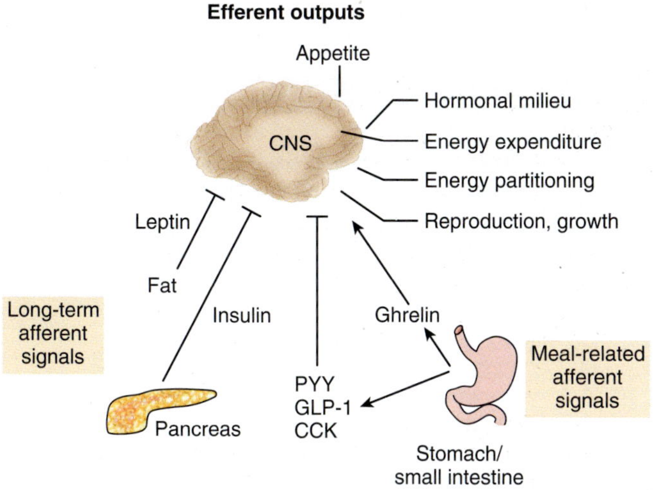

Fig. 9.18 Energy balance regulatory circuitry.

Leptin and ghrelin are two hormones that have been recognized to have a major influence on energy balance. Leptin is a mediator of long-term regulation of energy balance, suppressing food intake and thereby promoting weight loss. On the contrary, ghrelin is a fast-acting hormone, seemingly playing a role in meal initiation.

Leptin Leptin is a hormone secreted by adipocytes and its synthesis is tightly regulated by body fat stores. Leptin secretion is stimulated when the body's adipose tissue is abundant. It reduces food intake by stimulating POMC/CART neurons and inhibiting AgRP/NPY neurons. On the contrary, when the body fat stores are inadequate, leptin secretion is reduced which leads to increase in food intake. The gene responsible for production of leptin is the ob gene.

Ghrelin Ghrelin is a hormone produced by enteroendocrine cells of the gastrointestinal tract, especially the stomach, and is often referred to as the 'hunger hormone' because it increases food intake. Blood levels of ghrelin are highest before meals, when hungry, returning to lower levels after mealtimes. Ghrelin helps the body to prepare for food intake by increasing gastric motility and gastric acid secretion.

Adiponectin Adiponectin is an adipose tissue–specific protein, which is often referred to as 'fat-burning molecule'. It acts on its receptors AdipoR1 and AdipoR2 which are present in many tissues including brain, but are abundant in skeletal muscles and liver. Once these receptors are stimulated, cyclic adenosine monophosphate is activated which inactivates acetyl-CoA carboxylase, the crucial enzyme involved in fatty acid synthesis. Therefore, it proves to be a protective agent against obesity by promoting fatty acid oxidation and reducing fatty acid levels and hence fondly referred to as 'guardian angel against obesity'.

Apart from leptin, ghrelin and adiponectin, many other molecules are also involved in the pathogenesis of obesity including gut hormones such as PYY, GLP-1, adipose tissue (by releasing cytokines, chemokines, steroid hormones, etc.), and gut microbiome also participates in the pathogenesis of obesity.

Complications of Obesity

Obesity is associated with many of the most important diseases of humans, including insulin-resistant type 2 diabetes, cardiovascular disease, hypertension, dyslipidaemia, osteoarthritis and cancer. The complications of obesity are known since ages and Hippocrates quoted that 'sudden death is more common in those who are naturally fat than in lean'.

Obesity is associated with the following conditions:

- **Insulin resistance and hyperinsulinaemia** – insulin resistance is the result of inflammation induced by IL-1 and other factors.
- Hyperinsulinaemia causes sodium retention, expansion of blood volume, production of excess of norepinephrine and smooth muscle proliferation leading to **hypertension**.
- Hypertriglyceridaemia coupled with reduced levels of HDL seen in obese persons increases the risk of **coronary artery disease**. The coexistence of comorbid conditions such as diabetes, hypertension and dyslipidaemia increase the risk further.
- **Nonalcoholic fatty liver disease** (NAFLD) is a common disorder associated with obesity and diabetes.
- **Osteoarthritis** induced by the wear and tear of the joints because of the excess body weight is a commonly encountered problem in obese persons.
- **Cholelithiasis** is much more common in obese people when compared with lean people because of supersaturation of bile with cholesterol.
- **Obstructive sleep apnoea** with its consequent right heart failure and hypoventilation syndrome (Pickwickian syndrome) is commonly associated especially with morbidly obese persons.
- Inflammatory markers are commonly elevated in obese persons, the basis of which is still not clear. Activation of inflammasome by IL-1 triggered by the excess free fatty acids and lipids in tissues is central to induction of the **proinflammatory state**. Such chronic inflammatory state in obesity predisposes to other disorders such as cardiovascular complications and insulin resistance.
- The Centers for Disease Control and Prevention (CDC) includes obesity in the list of conditions that increase the likelihood of severe illness in persons with COVID-19. Obesity is associated with severe manifestations, higher incidence of hospitalization, intensive care requirement, mortality and post–COVID-19 sequelae.

Treatment

Various lifestyle modifications such as calorie restriction, physical activity and behaviour therapy have proven to help in obesity care. Pharmacological and surgical treatments are also available.

SELF-ASSESSMENT

Multiple Choice Questions

1. A 35-year-old man with a history of smoking and working in a battery manufacturing plant presents with symptoms of abdominal pain, constipation, and peripheral neuropathy. Which of the following is the most likely diagnosis?
   A. Chronic lead poisoning
   B. Nicotine addiction
   C. Alcoholic liver disease
   D. Diabetic neuropathy
2. A community near a coal power plant exhibits high rates of respiratory illnesses. Which pollutant is most likely contributing significantly to these health issues?
   A. Ozone
   B. Particulate matter
   C. Carbon monoxide
   D. Sulphur dioxide
3. A 50-year-old woman with a BMI of 42 kg/m^2 presents with dyspnoea, fatigue and obstructive sleep apnoea. Which obesity-related complication is she most likely experiencing?
   A. Hypertension
   B. Heart failure
   C. Type 2 diabetes
   D. Gastroesophageal reflux disease
4. A 10-year-old child from a low-income region presents with impaired wound healing, hair loss and diarrhoea. The child's diet is primarily corn-based. Which nutritional deficiency is most likely?
   A. Iron
   B. Vitamin C
   C. Protein
   D. Zinc
5. In a coastal town, several individuals present with symptoms of numbness, ataxia and impaired vision. The town's primary food source is seafood. Which environmental toxin exposure is most likely the cause?
   A. Mercury
   B. Lead
   C. Arsenic
   D. Cadmium
6. A 40-year-old woman with a sedentary lifestyle and high-stress job presents with central obesity, hypertension and high fasting blood sugar level. Which syndrome does this patient most likely have?
   A. Metabolic syndrome
   B. Polycystic ovary syndrome
   C. Cushing syndrome
   D. Hypothyroidism
7. Following a major earthquake, a population experiences increased respiratory problems due to dust inhalation. What is the most immediate public health measure to recommend?
   A. Antibiotics distribution
   B. Respiratory masks provision
   C. Vaccination campaign
   D. Relocation to shelters
8. A 30-year-old male presents with lethargy, muscle weakness and hyperpigmentation. Laboratory tests reveal hyponatraemia and hyperkalaemia. What is the most likely diagnosis?
   A. Addison disease
   B. Diabetic ketoacidosis
   C. Hypothyroidism
   D. Acute renal failure

9. In a city with high levels of air pollution, there is an observed increase in the incidence of which of the following diseases?
   A. Osteoporosis
   B. Asthma
   C. Hepatitis
   D. Gastroenteritis
10. A child living near an industrial area presents with developmental delays and a lower IQ. The child often plays in soil near a factory. What is the likely cause of the child's condition?
   A. Lead exposure
   B. Autism spectrum disorder
   C. ADHD
   D. Genetic factors
11. A middle-aged man who is a heavy smoker and lives in a high-pollution area presents with chronic cough and shortness of breath. What is the most likely diagnosis?
   A. Asthma
   B. Chronic obstructive pulmonary disease (COPD)
   C. Lung cancer
   D. Tuberculosis
12. In a community where rice is the staple food, several cases of peripheral neuropathy and skin lesions are reported. Which toxin is most likely the culprit?
   A. Mercury
   B. Arsenic
   C. Lead
   D. Cadmium
13. A woman living near a factory that emits large amounts of particulate matter develops a chronic skin condition characterized by inflammation and scaling. Which condition is she most likely to have developed?
   A. Psoriasis
   B. Eczema
   C. Urticaria
   D. Acne
14. A 45-year-old female with a BMI of 34 kg/m^2 presents with symptoms of chronic knee pain and difficulty in mobility. She has a sedentary lifestyle and a family history of type 2 diabetes. Which of the following is the most likely obesity-related complication she is experiencing?
   A. Osteoarthritis
   B. Gout
   C. Rheumatoid arthritis
   D. Fibromyalgia
15. A 38-year-old male with a BMI of 37 kg/m^2, working in a high-stress corporate job, experiences episodes of severe headaches, blurred vision and dizziness. He has been diagnosed with hypertension but is not on regular medication. What is the most likely immediate health risk associated with his obesity and symptoms?
   A. Diabetic retinopathy
   B. Migraine
   C. Stroke
   D. Glaucoma

Answers

1. (A); 2. (B); 3. (B); 4. (D); 5. (A); 6. (A); 7. (B); 8. (A); 9. (B); 10. (A); 11. (B); 12. (B); 13. (A); 14. (A); 15. (C).

Scenario-Based Questions

1. Air pollution and human diseases
2. Effects of tobacco on humans
3. Effects of alcohol
4. Severe acute malnutrition – causes, pathogenesis and morphology
5. Vitamin A – metabolism, functions and deficiency state
6. Vitamin D – metabolism, functions and deficiency state
7. Vitamin C – metabolism, functions and deficiency state
8. Role of antioxidants in health and diseases
9. Role of trace elements in health
10. Pathology of obesity

Topics for Self-Directed Learning

1. Menopausal hormone therapy
2. Cocaine abuse
3. Biomedical waste management
4. Hazards of plastic usage and waste
5. Obesity and cancer
6. Diet and diseases
7. Diet and cancer
8. Adverse drug reactions
9. Role of gut microbiome in obesity
10. Keshan disease

MIND MAP

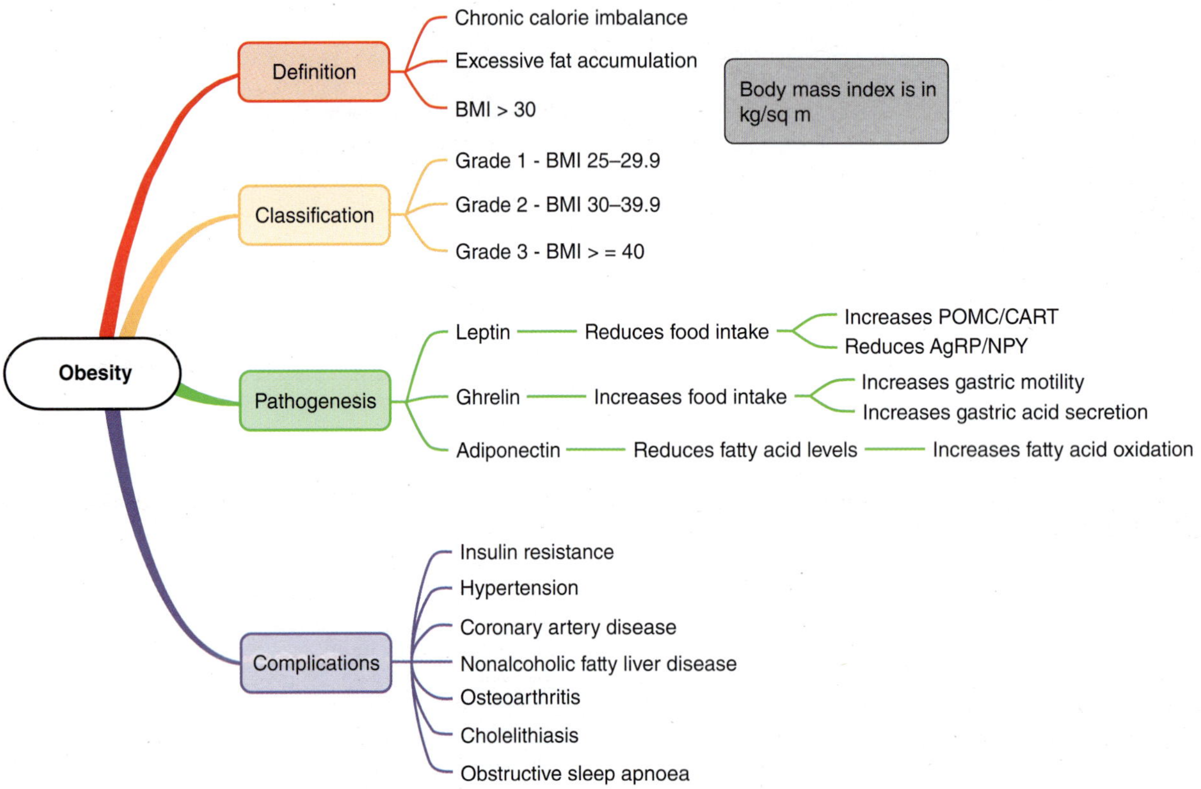
Obesity
Definition
Chronic calorie imbalance
Excessive fat accumulation
BMI > 30
Body mass index is in kg/sq m
Classification
Grade 1 - BMI 25–29.9
Grade 2 - BMI 30–39.9
Grade 3 - BMI > = 40
Pathogenesis
Leptin
Reduces food intake
Increases POMC/CART
Reduces AgRP/NPY
Ghrelin
Increases food intake
Increases gastric motility
Increases gastric acid secretion
Adiponectin
Reduces fatty acid levels
Increases fatty acid oxidation
Complications
Insulin resistance
Hypertension
Coronary artery disease
Nonalcoholic fatty liver disease
Osteoarthritis
Cholelithiasis
Obstructive sleep apnoea

Disorders of Infancy and Childhood

10

M Lavanya

PA 11.2 Describe the pathogenesis and pathology of **tumour and tumour-like conditions in infancy and childhood.**

CHAPTER OUTLINE

INTRODUCTION

Traditionally, the period of development from birth to childhood has been divided into several stages:

1. **Neonatal** (first 4 weeks)
2. **Infancy** (the first year)
3. **Early childhood** (1–4 years)
4. **Late childhood** (5–14 years)

At each stage, the anatomic, physiologic and immunologic characteristics of the child vary. Thus, at each stage, the child is vulnerable to a specific group of diseases. From the time of conception to birth and development, the child is exposed to varying challenges, which may result in mortality or significant morbidity. Some of the common causes of mortality for each stage are listed in Table 10.1.

With provision of better antenatal care for mothers, frequent monitoring of the fetus in utero and improved medical care, it has become possible to reduce perinatal mortality. This accomplishment is reflected in the global statistics by the World Health Organization (WHO) which shows the infant mortality rate (IMR) in the decreasing trend.

IMR in 1990 – 69/1000 live births
IMR in 2017 – 29/1000 live births

CONGENITAL ANOMALIES

Congenital anomalies are ***anatomical and functional defects*** present in the neonate at birth. Most of them are detected prenatally, at birth or later in infancy. Congenital anomalies are also known as ***birth defects, congenital disorders or congenital malformations.***

- These are the *most common cause for mortality in the first year* and contribute significantly to morbidity and mortality in early years.
- Congenital anomalies may be single or multiple; and it can be a minor or major anomaly.

TYPES AND DEFINITIONS OF CONGENITAL ANOMALIES

- **Major anomaly**: It refers to a severe defect with cosmetic and/or medical consequence and often requires surgical intervention.
  Examples: Cleft lip/palate, tracheoesophageal fistula, congenital heart defects.
- **Minor anomaly**: This has diagnostic importance but has little impact on the well-being of the individual.
  Examples: Anteverted nares, epicanthal folds, clinodactyly, single palmar crease.

Table 10.1 Common Causes of Death in Childhood

Stage of Development	Diseases
Neonate	**Congenital anomalies** Diseases related to prematurity and low birth weight Sudden infant death syndrome Complications of placenta, cord and membranes Neonatal infections Haemorrhage
Infancy	**Congenital anomalies** Diseases related to prematurity and low birth weight Sudden infant death syndrome Infections Accidents
Early childhood	Accidents, assaults Congenital anomalies Malignant neoplasms
Late childhood	Accidents, assault Malignant neoplasms Congenital anomalies

- **Functional anomaly**: The organs are normal structurally, but defective in their function.
  Examples: Congenital hearing loss, congenital blindness, inborn errors of metabolism.
- **Malformations**: These are defects in morphogenesis that results from intrinsically abnormal developmental process.
  Examples: Absent thumb, radial agenesis, anencephaly.
- **Disruptions**: These are due to extrinsic disturbances in morphogenesis. It results in secondary destruction of an organ or body region that had a previously normal development process.
  Example: Amniotic bands, which occur at site of rupture of amnion, may encircle the developing limb and cause distal hypoplasia or amputation of the limb.
- **Deformations**: These are also due to extrinsic disturbances in morphogenesis but are caused by abnormal mechanical force. Most deformities occur in the last trimester of pregnancy and get spontaneously corrected or are correctable with treatment in the postnatal period.
  Example: Clubfoot is caused by uterine wall compression in cases of oligohydramnios.
- **Sequence** is a cascade of anomalies arising from a single anomaly or pathogenetic mechanism.
  Example: Potter's sequence/oligohydramnios sequence. Oligohydramnios is a condition with reduced volume of amniotic fluid in the amnion, which normally acts as a cushion to the fetus. It is caused by maternal factors (chronic leakage of amniotic fluid, maternal hypertension) or fetal factors (bilateral renal agenesis, urethral obstruction). The lack of cushion effect causes compression of fetus by the uterine wall resulting in the classic spectrum of abnormalities – Potter's sequence (Table 10.2).

Table 10.2 Potter's/Oligohydramnios Sequence

Cause	Pathogenetic Mechanism	Anomalies
Fetal Renal agenesis Urethral obstruction	Oligohydramnios	Fetal compression Dysmorphic facies Abnormal position of hands and feet Breech presentation Pulmonary hypoplasia
Maternal Amniotic fluid leak		Amnion nodosum

- **Syndromes**: Multiple anomalies that affect various organ systems arising from a common pathogenetic mechanism but cannot be explained on the basis of a single initiating event are called syndromes.
  Examples: Chromosomal abnormalities (Down syndrome, Patau syndrome), viral infections (maternal TORCH infection, Zika virus)
- **Association**: It refers to multiple anomalies that arise concurrently but have different pathogenesis.
- **Agenesis**: It refers to the absence of an organ and its primordium.
- **Aplasia**: It refers to the absence of an organ because of failure of growth of existing primordium.
- **Atresia**: It refers to the absence of opening in a hollow organ like trachea and oesophagus.
- Hyperplasia, hypoplasia, hypertrophy and atrophy are same as defined in cellular adaptations.

CAUSES OF CONGENITAL ANOMALIES (TABLE 10.3)

The exact cause for congenital anomalies is not known in more than two-third of the cases. The known causes can be grouped into three major categories – genetic, environmental and multifactorial.

Pathogenesis

The pathogenesis of congenital anomalies is complex and still poorly understood. The various observations and researches have led to the formulations of general principles of teratology (study of developmental anomalies).

Susceptibility to teratogen is specific for each embryologic stage (Table 10.4).

Teratogenesis is ***dose-dependent and may be idiosyncratic.*** Hence, the absolute safe dose cannot be predicted for every woman. Moreover, susceptibility to teratogen is also

Table 10.3 Causes of Congenital Anomalies

Category	Examples
Genetic	Chromosomal aberrations Mendelian inheritance
Environmental	Maternal/placental infections TORCH infections Syphilis HIV Zika virus
Maternal disease states	Diabetes Hypertension/eclampsia Endocrinopathies – hypothyroidism
Drugs and chemicals	Alcohol Folic acid antagonist Phenytoin Sodium valproate Vitamin A
Multifactorial	Cleft lip Cleft palate Neural tube defects
Miscellaneous	Uterine factors Birth trauma/accidents
Unknown	

variable. It depends on complex interaction between the teratogen, maternal metabolism and fetal–placental unit.

DISEASES ASSOCIATED WITH PREMATURITY

OVERVIEW

Prematurity and Fetal Growth Restriction

Normal human pregnancy lasts 40 ± 2 weeks, and newborns on an average weigh 3300 ± 600 g. Prematurity or preterm babies are defined as babies born before 37 weeks of gestation. Low birth weight babies are those with birth weight less than 2500 g. Low birth weight may be because of prematurity or fetal growth restriction. In prematurity, the weight will be appropriate when adjusted for their gestational age. In contrast, some of the infants born at term have low birth weight and indicate fetal growth restriction (small for gestational age).

Both the conditions have similarities in the form of clinical presentation, risk factors and complications. Some of the differences between prematurity and fetal growth restriction are given in Table 10.5.

The common conditions affecting the neonate, especially preterm babies and their pathogenesis are discussed here.

DISEASES OF PREMATURITY

A. Neonatal respiratory distress syndrome (NRDS)
B. Necrotizing enterocolitis
C. Sepsis
D. Intraventricular haemorrhage

Neonatal Respiratory Distress Syndrome

NRDS is the most common cause for respiratory distress in newborns and if not treated, may lead to mortality (Table 10.6). This condition is also known as **hyaline membrane disease** because of the deposition of a layer of hyaline proteinaceous material in the alveolar spaces.

NRDS is usually associated with the following features:

1. **Prematurity:** Incidence of NRDS is inversely proportional to the gestational age. The lesser the gestational age, more the chances of developing NRDS.
2. **Male infant**
3. **Maternal diabetes:** High insulin level in fetus suppresses surfactant synthesis.
4. **Delivery by caesarean section:** Corticosteroids that play an active role in surfactant synthesis are produced by the fetus only during normal labour, and not in caesarean section.

Pathogenesis NRDS is due to ***immaturity of the lungs*** at the time of exposure to air, and the main factor responsible for the pathogenesis of NRDS is the ***pulmonary surfactant deficiency***. The surfactant is synthesized and stored by the type II pneumocytes in lung. The properties of surfactant are given in Table 10.7.

Table 10.4 Susceptibility to Teratogen and the Effects According to Stages of Development

Stage of Development	Period	Normal Development	Effect of Teratogen
Embryonic period – early	Fertilization to 3 weeks	Implantation, formation of bilaminar and trilaminar embryo	Spontaneous abortion
Embryonic period – late	3–9 weeks	Organogenesis	Highly susceptible to teratogenesis Abnormalities in various organ systems
Fetal period	10 weeks – birth	Maturation of organs	Growth retardation Deformations Disruptions

Table 10.5 Differences Between Prematurity and Fetal Growth Restriction

Factors	Prematurity	Fetal Growth Restriction
Birth weight	Low birth weight Appropriate for gestational age	Low birth weight Small for gestational age
Gestational age	<37 weeks Preterm	<37 weeks to 42 weeks Preterm to term
Risk factors	• Preterm premature rupture of membranes • Intrauterine infections caused by *Ureaplasma urealyticum*, *Gardenalla vaginalis*, *Trichomonas*, *Chlamydia* • Placental causes – placenta praevia, abruptio placentae • Multiple gestation **Maternal factors:** – Cervical incompetence – Uterine fibroids	• Congenital anomalies • Intrauterine infections – TORCH infection • Placental causes – single umbilical artery, placenta praevia, abruptio placentae, thrombosis and infarction of placenta • Multiple gestation **Maternal factors:** – Hypertensive disorders of pregnancy – Malnutrition – Drug (phenytoin) and substance abuse (narcotics, alcohol, cigarette smoking)
Pathogenesis for complications	• Immaturity of organs	• Mature organs, but defective development
Complications	• Neonatal respiratory distress syndrome • Necrotizing enterocolitis • Sepsis • Intraventricular haemorrhage	• Cerebral dysfunction, learning disability • Sequelae of birth defects • Disorders of prematurity

Table 10.6 Causes of Respiratory Distress in a Newborn

1. Neonatal respiratory distress syndrome (NRDS)
2. Excessive sedation of mother
3. Fetal head injury during delivery
4. Aspiration of blood/amniotic fluid
5. Intrauterine hypoxia due to prolonged labour/coiling of umbilical cord

Pathophysiology Before going to the pathophysiology, let us have a look at the changes that normally take place in the lungs at birth.

- In utero, at term, the lung alveoli are well developed and filled with amniotic fluid.
- At birth, during the first breath, high pressure is needed to force this fluid out of the lung and eventually fill it with air.
- This inspiratory stimulus causes the release of surfactant from type II pneumocytes.
- The surfactant acts on the alveolar wall and reduces its surface tension and keeps it patent during expiration.
- Patent alveoli requires less pressure to be inflated and hence subsequent respiration becomes effortless and rhythmic.

In surfactant deficiency

- The ***high surface tension in the alveolar walls*** causes the alveoli to collapse during expiration.

Table 10.7 Properties of Pulmonary Surfactant

Composition:	
Phospholipids: 90%	
Phosphotidylcholine (lecithin) – 75%	Starts appearing at 28 weeks, peaks at term
Phosphotidylglycerol – 10%	Starts appearing at 36 weeks
Sphingomyelin	High in immature lung and decreases towards term
Proteins: 10%	
Hydrophobic SAP: SP-B, SP-C	Reduces surface tension in alveoli; mutation in SFTPB, SFTPC causes respiratory insufficiency in neonate
Hydrophilic SAP: SP-A, SP-D	Regulate surfactant secretion and antimicrobial protection
Function: Reduces the surface tension and keeps the alveoli open at expiration	
Factors affecting surfactant synthesis:	
Stimulatory 1. Glucocorticoids 2. Thyroxine 3. Labour 4. Intrauterine stress and fetal growth restriction	Inhibitory 1. Insulin 2. Caesarean section

SAP, surfactant associated protein; SP, surfactant protein; SFTPB, gene for surfactant protein B; SFTPC, gene for surfactant protein C.

- The collapsed alveoli resist expansion during next breath.
- To overcome the stickiness within the alveoli and expand the lungs, considerable effort is needed.
- Hence, respiration becomes laboured, and this process damages the alveolar lining epithelium.
- The injured alveoli exude ***fibrin-rich exudate into the alveolar space***, impairing the gaseous diffusion and increasing the ***ventilation/perfusion mismatch***.
- The resulting hypoxia aggravates the damages to the alveolar epithelium, and the necrotic epithelial cells along with fibrin exudate form a hyaline membrane over the alveolar wall. This membrane further blocks the gaseous diffusion and a vicious cycle ensues.

Morphology

Gross The lungs appear normal in size, solid in consistency ***(airless)*** and reddish purple in colour. The consistency is liver-like, *as result of which* ***the lungs sink in water***, in contrast to normal spongy lungs which float in water.

Microscopy The lungs show normal development. The alveoli are collapsed and thick walled. The alveolar ducts and respiratory bronchiole are dilated and lined by characteristic conspicuous eosinophilic **hyaline membrane,** hence the name hyaline membrane disease (Fig. 10.1). The membrane is made up of protein-rich **fibrin exudate and necrotic cellular debris**. These changes are seen only in a neonate who dies early in the course of the disease. It is never seen in a stillborn infant.

Prevention Now with better understanding of the pathophysiology of the condition, focus is mainly on prevention than treatment. Careful intrauterine monitoring helps in identifying the fetus at risk of preterm labour, and appropriate preventive measures are taken which includes:

- Delaying labour until fetal lung achieves complete maturity
- Administration of steroids to mother to aid lung maturity
- Prophylactic administration of exogenous surfactant at birth to extremely premature babies (gestational age $<$28 weeks)

  The assessment of fetal lung maturity is done by *amniotic fluid analysis*. The ***indicators of fetal lung maturity in the amniotic fluid are as follows:***
  1. Lecithin–sphingomyelin ratio $>$ 2:1
  2. Presence of phosphotidylglycerol – best proof of optimal fetal lung maturity

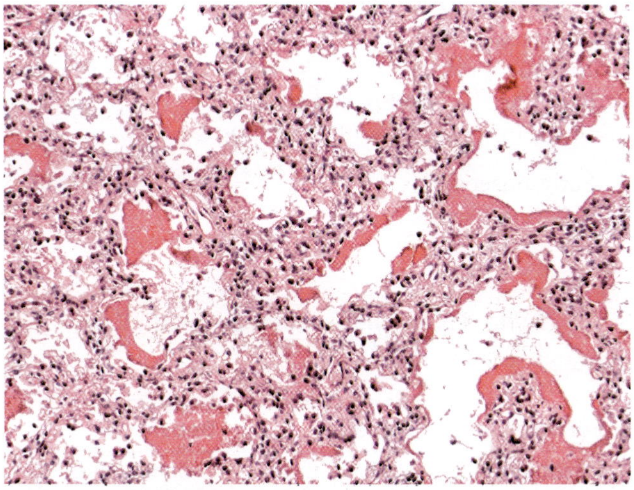

Fig. 10.1 Hyaline membrane disease: The lungs contained hyaline membranes (arrows), which are compacted proteinaceous material containing fibrin, other proteins and debris from necrotic epithelium, similar to the compacted exudates in adult diffuse alveolar damage. (*Source:* From Andrew J. Connolly, Walter E. Finkbeiner, Philip C. Ursell and Richard L. Davis. Microscopic Findings. In Autopsy Pathology: A Manual and Atlas 3rd edition. Elsevier 2016.)

Clinical Features and Management The characteristic clinical presentation is respiratory distress in the neonate. On examination, it was found that the baby is cyanotic with respiratory rate above 100 breaths/min. Fine rales can be heard in both the lung fields on auscultation and a chest X-ray reveals the characteristic **ground-glass granularity** (uniform minute reticulogranular densities).

Previously the standard treatment was to administer high oxygen (80%) under ventilatory support, which often fails and the child dies of respiratory failure. The neonates who are lucky enough to survive are usually affected by the complications of high oxygen therapy and other diseases of prematurity.

Complications of High Oxygen Therapy

- **Retrolental fibroplasia/retinopathy of prematurity**
  During oxygen therapy, the levels of proangiogenic vascular endothelial growth factor (VEGF) are suppressed. Once the baby is returned to air ventilation, the relative hypoxic state causes rebound increase in VEGF and induces new vessel proliferation in the retina.
- **Bronchopulmonary dysplasia**
  This condition is characterized by decrease in alveolar septations and dysmorphic capillary configuration due to arrest in lung development at the saccular stage. Hyperoxaemia, hyperventilation and inflammatory cytokines (TNF, IL-1β, IL-6, IL-8) play a role in the development of bronchopulmonary dysplasia.

In affected babies, oxygen therapy is required. Low tension oxygen is given with gentle ventilation techniques, to avoid the complications of high oxygen therapy.

Now the standard treatment for NRDS is as follows:

1. Low-tension oxygen with gentle ventilation support
2. Exogenous surfactant

In the era of treatment with exogenous surfactant, death due to NRDS has become uncommon. But the infants who recover are at increased risk of developing the other diseases of prematurity.

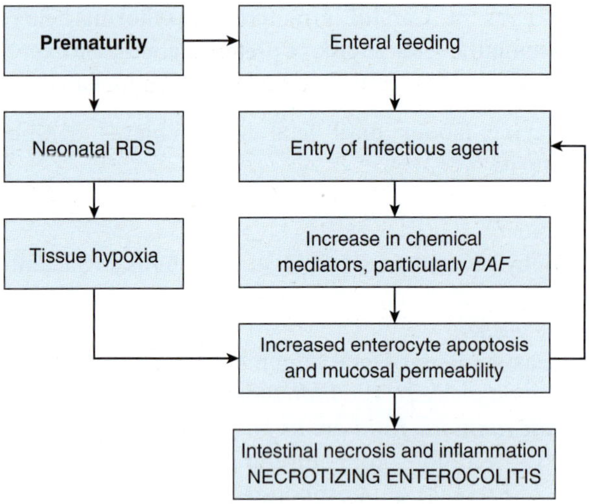

Fig. 10.2 Pathogenesis of necrotizing enterocolitis.

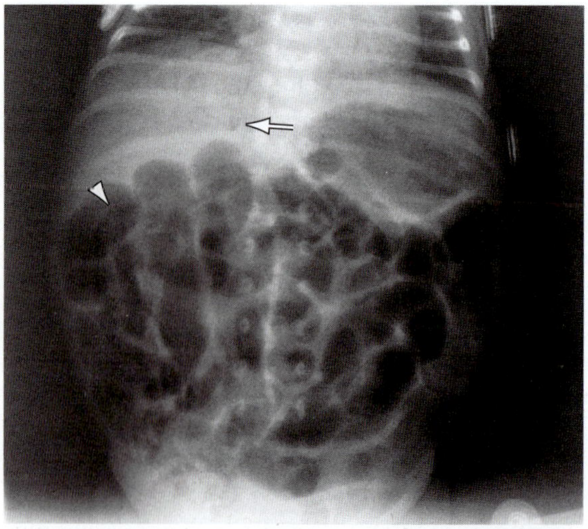

Fig. 10.3 Pneumatosis intestinalis. Abdominal X-ray demonstrates hepatic portal venous gas (arrow) and abdominal distention, with bubbly appearance of intestine (arrowhead; right lower quadrant). (*Source:* From Robert M. Kliegman, Joseph W. St Geme, Nathan J. Blum, Samir S. Shah, Robert C. Tasker and Karen M. Wilson. Digestive System Disorders. Nelson Textbook of Pediatrics. Elsevier 2020.)

Necrotizing Enterocolitis

Necrotizing enterocolitis may occur as a disease of prematurity or as a complication of NRDS. ***Its incidence is inversely proportional to the gestational age.*** It is considered as the most common cause of acquired gastrointestinal emergency in newborns.

Pathogenesis (Fig. 10.2) Pathogenesis of necrotizing enterocolitis is thought to be multifactorial. Most common associated findings are ***prematurity and enteral feeding***. Enteral feeding can introduce infectious agents into the gut and can initiate a cascade of events resulting in tissue destruction.

But no single infectious agent is associated with the condition. The chemical mediator *platelet-activating factor (PAF)* is found in increased concentration in affected baby's stool and serum samples.

Clinical Features The newborn characteristically presents with bloody stools, abdominal distension and circulatory collapse.

Abdominal radiograph may reveal air within the intestinal wall ***(pneumatosis intestinalis)*** or free air in the peritoneum (Fig. 10.3).

Morphology

Gross Common sites affected are the terminal ileum, cecum and right colon. The affected segment is distended, friable and congested to frankly gangrenous. Associated perforation or peritonitis may also be seen.

Microscopy The characteristic findings are as follows:

Mucosal/transmural coagulative necrosis
Ulceration
Bacterial colonization
Submucosal air bubbles
Reparative changes – granulation tissue and fibrosis may be seen

Management Most patients can be managed conservatively. Surgical intervention may be required depending on the severity.

- Conservative management – if detected early
- Surgical resection of the involved segment of the bowel in later stages

Necrotizing enterocolitis is associated with ***high mortality*** and most infants who survive develop ***strictures*** as the complication of the healing process.

Sepsis

Perinatal sepsis is because of infections acquired at or shortly before birth. The infections are acquired either by *transcervical* (ascending infection) or *transplacental* (haematogenous) route.

Based on the onset of symptoms, they can be grouped clinically into two types (Table 10.8):

1. Early-onset sepsis
2. Late-onset sepsis

Table 10.8 Differences Between Early- and Late-Onset Sepsis

Features	Early-Onset Sepsis	Late-Onset Sepsis
Onset of clinical symptoms	Within 7 days	7 days to 3 months
Common agent	Group B *Streptococcus*	*Listeria*, *Candida*
Latent period of the organism	Short	Long

These babies may present with signs and symptoms of pneumonia, sepsis or meningitis.

Intraventricular Haemorrhage

As the fetal brain is not fully mature, the periventricular germinal matrix contains dilated and thin-walled veins, which can rupture easily and result in intraventricular haemorrhage. Pathogenesis of this complication is believed to be hypoxic injury to the periventricular capillaries and impaired vascular auto regulation.

FETAL HYDROPS

Fetal hydrops refers to ***fluid accumulation in the fetus during intrauterine growth***. The amount of fluid accumulation can vary from severe generalized to mild localized collection. Fetal hydrops is the term used for severe generalized fluid accumulation, usually a ***lethal condition*** most commonly associated with ***Rh incompatibility*** (Table 10.9).

CLASSIFICATION

- **Based on aetiology:**
  a. Immune hydrops
  b. Nonimmune hydrops
- **Based on the distribution of fluid accumulation:**
  a. Generalized
     Fetal hydrops
  b. Localized
     Isolated pleural effusion
     Isolated peritoneal effusion (ascites)
     Postnuchal fluid accumulation (cystic hygroma)

Immune Hydrops

Immune hydrops is the haemolytic disease of newborn caused by the blood group incompatibility between the mother and fetus. The fetus can inherit blood group antigens from the father that are considered foreign to the mother. The mother's immune response against these foreign (fetal) blood group antigen results in breakdown of the RBCs (haemolytic reaction). Many blood group antigens (>60) can elicit antibody response, but significant haemolytic disease is caused by antibodies to

a. Rh antigen – D antigen
b. ABO blood group antigen

Table 10.9 Causes of Hydrops Fetalis

Immune hydrops
- Rh blood incompatibility
- ABO blood incompatibility

Nonimmune hydrops
- Cardiovascular
- Malformations, high-output failure
- Chromosomal
- Turner syndrome
- Trisomy 18, 21
- Fetal anaemia
- Homozygous α-thalassaemia
- Parvovirus B19 infection
- Twin gestation (twin-to-twin transfusion)
- Thoracic causes
- Cystic adenomatoid malformation
- Diaphragmatic hernia
- Infections
- Genitourinary malformations
- Metabolic disorders

Rh incompatibility

Aetiology The fetal hydrops/haemolytic disease of the newborn is caused by maternal antibodies against the fetal Rh (D) antigen.

Pathogenesis (Fig. 10.4) Immune hydrops typically occurs when an Rh-negative mother carries an Rh-positive fetus. The Rh-positive fetal RBCs enter the maternal circulation during the last trimester of pregnancy or at the time of delivery. The exposure to Rh-positive fetal RBCs results in sensitization of the mother (formation of anti-D antibodies). Sensitization can occur following abortion/ blood transfusion also.

The first fetus is usually not affected. The first child escapes because the sensitization of mother occurs usually at the time of delivery of first fetus only.

Also, the initial antibodies formed are of IgM type, which do not cross the placenta.

But in second and subsequent pregnancies, the fetuses are affected with increasing degree of severity. Second exposure of Rh-positive fetal RBCs results in increased production of ***IgG type anti-D antibodies*** (anamnestic response). The IgG antibodies *cross the placenta* and cause haemolysis of fetal RBCs (Table 10.10).

Factors which influence the immune response to Rh-positive cells in the mother:

1. Presence of additional ABO incompatibility offers protection against Rh immunization.
   The fetal RBCs which enter the maternal circulation are destroyed by anti-A or anti-B antibodies. These antibodies are of IgM type and do not cross the placenta.
2. The maternal Rh immunization (sensitization) depends on the dose of antigen exposure.
   For adequate sensitization, the mother must be exposed to more than 1 ML of fetal blood.
   The administration of Rhesus immunoglobulin containing ***anti-D antibodies*** to Rh-negative mothers at 28 weeks and within 72 hours of delivery prevents sensitization of the mother and the occurrence of haemolytic disease of newborn in subsequent pregnancies.

ABO incompatibility ABO incompatibility is *much more common* than Rh incompatibility. It occurs in 20%–25% of pregnancies. But *ABO haemolytic disease is very*

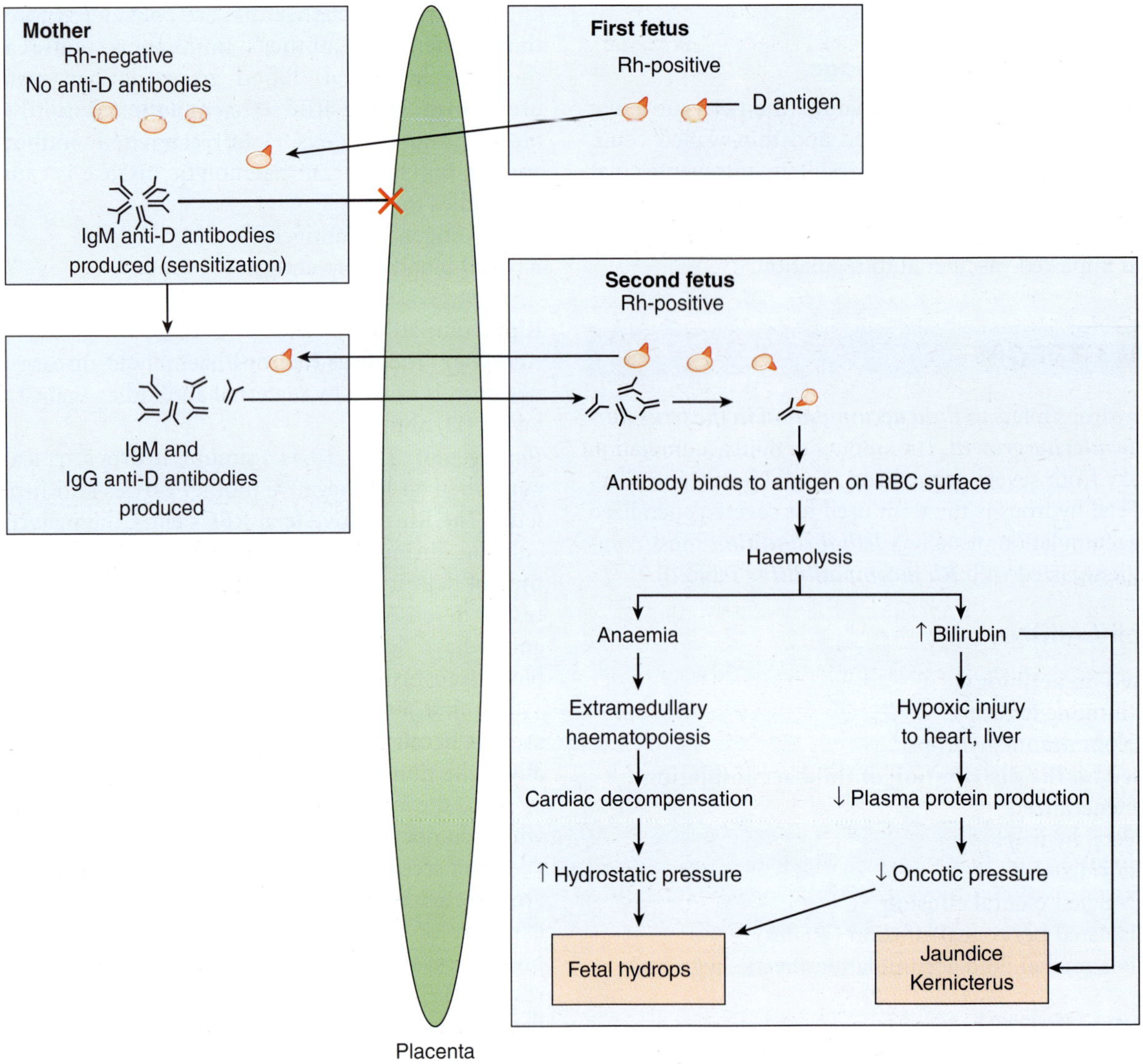

Fig. 10.4 Pathogenesis of immune hydrops.

Table 10.10 Immune Haemolytic Disease of Newborn

Features	Rh Incompatibility	ABO Incompatibility
Incidence	Most common	Very rare
Aetiology	Antibodies against Rh (D) antigen	Antibodies against A or B antigen
Mother's blood group	Rh-negative	O blood group
Antibodies in mother's plasma	No anti-D antibodies	Anti-A and anti-B antibodies (usually IgM); rarely some have IgG antibodies
First pregnancy	Sensitization with IgM anti-D antibodies occurs First child not affected	First child affected (only in females who have IgG antibodies against A and B antigen)
Second and subsequent pregnancies	IgG anti-D antibodies are formed Child is affected	Child is affected

rare (1 in 10 infants) and severe haemolysis requiring treatment is extremely rare (1 in 200 such infants).

Factors responsible for reduced haemolysis in ABO incompatibility:

- Anti-A and anti-B antibodies are mostly IgM type; do not cross the placenta.
- Fetal RBCs poorly express A and B antigens on their surface.
- Many cells other than RBCs express A and B antigens.

ABO haemolytic disease occurs exclusively in mothers with O blood group who have IgG antibodies against A or B or both blood group antigens. When they carry a fetus with A or B blood group, these IgG antibodies make their way across the placenta and affect the fetus. The first child will be affected, and not spared. Thus, even the first child can be exposed to the effect of haemolysis.

Consequences of Haemolysis

1. **Anaemia**
   It is due to direct immune-mediated destruction of fetal RBCs. The severity of anaemia may vary from mild to severe. Anaemia causes increased erythroid hyperplasia in bone marrow with immature cells appearing in the peripheral blood, including erythroblasts; hence, this condition is also known as ***erythroblastosis fetalis***. It also causes increased extramedullary haematopoiesis in various organs. Anaemia can cause hypoxic injury to fetal organs (heart, liver), which will result in the development of severe generalized oedema (fetal hydrops) or death of the child in utero (Fig. 10.5).

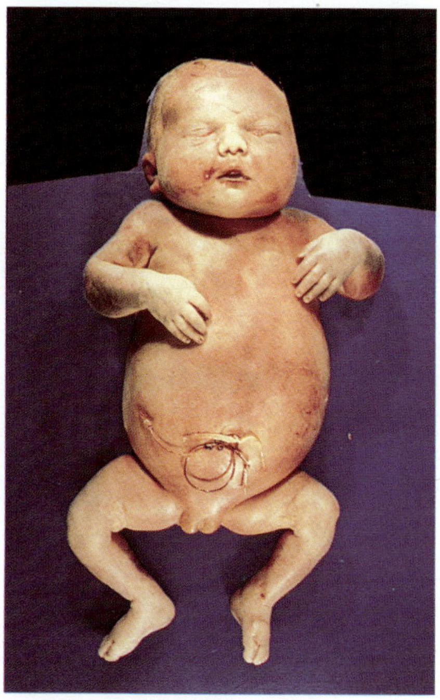

Fig. 10.5 Fetus with hydrops fetalis. (*Source:* From Lony C. Castro and Calvin J. Hobel. Rhesus Alloimmunization. Hacker & Moore's Essentials of Obstetrics and Gynecology. 6th edition. Elsevier 2016.)

2. **Jaundice**
   The unconjugated bilirubin formed as a result of haemolysis exceeds the capacity of the immature liver to conjugate. This results in increased levels of circulating unconjugated bilirubin, which crosses the blood–brain barrier and gets deposited in the brain causing CNS damage ***(kernicterus).***

Nonimmune Hydrops

Hydrops can also be due to nonimmune causes like:
- Cardiovascular defects
- Defects in other organ systems
- Dysmorphic features in some chromosomal anomalies

Morphology

The findings depend on the severity of the disease and the underlying aetiology. The fluid accumulation may be generalized and severe (fetal hydrops) leading to death of the infants in utero or in the first few days of life. Sometimes mild and localized collection (isolated pleural, peritoneal, postnuchal fluid collection) may occur that resolves completely within a few days.

- Fetus and placenta appear pale because of anaemia.
- Liver and spleen are enlarged and congested due to cardiac failure.
- Bone marrow show compensatory erythroid hyperplasia, with immature red cells in the peripheral blood including reticulocytes, normoblasts and erythroblasts, hence the name *erythroblastosis fetalis*.
- ***Extramedullary haematopoiesis*** is seen in liver, spleen, lymph nodes and other organs.
- ***Brain damage*** is the dreaded complication of fetal hydrops, known as kernicterus. The deposition of bilirubin (yellow discolouration) is seen in the area of basal ganglia, thalamus, cerebellum, cerebral grey matter and spinal cord.

Clinical Features Mild cases may present with pallor, jaundice and organomegaly, whereas severely affected infants present with generalized oedema, pallor, intense jaundice and signs of neurological damage.

Treatment

- *Phototherapy* converts the unconjugated bilirubin to dipyrroles, which are easily excreted from the body.
- *Total exchange transfusion* is done in severe cases to prevent brain damage.

INBORN ERRORS OF METABOLISM

Sir Archibald Garrod in 1908 coined the term 'Inborn Errors of Metabolism' to a group of genetically determined metabolic diseases caused by enzyme deficiency. Most these diseases are inherited as ***autosomal recessive trait***, rarely as X-linked trait or mitochondrial disorder. Many infants present with neurological signs and symptoms or failure to thrive. Some are lethal in early childhood whereas others are clinically insignificant. The list of inborn errors of metabolism is vast and beyond the scope of discussion. Here only three important, potentially lethal diseases are selected for discussion.

PHENYLKETONURIA

Phenylketonuria (PKU)/hyperphenylalaninaemia is caused by abnormality in phenylalanine metabolism that causes severe mental retardation in infants (Table 10.11).

Incidence: 1 in 10,000 live births
Inheritance: Autosomal recessive

Enzyme deficiency:
Type 1: Phenylalanine hydroxylase (PAH) (classic form)
Type 2: Dihydropteridine reductase (DHPR)
Type 3: Impaired tetrahydrobiopterin synthesis

Genetic defect:
- Mutation in the PAH gene on chromosome 12q22-24.1 – most common gene mutated in >95% of cases
- Mutation in DHPR gene on chromosome 4p
- Mutation causing impaired tetrahydrobiopterin synthesis

Pathogenesis (Fig. 10.6)

Phenylalanine is an essential amino acid derived exclusively from diet for protein synthesis. The phenylalanine in blood is oxidized in the liver to tyrosine by the enzyme PAH in the presence of cofactor tetrahydrobiopterin.

Table 10.11 Variants of Phenylketonuria (PKU)

Type	Enzyme Deficiency	Genetic Defect	Clinical Presentation
Type 1	Phenylalanine hydroxylase (PAH)	Mutation in PAH gene, chromosome 12q22 Mutation in PAH gene, chromosome 12q22	Classic form (PAH activity <1%) Benign form (PAH activity >5%)
Type 2	Tetrahydrobiopterin (cofactor for PAH)	Defect in synthesis of BH_4	Malignant PKU
Type 3	Dihydropteridine reductase (DHPR)	Mutation in DHPR gene, chromosome 4p	Malignant PKU

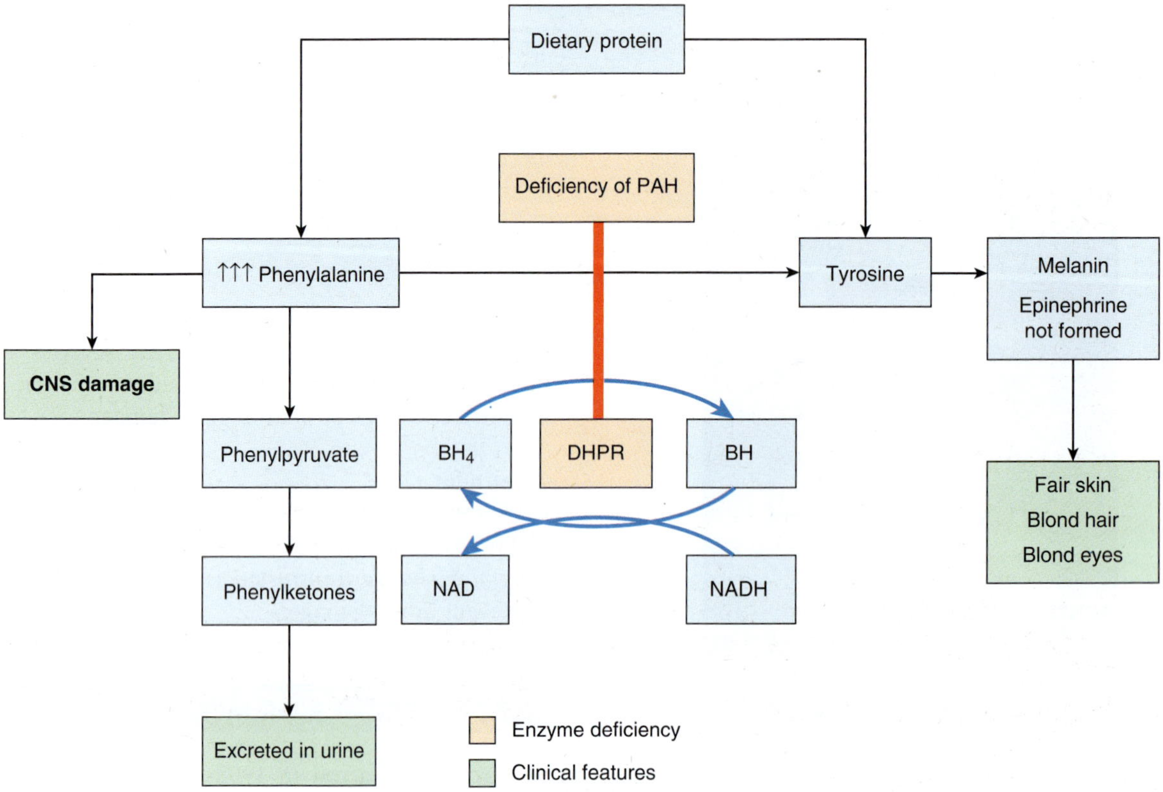

Fig. 10.6 Pathogenesis of phenylketonuria.

Deficiency of enzyme PAH causes:

1. Hyperphenylalaninaemia – neuronal damage
2. Formation of phenylketones – excreted in urine, causing the mousy/musty odour
3. Block in the tyrosine metabolism – decreased synthesis of melanin (fair skin, blond hair/eyes)

Clinical Features

PKU illustrates the interaction between genetic and environmental factors in the pathogenesis of the disease. It is caused by a genetic defect, but requires a dietary component for the expression of the disease. The affected infants are normal at birth and progressively develop neuronal damage. By restricting phenylalanine intake in the diet, the neuronal damage can be prevented. The classic form of PKU presents with the following:

1. ***CNS damage*** – mental retardation by 6 months of age, seizures
2. ***Skin changes*** – hypopigmentation of skin and hair, eczema
3. ***Urine*** – characteristic mousy/musty odour

PKU can present clinically with varying degree of severity depending on the level of enzyme activity. In classic form, the level of enzyme PAH activity is less than 1%. If the enzyme activity is greater than 5%, it results in a milder form of the disease with modest elevation of phenylalanine levels and no neurological damage. This is referred to as ***benign PKU.***

Malignant hyperphenylalaninaemia occurs in less than 5% of infants with the disease, where dietary restrictions do not arrest the neurological deterioration. They are caused by mutations that affect the synthesis or recycling of the cofactor tetrahydrobiopterin (type 2 and type 3 diseases).

Management

Early detection and prompt treatment has made the clinical phenotype of classic PKU, a historical event.

Early Detection

- Prenatal diagnosis can be done on chorionic villi sampling and amniotic fluid.
- Neonatal screening by a simple blood test (Guthrie test) to detect hyperphenylalaninaemia. The Guthrie test is based on the requirement of phenylalanine for the growth of *Bacillus subtilis.*

Treatment

Strict phenylalanine-restricted diet is recommended throughout life. These children usually grow into asymptomatic adults, but most of them discontinue dietary restrictions once they reach adulthood and have high phenylalanine levels in blood.

Children born to mothers with PKU are usually anomalous with mental retardation, microcephaly and cardiac anomalies. The *maternal hyperphenylalaninaemia* can affect the fetal development. To prevent this, maternal dietary restriction should be initiated before conception and continued throughout pregnancy.

GALACTOSAEMIA

Galactosaemia is a disorder of carbohydrate metabolism, resulting from accumulation of ***galactose-1-phosphate*** in tissues.

Incidence: 1 in 60,000 live births
Inheritance: Autosomal recessive

Genetic defects for the respective enzyme deficiencies in galactosaemia are listed in Table 10.12.

Pathogenesis

Main pathogenesis is due to accumulation of galactose in various tissues. Lactose, the milk protein is broken down by lactase into glucose and galactose at the intestinal microvilli. The galactose gets converted to glucose in three steps as shown in Fig. 10.7.

Deficiency of galactose-1-phosphate uridyl transferase (GALT) is more common and results in accumulation of galactose-1-phosphate in many tissues (Table 10.13). In addition, the galactitol and galactonate produced by the alternate metabolic pathway also accumulate.

Morphology

The major organs affected are the liver, eyes and brain. The pathologic changes in the liver are fatty change and progressive pseudoacinar change of hepatic architecture with ductular proliferation, cholestasis, focal necrosis and, finally, cirrhosis. Cataract in the eye is because of galactitol deposition in the lens, which absorbs water and swells causing lens opacity. The brain tissue shows loss of nerve cells, gliosis and oedema.

Clinical Features

Affected infants present with failure to thrive from birth. Ingestion of milk results in vomiting, diarrhoea, jaundice,

Table 10.12 Genetic Defect for Each Enzyme Deficiency in Galactosaemia

Type	Enzyme Deficiency	Genetic Defect
Classic	Galactose-1-phosphate uridyl transferase (GALT)	GALT gene on chromosome 9 (9p13.3)
Variant	Galactokinase (GALK)	GALK 1 gene on chromosome 17 (17q21-q22)
Variant	Uridine diphosphate galactose 4-epimerase (GALE)	GALE gene on chromosome 1 (1p36-p35)

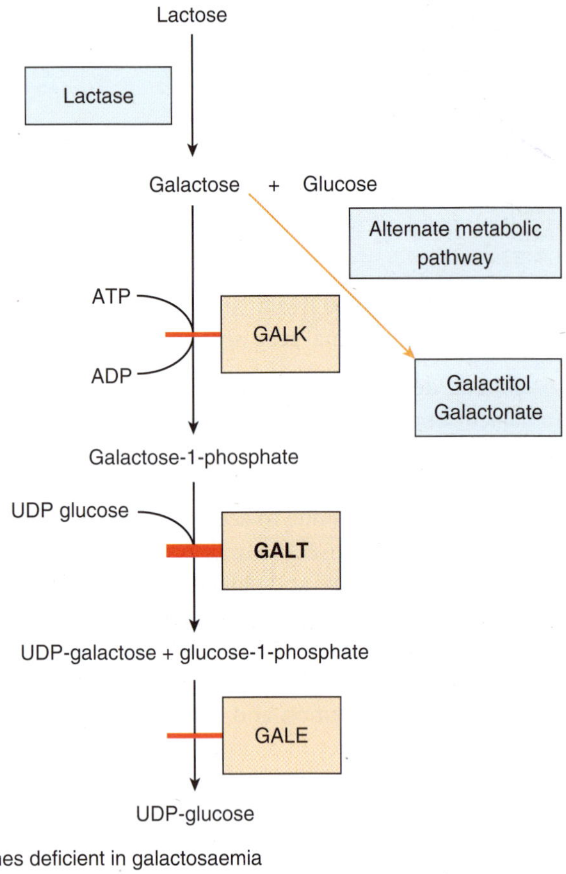

Fig. 10.7 Pathogenesis of galactosaemia.

Table 10.13 Clinical Features of Galactosaemia According to the Site of Accumulation

Site of Accumulation	Clinical Features
Liver	Hepatomegaly, cirrhosis
Eyes	Cataract
Brain	Mental retardation
Kidney	Aminoaciduria
Blood	Haemolysis, coagulopathy Fulminant *Escherichia coli* septicaemia (depressed neutrophil bactericidal function)

hepatosplenomegaly and cataract. Mental retardation is usually detected by 1 year of age, but even in untreated children, it is not as severe as in PKU.

Treatment

Early detection and *lactose-restricted diet* can prevent most of the damage caused by galactosaemia. Elderly patients usually develop speech disorder and gonadal failure (premature ovarian failure), as a long-term complication, even with strict diet restrictions.

Prenatal diagnosis can be done on chorionic villi sampling and amniotic fluid analysis.

Neonatal screening by testing blood for the presence of galactose can be done.

OTHER GENETIC DISORDERS

CYSTIC FIBROSIS (MUCOVISCIDOSIS)

Cystic fibrosis is the *most common lethal inherited disorder of metabolism caused by defect in ion transport protein.*
Incidence: 1 in 2500 live births *(most common lethal genetic disease)*
Inheritance: *Autosomal recessive*
Primary defect: Chloride channel – cystic fibrosis transmembrane conductance regulator (CFTR)
Genetic defect: Mutation in CFTR gene on chromosome 7 ***(7q31.2)***

Normal Structure and Functions of CFTR

Normally, chloride ions are transported across the membrane through an epithelial chloride channel protein called ***CFTR.***

The CFTR protein is made up of 1480 amino acids (Fig. 10.8). It consists of:

1. ***Transmembrane domains (TMDs):*** This has two domains – TMD1 and TMD2. Each TMD contains six α-helices that span through the cell membrane. Both the domains together form the channel through which chloride ion passes.
2. ***Cytoplasmic nucleotide-binding domains (NBDs):*** This also has two domains – NBD1 and NBD2. Each domain has binding site for ATP. When ATP binds the NBDs, the chloride channel opens.

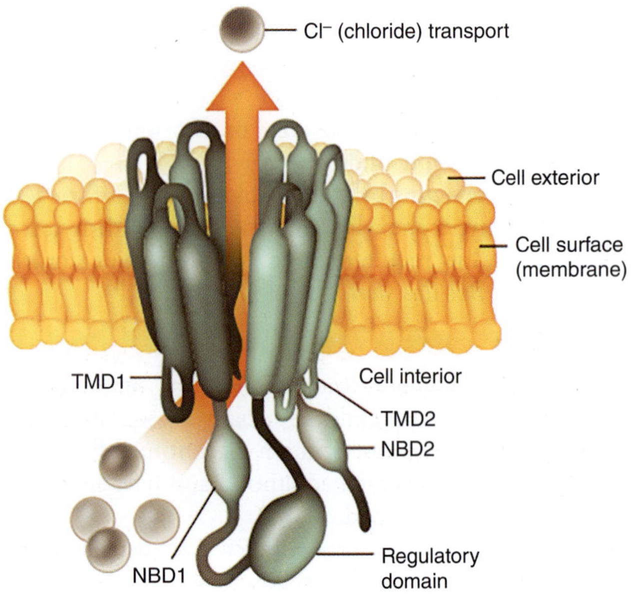

Fig. 10.8 CFTR structure.

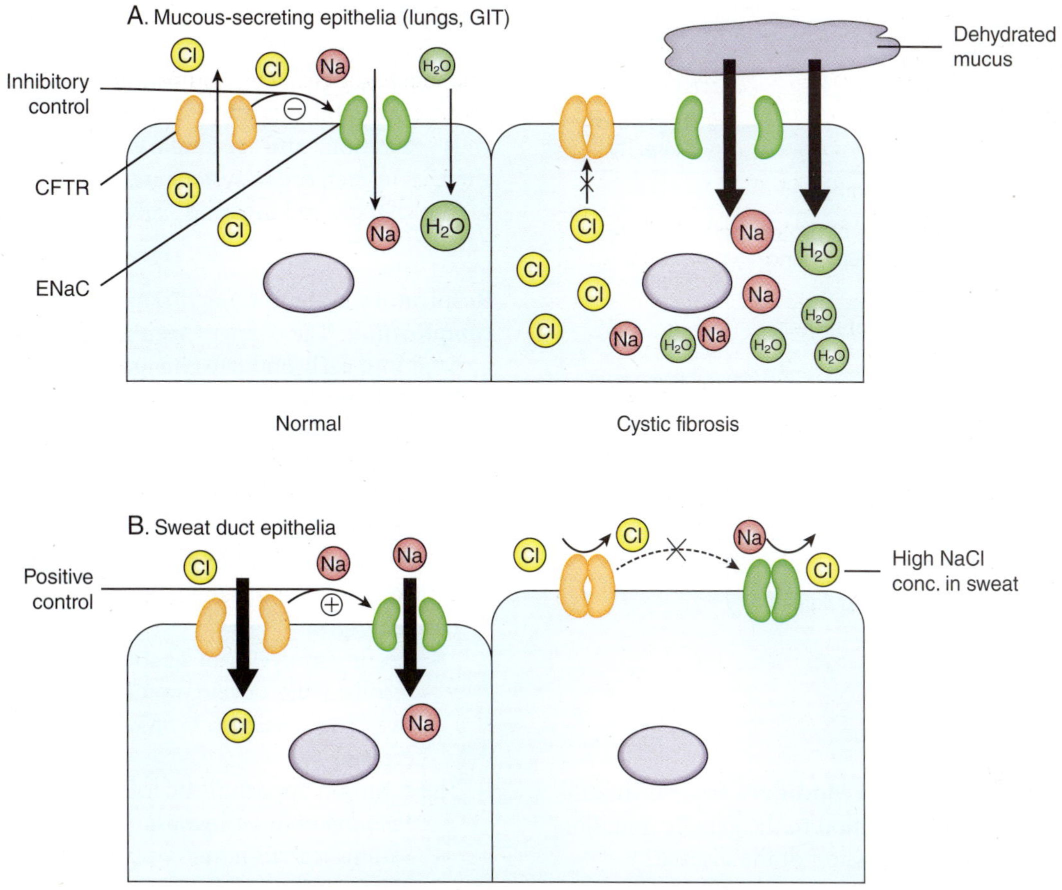

Fig. 10.9 Pathogenesis of cystic fibrosis.

3. ***Regulatory domain*** (R) – R domain contains protein kinase A and C phosphorylation sites. Phosphorylation of the R domains regulates ATP binding at NBD and opening of the chloride channel.

Functions

1. It regulates chloride ion transport in epithelial cells.
2. It also regulates many other ion channels:
   a. Epithelial sodium channel (ENaC)
   b. Potassium channel
   c. Gap junction channel
   d. Bicarbonate ion transport through SCL26 protein

Pathogenesis (Fig. 10.9)

CFTR regulates active secretion of chloride ions into the lumen in all mucous-secreting epithelium. It also inhibits ENaC. Regulation of ENaC causes low sodium uptake from the lumen. In cystic fibrosis, there is ***decreased chloride secretion and increased reabsorption of sodium*** (inhibitory control over ENaC is released) from the lumen. The movement of sodium into the cell causes passive water absorption (osmosis), making the *luminal secretion very thick and dehydrated*. This thick viscous secretion can ***obstruct the lumina*** (respiratory, pancreatic and biliary ducts and fetal intestine) causing damage in various organ systems.

The only exception to this rule occurs in human sweat duct, where normal CFTR augments ENaC. This allows uptake of chloride and sodium from the luminal secretion. Thus, in CFTR mutation, both chloride and sodium channels are closed, resulting in high sodium chloride content in the sweat secretions. Salty sweat is the compelling feature of classic cystic fibrosis.

CFTR Gene and Mutations CFTR gene encodes the chloride channel CFTR. It is located on long arm of chromosome 7 (7q31.2). Many mutations have been identified in this gene resulting in a spectrum of clinical presentations. In general, the mutations are classified into six classes listed in Table 10.14.

The most common mutation is Class II deletion of three nucleotides coding for phenylalanine (F) at amino acid position 508 (***FΔ508***). Presence of two severe mutations will result in a severe phenotype with all the classical features of the disease (pancreatic disease, sinopulmonary infection and gastrointestinal symptoms), whereas presence of two mild mutations will result in less severe disease (prevents pancreatic disease).

Table 10.14 Classes of Gene Mutation in Cystic Fibrosis

Class	Mutation	Degree of Severity
I	Defective protein synthesis	Severe
II	Defect in processing of protein in endoplasmic reticulum and Golgi apparatus	
III	Defect in transport of protein to the apical membrane	
IV	Decreased conductance through the ion channel (abnormality in TMD)	Mild
V	Reduced abundance; decreased number of normal proteins are formed	
VI	Altered function in regulation of ion channels	

TMD, transmembrane domain.

Genetic and Environmental Modifiers Several modifiers are present, which in addition to the genetic mutation can change the clinical expression of the disease.

Genetic modifiers: These are gene mutations that cause change in the neutrophil response to infection and thereby alter the severity of lung disease in cystic fibrosis.

Examples: Mannose-binding lectin 2 (MBL2), transforming growth factor β1 (TGF-β1)

Environmental modifiers: These influence the severity and progression of lung disease.

Examples: Infections with virulent organisms (*Pseudomonas aeruginosa*), efficacy of therapy, exposure to tobacco and other allergens

Morphology

The morphological changes common to all organs are obstruction and dilatation of the ducts by thick viscous secretion and secondary inflammation. The changes in each organ system are given in Table 10.15.

The changes in lungs and pancreas are discussed in detail.

Respiratory system: ***Lung disease is the most serious complication***. The changes seen in the lungs are categorized into early and late changes (Fig. 10.10).

Early changes:
- Thick viscous secretion causing obstruction of the bronchioles
- Secondary infection and inflammation of bronchiolar walls
- Hyperplasia and hypertrophy of bronchial mucous-secreting glands

Late changes:
- Recurrent cycles of obstruction and infection result in the development of chronic obstructive lung disease (chronic bronchitis, bronchiectasis)

The common opportunistic infections are caused by:
- *Pseudomonas aeruginosa*
- *Staphylococcus aureus*
- *Haemophilus influenzae*
- *Burkholderia cepacia*

Pancreas: Most patients (>85%) with cystic fibrosis have pancreatic abnormalities.

Early changes:
- Accumulation of mucous in small ducts
- Dilatation of exocrine glands

Late changes:
- Obstruction of ducts by thick mucus and calcium-containing debris

Table 10.15 Morphological Changes in Cystic Fibrosis

Organ	Early Changes	Late Changes
Lung	Obstruction of bronchioles Infection	Chronic obstructive pulmonary disease • Chronic bronchitis • Bronchiectasis
Pancreas	Obstruction of ducts dilation of exocrine glands	Exocrine gland atrophy Cystic dilatation of ducts with squamous metaplasia Fibrosis
Liver	Focal biliary cirrhosis	Diffuse biliary cirrhosis
Intestine	Meconium ileus	Distal intestinal obstruction syndrome Rectal prolapse
Reproductive system	Congenital bilateral absence of vas deferens	Azoospermia Infertility

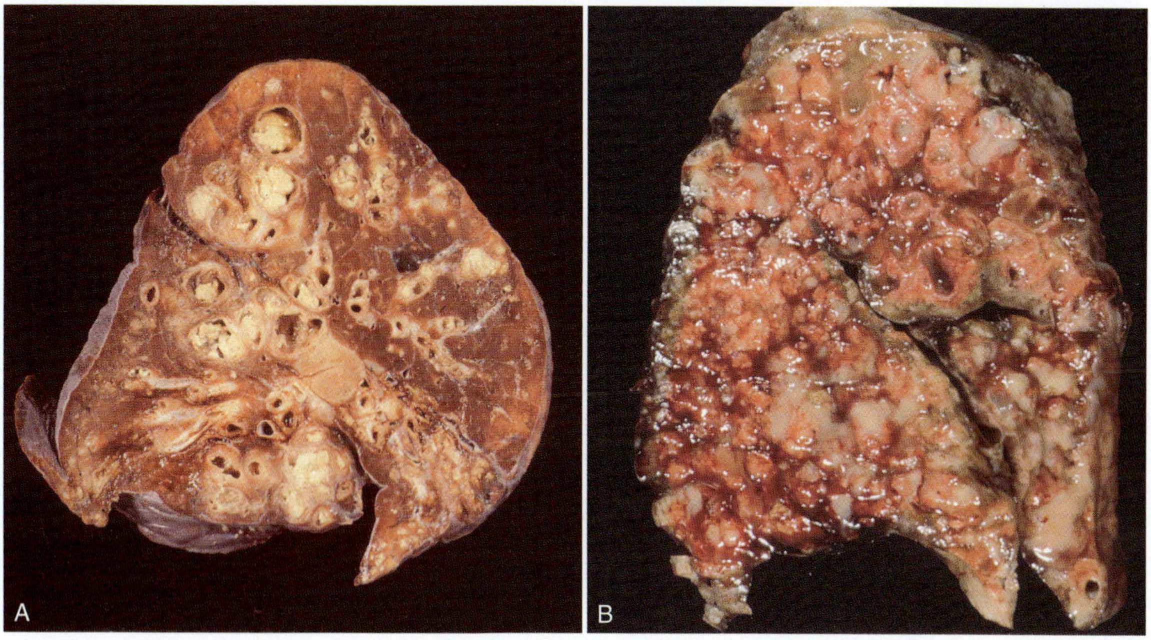

Fig. 10.10 Changes of cystic fibrosis in the lung. (A) Explant from a 13-year-old patient; (B) advanced disease at autopsy. (*Source:* From Ann E. McCullough and Kevin O. Leslie. Lung Infections. Cover of Practical Pulmonary Pathology: A Diagnostic Approach Practical Pulmonary Pathology: A Diagnostic Approach. 3rd edition. Elsevier 2018.)

- Atrophy with cystic dilatation and fibrosis of the exocrine glands, hence the name cystic fibrosis
- Chronic obstruction leads to squamous metaplasia of pancreatic duct; consequently, there is impaired fat absorption that also leads to vitamin A deficiency

Clinical Features

In classic cystic fibrosis, the mother usually makes the diagnosis by recognizing the ***salty sweat***. The diagnosis can be made based on the characteristic clinical features (Table 10.16), increased electrolyte concentration in sweat and confirmed by genetic testing for CFTR gene mutations.

Treatment

The management of acute and chronic complications of cystic fibrosis is by:

- Potent antimicrobial therapy
- Pancreatic enzyme replacement
- Bilateral lung transplantation

New treatment modalities aimed at restoring the mutant CFTR function are under trial. The major improvements in management has changed a lethal disease of childhood into a chronic disease of adults.

Table 10.16 Clinical Features of Cystic Fibrosis

Organ	Features
Respiratory system	Persistent colonization with pathogenic organisms Chronic obstructive lung diseases, commonly bronchiectasis Nasal polyps Clubbing of digits
Intestine	Meconium ileus at birth in 5%–10% of cases Distal intestinal obstruction syndrome
Pancreas	Pancreatic insufficiency Recurrent acute and chronic pancreatitis
Nutritional	Failure to thrive Protein–energy malnutrition Fat-soluble vitamin deficiencies
Male reproductive system	Azoospermia Congenital bilateral absence of vas deferens

SUDDEN INFANT DEATH SYNDROME

Sudden infant death syndrome (SIDS) is defined as 'the sudden death of an infant (<1 year of age), which could not be explained after a thorough investigation, that includes a detailed history, examination of the death scene and a complete autopsy'. If the cause for death can be explained after the investigations, then it is termed as ***sudden unexpected infant death (SUID).***

In SIDS, an apparently healthy infant goes to sleep at night and never wakes up, hence the name ***'cot death' or 'crib death'.***

Epidemiology

- SIDS is the leading cause of infant death in the United States.
- It is the third leading cause of death overall in infants, after congenital anomalies and diseases of prematurity.
- Most cases of SIDS (90%) occur during the first 6 months of life.

Morphology

SIDS is a diagnosis of exclusion. The autopsy usually fails to provide a clear cause of death. But its importance rests in identification of unsuspected causes of death in SUID and to rule out traumatic child abuse. The autopsy examination usually reveals the following findings:

In SIDS

- Multiple petechial spots on thymus, pleura and pericardium
- Lungs show congestion, with or without pulmonary oedema
- Upper respiratory tract (larynx, trachea) may show evidence of recent infection histologically
- CNS demonstrates brainstem abnormalities
  - Astrogliosis
  - Arcuate nucleus hypoplasia

In SUID

- Unsuspected infection – viral myocarditis, bronchopneumonia
- Unsuspected congenital anomaly
- Congenital aortic stenosis
- Genetic defects – fatty acid oxidation disorders
- Multiple fractures in traumatic child abuse

Nonspecific findings seen in SIDS and SUID:

- Persistent extramedullary haematopoiesis in liver
- Increased periadrenal brown fat

Pathogenesis

SIDS is generally accepted as a multifactorial condition. According to the triple-risk model of SIDS (Fig. 10.11), several factors make the infant vulnerable to sudden death during the critical period of development.

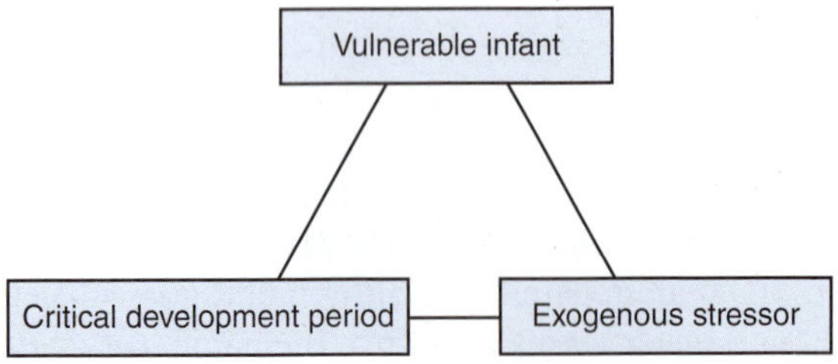

Fig. 10.11 Triple-risk model of SIDS.

Vulnerable Infants Vulnerability factors may relate to the parents or the infant.

Infant factors

- Brainstem abnormalities can cause delayed development of arousal and cardiorespiratory control.
- Prematurity and low birth weight.
- Male sex.
- SIDS in prior siblings.
- Mild respiratory tract infection in the infant can stimulate laryngeal chemoreceptors and elicit an inhibitory cardiorespiratory reflex.
- Survivors of apparent life-threatening events (combination of apnoea, marked change in colour or muscle tone, choking or gagging). Now they are proved to be unrelated entities by epidemiological studies.

Maternal factors

- Maternal smoking
- Young maternal age
- Short intergestational interval
- Inadequate antenatal care

Critical development period

- First 6 months of life.

Exogenous stressors

- Prone or side sleeping position. Supine position is considered as the safe sleeping position. The 'Back to Sleep' campaign by American Academy of Pediatrics, which recommends the supine sleeping position, has significantly reduced SIDS-related deaths in the United States.
- Sleeping with parents in the first 3 months.
- Sleeping on soft surfaces.
- Hyperthermia.

TUMOURS AND TUMOUR-LIKE LESIONS OF INFANCY AND CHILDHOOD PA 11.2

In childhood, *benign tumours are more common than malignant tumours. Malignant tumours, though uncommon (only 2%), account to be the second most common cause of death (9%)* next only to accidental trauma.

Any tumour can occur in children, but most commonly they arise from soft tissues of mesenchymal derivative (haematopoietic, nervous and soft tissue), unlike adults who commonly develop epithelial tumours. Tumour-like lesions are also common and have to be differentiated from true neoplasms. The common tumours and tumour-like lesions are listed in Table 10.17.

Childhood tumours may also develop as a part of developmental syndrome, e.g. deletion of short arm of chromosome 11 (11p13) results in WAGR syndrome (Wilms tumour, Aniridia, Genitourinary abnormalities and Mental Retardation).

Table 10.17 Common Tumour and Tumour-Like Lesions of Childhood

Tumour-Like Lesions	Benign Tumours	Malignant Tumours
Heterotopia (choristoma)	Haemangioma	Leukaemia
Hamartoma	Lymphatic tumours	Central nervous system tumours
	Fibrous tumours	Neuroblastoma
	Teratomas	Wilms tumour
		Lymphoma
		Rhabdomyosarcoma
		Retinoblastoma
		Bone tumours (Ewing sarcoma and osteogenic sarcoma)

TUMOUR-LIKE CONDITIONS

- **Hamartoma** refers to focal, unwarranted overgrowth of cells or tissues indigenous to the organ in which the lesion is seen. Although the lesion is composed of mature cells seen in the organ, they do not form the normal architecture and often show disorganized arrangement. It is difficult to differentiate hamartoma from benign tumours as both may be clonal.
  Example: Hamartoma of lung
- **Heterotopia (choristoma)** refers to normal cells or tissues that are present in abnormal location. They are of little significance, but can be confused clinically for neoplasms.
  Example: Pancreatic tissue found in stomach wall

BENIGN TUMOURS

- **Haemangioma**
  Haemangiomas are the most common tumours of childhood, frequently occurring on the skin of face and scalp.
  Morphologically they appear as flat to elevated, irregular bluish red masses. Microscopically both capillary and cavernous type of haemangiomas can be encountered. They commonly regress with growth. Multiple haemangiomas are seen associated with Von Hippel–Lindau syndrome.
  Example: Port wine stain
- **Lymphangioma**
  Lymphangiomas are hamartomas or benign tumours of lymphatic origin. They arise in the much deeper regions of neck, axilla, mediastinum and retroperitoneal tissue.
  Morphology: They are characterized by cystic and cavernous spaces.
  They increase in size after birth with accumulation of fluid, and cause compression of vital structures in the region.
  Example: Cystic hygroma in neck
- **Fibrous tumours**
  Fibrous lesions occurring in childhood include hamartomas, fibromatosis and infantile fibrosarcoma (malignant tumour). They may be sparsely cellular (fibromatosis) to highly cellular lesions.
- **Teratomas**
  Teratomas are tumours with derivatives from all three germ cell layers. These tumours represent the relation between histological maturity and biological behaviour. They are classified as follows:
  a. Mature teratoma – benign
  b. Immature teratoma – tumours of indeterminate potential
  c. Malignant teratoma

  Incidence: 1 in 20,000–40,000 live births.
  Age: It has two peaks in incidence – at 2 years of age and at early adulthood.
  Sex: Four times more common in girls than boys.
  Sites:
  Sacrococcygeal teratoma
  Testes, ovaries
  Midline locations: Mediastinum, retroperitoneum, head and neck.
  Sacrococcygeal teratomas are the most common teratomas of childhood; 10% of these teratomas are associated with congenital anomalies (meningocoele, spina bifida).

Morphology

They present as cystic to solid mass varying largely in size (1–30 cm).

Types:

A. **Mature teratomas** (75%) are most common, occurring in infants younger than 4 months. They present as cystic mass composed of benign (mature) cells.
B. **Immature teratoma** (13%) are composed of immature or primitive cells admixed with other mature components. Their malignant potential correlates with the amount of immature tissue, usually immature neuroepithelial elements. The more the immature component, higher is the risk of malignancy.
C. **Malignant teratomas** (12%) are solid tumours, usually yolk sac tumour. They occur in older children and are usually lethal.

Treatment

The treatment of mature and immature teratoma is surgical resection. Incomplete resection may lead to recurrence. Malignant teratomas require surgery with chemotherapy/radiotherapy.

MALIGNANT TUMOURS

Leukaemia is the most common malignant neoplasm in children younger than 10 years. The other malignant non-haematopoietic neoplasms are known as follows:

1. ***Blastoma*** (suffix): The tumour shows features of organogenesis specific to the site of origin, e.g. retinoblastoma and medulloblastoma.
2. ***Small round blue cell tumours:*** Histologically, they have primitive or undifferentiated appearance, characterized by sheets of cells with small, round nuclei (Table 10.18).

Neuroblastoma

Neuroblastic tumours are tumours of sympathetic ganglia and adrenal medulla. They arise from primordial neural crest cells in these sites.

Characteristic Features Their features include spontaneous or therapy-induced maturation (differentiation of primitive neuroblasts to mature elements), spontaneous tumour regression and wide range of clinical behaviour and prognosis.
Neuroblastoma is the most common extracranial solid tumour of childhood.
Incidence: 1 in 7000 live births.
Age: Median age of diagnosis is 18 months.

Pathogenesis Neuroblastomas are usually sporadic and rarely familial (1%–2%). Familial cases usually involve multiple autonomic sites or both adrenals and harbour germline mutations in anaplastic lymphoma kinase (ALK) gene.

Commonly Affected Sites
- Adrenal medulla (40%), most common
- Paravertebral region of abdomen (25%)
- Paravertebral region of mediastinum (15%)
- Others – pelvis, neck and within brain

Morphology

Gross Tumours vary in size from minute nodules (in situ lesions) to large masses. In situ lesions are more common and are clinically silent. They regress spontaneously and present as foci of fibrosis or calcification in adults. They are considered as developmental anomalies or rests.

Large neuroblastomas are tumour masses that are sharply demarcated by a fibrous pseudocapsule. They have infiltrative borders and invade adjacent structures – kidney, renal vein, vena cavae, aorta. Cut-section reveals soft, grey tan tissue with areas of necrosis, cystic change, haemorrhage and calcification.

Microscopy These tumours are ***'small blue round cell tumours'*** and have the following features:

- Sheets of small, blue, round cells (primitive neuroblast) (Fig. 10.12).
- Neuropil, a faintly eosinophilic fibrillar material in the background. They represent the neuritic processes of primitive neuroblast.
- Homer Wright pseudorossettes: Tumour cells, arranged concentrically around a central space filled with neuropil (Fig. 10.13).
- Pleomorphism, increased mitosis and nuclear breakdown (karyorrhexis) may be prominent.
- Presence of ganglion cell is a sign of maturation. They are large cells with abundant cytoplasm, large vesicular nuclei and prominent nucleolus. They are usually accompanied by Schwann cells.
  Ganglioneuroblastoma: Tumour with few ganglion cells admixed with primitive neuroblasts.
  Ganglioma: Tumour composed of ganglion cells with few, if any, residual neuroblasts.

Immunohistochemistry: Tumour cells are positive for *neuron-specific enolase (NSE).*

Electron microscopy: It shows dense core granules containing catecholamines in the cytoplasm.

Table 10.18 List of Paediatric Small Blue Round Cell Tumours

- Neuroblastoma
- Nephroblastoma (Wilms tumour)
- Lymphoma
- Rhabdomyosarcoma
- Ewing sarcoma/primitive neuroectodermal tumour
- Medulloblastoma
- Retinoblastoma

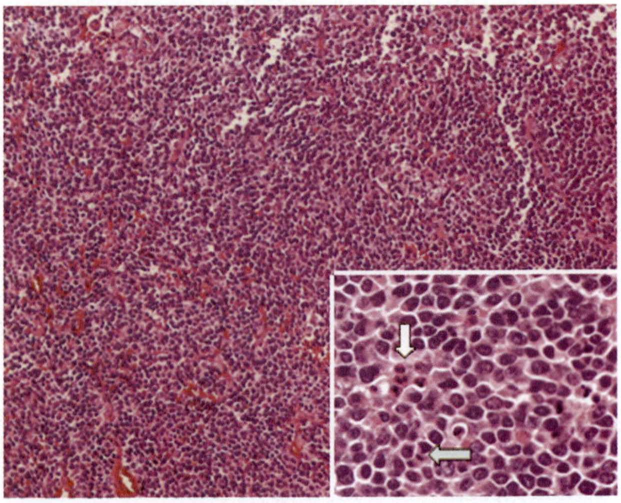

Fig. 10.12 Microscopy of neuroblastoma. A clump of karyorrhectic tumour cells (white arrow) and a tumour cell undergoing mitosis (grey arrow) are shown in the insert. (*Source:* From Andrew M. Davidoff and Jed G. Nuchtern. Neuroblastoma. Holcomb and Ashcraft's Pediatric Surgery. 7th edition. Elsevier 2020.)

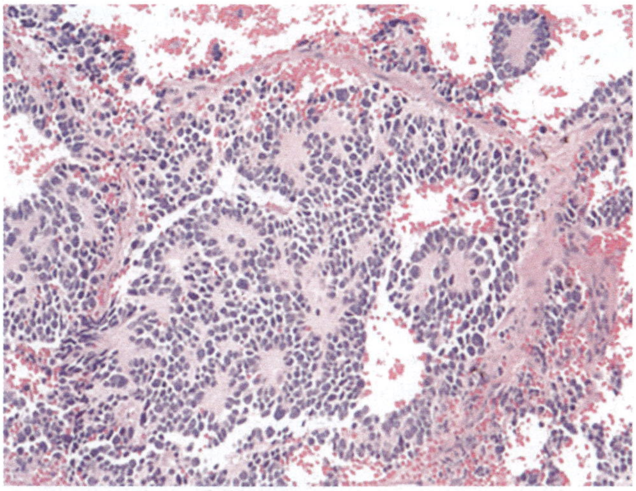

Fig. 10.13 Homer Wright rosettes in neuroblastoma. Note the absence of a central lumen. (*Source:* From Jesse K. McKenney. Adrenal Gland and Other Paraganglia. In Rosai and Ackerman's Surgical Pathology. 11th edition. Elsevier 2018.)

Metastasis Metastasis occur early and widely. They spread by bloodstream to liver, lungs, bone marrow and bones.

Staging The International Neuroblastoma Staging System is widely used. According to this system, there are four stages as listed in Table 10.19. Staging is important to determine the prognosis. Unfortunately, many children present with stage-3 or -4 tumours and have bad prognosis. Stages 1, 2 and 4S have a favourable prognosis.

Clinical Features In children younger than 2 years, neuroblastoma usually present with large intraabdominal mass, fever and weight loss. In neonates, disseminated neuroblastoma may present with multiple cutaneous metastasis causing deep blue discolouration of the skin ***(blueberry muffin baby)***. In older children, the tumour is silent and usually detected clinically by metastatic disease. The common sites of metastasis are as follows:

Site of Metastasis	*Symptoms*
Periorbital region	Proptosis, ecchymosis
Bone	Bone pain
Lung	Dyspnoea
GIT	Diarrhoea

Most of neuroblastomas (>90%) secrete catecholamines, which can be used in the detection of the tumour.

1. Increased blood catecholamines
2. Increased level of urine metabolites – vanillylmandelic acid (VMA) and homomandelic acid (HMA). This is widely used as **screening test** in asymptomatic children.

Prognostic Factors ***Age and stage*** are the most important determinants of outcome, followed by morphology. Several other factors have been identified, but the important ones used for risk stratification and therapeutic decisions are given in Table 10.20.

On the basis of these prognostic factors, the children are categorized into ***low, intermediate and high risk.*** Low-risk group has good prognosis. With improvements in therapy, long-term survival exceeds 90% in first two

Table 10.19 The International Neuroblastoma Staging System

Stage	Tumour	Regional Lymph Node	Metastasis
Stage 1	Localized tumour with complete gross excision	Ipsilateral nonadherent lymph nodes – negative Adherent lymph nodes may be positive	No
Stage 2A	Localized tumour with incomplete gross excision	Ipsilateral nonadherent lymph nodes – negative	No
Stage 2B	Localized tumour with or without complete gross excision	Ipsilateral nonadherent lymph nodes – positive	No
Stage 3	Unresectable tumour infiltrating across the midline	Ipsilateral nonadherent lymph nodes – positive	No
	Localized unilateral tumour	Contralateral lymph node – positive	
Stage 4	Any primary tumour	Any lymph node status	Positive – distant lymph nodes, bone, bone marrow, liver, skin and other organs
Stage 4S (S – special)	Localized tumour with or without complete gross excision	Ipsilateral nonadherent lymph nodes – negative/positive	Positive – skin, liver and/or bone marrow

Note: Stage 4S is limited to infants younger than 1 year.

Table 10.20 Prognostic Factors in Neuroblastoma

Prognostic Factors	Favourable	Unfavourable
1 Stage	Stages 1, 2A, 2B, 4S	Stages 3, 4
2 Age	<18 months	>18 months
3 Histology		
Evidence of maturation (presence of ganglion cells and Schwann cells)	Present	Absent
4 Mitosis-karyorrhexis index	<200/5000 cells	>200/5000 cells
5 DNA ploidy	Hyperdiploid	Near diploid
6 N-MYC expression	Not amplified	Amplified

groups. High-risk group has bad prognosis with less than 50% long-term survival.

Several other molecular variables with prognostic implications are as follows:

- Hemizygous deletion of short arm of chromosome 1
- Hemizygous deletion of long arm of chromosome 11
- Expression of neurotrophin receptors – TrkA and TrkB
- Mutations in neuritogenesis genes:
  - ATRX gene (alpha-thalassaemia/mental retardation, X-linked gene)
  - PTPRD gene (protein tyrosine phosphatase, receptor type D gene)

Treatment Mainstay of treatment is surgical resection. Administration of retinoids induce maturation and is used as an adjuvant therapy. Tumours with ALK mutation are amenable to treatment by target inhibitors of the encoded enzyme.

Wilms Tumour

Wilms tumour or nephroblastoma is the most common primary renal tumour of childhood and fourth most common paediatric malignancy.

Incidence: 1 in 10,000.

Age: 95% of cases occur before 10 years of age. Peak incidence is between 2 and 5 years.

It can be unilateral (>90%) or bilateral. Bilateral tumours occur earlier than unilateral tumours and they harbour germline mutations in one of the predisposing genes of Wilms tumour.

Pathogenesis Wilms tumour occurring in association with the three congenital syndromes constitute less than 10% of the cases but have provided insight into the biology of the tumour.

Syndromes associated with Wilms tumour (Table 10.21):

A. **WAGR syndrome** is characterized by Wilms tumour, aniridia, genitourinary abnormalities and mental retardation. Studies on these patients had led to the identification of first Wilms tumour–associated gene, WT1 gene on chromosome 11 (11p13) and better understanding of the two-hit hypothesis in tumourigenesis. WT1 protein is needed for normal renal and gonadal development.

B. **Denys–Drash syndrome** is characterized by gonadal dysgenesis (male pseudohermaphroditism) and early-onset nephropathy leading to renal failure. These patients are at increased risk of developing Wilms tumour and gonadoblastoma.

C. **Beckwith–Wiedemann syndrome** is characterized by enlargement of body organs (organomegaly), macroglossia, hemihypertrophy, omphalocoele and abnormal large cells in adrenal cortex (adrenal cytomegaly). This syndrome has led to the identification of WT2 gene, present distal to WT1 gene on chromosome 11. Patients with this syndrome are at increased risk of developing Wilms tumour and other tumours such as hepatoblastoma, pancreatoblastoma, adrenocortical tumours and rhabdomyosarcoma.

In sporadic tumours, gain of function mutations in β-catenin of the WNT (wingless) signalling pathway has been identified in addition to WT1 mutations, suggesting a synergistic role of both mutations in development of Wilms tumour.

Morphology

Gross Wilms tumour present as a solitary, large mass protruding over the surface of kidney. Approximately 10% cases are bilateral or multicentric. Cut-section

Table 10.21 Syndromes Associated With Wilms Tumour and the Associated Genes

Congenital Syndrome	Mutation	Wilms Tumour Associated Genes
A. WAGR	Deletion on chromosome 11 (11p13)	WT1 gene (tumour suppressor gene) PAX6 (gene for aniridia)
B. Denys–Drash syndrome	Dominant-negative missense mutation in zinc finger region of WT1 protein	WT1 gene
C. Beckwith–Wiedemann syndrome	Loss of genomic imprinting on band 11p15.5	WT2 gene IGF-2 gene

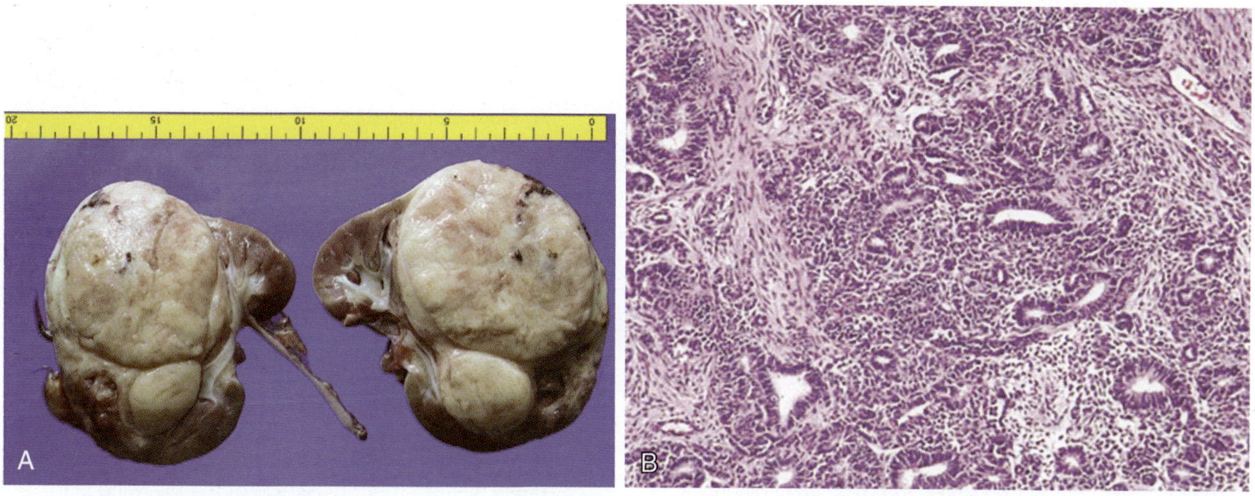

Fig. 10.14 Wilms tumour. (A) In gross examination, cut-surface of kidney shows an irregular mass, which has lobulated edges. (B) Microscopy of tumour shows triphasic histology composing of blastemal, stromal and epithelial component. (*Source:* From Jae Min Chung and Sang Don Lee. Wilms Tumor with dilated hypertensive cardiomyopathy, acute myocarditis, pulmonary edema, and heart failure. Urology Case Reports, 2020, 33. 2020; Jeffrey S. Dome, Elizabeth A. Mullen and Pedram Argani. Pediatric Renal Tumors. Nathan and Oski's Hematology and Oncology of Infancy and Childhood. 8th edition. Elsevier 2015.)

shows that tumour is soft, gelatinous, pale tan and bulging, surrounded by a thin rim of compressed renal cortex and capsule (Fig, 10.14A).

Microscopy The Wilms tumour resembles the different stages of nephrogenesis seen in fetal kidney. The classic triphasic combination of blastemal, stromal and epithelial cell types are seen in majority of tumours with varying proportions (Fig, 10.14B).

- **Blastemal component** – composed of sheets of small blue cells (small blue round cell tumour).
- **Epithelial component** – epithelial tumour cells tend to form abortive tubules or glomeruli.
- **Stromal component** – stromal cells are fibrocytic or myxoid in nature. Rarely heterologous elements like skeletal or smooth muscle, adipose tissue, cartilage, osteoid and neurogenic tissue are identified.

Presence of anaplasia (large hyperchromatic nuclei, atypical mitosis) is rare and seen in 5% of tumours with TP53 mutation.

Nephrogenic rests (precursor lesions of Wilms tumour) are composed of small nests of primitive blastemal cells. They are seen in the adjacent renal parenchyma in all cases of bilateral Wilms tumour and 25%–40% of unilateral tumours. Their presence is important to document in resected specimen as they are associated with high risk of developing Wilms tumour in contralateral kidney.

Clinical Features Most children with Wilms tumour present with a very large abdominal mass. The other presenting symptoms include haematuria, pain following abdominal trauma, intestinal obstruction and hypertension.

Prognosis and Treatment Wilms tumour has an excellent prognosis and most patients are considered cured of their malignancy, following surgical resection. Sometimes, recurrence and death can occur in cases that have had adverse prognostic factors like anaplasia, extrarenal spread of tumour or mutations in chromosomes 11q, 16q and 1q. The children who are cured are at increased risk of developing second primary tumours later in life, including bone and soft tissue sarcomas, leukaemia, lymphoma and breast cancer.

SELF-ASSESSMENT

Multiple Choice Questions

1. A 2-day-old neonate, born prematurely, presents with respiratory distress. Chest X-ray shows a ground-glass appearance. Which of the following is the most likely diagnosis?
   A. Asthma
   B. Bronchiolitis
   C. Neonatal respiratory distress syndrome (NRDS)
   D. Pneumonia
2. A 4-week-old infant develops vomiting and lethargy. The mother reports a 'mousy' odour. Which of the following conditions is most likely?
   A. Galactosemia
   B. Phenylketonuria
   C. Cystic fibrosis
   D. Gastroesophageal reflux

3. A 6-month-old infant presents with recurrent lung infections and steatorrhoea. Sweat chloride test is positive. Which of the following is the diagnosis?
   A. Asthma
   B. Bronchiolitis
   C. Cystic fibrosis
   D. Tuberculosis
4. A newborn has bilious vomiting and abdominal distension. X-ray shows a 'double bubble' sign. Which of the following is the likely diagnosis?
   A. Hirschsprung disease
   B. Intussusception
   C. Duodenal atresia
   D. Necrotizing enterocolitis
5. A 3-year-old child presents with an abdominal mass, hypertension, and haematuria. Ultrasound shows a renal mass. Which of the following is the most likely diagnosis?
   A. Neuroblastoma
   B. Wilms tumour
   C. Renal cyst
   D. Hydronephrosis
6. An infant presents with poor feeding, failure to thrive and hepatomegaly. Liver biopsy shows cirrhosis. Which of the following is the most likely diagnosis?
   A. Biliary atresia
   B. Hepatitis
   C. Galactosaemia
   D. Glycogen storage disease
7. A child presents with a firm, painless cervical mass. Biopsy shows small round blue cells. Which of the following is the most likely diagnosis?
   A. Hodgkin lymphoma
   B. Thyroid cancer
   C. Neuroblastoma
   D. Non-Hodgkin lymphoma
8. A neonate presents with projectile vomiting and a palpable 'olive' in the abdomen. Which of the following is the likely diagnosis?
   A. Pyloric stenosis
   B. Duodenal atresia
   C. Intussusception
   D. Gastroesophageal reflux
9. A 2-year-old child presents with developmental delay and cataracts. Mother's history reveals avoidance of dairy products. Which of the following is the likely diagnosis?
   A. Phenylketonuria
   B. Galactosemia
   C. Lactose intolerance
   D. Congenital hypothyroidism
10. An infant born at 32 weeks gestation presents with abdominal distension and bloody stools. Which of the following is the most likely diagnosis?
    A. Hirschsprung disease
    B. Necrotizing enterocolitis
    C. Intussusception
    D. Meconium ileus
11. A child presents with cherry-red spot on the macula and developmental regression. Which of the following is the most likely diagnosis?
    A. Tay–Sachs disease
    B. Retinoblastoma
    C. Neuroblastoma
    D. Lead poisoning
12. An infant has prolonged jaundice, hepatomegaly and poor feeding. Blood tests show conjugated hyperbilirubinemia. Which of the following is the likely diagnosis?
    A. Neonatal hepatitis
    B. Biliary atresia
    C. Breast milk jaundice
    D. Gilbert syndrome
13. A 6-month-old infant presents with a history of recurrent respiratory infections and failure to thrive. Immunoglobulin levels are low. Which of the following is the most likely diagnosis?
    A. Cystic fibrosis
    B. Primary immunodeficiency
    C. Asthma
    D. Bronchopulmonary dysplasia
14. A 1-year-old child presents with blue skin spells and a harsh systolic murmur. Which of the following is the likely congenital heart defect?
    A. Ventricular septal defect
    B. Tetralogy of Fallot
    C. Atrial septal defect
    D. Patent ductus arteriosus
15. A newborn presents with a high-pitched cry, microcephaly and overlapping fingers. Which of the following is the most likely chromosomal abnormality?
    A. Down syndrome
    B. Turner syndrome
    C. Klinefelter syndrome
    D. Cri du chat syndrome

Answers

1. (C); 2. (B); 3. (C); 4. (C); 5. (B); 6. (A); 7. (C); 8. (A); 9. (B); 10. (B); 11. (A); 12. (B); 13. (B); 14. (B); 15. (D).

Scenario-Based Questions

1. A 26-year-old woman (G2P1L1) came to hospital at term with labour pain for delivery of her second child. At birth, the baby was oedematous and icteric. The baby's haemoglobin level was 7 g/dL. The mother had not undergone routine antenatal check-up. Her first child is 2 years old, born at term by normal vaginal delivery with no significant medical history. What is the probable cause for the condition of the second baby?
2. A 32-year-old diabetic mother delivered a preterm infant. The baby was normal at birth but developed progressive respiratory distress after 1 hour and died despite resuscitation with mechanical ventilation. What is the probable cause of respiratory distress? Describe the microscopic finding of lung in this condition.
3. A 1-year-old child is brought to the clinic with complains of seizures and delayed neuronal milestones. On examination, it was found that the child has a fair complexion with white hairs. The mother gives history of mousy odour of urine. What is the diagnosis?
4. A 5-month-old infant is brought to the hospital with complains of failure to thrive, vomiting and diarrhoea since 1 month of age. On examination, it was found that the child has hepatomegaly and cataract in eyes. What is the probable diagnosis?
5. A 2-month-old infant is brought to the hospital with complains of abdominal distension. Ultrasound examination

reveals the presence of meconium ileus. The mother gives history of frequent respiratory infection and adds a note that she felt that the child's sweat was salty. Sweat chloride test is 120 mEq/L (normal <60 mEq/L). What is the diagnosis? Explain the pathogenesis of this condition.

6. A 6-month-old child was found dead in the bed in the morning. Detailed investigation revealed that the child was normal the previous night, had food and went to bed. On autopsy, no abnormal finding was found. What is the probable cause of death of this infant?
7. A 1-year-old child was brought to the hospital with complains of inadequate weight gain. On examination, it was found that the child's abdomen was distended and a firm mass was palpable in the left upper quadrant. Ultrasound revealed that the mass is arising from the left adrenal gland. Urine examination showed high levels of vanillylmandelic acid in urine. What is the diagnosis? Describe the gross and microscopic features of this condition.
8. A 5-year-old child is brought to the clinic with complains of abdominal distension and failure to thrive. On examination, it was found that a firm mass was palpable in the right side of the abdomen. Ultrasound revealed that the mass is arising from the upper pole of right kidney. What is the probable diagnosis? Describe the gross and microscopic features of this condition.

Answers

1. Hydrops fetalis due to Rh incompatibility
2. Acute respiratory distress syndrome due to surfactant deficiency
3. Phenylketonuria
4. Galactosaemia
5. Cystic fibrosis
6. Sudden infant death syndrome
7. Neuroblastoma
8. Wilms tumour

Topics for Self-Directed Learning

1. Congenital anomalies – malformation, disruptions, associations
2. TORCH group of infections
3. Congenital syphilis
4. Other inborn errors of metabolism
5. Other paediatric small blue round cell tumours

MIND MAPS

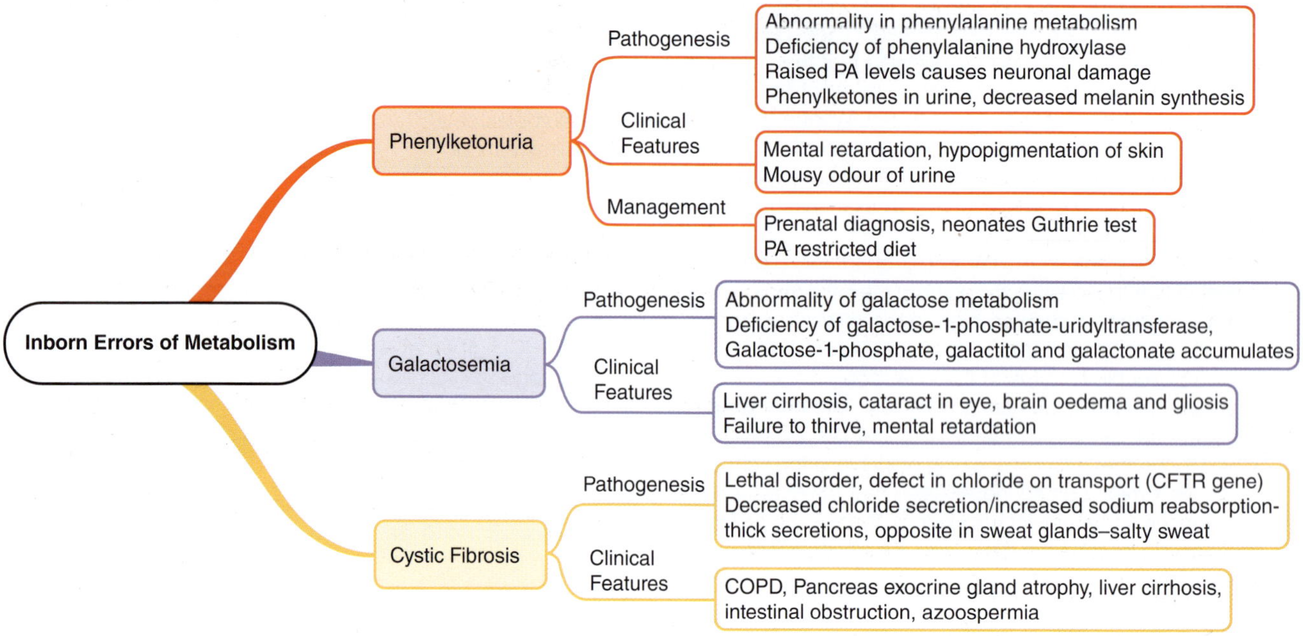
Inborn Errors of Metabolism
Phenylketonuria
Pathogenesis
Abnormality in phenylalanine metabolism
Deficiency of phenylalanine hydroxylase
Raised PA levels causes neuronal damage
Phenylketones in urine, decreased melanin synthesis
Clinical Features
Mental retardation, hypopigmentation of skin
Mousy odour of urine
Management
Prenatal diagnosis, neonates Guthrie test
PA restricted diet
Galactosemia
Pathogenesis
Abnormality of galactose metabolism
Deficiency of galactose-1-phosphate-uridyltransferase,
Galactose-1-phosphate, galactitol and galactonate accumulates
Clinical Features
Liver cirrhosis, cataract in eye, brain oedema and gliosis
Failure to thirve, mental retardation
Cystic Fibrosis
Pathogenesis
Lethal disorder, defect in chloride on transport (CFTR gene)
Decreased chloride secretion/increased sodium reabsorption-
thick secretions, opposite in sweat glands–salty sweat
Clinical Features
COPD, Pancreas exocrine gland atrophy, liver cirrhosis,
intestinal obstruction, azoospermia

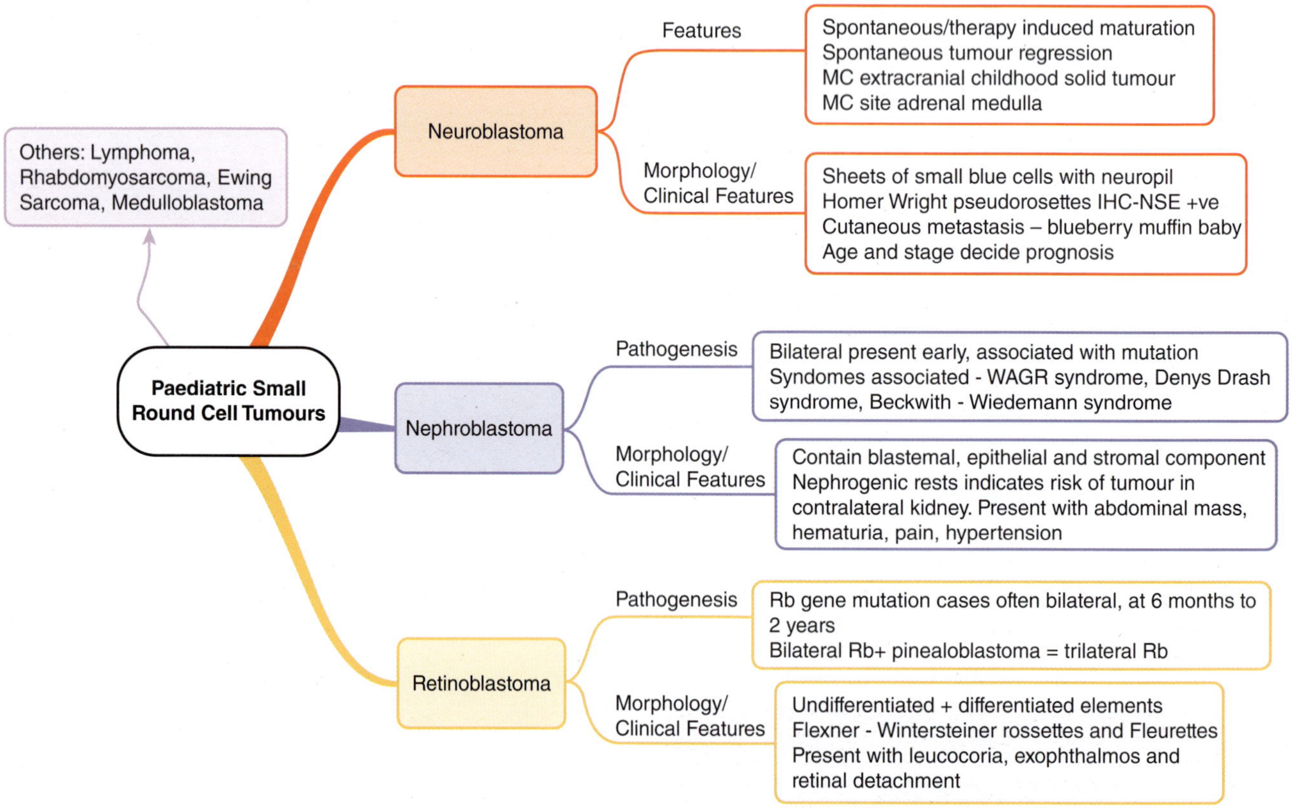
Paediatric Small Round Cell Tumours
Others: Lymphoma, Rhabdomyosarcoma, Ewing Sarcoma, Medulloblastoma
Neuroblastoma
Features
Spontaneous/therapy induced maturation
Spontaneous tumour regression
MC extracranial childhood solid tumour
MC site adrenal medulla
Morphology/ Clinical Features
Sheets of small blue cells with neuropil
Homer Wright pseudorosettes IHC-NSE +ve
Cutaneous metastasis – blueberry muffin baby
Age and stage decide prognosis
Nephroblastoma
Pathogenesis
Bilateral present early, associated with mutation
Syndomes associated - WAGR syndrome, Denys Drash
syndrome, Beckwith - Wiedemann syndrome
Morphology/ Clinical Features
Contain blastemal, epithelial and stromal component
Nephrogenic rests indicates risk of tumour in
contralateral kidney. Present with abdominal mass,
hematuria, pain, hypertension
Retinoblastoma
Pathogenesis
Rb gene mutation cases often bilateral, at 6 months to
2 years
Bilateral Rb+ pinealoblastoma = trilateral Rb
Morphology/ Clinical Features
Undifferentiated + differentiated elements
Flexner - Wintersteiner rossettes and Fleurettes
Present with leucocoria, exophthalmos and
retinal detachment

Basic Diagnostic Cytology and Clinical Pathology

11

Gayathri Devi Thanigaimani

Basic Diagnostic Cytology

PA 8.1 Describe the diagnostic role of **cytology** and its application in clinical care.

PA 8.2 Describe the basis of **exfoliative cytology** including the technique and stains used.

Clinical Pathology

PA 23.1 Describe abnormal **urinary findings** in disease states and identify and describe common urinary abnormalities in a clinical specimen.

PA 23.2 Describe abnormal findings in **body fluids** in various disease states.

PA 23.3 Describe and interpret the abnormalities in a panel containing **semen analysis, thyroid function tests, renal function tests or liver function tests**.

PA 35.3 Identify the aetiology of meningitis based on given cerebrospinal fluid (CSF) parameters.

PA 25.6 Interpret liver function and viral hepatitis serology panels. Distinguish obstructive from nonobstructive jaundice based on clinical features and **liver function tests**.

CHAPTER OUTLINE

I. BASIC DIAGNOSTIC CYTOLOGY

INTRODUCTION

Cytopathology is a branch of pathology in which cells obtained from tissues and fluids are studied to determine the cause and nature of the disease. This technique was invented by George Nicolas Papanicolaou in 1928 to study cells that were exfoliated from the cervical epithelium. This principle is now widely applied to many systems, with development of more techniques for obtaining optimal viable cells from the tissues. A cytopathologist is a pathologist who is trained to diagnose disease conditions by studying the cells which are obtained from the body. This field of pathology is gaining popularity nowadays due to its rapidity, simplicity, noninvasiveness and cost-effectiveness.

The technique dates back to early 1920s when Papanicolaou demonstrated its use in diagnosing cervical cancer, and the first scientific paper on cytopathology was published in 1930 from New York. This led to the establishment of cervical cancer screening clinics in 1940s. Since then, this field has been taken into serious consideration by the medical fraternity as a diagnostic modality. The first examination of the American Board of Cytopathology was started in the year 1989, making it a separate recognized branch of pathology.

COMPARISON OF CYTOPATHOLOGY WITH TISSUE BIOPSY

Although tissue biopsy is the final mode of definitive diagnosis, the degree of accuracy with cytopathology may be a bit lower. But this gap has been greatly reduced by newer and more sophisticated methods of sample collection and staining and by establishment of guidelines for diagnosis. The major differences between cytology and tissue biopsy are given in Table 11.1.

Table 11.1 Comparison of Cytology and Tissue Biopsy

Parameter	Cytology	Tissue Biopsy
Features studied	Cells – morphology	Tissue with architecture
Ideal for reporting	Dysplasia based on cellular details	Invasion across the basement membrane
Cost	Less costly	More costly
Sample collection	Can be done in the outpatient	May require admission
Anaesthesia	Not required	May be required
Patient tolerance	Better, as less invasive	Invasive, so pain perception more
Equipment	Minimal	Extensive
Scar	None	Will be formed
Reporting time	Lesser time required for preparing the slide	Processing is time consuming
Disadvantage	Cannot differentiate in situ vs. invasive carcinoma	Basement membrane invasion can be distinguished
Sampling error	Chances are higher when done without guidance	Chances are lesser

ROLE OF DIAGNOSTIC CYTOLOGY PA 8.1

The purposes of performing cytopathology are as follows:

- **Preliminary test before invasive investigation**
  In some instances, cytology may not give the final diagnosis but helps the clinician to justify further invasive investigations as a part of the diagnostic protocol.
- **To obtain a definitive diagnosis**
  The ultimate goal of the patient seeking medical help is to get cured of his or her ailment, and the first step towards that goal is arriving at a definitive diagnosis. So the clinician and the pathologist are, mutually, in favour of a test that can give an accurate diagnosis and thereby help in planning the treatment strategy. Cytopathology helps in achieving this in a majority of cases. The ability now to perform ancillary techniques in cytology specimens has increased the specificity of this modality.
- **Screening of large populations**
  Cytopathology as a screening investigation is well established, especially as cervical cancer screening programmes. The procedure is simple and less invasive and sample collection requires less expertise, enabling it to be performed in small establishments for a large population. This has greatly reduced the incidence and death due to cervical cancer worldwide.
- **Follow-up of patients**
  Patients treated for malignancies can be followed up for completion of treatment and recurrence by cytological evaluation. Fine-needle aspiration cytology (FNAC) of superficial and deep-seated lumps and sputum, bronchial lavage and urine cytology are examples of investigations done for follow-up.
- **For therapeutic and prognostic purposes**
  Performing ancillary studies on cytology specimens such as fine-needle aspirations (FNAs) may help in deciding treatment protocols and prognosis. For example, ER/PR/Her2 done on breast lump aspirate helps to decide on requirement of adjuvant chemotherapy and management of inoperable cases.

ADVANTAGES AND DISADVANTAGES OF CYTOLOGY

Cytopathology like any other speciality of pathology is heavily dependent on effective communication with the clinician and the radiologist. Providing the pathologist with relevant clinical information and radiological findings greatly contributes to the accuracy of results. The advantages and disadvantages of cytopathology are given in Table 11.2.

STAINING METHODS IN CYTOLOGY

Slides prepared from the collected material may be air-dried or alcohol-fixed. Many stains find utility on the

Table 11.2 Advantages and Disadvantages of Cytology

Advantages	Disadvantages
• Better appreciation of cell morphology • Simple outpatient procedure and does not require anaesthesia or special equipment • Patient anxiety is less and tolerance is good • Processing is very simple and quick – does not require much expertise • Result turnaround time is short • Can be done under imaging guidance • No significant complications • Cost-effective	• Tissue architecture cannot be studied, so **invasion in neoplasia cannot be checked over;** cannot distinguish carcinoma in situ from invasive carcinoma in the majority of cases • Expertise of the pathologist should be the prime factor for more accuracy of results • Sampling errors may occur in large or necrotic lesions, leading to incorrect diagnosis

smears, but the most common is Papanicolaou stain. The stains are classified as follows:

Air-dried smear stains
- Diff-Quick
- Romanowsky stain – May–Grünwald–Giemsa (MGG) stain

Alcohol-fixed smear stains
- Papanicolaou stain
- Haematoxylin and eosin (H&E)

Special stains
- Modified Ziehl–Neelsen (for acid-fast bacilli)
- Gram stain (for bacteria)
- Mucicarmine (for mucins)
- PAS (for glycogen, fungal wall, lipofuscin, etc.)
- Oil red O (for lipids)
- Perl's Prussian blue (for iron)

Immunocytochemistry
- Antibodies against certain cellular proteins are used to identify cells in the smear. The presence of certain proteins also helps in planning treatment of the patient before surgical excision.

DIFF-QUICK STAIN (FIG. 11.1)

Diff-Quick is a modified Romanowsky stain that is performed on air-dried slides. It can be done very quickly, approximately within a minute, hence the name. This stain is used to check adequacy of cell material in the specimen collected, especially in imaging/endoscopy-guided aspirations.

MAY–GRÜNWALD–GIEMSA STAIN (FIG. 11.2)

MGG stain is a Romanowsky stain that is done on air-dried slides. It is preferred for studying the cellular details

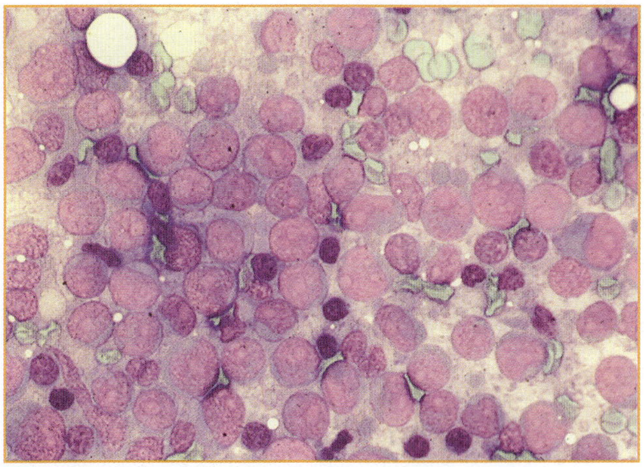

Fig. 11.1 Monomorphic pattern of large lymphocytes in high-grade non-Hodgkin thyroid lymphoma. Diff-Quick staining.

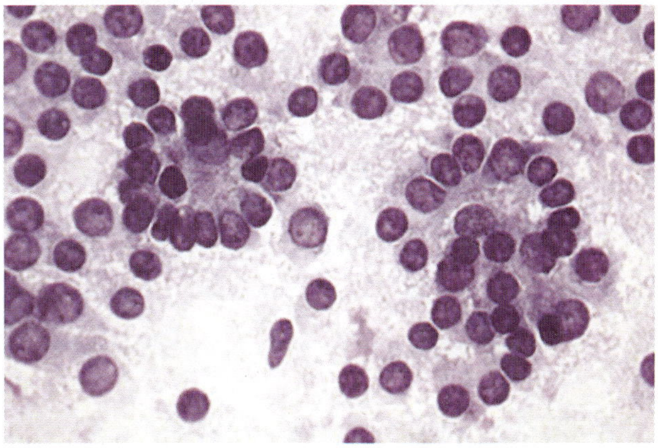

Fig. 11.2 Thyroid aspirate stained with MGG stain (papillary thyroid carcinoma). (*Source:* From Hugo Galera-Davidson and Ricardo González-Cámpora. Thyroid. Comprehensive Cytopathology. 4th edition. Elsevier 2015.)

including the cytoplasm, granules, vacuoles and basement membrane. Giemsa stain is made up of acidic eosin, alkaline methylene blue and Giemsa that provide azure. The methylene blue stains the acidic components of the cell such as nucleus into blue. The eosin stains the alkaline components of the cell such as cytoplasm into orange–red colour. The azure stains the basic cellular components into red and purple.

PAPANICOLAOU STAIN (FIG. 11.3)

Papanicolaou stain, also called Pap stain, is the most commonly used stain in cytology. It contains five dyes:

- Harris' haematoxylin – for optimal nuclear staining
- OG6 – Orange G with 6% phosphotungstic acid
- EA50 which contains three dyes – Eosin Y, Light Green SF yellowish and Bismarck brown – gives subtle ranges of green, blue and pink hues to the cell cytoplasm.

Cell nuclei are blue to black in colour, and the chromatin patterns of the nucleus are well defined. Pap stain is

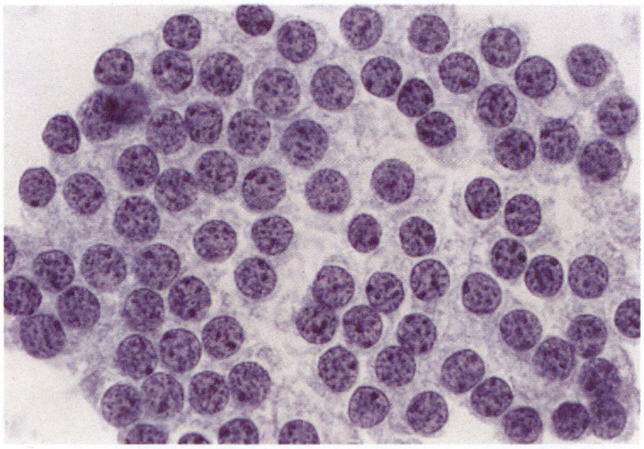

Fig. 11.3 Normal thyroid follicular cells in Pap stain. (*Source:* From Edmund S. Cibas. Thyroid. Cytology. 5th edition. Elsevier 2021.)

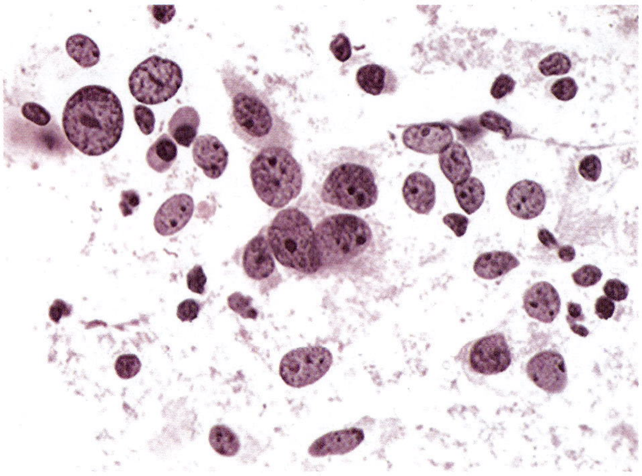

Fig. 11.4 Breast aspirate stained with H&E stain (medullary carcinoma). (*Source:* From Barbara S. Ducatman and Vaishali M. Pansare. Breast. Cytology. 5th edition. Elsevier 2021.)

the preferred stain for appreciating nuclear details. Cell cytoplasm in cervical smears stains blue to green, and keratin stains orange in colour.

HAEMATOXYLIN AND EOSIN (FIG. 11.4)

H&E stain that is commonly used in tissue biopsies may also be used for cytological slides. It contains haematoxylin for nuclear staining and eosin that gives different shades of pink for cytoplasm. H&E gives a tissue-like appearance to the slides, which makes the cellular characteristics more appreciable and easy to interpret for the pathologists.

TYPES OF DIAGNOSTIC CYTOLOGY

1. **Exfoliative cytology**
   Exfoliative cytology involves the study of cells that have exfoliated from the superficial surface, mucosal surface or serosa.
2. **Aspiration cytology**
   It is the study of cells aspirated from a lesion using a fine needle. It is also called FNAC.

EXFOLIATIVE CYTOLOGY **PA 8.2**

The exfoliated cells that are shed are collected from the fluid or by scraping the mucosa and examined under a microscope. The following are the areas in which exfoliative cytology is useful:

- **Gynaecology** – vaginal, cervical, endometrial and tubal cells
- **Respiratory cytology** – cells obtained from the bronchioalveolar tract
- **Urinary cytology** – cells shed from the bladder
- **Gastrointestinal tract** – gastric mucosal cells
- **Buccal smear** – squamous cells of the oral cavity
- **Body fluid cytology** – pleural, peritoneal, pericardial, synovial cavities and CSF

Smearing Techniques

The material that is collected may be converted into smears by the following techniques:

- **Direct smear:** This includes directly smearing the material on a slide.
- **Cytocentrifuge smears:** This is done using a cytocentrifuge to concentrate the cells and prepare the smears. It is useful when a large volume of fluids is received containing very few cells.
- **Monolayer liquid-based cytology (LBC):** This is an automated method preferred nowadays for cervical pap smear screening. The method gives a single sheet of cells on the slide with a clean background in contrast to the traditional direct smears in which cells overlap, making morphology deceptive.
- **Cell block technique:** Here, the cells are centrifuged and a cell button obtained at the bottom is subjected to formalin fixation and processed as a tissue biopsy. Also, the application of special stains or immunohistochemistry is an added benefit, thus contributing to more clarity on the arrangement/pattern and morphology of cells.

Female Genital Tract

The female genital tract specimens include vaginal smears for assessing hormonal status and cervical smears for cervical cancer screening. The former is not commonly done nowadays due to availability of tests to directly evaluate serum hormone levels. Cancer screening is the most common indication for cervical cytology studies, and this test has led to the early identification of precancerous lesions, reducing cancer-related mortality and morbidity. The screening protocol for women as per 'The American College of Obstetricians and Gynecologists' is given in Table 11.3. The sensitivity of the test varies from 30% to 80%, whereas the specificity is around 95%.

Table 11.3 Screening Protocol as per the American College of Obstetricians and Gynecologists Guidelines for Women of Average Risk

Age to begin screening	21 years
Age 21–30 years	Every 3 years
Age 30–65 years	Only pap smear – every 3 years Pap smear with HPV DNA testing – every 5 years
Age to stop testing	65 years if no history of CIN2 or greater lesion
Posthysterectomy	Not recommended if no history of CIN2 or greater

CIN2, cervical intraepithelial neoplasia grade 2.

Method of Collecting Specimen

Conventional smear: The specimen is collected by using brush and spatula and smeared on slides that are immediately fixed using alcohol.

Liquid-based cytology: The specimen is collected by using the LBC brush which is then dropped in a bottle of liquid fixative. This is then centrifuged to concentrate the cells and remove red blood cells (RBCs)/white blood cells (WBCs) and the cervical mucus. The cells obtained are spread as a monolayer sheet on a slide and stained.

Advantages of LBC

- Thin cell preparation with no overlapping of cells
- Clean background
- Opportunity to prepare duplicate slides
- Reduced chance of unsatisfactory smears
- Availability of material to perform human papillomavirus (HPV) DNA testing

Technique The fixed smears prepared by either method are stained using Papanicolaou stain and viewed by the cytopathologist. The PAP stain includes one nuclear stain, haematoxylin that stains the nucleus and two cytoplasmic stains, namely OG6, which stains keratin orange, and EA (Eosin Azure). EA comprises Eosin Y, which gives an orange to pink colour to the superficial epithelial squamous cells, nucleoli and RBCs, and Light Green SF stains the metabolically active cells turquoise blue, i.e. parabasal cells and intermediate cells. Superficial cells appear orange to pink. Intermediate and parabasal cells appear turquoise green to blue.

Interpretation of a Pap Smear The recommended reporting method is the Bethesda system. According to this system, the report should necessarily contain information about the following:

1. Satisfactory/unsatisfactory: A smear may be unsatisfactory because of labelling errors, scanty cellularity or the presence of contaminant such as blood.
2. Normal or abnormal cellular material: Abnormality may be squamous or glandular.
3. Additional information such as inflammation, infective organisms such as yeast and *Trichomonas*.

   Squamous cell abnormalities, which are the most common abnormalities detected, are classified into the following:

   i. Negative for intraepithelial abnormality
   ii. Atypical squamous cells of unknown significance (ASCUS)
   iii. Low-grade squamous intraepithelial lesion (LSIL)
   iv. High-grade squamous intraepithelial lesion (HSIL)
   v. Squamous cell carcinoma

Normal Smear (*Fig. 11.5*)

- The superficial cells, which are the most mature cells, are large polygonal cells with abundant pink or green cytoplasm and a small pyknotic nucleus.
- The intermediate cells are also large polygonal cells with abundant cytoplasm like superficial cells, but their nucleus is relatively larger with granular chromatin. These cells may be binucleate or multinucleate. The cells are often folded and hence called navicular cells.
- Parabasal cells are round or oval cells with a slightly larger nucleus.

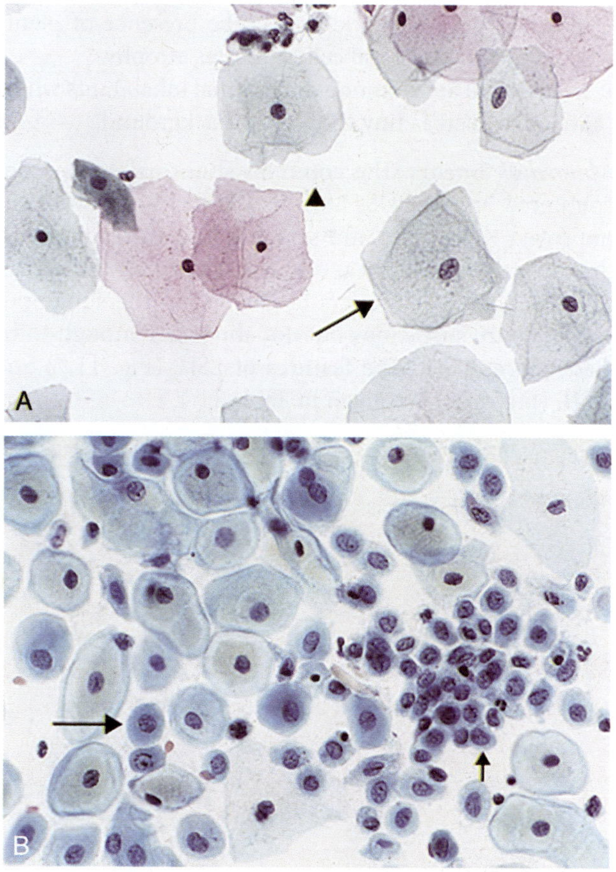

Fig. 11.5 Smear showing normal superficial cells (arrow head) and intermediate cells (arrow) (A), parabasal cells (large arrow) and basal cells (small arrow) (B). (*Source:* From Edmund S. Cibas. Cervical and Vaginal Cytology. Cytology. 5th Edition. Elsevier 2021.)

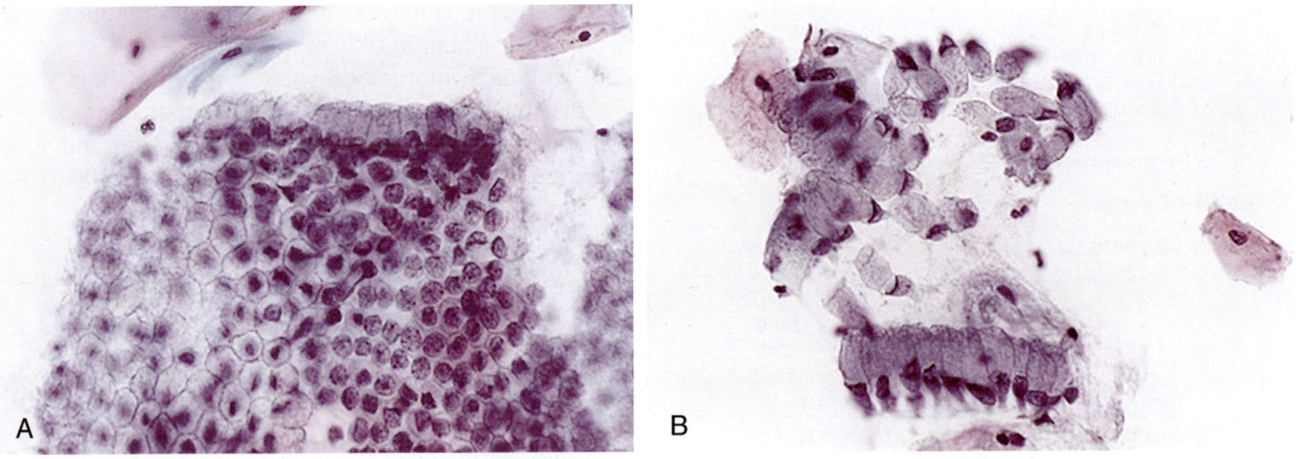

Fig. 11.6 Smear showing honeycomb appearance (A) and picket fence appearance (B) of endocervical cells. (*Source:* From Edmund S. Cibas. Cervical and Vaginal Cytology. Cytology. 5th Edition. Elsevier 2021.)

- Basal cells are smaller and have very less cytoplasm.
- Clusters of endocervical cells or sheets of endocervical cells which are columnar cells with an eccentric nucleus and abundant vacuolated cytoplasm may be seen (picket fence appearance) (Fig. 11.6).
- Background is usually clean.
- The presence of superficial cells indicates oestrogenic status, whereas the dominance of intermediate cells indicates progestogenic status. The presence of plenty of parabasal and basal cells indicates atrophy.
- Lactobacilli are common and normal inhabitants which are often seen as tiny rods in the background.

Abnormal Smears The common abnormal smears encountered are ASCUS, LSIL and HSIL. Because of the improved techniques and screening measures taken by the government, cervical cancer cases are in the downward trend. ASCUS refers to changes in the squamous cells that are suspicious but not abnormal enough to be classified as LSIL. The features of LSIL (Fig. 11.7) and HSIL (Fig. 11.8) are given in Table 11.4.

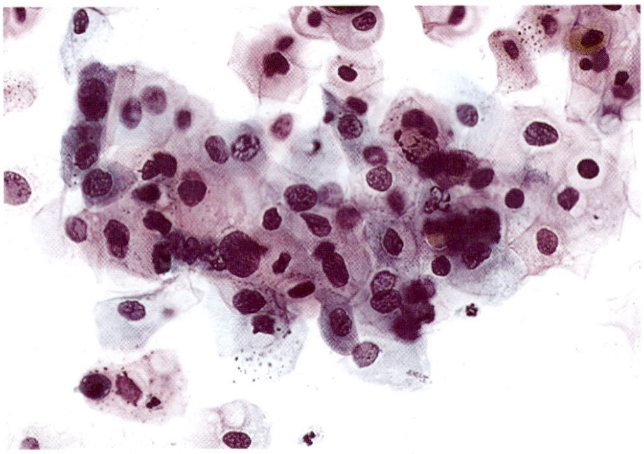

Fig. 11.7 Pap smear showing LSIL. (*Source:* From Edmund S. Cibas. Cervical and Vaginal Cytology. Cytology. 5th Edition. Elsevier 2021.)

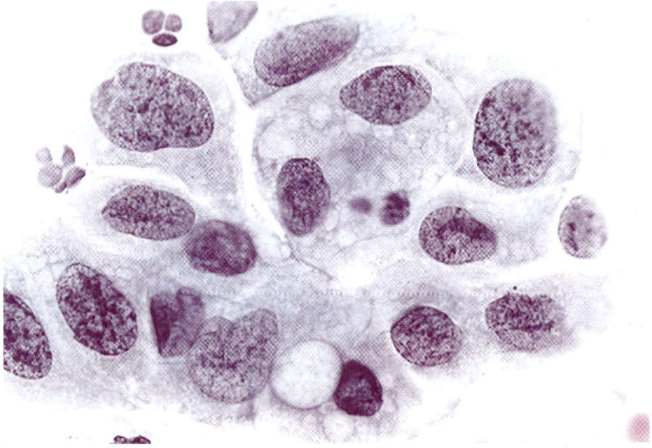

Fig. 11.8 Pap smear showing HSIL. (*Source:* From Edmund S. Cibas. Cervical and Vaginal Cytology. Cytology. 5th Edition. Elsevier 2021.)

Applications of Cervical Smears

- To screen cervical cancer.
- To study the hormone status.
- To identify the presence of infection and type of organism.
- To obtain a sample to perform HPV DNA testing.
- Endometrial cells that have exfoliated may be studied for neoplastic transformation. The presence of even normal endometrial cells in cervical smears above the age of 45 years is considered abnormal.
- Occasionally, tubal cells in tubal malignancy may be seen in cervical smears.

Urinary Tract

Urine cytology was introduced in 1940s to follow up patients with bladder cancer. It has been a very cost-effective method for studying bladder cancers since then.

Indications for Urine Cytology

- Haematuria
- Follow-up of patients who have been treated for bladder carcinoma

Table 11.4 Features of LSIL and HSIL

LSIL	HSIL

• Large, mature cells (equal in size to a normal superficial or intermediate squamous cell)
• Nuclear atypia such as
  • Enlargement
  • Irregular contour (slight)
  • Hyperchromasia
  • Slight chromatin coarseness
• Cytoplasmic cavities (koilocytes)
	• Usually parabasal-sized cells
	• Discrete cells or syncytium-like groups
	• Nuclear atypia
	  • Enlargement
	  • Marked irregularity in contour
	  • Usually marked hyperchromasia
	  • Marked chromatin coarseness

HSIL, high-grade squamous intraepithelial lesion; LSIL, low-grade squamous intraepithelial lesion.

- Screening of people who are at risk of developing bladder cancer

Methods of Collecting Specimen Several methods are used for collecting specimen depending on the case scenario. The methods with their advantage and disadvantage are given in Table 11.5.

Technique

- The urine specimen should be examined within 1–2 hours.
- The specimen is concentrated by sedimentation or centrifuge and smeared on slides.
- The slides are fixed in alcohol and stained.
- The most recommended stain is Papanicolaou stain.
- Using three samples of urine improves sensitivity of identifying cancer and hence is recommended.
- Sensitivity in identifying high-grade lesions is better than that of low-grade lesions.
- False-positive is rare, though low-grade lesions may be missed occasionally.

Normal Cytology Normal urine sample usually has scant cellularity. The commonly seen cells include the following:

- Urothelial cells (Fig. 11.9)
  - Intermediate and superficial ('umbrella') cells
  - Catheterized specimens may additionally have basal cells
- Squamous cells may be from urethra, bladder metaplasia or vaginal contamination.
- Degenerated intestinal epithelial cells may be seen in ileal conduit specimens.

The Paris system of reporting urinary cytology is the latest format accepted worldwide for reporting urine samples. This helps to maintain uniformity in the reporting terminologies worldwide and also makes it easy for histological correlation.

Information Obtained From Urine Cytology

- Urothelial carcinoma of bladder, ureter and renal pelvis
- Metastatic carcinoma
- Infections such as fungal, herpes simplex virus (HSV), cytomegalovirus (CMV), HPV, *Trichomonas vaginalis* and bacterial infections
- Malakoplakia, an inflammatory lesion of bladder due to bacteria
- Crystals and casts

Urothelial neoplasms are classified into flat and papillary lesions. In urothelial lesions, cells or papillary fragments shed into urine help in planning further

Table 11.5 Methods of Specimen Collection for Urinary Tract Cytology

Method	Advantage	Disadvantage
Voided urine • Not early morning specimen • Midstream catch	Noninvasive Easy to obtain	Vaginal contamination in women Low cellularity
Catheter specimen	Good cellularity	Specimen not fresh in patients with catheter Artefacts due to instrumentation
Bladder washing • Obtained by flushing saline into the bladder using a catheter	Good cellularity Cells well preserved	Invasive Artefacts due to instrumentation
Upper tract washing • Washing of the ureter and renal pelvis obtained using a catheter	Good cellularity Reliable method to evaluate this region in high-grade lesions	Invasive Artefacts due to instrumentation
Ileal loop • Ileal conduit is created to act as a bladder in patients operated for bladder carcinoma	Screening of patients for recurrence or second malignancy of ureters or kidney	Low cellularity Contamination with ileal epithelial cells Cells not preserved well

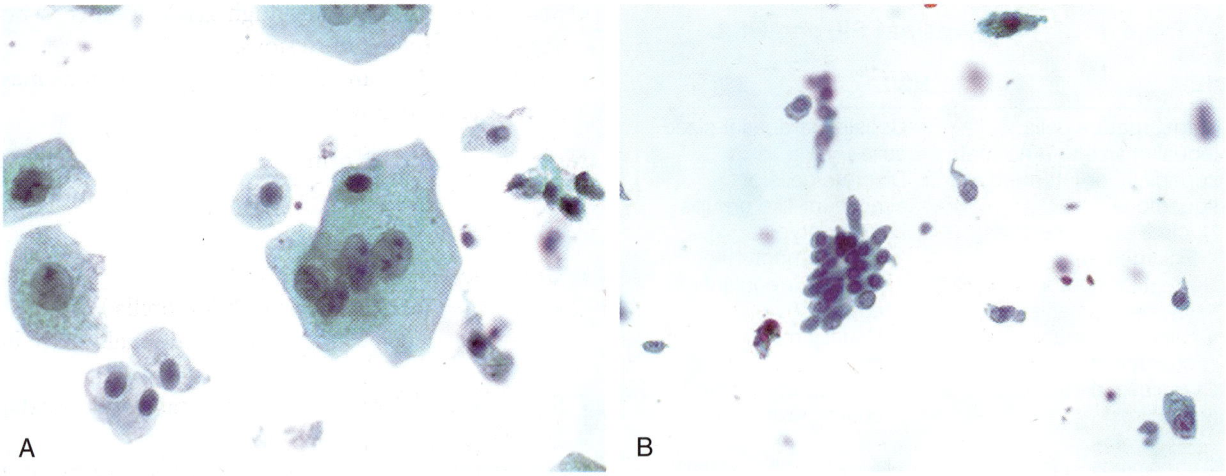

Fig. 11.9 Urine cytology of normal urothelial umbrella cells (A) and basal cells (B). (*Source:* From David G. Bostwick. Urine Cytology. Urologic Surgical Pathology. 4th edition. Elsevier 2020.)

investigation. The current WHO/ISUP classification is given as follows:

Flat lesions
- Dysplasia
- Carcinoma in situ

Papillary lesions
- Papilloma
- Papillary urothelial neoplasm of low malignant potential
- Low-grade urothelial carcinoma
- High-grade urothelial carcinoma

The term 'dysplasia' is avoided in urine cytology, as it is a nonspecific diagnosis. Papilloma is a rare lesion seen only in young patients. The diagnosis commonly reported in cytology based on cytological appearance of cells without information about the presence/absence of invasion is as follows:

- *Low-grade lesions*, which include papillary urothelial neoplasm of low malignant potential and low-grade urothelial carcinoma.
- *High-grade lesions*, which include high-grade papillary urothelial carcinoma and carcinoma in situ.

Features of Low-Grade Lesions (Fig. 11.10)
- Cytological features
  Increased nuclear to cytoplasmic ratio
  Homogeneous cytoplasm
  Irregular nuclear membrane
- Architectural features
  Papillary fragments containing a central fibrovascular core (diagnostic)
  Irregular cluster of cells

Features of High-Grade Lesions (Fig. 11.11)
- Cells scattered in singles
- Presence of nuclear atypia – pleomorphic hyperchromatic nucleus with an increased nuclear to cytoplasmic ratio

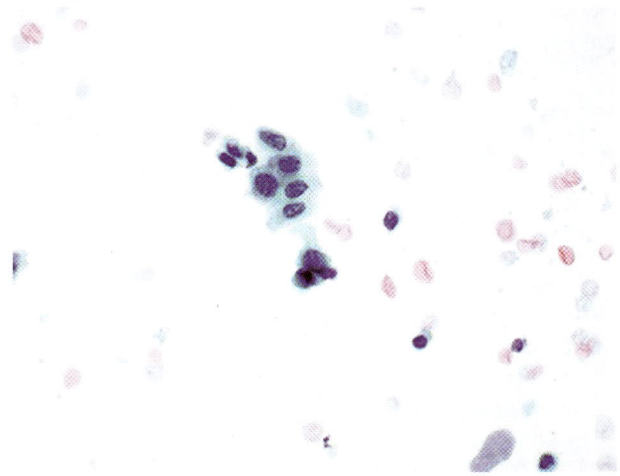

Fig. 11.10 Cytological features of low-grade urothelial neoplasm showing mild atypia. (*Source:* From David G. Bostwick. Urine Cytology. Urologic Surgical Pathology. 4th edition. Elsevier 2020.)

- Nuclear outline irregularity
- Chromatin coarse and granular
- Presence of large nucleoli

Respiratory Tract

The respiratory tract is a kaleidoscope with respect to epithelial lining. The upper respiratory tract is lined by squamous and ciliated columnar epithelium; in the lower tract, the trachea and bronchi have ciliated columnar; the terminal bronchioles have Clara cells (nonciliated columnar/cuboidal cells); and the alveoli have pneumocytes and alveolar macrophages. So familiarity with the normal appearance of different samples is critical for studying respiratory cytology.

Methods of Collecting Specimen
- **Sputum:** This is obtained by clearing the mucociliary apparatus. It is a noninvasive method of obtaining samples in symptomatic patients but is not useful in

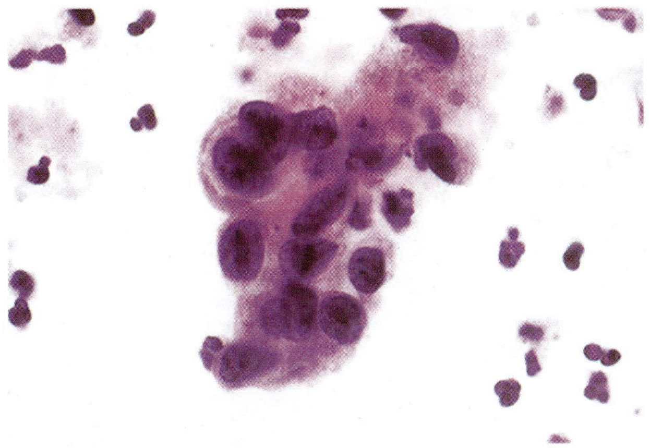

Fig. 11.11 Cytology showing high-grade urothelial neoplasm showing marked nuclear atypia. (*Source:* From David G. Bostwick. Urine Cytology. Urologic Surgical Pathology. 4th edition. Elsevier 2020.)

screening the population. Early morning samples and multiple samples over successive days give better yield.

- **Bronchial aspirate/bronchial aspirate:** The bronchial secretions are aspirated or saline is used to wash the bronchial mucosa and aspirated using a bronchoscope.
- **Bronchial brushing:** Using bronchoscopy, the bronchial tree is visualized and a brush is used to pick up cells, which are then smeared on a slide.
- **Bronchoalveolar lavage:** The distal part of the bronchoalveolar tree is washed with saline using the bronchoscope to reach as far as possible and aspirated.
- **Aspiration methods:** An FNA of the lesion may be done transbronchially, endobronchially, transoesophageally or percutaneously. This may give a more cellular yield from the lesion directly and is preferably performed under imaging guidance.

Advantages of Respiratory Tract Cytology **Helps in identification of the following:**

- Infections such as tuberculosis (TB), viral, bacterial, fungal and parasitic infections
- Pulmonary lesions such as amyloidosis and sarcoidosis
- Benign pulmonary lesions such as hamartoma
- Lung carcinoma
- Metastatic lung tumours

Gastrointestinal Tract

Gastrointestinal tract cytology is one of the useful tests done while performing endoscopy. The most common indication is a suspicion of malignancy.

Advantages of Cytology Over Biopsy

- Lesions occupying wide areas are better sampled by scraping with a brush than by performing multiple tissue biopsies.
- Lymphoma cells are better appreciated in cytology than small biopsies where they may be crushed, leading to artefacts.
- Less invasive
- Short turnaround time

Methods of Collecting

- Brush specimen of the lesion – smeared on the slide or dropped in a fixative
- FNA of submucosal lesions

Information Obtained Lesions of the oesophagus, stomach and duodenum can be studied.

- Metaplasia such as Barrett oesophagus
- Dysplastic changes
- Malignancies
- Infections

Buccal Smear

Buccal smears are obtained to investigate premalignant and malignant lesions. The buccal smears have long been used for studying DNA of the patients and for Barr body analysis.

Indications

- Screening of individuals at high risk of developing oral malignancies
- Suspicious lesions
- Follow-up of patients treated for oral carcinoma

Method of Collecting

- A disposable tongue depressor is used to scrape cells from the surface of the lesion and smeared on the slide, which is fixed and stained.
- A cytobrush similar to the one used in Pap smears may be used.

Information Obtained

- Dysplastic changes
- Malignant changes
- Cells for immunohistochemistry
- Material for DNA studies

Fluid Cytology

The fluids that are sent for cytological study include the following:

- Pleural fluid
- Peritoneal fluid/washing
- Pericardial fluid
- CSF
- Synovial fluid
- Cyst fluid such as ovarian/pancreatic cysts

Among these samples, peritoneal and pleural fluids are the most common samples received in the laboratory for cytological evaluation and are hence discussed here. The peritoneal, pleural and pericardial cavities are spaces lined by mesothelial cells that normally have minimal fluid for lubrication. Collection of fluid in these spaces may be a transudate or exudate. *Transudate* occurs because of disturbance in hydrostatic pressure or osmotic pressure, whereas *exudate* occurs because of an insult to the mesothelium by malignancies, trauma, pneumonia, autoimmune disorders, infections, etc. Identifying the nature of effusion is a preliminary investigation done in the laboratory by estimating the protein content of the fluid. This is very important because *only exudates need to be subjected to cytological evaluation for malignant cells.*

Methods of Sample Collection The fluids in these spaces are aspirated slowly by using a syringe and needle to create negative pressure.

- Pleurocentesis (from pleural space)
- Paracentesis (from peritoneal cavity through the abdominal wall)
- Culdocentesis (from peritoneal cavity through cul-de-sac via the vagina)
- Pericardiocentesis (from pericardial cavity)
- Suctioning during thoracic, abdominal or cardiac surgery
- Peritoneal washing with saline during abdominal surgery

Technique Fluid cytology provides a better sample to assess serosal malignancies than punch biopsy, giving a sensitivity of approximately 70% and specificity of almost 100%. Fluid is collected in heparinized containers to prevent clotting and sent unfixed to the laboratory. It can be stored in the refrigerator for up to a month till it is smeared on a slide. The specimen can be centrifuged to concentrate it when cells are scanty. The slides are fixed in alcohol and stained. The material can be used for immunohistochemistry to distinguish secondary tumours from mesothelioma or to identify the source of the primary tumour.

Normal Smear Normal fluid may contain mesothelial cells, occasional inflammatory cells and macrophages. The features of mesothelial cells are as follows (Fig. 11.12):

- Arranged in small clusters or singles
- Round cells with a single nucleus and a single nucleolus
- Small cluster of cells shows a window effect between them
- Cytoplasm is dense with peripheral clear rim (lacy skirt appearance)

Information Obtained

- Reactive effusions when there is an adjacent tumour or infection
- Infective conditions such as bacterial pneumonia involving adjacent pleura and TB
- Inflammatory conditions such as rheumatoid or lupus pleuritis

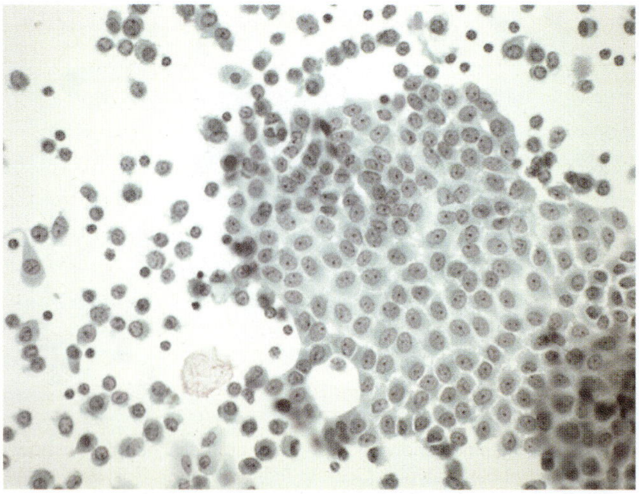

Fig. 11.12 Smear showing normal mesothelial cells in a two-dimensional sheet in peritoneal wash. (*Source:* From David C. Wilbur. Cytology in the Practice of Gynecologic Pathology. Gynecologic Pathology: A Volume in Foundations in Diagnostic Pathology Series. 2nd edition. Elsevier 2021.)

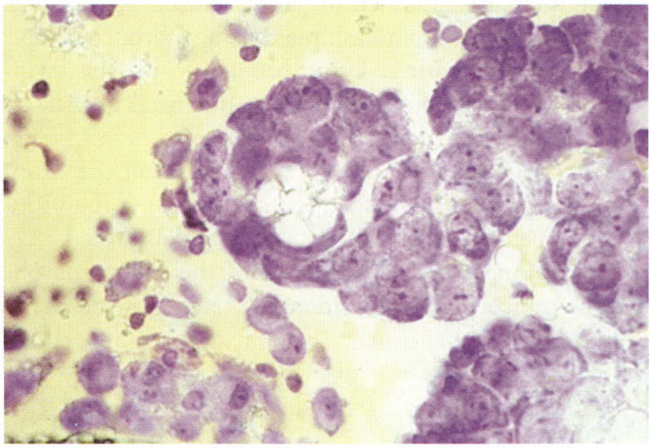

Fig. 11.13 Smear showing serous ovarian adenocarcinoma deposits in ascitic fluid cytology. (*Source:* From Marluce Bibbo, Rossitza Draganova-Tacheva and Bernard Naylor. Pleural, Peritoneal, and Pericardial Effusions. Comprehensive Cytopathology. 4th edition. Elsevier 2015.)

- Primary tumour: Mesothelioma is common in pleura than in peritoneum and is strongly associated with asbestos exposure.
- Metastatic deposits: The most common malignancies of serosa are metastatic carcinomatous deposits. Among secondaries, adenocarcinomatous secondaries are more common than squamous or small cell carcinomas.

  Features of adenocarcinomatous deposit cells are as follows (Fig. 11.13):
  - Arranged in large spheres or singles
  - Much larger with hyperchromatic pleomorphic nuclei
  - Have cytoplasmic vacuolation
  - In gastric/breast tumours, signet ring cells may be seen

FINE-NEEDLE ASPIRATION CYTOLOGY

Aspiration cytology involves removal of cells from tissues of the body by aspiration by using a syringe and studying the material after fixation and staining. This can be done for superficial palpable lesions and for deep lesions under imaging guidance. The skill of the person performing the aspiration is a main determinant of the quality of the material obtained. Hence, proper training under supervision to learn the technique and continuous performance to maintain the competency are crucial.

Steps for Performing Fine-Needle Aspiration

1. An adequate history should be obtained, the lesion examined and any imaging available should be studied to determine whether the FNA is required.
2. Procedure should be explained to the patient in understandable language, and consent of the patient should be obtained.
3. The patient should be conveniently positioned and the lesion immobilized.
4. An adequate number of pricks to cover the lesion should be done to obtain sufficient material.
5. Prepare slides, fix and stain them. If ancillary studies are to be conducted, allocate material appropriately.
6. After the procedure, instructions should be given to the patient regarding report collection.

Technique

The procedure is done by using a syringe attached to a 22-gauge needle or smaller. The two techniques are as follows:

- **Aspiration with negative pressure** (Fig. 11.14): Negative pressure may be created manually by using fingers to control the plunger or by using a syringe holder which produces a much more uniform suction.
- **Nonaspiration technique**: It is done passively by using only the needle or a needle with a syringe but without negative pressure. This yields quantitatively less material but is qualitatively superior one.

Complications of Fine-Needle Aspiration

- Pain, bleeding and bruising at the site may occur.
- Injury to adjacent organs may lead to complications such as pneumothorax in anterior chest wall FNA and carotid artery dissection in neck lesion FNA.
- Seeding of needle tract by malignant cells. This risk is much less in FNA than with needle biopsy.
- There is a risk of needle stick injury to the operator.

Squash Cytology

Squash cytology is an important investigation done for the analysis of lesions involving the central nervous system (CNS). Advantages of squash cytology include a quick and cheap intraoperative diagnostic test with a reasonably good accuracy. It is more useful for diagnosing neoplastic lesions than non-neoplastic lesions.

Indications

- To make intraoperative diagnosis of lesions
- To guide the extent of surgery
- To assess surgical margins
- To study tiny brain tissues obtained by stereotactic technique

Advantages

- Does not require sophisticated equipment
- Cheaper
- Requires less tissue
- Quicker, slides prepared for reporting within 10 minutes
- Can avoid contamination of equipment in viral infections
- Better appreciation of cytological features of lymphoma cells and cells of pituitary adenoma

Technique (Fig. 11.15) The brain tissue being soft makes this technique possible, while this consistency is a hindrance for performing frozen sections. A tiny fragment of unfixed tissue is compressed and smeared on the slide by giving adequate pressure to spread the tissue but avoiding excess pressure that might distort the cells. The slide is then fixed and stained for reporting.

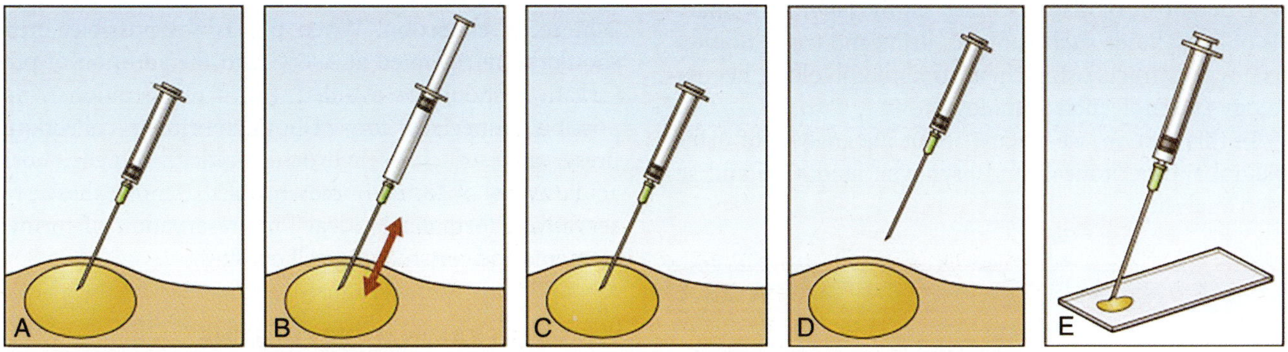

Fig. 11.14 Procedural technique with aspiration. The needle is inserted into the lesion, negative pressure is applied by withdrawing the plunger. After required material is obtained in the hub of the needle, the plunger is released and then needle is removed and material is transferred to the slide. (*Source:* From Svante R. Orell, Philippe Vielh. Orell and Sterrett's Fine Needle Aspiration Cytology. Elsevier 2012.)

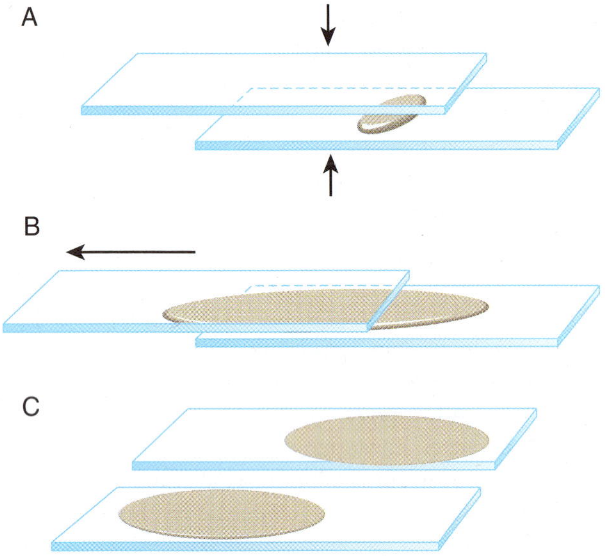

Fig. 11.15 Technique of squash cytology.

Imprint Cytology

Imprint cytology is a quick, inexpensive method to study solid lesions. It is very useful in underdeveloped infrastructure where expensive equipment and trained personnel are not available. It may also be used in intraoperative diagnosis.

Advantages of Imprint Cytology

- To make intraoperative diagnosis and margin assessment
- To study lymph nodes
- To study CNS tumours
- To study basal cell carcinoma of skin which presents as ulcers

Technique Freshly cut unfixed specimen is gently dabbed on the slide without gliding. The slides are then fixed in alcohol and stained.

II. CLINICAL PATHOLOGY

Clinical pathology is a branch of pathology that deals with diagnosis of diseases based on the laboratory analysis of body fluids such as blood, urine and tissue homogenates or extracts using chemistry, microbiology, haematology and molecular pathology.

In this section, we discuss about the analysis of urine, pleural and peritoneal fluids, synovial fluid, CSF and semen analysis.

URINE ANALYSIS PA 23.1

Urine is the fluid excreted by the kidneys, aiding in the removal of various toxic substances from our blood. Urine analysis not only helps us to identify diseases of the urinary tract but also hints on the underlying possibility of systemic diseases. A urine dipstick can give a quick preview at the bedside as to what immediate measures can be taken till the blood investigations are ready. The most familiar example can be a urine pregnancy test. Also to keep in mind, the timing and method of collection have a profound influence on the interpretation and hence should be done with proper knowledge.

URINE SAMPLING METHOD

Single specimen: A single specimen of urine is collected preferably in the early morning except for postprandial sugar detection when it is collected postprandially. Early morning specimen is more acidic because of its higher concentration and is useful for studying formed elements. It also has a higher concentration of various constituents and hormones, thereby gives better sensitivity. But a random specimen of urine can be collected any time of the day and hence is more convenient for screening purposes.
Twenty-four–hour specimen: This is the ideal method for quantitative estimation of proteins and hormones. Urine is collected over a period of 24 hours in a container kept at 4–6°C in the refrigerator.

URINE COLLECTION METHODS

- **Midstream specimen:** The mid part of the stream is collected after discarding the initial urine stream, which is more likely to be contaminated by the exfoliated cells and commensal organisms. It is used for all routine urine examinations.
- **Clean catch specimen:** For bacteriological examination, it is important to reduce chances of contamination by flora in the genitalia. The genitalia are cleaned with soap and water and the sample is collected midstream.
- **Catheter specimen:** This is done in catheterized patients and patients unable to pass urine such as in urinary obstruction. Fresh specimen should be considered, whereas stagnant urine in the Urobag is avoided.

TRANSPORTATION OF URINE SAMPLE

Urine sample that is collected should be evaluated within 2 hours of collection. When this is not possible, urine should be refrigerated at 4–6°C and the addition of preservatives should be avoided. But if refrigeration is not possible, especially for 24-hour–specimen collections, preservatives such as hydrochloric acid, toluene, boric acid, thymol or formalin may be used. Among these preservatives, formalin is ideal for preservation of formed elements and for studying cell cytology.

PHYSICAL EXAMINATION OF URINE

This includes assessment of the parameters given in Table 11.6.

Table 11.6 Normal Parameters in Physical Examination of Urine

Parameter	Normal Value
Volume	600–2000 mL
Appearance	Clear
Reaction	Acidic
Colour	Pale yellow
Odour	Mildly aromatic
Specific gravity	1.003–1.030

Volume

Volume of urine is committed in the report only in 24-hour specimen. The normal volume of urine is between 600 and 2000 mL but depends on various factors such as water intake and climate. The abnormalities in volume and their causes are given in Table 11.7.

Appearance

Normal urine is clear in appearance. The presence of phosphates, urates and protein may make it to appear cloudy. Turbidity in the urine sample may be seen when it contains pus cells or bacteria.

Reaction (Table 11.8)

Normal urine is slightly acidic due to the hydrogen ion maintenance function of kidney. The average urine pH is 6.0, but this is influenced by the diet, acid–base balance, concentration of urine, renal tubular function and water balance. The pH of urine should be tested in the fresh sample to avoid errors as long-standing urine tends to turn alkaline due to ammonia formation from urea. The pH of urine is tested using a litmus paper, pH meter or reagent strip test, the first being the simplest one.

Colour

Normally, urine is pale yellow or amber-coloured but is influenced by the water intake as well.

The common colours of urine are mentioned in Table 11.9.

Odour

Freshly passed urine has a typical aromatic smell due to the presence of few organic compounds that are volatile and disappear on standing. In the meantime, urea gets converted to ammonia and so the standing urine sample develops an ammoniacal odour. The commonly encountered odours are enlisted in Table 11.10.

Specific Gravity

Specific gravity of urine helps to measure the quantity of dissolved solids in the urine sample. The normal specific gravity is between 1.003 and 1.030 and is mainly due to the presence of urea and sodium in it. It reflects the urine-concentrating ability of the tubules of the kidney. It is measured using a urinometer, a refractometer or automated machines that interpret reagent strips. The abnormalities of specific gravity and their causes are given in Table 11.11.

Table 11.7 Abnormalities in Volume of Urine

Abnormality	Definition	Physiological Cause	Pathological Cause
Oliguria	Urine output < 400 mL in 24 h	Reduced water intake Hot climate	Dehydration Fever Acute glomerulonephritis Congestive cardiac failure
Anuria	Urine output < 100 mL in 24 h	–	Acute tubular necrosis (acute renal failure) Complete obstruction of the urinary tract
Polyuria	Urine output > 2000 mL in 24 h	Excess water intake Cold climate	Diabetes mellitus Diabetes insipidus Chronic renal failure Diuretic therapy

Table 11.8 Relevance of Reaction of Urine Specimen

	Litmus Paper Test	Physiological Causes	Pathological Causes
Acidic pH	Blue litmus → turns red	High protein diet Reduced water intake	Urinary infection with *Escherichia coli* Ketosis
Alkaline pH	Red litmus → turns blue	Vegetarian diet High water intake	Urinary infection with *Proteus*, *Pseudomonas* Severe vomiting Chronic renal failure

Table 11.9 Causes for Change in Urine Colour

Physiological Causes	
Yellow Colourless Red Orange	Concentrated urine (reduced water intake, early morning specimen), vitamin B tablet High water intake Beetroot ingestion Rifampicin (antituberculosis drug) intake
Pathological Causes	
Colourless Red Brown Black Dark yellow with yellow foam Greenish yellow Milky white	Diabetes mellitus, diabetes insipidus Haematuria, haemoglobinuria, myoglobinuria Haemoglobinuria Alkaptonuria Bilirubin (jaundice) Biliverdin Chyluria

Table 11.10 Commonly Encountered Odours and Their Cause

Odour	Cause
Physiological Causes	
Ammoniacal odour	Old urine sample
Pathological Causes	
Fruity odour	Ketonuria
Ammoniacal odour	Urinary tract infection with *E. coli*
Mousy odour	Phenylketonuria
Fishy odour	Urinary infection with *Proteus*
Foul smell	Urinary infection with other organisms

Table 11.11 Abnormal Specific Gravity and Its Causes

Abnormality	Value	Cause
High specific gravity	Above 1.030	Diabetes mellitus (glucose in urine) Nephrotic syndrome (protein in urine) Fever, dehydration
Low specific gravity	<1.003	Diabetes insipidus
Fixed specific gravity	1.010, which is the specific gravity of the glomerular filtrate	Chronic renal failure (due to loss of concentrating ability of tubules)

CHEMICAL EXAMINATION

Chemical examination of urine is done to detect the presence of proteins, sugar, blood, ketones, bile salts, bile pigments, urobilinogen or nitrite. Let us consider the significance of each one of these components before summarizing the urine parameters in common disease processes.

Proteins

The amount of protein present in normal urine is less than 150 mg/24 h. This is mainly contributed by albumin from plasma and proteins such as Tamm–Horsfall protein and IgA by the renal tubules. Any increase in this amount is pathological and is termed proteinuria. The types of proteinuria and their relevance are as follows:

1. **Microalbuminuria:** Urinary excretion of albumin is approximately 30–300 mg/24 h. The presence of microalbuminuria indicates early renal damage in diabetic and hypertensive patients.
2. **Highly selective proteinuria:** Loss of low-molecular-weight proteins, such as albumin and transferrin, with the sparing of high-molecular-weight proteins that are retained by the kidney, indicates the early stage of glomerular damage.
3. **Nonselective proteinuria:** Loss of low- and high-molecular-weight proteins in urine indicates a significant glomerular damage.
4. **Bence–Jones proteinuria:** Bence–Jones proteins are light chains of monoclonal immunoglobulin produced in plasma cell tumours that overflow from blood into urine due to their high concentration in blood. These proteins have a characteristic response to heating, which makes them unique (and a favourite question to examiners). These precipitate between 40°C and 60°C on heating and dissolve on further heating up to 85–100°C. The methods for estimation of protein are as follows:
   - **Qualitative test**
     1. Heat and acetic acid test
     2. Sulphosalicylic acid test
   - **Semiquantitative test**
     1. Reagent strip test
   - **Quantitative test**
     1. Estimating 24-hour urine protein content
     2. Protein to creatinine ratio estimation

   Common causes of proteinuria
   - Nephrotic syndrome (>3.5 g/24 h)
   - Acute glomerulonephritis
   - Pyelonephritis
   - Heavy metal poisoning
   - TB of kidney
   - Interstitial nephritis
   - Plasma cell dyscrasias
   - Intravascular haemolysis
   - High fever
   - Heavy exercise
   - Congestive cardiac failure

Glucose

Glucose is not usually present in urine in easily detectable levels because it is almost completely reabsorbed by the renal tubules. A small amount of less than 500 mg/24 h is only usually lost in urine. The presence of a significant amount of glucose in urine is called *glycosuria*. This usually happens when the blood glucose level is greater than the renal threshold of 180 mg/dL. Renal threshold is the blood glucose level up to which the kidney can withhold loss of glucose in urine. Glycosuria can be due to blood glucose levels above the renal threshold (hyperglycaemic state) or due to lowering of renal threshold.

Tests for detection of glucose in urine

1. Benedict's copper reduction test
2. Reagent strip test

Causes for glycosuria

1. Diabetes mellitus
2. Other endocrine disorders such as acromegaly, Cushing syndrome
3. Drugs such as adrenocorticotrophic hormone (ACTH), corticosteroids
4. Alimentary glycosuria due to rapid intestinal absorption of glucose
5. Renal glycosuria due to lowering of renal threshold

Ketones

The presence of ketone bodies such as acetone, acetoacetic acid and β-hydroxyl butyric acid in urine is called ketonuria. Ketones are by-products of fatty acid metabolism and are produced in excess when the body is unable to derive the required energy from carbohydrate metabolism. Ketones cross the blood–brain barrier and may affect the brain, causing irritability and confusion. The presence of ketonuria in diabetic patients may be an indicator of a serious complication called *diabetic ketoacidosis* and requires immediate management.

Tests for deduction of ketonuria

- Rothera's test
- Acetest tablet test (Rothera's test in a tablet form)
- Gerhardt's test
- Reagent strip test

Causes of ketonuria

- Diabetic ketoacidosis – occurs because of inability to utilize glucose for energy production
- Starvation, weight-reduction diets – due to reduced consumption of glucose
- Fever, pregnancy, thyrotoxicosis – due to increased energy requirement

Bile Pigments (Bilirubin)

Bilirubin is of two types – unconjugated and conjugated. Bilirubin derived from haemolysis of RBCs is unconjugated. It is insoluble in water and found in blood as a complex with albumin. On the other hand, conjugated bilirubin is soluble in water and can be filtered by the kidney. So the presence of bilirubin in urine implies conjugated hyperbilirubinaemia.

Tests for detection of bilirubin

- Foam test
- Gmelin's test
- Lugol's iodine test
- Fouchet's test
- Reagent strip test

Causes for bilirubin in urine

1. Obstructive jaundice
2. Hepatocellular jaundice

Bile Salts

Bile salts are substances produced by the liver that act as natural detergents and help in the emulsification of fats in the intestine before their enzymatic breakdown. These are reabsorbed from the intestine to go to the liver for enterohepatic circulation. Bile salts include glycine and taurine salts of the four bile acids – cholic, deoxycholic, chenodeoxycholic and lithocholic acids.

Tests to detect bile salts

Hay's test

Causes for bile salts in urine

In obstructive jaundice, the increased pressure within the biliary canaliculi due to the distal obstruction leads to the entry of bile salts into blood, leading to its appearance in urine.

Urobilinogen

The conjugated bilirubin on entering the intestine is converted into urobilinogen by the bacterial flora. Urobilinogen gets reabsorbed in the intestine and undergoes enterohepatic circulation. During its circulation in the blood, small quantities pass into urine in the range of 0.5–4 mg/24 h. It is colourless but on standing in urine, it undergoes oxidation and turns orange–yellow. Disease processes may cause an increase or decrease of urobilinogen in urine.

Tests to detect urobilinogen

- Ehrlich's aldehyde test
- Reagent strip test

Causes for increased urobilinogen in urine

- Haemolytic jaundice
- Internal haemorrhage

Causes for decreased urobilinogen in urine

- Obstructive jaundice
- Reduced bacterial flora in intestine

Blood

The presence of blood in urine refers to the presence of RBCs in urine. This commonly indicates bleeding arising from the urogenital tract. The presence of blood in urine leading to reddish discolouration of urine is called gross haematuria, whereas RBCs detected only on microscopic examination of urine specimen is called microscopic or occult haematuria. Care should be taken to avoid contamination of urine with menstrual blood to avoid a false-positive test. Similarly, the presence of high quantities of ascorbic acid or use of formalin as preservative yields false-negative results in chemical methods.

Tests to detect blood in urine

- Chemical tests – Benzidine test – *ortho*-Toluidine test – Reagent strip test
- Microscopic examination of urinary sediment: This reveals the presence of intact RBCs and helps to identify the minimal blood loss (microscopic haematuria). Sometimes, microscopic haematuria may be an early marker of renal damage.

Causes of haematuria

- Glomerular diseases such as glomerulonephritis, IgA nephropathy and lupus nephritis
- Nonglomerular diseases such as renal calculi, urinary tract infection, TB, pyelonephritis and polycystic renal disease
- Tumours such as renal cell carcinoma, urothelial carcinoma and prostatic carcinoma
- Haematological conditions such as sickle cell disease

Haemoglobin

Free haemoglobin may be detected in urine in cases of intravascular haemolysis and this is called haemoglobinuria. Chemical tests used to detect haemoglobinuria are similar to those for blood. The methods used to differentiate haemoglobinuria from haematuria are as follows:

1. Centrifuging a sample of red-coloured urine yields a clear supernatant with red deposit in haematuria as the RBCs settle down, whereas in haemoglobinuria it yields a pink supernatant as a result of the dissolved free haemoglobin.
2. Microscopic examination shows intact RBCs in haematuria, whereas RBCs are absent or few in haemoglobinuria.

   Causes of haemoglobinuria
   - Infections such as severe *falciparum* malaria
   - Trauma to RBCs such as march haemoglobinuria, prosthetic heart valves
   - Glucose-6-phosphate dehydrogenase deficiency
   - Immune haemolysis such as mismatched blood transfusion, paroxysmal cold haemoglobinuria
   - Paroxysmal nocturnal haemoglobinuria
   - Haemolytic uraemic syndrome
   - Disseminated intravascular coagulation

MICROSCOPIC EXAMINATION OF URINE

The urine may contain many suspended undissolved solid elements that can be studied using a microscope. These are classified into organized substances, which include cells and organisms (Fig. 11.16), and unorganized substances, which are structureless crystalline or amorphous substances (Fig. 11.17). Early morning midstream urine is preferred because acidic pH helps in preserving the cells.

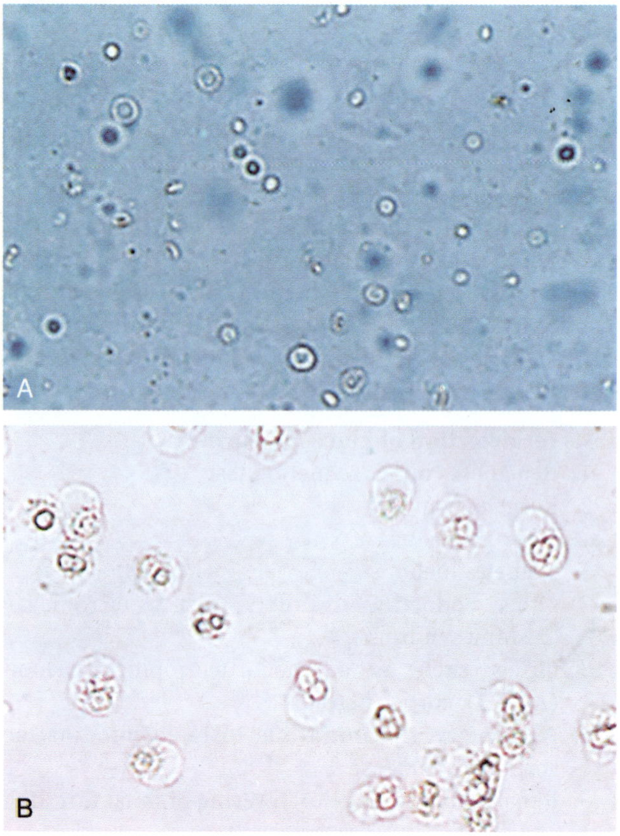

Fig. 11.16 Demonstration of RBCs (A) and neutrophils (B) in urine sediment. (*Source:* From Roger S. Riley, Richard A. McPherson, Henry's Clinical Diagnosis and Management by Laboratory Methods, Elsevier 2017.)

The specimen should be examined within an hour of collection. The urine sample is centrifuged at 1500 rpm for 5 minutes, and the sediment at the bottom is examined under a microscope. The structures that may be seen are given in Table 11.12.

Urine casts (Table 11.13) help us to identify renal damage and also give a clue regarding the cause of renal damage. Casts are formed in the distal renal tubules (Fig. 11.18), thereby taking a cylindrical shape of the lumen of the tubule. The presence of casts thus indicates that the cause is higher up within the renal parenchyma.

URINARY FINDINGS IN VARIOUS DISEASE PROCESSES

1. Diabetes mellitus with ketoacidosis

Physical examination	Volume	Increased (polyuria)
	Appearance	Clear
	Reaction	Acidic
	Colour	Pale yellow
	Odour	Fruity odour (due to ketones)
	Specific gravity	Increased (due to glucose)
Chemical examination	Glucose	Positive (3+ to 4+)
	Ketones	Positive

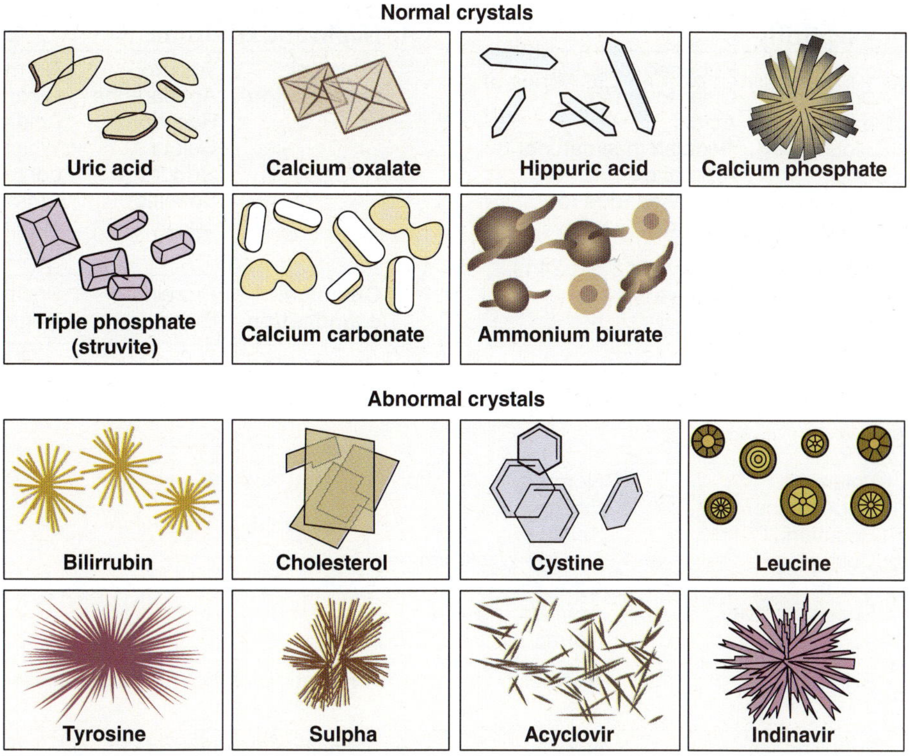

Fig. 11.17 Morphology of urinary crystals.

Table 11.12 Structures Seen in Microscopic Examination of Urine

Category		Structure
Cells		RBCs WBCs Epithelial cells
Organisms		Bacteria *Trichomonas vaginalis* Schistosoma haematobium Yeast Microfilaria
Casts	**Cellular casts**	RBC cast WBC cast Renal epithelial cast
	Noncellular cast	Hyaline cast Granular cast Fatty cast Waxy cast
Crystals	**Physiological**	Amorphous urate Calcium carbonate Uric acid Phosphate Calcium oxalate
	Pathological	Cysteine Cholesterol Bilirubin Tyrosine Leucine Sulphonamide
Others		Sperm

Table 11.13 Causes of Urinary Casts

Cast	Common Cause
RBC cast	Acute glomerulonephritis
WBC cast	Pyelonephritis
Renal epithelial cast	Acute tubular necrosis, acute graft rejection
Hyaline cast	Physiological, many in glomerular proteinuria
Granular cast	Strenuous exercise, fever, acute glomerulonephritis
Fatty cast	Nephrotic syndrome
Waxy cast	End-stage renal failure

2. **Diabetes insipidus**

Physical examination	Volume Appearance Reaction Colour Odour Specific gravity	Increased (polyuria) Clear Alkaline (due to increased output) Pale yellow to colourless Aromatic Reduced (dilute urine)
Chemical examination	Glucose Ketones	Negative Negative

3. **Acute glomerulonephritis**

Physical examination	Volume Appearance Reaction Colour Odour Specific gravity	Reduced (oliguria) Clear to turbid Acidic Reddish (haematuria) Aromatic Increased (due to proteins)
Chemical examination	Proteins Blood	Positive (<3.5 g/24 h) Positive

4. **Nephrotic syndrome**

Physical examination	Volume Appearance Reaction Colour Odour Specific gravity	Normal Clear to turbid Acidic Whitish (due to protein content) Aromatic Very high (due to massive proteinuria)
Chemical examination	Proteins Blood	Positive (>3.5 g/24 h) Negative

5. **Jaundice**

Physical examination	Volume Appearance Reaction Colour Odour Specific gravity	Normal Frothy Acidic Dark yellow (foam also yellow coloured) Aromatic Normal		
Chemical examination	Bilirubin	Haemolytic jaundice	Hepatic jaundice	Obstructive jaundice
	Urobilinogen	Negative (unconjugated hyperbilirubinaemia) Positive	Positive (conjugated hyperbilirubinaemia) Positive	Positive (conjugated hyperbilirubinaemia) Negative (entry of bilirubin into the intestine for bacterial action blocked)

6. **Pyelonephritis/urinary tract infection**

Physical examination	Volume	Normal
	Appearance	Turbid (due to WBCs and bacteria)
	Reaction	Acidic – *Escherichia coli* infection Alkaline – *Proteus, Pseudomonas* infection
	Colour	Pale yellow Foul – severe infection
	Odour	Fishy – *Proteus* infection
	Specific gravity	Normal
Chemical examination	Proteins	Trace positive
	Blood	May be positive
Microscopic examination	RBCs	Few
	WBCs	Numerous
	Bacteria	Present
	Casts	WBC casts seen in pyelonephritis – indicate the renal origin of infection

EXAMINATION OF BODY FLUIDS PA 23.2

PLEURAL FLUID

Pleural space is the space between the visceral and parietal pleural membranes of the lungs. The fluid in this space is usually less than 10 mL and resembles plasma in its composition except that it has a lower protein content (<1.5 g/mL). Accumulation of excess fluid in this space is called pleural effusion.

Collection of pleural fluid: The fluid is collected for diagnostic purpose or sometimes for therapeutic purpose to decompress the pressure it exerts on the lungs. The method of collection is called thoracocentesis. The fluid that is collected is taken in the following containers:

- EDTA tubes for cell counts
- Sterile tube for microbiological studies
- Blood culture bottles for culture
- Clean tubes for cytology (formalin may be added as a fixative if fluid cannot be analysed immediately)

Causes of Pleural Effusion

Pleural effusion may be transudate or exudate. Recall the differences between transudate and exudate studied in Chapter 4. The causes are given in Table 11.14.

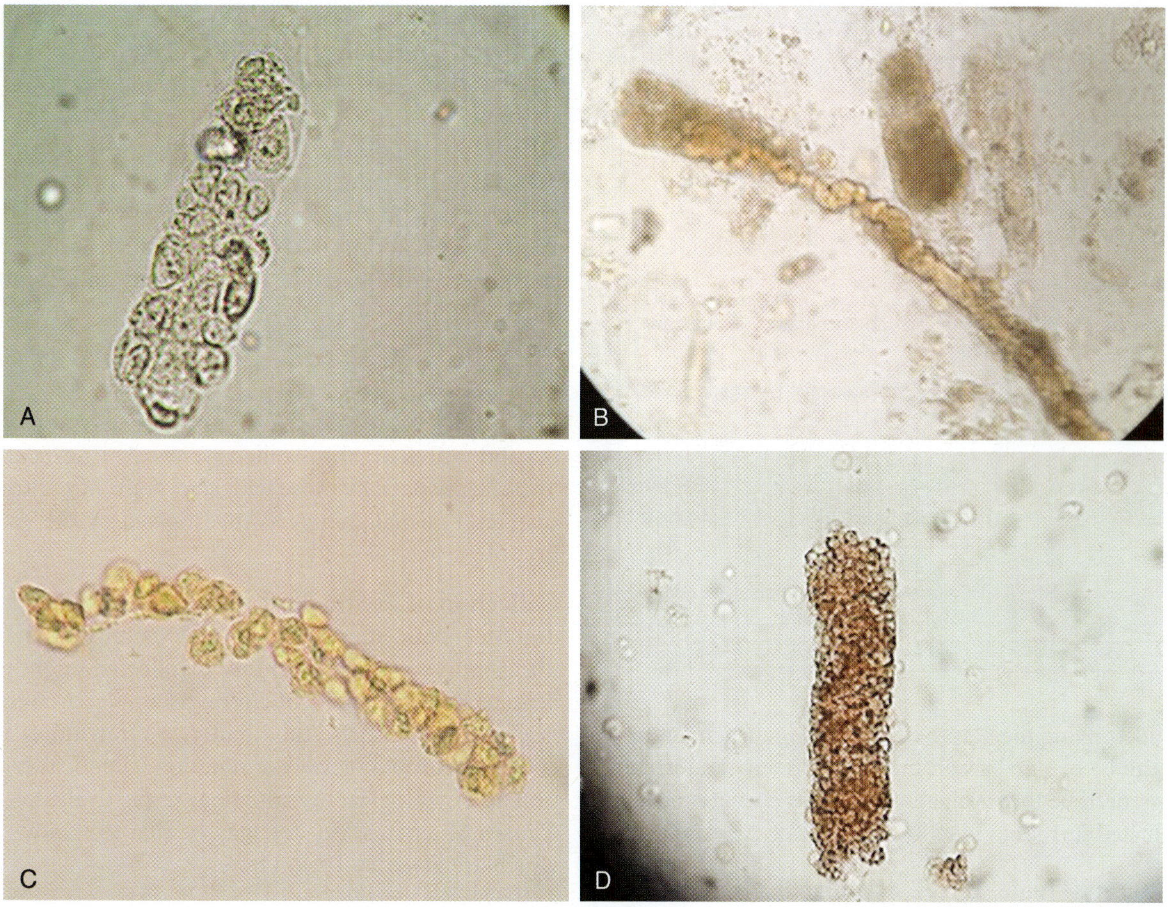

Fig. 11.18 Morphology of urinary casts, renal tubular epithelial cell cast (A), granular cast (B), WBC cast (C) and RBC cast (D). (*Source:* From Mark A. Perazella, American Journal of Kidney Diseases, Elsevier 2015.)

Table 11.14 Causes of Exudate and Transudate

Exudate	Transudate
1. Infections such as tuberculosis, bacterial pneumonia 2. Autoimmune disorders such as rheumatoid arthritis, SLE 3. Pulmonary infarction 4. Chest wall trauma 5. Malignancies – secondaries from bronchogenic carcinoma, breast carcinoma • Mesothelioma • Lymphoma	1. Congestive cardiac failure 2. Liver cirrhosis, failure 3. Hypoproteinaemia due to various causes 4. Pulmonary embolism

SLE, systemic lupus erythematosus.

Examination of Pleural Fluid

- Colour and appearance
- Chemical examination
- Cell counts
- Microbiological examination
- Cytological examination

Colour and Appearance The colour and appearance of pleural fluid give a clue as to the underlying pathology (Box 11.1).

Chemical Examination The first important finding in pleural fluid is categorizing the nature of effusion as exudate or transudate. This is done by Light's criteria. The presence of one or more of the following indicates effusion as exudate:

1. The ratio of pleural fluid protein to serum protein is greater than 0.5.
2. The ratio of pleural fluid lactate dehydrogenase (LDH) to serum LDH is greater than 0.6.
3. The pleural fluid LDH level is greater than two-thirds of the upper limit of normal for serum LDH.

Box 11.1 Classification of Fluid Based on Appearance

Clear, pale yellow, does not clot on standing	Transudate
Turbid (due to proteins and cells), clots on standing	Exudate
Haemorrhagic fluid	Traumatic tap, malignancy, pulmonary infarction
Milky effusion	True chylous effusion – lymphatic block • TGL – 110 mg/dL • Fat droplets present that stain with Sudan black • Chylomicrons present Pseudochylous effusion – long-standing effusion as in TB • TGL – 50 mg/dL • Microscopy shows cholesterol crystals • Chylomicrons absent

On identifying the nature of effusion, management protocols can be planned accordingly. Transudate fluid usually does not need further evaluation, whereas exudates need to be evaluated further to identify the cause of the exudate.

Cell Counts (Table 11.15) RBCs and WBCs can be counted in effusion fluids. Transudates may contain normal small lymphocytes, but these are less than 1000/mL. Exudates may contain neutrophils, indicating an acute infectious pathology, or lymphocytes, indicating chronic infectious pathology.

Microbiological Examination
- Gram staining and culture for bacteria
- Ziehl–Neelsen stain, culture and if required polymerase chain reaction (PCR) for TB

Table 11.15 Cell Counts and Interpretation in Pleural Fluid

WBC count >50,000/mL with neutrophilic predominance	Parapneumonic effusion
Plenty of small mature lymphocytes	Tuberculosis
Plenty of RBCs >100,000/mL	Haemorrhagic effusion as in malignancy, pulmonary infarction
Presence of RBCs but no haemosiderin-laden macrophages	Traumatic aspiration (a gradual reduction in red colour while drawing pleural fluid is an important finding)
Atypical WBCs	Leukaemia/lymphoma – refer to cytology

Cytological Examination The fluid is centrifuged and the fluid containing cells at the bottom is smeared, stained commonly with Papanicolaou stain or other stains such as H&E or MGG and examined under the microscope. If cellularity is good, the cell button at the bottom of the centrifuge can be fixed in formalin and processed as that for the tissue. This is called cell block and may give additional information such as architecture and also may be used for special stains and immunocytochemistry.

PERITONEAL FLUID

Fluid collected within the peritoneal cavity surrounding the abdominal organs is called ascites. Any new collection of ascites, especially those with symptoms of peritonitis or suspicion of malignancy, is investigated by the examination of peritoneal fluid.

Collection of ascitic fluid: The fluid is aspirated by abdominal paracentesis usually after confirmation by the ultrasound scan. The fluid that is collected might need to be heparinized to prevent clotting. Samples are sent in an EDTA tube, a sterile tube and two clean tubes for cell counts, microbiological examination, chemical examination and cytological examination, respectively.

Causes of ascites: Ascites may be due to various causes which are given in Table 11.16.

Examination of Ascitic Fluid

- Colour and appearance
- Chemical examination
- Microbiological examination
- Cytology

Colour and Appearance

Normal peritoneal fluid is pale yellow in colour. The other commonly seen appearances are chylous ascites and haemorrhagic ascites. Abdominal malignancy is an important cause of chylous ascites in adults, whereas it is considered to be congenital lymphatic abnormalities in children.

The presence of chylomicrons and high triglyceride concentration helps to differentiate chylous from pseudochylous collections, which may occur because of infections and perforation.

Haemorrhagic ascites is a common feature of malignant effusions but may also be seen in perforation.

Chemical Examination

- **Serum ascites to albumin gradient (SAAG):** It is the difference between the albumin content of serum and the albumin content of ascitic fluid. SAAG is low (<1.1 g/dL) in ascites because of infection or malignancy, whereas it is high (≥1.1 g/dL) in portal hypertension-related ascites. It is a good parameter to differentiate transudate and exudate.

Table 11.16 Causes of Ascites

Type of Ascites	Primary Disease
Hepatic	Cirrhosis
	Budd–Chiari syndrome
	Portal vein occlusion
	Inferior vena cava obstruction
	Hepatic cancer
Cardiogenic	Congestive cardiac failure
	Constrictive pericarditis
Nephrogenic	Nephrotic syndrome
Malignant	Secondaries from the abdominal, pelvic and thoracic organs, most common being gastrointestinal and ovarian origin
	Primary peritoneal cancer
Infectious ascites	Tuberculous peritonitis
	Spontaneous bacterial peritonitis
	Fungal infection
Miscellaneous causes	Chylous ascites
	Pancreatic ascites
	Ovarian disease (Meigs syndrome, struma ovarii, ovarian hyperstimulation)
	Systemic lupus erythematosus

- **Lactate dehydrogenase:** Effusions due to malignant causes have high LDH values, whereas effusions caused by portal hypertension have lower values. So a scale similar to Light's criteria for differentiating transudate from exudate involving three values is under evaluation. The presence of any two of the three, **LDH of 400 SU, fluid/serum LDH ratio of 0.6 and fluid to serum total protein (TP) ratio of 0.5**, indicates a nonhepatic cause, whereas the absence of all three favours a hepatic cause.
- **Glucose and adenosine deaminase:** Ascitic fluid glucose levels are low in TB and bacterial infections due to the consumption of glucose by bacteria. Though this phenomenon is helpful in the diagnosis of TB, it is not used because of low sensitivity and specificity. But adenosine deaminase levels are more sensitive and specific and are more useful in the diagnosis of TB. A higher value of 36–40 IU/L is seen in TB. A value less than that indicates nontubercular effusion.
- **Amylase:** Ascitic fluid amylase levels are significantly elevated in pancreatic conditions such as inflammation, duct damage and trauma. But it is also seen in other conditions such as malignancy (elevated amylase levels have been detected in pancreatic, ovarian and few other malignancies) and perforation and hence cannot be considered as a specific marker of pancreatic disease.

Microbiological Examination

- Gram stain and culture for bacteria
- Ziehl–Neelsen stain, culture and if required PCR for TB
- Fungal staining

Cytology

The peritoneal fluid is processed just as pleural fluid for smearing and cell block preparation. Larger volumes yield better results. Cell blocks can also be used for immunohistochemistry for the identification of primary disease when it could not be identified by clinical and radiological examinations.

CEREBROSPINAL FLUID PA 35.3

CSF is an ultrafiltrate of plasma, produced by the choroid plexus of the ventricles of the brain, and is usually approximately 100–160 mL. It moves within the ventricles, spinal canal and subarachnoid space, providing nutrients to the brain, removing the waste and acting as a shock absorber to the brain. This fluid is collected from the subarachnoid space to help in diagnosing various conditions of the brain and in treating few diseases.

Method of Collection

CSF is collected from the subarachnoid space by inserting a lumbar puncture needle in the intervertebral space either between L3 and L4 or between L4 and L5. This site is selected to avoid injury to the spinal cord, which ends at the level of T12. This procedure is called lumbar puncture. The technique is similar to the one used by an anaesthetist to administer spinal block. Once the needle is in place, the opening pressure of CSF is measured, which is then followed by collection of CSF in four tubes in the following order:

Tube 1: Chemistry and serology – should be done within 1 hour
Tube 2: Microbiology
Tube 3: Haematology – cell counts should be done within 30–60 minutes
Tube 4: Cytology and special studies

Indications for Lumbar Puncture

- **Diagnostic**
  - Examination of CSF for diagnosis of the following:
    - CNS infections (meningitis, encephalitis)
    - Subarachnoid haemorrhage
    - Inflammatory diseases (multiple sclerosis, Guillain–Barré syndrome)
    - CNS neoplasms
    - Malignancy involving meninges
  - Introduction of radiographic contrast media for myelography
  - For Queckenstedt's test to help diagnose subarachnoid block or a tumour or a sinus thrombosis

- **Therapeutic**
  - In benign intracranial hypertension to reduce CSF pressure
  - Administration of medications such as anaesthetic and antibiotics

Cerebrospinal Fluid Analysis

Concentration of constituents of CSF depends on their plasma levels and hence should be studied along with plasma values.

1. **Opening pressure** (Table 11.17)
   A manometer is attached to the hub of the needle to record the opening pressure. The patient's neck should be brought to neutral and legs extended. A false increase may be noted on straining, holding breath or if tensed. False low values may be obtained if the patient hyperventilates (Table 11.18).
2. **Gross appearance**
   CSF is normally clear and colourless. It does not clot spontaneously because of low protein content. The abnormal colours of CSF and their causes are given in Table 11.19.
3. **Cell counts**
   a. **Total WBC count:** It is performed manually in all samples of undiluted CSF. The increase in CSF leucocyte count is called pleocytosis. If turbid, it is diluted with Turk's fluid; else, the undiluted fluid is charged into the Fuchs–Rosenthal counting chamber and five large squares are counted, which gives the total count per cubic millimetre of CSF. Common causes of increased leucocyte count in CSF include meningitis, encephalitis, intracranial haemorrhage and meningeal tumours.

Table 11.17 Normal CSF Pressure

Age	Normal Value
<8 years	10–100 mm of water
>8 years to adulthood	60–180 mm of water

Table 11.18 Causes of CSF Pressure Changes

Causes of Decreased Pressure	Causes of Increased Pressure
• Trauma or lumbar puncture–related CSF leak • Complete spinal block by tumour, abscess that may obstruct the spinal subarachnoid space	• Intracranial mass lesion such as neoplasm, abscess, etc. • Intracranial/subarachnoid haemorrhage • Meningitis • Cerebral oedema • Benign intracranial hypertension

Table 11.19 Abnormalities in CSF Colour

Appearance	Common Causes
Turbid	Increased RBCs (>400/mm^3) Increased WBCs (>200/mm^3) Increased protein Presence of microorganisms
Haemorrhagic	Traumatic tap (blood decreases in successive tubes, blood clots on standing, CSF pressure and protein normal) Subarachnoid haemorrhage (blood constant in all tubes, blood does not clot on standing, CSF pressure and protein increased)
Xanthochromasia (yellow)	• Old subarachnoid haemorrhagic (>12 h) • Jaundice (serum bilirubin >6.0 mg/dL)
Brown colour	Metastatic melanoma
Orange colour	Excess ingestion of carotene
Clot formation	Increased protein content • Tuberculous meningitis (cobweb) • Pyogenic meningitis
Thick viscous CSF	Cryptococcal meningitis Secondary meningeal deposit of mucinous adenocarcinoma Severe meningitis

   b. **Differential count:** A smear prepared from CSF, after centrifuging if the total count is low, is stained with Romanowsky stain and viewed under the microscope. Normally, the CSF contains 70% lymphocytes and 30% monocytes in adults.
   c. **Other cells:** Immature WBCs may be seen in acute lymphocytic leukaemia (ALL) and atypical neoplastic cells may be seen in malignancy.
4. **Chemical examination**
   a. **Proteins:** Increased protein levels in CSF are an early marker of CNS disease but have low specificity. Normal CSF protein level in adults is 15–45 mg/dL. The following are the causes of increased protein content in CSF:
   - Meningitis due to an increase in permeability of blood–brain barrier
   - Spinal cord tumour that obstructs CSF circulation, leading to stasis
   - Multiple sclerosis and subacute sclerosing panencephalitis due to local IgG production
   - Guillain–Barré syndrome due to increased permeability of blood–brain barrier and local IgG production
   - Subarachnoid haemorrhage

   The proteins in the CSF may be albumin or immunoglobulin IgG. Albumin is not synthesized in the CNS, so it is purely derived from plasma by crossing the blood–brain barrier. On the contrary, IgG is synthesized in the CNS and its increased levels may be due to increased blood–brain barrier permeability or de novo synthesis. Hence, the analysis of their ratio helps to identify the pathology.

b. **Glucose:** CSF glucose is derived from plasma and is usually two-thirds of the plasma value. It should be tested immediately, as glucose may be lost on standing because of glycolysis. Its normal value is 45–80 mg/dL. Reduction of CSF glucose to less than 40 mg/dL is seen in the following conditions:
   - Acute bacterial meningitis
   - Tuberculous meningitis
   - Fungal meningitis
   - Tumour involvement of meninges
   - Hypoglycaemia

5. **Microbiological examination**
   Various techniques and stains are used to identify the presence of microorganisms in CSF. These are outlined in Table 11.20.

Table 11.20 Procedure Adopted to Identify Various Microorganisms

Procedure	Suspected Organism
Direct wet mount	Cryptococcosis Amoebic meningoencephalitis *Candida* infection Trypanosomiasis
Gram stain	Increased neutrophils, indicating bacterial infection
Ziehl–Neelsen stain	Tuberculous meningitis
Serological tests	Syphilis
Culture	Bacteria *Mycobacterium tuberculosis*
PCR	*Mycobacterium tuberculosis* Viruses

6. **Cytology**
   Like any other body fluid, CSF is processed in cytocentrifuge, smeared and stained with Papanicolaou stain for microscopic examination. This is mainly done for identifying malignant cells (Table 11.21).

ORGAN FUNCTION TESTS — PA 23.3

RENAL FUNCTION TEST

The investigations done in an individual to assess the function of the kidney are called renal function tests. These may include blood investigations and urine investigations. These investigations may be broadly classified into tests that assess glomerular function and those that assess tubular function (Table 11.22). These may be complimented by imaging and biopsy which help to assess the morphological changes in the kidney.

The indications for renal function tests include:

- To screen for impairment of renal function
- To diagnose renal impairment
- To follow up patients with renal disease
- To plan dialysis/renal transplant
- To adjust dosage of drugs eliminated by renal route

In this chapter, the blood biochemistry parameters used to assess renal function are discussed along with a brief note about the clearance assays.

Clearance Tests

Glomerular filtration rate (GFR) is the rate in millilitres per minute at which a substance is cleared by the glomeruli from the circulation. Normal GFR in young adults is 120–130 mL/min per 1.73 m^2 of body surface area and it declines at the rate of 1 mL/min per year after the age of 40 years. Chronic renal disease is classified into five stages based on the GFR (Table 11.23), which implies the importance of measuring GFR but still these investigations are cumbersome and not easily available.

Inulin clearance: This is the gold standard test for measuring GFR because inulin is an inert exogenous substance

Table 11.21 CSF Findings in Various Diseases

Condition	Appearance	Leucocytes	Proteins (mg/dL)	Glucose (mg/dL)	Additional Investigations
1. Normal	Clear, colourless	<5/μL (mostly lymphocytes)	15–45	45–80	–
2. Acute pyogenic meningitis	Turbid or purulent	Increased (>1000/μL); mostly neutrophils	Increased; 50–1500	Decreased; <40	Gram stain; culture; latex agglutination test
3. Tuberculous meningitis	Clear or cloudy	Increased (100–600/μL); mostly lymphocytes or both lymphocytes and neutrophils	Increased; 45–300	Decreased; 10–45	AFB stain; culture; polymerase chain reaction
4. Viral meningitis	Clear or cloudy	Increased (6–300/μL); lymphocytes	Increased	Normal	Polymerase chain reaction

Table 11.22 Investigations to Assess Renal Function

To Assess Glomerular Function	To Assess Tubular Function
1. Clearance tests (creatinine, inulin clearance) to assess glomerular filtration rate 2. Blood parameters: Serum creatinine, blood urea nitrogen (BUN) and BUN/serum creatinine ratio 3. Albuminuria and microalbuminuria	1. Tests to assess proximal tubular function: • Glycosuria, phosphaturia, uricosuria and generalized aminoaciduria • Tubular proteinuria • Fractional sodium excretion 2. Tests to assess distal tubular function: • Specific gravity and osmolality of urine • Water-deprivation test and water-loading test • Ammonium chloride loading test

Table 11.23 Stages of Chronic Renal Disease

Stage	Description	GFR (mL/min/1.73 m²)
1	Kidney damage with normal or ↑ GFR	≥90
2	Kidney damage with mild ↓ GFR	60–89
3	Moderate ↓ GFR	30–59
4	Severe ↓ GFR	15–29
5	Kidney failure	<15 (or dialysis)

that when administered is secreted by the glomeruli and is unaffected by tubular factors. But the test is expensive and difficult to perform and hence used only for research purposes.

Creatinine clearance: This is the most commonly used test to assess GFR. Creatinine is produced constantly by our body by breakdown of muscle creatinine. It is filtered by the glomeruli but is not a perfect test because a small amount is secreted by the tubules, which makes the test to overestimate the GFR by 10%. The value is calculated by using the urine creatinine levels, volume of urine excreted in 24 hours and blood creatinine levels. The values can be altered by intake of meat and certain drugs such as cimetidine and trimethoprim.

In conclusion, the clearance tests are difficult to perform and are indicated in patients in whom renal impairment is suspected in spite of normal blood parameters. If blood parameters are abnormal, then there is no need to perform clearance assays.

Blood Biochemistry

The clinically used blood parameters of renal function are blood urea nitrogen (BUN) and serum creatinine levels. These are insensitive markers but used for the sake of convenience.

- **BUN:** Urea is one of the body wastes that is produced by the liver and excreted by the kidney. Amino acids break down into ammonia and liver converts the ammonia into urea. The blood levels of urea are expressed in terms of nitrogen because it is the measurable component. Each molecule of urea of molecular weight 60 g contains 28 g of nitrogen. The blood urea values can hence be derived by multiplying BUN with 60/28.
  Blood urea = BUN × 60/28 = BUN × 2.14
  BUN value is not an accurate predictor of glomerular function because urea is reabsorbed by the tubules and various factors such as diet and liver function may affect the values. Furthermore, BUN levels rise only after much destruction of renal parenchyma. Increase in BUN levels beyond normal is called azotaemia, and the causes of azotaemia include:
  - Pre-renal azotaemia – shock, cardiac failure, water and salt deprivation
  - Renal azotaemia – renal failure
  - Postrenal azotaemia – urinary tract obstruction
  - Increased rate of production of urea – high-protein diet, increased protein catabolism (trauma, burns, fever)

  The tests performed to assess BUN levels include diacetyl monoxime urea method and urease–Berthelot reaction, the details of which are beyond the scope of the book.
  The normal values for BUN in adults are 7–18 mg/dL and 8–21 mg/dL in those older than 60 years.
- **Serum creatinine levels:**
  Creatinine is also a waste that is produced in muscle from creatinine phosphate. Its production depends on muscle mass, age and sex, and hence the values need correlation with these factors. It is a better indicator of renal function than BUN because it is produced at a constant rate by the muscles. It is not affected by exogenous factors and is not altered much by the tubular function. But still the sensitivity is low for serum creatinine because it is not elevated in minor renal impairment.
  The causes for increased creatinine include:
  - Pre-renal, renal and postrenal azotaemia
  - Active acromegaly and gigantism

  The causes for decreased levels include:
  - Pregnancy
  - Reduction in muscle mass, such as in old age

  Methods to measure serum creatinine levels:
  - Alkaline picrate method (Jaff's reaction)
  - Enzymatic method

  The normal value of serum creatinine in adults: Males, 0.7–1.3 mg/dL; females, 0.6–1.1 mg/dL.
- **BUN/serum creatinine ratio:**
  BUN/creatinine ratio is calculated to discriminate pre-renal and postrenal azotaemia from renal azotaemia.

Table 11.24 Causes of Variation in BUN/Creatinine Ratio

Increased BUN/ Creatinine Ratio (>20:1)	Decreased BUN/ Creatinine Ratio (<10:1)
1. Increased BUN with normal serum creatinine: Pre-renal azotaemia (reduced renal perfusion) High-protein diet Increased protein catabolism Gastrointestinal haemorrhage 2. Increase of both BUN and serum creatinine (disproportionately higher BUN): Postrenal azotaemia (obstruction to the outflow of urine)	1. Acute tubular necrosis 2. Low-protein diet 3. Starvation 4. Severe liver disease

Normal ratio is 12:1 to 20:1. The causes of increased and decreased ratios are given in Table 11.24.

Sample scenarios for interpretation of blood biochemistry in renal impairment are given as follows.

Interpretation of Abnormal Renal Function Test

Most often the investigations performed to assess renal function include blood test for serum creatinine, BUN, BUN/serum creatinine ratio and serum electrolytes along with urine routine investigation. The kidneys play a major role in maintenance of electrolyte levels in the serum and hence help to identify disturbance in renal function. The electrolytes measured are sodium, potassium, chloride and bicarbonate. The normal values of the renal function tests are given in Table 11.25.

Table 11.25 Normal Values of Renal Function Tests

Parameter	Reference Range
Blood urea	15–40 mg/dL
Serum creatinine	0.6–1.2 mg/dL
Serum uric acid	M: 4–7 mg/dL; F: 3–6 mg/dL
Sodium	135–145 mmol/L
Potassium	3.5–5.0 mmol/L
Chloride	96–106 mmol/L
Bicarbonate	23–27 mmol/L
Arterial blood pH	7.35–7.45
Arterial pCO_2	35–45 mm Hg
Arterial pO_2	80–100 mm Hg

Laboratory Values in Acute Renal Failure

Laboratory Test	Values if Pre-renal Cause of Acute Renal Failure	Values if Intrarenal Cause of Acute Renal Failure
BUN/creatinine ratio	>20:1	10:1 to 20:1
Urine specific gravity	>1.020	1.010–1.020
Urine osmolality (mOsm/kg)	>500	300–500
Urine sodium concentration; mEq/L (mmol/L)	<10 (10)	>20 (20)
Urine sediment	Hyaline casts	Granular casts

Laboratory Values in Chronic Kidney Disease (CKD)

Parameter	Change Noted in CKD
BUN	Increased
Creatinine	Increased
BUN/creatinine ratio	Increased
Potassium	Increased
Sodium	Decreased
Bicarbonate	Decreased

LIVER FUNCTION TESTS PA 25.6

Liver function tests are tests performed to identify liver disease, its severity and type. They are performed as a set of investigations that need to be assessed along with the clinical picture to identify the type of liver disease. An isolated abnormality of one parameter usually indicates an aetiology outside the liver such as haemolytic anaemia reflecting as raised bilirubin and malabsorption reflecting as low albumin. The liver function tests are classified on the basis of the function of the liver they assess and are given in the following table:

Function	Test
Excretory function	Serum bilirubin Urine bilirubin Urine urobilinogen Faecal urobilinogen
Synthetic and metabolic function	Serum proteins Serum albumin Serum albumin/globulin (A/G) ratio Prothrombin time (PT) Blood ammonia level
Liver injury	Serum alanine aminotransferase (ALT) Serum aspartate aminotransferase (AST) Serum alkaline phosphatase Serum γ-glutamyl transferase (GGT) 5′-Nucleotidase (5′-NT)
Clearance of exogenous substance	Bromosulphthalein excretion test

The indications of liver function tests:

- To screen for liver disease
- To identify the type of liver disease (hepatocellular, cholestatic or infiltrative)
- To assess the severity of liver disease
- To follow the course of liver disease and response to treatment

To understand the interpretation of these tests, it would be ideal to revise the bilirubin metabolism and pathophysiology of jaundice in Chapter 22: Liver and Gallbladder. The interpretation of liver enzyme is elucidated clearly in that chapter and urine investigations are dealt with in the urine analysis part of this chapter. Hence, now we will proceed to the blood investigation that assesses the functions of the liver.

Markers of Hepatocellular Injury

Alanine aminotransferase (ALT), found predominantly in the liver, is a relatively more specific marker of liver injury. Aspartate aminotransferase (AST) is present in several other tissues including the heart, skeletal muscle, intestines and kidney and is thus elevated in myocardial infarction besides liver injury. Zone 3 hepatocytes have a higher concentration of AST, and ALT is more notable in zone 1 (periportal) hepatocytes. Thus, acute viral hepatitis or autoimmune hepatitis that predominantly involves zone 1 hepatocytes results in ALT elevation, whereas zone 3 hepatocytes which are more vulnerable to ischaemic and toxic insults are more likely to cause AST elevation.

The AST/ALT ratio is another important parameter in assessing liver disease. An AST/ALT ratio of 2:1, in which the AST levels are twice more than that of ALT, is highly predictive of alcoholic liver disease (ALD). In conditions such as nonalcoholic fatty liver disease (NAFLD), ALT levels are significantly higher than those of AST and lower the AST/ALT ratio to less than 1.

Markers of Cholestasis

The majority of serum alkaline phosphatase (ALP) is contributed by the liver and bone and in minor quantities by the intestine and placenta. Though an important biomarker of hepatic disease, an increase in ALP levels warrants an exclusion of a bone disease. In the LFT panel, ALP is often complemented by γ-glutamyl transferase (GGT). Raised GGT levels corroborate an increased ALP level to be of liver origin rather than being extrahepatic. Thus, a concurrent elevation of GGT and ALP levels is highly suggestive of biliary tract obstruction (results in cholestasis – stagnation of bile) and primary biliary diseases. Physiological isolated ALP elevations may be seen in pregnancy, children (during rapid bone growth) and elderly individuals.

Markers of Synthetic And Metabolic Functions

Serum Bilirubin You may recall raised serum bilirubin levels present in patients with jaundice. The total normal bilirubin level in blood is less than 1 mg/Dl, of which 10% constitutes conjugated bilirubin and remaining 90% is unconjugated bilirubin. The main source of unconjugated bilirubin is from destruction of RBCs. It is tightly bound to albumin and water insoluble and hence not excreted in urine. On the other hand, bilirubin after conjugation in the liver gets converted into bilirubin glucuronide, bilirubin diglucuronide, that is weakly bound to albumin and water soluble, and hence is excreted by the kidney into urine.

The two methods used for estimation of serum bilirubin:

1. Diazo method: This method is used to estimate total bilirubin and conjugated bilirubin. The unconjugated component is obtained by subtracting the latter from the former. Because conjugated bilirubin is estimated directly by this test, it is also called direct bilirubin, whereas unconjugated bilirubin which is a calculated value is named as indirect bilirubin. The role of bilirubin in identifying the type of jaundice is given in the following table:

Type of Jaundice	Bilirubin Levels
Prehepatic/haemolytic jaundice	Direct bilirubin is <15% of the total
Intrahepatic/hepatocellular jaundice	Direct bilirubin is 20%–50% of the total
Posthepatic/obstructive jaundice	Direct bilirubin is >50% of the total

2. Direct spectroscopic method: This method is based on the colour of the plasma which correlates to the absorption of light passed through it by the spectrophotometer at 454 nm. This method can be used only in newborns and infants who do not have any other pigment in their plasma.

Serum Proteins Liver is the major source of serum proteins such as albumin and globulin. A small fraction of the gamma globulins or immunoglobulins are produced by plasma cells. Hence, measuring the protein levels in blood helps to assess the synthetic function of the liver.

1. Total proteins:
   The normal total protein level in adults is 5.5−8.0 g/dL. It can be measured either by using the refractometer method which measures the refractive index of plasma or the biuret method. The major component of the proteins in adults is albumin. But in conditions such as cirrhosis, the reduction in albumin synthesis is compensated by increase in globulin synthesis, thereby giving a normal value for total proteins. Hence, this test should be interpreted along with serum albumin and serum protein electrophoresis results.
2. Serum albumin:
   Albumin is the major protein of human body and is produced solely by the liver. Its estimation is a good indicator of liver function, making this test sensitive but other factors such as malabsorption and

proteinuria may cause decrease in its levels, making the test less specific. Another important point to note is that albumin has a long half-life of approximately 20 days; hence, its values are not altered in acute liver illness. But it is a good indicator of severity and progression of disease in chronic liver impairments. Serum albumin is measured by spectrophotometry by using bromocresol green method. The causes of reduced albumin (hypoalbuminemia) level are given in the following table:

Causes of Hypoalbuminemia

Causes	Conditions
Decreased intake	Malnutrition
Decreased absorption	Malabsorption syndromes
Decreased synthesis	Liver disease, chronic infections
Increased catabolism	Thyrotoxicosis, fever, malignancy, infections
Increased loss	Nephrotic syndrome, severe burns, protein-losing enteropathies, ascites
Increased blood volume	Pregnancy, congestive cardiac failure

3. Serum albumin/globulin ratio:
   Liver conditions associated with inflammation show an increase in gammaglobulin levels along with the decrease in albumin levels. In such cases, there is a reversal of the normal >1.5 ratio. This includes cirrhosis and chronic active hepatitis.

Prothrombin Time Prothrombin time is a coagulation assay that helps to identify deficiency of factors I, II, V, VII and X. It is the time taken by plasma to clot by the extrinsic pathway and is normally 11−13.5 seconds. These factors are produced by the liver and hence in liver disease, deficiency of these factors prolongs the PT. Apart from liver disease, vitamin K deficiency also affects PT because vitamin K is necessary for synthesis of factors II, VII, IX and X. The causes for increased PT hence include the following:

- Obstructive jaundice in which absence of bile in the intestines causes vitamin K deficiency. This can be corrected by administration of vitamin K.
- Hepatocellular jaundice in which liver cells are unable to synthesize clotting factors. PT does not get corrected with vitamin K supplementation in these patients.

Blood Ammonia Ammonia is produced in the intestine by the action of bacteria on the food-containing nitrogen. It is then carried to the liver by the portal circulation for detoxification into urea and urea is eliminated from the body by the kidney. Any factor that affects this cycle causes elevation of ammonia levels and hepatic encephalopathy. The factors that cause raised ammonia levels are given in the following table and the commonest among them is the failure of liver to convert ammonia into urea.

Causes of Raised Ammonia in Blood

- Fulminant hepatic failure
- Cirrhosis
- Reye syndrome
- Entry of portal blood into systemic circulation bypassing the liver
- Gastrointestinal haemorrhage which leads to increased ammonia production in the intestine
- Inherited deficiencies of urea cycle enzymes

No single test can indicate any specific disease. Thus, LFTs routinely are ordered as a panel. Also, it is important to remember that healthy individuals can have abnormal results. A simple and practical approach to abnormal liver function tests is shown in Flowchart 11.1

Interpretation of Liver Function Test in Jaundice

The liver function tests should be analysed along with clinical symptoms and urine investigations to get a better understanding. Imaging also gives a better understanding of the aetiology of jaundice. The normal reference ranges for liver function test are given in the following table:

Normal Ranges for Liver Function Test

Parameter	Range
Total serum bilirubin	0.3−1.0 mg/dL
Direct (conjugated) bilirubin	0−0.2 mg/dL
Serum protein total	5.5−8.0 g/dL
Serum albumin	3.5−5.0 g/dL
Serum globulins	1.8−3.5 g/dL
Albumin/globulin (A/G) ratio	>1.5
Prothrombin time	11−15 s
Plasma ammonia	9−33 μmol/L
Serum alanine aminotransferase (ALT, SGPT)	5−42 U/L
Serum aspartate aminotransferase (AST, SGOT)	5−40 U/L
Serum alkaline phosphatase (ALP)	• Children: 25−350 U/L • Adult males: 25−120 U/L • Adult females: 25−90 U/L
AST/ALT ratio	0.7−1.4

Jaundice, the common presentation of many liver disorders, is diagnosed by raised serum bilirubin levels. The type of bilirubin in blood and the level of liver enzymes complemented by urinary findings help in differentiating the type of jaundice and identifying the cause. It also helps

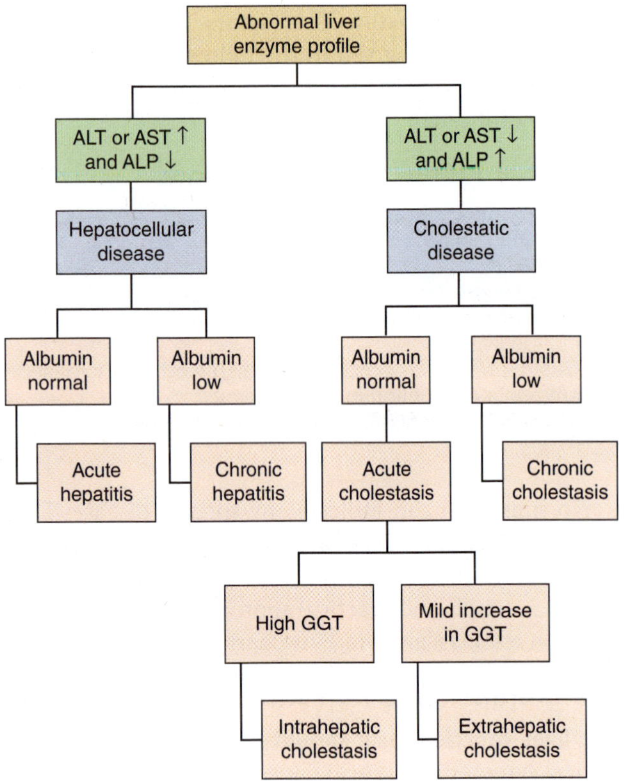

Flowchart 11.1 A simple pragmatic approach to abnormal liver function tests.

in follow up of patients and assessing response to treatment. The blood and urine findings of haemolytic, hepatic and obstructive jaundice are given in the following table:

The pattern of increase in liver enzymes helps in guiding the investigation and management of patients with hepatic injury. The common causes of raised liver enzyme levels and the specific investigations for confirming the diagnosis are given in the following table:

Causes of Raised Liver Enzymes

Cause	Diagnostic Factor
Viral hepatitis A	IgM antihepatitis A antibodies
Viral hepatitis B	IgM antihepatitis B core antigen antibodies, hepatitis B surface antigen
Viral hepatitis C	Hepatitis C-RNA, antihepatitis C antibodies
Viral hepatitis E	Anti-HEV
Nonalcoholic steatohepatitis	Liver biopsy
Alcoholic liver disease	AST/ALT ratio > 2.0, raised GGT

THYROID FUNCTION TEST

Thyroid gland is an endocrine gland that is under the control of the pituitary gland by a feedback mechanism. The hypothalamus produces thyrotrophin-releasing hormone (TRH) that potentiates the pituitary hormone production. Thyroid-stimulating hormone (TSH) thus secreted by the anterior pituitary gland stimulates thyroid hormone (T3 and T4) production, which in turn can lower TSH production forming a negative feedback mechanism. This T3 and T4 production requires iodine which is a mineral in the diet and its deficiency can lead to hypothyroidism.

Indications for thyroid function test:

- To confirm euthyroid state
- To screen for thyroid function in newborns (especially TSH)
- To diagnose clinical and subclinical hypo- and hyperthyroidism
- To follow up T3 and T4 replacement therapy

Thyroid Hormones

The thyroid gland secretes T4 and small quantities of T3 into the circulation creating a higher level of T4 in circulation. But a part of the T4 that is secreted is converted peripherally to T3 by removal of an iodothyronine unit. These hormones are in circulation in free and bound form, in which they are bound to carrier proteins such as thyroxine-binding globulin (TBG), thyroxine-binding pre-albumin and albumin. The free form, though less, is

Urine and Blood Parameters in Types of Jaundice

	Urine			Blood		
	Urobilinogen	**Bilirubin**	**Unconjugated Bilirubin**	**Conjugated Bilirubin**	**ALT and AST**	**GGT and ALP**
Normal	Trace	Nil	N: 0.2–1 mg/dL	N: 0–0.2 mg/dL	Normal	Normal
Haemolytic jaundice	**Increased**	Nil	**Increased**	N: 0–0.2 mg/dL	Normal	Normal
Obstructive jaundice	**Decreased or absent**	**Present**	N: 0–0.2 mg/dL	**Increased**	Normal or mild increase	**Marked Increase**
Hepatocellular jaundice	**Decreased or absent**	**Present**	**Increased**	**Increased**	**Marked Increased**	Normal or mild increase

the biologically active form. The bound form of thyroid hormones also shows variation when there is an alteration in the TBG levels. Factors that increase TBG level increase total T3 and T4 levels by increasing the bound fraction and similarly factors that decrease TBG levels may reduce total T3 and T4 levels. In both these conditions, the levels of free T3 and T4 which are actually the required functional component are not affected. Hence, measurement of free values gives a better clue of the patient's condition.

The important investigations to assess thyroid function include TSH, total T3 or free T3 and total T4 or free T4. Because the value of these hormones may be altered in acute conditions such as fever, infections, trauma, surgery, cardiac/renal failure, it is better to perform this investigation after the acute episode subsides.

1. **TSH:** This is the most important and sensitive test for the thyroid gland. A normal value indicates a normal functioning thyroid gland. The test performed for TSH levels is an immunoassay test and the latest third- and fourth-generation kits are sensitive in picking up low values too.
   TSH values in primary thyroid disorders: Primary hyperthyroidism presents with low TSH because of negative feedback inhibition; on the contrary, high value of TSH is seen in primary hypothyroidism in which the pituitary tries to stimulate the thyroid gland to increase the hormone production.
   TSH values in pituitary disorders: Secondary hyperthyroidism is due to elevated TSH level and secondary hypothyroidism is due to reduced TSH secretion by the pituitary because of various reasons.
   In these conditions, TSH value is interpreted along with values of T3 and T4.
2. **Total and free thyroxine (T4):** The levels of free T4 and total T4 are measured by competitive immunoassay method. Normal level of total T4 is 5.0–12.0 μg/dL and free T4 is 0.7–1.9 ng/dL in adults. As mentioned earlier, free T4 measurement is a better indicator of hormonal status than total T4 and is used in conjunction with TSH for diagnosis. The causes of total T4 variations are given in the following table:

Causes of Increase/Decrease in Total T4 Levels

Increase in Total T4	Decrease in Total T4
Endocrine related: • Hyperthyroidism due to hyperfunctioning of thyroid gland (associated with reduced TSH due to negative feedback) • Pituitary TSH-secreting tumour (increased TSH levels) • Factitious hyperthyroidism	Endocrine related: • Primary hypothyroidism (associated with elevated TSH) • Secondary or pituitary hypothyroidism (reduced TSH levels) • Tertiary or hypothalamic hypothyroidism (reduced TSH levels)
Others: • Increase in thyroxine-binding globulin levels	Others: • Hypoproteinaemia, e.g. liver disorders and nephrotic syndrome • Drugs: Oestrogen, danazol • Severe nonthyroidal illness

3. **Total and free triiodothyronine (T3):** This parameter is not useful in routine assessment of thyroid function because its level in blood is very small and may be low even in normal individuals. However, an increased T3 with normal T4 along with lowered TSH levels is the diagnostic feature when T3 toxic thyrotoxicosis is suspected. Raised T3 levels may also help in early diagnosis of hyperthyroidism when T4 levels have not yet started to rise. Normal total T3 level is 80–180 ng/dL and free T3 forms 0.5% of the total T3.

The other investigations performed for evaluation of thyroid include the following:

- Antithyroid antibodies: They are used in diagnosis of autoimmune thyroid disorders. Hashimoto thyroiditis shows antimicrosomal and antithyroglobulin antibodies, whereas TSH receptor antibodies are present in Graves disease.
- Radioactive iodine uptake test: This test assesses the amount of iodine taken up by the thyroid gland and hence to assess the functioning of the gland.
- Thyroid scintiscanning: In this test, an isotope, ^{99m}Tc-pertechnetate, is used to differentiate the various causes which show increased radioiodine uptake.

Interpretation of Thyroid Function Tests in Thyroid Disorders

Thyroid function tests when interpreted along with clinical symptoms help to find the thyroid status of the individual and also identify the cause of the abnormality. Imaging of thyroid gland by ultrasound gives additional information regarding the size, nodularity and the contents of the nodule. FNA of the thyroid performed with or without ultrasound guidance helps in confirmation of the diagnosis and appropriate management of patients with structural abnormality. An outline for interpretation of thyroid function test is given in the following table:

Interpretation of Thyroid Function Tests

TSH	Free T4	Total or Free T3	Most Likely Diagnosis
Normal	Normal	Normal	Euthyroid status (normal functioning thyroid)

Interpretation of Thyroid Function Tests—cont'd

TSH	Free T4	Total or Free T3	Most Likely Diagnosis
Increased	Normal	Normal	Subclinical hypothyroidism (no symptoms)
Increased	Decreased	Decreased	Primary hypothyroidism (thyroid problem)
Decreased	Decreased	Decreased	Secondary/ tertiary hypothyroidism (pituitary or hypothalamus problem)
Decreased	Normal	Normal	Subclinical hyperthyroidism (no symptoms)
Decreased	Increased	Increased	Primary hyperthyroidism (thyroid hyperfunction)
Increased	Increased	Increased	Secondary hyperthyroidism (pituitary tumour) or thyroid hormone resistance
Decreased	Normal	Increased	T3 thyrotoxicosis

SEMEN ANALYSIS

Semen is a combination of secretions of the testis and the male reproductive glands that contain sperm for fertilization of the egg to form a zygote. All parts of the male reproductive system contribute to the production of seminal fluid. The sperms produced by the testes mature in the epididymis and after addition of secretions from seminal vesicles, prostate and Cowper's glands are ready for ejaculation.

INDICATION OF SEMEN ANALYSIS

- **Fertility related:** For investigation of infertility
  For obtaining sperms for assisted reproduction techniques
  For assessment of sperm donors
- **Medicolegal:** For paternity-related issues
  For confirmation of semen in vagina/clothing in rape cases
- **For confirmation of the absence of sperm after vasectomy**

COLLECTION OF SPECIMENS

The specimen is collected by masturbation in a clean sterile container after 3 days of abstinence and examined immediately.

EXAMINATION OF SEMEN

The following tests are done on seminal fluid:

1. **Physical examination:** Time taken **for** liquefaction, viscosity, volume, pH, colour, etc. The normal values are given in Table 11.26 and the terminologies used to describe abnormal values are given in Table 11.27.
2. **Microscopic examination:** Sperm count, vitality, motility, morphology and the number of WBCs (Fig. 11.19).

Table 11.26 Normal Values of Semen Analysis as per WHO 2010 Guidelines for Semen Analysis Test

Parameter	Definition	Reference Range
Semen volume	Total amount of fluid ejaculated	≥1.5 mL
Sperm count	Total number of sperms in the measured volume of ejaculate	≥15 million/mL
Total sperm number	Total number of sperms in the ejaculate	≥39 million
Sperm motility	Number of motile sperms compared to nonmotile sperms and is reported as the percentage	Total motility ≥40% motile sperms within 60 min of ejaculation Progressive motility ≥32%
Sperm viability or vitality	The number of sperms in the sample that are alive as a percentage of the total number of sperms	≥58%
Sperm morphology	Number of ideally shaped sperms as compared to imperfectly shaped sperms and reported as a percentage of the total number of sperms	≥4%
WBCs	A large number of WBCs can be a sign of infection in the reproductive tract	<1 million/mL
Semen pH	Measured to test if the semen is acidic or alkaline	≥7.2
Sperm antibodies	Normally done in specialized laboratories using methods approved by WHO	≥50% motile sperms showing antibody activity

Table 11.27 Terminologies Commonly Used in Semen Analysis

Semen Analysis – Abnormal Results	
Abnormalities	**Definition**
Aspermia	Absence of semen
Azoospermia	Absence of sperm in the semen
Hypospermia	Low semen volume
Hyperspermia	High semen volume
Oligozoospermia	Very low sperm count
Polyzoospermia	Abnormally high sperm count in the ejaculate
Asthenozoospermia	Poor sperm motility
Teratozoospermia	Sperms that have morphological defects
Necrozoospermia	All sperms in the ejaculate are dead
Leucospermia	A high level of white blood cells presents in the semen
Haematospermia	Presence of red blood cells in the ejaculate

3. **Immunological analysis:** To detect **antisperm** antibodies.
4. **Bacteriological analysis:** When infection is suspected.

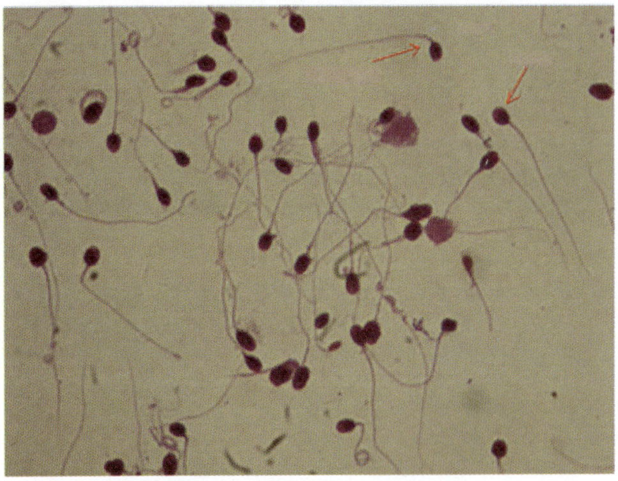

Fig. 11.19 Semen analysis showing normal sperm morphology (→). (*Source:* From C.A. Zambrano Serrano, A. Carvajal Obando, Actas Urológicas Españolas (English Edition), Elsevier 2020.)

5. **Biochemical analysis:** Fructose, zinc, acid phosphatase, carnitine, etc.
6. **Sperm function tests:** These are specialized tests done in cases of infertility – postcoital test, cervical mucus penetration test and hamster egg penetration assay.

Recently, newer techniques for semen analysis such as computer-assisted semen analysis have been developed to get more accurate results.

SELF-ASSESSMENT

Multiple Choice Questions

1. A 40-year-old male with a history of chronic alcoholism presents with ascites and spider naevi. Laboratory tests show elevated serum ammonia. What is the most likely diagnosis?
   A. Pancreatitis
   B. Hepatic encephalopathy
   C. Cholecystitis
   D. Peptic ulcer disease
2. A patient presents with a cherry-red spot on the macula and hepatosplenomegaly. Which of the following is the most likely diagnosis?
   A. Tay–Sachs disease
   B. Niemann–Pick disease
   C. Gaucher disease
   D. Krabbe disease
3. A 55-year-old woman presents with a thyroid nodule. Fine-needle aspiration shows papillary structures. What is the most likely diagnosis?
   A. Papillary carcinoma
   B. Follicular adenoma
   C. Medullary carcinoma
   D. Anaplastic carcinoma
4. A patient with recurrent respiratory infections and infertility undergoes a sperm analysis, which shows immotile sperms. Which of the following is the most likely associated condition?
   A. Klinefelter syndrome
   B. Kartagener syndrome
   C. Cystic fibrosis
   D. Sertoli cell-only syndrome
5. A 45-year-old woman presents with fatigue, weight gain and constipation. Laboratory tests reveal elevated TSH and decreased T4. What is the most likely diagnosis?
   A. Graves disease
   B. Hashimoto thyroiditis
   C. Thyroid adenoma
   D. Pituitary adenoma
6. In a patient with suspected acute pancreatitis, which of the following laboratory findings is most indicative of a severe prognosis?
   A. Elevated serum amylase
   B. Elevated serum lipase
   C. Increased haematocrit
   D. Hypocalcaemia
7. A patient presents with fever, headache and a petechial rash. CSF analysis shows increased WBCs, predominantly neutrophils. Which of the following is the most likely diagnosis?
   A. Viral meningitis
   B. Bacterial meningitis

C. Tuberculous meningitis
D. Fungal meningitis

8. A 60-year-old smoker presents with a persistent cough and weight loss. A biopsy of a lung nodule shows small cells with neuroendocrine markers. What is the diagnosis?
A. Small cell lung carcinoma
B. Squamous cell carcinoma
C. Adenocarcinoma
D. Large cell carcinoma

9. A newborn presents with hypoglycaemia, hepatomegaly and a doll-like face. Which enzyme deficiency is most likely?
A. Glucose-6-phosphatase
B. Pyruvate kinase
C. Hexokinase
D. Glucokinase

10. A patient with a history of IBD develops a liver mass. Alpha-fetoprotein levels are normal. What is the most likely diagnosis?
A. Hepatocellular carcinoma
B. Cholangiocarcinoma
C. Hepatic adenoma
D. Metastatic colorectal cancer

11. A patient presents with a hard, irregular breast mass and axillary lymphadenopathy. Biopsy shows ductal carcinoma in situ. What is the next best step in management?
A. Total mastectomy
B. Lumpectomy and radiation
C. Chemotherapy
D. Hormonal therapy

12. In a patient with jaundice, LFTs reveal elevated bilirubin, predominantly conjugated, and normal AST and ALT. What is the most likely diagnosis?
A. Haemolytic anaemia
B. Dubin–Johnson syndrome
C. Viral hepatitis
D. Cirrhosis

13. In a patient with jaundice, liver function tests reveal elevated direct bilirubin and alkaline phosphatase. Which of the following is the most likely cause?
A. Hepatic cirrhosis
B. Hepatocellular carcinoma
C. Cholelithiasis causing biliary obstruction
D. Viral hepatitis

14. A patient with a history of chronic cough and dyspnoea is diagnosed with interstitial lung disease. What is the most likely associated condition?
A. Chronic bronchitis
B. Asthma
C. Sarcoidosis
D. Pulmonary embolism

15. A patient presents with a firm, painless testicular mass. Serum markers show elevated AFP and hCG. What is the most likely diagnosis?
A. Testicular seminoma
B. Leydig cell tumour
C. Testicular teratoma
D. Sertoli cell tumour

16. A 65-year-old smoker presents with chronic cough and weight loss. Sputum cytology reveals atypical cells with enlarged nuclei. Which of the following is the most likely diagnosis?
A. Bronchitis
B. Small cell lung carcinoma
C. Tuberculosis
D. Asthma

17. A patient with a history of asbestos exposure presents with shortness of breath. Sputum cytology shows pleomorphic cells and 'ferruginous bodies'. What is the most likely diagnosis?
A. Mesothelioma
B. Adenocarcinoma
C. Squamous cell carcinoma
D. Bronchial asthma

18. A patient presents with weight loss, heat intolerance and palpitations. TFTs show decreased TSH and increased T4. What is the most likely diagnosis?
A. Primary hypothyroidism
B. Secondary hypothyroidism
C. Primary hyperthyroidism
D. Secondary hyperthyroidism

Answers

1. (B); 2. (B); 3. (A); 4. (B); 5. (B); 6. (D); 7. (B); 8. (A); 9. (A); 10. (B); 11. (B); 12. (B); 13. (C); 14. (C); 15. (C); 16. (B); 17. (A); 18. (C).

Self-Assessment Questions

1. An 8-year-old male child is brought to paediatric outpatient department (OPD) with a history of reduced urine output, fever and passing cola-coloured urine. His blood pressure is 160/110 mm Hg and skin shows many healing pustules. What is your provisional diagnosis? What will be his expected urinary profile?
2. A 5-year-old male child brought to the OPD with puffiness of face and a history of passing white-coloured urine. His blood pressure is normal, but his lipid profile shows increased cholesterol. What is your diagnosis and what will his urine examination reveal?
3. A 55-year-old man has polyuria, polydipsia and polyphagia. This morning he appears a bit confused and does not respond well to questions? What is your diagnosis and what will his urine examination reveal?
4. A 55-year-old woman from a nearby rural area visits a primary health centre with complaints of irregular vaginal spotting and loss of weight. She is postmenopausal and has never been to a hospital before. What is the first investigation you can do in the OPD? What will you look for?
5. A 60-year-old man complains of frank haematuria for past few days. He has been having lower abdominal pain recently and on enquiring he says he has lost weight because he does not feel hungry nowadays. What urine investigation will you order?
6. A 25-year-old man presents with confusion and delirium. He had been having fever and headache for past few days. On examination, neck stiffness is present. What will you suspect and how will the CSF findings help you?
7. A man being investigated for infertility gives his semen for analysis. His doctor gives him the following report. What is your diagnosis?

Parameter	Report
Volume (mL)	1.5
Liquefaction time (min)	40

Parameter	Report
Viscosity	**Increased**
pH	7.6
Sperm count (millions/mL)	05
Motility	
Active (%)	40
Sluggish (%)	40
Nonmotile (%)	20

8. A 45-year-old woman presents to the OPD with yellowish discolouration of stools. She has intermittent right hypochondrial pain for past 6 months. She gives a history of pale stools and generalized pruritus. What is your diagnosis? What is the expected urinary profile?

Answers

1. Acute glomerulonephritis
2. Nephrotic syndrome
3. Diabetic ketoacidosis
4. Pap smear to look for carcinoma of cervix
5. Urine cytology
6. Meningitis
7. Oligozoospermia
8. Obstructive jaundice

Topics for Self-Directed Learning

1. Liquid-based cytology
2. Colposcopy in diagnosis and treatment
3. Role of cystoscopy in evaluating bladder lesions
4. Pleural fluid cytology in various malignancies
5. Immunohistochemistry in ascitic fluid cytology
6. Liver function test
7. Renal function test
8. Abnormalities in sperm morphology
9. Method of urine chemical examination
10. Synovial fluid analysis

12 Advanced Diagnostic Techniques

Rajeswari Kathiah, V Rajalakshmi

CHAPTER OUTLINE

INTRODUCTION

The practice of pathology has seen several milestones and is currently undergoing significant changes in many ways because of advances in techniques for DNA, RNA and tissue protein analyses. Such advances have permitted improved biological insights into many developmental, inflammatory, metabolic, infectious and neoplastic diseases. Also, molecular analysis has led to improvements in the accuracy of disease diagnosis and classification. It is likely that in the near future, these methods will increasingly enter the day-to-day diagnosis and management of patients. Pathologists will play a key role in guiding the implementation and interpretation of these tests, as they ascend from the research laboratory into diagnostic pathology.

Many techniques are mentioned in the respective chapters under relevant topics. This chapter discusses the common advanced diagnostic techniques and their applications in brief.

IMMUNOHISTOCHEMISTRY

Immunohistochemistry (IHC) is a widely used diagnostic technique that allows the localization of antigens in tissue preparations and permits morphological evaluation by light microscopy.

Conventional IHC is also referred to as chromogenic IHC, in which an antibody is conjugated to an enzyme, such as peroxidase, that can catalyse a colour-forming reaction. Immunofluorescence is a slight variant of IHC and is discussed later.

PRINCIPLE (FIG. 12.1)

Localization of the desired antigen or the antigen of interest (the proteins) can be achieved with the use of a corresponding antibody in a tissue sample while maintaining the spatial context and tissue architecture. Detection at the microscopic level of antigen–antibody interactions can be achieved by labelling the antibody with a substance that can be visualized by conjugation either to a fluorescent marker or to an enzyme, followed by colorimetric detection.

The major steps are as follows:

1. Fixation and embedding of tissue
2. Retrieval of antigens by application of heat or proteolytic enzymes
3. Binding of primary antibody to a specific antigen
4. Formation of antigen–antibody complex by incubation with a secondary enzyme-conjugated antibody
5. Generation of coloured deposits at the sites of antigen–antibody binding because of the presence of substrate and chromogen

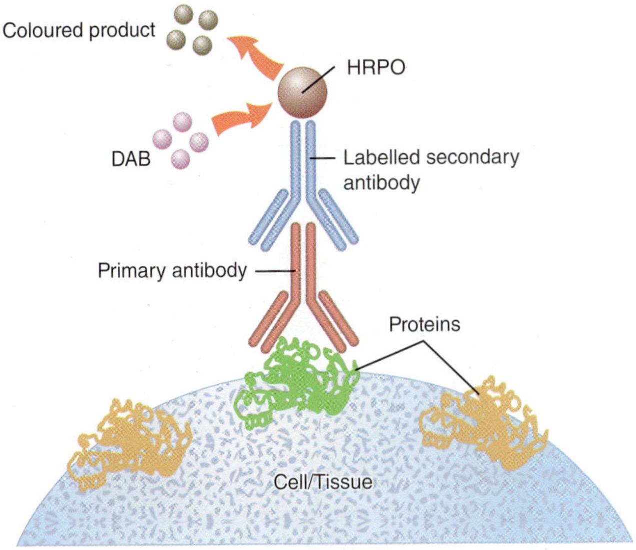

Fig. 12.1 Principles of indirect immunohistochemistry (IHC). DAB, 3,3′-diaminobenzidine used as a chromogen; HRPO, horseradish peroxidase used for conjugation of antibody.

LOCATION OF THE ANTIGENS

The antigen of interest can be located within the nucleus, cytoplasm or membrane (Figs 12.2–12.4).

APPLICATIONS (TABLE 12.1)

IHC has a wide range of applications. The antigens traced and detected could be of diagnostic, prognostic or theranostic importance.

IHC helps at many levels in the workup of diseases:

- To identify the lineage of the tumour cells
- To differentiate benign tumours and reactive proliferations
- To differentiate benign and malignant tumours
- To identify the level of differentiation of tumour cells
- To identify the cell of origin in metastatic deposits of an unknown primary
- To identify markers to indicate prognosis
- To identify markers to guide therapy – theranostic markers

Immunohistochemical markers used routinely in disease workup have already been mentioned under the relevant chapters and topics. Here is a brief list of markers categorized empathetically to describe their purpose.

LIMITATIONS

IHC can never be an alternative to routine histopathological studies but can add much value to the final diagnosis only when used as an adjunct. Choice of markers should be decided based on the morphological appearance of the

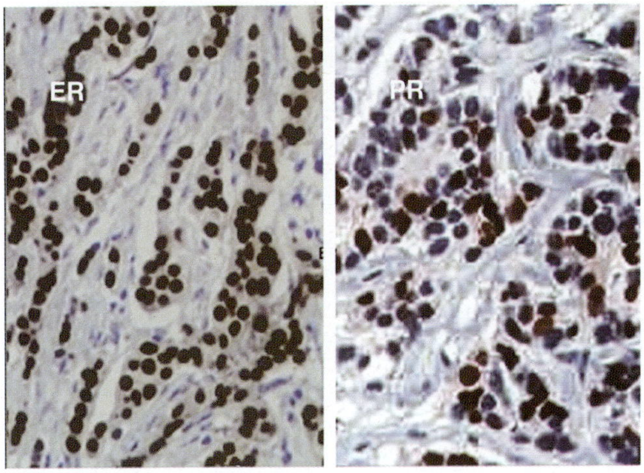

Fig. 12.2 Nuclear staining pattern of IHC for ER and PR. ER, oestrogen receptor; PR, progesterone receptor. (*Source:* https://breast-cancer.ca/6c-er-pr-her2/)

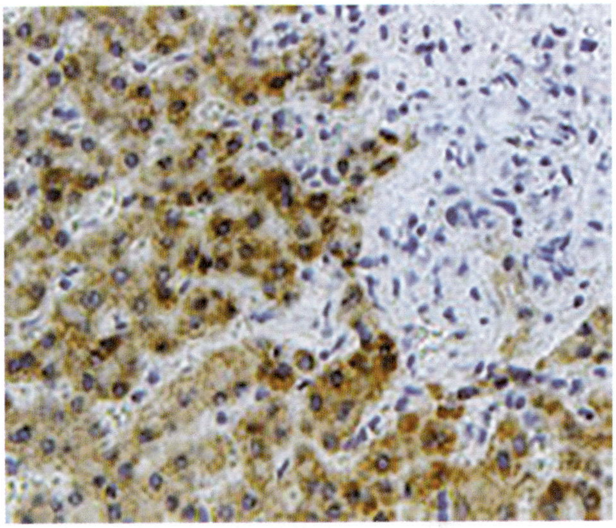

Fig. 12.3 Cytoplasmic staining pattern of IHC for α-fetoprotein. (*Source:* https://biocare.net/product/ck7-antibody-mouse/)

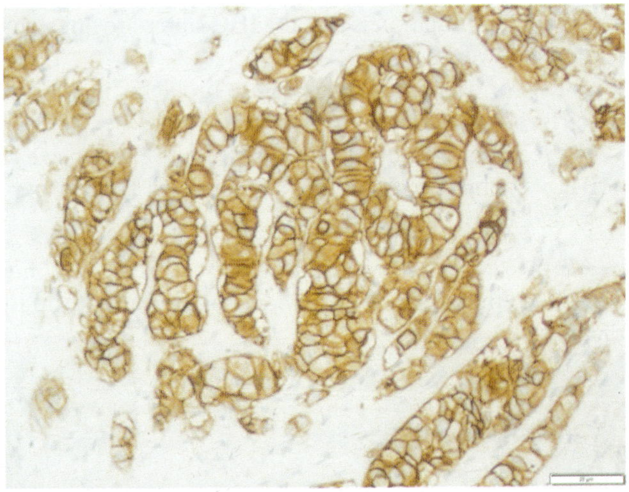

Fig. 12.4 Membranous location of HER2/neu antigens highlighted as fishnet pattern with IHC.

Table 12.1 Applications of IHC

Category	Markers	Application
Diagnostic markers	Cytokeratin	To differentiate carcinomas from other malignancies
	Vimentin	To differentiate sarcomas from other malignancies
	CD45	To differentiate lymphomas from other malignancies
	CD20	To differentiate B-cell lymphomas from T-cell lymphomas
	CD3	To differentiate T-cell lymphomas from B-cell lymphomas
	CD10	To differentiate pre-B lymphomas from other B-cell lymphomas
	PSA	If positive in metastatic deposits, it indicates prostatic primary
	P63	Absence in breast tumours is a characteristic feature of malignant lesions
	α-Fetoprotein	Yolk sac tumours, hepatocellular carcinoma
Prognostic markers	Ki-67	If the labelling index is high, it indicates a high proliferative status and thus marks a higher grade
Theranostic markers	ER	Decision on starting tamoxifen
	HER2/neu	Decision on starting trastuzumab (Herceptin)
	KIT	Decision on starting imatinib

tumour. Blind usage of multiple markers without morphological examination leads to confusions.

- The major limitation is that the IHC stains are not standardized worldwide.
- Under- or overfixation can lead to problems in antigen retrieval and results.
- The technique requires reagents which are expensive.
- IHC is subject to human error, and well-trained personnel are paramount.

All the aforementioned limitations can be overcome and this is the reason IHC is widely used in the world of diagnosis.

IMMUNOFLUORESCENCE

Immunofluorescence is a technique that follows the same principles of IHC but uses an antibody that is tagged to a fluorophore, such as fluorescein or rhodamine (Fig. 12.5). Fluorescence microscope is used for immunofluorescence technique. This test is widely used in skin (Fig. 12.6) and renal lesions and has been discussed in Chapters 24 and 29.

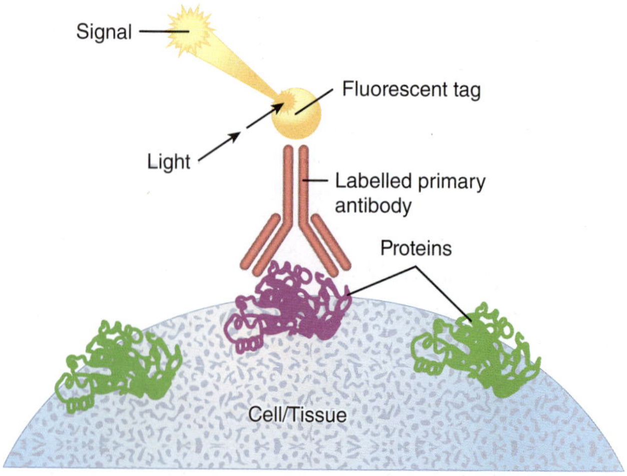

Fig. 12.5 Principles of immunofluorescence. Note the tagging of the antibody with a fluorescent material and the generation of signals following antigen–antibody interaction.

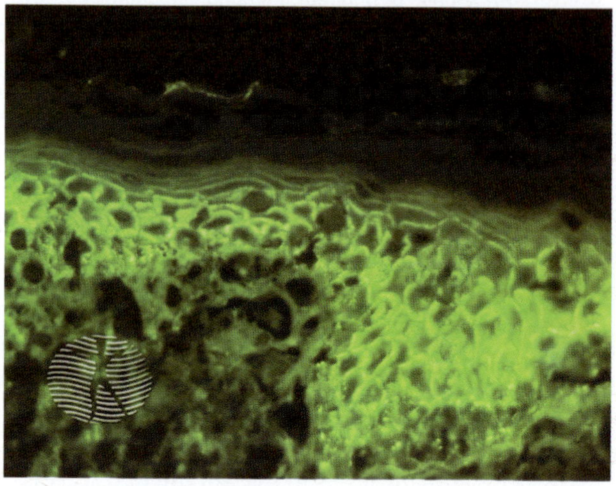

Fig. 12.6 Intercellular space staining pattern (chicken-wire), pemphigus vulgaris. (*Source:* https://dermnetnz.org/topics/direct-immunofluorescence/)

FROZEN SECTION

The frozen section is a laboratory procedure to perform rapid microscopic analysis of a specimen. The technical name for frozen section is cryosection. It is most often used in oncological surgeries.

It is also referred to as 'intraoperative consultation' by the pathologists which includes not only frozen section but also gross examination of the specimen sent, examination of the cytological preparations taken from the specimen and aliquoting of the specimen for special studies like molecular pathology techniques and others. Rapid diagnosis can guide intraoperative patient management.

PRINCIPLE

The excised fresh tissue is rapidly frozen. The tissue turns into ice and becomes firm with water, which acts as an embedding medium. Rapid freezing of fresh tissue converts water to ice. The firm ice formed within the tissue acts as embedding media to cut the tissue.

PROCEDURE

The main instrument in frozen section procedure is the cryostat, which is a microtome placed inside a refrigerator (Fig. 12.7). Microtome is the equipment used for making tissue sections of required thickness ranging from 1 to 10 µm. The specimen (sent fresh without formalin) after gross examination and taking bits from representative areas is placed on a metal disc which is then secured in a chuck and frozen rapidly to approximately −20°C to −30°C. The specimen is then embedded in a gel-like medium called OCT, optimum cutting temperature compound or similar embedding media. At this temperature, most tissues become rock hard, but each type of tissue has a preferred temperature for processing. Following this step, the sections are taken by the cryostat and are stained with haematoxylin and eosin or any other indicated stain.

The preparation of the slides is much more rapid than with conventional histology technique. The entire procedure usually takes a minimum of 10–20 minutes, which is variable according to the number and size of the specimen. However, the quality of the tissue sections is much lower than the conventional sections, with much less clarity on the cellular details.

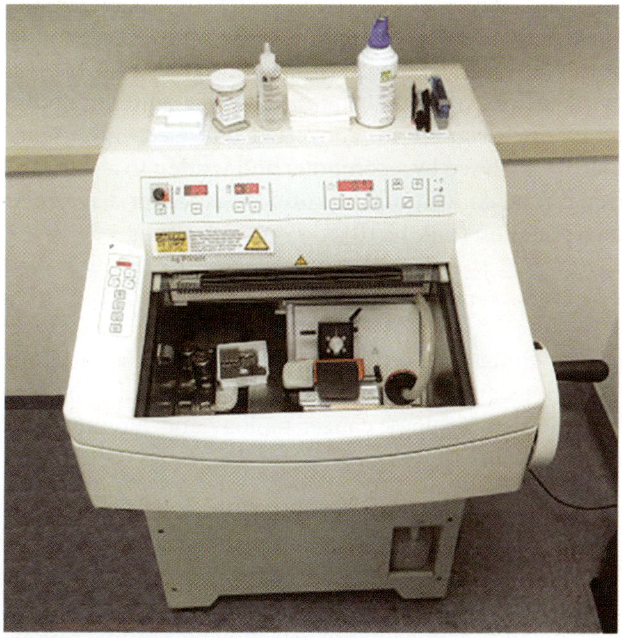

Fig. 12.7 Cryostat. (Source: From Stephen Bullock, Bonnie Balzer and Alberto M. Marchevsky. Guide to the Preparation of Frozen Sections. Intraoperative Consultation: Foundations in Diagnostic Pathology. Saunders. 2015.)

APPLICATIONS

The major application of frozen section is the examination of tissue while the surgery is taking place. The following are the uses of frozen section:

- For providing rapid gross and microscopic diagnoses
  - To identify an unknown pathological process
  - To identify the extent of disease or to evaluate the margins
  - To identify lymph node metastases
  - To confirm the presence of representative tissue for diagnosis on permanent sections
- For demonstrating labile enzymes, e.g. lipids and some carbohydrates
- For immunofluorescence procedure
- For IHC technique to demonstrate heat-sensitive antigens

LIMITATIONS

It should be remembered that frozen section can never be an alternative for conventional tissue sections, as the quality of the slides of frozen sections is inferior to the formalin-fixed paraffin section slides and artefacts are also quite frequent.

FLOW CYTOMETRY

Flow cytometry is a technique that provides rapid multiparametric analysis (physical and chemical properties) of single cells in a liquid medium.

PRINCIPLE (FIG. 12.8)

Flow cytometers analyse single cells or particles as they flow past single or multiple lasers while suspended in a buffered salt-based solution.

PROCEDURE

In the process, a sample containing cells or particles is suspended in a fluid and injected into the flow cytometer (Fig. 12.9). Each particle is analysed for visible light scatter and one or more fluorescence parameters. Visible light scatter is measured in two different directions: the forward direction (the forward scatter), which indicates the relative size of the cells; and at 90° (side scatter), which indicates the internal complexity or granularity of the cells. Light scatter is independent of fluorescence.

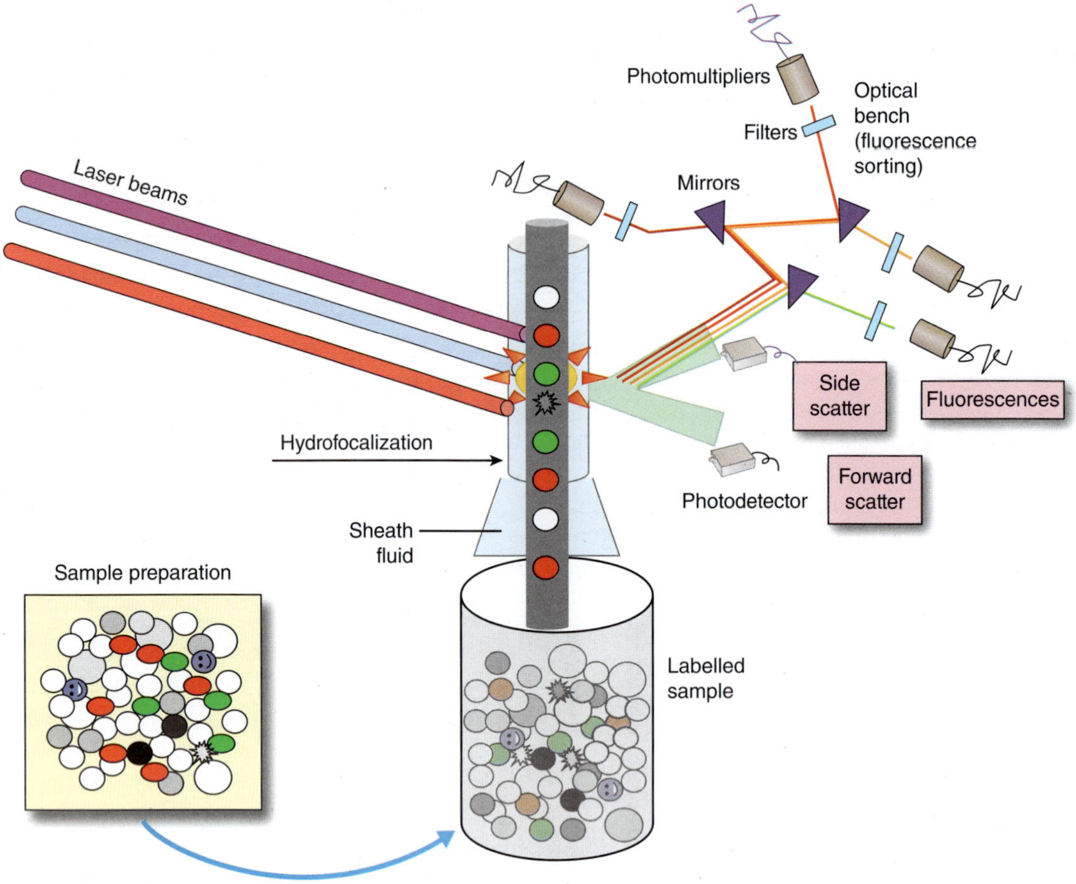

Fig. 12.8 Principles of flow cytometry. (*Source:* Reproduced from https://www.researchgate.net/figure/Principles-of-flow-cytometry-in-a-sample-cells-of-interest-are-labeled-with_fig2_304613284)

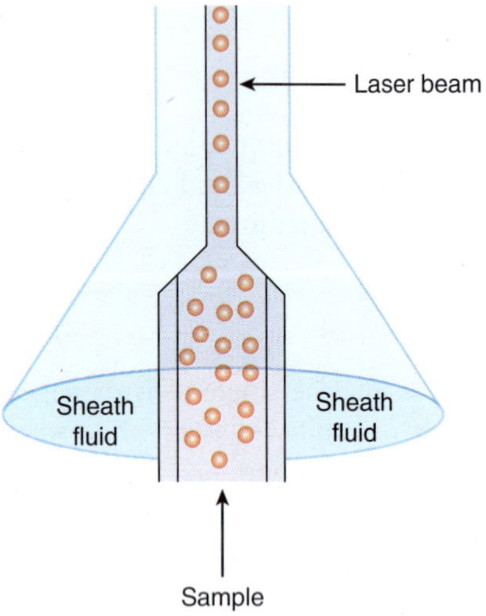

Fig. 12.9 Hydrodynamic focussing of a sample for flow cytometry. (*Source:* Reproduced from https://aws.labome.com/figure/te-125-2.png)

Samples are prepared for fluorescence measurement by the addition of fluorescent reagents. Many types of fluorescent reagents are used in flow cytometry. This includes fluorescently conjugated antibodies, DNA-binding dyes, viability dyes, ion indicator dyes and fluorescent expression proteins.

Cell populations can be analysed and/or purified based on their fluorescent or light scattering characteristics. Flow cytometers use lasers as light sources to produce both scattered and fluorescent light signals that are read by detectors such as photodiodes or photomultiplier tubes. Such signals are converted into electronic signals that are analysed by a computer and written to a standardized format data file and reproduced as scatter diagram for interpretation (Fig. 12.10).

APPLICATIONS

Flow cytometry is a powerful tool that has applications in various fields like immunology, molecular biology, bacteriology, virology, cancer biology and monitoring of infectious diseases.

- By studying the protein expression of cells (CD markers), lineage and differentiation of cells can be established and thus flow cytometry has a major role in the workup of haematological malignancies. The same principle is applied in the detection of minimal residual disease following treatment.
- DNA content of cells can be measured and thus ploidy status of the tumour population can be determined.

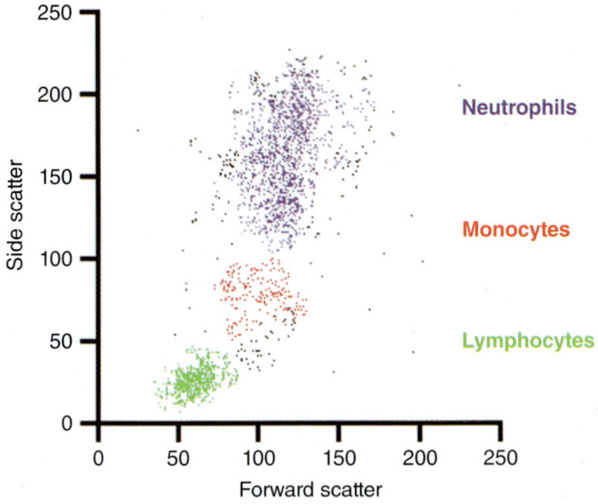

Fig. 12.10 Two-dimensional scatter plot of a peripheral blood sample. (*Source:* https://aws.labome.com/figure/te-125-5.png)

- Flow cytometers can also analyse the replication of cells by using fluorescent dyes for four different stages of the cell cycle.
- Cytometers can be used to sort cells of interest in separate collection tubes physically.
- Multidrug-resistant bacteria in the blood and other samples can be studied using flow cytometers.
- The different stages of cell death, apoptosis and necrosis can be detected based on the differences in the morphological and biochemical changes using flow cytometry.

LIMITATIONS

- Flow cytometry cannot provide information about the intracellular location or distribution of proteins.
- Certain factors like accumulation of debris can lead to false-positive or false-negative results.
- It is a time-consuming and expensive process that requires highly qualified technicians and pathologists.

ELECTRON MICROSCOPY

An electron microscope is a special type of microscope that uses a beam of accelerated electrons as a source of illumination. The wavelength of an electron can be up to 10,000 times shorter than that of visible light photons, so electron microscopes have a higher resolving power than light microscopes and can reveal the structure of smaller objects. The major application of electron microscope is to investigate the ultrastructure of a wide range of biological and inorganic specimens.

PRINCIPLE

An electron microscope uses signals arising from the interaction of an electron beam with the sample to obtain information about structure, morphology and composition.

Electron microscopes use shaped magnetic fields to form electron optical lens systems that are analogous to the glass lenses of an optical light microscope. Specimen to be examined with electron microscopy must be fixed using special fixatives like glutaraldehyde or osmium tetroxide. Specimen can also be frozen and then examined with an electron microscope. This is referred to as cryo-electron microscopy.

An electron microscope has four major parts – the electron gun, electromagnetic lenses, specimen holder, and image viewing and recording system.

TYPES

- Transmission electron microscope (Fig. 12.11)
- Scanning electron microscope

APPLICATIONS

The following are some of the common applications:

- To study the ultrastructure of nephrons in renal lesions (Fig. 12.12)
- To look for the presence of microvilli over the mesothelial cells (Fig. 12.13)
- To look for the presence of neurosecretory granules in tumours of neuroendocrine origin (Fig. 12.14)

LIMITATIONS

- The equipment is huge; hence, it needs much space and is expensive.

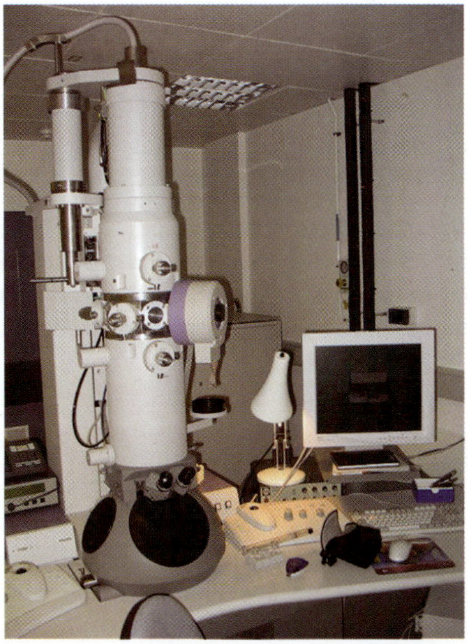

Fig. 12.11 A modern transmission electron microscope. (*Source:* https://en.wikipedia.org/wiki/Electron_microscope)

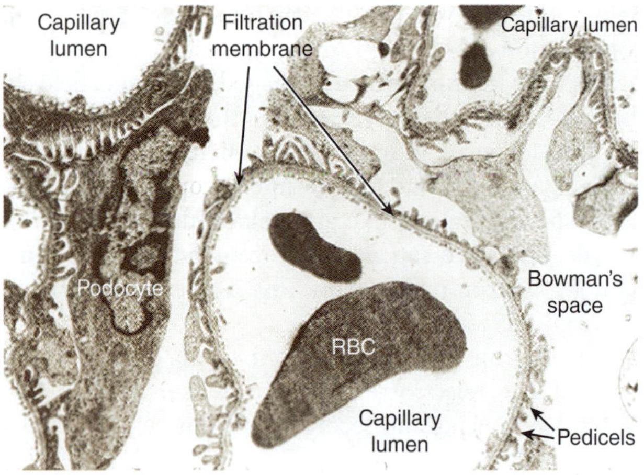

Fig. 12.12 Electron microscopic picture of glomerular filtration membrane.

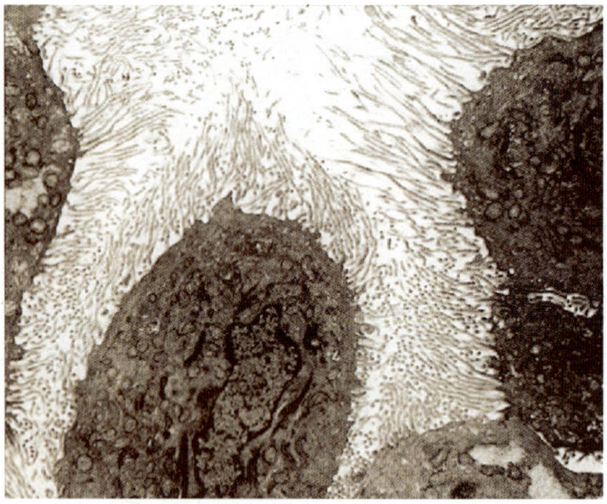

Fig. 12.13 Electron microscopy of mesothelioma cells with the presence of long villi along the apical and lateral surfaces. (*Source:* https://www.researchgate.net/figure/Electron-micrograph-showing-a-group-of-mesothelioma-cells-with-a-profusion-of-long_fig21_6326658)

- Researchers need intensive training to interpret the result.

The use of an electron microscope should be restricted to specific lesions which need the ultrastructural details of cells after examining the morphological features with tissue sections. Indiscriminate use of electron microscopy should be avoided.

POLARIZING MICROSCOPY

Polarizing light microscopy means any of the optical light microscopy techniques that involve the polarized light. Simple techniques include illumination of the sample with polarized light in which the directly transmitted light can optionally be blocked with a polarizer oriented at 90° to the illumination.

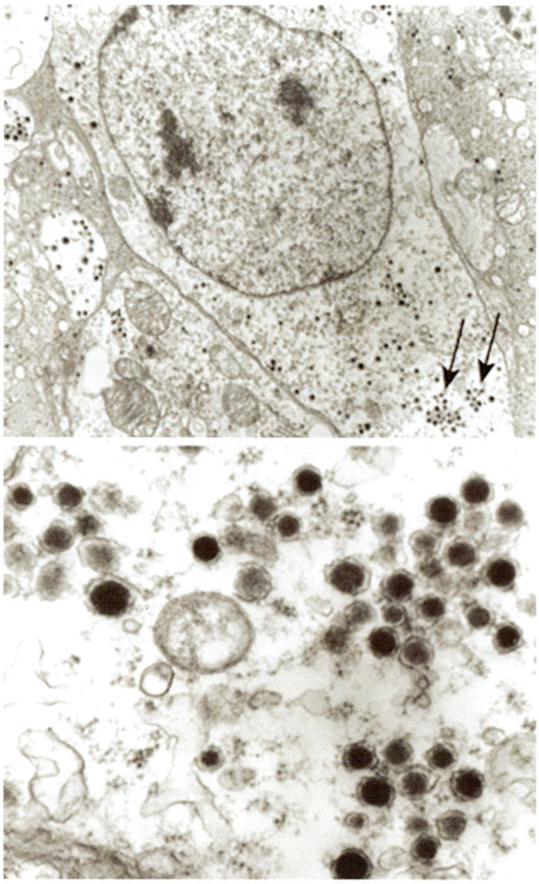

Fig. 12.14 Electron-dense neurosecretory granules seen in neuroendocrine tumours. (*Source:* https://thoracickey.com/neuroendocrine-lesions-of-the-lung/)

More complex microscopy techniques include differential interface contrast microscopy and interference reflection microscopy.

Polarizing microscopy is mostly used on birefringent samples when polarized light interacts strongly with the sample and thus generating contrast with the background. Recall the role of polarizing microscope in amyloidosis (Chapter 6), where it demonstrates the apple green birefringence of amyloid fibrils after Congo red staining (Fig. 12.15).

FLUORESCENCE IN SITU HYBRIDIZATION

Fluorescent in situ hybridization (FISH) is a laboratory technique used for detecting and locating a specific DNA sequences on a chromosome. It is used in the detection of large deletions, duplications or complex rearrangements.

PRINCIPLE

FISH uses DNA probes that recognize specific sequences in the chromosomes. In Human Genome Project, a library of bacterial chromosomes that span the entire length of

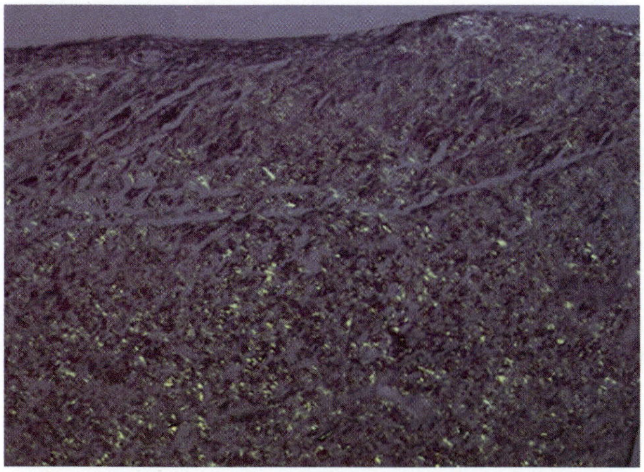

Fig. 12.15 Apple green birefringence of amyloid deposits shown by the polarizing microscope. (*Source:* From Amy Y. Lin. Tumors of the conjunctiva. McKee's Pathology of the Skin. 5th edition. Elsevier 2020.)

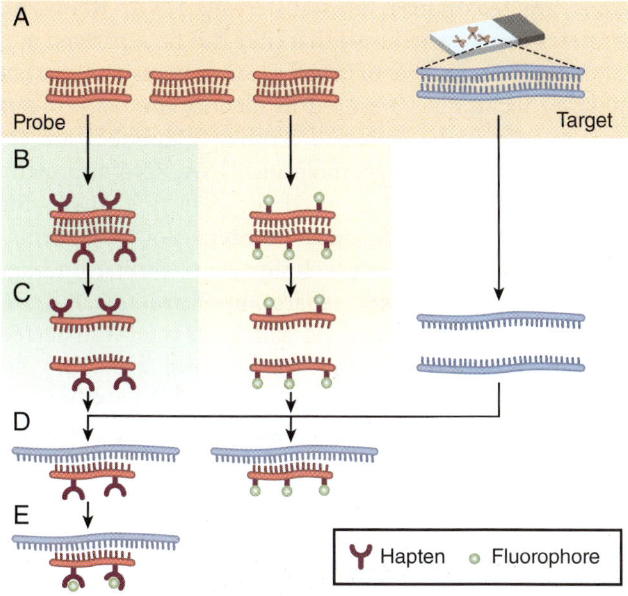

Fig. 12.16 Steps involved in FISH. (*Source:* https://www.nature.com/scitable/topicpage/fluorescence-in-situ-hybridization-fish-327/)

human genome was created. Bacterial chromosomes can be used to create the DNA probes and labelled with fluorescent dye.

PROCEDURE (FIG. 12.16)

When fluorescent-labelled DNA probes are applied to chromosomes, they hybridize with their complementary sequence on the chromosome and label the region with fluorescent dye. The labelled region can then be visualized under a fluorescent microscope.

The probes can be used to paint the entire chromosome or the centromeric region or a specific sequence in the chromosome.

Advantages of FISH include rapid diagnosis and the procedure can be done on any sample such as prenatal samples, peripheral blood leucocytes, cytological specimens, fresh frozen or fixed tissue.

(a) The basic elements of FISH are a DNA probe and a target sequence. (b) Before hybridization, the DNA probe is labelled by various means such as nick translation, random primed labelling and polymerase chain reaction (PCR). Two labelling strategies are commonly used: indirect labelling (left panel) and direct labelling (right panel). For indirect labelling, probes are labelled with modified nucleotides that contain a hapten, whereas direct labelling uses nucleotides that have been directly modified to contain a fluorophore. (c) The labelled probe and the target DNA are denatured. (d) Combining the denatured probe and the target allows the annealing of complementary DNA sequences. (e) If the probe has been labelled indirectly, an extra step is required for visualization of the nonfluorescent hapten that uses an enzymatic or immunological detection system.

APPLICATIONS

1. Chromosomal aberrations: numerical and structural
2. Gene mutation

   Examples
   a. Translocation: BCR–ABL fusion gene in chronic myeloid leukaemia (Fig. 12.17)
   b. Amplification: HER2 amplification in breast cancer (Fig. 12.18)

Spectral karyotyping (Fig. 12.19) is a type of FISH where the entire human genome can be visualized with a distinct colour label for each chromosomal pair. The different colours are produced by different mixtures of five fluorochromes used to tag the DNA probe. In contrast to conventional karyotyping, this method appears spectacular with easy detection of chromosomal abnormalities and complex translocations.

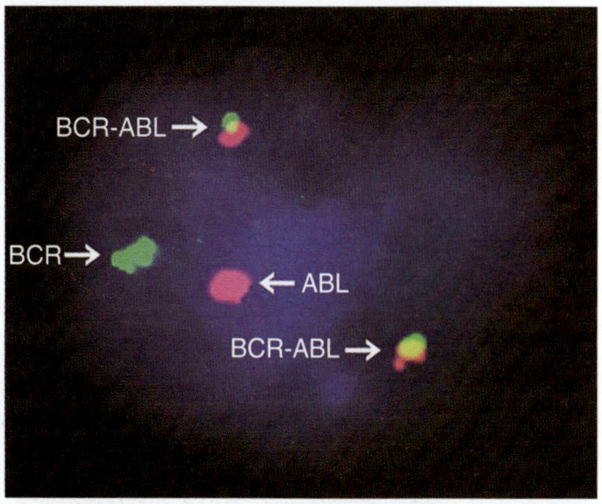

Fig. 12.17 BCR–ABL fusion highlighted by FISH. (*Source:* https://www.sysmex-europe.com/media-center/bcr-abl-fusion-gene-detected-by-fluorescence-in-situ-hybridisation-1286.html)

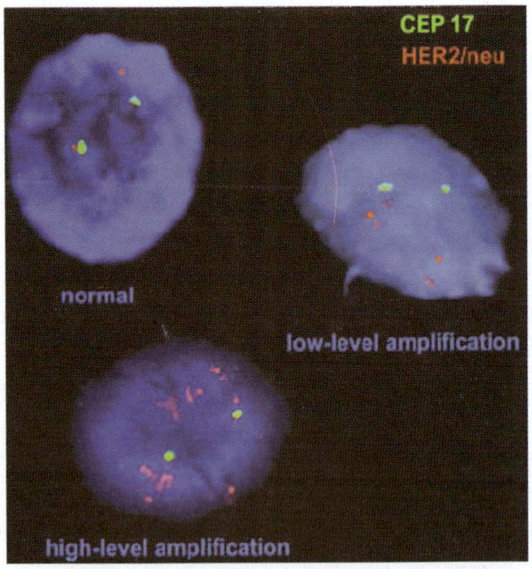

Fig. 12.18 HER2/neu amplification highlighted by FISH. (*Source:* https://www.researchgate.net/figure/A-picture-showing-the-differences-in-level-of-HER2-neu-gene-amplification-in-tumor_fig1_23134004)

ELECTROPHORESIS

Though electrophoresis is not an advanced diagnostic technique, it is one of the steps involved in techniques like blotting and PCR, and hence briefly mentioned here along with its illustration (Fig. 12.20).

Electrophoresis is a laboratory technique that is used to separate DNA, RNA and protein molecules based on their size and electrical charge. Electrophoresis is the motion of dispersed particles relative to a fluid under the influence of a spatially uniform electric field. In simple words, an electric current is used to move molecules to be separated (Fig. 12.21). Such separation happens through a gel whose pores work like a sieve, allowing smaller molecules to move faster than larger molecules. The conditions used during the procedure can be adjusted to separate molecules in a desired size range.

Electrophoresis of positively charged particles is called cataphoresis, while that of the negatively charged particles is referred to as anaphoresis.

APPLICATIONS

- DNA sequencing
- Separation and purification of DNA, RNA, proteins and nucleic acids
- Separation of organic acids, alkaloids, carbohydrates, amino acids and alcohol
- Medical research

BLOTTING TECHNIQUES

Blots are techniques for transferring DNA, RNA and proteins on to a carrier so that they can be separated and often follow the use of a gel electrophoresis. Different blotting techniques are used to identify unique proteins and nucleic acid sequences. Blotting techniques are selected based on the target molecule: DNA, RNA or protein.

The Southern blot is used for detecting DNA, the northern blot for RNA and the western blot for proteins.

All the three blotting techniques are similar and begin with electrophoretic separation of proteins and nucleic acid fragments on a gel which are then transferred to a membrane where they are immobilized. This enables radiolabelled or enzymatically labelled antibody or DNA probes to bind the immobilized target, and the molecules of interest may then be visualized using different methods.

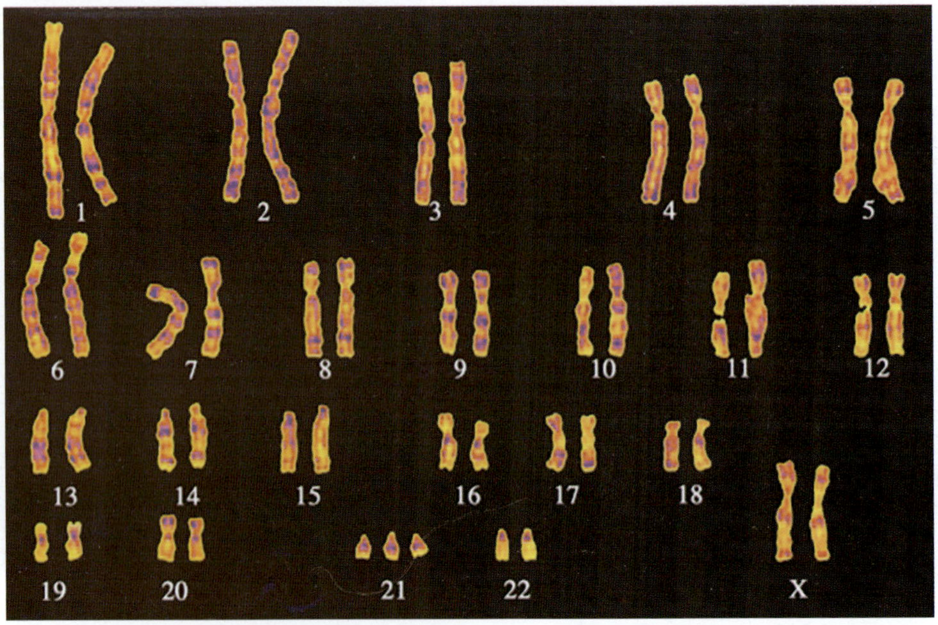

Fig. 12.19 Spectral karyotype of Down syndrome. (*Source:* https://the-gist.org/2016/03/tale-of-the-tiny-chromosome/)

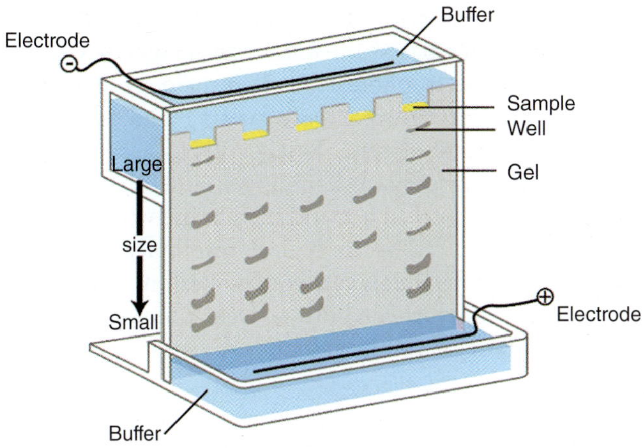

Fig. 12.20 Illustration of electrophoresis.

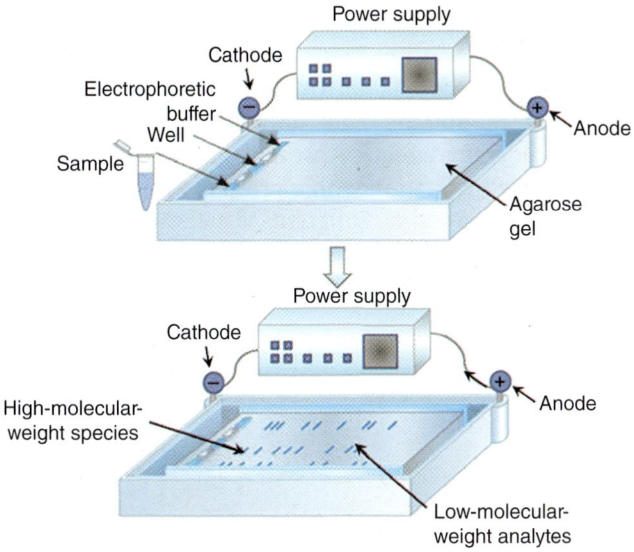

Fig. 12.21 Illustration of agarose gel electrophoresis. DNA samples are pipetted into the sample wells, seen as dark slots. Application of an **electric current** at the top (anodal, negative) end causes the negatively charged **DNA** to migrate (electrophorese) towards the bottom (cathodal, positive) end. The rate of migration is proportional to the size – smaller fragments move more quickly and wind up at the bottom of the gel. DNA is visualized by including an intercalating dye, ethidium bromide, in the gel. DNA fragments take up the dye as they migrate through the gel. Illumination with ultraviolet light causes the intercalated dye to fluoresce with a pale pink colour. (*Source:* sciencedirect.com/topics/biochemistry-genetics-and-molecular-biology/agarose-gel-electrophoresis)

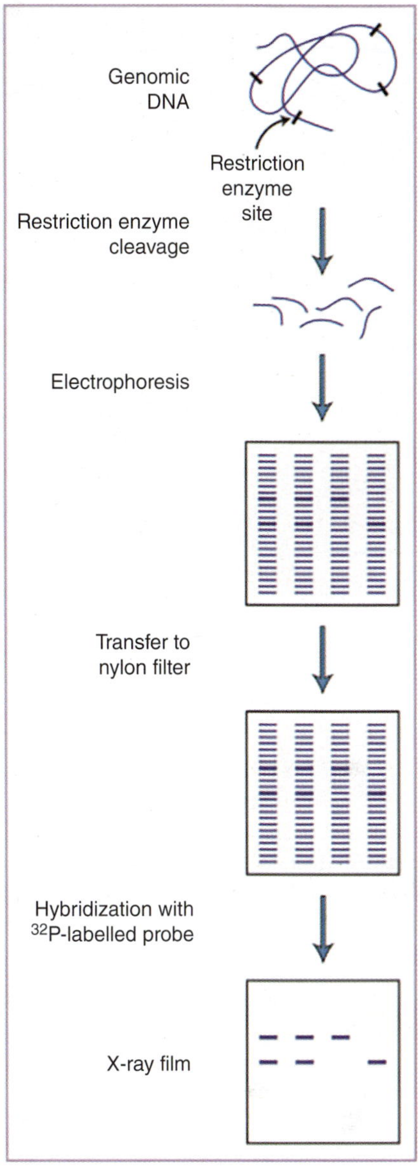

Fig. 12.22 Southern blot technique. (*Source:* From Jennifer Gilner, Aleksandar Rajkovic and Jeffrey A. Kuller. Molecular Genetic Technology. Creasy and Resnik's Maternal-Fetal Medicine: Principles and Practice. 8th edition. Elsevier 2019.)

SOUTHERN BLOT TECHNIQUE (FIG. 12.22)

Southern blot is used to determine the identity, size and abundance of specific **DNA** sequences. This technique begins with extraction of DNA from cells and tissues from which DNA fragments are then extracted by enzymatic digestion. The fragments are then separated by size on an agarose or polyacrylamide gel via electrophoresis. Following gel electrophoresis, DNA on the gel is transferred to a nylon membrane. The membrane is incubated with a nucleic acid probe that has a sequence and is labelled with radioactivity, fluorescent dye or an enzyme capable of generating a chemiluminescent signal. Hybridization of complementary sequences happens during incubation, and the unbound probe is removed by washing with buffer. The hybridized labelled probe molecules will remain bound to the blot. Choice of detection method is based on the probe label. Enzymatically labelled probes are visualized with a chemiluminescent substrate, and radiolabelled probes are visualized with X-ray film or phosphorimaging.

NORTHERN BLOT TECHNIQUE (FIG. 12.23)

Northern blots are used to determine the identity, size and abundance of specific **RNA** sequences. This

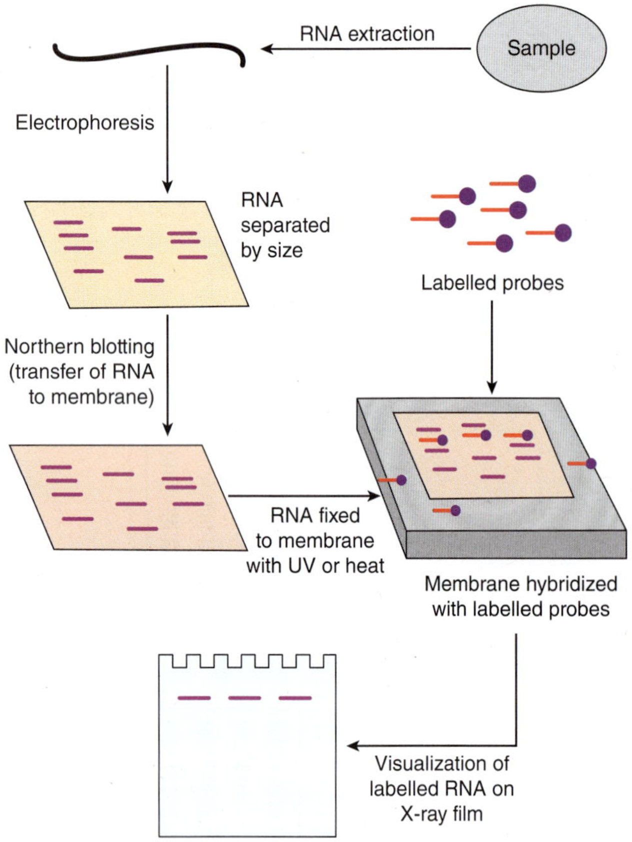

Fig. 12.23 Northern blot technique. (*Source:* Reproduced from MyBioSource Learning Center.)

technique begins with RNA isolation, and separation techniques differ based on RNA size. Larger RNAs are separated by electrophoresis on a formaldehyde agarose gel that prevents normal base pairing and maintains RNA in a denatured state. Smaller RNAs are separated on a denaturing polyacrylamide gel, and RNA is then transferred from gel to a nylon membrane which is then incubated with a radioactively or nonisotopically labelled RNA, DNA or oligodeoxynucleotide. Washing with buffer removes the unhybridized probe. Detection methods are similar to those of Southern blot.

WESTERN BLOT TECHNIQUE (FIG. 12.24)

Western blots are used to determine the identity, size and abundance of specific **proteins** within a sample. This technique begins with sample lysate preparation from tissue or cell culture and separation on a polyacrylamide gel via electrophoresis. The separated proteins are then transferred to a nitrocellulose or polyvinylidene difluoride membrane, and the membrane is incubated with a blocking agent to prevent nonspecific binding, followed by incubation with a primary antibody to bind the desired protein. Different visualization methods are available such as colorimetric assays in which a coloured precipitate is produced, chemiluminescence and fluorescence.

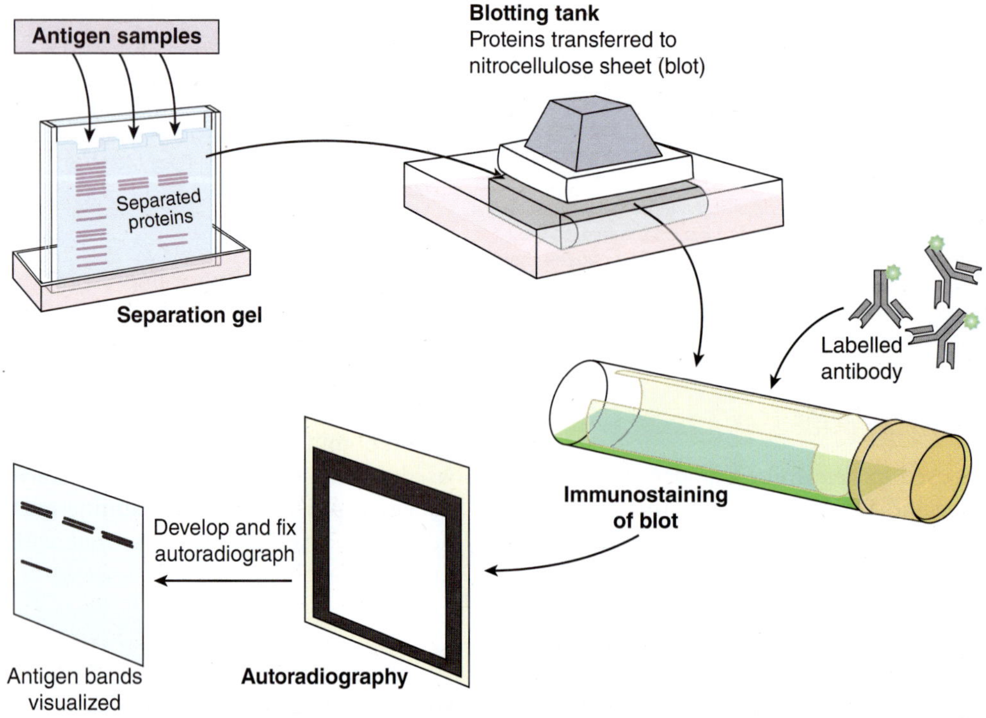

Fig. 12.24 Western blot technique. (*Source:* Reproduced from MyBioSource Learning Center.)

APPLICATIONS

Southern blot

- Identification of a single gene in a pool of DNA fragments
- Gene mapping
- Analysis of genetic patterns of DNA
- Detection of specific DNA sequences in a genome
- Study of gene deletions, duplications and mutations that cause various diseases

Northern blot

- Observation of the gene expression pattern between tissues, organs, developmental stages, environmental stress levels, pathogen infection and over the course of treatment.
- Identification of overexpression of oncogenes and downregulation of tumour suppressor genes in cancerous cells when compared to normal tissue.

Western blot

- Determine the size and amount of protein in a given sample.
- Disease diagnosis – detects antibody against virus or bacteria in serum.
- Western blotting technique is the confirmatory test for HIV infection. It detects anti-HIV antibody in a patient's serum.
- Useful to detect defective proteins, e.g. prion disease.

POLYMERASE CHAIN REACTION

PCR is a widely used method to rapidly make millions to billions of copies of a specific DNA sample, permitting scientists to take extremely small sample of DNA and amplify it to a large enough amount to study in detail. PCR is indicated when amplification of a known DNA sequence is desired.

PCR involves exponential amplification of a short segment of DNA carrying the mutation so that the mutations can be easily detected and measured by secondary sequence analysis.

Basic components of PCR are as follows:

- Template DNA strand
- Two DNA primers (oligonucleotide strand), which flank the area of interest
- DNA polymerase (heat resistant)
- Nucleotides – deoxynucleotide triphosphate (dATP, dTTP, dCTP, dGTP)
- Buffer solution

The three basic steps in each cycle of PCR are as follows (Fig. 12.25):

1. **Denaturation:** Double-stranded DNA is denatured by heat (90–95°C) to form single-stranded DNA.
2. **Annealing:** DNA primers attach to complementary bases on the single-stranded DNA at cooler temperature.

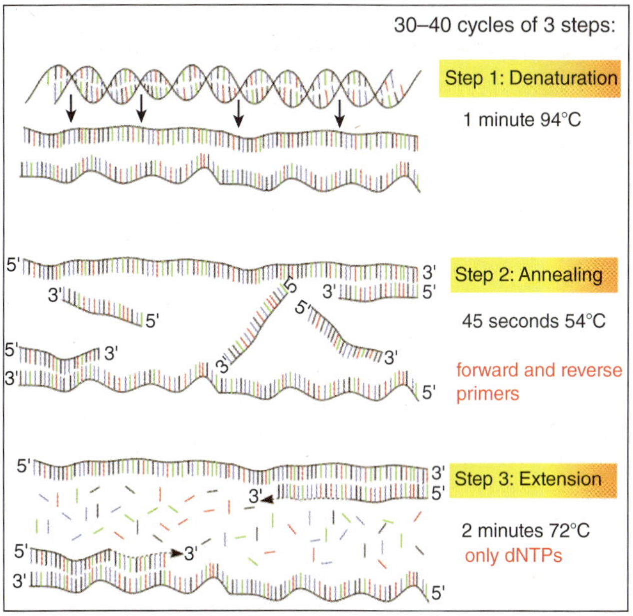

Fig. 12.25 Steps involved in PCR. (*Source:* https://users.ugent.be/~avierstr/principles/pcr.html)

3. **Extension:** DNA polymerase causes extension of the primer strand by adding nucleotides complementary to the template strand. This results in the formation of two identical copies of the template DNA strand.

At the end of each cycle, the number of copies doubles up. After 30–40 cycles, million copies of the original DNA sequence are formed (Fig. 12.26).

The PCR product can be used for **secondary analysis** such as electrophoresis or sequence studies.

a. **Electrophoresis:** It is used to determine the charge and migratory patterns of PCR products. Because all the copies are identical, these migrate simultaneously to form a single band during gel electrophoresis. If the primers are tagged with fluorescent label, capillary electrophoresis can be used to capture the fluorescence at the migrated location of PCR copies.
b. **Restriction fragment length analysis:** The PCR products are treated with restriction endonucleases, which cleave the DNA at specific sites. The length of the fragments is altered in case of mutation which affects the splicing sites.
c. **Sequence studies:**
   Sanger sequencing consists of the following steps:
   1. Production of DNA fragments of varying lengths tagged with fluorescent labels – using DNA polymerase, DNA primers, nucleotides and four fluorescent-labelled end nucleotides
   2. Capillary electrophoresis – to separate DNA fragments based on size
   3. Sequence studies of individual bands are analysed and compared with normal to detect the presence of mutations

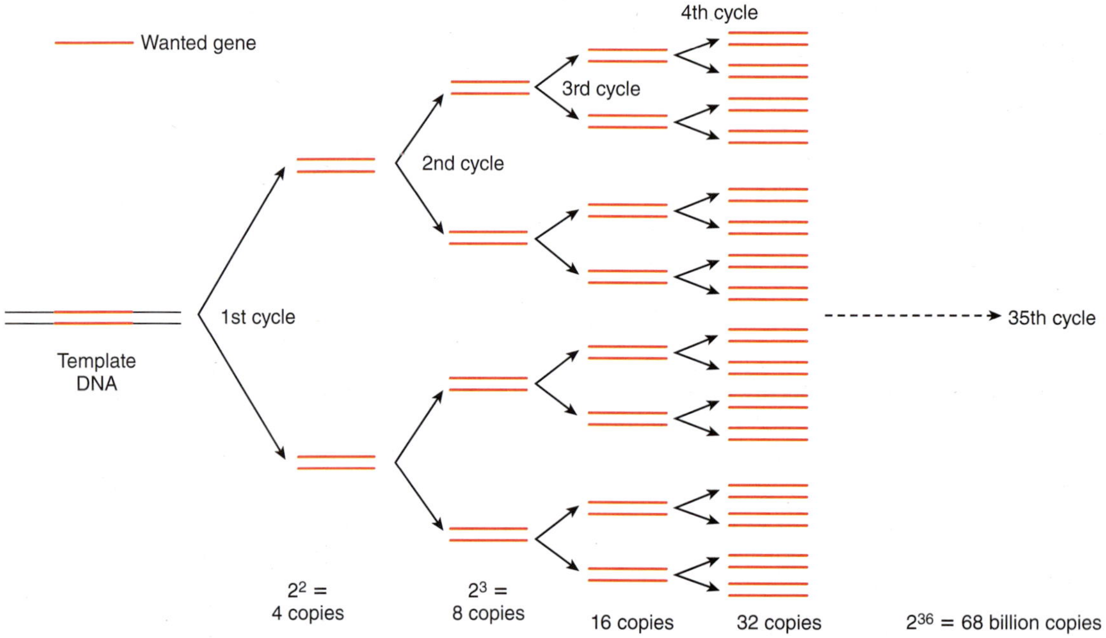

Fig. 12.26 Exponential amplification of the genome in PCR. (*Source:* https://users.ugent.be/;avierstr/principles/pcr.html)

Pyrosequencing: It is most often used to check for variants of a particular sequence. It involves release of a pyrophosphate molecule.

VARIOUS MODIFICATIONS OF POLYMERASE CHAIN REACTION

1. RT-PCR: It is used for the amplification of RNA sequence. It uses reverse transcriptase enzyme to convert RNA to DNA strand and then amplifies the fragment.
2. Nested PCR: Multiple DNA primers are used together to study different fragments in the same template strand.
3. Real-time PCR: It allows quantitation of PCR product with each cycle using a fluorescent dye intercalated to the DNA strand.

APPLICATIONS

Applications of polymerase chain reaction are given in Flowchart 12.1.

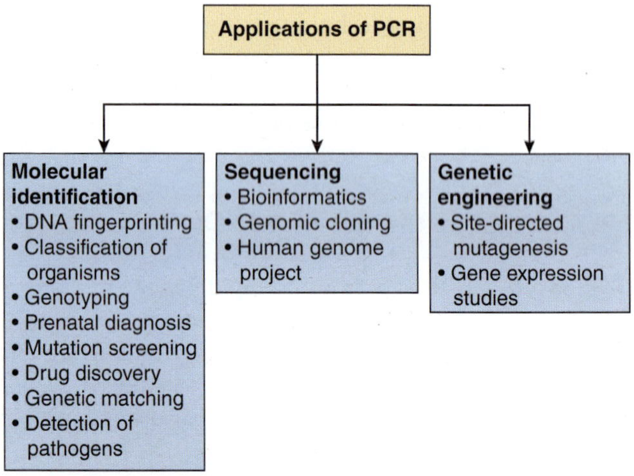

Flowchart 12.1 Applications of polymerase chain reaction.

NEXT-GENERATION SEQUENCING

Next-generation sequencing (NGS) is a group of DNA sequencing technologies that produce large amounts of sequence data in a massively parallel manner. It can sequence the entire human genome within a single day. It allows rapid sequencing at low cost.

PRINCIPLE

NGS uses the same principle as Sanger sequencing but on a microarray platform. This enables processing of millions of DNA fragments at the same time.

PROCEDURE

Basic steps of NGS are as follows:

1. **DNA fragmentation and spatial separation:** The DNA strand is enzymatically fragmented and ligated to an adaptor molecule. The fragments are spatially separated and attached to a platform in an array fashion with the help of an adaptor molecule. This is called library preparation.
2. **Amplification:** PCR amplification is done using fluorescent-labelled nucleotides. Four separately labelled nucleotides (A, T, C, G) are added one at a time in a controlled manner. Amplification is needed to generate enough signals for detection.
3. **Parallel sequencing:** Sequencing of all the amplified fragments in the microarray platform is done simultaneously, yielding massive data (180 billion base pairs).

4. **Bioinformatics:** The enormous data generated are analysed by using computer program and carefully interpreted.

TYPES OF NEXT-GENERATION SEQUENCING

- **Targeted sequencing:** Here one gene or a panel of genes is sequenced. This minimizes the time and expertise needed for interpretation and reporting.
- Whole exome sequencing: It is a type of targeted sequencing where only the protein-coding regions of the genome are sequenced.
- Whole genome sequencing: Here the entire human genome is sequenced.

USES OF NEXT-GENERATION SEQUENCING

- Diagnosis of common genetic diseases by using a panel of genes
- Diagnosis and treatment of orphan disease
- Cancer detection and treatment
- Microbiome analysis and screening for early markers of disease

DIFFERENCES BETWEEN SANGER SEQUENCING AND NGS

Features	Sanger Sequencing	NGS
General	Time-consuming, costly, accurate	Rapid, cheap, less accurate
Sequencing volume	Single DNA strand	Millions of short DNA fragments
Length of sequence amplified	Long: 700–1000 base long	Short: 100–200 base long
Test done in	Test tube	Microarray platform
Interpretation	Simple	Complex – requires advanced bioinformatics technologies

MULTIPLEX LIGATION-DEPENDENT PROBE AMPLIFICATION

Multiplex ligation-dependent probe amplification (MLPA) is a variation of multiplex PCR that allows amplification of multiple targets with only a single primer pair. It detects copy number changes at the molecular level, and software programs are used in the analysis. It is usually indicated in the detection of deletions and duplications of any size.

PRINCIPLE

It uses DNA hybridization, DNA ligation and PCR amplification.

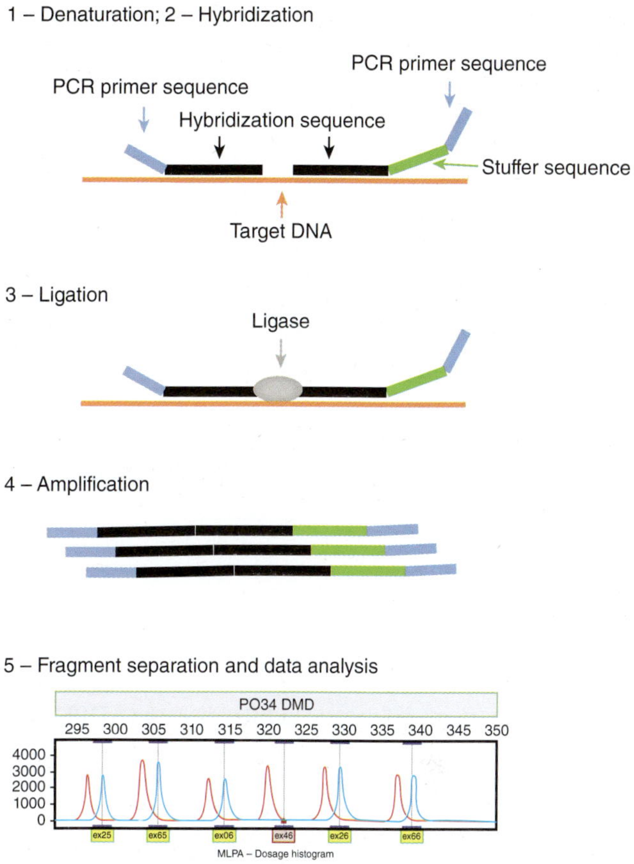

Fig. 12.27 Steps involved in multiplex ligation-dependent probe amplification.

PROCEDURE (FIG. 12.27)

1. **DNA hybridization:** A pair of DNA probes is used to hybridize with the target DNA strand. One of the probes from the pair contains a stuffer sequence, which is different in length for each target site. The length of the stuffer sequence changes between different probes, allowing multiplexing. Hence, each amplification product has a unique length.
2. **DNA ligation:** DNA ligase is used to covalently bind the probes.
3. **PCR amplification:** The ligated probe creates a template DNA strand, which is amplified by PCR.
4. **Analysis:** Quantification of the amplified DNA yields accurate information about the genetic material.
   Example:
   Homologous deletion of the gene produces no signal, whereas heterologous deletion produces 50% of signal when compared to normal.

LINKAGE ANALYSIS

Linkage analysis in simple words is a study aimed at establishing linkage between genes. The phenomenon of linkage is used to study the transmission of disease whose disease-specific genes/mutations are not known. Here, a known polymorphic marker close to the disease gene loci is used to study the transmission of the disease gene. Nowadays, linkage analysis serves as a way of gene hunting and genetic testing.

PRINCIPLE

The fundamental principle of linkage analysis is that any two genes in the same chromosome, situated close together, segregate together during meiosis and are transmitted together in the family degree.

Polymorphic markers commonly used for linkage analysis are as follows:

- Single nucleotide polymorphism (SNP)
- Repeat length polymorphism (microsatellite/minisatellite)

APPLICATIONS

1. For detection of disease-specific genes, which are difficult to sequence:
   - Detection of PKD gene for the diagnosis of autosomal dominant polycystic kidney disease (ADPKD) is done by using microsatellite linkage analysis.
   - It is found that the longest microsatellite allele is associated with PKD gene mutation.
   - Hence, checking the transmission pattern of longest microsatellite allele helps in detection of familial cases of ADPKD.
2. Genome-wide analysis
   a. SNP genotyping array technology is used to perform large-scale linkage studies of polygenic diseases (hypertension, diabetes mellitus).
   b. **Genome-wide association studies (GWAS):** Here, two large cohorts (groups) of participants with and without the disease to be studied are selected. Then their entire genome is checked for polymorphisms that are overrepresented in the diseased group. This helps to identify the region of the genome harbouring the disease susceptibility genes. The exact gene responsible can be identified by further research.

GWAS can be used to identify genes that modulate physical traits in the population (height, weight, hair, eye colour, etc.).

TISSUE MICROARRAY

Tissue microarray is a recent innovation in the field of pathology which is used in the detection of unknown genetic abnormalities by simultaneous assessment of the entire genome by using a microarray (Fig. 12.28).

Microarray is a glass slide with thousands of premarked slots. Each slot is coated with a DNA probe that spans the entire genome at a regular interval. Microarray is referred to as gene chip or DNA chip. The difference between traditional method and the tissue microarray is shown in Fig. 12.29.

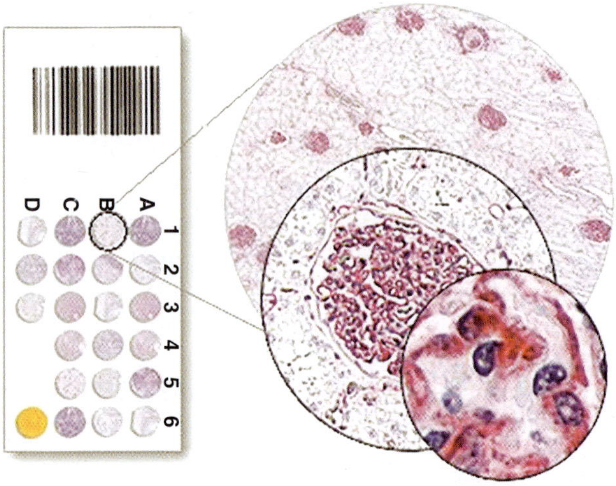

Fig. 12.28 Tissue microarray, a sample. (*Source:* https://usbiolab.com/tissue-array)

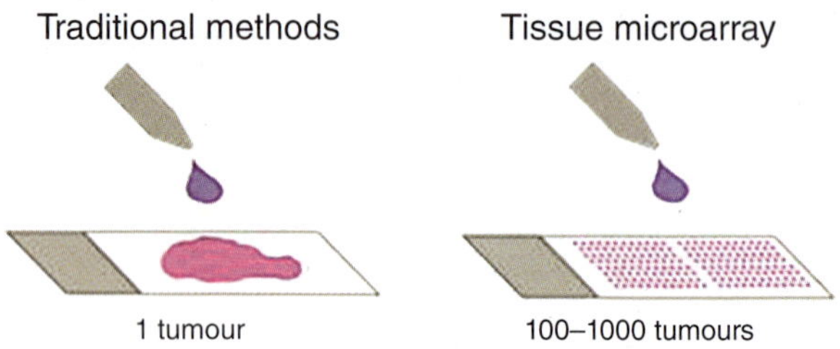

Fig. 12.29 Traditional methods versus tissue microarray.

TYPES

1. Array-based comparative genomic hybridization (array CGH)
2. SNP genotyping arrays

Array Comparative Genomic Hybridization

The genetic sequences are compared between test DNA and normal reference DNA for detecting genetic alteration.

Procedure

1. Labelling: Both test DNA and reference DNA are labelled with different coloured fluorescent dyes (red for test and green for control).
2. Cohybridization of test DNA and reference DNA in DNA arrays.
3. Analysis: At each slot, the binding of DNA probes with test DNA and the reference sample is compared.
   Yellow colour in the slots: Equal binding of test DNA and the reference probe.
   Skewing towards red colour: Duplication or gain of function at the particular probe spot.
   Skewing towards green colour: Deletion or loss of function at the particular probe spot.

Uses: Accurate determination of copy number variations across the genome.

Single Nucleotide Polymorphism Genotyping Arrays

Principle It uses the same concept as array CGH, but the probes are designed to identify the SNP sites across the genome.

Uses

- To identify SNP across the genome
- To detect copy number variations in paediatric patients with suspected (structural) chromosomal abnormality and normal karyotype
- To conduct genome-wide association studies

DIGITAL PATHOLOGY

The aim of technological advances in diagnostic pathology is to provide improved quality patient care. Digital pathology, with its ready access to pathologists, ensures better patient care.

EVOLUTION OF DIGITAL PATHOLOGY

The trajectory of diagnostic pathology began with the microscope, glass slides and staining techniques, progressing to multiheaded immunofluorescence and electron microscopes, where the glass slides with tissues are viewed for diagnosis.

Digital pathology has evolved since the 1990s. During and after the COVID era, digital pathology has proven to be a boon to medical consultants and patients alike. It has replaced the traditional microscopic viewing of glass slides and employs scanned digital images that can be accessed through the internet.

PRINCIPLE

What is digital pathology?

Glass slides are digitized, and the digitized slides with the data can be stored on servers and in clouds, which can be accessed by pathologists in distant geographical areas. This makes it possible to obtain expert opinions from around the globe within a few hours, benefiting patients. This eliminates the difficult task of transporting glass slides to distant sites, which involves arduous logistics.

PROCEDURE

How can a glass slide be digitized?

The basic requirement for digitizing glass slides is whole-slide imaging scanners (Fig. 12.30A). The slides are scanned by the scanners, and the data are stored in servers and clouds. The digitized slides can be viewed on monitors or cellphone screens through the internet (Fig. 12.30B).

APPLICATIONS

- Digital pathology, coupled with artificial intelligence algorithms, aids in organizing samples, cell counting, image analysis and counting mitosis, thereby expediting diagnosis.
- Pathologists can now allocate more time to important tasks such as diagnosis, research and education.

ADVANTAGES

- Digital pathology provides images with very high resolution, enabling viewing at desired focus and magnification.
- Remote work is now possible for pathologists in areas with fewer pathologists.
- Expert opinions can be obtained without hassle, avoiding time delays.
- Clinicopathological conferences can cover large areas, facilitating collaboration with other specialty consultants.
- Images can be annotated for undergraduate and postgraduate classes.

LIMITATIONS

- Data usage for downloading digitized images is high.
- Stable and high-speed internet access is required, posing concerns in rural areas.
- Scanners are expensive, and not all centres can afford them.

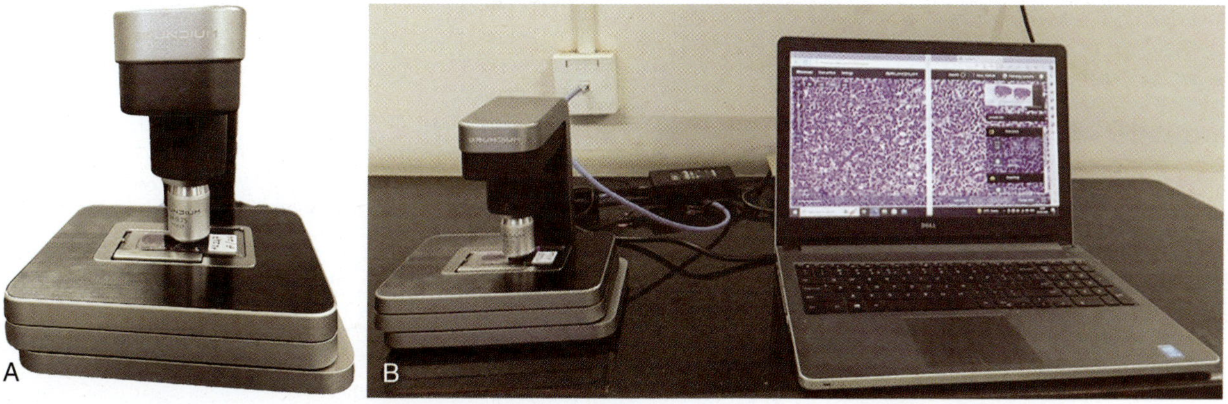

Fig. 12.30 (A) Whole-slide imaging scanner. (B) Digitized images.

- Familiarity with newer technologies is mandatory and requires practice.

The future of diagnostic pathology is heavily reliant on modern technological advances, with digital pathology coupled with artificial intelligence leading the way. Digital pathology, with its numerous advantages, is here to stay, promising better health care.

SELF-ASSESSMENT

Multiple Choice Questions

1. A pathologist uses immunohistochemistry (IHC) to identify the presence of specific tumour markers. Which component is essential in the IHC technique for visualizing the antigen-antibody interaction?
   A. Fluorophore
   B. Chromogen
   C. Electrophoresis gel
   D. PCR primers
2. In a case of nephrotic syndrome, electron microscopy is employed to study the glomerular filtration membrane. What is the main advantage of using electron microscopy in this scenario?
   A. High throughput
   B. Real-time analysis
   C. High-resolution imaging
   D. Rapid processing time
3. During a frozen section procedure, a surgeon awaits rapid diagnostic information for intraoperative decision-making. What is the primary purpose of this technique?
   A. Detailed molecular analysis
   B. Long-term storage of tissue samples
   C. Immediate microscopic examination of a specimen
   D. Identifying genetic mutations
4. Flow cytometry is used for the analysis of a blood sample. What characteristic of the cells is primarily analysed using this technique?
   A. Morphology under a light microscope
   B. Size and granularity by light scattering
   C. Histological staining patterns
   D. Tissue architecture
5. A patient's biopsy is analysed using fluorescence in situ hybridization (FISH) to detect chromosomal abnormalities. What is FISH primarily used to identify?
   A. Protein expressions
   B. DNA sequences on chromosomes
   C. RNA sequences
   D. Enzymatic activity
6. In assessing a tumour's proliferative index, a pathologist uses Ki-67 marker in IHC. What does a high Ki-67 index indicate about the tumour?
   A. Low malignancy potential
   B. High rate of cell division
   C. Hormonal responsiveness
   D. Viral infection association
7. A researcher uses PCR to amplify a segment of DNA. What is the purpose of the annealing step in PCR?
   A. Denaturing the DNA strands
   B. Extending the new DNA strand
   C. Attaching primers to the template DNA
   D. Visualizing the DNA fragments
8. In a case of suspected lymphoma, a pathologist utilizes flow cytometry. What aspect of the cells is most crucial for the diagnosis in this scenario?
   A. Mitochondrial DNA
   B. Cell surface markers
   C. Cytoplasmic enzymes
   D. Nuclear morphology
9. A patient with suspected mesothelioma undergoes an examination by using electron microscopy. What key feature would support the diagnosis?
   A. Presence of neurosecretory granules
   B. Long villi on mesothelial cells
   C. Amyloid deposits
   D. Lipid accumulation
10. In a study of gene expression, northern blotting is used. What is this technique primarily used to analyse?
    A. DNA fragmentation patterns
    B. RNA size and abundance
    C. Protein folding structures
    D. Enzyme kinetics
11. A Southern blot is performed to detect gene mutations. What type of genetic material is analysed using this technique?
    A. mRNA
    B. tRNA
    C. DNA
    D. Proteins
12. A laboratory uses next-generation sequencing (NGS) for a patient's genetic analysis. What is the primary advantage of NGS over traditional sequencing methods?
    A. Lower cost per base sequenced
    B. Shorter time for protein expression analysis
    C. Ability to visualize chromosomes
    D. Simplicity in sample preparation
13. In assessing a tumour for targeted therapy options, a pathologist uses western blotting to detect specific proteins. What does this technique primarily identify?
    A. Gene mutations
    B. Protein size and presence
    C. RNA transcription levels
    D. Chromosomal anomalies
14. For detecting subtle copy number changes in a patient's genome, which technique would be the most appropriate?
    A. PCR
    B. Electrophoresis
    C. MLPA
    D. Immunofluorescence
15. During a linkage analysis, what is primarily being investigated?
    A. The physical location of genes on a chromosome
    B. The relationship between different proteins
    C. The association between genetic markers and diseases
    D. The structural differences in DNA

Answers

1. (B); 2. (C); 3. (C); 4. (B); 5. (B); 6. (B); 7. (C); 8. (B); 9. (B); 10. (B); 11. (C); 12. (A); 13. (B); 14. (C); 15. (C).

Self-Assessment Questions

1. A pathologist receives a biopsy sample from a patient with a suspected breast tumour. The clinical team is particularly interested in determining the hormonal receptor status of the tumour. Describe the process the pathologist would use to apply immunohistochemistry (IHC) for identifying oestrogen and progesterone receptors in the tissue sample. Include details about the types of antibodies used and how the results would inform treatment decisions.
2. A nephrologist encounters a case of a patient with suspected glomerular disease. The standard light microscopy has not provided conclusive results. The nephrologist decides to refer the case for electron microscopy analysis. Explain how electron microscopy can contribute to the diagnosis of glomerular diseases and what specific ultrastructural details the nephrologist should expect to see in conditions like minimal change disease or focal segmental glomerulosclerosis.
3. A haematologist is evaluating a patient with enlarged lymph nodes and a high white blood cell count. To determine the type of lymphoma, a sample is sent for flow cytometry analysis. Outline the steps involved in flow cytometry and discuss how this technique helps in differentiating between various types of lymphomas based on cell surface markers.
4. A geneticist is presented with a case of a child with developmental delays and multiple congenital anomalies. Suspecting a chromosomal abnormality, the geneticist orders a fluorescence in situ hybridization (FISH) test. Describe the FISH technique and explain how it can be used to identify specific chromosomal abnormalities, such as deletions or duplications, that might be responsible for the child's condition.
5. In a clinical setting, a patient presents with symptoms suggestive of a viral infection. The infectious disease specialist decides to utilize PCR for rapid identification of the viral pathogen. Describe the PCR process, focusing on how this technique can amplify specific segments of viral DNA or RNA, and how it aids in the rapid and precise diagnosis of viral infections.
6. A researcher is studying a form of hereditary cancer. To better understand the genetic basis of the disease, they decide to use next-generation sequencing (NGS). Detail the process of NGS and discuss how it can be used to analyse the entire genome of cancer patients, leading to insights into genetic mutations and variations that contribute to the cancer's development and progression.

Topics for Self-Directed Learning

1. Epigenetics
2. Applications of RT-PCR
3. Quantiferon gold
4. Nucleic acid amplification test
5. ELISA
6. Phase-contrast microscopy
7. Laser capture microdissection
8. Morphometry

13 Blood Vessels

Indhu Kannan

PA 27.1 Distinguish arteriosclerosis from atherosclerosis. Describe the pathogenesis and pathology of various causes and types of **arteriosclerosis.**

PA 27.2 Describe the aetiology, dynamics, pathology types and complications of **aneurysms** including aortic aneurysms.

CHAPTER OUTLINE

OVERVIEW OF VASCULAR SYSTEM

Blood vessels are a network of channels or conduits responsible for the dynamic transportation of blood and blood products to every cell in the body. The vascular network begins at the aortic valve, courses the entire body and ends with the openings of the venae cavae into the right atrium. Vascular disease refers to any abnormal condition of the blood vessels. Pathologies concerning this vast network can cause a spectrum of severe disability and death.

Before exploring the details of the pathology, let us briefly discuss the components of vessels and their function.

VASCULAR STRUCTURE AND FUNCTION

In general, the blood vessels of the circulatory system may be broken down into five different types: The arteries and arterioles comprising the arterial system, the veins and the venules constituting the venous system and the capillaries that connect the arterioles and the venules forming the vascular bed within each organ (Fig. 13.1). The structure of each of these vessels is naturally customized to suit their individual function and anatomic relationships. Despite their varied functions, blood vessels, except the capillaries, share a common trilaminar structure composed of the tunica intima, tunica media and tunica adventitia.

- **Tunica intima**: The innermost layer of the vessel wall is primarily defined by a single layer of endothelial cells resting upon an incomplete basement membrane, also known as the extracellular matrix. The intima is enveloped by the internal elastic membrane, a layer of elastic fibres separating it from the media. It is thickest in the arterial system, specifically the muscular arteries and attenuated throughout the entire venous system. The integrity of the endothelial layer is critical as any damage can lead to initiation of thrombus formation at that site.

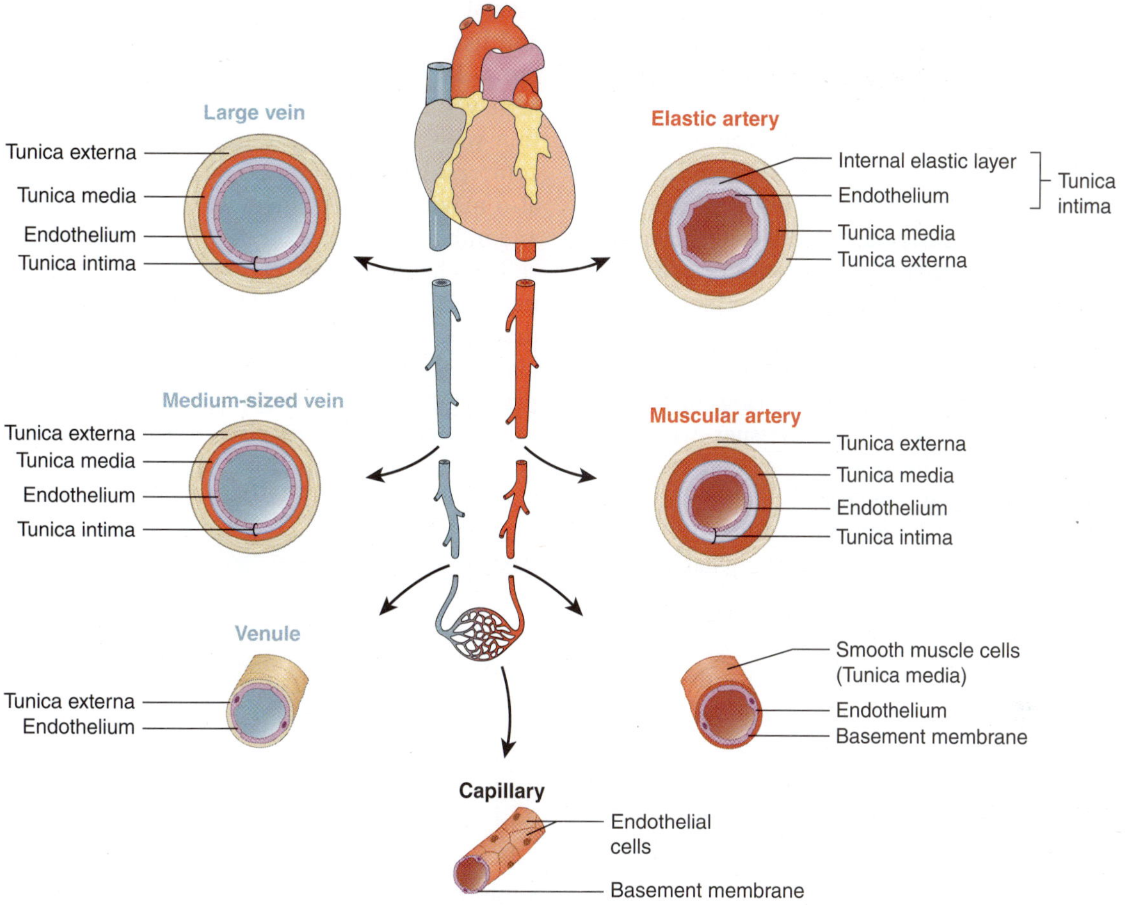

Fig. 13.1 Schematic representation of the vascular system eliciting the functional and structural interrelationship of the different classes of blood vessels.

- **Tunica media**: The middle layer of the vessel wall is composed of smooth muscle cells and elastic fibres. Blood flows within the arteries at very high pressure, and hence the tunica media is composed of multiple layers of smooth muscle cells that are arranged concentrically to help propel the blood to the tissues. The venous system that operates at a relatively lower pressure has a relatively thinner media with smooth muscle cells arranged haphazardly. Externally, the tunica media is enveloped by an external elastic membrane that separates the media from the adventitia.
- **Tunica adventitia:** It is the outermost layer composed entirely of connective tissue fibres. This layer anchors the vasa vasorum, 'vessels of the vessels', a vascular bed designed to perfuse the vessel wall itself. These are composed of small arterioles that perfuse the outer two-thirds of the media and adventitia, whereas the tunica intima and inner third of the media are nourished by direct diffusion from the blood present within the lumen. The adventitia is also responsible for the vessel integrity and takes up most part of the venous wall, especially in the larger veins. Thus, the tunics are optimized according to their function.

Elastic arteries: These are the largest arteries and lie closest to the heart, e.g. aorta, subclavian, common carotid and major pulmonary artery. The media of these arteries contains large amount of elastin fibres to allow expansion during ventricular systole and passive recoil during diastole. Ageing-related degeneration of these central elastic arteries decreases the compliance leading to '**arterial stiffness**'. This often preludes hypertension and cardiovascular diseases (CVDs).

Muscular arteries: These are branches of elastic artery. Examples include coronary, renal and femoral arteries. These vessels function to precisely control and regulate the blood flow to the organs. Their tunica media is composed of several layers of predominantly smooth muscle fibres arranged in concentric fashion that allow them to undergo vasoconstriction and vasodilation on stimulation by the autonomic nervous system and local metabolic factors, according to the demand of the organ they supply.

Arterioles: The importance of the arterioles is that they are key players in offering physical resistance to blood flow. With a small lumen (20–100 μm), they help in slowing down or resisting blood flow, and thus cause a substantial drop in blood pressure (BP). Owing to this effort, they are sometimes referred to as resistance vessels. The muscle fibres in arterioles comprise one or two layers of smooth muscle cells. The external elastic lamina is absent, and the adventitia is also thinned out.

Capillaries: These are extremely narrow segments of the vasculature, some just about the size of an RBC (7–8 μm). Capillaries are grouped together to form capillary beds that perfuse organs and tissues. Blood flows slowest within the capillaries also because of their small cross-sectional area, enabling the exchange of gases, nutrients, hormones and wastes between the bloodstream and the tissues. To further facilitate their function, the vessel wall is composed of only endothelium surrounded by connective tissue and a few pericytes (Fig. 13.4). Pericytes are isolated contractile cells. Tissues with high metabolic rate such as the myocardium and the brain have the richest density of capillaries.

Capillaries can be divided into three different types on the basis of the morphology of their endothelial layer:

- ***Continuous capillaries*** have an uninterrupted endothelium capable of performing transcytosis. These capillaries are present in muscle, connective tissue, skin, lung and central nervous system. In the nervous system particularly, these tight junctions forming the blood–brain barrier are important because they limit the movement of cells, toxins and large molecules between the blood and the cerebrospinal fluid.
- ***Fenestrated capillaries*** have circular pores in the capillary wall but with a continuous basal lamina. These are found in locations of metabolic absorption such as renal glomeruli, intestinal villi, pancreas and endocrine glands.
- ***Discontinuous capillaries*** also referred to as sinusoidal capillaries have large gaps between the endothelial cells as well as a discontinuous basement membrane. Such capillaries allow the passage and macromolecules and even blood cells causing continuous exchange. Thus, these sinusoids are found in the liver and sites of blood formation and lymphoid organs.

From the capillaries, the blood flows into the **postcapillary venules** that join multiple capillaries exiting from a capillary bed. The blood then flows into **small veins** followed by the medium veins. Characteristically, **medium veins** have semilunar valves formed by intimal infoldings projecting into the lumen. These one-way valves help to prevent retrograde flow of blood and particularly predominant in the lower extremities. A common disorder that takes reference here is, *varicose veins*, that arises when defective valves allow blood to accumulate within the veins, causing them to distend and become visibly tortuous. Medium veins have a much thinner tunica media than is seen in parallel arteries. The adventitia is the predominant layer in the medium veins comprising collagen and elastin fibres.

Following are the **large veins:** The portal vein, inferior vena cava and superior vena cava. They lack a clear demarcation between the tunica intima and tunica media, and like medium veins, they contain a thick tunica externa. These large veins are capable of distending to hold large volumes of blood at any given time. The relatively thin walls of veins make them far more distensible and compressible than arteries of their corresponding size also making them vulnerable to infiltration by tumours and inflammation.

Lymphatics are also endothelium-lined vascular channels, relatively thin walled, that are responsible for the drainage of lymph from the organs and the interstitium via the thoracic duct to the lymph nodes. Though the primary function of the lymph channels is to transport inflammatory cells, they also serve to disseminate tumour cells and infectious microbes to distant sites.

VESSEL WALL RESPONSE TO INJURY

The endothelial cells have a pivotal role in regulating vessel stability and in maintaining vascular homeostasis. Under resting conditions, the endothelial cells inertly inhibit excessive platelet aggregation to maintain blood fluidity, and promote fibrinolysis. The quiescent endothelium is a potent source of antioxidant enzymes and synthesizes TGF-1β that inhibits leucocyte adherence maintaining an anti-inflammatory status. Endothelium-derived factors produce a balance of vasoconstrictive and vasodilatory effects that coordinate vascular tone. In addition, endothelial cells also regulate smooth muscle cell proliferation, vascular growth and remodelling. This nonadhesive, nonthrombogenic state of the physiological endothelium is maintained most importantly by the laminar flow of blood along with the other various chemical mediators mentioned in Fig. 13.2.

Located strategically at the interface of the bloodstream and the vessel wall, the endothelial cells are constantly exposed to countless number of stimuli such as bacterial products, complement proteins, hypoxia, turbulent blood flow, oxidative stress, advanced glycation end products in diabetes and irritants such as tobacco. When the impact tips the fine homeostatic balance, the endothelial cells undergo dramatic functional modifications, a process known as **endothelial cell activation.** The exact mechanism by which endothelial cells become 'active' is multifactorial, but has been postulated to be predominantly due to oxidative stress and reduced nitric oxide (NO) availability.

The core changes that occur in the 'active endothelial cells' include a transition from a quiescent to **prothrombotic, proinflammatory phenotype, increased vascular permeability, leucocyte recruitment and upregulation of HLA molecules** (Fig. 13.3).

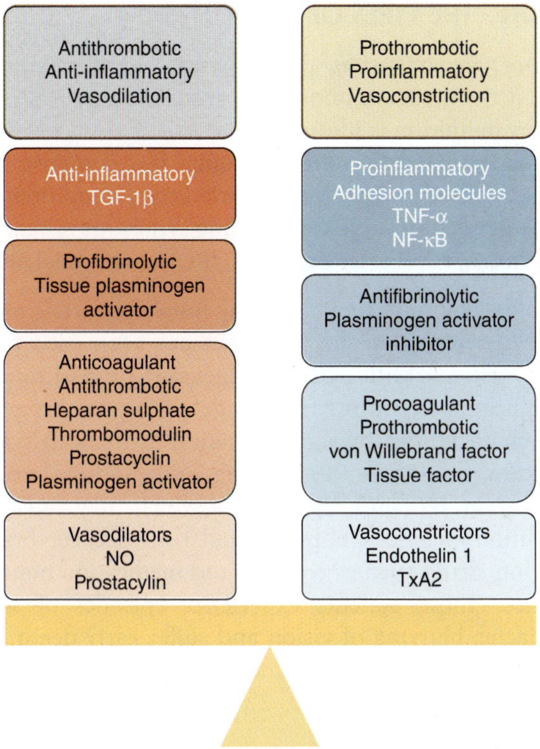

Fig. 13.2 Endothelial mediators of vascular homeostasis.

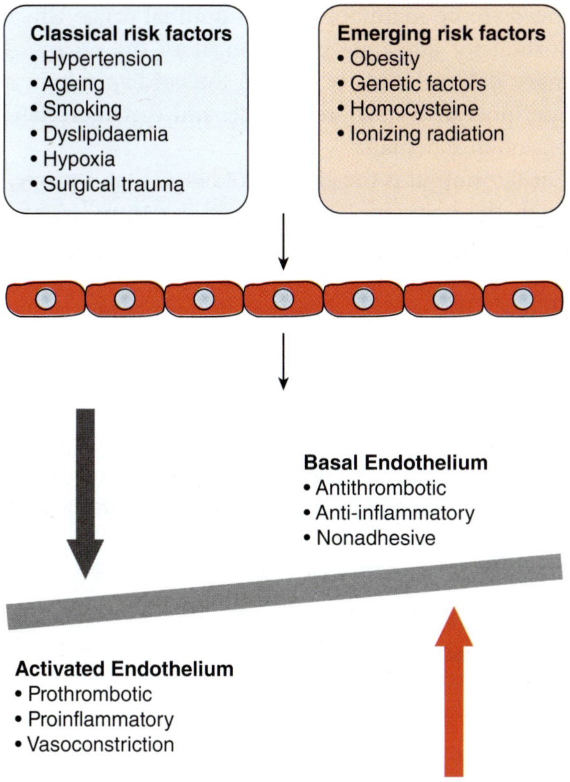

Fig. 13.3 Fundamentals of basic and activated endothelium.

Endothelial dysfunction refers to the diverse syndromes that involve the switch over of the basal endothelium to an active endothelium. The fluctuating imbalances in the endothelial mediators result in altering the permeability allowing transport of plasma proteins, transendothelial migration of leucocytes, expression of adhesion molecules for the inflammatory cells and growth factors for endothelial proliferation. Endothelial dysfunction has been linked to a variety of disease states, including atherosclerosis, coronary artery disease (CAD), hypertension and a myriad of consequences (Fig. 13.4). Although several forms of endothelial dysfunction are rapid in onset and reversible, other forms have delayed onset and involve genetic alterations.

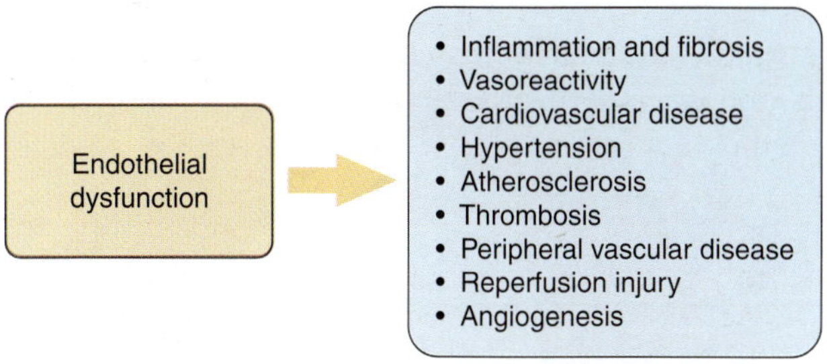

Fig. 13.4 Consequences of endothelial dysfunction.

The vascular smooth muscle cells, like the endothelial cells, are responsive to stimuli and undergo 'activation'. In health, vascular smooth muscle cells are specialized with a contractile phenotype composed of smooth muscle actin to maintain the BP amidst the pulsatile strain. Vascular injury causing endothelial dysfunction, along with endothelial-derived growth factors, and cytokines promote the phenotypic switch from contractile to an activated state. On activation, the smooth muscle cells attain the ability to migrate to the intima, proliferate and synthesize extracellular matrix. The resultant intimal hyperplasia is also referred to as neointima or intimal thickening. Endothelial cells migrate from adjacent uninjured areas or are recruited from the endothelial cell progenitor (EPC) pool in the bone marrow and typically cover the luminal surface of the **neointima.** ***Intimal thickening is the stereotypical response of the vessel walls to any insult.***

Regrowth of the endothelium appears to downregulate intimal smooth muscle cell proliferation. In most outcomes of the healing process, the luminal area is patent and only rarely, the intimal thickening causes obstruction with downstream ischaemia. However, once the endothelial cells normalize, the smooth muscle cells reverse to a nonproliferative state (Fig. 13.5).

Intimal thickening has a physiological role as well, most notably in the closing of the ductus arteriosus at birth. It is involved in a number of known organ pathologies such as pulmonary hypertension and atherosclerosis, and may also be a sequalae of procedures such as balloon angioplasty and stenting.

HYPERTENSIVE VASCULAR DISEASE

BP is the measure of the force generated by the blood pushing against the walls of blood vessels (arteries) during

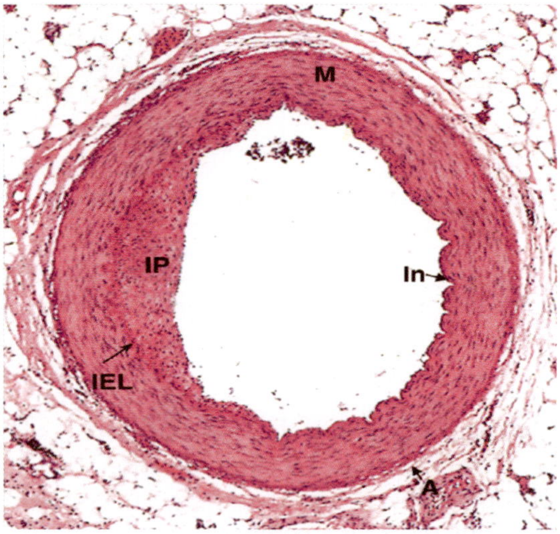

Fig. 13.5 A small artery with eccentric intimal hyperplasia. (In) represents the unremarkable intima. The media is denoted by M. Note the internal elastic lamina (IEL) clearly defined from the intimal proliferation (IP). (*Source:* From Geraldine O'Dowd, Sarah Bell and Sylvia Wright. Atherosclerosis. In Wheater's Pathology: A Text, Atlas, and Review of Histopathology. 6th edition. Elsevier 2020.)

each systole (systolic BP) and diastole (diastolic BP). It is determined primarily by the amount of blood pumped by the heart and the amount of resistance that hampers the blood flow. Thus, higher the pressure, more will be the force exerted by the heart to propel the blood.

Hypertension or raised BP is a serious medical condition and remains one of the most significant causes of mortality worldwide. According to WHO, over 1.13 billion people suffer from hypertension mostly in the middle- and low-income countries. On the basis of data from the study, 90% of people older than 55 years are certain to develop hypertension during their lifetime.

Hypertension is characterized by a sustained diastolic pressure more than 80 mm Hg or sustained systolic pressure more than 130 mm Hg. Associated complications of hypertension include CVD, atherosclerosis, kidney disease, diabetes mellitus, being the most significant. Also, incidental prevalence of metabolic syndrome, preeclampsia, erectile dysfunction and eye disease are on record. Broadly, hypertension increases chances of end-organ damage, whereas hypotension (low BP) results in poor perfusion of the organs.

The pathophysiology of hypertension over years has been linked to environmental and genetic factors. Lifestyle habits that include obesity, physical inactivity, chronic stress and excess sodium intake have been attributed to hypertension. Similarly, familial aggregation of hypertension is now a well-recognized phenomenon. Undoubtedly, evidence-based data suggest that reducing modifiable risk factors such as unhealthy diets, physical inactivity, consumption of tobacco and alcohol and obesity, is the best way to prevent hypertension and its accompanying complications.

AMONG THE TYPES OF HYPERTENSION

Primary hypertension, also known as essential hypertension, is the most common type, accounting to 90%−95% and by definition is idiopathic.

Secondary hypertension is a much less common form (<5%) caused by an identifiable primary condition such as primary aldosteronism, Cushing syndrome, pheochromocytoma, renal artery stenosis, tumours or renal failure.

A less common type requiring more concern is ***malignant hypertension***, the term that has been used to describe patients with extremely elevated BP and multiple complications (end-organ damage) with poor prognosis. It is characterized by rapid elevation of BP with systolic pressure more than 180 mm Hg, and diastolic pressure more than 120 mm Hg. Factors which may cause this condition include SLE, renovascular disease, cerebral infarction, drugs such as cocaine, and medication noncompliance. These patients experience episodes of severe headache, blurring of vision and suffer early death from cerebral and brainstem haemorrhages. If left untreated, it may lead to death within 1–2 years.

BLOOD PRESSURE REGULATION

BP needs to be maintained at an optimal range which is important for adequate perfusion of all the organs. The primary determinants of BP are the cardiac output and the peripheral vascular resistance, and the interrelationship is often schematic.

Cardiac output is the amount of blood that is propelled through the heart in 1 minute and is controlled by the stroke volume and the heart rate. Peripheral resistance reflects the change in vessel diameter and the viscosity of the blood. The central dictation of peripheral resistance occurs at the level of the arterioles because they account for the greatest pressure drop and are the compliance vessels that can respond to the changes in resistance by selectively constricting or relaxing. The BP fluctuates moment to moment to adapt to the demands of the body, such as in exercise, change in body position or emotional disturbances. Such regulation is achieved by the interdependent adjustments of the above-described parameters through regulatory mechanisms showed in Fig. 13.5.

Local factors: As we already know, the endothelial cells regulate vascular tone by a fine balance of local vasoconstrictive and vasodilatory agents. Endothelial dysfunction is one of the important precipitating factors for hypertension because it impairs the vasomotor responses and promotes a proinflammatory phenotype.

Neural mechanism: The vasomotor and cardiac control centres for the regulation of BP are located in the medulla. Stretch-sensitive nerve endings, called baroreceptors, are located on the carotid artery and the aortic arch. These sensors respond strategically to changes in the BP. The stretching of the arterial wall sends prompt signals to the control centres in the brainstem to affect appropriate sympathetic or parasympathetic nerve impulses to balance vascular and muscle tone. Sympathetic activity in instances of drop in pressure effectively cause arteriolar vasoconstriction and increase in heart rate. Conversely, when the BP rises, parasympathetic response is accelerated with inhibition of sympathetic activity leading to vasodilation and decrease in heart rate. In addition to the baroreceptors, chemoreceptors are chemosensitive cells that monitor carbon dioxide and hydrogen ion (pH) levels, and also signal the vasomotor centre for necessary action.

Hormonal factors: The endocrine control over BP is multifold. Among the most considerable are the catecholamines, epinephrine and norepinephrine released by the adrenal medulla in instances such as exercise or during a 'fight-or-flight' response. When the sympathetic system is activated, catecholamines exert vasoconstrictive effects through the α-adrenergic receptors on the smooth muscle cells. Also, note that catecholamines meditate dilator responses through the β_2 receptors. Aldosterone also secreted from the adrenal glands takes part in the renin–angiotensin system (described in detail below). Vasopressin is secreted from the posterior pituitary usually in response to significant blood or fluid loss. To restore the blood volume, vasopressin works by increasing the reabsorption of water in the kidney and vasoconstriction. Counteractively, when the BP raises because of volume overload, the cardiac myocytes release atrial natriuretic peptide (ANP), a peptide hormone. ANP instantly increases the renal excretion of salt and water, increases the vascular permeability and systemic vasodilation, all of which contribute to lower the BP (Fig. 13.6).

Interestingly, the resistance vessels also self-regulate themselves to the changes in the BP by a process known as autoregulation. This can be explained by two responses. The myogenic response, an intrinsic property of the vascular smooth muscle triggers passive stretching of the vessel wall when BP abruptly rises. Similarly, when the BP falls, vascular smooth muscles contract to maintain steady state flow. Secondly, the metabolic mediator, oxygen, which is when insufficient causes vasodilation to improve the blood flow to the particular organ. Autoregulation protects most of the important organ systems, including the coronary, cerebral and renal blood flow.

These mechanisms work coordinately for **short-term regulation** of BP and are also the saviours in life-threatening conditions such as acute blood loss.

Baroreceptors cannot regulate BP for long because they reset themselves once BP returns to normal. **Long-term regulation** of pressure is carried out by many physiological mechanisms, the most significant being the **renin–angiotensin–aldosterone system** (Fig. 13.7).

Renin is an initiative enzyme for the renin–angiotensin system that is synthesized and released by the granular

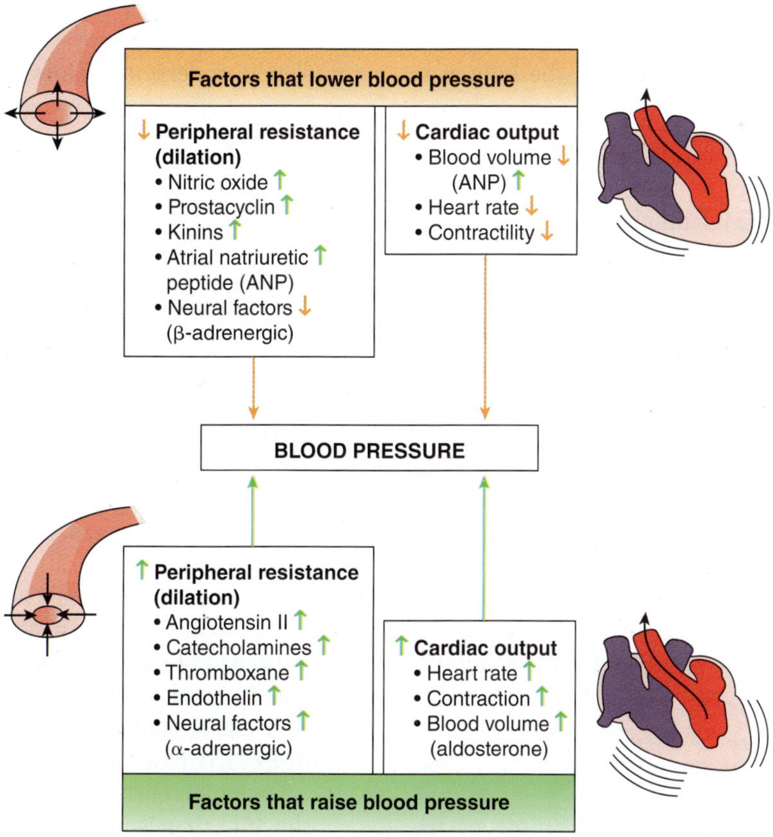

Fig. 13.6 Mediators in regulation of blood pressure.

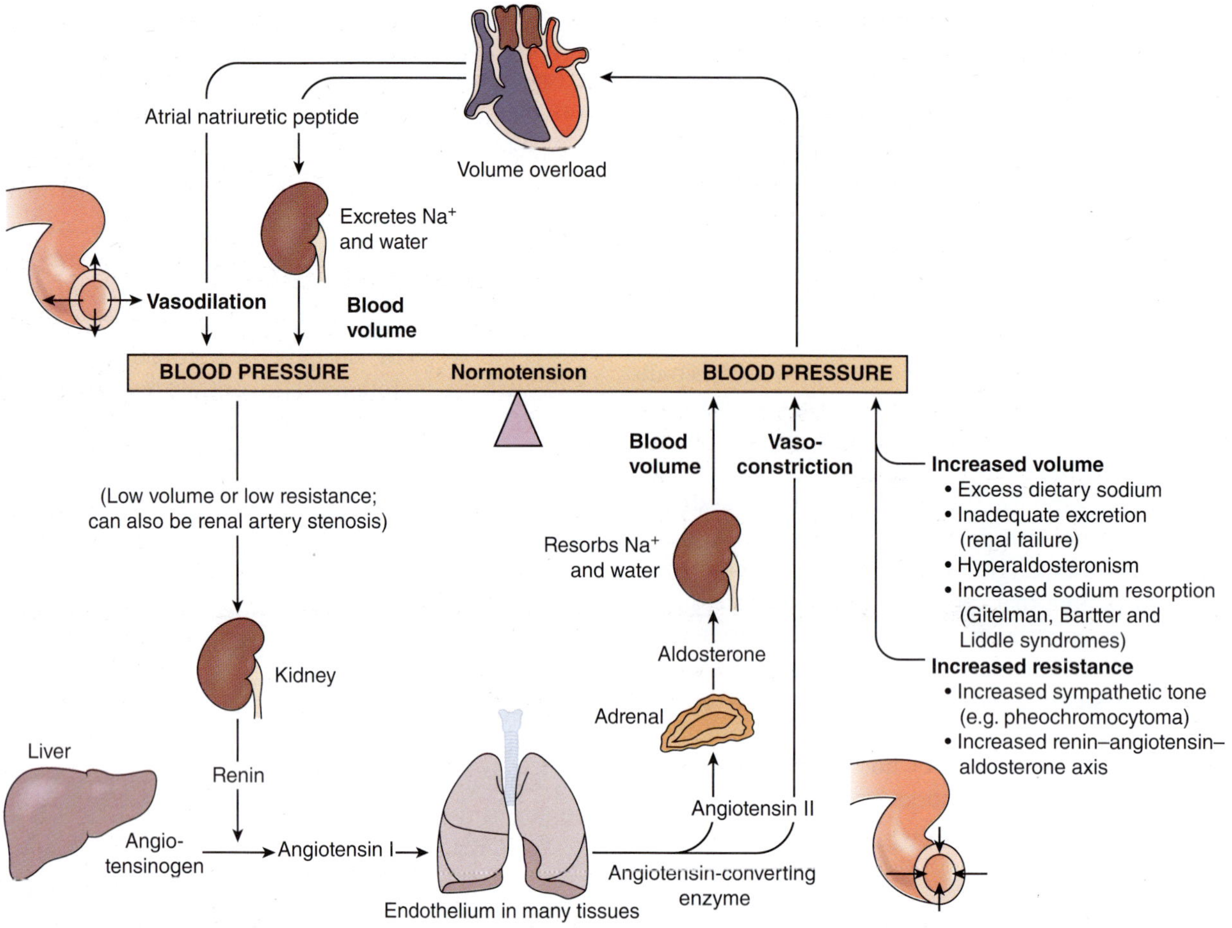

Fig. 13.7 Long-term regulation of blood pressure with the working physiological model of the renin–angiotensin system.

cells of the *juxtaglomerular apparatus* in the kidney in response to

- Low blood volume
- Hypotension
- Sympathetic nervous stimulation
- Reduced sodium levels in the distal convoluted tubule
- Decreased renal perfusion

Renin enables the conversion of angiotensinogen that is released by the liver to angiotensin I, which is further converted to angiotensin II by using angiotensin-converting enzyme (ACE) that is found in the lungs. Angiotensin II has profound effects on the sodium retention by the kidney, a potent vasoconstrictor by itself and also stimulates the release of aldosterone from the renal cortex. Aldosterone promotes sodium reabsorption in the proximal convoluted tubule which in turn increases the blood volume, thereby BP. Note that ACE also breaks down bradykinin which is a potent vasodilator further enhancing the vasoconstrictive effect.

AETIOPATHOGENESIS OF HYPERTENSION

Essential hypertension: The pathophysiological mechanisms underlying essential (primary) hypertension is not completely understood. However, as in other common conditions, hypertension is speculated to be triggered by environmental influences in a genetically susceptible individual. Table 13.2 categorically shortlists the various causative factors of hypertension. The probable summation of the pathogenesis of hypertension is elucidated in Fig. 13.13.

- **Environmental factors:** Lifestyle modifications, excess salt intake, obesity, diabetes, physical inactivity, stress and many more factors have been known to contribute to hypertension.
- **Genetic factors:** Essential hypertension is a complex trait with inheritable epigenetic changes. Presently approximately 20 different genes causing hypertension have been uncovered, some immune related, and some being biochemical factors influencing the renal salt reabsorption mechanisms. Novel genes involving DNA methylation and histone modification have been attributed to hypertension triggered by excess salt intake, mental stress and pregnancy. Evidence-based data claim higher rate of elevated BP among first-degree relatives and high concordance between identical twins supporting the role of inheritance. However, the inheritance pattern is polygenic and a single consistent genetic marker is difficult to establish.

- Role of pressure natriuresis and renal damage – pressure natriuresis is the effect of renal arterial pressure on sodium excretion. In individuals with no hypertension, any increase in the BP is balanced by an equivalent increase in sodium and water excretion, in an attempt to normalize the BP. However, in patients with hypertension, the pressure natriuresis seems to be reset at a higher threshold, in which a disproportionate normal sodium excretion occurs despite the high BP. Renal damage in patients with hypertension augments the process through a vicious cycle of nephron loss and impairment of pressure natriuresis preluding chronic hypertension. Thus, the 'resetting of pressure natriuresis' can be considered as an initiating factor and a consequence of essential hypertension.
- Vasoconstrictive factors: Blood vessels exhibiting constrictive responses to increased sympathetic activity and abnormal regulation of vascular tone by local factors, contribute to increase in peripheral resistance and lead to essential hypertension.

Secondary hypertension: This involves well-established mechanisms. Regardless of the cause, increased cardiac output and/or peripheral resistance is responsible for secondary hypertension. The common causes are as follows (Table 13.1):

- Renovascular hypertension is caused by virtue of renal ischaemia due to chronic renal disease. This induces renin secretion, which acts via the angiotensin–aldosterone pathway causing increased vascular tone and blood volume.
- Primary hyperaldosteronism is the most common cause of secondary hypertension. The excess aldosterone is contributed by idiopathic adrenal hyperplasia or by aldosterone-producing tumours. Note that primary aldosteronism also accounts for a considerable proportion of resistant/refractory hypertension.
- Another common cause of secondary hypertension is oral contraceptive use, involving a minimal of 5% women following exposure. The oestrogen provokes the synthesis of angiotensinogen by the liver, in turn activating the renin–angiotensin system. The hypertension usually wanes off within 6 months of discontinuation of the drug.
- Rare single-gene disorders capable of causing severe forms of hypertension include Liddle syndrome with mutations in the epithelial sodium channels interfering with sodium and water reabsorption. Other causes include gene defects affecting enzymes involved in aldosterone metabolism (e.g. aldosterone synthase, 11β-hydroxylase and 17α-hydroxylase).

VASCULAR PATHOLOGY IN HYPERTENSION

Vascular changes due to hypertension are both a cause and a key to target organ damage, especially in vital organs such as the brain, the heart and the kidney. Hypertension-induced morphological changes begin with initial thickening of the vessel wall, which over time leads to reactive changes referred to as arteriosclerosis (that involve the arteries) and arteriolosclerosis (when arterioles are involved).

- **Hyaline arteriolosclerosis**
  As that can be speculated, in patients with long-term modest elevation of BP, chronic haemodynamic stress can result in endothelial dysfunction followed by smooth muscle cell proliferation and matrix synthesis. This excess matrix along with the plasma proteins that have leaked across the damaged endothelium form a pink homogenous hyaline deposition in the walls of the arterioles thereby causing luminal narrowing (Fig. 13.8). Notably, hyaline arteriolosclerosis is also seen in the elderly individuals even without hypertension but are less widespread and less severe.
  Similar changes are also seen in diabetic patients, due to endothelial injury by glycation end products. Hyaline arteriosclerosis of the renal vessels in chronic hypertension is called benign nephrosclerosis and it causes glomerular scarring and diffuse renal ischaemia.
- **Hyperplastic arteriosclerosis**
  Hyperplastic arteriosclerosis is often manifested in patients suffering from extreme elevations of BP, as in the context of hypertensive emergencies *malignant hypertension*. In response to the intensely high luminal pressure, the smooth muscle in the media undergoes hypertrophy in a concentric, laminated pattern along with the reduplication of basement membrane, resulting

Table 13.1 Secondary Causes of Hypertension

Renal	Endocrine	Vascular	Neurogenic	Drug Induced
• Renal artery stenosis • Glomerulonephritis • Chronic renal disease • Adult polycystic kidney disease • Renin-producing tumours • Diabetic nephropathy	• Cushing syndrome • Primary hyperaldosteronism • Pheochromocytoma • Exogenous hormones (glucocorticoids administration) • Pregnancy induced • Hyperthyroidism • Carcinoid	• Coarctation of aorta • Vasculitis • Rigidity of the aorta • Increased cardiac output	• Psychogenic • Sleep apnoea • Increased intracranial pressure	• Contraceptives • Cocaine • Alcohol • Erythropoietin • Nonsteroidal anti-inflammatory drugs

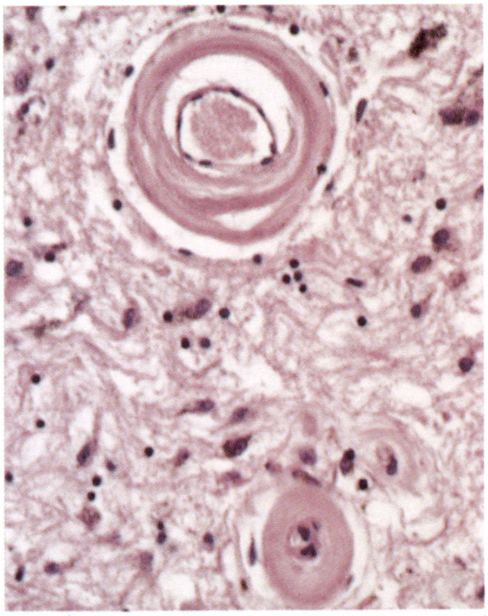

Fig. 13.8 Small arteries affected by mural hyaline thickening. (*Source:* From David Ellison, Seth Love, Leila Chimelli, Brian N. Harding, James S. Lowe, Harry V. Vinters, Sebastian Brandner and William H. Yong. Hemorrhage. Neuropathology. 3rd edition. Elsevier 2013.)

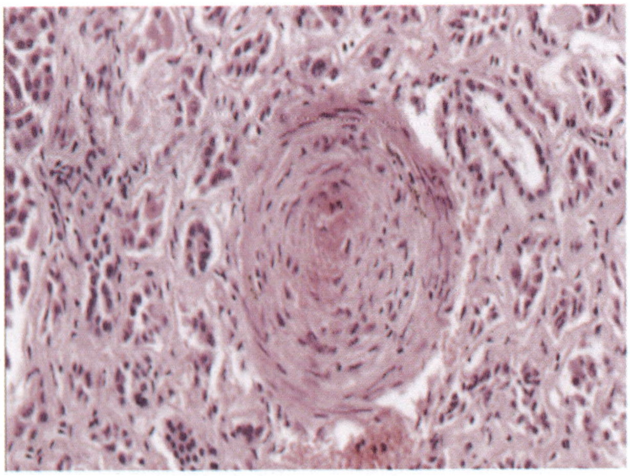

Fig. 13.9 Onion skin appearance in a small renal arteriole with severe compromise of the vascular lumen. (*Source:* From David Ellison, Seth Love, Leila Chimelli, Brian N. Harding, James S. Lowe, Harry V. Vinters, Sebastian Brandner and William H. Yong. Hemorrhage. Neuropathology. 3rd edition. Elsevier 2013.)

in the characteristic **'onion skin'**-like appearance (Fig. 13.9). The arteriolar wall is thus thickened or rather stiffened restricting its capacity to dilate. Because end-organ damage is an expected sequelae in malignant hypertension, morphology can also reveal fibrinoid necrosis of the vessel wall (necrotizing arteritis) chiefly in the kidney.

Long-standing poorly treated hypertension can lead to complications such as left ventricular hypertrophy, CAD, aortic dissection, cerebral infarctions or renal failure and are dealt with in detail in the subsequent chapters.

ARTERIOSCLEROSIS PA 27.1

The name arteriosclerosis is a term of Greek origin meaning *'hardening of the arteries'*. The condition is described by features that include thickening and hardening of the arterial walls with loss of the intrinsic elasticity of vessels.

The following morphologic entities are included under arteriosclerosis:

- Arteriosclerosis which may be due to ageing (senile) or hypertension
- Mönckeberg arteriosclerosis (medial calcific sclerosis)
- Atherosclerosis

Arteriosclerosis: Senile arteriosclerosis is the thickening of media and intima as a part of age-related degeneration probably due to wear and tear of the vessel wall. The changes are nonselective and affect most of the arteries. Morphological changes include fibroelastosis of the intima and media with reduplication of the internal elastic lamina. Eventually, the intense fibrotic changes set in.

Hypertensive arteriosclerosis: As explained earlier, hyaline arteriosclerosis may be seen physiologically in ageing and pathologically in patients with hypertension as benign nephrosclerosis and microangiopathy in diabetes patients. Hyperplastic arteriosclerosis is a characteristic lesion of malignant hypertension.

Mönckeberg arteriosclerosis: Mönckeberg medial calcific sclerosis, as its name implies, is a calcification process that affects the media of large- and medium-sized arteries, most commonly of the extremities and genital tract. The calcium deposits collect within the tunica media but do not cause luminal narrowing (Fig. 13.10). The exact pathogenesis is largely unknown but is considered as an age-related degenerative process, a typical

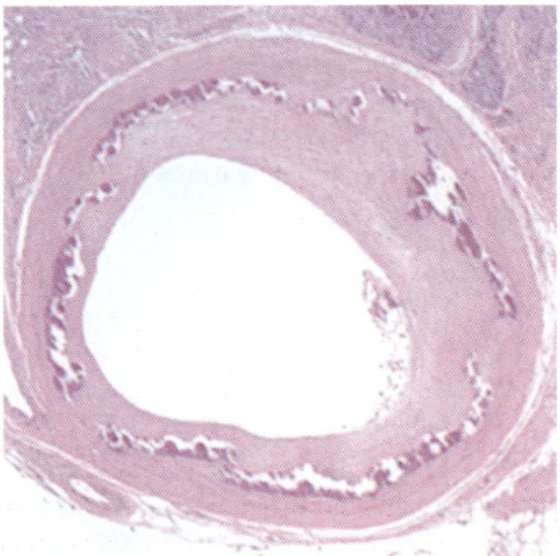

Fig. 13.10 Blood vessel wall showing coarse calcium deposits within the media (arrow) – Mönckeberg medial sclerosis. (*Source:* From Lanfroi Graziani. Crossing the Rubicon: A Closer Look at the Pedal Loop Technique. Annals of Vascular Surgery. 2017;45:315-323.)

example of dystrophic calcification but has no clinical significance.

Atherosclerosis: By no doubt, atherosclerosis is the most important type of arteriosclerosis explained in detail as follows, though sometimes the terms are used interchangeably.

ATHEROSCLEROSIS PA 27.1

Atherosclerosis is the culprit lesion behind many life-threatening conditions such as acute myocardial infarction, stroke, gangrene, aortic aneurysms and ischaemic heart disease (IHD). Alarmingly, atherosclerosis-induced CVD represent an enormous burden on the health care system accounting to nearly 50% of all deaths in the western world. Atherosclerosis is caused by progressive fatty deposits called *atherosclerotic plaques* (also referred to as atheroma) occurring within the inner layers of the artery. Over time, the plaque hardens and causes clinical disease through luminal narrowing or by disintegration of the plaque resulting in distal emboli. Likewise, it impedes the blood flow, compromising the oxygen diffusion across the wall leading to ischaemic changes. When this occurs in the coronary arteries, the most common manifestation of atherosclerosis - CAD - occurs leading to myocardial infarction (the '*heart attack*'). When the blockage occurs in the brain, the individual is likely to experience a stroke. Thus, it is the severity of the occlusion and the vessel affected that determine the symptoms and the associated consequences.

Peripheral artery disease (PAD) is a broader condition which includes atherosclerosis causing occlusions within the arteries of the lower limbs. Similar pathology follows kidney disease and carotid artery disease due to atherosclerosis. Beyond doubt, atherosclerosis represents a grave health problem, contributing to significant mortality and morbidity worldwide.

EPIDEMIOLOGY (FIG. 13.11)

Because atherosclerosis is predominantly an asymptomatic condition, it is difficult to determine the incidence accurately. Worldwide, atherosclerosis causing IHD and ischaemic stroke remain the world's first and fifth causes of death, respectively.

Many studies infer that the prevalence of CAD is higher among the Indians as compared with Americans. The last 3 decades have recorded a surge in CAD cases in India owing to the rapid lifestyle changes, stress, smoking, diabetes and many more factors. According to WHO, 45 million people suffer from CAD contributing to approximately one-third of deaths also involving the younger population. It is estimated that in few years, CVD, mainly atherosclerosis, will become the leading cause of total global disease burden.

ATHEROSCLEROSIS RISK FACTORS AND INDICATORS

Atherosclerosis is a complex multifactorial arterial disease caused by genetic and environmental influences. Hence, the risk factors can be categorized into modifiable and nonmodifiable risk factors (Table 13.2).

Modifiable risk factors: A huge proportion of atheromatous lesions is associated with several risk factors such as dyslipidaemia, hypertension, diabetes, smoking, obesity and inactive lifestyle; all of which are modifiable. The four **major risk factors** are discussed as follows.

- **Dyslipidaemia:** Dyslipidaemia is the *elevation* of plasma cholesterol, triglycerides, or both or a low high-density lipoprotein (HDL) cholesterol level that contributes to the development of atherosclerosis. The interaction between hypercholesterolaemia and other risk factors (e.g. smoking, hypertension and diabetes) can further accelerate atherogenesis. Cholesterol, an important constituent of the cell membrane is required for the biosynthesis of hormones. Because the daily requirement for cholesterol cannot be met from dietary intake, the majority (80%) is derived from biosynthesis in the liver. Triglycerides are the storage form of fatty acids. Cholesterol and triglycerides that circulate in blood plasma are transported in globules known as lipoproteins.

  Among these are low-density lipoprotein (LDL), often referred to as 'bad' cholesterol, which delivers cholesterol to tissue, has been associated with the progression on atherosclerosis. On the contrary, HDL, also referred to as 'good' cholesterol, offers protection against atherosclerosis by removing the excess cholesterol from the tissues and returning it to the liver for breakdown. The effect of triglyceride on atherosclerosis is controversial. Thus, our lifestyle modification should focus on improving blood HDL levels.

  Modest physical activity, avoidance of trans fat (found in commercial baked food and fried food), switching to a diet rich in monosaturated and polyunsaturated fats, omega-3 fatty acids (fish, avocados, nuts, seeds, peanuts) and cessation of smoking contribute to increase in HDL levels significantly. Among the most powerful cholesterol-lowering drugs available, statins suppress cholesterol biosynthesis in the liver by inhibiting the enzymatic activity of HMG-CoA reductase, as well as by increasing the number of hepatic LDL receptors to help clear the plasma LDL and have been in use for a long time.
- **Hypertension:** *Hypertension is a major, independent risk factor for atherosclerotic CVD.* High pressure can probably damage the arterial lining, making arteries more vulnerable to the narrowing and plaque build-up associated with atherosclerosis. The narrowed artery limits or blocks the flow of blood to the heart

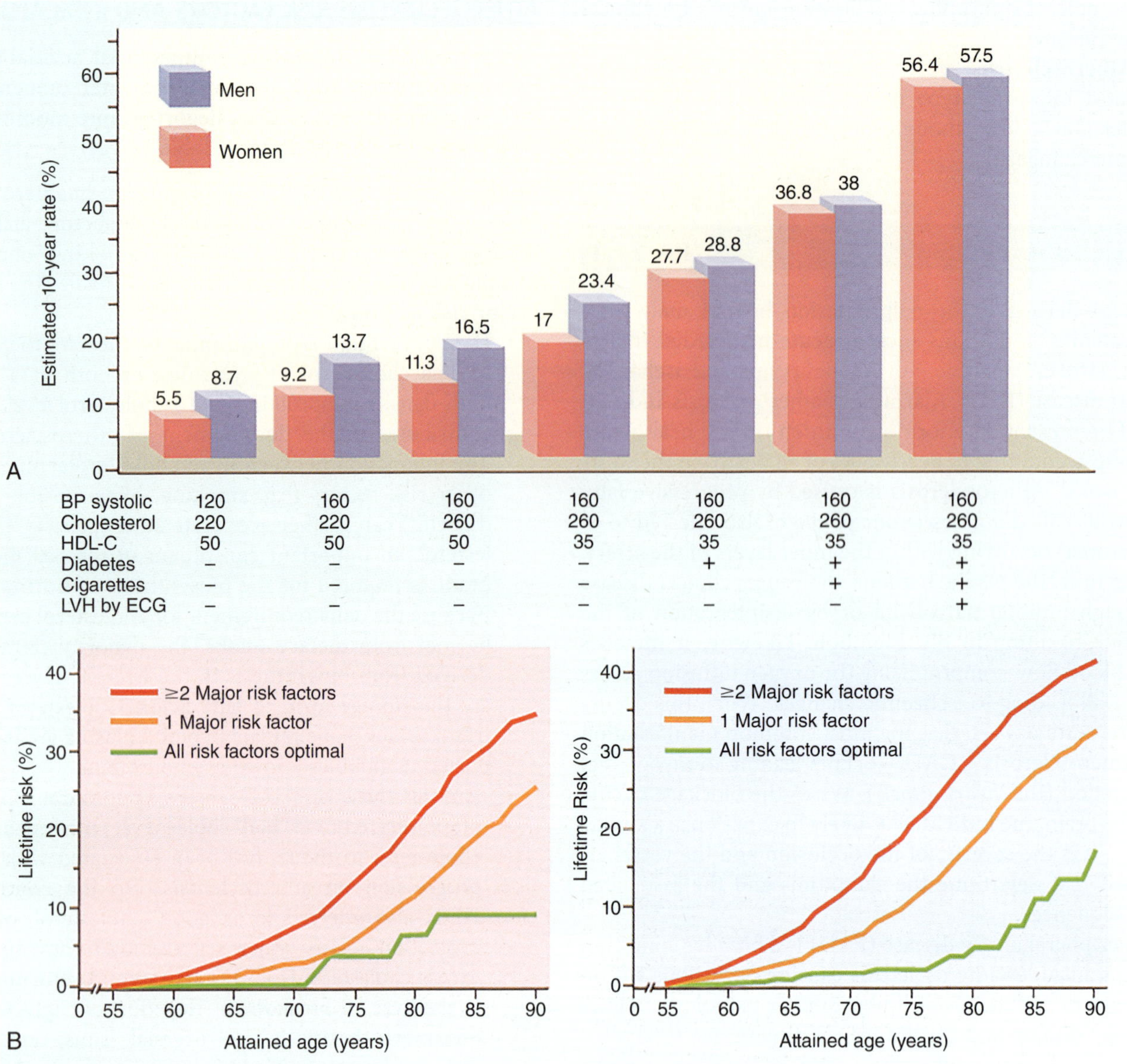

Fig. 13.11 Graph demonstrates the epidemiology of atherosclerosis.

Table 13.2 Risk Factors for Atherosclerosis

Nonmodifiable	Modifiable	Additional Risk Factors
• Gender • Age • Genetic factors	• Dyslipidaemia • Hypertension • Smoking • Diabetes	• Inflammation • Hyperhomocysteinaemia • Metabolic syndrome • Obesity • Physical inactivity • Alcohol • Hormones – oestrogen, OCP intake • Lipoprotein

muscle, depriving the heart of oxygen. On its own, hypertension can increase the risk of developing IHD by approximately 60%.

- **Smoking:** Smoking is an agreeably preventable risk factor involved in the development of CAD. The primary effect of smoking is initiated by oxidative stress causing vascular dysfunction and generation of systemic inflammatory signals predisposing to a prothrombotic state and atherogenesis. Relative to nonsmokers and long-term smokers who have quit smoking over a considerable period of time, the risk of progression and complications of atherosclerosis remains inevitably high among heavy smokers.
- **Diabetes mellitus:** Prolonged exposure to hyperglycaemia and insulin resistance potentially induces the progression of atherosclerosis, especially when

associated with other risk factors. Evidently, the incidence of CAD, stroke and atherosclerosis-induced gangrene is relatively more common in individuals suffering from long uncontrolled diabetes. The mortality in approximately 65% of diabetic patients is related to atherosclerosis.

Nonmodifiable risk factors: Apart from the above-mentioned modifiable risk factors, **nonmodifiable genetic and other factors** that may represent consequential determinants of atherosclerotic cardiovascular risk are discussed as follows:

- ***Genetic:*** Research on the genetic factors cornering the inheritance patterns in atherosclerosis and its manifestations are starting to unravel. Mutations or common polymorphisms identified have been associated with the host response to risk factors, such as plasma lipoprotein levels, inflammation and vascular remodelling. Familial hypercholesterolaemia is an autosomal dominant disorder primarily due to mutations causing reduction or defect in the LDL receptor, leading to high cholesterol levels in the blood and consequent pathologies. Thus, a family history of atherosclerosis is an independent risk factor that significantly influences the progression of CVDs.
- ***Age:*** Atherosclerosis is an age-related disease. Although genetic influences and family history may predispose the individual to early lesions of atherosclerosis, clinically significant lesions are observed in the middle age and beyond. This is evidenced by the high death rate from IHD in older age groups.
- ***Gender:*** Atherosclerosis presents more commonly in men, older than 45 years than in women, in whom it presents much later (>55 years). The lower incidence of IHD in women, especially in the premenopausal age group, has been attributed to high oestrogen levels which are protective against atheromatous lesions. This is further evidenced by studies indicating that the incidence of atherosclerosis double in postmenopausal women because of declining oestrogen levels. However, research on oestrogen replacement therapy in older women (>65 years) with preexisting coronary artery atherosclerosis revealed no beneficial effects, whereas in younger postmenopausal women with early stages of atherosclerosis, oestrogen replacement therapy proved beneficial.

Additional risk factors: It is noteworthy that many patients develop atherosclerosis even in the absence of conventional risk factors. Thus, research has been focused on the **additional risk factors** that may cause progression to atherosclerosis, which are as follows:

- ***Inflammation:*** Current evidence supports a central role for inflammation in all phases of the atherosclerotic process. Clinical studies affirm the correlation of circulating markers of inflammation with progression of the disease. Among those inflammatory markers is **C-reactive protein,** an acute phase reactant. Plasma CRP levels predict the extent and severity of atherosclerotic vascular disease as well as the risk of future coronary events. Thus, these inflammatory markers can independently be used nowadays for risk stratification.
- ***Lipoprotein(a):*** It is a modified LDL particle with an additional apolipoprotein(a) [apo(a)] moiety bound to apolipoprotein B100 by a disulphide bond. Elevated plasma concentration of lipoprotein(a) is an independent predictor for atherosclerotic CVD, also of myocardial infarction and ischaemic stroke. The association is continuous, and is independent of the serum cholesterol and HDL levels. Nonetheless, the use of Lp(a) as a screening tool has some limitations requiring extensive research.
- ***Homocysteine:*** Several studies have established the emergence of elevated homocysteine levels as an important risk factor in the pathogenesis of atherosclerosis. Curiously, the rare hereditary disease homocystinuria is also associated with premature vascular disease.
- ***Metabolic syndrome:*** It is characterized by a constellation of interrelated metabolic abnormalities (namely obesity, dyslipidaemia, hyperglycaemia and hypertension), all of which are individual contributors to CVD.

Other significant risk factors include prothrombotic factors and elevated fibrinogen levels that favour formation of thrombus which is one of the hideous complications of atherosclerosis. Role of infections, particularly of *Chlamydia pneumoniae* and viruses such as herpesvirus and cytomegalovirus, in the predisposition to atherosclerotic lesions are also being currently established.

PATHOGENESIS

The most widely accepted mechanistic basis of the pathogenesis of atherosclerosis is the 'response to injury' hypothesis, which also stands as an integrated model of all the risk factors discussed earlier. Accordingly, atherosclerosis is recognized as a chronic inflammatory disease of the large- and the medium-sized arteries, characterized by endothelial dysfunction followed by subendothelial accumulation of lipoproteins that undergo subsequent oxidation, immune cells and extracellular matrix. The immune cells, particularly the macrophages, neutrophils, T and B lymphocytes and mast cells, operate through a complex network of interactions with the other cellular constituents impacting the plaque progression and stability. The pathophysiological sequence in the development of atherosclerotic lesions is summarized in Flowchart 13.1 and is schematically represented in Fig. 13.12.

Endothelial cell dysfunction is the initial, provocative step in the formation of atheromas. It has been demonstrated that endothelial dysfunction is one of the earliest signs of atherosclerosis and can be detected even before

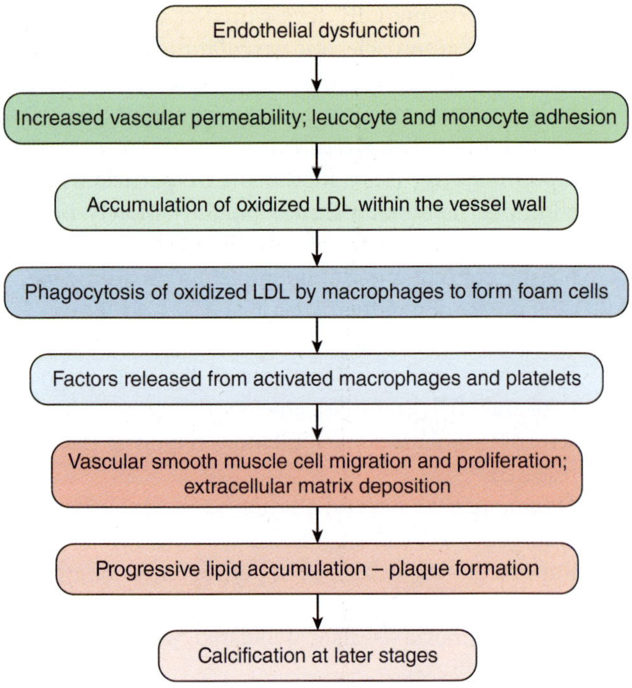

Flowchart 13.1 Pathogenesis of atherosclerosis.

angiographic structural changes of the vessel wall are apparent. Endothelial cell damage enhances intimal permeability, leucocyte recruitment and also contributes to thrombus formation, marking its role in disease progression as well.

Endothelial cell dysfunction and damage in the form of oxidative injury may occur because of conditions such as smoking and hypertension, advanced glycation end products in diabetes mellitus and all the above-explained risk factors, but the most significant are haemodynamic stress, hypercholesterolaemia and inflammation.

- ***Haemodynamic stress:*** Turbulent flow observed at the ostia of the exiting vessels, branching points, bends and bifurcations in the arterial vessels, comprise the arterial sites prone to atherosclerotic lesions. The nonbranching straight vessels with laminar nonturbulent blood flow are usually spared. This is attributed to the fact that exposure of the endothelial cells to nonturbulent flow increases the transcription of Kruppel-like factor 2 (KLF2) which helps to maintain the endothelial cells in a nonactive state (atheroprotective). With disturbed laminar flow, KLF2 expression is decreased in the endothelial cells switching them into an active phonotype promoting atherogenesis.
- ***Hypercholesterolaemia:*** It is caused by inherited defects or acquired conditions such as dyslipoprotinaemias, nephrotic syndrome, alcoholism, hypothyroidism or diabetes mellitus; all of these are associated with an increased risk of atherosclerosis. The raised cholesterol, LDL and Lp(a) levels exert endothelial cell injury by increasing release of reactive oxygen species which causes DNA and mitochondrial damage and endothelial

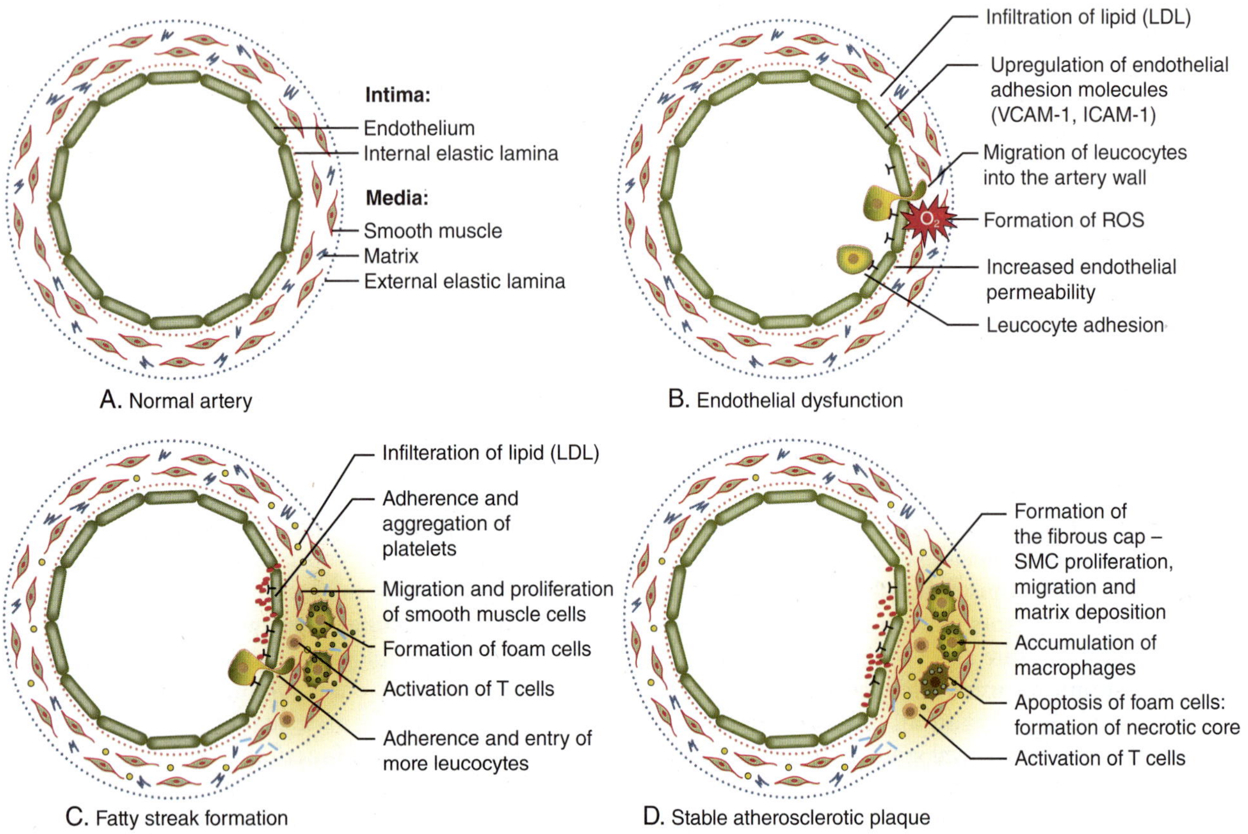

Fig. 13.12 Atheroma formation.

cell apoptosis. The cholesterol esters also have the ability to scavenge NO, impairing the vasodilatory activity. Continued endothelial compromise with chronic hyperlipidaemia causes the circulating LDL to increasingly migrate from the plasma into the extracellular matrix of the tunica intima. Once within the blood vessel, LDL undergoes oxidative modification to form ox-LDL by the action the reactive oxygen species produced by the inflammatory cells. The activated endothelium generates a range of chemokines and other cytokines and increases the expression of adhesion molecules on their cell surface. This paves way for the recruitment and infiltration of monocytes and immune cells into the vessel wall. The monocytes differentiate into macrophages and internalize the ox-LDL via the so called 'scavenger receptors'. Unable to degrade the modified lipoproteins entirely, the macrophages retain the lipid giving rise to lipid-laden cells, also called foam cells. With progressive lipoprotein accumulation, the macrophages eventually die by apoptosis. Under similar influences, the smooth muscle cells migrate from the media towards the intima and progressively transform into lipid-laden foam cells by engulfing ox-LDL. The foam cells constitute the fatty streak, the earliest visible lesion of the atherosclerosis, also the precursor of a fully formed atheromatous plaque.

- *Inflammation:* It is now established to have a fundamental role in mediating all the stages of atheroma development. The accumulation and retention of cholesterol and lipoproteins within the macrophages are one hypothetical trigger factor for inflammation in atherosclerotic lesions. Proinflammatory cytokines such as IL-1 and TNF regulate the expression of adhesion molecules for leucocyte, T lymphocyte and monocyte recruitment. The activated macrophages and leucocytes in turn produce reactive oxygen species that effect LDL oxidation and also induce the production of growth factors that attract smooth muscle migration to the intima. The accumulation, retention and oxidative modification of LDL continue to generate the expression of adhesion molecules, cytokines, chemokines, and other macrophage inflammatory mediators forming a self-perpetuating positive feedback loop contributing to the growth of the lesion.
- *Smooth muscle cell (SMC) proliferation and matrix synthesis:* Potential mediators elaborated by the activated macrophages such as fibroblastic growth factor (FGF) and platelet-derived growth factor (PDGF) are responsible for smooth muscle migration and proliferation. Transforming growth factor β (TGF-β), among other mediators, stimulates interstitial collagen synthesis by the smooth muscle cells and the production of extracellular matrix. This process typifies the more advanced atherosclerotic lesion. Other cytokines such as interferon-γ produced by activated T lymphocytes limit the collagen synthesis by smooth muscle cells. Cholesterol derived from the insudated blood lipid or extruded from the dying foam cells gets entrapped within this matrix contributing to the lipid necrotic core. Within the atherosclerotic plaque, smooth muscle cells deposit extracellular matrix to form a fibrous cap that walls off the plaque on the luminal side. The plaque stability is inherently dependent on the lipid core, thickness of the fibrous cap and inflammation within the cap.

Morphology

Fatty streaks: Grossly, they appear as multiple slightly elevated or flattened streaks approximately 1 cm or longer. They are composed of lipid-laden foam cells. Fatty streaks do not deform the vessel or obstruct the lumen. Notably, not all fatty streaks progress to form plaques. Some may in fact disappear from the intima overtime. Aortic fatty streak areas may also be observed in early childhood and even in neonates or adolescents with no predisposing risk factors. Studies indicate that most lesions of early infancy reverse, but those that lead into childhood persist.

Atherosclerotic plaque: The raised lesion or fibrolipid plaque is the prototypical lesion of atherosclerosis. The most extensively involved vessels are the muscular and elastic arteries, the branch point being the most favourable sites. In decreasing order of frequency, the involved vessels are the lower abdominal aorta and iliac arteries, the coronary arteries, the popliteal arteries, the internal carotid arteries and the vessels of the circle of Willis. The severity of the disease varies according to the location of the affected vessel.

Grossly, atherosclerotic plaques are elevated, pale yellow, smooth-surfaced lesions, though may sometimes show surface ulceration. The plaque is often eccentric, i.e. it occupies only part of the circumference of the lumen. On cut section, the luminal surface is often firm, owing to the fibrous cap and a central core composed of yellowish white, soft, fluid material, hence the name atheroma (Fig. 13.13).

At the microscopic level, atherosclerotic plaques comprise four principal components, namely the cells (SMCs, macrophages and T cells), ECM (collagen, elastic fibres and proteoglycans), the lipids (intra- and extracellular) and calcifications at later stages. The parts of the plaque include the following:

Fibrous cap: It is a thick layer of fibrous connective tissue, usually covered by a layer of regenerating endothelium, composed of dense connective tissue, predominantly collagen and smooth muscle cells, along with macrophages and T lymphocytes clinging onto the sides of the cap which is referred to as the shoulders.

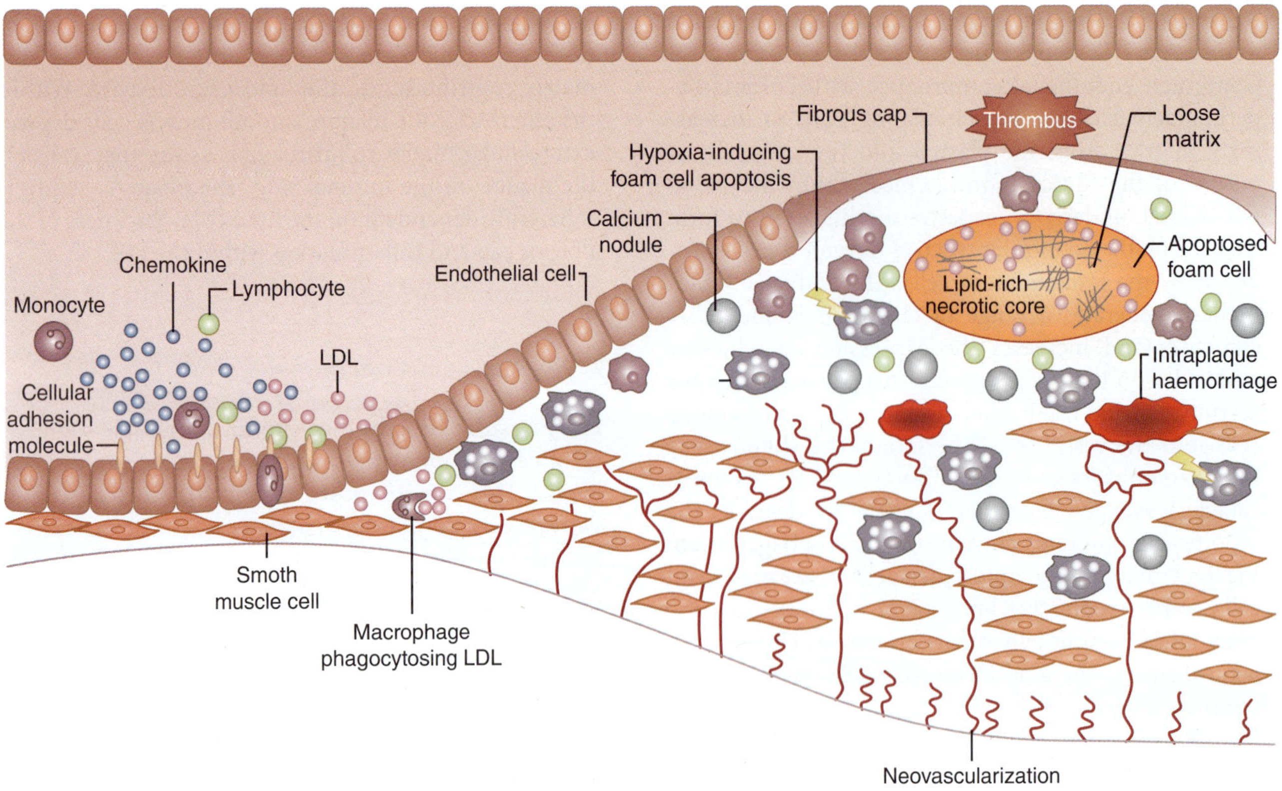

Fig. 13.13 Overview of complicated plaque.

Necrotic mass of lipid material: They are found deep to the fibrous cap and form the core the atheroma. This lipid-rich core comprises predominantly cholesterol and cholesterol esters, foam cells, cellular debris and variable inflammatory infiltrate. A few atheromas may demonstrate less cellularity and predominance of smooth muscle cells and fibrous tissue, often referred to as fibrous plaques. The periphery of the lesions demonstrates *neovascularization* (proliferating small blood vessels) that are probably derived from the vasa vasorum.

Calcification: This most commonly involves the coronary and aortic blood vessels. Calcium deposition occur typically within the central necrotic core and the intima. Recollecting Mönckeberg arteriosclerosis that involves only the tunica media.

Complicated atheromatous plaque: The complications that tend to occur within the atheromatous plaques draw special attention owing to the dramatic clinical events that follow (Fig. 13.14).

Rupture, ulceration and thrombosis: In response to haemodynamic forces on the atheroma, the fibrous cap may undergo thinning and rupture. Plaque disruption initiates platelet adhesion and aggregation and activation of the clotting cascade, predisposing to thrombus formation. The so called 'atherothrombotic process' capable of lumen occlusion is the hallmark feature implicated in stroke and myocardial infarction. However, a nonocclusive thrombus most often triggers a healing response resulting in the fibrous plaque getting incorporated into the vessel wall with a compromised lumen.

Atheroembolism: In certain scenarios, plaque rupture releases the underlying cholesterol-rich matrix into circulation and eventually lodges into a distal site causing occlusion. Atheroembolism is characterized by showering of numerous cholesterol microemboli to a variety of tissues and organs (Fig. 13.15).

Haemorrhage: Haemorrhage of the fibrous cap or of the vessels of neovascularization can cause a contained intraplaque haematoma. Neoangiogenesis and its associated intraplaque haemorrhages provide the lesion all the blood components, such as macrophages, platelets and plasma proteins to participate in necrotic core enlargement.

Aneurysm formation: Atherosclerosis-induced pressure causes degenerative ischaemic changes in the blood vessel wall. This leads to progressive weakening and loss of elastic recoil of the wall contributing to aneurysm formation (explained in detail later).

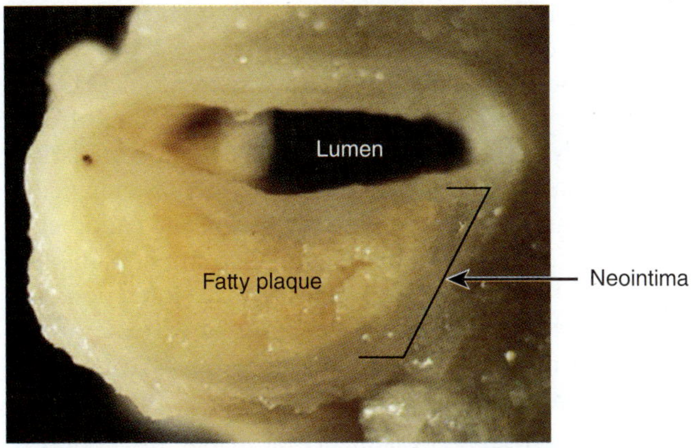

Fig. 13.14 Atherosclerotic plaque within the vessel wall in a patient who died of myocardial infarction. Note the reduction in vessel lumen diameter. (*Source:* From Roy L. Silverstein. Atherothrombosis. Hematology: Basic Principles and Practice. 7th edition. Elsevier 2018.)

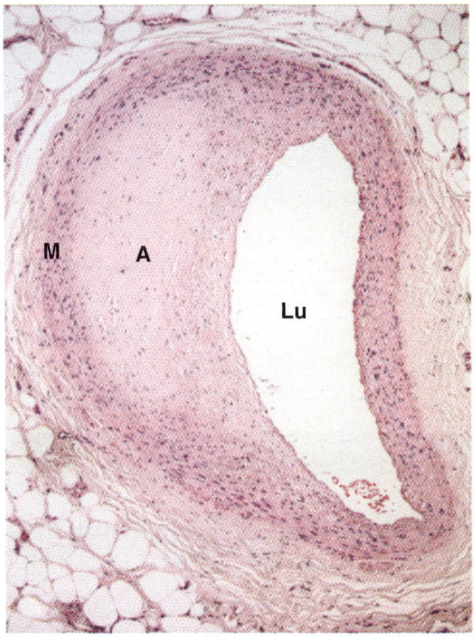

Fig. 13.15 Branch of coronary artery showing an atherosclerotic plaque (A) seen within the intima encroaching into the luminal space (Lu). Note the compressed thinned media (M). (*Source:* From Geraldine O'Dowd, Sarah Bell and Sylvia Wright. Atherosclerosis. In Wheater's Pathology: A Text, Atlas, and Review of Histopathology. 6th edition. Elsevier 2020.)

Clinical Consequences Atherosclerosis is clinically silent until there is sufficient stenosis (Fig. 13.16) or catastrophic occlusive thrombosis of the vasculature. The important question, therefore, is not the absolute prevalence of atherosclerosis, but the degree to which it causes clinically significant disease. Following are the vessels which are particularly predisposed and whose involvement forms the basis of most atherosclerotic clinical consequences:

- **Prone vessels**
  - Coronary arteries: Responsible for myocardial infarction
  - Renal artery: Can result in renal artery stenosis
  - Carotid artery: Can result in stroke

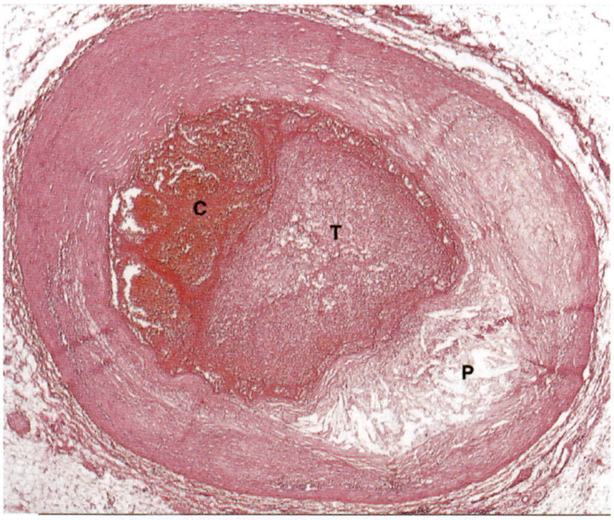

Fig. 13.16 Thrombus (T) formation on the surface of an ulcerated atheromatous plaque (P). The residual lumen is filled with bright red postmortem clot (C). (*Source:* From Geraldine O'Dowd, Sarah Bell and Sylvia Wright. Atherosclerosis. In Wheater's Pathology: A Text, Atlas, and Review of Histopathology. 6th edition. Elsevier 2020.)

  - Aorta: Can result in abdominal aortic aneurysm (AAA), the most common form of atherosclerotic aneurysms

Most of these clinical manifestations of atherosclerosis are because of atherosclerotic stenosis or plaque rupture followed by vascular thrombosis.

Atherosclerotic stenosis: The blood vessels can enlarge radially (outward remodelling) to accommodate atheromatous plaques without narrowing the lumen, producing silent plaques. In a majority of cases, the remodelling effect is exhausted and plaque eventually begins to expand inwardly, reducing the luminal diameter. This results in arterial stenosis which can manifest clinically as downstream tissue hypoperfusion. In these patients, though the plaque is generally stable and does not rupture, the reduction in blood flow to the distal tissues causes symptoms in patients. The extent of occlusion at which the atheroma causes tissue ischaemia is called critical stenosis.

When such an event occurs in the coronary artery causing luminal narrowing beyond the critical value (>70% of the luminal space), the myocardial tissue suffers from ischaemia particularly during times of increased oxygen demand and is referred to as '**demand ischaemia', exertional angina or chronic stable ischaemia.**

Similarly, flow-limiting stenosis can manifest as *ischaemic encephalopathy, intermittent claudication* (in PAD), bowel ischaemia (mesenteric vessel occlusion) or sudden cardiac death, later in the course of the disease.

Acute plaque change: It is displayed by plaque erosion or rupture with superimposed thrombus. It is the main cause of acute coronary syndromes, especially myocardial infarction, unstable angina and sudden cardiac death. Large acellular plaques with lipid-rich necrotic core, relatively thin fibrous cap and with ongoing inflammation constitute the high-risk type prone to acute changes.

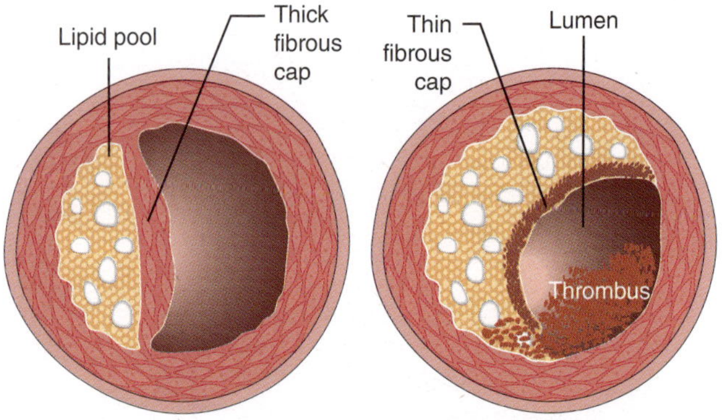

Fig. 13.17 Stable versus vulnerable plaque.

Mildly or moderately stenotic plaques can also undergo abrupt episodes of plaque disruption and eventually progress to totally occlusive lesion. Furthermore, the plaque changes occur at sites where the plaque surface is the weakest, corresponding to locations where the haemodynamic and mechanical forces have their maximal impact. Thus, the risk of plaque disruption is related to the vulnerability of the individual plaques (intrinsic factors) and to the dynamic extrinsic forces that precipitate it.

- **Intrinsic factors:** The fibrous cap overlying the lipid necrotic core is principally composed of collagen produced by the vascular smooth muscle cells. Vulnerability of the fibrous cap to rupture depends on the collagen turnover that is controlled by metalloproteinases (MMPs), collagen degradation enzymes synthesized mostly by macrophages and smooth muscle cells within the plaque and their inhibitor (tissue inhibitor of matrix metalloproteases) produced by endothelial and smooth muscle cells. Stable plaques are maintained by a relative balance, whereas tilting of the balance towards increased collagen degradation results in plaque instability. Also, active inflammation within the plaque reflecting the enhanced recruitment of macrophages and T lymphocytes further contributes to plaque vulnerability (Fig. 13.17). Statin drugs are beneficial in reducing plaque inflammation apart from lowering cholesterol and are being increasingly used in the therapeutic regimen.
- **Extrinsic forces:** Several factors such as increase in systemic BP, acute infection, exposure to illicit drugs, haemodynamic shear stress and adrenergic stimulation can stimulate local vasoconstriction thereby enhancing platelet activation, thrombus formation and endothelial dysfunction potentiating plaque disruption. Nonetheless, approximately 5% of all myocardial infarctions are triggered by severe emotional stress or extreme physical activity. Of note, avoiding or reducing trigger activities may prevent plaque disruption.

The most feared consequence of plaque disruption is thrombotic occlusion. Importantly, thrombus formation is not the end point in all plaque disruptions. Also, in certain scenarios, luminal obstruction by thrombus may be incomplete or may lyse or organize into a mural thrombus without occluding the vessel. The subsequent thrombin-induced fibrosis and healing generate a fibroproliferative response predisposing to a more fibrotic lesion that can cause haemodynamically significant luminal narrowing. However, considering that plaque disruption is dangerous and is responsible for acute myocardial infarction, more research in detecting vulnerability of the plaques and preventive intervention protocols can be rewarding. The resultant changes in the vulnerable plaque may be of four types as described in Table 13.3 and a summary of the clinical consequences of atherosclerotic plaques is elucidated in Fig. 13.18.

ANEURYSMS AND DISSECTION PA 27.2

An aneurysm is a localized abnormal dilation of a blood vessel or the heart. It is often referred to as 'ballooning of the blood vessel'. Aneurysms may occur in any part of the aorta or major arteries of brain (cerebral aneurysm), with much predilection to the vessels of the intestine, kidney, spleen and the extremities (iliac, femoral and popliteal aneurysms). Dissection is initiated through a tear in the lumen or less commonly by the rupture of the vessels of the vasa vasorum. The blood dissects through the vessel wall and separates the layers forming an illusional false lumen within the wall.

Table 13.3 Acute Plaque Change

Type of Change	Effect on Plaque	Consequence
Rupture/fissuring	Exposes highly thrombogenic plaque constituents	Occlusive thrombosis (common)
Erosion/ulceration	Exposes the thrombogenic subendothelial basement membrane	Occlusive thrombosis (less frequent)
Haemorrhage into the atheroma	Increase in size of the necrotic core	Occlusion of vessel
Microembolization	Cholesterol microemboli detach from disrupted plaque	Obstruct distal intramural vessels

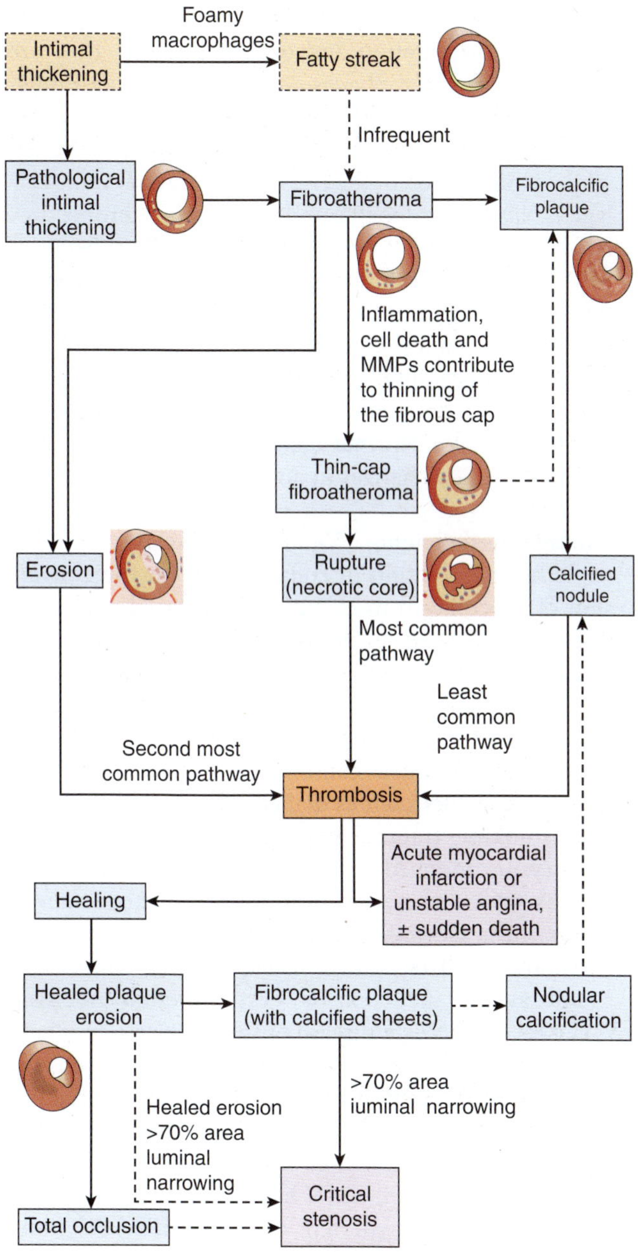

Fig. 13.18 The clinical course of atherosclerotic plaques.

TYPES OF ANEURYSMS (FIG. 13.19)

- **True versus pseudoaneurysms**
  - True aneurysms are bounded by all three layers of the blood vessel: the tunica intima, media and adventitia.
  - Pseudoaneurysms are generated when blood leaks into the vascular wall or surrounding tissues and forms a perfused sac that communicates with vascular lumen. The perfused sac is bound by media or adventitia or in some cases by the connective tissue structures surrounding the injured vessel. The clinical presentation of a pseudoaneurysm is usually a tender, pulsatile mass in the region of the affected artery. Pseudoaneurysms arise as a result of inflammation, trauma or surgical procedures such as angiography and vascular grafting.

    For example, left ventricular aneurysms following myocardial infarction are true aneurysms as defined by areas of thinned myocardium comprising all three layers: the endocardium, myocardium and pericardium. Conversely, left ventricular pseudoaneurysms develop as a result of rupture of the ventricular wall and the perfused sac is contained by an overlying adherent pericardium.
- **Fusiform versus saccular aneurysms**
  - Fusiform aneurysms appear as concentric dilations of the blood vessel involving full circumference of the vessel wall.
  - Saccular aneurysms are focal protrusions involving only a portion of the circumference of the vessel wall. These arise from focal defects of the vessel causing the wall to focally bulge outward. Saccular cerebral aneurysms, referred to as *berry aneurysms*, account for the majority of intracranial aneurysms and are the most common cause of nontraumatic subarachnoid haemorrhage (Fig. 13.20).

AETIOPATHOGENESIS

Aneurysms are principally caused by factors which tend to damage and compromise the structure and the function

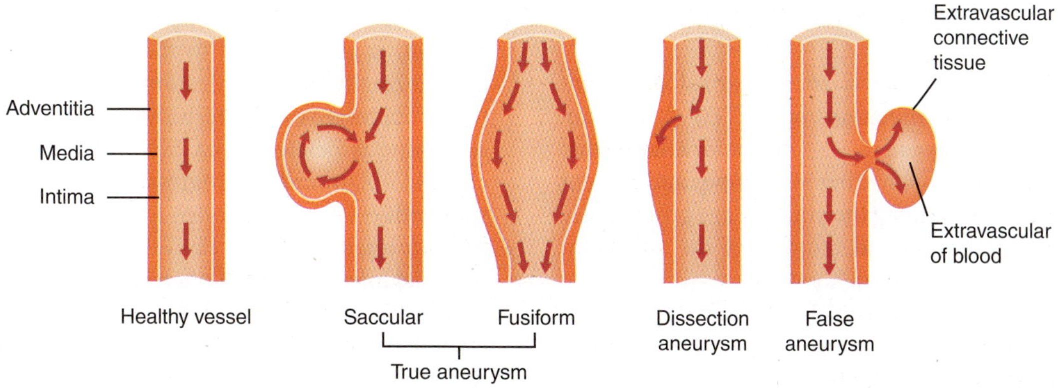

Fig. 13.19 Types of aneurysm.

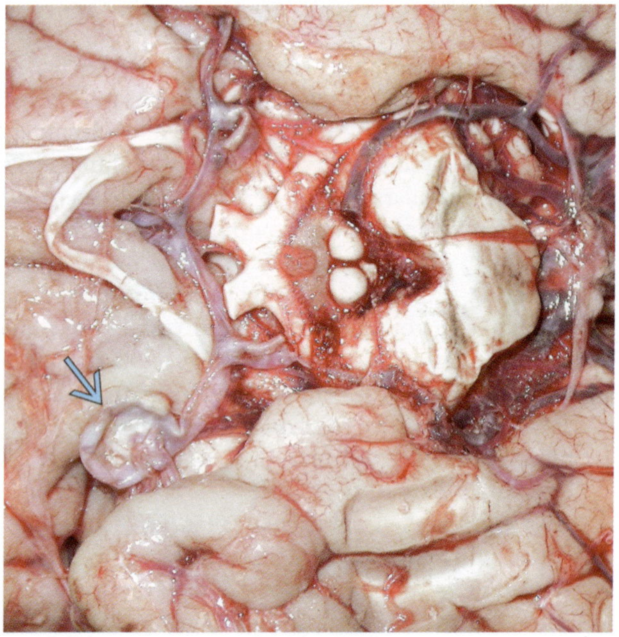

Fig. 13.20 Berry aneurysm: An unruptured berry aneurysm is present in this brain. This was an incidental finding.

of the connective tissue within the vascular wall. Although pathogenesis of aneurysms is multifactorial, the most important triggers would be loss of vessel wall integrity, inflammation and degenerative changes.

- Among the **heritable factors: Mutations** affecting the intrinsic quality of the vascular wall are an important cause of aneurysms.
  - ***Marfan syndrome (MFS)*** is an autosomal dominant connective tissue disorder characterized by mutations of the fibrillin 1 gene. Fibrillin, a scaffolding protein is an essential constituent of the extracellular matrix. The mutations result in defective synthesis of fibrillin or defective incorporation into the connective tissue. Resultant vessel wall fragility predisposes to aneurysm formation particularly in the aorta.
  - ***Ehlers–Danlos syndrome (EDS)*** is a heterogeneous group of six connective tissue disorders with variable inheritance. The syndrome is characterized by mutations that result in defective synthesis and processing of collagen, especially type III collagen, predisposing to aneurysm formation, the hallmark feature of the vascular from of EDS (refer to Chapter 5 for detailed description).
  - ***Loeys–Dietz syndrome*** is an autosomal dominant disorder involving mutations of the TGF-β receptor. These patients show an increased risk for aneurysmal rupture compared with other syndromes and present more commonly among the younger age group. Early surgical intervention and removal of the aneurysm can prove beneficial in such patients.
- **Inflammation and proteases:** Proteolytic degradation of vascular wall connective tissue by matrix metalloproteinases (MMPs) are integral to aneurysm formation. MMPs are prominent in pathologic conditions such as *atherosclerosis and vasculitis, neoplasia*, other states of inflammation and oxidative stress. They are derived from macrophages and vascular smooth muscle cells and are secreted into the extracellular matrix. These enzymes have the capacity to degrade virtually all the components of the ECM in the arterial wall (collagen, elastin, proteoglycan, laminin and fibronectin). Also, the balance of vessel wall remodelling between MMPs and their inhibitors, tissue inhibitors of metalloproteinases (TIMPS), is lost which further favours elastin and collagen degradation. Consequently, the vessel loses its ability to distend normally with left ventricular contraction, and instead abnormally bulges to form aneurysms. Normal ageing process also may contribute to subtle changes in aortic structure promoting aneurysm.
- **Vitamin C deficiency:** Vitamin C is relevant for the triple helix formation of collagen and for the conversion of procollagen to collagen. Nutritional deficiency of vitamin C, *scurvy*, impairs collagen synthesis and weakens the vessel wall defining the **nutritional basis of aneurysms.**
- **Atherosclerosis and hypertension:** These constitute the two most frequent causes of aneurysms apart from other risk factors such as diabetes, hypercholesterolaemia, smoking trauma, vasculitis and advanced age. Aneurysms induced by atherosclerosis are common such as AAAs, whereas hypertension is related to aneurysms of the ascending aorta.
  - Another well-recognized cause of aortic dissection and aortic aneurysm is **cystic medial necrosis** (CMN). CMN is a disease of the large arteries characterized by degenerative breakdown of collagen and increased deposition of ground substance, creating cyst-like lesions, weakening the vessel wall. Although the exact reason for their development is yet to be completely elicited, CMN has been linked to ageing, atherosclerosis, hypertension and MFS. Of note, CMN marks the hallmark histological feature of dissection in patients with MFS (Fig. 13.21). Atherosclerosis and hypertension are believed to contribute by causing narrowing of the vasa vasorum causing outer medial ischaemia predisposing to CMN.
- ***Syphilitic aneurysms, with particular affinity for aortic root, is*** encountered in the tertiary syphilis stage. This normally follows infection of the aorta secondary to the obliterative endarteritis of the vasa vasorum. It is sometime associated with CMN (explained below). The chronic inflammation progressively weakens the vessel wall with eventual aneurysm formation.
- ***Mycotic aneurysms*** are relatively rare and are caused by bacterial infections. Most often an atherosclerotic plaque acts as the nidus for microbial infection. Alternatively, emboli of contaminated particles from vegetations of infective endocarditis may lodge in the vasa vasorum and cause ischaemic changes in vessel wall. The culprit

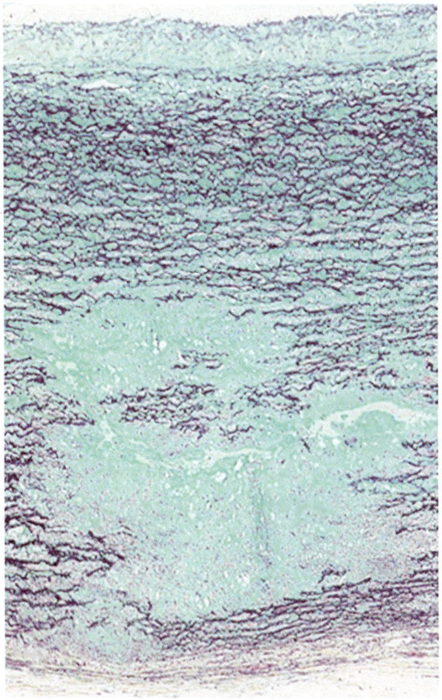

Fig. 13.21 Histological image of a patient with aortic dissection due to Marfan syndrome. The affected region shows marked loss of elastic fibres, cystic change with increased ground substance – cystic medial necrosis (Movat's stain). (*Source:* From E. Ladich, J. Butany and R. Virmani. Aneurysms of the Aorta: Ascending, Thoracic and Abdominal and Their Management. Cardiovascular Pathology. 4th edition. Elsevier 2016.)

organisms in such conditions are mostly *Staphylococcus aureus, Streptococcus pyogenes or Salmonella.*

- ***Ventricular aneurysms*** usually occur in the left ventricle following a myocardial infarction in which the myocardium is fragile and dyskinetic. Over time, these weak areas of the myocardium bulge out by reflex during each ventricular contraction evolving into true aneurysms. A schematic representation of the preferred sites of aneurysms is provided in Fig. 13.22.

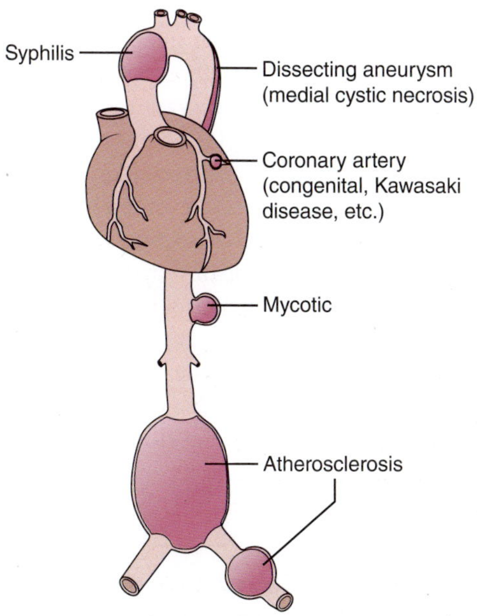

Fig. 13.22 Preferred sites of aneurysms.

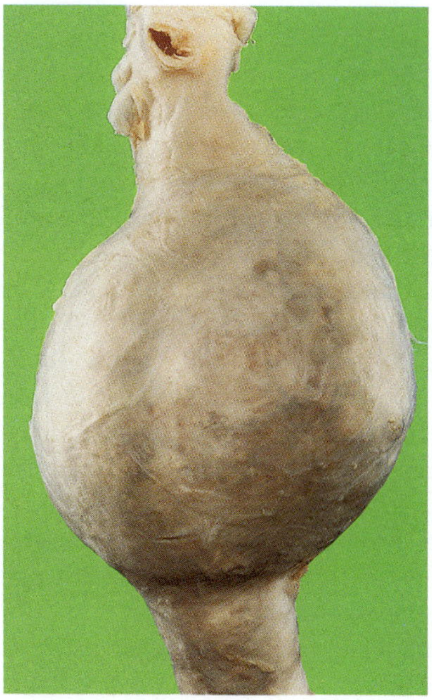

Fig. 13.23 A large unruptured atherosclerotic abdominal aortic aneurysm. (*Source:* From S. Kim Suvarna. Cardiovascular system. Underwood's Pathology. 7th edition. Elsevier 2019.)

Abdominal Aortic Aneurysms

These are true aneurysms of the abdominal aorta which generally occur below the level of the renal arteries and above the aortic bifurcation (Fig. 13.23).

Pathogenesis By large, atherosclerotic type aneurysms manifest as AAAs and can also involve the common iliac arteries. Apparently, the inflammation associated with atherosclerosis leads to destruction, thinning and thus weakening of the vascular wall, specifically the tunica media, which contributes to aneurysmal dilation of the vessel. Other risk factors include advanced age, tobacco use, hypercholesterolaemia, chronic obstructive pulmonary disease and male gender. Thus, the incidence of AAA considerably increases in elderly men older than 60 years and in people who are smokers.

Morphology

AAAs are usually >3 cm in diameter, sometimes reaching a maximal of 5.5 cm, and up to 25 cm in length. They display both fusiform and saccular forms. Morphological features rationally reveal evidence of severe complicated atherosclerosis with marked degeneration of the media and in most instances an ill-organized mural thrombus. Although AAA frequently involves the infrarenal segment of the abdominal aorta, approximately 5% of cases may show suprarenal segment involvement. Also, simultaneous presentation in the smaller iliac, thoracic and femoropopliteal arteries is being increasingly detected.

Inflammatory AAAs, a variant of the classical AAA, is characterized by inflammatory thickening of the aneurysmal wall evidenced by dense lymphoplasmacytic infiltrate microscopically. Inflammation and fibrosis extend into the periaortic zone causing severe adhesion and scaring. Most cases, however, are confined to the aorta and do not involve the other arteries. The condition typically occurs in young patients and accounts for approximately 5%–10% of all AAAs.

Immunoglobulin G4-related disease (IgG4-RD)-associated aneurysms are a subset of inflammatory AAAs, which is gaining rapid momentum of research and recognition. The disease is characterized by high detectable levels of IgG4 with microscopic evidence of storiform fibrosis and plasma cells that are IgG4-positive. Patients usually respond well to steroids and anti-B cell therapies.

Mycotic aneurysms are another variant caused by bacterial infection and associated inflammation. A painful, rapidly growing, often presenting as a ruptured aneurysm at the time of diagnosis typifies a mycotic aneurysm, probably provoked by the localized suppurative process.

COURSE OF THE DISEASE

AAAs generally grow slowly and produce no symptoms and can be found incidentally on physical examination as a pulsatile abdominal mass. When large, they tend to impinge on the adjacent viscera and cause gastrointestinal (GI) or renal manifestations or may cause obstruction of branching vessels resulting in ischaemia. In 75%–80% of cases, the vessel wall is often obscured by an intraluminal thrombus which may cause distal embolization. The frequent fatal complication of AAAs is the event of sudden rupture, leading to a catastrophic haemoperitoneum. The risk of rupture is directly proportional to the size of the aneurysm. Once an AAA ruptures, the prognosis is grim. More than 50% of patients die before they reach the hospital.

The treatment of large aneurysms involves the surgical removal of the damaged section of the aorta and replacing it with a synthetic tube (graft).

Thoracic Aortic Aneurysm

A thoracic aortic aneurysm (TAA) predominantly involves the ascending aorta or aortic root. Although thoracic aneurysms are less common than AAAs, they are associated with high mortality.

The most important risk factor for developing TAA is hypertension, followed by connective tissue disorders such as MFS or EDS, and aortitis. Owing to their location, TAA tends to compress the structures of the neck and chest causing symptoms such as dyspnoea or cough, symptoms of heart failure and hoarseness of voice. Thoracic aneurysms stand a risk of rupture and dissection, which are both potentially lethal. Management of thoracic aneurysm depends on the location and usually involves graft placement.

Aortic Dissection

Aortic dissection occurs when a tear in the intima allows blood to seep in and separate the laminar planes of the media to form a blood-filled channel within layers of the vascular wall.

Aetiology The highest attributable risk population include elderly men with long-standing hypertension and preexisting aortic aneurysm. MFS, Loeys–Dietz or EDS contribute to the increased risk of aortic dissection but the presentation is usually at a much younger age. Dissections may also follow arterial cannulations during coronary catheterization procedures or cardiopulmonary bypass. Rarely, pregnancy is associated with aortic dissection usually manifesting in the second or third trimester. Interestingly, in conditions such as atherosclerosis and *Treponema pallidum* infection (syphilis), dissection is usually less prevalent, probably because of the associated fibrosis and calcification.

Pathogenesis A classic aortic dissection is initiated by a tear of the aortic intima, following which blood enters the vessel wall and causes medial dissection and haematoma. The exact trigger mechanisms involving intimal tear has not been resolved till date. It is hypothesized that haemodynamic factors, chiefly in hypertension, cause tears in the intima and initiate these dissecting aneurysms. The intimal tear more frequently occurs in segments exposed to the greatest shear stress such as the proximal descending aorta or the right lateral wall of the ascending aorta. In patients with hypertension and connective tissue disorders, degenerative changes within the media and the loss of the elastic tissue cause CMN prompting aortic dissection. However, recent studies have revealed that in approximately 10% of patients, dissections present without an intimal tear probably because of disruption of the vasa vasorum.

Once the dissection erupts, because of the systemic pressure, when the vessel contracts, the blood collects between the layers of the media eventually progressing to haematoma formation. The dissecting haematoma often spreads in an either antegrade or retrograde fashion creating a false lumen within the vascular wall. With further progression, the dissection may rupture through a second distal intimal tear into the true lumen (double-barrel aorta), or through the adventitia into the pericardium. These vascular channels may develop an endothelial lining to become chronic dissections.

Morphology

Approximately 60% of aortic dissections occur with an intimal tear along the ascending aorta, usually **within**

10 cm of the aortic valve. The next most common site is the descending thoracic aorta immediately distal to the origin of the left subclavian artery. The intimal tear is usually 4–5 cm in length, sharply defined, transverse or oblique. The frequently encountered histological lesion is **cystic medical necrosis** that is characterized by degeneration and fragmentation of the fibromuscular components of the media along with the development of small, cystic spaces between them. Associated inflammation is characteristically absent. The dissecting haematoma spreads typically along the laminar planes of the aorta, usually between the middle and adventitial layers.

Classification (Fig. 13.24)

DeBakey classification classifies aortic dissection depending on the extent of involvement:

- *Type I* involves the ascending aorta, aortic arch and descending thoracic aorta and may progress to involve the abdominal aorta. It is the most common type comprising 75% of cases.
- *Type II* involves only the ascending aorta.
- *Type IIIa* involves the descending thoracic aorta distal to the origin of the left subclavian artery up to the diaphragm.
- *Type IIIb* dissection extends further to involve the thoracic and abdominal aorta distal to the left subclavian artery beyond the diaphragm.

Along with the DeBakey classification, the ***Stanford classification*** is used to plan the treatment protocols, to differentiate those that require surgical intervention and those that can be medically managed.

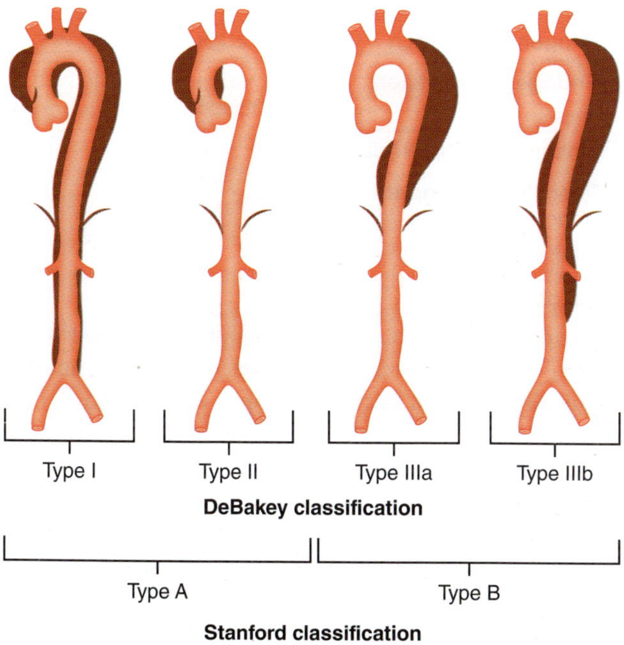

Fig. 13.24 Classification of aortic aneurysms.

Stanford classification

- Type A includes all dissections involving the ascending aorta, regardless of the exact site.
- Type B involves the descending thoracic or thoracoabdominal aorta distal to the left subclavian artery, or rather all dissections not involving the ascending aorta.

Clinical Features and Consequences Patients with aortic dissection initially present with intense chest pain which often radiates to the back. Rupture of the dissection can cause haemopericardium and cardiac tamponade which may be fatal. As mentioned earlier, the dissection may extend proximally or distally or both. Extension into the aortic root can result in aortic regurgitation, whereas extension into the coronary arteries can result in myocardial infarction.

Type A dissections usually require surgical management and antihypertensive treatment but haemorrhage and ischaemia can cause disastrous implications. Most type B dissections can be managed conservatively, but regardless of the treatment plan, the survival rate is only 75%.

VASCULITIS

Vasculitis refers to the inflammation of the blood vessel wall that can manifest as a primary disease by itself or as secondary to other pathological disease processes. Vasculitic syndromes can involve vessels of any segment of the vasculature and the clinical consequences usually depend on the blood vessels involved.

The inflammation often induces damage to the vessel wall with fibrinoid necrosis and wall thickening causing narrowing of the lumen which may worsen up to complete occlusion in some cases. Occasionally, thrombosis resulting in tissue ischaemia and necrosis may occur. Moreover, the inflammation weakens the vessel wall predisposing to the development of aneurysms that may rupture with bleeding eventually.

When the vasculitic process affects one organ predominantly, it is referred to as single-organ vasculitis, whereas the involvement of multiple organ system defines systemic vasculitis.

Systemic vasculitis can be **primary** when no aetiological factor is identified or **secondary** to pathologies such as infections (e.g. secondary to hepatitis C or HIV infection), drugs (e.g. propylthiouracil and hydralazine), irradiation, mechanical trauma, toxins, systemic autoimmune diseases (e.g. systemic lupus erythematosus, rheumatoid arthritis and Sjögren syndrome) or cancer (Fig. 13.25).

PATHOGENESIS

Vasculitis is induced by a variety of aetiologies and pathogenetic mechanisms, all of which mediate vascular inflammatory injury. The two most common mechanisms

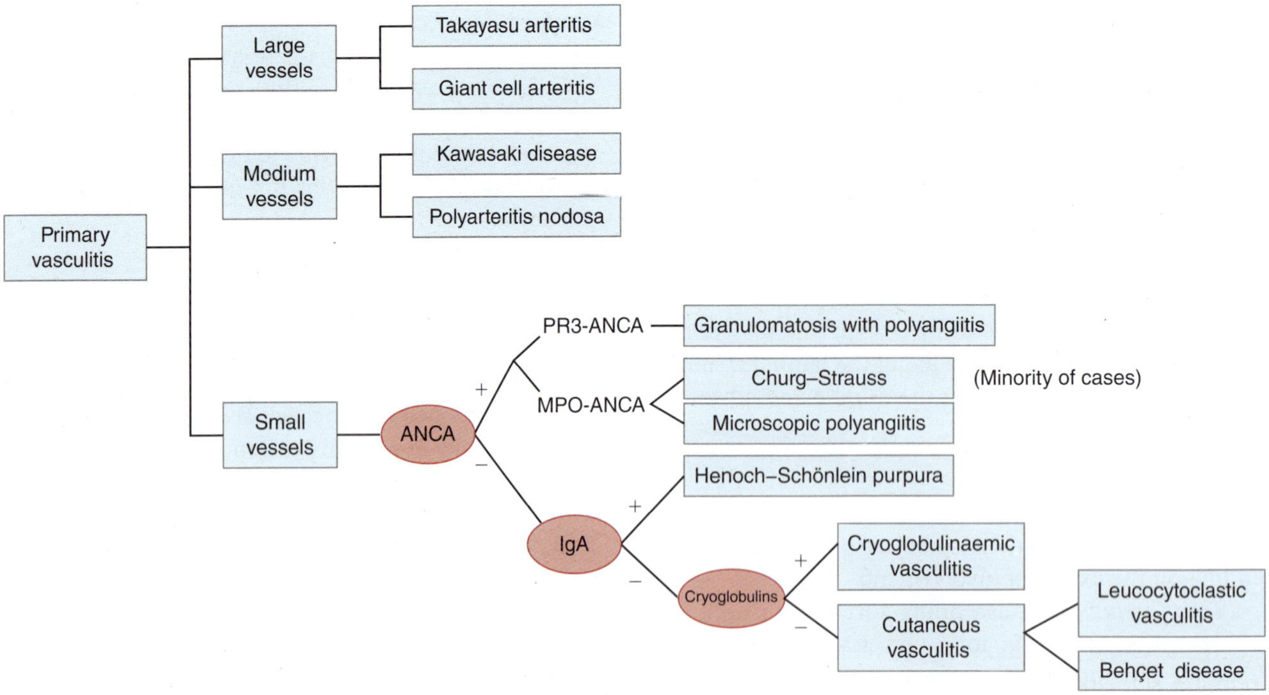

Fig. 13.25 Classification of vasculitis – the Chapel Hill Consensus criteria, nomenclature update 2012.

are direct injury of the vessel wall by infectious pathogens and immune-mediated inflammation. The inflammatory response in infectious vasculitis involves both nonimmune and immune mechanisms. The former is due to direct invasion of the vessel wall by the organisms, whereas the latter is due to the immune mechanisms that fight the pathogen. For example, systemic vasculitis in rickettsial infection results from proliferation of the pathogen in the vessel wall causing vascular necrosis and inflammation. On the contrary, hepatitis B virus (HBV) infection of liver can cause systemic vasculitis by the deposition of immune complexes (viral antigen and corresponding antibody) on the vessel wall.

Clinically, differentiating infectious vasculitis and immune-mediated vasculitis holds utmost importance because immunosuppressive therapy can be relevant in immune-mediated vasculitis and proves hazardous in infectious vasculitis (Table 13.4).

Table 13.4 Vasculitis Classification Based on Aetiological Factors

Infectious Vasculitis	
Bacterial	Bacterial endocarditis, septicaemia, mycobacterial infection
Viral	Herpes virus, HIV cytomegalovirus, HTLV
Rickettsial	Ehrlichiosis
Immune-Mediated Vasculitis (Noninfectious Vasculitis)	
Exogenous antigen	Drugs, food additives
Endogenous antigen	Neoplasia, connective tissue diseases
Unknown antigen (idiopathic)	
Vasculitis secondary to infections	

IMMUNE-MEDIATED VASCULITIS

The immunological mechanisms that underlie vasculitis include:

- Immune complex deposition
- Antineutrophil cytoplasmic antibodies (ANCAs)
- Antiendothelial cell antibodies (AECAs)
- Autoreactive T cells
- **Immune complex deposition:**

Immune complex–associated vasculitis is typically triggered by adverse drug reactions (antibiotics, nonsteroidal anti-inflammatory medications, vaccines, therapeutic injections of sera), or underlying internal diseases (neoplasia, infections) or autoimmune diseases (connective tissue diseases such as systemic lupus erythematosus).

Pathogenic preformed immune complexes may be deposited in blood vessels from the circulation as in SLE or occasionally immune complexes may be formed by antibodies against deposited antigens. Serum sickness is considered a prototype of immune complex–associated vasculitic syndromes, thus attributing most cases to type III immune complex–mediated hypersensitivity. Immune complexes fix complement and deposit in the vascular endothelium or in

Table 13.5 Pathological Mechanisms Underlying Different Types of Vasculitis

Immune Complex Mediated	ANCA-Associated Diseases
Goodpasture disease	Granulomatosis with polyangiitis
Cutaneous leucocytoclastic vasculitis (hypersensitivity vasculitis)	Microscopic polyangiitis
Essential cryoglobulinaemia	Churg–Strauss syndrome
Polyarteritis nodosa	Renal-limited vasculitis

ANCA, antineutrophil cytoplasmic antibody.

capillary beds, such as those found in the skin, kidneys or lungs. Cryoglobulinaemia vasculitis is a recognized entity, most commonly due to HCV-induced immune complex–mediated vasculitis involving small vessels. The most common skin manifestation of small vessel vasculitis is palpable purpura. Identifying drug hypersensitivity vasculitis is particularly important because removal of the offending agent can reverse the condition (Table 13.5).

- **Antineutrophil cytoplasmic antibodies:**
  ANCAs are autoantibodies which react with antigens in the cytoplasm of the neutrophils. Their presence is associated with several vasculitic syndromes, although their origin or role in pathogenesis is poorly understood. They are detected by immunofluorescence and distinguished by their pattern of staining. ANCAs are classified according to their differential specificity to neutrophilic antigens.
  - ***Antiproteinase-3 (PR3-ANCA, previously c-ANCA):*** PR3 is a neutrophil azurophilic granule constituent that is speculated to provide molecular mimicry against microbes. The antibody stains neutrophils in a cytoplasmic pattern and is observed in granulomatosis with polyangiitis (GPA) (previously known as Wegener granulomatosis) (Fig. 13.26).
  - ***MPO-ANCA (previously p-ANCA):*** MPO is a lysosomal granule constituent involved in oxygen free radical generation. MPO-ANCAs are induced by several therapeutic agents, particularly propylthiouracil. MPO-ANCAs stain neutrophils in a perinuclear pattern and are observed in microscopic polyangiitis and Churg–Strauss syndrome.

  ANCA-associated vasculitis is often referred to as 'pauci-immune' because it does not trigger immune complex formation in circulation. Pauci-immune indicates the relative lack of immunoglobulin and complement deposition on the vessel wall as demonstrated by indirect immunofluorescence techniques. Note that atypical patterns of ANCA may be observed in conditions other than vasculitis (e.g. inflammatory bowel disease).

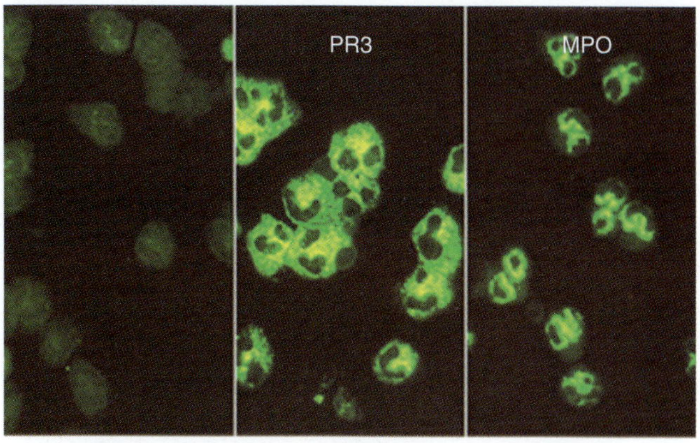

Fig. 13.26 Immunofluorescence studies on ethanol-fixed neutrophils. Note, PR3-ANCA shows a characteristic cytoplasmic granularity (middle) and MPO-ANCA shows a perinuclear pattern (right). (*Source:* From David A. Cabral and Kimberly A. Morishita. Antineutrophil Cytoplasmic Antibody Associated Vasculitis. Textbook of Pediatric Rheumatology. 8th edition. Elsevier 2021.)

- **Antiendothelial cell antibodies:** These antibodies are demonstrable in cases of SLE, Kawasaki disease and Buerger disease.

  The above-mentioned pathogenetic mechanisms can give rise to many vasculitic syndromes. The following discussion briefly explains the most recognized forms.

Giant Cell Arteritis

Overview Giant cell arteritis is a primary vasculitis which traditionally affects large- to small-sized arteries. The extracranial arteries, especially **temporal arteries**, are preferentially involved in GCA along with the vertebral and ophthalmic arteries.

Epidemiology Ageing is the most important risk factor for giant cell arteritis because this disease almost exclusively affects people older than 50 years. The disease risk is highest among those aged between 75 and 85 years with high prevalence among European and American populations.

Pathogenesis The pathogenesis of giant cell arteritis is poorly understood, but a possible bacterial or viral trigger has been speculated. Dendritic cells (DCs) migrate to the inflamed wall to initiate and maintain activation of T cells. $CD4^+$ T cells produce IFN-γ and induce macrophages to carry out their effector functions that result in vascular injury. The formation of granulomas within the media is also a T-cell–dependent phenomenon.

Morphology

The histological findings include **panarteritis** with T cells and macrophages infiltrating the arterial wall associated with intimal hyperplasia. Classically, giant cell arteritis is characterized by granulomatous

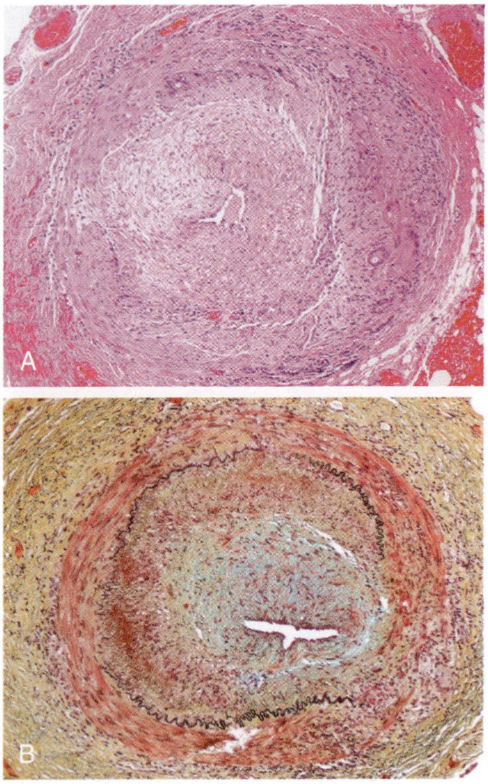

Fig. 13.27 Giant cell arteritis. (A) A temporal artery biopsy shows transmural granulomatous inflammation with giant cells in the media and adventitia of this muscular artery. (B) Movat's stain shows disruption of the internal elastic lamina in the areas with inflammation and marked intimal hyperplasia. Fibrinoid necrosis is occasionally observed.

inflammation organized around the internal elastic membrane causing fragmentation of the elastic laminae (Figs 13.27 and 13.28). Multinucleated giant cells can be frequently seen in approximately 75% of biopsies often accompanied by lymphocytes ($CD4^+ > CD8^+$). Inflammation results in thickening and narrowing of the arterial lumen which can additionally undergo thrombosis. Subsequent fibrotic organization of the thrombosis can convert the artery into a solid cord.

Clinical Consequences Headache is usually the predominant feature along with intense pain over the temples, jaw pain while talking and chewing, and scalp tenderness. The temporal artery on palpation may show signs of tenderness and mild nodularity. Patients may present with constitutional symptoms because of hypoperfusion caused by stenosis or obliteration of the involved vessels. A feared complication is visual impairment or blindness which can occur because of involvement of the ophthalmic artery in at least 50% of patients.

Takayasu Arteritis

Overview Takayasu arteritis (TA) is a primary vasculitic syndrome which predominantly affects large- and medium-sized arteries. The disease has high predilection for the aortic arch and its branches. The pulmonary arteries, coronary and the renal arteries are also frequently involved.

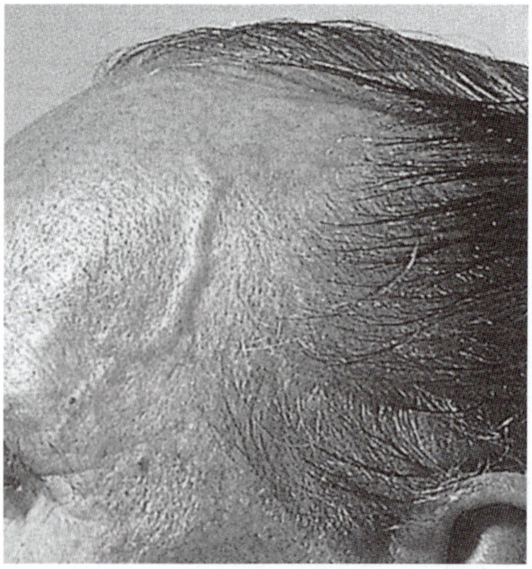

Fig. 13.28 Photograph showing the prominence of the temporal artery in temporal arteritis. (*Source:* From David S. Younger. Giant Cell Arteritis. Neurologic Clinics. 2019;7:335-344.

Epidemiology TA most commonly affects women of the adolescent age group and shares many common clinical and histological features with that of giant cell arteritis. It is a generic consideration that the diagnosis of giant cell aortitis is made in patients older than 50 years, whereas it is TA in those younger than 50 years.

Pathogenesis In the past, TA was believed to be prevalent only among the Japanese population, associated with only a subset of human leucocyte antigen (HLA) alleles. However, TA has now been identified to have a wider distribution, among different populations, and has been linked to autoimmune and genetic aetiology.

Morphology

Involved arteries display mononuclear cell infiltrate most commonly observed centred around the tunica adventitia, particularly near the vasa vasorum or in the tunica media. One of the important features is the formation of **granulomas that may contain giant cells, marking the difficulty in distinguishing from giant cell arteritis. The inflammation causes significant intimal hyperplasia and thickening of the vascular wall which is often evident macroscopically.** Eventually, in some cases, the proliferative or fibrotic thickening of the tunica intima may cause narrowing or obliteration of the vascular lumen.

Clinical Consequences The inflammation initially causes constitutional symptoms, which is followed by the painful ischaemic phase. The final 'burnt-out disease' stage elicits decreased or absent pulse in the upper extremities, the most characteristic feature, hence the name **'pulseless disease'**. This is seen in 80%–90% of the patients and is usually associated with limb claudication and BP discrepancies. The other common symptoms include ocular disturbances, such as visual defects, retinal haemorrhages, progressing up to total blindness and neurologic deficits. Arterial hypertension may result from stenosis of renal arteries or abdominal aorta. Takayasu retinopathy, neurological manifestations especially stroke and myocardial infarction are the serious consequences of Takayasu vasculitis.

Polyarteritis Nodosa

Overview Polyarteritis nodosa (PAN) is a systemic vasculitis characterized by necrotizing inflammation primarily affecting the medium-sized blood vessels of the kidney and other organs but the pulmonary vasculature, regardless of the vessel size, is completely spared.

Epidemiology PAN is a protracted, recurring disease, typically affecting young adults but can affect individuals of any all age.

Pathogenesis The pathogenesis of PAN is yet to be fully understood. Although the primary cases of PAN are idiopathic, secondary PAN is much less frequent and is believed to be associated with hepatitis B infection, hepatitis C infection and hairy cell leukaemia. It is one of the rare associates with hepatitis B virus infection, supported by the fact that after the decline in HBV infection because of vaccination and appropriate antiviral therapy, the prevalence of PAN has significantly reduced. Up to 30% of patients with classical PAN are known to have circulating hepatitis B antigen in their serum. Other infectious agents associated with PAN include HIV, cytomegalovirus, parvovirus B19, human T-lymphotropic virus type I (HTLV-I) and HCV. In general, no association between PAN and ANCAs has been observed.

Morphology

Most patients show positive angiographic evidence of the disease in the visceral arteries, arteries of the extremities and the smaller branches of the aorta. Angiographically, a well-recognized feature is the presence of microaneurysms which are characteristic but not pathognomonic (Fig. 13.29).

Microscopically, PAN is defined by a necrotizing inflammation involving all layers of the vessel wall. The inflammatory infiltrate initially is predominantly neutrophilic but evolves to become dominated by mononuclear cells later. **Fibrinoid necrosis** is frequently observed owing to immune complex deposits. The inflammation and fibrinoid necrosis can weaken the vascular wall and thus render it prone to aneurysmal dilations which in some cases may rupture, leading to haemorrhage (Fig. 13.30). In addition, thrombosis is a frequent finding in the involved segments usually causing downstream hypoperfusion. Over time, a healing phase results in fibrotic remodelling of the vascular wall and may worsen the luminal occlusion. Uniquely, different morphological stages of the disease can be observed simultaneously in the same vessel.

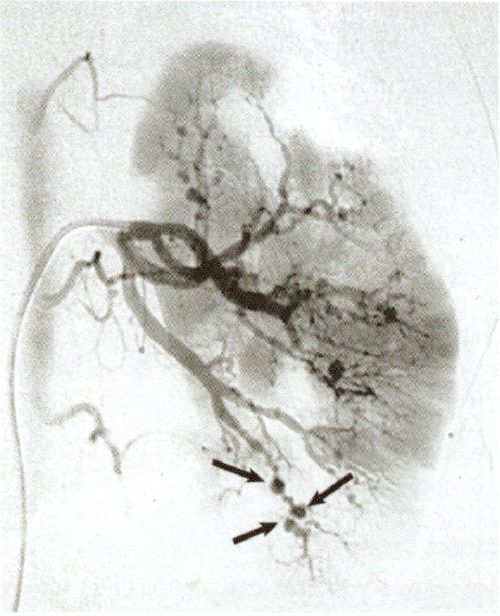

Fig. 13.29 Renal angiogram showing multiple small aneurysms (arrows) in a patient with polyarthritis nodosa. Note the characteristic string of beads appearance. (*Source:* From Nicole B. Yang, Anthony M. Reginato, Sarah Aziz, Syeda M. Sayeed. Vasculitis, Systemic. Elsevier 2022.)

Clinical Consequences PAN presents with nonspecific constitutional symptoms such as fever, myalgia, abdominal pain and headache. At the most, organ-specific symptomology may manifest because of occlusion-induced

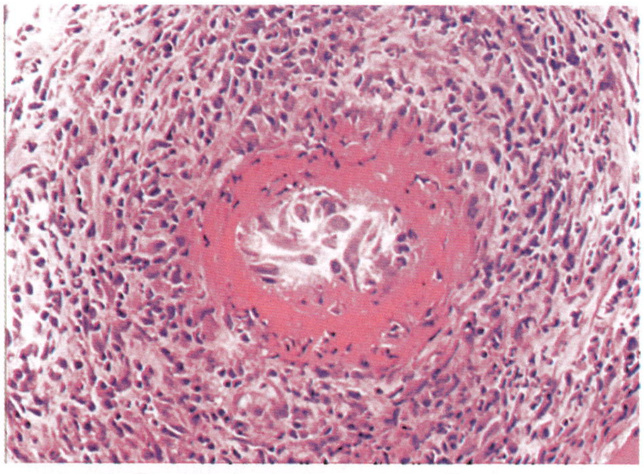

Fig. 13.30 Polyarteritis nodosa. The affected medium-sized blood vessel shows dense inflammatory cell infiltrate with fibrinoid necrosis. (*Source:* From Nicole B. Yang, Anthony M. Reginato, Sarah Aziz, Syeda M. Sayeed. Vasculitis, Systemic. Elsevier 2022.)

hypoperfusion of the specific vascular beds. The kidneys are the most commonly affected organs.

- Kidney – characteristically inflammation is confined to the renal arteries with relative sparing of the glomeruli causing hypertension
- Heart – affected coronary arteries can predispose to myocardial infarction
- Muscles and joints – inflammation can manifest as myalgia and arthritis
- GI system – GI bleeding and abdominal pain
- Peripheral nervous system – peripheral neuritis
- Skin – palpable purpura

Untreated PAN is usually fatal. In cases detected early, immunosuppression can be particularly helpful.

Kawasaki Disease

Overview Kawasaki disease is a vasculitis which affects medium- and small-sized arteries, although fatalities are solely due to consequences of coronary artery inflammation.

Epidemiology The vast majority of patients are infants and children younger than 5 years. Kawasaki disease is one of the leading causes of acquired heart disease in children.

Pathogenesis The aetiology of Kawasaki disease is still unknown, but there is some evidence that infectious agents could play a role in the pathogenesis. It is hypothesized that the possible pathogen could enter the body via the respiratory tract or the digestive tract and would be processed by lymphoid tissues within those organs. Thus, activated T cells and macrophages mediating a delayed-type hypersensitivity reaction are attributed to play a role in Kawasaki disease.

Morphology

The morphology of Kawasaki disease is similar to that of PAN with a **necrotizing inflammation** of the entire vascular wall. Although the inflammation is self-limited, the healing phase may present with aneurysmal dilation, thrombosis and intimal proliferation.

Clinical Consequences Kawasaki disease is characterized by an acute, self-limited febrile illness of infants and children, which is benign on its own but can yield serious coronary complications during its healing phase.

Kawasaki disease typically presents with erythematous cracked lips and conjunctiva, strawberry tongue, extremity changes such as oedema of the hands and feet, erythema of the palms and soles, a desquamative rash and cervical lymphadenopathy, hence its other name, ***mucocutaneous lymph node syndrome*** (Fig. 13.31).

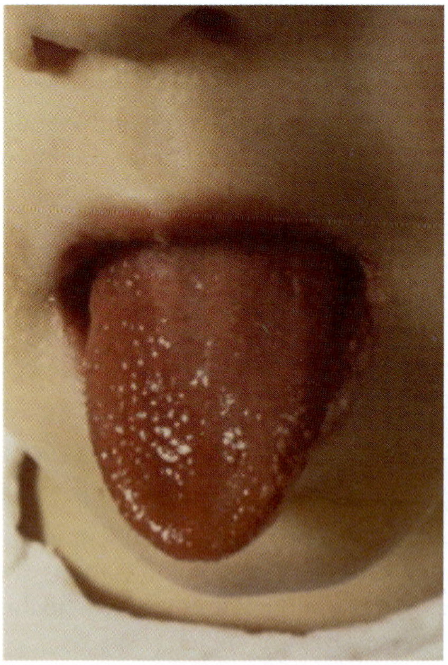

Fig. 13.31 Clinical manifestations of Kawasaki disease: **(A)** bulbar conjunctivitis; **(B)** red cracked erythematous lips; **(C)** strawberry tongue. (*Source:* From Rosie Scuccimarri. Kawasaki Disease. Pediatric Clinics of North America. 2012:59:425-445.)

The most feared complication of Kawasaki disease is **myocardial infarction**. However, long-term complications such as coronary artery aneurysms, heart failure, myocardial infarction, arrhythmias and PAD worsen the prognosis, leading to an increased morbidity and mortality.

Proper treatment of Kawasaki disease is important because a significant percentage of untreated children may develop permanent coronary damage. The administration of intravenous immunoglobulin with aspirin during the acute phase of the disease can reduce the incidence of coronary aneurysms.

Microscopic Polyangiitis

Overview Microscopic polyangiitis is a vasculitis of small- to medium-sized vessels including arterioles, capillaries and venules. The most commonly involved tissues include skin, mucous membranes, lungs, brain, heart, GI tract, kidneys and muscle. Microscopic angiitis can be a feature of a number of immune disorders such as Henoch–Schönlein purpura, essential mixed cryoglobulinaemia and vasculitis associated with connective tissue disorders.

Epidemiology This disease primarily affects the elderly and has a slight predilection for men.

Pathogenesis The condition results from immunologic response to an identifiable antigen that may be microorganisms (e.g. mycobacteria, HBV, CMV), certain drugs, chemicals or connective tissue diseases such as rheumatoid arthritis and SLE. These may give rise to immune complex deposition or trigger secondary immune response, i.e. development of ANCAs. Most cases are associated with MPO-ANCA. Recruitment and activation of neutrophils within the affected vascular beds cause easy access for the antibodies.

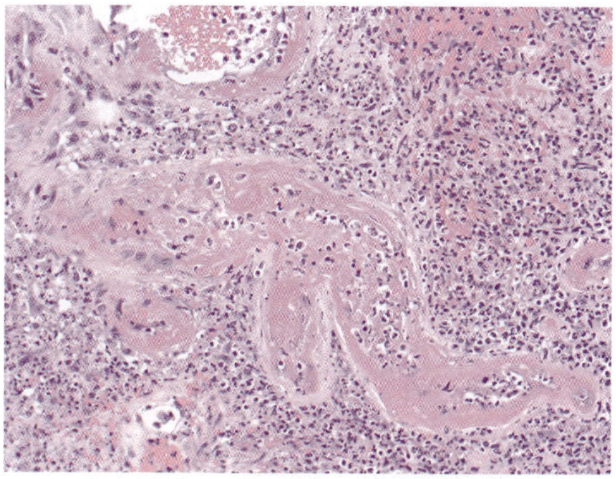

Fig. 13.32 Microscopic polyangiitis. Neutrophils seen infiltrating the vessel wall causing degeneration – leucocytoclastic vasculitis. (*Source:* From Aliya N. Husain. Microscopic Polyangiitis. High-Yield Thoracic Pathology. Saunders 2012.)

Morphology

Microscopic polyangiitis is characterized by a **necrotizing vasculitis** and segmental fibrinoid necrosis of the media similar to that of PAN, but in contrast spare the medium- and large-sized blood vessels. In a few cases, infiltrated neutrophils in the small vessel walls undergo degeneration, known as leucocytoclasis with nuclear dust (karyorrhexis) giving rise to ***leucocytoclastic vasculitis, typically in the postcapillary venules*** (Fig. 13.32). Immunoglobulins can be demonstrated only rarely in the early lesions because most cases are pauci-immune.

Clinical Course Most importantly, involvement of the glomerular capillaries results in a pauci-immune glomerulonephritis which manifests as nephritic syndrome with haematuria and hypertension. Involvement of the pulmonary circulation may lead to haemorrhage from the pulmonary capillaries, resulting in haemoptysis. *Glomerulonephritis and pulmonary capillary involvement* are undoubtedly the most significant and common complications of microscopic polyangiitis.

Granulomatosis With Polyangiitis (Wegener Granulomatosis)

Overview GPA is a vasculitis of small- to medium-sized vasculature, including arterioles, capillaries and venules. Previously called Wegener granulomatosis, GPA is a necrotizing vasculitis characterized by a clinicopathological triad of

- *Necrotizing granulomas involving the* upper respiratory tract (ear, nose, sinuses, throat and the lung
- *Necrotizing or granulomatous vasculitis particularly of the* lungs and upper airways
- *Focal necrotizing, often crescentic, glomerulonephritis*

'Limited' forms of this disease may be restricted to the respiratory tract, whereas a widespread form of the disease can affect eyes, skin, heart and other organs.

Epidemiology The disease can manifest at any age, although there is a predilection for middle-aged individuals. There does not appear to be a gender bias.

Pathogenesis GPA is postulated to result from T-cell–mediated hypersensitivity response to inertly inhaled microbial or other environmental agents. In approximately 95% of cases, **PR3-ANCA** is detected which makes it an important marker to predict the disease activity.

Morphology

Respiratory Lesions Granulomatosis with polyangiitis is characterized by necrotizing vasculitis involving both the upper and lower respiratory tract. Most often inflammation is associated with formation of intravascular or extravascular **granulomas** that contain geographic patterns of central **necrosis (due to high turnover of cells forming nuclear debris)** and giant cells (Fig. 13.33). Away from the areas of large necrosis, other arteries show inflammatory cells, predominantly lymphocytes, infiltrating the media. Coalescence of granulomas in the lung can be visualized as nodules which may undergo **cavitation** on chest radiography. As the disease progresses, the necrosis may become more widespread with alveolar haemorrhages and may later undergo organization and fibrosis.

Renal Lesions Initially there is **focal, segmental inflammation** of the glomerulus which may later advance to a rapidly progressive glomerulonephritis. As no immune complexes are observed by immunofluorescence, glomerular lesions are considered as pauci-immune glomerulonephritis.

Clinical Consequences The disease affects males more than females of an average age of 40 years. Most patients display an array of respiratory and renal symptoms. Respiratory tract shows chronic sinusitis, ulcerations of the nasopharyngeal mucosa, epistaxis and haemoptysis. With renal involvement, signs of nephritic syndrome become apparent. If left untreated, most patients die within a year of diagnosis. With treatment (steroids, anti-B cell antibodies) also, GPA is known for its relapsing and remitting status.

Thromboangiitis Obliterans (Buerger Disease)

Overview Thromboangiitis obliterans (TO) is a vasculitis of small- and medium-sized arteries which can extend into contiguous veins and nerves. It typically involves the vessels of the extremities, specifically the tibial and radial artery with features of segmental, thrombosing acute and chronic inflammation.

Epidemiology TO is considered to be an exclusive disease of heavy chronic smokers, especially in men younger than 35 years.

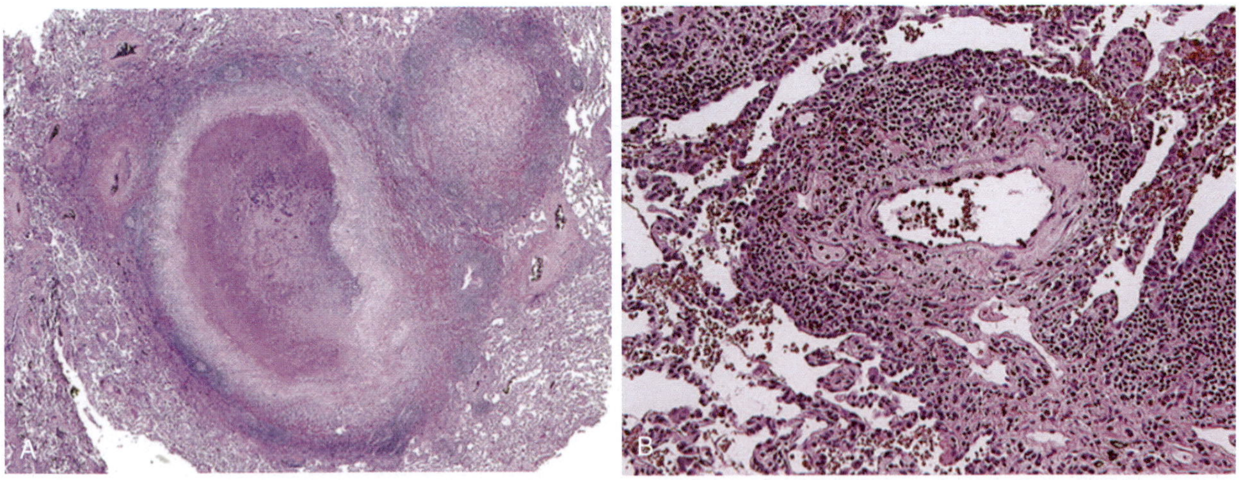

Fig. 13.33 Granulomatosis with polyangiitis. **(A)** Lung biopsy showing well-formed granulomas, large areas of 'geographical necrosis' that appear basophilic because of the abundance of necrotic debris, with a rimming of lymphocytes. **(B)** Blood vessel with extensive medial inflammation. (*Source:* From Michael A. Seidman and Richard N. Mitchell. Surgical Pathology of Small- and Medium-Sized Vessels. Surgical Pathology Clinics. 2012; 5:435-451.)

Pathogenesis The **strong association with cigarette** leads to the speculation that endothelial cell injury caused by smoking, or an immune response to the components of tobacco smoke can trigger the disease. Association with particular HLA haplotypes have also been reported.

Morphology

TO is characterized by an initial infiltration of the vascular wall with neutrophils. Over time, the inflammatory infiltrate is replaced by mononuclear cells and occasionally thrombus may appear. The thrombus may contain small microabscesses composed of neutrophils surrounded by granulomatous inflammation. This is often followed by thrombosis of the vascular lumen. Over time, vascular fibrosis develops followed by recanalization of the obstructed vessel.

Clinical Consequences The vascular insufficiency caused by TO often manifests initially as Raynaud phenomenon (explained later) and claudication pain induced by exercise and superficial nodular phlebitis. Later, inflammatory involvement of adjacent peripheral nerves leads to severe pain even at rest. The ischaemia can cause chronic ulcerations of hands and feet and in severe cases gangrenous necrosis. Abstinence from smoking can prevent disease progression in the early stages, but once the vascular pathology commences, smoking abstinence is of no help.

Churg–Strauss Syndrome

Overview Churg–Strauss syndrome is a small-vessel necrotizing vasculitis capable of involving virtually any organ, with a high predilection for the lung. Likewise, the syndrome is most often associated with asthma, allergic rhinitis and lung infiltrates and is hence referred to as allergic granulomatosis and angiitis.

Epidemiology Although Churg–Strauss syndrome tends to affect individuals of all age groups, with no particular gender bias, most cases are seen to occur in men around the age of 30–40 years.

Pathogenesis The disease is postulated to be a likely consequence of allergic reactions to certain innocuous stimuli. A minor fraction of cases has seen associated with **MPO-ANCA as well.**

Morphology

The lung and the extrapulmonary sites involved (heart, skin, GIT, brain) show characteristic necrotizing inflammation of the vascular wall accompanied by focal granulomas. Prominent eosinophilic infiltrate is seen usually around the necrotic foci. Also, areas of fibrosis, eosinophilic microabscesses and oedema can be observed. This is often reflected by peripheral blood eosinophilia.

Clinical Consequences Long-term treatment with glucocorticoids can be useful in reducing symptoms. Many patients rather enter a phase of chemical remission through drug therapy. The disease is usually chronic and lifelong.

Behçet Disease

Behçet disease is a type of neutrophilic vasculitis involving the medium- to small-sized blood vessels classically presenting as a clinical triad of genital ulcers, recurrent oral aphthous ulcers and uveitis. Although infectious, environmental, genetic and immunological factors have been attributed to the disease, its exact pathogenic mechanism still remains obscure. Treatment usually follows corticosteroids therapy.

Henoch–Schönlein Purpura

Henoch–Schönlein purpura, also known as **IgA vasculitis,** is a disorder that affects the small blood vessels in the skin, joints, intestines and kidneys (Fig. 13.34).

The hallmark feature of Henoch–Schönlein purpura is a purple-coloured rash, typically occurring on the lower legs and buttocks, most common in children aged between 2 and 6 years. The condition usually improves on its own. Medical care is generally needed if the disorder affects the kidneys (the topic is dealt with greater detail in Chapter 24).

Vasculitis Associated With Other Noninfectious Disorders

Vasculitis can sometimes be associated with other disorders such as rheumatoid arthritis, systemic lupus erythematosus, malignancy, or systemic illnesses such as mixed cryoglobulinaemia, and antiphospholipid antibody syndrome.

Infectious vasculitis

As mentioned earlier, arteritis can be caused by the direct infiltration of the infectious agent, usually bacteria (*Pseudomonas, a prototypical* example) or fungi, especially ***Aspergillus* and *Mucor* species.** Vascular invasion can arise from adjacent abscesses, or through haematogenous spread in septicaemia or embolization from infective endocarditis. The following are of interest:

- **Rheumatoid vasculitis** affects chiefly the small- and medium-sized arteries of multiple visceral organs in patients who have rheumatoid nodules of long duration. Vasculitis in SLE affects mainly the small arteries of the skin.
- **Rheumatic vasculitis** involves the aorta, carotid and coronary arteries and the visceral vessels. Usually, fibrinoid change and perivascular inflammation are seen rather than typical Aschoff nodules.

Raynaud Phenomenon

Raynaud phenomenon is caused by episodic vasoconstriction of arteries and arterioles because of hyperactivity to cold and emotional stress. This is believed to be a thermoregulatory mechanism to prevent the loss of

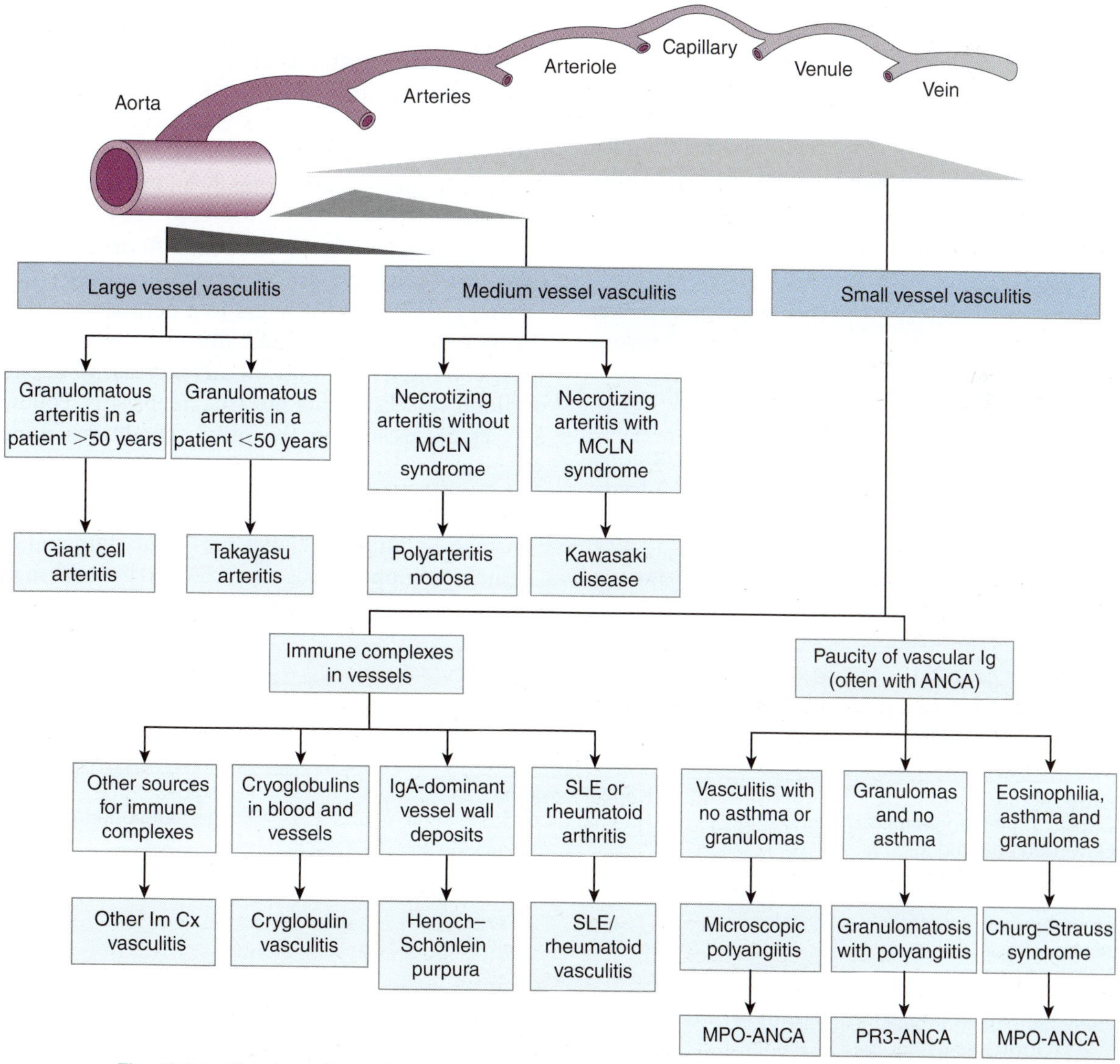

Fig. 13.34 Structure of vasculitis workup. MCLN syndrome, mucocutaneous lymph node syndrome.

heat from the body and to maintain core body temperature. The reduced blood flow often manifests as well-demarcated areas of pallor or sometimes even cyanosis. The pallor typically sustains for roughly 20 minutes following which rewarming results in erythema (reactive hyperaemia).

Raynaud phenomenon often manifests in the extremities especially in the fingers and toes, but occasionally may be seen to involve nose, lips and earlobes. The attack is seen mostly symmetrically on both hands with typical sparing of the thumb.

As with other disorders, Raynaud phenomenon can be primary or secondary.

Primary Raynaud phenomenon accounts for a total of 3%–5% of the general population. Although the exact cause is not fully elucidated, patients with primary Raynaud phenomenon tend to have increased $\alpha 2$ adrenergic sensitivity in the digital vessels showing exaggerated responses to stimuli. The disease usually follows a benign course but over a period of time, atrophy of the skin, muscle and subcutaneous tissue may develop.

Secondary Raynaud phenomenon can follow conditions such as SLE, Buerger disease, systemic sclerosis and drugs (antimigraine medications, cyclosporine).

Patients with Raynaud phenomenon usually show spontaneous remission with avoidance of the provoking stimuli. Few patients may require medications to induce vasodilation, such as in calcium channel blockers. However, spontaneous remission is not seen with secondary Raynaud disease.

VASCULAR TUMOURS

Vascular tumours are neoplasms that feature high endothelial cell turnover. These tumours of the vascular system can be broadly categorized into benign lesions, tumours of intermediate grade and malignant neoplasms (Table 13.6).

Benign tumours constitute the majority and are predominantly seen in the paediatric and adolescent age group. Tumours belonging to the intermediate-grade category are relatively less common and include tumours that may be locally aggressive but show no or low metastatic potential.

Two general rules pertaining to vascular tumours are as follows:

- Benign tumours usually follow a lobular architecture and show distinct well-formed vessels lined by monolayered endothelial cells that appear near normal.
- Malignant tumours on the contrary, are more proliferative, display cytological atypia and do not form organized vessels. Thus, determination of endothelial origin of these tumour cells require immunohistochemical staining with endothelial cell-specific markers such as CD31, CD34 or von Willebrand factor.

BENIGN TUMOURS AND TUMOUR-LIKE CONDITIONS

Benign vascular tumours are the most common childhood tumours. Importantly, these benign tumours need to be differentiated from vascular malformations because they follow different clinical courses and require different management protocols. This is partly because of the confusion that prevails in using these terms interchangeably. Vascular malformations arise from dysmorphogenesis and are present at birth. They do not have an increased endothelial turnover and expand slowly over time. All vascular tumours except congenital haemangioma present later in life, and grow rapidly and may spontaneously involute.

Vascular ectasia is the term used to describe any local dilatation of the preexisting normal blood vessels. On the contrary, telangiectasia refers to a permanent dilation of the vessels of the skin and mucous membranes. Both these conditions do not show any increase in the number of blood vessels and are not true neoplasms. Following is a brief discussion on the prime conditions under the spectrum of vascular ectasia:

- Naevus flammeus: Also referred to as the 'birthmark', naevus flammeus includes port-wine stain and salmon patch. Salmon patch is characterized by reddish macule in the head and neck areas that curiously involutes with

Table 13.6 Categories of Vascular Tumours

Benign Neoplasms	Intermediate-Grade Neoplasms	Malignant Tumours

• Haemangioma
  • Capillary haemangioma
  • Cavernous haemangioma
  • Pyogenic granuloma
• Lymphangioma
• Glomus tumour
• Vascular ectasia
  • Naevus flammeus
  • Spider telangiectasia
  • Hereditary haemorrhagic telengiectasis
	• Kaposi sarcoma
	• Haemangioendothelioma
		• Angiosarcoma
		• Haemangiopericytoma

time. Port-wine stain is now accepted to be a vascular malformation that manifests as an elevated red to purple discolouration of the skin often in the facial areas, that turns darker with time. Sturge–Weber syndrome, also referred to as encephalotrigeminal angiomatosis, is a rare congenital neurological disorder that is associated with port-wine stain and ipsilateral venous angiomas in the brain, meninges and retina. Both syndromic and nonsyndromic port-wine stains have been recognized to be caused by activating somatic mutations in GNAQ (the alpha subunit of heterometric transmembrane signalling molecule).

- Angiokeratoma: It represents a vascular ectasia of the papillary dermis overlying warty epidermal changes and is not a true neoplasm. Patient present with red to purple papule with superficial crusting. Histologically, the dermis is occupied by distended capillaries accompanied by epidermal acanthosis, hyperkeratosis and papillomatosis.
- Spider naevus: Also known as spider telangiectasia, it is characterized by anomalous, torturous, dilatation of the superficial end arteries. The lesion is often described as a red pinhead papule with radiating blood vessels resembling a spider's web. They may be solitary or multiple and are mostly occur on the face, upper chest and the arms. Spider naevus has been associated with pregnancy, chronic liver disease, oral contraceptive intake and hyperthyroidism. However, they tend to disappear after delivery or cessation of the inducing drug.
- Hereditary haemorrhagic telangiectasia (Osler–Weber–Rendu syndrome) is an inheritable autosomal dominant condition. Molecular studies have demonstrated mutations in the genes involved in the TGF-β signalling pathway in the endothelial cells. The condition is characterized by multiple telangiectasias of the skin and mucous membranes, especially of the GI tract, urinary tract, liver and the lungs. Patients exhibit high risk of spontaneous rupture causing epistaxis, haematuria or GI bleeding.

Haemangioma

Haemangiomas are among the most common benign soft tissue tumours next to lipoma. They account for 7% of all benign childhood tumours. Haemangiomas are classified by different parameters including:

- Vessel type involved – capillary, cavernous and venous haemangiomas
- Location – cutaneous, intramuscular, synovial haemangioma are some among many others
- Characteristic cell type – epithelioid, spindle, hobnail, etc.
- Patient's age – juvenile and senile haemangioma

Capillary Haemangioma

Capillary haemangiomas are the most common type, especially in infancy, affecting 1 in every 100 live births. Clinically, haemangiomas present as flat or slightly elevated, red to purple, soft lobulated lesions of varying sizes. They may affect almost any organ, but commonly manifests in the head and neck region (Fig. 13.35).

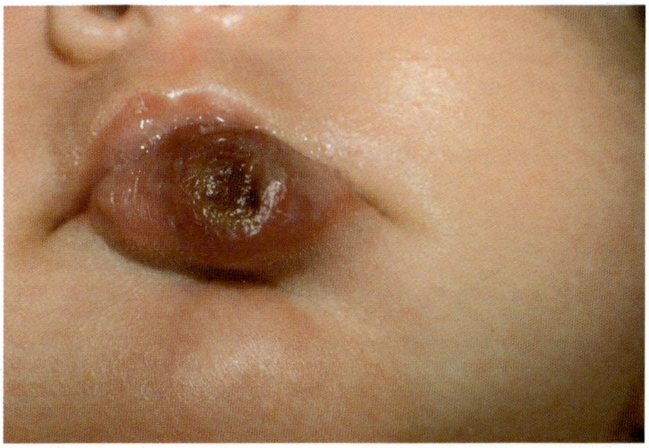

Fig. 13.35 Capillary haemangioma of the lower lip. (*Source:* From Diaz L et al: Neonatal mucous membrane disorders. In: Eichenfield LF et al, eds: Neonatal and Infant Dermatology. 3rd ed. Philadelphia, PA: Saunders; 2015:497-509, Figure 30.8.)

Morphology

Macroscopically, capillary haemangiomas are well-defined encapsulated tumours. ***Microscopically***, lobules of highly cellular, plump endothelial cells can be seen forming capillary-sized, thin-walled, blood-filled vessels embedded in scant connective tissue stroma (Fig. 13.36). A small feeding vessel is often notable in the vicinity of the tumour.

Many of the capillary haemangiomas regress spontaneously within a few years. Although most haemangiomas typically are localized lesions confined to the skin, they can occasionally be more extensive (***angiomatosis***) and can occur internally. Roughly one-third of these internal lesions occur in the liver. Malignant transformation is rare.

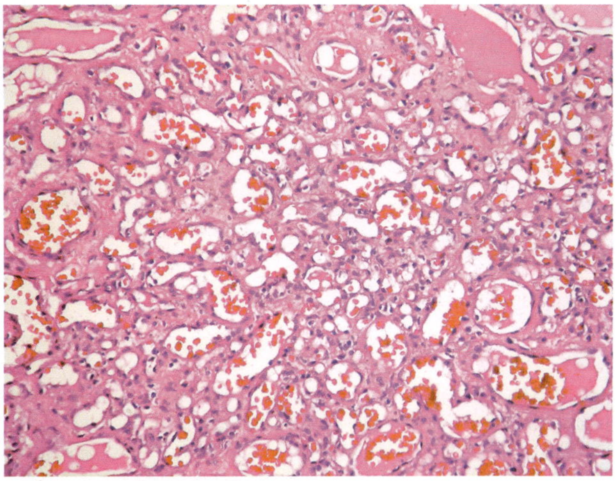

Fig. 13.36 Microscopic image of capillary haemangioma showing numerous small capillary channels containing RBCs.

Juvenile Haemangiomas

Juvenile haemangiomas are extremely common lesions affecting the newborn. In the early stages, it may resemble a birthmark, but over time, it rapidly proliferates into an elevated, red, protruding lesion, fancily recognized as the 'strawberry naevus'. Following the proliferative phase, these tumours enter into a phase of spontaneous regression and almost completely regress by the age of 7 years in most cases.

Cavernous Haemangioma

Cavernous haemangiomas are tumours composed of large, dilated vascular channels appearing as discrete or diffuse, red to blue, soft spongy masses. Like capillary haemangiomas, cavernous haemangiomas also show predilection for the head and neck areas with lesser involvement of other sites such as oral cavity, stomach and small intestine, liver and spleen. Multiple cavernous haemangiomas are often seen associated with von Hippel–Lindau disease, particularly involving the cerebellum, brainstem, liver, retina and the pancreas.

Morphology

Histologically, cavernous haemangiomas are unencapsulated lesions with infiltrative borders and are composed of thin-walled cavernous vascular spaces, filled partly or completely with blood. The vascular spaces are lined by flattened endothelial cells (Fig. 13.37). *Cavernous haemangiomas* are **more infiltrative**, frequently involving deep structures and do not regress spontaneously.

Haemangiomas on the whole are less troublesome. Certain features such as intravascular thrombosis and associated dystrophic calcification, traumatic bleeding or ulceration or cosmetic issues may require surgery.

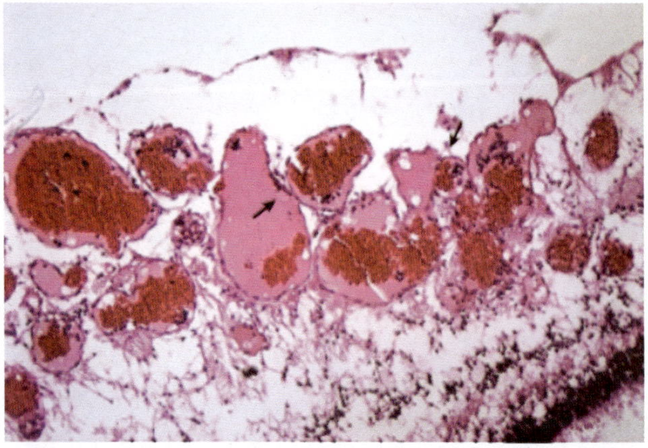

Fig. 13.37 Cavernous haemangioma of the retina. Note the large vascular channels (arrow) filled with blood and lined by flat endothelial cells. (*Source:* From Sudheer Ambekar, Venkatesh Madhugiri, Mayur Sharma, Hugo Cuellar and Anil Nanda. Evolution of Management Strategies for Cavernous Carotid Aneurysms: A Review. World Neurosurgery. 2014;82:1077-1085.)

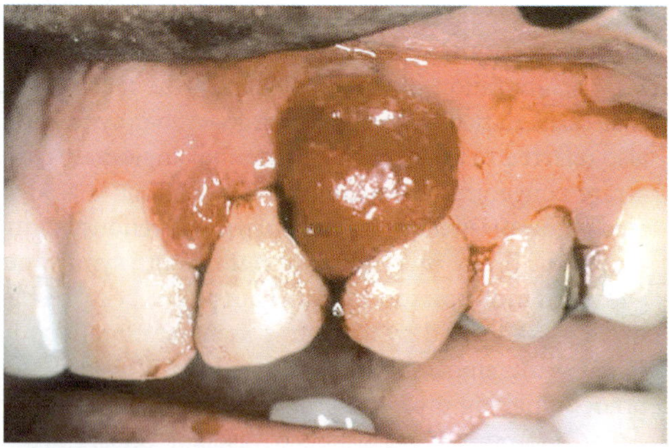

Fig. 13.38 Pyogenic granuloma in the gingiva of a 27-year-old pregnant female. (*Source:* From Brad W. Neville, Douglas D. Damm, Carl M. Allen and Angela C. Chi. Soft Tissue Tumors. Oral and Maxillofacial Pathology. 4th edition. Elsevier 2016.)

Pyogenic Granuloma

Pyogenic granulomas are capillary haemangiomas that present as rapidly growing exophytic, red pedunculated, granulation tissue–like nodule, most often involving skin and mucosa of gingiva or oral cavity. **Pregnancy tumour or granuloma gravidarum** is a variant occurring on the gingiva during pregnancy which regresses after delivery (Fig. 13.38). Pyogenic granulomas often develop following trauma.

Morphology

Histologically, proliferating capillaries similar to capillary haemangioma are seen but the capillaries are separated by abundant oedema and inflammatory infiltrate, thus resembling inflammatory granulation tissue (Fig. 13.39).

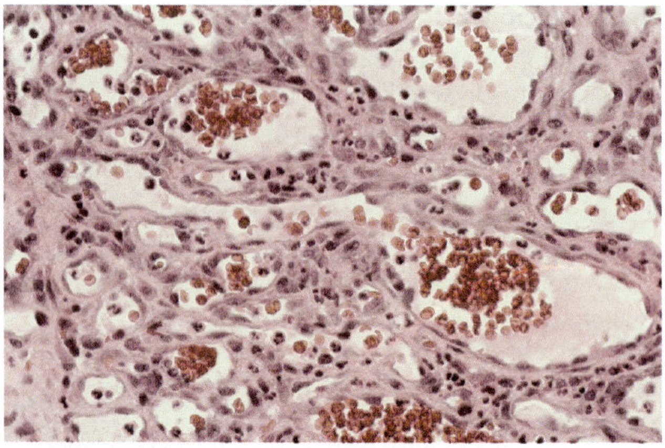

Fig. 13.39 High-power view of pyogenic granuloma showing vascular spaces with blood and inflammatory cell infiltrate. (*Source:* From Brad W. Neville, Douglas D. Damm, Carl M. Allen and Angela C. Chi. Soft Tissue Tumors. Oral and Maxillofacial Pathology. 4th edition. Elsevier 2016.)

Lymphangioma

Lymphangiomas are benign lymphatic counterparts of vascular angiomas. Lymphangiomas are congenital lesions which can be classified into capillary and cavernous types.

Morphology

Capillary lymphangioma: It presents as small, circumscribed, slightly elevated lesions most often involving skin of head and neck, axilla and mucous membranes (Fig. 13.40). Histologically, capillary lymphangiomas are composed of a network of endothelium-lined, capillary-sized spaces containing lymph and often separated by lymphoid aggregates (Fig. 13.41).

Cavernous lymphangioma: It is also called cystic hygroma and occurs predominantly in infants in the neck and axilla and rarely in the retroperitoneum. Patients with Turner syndrome manifest with cystic hygromas of the neck. The tumour is capable of growing up to huge sizes causing compression symptoms.

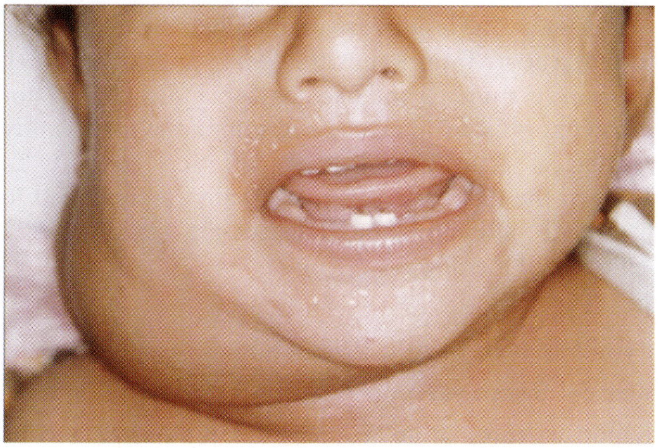

Fig. 13.40 Swelling in the neck – lymphangioma. (*Source:* From Joseph A. Regezi, James J. Sciubba and Richard C.K. Jordan. Clinical overview. Oral Pathology. 7th edition. Elsevier 2017.)

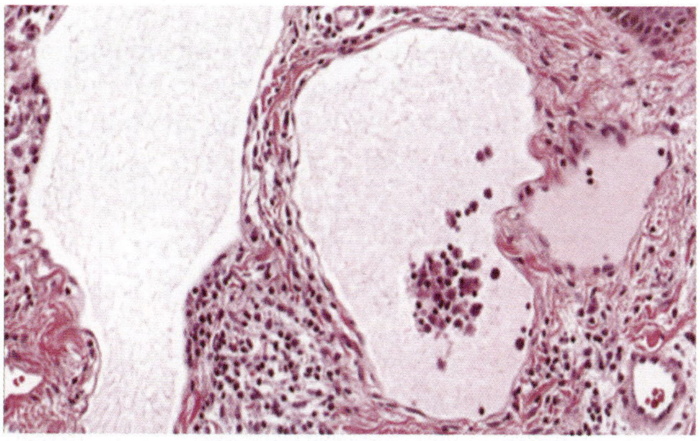

Fig. 13.41 High-power view of lymphangioma showing large lymphatic spaces filled with proteinaceous fluid, lined by flattened endothelial cell and lymphocytes. (*Source:* From Andrew E. Horvai, High-Yield Bone and Soft Tissue Pathology, Elsevier 2012.)

Histologically, cavernous lymphangioma consists of large dilated lymphatic spaces lined by flattened endothelial cells and are filled with lymph. Scanty intervening stromal connective tissue often contains lymphoid aggregates. These lesions, though benign, are often difficult to remove because of infiltration into adjacent tissues.

Glomus Tumour (Glomangioma)

Glomus tumours are benign but exquisitely painful tumours ***arising from modified smooth muscle cells of the glomus bodies***, arteriovenous structures involved in thermoregulation. The terminologies differ on the basis of morphology as glomus tumour, glomangiomyoma or glomangiomatosis and the malignant counterpart – glomangiosarcoma. These tumours are found most often in the dermis of the fingers or toes, especially under the nails (Fig. 13.42).

Morphology

They may be single or multiple, small, often less than 1 cm in diameter, flat or slightly elevated, red-blue, painful nodules. Histologically, the tumours are composed of branching capillary-sized vessels surrounded by aggregates, collars and masses of glomus cells, in a myxoid or hyalinized stroma (Fig. 13.43). Glomus cells can be described as small, round cells, with basophilic nucleus, inconspicuous nucleoli and scanty cytoplasm. Nuclear atypia and mitotic figures are rare findings.

The most common presenting symptom would be a painful fingertip. Benign tumours are curative by excision but 10% cases recur probably because of incomplete resection.

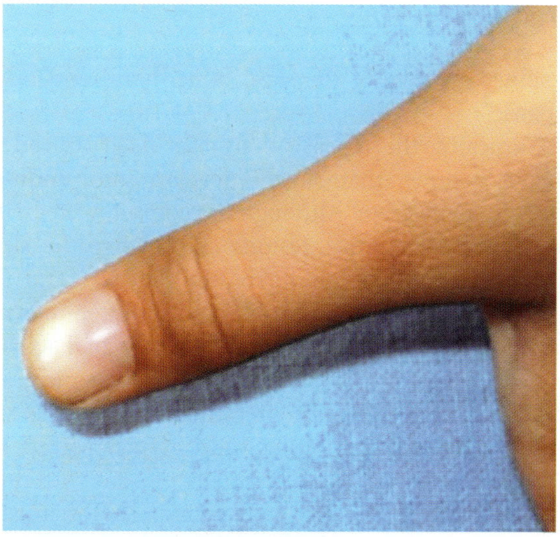

Fig. 13.42 Glomus tumour seen as a bluish-pink discolouration in the nail bed in a 21-year-old female patient. (*Source:* From Andrew E. Horvai and Thomas Link. Lymphangioma. High-Yield Bone and Soft Tissue Pathology. Saunders 2012.)

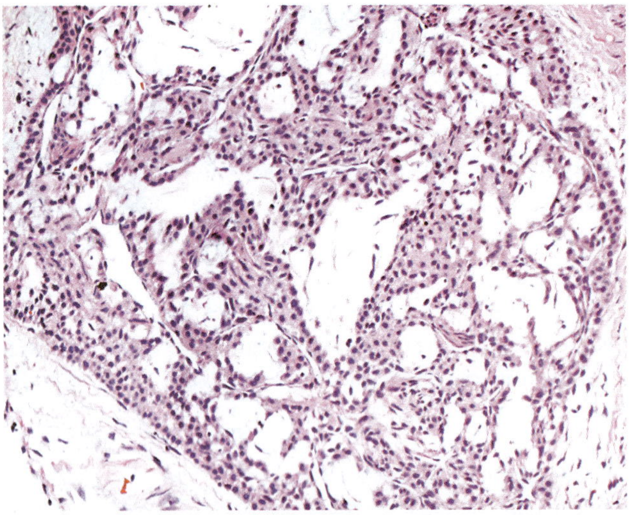

Fig. 13.43 Glomus tumour. Nodular proliferation of uniform round cells with central nuclei and pale cytoplasm. Pale areas of myxoid stromal change and endothelial-lined vascular lumina are present.

Bacillary Angiomatosis

Bacillary angiomatosis, also referred to as epithelioid angiomatosis, is a tumour-like lesion caused by opportunistic infection with Gram-negative bacilli, *Bartonella henselae* or *Bartonella quintana*. It has been frequently reported in association with immunocompromised states, especially, **HIV/AIDS** when the CD4$^+$ T-cell counts dip below 100/μL. The disease is only rarely encountered in immunocompetent individuals.

The causative infectious organism *B. henselae* probably spreads by fleas from the household domestic cat, the principal reservoir of the bacteria. Infection with *B. quintana* spreads by lice. Trench fever or rather 'quintain fever' was a disease caused by *B. quintana* that spread rapidly among the troops in World War I.

Morphology

Lesions can involve the skin, bone, brain and other organs.

Clinically, the disease manifests itself as red to purple papules that slowly develop into nodules, which may ulcerate. Although the common site being the upper extremities, lesions can involve the skin, bone, brain and other organs. In the liver and the spleen, this neovascular proliferation is often referred to as peliosis. The microscopic picture of bacillary angiomatosis closely resembles that of pyogenic granuloma, with lobules of proliferating blood vessels and endothelial cells exhibiting mild atypia. Mixed inflammatory cell infiltrate is usually present with multiple foci of nuclear dust and debris. The organisms can be demonstrated by using Warthin–Starry stain, especially useful in difficult cases to confirm diagnosis (Fig. 13.44).

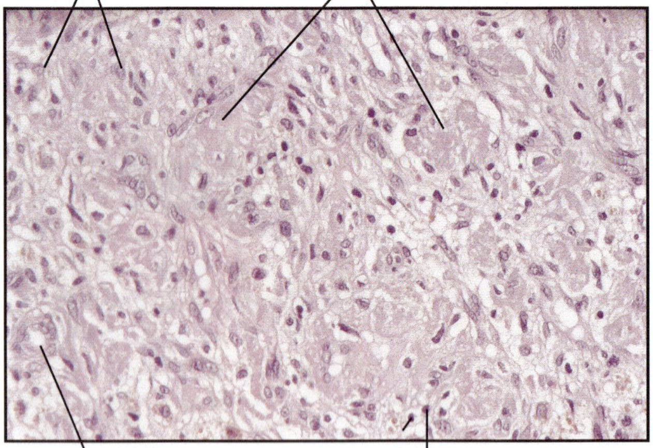

Fig. 13.44 Bacillary angiomatosis. **(A)** High magnification showing neovascularization, areas of necrotic debris (smudge areas) and mixed inflammatory cells. **(B)** Warthin–Starry silver stain demonstrating clumps of bacteria amidst the blood vessel proliferation. (*Source:* From Glenn G. Fort. Cat-Scratch Disease. Elsevier 2022.)

Clinically, the lesions are practically indistinguishable to differentiate from Kaposi sarcoma (described below), pyogenic granuloma and haemangioma. Although histopathology is useful in most cases, some cases may require serological analysis and PCR detection methods to confirm the diagnosis. Patients usually respond well to macrolide antibiotics, but relapses are common after cessation of therapy.

INTERMEDIATE-GRADE TUMOURS

Kaposi Sarcoma

Kaposi sarcoma is an angiomatous tumour caused by **human herpesvirus 8 (HHV-8), also called Kaposi sarcoma–associated herpes virus (KSHV).** Its close association with HIV/AIDS has been well recognized, especially in patients with HIV infection with CD4 count less than 200 cells/mm^3 (Fig. 13.45).

The disease was first described by Moritz Kaposi in the year 1872, when five of his patients developed the multifocal disease. During the AIDS epidemic in 1980, HHV-8 was reported as the causative agent. Furthermore, epidemiological studies have recognized four forms of Kaposi sarcoma which are as follows:

- *Classic (European) Kaposi sarcoma:* It is common in men older than 60 years of Eastern European descent. Of note, these patients are more prone to develop secondary malignancies, but are not associated with HIV infection. Clinically, the disease is slow growing and manifest as multiple, small, reddish purple nodules in the skin with more predilection for the lower extremities which later spread proximally. These lesions

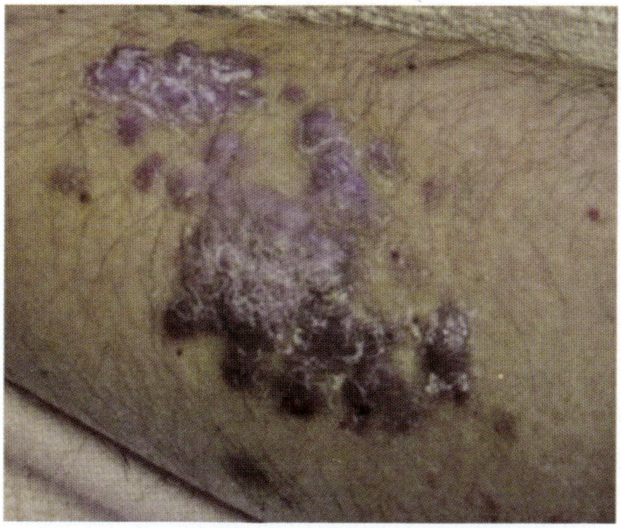

Fig. 13.45 Kaposi sarcoma on the leg in an HIV-positive patient. (*Source:* From Rathore, Ritesh. Kaposi Sarcoma. Elsevier 2022.)

typically have no associated symptoms and mostly chronically persistent.

- *African (endemic) Kaposi sarcoma:* It is more prevalent among individuals younger than 40 years, and mirrors HHV-8 seropositivity. The disease is common in equatorial Africa and follows a more aggressive course than the classic form with extensive lymph node and visceral involvement. Endemic Kaposi sarcoma is now one of the most common cancers in Uganda and Zimbabwe.
- *Epidemic (AIDS-associated) Kaposi sarcoma:* It is the second most common tumour in patients with HIV infection with low CD4 count and is now considered an AIDS-defining illness. High prevalence has been recorded especially among young male homosexuals, and approximately 30% of patients with HIV infection refuse therapy. The cutaneous lesions are not localized to lower legs but are more extensively distributed involving mucous membranes, lymph nodes and internal organs early in the course of disease. Most patients eventually die of opportunistic infections rather than Kaposi sarcoma.
- *Kaposi sarcoma in renal transplant cases:* The increased incidence of Kaposi sarcoma among patients with renal transplant can be partly attributed to the immunosuppression therapy that is being administered over prolonged periods of time. The lesions may be localized to the skin or may have widespread systemic involvement. Lesions often regress with cessation of immunosuppressive therapy, but the risk of organ rejection prevails.

Pathogenesis Pathogenesis of Kaposi sarcoma is complex. Nearly all patients show infection with ***HHV-8** which is a double-stranded enveloped DNA virus.* HHV-8 is transmitted sexually and by poorly understood nonsexual routes. Interestingly, the prevalence of cutaneous endemic African Kaposi sarcoma is inversely related to the wearing of shoes. Once within the endothelial cells, the virus controls immune suppression and inflammation to proliferate and persist. The defective immunoregulation also supports the occurrence of secondary malignancies (e.g. leukaemia, lymphoma and myeloma) in approximately one-third of patients with Kaposi sarcoma.

Morphology

Pathologically, all forms of Kaposi sarcoma show similar features and progress through three clinical phases:

- **Patches:** Morphology resembles granulation tissue with dilated vascular spaces with interspersed inflammatory cells. Extravasated RBS and haemosiderin-laden macrophages are frequent findings (Fig. 13.46A).
- **Raised plaques:** Over time, the patches progress to the plaque stage that is characterized by larger vascular channels extending into the subcutis. The stroma often shows the prominence of hyaline globules that can be well demonstrated by periodic acid–Schiff stain (Fig. 13.46B).
- **Nodular stage:** The plaques eventually grow to form large neoplastic nodules composed of sheets of

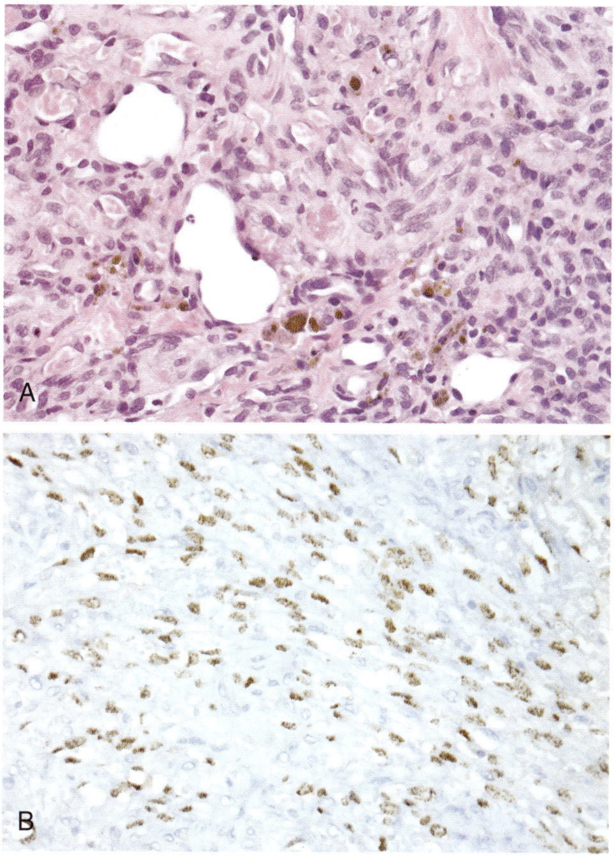

Fig. 13.46 Kaposi sarcoma. **(A)** Plump, spindle tumour cells seen abutting vascular spaces. Eosinophilic globules and abundant haemosiderin can be seen. **(B)** Immunohistochemical studies showing positive nuclear staining for HHV-8. (*Source:* From Sook-Bin Woo. Vascular, Neural, Muscle, and Myofibroblastic Tumors. Oral Pathology. 2nd edition. Elsevier 2017.)

plump, proliferating spindle cells that are of probably endothelial origin. Tumour cells often display features of atypia and mitotic figures. The nodular stage indicates nodal and visceral involvement, particularly in the African and AIDS-associated variants.

Clinical Course The clinical course of Kaposi sarcoma is wide. Although primary KSHV infections are mostly asymptomatic, the classic form of Kaposi sarcoma features a slow-growing disease largely confined to skin. A skin biopsy is often required to make a definitive diagnosis of Kaposi sarcoma. Immunohistochemical studies with LANA-1 (a surrogate marker for HHV-8) are particularly useful in differentiating Kaposi sarcoma from other spindle cell tumours.

Excision is usually curative in cutaneous Kaposi sarcoma, though some patients may require chemotherapy. Patients with HIV-associated Kaposi sarcoma respond well to HAART therapy. Classical Kaposi sarcoma is radiosensitive and radiation doses are useful particularly in the early stages. Prognosis is generally poor in patients with extensive visceral involvement, especially the lung.

Haemangioendothelioma

Haemangioendothelioma is the term used for vascular tumours that show 'borderline' behaviour, intermediate between benign haemangiomas and malignant angiosarcomas (described below). Epithelioid haemangioendothelioma is a tumour of the medium- and large-sized veins. Haemangioblastoma is the term used for a similar tumour occurring in the cerebellum. Haemangioendotheliomas occur relatively commonly in males with no age predilection. Skin and subcutis of the lower extremities, the liver, the lung and the bone are the most preferred sites.

Morphology

Grossly, the tumour is usually well defined, solitary or multiple, grey-red and polypoid with infiltrative borders. Microscopically, ill-defined vascular channels are seen surrounded by neoplastic cells, morphologically epithelioid or spindled. The epithelioid type sometimes exhibit an intracellular lumen, which forms the hallmark feature of epithelioid haemangioendothelioma. Tumour cells show mild to moderate atypia and variable mitotic activity. Although most cases are cured by excision, their clinical course is highly variable. Recurrence is possible in approximately 40% of patients. Although 20%–30% bear the risk of metastasis, 15% of patients succumb to the disease.

MALIGNANT TUMOURS

Angiosarcoma

Angiosarcoma/haemangiosarcoma is a malignant vascular tumour comprising 1% overall soft tissue sarcomas. Although any part of the body may be affected, it commonly manifests as a cutaneous disease in the elderly age group, or may involve the liver, breast, spleen, bone, lung and retroperitoneal tissues. Hepatic angiosarcomas in particular have been associated with carcinogens such as polyvinyl chloride, arsenical pesticides and Thorotrast (a radioactive contrast material used in the past).

Stewart–Treves syndrome (previously referred to as lymphangiosarcoma) is a rare and fatal disease defined by angiosarcomas presumably arising from lymphatic vessels in a setting of chronic lymphedema. It is prototypically seen in women who undergo radical mastectomy (with lymph node resection) or radiation therapy for breast carcinoma.

Morphology

Macroscopically, angiosarcomas are red to grey fleshy masses, devoid of capsule, with infiltrative margins. Areas of haemorrhage and central necrosis are frequent findings.

Microscopically, tumour cells display wide variations in differentiation. Well-differentiated areas feature organized vascular channels with abnormal endothelial cells. The architecture is distorted in many areas and the tumour cells form papillary fronds that project into the lumen. The poorly differentiated foci are composed of pleomorphic, anaplastic clusters of endothelial cells. Abundant areas of haemorrhage and necrosis are often seen. Often, the endothelial origin of the tumours needs to be demonstrated by immunohistochemical staining by using CD31 or von Willebrand factor (Fig. 13.47).

Angiosarcomas are typically a multifocal disease. They invade locally with frequent metastasis to the lung, bone and other soft tissue structures. Management protocols definitively include surgery and intensive chemotherapy. Prognosis is usually dim with a mean survival rate of less than 60% in most patients.

Haemangiopericytoma

Haemangiopericytomas are rare tumours that are derived from the pericytes. Pericytes are cells present external to the endothelial cells of capillaries and venules having myofibroblastic-like activity. Recent updates in classification of tumours of pericytes include solitary fibrous tumour of the pleura.

Morphology

Microscopically, haemangiopericytomas are composed of capillaries surrounded by whorls of spindle-shaped pericytes. These tumour cells may have high mitotic rate and areas of necrosis.

Local recurrences are common, and distant spread occurs in approximately 20% of cases.

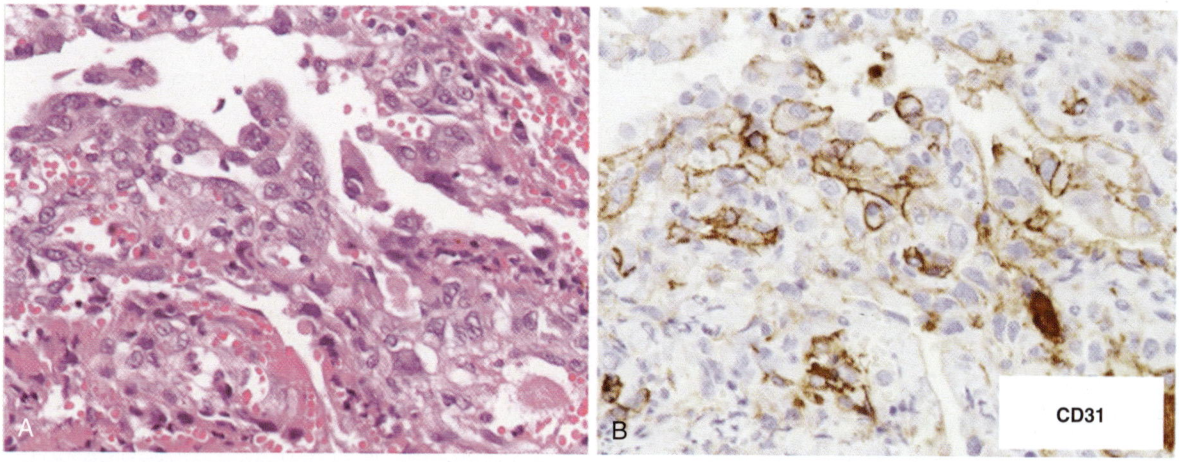

Fig. 13.47 **(A)** Angiosarcoma of the synovial tissue. Note the pleomorphic, hyperchromatic tumour cells amidst primitive vascular channels. **(B)** Immunohistochemical studies showing tumour cell positivity for CD31. (*Source:* From Bharti Rathore. Bone Tumor, Primary Malignant . Elsevier 2022.)

SELF-ASSESSMENT

Self-Assessment Questions

1. A 40-year-old woman complains of a 4-week history of headache and visual disturbances. On examination, it was found that her BP was recorded to be 220/170 mm Hg. What is the likely diagnosis and what are the characteristic histological features associated with the lesion?
2. An 86-year-old woman presents with complains of severe headache, facial pain, scalp tenderness and blurring of vision. She is diagnosed with vasculitis. What type of vasculitis could she be suffering from and what are the expected histological findings?
3. A 25-year-old man presents to the OPD with complaints of fever, abdominal pain, malaise and multiple cutaneous nodules. On examination, it was found that the lung was clear of any significant pathology. Laboratory tests were negative for ANCA but patient's serum was found to be positive for HBsAg. Further evaluation revealed inflammation of predominantly the medium-sized blood vessels sparing the smaller vasculature. What does the workup reveal?
4. An elderly male patient complains of oliguria and occasional episodes of haematuria. On examination, it was found that other features of renal failure were evident accompanied with necrotizing inflammation of the glomerular capillaries. Laboratory tests revealed positivity for MPO-ANCA. What is the diagnosis and what are its differentials?
5. A 40-year-old woman presents with complaints of abrupt onset of purpuric skin lesions. Patient has been diagnosed with asthma and mild hypertension since 3 years. Laboratory tests revealed eosinophilia, but the tests were negative for ANCA IgA. Biopsy from the lesion shows predominantly neutrophils infiltrating the blood vessel wall admixed with eosinophils. What is the best diagnosis for this patient?
6. A 1-year-old child is brough to the OPD with a huge swelling protruding from the nape of her neck. On evaluation, chromosomal analysis revealed a 45X karyotype. What is the likely association?
7. A 25-year-old HIV-positive patient developed irregular reddish-brown lesions on his forearm. The histopathological examination of the biopsy revealed proliferating spindle-shaped cells and extravasated RBCs. What is the likely diagnosis for this patient?
8. A 56-year-old man complains of reduced exercise tolerance over the past 3 years. Also, occasionally he has experienced chest pain on climbing stairs. He is a smoker since many years and on examination his BP was recorded to be 190/110 mm Hg. Laboratory findings revealed high serum cholesterol levels with low levels of HDL cholesterol. What is the probable predisposing factor causing the symptoms and what are the health risks associated with it?
9. Describe the role of endothelial cells in heath and disease.
10. What are the cardiovascular risks of hypertension?

Answers

1. Malignant hypertension – onion skin pattern of hyperplastic arteriosclerosis
2. Temporal arteritis; fragmentation of the internal elastic lamina with giant cells and granuloma
3. Polyarteritis nodosa
4. Microscopic polyangiitis; Churg–Strauss syndrome can also show MPO-ANCA positivity
5. Churg–Strauss syndrome
6. Cystic hygroma in Turner syndrome
7. Kaposi sarcoma
8. Atherosclerosis

Topics for Self-Directed Learning

1. Genetic factors and inheritable mutations causing atherosclerosis
2. Role of definitive predictive markers in assessing risk of atherosclerosis progression
3. Pathogenesis of ANCA-associated vasculitis
4. Congenital vascular tumours
5. Vascular intervention
6. Leucocytoclastic vasculitis
7. Cardiac transplant
8. Immunohistochemical markers' usefulness in vascular tumours
9. Vascular ectasias

14 The Heart

Indhu Kannan

PA 27.3 Describe the aetiology, types, stages, pathophysiology, pathology and complications of **heart failure.**

PA 27.4 Describe the aetiology, pathophysiology, pathology, gross and microscopic features, criteria and complications of **rheumatic fever.**

PA 27.5 Describe the epidemiology, risk factors, aetiology, pathophysiology, pathology, presentations, gross and microscopic features, diagnostic tests and complications of **ischaemic heart disease.**

PA 27.6 Describe the aetiology, pathophysiology, pathology, gross and microscopic features, diagnosis and complications of **infective endocarditis.**

PA 27.7 Describe the aetiology, pathophysiology, pathology, gross and microscopic features, diagnosis and complications of **pericarditis and pericardial effusion.**

PA 27.9 Classify and describe the aetiology, types, pathophysiology, pathology, gross and microscopic features, diagnosis and complications of **cardiomyopathies.**

PA 27.10 Describe the aetiology, pathophysiology, pathology features and complications of **syphilis** on the cardiovascular system.

CHAPTER OUTLINE

INTRODUCTION

The heart is the first organ to develop in the embryo and the circulatory system is the first system to mature in the human body. This fist-sized hollow muscular organ beats up to 100,000 times a day circulating about 5.6 L of blood each minute. Knowing that it is one of the most vital organs of the body with a central role in maintaining homeostasis, it is important to treat it as a precious commodity that it is. Undeniably, any disorder that affects the adequate functioning of the heart can bring forth catastrophic results. According to the data reported by the World Health Organization (WHO), cardiovascular diseases (CVDs) claim approximately 31% of all global deaths. Most diseases, though chronic, are often preventable and are rapidly overtaking infectious diseases worldwide. Yes! Heart disease prevention is to some extent possible by regular exercise, tobacco abstinence and a watchful diet. The challenge remains before us as to how we are to manage the factors that are under our control.

Heart disease is the blanket term for any disease affecting the heart, such as hypertension, myocardial infarction (MI) and coronary heart disease, diseases of the heart valves and many more. Before discussing them in detail, let us take a brief tour on the anatomy and physiological functioning of the heart.

OVERVIEW OF CARDIAC STRUCTURE AND PHYSIOLOGY

The average weight of the adult heart is 300–350 g in men and 250–320 g in females. It is located centrally within the mediastinum, anteriorly overlaid by the lungs covering its lateral borders. The cardiac apex is directed inferiorly, slightly leftwards. In the normal anatomic position, the right ventricle forms the anterior border and lies just behind the sternum. The left ventricle forms the posterior, inferior and the left lateral surfaces of the heart. The right lateral border is formed by the right atrium that receives the venae cavae. The left atrium is the most superior and posterior structure, lying anterior to the vertebral column. Of note, the position of the heart in the torso between the vertebral column and the sternum makes it practicable to exercise the popular technique of cardiopulmonary resuscitation (CPR). The external chest compressions, in cases of cardiac arrest, can help to push the blood within the heart into the pulmonary and systemic circuits to particularly reach the brain.

The interatrial and the interventricular septa divide the right and left atria and ventricles, respectively. The normal thickness of the left ventricular wall in an adult heart is 0.8–1.2 cm. The right ventricular wall which operates at a relatively lower pressure and lesser afterload measures 0.3–0.5 cm. The ratio of the interventricular septum to the left ventricular wall thickness is normally less than 1.3. A ratio of more than 1.3 may raise the concern of hypertrophic cardiomyopathy (HCM).

The wall of the heart is made up of three distinct layers – endocardium, myocardium and pericardium. The endocardium is the innermost layer and consists of a single layer of endothelial cells (similar to those within the blood vessel) lining the cardiac chambers. The subendothelial space between the myocardium and the endocardium houses the impulse conduction system of the heart. Any damage to this layer, hence can result in arrhythmias (explained later).

The myocardium is the middle layer, enveloped externally by a double-layered, fluid-filled sac, the pericardium. The two layers of the pericardium include the outer parietal pericardium and the internal visceral pericardium (also known as the epicardium).

The myocardium contributes to the bulk of the heart wall and is constituted by billions of cardiomyocytes. The left ventricular myocardium is significantly thicker with the cardiomyocytes arranged obliquely with a spiral circumferential orientation. Comparatively, the myocytes of the right ventricle are relatively poorly organized because it operates with a much lesser contractile force. The cardiomyocytes are striated muscle cells, each of which contains numerous myofibrils which run the length of the fibre. The myofibrils are composed of repetitive units of sarcomeres, the contractile unit of the muscle fibre. Between the myofibrils, the sarcoplasm (cytoplasm of the muscle cells) accommodates numerous mitochondria, a centrally located nucleus and intracellular membrane systems.

Apart from the contractile function, the myocardium also elicits endocrine functions. Atrial natriuretic peptide (ANP) and β-natriuretic peptide (BNP) are synthesized mainly by the cardiomyocytes. Their biological actions are similar and help in regulation of circulating plasma volume and blood pressure.

The unidirectional flow of blood through the heart is maintained by the four cardiac valves namely the tricuspid, the mitral, the pulmonary and the aortic valves. Blood enters the ventricles across the atrioventricular (AV) valves, the tricuspid on the right and the mitral valve on the left. The pulmonary and the aortic valves are the semilunar valves that guard the openings of the pulmonary artery and the aorta, respectively. The papillary muscles of the ventricles attach to the cusps of the AV valves via the chordae tendineae. This anatomy prevents the inversion of the valves during ventricular contraction. To further promote their functional behaviour, and to withstand the constant cyclical shear stress, cardiac valves are lined by endothelial cells and possess a distinct trilaminar architecture comprising the external fibrosa, middle spongiosa and the inner ventricularis layers.

Malfunctioning cardiac valves dramatically disrupt homeostasis and eventually cause heart failure. Left ventricular dilation, ruptured papillary muscle or chord, aortic root dilation and congenital malformations are among the few causes that can contribute to valvular insufficiency.

CONDUCTION SYSTEM (FIG. 14.1)

The cardiac conduction system is responsible for the rhythmic contractions of the atria and ventricles and holds a tight control over the electrical impulse propagation. The main components of the conduction system include the sinoatrial (SA) node, the AV node, the bundle of His, the left and right bundle branches and the Purkinje fibres. The action potentials are generated by the SA node, which is positioned at the junction of the atrial appendage and the interatrial septum. The impulse travels through the atria, via the gap junctions of the intercalated discs and the internodal tracts to reach the AV node, which is located in the right atrium along the interatrial septum. The AV node conducts slowly and there is delay of approximately 0.1 second before the stimulus is transmitted to the bundle of His. The slow conduction at the AV node delays ventricular contraction and facilitates ventricular filling. From here, the impulse is rapidly conducted through the right and left bundle branches, the interventricular septum and the Purkinje fibres, also known as the peripheral ventricular conduction system.

The electrocardiogram (ECG) represents a recording of the electric activity of the heart. The conventional ECG machine consists of 12 leads, electrodes that are placed on the skin, configured to record the changes in depolarization and repolarization activity by drawing a trace on moving electrocardiograph paper. It is basically a noninvasive diagnostic modality and has a substantial clinical impact in assessing the severity of the CVDs.

THE CORONARY CIRCULATION

The coronary circulation is distinctive in its anatomy encircling the heart like a crown and hence the name. The coronary arteries originate at the aortic valves, course

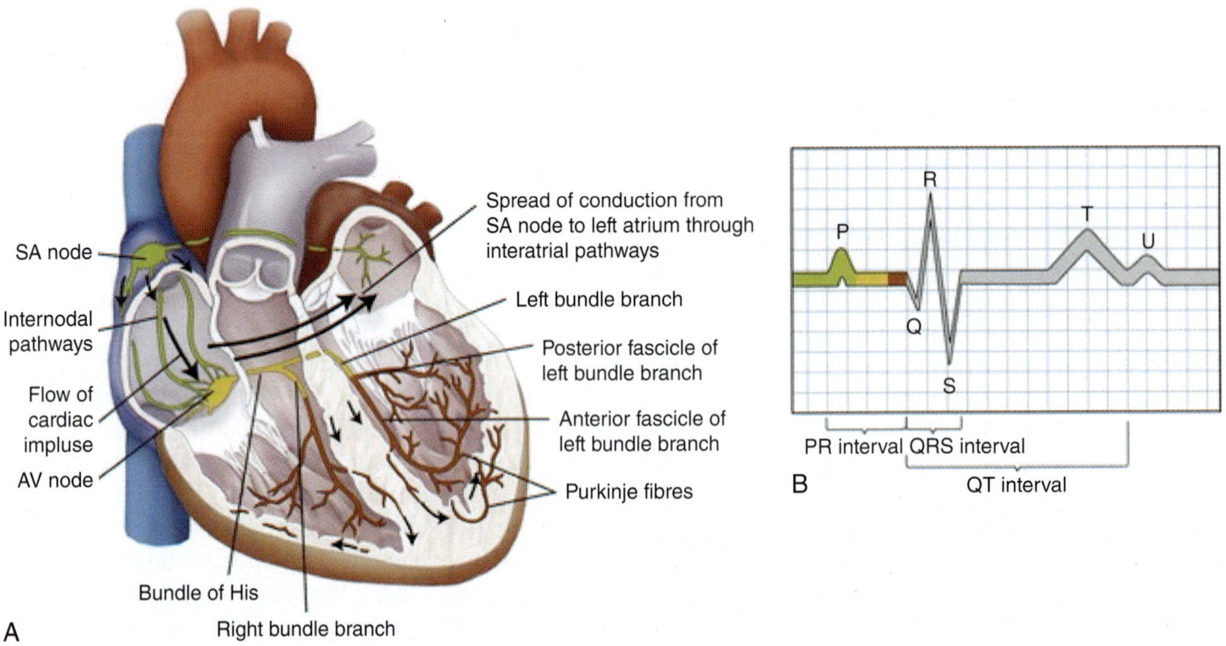

Fig. 14.1 Conduction system of the heart. (*Source:* From Tyerman, J., & Cobbett, S. [Eds.]. [2023]. Lewis's medical-surgical nursing in Canada: Assessment and management of clinical problems [5th ed.]. Elsevier.)

along the external surface of the heart as epicardial coronary arteries, before piercing into the myometrium as intramural arterioles and breaking into a dense network of capillaries. The left coronary artery bifurcates into the left anterior descending (LAD) and left circumflex (LCX) coronary arteries and supplies the lateral and anterior walls of the left ventricle and the anterior two-thirds of the interventricular septum. The right coronary artery (RCA) gives off the posterior left ventricular branch and the posterior descending artery (PDA) supplying the right ventricle, posterior wall of the left ventricle and the posterior-third of the septum. Most of the cardiac veins run parallel to the coronary arteries and drain into the coronary sinus and eventually into the right atrium. The RCA supplies the posterior-third of the interventricular septum and the posterior and the inferior wall of the left ventricle. The majority of the cardiac blood flow occurs during the diastole. During systole, the heart throttles its own blood supply compressing the vessels by the contracting cardiac muscle. The coronary arteries have been known to be functional end arteries since decades. Although collateral arteries have been identified interconnecting the epicardial coronary vessels, their relevant protective role on coronary artery disease (CAD) is yet a matter of debate.

CARDIAC REGENERATION

The cardiomyocytes of the human heart have been traditionally known to be terminally differentiated, with no regenerative capacity during adulthood. The embryonic and fetal cardiomyocytes avidly proliferate to accommodate the increasing workload during organ development. Soon after birth, the subsequent growth of the heart is attributed to myocyte hypertrophy rather than hyperplasia.

However, the dogma that the adult heart is a postmitotic organ has been challenged many times. A few recent studies have claimed evidence of cardiomyocyte turnover, averaging of about 0.1%–0.3% per year. Rationally, this slow turnover rate is insufficient to replace the large number of myocytes lost during cardiac injury.

Another concept gaining tremendous enthusiasm for research is stem cell–based cardiac repair. Among the most promising transplantable cell types capable of cardiomyogenesis, skeletal myoblasts, haematopoietic stem cells, endothelial progenitor cells and the pluripotent stem cells have been incorporated into repeated experiments for cardiac regeneration. Despite substantial progress in the understanding of the strong regenerative potential of stem cells, strategies for stem cell transplant have so far been intriguing but disappointing. The effectiveness of the stem cells is often reduced by the hostile cardiac microenvironment and poor cell grafting. Moreover, clinical hurdles regarding tumourigenesis, frequently induced arrhythmias, graft cell death, immune rejection have limited its use in clinical practice.

OVERVIEW OF CARDIAC PATHOPHYSIOLOGY

Although CVDs are attributable to a multitude of risk factors, the core mechanisms that underlie cardiovascular dysfunction are as follows:

- ***Pump failure***: It occurs commonly in conditions when the cardiac muscle contracts weakly and systolic dysfunction results in reduced ejection fraction. Conversely, the cardiac muscle may relax insufficiently offering resistance to ventricular filling, resulting in diastolic dysfunction.
- ***Obstruction to flow***: Valvular lesions such as aortic stenosis (AS), in which the valve fails to open completely, obstructive lesions at the level of the vessels, e.g. atherosclerotic plaques, hypertension, coarctation of aorta are some of the common conditions that cause outflow tract obstruction. Obstructive lesions usually result in a clinical scenario that correlates with the severity of the obstruction, with an audible murmur and/or ECG changes.
- ***Regurgitant flow***: Another functional outcome of cardiac valve injury apart from the stenosis mentioned earlier is valvular regurgitation, in which the blood flows in the reverse direction owing to the failure of the valve to close properly. The regurgitated blood adds to the volume workload impeding the pumping capacity of the affected chambers.
- ***Shunted flow***: Shunting refers to the diversion of blood abnormally from one chamber to another or between vessels, resulting in pressure and volume overload. Defects may be congenital (e.g. patent foramen ovale [PFO]) or acquired (e.g. MI).
- ***Disorders of conduction***: Conduction defects include conditions interfering with the improper generation of impulses (arrhythmias) and with improper transmission of impulses (atrial and ventricular fibrillation). These disorders often lead to uncoordinated, poorly timed, mechanically inefficient myocardial contractions which may be fatal.
- ***Rupture of the heart or a major vessel***: Traumatic rupture such as in gunshot injury can result in massive bleeding externally or into the body cavities, hypotensive shock and death.

On a general consensus, environmental and epigenetic factors are believed to influence most CVDs. Lifestyle factors themselves are partly determined by genetic factors. This interaction can also be termed as 'context dependency' of any genetic effect on the CVD risk itself. Moreover, ageing-related changes have also been associated with genetic polymorphisms. Curiously, several gene–environment interactions have been shown to impact individual response to therapy. However, further expansive research would be required to broaden our knowledge on the genetic and molecular underpinnings of CVD to determine the genetic susceptibility of an individual.

HEART FAILURE PA 27.3

The ventricles are normally compliant at low atrial pressure during diastolic filling and then propel the blood forward at higher pressure during systole. Heart failure, is a complex clinical syndrome, in which the heart is unable to pump blood adequately to meet the body requirements, or can do so only at abnormally high pressure.

Any cardiac disorder that may impair the ability of ventricular filling or ejection can give rise to heart failure. The cardinal manifestations of heart failure include fatigue, dyspnoea, exercise intolerance and fluid retention prompting pulmonary and peripheral oedema. Because congestion is a common but not a universal feature, the term heart failure is preferred to the older term, congestive cardiac failure.

Heart failure syndrome had been described as an emerging pandemic 25 years ago. Nowadays, it is estimated that about 64.3 million people are living with heart failure worldwide and the numbers continue to rise.

AETIOLOGY OF HEART FAILURE (TABLE 14.1)

A wide range of cardiac diseases, systemic diseases and genetic defects can give rise to the pathophysiological state of heart failure. It is a common end stage of nearly every heart disease including valvular diseases, hypertension, MI, congenital heart diseases (CHDs) and the cardiomyopathies. Most patients have mixed aetiologies that culminate to cause direct damage to the myocardium or cause chronic stress resulting in functional/anatomical alterations of the cardiomyocytes. Although a multitude of factors have been associated with heart failure, by far, CAD and hypertension are the most prominent. Patients with uncontrolled hypertension carry a 40% lifetime risk of developing heart failure. In industrialized countries, nearly 60%–75% of patients with heart failure have CAD, which is a strong predictor of mortality in patients with acute heart failure.

In recent years, several lines of evidence state obesity, diabetes mellitus and metabolic syndromes that are strongly correlated to insulin resistance, to be independent risk factors for heart failure. Studies conclude that a vast majority of incidents of heart failure cases, close to 90%, are attributable to the modifiable risk factors of obesity, diabetes, hypercholesterolaemia and smoking. Prior viral infection or toxin exposure has been studied to have acute effects on the myocardial contractility, with long-term effects of permanent mitochondrial dysfunction. Alcohol consumption also has a dose-dependent risk of heart failure.

Heart failure can be classified as left ventricular, right ventricular or biventricular on the basis of the location of the deficit. Depending on the time of onset, it can be classified as acute or chronic.

Clinically, however, heart failure is specified on the basis of functional status of the heart. Although in the past, it was believed that heart failure manifests in patients with depressed ventricular ejection fraction, more recent studies suggest that over one-half of patients who develop heart failure have a normal or rather preserved ejection fraction of ≥50%. Thus, heart failure can be functionally categorized into heart failure with preserved ejection fraction (formerly known as diastolic heart failure) and heart failure with reduced ejection fraction (formerly systolic failure).

In heart failure with reduced ejection fraction, owing to the progressive decline in the myocardial contractile ability, the percentage of the volume of blood ejected during systole reduces to less than 40% (normal range being 45%–65%). This may be due to primary myocardial factors such as CAD and cardiomyopathies or hypertension and valvular diseases that cause systolic dysfunction.

Heart failure with preserved ejection fraction: It is more common among older patients and women and results from abnormalities involving ventricular relaxation and compliance during diastolic filling. In such patients, exercise intolerance is nearly a universal hallmark feature. Primary diastolic dysfunction is typically seen in patients with hypertension because of the associated left ventricular hypertrophy that reduces diastolic capacity of the ventricle. Factors that cause increased resistance to diastolic filling externally (e.g. constrictive pericarditis) and those that cause internal resistance (e.g. ventricular hypertrophy, myocardial fibrosis, infiltrative myopathies such as amyloidosis) are the other attributable causes of diastolic heart failure.

Table 14.1 Aetiology of Heart Failure

Table 14.1 Aetiology of Heart Failure
Volume Overload
• Valvular regurgitation (mitral or aortic) • High-output states: Anaemia, hyperthyroidism • Arteriovenous shunts
Pressure Overload
• Hypertension • Outflow obstruction (aortic stenosis) • Chronic lung diseases
Restricted Filling
• Pericardial diseases (constrictive pericarditis) • Mitral stenosis • Infiltrative diseases (amyloidosis)
Myocyte Loss
• Ischaemic heart disease (postmyocardial infarction) • Connective tissue disorders (systemic lupus erythematosus)
Impaired Myocyte Contractility
• Genetic mutations • Viral/bacterial infection – myocarditis • Toxin/drug induced (alcohol)

PATHOPHYSIOLOGY

Heart failure can be viewed as a progressive disorder that is initiated by an index event that causes (1) inappropriate pressure or volume overload, (2) restricted ventricular filling, (3) myocyte loss or (4) impaired myocyte contractility. Irrespective of the mechanism, a common ultimatum to each of these index events is the decline in the pumping capacity of the heart. The circulatory changes arising as a result of the cardiac dysfunction are sensed by the baroreceptors as 'underfilling' of the circulation. These signal the activation of a variety of compensatory mechanisms with an attempt to restore the cardiovascular function to a normal homeostatic range. These compensations include:

- ***Frank–Starling mechanism:*** The Frank–Starling law states that the increased stretch on the myocytes increases their force of contraction. Heart failure and impaired contractile function of the myocardium lead to incomplete ventricular emptying, thereby decreasing the stroke volume, such that the volume of blood that collects during diastole is more than normal. The amplified residual volume stretches the myocardium, causing the myocytes to exert forceful contraction via the Frank–Starling mechanism allowing better ventricular emptying as an attempt to maintain the cardiac output.
- ***Activation of neurohormonal systems:*** Neurohormonal systems are composed of the adrenergic nervous system and the renin–angiotensin–aldosterone system (RAAS). The release of norepinephrine by the adrenergic nerves of the autonomic nervous system augments myocardial contractility and increases vascular resistance. The RAAS promotes vasoconstriction and sodium water retention by the kidney. The net effect of these processes aims to preserve the central arterial pressure to maintain vital organ perfusion. In addition, to counterbalance any excessive vasoconstrictive effect of the RAAS, natriuretic peptides, the natural 'beneficial' hormones are released by the atrial cells in response to atrial stretch. Both atrial and brain natriuretic peptides, ANP and BNP, antagonize the activated hormonal systems by promoting diuresis and vascular smooth muscle relaxation.

Owing to the heart's capacity to compensate, heart failure is often tolerated asymptomatically or minimally symptomatically for months to years. However, these adaptive responses are eventually overwhelmed, producing a downward spiral of deterioration with progressive heart failure symptomatology. Although the exact mechanism for this transition is unknown, sustained neurohormonal activation (neurohormones; angiotensin II), hyperadrenergic state, inflammatory cytokines (TNF), growth factors (endothelin) along with the persistent pressure and volume overload status are believed to cause detrimental effects, leading to cellular and molecular changes within the myocardium, collectively known as ***ventricular remodelling.***

Remodelling is associated with myocardial alterations that include (1) cardiomyocyte hypertrophy, (2) alterations in the contractile properties of the myocyte, (3) myocyte loss by apoptosis and necrosis and (4) myocardial fibrosis.

Cardiac Hypertrophy: Pathophysiology and Progression to Heart Failure (Flowchart 14.1)

The onset of heart failure is typically preceded by cardiac hypertrophy. At the cellular level, cardiac hypertrophy is characterized by increase in the cell size, elevated protein synthesis and changes in the sarcomere organization within the cells. Although initially the hypertrophy acts as an adaptive response to maintain cardiac function, chronic cardiac hypertrophy turns maladaptive promoting heart failure.

Classically, two patterns of hypertrophy can be distinguished on the basis of nature of the stimulus (Fig. 14.2):

Pressure overload: AS or hypertension mediates hypertrophy through thickening of the ventricular wall with little or no increase in chamber size. The newly synthesized

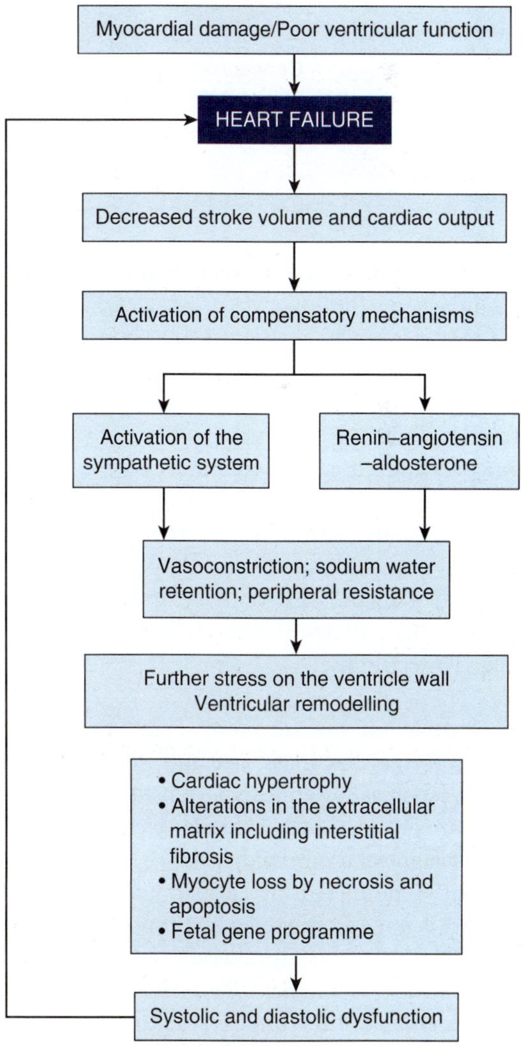

Flowchart 14.1 Schematic representation of the pathophysiological mechanism that underlies heart failure.

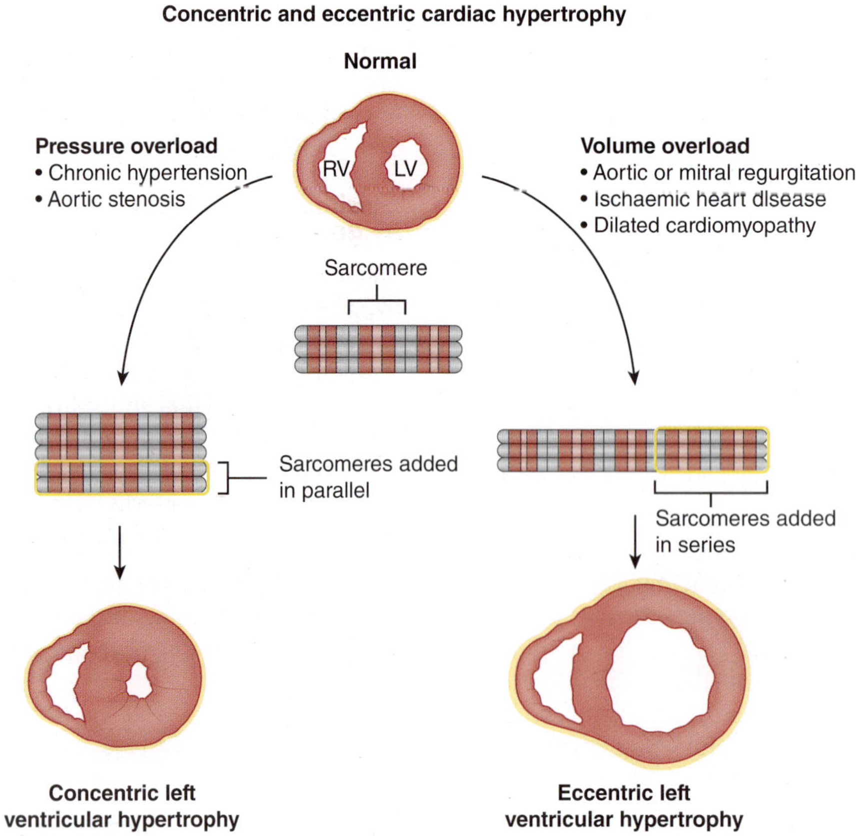

Fig. 14.2 Patterns of cardiac cellular remodelling in response to haemodynamic overload.

sarcomeres are added in parallel to the existing sarcomeres, increasing the myocyte cross-sectional area. This pattern of hypertrophy is referred to as concentric hypertrophy, in which the ventricle is capable of generating greater forces to combat the increased workload, while substantially reducing wall stress.

Volume overload: It is seen secondary to conditions such as valvular regurgitation, which results primarily in the assembly of new sarcomeres in series to the existing sarcomeres, with individual cardiomyocytes undergoing longitudinal growth. The ventricular chamber thereby dilates and this pattern of remodelling is referred to as eccentric hypertrophy.

Hypertrophy of the cardiomyocytes also reflects an increase in the cardiac mass, size and weight of the heart. Conditions such as systemic hypertension or aortic regurgitation can produce heavy hearts, weighing double or triple the weight of a normal heart.

Inherently, the increasing cardiac mass in a hypertrophied heart is not accompanied by proportionate capillary growth. The cardiomyocytes thereby suffer by inadequate perfusion which is further provoked by the increased metabolic demand of the proliferating muscle cells resulting in ischaemic necrosis. Furthermore, a smaller fraction of cardiac myocytes is lost by apoptosis, activated by the release of pro-apoptotic factors in response to stress. In parallel to the ventricle remodelling, the extracellular matrix also undergoes substantial change with increase in the number of fibroblasts that synthesize excessive amounts extracellular proteins, especially collagen. The resultant interstitial fibrosis renders the ventricle 'stiff', albeit less compliant for diastolic filling contributing to diastolic dysfunction, soon followed by systolic dysfunction.

Physiological stimuli, such as pregnancy or strenuous exercise, may also produce cardiac hypertrophy. This form of physiological hypertrophy, unlike pathological hypertrophy in heart failure, is characterized by conserved or improved cardiac function, negligible alterations of the cardiac gene expression pattern, and is also reversible on cessation of the stimuli. Note that remodelling causing interstitial fibrosis does not occur in the physiological form.

Overall, the final outcome of the disease process of chronic heart failure manifests as either forward failure in which the ventricles are unable to propel the blood into the arterial system, or backward failure in which inadequate ventricular filling poses back pressure on the atria and venous system resulting in pulmonary oedema and venous pooling of blood.

Currently, it is well accepted that cardiac remodelling contributes to the development of heart failure. Patients with any increasing degree of cardiac remodelling exhibit poorer prognosis in terms of increasing mortality and morbidity. Rationally, therapeutic antagonism of the neurohormonal system has become the cornerstone of contemporary pharmacotherapy of heart failure.

Although the disease process can involve the right and left side of the heart separately, eventually, the heart fails as a whole. This is because both the ventricles are connected by circulation and failure of one side causes excessive strain on the other. The terminologies are still useful in determining the location of the deficit for initial evaluation and treatment.

Left Heart Failure

The most significant initiating factors of left heart failure include:

- Hypertension
- CAD
- Valvular disease (aortic and mitral)
- Intrinsic myocardial diseases

Left heart failure is usually the dominant picture of the heart failure syndrome. The morphological and clinical sequels of left heart failure stem primarily from the inadequate cardiac output causing hypoperfusion of the vital organs. In addition, the increased pressure overload that is associated with left heart failure is transmitted through the pulmonary veins into the pulmonary vasculature, resulting in passive pulmonary congestion.

Morphology

Heart: The morphological features first describe the underlying index event, such as myocardial infarcts or valvular deformities. Except in cases of mitral stenosis and restrictive cardiomyopathy, in most cases, ventricular hypertrophy is prominent, and may be sometimes massively dilated. Ventricular hypertrophy is seldom accompanied by secondary enlargement of the left atrium increasing the risk of atrial fibrillation (described by rapid atrial contractions). In turn, atrial fibrillation can cause blood stasis within the atrial appendage predisposing to thrombus formation and is a substantial risk of embolic stroke. Microscopically, cardiomyocytes show features of hypertrophy with enlarged nuclei. Fibrosis of the interstitial and perivascular regions of the myocardium is another common feature in the failing heart (Fig. 14.3).

Lung: Among the extracardiac effects of left heart failure, lung holds most significant. Acute heart can be dramatic when the rising pressure within the ventricle is transmitted via the pulmonary veins to the pulmonary vasculature causing pulmonary congestion and oedema. These 'wet and heavy' lungs may have a combined weight of more than 1000 g in adults. Microscopically, fluid accumulation within the alveolar spaces, perivascular and interstitial transudates and alveolar septal oedema can be evidenced. With chronicity, red blood cells extravasate through the leaky capillaries into the alveolar spaces where they are phagocytosed by the macrophages. The haemoglobin within the RBCs is subsequently broken down into haemosiderin giving rise to pigment-laden macrophages (heart failure cells), reflecting prior episodes of pulmonary oedema.

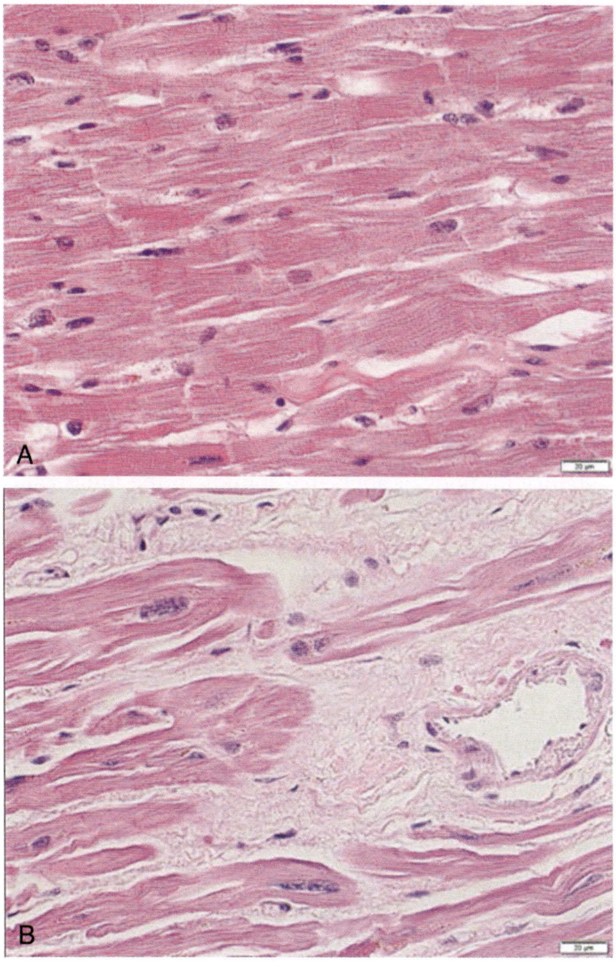

Fig. 14.3 Photomicrograph of (A) normal myocardium in comparison with (B) hypertrophied myocardium. Note the enlargement in the cell size and the nuclear size. This is accompanied by foci of fibrosis adjacent to the arteriole in the image. (*Source:* From David Ben-Nun, L. Maximilian Buja and Francisco Fuentes. Prevention of heart failure with preserved ejection fraction (HFpEF): reexamining microRNA-21 inhibition in the era of oligonucleotide-based therapeutics. Cardiovascular Pathology, 2020;49.)

Clinical Features Patients commonly present with cough and dyspnoea (shortness of breath), often on exertion, early in the course of the disease primarily due to pulmonary venous congestion. With further cardiac impairment, orthopnoea, paroxysmal nocturnal dyspnoea (PND) and other symptoms of volume overload such as pedal oedema and abdominal distention ensue. Orthopnoea is the sensation of laboured breathing on lying flat and is typically relieved by sitting or standing. This is because, in supine position, increased venous return from the lower extremities cause marked increase in the ventricular pressure. PND is a quiet frightening experience of sudden shortness of breath that awaken the patient often after 1–2 hours of sleep. PND probably occurs because of the normal nocturnal depression of the respiratory centre during sleep and the increase in the blood return as previously described. The symptoms are often relieved on sitting but takes much longer to resume normal breathing.

On physical examination, tachycardia and tachypnoea are apparent. Imaging reveals an enlarged heart. The auscultatory findings of abnormal sounds in the lungs called rales, resembling 'crackling leaves', are created by the popping open of the small airways during inspiration that had been closed off by the oedema fluid. On cardiac auscultation, a third and fourth heart sound (S3 and S4) may be heard. S3 indicates increased end-systolic volume and is almost pathognomonic of ventricular failure, whereas S4 is due to the forceful contraction of the atria against a stiff and hypertrophied ventricle. In patients with long-standing heart failure, murmurs of mitral and tricuspid regurgitation can be observed. As stated earlier, cardiac failure may predispose to atrial fibrillation and thromboembolism.

Among features related to decreased cardiac output, renal hypoperfusion activates the RAAS, causing salt and water retention, increasing the intravascular volume and pressure. In far advanced cases of heart failure, reduced renal function may lead to azotaemia, and hypoxic encephalopathy may manifest with marked irritability, confusion and restlessness. In addition, patients may present with haemoptysis and nocturia.

Right Heart Failure

Right heart failure, most commonly, is a consequence of left heart failure. This is attributed to the rationale that the elevated pulmonary vascular pressure that results from left ventricle dysfunction taxes the right ventricle with an intolerable afterload. Thus, causes of left heart failure can predispose to right heart failure as well.

Isolated right heart failure is less common and is usually caused by intrinsic lung diseases. Cor pulmonale, also referred to as pulmonary heart disease, is the term used to define the alteration in the right ventricle structure and function by chronic lung diseases, primarily triggered by the onset of pulmonary hypertension. Although chronic obstructive pulmonary disease (COPD) and chronic bronchitis account for about 50% of cases of cor pulmonale, lung parenchymal diseases and pulmonary vascular disorders such as primary pulmonary hypertension or pulmonary thromboembolism also contribute to cor pulmonale.

Pulmonary hypertension creates resistance to blood flow through the lung, in turn elevating the right atrial pressure. This pressure when transmitted retrograde causes subsequent congestion of the systemic and portal veins. Furthermore, the increased pressure on the right side of the heart causes bending of the interventricular septum towards the left, decreasing left ventricular stroke volume. This effects the morphological and clinical consequences of right heart failure.

Morphology

Liver: Secondary to right heart failure, the elevated venous pressure results in passive congestion of the liver, leading to sinusoidal dilation and oedema. In the case of congestive hepatopathy, the liver appears as an enlarged purplish organ with blunted edges and prominent hepatic veins. On sectioning, the liver often conforms to the classical description of the so called 'nutmeg liver' described by the alternating dark centrilobular zones reflecting sinusoidal congestion and the yellowish paler periportal areas representing the normal or mildly fatty liver. In addition, when left-sided heart failure occurs, impaired perfusion and tissue hypoxia can precipitate ischaemic hepatopathy in the form of centrilobular necrosis. Over time, chronic congestion can lead to perivenular fibrosis and eventually cirrhosis – cardiac cirrhosis.

Also, progressive congestive hepatopathy can cause portal hypertension leading to ascites. Congestive splenomegaly may occur as a result of increased portal venous resistance.

Oedema of the subcutaneous tissue: Pleural and pericardial spaces – oedema is one the fundamental features of right heart failure, the spectrum ranging from transudative, pleural and pericardial effusions to gross peripheral oedema (anasarca). Pericardial effusions form only with elevation of right-sided filling pressure. Pleural effusions in patients, however, can manifest with both right and left heart failure. More prominently, oedema of the dependent regions, the lower extremities, marks the hallmark feature of right heart failure.

Clinical Features In patients with isolated right heart failure, dyspnoea may be a manifestation of the underlying lung disease (e.g. COPD). Swelling of the ankles and feet, abdominal bloating (ascites), and loss of appetite with anorexia and nausea are some of the common complaints related to the oedema and congestion. Congestion of the liver and stretching of the capsule may cause right upper quadrant pain. In addition, venous congestion of the vital organs such as the brain and kidney can produce deficits similar to those produced by left heart failure. Clinical examination of the jugular vein pressure provides an estimation of the right atrial pressure.

At this point, it is important to reiterate that both the processes of right and left heart failure are interdependent and most cases of chronic cardiac decompensation encompass features of biventricular dysfunction. Circulating levels of biomarkers such as BNP are relatively sensitive markers for the presence of heart failure. Moreover, BNP levels also aid in assessing the severity of the disease and can be useful in planning optimal dosage of medical therapy. According to the current rationale, the management of heart failure requires a multimodal approach. A combination of drugs to combat the fluid overload (e.g. diuretics), drugs to hamper the effect of the RAAS, and adrenergic blockers have proved beneficial in most patients. In patients refractory to medical treatment, newer approaches include resynchronization therapy, ventricular assist devices or cardiac transplant depending on the severity. Despite these recent advances, the prognosis of patients with chronic heart failure remains bleak with over 50% of patients suffering mortality because of ventricular arrhythmias.

CONGENITAL HEART DISEASES

The term CHDs is used to accommodate the structural abnormalities of the heart and the great vessels that occur during fetal development. These malformations arise from defective morphogenesis, either as misplaced structures or arrested progression of normal structures. The resultant phenotype can range from severe anomalies that are incompatible with life, to symptomatic lesions and defects that go unnoticed throughout life. Although many of the malformations develop in utero, only when detached from the maternal circulation, the impact of the defects becomes apparent. The unique features of the prenatal circulation, particularly, the placenta and the foramen ovale, allow compensation for the structural cardiac defects that develop in utero, such that, most fetuses with isolated CHD thrive to survive until delivery.

INCIDENCE

CHD complicates about 1% of all live births, i.e. around 40,000 births/year among the general population. The true incidence may be still higher because the CHDs occur much more frequently in stillborns and premature infants. Accounting for almost 20%–30% of all birth defects, CHDs are the most common congenital malformations of infancy and the most common cause of birth defect associated with mortality. Improvement in the survival and quality of life of infants born with CHD claimed to be one of the biggest achievements of contemporary medicine. Fortunately, in the past half century, there has been remarkable advancement in the diagnostic techniques, such as in echocardiography, cardiac catheterization, electrophysiology and surgical alternatives, such that more than 90% of the afflicted neonates are now able to survive into adulthood. However, most patients, following repair would require lifelong monitoring and expert surveillance.

The spectrum of anatomic defects associated with CHD is broad; however, overall, a few discrete lesions account for almost 90% of reported cases. Their relative frequencies, a range derived from several sources, have been listed in Table 14.2. Note that this does not include, the two, probably, common conditions – the congenital, functionally normal bicuspid aortic valve and the myxomatous mitral valve prolapse (MVP).

Table 14.2 Relative Incidence of Specific Anomalies in Patients With CHDs

Ventricular septal defects (VSDs)	25%–30%
Atrial septal defects (ASDs)	10%–15%
Patent ductus arteriosus (PDA)	8%–10%
Tetralogy of Fallot (TOF)	5%–7%
Pulmonary stenosis	5%–7%
Coarctation of aorta	5%–7%
Aortic stenosis	4%–6%
Complete transposition of the great arteries	3%–5%
Truncus arteriosus	1%–2%
Tricuspid atresia	1%–2%
Atrioventricular septal defect	2%–4%
Total anomalous pulmonary venous connection	1%–2%

AETIOLOGY AND PATHOGENESIS

A multitude of environmental and genetic factors have been attributed to the development of CHD, yet, the fundamental aetiology in majority of cases remains unknown. Epidemiological studies, by large, suggest sporadic genetic abnormalities to be the most predominant cause, supported by the increase in the occurrence of the disease among siblings of the affected children or children of the affected parent.

About 20%–40% children with CHD manifest with extracardiac anomalies or more so as a part of an identified syndrome. Chromosomal aneuploidy, the first recognized cause of CHD, continues to contribute to a significant portion of cases. In particular, 50% of patients with trisomy 21, Down syndrome, present with atrial and ventricular septal defects (VSDs). The incidence increases up to 80% in patients with trisomy 13 manifesting additionally with malposition complexes. Almost all patients with trisomy 18 present with septal defects. CHD occurs in approximately 30% of patients with Turner syndrome, most commonly with bicuspid aortic valve, AS or coarctation of aorta (explained later).

Apart from aneuploidy, chromosomal deletion, classically, DiGeorge syndrome (22q11 deletion syndrome) leads to cardiac malformations along with thymic and parathyroid hypoplasia and the characteristic dysmorphic facies. The phenotypes associated with the syndrome are believed to be caused by the mutations of the TBX1 gene, contained within the 22q11 interval. The gene TBX1 encodes for a transcription factor that promotes cell proliferation in the second heart field, from which the outflow tract and the right ventricle develop.

More recently, single-gene defects have been found to be associated with syndromic, and nonsyndromic or isolated CHDs. These genes include members of a core group of cardiac transcription factors, signalling molecules or important structural proteins involved in cardiac embryogenesis such as transcription factor genes NKX2-5, GATA4, TBX5. In addition, mutations of similar functional genes, TBX20, have been subsequently described in adult-onset CHDs and cardiomyopathies, suggesting that these genes also play a vital role in postnatal heart function. The gene NOTCH1 encodes for receptors involved in the highly conserved signalling pathway critical for cardiovascular development. NOTCH1 mutations typically cause malformations of the aortic valve (bicuspid aortic valve). Kindred mutations of NOTCH2 and JAG1 have been associated with tetralogy of Fallot (TOF). Rare missense mutations in structural proteins of the cardiac muscle, such as MYH6, are believed to give rise to isolated cases of CHD. Fibrillin, an important structural protein of the ECM, acts as a negative regulator of TGF-β signalling. Dysregulated TGF-β signalling is known to be responsible for cardiovascular manifestations in Marfan and Loeys–Dietz syndrome.

Although epidemiological studies suggest the predominance of genetic factors in the causation of CHD, environmental factors are also relevant. Casual links have been established with factors such as maternal diabetes, congenital rubella infection, toxin exposure, alcohol consumption during pregnancy and maternal viral infection. A host of cardiac teratogens has been identified and includes drugs such as thalidomide, lithium and other anticonvulsants. On the contrary, periconceptional folate or multivitamin supplements have been beneficial in reducing the risk of CHDs in the fetus. Despite the extending list of environmental risk factors, definitive aetiology can be determined only in about 10% of cases. The much-accepted rationale is that the aetiology of CHDs follows a multifactorial inheritance model, involving both genetic and environmental risk factors.

CLINICAL FEATURES AND CONSEQUENCES

The pathological features and the clinical correlates of the specific forms of CHDs can be presented on the basis of a classification into three major categories:

- Left to right shunt
- Right to left shunt
- Obstruction

Shunt refers to an abnormal channel of communication between the chambers of the heart, the blood vessels or both. The flow and direction of blood through the channel is determined by the pressure gradients across the chambers involved. In conditions where there is shunting of blood from the right side to the left, deoxygenated blood directly enters systemic circulation bypassing the lungs. The resulting hypoxaemia manifests clinically as cyanosis. Persistent cyanosis over a period of time results in polycythaemia as an attempt to increase the oxygen saturation of blood. Polycythaemia is often accompanied by clubbing of the tips of the fingers and toes and hypertrophic osteoarthropathy. Also, right to left shunts provide an abnormal conducive pathway for bland or septic venous thrombi to embolize into systemic circulation, causing potential risk for cerebral infarcts and abscesses. Common CHDs encountered with a right to left shunt include the 5 Ts, **T**OF, **T**ransposition of great vessels, persistent **T**runcus arteriosus, **T**ricuspid atresia and **T**otal anomalous pulmonary venous connection. Collectively, these conditions are also referred to as cyanotic congenital heart defects. The right to left shunts are often diagnosed prenatally, or manifest soon after birth, and require urgent surgical intervention.

On the contrary, left to right shunts include the so called 'holes of the heart', atrial septal defect (ASD), VSD and PDA, which are of clinical significance only after birth. These conditions are not associated with cyanosis, at least initially, hence referred to as the acyanotic or the late cyanotic group. The shunting of oxygenated blood from the left to the right side exposes the low-resistance, low-calibre pulmonary vasculature to increased blood flow and the potentially higher pressures. The initial response of the muscular pulmonary arterioles to the increased pulmonary blood flow includes intimal proliferation, medial hypertrophy and vasoconstriction. Although these changes are partially reversible, over time, pulmonary arterial hypertrophy and persistent vasoconstriction eventually lead to elevated pulmonary vascular resistance and pulmonary hypertension. The increased afterload associated with pulmonary hypertension reflects on the right ventricle causing right ventricular hypertrophy. This causes a shift in the pressure gradient reversing the left to right shunt to a bidirectional and ultimately to a right to left shunt – Eisenmenger syndrome. Patients with this condition display late-onset cyanosis and right heart failure.

Obstructive forms of CHDs include conditions causing abnormal narrowing of the blood vessels, valves or chambers and are collectively referred to as obstructive congenital heart defects. Coarctation of aorta, valvular stenosis (partial narrowing) and atresia (complete narrowing) are some examples under this category.

The chronic haemodynamic stress caused by the CHDs induce compensatory myocardial hypertrophy or chamber dilatation or both of one or more cardiac chambers. A significant portion of patients also suffer from arrhythmias due to the underlying congenital defect or as a sequel of interventional cardiac repair. Infants may also present with recurrent pneumonia, failure to thrive and growth retardation depending on the severity of the defect. The following sections cover more details pertaining to the specific forms of CHD.

LEFT TO RIGHT SHUNTS

The left to right shunt lesions that include ASD, VSD and PDA are the most common congenital heart defects and are the most common cause of high-output heart failure. In general, shunting at the level of the atria (ASD) produces minimal alterations of the volume and pressure changes on the right side. Large shunts at the level of the ventricles (VSD) and at the level of the great vessels (PDA) are often more problematic causing dramatic changes in the pulmonary flow and pressure.

ATRIAL SEPTAL DEFECT

ASDs are true defects of the interatrial septum allowing abnormal blood flow between the atria. Any defect in the septum other than the PFO (explained later) represent an ASD. These defects are commonly recognized among the adult population, as most patients remain asymptomatic until adulthood, and are much more frequent in females. The development of the interatrial septum is a complex process and deficiencies within the septum constituting ASDs arise from derangements of the septum during embryogenesis.

The atrial septation process begins around the 5th week of gestation, with the septum primum, a crescent-shaped membranous tissue that originates from the posterior superior atrial roof. The septum primum grows caudally towards the AV canal lined by endocardial cushions. The progressively diminishing space between the septum primum and the endocardial cushion is known as the ostium primum. Before the ostium primum is completely closed, small perforations develop in the superior end of the septum primum, which coalesce together to form the ostium secundum. Simultaneously, another infolding begins to appear in the atrial roof, a little right to the septum primum, known as the septum secundum. This septum stretches across the atria overlapping the ostium secundum, leaving a small opening called the foramen ovale. While the superior segment of the septum primum gradually regresses, the lower segment serves as a small flap valve that controls the blood flow across the foramen ovale. The valve operates according to the pressure gradient within the atrial chambers. During intrauterine life, the lung being nonfunctional, most of the gas exchange occurs via the placenta. As most of the blood from the umbilical arteries reaches the right atrium through the inferior vena cava, the right atrial pressure is higher than the left atrial pressure allowing right to left shunting of blood through the foramen ovale. After birth, lung inflation and expansion of the pulmonary blood flow increase the left atrial pressure, causing functional closure of the foramen ovale, making a complete interatrial septum.

Although ASDs can occur anywhere along the septum, the main forms are discussed as follows (Fig. 14.4):

- Secundum ASD accounts for nearly 75% of cases. The defect arises over the midportion of the septum secundum either because of excessive resorption of the septum primum resulting in a large ostium secundum or inadequate septum secundum formation. This variant is generally not associated with other CHDs and may be of any size, occurring in multiples or may be fenestrated.
- Primum ASD is a less common variant of ASD that appears in the inferior portion of the interatrial septum, adjacent to the AV valves. This results from a defect in the formation of the endocardial cushion. In cases of severe endocardial cushion defect, ostium primum ASD can be associated with other abnormalities such as membranous VSD, and abnormal AV valve that may straddle across the common atrioventricular canal.
- The sinus venous ASD (10% of cases) is located high on the interatrial septum, at the superior end, close to the entry of the superior vena cava. Rarely, it may occur at the entry of the inferior vena cava (inferior vena caval type).

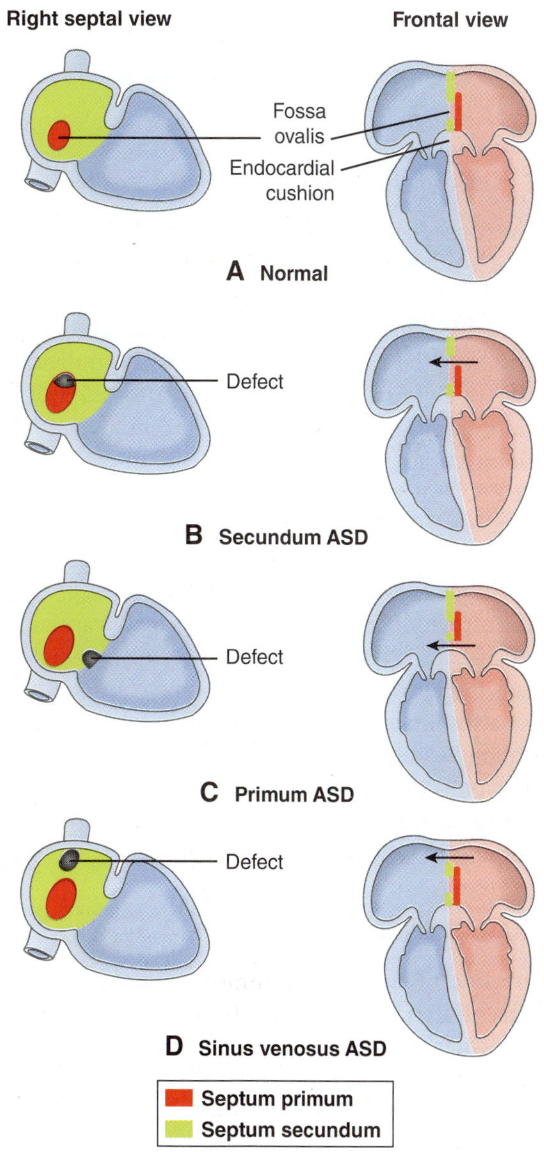

Fig. 14.4 Arterial septal defects.

Clinical Features

Although most infants, children and young adults are asymptomatic, symptoms become apparent with advancing age, usually in adulthood. Blood flow through the defect is largely determined by the size of the defect and the relative atrial pressures, reflected by the compliance of the ventricles. In case of an uncomplicated ASD, blood is shunted from the left to the right atrium more often because of the relatively high right ventricular compliance, in comparison with the left ventricle and low pulmonary vascular resistance. The shunting, in due course, causes diastolic overloading of the right ventricle and pulmonary overflow. The increased blood flow across the pulmonary valve often creates a murmur that can be heard during physical examination. This may be worsened by pulmonary hypertension and atrial arrhythmias. However, complications such as paradoxical embolism, heart failure or irreversible pulmonary hypertension are rare.

Operative repair usually with a pericardial or prosthetic patch, or a percutaneous transcatheter device closure is advised for patients to prevent complications. In most patients, morphological changes in the right ventricle return to normal postrepair and show good survival rates (96.2%).

PATENT FORAMEN OVALE

PFO is a consequence of failed closure of the foramen ovale, which otherwise, as explained earlier, is a normal structure that allows right to left shunting of blood during intrauterine life. The foramen ovale is permanently sealed by the fusion of the atrial septum in over 75% individuals by the age of 2 years. In the remaining 20%–25% of the population, the PFO may persist as a haemodynamically insignificant communication through the interatrial septum. The PFO is usually a clinically silent flap valve, which, though not sealed, is functionally closed because the left atrial pressure is higher than the right atrial pressure. However, conditions that may increase the right atrial pressure, for instance, pulmonary hypertension or right heart failure, or events such as bowel movements, sneezing or coughing, may result in pathological right to left intercardiac shunting. PFO also implicates a potential route for paradoxical embolization, leading to stroke and death. Almost 61% of cases of cryptogenic stroke have been associated with PFO. Percutaneous closure of PFO has been significantly beneficial in patients in preventing complications.

VENTRICULAR SEPTAL DEFECT (FIG. 14.5)

VSDs are one of the most common congenital cardiac defects in children, defined as an abnormal opening in the interventricular septum. The septum develops around the 5th week of intrauterine life and VSDs result from any disruptions in the septum formation during embryonic morphogenesis.

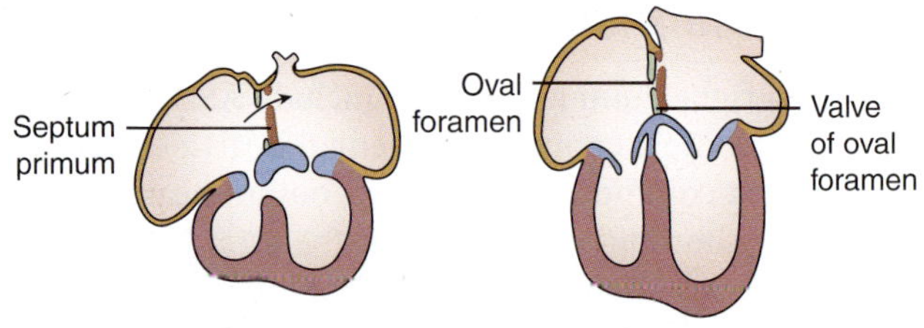

Fig. 14.5 Development of the interventricular septum.

The interventricular septum is constituted by the muscular portion that grows upwards from the apex towards the endocardial cushion and the membranous portion that grows downwards from the endocardial cushion. Deficient contributions of these embryonic structures lead to the development of VSDs. VSDs can be thus categorized into the following types:

Membranous VSD: It is by far the most common, involving about 90% of cases. It is located at the base of the heart in the membranous part of the interventricular septum.
Infundibular VSD: It is among the less common variety representing 6% of the cases, and is located below the semilunar valves.
Muscular VSD: It is located in the muscular septum and may be multiple. Muscular VSDs contribute to 20% of cases in children, whereas the occurrence is much lesser among adults because of tendency of spontaneous closure.

Clinical Features

VSDs manifest both in children and adults. Children mostly present with associated anomalies such as TOF, whereas adults present with isolated VSDs more commonly. The pathophysiological consequences of VSD depend largely on the size and location of the defect and the pulmonary vascular resistance. Small-sized defects are usually functionally insignificant because at least 50% of these close spontaneously, and even if persistent, these are well tolerated for years. Larger defects that cause significant left to right shunting eventually lead to right ventricular hypertrophy, increase in pulmonary vascular resistance and pulmonary hypertension. Additional complications include infective endocarditis (IE) at the lesion site and paradoxical emboli. Thus, larger defects mostly demand surgical repair or catheter-based closure to prevent complications.

PATENT DUCTUS ARTERIOSUS (FIG. 14.6)

Ductus arteriosus is a vessel that connects the pulmonary artery to the descending aorta just distal the left subclavian artery. The channel is normally open in the fetus and closes after birth. During intrauterine life, the ductus conveys most of the pulmonary outflow to the aorta bypassing the unoxygenated lung. In a newborn, as the lungs begin to function, oxygen tension rises and pulmonary vascular resistance decreases. This, along with the withdrawal of the maternal prostaglandins synthesized by the placenta, the ductus shrinks and becomes occluded by

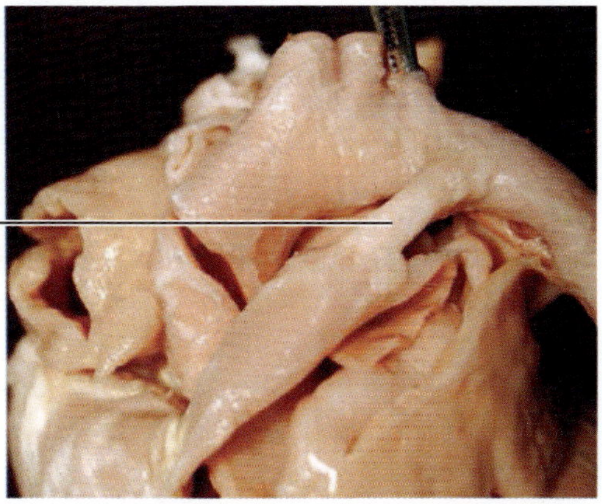

Fig. 14.6 Patent ductus arteriosus. (*Source:* From Craig L. Basman, Rebecca Jonas. Patent Ductus Arteriosus. Elsevier 2022.)

fibrosis, 12–24 hours after birth, and is completely sealed by the first few months of life, which is then referred to as ligamentum arteriosus.

Persistent ductus arteriosus refers to the condition in which the ductus fails to close after birth. Rubella infection during the first trimester of pregnancy has been associated with a high incidence of PDA. Also, premature infants, in particular those with respiratory distress, experience prematurity preluded closure. In such patients, the ductus however, closes spontaneously later in life. In full-term infants, PDA only rarely closes spontaneously.

Children with small PDAs and low-pressure PDAs are usually asymptomatic. However, larger defects typically produce a characteristic continuous 'machine-like' murmur. Most patients though otherwise initially clinically asymptomatic, develop symptoms as the pulmonary vascular pressure and resistance increase, causing pulmonary obstruction and reversal of flow.

Isolated PDAs require immediate closure. A frequent complication among untreated patients with PDA is IE involving the pulmonary artery side of the ductus. Conservative medical treatment includes administration of cyclooxygenase inhibitors or more recently, acetaminophen. On the contrary, in children with associated congenital malformations that cause systemic and pulmonary obstruction, administration of prostaglandin E1 to maintain ductal patency can be beneficial. Surgery is preferred in patients in whom medical treatment fails.

RIGHT TO LEFT SHUNTS

This category includes disorders in which there is right to left shunting of blood causing the entry of poorly oxygenated blood into systemic circulation leading to the development of early cyanosis. Following conditions are some of the common cyanotic CHDs.

TETRALOGY OF FALLOT

TOF is the most common cyanotic CHD among infants, also accounting for the highest proportion of in-hospital mortality due to congenital defects. Embryologically, TOF is a resultant of an abnormal anterosuperior displacement of the infundibular portion of the interventricular septum, consequently producing the following major anomalies:

- Pulmonary stenosis
- VSD
- Dextropositions of the aorta so that it overrides the VSD
- Right ventricular hypertrophy primarily because of high pressure overload caused by the above-mentioned defects

Morphology

VSD may involve both the muscular septum and the endocardial cushions. The aorta is displaced and overlies the VSD. Pulmonary stenosis is often resultant of subpulmonary muscular hypertrophy, accompanied by an enlarged infundibular muscle obstructing the pulmonary blood flow. In about 30% of cases, the pulmonary valve itself is defected, being funnel shaped, causing stenosis or there may be a complete pulmonary atresia (Fig. 14.7).

The right ventricular hypertrophy and the decrease in the luminal diameter of the pulmonary artery segments gives the heart a typical 'boot shape' which can be appreciated on a chest radiography. Most patients with TOF also present with associated cardiac anomalies such as ASD (ostium secundum variant), PDA, endocardial cushion defects or a right-sided aortic arch (in 25% of cases).

Clinical Features

Patients with mild pulmonary stenosis, generally survive into adulthood. The symptoms pertain to an isolated VSD, with left to right shunting of blood, thereby no cyanosis, also referred to as pink tetralogy. In patients with severe pulmonary stenosis, the blood from the right ventricle

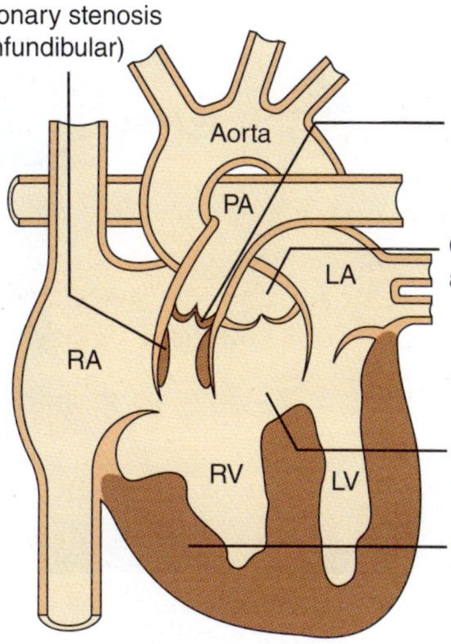

Fig. 14.7 Tetralogy of Fallot – components. (*Source:* From Davidson's Principles & Practice of Medicine, 22ed. Churchill Livingstone; Elsevier: 2014 {Fig. 18.102/634].)

takes route through the VSD mixing with the oxygenated blood in the aorta, causing dyspnoea on exertion and cyanosis – the classic TOF. In patients presenting with associated PDA, the patency of the ductus can prove beneficial because the ductus provides a source of blood to the otherwise deprived pulmonary vascular bed. However, in these cases, the patients become prone to cerebral thrombosis, bacterial endocarditis and brain abscess due to marked polycythaemia.

Surgical correction is requisite and is recommended to be performed electively in infants at 6 months to 1 year of age, to prevent complications. Surgical repair aims at complete closure of the VSD and expansion of the subpulmonic infundibulum by using a pericardial patch. Although total correction is not possible, most patients show excellent long-term prognosis.

TRANSPOSITION OF GREAT ARTERIES

As the term implies, transposition of great arteries (TGA) refers to a complex malformation arising from an embryological discordance in reference to the position of the aorta and the pulmonary artery. In typical cases, the most common variant is the dextro-TGA or d-TGA, in which the aorta arises from the right ventricle and the pulmonary artery arises from the left ventricle, leading to the formation of two parallel circuits that are incompatible with life (Fig. 14.8). Many cases have been associated with maternal diabetes and also show slight male predominance.

During cardiac development, the embryological discordance of the conotruncal septum which fails to ensure its spiral course and instead follows a linear orientation, is believed to produce these aberrant placing of the great vessels. This arrangement that forces deoxygenated blood in systemic circulation and oxygenated blood into pulmonary circulation can cause extreme cyanosis and hypoxia, unless a shunt exists to allow communication between the two circuits and adequate mixing of blood. In utero, the ductus arteriosus and the foramen ovale provide channels for interchange of blood. Postnatally, after physiological closure of these shunts, intervention would be necessary to create a new shunt by using a balloon catheter, referred to as the Rashkind procedure.

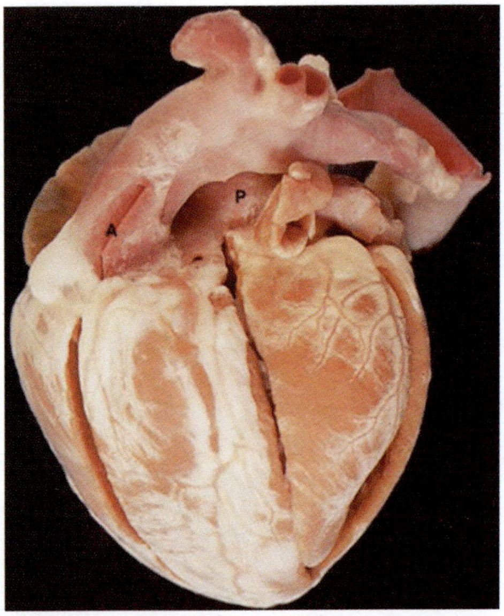

Fig. 14.8 Specimen of heart with d-transposition of great vessels. Note that the aorta is anterior to the pulmonary artery arising from the right ventricle. (*Source:* From Andrew J. Connolly, Walter E. Finkbeiner, Philip C. Ursell and Richard L. Davis. Atlas of Gross Autopsy Pathology. Autopsy Pathology: A Manual and Atlas. 3rd edition. Elsevier 2016.)

TRICUSPID ATRESIA

Tricuspid atresia refers to a condition characterized by congenital absence of the tricuspid valve. The defect results from unequal division of the AV canal during cardiac morphogenesis. Likewise, affected patients develop an enlarged mitral valve and frequently hypoplasia of the right ventricle and the pulmonary artery. This obligates survival only by means of a right to left shunt through the foramen ovale or an ASD. In most patients, in addition, an associated VSD helps to deviate the blood into the pulmonary circulation.

Three variants of tricuspid atresia have been identified, on the basis of its associated relationship with TGA:

Type I – most common, involving >75% patients, in which the great vessels are normal functionally and anatomically
Type II – the great vessels exhibit d-transposition
Type III – rare type with l-TGA.

Patients with TA present with cyanosis due to the right to left shunting of blood which can be worsened if the associated VSD is small in size. If so, a cardiac murmur may be heard on examination. Surgical intervention aims to bypass the atretic valve and ease circulation. However, most cases endure high early mortality.

OBSTRUCTIVE LESIONS

Congenital malformations that can cause obstruction to blood flow commonly include obstruction at the level of the aorta (coarctation of aorta), obstruction at the level of the right ventricle (pulmonary stenosis) and at the level of the left ventricle (AS).

COARCTATION OF AORTA (FIG. 14.9)

Coarctation of aorta is simply a narrowing of the aorta, that almost always occurs immediately below the origin of the left subclavian artery, at the site of the ductus arteriosus. About two-third of the patients present with an associated bicuspid aortic valve and is much more common in males than females. However, females with Turner syndrome, in particular, commonly manifest with coarctation

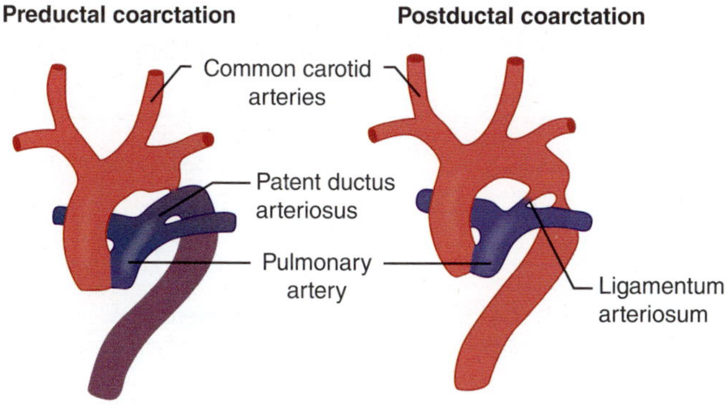

Fig. 14.9 Coarctation of aorta.

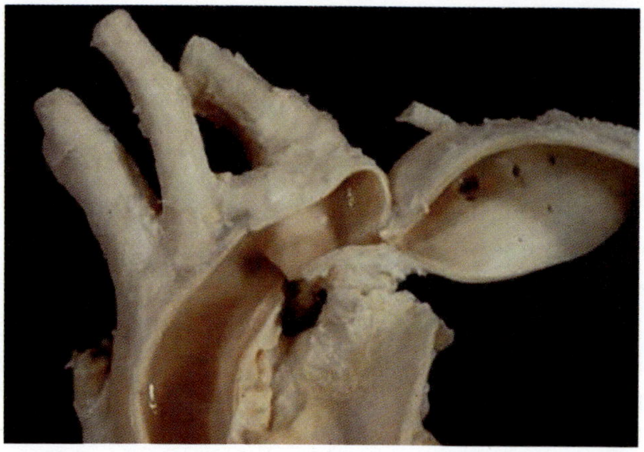

Fig. 14.10 Anatomical specimen showing heart with severe aortic coarctation, postductal type. (*Source:* From Stephani C. Wang, Pranav M. Patel. Aortic Coarctation. Elsevier 2022.)

of aorta. Apart from these, coarctation of aorta may be associated with berry aneurysms in the brain, ASD, VSD or mitral regurgitation.

Two forms of coarctation of aorta that have been identified in the past on the basis of location of the defect and the patency of the ductus arteriosus.

- Preductal/infantile form, in which patients present with tubular hypoplasia of the aortic arch proximal to a PDA
- Also, an adult form characterized by a ridge-like infolding of the aorta just opposite to the closed ductus arteriosus distal to the arch vessels

In any case, the narrowing of the aortic lumen is variable ranging from a small opening to minimal narrowing.

Morphology

The infantile type, as previously described, is accompanied by a PDA and the narrowing 'coarct' occurs between the left subclavian artery and the PDA. The PDA serves as a channel for blood entry into the pulmonary artery, thereby compelling perfusion of poorly oxygenated blood to the organs distal to the narrowed segment. The pulmonary artery undergoes dilatation owing to increased blood flow and eventually, right ventricular hypertrophy.

The adult/postductal type is relatively more common (Fig. 14.10). The aorta is narrowed by means of a constriction contained of a discrete tissue ridge in close proximity to the resolved ductus. In view of the increased afterload, the left ventricle faces a hypertrophy supplemented by dilatation of the aortic branch vessels proximal to the defect.

Clinical Features

The clinical presentation of infants with coarctation of aorta varies according to the degree of impedance of the aortic narrowing and the persistence of the ductus. Newborns with PDA typically present with differential cyanosis which involves cyanosis of the lower half of the body, whereas the upper half of the body is spared because the vessels supplying these areas branch off from the aorta proximal to the defect. Such infants struggle to survive into the neonatal period and require mandatory surgery to seal the PDA.

Infants without a PDA are mostly asymptomatic and survive into adulthood. Patients present classically with hypertension in the upper limbs and hypotension in the lower extremities, accompanied by claudication pain (due to arterial insufficiency).

In untreated patients, as a compensatory mechanism, the intercostal and internal mammary arteries contribute to the development of collaterals connecting the before and after segments of the coarct. These can be evident on chest radiography as erosions or 'notching' that erode the inferior surface of the posterior ribs.

On examination, murmurs can be heard throughout systole, in some cases, accompanied by a vibratory thrill. ECG may reveal a hypertrophied left ventricle resulting from the pressure overload. Among the several surgical interventional procedures that are available, excision of the affected segment and replacement by a prosthetic graft with end-to-end anastomosis yield direct repair of the defect and are usually successful.

PULMONARY STENOSIS AND ATRESIA

Pulmonary stenosis refers to a condition of obstruction at the level of the pulmonary valve. The spectrum of the disease may range from mild to severe and may be associated commonly with a TGA or a TOF. Forceful contractions against the stenotic valve rationally give rise to increased right ventricular pressures and chamber hypertrophy, sometimes followed by pulmonary artery dilatation due to arterial wall injury and right heart failure.

Pulmonary atresia on the other hand is characterized by complete occlusion of the pulmonary valve. Frequently such patients manifest with an associated hypoplastic right ventricle and an ASD, through which the blood bypasses the right ventricle and enters the lung through a PDA.

Patients with mild stenosis are generally asymptomatic and tolerate well. Symptomatic cases may require surgical correction.

AORTIC STENOSIS AND ATRESIA

Likewise, congenital narrowing of the aortic valve refers to AS. The defect may be present at birth (congenital) or may develop later in life (acquired). More commonly (>80%), cases occur as an isolated lesion. AS may be classified according to the level of obstruction into valvular, subvalvular and the supravalvular sites.

The severe forms of AS are followed by hypoplasia of the left ventricle and ascending aorta. In long-standing cases, the left ventricle may undergo dense calcification, porcelain like, which is when referred to as ***endocardial fibroelastosis*** (Flowchart 14.2). Such patients would require a patent ductus arteriosus for survival. These findings constitute the hypoplastic left heart syndrome. Closure of the valve after birth can be lethal.

Subvalvular stenosis is a resultant of a thickened ring of dense endocardial fibrous tissue below the level of the cusps. It roughly contributes to 10% of cases and is more common in males. Patients sometimes display a systolic murmur and a 'vibratory' thrill.

Supravalvular stenosis is the least common variant. It is usually caused by elastin gene mutations that interfere with the elastin–smooth muscle interaction during morphogenesis.

The survival rate following surgical repair in these patients is usually excellent.

ISCHAEMIC HEART DISEASE PA 27.5

Ischaemic heart disease (IHD) includes a spectrum of diseases reflecting the imbalance between the myocardial blood supply and the perfusion demand. William Heberden, a British physician, was the first to report on this condition in 1772. Although he did not comprehend the aetiology, he described the symptoms as an uncomfortable feeling in the chest while walking or on exertion. The difficulty is relieved on standing still but would recur with activities. He also coined the term angina pectoris. IHD is by far the most common type of heart disease and also the leading cause of death, accounting for about 80% of all deaths in the modern industrialized nations.

Most cases of IHD are a resultant of obstruction or reduced blood flow through the epicardial vessels due to atherosclerotic lesions. Thus, the terms CAD and IHD are often used interchangeably, though from the pathophysiological perception, IHD is the more preferred term. These coronary lesions are slow growing and produce

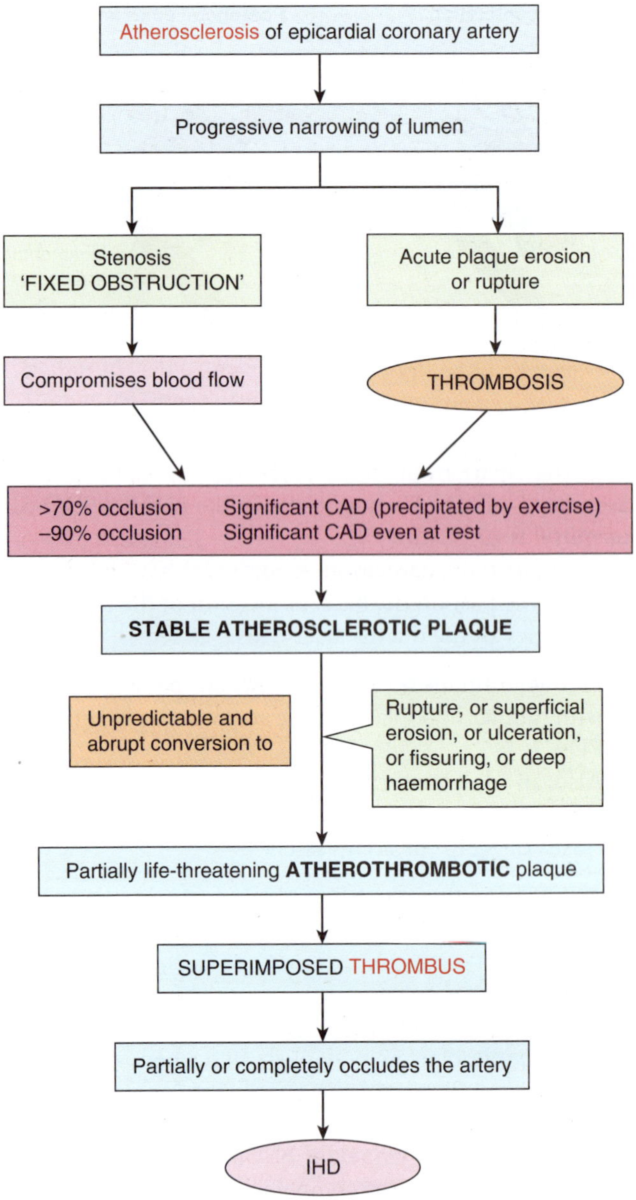

Flowchart 14.2 Pathogenesis of ischaemic heart disease – summarized.

clinical symptoms only after a long period of time. Ischaemia due to any cause, that is persistent for a considerable duration and magnitude to an extent that irreversible ischaemic injury occurs, leads to myocardial necrosis, in other words, infarction.

EPIDEMIOLOGY

In the recent years, there has been a proportional increase in the number of newly diagnosed cases of type 2 diabetes, reflecting on the prevalence of obesity and IHD. The global burden of the disease is largely blamed on the energy-rich western food and the rapid urbanization. However, progress in the preventive strategies, diagnostic advances and evidence-based treatment has succeeded in producing a downfall in the death rate because of the

IHD, worldwide. Clinical and public health efforts in thwarting significant risk factors such as smoking, poor glycaemic control, high blood cholesterol levels and hypertension have contributed to a great degree to the declining trends of events. In addition, early diagnostic tests such as blood tests for cholesterol, ECG, ECHO, and preventive strategies such as in statin administration to combat the cholesterol levels, thrombolysis in the patient experiencing MI, coronary artery bypass graft, revascularization procedures and many more have proved effectively beneficial.

PATHOGENESIS

The most common attributable factors causing IHD syndromes include chronic vascular occlusion in the form of atherosclerotic plaque, the events following 'acute plaque change' and the other nonatherosclerotic causes (Flowchart 14.2).

CHRONIC VASCULAR OCCLUSION

The epicardial coronary arteries are the most sought over vessels involved in the pathogenesis of IHD. The haemodynamic significance of the vessel narrowing depends largely on the degree of stenosis and the capacity of the resistance vessels that undergo compensatory vasodilatation. When the vessel wall is narrowed by 60%, though the maximal flow within the vessel is decreased, the resistance vessels help to maintain perfusion in situations of increased demand. When more than 70% of the vessel lumen is compromised, it is referred to as 'critical stenosis', the point at which the maximal blood flow is reduced even with full dilatation of the resistance vessels, but the resting blood flow is normal. This marks the cut-off value, at which patients present with exertional angina (angina on exertional activity such as exercise or lifting heavy weights). At the time of more than 90% occlusion of vessel lumen, the blood flow is inadequate to meet the basic requirements and patients manifest angina even at rest. To save the at-risk myocardium, collateral vessels begin to develop to help perfusion bypassing the incompetent vessel.

Among the three epicardial vessels, namely, the LAD, the LCX and the RCA, a single vessel may be affected at a time or frequently two or all three vessels may be involved. However, the most preferential site for symptomatic plaque formation includes the proximal portion of the LAD and LCX in the decreasing order, followed by the LAD diagonal branches, LCX obtuse marginal branches and the posterior descending branch of the RCA.

ACUTE PLAQUE CHANGE

This phenomenon explains the sequel that forces an otherwise stable atherosclerotic plaque to a life-threatening lesion, which manifests as a catastrophic MI or sudden cardiac death (SCD). In most patients, the event is precipitated by a spontaneous rupture of the plaque usually at a site weakened by chronic inflammation. Other sudden changes include superficial erosion, ulceration or deep haemorrhage that result in thrombotic embolization of the atheromatous debris and thromboembolic events that partially or completely occlude the vessel wall.

Other nonatherosclerotic causes:

Apart from the traditional view of coronary atherosclerosis causing IHD, other causes such as inflammation of the myocardial vessel wall, aneurysms, stenosis of the coronary ostia caused by syphilitic aortitis or vascular spasm have also been demonstrated to contribute to MI. Likewise, in patients with reserved luminal narrowing, disease progression occurs in instances of increased cardiac workload, such as hypoxaemia, systemic hypertension, cardiac hypertrophy and coarctation of aorta. The common sign tachycardia is mechanized by increased contractions per unit time that increases the oxygen demand while decreasing the functional supply (shorter diastole). Last in order, conditions in which the blood cannot deliver adequate oxygen to the myocardial tissue putting the myocardium at risk for ischaemia include severe, chronic anaemia and carbon monoxide poisoning. Notably, cigarette smoking provides high levels of carbon monoxide polluting the blood with carboxyhaemoglobin.

CONSEQUENCES OF ISCHAEMIA

Depending on the severity of the ischaemic insult, a variety of clinical syndromes may result, which are as follows:

Stable (typical) angina: It is usually caused by a fixed atherosclerotic plaque involving one or more coronary arteries. It is usually not associated with plaque disruption. Also called 'chest pain', angina pectoris remains the most common symptom of IHD and refers to a condition in which the ischaemia is not severe enough to cause frank necrosis. Patients classically present with a transient chest discomfort, a crushing or a squeezing sensation substernally that radiates to the left arm or the jaw, during emotional or physical stress. As explained earlier, this is due to the increased oxygen demand that exceeds the reduced supply through the stenosed vessels. The symptoms last for 15–20 minutes and are usually relieved by rest, or till the demand is alleviated, and the oxygen balance is restored. Rationally, patients experiencing angina are administered with vasodilators such as nitroglycerine and calcium channel blockers to increase the perfusion.

Prinzmetal angina: It is much less frequent and is characterized by episodic focal coronary artery spasm causing myocardial ischaemia. The vasospasm is postulated to be resultant of endothelial cell dysfunction and is not always associated with coronary atherosclerosis. The angina does not follow any exertional activity and occurs even at rest. Vasodilators have been beneficial in relieving symptoms in such patients.

Unstable or crescendo angina: It describes a condition where the patients experience the chest pain at rest or even during sleep or following minimal physical activity and the pain persists for more than 20 minutes. The accelerated symptoms could serve as a precursor lesion for MI and hence unstable angina is also referred to as crescendo angina, preinfarction angina or accelerated angina. It is mostly a resultant of an acute plaque with subsequent thrombosis and vasoconstriction. Rarely, microinfarcts can be seen distal to the disrupted plaques.
MI: As we already know, the infarct is a discrete area of ischaemic necrosis that follows an abrupt occlusion of the vessel wall usually because of rupture of the plaque and thrombosis. MIs may present as a 'silent' MI or lead to catastrophic events leading to haemodynamic deterioration and sudden death. The so called 'silent' MIs are particularly common among the elderly age group and in patients with diabetic neuropathy.
SCD: In some cases, the acute plaque change or fixed plaques may give rise to spontaneous ventricular tachycardia that degenerates into ventricular fibrillation causing SCD.

MYOCARDIAL INFARCTION

The more commonly used term, 'heart attack', refers to MI which marks the end result of acute or chronic myocardial ischaemia. Although a host of factors may lead to MI, coronary heart disease is one of the major causes of the disease burden and deaths. In India, cross-sectional epidemiological studies performed reveal increased incidence of the disease among both the urban and the rural populations. Also, the patients experiencing MI are much younger in India in comparison to the western world. In terms of absolute number, around 30 million CHD patients are diagnosed per year.

The traditional risk factors, the commonly studied and the well-known factors that have been linked to IHD include obesity, increased age, sedentary lifestyle, smoking, male sex and agreeably the emotional and physical stress. Women are generally protected from IHD in their reproductive years, whereas female patients suffering from IHD belong to the postmenopausal age group. Thus, the lack of hormones has been thought to potentiate the risk.

Pathogenesis

The likely pathway paving way for MI can be briefly explained as a disease sequence that is mostly initiated with an acute plaque change within a vulnerable atherosclerotic plaque, causing endothelial dysfunction and consequent platelet aggregation and vasospasm. This is followed by activation of coagulation pathway by circulating tissue factor and other factors, giving rise to thrombus formation. The resultant acute thrombotic occlusion of the vessel wall of the coronary artery, forms an integral part of the MI syndrome.

Curiously, most patients who undergo angiography after the MI reveal evidence of coronary thrombus at a site that previously did not have fixed critical stenosis. Also, although 90% of patients show coronary thrombus on the angiogram performed 4 hours after the onset of symptoms, only 60% show thrombus formation in angiographies performed 12 hours later with no intervention. This is explained by the possible spontaneous dissolution, thrombolysis of some part of the thrombus or relaxation of the blood vessel. This phenomenon has been implicated in the latest therapeutic regimens, targeting acceleration of spontaneous thrombolysis to limit the extent of the infarct.

In addition, nonatherosclerotic causes of MI contribute through one of the following possible mechanisms. Note that the occurrences of such events are relatively infrequent and is generally suspected in younger patients (<50 years).

Vasospasm: Coronary vasospasm is mostly a resultant of hyperactive vascular smooth muscle probably due to endothelial dysfunction. It may or may not be associated with coronary atherosclerosis. Drugs such as cocaine or ephedrine have been associated with vasospasm-induced MI. Cocaine enhances the release of adrenal catecholamines and increases the myocardial sympathetic tone leading to vasospasm followed by MI.

Emboli: Atrial fibrillation is among the most common nonatherosclerotic cause of MI, carrying the highest risk for thromboembolism. However, thromboembolism causing MI is a rare phenomenon. Other causes that could give rise to coronary emboli include paradoxical emboli from the right heart or IE, intracardiac prosthetic material, aneurysm or dilated cardiomyopathy (DCM).

Other uncommon causes of MI described are vasculitis, amyloid deposition, AS and shock and some cases following cardiac surgery.

Myocardial Response

By all means, the reduced blood supply because of arterial obstruction initiates myocardial dysfunction followed by myocyte necrosis. The response of the 'at-risk myocardium' depends largely on the duration and the severity of the diminished blood flow.

The foremost change within the ischaemic myocardium is the loss of myocardial contractility that quickly leads to ventricular dysfunction. The abrupt loss of blood supply causes complex biochemical changes within the myocardium, the most significant being termination of aerobic metabolism leading to virtually complete loss of ATP. This causes a switch over to the anaerobic metabolism through glycolysis, leading to accumulation of lactic acid thereby lowering the pH. Also, the paucity of ATP interferes with functioning of the membrane pumps, causing release of intracellular potassium and magnesium, with entry of water and sodium. Collectively, these changes hamper the myocardial contractility that almost occur instantaneously within minutes. Thus, even before myocardial death, systolic function of the myocardium is disturbed.

At this stage however, the changes are reversible and without intervention irreversible damage ensues. Studies show that only severe ischaemia, in which the myocardium receives less than 10% of the usual supply and that which lasts for more than 20–30 minutes, can lead to necrosis or irreversible damage. An infarct is usually completely developed within 3–4 hours. Thus, the need for early diagnosis and intervention within the 'critical widow' helps to save the myocardium before irreparable damage sets in.

Ultrastructurally, disruption of the cellular membrane marks the initial detectable features of necrotic myocytes. This causes leakage of intracellular contents, importantly proteolytic enzymes and certain macromolecules into circulation. These serve as clinical markers of acute inflammation because they can be detected by blood tests. The irreversible injury typically initiates in the subendocardial zone. This zone is particularly susceptible to ischaemia because it is the last area to receive blood supply, has very few collateral channels, and is also subjected to high intramural pressures. Prolonged ischaemia activates a wavefront of cardiomyocyte death that extends from the subendocardium to the subepicardium. However, in almost every case of transmural infarct that progressively encloses the entire thickness of the perfused area of the involved vessel, approximately 0.1 mm of the ventricular wall is preserved with viable myocytes, the subendocardial region that is perfused by the luminal contents.

Patterns of Infarct

The distribution and the location of the infarct within the myocardium depend on the vessel involved and the anatomical area that it perfuses (Fig. 14.11). Infarcts may manifest as transmural or subendocardial infarcts according to the extent of involvement of the ventricular wall (Fig. 14.12). Transmural infarcts span the entire thickness of the ventricular wall and are usually caused by chronic coronary atherosclerosis undergoing acute plaque change with superimposed thrombus, causing complete occlusion of the vessel lumen. Thus, the location of the transmural infarcts correlates with the distribution of the main coronary vessels.

LAD: LAD is the most common vessel that undergoes obstruction comprising about 40%–50% cases. The event primarily leads to an 'anterior' infarct, where the anterior and the anteroseptal walls of the left ventricle are affected, along with circumferential involvement of the apex.
RCA: It is next in frequency (30%–40%). The occlusion results in an 'inferior' or posterior infarct involving the posterior lower region of the left ventricle and the posterior half of the interventricular septum. In about 15%–20% of cases, the infarct may extend into the posterior free wall of the right ventricle.
Left circumflex artery: This is the least frequent vessel to be involved and affects the lateral left ventricle wall.

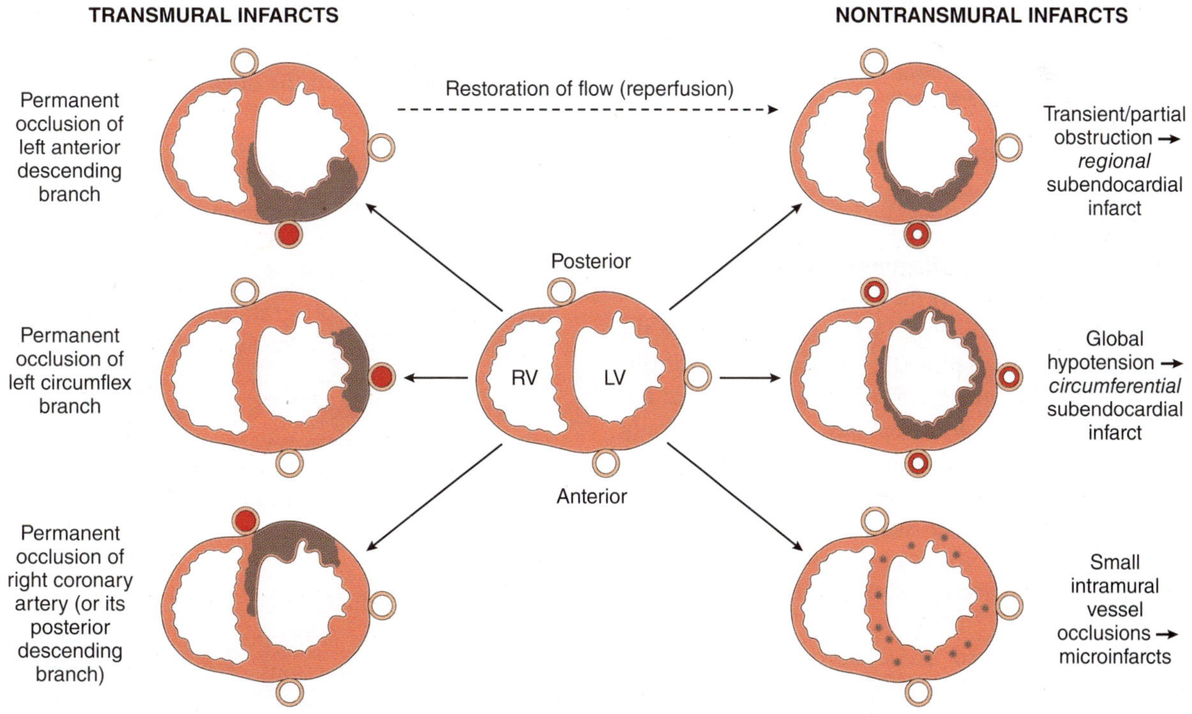

Fig. 14.11 Pattern of distribution of myocardial ischaemic necrosis according to the vessel involved and their area of perfusion. (*Source:* From Richard N. Mitchell and Andrew J. Connolly. The Heart . Robbins & Cotran Pathologic Basis of Disease. 10th edition. Elsevier 2021.)

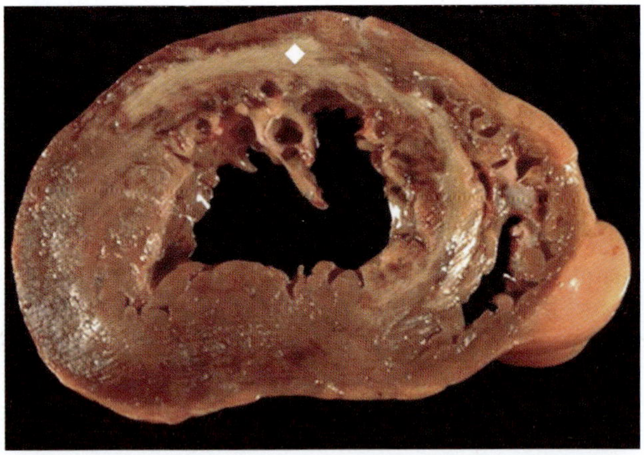

Fig. 14.12 Transmural infarct of the myocardium in a patient with acute myocardial infarction (marked with |). (*Source:* From Gangadhara Rao Golla, Maheswara Satya. Myocardial Infarction. Elsevier 2022.)

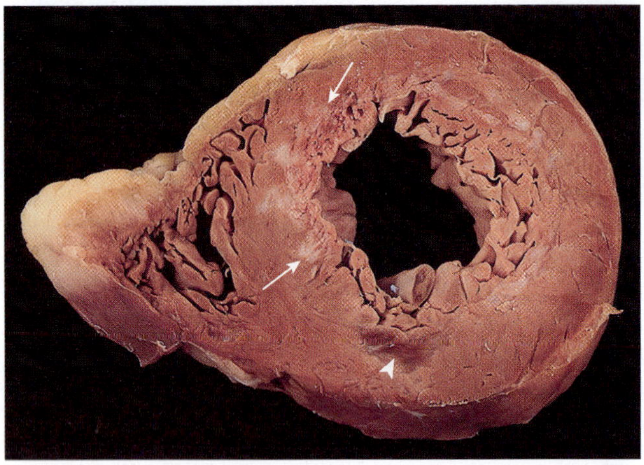

Fig. 14.13 Gross photograph showing several subendocardial infarcts, some acute and some healed. The arrowhead points to a fresh infarct. The arrows indicate healed fibrous scars. (*Source:* From Andrew J. Connolly, Walter E. Finkbeiner, Philip C. Ursell and Richard L. Davis. Atlas of Gross Autopsy Pathology. Autopsy Pathology: A Manual and Atlas. 3rd edition. Elsevier 2016.)

Other less commonly involved vessels include the left main coronary artery, the diagonal branches of the LAD or the marginal branches of the LCX.

Subendocardial infarcts (Fig. 14.13): These involve the inner one-third or one-half of the ventricular myocardial wall. It may arise following coronary thrombus that has undergone lysis either spontaneously or therapeutically, and the myocardial wall has been salvaged from full-thickness necrosis. As only one inner layer of the ventricular wall undergoes necrosis, subendocardial infarcts are not followed by complications as in a transmural infarct, such as constrictive pericarditis or ventricular rupture.

Multifocal microinfarcts: These occur when only the smaller transmural vessels are involved by microembolization, vasculitis or vasospasm. This also occurs in response to increase in endogenous catecholamines which also increase the pulse rate and myocardial contractility, further exacerbating the ischaemia. The fatal outcome of such vasospasm can be SCD or an ischaemic DCM.

Morphology

The morphological changes within the myocardium in an event of acute MI are detailed in the Table 14.3.

The affected myocardium undergoes a spectrum of morphological changes from the onset of ischaemia till myocardial death that is further followed by inflammation and repair.

The detectable morphological changes however depend on the time interval between the onset of ischaemia and the occurrence of myocardial death. In cases where the individual dies within few hours of the ischaemic attack, the morphological changes are difficult to detect because the body stops responding to the ischaemia.

Grossly, most infarcts occur singly and vary in size.

Infarcts that are 6–12 hours old show no discernible changes grossly and may be slightly paler and drier than normal. Early infarcts that are 3–6 hours old can be subjected to histochemical staining by using **triphenyltetrazolium chloride** (TTC). Here, an unfixed slice of the affected myocardium is placed in a solution containing the TTC dye. The dye imparts a red-brown colour to the normal myocardium with preserved lactate dehydrogenases, whereas the infarcted myocardium has lowered levels of dehydrogenases because they are lost by the leakiness of the myocardium, and hence stains pale with the dye. Similarly, another stain used to detect the viability of the myocardium is the **nitroblue tetrazolium dye** which stains the unaffected myocardium blue and the does not stain the infarcted myocardium.

By about 12–24 hours following infarction, the affected myocardium grossly develops a reddish-blue cyanotic area of discolouration because of congestion and stagnation of blood.

By 3–7 days, the affected area is often rimmed by a hyperaemic zone of granulation tissue indicating wound healing. Progressively, the infarct appears more well defined with a soft yellow tan and eventually as a fibrous scar by the end of 6 weeks. However, the time taken for scar formation vary according to the size of the infarct and the collateral circulation.

Microscopically, no detectable changes can be seen within the first 6 hours on light microscopy. The changes become apparent around 6–12 hours following infarction. Initially, the muscle fibres in the infarcted zone appear 'wavy' at the periphery of the infarct. This is due to the contractions of the viable myocardium causing the stretching strain over the dead fibres (Fig. 14.14).

Table 14.3 Changes Observed in the Infarcted Muscle Tissue

Time	Gross Features	Light Microscope Findings	Electron Microscope Findings
First half an hour	Stretched wavy muscle fibres	None	Myocyte relaxation, loss of myocyte glycogen granules and mitochondrial swelling
Half to 4 h	None	Usually none	Sarcolemmal disruption
4–12 h	Dark mottling	Early coagulative necrosis	
12–24 h	Dark mottling	Ongoing coagulative necrosis	
1–3 days	Mottling with a central yellow tan-coloured centre	Coagulation necrosis with heavy neutrophilic infiltration at the periphery	
3–7 days	Congested periphery with yellow tan centre – softening	Macrophage infiltration to clear the debris	
7–10 days	Diminished congestion, predominantly yellow tan	Granulation tissue formation at the periphery	
10–14 days	Red-grey depressed infarct borders	Granulation tissue with blood vessels and minimal collagen disposition	
2–8 weeks	Grey-white scar	Increased collagen deposition	
After 2 months	Complete healing with scar formation	Dense fibrocollagenous scar	

The loss of functioning of the ion channels that result in salt and water imbibement into the dead myocardium can be seen as myocardial vacuolization microscopically, called myocytolysis. It implies that the myocytes may be viable but have lost their contractile function.

Around 1–3 days after the infarction, coagulative necrosis of the myocytes begins to appear provoking an acute inflammatory response. Neutrophils begin to appear at the periphery of the infarct. Progressively, the coagulative necrosis may be apparent by loss of striations and hyaline appearance of the myocytes, with nuclear changes (karyolysis and pyknosis) and intense neutrophilic infiltrate. By the next 3–7 days, this is followed by a wave of macrophages that aid in the process of resorption of the necrotic debris and the neutrophilic fragments. Granulation tissue begins to form around the 7–10 days post-MI. The granulation tissue forms the scaffolding for the deposition of collagenous material for scar formation, marking the healing phase. The infarct heals from the periphery towards the centre because the healing process would require new growth components from the viable myocytes. Subsequently, the necrotic muscle fibres from the infarcted area are removed and are replaced by collagen fibres with continuous ingrowth of fibrovascular tissue from the periphery towards the centre. By the end of 6 weeks, a contracted fibrocollagenous scar, with diminished vascularity replaces the infarcted area (Table 14.3).

REPERFUSION AND THE ISCHAEMIC MYOCARDIUM

Reperfusion implies the restoration of blood flow to the ischaemic myocardium. The ultimatum of treatment of MI lies in limiting the extent of the infarct and salvaging the injured myocardium by restoration of perfusion. In almost every patient of MI, timely thrombolytic therapy needs to be initiated, but as described earlier some patients may undergo spontaneous thrombolysis such as in the cases of small-sized infarcts. Although within 6 hours a complete transmural infarct may develop, with successful reperfusion therapy the risk may be reduced by a significant 60%. Current guidelines suggest that reperfusion therapy must be performed within 6 hours of the ischaemic attack. Thus, benefits of reperfusion depend on the timeliness of thrombolysis and the extent of reestablishment of blood flow.

However, whether reperfusion therapy is purely beneficial is arguable because of the existence of the phenomenon of 'reperfusion injury'. This relates to the concept that the ischaemic myocardium is composed of irreversibly damaged cells, along with cells with varying degrees of reversible injury. With reperfusion, the irreversibly damaged cells by virtue die, although one portion of the reversibly damaged cells are salvaged, the marginal cells (at the periphery of the infarct) undergo further damage. The postulation that underlies this event include mitochondrial dysfunction, calcium influx by the injured cardiomyocytes, the so called, no-reflow process and the potential culprit, the oxygen free radicals. These are explained as follows:

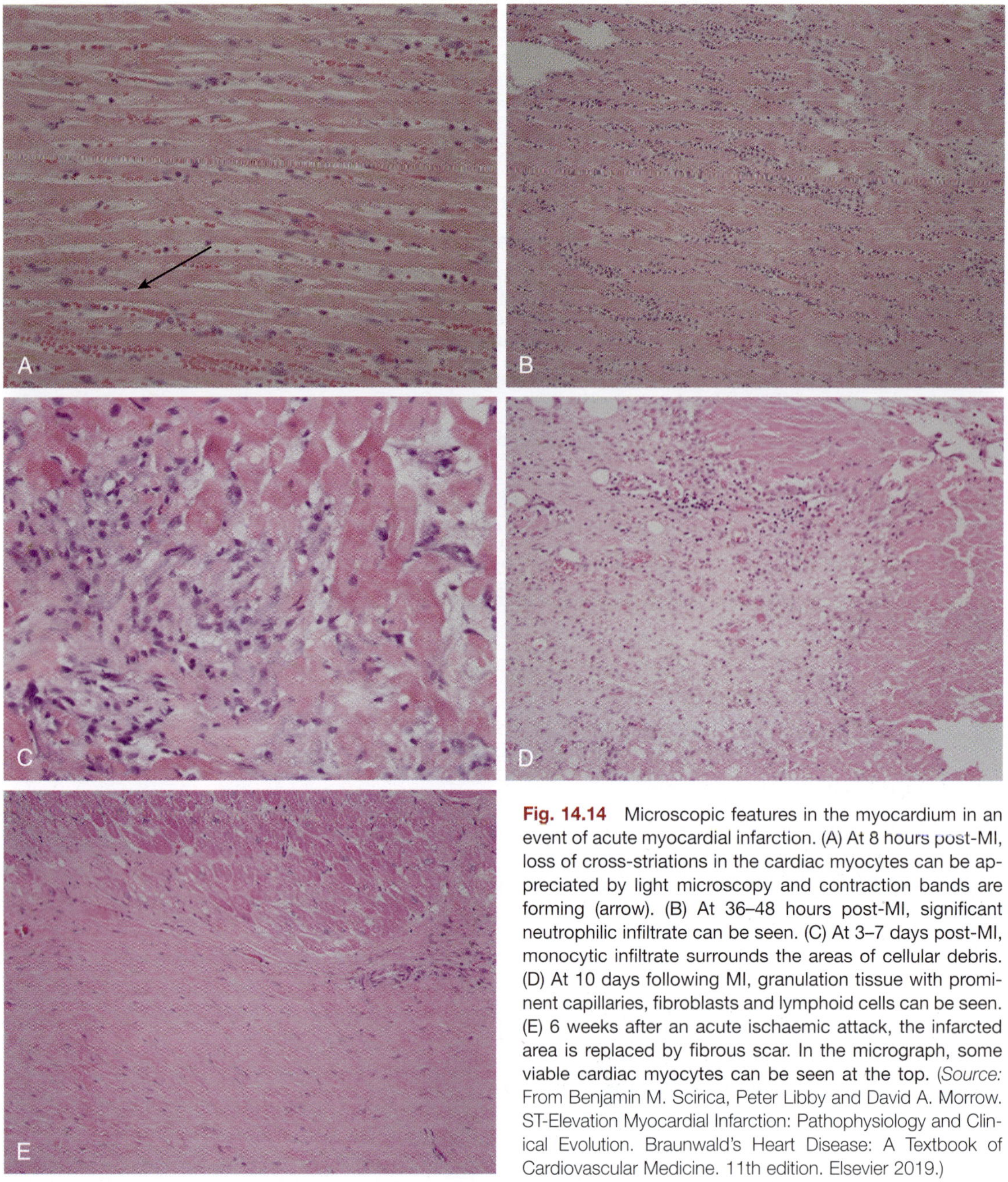

Fig. 14.14 Microscopic features in the myocardium in an event of acute myocardial infarction. (A) At 8 hours post-MI, loss of cross-striations in the cardiac myocytes can be appreciated by light microscopy and contraction bands are forming (arrow). (B) At 36–48 hours post-MI, significant neutrophilic infiltrate can be seen. (C) At 3–7 days post-MI, monocytic infiltrate surrounds the areas of cellular debris. (D) At 10 days following MI, granulation tissue with prominent capillaries, fibroblasts and lymphoid cells can be seen. (E) 6 weeks after an acute ischaemic attack, the infarcted area is replaced by fibrous scar. In the micrograph, some viable cardiac myocytes can be seen at the top. (*Source:* From Benjamin M. Scirica, Peter Libby and David A. Morrow. ST-Elevation Myocardial Infarction: Pathophysiology and Clinical Evolution. Braunwald's Heart Disease: A Textbook of Cardiovascular Medicine. 11th edition. Elsevier 2019.)

Within the ischaemic myocardium, the electron transport across the mitochondria is cessed because of loss of ATP. The components of the electron transport chain are primed to produce oxygen free radicals on perfusion. This leads to an oxidative burst with reperfusion.

Another postulated mechanism is the increased Ca ion influx into the damaged myocardium from plasma during the period of ischaemia probably because of the loss of the membrane integrity. Following perfusion, the myofibrils contract uncontrollably causing cytoskeletal damage and cell death. The associated biochemical and morphological changes due to reperfusion injury include tissue water and calcium increase and massive loss of myocardial enzymes and proteins (washout phenomenon). The calcium overload can be visibly seen on light microscopy as contraction bands marking the hallmark feature of reperfusion injury.

The no-reflow phenomenon is explained by leucocyte aggregates that may occlude the microvasculature contributing to cell death. This can be further accelerated by platelet and complement activation that injures the endothelium.

The apparent gross and microscopic appearance of a reperfused myocardium include a large, densely haemorrhagic infarct that follows fibrinolytic therapy consequence by vascular injury and leakiness. Microscopically, as already described, contraction bands are evident.

Sometimes, following reperfusion therapy, the injured myocardium may go into a state of prolonged contractile dysfunction with slow gradual recovery – also referred to as **stunned myocardium**. **Hibernation** is the term used to describe myocardial segments with slow metabolism and function, that are subjected to chronic, sublethal ischaemia. However, revascularization procedures, such as CABG or stenting, often revive function in such conditions.

Clinical Features

Patients present with typical clinical symptoms of prolonged chest pain (angina) that is described as a crushing, stabbing or squeezing type of pain in the anterior chest wall radiating to the left arm and the back. Patients often experience nausea, vomiting, profuse sweating and dyspnoea, probably because of pulmonary congestion and oedema caused by the ischaemic myocardium. In some cases, acute MI is preceded by episodes of unstable angina.

The initial investigation in such a patient would be an ECG. The findings on the ECG can distinguish the two types of infarcts, namely, a transmural infarct or an ST-elevation MI (STEMI) and a subendocardial infarct, also known as a non-ST-elevation infarct (NSTEMI).

The laboratory investigations include the detection of the protein levels that have leaked out of the damaged myocardial cells (Fig. 14.15). The most clinically significant among these are the cardiac-specific troponins T and I (cTnT and cTnI). Cardiac troponins begin to increase around 2–4 hours post-MI and peak levels can be observed at 24–48 hours after an acute attack. Because these troponins are not normally detected in the blood, their elevation in a setting of possible MI is highly specific and are thus the preferred biochemical markers for MI. Apart from cardiac troponins, another marker, creatinine kinase, especially its isoenzyme, CK-MB is of particular importance because it aids in differentiating unstable angina from STEMI. CK rises within 4–8 hours and follows a declining course earlier than troponins. The pitfall concerning CK is its lack of specificity because it is elevated

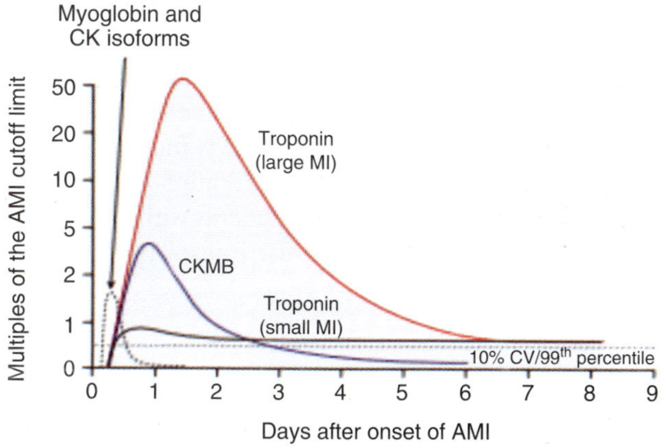

Fig. 14.15 The proteins that spill over from the damaged myocardium are cleared by the lymphatic and the venous system to be detected on laboratory tests. The cytoplasmic markers such as myoglobin rise quickly and disappear, whereas the troponins follow a more protracted course.

Table 14.4 Enzyme Levels in Myocardial Infarction

Enzyme	Begins to Rise At	Peak	Returns to Normal	Usefulness
Troponin I	3–12 h	24 h	5–10 days	Sensitive and specific
Troponin T	3–12 h	12–48 h	5–14 days	Sensitive and specific
CK-MB	3–12 h	24 h	2–3 days	Sensitive but not specific

in conditions of skeletal muscle disease or trauma as well. However, its isoenzyme CK-MB is relatively specific because its concentration in the extracardiac tissues is low but often misleadingly elevated in conditions of cardiac surgery and myocarditis. The major application of CK-MB is to diagnose a second ischaemia that occurs during the recovery stage of first MI because their levels reach normal values within 3 days and a second rise may indicate another occlusive episode. To conclude, in most cases, troponins are used as routine markers for MI diagnosis and likewise, it is not cost-effective to measure troponins and CK levels in all patients. Summary of the enzyme levels is given in Table 14.4.

Recommended Initial Therapies for Acute Myocardial Infarction

Oxygen supplementation
Nitrates – induce vasodilation and reverse vasospasm
Antiplatelet agents – aspirin, ADP receptor inhibitors
Anticoagulant therapy – with heparin, thrombin inhibitors
Beta-blockers – to decrease myocardial oxygen demand
Prompt reperfusion – to save the myocardium
Percutaneous coronary intervention (PCI) – dilatation of the narrowed vessel can be achieved by using inflation of a balloon catheter when thrombolytic therapy fails
Coronary artery bypass grafting

Complications of Myocardial Infarction

The clinical course of an acute MI is often dominated by the functional or mechanical complications that follow.

Contractile dysfunction: Rationally, almost every patient experiences some degree of left ventricular failure in the form of hypotension, pulmonary congestion or pulmonary oedema. In approximately 10% of patients, cardiogenic shock may manifest especially when more than 40% of the left ventricle is apparently damaged.
Papillary muscle dysfunction: In the setting of ischaemia, papillary muscle dysfunction can result in mitral regurgitation. In due course, the papillary muscle may undergo shortening and fibrosis or in worse cases rupture (Fig. 14.16).
Myocardial rupture: Although much less common, comprising only 1%–5% of MIs, it is often fatal. Anterior

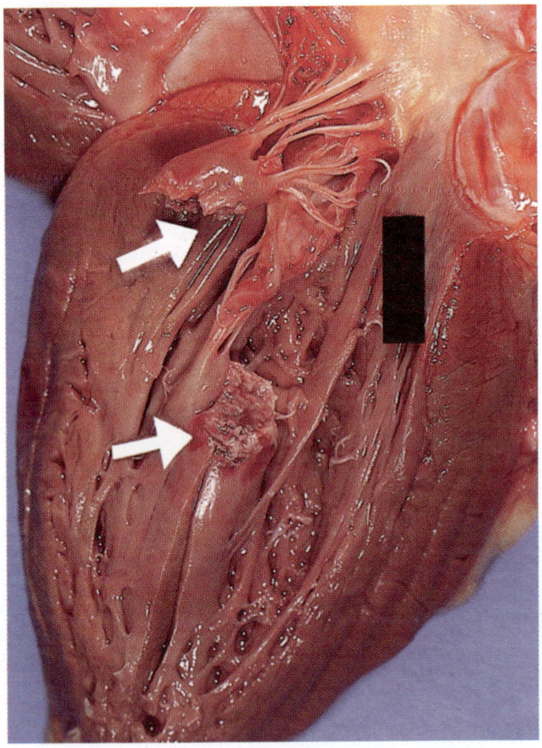

Fig. 14.16 Gross photograph showing papillary muscle rupture (arrows) postacute myocardial infarction. (*Source:* From Andrew J. Connolly, Walter E. Finkbeiner, Philip C. Ursell and Richard L. Davis. Atlas of Gross Autopsy Pathology. Autopsy Pathology: A Manual and Atlas. 3rd edition. Elsevier 2016.)

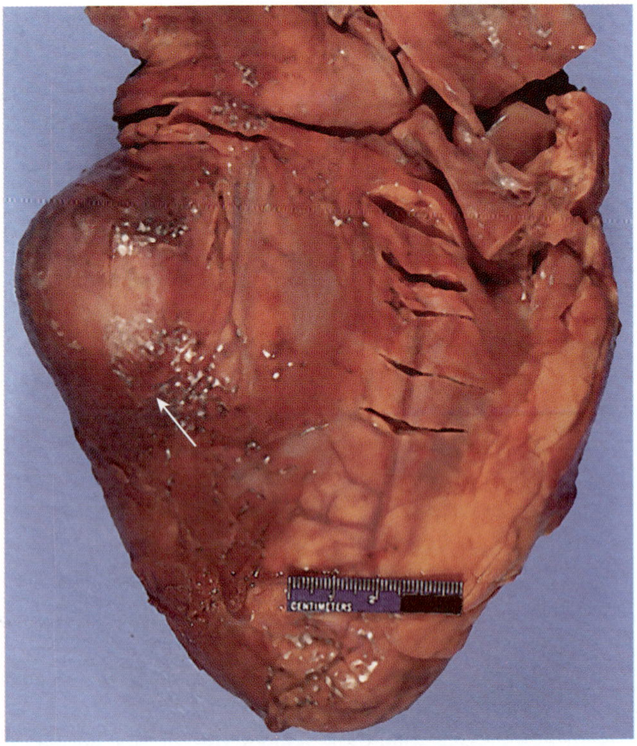

Fig. 14.17 Gross photograph of the heart showing a ventricular aneurysm (arrow) following myocardial infarction. (*Source:* From Andrew J. Connolly, Walter E. Finkbeiner, Philip C. Ursell and Richard L. Davis. Atlas of Gross Autopsy Pathology. Autopsy Pathology: A Manual and Atlas. 3rd edition. Elsevier 2016.)

infarcts and the left ventricular wall are most prone to rupture and results in pericardial effusion and cardiac tamponade. It mostly occurs 3–7 days post-MI when the myocardium is weak with necrosis or granulation tissue. Newer scars are more prone to rupture than the old scars owing to the lesser collagen content.

Arrythmias: As a rule, almost all patients with MI develop rhythm abnormalities, which may lead to SCD in a significant number of patients. A number of conditions such as bradycardia, supraventricular tachyarrhythmias or ventricular fibrillation marks the most serious risk of fatality.

Chamber dilation: The myocardial wall may undergo disproportionate stretching because of weakening of the wall by the infarct.

Mural thrombus: All the above-mentioned complications make way for mural thrombus development which may lead occurrence with a potential fate of embolism.

Ventricular aneurysm (Fig. 14.17): Although a late complication of MI, ventricular aneurysms frequently lead to the development of mural thrombus, heart failure and arrhythmias.

Pericarditis – inflammation of the pericardium following MI can occur in 10%–20% patient. Pericarditis manifests as pericardial friction rub on auscultation.

Post-MI syndrome (Dressler syndrome) – it refers to a delayed form of pericarditis that develops 2–3 weeks post-MI. The syndrome is postulated to have an immunologic aetiology, as patients respond well to corticosteroids. A similar scenario follows cardiac surgery.

The extent of myocardial damage is an important predictor of the outcome in terms of morbidity and mortality. Procedures to restore perfusion need to be initiated within the first few hours of symptoms beyond which the myocardium is lost to permanent damage.

CHRONIC ISCHAEMIC HEART DISEASE

In a small proportion of patients, accumulated ischaemic myocardial damage can result in progressive congestive heart failure. In most instances, a previous MI or cardiac surgery, such as in coronary arterial interventions and bypass surgery, is present. Chronic IHD is mostly a result of functional decompensation of the noninfarcted myocardium following acute MI. In fact, patients with chronic IHD contribute to at least 50% of cardiac transplant procedures.

Morphology

Chronic IHD is also referred to as ischaemic cardiomyopathy. Left ventricular hypertrophy and dilation and evidence of atherosclerosis is a common finding. Discrete scars representing healed infarcts is usually apparent. The mural endocardium often exhibits patchy fibrous thickening and mural thrombi.

ARRHYTHMIAS

Arrhythmias may result from disorders of impulse formation or impulse conduction or both. The only normal rhythm of the heart is the sinus rhythm in which the impulse is generated in the SA node and follows the usual course through the AV node, bundle of His and the Purkinje fibres. Any deviation from this conduction pathway can cause arrhythmias. The common categories of arrhythmias on the basis of rate of conduction include:

Bradyarrhythmias: These develop because of decreased intrinsic pacemaker function or blocks in conduction, and are characterized by heart rate lesser than 60 beats per minute.
Tachyarrhythmias: They develop because of increased automaticity and are characterized by heart rate higher than 100 beats per minute.

Tachyarrhythmias are further categorized into supraventricular type when the pathophysiology involves the AV node, and ventricular type when the arrhythmias are initiated at the level of the His–Purkinje system or the ventricles.

Other types of arrhythmias include irregular rhythm with normal ventricular contraction, chaotic depolarization without functional ventricular contraction and no electrical activity referred to as asystole. The common causes of arrhythmias include:

A frequent cause of arrhythmias is CAD causing myocardial ischaemia. In a situation of low oxygen supply, the myocardial cells depolarize leading to altered impulse formation or signal conduction. Structural deficiencies in the conduction system can be caused by conditions such as IHD or cardiomyopathies and give rise to arrhythmias.
Sick sinus syndrome, also known as sinus node dysfunction, is a disorder that results from the altered pacemaker functioning and conduction at the level of the SA node. Although the most common intrinsic factor leading to sick sinus syndrome is age-related degeneration, congenital disorders and surgery are the other less common aetiologies. Patients experience acute, severe bradycardia, probably because the AV node takes over the pacemaker functioning, slowing down the heart rate.
Atrial fibrillation is the most common type of sustained arrhythmia that increases with age and manifests with a wide range of symptoms and severity. It is attributed to various heart diseases that cause stretching and scarring of the myocardium (cardiac remodelling), resulting in some form of disorganization of atrial depolarization. The condition is rather a predictable outcome of heart failure or rather synergistically contributing to it. Such patients usually record an 'irregularly irregular heartbeat' due to uncoordinated chaotic atrial contractions. These ineffectual atrial contractions potentially reduce the cardiac output, causing stasis of blood increasing the risk of thrombus formation.
Heart block manifests in conditions of AV node dysfunction. Subclinical disease, overtly picked up on ECG, comprises the first-degree heart block. Second-degree heart block refers to intermittent transmission of impulses. Complete failure represents the third-degree heart block.
Re-entry circuits: Spontaneous aberrant myocyte depolarization may be triggered by myocarditis, myocyte hypertrophy, ischaemia or sarcoidosis, resulting in abnormal electric circuits, also called re-entry circuits, and cause ventricular tachycardia which may progress to fatal ventricular fibrillation. The process can be accelerated by the deposition of abnormal substances such as amyloid that may cause disruption of the myocyte–myocyte signalling.
Rarely, congenital cardiac disease may give rise to arrhythmias. HCM, MVP and other congenital anomalies have been associated with arrhythmias and the cause of sudden death. The occurrence of such events in the absence of any anatomical cardiac abnormalities are referred to as primary electrical disorders. The most common entity among this category is channelopathies in which gene mutations cause abnormal functioning of the ion channels namely the sodium (Na^+), potassium (K^+) and calcium (Ca^{2+}) in the myocyte cellular membrane and can give rise to life-threatening arrhythmias. The typical presentation follows that of the congenital long QT syndrome, characterized by prolongation of the QT interval on ECG, and also represents the leading cause of sudden death in the young.

SUDDEN CARDIAC DEATH

SCD refers to the death of an individual caused by a cardiac condition, occurring within 1–24 hours of onset of symptoms. The most predictable underlying mechanism includes a lethal arrhythmia manifesting as ventricular fibrillation. As one can expect, CAD is one of the leading causes of SCD responsible for nearly 80% of cases. The most common nonischaemic causes of SCD include conditions causing cardiac hypertrophy, myocardial fibrosis, hypertension, obesity and alcoholism.

The major concern arises over the occurrence of SCD in young patients, younger than 35 years. The common aetiologies include:

- Cardiac conduction abnormalities, congenital or acquired
- DCM or HCM
- Anomalous coronary origin
- Channelopathies – long QT syndrome, short QT syndrome and Brugada syndrome
- Myocarditis
- MVP
- Pulmonary hypertension
- Heart failure

- Other causes – cardiac tamponade; pulmonary embolism; drug abuse, in particular cocaine and methamphetamine

Interventions by modern techniques, especially implantable cardioverter defibrillator, that can sense and electrically counteract episodes of ventricular fibrillation have proved particularly useful in preventing sudden death in patients who have previously experienced arrhythmia-induced syncope or survived a cardiac arrest.

HYPERTENSIVE HEART DISEASE

Hypertensive heart disease refers to a constellation of structural and functional changes occurring in the myocardium and the coronary arteries in response to chronically elevated blood pressure. As discussed in Chapter 13, hypertension is a common disorder with considerable morbidity and mortality, affecting most of the systemic organs. The discussion here focuses on the cardiac pathology pertaining to systemic hypertension, and pulmonary hypertension that can cause right-sided hypertension and 'cor pulmonale'.

SYSTEMIC (LEFT-SIDED) HYPERTENSIVE HEART DISEASE

Currently, the American Cardiology Association/American Heart Association (AHA) guidelines define hypertension as a record of systolic blood pressure more than 120 mm Hg or a diastolic pressure more than 80 mm Hg. These recent recommendations have driven over one-half of the general population into the hypertensive category and at risk of hypertensive heart disease.

High systemic arterial pressure causes pressure overload and increased wall tension on the left ventricle which is compensated by myocardial hypertrophy. Although initially the hypertrophy serves as an adaptive response, over time, the left ventricle mass may be insufficient to balance the high wall tension. This leads to systolic dysfunction which along with the increased oxygen demand of the hypertrophied myocardium results in 'demand' ischaemia. The degree of hypertrophy correlates with the development of congestive cardiac failure, arrhythmias, MI and in some cases SCD. Thus, left ventricular hypertrophy is one of the strong predictors of cardiac mortality and morbidity in the hypertensive patients.

Morphology

As explained earlier, the left ventricular wall undergoes hypertrophy owing to the pressure overload. The left ventricular free wall and the interventricular septum become thickened uniformly and concentrically. Concentric hypertrophy without ventricular dilation is the usual pattern of compensation, until very late in the process (Fig. 14.18). The heart increases in weight exceeding – 375 g in men and 350 g in women. In due course, the ventricular thickening imparts a wall stiffness that impairs diastolic filling, causing elevated diastolic filling pressures. This is manifested by pulmonary congestion. In such patients, atrial dilation may be evident.

In long-standing cases of hypertension, decompensation supervened by congestive cardiac failure may develop and the left ventricle displays an eccentric hypertrophy with dilation.

Microscopically, myocardial cells appear thicker with enlarged, hyperchromatic and rectangular ('box-car') nuclei (Fig. 14.19). Also, areas of myocyte degeneration and focal areas of interstitial and perivascular fibrosis can be seen.

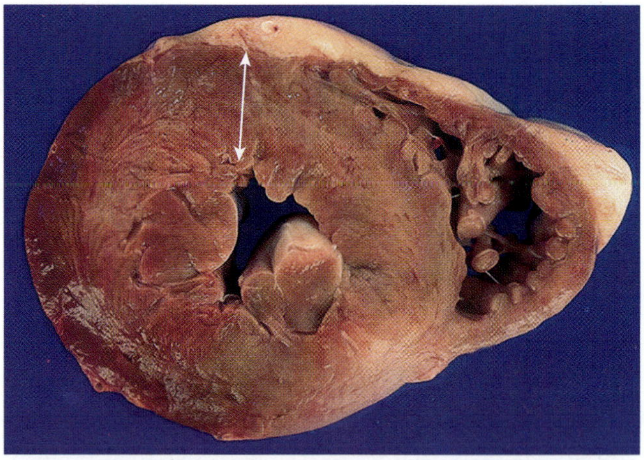

Fig. 14.18 Gross image of the short-axis plane section of the cardiac specimen of hypertensive heart disease showing concentric hypertrophy of the left ventricular wall and the papillary muscle reducing the cavity space. At autopsy, the myocardial thickness is measured excluding the epicardial fat pad (arrow). (*Source:* From Andrew J. Connolly, Walter E. Finkbeiner, Philip C. Ursell and Richard L. Davis. Atlas of Gross Autopsy Pathology. Autopsy Pathology: A Manual and Atlas. 3rd edition. Elsevier 2016.)

Clinical Features

Meta-analysis has demonstrated a log-linear relationship between elevated blood pressure and risk of CVD, which increases substantially with age. Interestingly, hypertensive heart disease manifests more commonly in women with an associated increased risk of heart failure in comparison to men. This may be attributed to the fact that women are more likely to have uncontrolled blood pressure and further recent studies have suggested certain classes of antihypertensive medications to be less effective in women. Compensated hypertensive heart disease is usually asymptomatic. However, ECG or ECHO may show evidence of left ventricular hypertrophy. Some patients may manifest only after the onset of congestive

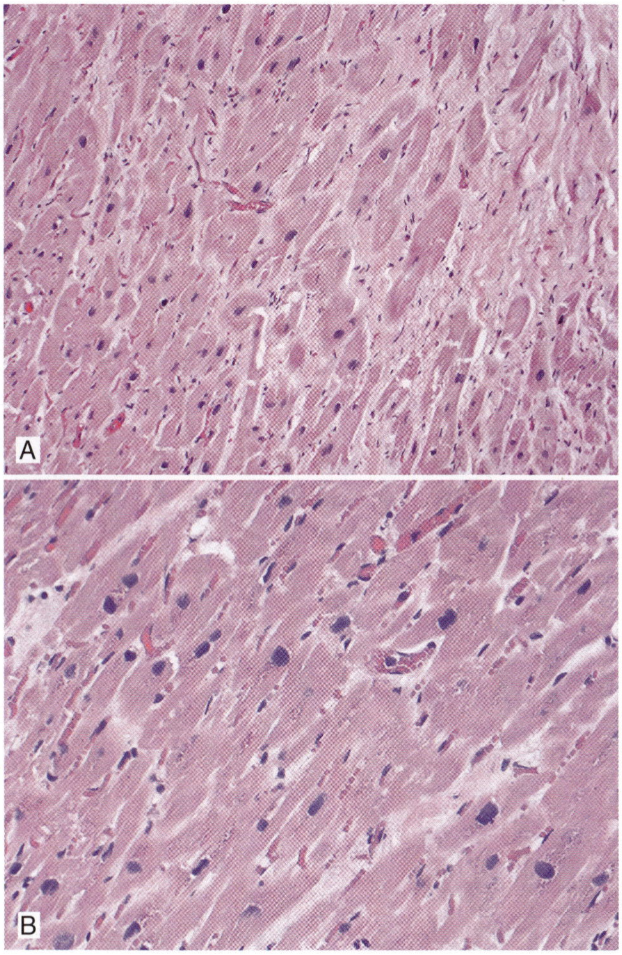

Fig. 14.19 Histomicrograph showing cardiac myocytes in a patient with hypertensive heart disease. (A) Enlarged cardiomyocytes with areas of fibrosis. (B) High power view showing 'box-car'–shaped nucleus. (*Source:* From Aliya N. Husain. Hypertensive Heart Disease. High-Yield Thoracic Pathology. Saunders 2012.)

cardiac failure or atrial fibrillation due to atrial enlargement. Aggressive control of hypertension with antihypertensives can help in regression of the left ventricular mass and reduction in the risk of complications.

PULMONARY (RIGHT-SIDED) HYPERTENSIVE HEART DISEASE: COR PULMONALE

Pulmonary hypertension attributable to primary lung parenchymal disorders and disorders pertaining to the pulmonary vasculature may cause right ventricular hypertrophy, frequently accompanied by right heart failure. This comprises the complex of cor pulmonale.

Acute cor pulmonale can be precipitated by sudden, massive pulmonary embolization and can be life threatening, whereas chronic cor pulmonale develops over many years because of chronic bronchitis or emphysema and contributes to 30%–40% cases. The right ventricle is normally more compliant and thinner than the left ventricle. As a consequence of the pressure overload caused

Table 14.5 Aetiological Factors of Cor Pulmonale

Diseases of the Pulmonary Parenchyma

- Chronic bronchitis and emphysema
- Pulmonary fibrosis (from any cause)
- Pneumoconiosis
- Cystic fibrosis
- Bronchiectasis

Diseases of the Pulmonary Vasculature

- Recurrent pulmonary thromboembolism
- Primary pulmonary hypertension
- Peripheral pulmonary stenosis
- Extensive pulmonary arteritis (granulomatosis with polyangiitis)
- Intravenous drug abuse
- Radiation-induced vascular obstruction
- Schistosomiasis

Disorders Affecting Chest Movement

- Kyphoscoliosis
- Marked obesity (Pickwickian syndrome)
- Neuromuscular disease
- Pleural fibrosis
- Neuromuscular disorders

by factors elaborated in Table 14.5, the right ventricle undergoes hypertrophy and dilation, leading to right heart failure. Note that many cases of pulmonary hypertension stem from long-standing left-sided heart disease.

Morphology

In acute cor pulmonale, the right ventricle is characteristically ovoidly dilated owing to the excessive dilation without hypertrophy. Sometimes, right atrial dilation may be evident. In chronic cor pulmonale, the right ventricle may be thickened up to 1 cm or more from its normal range of 3–5 mm (Fig. 14.20). In most instances, the ventricular wall only minimally expresses the hypertrophy, but the pectinate muscles are enormously thickened and can be considered to be a reasonable sign of right ventricular hypertrophy. Sometimes, the right ventricle hypertrophy may also cause fibrous thickening of the tricuspid valve probably due to the high right ventricular systolic pressure. The ventricular septum may also be thicker than the left or right ventricular free walls.

SYPHILITIC HEART DISEASE **PA 27.10**

Syphilitic heart disease once accounted for 5%–10% all cardiovascular deaths, and is a late form of the disease presenting with a latent period of 1–25 years. Before the discovery of penicillin, tertiary syphilis was the most common cause of thoracic aortic aneurysm. It is uncommon in

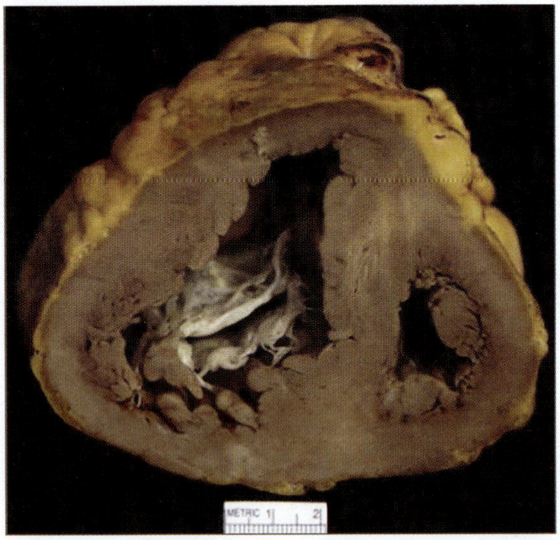

Fig. 14.20 Transverse section of the heart in a patient with cor pulmonale. The right ventricular wall is dilated but as about as thick as the left ventricular wall. Note the thickened wall of the tricuspid valves in this patient. (*Source:* From William Clifford Roberts, Alexis E. Shafii, Paul A. Grayburn, Jong Mi Ko, Matthew R. Weissenborn, Randall L. Rosenblatt and Joseph M. Guileyardo. Clinical and Morphologic Features of Acute, Subacute and Chronic Cor Pulmonale (Pulmonary Heart Disease). The American Journal of Cardiology. 2015;115:697-703.)

today's era, but is worth a mention here because it is considered a differential in the evaluation of aortic valve disease or aortic aneurysm. Cardiovascular syphilis is estimated to occur in about 10% of patients with untreated syphilis.

PATHOGENESIS

The aetiopathogenesis and the forms of syphilis are discussed in detail in Chapter 8.

The major pathological cardiac changes in cardiovascular disease can be categorized into four forms, namely:

- Syphilitic aortitis
- Syphilitic aortic aneurysm
- Syphilitic aortic vasculitis with aortic regurgitation
- Syphilitic coronary ostial stenosis

MORPHOLOGY

The primary lesion of cardiovascular syphilis is aortitis, an inflammatory response to the invasion of the aortic wall by the causative organism *Treponema pallidum* that evolves to obliterative endarteritis of the vasa vasorum and results in necrosis of the elastic fibres and connective tissue in the aortic media. This leads to weakening of the aortic wall and progresses to the late vascular manifestations of syphilis.

Syphilitic aortitis is reported in 70%–80% of untreated cases after the primary infection, and in 10% of these patients, significant cardiovascular complications will occur, such as aortic aneurysm, aortic regurgitation and coronary ostia stenosis. However, extensive involvement of the tubular portion of the thoracic aorta is a constant finding in the syphilitic process. The ascending aorta is the segment most commonly affected (50%), followed by the arch (35%) and the descending aorta (15%). The aortitis does not involve the distal aorta and is restricted to the proximal portion probably because of the rich vascular and lymphatic drainage in the ascending aorta.

The inflammation may extend into the aortic root causing aortic regurgitation due to the dilation of the aortic annulus. Aortic incompetence and coronary stenosis are due to the mesaortitis of the proximal portion of the aorta. The various changes in the syphilitic heart such as ischaemia, fibrosis, hypertrophy, dilatation, cardiac degeneration, angina pectoris are the end results of aortitis which increases the heart's workload and diminishes its blood supply.

The finding of a massive aortic root dilatation with thinning of the aortic wall due to inflammation is most commonly an evidence of syphilitic infection. Syphilis may also involve other large arteries, cerebral vessels or myocardium.

CLINICAL FEATURES

Manifestations are more common in patients with insufficient treatment in early stages of infection than in those who had late treatment. Cardiovascular syphilis may become symptomatic with thoracic pain or symptoms of compression of the surrounding structures, but can enlarge asymptomatically until incidental finding in a chest X-ray or a catastrophic and often fatal aneurysmal rupture. Chest X-ray may show an irregular dilatation and linear calcification of ascending aorta, whereas CT angiogram is best imaging study to define the size and anatomy of the aneurysm.

LABORATORY DIAGNOSIS

In the absence of a clinical history, positive serology is a prerequisite for the diagnosis. *Treponema*-specific tests such as TPHA, micro-haemagglutination test and fluorescent treponemal antibody absorption test are more sensitive than nontreponemal tests such as VDRL and RPR tests.

Management and Prognosis

Prognosis is better in patients with uncomplicated aortitis than in those with aortic insufficiency, aneurysmal dilatation or myocardial degeneration. Once the aorta is damaged or it has damaged the heart, antisyphilitic treatment with penicillin may at best arrest the advance of the disease, increase life expectancy and ease symptoms.

DISEASES OF THE VALVES

Valvular heart diseases are the third most common cause of CVD. Interestingly, the types of valvular heart diseases seen in different parts of the world are increasingly different. In developed countries, rheumatic heart disease (RHD) has been declining, whereas infectious diseases and rheumatic diseases are still common in the developing countries.

Various forms of congenital and acquired diseases cause valvular deformities. Among the acquired conditions, RHD is the most common. Likewise, valvular deformities of the left-side valves are much more frequent than the right-side valves. The mitral valves are the most commonly affected valves followed by the aortic valves.

The valvular deformities may be one of types described as follows:

- ***Valvular stenosis***: The clinical picture of valvular stenosis results from the failure of the valve to open completely during diastole causing obstruction to forward flow of blood. They can be both congenital and acquired. The two most common causes for stenosis particularly at the valvular level are fibrosis or calcifications of the leaflets or the cusps or the commissures, either alone or in combination. Rare causes include vegetations, thrombus or neoplasm that cause obstruction by external compression. Stenotic valves are generally more common than the regurgitant valves encountered in surgical practice.
- ***Regurgitation or incompetency of the valve***: This refers to the condition where the valve fails to close completely during systole resulting in back flow or regurgitation of blood. Also referred to as valvular insufficiency, valvular regurgitation can be caused by intrinsic defect of the valve such as in endocarditis or damage of the supporting structures such as the papillary muscles, tendinous cords, the aorta or the ventricular wall.

Both the conditions may coexist also within the same valve and may also involve multiple valves. The clinical manifestations depend on the valve involved, the severity of the disease, and the rate and quality of the compensatory mechanisms that help to maintain the blood flow. Valvular insufficiencies for instance, IE that affects the aortic valve cusps causes an acute, rather severe, rapidly developing aortic regurgitation, whereas stenosis such as rheumatic mitral stenosis is a slower chronic process that develops over the years and is generally tolerated well. The condition can be complicated by a state of increased oxygen demand, such as pregnancy or anaemia. Also, valvular heart diseases, especially stenotic valvular disease may give rise to secondary changes such as pressure overload ventricular hypertrophy and heart failure, and endothelial dysfunction due to the forceful ejections of blood through the diseased valve into the vessel injuring the endothelium. On physical examination, it is found that the abnormal blood flow within the valves produces characteristic murmurs and more severe lesions may give rise to an externally palpable thrill. The murmurs may be heard on different locations depending on the valve involved and may be a systolic or diastolic murmur depending on the type of defect.

The most common causes of the clinically significant valvular heart diseases are as follows:

- AS – calcification or sclerosis of the normal or congenitally bicuspid aortic valve
- Aortic regurgitation – dilatation of the ascending aorta mostly due to hypertension or ageing
- Mitral stenosis – RHD
- Mitral regurgitation – myxomatous degeneration of the valve

The common acquired causes of valvular heart diseases are mentioned below:

Mitral Valve Disease	Aortic Valve Disease
Mitral Stenosis	**Aortic Stenosis**
Rheumatic heart disease (most common cause) Atrial tumours Prior exposure to chest radiation Ball-valve thrombus	Rheumatic heart disease Senile calcific aortic stenosis Congenital deformed valve calcification
Mitral Regurgitation	**Aortic Regurgitation**
Abnormalities of the leaflets and the commissures Postinfective scarring Infective endocarditis Mitral valve prolapse Abnormalities of tensor apparatus Rupture/fibrosis of the papillary muscle Rupture of the chordae tendineae Abnormalities of the left ventricular cavity Left ventricular enlargement due to myocarditis or cardiomyopathy Calcification of the mitral ring	Intrinsic valve disease Rheumatic heart disease Infective endocarditis Traumatic rupture of the aortic valve Aortic disease Aortic dissection Syphilitic aortitis Ankylosing spondylitis Rheumatoid heart disease Marfan syndrome Severe hypertension Bicuspid aortic valve

CALCIFIC VALVULAR DEGENERATION

Calcific valvular degeneration is the most common type of valvular abnormalities encountered. This is not surprising because the valves are chronically exposed to high levels of mechanical stress over the years, owing to the number of contractions per day cumulating over the years, and the persistent remodelling due to the constantly altered transvalvular pressure gradients.

Calcific Aortic Stenosis

As previously mentioned, calcific degeneration of a previously normal aortic valve is the most common valvular abnormality, accounting for about 2% of cases among the elderly population. Degenerative AS is the most common cause of AS. The so called senile degeneration results from the age-related wear and tear of the valve with progressive calcium phosphate deposition. Congenital bicuspid valves undergoing calcific degeneration account for approximately 1%. Patients usually present in the seventh to ninth decades of life.

The risk factors for calcific degeneration are much similar to that of atherosclerosis and include the following:

- Chronic injury due to hyperlipidaemia, hypertension, inflammation and smoking. The injury is caused by the risk factors that progressively, cause valvular degeneration and provoke the deposition of calcium.
- Mechanical forces of forceful ejection of blood promote the accumulation of LDL and other cellular components causing inflammation.
- Another theory postulates that aortic valvular calcification is not due to passive deposition of calcium over devitalized tissue, but is rather an active process that modifies the valvular interstitial cells into cells that functionally resemble osteoblasts which synthesize bone material and lead to cell-mediated mineralization of the extracellular matrix.

Despite these similarities with atherosclerosis, effective prevention of the latter does not help prevent the development of calcific AS.

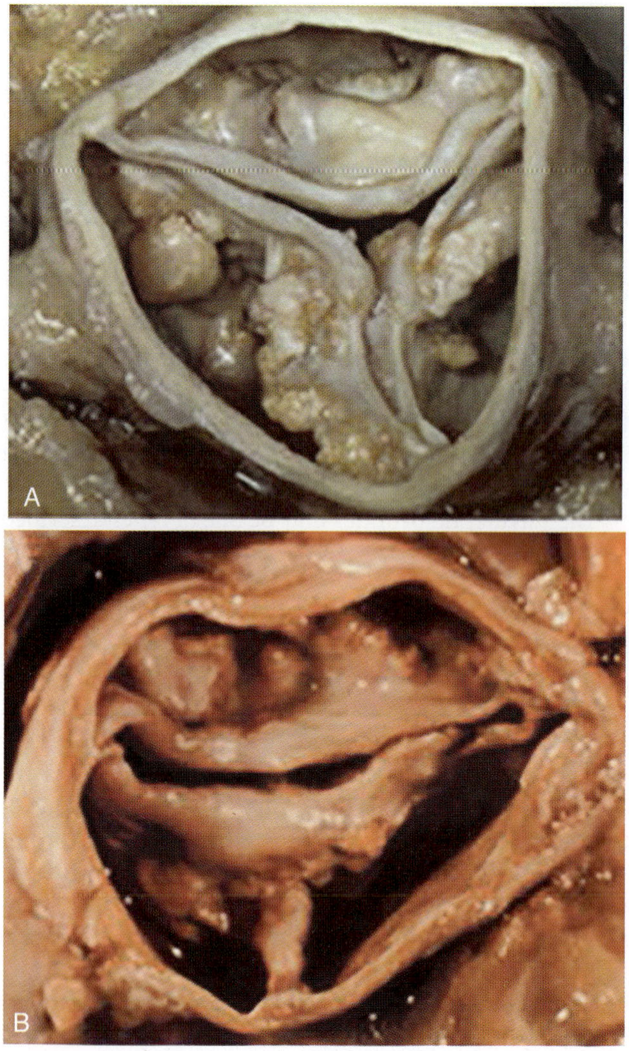

Fig. 14.21 (A) Aortic valve stenosis. (B) Calcific stenosis in a bicuspid valve. (*Source:* From Richard N. Mitchell and Andrew J. Connolly. The Heart . Robbins & Cotran Pathologic Basis of Disease. 10th edition. Elsevier 2021.)

Morphology

The gross hallmark feature of calcific AS is the presence of moulded calcific deposits found predominantly on the outflow surfaces, i.e. the aortic surface of the cusps preventing the cuspal opening (Fig. 14.21). Free edges of the valve are usually spared. There is no commissural fusion and that distinguishes degenerative AS from postinflammatory valvular disease (rheumatic valvular disease). Microscopically, the layered anatomy of the valve is preserved. The degenerated aortic valve shows nodular calcific deposits on the valvular fibrosa, outflow surface of the valve near the margins of attachment. The inflammation is variable and sometimes metaplastic bone formation can be seen.

Clinical Features The obstruction to the ventricular outflow tract causes an increased pressure overload hypertrophy on the left ventricle. The hypertrophy predisposes to reduced microcirculatory perfusion often complicated by atherosclerosis leading to ischaemic myocardium and angina pectoris. Untreated patients eventually develop cardiac decompensation and congestive heart failure within 2 years of onset of symptoms.

The mortality rate is as high as 57% at the end of 3 years. In severe cases, medical treatment is not much beneficial. Thus, patient with symptomatic AS would require surgical valve replacement.

Calcific Stenosis of the Congenital Bicuspid Valve

Congenital bicuspid valve (BAV) (Fig. 14.21) accounts for approximately 50% of AS in adults. Genetic studies have revealed NOTCH1 to be specifically associated with BAV. In a congenital bicuspid valve, the cusps are mostly of an unequal size with the larger cusp possessing a midline raphe. The raphe is the most preferred site for calcific deposits. Most BAV are well tolerated until the calcific deposits cause haemodynamic instability. Other complications of BAV include aortic regurgitation and IE.

Mitral Annular Calcification

The degenerative calcific deposits in a mitral valve typically occur in the fibrous annulus as opposed by the cuspal deposits in aortic calcific stenosis. The calcification is stony hard, initially developing over the connective tissue of the valve and eventually extending over base of the leaflets and the interventricular septum. The calcific deposits transform the valve into a rigid curved structure that is evident radiologically. However, mitral annular calcifications do not cause any functional disturbance, although murmurs can be apparent. It is also common among the elderly population and is more common in women than men. Rarely, regurgitation, stenosis, arrhythmias and sudden death may occur because of penetrance of the calcific deposits such that they may impinge on the AV conduction system.

Complications arise when the calcific deposits predispose to thrombus formation or IE. Thus, virtually all patients with mitral annular calcification carry a mild risk of embolic stroke.

MITRAL VALVE PROLAPSE (MYXOMATOUS DEGENERATION OF THE MITRAL VALVE)

MVP is one of the common incidental findings detected during routine physical examination. It refers to a condition in which the mitral valves become 'floppy' causing an abnormal billowing of one or more leaflet into the left atrium during systole. The condition is frequently accompanied by mitral regurgitation. MVP occurs in about 2%–3% of the population and is much more common in females.

Pathogenesis

MVP is believed to rise from any condition that causes weakening of the leaflets and its supportive structures. Rare heritable causes are Ehlers–Danlos syndrome or Marfan syndrome caused by fibrillin-1 mutations and dysregulation of TGF-β signalling. More evidence has been aligning in view of TGF-β overactivity in the causation of the laxity of the valvular wall.

Morphology

Apart from the mitral valve, tricuspid, aortic and pulmonary valves may be affected. Pathologically, the leaflets, particularly the posterior leaflets, are often enlarged, rubbery and redundant. A significant anatomical alteration is the ballooning or aneurysmal protrusion of the affected valve (Fig. 14.22).

Microscopically, the collagen and elastin matrix of the valvular fibrosa is disintegrated and replaced by loose myxomatous connective tissue. In more severe lesions, the chordae tendineae may rupture or elongate with annular enlargement or thickening of the leaflet.

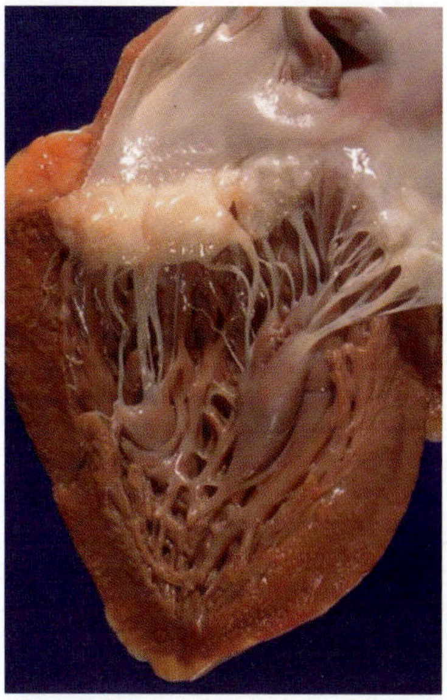

Fig. 14.22 Gross specimen of myxomatous degeneration of the mitral valve. (*Source:* From Mitral Regurgitation. Elsevier Point of Care. Elsevier 2021.)

Pronounced mechanical stress on the affected valve can cause thrombi on the atrial surface of the leaflets and calcifications on the posterior part of mitral leaflet. Note that regurgitation in instances such as ischaemic dysfunction can also give rise to myxomatous valvular degeneration.

Clinical Features

Most cases are diagnosed incidentally, following auscultation of midsystolic click and a late systolic murmur. The midsystolic click is believed to correspond to the sudden tension developing in the mitral leaflet or the chordae tendineae when the valve attempts to close. The murmur is caused by the regurgitant blood flow through the incompetent valve. The diagnosis is often confirmed by echocardiography. On the contrary, the ECG and the chest X-ray do not show any significant findings unless left atrial or left ventricular enlargement sets in.

Although a small minority of patients present with angina-like symptoms and dyspnoea, the clinical course is generally benign. These symptomatic patients may require valve replacement surgery to prevent complications such as IE, arrhythmias, mitral insufficiency or very rarely, SCD.

RHEUMATIC FEVER AND RHEUMATIC HEART DISEASE PA 27.4

Rheumatic fever (RF) is an acute, immunologically mediated, recurrent, nonsuppurative inflammatory disease that typically follows a group A streptococcal pharyngitis within few weeks (approximately 10 days to 6 weeks). Rarely, RF can follow streptococcal infections at other sites such as the skin. During prior epidemics, approximately 3% of the population developed RF preceded by an initial throat infection.

Approximately 50%–70% of patients usually present with several episodes of acute carditis implying active RF before manifesting with chronic RHD.

RHD is a condition characterized by **deforming fibrotic valvular disease**, in particular the mitral valve. Indeed, mitral valve stenosis is overwhelmingly caused by chronic RHD.

Undoubtedly, the incidence of RF and RHD has significantly declined in the developed nations. Credits are to the public awareness efforts and the frequent sanitization protocols that have decreased the prevalence of the causative condition, streptococcal pharyngitis. However, RHD and RF continue to be rampant in the developing and underdeveloped nations.

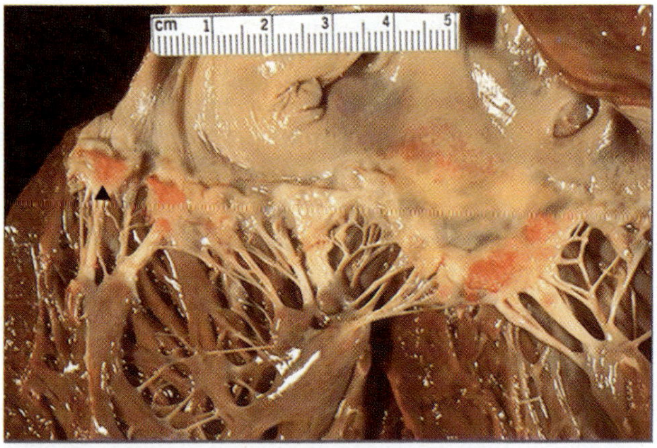

Fig. 14.23 Gross image of rheumatic heart disease. Note the vegetations at the line of closure of the valves. (*Source:* From Jorge Mercado. Acute Respiratory Failure (ARF). Elsevier 2022.)

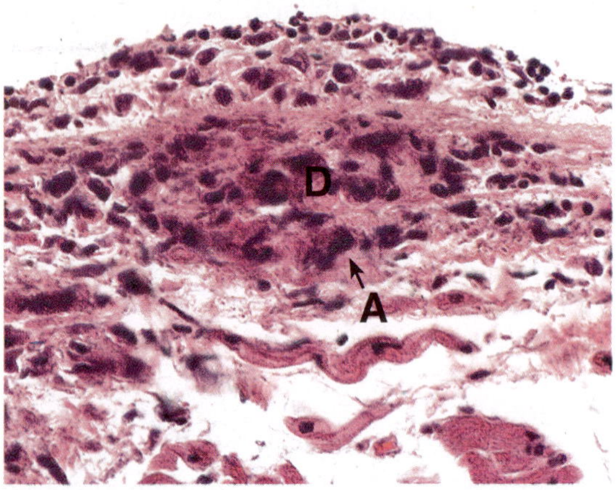

Fig. 14.24 Microscopy image of rheumatic carditis showing a well-organized Aschoff body with inflammatory cells and Anitschkow cell (A) described by the ribbon-like nucleus and extensive eosinophilic cytoplasm. (*Source:* From Jorge Mercado. Acute Respiratory Failure (ARF). Elsevier 2022.)

Aetiopathogenesis

Acute RF is a resultant of the abnormal humoral and cellular response to the streptococcal antigens. This explains the 10 days to 6 weeks time which is probably the time taken to generate the immune response. The antibodies thus produced are directed against the bacterial cell wall proteins, but also cross-react with the tissue glycoproteins in the cardiac and the extracardiac tissue probably due to **molecular mimicry**. The most important among the streptococcal antigens includes the M protein, a constituent of the cell wall. The M protein also shares a structural homology and antibody cross-reactivity with host proteins such as myosin, tropomyosin, and the endothelial cell basement membrane. The resultant cytotoxicity and the acute phase damage promote a granulomatous response, which is referred to as **Aschoff body**. It is notable that because of the intense immunological response, streptococci are virtually absent in the lesions. The role of genetic influence on the development of RHD is derived from the fact that only a small proportion of infected patients develop RHD.

Morphology

The cardinal morphological features of RHD include **pancarditis,** in which inflammation affects all layers of the heart (Fig. 14.23).

Myocarditis is the frequent cause of mortality in such patient. Characteristic Aschoff bodies can be demonstrated, accompanied by areas of fibrinoid necrosis surrounded by inflammatory cells which may in due course resolve to form fibrous scar tissue. The inflammatory cells comprise T lymphocytes and activated macrophages which are referred to as Anitschkow cells (Fig. 14.24). These cells have round to ovoid nucleus and abundant eosinophilic cytoplasm in which the nucleus condenses to form central, slender, wavy ribbon which is when it is referred to as caterpillar cells. Anitschkow cells fuse to form giant cells and are likely to remain in the tissue for 3–6 months or even longer. Similar lesions tend to occur in the joints, skin and connective tissue of the brain and the lung.

Consequently, the fibrinoid necrosis is replaced by inflammatory cells and fibrous tissue. At this stage, morphologically perivascular scar and onion skin appearance are the only tell-tale signs of past inflammation.

Endocarditis: In the acute phase, valve leaflets are often oedematous and inflamed. Although all valves may be involved, left-sided valves are more prone because they are subjected to greater pressures than the right-sided valves. The resultant damage of the endothelium leads to the deposition of tiny nodules of fibrin, grossly referred to as 'verrucae' and are mostly observed along the line of closure.

Sometimes, subendocardial lesion, probably precipitated by regurgitant jets, leads to irregular thickenings, also called MacCallum patches.

Pericarditis: Tenacious irregular deposits of fibrin are usually seen on both the visceral and the parietal surfaces of the pericardium. When the two surfaces may be pulled apart, the shaggy appearance is due to the dense fibrin deposition in the valve. This is often referred to as 'bread and butter appearance'. If the fibrinous pericarditis fails to resolve, chronic adhesive pericarditis develops.

Among the valvular involvement, mitral valve is commonly affected in chronic RHD, along with the aortic valve in about 25% of cases. The anatomic changes within the valve include commissural fusion and shortening and thickening of the tendinous cords. The calcification and fibrous bridging of the commissural walls in the mitral valve produce the characteristic 'fish-mouth' stenosis. Microscopically, the valves show organized acute inflammation, neovascularization and transmural fibrosis that contributes to the stenosis.

Clinical Features

The disease primarily affects children with onset of febrile illness usually associated with migratory arthritis. The clinical diagnosis is however made in accordance with the revised Jones criteria which elaborate major and minor criteria.

Major Criteria	Minor Criteria
• Carditis • Polyarthritis • Chorea (Sydenham chorea) • Erythema marginatum • Subcutaneous nodules	• Fever • Arthralgia • Previous history of RF • Laboratory findings of elevated ESR, raised C-reactive protein and leucocytosis

A minimum of 2 major criteria or 1 major and 2 minor criteria have to be met to make a diagnosis of RF. The symptoms usually begin 2–3 weeks after infection with *Streptococcus pyogenes*. The throat cultures are negative by then but blood investigations can reveal increased levels of serum antibodies to group A streptococcal antigens, such as antistreptolysin-O, anti-DNase B and antihyaluronidase. During an acute episode, patients may experience tachycardia and transient heart murmurs that reflect the turbulent flow across the inflamed valve. The main cause of death is heart failure due to myocarditis.

Medical line of management includes administration of aspirin to reduce the inflammation and penicillin to treat the residual streptococcal infection. ARF often draws a lot of clinical attention because chronic RHD is characterized by permanent deformity and functional impairment of the valves. Symptoms of RHD do not develop until 10–30 years postacute RF. Thus, the management of RHD includes vigorous prophylaxis against streptococcal infections and treatment of chronic valvular disease.

ENDOCARDITIS

Infective Endocarditis **PA 27.6**

IE is a microbial infection of the heart valves or the mural endocardium, in which the organisms incorporate and proliferate in thrombotic vegetations attached to an injured endocardium caused by congenital or acquired aetiologies. The microorganisms provoke an inflammatory response in both the valve and the vegetations exacerbating the damage. IE affects individuals of all age groups, although infants are mostly spared. The disease is also more common in males than females and also involves the left heart valves more than the right heart valves.

Aetiology The classical risk factors involved in the development of IE include RHD and some types of CHDs such as VSDs, PDA, coarctation of aorta and ASDs. The newly identified risk factors include ageing, immunosuppression due to the use of immunosuppressant drugs and immunodeficient diseases. In addition, aneurysms, prosthetic devices, end-stage renal disease, chronic haemodialysis and intravenous drug abuse predispose to IE. IE of the right-side valves is almost always caused by intravenous drug abuse. The most common organisms responsible for IE are bacterial (bacterial endocarditis), whereas fungal and viral infections are less common. Notably, *Staphylococcus aureus* is the major offender in intravenous drug abuse. Streptococcal infections predominate with staphylococcal infections next in order. Among the fungal infections, *Candida* IE has been encountered.

Other bacterial causes belong to the HACEK group – *Haemophilus*, *Actinobacillus*, *Cardiobacterium*, *Eikenella* and *Kingella*; all of which are commensals of the oral cavity. IE of the prosthetic valves typically involves skin flora organisms – *S. aureus* and *Staphylococcus epidermidis*.

The microorganisms often find their way into the bloodstream during dental or surgical procedures, precipitated by the usage of contaminated needle and intravenous drug abuse.

Pathogenesis Overall, the development of IE would require prodromal endothelial injury with a period of significant bacteraemia. The preliminary endothelial disruption leads to platelet deposition creating small sterile vegetations. Microorganisms that gain entry into the bloodstream and that overcome the body's defence mechanisms adhere to these sterile vegetations and infect them. Besides, the organisms also produce enzymes such as matrix metalloproteases that cause additional destruction of valves.

Over the many years, bacterial endocarditis has been classified on the basis of clinical course into acute and subacute forms. Acute bacterial endocarditis (ABE) is when the syndrome presents as an acute and fulminant infection caused by highly virulent organisms such as *S. aureus*. As the responsible organisms are highly aggressive, the disease may precipitate in normal cardiac valves as well. Antibiotic alone may not be beneficial and such patients would require surgery. Despite prompt treatment, morbidity and mortality are yet significantly high. On the contrary, subacute bacterial endocarditis (SBE) is caused by low-virulence organisms (e.g. *Streptococcus viridans*) and is more insidious in onset. SBE involves valves with prior damage. Patients usually respond well to antibiotics alone. However, clear demarcation between acute and subacute cases is not always possible and most patients fall under an intermediate category instead.

Morphology

The vegetations in cases of IE are described as grey, yellow to brown, soft to slightly friable tissue masses that occupy large areas over the leaflet or the cusp. The size of the vegetations is generally variable with the fungal infections causing larger ones. The mitral valve is the most commonly involved followed by the aortic, tricuspid and the pulmonary valves. The involved valves may also exhibit features implying the pre-existing pathology or may be normal.

Histologically, vegetations contain platelet or fibrin thrombin superimposed by neutrophilic infiltrate. Older lesions may show features of hyalinization. Bacterial or fungal organisms may be found at the edge or within the vegetation. Occasionally, the organisms may erode the underlying myocardium producing an abscess.

Vegetations larger than 1 cm carry a higher risk for embolization. Decisively, as the embolic fragments contain virulent organisms, they tend to develop abscesses where they lodge, also contributing to septic infarcts and mycotic aneurysms.

Cases of subacute vegetations apparently show lesser valvular damage with microscopy revealing granulation tissue with variable fibrosis and chronic inflammatory infiltrate.

Clinical Features A patient with acute onset of IE is likely to manifest with rapidly progressive illness with high-grade fever, chills and rigors, whereas patients with subacute IE generally present with nonspecific flu-like symptoms, fatigue, myalgia and weakness. On cardiac examination, a murmur may be apparent implying a prior valvular pathology. In routine clinical practice, to facilitate diagnosis, the ***modified Dukes criteria*** are used, which are as follows:

Modified Duke Criteria for the Diagnosis of Endocarditis

Major criteria	Two separate positive blood cultures with microorganisms typical for infective endocarditis (viridans streptococci, *Streptococcus bovis*, HACEK group, *Staphylococcus aureus*, enterococci)
	Echocardiographic evidence of endocardial involvement (typical valvular lesions: vegetations, abscess or partial dehiscence of a prosthetic valve)
Minor criteria	Predisposition: Predisposing heart condition or i.v. drug use
	Temperature > 38°C
	Vascular phenomena: Major arterial emboli, septic pulmonary infarcts, mycotic aneurysm, intracranial haemorrhage, conjunctival haemorrhage, Janeway lesions
	Immunological phenomena: Glomerulonephritis, Osler nodes, Roth spots, rheumatoid factor
	Microbiological evidence: Positive blood culture but not meeting major criterion, or serologic evidence of active infection with organism consistent with infective endocarditis

For the diagnosis of endocarditis to be made, the following must be present:

- 2 major criteria
- 1 major criterion and 3 minor criteria
- 5 minor criteria

Complications of IE begin to manifest within the first few weeks of onset of the disease. The circulating organisms may give rise to glomerulonephritis, including glomerular antigen–antibody complex deposition, sepsis and systemic embolization. The presence of arrhythmias in such patients indicates myocardial penetration and impingement over the conduction system.

In untreated cases, the mortality is usually high, particularly with fungal infection. However, with appropriate antibody regimens and surgical therapy, the mortality rate is slowing down.

Noninfected Vegetations

Noninfected vegetations may occur in a setting of nonbacterial thrombotic endocarditis (NBTE) and endocarditis of SLE.

Nonbacterial Thrombotic Endocarditis NBTE, also known as marantic endocarditis refers to the deposition of noninfected vegetations over the normal cardiac valve, as a rule, always associated with malignancy or some other wasting disease. Histologically, early vegetations of NBTE consist of fibrin and entangles leucocytes and platelets. The vegetations are generally bland and do not contain microorganisms or inflammation. No associated significant valvular damage is evident.

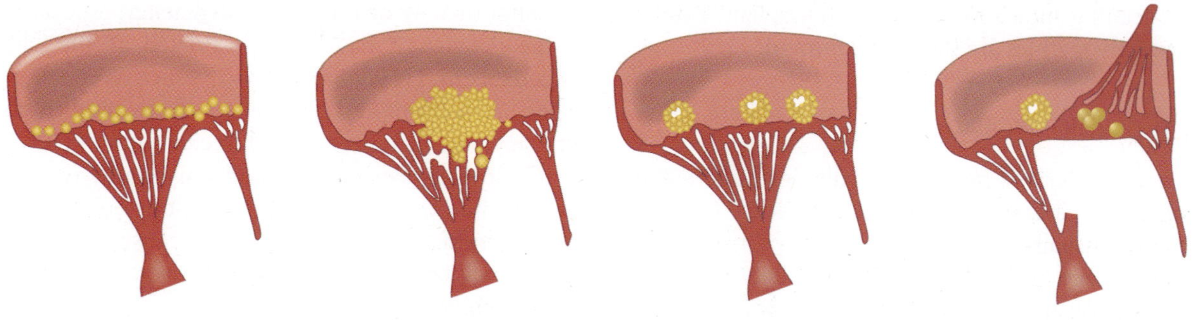

Fig. 14.25 Schematic representation of the major forms of vegetative endocarditis. Note the warty, small vegetations along the lines of closure of the valve leaflets in rheumatic heart disease. Infective endocarditis is described by aggregated irregular masses predominantly on the valve cusps. Lesions comprising nonbacterial endocarditis attach as small masses typically at the line of closure. Libman–Sacks endocarditis (LSE) lesions on the other hand attach to either side of the valve leaflets.

Although the exact aetiopathogenesis of NBTE is unknown, the condition has been frequently associated with hypercoagulable state due to advanced cancer, in particularly mucinous adenocarcinoma and in cases of deep vein thrombus, vitamin C deficiency and endocardial trauma.

Endocarditis of Systemic Lupus Erythematosus (Libman–Sacks Disease [Fig. 14.25]) It is recognized as a sterile vegetation that occurs as bland, dry pinkish single or multiple vegetations often located on the nonflow surfaces of the valves. Mural endocardium and the chordae tendineae may also be involved in some cases. This is mostly a consequence of immune complex–mediated deposition and recruitment of the Fc-bearing cells. Such vegetations are seen in about 35%–65% of lupus patients in autopsy studies.

CARDIOMYOPATHIES PA 27.9

Cardiomyopathies are a diverse set of heart muscle disorders that cause myocardial dysfunction. Excluded from this category are conditions that cause heart muscle impairment as secondary consequences, such as loss of pump function due to MI or an incompetent valve causing pressure volume overload. Thus, a more precise definition of cardiomyopathies as suggested by the AHA is as follows: 'Cardiomyopathies are a heterogenous group of diseases of the myocardium associated with mechanical and/or electrical dysfunction that usually but not invariably, exhibits inappropriate ventricular hypertrophy or dilatation, and are due to a variety of causes that are frequently genetic'. These conditions can evolve as a disease confined to the heart or may be a part of a systemic syndrome.

On the basis of causative factors, cardiomyopathies can be classified into two categories:

- Primary cardiomyopathies are mostly genetic abnormalities involving the heart muscle predominantly. Acquired causes such as viral infection or anthracycline toxicity affecting the myocardium also falls into this category.

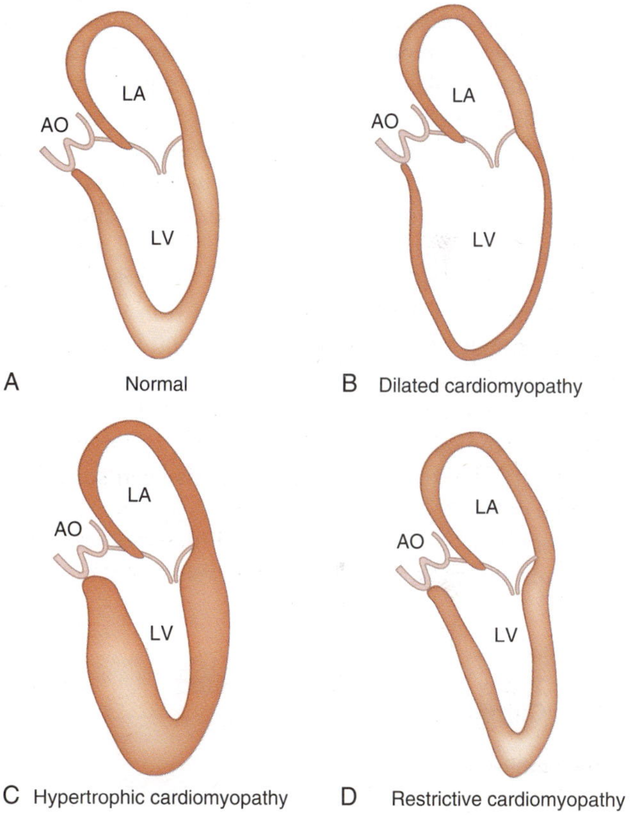

Fig. 14.26 Types of cardiomyopathies.

- Secondary cardiomyopathies are conditions that involve the myocardium as a part of a systemic syndrome, e.g. haemochromatosis and amyloidosis.

Another classification of cardiomyopathies on the basis of anatomical appearance and abnormal physiology of the ventricle is as elucidated as follows (Fig. 14.26):

- DCM
- HCM
- Restrictive cardiomyopathy

Among the three varieties, dilated cardiomyopathies are the most common, accounting for 90% of cases and is also the leading indication for heart transplant. Restrictive cardiomyopathies are the least common.

DILATED CARDIOMYOPATHY

DCM is characterized morphologically and functionally by progressive cardiac dilation and contractile (systolic) dysfunction, usually with concomitant hypertrophy. The myocyte damage in DCM can be the resultant of a range of genetic, toxic and metabolic causes; a few are given in Table 14.6.

Genetic or familial causes: These account for 20%–30% of cases of DCM. Before the molecular era, these cases were classified as idiopathic. However presently, autosomal dominant, autosomal recessive, X-linked and mitochondrial patterns of inheritance have been demonstrated, among which autosomal dominant is predominant. Mitochondrial defects typically present in infants and children, whereas the X-linked DCM manifests after puberty.

Mutations in more than 50 genes have been identified. Genes encoding cytoskeletal proteins such as laminin A/C and desmin, anchoring proteins in particular δ-sarcoglycan and dystrophin, and genes encoding the sarcomeric proteins such as actin, titin, troponin T and β- or α-heavy chain mutations account for 35%–45% of the genetic causes of DCM. Mutations in titin, the largest known human protein with almost 30,000 amino acids, alone constitutes 20% of all DCM (Fig. 14.27).

Myocarditis: The progression of myocarditis to DCM has been studied in substantial number of cases. Viral myocarditis due to coxsackie B virus has been suggested in some cases.

Alcohol and other toxins: Alcohol toxicity is virtually very commonly associated with the development of DCM. Ethanol toxicity or nutritional deficiency, especially thiamine deficiency, has been postulated as the causative mechanisms. Heavy metal toxicity, such as cobalt used in beer production, and cardiotoxic drugs used in chemotherapy have also been linked to causation of DCM.

Childbirth: Peripartum cardiomyopathy refers to the occurrence of DCM in late pregnancy or up to 5 months postpartum. This is probably because of nutritional deficiency, pressure or volume overload, or genetic susceptibility.

Iron overload: DCM is one of the most common manifestations of iron overload. Excess iron because of any cause, hereditary haemochromatosis or multiple transfusions can, over the course of time, give rise to DCM. Iron-dependent enzyme processes and reactive oxygen species derived from iron-mediated reactions are believed to be the pavement for DCM.

Table 14.6 Causes of Dilated Cardiomyopathy

Idiopathic
Genetic Causes
Inflammatory causes Viral infection (coxsackievirus, parvovirus B19) Connective tissue diseases Peripartum cardiomyopathy Sarcoidosis
Toxic Chronic alcoholism Immunosuppressive drugs Chemotherapeutic agents (e.g. doxorubicin, trastuzumab)
Metabolic Hypothyroidism Chronic hypocalcaemia
Neuromuscular Muscular or myotonic dystrophy

Morphology

As a rule, the heart is enlarged weighing around 3 times its normal weight (>900 g). All the cardiac chambers are dilated, the ventricles affected more than the atria. The myocardium appears flabby and pale (Flowchart 14.3). In some cases, endocardial scars may be evident. The condition also predisposes to an increased risk of mural thrombi.

Microscopically, DCM is characterized by predominantly hypertrophic myocardial fibres. Variable degrees of interstitial and endocardial fibrosis can be observed. Some of the enlarged myocytes show attenuated, stretched, irregular-shaped nucleus (Fig. 14.28). Interestingly, DCM with titin mutations often exhibit a hyperchromatic, highly distorted 'ninja-like' nucleus. Identifying more than 5% of myocytes with such nucleus points the possibility of titin truncation mutation. Note that none of these findings are specific for DCM (Figs 14.29 and 14.30).

Clinical Features

DCM can occur at any age but most affected individuals belong to the age group of 20–50 years. The disease is insidious in onset and patients usually present with symptoms of dyspnoea, easy fatigability and secondary mitral regurgitation. The principal defect in DCM, however, is defective contraction. The exercise intolerance progresses relentlessly to cause congestive cardiac failure and lowered cardiac ejection fraction, that even drops to less than 25%.

Electrical resynchronization (biventricular spacing) and pharmacological treatment have been beneficial in some patients, yet, the annual mortality is high, around 10%–15%. In at least half the patients, mortality is due to ventricular arrhythmias and heart failure. Cardiac transplant or a ventricular assist device can be tried in the end-stage disease to prevent mortality.

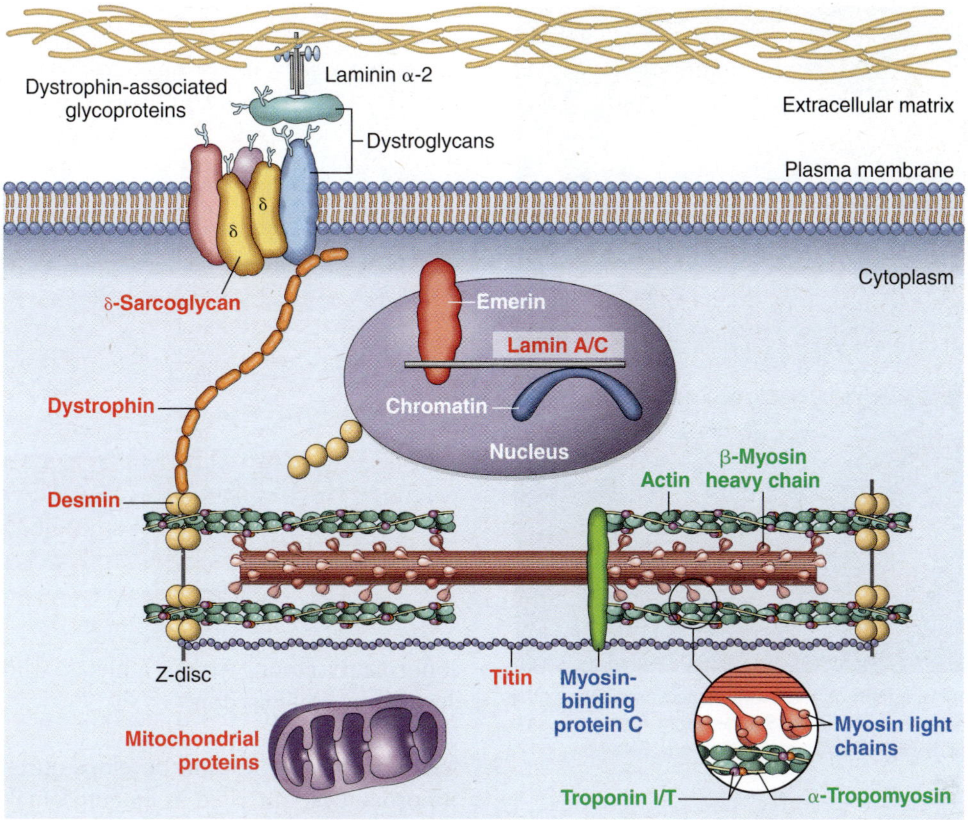

Fig. 14.27 Schematic representation of the important proteins and cellular components of the myocyte. The vital proteins involved in the pathogenesis of DCM are highlighted in red, whereas mutations giving rise to hypertrophic cardiomyopathy are highlighted in blue and proteins involved in both the disease processes are elucidated in green. (*Source:* From Richard N. Mitchell and Andrew J. Connolly. The Heart . Robbins & Cotran Pathologic Basis of Disease. 10th edition. Elsevier 2021.)

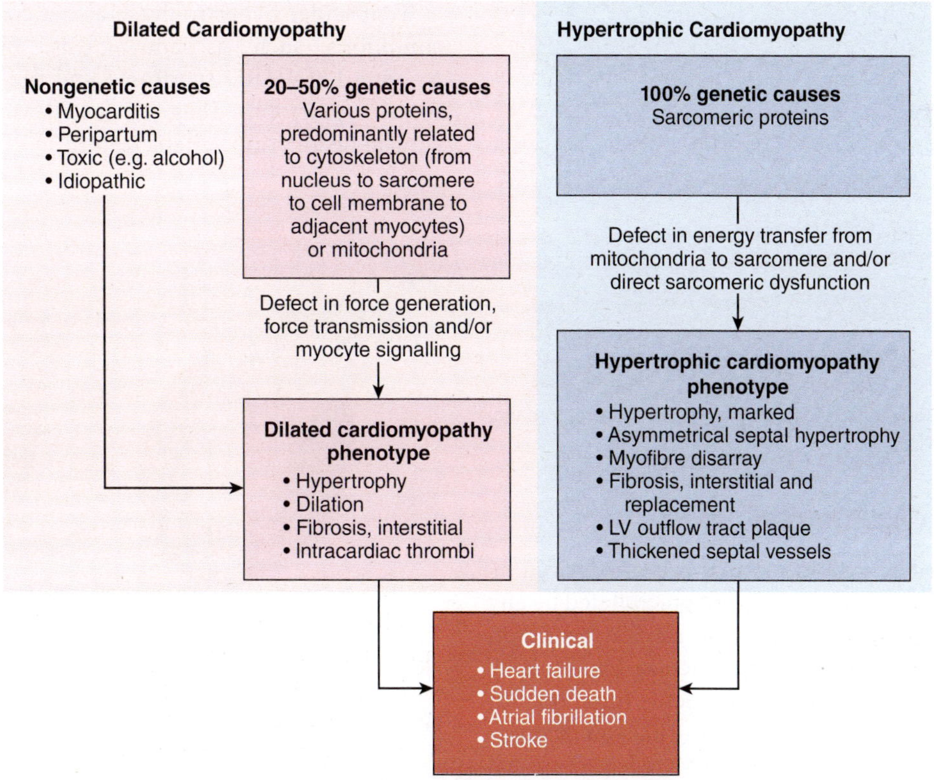

Flowchart 14.3 Causes and clinical outcomes of dilated and hypertrophic cardiomyopathies.

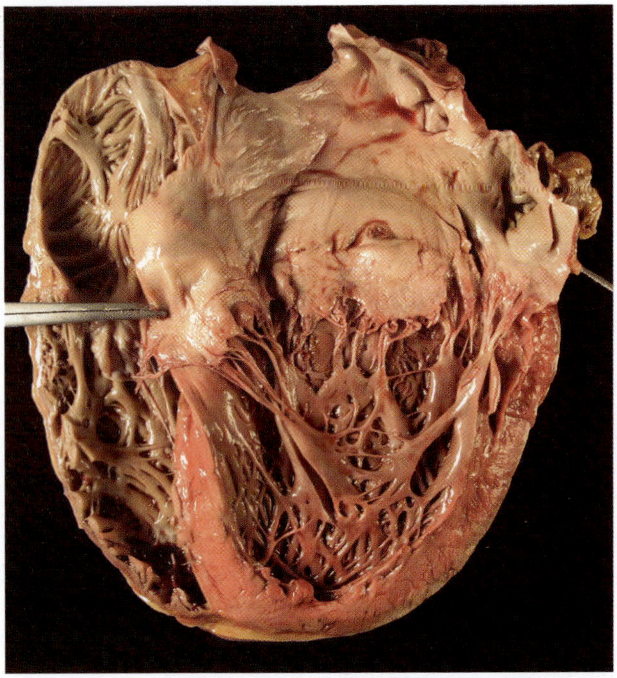

Fig. 14.28 Gross photograph of heart with dilated cardiomyopathy. Note the thinned-out ventricular wall. (*Source:* From Aliya N. Husain. Dilated Cardiomyopathy. High-Yield Thoracic Pathology. Saunders 2012.)

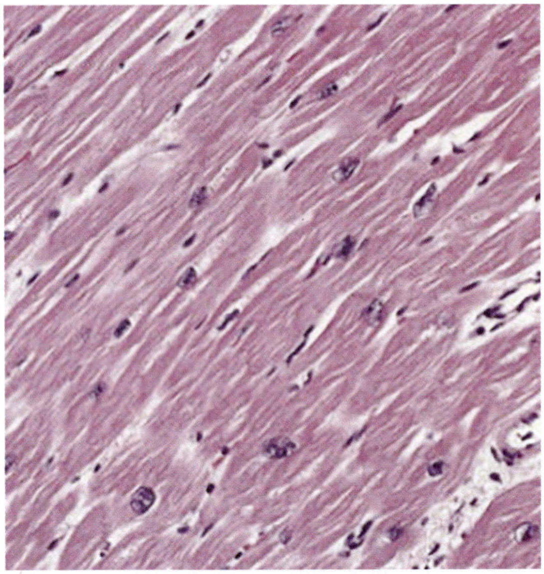

Fig. 14.29 Microscopy in DCM showing enlarged, hyperchromatic, irregular-shaped nucleus.

HYPERTROPHIC CARDIOMYOPATHY

HCM is described as a condition that is characterized by left ventricular hypertrophy that is not precipitated by any pressure overload–associated chronic cardiac condition (e.g. hypertension or AS). The ventricular hypertrophy results in above optimal systolic contractile function, but the muscle being stiff fails to relax during diastole, thereby increasing the diastolic pressure. HCM received special attention years back when it occurred as a common abnormality among young athletes, who died suddenly during physical exertion.

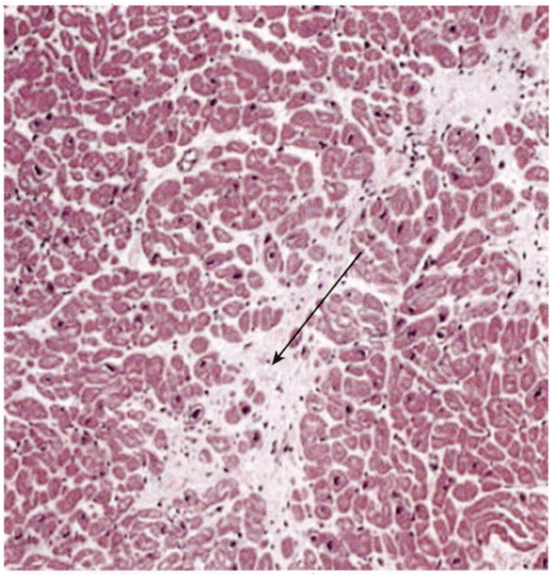

Fig. 14.30 Interstitial fibrosis (arrow) in a case of DCM.

Aetiology The condition develops purely out of genetic abnormalities, inherited as an autosomal dominant trait. The proteins encoded by the involved mutated genes are all a part of the sarcomere complex which includes β-myosin heavy chain (β-MHC), cardiac troponins and myosin-binding protein C. The resultant loss of contractile functions eventually leads to cardiac hypertrophy accompanied by fibroblastic proliferation (Fig. 14.31).

Ventricular hypertrophy is also a common finding in conditions such as amyloidosis, Friedreich ataxia, Noonan/LEOPARD syndrome and age-related subaortic septal hypertrophy. Diagnosis of HCM is often based on clinical history and genetic testing.

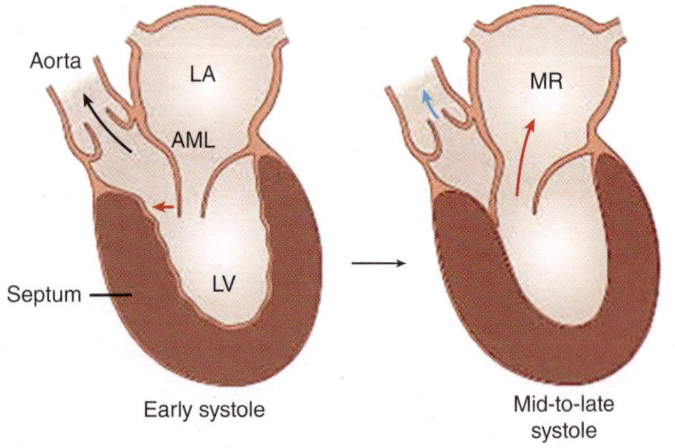

Fig. 14.31 Pathophysiology of HCM with left ventricular outflow tract obstruction. The left outflow tract is narrowed by virtue of the hypertrophied myocardium. During systole, the anterior mitral leaflet is abnormally drawn towards the septum, causing obstruction of flow through the aorta. Simultaneously, mitral regurgitation occurs as the mitral valve leaflets do not promptly close during systole.

Morphology

The hallmark features of HCM include a massively enlarged myocardium with signs of hypertrophy (Fig. 14.32). Typically, this is followed by asymmetric relative thickening of the interventricular septum. Although hypertrophy may involve the entire septum, it is most prominent at the subaortic region. Approximately one-third of the patients manifest with HCM with outflow obstruction. During ventricular contraction, the ejection of blood is more forceful than usual as the outflow tract is narrowed by the thickened septum. This draws the anterior mitral leaflet towards the hypertrophied septum causing transient obstruction to blood flow into the aorta. Thus, the ventricular systolic pressure raises, further increasing the wall stress, resulting in angina. Because the anterior mitral leaflet is undergoing an abnormal motion, the posterior leaflet does not close properly resulting in mitral regurgitation which may lead to atrial fibrillation.

The hypertrophied segment shows the following features:

- Increased diameter of myocytes
- Haphazard arrangement of myocyte bundles, the contained individual myocytes and the intracellular sarcomeres, all together termed myofibre disarray (Fig. 14.33)
- Interstitial fibrosis later, sometimes with replacement fibrosis

Clinical Features The symptoms among patients with HCM are highly variable. One of the constant complaints is dyspnoea due to the elevated diastolic pressures. Angina is a frequent complaint among patients, notably in the absence of a CAD. The structurally abnormal fibres may

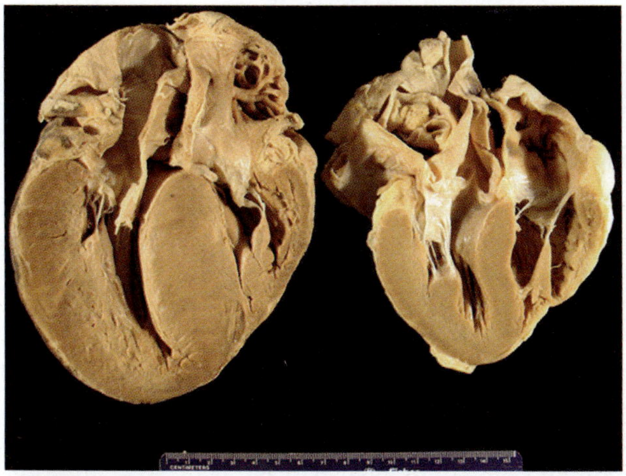

Fig. 14.32 Gross specimen showing two cases of hypertrophic cardiomyopathy. Note the asymmetric septal hypertrophy. (*Source:* https://www.clinicalkey.com/#!/content/undefined/1-s2.0-S155171360900110X?scrollTo=%231-s2.0-S155171360900110X-gr1)

give rise to cardiac arrhythmias manifesting as syncope. Patients with outflow tract obstruction have lowered cardiac output and increased pulmonary venous pressure, manifesting as exertional dyspnoea. A harsh systolic ejection murmur can be apparent in such patients.

HCM responds paradoxically to medical treatment with β-adrenergic blockers and Ca^{2+} channel blockers that reduce contractility. Surgical removal of the hypertrophied septum is usually achieved by injecting ethanol through a septal artery to cause localized infarction. However, the risk of sudden death persists.

RESTRICTIVE CARDIOMYOPATHY

Restrictive cardiomyopathy is the least common type of cardiomyopathies, and is characterized by abnormally rigid ventricle with diminished ventricular compliance, in turn causing improper diastolic filling. The systolic function of the myocardium is usually unaffected and is normal or near normal.

The primary aetiological factors associated with restrictive cardiomyopathy include fibrosis or scarring of the endomyocardium and amyloidosis, the latter being the most recognized cause. The pathophysiological consequences of reduced compliance of the ventricle, leading to raised diastolic pressure are atrial dilation, elevated venous pressure and venous congestion. The clinical picture is similar to that of constrictive pericarditis (explained later) which is an important differential.

The morphological features of restrictive cardiomyopathy are highly nonspecific. Grossly, biatrial dilation is a common occurrence, as explained earlier, due to high diastolic pressure. The ventricles, however, maintain normal size and dimensions. Microscopically, patchy to diffuse interstitial fibrosis may be the only finding and it may vary from subtle to extensive scarring.

Restrictive cardiomyopathy typically exhibits very poor prognosis and the disease invariably progresses to congestive cardiac failure. Only 10% of patients survive for 10 years.

Three restrictive entities of the heart that are considered to be manifesting forms of restrictive cardiomyopathy are briefly explained as follows.

CARDIAC AMYLOIDOSIS

Cardiac amyloidosis can occur as a part of systemic amyloidosis or as isolated cardiac amyloidosis in the aged, also termed as senile cardiac amyloidosis. Restrictive cardiomyopathy is a frequent association of cardiac amyloidosis, and is the major cause of morbidity in such patients.

Amyloid infiltration results in cardiac enlargement without concomitant ventricular dilatation. The chambers are usually of normal size and the macroscopic appearance often resembles that of HCM. The ventricular

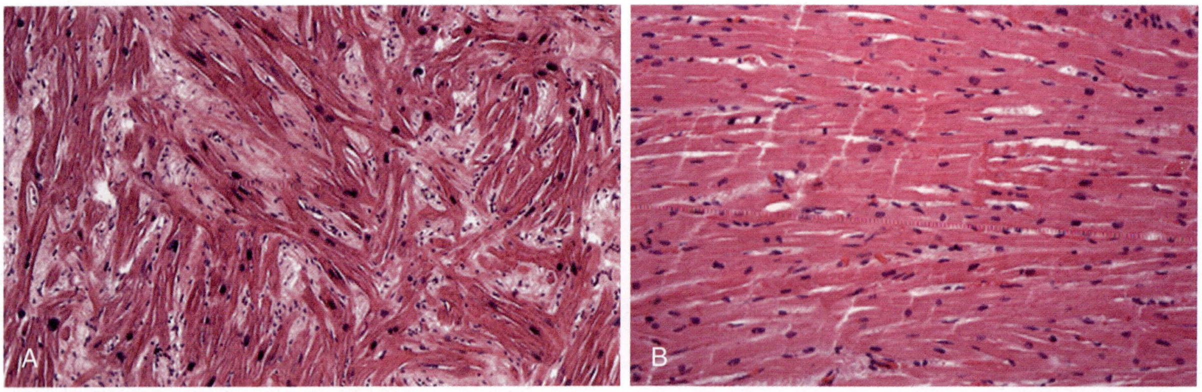

Fig. 14.33 Histological sections demonstrating myocyte disarray with the myocardial fibres being haphazardly arranged (A) in comparison with the normal myocardium (B).

walls are typically thickened, firm and rubbery. Histologically, amyloid deposition can be seen as hyaline, eosinophilic accumulations predominantly seen within the interstitium, also involving the perivascular, endocardial regions, cardiac valves and sometimes small coronary arteries. Special stains, such as Congo red, produce apple-green birefringence under polarized light.

Clinically, cardiac amyloidosis is most often a restrictive cardiomyopathy with progressive diastolic and eventually systolic dysfunction.

Endocardial Fibroelastosis It is a rare condition of the heart primarily occurring in infants and children, younger than 2 years. The disease is more prevalent in Africa and other tropical countries. The *infantile form* is postulated to occur because of intrauterine endocardial anoxia. Some cases contain mural thrombi. One-third of cases show associated aortic valve obstruction or other congenital abnormalities. Progressively myocardial failure may develop. This condition generally carries a poor prognosis.

Loeffler Endomyocarditis This condition is known by a more appropriate term, fibroblastic parietal endocarditis with peripheral blood eosinophilia. This cardiac disorder is similar to endomyocardial fibrosis morphologically, with additional hypereosinophilia and multisystem eosinophilic infiltrates that may involve the heart also. The release of cytoplasmic proteins of eosinophils, such as major basic protein, and other toxin products are believed to cause endomyocardial necrosis. This is eventually followed by fibrosis or organized thrombus formation. This condition has a worse prognosis.

PERICARDIAL DISEASES PA 27.7

Diseases of the pericardium range from a benign hyperplastic condition to life-threatening cardiac tamponade. The pericardium is a two-layered sac that encircles the heart. The visceral pericardium (inner layer) adheres to the outer layer of the heart and is enveloped by the parietal pericardium (outer layer) externally.

The pericardium serves to fix the heart within the mediastinum, to prevent extreme dilation of the heart in conditions that raise the intracardiac volume, and functions as a barrier to prevent infections. In a healthy individual, the pericardiac sac contains less than 50 mL of thin clear straw-coloured fluid. Pericardial effusion refers to a condition in which the parietal pericardium is distended by serous fluid. If the effusion is contaminated by blood, it is called haemopericardium, and if purulent exudate is present, it is referred as purulent pericarditis. Less frequent are chylous effusions caused by lymphatic obstruction, by tumour or infection. Slow, long-standing effusions may lead to pericardial remodelling, such that it can accommodate even up to 2 L of fluid, without significant haemodynamic alterations. However, in events of rapid accumulation of fluid or blood, such as in ruptured MI or aortic dissection, even lesser amount such as 150–200 mL, can significantly raise the intrapericardial pressure. This may cause compression of the atria, vena cava or the ventricles, and interfere with cardiac filling, causing reduced cardiac output. Unless the pressure is relieved by removing the pericardial fluid, acute cardiac tamponade is almost always fatal.

PERICARDITIS

Inflammation of the pericardium can be a primary or a secondary event. The major causes of pericarditis are listed in Table 14.7.

Acute Pericarditis

Acute pericarditis is mostly idiopathic in origin or caused by viral infections. Among infections causing pericarditis, viral origin has been much prevalent. Pericarditis is also a common manifestation in patients with HIV infection. Bacterial pericarditis has been less frequent in the antibiotic era and is likely to occur only in immunocompromised patients. However, the primary focus of bacterial or

Table 14.7 Causes of Pericarditis

Infections	Viruses (coxsackievirus, adenovirus, HIV) Bacteria (diphtheria, staphylococcal, streptococcal infections) Fungi (*Candida*, aspergillosis) Tuberculosis Parasites (Chagas disease)
Immunological Causes	Rheumatic fever SLE Scleroderma Postmyocardial infarction (Dressler syndrome) Drug reaction (penicillin, sulphonamide)
Others	Myocardial infarction Uraemia Tumours Trauma Radiation Sarcoidosis

viral infection in most cases lie elsewhere, probably the upper respiratory tract, lung or the parotid. Acute pericarditis may be serous, serofibrinous, purulent or haemorrhagic (Fig. 14.34). The most common forms are, however, fibrinous and serofibrinous pericarditis.

Macroscopically, the normal glistening smooth pericardial surface is replaced by a rough texture of inflamed pericardium, with obvious surface exudates (Fig. 14.35). This may also produce a friction rub that may be heard on auscultation.

On examination, the effusion fluid is generally rich in protein and the pericardial surface usually contains mononuclear inflammatory cells, also infiltrating the epicardial fat. This fibrinous pericarditis is more common with uraemic conditions and viral infections post-MI. Also, patients receiving radiation for breast or lung cancers are prone to develop fibrinous pericardial effusions. Most patients complain of a sharp, pleuritic type pain and sometimes with congestive failure.

Bacterial infections on the contrary produce purulent pericarditis. The effusion contains large amounts of neutrophils, as evidenced by microscopic examination. The infections may stem from direct extension from the surrounding organs or may reach the pericardium through the vascular or lymphatic channels. Rarely they may be iatrogenic.

Haemorrhagic pericarditis refers to gross blood within the pericardial effusion and can be seen in conditions such as tuberculosis and malignancy.

Chronic or Healed Pericarditis

Recurrent episodes of acute pericarditis may lead to organization of the pericardial inflammation, producing

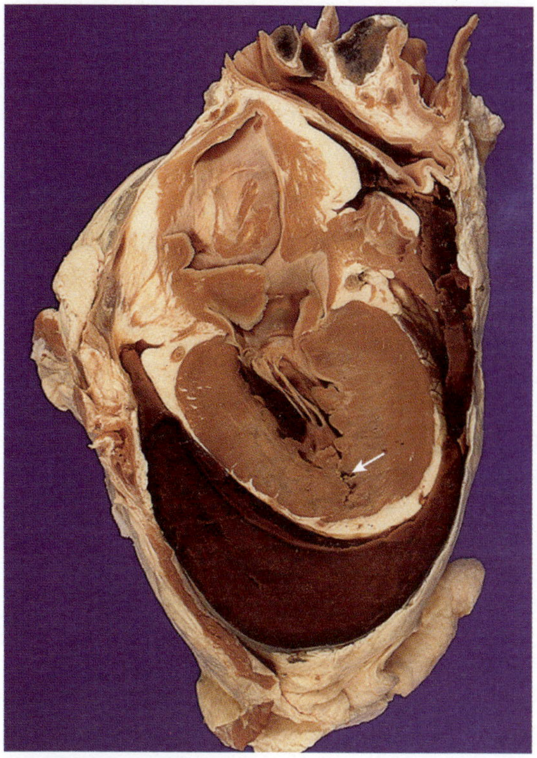

Fig. 14.34 Massive haemopericardium in a patient with ruptured myocardial infarction. Arrow indicates the site of the rupture. (*Source:* From Andrew J. Connolly, Walter E. Finkbeiner, Philip C. Ursell and Richard L. Davis. Atlas of Gross Autopsy Pathology. Autopsy Pathology: A Manual and Atlas. 3rd edition. Elsevier 2016.)

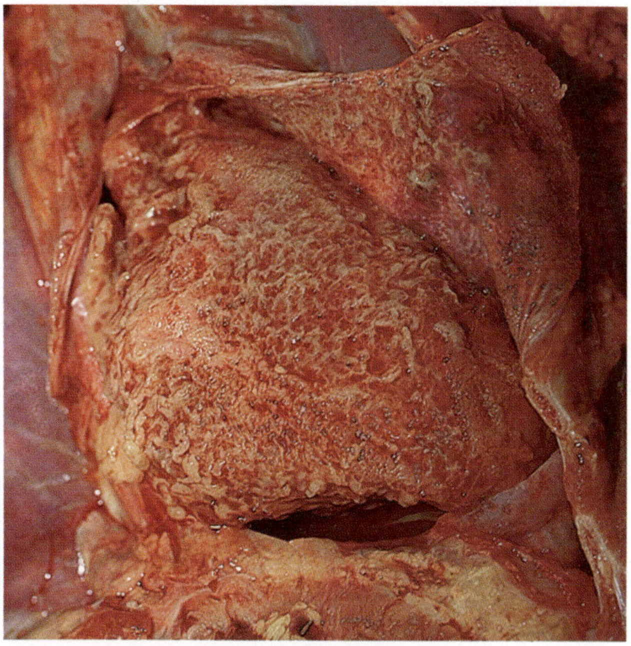

Fig. 14.35 Suppurative pericarditis following infectious aetiology. The pericardial surfaces appear red, granular and are coated with exudate. (*Source:* From Andrew J. Connolly, Walter E. Finkbeiner, Philip C. Ursell and Richard L. Davis. Atlas of Gross Autopsy Pathology. Autopsy Pathology: A Manual and Atlas. 3rd edition. Elsevier 2016.)

plaque-like fibrous thickenings of the serosal membranes, also known as soldiers' plaques. These may be in the form of thin delicate adhesions that develop between the pericardial surfaces and do not impair cardiac function, or may be mesh-like stringy adhesions that obliterate the pericardial space. The following are the clinically significant forms of chronic pericarditis.

Adhesive pericarditis: Here, the pericardial sac is obliterated by fibrous adhesions that not only involve the pericardial layers but also the surrounding structures. With each contraction, the heart pulls on the adhering pericardial layers and the attached structures causing systolic retraction of the rib cage and the diaphragm. Eventually cardiac hypertrophy supervenes with increased workload.

Constrictive pericarditis is another potential complication of pericardial diseases. Although not frequently encountered, constrictive pericarditis is important to understand because it causes profound symptoms. In this condition, the heart is enclosed within a dense, fibrous stiff pericardium that restricts diastolic expansion. The fibrous scar may sometimes undergo calcification, further worsening the symptoms. Patients may or may not have a history of pericarditis. On examination, muffled heart sounds may be apparent along with elevated jugular venous pressure and peripheral oedema. Patients may require pericardiectomy.

CARDIAC TUMOURS

PRIMARY CARDIAC TUMOURS

Cardiac tumours can be primary or secondary. Primary cardiac tumours are uncommon, but are frequently benign. Secondary cardiac tumours are considerably more common than primary tumours. The five common benign primary tumours of the heart in decreasing order of frequency are myxomas, fibromas, lipomas, papillary fibroelastosis and rhabdomyoma. Although these benign tumours account for 90% of cardiac tumours, a rare 10% of primary tumours may be malignant, which includes sarcomas such as angiosarcoma.

MYXOMA

Myxomas are the most common primary tumour of the heart. They are believed to arise from the pluripotent stem cells. Although most cases are sporadic in origin, about 7% of tumours are familial with an autosomal dominant inheritance. Activating mutations in the GNAS1 gene, encoding a subset of the G protein (Gsα) as a part of the McCune–Albright syndrome or null mutations in the PRKAR1A gene that encodes for a subunit of cyclic CMP–dependent protein kinase, as a part of Carney complex, have all been associated with atrial myxoma.

Morphology

Myxomas draw major clinical attention because of the valvular 'ball-valve' obstruction they cause, and their potential for fragmentation and embolization. Patients present with constitutional symptoms such as fever and malaise, probably due to the cytokine elaboration by some myxomas. The tumour is detected in routine echocardiogram. Surgical removal is curative. Recurrence is possible within months or years of excision because complete excision of tumour is not always possible.

Cardiac myxomas usually occur in singles but can also be multiple. They can occur in any chamber and any valve but the fossa ovalis in the atrial septum is the most favoured site. Macroscopically, they appear as round to oval, glistening masses, with a slightly bosselated surface, sized between 1 and 10 cm (Fig. 14.36). They may be pedunculated or sessile. The pedunculated forms are mobile and often obstruct the AV valve during systole. One-third of these tumours are soft with an irregular surface, comprising villi-like projections posing a risk for embolization. Calcifications are common, particularly in the right atrial myxomas. The differential diagnoses of cardiac myxoma include papillary fibroelastoma (explained later), organized thrombus and other sarcomas. Immunohistochemistry may help to distinguish myxomas from other cardiac malignancies.

Histologically, myxoma cells (the so called lepidic cells) are polygonal or stellate syncytial cells arranged in nests or cords, embedded in a proteoglycan-rich myxoid stroma (Fig. 14.37). Large, thick-walled blood vessels are found at the base, near the stalk of the lesion. Haemorrhage and organizing thrombus, accompanied by

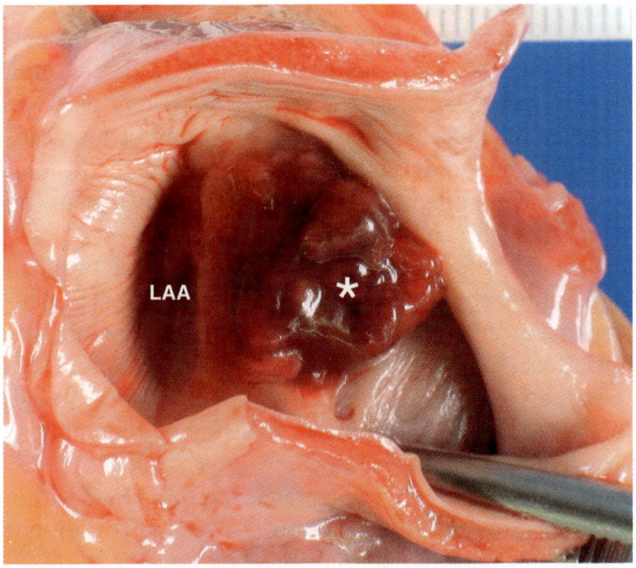

Fig. 14.36 An atrial myxoma marked by an asterisk, appearing similar to that of an organizing thrombus owing to the gelatinous appearance. (*Source:* From Andrew J. Connolly, Walter E. Finkbeiner, Philip C. Ursell and Richard L. Davis. Atlas of Gross Autopsy Pathology. Autopsy Pathology: A Manual and Atlas. 3rd edition. Elsevier 2016.)

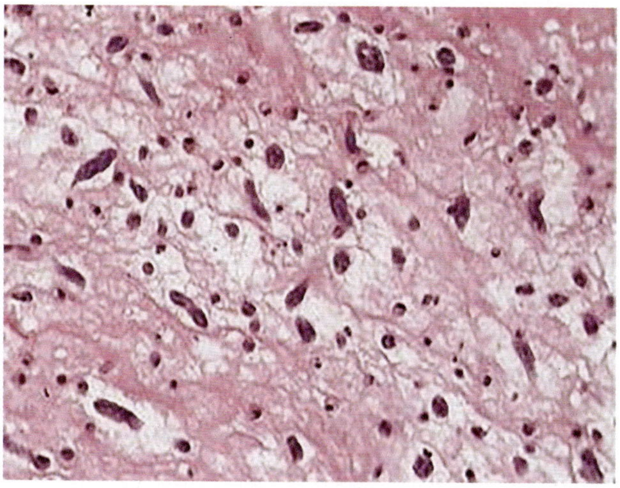

Fig. 14.37 Histological sections showing myxoma cells, stellate cells in cords embedded in a myxoid stroma. (*Source:* From Pradeep Vaideeswar and Jagdish W. Butany. Benign cardiac tumors of the pluripotent mesenchyme. Seminars in Diagnostic Pathology.2008;25:20-28.)

haemosiderin-laden macrophages, are almost always present and are a useful diagnostic clue.

Myxomas draw major clinical attention because of the valvular 'ball-valve' obstruction they cause, and their potential for fragmentation and embolization. Surgical removal is curative. Recurrence is possible within months or years of excision, as complete excision of tumour is not always possible.

PAPILLARY FIBROELASTOSIS

Also called endocardial papilloma, the tumour occurs most frequently within the valves of the heart. The aortic valve is the most common site, accounting for 75% of the cases, and is followed by the mitral valve, next in frequency. Macroscopically, papillary fibroelastomas often appear as round soft masses usually attached to the endocardium by means of a small stalk. Interestingly, when placed in a bowl of water, multiple delicate fronds unfurl from the tumour which is why it is said to resemble a sea anemone.

Microscopically, complexly branching central avascular cores can be seen lined by endothelial cells. The papillary cores contain abundant myxoid connective tissue with abundant mucopolysaccharide matrix, proteoglycans and elastic fibres. The cells lining the cores express vimentin, factor VIII–related antigen and CD34, demonstrated by immunohistochemistry, differentiating it from myxomas.

RHABDOMYOMAS

Rhabdomyomas are frequent tumours of the paediatric age group. About 50% of the tumours are sporadic, whereas the rest are associated with tuberous sclerosis. In such patients, mutations of the tuberous sclerosis complex genes TSC1 and TSC2 can be demonstrated. Both genes are tumour suppressor genes that regulate embryonic and neonatal growth and differentiation of cardiomyocytes. Rhabdomyomas are often considered as hamartomas than true neoplasms because they undergo spontaneous regression, a topic still under debate.

Grossly, rhabdomyomas present almost always as multiple small grey-white masses involving the ventricles and the atria. In about half the cases, the tumours project into the cardiac chambers and sometimes cause obstruction. Microscopically, tumour cells have small central nucleus surrounded by glycogen-rich cytoplasm that appears clear because of artefactual loss of glycogen in routine processing of histopathological tissue. In the cytoplasm, radiating fibrillar processes are usually evident; hence, these cells are also called spider cells.

SELF-ASSESSMENT

Multiple Choice Questions

1. In a case of myocardial infarction, which histological change is most likely to be seen 24 hours postinfarction?
   A. Coagulative necrosis
   B. Neutrophilic infiltration
   C. Granulation tissue formation
   D. Fibrosis
2. A pathology report of a heart shows asymmetric septal hypertrophy and myofibrillar disarray. These findings are characteristic of:
   A. Dilated cardiomyopathy
   B. Hypertrophic cardiomyopathy
   C. Restrictive cardiomyopathy
   D. Myocarditis
3. In rheumatic heart disease, Aschoff bodies are primarily found in which part of the heart?
   A. Myocardium
   B. Endocardium
   C. Pericardium
   D. Valves
4. A heart biopsy shows extensive deposition of amyloid protein. This finding is characteristic of:
   A. Amyloidosis affecting the heart
   B. Dilated cardiomyopathy
   C. Hypertrophic cardiomyopathy
   D. Myocarditis
5. A patient with a heart valve replacement develops a fever and heart murmur. Histopathology of the valve shows vegetations composed of fibrin and bacteria. This is indicative of:
   A. Rheumatic heart disease
   B. Infective endocarditis
   C. Nonbacterial thrombotic endocarditis
   D. Libman–Sacks endocarditis
6. An autopsy of a young athlete who died suddenly shows cardiac hypertrophy with no coronary artery obstruction. This is most likely:
   A. Hypertrophic cardiomyopathy
   B. Dilated cardiomyopathy
   C. Myocarditis
   D. Restrictive cardiomyopathy

7. In atherosclerosis, foam cells in the arterial wall are primarily derived from:
   A. Endothelial cells
   B. Smooth muscle cells
   C. Macrophages
   D. Fibroblasts
8. A patient with long-standing hypertension is likely to show which of the following changes in the heart?
   A. Myocardial thinning
   B. Dilated cardiomyopathy
   C. Concentric left ventricular hypertrophy
   D. Myocardial infarction
9. Which of the following is a characteristic feature of cardiac tamponade?
   A. Hypertrophied myocardium
   B. Compression of the heart by fluid in the pericardial sac
   C. Thickening of the pericardial layers
   D. Calcification of the pericardium
10. A patient with a history of lung cancer develops a pericardial effusion. The effusion is most likely:
    A. Serous
    B. Serosanguineous
    C. Chylous
    D. Haemorrhagic
11. Which of the following is a hallmark feature of chronic constrictive pericarditis?
    A. Myocardial fibrosis
    B. Pericardial calcification
    C. Valvular vegetations
    D. Myocardial infarction
12. A pathology report of an explanted heart shows 'onion-skin' fibrosis around coronary arteries. This is typical of:
    A. Hypertensive heart disease
    B. Restrictive cardiomyopathy
    C. Cardiac sarcoidosis
    D. Chronic pericarditis
13. A heart with extensive fatty infiltration, particularly in the right ventricle, is indicative of:
    A. Arrhythmogenic right ventricular cardiomyopathy
    B. Dilated cardiomyopathy
    C. Hypertrophic cardiomyopathy
    D. Myocarditis
14. In a patient with Marfan syndrome, which cardiac pathology is most likely?
    A. Mitral valve prolapse
    B. Aortic dissection
    C. Pulmonary valve stenosis
    D. Tricuspid regurgitation
15. A microscopic examination of heart tissue shows iron deposition within the myocardial cells. This is characteristic of:
    A. Haemochromatosis
    B. Amyloidosis
    C. Sarcoidosis
    D. Lipofuscinosis
16. The presence of 'tree-bark' appearance of the aorta is most commonly associated with:
    A. Syphilitic aortitis
    B. Aortic aneurysm
    C. Takayasu arteritis
    D. Aortic dissection
17. In myocarditis, which of the following is the most common causative agent?
    A. Bacterial infection
    B. Viral infection
    C. Fungal infection
    D. Autoimmune reaction
18. A heart biopsy in a patient with heart failure shows interstitial fibrosis and myocardial hypertrophy. These findings are most characteristic of:
    A. Dilated cardiomyopathy
    B. Hypertrophic cardiomyopathy
    C. Restrictive cardiomyopathy
    D. Ischaemic cardiomyopathy
19. In a patient with acute myocardial infarction, which of the following changes is likely to be seen in the first 12 hours?
    A. Coagulative necrosis
    B. Contraction band necrosis
    C. Neutrophilic infiltration
    D. Granulation tissue
20. A pathology report shows endocardial fibroelastosis. This condition is most commonly associated with:
    A. Paediatric heart disease
    B. Elderly heart disease
    C. Hypertensive heart disease
    D. Ischaemic heart disease
21. In cardiac amyloidosis, the amyloid protein is most often derived from:
    A. Immunoglobulin light chains
    B. Transthyretin
    C. Serum amyloid A protein
    D. Fibrinogen
22. A patient with Loeffler endocarditis is likely to show which of the following on histopathological examination?
    A. Myocardial fibrosis with eosinophilic infiltration
    B. Aschoff bodies in the myocardium
    C. Caseating granulomas in the myocardium
    D. Amyloid deposition in the myocardium

Answers

1. (B); 2. (B); 3. (A); 4. (A); 5. (B); 6. (A); 7. (C); 8. (C); 9. (B); 10. (D); 11. (B); 12. (A); 13. (A); 14. (B); 15. (A); 16. (A); 17. (B); 18. (D); 19. (B); 20. (A); 21. (A); 22. (A)

Self-Assessment Questions

1. A 3-year-old child with normal development of milestones presents with mild fever. On cardiac examination, a harsh machine-like murmur is heard. Patient also gives history of high-fever episode a year back, recovering after a course of antibiotics. ECHO reveals the presence of normal cardiac valves. What is the child probably suffering from?
2. A 45-year-old male patient presents to the OPD with complaints of repeated episodes of chest pain, especially on jogging. On examination, it was found that he is afebrile, pulse is regular and no murmurs are heard. Laboratory tests for the patient reveal high serum cholesterol. What is the likely diagnosis?

3. A 55-year-old patient, chronic diabetic on medications, complaints of substernal pain radiating to the left shoulder with dyspnoea. He also reveals on questioning that he has been experiencing these symptoms since 8 hours and the pain has been persisting until then. What parameters do you expect to be raised in such a situation, to support the diagnosis in your mind?
4. A 56-year-old patient with complaints of severe chest pain radiating to the neck presents at the medicine OPD. On examination, it was found that the patient is tachycardic and hypotensive but with no murmurs. ECHO reveals 80% atherosclerotic narrowing of the left coronary artery. What is the expected complication to occur in such a patient within 1 hour following these events?
5. A 70-year-old woman undergoes a master health checkup. All laboratory parameters are within range with may be minimal derangement. On auscultation, however, a midsystolic click is heard. ECHO shows mitral regurgitation from a prolapsed leaflet. What pathological changes can one expect in a such a scenario?
6. A 7-year-old boy presents to the OPD with recently developed subcutaneous nodules over the arms. On questioning, the parents reveal a history of acute pharyngitis 3 weeks back. The patients also complain of pain over the knee joints and the hips. What is the likely diagnosis?
7. A 22-year-old man suffers a sudden cardiac arrest. On examination, it was found that the vitals are normal. Autopsy revealed an enlarged heart with dilated right ventricle with thinned walls. The left ventricle is relatively normal. No signs of inflammation were evident. What is the probable cause of death?
8. A 7-year-old male patient complains of syncope and easy fatiguability. On examination, it was found that the vitals are normal. ECHO reveals normal cardiac size and valve function. With vagal stimulation, the heart is irregular. Where is the abnormality located in the patient?
9. A 58-year-old woman presents with complaints of increasing dyspnoea for the past 2 years. On examination, rales can be heard over the lung fields. ECHO shows a decreased ejection fraction with concentric hypertrophy of the left ventricular wall. The valve function is normal. What is the likely diagnosis?
10. A doctor examining a newborn documents the presence of a systolic murmur on examination. ECHO reveals a muscular defect in the interventricular septum. The parents are warned of the possibility of a congenital heart disease. Thirty years later, on examination, the murmur and the defect are not evident. What is the likely process behind the event?

Answers

1. PDA
2. MI/CAD
3. CK-MB
4. Sudden cardiac death
5. Myxomatous degeneration of the mitral valve
6. Acute rheumatic fever
7. Cardiomyopathy
8. Sinoatrial node
9. Hypertension
10. Spontaneous closure by stem cells

Topics for Self-Directed Learning

1. Emerging biomarkers of acute heart conditions
2. Mechanisms of CaMKII activation in the heart
3. Endogenous cardiac stem cell therapy for cardiac diseases
4. Resynchronization therapy, ventricular assist devices
5. Echocardiography, cardiac catheterization, electrophysiology
6. Life after surgery for patients with CHD
7. Genetic basis of CHD
8. Re-entrant arrhythmias, congenital heart diseases
9. Cardiac transplantation pathology
10. Recent advances in cardiac stem cells

15 Red Cell Disorders

Rajeswari Kathiah

PA 13.1 Describe **haematopoiesis and extramedullary haematopoiesis.**

PA 17.2 Enumerate the indications and describe the findings in **bone marrow aspiration and biopsy.**

PA 13.3 Define and classify **anaemia.**

PA 13.4 Enumerate and describe the **investigation of anaemia.**

PA 14.1 Describe **iron metabolism.**

PA 14.2 Describe the aetiology, investigations and differential diagnosis of **microcytic hypochromic anaemia.**

PA 15.1 Describe the metabolism of vitamin B_{12} and the aetiology and pathogenesis of vitamin **B_{12} deficiency.**

PA 15.2 Describe laboratory **investigations of macrocytic anaemia.**

PA 15.4 Enumerate the differences and describe the aetiology and distinguishing features of **megaloblastic and nonmegaloblastic macrocytic anaemias.**

PA 16.1 Define and classify **haemolytic anaemia.**

PA 16.2 Describe the pathogenesis and clinical features and haematological indices of **haemolytic anaemia.**

PA 16.3 Describe the pathogenesis, features, haematological indices and peripheral blood picture of **sickle cell anaemia and thalassaemia.**

PA 16.4 Describe the aetiology, pathogenesis, haematological indices and peripheral blood picture of **acquired haemolytic anaemia.**

PA 16.5 Describe the **peripheral blood picture** in different haemolytic anaemias.

PA 17.1 Enumerate the aetiology, pathogenesis and findings in **aplastic anaemia.**

CHAPTER OUTLINE

INTRODUCTION AND BASIC HAEMATOLOGY

Red cell disorders are one of the most common diseases affecting human beings. We briefly discuss the process of haematopoiesis and basics of haematology under the following headings before delving into the individual disorders:

A. Haematopoiesis
B. Extramedullary haematopoiesis
C. Morphology of bone marrow

D. Normal reference ranges for blood cells
E. Reticulocyte count
F. Common red cell terminologies

HAEMATOPOIESIS PA 13.1

Haematopoiesis is a physiological process of formation of blood cells that begins during embryonic development and continues throughout life to produce and replenish the blood system. All cellular blood elements are derived from the haematopoietic stem cells (HSCs) that reside in the medulla of the bone marrow in a healthy adult. On an average, 10^{11}–10^{12} new blood cells are produced every day to maintain steady-state levels in the peripheral circulation.

Development and Maintenance of Haematopoietic Tissues

The sequence in which the haematopoietic cells appear and mature is described as follows:

- By the third week of intrauterine life, blood cell progenitors appear in the yolk sac.
- After few weeks, HSCs arise from the mesoderm of the aorta, gonads and mesonephros region.
- By the third month till birth, HSCs populate the liver, which is the major site of haematopoiesis.
- A fraction of HSCs also resides in the placenta as the source of stem cells in umbilical cord blood.
- By birth, the marrow throughout the skeleton is haematopoietically active.
- By postpuberty, haematopoietically active marrow is restricted to the axial skeleton.
- In normal adults, only half of the marrow space is haematopoietically active.

Components of the haematopoietic system can be broadly divided into two types – **myeloid** tissues (which are composed of bone marrow and its derivatives) and **lymphoid** tissues (which are composed of the thymus, lymph nodes and spleen). Pluripotent stem cells in the marrow give rise to two types of multipotent stem cells – trilineage myeloid stem cells and lymphoid stem cells. The trilineage myeloid stem cells further differentiate to form three types of cell lines:

- *Erythroid progenitor cells*
- *Megakaryocytic progenitor cells*
- *Granulocyte–monocyte progenitor cells*

The lymphopoietic precursor cells give rise to B lymphocytes, T lymphocytes and natural killer (NK) cells, which undergo further maturation in peripheral lymphoid organs and thymus.

Haematopoiesis: The Process HSCs reside at the apex of the haematopoiesis hierarchy and have the capacity of self-renewal and multipotent differentiation (Fig. 15.1). As per the current research, all blood cells are said to be derived from these pluripotent HSCs. The myeloid and lymphoid stem cells originate from the pluripotent HSCs, which further give rise to more committed progenitors

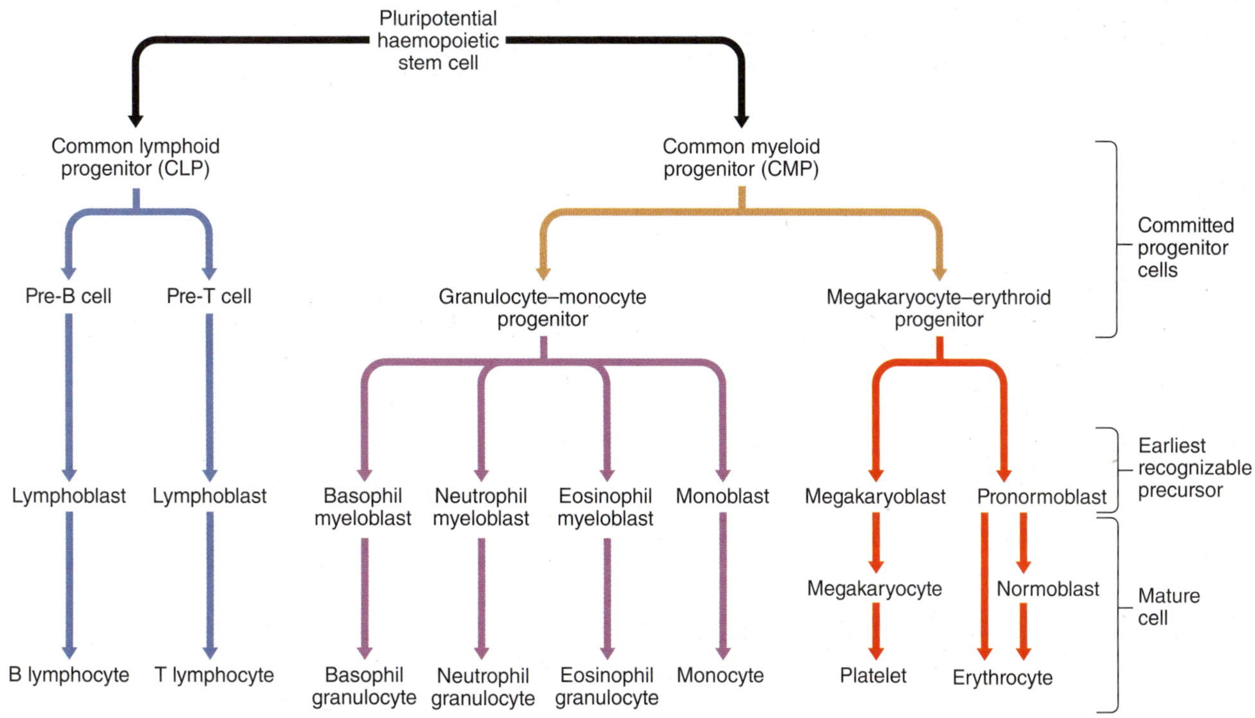

Fig. 15.1 Differentiation of blood cells. *(Source:* From Dominic Culligan and Henry G. Watson. Blood and bone marrow. Underwood's Pathology. 7th edition. Elsevier 2019.)

downstream. These progenitors are committed to generate only a single type of cell, and these single-lineage progenitors further differentiate to produce morphologically identifiable mature blood cells.

Red cells, granulocytes, monocytes and platelets are derived from myeloid stem cell, whereas B and T lymphocytes are formed from lymphoid stem cells.

The growth and differentiation factors, which influence the commitment of stem cells and progenitor cells to different lineages, are not clearly understood yet. The bone marrow microenvironment and responsiveness of progenitors to haematopoietic growth factors (HGFs) appear to have an impact.

HGFs help in the differentiation and proliferation of haematopoietic cells at different levels and are listed in Table 15.1.

HGFs can be multilineage or lineage restricted. Recombinant erythropoietin, GM-CSF and G-CSF are currently used for many disorders. Many other HGFs are being produced by the recombinant DNA technology and are currently in clinical trials for many disorders.

Microenvironment of the Marrow The bone marrow microenvironment plays a key role in regulating haematopoiesis and is the reason behind the restriction of blood cell formation in the bone marrow, but its molecular complexity and stress response are not yet completely understood. The exact composition has not been studied entirely but seems to be composed of vascular endothelial cells, fibroblasts, adipocytes, macrophages and extracellular matrix. The bone marrow microenvironment offers the stromal support and growth factors for haematopoiesis. Stem cells and haematopoietic progenitors are bound either to the stromal cells or to the adhesion molecules expressed by the matrix. The microenvironment also regulates the release of mature blood cells from the marrow.

Maturation of Erythroid Series

Stages of Erythropoiesis (Fig. 15.2) Within the bone marrow, erythroid cells are arranged in the form of islands.

- The earliest morphologically identifiable erythroid cell in the bone marrow is the **proerythroblast** (also called pronormoblast), a large cell with a fine, uniform chromatin pattern, one or more nucleoli and dark blue cytoplasm. Haemoglobin synthesis starts at this stage but is not stainable and cannot be demonstrated.
- The next cell in the maturation process is the **basophilic (early) normoblast**. This cell is smaller in size and has a coarser nuclear chromatin with barely visible nucleoli. The cytoplasm is deeply basophilic.
- The better differentiated erythroid cell is the **polychromatic (intermediate) normoblast.** The nuclear size is smaller and the chromatin becomes clumped. Polychromasia of cytoplasm results from the admixture of blue ribonucleic acid and pink-stainable haemoglobin. This is the last erythroid precursor capable of cellular division.
- The **orthochromatic (late) normoblast** is the next stage in the erythroid series. The nucleus is small, dense pyknotic and commonly eccentrically located. The cytoplasm stains mostly pink due to haemoglobinization. The term 'orthochromatic' is used because cytoplasmic staining is largely similar to that of erythrocytes. The nucleus is ultimately expelled from the orthochromatic normoblast with the formation of a reticulocyte.

Table 15.1 Growth Factors Involved in Haematopoiesis and Their Sources and Actions

Growth Factor	Source	Action
Interleukin-1 (IL-1)	Activated macrophages	Mediates synthesis and release of acute-phase proteins by liver cells; synthesis of other cytokines
Interleukin-2 (IL-2)	T lymphocyte	Growth factor for activated T cells
Interleukin-3 (IL-3)	T lymphocyte	Growth factor for haematopoietic stem cells
Interleukin-6 (IL-6)	T lymphocyte, monocytes, macrophages	Growth factor for B and T lymphocytes; mediates acute-phase response
C-kit ligand		Acts along with other growth factors to stimulate pluripotent stem cells
GM-CSF	T cells, fibroblasts, endothelial cells	Multilineage growth factor for neutrophils, monocyte/macrophage, eosinophils, red cells, platelets
G-CSF	Monocytes/macrophages, fibroblasts	Lineage-restricted growth factor for neutrophils
M-CSF	Monocytes/macrophages, fibroblasts, endothelial cells	Lineage-restricted growth factor for monocytes and macrophages
Erythropoietin	Kidneys and liver	Lineage-restricted growth factor for erythrocytes
Thrombopoietin	Kidneys and liver	Lineage-restricted growth factor for platelets

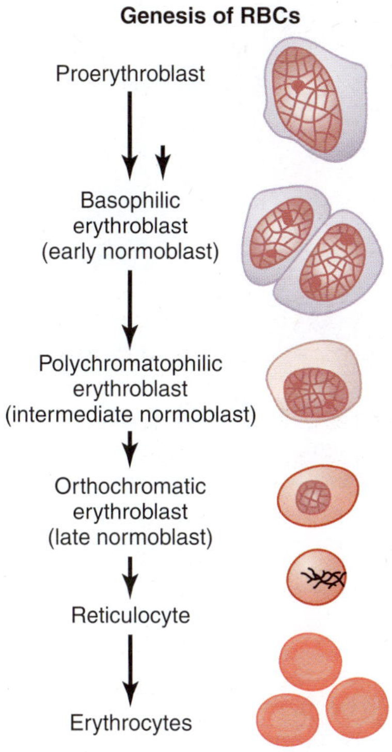

Fig. 15.2 Stages in the maturation of erythroid series. (*Source:* From John E. Hall and Michael E. Hall. Red Blood Cells, Anemia, and Polycythemia. Guyton and Hall Textbook of Medical Physiology. 14th edition. Elsevier 2021.)

- **The reticulocyte** still has remnants of ribosomal RNA in the form of a cytoplasmic reticulum. After 1–2 days in the bone marrow and 1–2 days in peripheral blood, reticulocytes lose RNA and become mature pink-staining erythrocytes. This is the earliest stage red blood cell (RBC) in the peripheral blood.
- In conjunction, about four mitotic divisions and continued differentiation lead to the generation of 16 mature erythrocytes from each pronormoblast.

Maturation of Myeloid Series

Stages of Granulopoiesis (Fig. 15.3)

Myeloblast: It is the earliest recognizable cell in the granulocytic maturation process. It is about 15–20 μm in diameter, with a large round to oval nucleus, and scant basophilic cytoplasm. The nucleus has two to five nucleoli, and nuclear chromatin is fine and reticular.

Promyelocyte: *Following the myeloblast,* the promyelocyte is generated that is slightly larger in size than its precursor. Primary or azurophil granules appear at this stage. The nucleus contains nucleoli as in the myeloblast, but nuclear chromatin shows slight condensation.

Myelocyte: Myelocytes are characterized by the appearance of secondary or specific granules (neutrophilic, eosinophilic or basophilic). They are smaller cells with a round to oval eccentrically placed nucleus and more condensed chromatin than the promyelocyte, with absence of nucleoli and relatively more cytoplasm. Myelocyte is the last stage capable of mitotic division.

Metamyelocyte: Sequentially, in the metamyelocyte, the nucleus becomes indented and kidney shaped, with nuclear chromatin being moderately coarse. Cytoplasm has both primary and secondary granules as in the myelocyte.

Band forms (stab form): Band forms, as they are referred to, have a band-like shape of the nucleus with constant diameter throughout and condensed nuclear chromatin. These are the earliest cells of this series to appear in peripheral blood.

Segmented neutrophil (polymorphonuclear neutrophil): These are the mature cells that are found in circulating blood. With Leishman's stain, the nucleus appears deep purple with two to five lobes that are joined by thin filamentous strands. Nuclear chromatin pattern is coarse; the cytoplasm stains light pink and has small, specific granules.

Primary and secondary granules: The neutrophil granules are of two types – primary or azurophilic granules and secondary or specific granules. Azurophil granules contain myeloperoxidase, lysozyme, acid phosphatase, elastases, collagenases and acid hydrolases. Specific granules contain lysozyme, lactoferrin, alkaline phosphatases, vitamin B_{12}–binding protein and other substances. Maturation of lymphoid series is discussed in Chapter 6. Morphology and functions of individual mature myeloid cells are discussed in Chapter 16. Morphology of cells in a normal peripheral smear is shown in Fig. 15.4.

EXTRAMEDULLARY HAEMATOPOIESIS PA 13.1

Extramedullary haematopoiesis refers to haematopoiesis that occurs outside the marrow in physiological or pathological conditions. Other than the embryonic and fetal periods of life, extramedullary haematopoiesis is

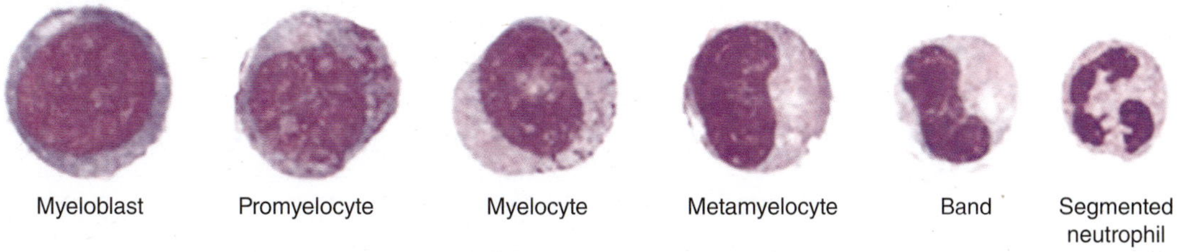

Fig. 15.3 Stages in the maturation of myeloid cells. (*Source:* From Arati Khanna-Gupta and Nancy Berliner. Granulocytopoiesis and Monocytopoiesis. Hematology: Basic Principles and Practice. 17th edition. Elsevier 2018.)

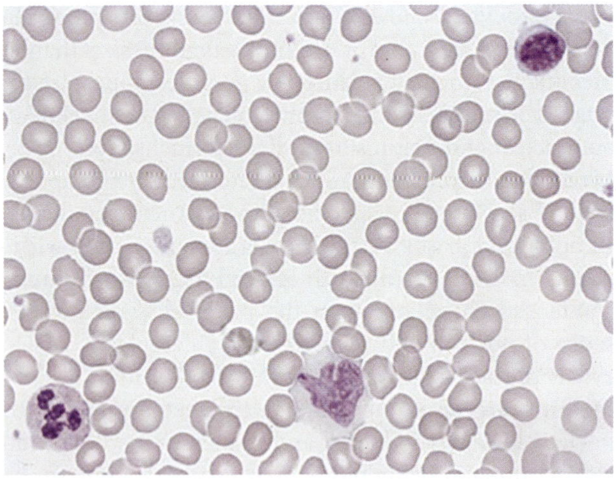

Fig. 15.4 Normal peripheral blood smear showing RBCs, a neutrophil, a lymphocyte, a monocyte and platelets. *(Source:* From Patrick G. Gallagher. Hemolytic Anemias: Red Blood Cell Membrane and Metabolic Defects. Goldman-Cecil Medicine. 26th edition. Elsevier 2020.)

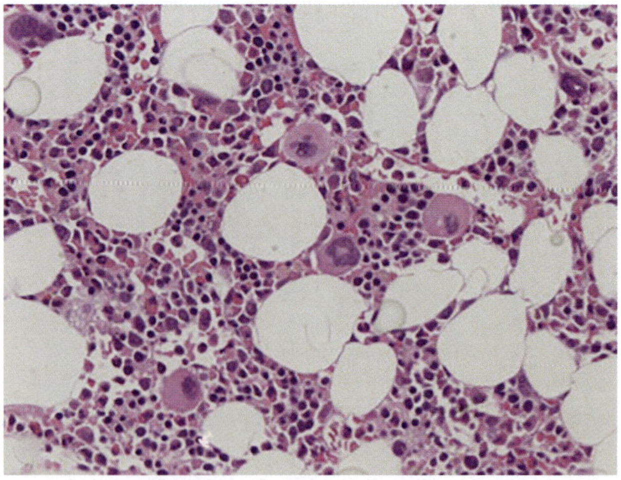

Fig. 15.5 Histology of bone marrow. *(Source:* From Vajpayee Neerja, Graham Susan S. and Sylva Bem. Basic Examination of Blood and Bone Marrow. Henry's Clinical Diagnosis and Management by Laboratory Methods. 24th edition. Elsevier 2022.)

always pathological. When the requirement of blood cells exceeds the capacity of the marrow or when the marrow is subfunctional or nonfunctional (failed marrow haematopoiesis) due to fibrosis or sclerosis, extramedullary haematopoiesis takes place. Extramedullary haematopoiesis occurs in secondary lymphoid organs like the spleen, liver and lymph nodes by ***migration of HSCs*** *from the marrow to these organs.*

Common conditions causing extramedullary haematopoiesis are as follows:

- Thalassaemia
- Sickle cell anaemia
- Hereditary spherocytosis (HS)
- Idiopathic thrombocytopenia
- Myeloproliferative disorders
- Osteopetrosis

Haematopoiesis in extramedullary sites also requires the same growth factors like medullary haematopoiesis but results in disordered maturation.

BONE MARROW SAMPLING **PA 17.2**

Bone marrow is sampled in many haematological and nonhaematological conditions to evaluate the disease process and is helpful for clinicians to arrive at the correct diagnosis. Before discussing the sampling methods, a brief review is presented for a better understanding of bone marrow histology.

Morphology of Bone Marrow (Fig. 15.5)

Bone marrow is the spongy portion inside the bones and consists of a meshwork of bony trabeculae containing haematopoietic marrow elements and fat cells. The ratio of haematopoietic elements and fat cells depends on the age and activity of the bone marrow in response to various physiological stimuli, and the marrow cellularity is roughly inversely proportional to the age of the person. Thus, newborns have nearly 100% cellular marrow, whereas older individuals in their eighth decade of life or later have only 20%–30% cellularity. The bone trabeculae provide a supportive framework for haematopoiesis to occur.

A normal bone marrow is said to show **trilineage haematopoiesis**, meaning that all the elements of three major cell lines are represented. The trilineage includes myelomonocytic cells, erythroid cells and megakaryocytic cells.

Normal Adult Bone Marrow Counts: Myelogram

Parameter	Normal range
Fat/bone marrow cell ratio	50:50
Myeloid to erythroid ratio	2–4:1 (mean 3:1)
Myeloid series 1. Myeloblasts 2. Promyelocytes	30%–45% 0.1%–3.5% 0.5%–5%
Erythroid series	10%–15%
Megakaryocytes	0.5%
Lymphocytes	5%–20%
Plasma cells	≤3%
Reticulum cells	0.1%–2%

Sampling Methods and Indications

Examination of the bone marrow provides an invaluable diagnostic help in some diseases, whereas in other cases, it is of value in confirming a diagnosis suggestive of clinical examination or peripheral blood examination. However, peripheral smear examination should always precede bone marrow examination.

Examination of marrow can be performed by two methods – aspiration cytology and trephine biopsy.

Bone Marrow Aspiration In this method, *Salah bone marrow aspiration needle* is used to aspirate the marrow, following which smears are prepared immediately and fixed in 95% methanol after air drying. The marrow smears are studied under the microscope to assess cellularity, analyse the development of blood cells, calculate myeloid to erythroid ratio, and detect the presence of storage diseases, metastatic deposits, granulomatous conditions, fungi (e.g. histoplasmosis) and parasites (e.g. malaria, leishmaniasis, trypanosomiasis). The marrow aspirate material can also be used for more specialized tests like cytogenetics, microbiological culture, biochemical analysis, immunological and cytological markers.

Bone Marrow Biopsy: Trephine Biopsy This method involves the use of *Jamshidi trephine needle*, with which a core of tissue can be obtained from the periosteum to the marrow cavity. The tissue is then fixed, decalcified and processed for histopathological sections and stained with haematoxylin and eosin and for reticulin to check marrow fibrosis. Trephine biopsy is preferred over aspirations to examine the overall marrow architecture, cellularity and the presence and pattern of infiltrates. The differences between bone marrow aspiration and trephine biopsy are given in Table 15.2.

Bone marrow findings in individual diseases are discussed under the individual disorders.

NORMAL REFERENCE RANGES FOR BLOOD CELLS

Adult Reference Ranges for Red Cells and Platelets

Parameter	Unit	Men	Women
Haemoglobin	g/dL	13.6–17.2	12.0–15.0
Haematocrit	%	39–49	33–43
Red cell count	$\times 10^6/\mu L$	4.3–5.9	3.5–5.0
Reticulocyte count	%	0.5–1.5	
MCV	fL	90 ± 6	
MCH	Pg	30 ± 3	
MCHC	g/dL	33–37	
RDW		11.5–14.5	
Platelets	$\times 10^3/\mu L$	150–450	

Table 15.2 Comparison of Bone Marrow Aspiration and Trephine Biopsy

Feature	Aspiration	Trephine
Site	Sternum, posterior iliac crest, tibial heads in infants	Posterior iliac crest
Instrument used	Salah bone marrow aspiration needle	Jamshidi trephine biopsy needle
Common stains used	Romanowsky, Perl's reaction for iron	H&E, reticulin
Time taken for the report	1–2 h	1–7 days
Preferred for	Better cellular morphology	Better marrow architectural pattern
Indications	• Anaemias • Suspected leukaemias • Neutropenia • Thrombocytopenia • Polycythaemia • Myeloma • Lymphomas • Lipid storage disorders • Granulomatous diseases • Parasitic infestations • Fungal infections • Unexplained hepatomegaly, splenomegaly or lymphadenopathy	• Myelofibrosis • Aplastic anaemia • Hairy cell leukaemia

H&E, haematoxylin and eosin.

Normal White Blood Cell Counts in Health

	Absolute Count
Total Leucocyte Count	
Adults	4000–11,000/µL
Infants (full term at birth)	10,000–25,000/µL
Infants (1 year)	6000–16,000/µL
Children (4–7 years)	5000–15,000/µL
Children (8–12 years)	4500–13,500/µL
Differential Count in Adults	
Neutrophils: 40%–75%	2000–7500/µL
Lymphocytes: 20%–50%	1500–4000/µL
Monocytes: 2%–10%	200–1000/µL
Eosinophils: 1%–6%	40–400/µL
Basophils: <1%	10–100/µL

Red Cell Indices

- **Mean corpuscular volume (MCV):** Average size/volume of a red cell – expressed in femtolitres
- **Mean corpuscular haemoglobin (MCH):** Average content of haemoglobin per red cell – expressed in picograms
- **Mean corpuscular haemoglobin concentration (MCHC):** Average concentration of haemoglobin in a given volume of packed red cells, expressed in grams per decilitre
- **Red cell distribution width (RDW):** Coefficient of variation of red cell volume

RETICULOCYTES

Reticulocytes are immature RBCs. In the process of erythropoiesis, reticulocytes develop and mature in the bone marrow and then circulate for about a day in the peripheral blood before developing into mature RBCs. Like mature red cells, reticulocytes are **non-nucleated**. They are called reticulocytes because they contain reticular network of ribosomal RNA that become more evident with supravital stains like new methylene blue and brilliant cresyl blue (Fig. 15.6).

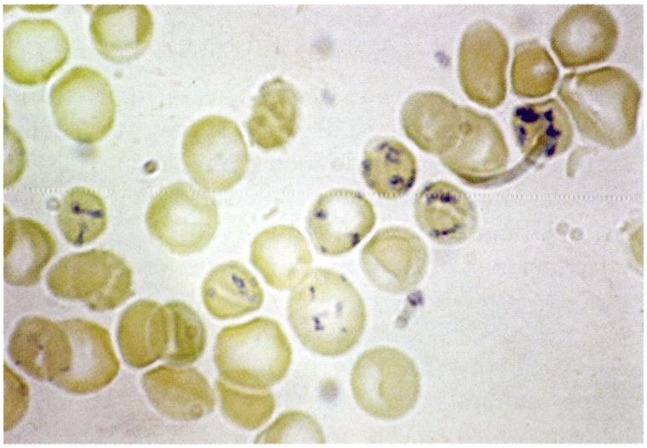

Fig. 15.6 Reticulocyte with supravital staining show intracellular RNA. *(Source:* From S. David Hudnall. Colour insert. Hematology. Mosby 2012.)

The number of reticulocytes is a good indicator of bone marrow activity because it represents recent production and allows for the determination of reticulocyte count. When there is an increased production of RBCs to overcome chronic or severe loss of mature RBCs, such as in a haemolytic anaemia, there is often a markedly high number and percentage of reticulocytes. A very high number of reticulocytes in the blood can be described as reticulocytosis. An abnormally low number of reticulocytes are referred to as reticulocytopenia, which is due to reduced red cell production by the marrow.

Conditions associated with reticulocytosis and reticulocytopenia are listed in Table 15.3.

Table 15.3 Conditions Causing Reticulocytosis and Reticulocytopenia[a]

Reticulocytosis	Reticulocytopenia
• Acute blood loss • Haemolytic anaemias • Response to specific therapy in nutritional anaemia	• Aplastic anaemia • Nutritional deficiency • Iron-deficiency anaemia • Megaloblastic anaemia • Marrow infiltration

[a]Normal reticulocyte count is 0.5%–2%.

Corrected Reticulocyte Count

Reticulocyte count is reported as reticulocyte percentage per 100 RBCs. Thus, the raw reticulocyte count is not a count but rather a percentage. In conditions like anaemia, the number of RBCs decreases and therefore the reticulocyte percentage appears spuriously high and may not reflect the true bone marrow response to anaemia. Hence, the value needs to be adjusted to corrected reticulocyte count on the basis of the patient's haematocrit or absolute reticulocyte count may be used.

Corrected reticulocyte count, also called reticulocyte production index, is a calculated value. The formula for calculation of corrected reticulocyte count is as follows:

$$\textbf{Corrected reticulocyte count} = \textbf{Reticulocyte (\%)} \times \frac{\textbf{Haematocrit}}{\textbf{Normal haematocrit}}$$

A value of 45 is commonly used as normal haematocrit for adults.

With automated haematology analysers, absolute reticulocyte count is reported easily. The normal absolute reticulocyte count is 50 × 10^9/L to 100 × 10^9/L.

Table 15.4 Common Red Cell Terminologies and Their Description

Terms	Description
Anisocytosis	Variation in the size of RBCs
Poikilocytosis	• Variation in the shape of RBCs • Different poikilocytes are listed in Table 15.5
Polychromatophilic red cells	• Red cells with slightly increased size and faint blue-grey tint due to the presence of ribosomal RNA • They are actually reticulocytes seen in the peripheral smear
Basophilic stippling	Presence of fine or coarse purple-blue granules
Howell–Jolly bodies	Round purple nuclear remnants
Dimorphic red cells	Presence of two populations of red cells

RBC, red blood cell.

Table 15.5 List of Different Poikilocytes and the Conditions Causing Them

Poikilocyte	Seen in
Spherocytes	• Hereditary spherocytosis • Autoimmune haemolytic anaemia • Haemolytic disease of newborn • Burns
Sickle cells	Sickle cell anaemia
Target cells	• Iron-deficiency anaemia • Thalassaemia • Liver disease • Hypothyroidism • Alcoholism
Schistocytes	Microangiopathic haemolytic anaemia
Teardrop cells	Myelophthisic anaemia
Burr cells	Uraemia
Bite cells	G6PD deficiency
Acanthocytes	Hereditary acanthocytosis
Basophilic stippling	• Lead poisoning • Thalassaemia • Megaloblastic anaemia
Howell–Jolly bodies	• Postsplenectomy • Thalassaemia • Megaloblastic anaemia

G6PD, glucose-6-phosphate dehydrogenase.

Reticulocyte count is a valuable tool in the evaluation of haematological disorders such as severity of anaemia and also in assessing the bone marrow response to treatment.

COMMON RED CELL TERMINOLOGIES

Familiarity with common terminologies used in red cell disorders is essential before discussing the diseases. Common terminologies are listed and described in Table 15.4.

Different poikilocytes are described and discussed under the relevant diseases (Fig. 15.7).

ANAEMIAS PA 13.3

Anaemia is the most common blood disorder, affecting about one-third of the global population. Iron-deficiency anaemia affects nearly 1 billion people worldwide.

Definition: Anaemia is defined as the reduction in the total circulating red cell mass or haemoglobin. It represents the lowered ability of the blood to carry oxygen below normal limits. In practice, anaemia is diagnosed by measuring the haemoglobin concentration and haematocrit, because the measurement of red cell mass is not simple.

There are many ways of classifying anaemia. The common method of classification is based on the underlying causative mechanisms (Table 15.6).

The other way of classifying anaemia is based on the morphology of red cells that includes the red cell size and colour. Red cells, according to their size, are categorized into normocytic (normal sized)/microcytic (small sized)/macrocytic RBCs (enlarged) and into normochromic/hypochromic on the basis of the degree of haemoglobinization. Normochromic RBCs are salmon pink in colour, whereas hypochromic RBCs appear paler due to enlargement of the central pallor.

Although the size and colour of the RBCs can be checked and compared by the visual examination of the peripheral smears, a more objective way of assessing them is by the red cell indices measured by automated haematology analysers.

On the basis of the red cell indices, anaemia can be morphologically classified into three categories as shown in Table 15.7.

Features of anaemia: Patients appear pale and complain of fatigue, weakness and malaise. In severe anaemia, patients may experience difficulty in breathing on mild exertion. In response to anaemia, hypoxia can cause fatty change in the liver, myocardium and kidney. If anaemia and the hypoxic changes are extensive, it could precipitate cardiac failure. Patients with acute blood loss causing anaemia present with acute renal failure. Features specific for specific types of anaemia are discussed under the individual disorders.

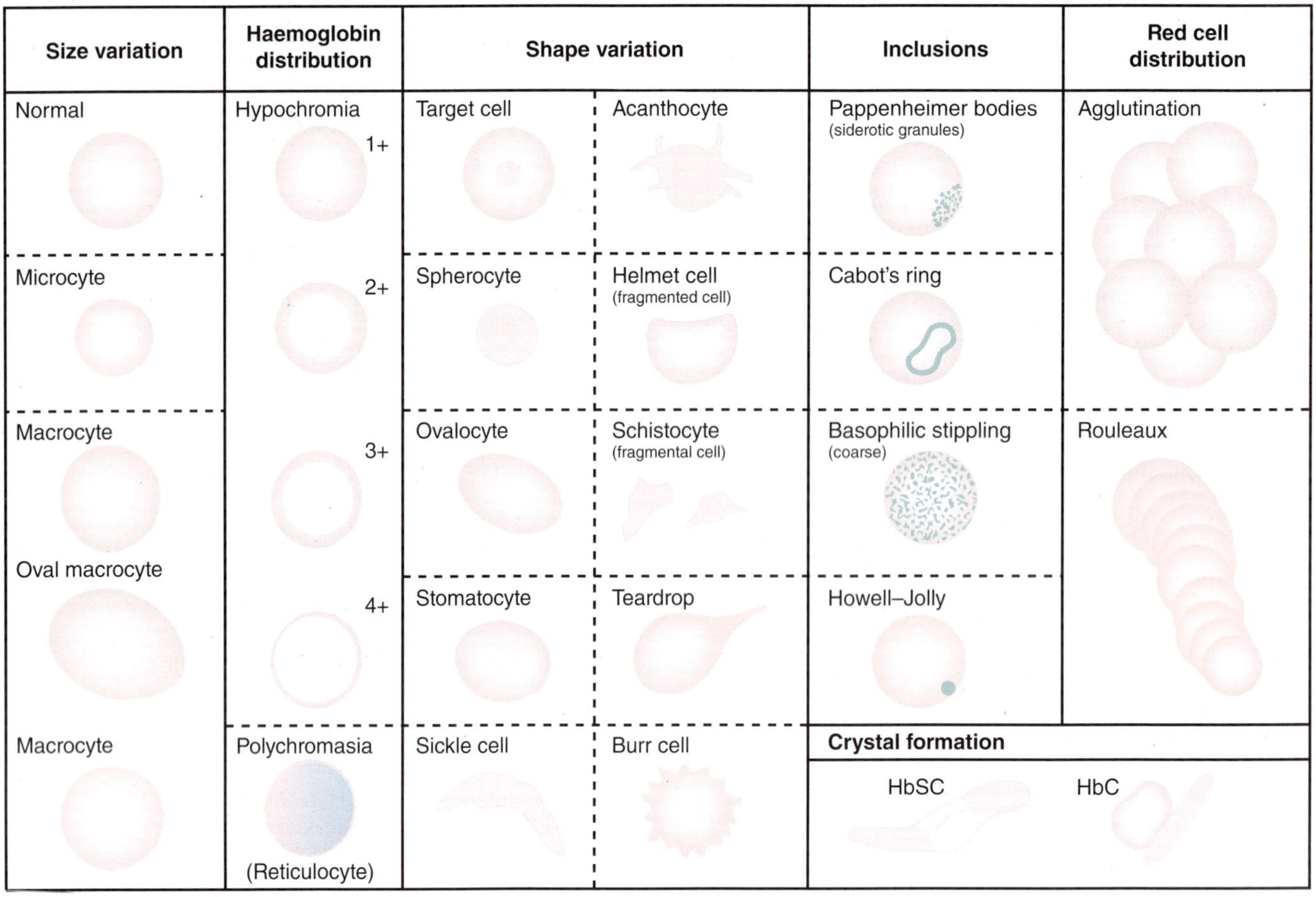

Fig. 15.7 Red blood cell morphology: Diagrammatic representation of different poikilocytes. (*Source:* Reproduced from https://theartofmed.wordpress.com)

ANAEMIA OF BLOOD LOSS

Anaemia due to blood loss is divided into two categories depending on the duration of blood loss:

- Acute blood loss
- Chronic blood loss

Pathophysiology, clinical presentation, consequences, investigations and treatment are completely different for both the categories and hence discussed separately.

Acute Blood Loss

Anaemia due to acute blood loss is also called posthaemorrhagic anaemia. Acute blood loss can be external (due to trauma, obstetric causes) or internal (due to gastrointestinal bleeding, rupture of ectopic pregnancy or rupture of the spleen). Clinical features depend on the severity and rate of blood loss and whether the blood is lost externally or internally.

Acute severe loss of blood is followed by three clinical stages:

1. The predominant feature in the beginning is **hypovolaemia**, which endangers the organs that require high blood supply such as the brain and kidneys, resulting in loss of consciousness and acute renal failure. At this stage, complete blood cell count does not reveal anaemia because haemoglobin concentration is not affected.
2. As an emergency response, baroreceptors and stretch receptors cause the release of vasopressin and other peptides, causing shift of fluid from extravascular space to intravascular space. At this stage, hypovolaemia gradually gets converted to anaemia because there is dilution of blood.
3. If the bleeding stops, compensatory erythropoiesis by the bone marrow gradually improves the anaemia. At this stage, reticulocyte count and erythropoietin levels are elevated.
4. If the bleeding continues, patients progress into hypovolaemic shock, which is discussed in greater detail in Chapter 4.

Blood loss causes significant changes in RBCs, leucocytes and platelets.

Significant bleeding induces changes in the blood such as leucocytosis, thrombocytosis and reticulocytosis.

If the blood loss is external, iron is lost and the restoration of normal red cell count is difficult without replacement of lost iron.

Chronic Blood Loss

Chronic blood loss induces anaemia only when the loss exceeds the regenerative capacity of the marrow or when

Table 15.6 Classification of Anaemia According to Underlying Mechanisms

Type of anaemia	Mechanism	Subcategories	Specific examples
Blood loss	Acute		Trauma
	Chronic		• GI bleeding • Genitourinary bleeding
Increased red cell destruction – haemolytic anaemia	Inherited genetic defects	Red cell membrane disorders	• Hereditary spherocytosis • Hereditary elliptocytosis
		Enzyme deficiency	• G6PD deficiency • Pyruvate kinase deficiency
	Haemoglobin abnormalities	Quantitative haemoglobinopathy	Thalassaemias
		Qualitative haemoglobinopathy	Sickle cell disease
	Acquired genetic defects	Deficiency of GPI-linked proteins	Paroxysmal nocturnal haemoglobinuria
	Antibody-mediated destruction		• Haemolytic disease of newborn • Transfusion reactions • Drug-induced autoimmune reactions
	Mechanical trauma		• Haemolytic uraemic syndrome • Thrombotic thrombocytopenic purpura • DIC
	Infections of red cells		• Malaria • Babesiosis
	Toxic or chemical injury		• Clostridial sepsis • Snake venom • Lead poisoning
	Membrane lipid abnormalities		Abetalipoproteinaemia
	Sequestration		Hypersplenism
Decreased red cell production	Inherited genetic defects	Defects due to stem cell depletion	Fanconi anaemia
		Defects affecting erythroblast maturation	Thalassaemia syndromes
	Nutritional deficiencies	Affecting DNA synthesis	Megaloblastic anaemias
		Affecting haemoglobin synthesis	Iron-deficiency anaemia
	Erythropoietin deficiency		• Renal failure • Anaemia of chronic disease
	Immune-mediated injury of the progenitors		• Aplastic anaemia • Pure red cell aplasia
	Inflammation-mediated sequestration of iron		Anaemia of chronic disease
	Primary haematopoietic neoplasms		• Acute leukaemia • Myelodysplasia • Myeloproliferative disorders
	Space-occupying marrow lesions		• Metastasis • Granulomatous diseases
	Infections of red cell progenitors		Parvovirus B19 infection

DIC, disseminated intravascular coagulation; G6PD, glucose-6-phosphate dehydrogenase; GI, gastrointestinal; GPI, glycosylphosphatidylinositol.

Table 15.7 Morphological Classification of Anaemia

Category of Anaemia	Common Causes
Normocytic normochromic anaemia	• Aplastic anaemia • Recent blood loss • Myelophthisic anaemia • Chronic renal failure
Microcytic hypochromic anaemia	• Iron-deficiency anaemia • Anaemia of chronic disease • Thalassaemia • Sideroblastic anaemia
Macrocytic anaemia	• Megaloblastic anaemia • Liver disease • Alcoholism

iron reserves are exhausted. The reason for the development of anaemia in chronic blood loss is loss of iron externally and the picture is that of iron-deficiency anaemia. Serological findings, peripheral smear morphology and clinical features are similar to those of iron-deficiency anaemia and discussed in detail in the section 'Iron-deficiency anaemia'.

ANAEMIAS OF DIMINISHED ERYTHROPOIESIS

Anaemias of diminished erythropoiesis are a category of disorders characterized by inadequate production of blood cells due to varied reasons.

The following are the common disorders that are characterized by reduced RBC production:

- Iron-deficiency anaemia
- Megaloblastic anaemias
- Anaemia of chronic disease
- Sideroblastic anaemia
- Aplastic anaemia

Iron-Deficiency Anaemia PA 14.1, PA 14.2

Iron-deficiency anaemia is the most common nutritional disorder in the world and is more common in developing countries, commonly affecting toddlers, adolescents, women of childbearing age and the elderly. The symptoms are mostly due to inadequate synthesis of haemoglobin.

Let us take a brief look into normal iron metabolism before discussing iron deficiency.

Iron Metabolism A normal Western diet contains 10–20 mg of iron, but the iron content in the diet consumed by people in the developing countries is much lesser. Haem iron derived from animal sources is better absorbed at around 20%. In contrast, only 1%–2% of nonhaem iron that is consumed is absorbed and also absorption is influenced by enhancers and inhibitors in the food.

Body iron exists in three compartments – functional, transport and storage iron (Fig. 15.8).

The distribution of iron is shown in Table 15.8.

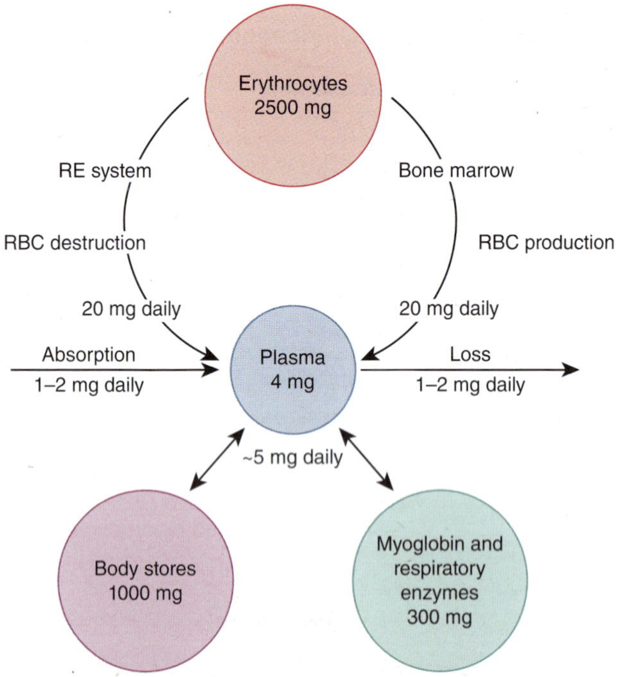

Fig. 15.8 Distribution of iron in the body.

Table 15.8 Distribution of Iron in the Functional, Transport and Storage Forms

Functional Iron – 80%	Transport Iron	Storage Iron* – 15%–20%
• Haemoglobin • Myoglobin • Catalase • Cytochrome	Transferrin	• Ferritin • Haemosiderin

Daily iron requirement:
- Men, 7–10 mg
- Women, 7–20 mg

Total body iron:
- Men, 6 g
- Women, 2.5 g

Serum iron:
- Men, 120 mg/dL
- Women, 100 mg/dL

*Iron is recycled between the compartments
Transferrin is one-third saturated with iron
Serum ferritin correlates with storage iron

The function of transferrin is to deliver iron to cells that require it, mainly erythroid precursors. Erythroid precursors possess high-affinity receptors for transferrin for iron uptake.

Storage iron is sequestered, because free iron is highly toxic. Iron is stored as **ferritin** in the macrophages of the bone marrow, spleen and liver, whereas **haemosiderin** is the major form of storage iron in the iron-overloaded state. Iron in haemosiderin is chemically reactive – stained by **Perl's Prussian blue** stain.

Iron is absorbed from the **proximal duodenum**, and iron balance is maintained by regulating its absorption, because excretion is not well regulated. Iron levels have to be meticulously regulated, because iron is essential for cellular metabolism and at the same time highly toxic when its level exceeds the specified amount.

Steps involved in the regulation of iron absorption (Fig. 15.8):

1. Haem iron is transported into the duodenal epithelial cells by haem transporter.
2. Nonhaem iron requires conversion from the ferric to the ferrous form, which is done by the enzyme duodenal cytochrome B found in brush border of duodenal epithelial cells.
3. The converted ferrous iron is transported into the mucosal epithelial cells by divalent metal transporter 1 (DMT1).
4. Although a part of this iron is stored in the mucosal epithelial cells as mucosal ferritin, a portion exits the mucosal cells through ferroportin, a transporter found on the basal side of duodenal epithelium.
5. The iron that is released from the epithelial cells in the ferrous form is further converted to the ferric form by hephaestin and ceruloplasmin, which are also mucosal enzymes.
6. Iron that exits mucosal cells after conversion is transported by transferrin to the sites of requirement.
7. A fraction of the absorbed iron that is stored in the mucosal epithelial cells is lost with shedding of the mucosa.

Iron that has entered the mucosal epithelial cell can follow one of the following two pathways: it can either be transported into the blood or stored as mucosal ferritin and lost with shedding of the mucosa. The pathway is decided by the body iron stores.

When serum iron levels reduce, iron absorption increases, and when the serum iron levels increase, absorption decreases, and this process is under the control of **hepcidin**, a protein synthesized by the liver (Fig. 15.9). In iron-replete situations, more hepcidin is produced by the

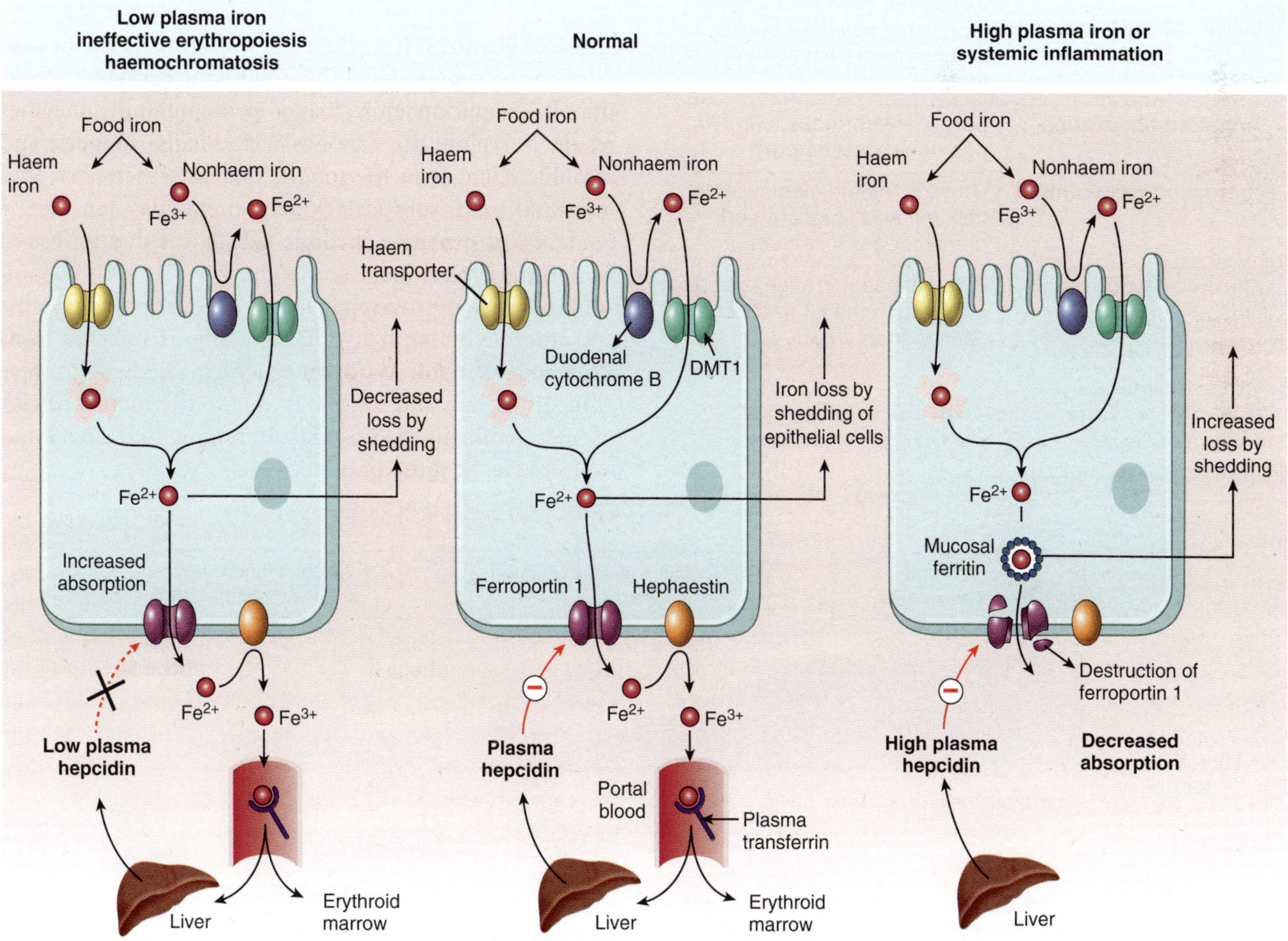

Fig. 15.9 Regulation of iron absorption. In the normal setting, plasma hepcidin balances iron uptake and loss by downregulating ferroportin and limiting iron uptake (middle panel). Hepcidin rises in the setting of systemic inflammation or when liver iron levels are high, decreasing iron uptake and increasing iron loss during the shedding of duodenocytes (right panel). Conversely, hepcidin levels fall in the setting of low plasma iron, primary haemochromatosis or ineffective haematopoiesis (left panel), leading to a rise in iron absorption. DMT1, divalent metal transporter 1. (*Source:* From Vinay Kumar, Abul K. Abbas and Jon C. Aster. Red Blood Cell and Bleeding Disorders. Robbins & Cotran Pathologic Basis of Disease. 10th edition. Elsevier 2021.)

liver, which prevents transfer of iron from enterocytes into the circulation by downregulating ferroportin. It also inhibits iron release from macrophages to erythroid precursors and thus acts to bring down the levels of serum iron. In iron-depleted situations, the hepcidin level comes down, which removes its negative control on ferroportin, and increases the iron absorption. Alterations in hepcidin levels play a major role in disorders involving iron metabolism.

Pathogenesis (Table 15.9) In conditions causing chronic blood loss, at the initial stage, storage iron may be adequate to maintain normal haemoglobin, along with normal serum iron and transferrin saturation levels. Thus, in this stage, only the storage iron is compromised and is reflected by a fall in serum ferritin levels, which is the earliest marker for detecting anaemia. Progressive depletion of reserves then lowers serum iron and transferrin saturation levels without producing anaemia. In this stage, there is increased erythroid activity in the marrow. In the third stage, anaemia appears because iron stores are completely depleted and is manifested by microcytic hypochromic RBCs. At this stage, there are reduced levels of serum iron, ferritin and transferrin saturation along with low haemoglobin, MCV and MCH and increased total iron-binding capacity (TIBC) and RDW (Fig. 15.10).

Table 15.9 Aetiology of Iron-Deficiency Anaemia

Category of Disorder	Common Causes
Dietary lack	Food that is poor in iron, inhibitors of iron absorption, exclusively breastfed infants, impoverished, older adults and teenagers eating junk food
Impaired absorption	Sprue, steatorrhoea, chronic diarrhoea, gastrectomy
Increased requirement	Growing infants, adolescents, children and pregnant and premenopausal women
Chronic blood loss	External haemorrhage, bleeding through the GI tract[a] and genitourinary tract

GI, gastrointestinal.
[a]Iron-deficiency anaemia in adult men and postmenopausal women is attributed to GI blood loss, until proven otherwise.

Morphology

Peripheral smear reveals microcytic hypochromic RBCs with anisopoikilocytosis. Pencil cells and target cells may be seen (Fig. 15.11).

Bone marrow displays mild to moderate increase in erythroid progenitors with lack of stainable iron in the macrophages detected with the use of Perl's Prussian blue stain.

Clinical Features Iron-deficiency anaemia is a sign with dominating symptoms of the underlying causative condition. In chronic anaemia, loss of iron-containing enzymes results in koilonychia (spoon-shaped nails), alopecia and atrophic changes in the tongue and gastric mucosa and intestinal malabsorption. Some patients develop pica, a tendency to consume inedible substances due to loss of iron in the central nervous system.

The triad of oesophageal webs, atrophic glossitis and microcytic hypochromic anaemia is referred to as **Plummer–Vinson syndrome**, which needs aggressive clinical workup and follow-up due to the increased risk of malignancy in the postcricoid region, oral cavity and oesophagus in these patients.

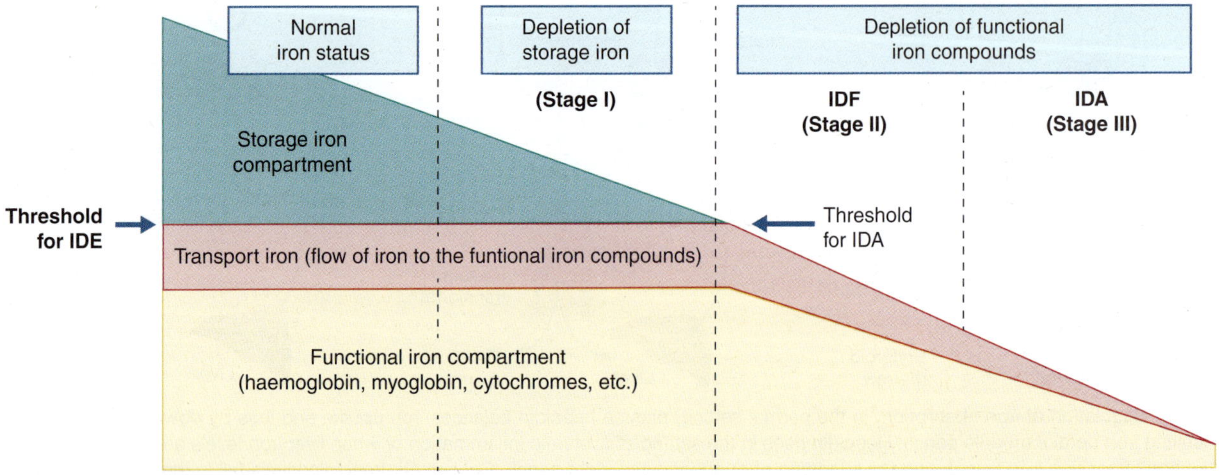

Fig. 15.10 Stages of development of iron-deficiency anaemia. Note that the first to get depleted is the storage iron and the first serum marker to reflect it is serum ferritin. *(Source:* From Jeffrey S. Durmer. Restless Legs Syndrome, Periodic Leg Movements and Periodic Limb Movement Disorder. Principles and Practice of Pediatric Sleep Medicine. Second edition. Elsevier 2014.)

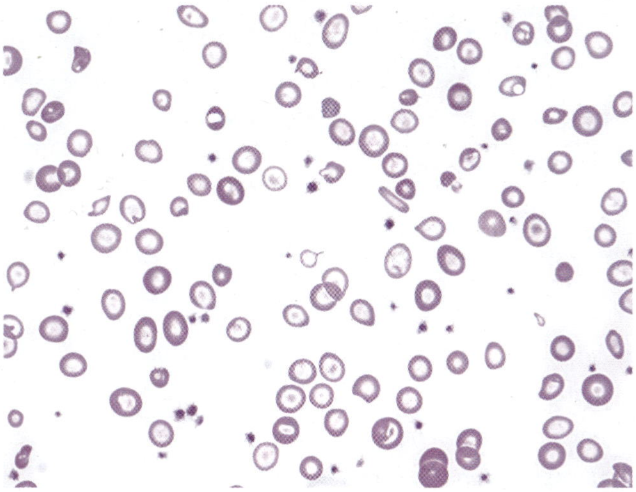

Fig. 15.11 Peripheral smear of iron-deficiency anaemia showing microcytic hypochromic cells with anisopoikilocytosis. An elongate elliptocyte (pencil cell) is visible slightly to the right and above the centre of the field. *(Source:* From Richard N. Mitchell and Andrew J. Connolly. The Heart. Robbins & Cotran Pathologic Basis of Disease. 10th edition. Elsevier 2021.)

Management

Laboratory Investigations In patients with iron-deficiency anaemia, haemoglobin, haematocrit and red cell indices like MCV and MCH are low with elevated RDW. Biochemical parameters like serum iron, ferritin and transferrin saturation are also reduced, whereas TIBC is elevated as a compensatory measure by the body.

In a patient with signs and symptoms of anaemia, findings of **low serum iron and increased serum iron-binding capacity** clinch the diagnosis of iron-deficiency anaemia.

Reticulocyte count is generally low or normal in an untreated case of iron deficiency. In uncomplicated iron deficiency, oral iron supplements result in brisk reticulocytosis in 5–7 days, followed by an increase in red cell counts and then red cell indices.

Treatment Iron-deficiency anaemia is treated with oral and parenteral iron supplements, and blood transfusion in severe cases. Treating the underlying cause is essential.

Megaloblastic Anaemias

PA 15.1, PA 15.2, PA 15.4

Megaloblastic anaemias are a group of disorders characterized by the deficiency of vitamin B_{12} or folic acid levels, resulting in ineffective haematopoiesis and associated with distinctive morphological changes in the haematopoietic cells due to defective DNA maturation.

Anaemias of Vitamin B_{12} Deficiency

Normal Vitamin B_{12} Metabolism

Daily requirement: 2–3 μg

Vitamin B_{12} is a complex organometallic compound also known as cobalamin. Humans are completely dependent on the dietary supply of vitamin B_{12}. Animal products are the chief source because vegetables and fruits contain only traces of this vitamin. Vitamin B_{12} is absorbed in the **terminal ileum**, and **intrinsic factor** secreted by the gastric parietal epithelial cells is required for the absorption of oral vitamin B_{12}.

The steps involved in the absorption (Fig. 15.12) **and metabolism of vitamin B_{12} are as follows:**

1. Haptocorrin, a salivary protein, binds to vitamin B_{12} after it is freed from binding proteins by the action of pepsin in the stomach.
2. Pancreatic proteases release vitamin B_{12} from haptocorrin in the duodenum.
3. In the duodenum, it binds to intrinsic factor and this complex is endocytosed by the ileal enterocytes that express a receptor for intrinsic factor, called cubilin, on their surface.

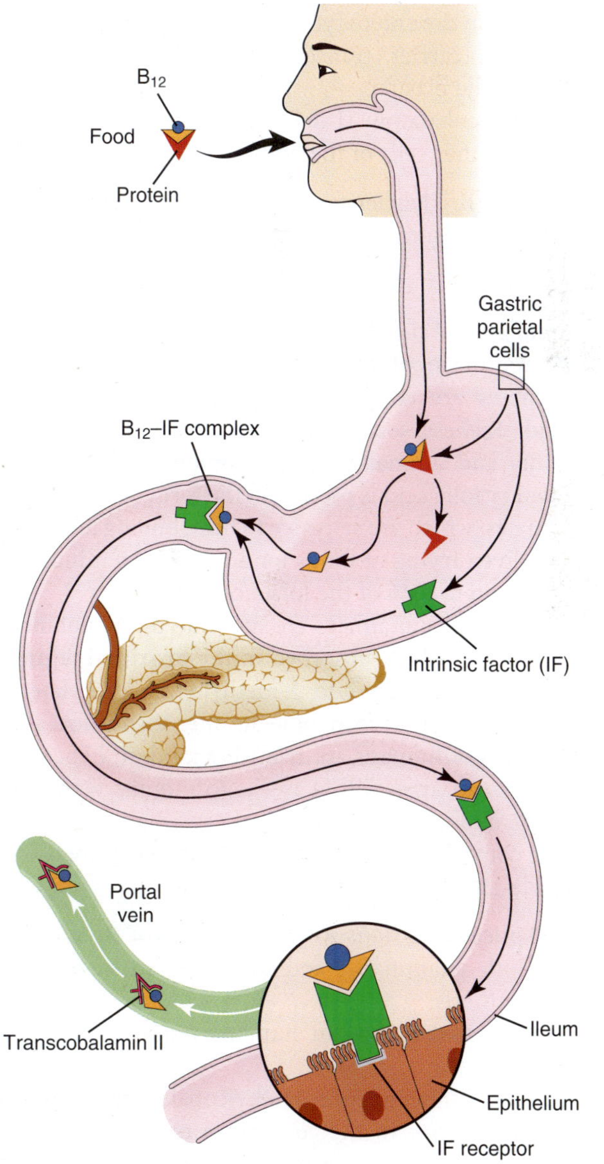

Fig. 15.12 Illustration of vitamin B_{12} absorption. *(Source:* From Vinay Kumar, Abul K. Abbas and Jon C. Aster. Red Blood Cell and Bleeding Disorders. Robbins & Cotran Pathologic Basis of Disease. 10th edition. Elsevier 2021.)

Table 15.10 Common Causes of Vitamin B_{12} Deficiency

Category	Common examples
Decreased intake	Inadequate diet Vegetarianism
Impaired absorption	Intrinsic factor deficiency • Pernicious anaemia • Gastrectomy Malabsorption states Diffuse intestinal disease • Lymphoma • Systemic sclerosis Competitive parasite uptake • Tapeworm infestation Bacterial overgrowth in blind loops

4. Within the enterocytes, vitamin B_{12} gets bound to its major carrier, transcobalamin II, and is secreted into the plasma.
5. Transcobalamin II delivers vitamin B_{12} to the liver and other cells of the body.

Vitamin B_{12} deficiency can be due to a decreased intake or impaired absorption, and the common causes are listed in Table 15.10.

Normal Folic Acid Metabolism

Daily requirement: 50–200 μg

Humans are completely dependent on dietary folic acid. Richest sources are green vegetables, whereas fruits and animal products contain lesser amounts. Dietary folic acid is present in the form of folylpolyglutamates, which are sensitive to heat, boiling and steaming. Even frying of foods for a mere 5–10 minutes destroys up to 95% of the folate content.

Dietary polyglutamates are split into monoglutamates, which are readily absorbed in the **proximal jejunum**. These are modified to 5-methyltetrahydrofolate, the normal transport form of folate after absorption. Folate reserves of humans are relatively modest; hence, deficiency can arise within weeks to months with inadequate intake.

The common causes of folic acid deficiency are listed in Table 15.11.

Biochemical Reactions Requiring Vitamin B_{12} and Folic Acid Both vitamin B_{12} and folic acid are required for DNA synthesis.

Only two reactions in humans require vitamin B_{12} (Fig. 15.13).

In one of the reactions, methylcobalamin serves as an essential cofactor in the conversion of homocysteine to methionine by methionine synthase. In the process, methylcobalamin yields a methyl group that is recovered from N5-methyltetrahydrofolic acid (N5-methyl-FH_4), the principal form of folic acid in plasma. In the same

Table 15.11 Common Causes of Folic Acid Deficiency

Category	Common examples
Decreased intake	Inadequate diet Alcoholism
Impaired absorption	Malabsorption states Intrinsic intestinal disease
Increased requirement	Pregnancy Infancy Disseminated cancer
Increased loss	Haemodialysis
Impaired utilization	Folic acid antagonists
Unresponsive to vitamin B_{12} or folic acid therapy: Metabolic inhibitors of DNA synthesis or folic acid metabolism – e.g. methotrexate	

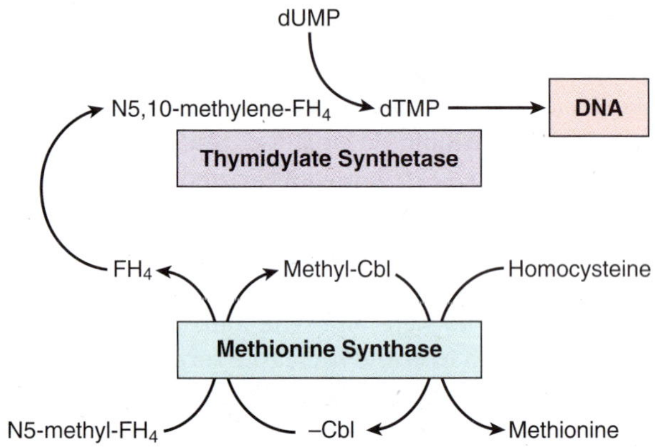

Fig. 15.13 Reactions that require vitamin B_{12} as a cofactor. In cobalamin (Cbl) deficiency, folate is sequestered as N5-methyl-FH_4, depriving thymidylate synthetase of its folate coenzyme (N5,10-methylene-FH_4), and thereby impairing DNA synthesis. dTMP, deoxythymidine monophosphate; dUMP, deoxyuridine monophosphate; FH_4, tetrahydrofolic acid. *(Source:* From Vinay Kumar, Abul K. Abbas and Jon C. Aster. Red Blood Cell and Bleeding Disorders. Robbins & Cotran Pathologic Basis of Disease. 10th edition. Elsevier 2021.)

reaction, N5-methyl-FH_4 is converted to tetrahydrofolic acid (FH_4).

The functions of FH_4 are crucial, because it is required for the conversion of deoxyuridine monophosphate (dUMP) to deoxythymidine monophosphate (dTMP), the building blocks for DNA (Fig. 15.14).

Pathogenesis It is clear that the functions of vitamin B_{12} and folic acid are required for the synthesis of thymidine, one of the four bases of DNA. Thus, megaloblastic anaemias are characterized by **defective nuclear maturation** due to inadequate DNA synthesis, causing delay in cell division. This results in abnormal morphological changes in cells and ineffective haematopoiesis in the marrow.

The basis of impaired DNA synthesis in vitamin B_{12} deficiency is the reduced availability of FH_4, most of

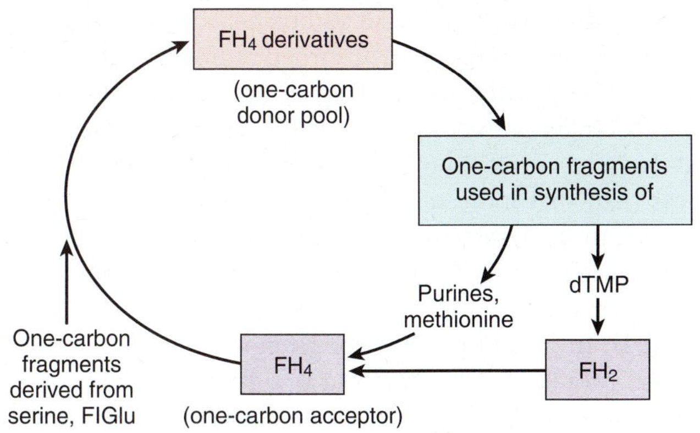

Fig. 15.14 Role of folate derivatives in the transfer of one-carbon fragments for the synthesis of biological macromolecules. dTMP, deoxythymidine monophosphate; FH_2, dihydrofolic acid; FH_4, tetrahydrofolic acid; FIGlu, formiminoglutamate. *(Source:* From Vinay Kumar, Abul K. Abbas and Jon C. Aster. Red Blood Cell and Bleeding Disorders. Robbins & Cotran Pathologic Basis of Disease. 10th edition. Elsevier 2021.)

which is 'trapped' as N5-methyl-FH_4. The FH_4 deficit may further be exacerbated by an internal folate deficiency caused by the failure to synthesize metabolically active polyglutamylated forms. This stems from the requirement of vitamin B_{12} for the synthesis of methionine from homocysteine, which contributes a carbon group needed in the metabolic reactions that create polyglutamates.

Pathogenesis of Neurological Complications Adenosyl cobalamin is the cofactor for the enzyme methylmalonyl-coenzyme A (CoA) mutase in the conversion of methylmalonyl-CoA to succinyl-CoA, as shown in Fig. 15.13. In the setting of vitamin B_{12} deficiency, this step gets blocked, resulting in the accumulation of methyl malonate and propionate (a precursor) and incorporation of these abnormal fatty acids into neuronal lipids is the suggested mechanism for neurological complications of vitamin B_{12} deficiency.

Morphology

Morphological changes are similar for all megaloblastic anaemias and are commonly described here.

Peripheral Smear All the blood cells are reduced in number with the resultant **pancytopenia.** Macrocytic and oval red cells, **macro-ovalocytes**, are characteristic with marked aniospoikilocytosis. Neutrophils are larger in size with **hypersegmentation** of the nuclear lobes (five to six lobes instead of normal three to four lobes) (Fig. 15.15).

Normoblasts, which are nucleated red cell progenitors, are sometimes seen in the peripheral blood. **Reticulocytopenia** is a consistent finding, because the erythropoiesis is ineffective.

Bone Marrow Bone marrow is markedly hypercellular with the following changes in the lineages:

Erythroid series: Megaloblastic changes of the pronormoblasts with deeply basophilic cytoplasm, fine nuclear chromatin and prominent nucleoli, which are the gold standard findings (cytoplasmic maturation is normal with the accumulation of haemoglobin, whereas nuclear maturation lags behind, which is referred to as 'nuclear cytoplasmic asynchrony')
Granulocytic series: Giant metamyelocytes and bands
Megakaryocytic series: Giant megakaryocytes with bizarre multilobated nuclei

In spite of the marrow cellularity, pancytopenia is the result of ineffective haematopoiesis. Owing to maturation defect, the abnormal cells undergo apoptosis in the marrow itself.

Management

Laboratory Investigations Pancytopenia along with reduced levels of haemoglobin and haematocrit values is a characteristic finding. Elevated levels of MCV, MCH and normal MCHC are consistent findings. Reticulocyte count is invariably depressed. Indirect hyperbilirubinaemia and elevated lactate dehydrogenase (LDH) levels are due to mild haemolysis of an unknown mechanism. Formiminoglutamate (FIGlu) excretion test is performed and is described later. Serum homocysteine and methylmalonic acid levels are elevated. Specific tests include measurement of serum vitamin B_{12} and folic acid levels, which are reduced depending on the aetiology.

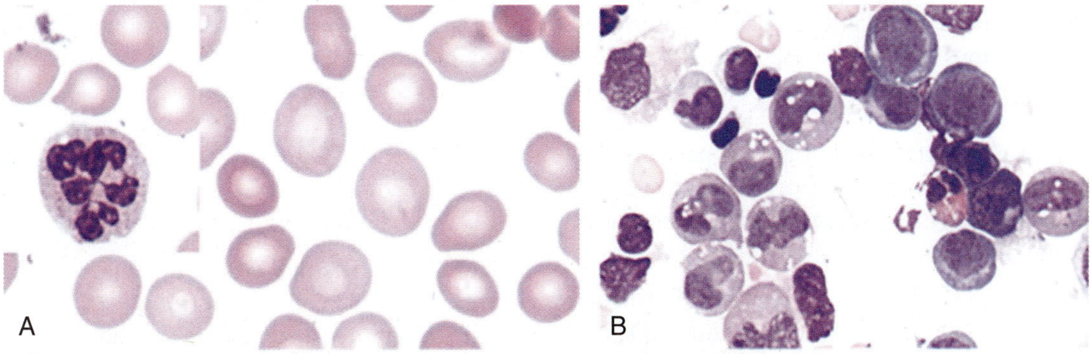

Fig. 15.15 Peripheral smear (A) exhibits macro-ovalocytosis and hypersegmented neutrophils (inset). Bone marrow aspirate (B) shows megaloblastic changes in both granulopoiesis and erythropoiesis.

Morphological features seen in peripheral smear and bone marrow are characteristic.

FIGlu excretion test: FIGlu is excreted in excessive amounts in folate deficiency. In this test, a 15-g oral dose of histidine is given to the patient and urinary excretion of FIGlu is measured by spectrophotometry. Increased excretion of FIGlu occurs in vitamin B_{12} deficiency.

Treatment Megaloblastic anaemia due to vitamin B_{12} and folic acid deficiency is treated with oral or parenteral vitamin B_{12} or folic acid depending on the deficient vitamin. Diagnosing and treating the underlying cause are crucial.

Pernicious Anaemia Pernicious anaemia is a disease of older adults with autoimmune destruction of the gastric mucosa. This disorder is commonly associated with other autoimmune disorders like autoimmune thyroiditis and adrenalitis. It is characterized by the **lack of intrinsic factor** due to destruction of gastric parietal epithelial cells, leading to vitamin B_{12} deficiency.

Autoreactive T cells initiate mucosal injury and also trigger the formation of autoantibodies.

Autoantibodies are of diagnostic importance.

Types of Autoantibodies in Pernicious Anaemia

A. Type 1: Blocks the binding of vitamin B_{12} with intrinsic factor
B. Type 2: Blocks the binding of vitamin B_{12}–intrinsic factor complex with ileal receptor
C. Type 3: Against the α and β subunits of the gastric proton pump of the parietal epithelial cells

Morphology of Stomach

It shows chronic atrophic gastritis with intestinalization (intestinal metaplasia) of the gastric mucosa and megaloblastic changes in the nuclei.

Clinical Features Clinical features are those of megaloblastic anaemias with gastritis. Features of other associated autoimmune diseases may dominate the clinical picture.

Investigations Pernicious anaemia was diagnosed in the past using the Schilling test, but nowadays serum vitamin B_{12} levels, autoantibody titres and gastric biopsy are used to diagnose pernicious anaemia.

Schilling Test Schilling test is used in the evaluation of absorption of vitamin B_{12} in the gastrointestinal tract and is performed in two parts – parts I and II; part I is performed to identify the presence of defect in vitamin B_{12} absorption, and part II is performed to identify the cause of defective absorption.

Part I: In this part of the test, 0.5–1 μg of radiolabelled vitamin B_{12} is given orally. An intramuscular dose of 1000 μg of unlabelled vitamin B_{12} is given after 2 hours to saturate the vitamin B_{12}–binding sites of transcobalamin I and II and to displace any bound radiolabelled vitamin B_{12} to allow urinary excretion of absorbed radiolabelled vitamin B_{12}. Subsequently, urine samples are collected and the radioactivity is measured as a percentage of total oral doses. The cutoff value is 7%, above which is normal and less than that indicates impaired absorption, which may be due to small intestinal malabsorption or due to the lack of intrinsic factor. If part I has abnormal results, then part II is performed.

Part II: In part II, patients are given intrinsic factor along with oral radiolabelled vitamin B_{12}. The remaining part is carried out as in part I. If excretion of radiolabelled vitamin B_{12} is greater than 7%, then the cause is concluded as pernicious anaemia, whereas if the values remain lower than 7%, then small intestinal malabsorption is the probable cause.

The test results are unreliable in chronic renal disease due to impaired excretion. This test should be performed after blood samples are obtained for vitamin B_{12} assay, because the large parenteral dose of vitamin B_{12} alters the serum levels of vitamin B_{12}.

Owing to the introduction of much simpler, noninvasive and specific tests, Schilling test is not being performed nowadays.

Treatment Vitamin B_{12} deficiency is managed with parenteral vitamin B_{12}. Patients with pernicious anaemia are at a higher risk of gastric carcinoma development due to the chronic inflammation and the metaplastic and dysplastic changes of the gastric mucosa and hence require close follow-up.

Anaemia of Chronic Disease

Anaemia of chronic disease or anaemia of chronic systemic inflammation is due to chronic diseases associated with inflammation causing impairment of red cell production. This type of anaemia is emerging as a common cause of anaemia, especially in developed countries. It is difficult to estimate its actual incidence and it is often diagnosed as a disease of exclusion because it is often confused with iron-deficiency anaemia.

Common disorders causing this type of anaemia are listed in Table 15.12.

Pathogenesis Pathogenesis of anaemia of chronic disorders is still not very clear. The major mechanism postulated includes the suppression of erythroid progenitors and impaired utilization of iron.

- **Decreased red cell survival**
  Diseases associated with anaemia of chronic disorders cause enhancement of phagocytic activity of macrophages and exaggerated sensitivity to mild alterations in red cells, leading to their premature destruction.
- **Decreased red cell production**
  The reasons for anaemia are as follows:
  - Inflammatory mediator-induced suppression of erythropoietin levels

Table 15.12 Common Causes of Anaemia of Chronic Disease

Category of Disorder	Common Examples
Chronic infections	Osteomyelitis Bacterial endocarditis Lung abscess Chronic urinary tract infections
Chronic immune disorders	Rheumatoid arthritis Ulcerative colitis
Neoplasms	Carcinoma of breast Carcinoma of lung Hodgkin lymphoma
Miscellaneous	Chronic rejection after solid-organ transplantation Chronic kidney disease and inflammation

- Production of hepcidin induced by raised **IL-6** associated with systemic inflammation, which impairs iron absorption and leads to reduced production of red cells
- **Impaired metabolism of iron**
  Sequestration of iron in macrophages under the influence of hepcidin results in low availability of iron for erythropoiesis. Some cytokines act by directly inhibiting erythropoietin production in the kidneys and also inhibit proliferation of erythroid progenitors.

Clinical Features Mild anaemia occurs with predominant symptoms of the underlying disease. Differentiating anaemia of chronic disease from iron-deficiency anaemia is a common clinical dilemma and is extremely essential because the treatment of both the conditions is entirely different. Differences between the two are listed in Table 15.13.

Morphology

Peripheral smear shows normocytic normochromic or microcytic hypochromic anaemia.

Bone marrow reveals the increased storage iron in marrow macrophages.

Laboratory Investigations Laboratory investigations reveal reduced levels of haemoglobin, MCV, MCH, serum iron, serum iron-binding capacity, erythropoietin and reticulocyte count. Serum ferritin, which is an indicator of bone marrow iron stores, is elevated. Apart from these parameters, erythrocyte sedimentation rate and C-reactive protein are elevated due to the underlying disorders and elevated cytokines.

Treatment Treating the underlying cause corrects the anaemia. In some cases, administration of erythropoietin may be beneficial.

Table 15.13 Differences Between Anaemia of Chronic Disease and Iron-Deficiency Anaemia

Feature	Anaemia of Chronic Disease	Iron-Deficiency Anaemia
MCV	Reduced or normal	Reduced
Serum iron	Reduced or normal	Reduced
Transferrin saturation	Reduced or normal	Reduced
TIBC	Reduced	Increased
Serum ferritin	Increased or normal	Reduced
Serum transferrin receptor	Normal	Increased
Serum transferrin/ serum ferritin index	Low, <1	High, >1
Bone marrow storage iron	Normal or increased	Reduced or absent
Degree of anaemia	Mild	Variable
Manifestations of underlying disease	Chronic infection Chronic inflammation	Malnutrition Chronic blood loss
Neoplasms	Present or absent	Present or absent

MCV, mean corpuscular volume; TIBC, total iron-binding capacity.

Sideroblastic Anaemia

Sideroblastic anaemia is a group of inherited and acquired bone marrow disorders due to abnormal utilization of iron during erythropoiesis. There are different types of sideroblastic anaemias, and the common feature they share is the presence of sideroblasts. This group of anaemia is characterized by dimorphic or microcytic hypochromic anaemia, the presence of ring sideroblasts in the bone marrow and ineffective erythropoiesis. Causes of sideroblastic anaemia are listed in Table 15.14.

Pathogenesis Pathogenesis of sideroblastic anaemia is yet to be completely understood. Primary pathology is at the level of haem synthesis in the mitochondria, which is impaired, thus leading to its accumulation in the mitochondria and resulting in the formation of sideroblasts.

Iron uptake within erythroblasts is regulated by intracellular levels of haem and in sideroblastic anaemia, defective haem synthesis is coupled with an increased iron uptake due to the absence of feedback inhibition.

Morphology

Sideroblastic anaemia is primarily a pathological diagnosis made on the basis of bone marrow examination

Table 15.14 Causes of Sideroblastic Anaemia

Type	Subtypes	Causes
Hereditary		
Acquired	Primary	Refractory anaemia with ringed sideroblasts
	Secondary	Haematological malignancies • Myeloproliferative disorders • Multiple myeloma • Acute myeloid leukaemia – M6 Drugs • Isoniazid • Pyrazinamide • Cycloserine • Chloramphenicol Alcoholism Lead poisoning Others • Collagen vascular disorders • Carcinoma

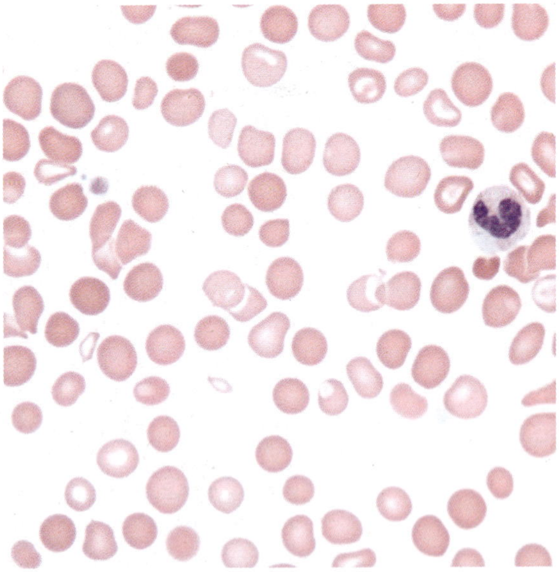

Fig. 15.17 Peripheral smear with dimorphic blood picture in sideroblastic anaemia. *(Source:* From Dita Gratzinger and Peter L. Greenberg. Update on Myelodysplastic Syndromes Classification and Prognosis. Surgical Pathology Clinics. 2013;6:693-728.)

with Prussian blue stain. Sideroblasts are erythroblasts containing aggregated iron in their mitochondria (Fig. 15.16). In Prussian blue–stained smear, abnormal iron–laden mitochondria appear to encircle erythroblast nuclei, giving rise to the defining morphological feature of the ring sideroblasts. Sideroblasts are not pathognomonic of any particular disease but rather are a manifestation of varied disorders. Peripheral smear shows dimorphic anaemia with a dual population of normocytic normochromic anaemia and microcytic hypochromic anaemia (Fig. 15.17).

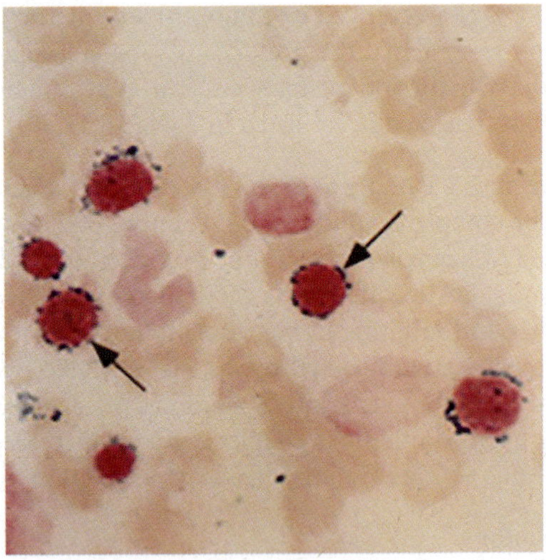

Fig. 15.16 Bone marrow smear stained with Prussian blue demonstrating the presence of sideroblasts. *(Source:* From Sylvia S. Bottomley and Mark D. Fleming. Sideroblastic Anemia. Hematology/Oncology Clinics of North America. 2014;28:653-670.)

Treatment Treatment of sideroblastic anaemia is based on the primary cause and includes removal of toxic agents; administration of pyridoxine, thiamine or folic acid; transfusion; and bone marrow or liver transplantation.

Aplastic Anaemia **PA 17.1**

Aplastic anaemia is a syndrome of **chronic primary haematopoietic failure** with resultant pancytopenia in the absence of any underlying neoplasia or reticulin fibrosis. The term 'aplastic anaemia' is a misnomer, because the disease causes pancytopenia and not just anaemia.

Aetiology There are varied aetiological factors for aplastic anaemia. The common causes are listed in Table 15.15.

Most cases are sporadic with an autoimmune basis but can be congenital or occur as a consequence of different germline genetic defects.

Pathogenesis (Fig. 15.18) It is not completely understood, but two major causative mechanisms have been proposed:

1. Extrinsic immune-mediated suppression
2. Intrinsic abnormality of stem cells

Both the mechanisms work independently and affect the stem cells by inducing the expression of neoantigens that evoke autoimmune reaction or give rise to a clonal population with **reduced proliferative capacity**. Both the pathways lead to marrow aplasia. In some cases, the presence of karyotypic abnormalities supports stem cell defects as the fundamental cause.

Table 15.15 Causes of Aplastic Anaemia

Category	Subcategory	Examples
Acquired	Idiopathic	
	Acquired stem cell defects	
	Infectious agents	Hepatitis – non-A, non-B, non-C, non-G type Cytomegalovirus Epstein–Barr virus Herpes zoster
	Chemical agents	**Dose related** • Alkylating agents • Antimetabolites • Benzene • Chloramphenicol • Inorganic arsenicals **Idiosyncratic** • Chloramphenicol • Phenylbutazone • Organic arsenicals • Penicillamine
	Physical agents	Whole-body irradiation
	Other conditions	Pregnancy Thymoma Autoimmune diseases
Constitutional	• Fanconi anaemia • Telomerase defects • Dyskeratosis congenita • Shwachman–Diamond syndrome • Congenital amegakaryocytic thrombocytopenia	

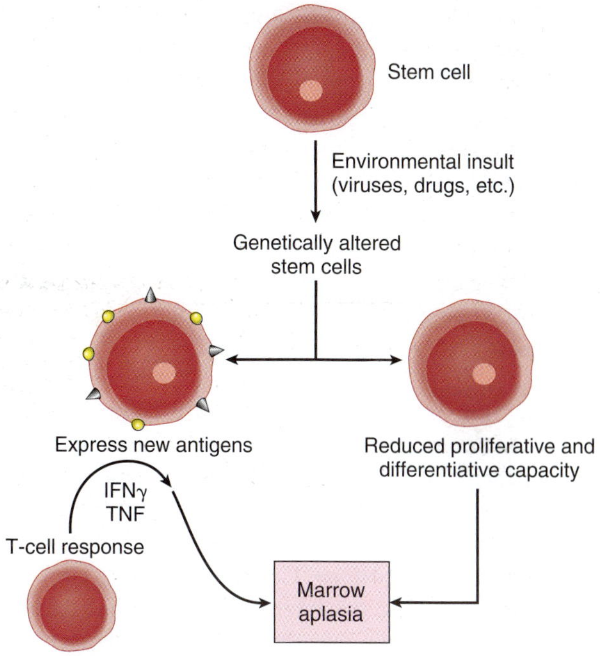

Fig. 15.18 Pathogenesis of aplastic anaemia. (*Source:* Vinay Kumar, Abul K. Abbas and Jon C. Aster. Red Blood Cell and Bleeding Disorders. Robbins & Cotran Pathologic Basis of Disease. 10th edition. Elsevier 2021.)

Morphology

Peripheral smear examination reveals pancytopenia with macrocytic or normocytic normochromic anaemia. **Reticulocytopenia** is the rule.
Bone marrow aspiration yields a typical 'dry tap'.
Bone marrow biopsy (best investigation for aplastic anaemia) shows **hypocellular marrow** devoid of haematopoietic cells with the predominance of fat cells and scattered lymphocytes and plasma cells (Fig. 15.19).

Clinical Features Early manifestations depend on the predominant lineage affected, but ultimately pancytopenia ensues. Fatigue, recurrent infections and spontaneous superficial bleeding due to anaemia, leucopenia and

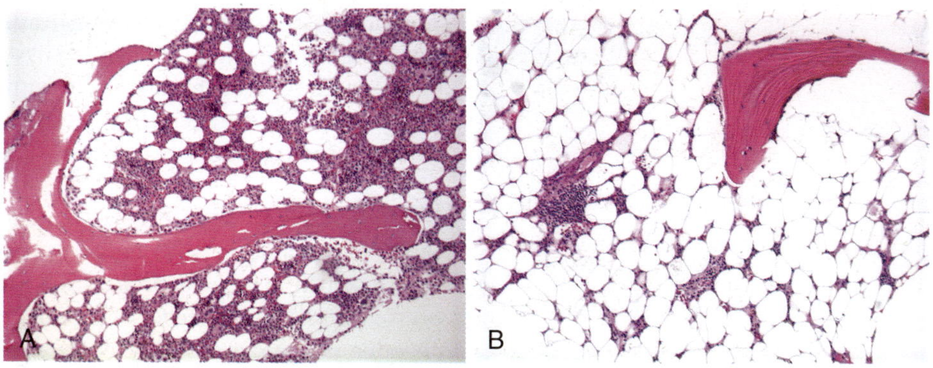

Fig. 15.19 Bone marrow hypocellularity on the right (B) in contrast with normal bone marrow on the left (A) on bone marrow biopsy. (*Source:* From Grover C. Bagby. Aplastic Anemia and Related Bone Marrow Failure States. Goldman-Cecil Medicine. 26th edition. Elsevier 2020.)

thrombocytopenia manifest. **Splenomegaly is typically absent**; if present, the diagnosis of aplastic anaemia is seriously doubted.

Differentiating aplastic anaemia from other disorders causing pancytopenia is crucial because the treatment is completely different. Hence, bone marrow aspiration or biopsy is essential in the evaluation of every case of pancytopenia, especially if the clinical findings are demanding and the anaemia is refractory. Diseases associated with pancytopenia may have hypocellular or hypercellular marrow and are listed in Table 15.16.

Complications Aplastic anaemia might complicate with transformation to myelodysplastic syndrome or acute myeloid leukaemia by acquiring additional genetic insults.

Management

Laboratory Investigations Complete blood cell count parameters are reduced – haemoglobin and haematocrit, total count, absolute neutrophil count and platelets. Reticulocytopenia is a striking feature. Levels of serum iron and ferritin are elevated because they are not used due to suppression of haematopoiesis. Aplastic anaemia is graded as nonsevere, severe and very severe on the basis of peripheral blood counts and corrected reticulocyte count.

Nonsevere aplastic anaemia:
- Haemoglobin <10 g/dL
- Absolute neutrophil count <1500/mm^3
- Platelet count <50,000/mm^3

Severe aplastic anaemia: Any two of the following three parameters are required for the diagnosis:
- Absolute neutrophil count <500/mm^3
- Platelets <20,000/mm^3
- Corrected reticulocyte counts <1.0%

Table 15.16 Causes of Pancytopenia

Pancytopenia with Hypocellular Marrow	Pancytopenia with Cellular Marrow
Aplastic anaemia[a]	Megaloblastic anaemia
Hypocellular MDS (uncommon presentation)	Myelodysplastic syndrome
Hypocellular acute leukaemia (uncommon presentation)	Acute leukaemia
Paroxysmal nocturnal haemoglobinuria	Lymphoma
Hairy cell leukaemia (due to reticulin fibrosis)	Storage disorders
Lymphoma	Hypersplenism
Myelofibrosis	Autoimmune disorders

MDS, myelodysplastic syndrome.
[a]Most common cause.

Very severe aplastic anaemia:
- Absolute neutrophil count <200/mm^3
- Platelets <20,000/mm^3
- Corrected reticulocyte counts <1.0%

Treatment In patients with nonsevere aplastic anaemia, the main form of treatment is supportive in the form of blood transfusion with the hope of achieving spontaneous recovery. There are two forms of treatment of severe and very severe aplastic anaemias – allogenic HSC transplantation and immunosuppression. Younger patients (younger than 40 years) can be cured with HSC transplantation, and older patients can be treated with transfusion support and immunosuppressive therapy with close follow-up.

OTHER FORMS OF MARROW SUPPRESSION

Anaemia of Chronic Renal Failure

Anaemia is a common feature of patients with chronic renal failure occurring due to the following mechanisms:

a. Failure of erythropoietin production by the kidneys
b. Uraemia leading to inhibition of differentiation and proliferation of erythroid progenitors
c. Red cell life span shortened due to inhibition of hexose monophosphate (HMP) shunt and membrane Na^+–K^+ pump
d. Bleeding due to defective platelet function
e. Microangiopathic haemolytic anaemia (MAHA) in some cases

Clinical Features Signs and symptoms of chronic renal failure dominate the clinical picture in the majority of cases, whereas in some patients, anaemia may be the predominant cause of symptoms.

Laboratory Findings Anaemia is typically normocytic and normochromic with a normal or reduced reticulocyte count. **Burr cells**, red cells with regularly spaced tiny projections on the surface, are a common finding in anaemia due to chronic renal failure. Serum erythropoietin levels are lower for the degree of anaemia.

Treatment Renal transplantation leads to rapid correction of anaemia, whereas haemodialysis offers some improvement. Androgens are used with partial benefits. Recombinant human erythropoietin is effective and is currently the treatment of choice.

Pure Red Cell Aplasia

Pure red cell aplasia (PRCA) is a primary marrow disorder in which erythroid progenitors are selectively suppressed, with other lineages being unaffected. This type of anaemia is characterized by normocytic normochromic anaemia and reticulocytopenia. The common causes of PRCA are listed in Table 15.17.

Table 15.17 Causes of Pure Red Cell Aplasia

Category	Causes
Constitutional	Diamond–Blackfan syndrome
Neoplasms	Thymoma Large granular lymphocytic leukaemias 5q-myelodysplastic syndrome
Infections	Parvovirus B19 infection
Autoimmune disorders	Collagen vascular disorders Myasthenia gravis
Drugs	Phenytoin, azathioprine and isoniazid

PRCA Due to Parvovirus B19 Infection PRCA occurs during the course of chronic haemolytic anaemias in children with sickle cell anaemia, thalassaemia and glucose-6-phosphate dehydrogenase (G6PD) deficiency. Parvovirus B19 acts by causing selective cytopathic effect on erythroid precursors. In normal individuals, anaemia does not manifest due to the transient viral cytopathic effect and long life span of red cells. In patients with haemolytic anaemias, owing to the shortened life span of RBCs, patients present with sudden worsening of anaemia with reticulocytopenia and depletion of erythroid precursors in the bone marrow. In immunocompromised individuals, parvovirus B19 causes chronic PRCA, because the antibody response against the virus is poor. Children with PRCA have a self-limited illness, whereas adults tend to have a chronic course.

In patients with haemolytic anaemias presenting with haemolytic crisis due to parvovirus infection, blood transfusion is the main form of treatment. Immunosuppressive therapy can be tried with partial response, whereas treating the underlying illness is the main from of treatment.

Congenital Dyserythropoietic Anaemia

Congenital dyserythropoietic anaemia (CDA) is a rare group of inherited anaemias characterized by abnormal nuclear morphology of red cell precursors. The common features of this group of disorders are as follows:

- Presentation in childhood with anaemia, splenomegaly and jaundice
- Dyserythropoiesis with abnormal nuclear morphology of red cell precursors
- Ineffective erythropoiesis
- Iron accumulation

There are three types of CDA – types I, II and III – depending on the red cell nuclear morphology.

Red cell nuclear features include megaloblastoid features, bi- and multinucleated erythroblasts, giant erythroblasts, internuclear chromatin bridges, pleuripolar mitoses and karyorrhexis.

Dyserythropoiesis is seen in association with many other causes of anaemia such as megaloblastic anaemia, thalassaemia, alcoholism, drugs, acute myeloid leukaemia and certain infections. In CDA, dyserythropoiesis is primary (or congenital) and inborn.

Myelophthisic Anaemia

Myelophthisic anaemia is a group of disorders due to extensive space-occupying lesions of the marrow resulting in marrow failure. Common causes are listed in Table 15.18.

Morphology

Anaemia is mild to moderate with normocytic normochromic blood picture. Peripheral blood smear shows features like shift to the left of myeloid and erythroid series termed leucoerythroblastosis (Fig. 15.20) – **leucoerythroblastosis** along with teardrop-shaped red cells is an important blood smear finding. Total leucocyte count (TLC) and platelet count may be normal or reduced. Bone marrow studies are essential in all the cases to detect the underlying cause.

Clinical picture is dominated by the underlying illness. Treatment consists of management of the underlying primary disorder.

HAEMOLYTIC ANAEMIAS

PA 16.1, PA 16.2, PA 16.5

Haemolysis is the **premature destruction of erythrocytes**, and haemolytic anaemia develops when the bone marrow compensatory response is overcome by the loss of RBCs.

Table 15.18 Causes of Myelophthisic Anaemia

Category	Causes
Malignant Diseases	**Haematological** • Acute leukaemias • Chronic leukaemias • Myeloproliferative disorders • Multiple myeloma **Nonhaematological metastatic deposits from** • Lung carcinoma • Breast carcinoma • Gastric carcinoma • Prostatic carcinoma
Lipid Storage Diseases	Gaucher disease Niemann–Pick disease
Infectious Diseases	Miliary tuberculosis
Miscellaneous	Osteopetrosis Myelofibrosis

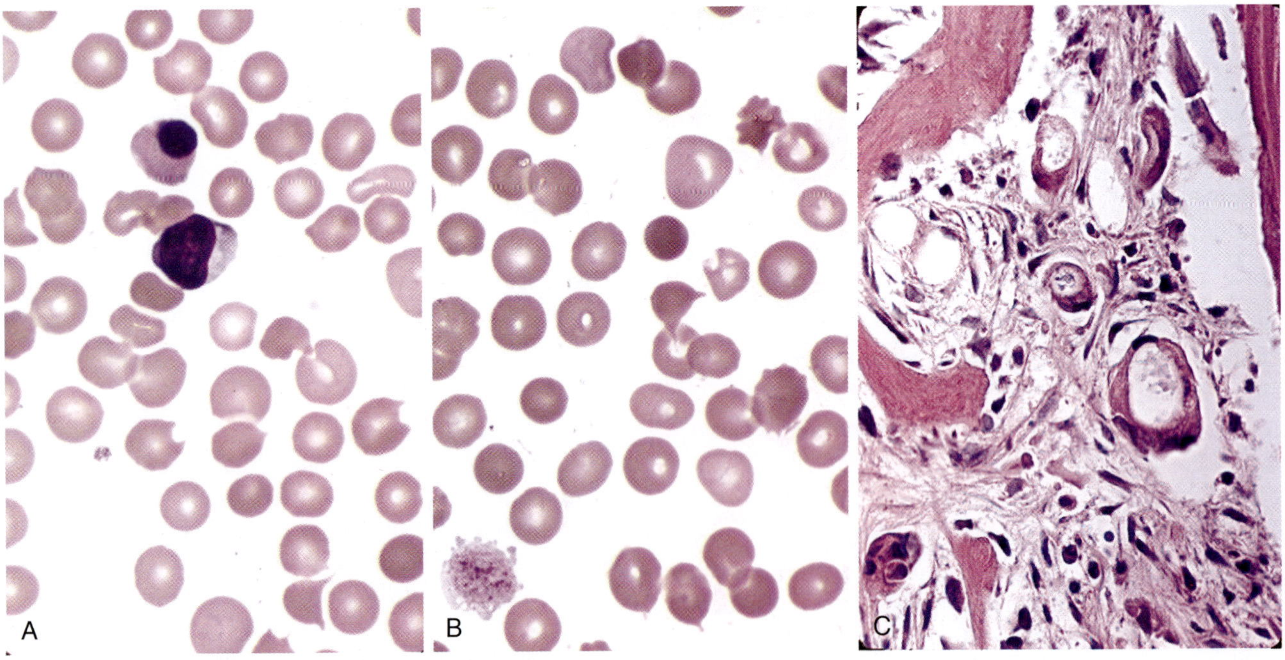

Fig. 15.20 Peripheral smear with leucoerythroblastic picture (A), giant platelet (B) in bone marrow showing metastatic adenocarcinoma (C) that had caused this effect. *(Source:* From Carla S. Wilson, Maria E. Vergara-Lluri and Russell K. Brynes. Evaluation of Anemia, Leukopenia, and Thrombocytopenia. Hematopathology. 2nd edition. Elsevier 2017.)

All haemolytic anaemias share the following features:

- **Shortened red cell life span**
- **Elevated erythropoietin + compensatory erythropoiesis**
- **Accumulation of haemoglobin degradation products**

Normally, senescent red cells undergo physiological destruction by macrophages of the spleen, liver and bone marrow after surviving for an average 120 days. This process is stimulated by age-dependent changes in RBC surface proteins, followed by their recognition and phagocytosis by macrophages. In haemolytic anaemias, the life span of red cells is significantly reduced to as low as 10 days in severe cases.

On the basis of the site of premature destruction of RBCs, haemolytic anaemias are classified into two categories – extravascular haemolytic anaemia and intravascular haemolytic anaemia (Fig. 15.21).

Extravascular haemolysis: Red cells are subjected to extreme changes in shape to navigate through splenic sinusoids. Owing to alterations that make red cells less deformable, these cells get trapped in splenic sinusoids and undergo premature phagocytosis by splenic macrophages. Hence, the triad of extravascular haemolytic anaemias includes ***anaemia, jaundice and splenomegaly***. Jaundice in haemolytic anaemias does not occur unless the haemolysis is severe or the liver function is compromised, and it is always due to unconjugated bilirubin. Excessive unconjugated bilirubin leads to the development of pigmented gallstones, which may be the first manifestation in some cases.

Example: HS

Intravascular haemolysis, which is less common, is seen in red cells that are destroyed by complement fixation, mechanical injury, parasites and toxins.

The sequence of events in intravascular haemolysis is as follows:

1. Lysis of red cells → haemoglobinaemia, haemoglobinuria
2. Oxidation of free haemoglobin → methaemoglobin, methaemoglobinuria
3. Free haemoglobin bound by haptoglobin synthesized by the liver to promote its clearance → reduction in the levels of serum haptoglobin
4. Iron released from haemoglobin taken in and catabolized by proximal tubular epithelial cells and then stored as haemosiderin; the cells later shed in urine → renal haemosiderosis and haemosiderinuria
5. Breakdown of haemoglobin to degradation products → unconjugated bilirubinaemia

Splenomegaly is not a feature of intravascular haemolysis.

Example: Paroxysmal nocturnal haemoglobinuria (PNH)

Morphology (Fig. 15.22)

Bone marrow shows an increased number of erythroid precursors.

Peripheral blood shows anaemia and reticulocytosis. Polychromatophilic red cells in peripheral smear are

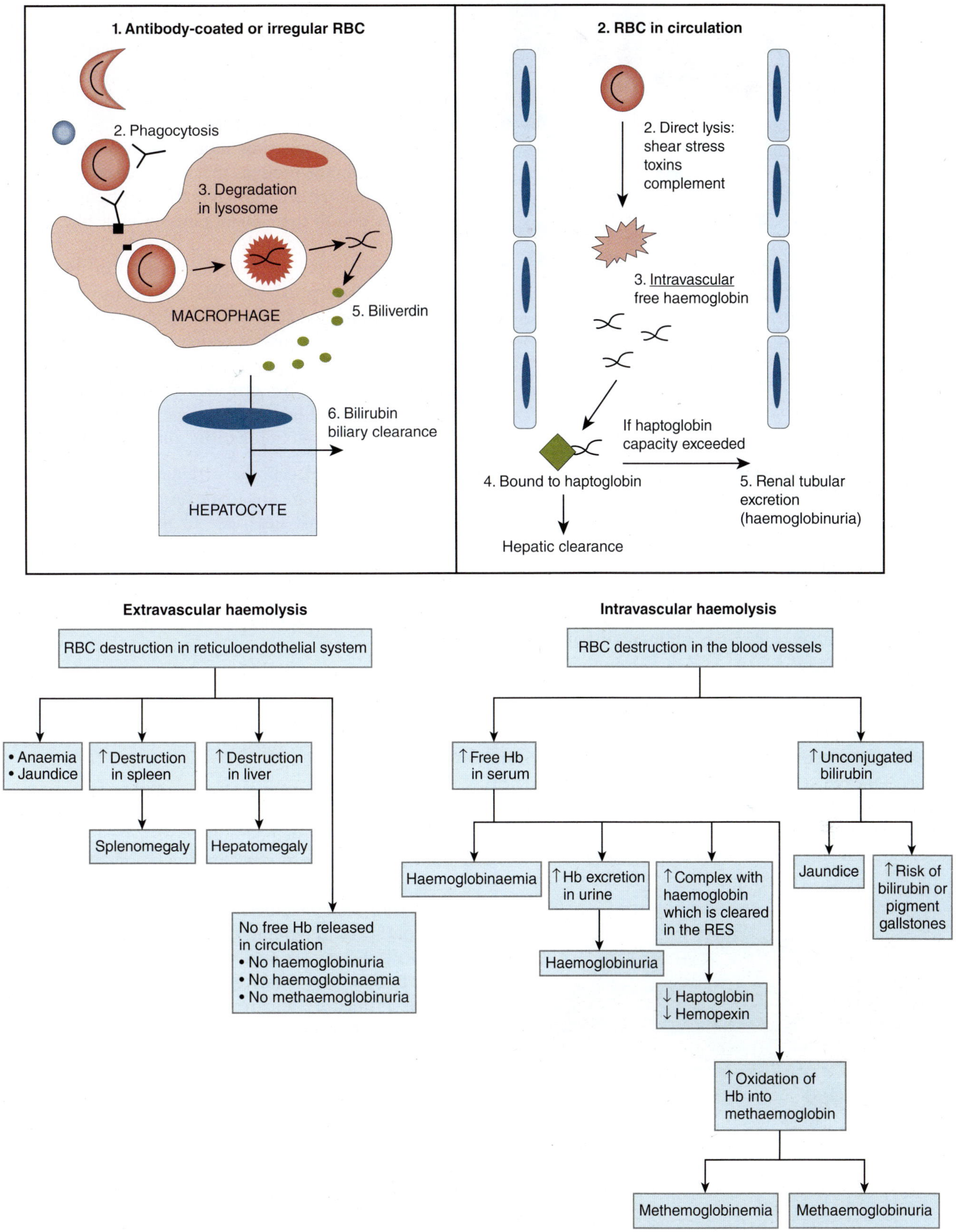

Fig. 15.21 Sequence of events in intravascular versus extravascular haemolysis.

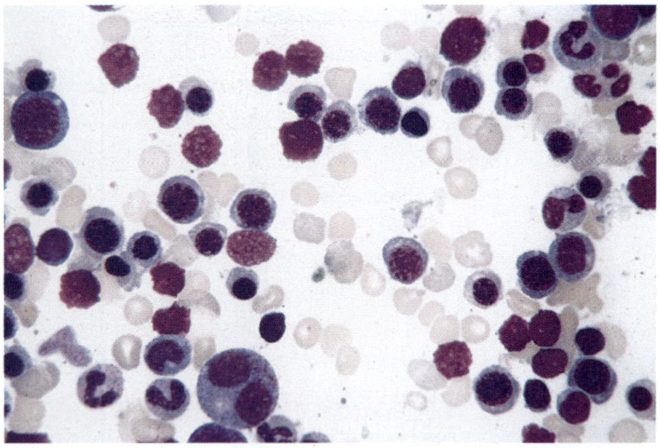

Fig. 15.22 Bone marrow morphology in haemolytic anaemia showing compensatory erythroid hyperplasia. *(Source:* From Vinay Kumar, Abul K. Abbas and Jon C. Aster. Red Blood Cell and Bleeding Disorders. Robbins & Cotran Pathologic Basis of Disease. 10th edition. Elsevier 2021.)

equivalent to reticulocytes and are stained with supravital stains like brilliant cresyl blue and new methylene blue.

The liver, spleen and marrow may show features of **haemosiderosis**.

Liver, spleen and lymph nodes may exhibit features of **extramedullary haematopoiesis**. The gall bladder may develop **pigmented gallstones** (Fig. 15.23).

Hereditary Spherocytosis

HS is an inherited haemolytic disorder with an intrinsic defect of the red cells along with alterations in the red cell membrane and shape. The disease is commonly transmitted as **autosomal dominant** inheritance and was first described in 1871. It is the most common cause of inherited haemolysis in some parts of the world such as the European and North American Caucasian population, with an incidence of 1 in 5000 births. The clinical spectrum of HS ranges from symptom-free carrier state to severe haemolysis, because the disease manifests with incomplete penetrance and varied expression like other autosomal dominant disorders.

The disease is caused by mutations in genes related to red cell membrane proteins that allow red cells to change shape. Normal red cells have remarkable physicochemical properties due to their membrane skeleton that renders them extremely deformable and durable. The abnormal erythrocytes in HS are spherical instead of the normal biconcave disc-shaped. The defect in the membrane proteins makes the red cells nondeformable and rigid with a spherical shape because of which they are vulnerable to sequestration in the spleen and extravascular haemolysis. Investigation of HS has provided important insights into the structure and function of cell membranes and the role of the spleen in maintaining RBC integrity.

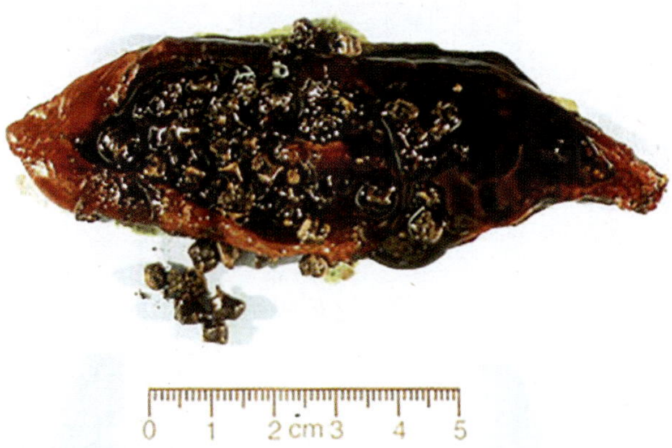

Fig. 15.23 Pigmented gallstones in extravascular haemolytic anaemia. *(Source:* From James M. Crawford. Gallbladder, Extrahepatic Biliary Tract, and Pancreas Tissue Processing Techniques and Normal Histology. In Odze and Goldblum Surgical Pathology of the GI Tract, Liver, Biliary Tract and Pancreas. 3rd edition. Elsevier 2015.)

Pathogenesis Red cells have remarkable deformability and flexibility that are due to the properties of their membrane skeleton that lies close to the inner side of the plasma membrane. Red cell membrane skeleton is supported by many protein complexes, all of which function to provide the red cells with their magical property of flexibility. The major ones are as follows:

- **Ankyrin**
- **Spectrin**
- **Band 3**
- **Band 4.2**
- **Band 4.1**
- **Actin**

Spectrin is composed of two polypeptide chains, α and β, which are intertwined and form helical heteromers. The head portions of spectrin dimers self-associate and form tetramers, whereas the tail portions attach themselves with actin oligomers. Every actin molecule binds to multiple spectrin tetramers, thus forming spectrin–actin cytoskeletal complex that is attached to the cell membrane by two other complexes of proteins. One such complex is formed by ankyrin and band 4.2, which binds spectrin with band 3. The other one is formed by protein 4.1, which connects the tail of spectrin to glycophorin, a transmembrane protein of red cells.

The complexes formed by interaction between these proteins are shown in Fig. 15.24.

The primary defect in HS is the deficiency of membrane surface area. Decreased surface area is the result of two different mechanisms (Fig. 15.25):

1. Defects of spectrin, ankyrin and protein 4.2, resulting in reduced density of membrane skeleton and destabilization of the overlying lipid layer
2. Defects of band 3, leading to loss of its lipid-stabilizing effect

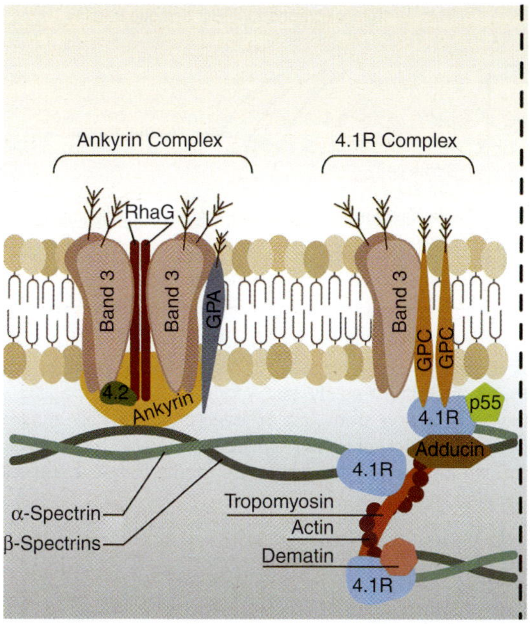

Fig. 15.24 Schematic representation of structure of red cell membrane skeleton. The skeleton network is composed of α-spectrin and β-spectrin tetramers linked to the 4.1R junctional complex containing actin, protein 4.1R, tropomyosin, adducin, dematin and p55. This network is tethered to the overlying lipid bilayer via vertical linkages involving ankyrin (ankyrin complex) and protein 4.1R (4.1R complex) that interact with different transmembrane proteins such as glycophorin A (GPA), glycophorin C (GPC), band 3 and Rh-associated glycoprotein (RhAG). (*Source:* From M. Tarek Elghetany and Katalin Banki. Erythrocytic Disorders. Henry's Clinical Diagnosis and Management by Laboratory Methods. 24th edition. Elsevier 2022.)

Both the mechanisms result in membrane loss, leading to decreased surface area with the formation of spherocytes that have reduced deformability.

HS occurs due to deficiency of any of these proteins; the commonest one is **ankyrin**.

The spleen targets and attacks any abnormally shaped RBCs, so it also destroys spherocytes. In the spleen, red cells need to be extremely flexible to pass through the narrow passage from the cords of Billroth into the sinusoids. In HS, red cells fail to pass through this bottleneck passage and get trapped and phagocytosed by splenic macrophages, resulting in extravascular haemolysis.

The sequence of events can be explained as follows: red cells are born with biconcave disc shape but have membrane protein deficiency → membrane stability is lost → partial loss of membrane → rearrangement of red cell structure with the remaining membrane → spherical shape → loss of deformability → sequestration of spherocytes in the splenic sinusoids → loss of water, potassium, glucose and pH → dehydration → exaggeration of spherocytosis → premature phagocytosis – **extravascular haemolysis.**

Morphology

Peripheral smear shows the presence of **microspherocytes** with reduced cell size and loss of central pallor (Fig. 15.26). Microspherocytosis is the striking feature, though not an exclusive feature of HS.

Features common to haemolytic anaemias like anaemia, unconjugated hyperbilirubinaemia, reticulocytosis and marrow erythroid hyperplasia are seen.

Pigmented cholelithiasis and moderate splenomegaly as features of extravascular haemolysis are characteristic.

Clinical Features Diagnosis of HS is based on family history, clinical features, haematological findings and laboratory evidence. Anaemia, splenomegaly and jaundice with variable severity are the common clinical features. Most patients with HS have a positive family

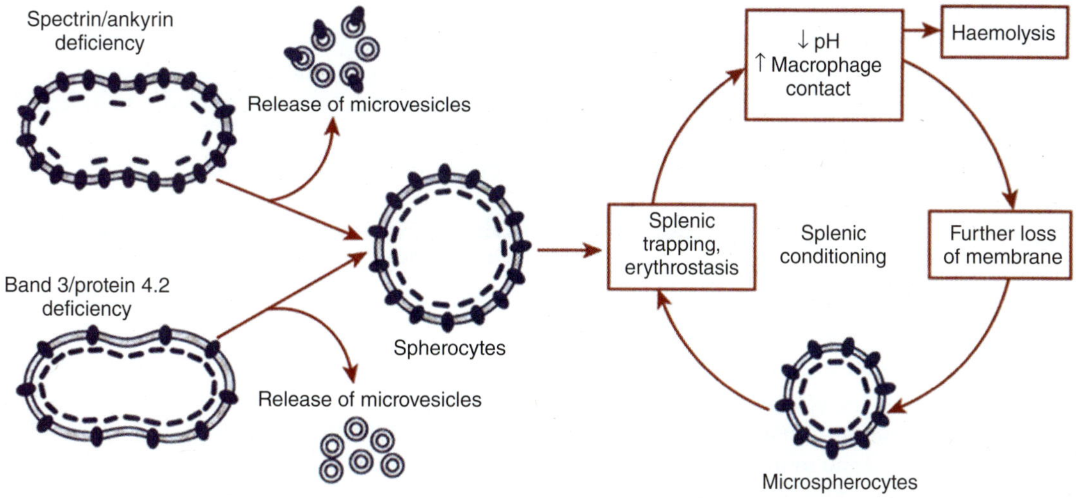

Fig. 15.25 The process of haemolysis in hereditary spherocytosis. Decreased surface area may occur due to (1) defects of spectrin, ankyrin or protein 4.2 and result in the release of band 3–containing microvesicles. (2) Band 3 deficiency and loss of its lipid-stabilizing effect result in the loss of band 3–free microvesicles. Both result in membrane loss, decreased surface area and the formation of spherocytes with decreased deformability that get trapped in the hostile environment of the spleen where splenic conditioning inflicts further membrane damage, amplifying the injury. (*Source:* From Patrick G. Gallagher. Red Blood Cell Membrane Disorders. Hematology: Basic Principles and Practice. 7th edition. Elsevier 2018.)

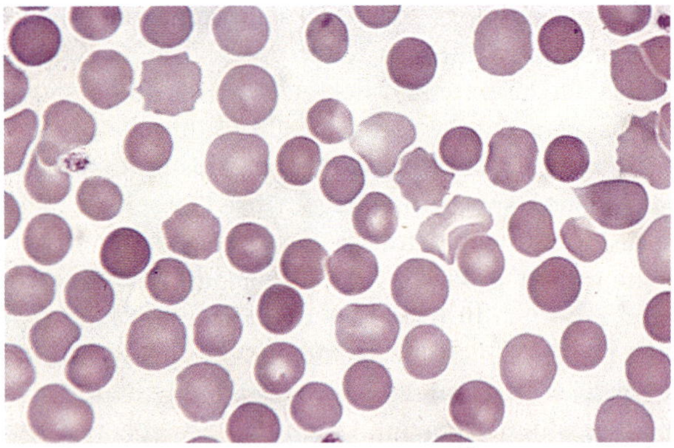

Fig. 15.26 Peripheral smear showing the presence of microspherocytes in HS. (*Source:* From Barbara J. Bain. Blood Cell Morphology in Health and Disease. Dacie and Lewis Practical Haematology. 12th edition. Elsevier 2017.)

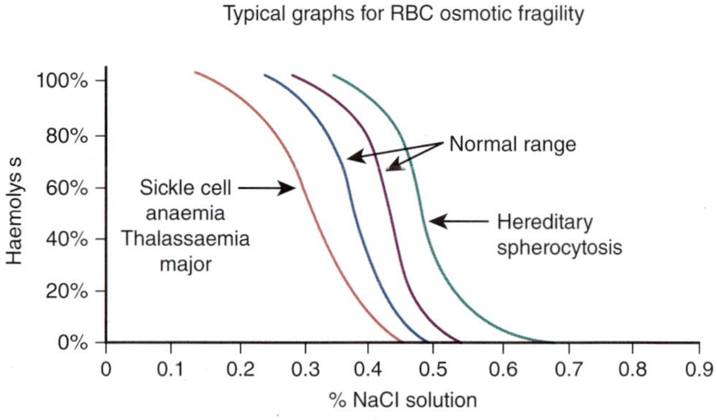

Fig. 15.27 Osmotic fragility test – graph. Osmotic fragility curves of patients suffering from the following: sickle cell anaemia, β-thalassaemia major, hereditary spherocytosis and 'idiopathic' warm autoimmune haemolytic anaemia. The normal range is indicated by the unbroken lines.

history. HS should be suspected in any child presenting with splenomegaly, anaemia and hyperbilirubinaemia. Patients may also present with asymptomatic cholelithiasis of undetermined aetiology, commonly with a positive family history. In up to 30% of patients, the disease remains clinically silent.

Features of chronic haemolysis are absent in neonates in whom the most common presentation is jaundice. HS should be suspected in neonates with hyperbilirubinaemia of an unknown cause. In a small percentage of children with HS, the disease manifests with severe jaundice and requires exchange transfusion.

About one-third of patients are well compensated with compensatory erythropoiesis. The remaining patients present with chronic haemolytic anaemia.

Episodes of **aplastic crisis** punctuate the course of disease due to infection by parvovirus B19, which preferentially infects erythroid progenitors. Transfusion support is needed till the marrow returns to function, with the immune response clearing the virus. **Haemolytic crisis** is precipitated by splenomegaly due to intercurrent infections like infectious mononucleosis.

Management

Laboratory Investigations **Osmotic fragility test** is performed in which the red cells are dropped into hypotonic saline solutions of descending concentration and checked for haemolysis. Normal red cells that are biconcave disc-shaped become spherical by imbibing water before they undergo lysis. In blood samples containing spherocytes, these cells have less margin for expansion and hence undergo premature lysis. Target cells undergo delayed lysis because they have membrane surface area to volume ratio opposite to that of spherocytes and more space to resist lysis.

Normally, the highest concentration of saline at which the haemolysis starts is 0.5% and the highest concentration of saline at which the haemolysis is complete is 0.3%. Fifty per cent lysis is seen with 0.4%–0.45% NaCl. Lysis of red cells before this concentration denotes increased fragility. A graph may be plotted with the amount of haemolysis on the *Y* axis and saline concentration on the *X* axis (Fig. 15.27).

Interpretation of Osmotic Fragility Test As shown in Fig. 15.27, the normal curve is sigmoid; a shift to the right indicates the presence of spherocytes and increased fragility, and a shift to the left occurs with target cells with relative resistance to haemolysis induced by osmosis. The curve may display a shift to the right with the presence of target cells in the blood sample as in thalassaemia and iron-deficiency anaemia.

This can be used as a screening test but not a confirmative test, because this proves the presence of spherocytes in blood and not HS. Remember that spherocytes are also seen in autoimmune haemolytic anaemia (AIHA), G6PD deficiency, pyruvate kinase deficiency, haemolytic disease of newborns and few other conditions.

Treatment Patients with symptomatic HS are managed with blood transfusion and the crisis is managed accordingly. **Splenectomy** is offered as the treatment of choice in symptomatic patients, refractory to conservative management. It is beneficial in such patients because the site of red cell destruction is removed, but splenectomy comes with its own price of depressed immunity and risk of recurrent infections and sepsis.

Glucose-6-Phosphate Dehydrogenase Deficiency

Haemolytic Anaemia Due to Red Cell Enzyme Defects

G6PD deficiency is the most common enzymatic disorder of red cells affecting 400 million people across the globe and is particularly prevalent in certain parts of Africa, Asia, Mediterranean countries and the Middle East. It was first reported in 1956 in a patient previously diagnosed as a case of 'primaquine sensitivity'.

G6PD is an enzyme involved in pentose monophosphate pathway and its function is to generate nicotinamide adenine dinucleotide phosphate hydrogen (NADPH), which is essential for the conversion of glutathione to its reduced form. Reduced glutathione is the major antioxidant of red cells.

Genetics The disease is commonly transmitted as **X-linked recessive** trait and therefore males are more commonly affected. G6PD deficiency is polymorphic, with more than 400 variants. Several hundred variants exist, but the majority of them are harmless.

Normal variant: **G6PD B**
Abnormal variant: **G6PD$^-$** (moderate reduction) and **G6PD Mediterranean** (marked reduction)

Mutation → misfolding of protein → proteolytic degradation → half-life of the enzyme reduced → deficiency of G6PD in older RBCs

Pathophysiology (Fig. 15.28) RBCs carry oxygen and are metabolically active, so these cells are susceptible to oxidative stress that is generally regulated by the normally functioning G6PD/NADPH pathway.

G6PD/NADPH pathway is the only source of reduced glutathione in the red cells, which is the major antioxidant of red cells. G6PD enzyme catalyses the oxidation of glucose-6-phosphate and the reduction of nicotinamide adenine dinucleotide ($NADP^+$) to NADPH in the pentose monophosphate shunt, which is an essential element in the maintenance of glutathione in its reduced form. **Glutathione protects the red cells from oxidative stress** only in this **reduced form.**

In patients with G6PD deficiency, red cells undergo oxidative stress and premature lysis. Mature red cells cannot synthesize new proteins, so enzyme activities of G6PD$^-$ or G6PD Mediterranean variants fall sharply. Thus, older cells are much more prone to undergo haemolysis than the younger red cells.

Haemolysis is precipitated with exposure to oxidative stress such as infections, drugs and certain food (Table 15.19). It is **episodic and self-limiting**, because only the older red cells are at risk of lysis, and comes to a halt when all the older cells are lysed; the sequence of events in G6PD deficiency can be explained as follows:

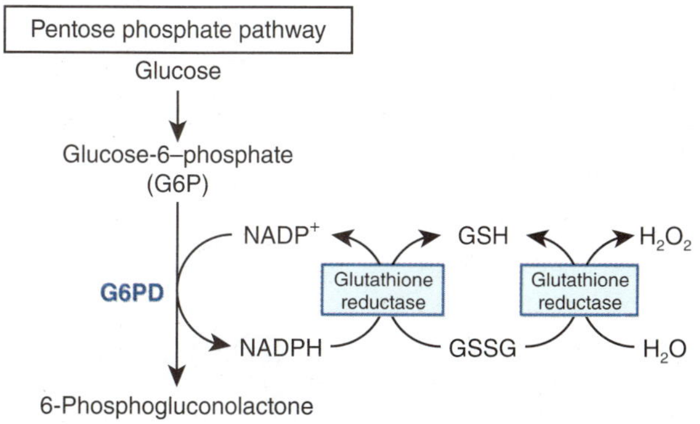

Fig. 15.28 Role of G6PD. G6PD, glucose-6-phosphate dehydrogenase. (*Source:* From Anna D. Cunningham, Sunhee Hwang and Daria Mochly-Rosen. Glucose-6-Phosphate Dehydrogenase Deficiency and the Need for a Novel Treatment to Prevent Kernicterus. Clinics in Perinatology. 2016;43:341-354.)

Table 15.19 Common Triggers of Haemolytic Crisis in G6PD-Deficient Persons

Category	Common causes
Infections	Viral hepatitis Pneumonia Typhoid fever
Drugs	Primaquine Chloroquine Sulphonamides Nitrofurantoins
Foods	Fava beans (favism is common in the Mediterranean region)

G6PD, glucose-6-phosphate dehydrogenase.

1. Red cells with G6PD deficiency → exposure to oxidants → denaturation of haemoglobin → precipitation of haemoglobin inside the cell (Heinz bodies) → failure of Heinz bodies to take up Romanowsky stain → unstained region in red cell makes it appear as **bite cells** → membrane damage → **intravascular haemolysis**
2. Red cells with G6PD deficiency → exposure to oxidants → denaturation of haemoglobin → precipitation of haemoglobin **(Heinz bodies)** → removal of inclusions in the periphery of red cells by splenic macrophages → rearrangement of remnant red cell membrane → **spherocytes** → splenic trapping → premature phagocytosis → **extravascular haemolysis**

Morphology

Peripheral smear shows evidence of haemolytic anaemia such as polychromatophilic red cells. Specific findings include the presence of **bite cells** or blister cells and **spherocytes** (Fig. 15.29).

Heinz bodies, the denatured haemoglobin, can be stained by supravital stains like crystal violet.

Reticulocytosis is demonstrated by supravital stains on peripheral smear.

The haemolysis is episodic and self-limiting, so **features of chronic haemolysis are absent.**

Clinical Features The diagnosis is usually suspected in patients who come from certain ethnic groups and present with anaemia, jaundice and symptoms of haemolysis after exposure to the triggering factors mentioned earlier, especially when there is a positive family history.

Management

Laboratory Investigations Apart from the routine tests performed for haemolytic anaemia workup, specific tests are needed to confirm the diagnosis that include Heinz

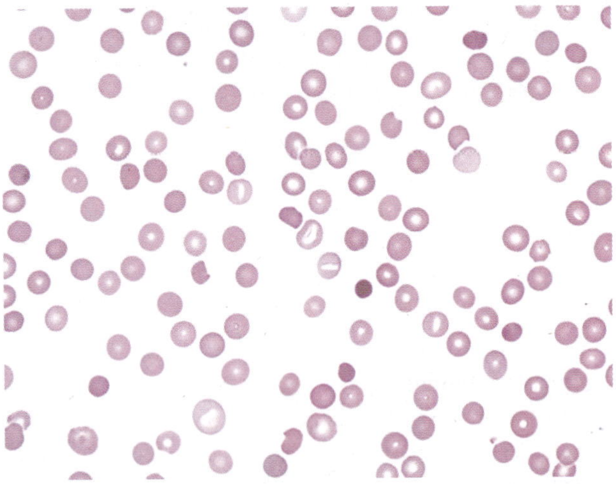

Fig. 15.29 Peripheral smear of G6PD deficiency with bite cells and spherocytes. *(Source:* From Juehua Gao and Sara A. Monaghan. Red Blood Cell/Hemoglobin Disorders. Hematopathology. 3rd edition. Elsevier 2018.)

body preparation, **NADPH assay**, G6PD assay and genetic testing for mutational analysis.

Treatment Most patients with G6PD deficiency do not require treatment. Acute episodes of haemolytic anaemia in these patients are largely preventable by avoiding exposure to the triggers. Identification and discontinuation of the precipitating factor are critical in the management of haemolytic episodes in such patients. Anaemia due to mild to moderate haemolysis is usually self-limiting and resolves within 2 weeks. Transfusion support is rarely needed in cases of severe anaemia.

Sickle Cell Disease **PA 16.3**

Sickle cell disease (SCD) is a group of common inherited haemoglobinopathies due to point mutation in β globin gene that alter the physicochemical properties of the haemoglobin, resulting in red cell distortion, sickling, haemolytic anaemia, microvascular obstruction and ischaemic tissue damage. Although SCD had been present in Africa for at least 5000 years and has been known by many names, it was only in 1910 that Dr Herrick named it 'the disease with sickle-shaped cells', after examining the blood smear of one of his patients. SCD is prevalent in Africa and also to a lesser extent in India, Mediterranean regions and the Middle East.

Genetics Haemoglobin is a tetrameric protein composed of two pairs of globin chains, each with a haem group. Normal red cells of adults contain mainly haemoglobin A (HbA), which is composed of two α chains and two β chains – $\alpha2\beta2$. In SCD, haemoglobin S (HbS) replaces HbA. HbS arises from **point mutation** substituting thymine for adenine in the sixth position of β globin gene, causing **replacement of glutamate by the valine residue**.

Approximately 8%–10% of African Americans are heterozygous for HbS and are predominantly affected by the condition called sickle cell trait, with 40% of haemoglobin composed of HbS.

In the homozygous state, there is 100% HbS – symptomatic SCD. A high prevalence is seen in areas with *falciparum* endemicity, due to Darwinian selection, because the red cells with HbS are relatively resistant to infection by *Plasmodium falciparum* and its related complications.

Pathophysiology (Fig. 15.30) HbS has physical properties different from those of HbA and forms polymers under deoxygenated conditions. It also exhibits changes in solubility and molecular stability. These altered properties of HbS are responsible for the profound clinical expression of the sickling disease (Fig. 15.31).

Under oxygenated state, HbS is in a free-flowing liquid state like HbA. With deoxygenation, HbS undergoes a marked decrease in solubility and an increase in viscosity, leading to polymer formation. Thus, it gets transformed into a viscous gel-like substance containing haemoglobin crystals called **tactoids**. The herniation of HbS from the red cell membrane occurs when deoxygenation persists and red cells become **sickled**. This is associated with influx of calcium and efflux of water and potassium. This is partly due to impairment in the Ca^{2+} pump, which is dependent on ATPase. With an extended period of deoxygenation, red cells are further dehydrated and become dense and rigid. However, these cells regain their normal shape, which is referred to as reversible sickling.

The repeated changes in RBC shape during cycles of oxygenation and deoxygenation damage the cell membrane, making it rigid with alterations in the cytoskeletal protein interactions. Hence, RBCs assume the characteristic sickle shape permanently and are no longer capable of resuming their normal biconcave shape even with reoxygenation, referred to as irreversibly sickled RBCs.

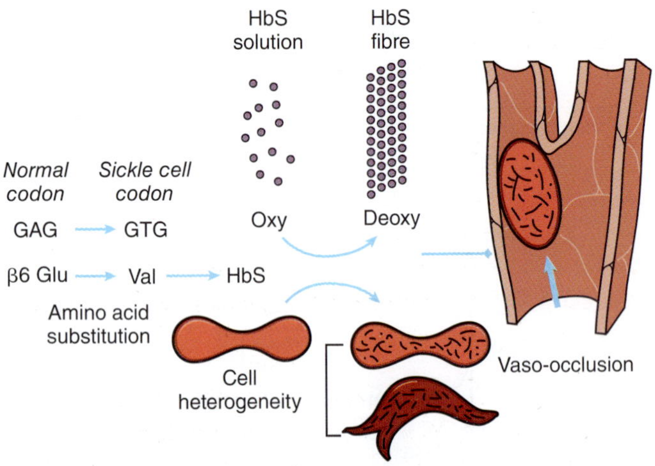

Fig. 15.30 Pathogenesis of sickle cell anaemia. *(Source:* From Robert L. Nussbaum, Roderick R. McInnes and Huntington F. Willard. The Molecular Basis of Genetic Disease: General Principles and Lessons from the Hemoglobinopathies. Thompson & Thompson Genetics in Medicine. 8th edition. Elsevier 2016.)

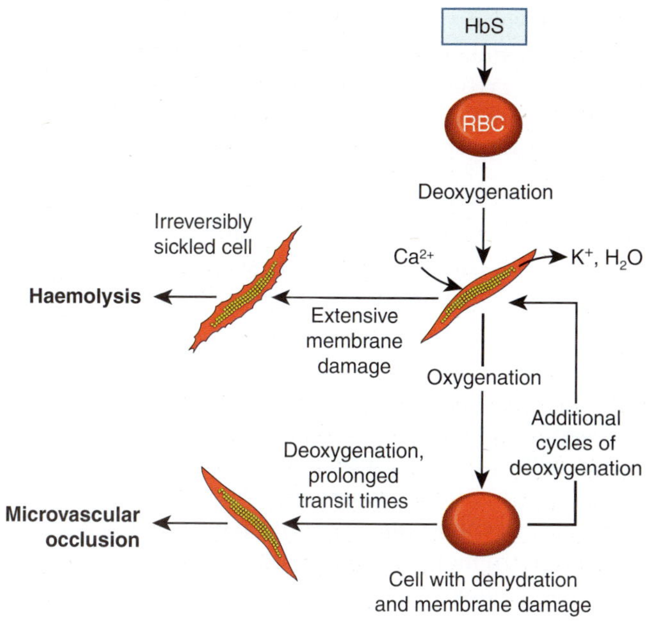

Fig. 15.31 Consequences of sickling. *(Source:* From Vinay Kumar, Abul K. Abbas and Jon C. Aster. Red Blood Cell and Bleeding Disorders. Robbins & Cotran Pathologic Basis of Disease. 10th edition. Elsevier 2021.)

One of the complications of SCD is microvascular occlusion. Characteristically, sickle cells express more adhesion molecules than normal cells. Thus, in a setting of inflammation or when there is slowing down of circulation in microvascular beds, there is a local generation of more reversibly sickled red cells. These reversibly sickled red cells are the cause of **microvascular occlusion**, which is responsible for serious consequences like tissue ischaemia and infarction. Furthermore, a minor fraction of the cells undergoes **intravascular haemolysis**, releasing free haemoglobin. This haemoglobin binds to nitric acid and inactivates it, resulting in the accentuation of vasoconstriction and platelet aggregation, because nitric oxide is a powerful vasodilator and an inhibitor of platelet aggregation.

On the other hand, irreversibly sickled red cells get stuck in the splenic microcirculation and get phagocytosed by the splenic macrophages, resulting in **extravascular haemolysis**. Up to 50% of red cells permanently remain in the altered sickle shape.

In addition to these changes, disturbances are seen at the lipid bilayer. The outer leaflet has increased amounts of phosphatidylethanolamine and contains phosphatidylserine, and this contributes to thrombosis by acting as a catalyst for clotting factors.

Factors Influencing Sickling in Sickle Cell Disease

- **Interaction of HbS with other haemoglobins:**
  HbA interferes with sickling. Hence, people with sickle cell trait, who have only 40% HbS, do not show sickling except in profound hypoxic states.
  Haemoglobin F (HbF) also prevents sickling and hence children do not present with symptoms until their HbF is cleared, which takes at least 6 months from birth.
  Haemoglobin C (HbC) aggravates sickling and hence HbSC disease, which is a compound heterozygous state, presents with more sickling episodes than sickle trait but less than SCD.
- **MCHC:** Intracellular dehydration, which increases MCHC, precipitates sickling. In α-thalassaemia, in which MCHC is less due to deficiency of haemoglobin, the disease is mild.
- **Intracellular pH:** Reduction in pH reduces the oxygen affinity of haemoglobin and hence promotes sickling.
- **Transit time of red cells in microvascular beds:** Transit time is prolonged in the microvascular beds of the spleen and bone marrow, making these sites the commonly affected parts in sickle cell anaemia. Furthermore, transit time is more in other vascular beds under the influence of inflammation and so inflammation accentuates sickling.

Morphology

Peripheral smear examination shows the presence of variable numbers of irreversibly **sickled cells** (Fig. 15.32). In addition to this, reticulocytosis, nucleated red cells and target cells are seen. **Howell–Jolly bodies**, nuclear remnant in red cells, may be seen in patients with postautosplenectomy status.

Compensatory marrow expansion leads to resorption of bone with new bone formation on the outer surface, resulting in the prominence of cheek bones and changes in skull bone that resembles a **'crew cut'** also referred to as '**hair on end**' appearance on radiographs (Fig. 15.33).

Apart from these, other features of extravascular haemolysis are present. In preadolescent children, there is splenomegaly due to congestion. In postadolescent children, due to repeated sickling, ischaemia and infarcts, the spleen gets converted into a thin fibrotic cord. This is called **autosplenectomy** and is caused by splenic infarction due to chronic erythrostasis.

Other organs including bones, brain, kidney, liver, retina and pulmonary vessels are affected by **infarction** caused by microvascular occlusion.

Clinical Features Signs of SCD usually begin in early childhood, and the severity of symptoms can vary from person to person. A majority of the affected patients present with moderate to severe anaemia, and it is associated with a high mortality rate. The clinical course is often punctuated by several crises:

A. **Vaso-occlusive crisis – 'pain crisis'** – occurs due to hypoxia and infarction in the organs involved. This is the most common cause of morbidity and mortality. Commonly affected organs are bones, lungs, liver,

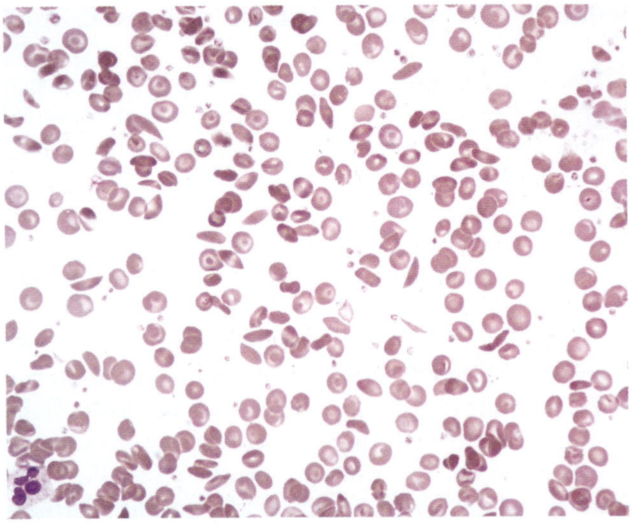

Fig. 15.32 Peripheral smear showing the presence of sickle cells in SCA. *(Source:* From Juehua Gao, Sara A. Monaghan, Hematopathology, Elsevier 2018.)

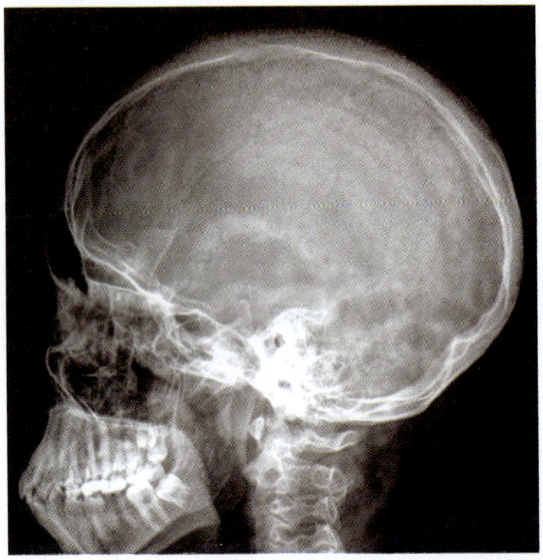

Fig. 15.33 Crew cut appearance on the X-ray in SCA. *(Source:* From A. Carlson Merrow and Selena Hariharan. Sickle Cell Disease, Musculoskeletal. Imaging in Pediatrics, 287-287.)

brain, spleen and penis. It is clinically difficult to distinguish from osteomyelitis. Its common manifestations are as follows:

- Hand–foot syndrome (dactylitis of the bones of hands and feet) seen in children
- Acute chest syndrome – lungs
- Priapism – painful penile erection
- Stroke
- Retinopathy

Vaso-occlusive crisis involving organs such as the penis and lungs is considered an emergency and is treated with exchange transfusions.

B. **Sequestration crisis:** This crisis affects preadolescent children with an intact spleen, which enlarges markedly due to massive entrapment of sickle cells, resulting in hypovolaemia and shock. This may be fatal in some children and needs immediate intervention.

C. **Aplastic crisis** due to parvovirus B19 infection of the red cell progenitors causing a sudden drop in the haemoglobin levels is a medical emergency.

Apart from these crises, patients with sickle cell anaemia have other manifestations of chronic tissue hypoxia, including impairment of growth and development, hyposthenuria due to renal medullary ischaemia and recurrent infections due to autosplenectomy.

Laboratory Findings The diagnosis is suspected based on family history, clinical features and the presence of sickle cells in the peripheral smear, especially in patients from certain ethnic background. Metabisulphite test is used for screening, and the confirmatory test is haemoglobin electrophoresis. Genetic tests are indicated for genetic counselling.

Screening test (Fig. 15.34): Sickling test is performed with metabisulphite, which is a hypoxia-inducible agent. It is added to a drop of blood on a slide to deoxygenate it, and the smear is checked for the presence of sickle cells.

Haemoglobin electrophoresis (Fig. 15.35): It shows the presence of HbS in the blood.

High-performance liquid chromatography: This is the gold standard investigation now to quantify the different types of haemoglobins.

Prenatal diagnosis: Testing is performed for point mutation in fetal DNA obtained by amniocentesis and chorionic villus sampling.

Treatment Hydroxyurea, which acts by inhibiting DNA synthesis, helps by many mechanisms like increasing the HbF and also by its anti-inflammatory effects.

HSC transplantation offers ray of hope for cure in selected patients.

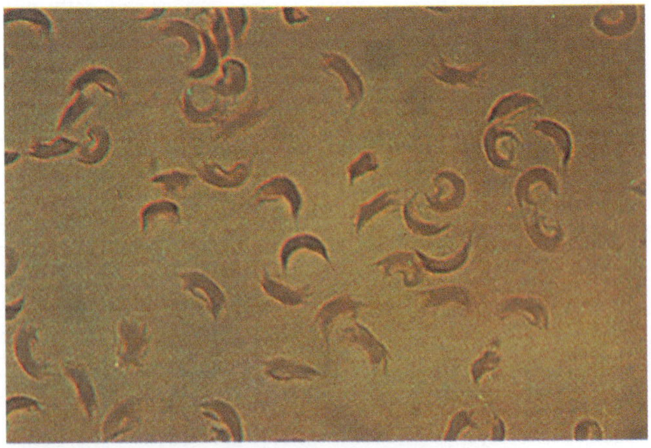

Fig. 15.34 Sickling test – peripheral blood film. Sickle cell preparation in sodium metabisulphite. Even in sickle cell trait, all cells eventually sickle. *(Source:* From M. Tarek Elghetany, Katherine I. Schexneider and Katalin Banki. Erythrocytic Disorders. Henry's Clinical Diagnosis and Management by Laboratory Methods. 23rd edition. Elsevier 2017.)

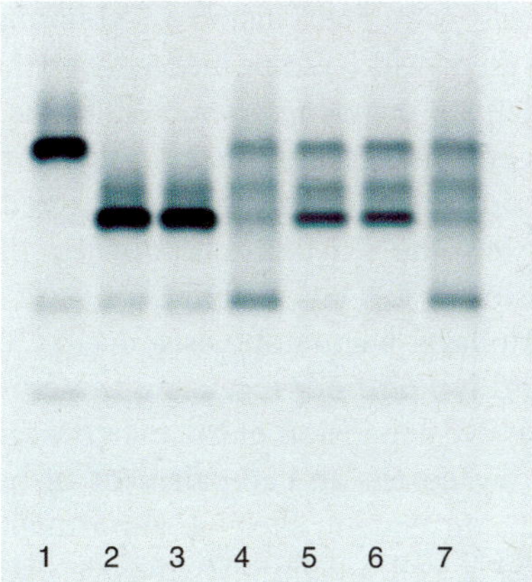

Fig. 15.35 Haemoglobin electrophoresis in SCA. Electrophoretic separation of haemoglobins at alkaline pH. 1, A normal adult; 2 and 3, a 17-year-old with sickle cell anaemia; 5 and 6, a patient with sickle cell anaemia, recently transfused; 4 and 7, haemoglobins A/F/S/C standard. *(Source:* From M. Tarek Elghetany, Katherine I. Schexneider and Katalin Banki. Erythrocytic Disorders. Henry's Clinical Diagnosis and Management by Laboratory Methods. 23rd edition. Elsevier 2017.)

Thalassaemia Syndromes **PA 16.3**

Thalassaemia syndromes are a group of inherited disorders associated with **deficiency of either α or β globin chain** of adult haemoglobin, HbA. This deficiency of globin chains results in an imbalance in globin synthesis, resulting in haemolysis, tissue hypoxia and iron-overloaded state. This disease is prevalent in the Mediterranean belt.

Before discussing the aetiopathogenesis of thalassaemia syndromes, let us discuss the genetics and composition of normal adult haemoglobin.

Genetics and Composition of Adult Haemoglobin (Table 15.20) Haemoglobin is a tetramer containing two α subunits and two β subunits. HbA, also known as adult haemoglobin, haemoglobin A1, composed of α2β2, is the most common human haemoglobin tetramer, accounting for greater than 97% of the total RBC haemoglobin.

Haemoglobin A2 is a less common adult form of haemoglobin and is composed of two α and two δ globin subunits, α2δ2. This haemoglobin makes up 1%–3% of adult haemoglobin.

The other haemoglobin is fetal haemoglobin (HbF), which is composed of α2γ2 and is the predominant haemoglobin during the fetal period. In the newborn, levels of HbF gradually decrease and reach adult levels (less than 1% of total haemoglobin) usually within 1 year of life.

α chains are coded by four α genes located on **chromosome 16**, and **β chains** are coded by two β genes located on **chromosome 11**.

α-Thalassaemia is due to deficient α chains, and β-thalassaemia is due to deficient β chains.

Deficiency of globin chains is the cause for anaemia, whereas the precipitation of excess unpaired globin chains is the cause for haemolysis.

β-Thalassaemias β-Thalassaemias are associated with deficiency in β globin chains and excess of unpaired α chains, usually due to mutation in the β globin locus. The relative excess of α globin results in the formation of insoluble aggregates, causing ineffective erythropoiesis and haemolysis.

Genetics of β-Thalassaemia *(Table 15.21)* As β chains are coded by two genes on chromosome 11, the clinical syndromes are dependent on the number of mutated genes and the type of mutation.

Mutated alleles are called β^+, when the partial function is preserved (either the protein has a decreased function or it is produced in lesser quantity), and β^0, when no protein is produced. The type of allele in the two genes determines the clinical syndrome.

Mutations in β-Thalassaemia Reduction in β chain synthesis is due to more than 100 different mutations, with **point mutation** being the predominant type:

A. Splicing mutation – β^+
B. Promotor region mutation – β^+
C. Chain terminator mutation – β^0

Pathogenesis *(Fig. 15.36)* The major events for the development of clinical features and complications of β-thalassaemia are anaemia, extramedullary haematopoiesis and excess iron absorption.

A. **Anaemia in β-thalassaemia is due to three mechanisms:**
   1. Deficient β globin chains with the resultant deficiency of haemoglobin are present.

Table 15.20 Types of Normal Haemoglobin in Adults

Globin Genes in Chromosome		Gene Product (Globin) in RBCs	Tetramers	Name of Haemoglobin	Concentration in Adult
16	11				
α	β	α, β-chain	α2 β2	Hb A	96–97
α	δ	α, δ-chain	α2 δ2	Hb A2	2.3–3.5
α	γ	α, γ-chain	α2 γ2	Hb F	<1.0

HbA, haemoglobin A; HbF, haemoglobin F; RBC, red blood cell.

Table 15.21 Clinical and Genetic Classification of β-Thalassaemia

Clinical Syndromes	Genotypes	Clinical Features
β-Thalassaemia major	$\beta^0\beta^0/\beta^+\beta^+/\beta^0\beta^+$	Severe anaemia requiring transfusion
β-Thalassaemia intermedia	$\beta^0\beta^+/\beta^+\beta^+/\beta^0\beta/\beta^+\beta$	Severe anaemia but is not transfusion dependent
β-Thalassaemia minor	$\beta^0\beta/\beta^+\beta$	Asymptomatic with mild or absent anaemia; red cell abnormalities

- β^+ is diminished in β globin production
- β^0 is absent in β globin production

2. The immature red cells in the marrow with excess, unpaired α chains, as insoluble inclusions in the red cells, undergo apoptotic cell death triggered by membrane damage induced by the inclusions – **ineffective erythropoiesis.** In β-thalassaemia major, this mechanism contributes to up to 80% of haemolysis.
3. Red cells with precipitation of abnormal inclusions within them, which escape ineffective erythropoiesis, are picked up for premature haemolysis by the splenic macrophages. This contributes to **extravascular haemolysis.**

B. **Extramedullary haematopoiesis** triggered by haemolysis worsens the existing situation by the following mechanisms:
Extramedullary haematopoiesis occurs in the liver, spleen and lymph nodes, causing these organs to enlarge. Massive expansion of the marrow causes erosion of the bony cortex and impairment of bone growth, with the consequent skeletal abnormalities in full-blown sickle cell anaemia. Extensive extramedullary haematopoiesis induces changes in the facial bones, referred to as **thalassaemia facies** (Fig. 15.37).

C. **Excess iron accumulation** occurs by the following mechanisms:
1. Exaggerated erythropoietic drive stimulated by extramedullary erythropoiesis leads to increased iron absorption from the gut, which is aided by low hepcidin levels.
2. Repeated blood transfusions done to treat severe anaemia also lead to iron accumulation. These two mechanisms result in a syndrome called **secondary haemochromatosis** or iron-overloaded state.

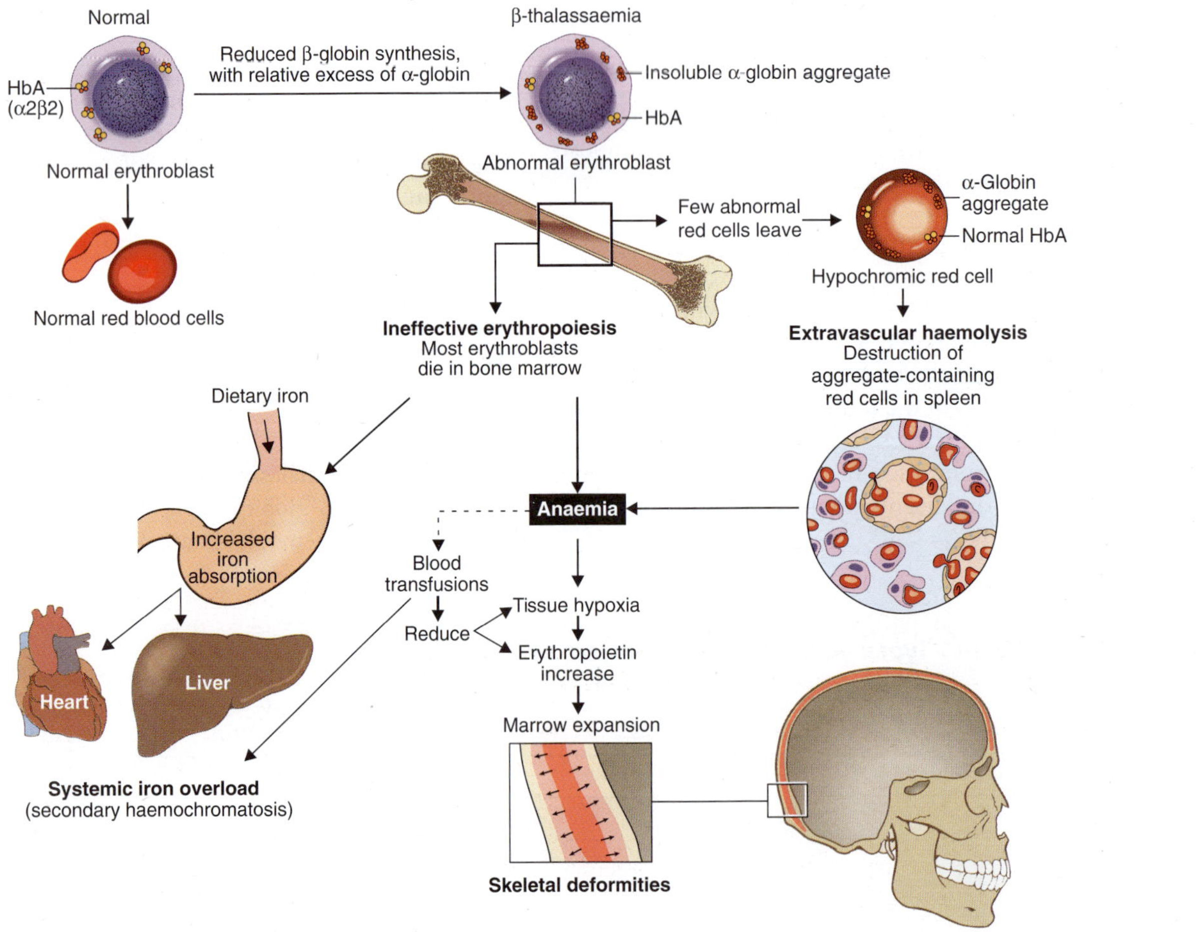

Fig. 15.36 Pathogenesis of β-thalassaemia. *(Source:* From Vinay Kumar MBBS, MD, FRCPath, Abul K. Abbas MBBS and Jon C. Aster MD, PhD. Red Blood Cell and Bleeding Disorders. Robbins & Cotran Pathologic Basis of Disease. 10th edition. Elsevier 2021.)

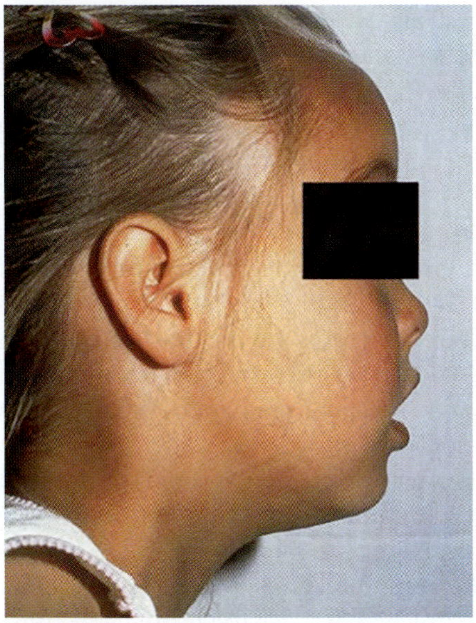

Fig. 15.37 Thalassaemia facies in a child with β-thalassaemia major. *(Source:* From Martin R Howard and Peter J Hamilton. The thalassaemias. Haematology: An Illustrated Colour Text. 4th edition. Elsevier 2013.)

Morphology

Peripheral smears show severe red cell abnormalities like severe **microcytic hypochromic** anaemia, anisocytosis and poikilocytosis. **Target cells**, basophilic stippling and fragmented red cells are also seen. Polychromatophilic red cells equivalent to reticulocytes are seen; in severe anaemia, normoblasts (nucleated red cell precursors) are also seen in the peripheral smear.

Reticulocytosis is present, but lesser than expected for the degree of anaemia, due to ineffective erythropoiesis.

Facial and skull bones show changes induced by extramedullary haematopoiesis in the absence of blood transfusion. The active marrow erodes the existing cortical bone and stimulates new bone formation, giving rise to the aforementioned **'crew cut'** appearance on radiographs. The orofacial features are collectively referred to as 'thalassaemia facies' (Fig. 15.37).

Splenomegaly is due to phagocyte hyperplasia and extramedullary haematopoiesis, which also occurs in the liver and lymph nodes.

Organs like the **heart, liver and pancreas** show parenchymal iron deposition as a part of **secondary haemochromatosis.**

Clinical Features As shown in Table 15.21, clinical picture is dictated by the genetic dosage. On the basis of the genotype and severity of clinical syndromes, β-thalassaemia is classified into the following three types:

1. **β-Thalassaemia major:** It is also referred to as **Cooley anaemia or Mediterranean anaemia.** Patients on this end of the spectrum present with severe anaemia and compensatory extramedullary haematopoiesis. The clinical course is punctuated by the recurrent need for transfusions, causing an iron-overloaded state as the expected long-term complication. Facial deformities, hepatosplenomegaly and growth retardation are present. X-ray of the skull shows 'crew cut' appearance. Cardiac failure due to secondary haemochromatosis is an important cause of death in patients treated with repeated blood transfusions. Outlook for these patients is still guarded. HSC transplantation is curative in selective patients.
2. **β-Thalassaemia intermedia:** Patients present with symptoms milder than those of β-thalassaemia major but severe than those of β-thalassaemia minor.
3. **β-Thalassaemia minor:** Patients with this disorder are predominantly asymptomatic or may present with features of mild anaemia. They may clinically be confused with iron-deficiency anaemia due to the microcytic hypochromic blood picture. Peripheral smear may also show numerous target cells and basophilic stippling (Fig. 15.38).

Differentiating thalassaemia from iron-deficiency anaemia is critically important, because the treatment for both these disorders is completely different.

Parameters that help differentiate these two complications are as follows:

- **Mentzer index:** MCV/RBC count (if the value is less than 13, thalassaemia minor/trait; if the value is more than 13, iron-deficiency anaemia)
- Serum iron, ferritin and TIBC levels
- MCHC and RDW normal in thalassaemia but abnormal (MCHC is reduced and RDW is increased) in iron-deficiency anaemia

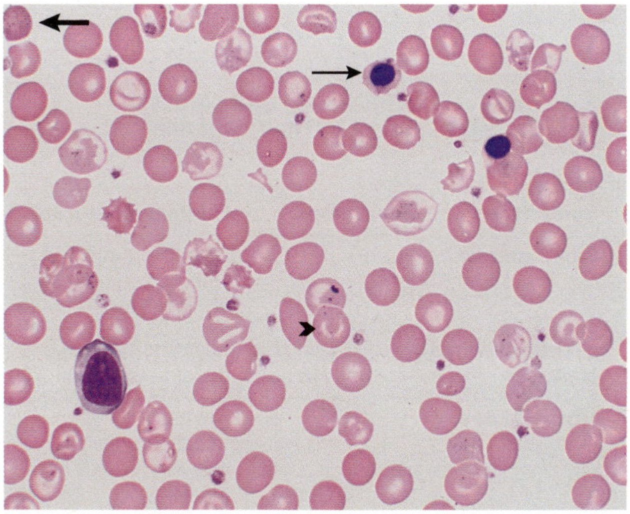

Fig. 15.38 Peripheral smear of β-thalassaemia major showing numerous target cells (arrow head), polychromatophilic red cells (thick arrow) and nucleated red cells (thin arrow). *(Source:* From Meenakshi Garg Bansal and Genevieve Marie Crane. Hypochromic and Hemolytic Anemias. Atlas of Diagnostic Hematology, 3, 22-46.)

α-Thalassaemia α-Thalassaemias are caused by inherited genetic mutations causing deletion of one or more α genes that code for α chains of haemoglobin. As discussed earlier, two α chains are coded by four genes on chromosome 16.

Like β-thalassaemia, anaemia in α-thalassaemia is due to reduced synthesis of α chains of haemoglobin; ineffective erythropoiesis and extravascular haemolysis are due to precipitation of excess unpaired β chains in the red cells.

The clinical manifestations vary according to the age.

In newborns with α-thalassaemia, a compensatory increase in γ globin chain production causes precipitation of excess unpaired γ4 chains, forming γ4 tetramers known as **haemoglobin Barts**.

In older children and adults, compensatory increase in β globin chain production causes precipitation of β4 tetramers known as **HbH** disease. The free β and γ chains are more soluble than free α chains and form relatively stable homotetramers, so haemolysis and ineffective erythropoiesis and excess iron deposition are less severe than in β-thalassaemia.

Clinical Features Clinical features of α-thalassaemia are dependent on the genotypes and are listed in Table 15.22.

We describe here the features of hydrops fetalis, the most severe form, because other states are explained in Table 15.22.

Hydrops Fetalis Hydrops fetalis is a serious, fatal condition defined by abnormal accumulation of fluid in two or more fetal compartments, such as ascites, pleural effusion, pericardial effusion and skin oedema. It is the most severe form of α-thalassaemia caused by the deletion of all the four α genes. In the fetus, a compensatory increase in the γ globin chains forms tetramers, haemoglobin Barts, which have a very high affinity for oxygen and hence deliver very less oxygen to the tissues.

Table 15.22 Clinical and Genetic Classification of α-Thalassaemia[a]

Clinical Syndromes	Genotypes	Clinical Features
Silent carrier	−α/αα	Asymptomatic with no red cell abnormality
α-Thalassaemia trait	−α/−α (African) − −/αα (Asian)	Asymptomatic like thalassaemia minor
HbH disease	− −/−α	Severe with thalassaemia intermedia–like features
Hydrops fetalis	− −/− −	Lethal in utero without transfusions

Hb, haemoglobin.

Fetal distress usually becomes evident in the third trimester of pregnancy. This condition used to be fatal earlier but with intrauterine transfusion, many infants are now saved. The affected fetus shows severe pallor, generalized oedema and massive hepatosplenomegaly. The infants who survive the hydrops fetalis are dependent on repeated blood transfusion and its associated complications.

HSC transplantation offers ray of hope for cure.

Prenatal Genetic Testing for Prevention of Thalassaemia Haemoglobin disorders are the most common worldwide inherited conditions, especially thalassaemias. It is estimated that 307,900 children are born annually with a severe haemoglobin disorder, and 60%–70% of births occur in sub-Saharan Africa. Thalassaemia is prevalent in the Mediterranean area, the Middle East, Southeast Asia and the Pacific region. The carrier rates range from 2% to 19% in the different populations. Hence, it is extremely important to opt for prenatal genetic testing and counselling to prevent the birth of children with severe form of thalassaemias.

Prenatal diagnosis offers new options to couples at risk of a major haemoglobinopathy and changes the perspective of screening and counselling for thalassaemias. Prenatal diagnosis of thalassaemias is still carried out by the traditional methods such as amniocentesis, chorionic villus sampling and cordocentesis. Although the prenatal testing has the risk of fetal loss by 1%, its benefits cannot be overseen.

Paroxysmal Nocturnal Haemoglobinuria PA 16.4

PNH is a rare, acquired, life-threatening disease characterized by haemolytic anaemia, bone marrow failure and a predisposition to thrombosis. It stems from a somatic mutation in the PIGA gene in hematopoietic stem cells, leading to a deficiency of glycosylphosphatidylinositol (GPI)-anchored proteins on the cell surface. This deficiency makes RBCs susceptible to complement-mediated lysis.

Pathogenesis PIGA gene codes for an enzyme that is essential for the synthesis of certain membrane-associated **complement regulatory proteins**, anchored by GPI anchors. *PNH is the only intrinsic haemolytic anaemia caused by acquired genetic defect.*

Proteins are anchored on the lipid bilayer by any of the following two ways: either as transmembrane proteins or attached through a specialized phospholipid anchors called GPI. In patients with PNH, these **GPI anchors are deficient** due to mutations affecting PIGA gene.

As the mutation affects the HSC, all its derivatives are GPI deficient. Typically, the mutant clone coexists with the normal clones that have GPI anchors intact. Strikingly, most of us harbour small numbers of bone marrow cells with PIGA gene mutations similar to PNH, and in rare situations, these gain selective advantage and develop into overt haemolytic anaemia.

The following membrane proteins are absent on the surface of haematopoietic cells in PNH:

- **Decay accelerating factor – CD55**
- **Membrane inhibitor of reactive lysis – CD59**
- **C8-binding protein**

These proteins are responsible for the prevention of lysis of haematopoietic cells by activated complements by inhibiting them. In their absence, lysis of blood cells by complement overactivity is not prevented. Predominant manifestation is **intravascular haemolysis** due to C5–C9 membrane attack complex.

Depending on the degree of sensitivity to complement-mediated lysis, three different types of red cells are found in PNH:

PNH I: Red cells with normal sensitivity to complement
PNH II: Red cells with intermediate sensitivity to complement-mediated lysis
PNH III: Red cells with marked sensitivity to complement-mediated lysis

Severity of haemolysis depends on the proportion of PNH III red cells.

Clinical Features The name of the disorder is a descriptive term for the clinical consequence of red cell breakdown with release of haemoglobin into the urine, which manifests as dark-coloured urine in the morning. The term 'nocturnal' refers to the belief that haemolysis is triggered by acidosis during sleep and activates complement to haemolyse unprotected red cells. However, this belief was later disproved. Haemolysis has been shown to occur throughout the day and is actually not paroxysmal, but the concentration of the urine overnight and slightly increased haemolysis due to the mild acidosis during sleep produce the dramatic change in its colour. Chronic haemolysis without dramatic haemoglobinuria is the commonest manifestation. The haemolysis is paroxysmal and nocturnal in only 25% of cases. The other causes that increase haemolysis are stress, surgery and strenuous exercise.

On the basis of the clinical presentations, the presence or absence of another specific bone marrow disorder and the size of PNH clones, PNH is classified into three categories as shown in Table 15.23.

Venous thrombosis is the leading cause of death in patients with PNH because 40% of patients present with deep vein thrombosis. The tendency of patients with PNH to suffer thrombosis has been recognized as a major part of the disease and is interpreted as a very bad prognostic sign.

Complications Patients with PNH develop any of the following complications when the HSCs suffer additional mutations:

- Aplastic anaemia
- Acute myeloid leukaemia
- Myelodysplastic syndrome

Table 15.23 Classification of PNH

Type	Features
Classic	Severe intravascular haemolysis, cellular marrow with erythroid hyperplasia; large PNH clones
PNH in the setting of another specific bone marrow disorder	Mild to moderate intravascular haemolysis; evidence of another specific bone marrow disorder (aplastic anaemia, myelodysplastic syndrome); moderate-sized PNH clones
Subclinical PNH	No evidence of intravascular haemolysis; evidence of another specific bone marrow disorder (aplastic anaemia, myelodysplastic syndrome); small PNH clones detected by flow cytometry

PNH, paroxysmal nocturnal haemoglobinuria.

Management

Screening Tests In a typical patient presenting with the classical triad of haemolytic anaemia, pancytopenia and thrombosis, the following screening tests were performed routinely before the invention of flow cytometry:

1. **Sucrose lysis test**
   This is the standard screening test in which the patient's red cells are added to ABO-compatible normal serum and isotonic sucrose solution, which provides the low ionic strength medium and favours attachment of IgG and complement to red cells. The amount of haemolysis is measured by spectrophotometer following incubation at 37°C and centrifugation. More than 10% haemolysis indicates PNH.
2. **Acidified serum test, Ham test**
   Ham test is a more sensitive screening test performed in PNH if the sucrose lysis test is positive. Fresh normal ABO-compatible serum is acidified and red cells from patients are added. Acidification of serum to pH 6.5 activates complement via alternate pathway and causes haemolysis of red cells sensitive to complement. The amount of haemolysis is measured, and the test result is interpreted as positive if more than 10% haemolysis is observed.

Investigation of choice

Flow cytometry (Fig. 15.39) confirms the absence of GPI-linked proteins on the surface of haematopoietic cells and is the investigation of choice. It measures the percentage of cells that are deficient in the GPI anchors and identifies discrete populations with different degrees of deficiency.

Treatment Symptomatic patients are treated with blood transfusion. Recent advancements in PNH treatment have been significant. Ravulizumab, a long-acting C5

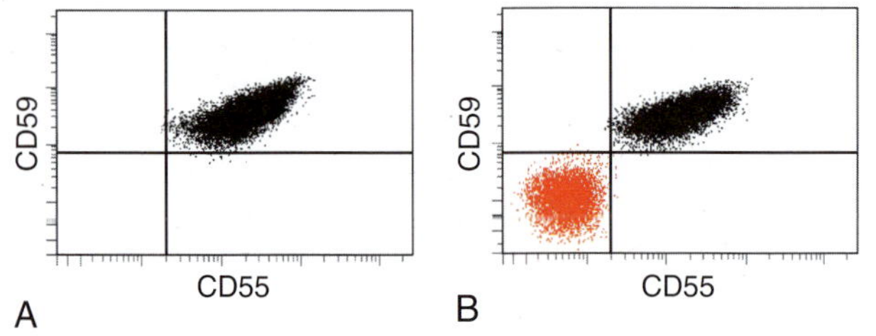

Fig. 15.39 Flow cytometry for PNH. (A) Flow cytogram of blood from a normal individual shows that the red cells express two phosphatidylinositol glycan (PIG)–linked membrane proteins – CD55 and CD59 – on their surfaces. (B) Flow cytogram of blood from a patient with PNH shows the population of red cells that is deficient in both CD55 and CD59. As is typical of PNH, a second population of $CD55^+/CD59^+$ red cells that are derived from residual normal haematopoietic stem cells also is present. PNH, paroxysmal nocturnal haemoglobinuria. *(Source:* From Vinay Kumar, Abul K. Abbas and Jon C. Aster. Red Blood Cell and Bleeding Disorders. Robbins & Cotran Pathologic Basis of Disease. 10th edition. Elsevier 2021.)

complement inhibitor, has emerged as a promising therapeutic option. Clinical trials have demonstrated its efficacy in reducing haemolysis, improving quality of life and decreasing the risk of thrombosis in patients with PNH. This development represents a crucial step forward in the management of this condition, offering an alternative to eculizumab, the first-in-class complement inhibitor. Immunosuppressive drugs are also beneficial. HSC transplantation is curative.

Immunohaemolytic Anaemias **PA 16.4**

Immunohaemolytic anaemias encompass a range of disorders characterized by the immune system's destruction of RBCs. These conditions include AIHA, alloimmune haemolytic anaemia and drug-induced immune haemolytic anaemia. AIHA, in particular, has seen notable advancements in its understanding and management. The disease is also referred to as '**Coombs-positive haemolytic anaemia**' because all the subtypes of this disorder are Coombs test positive.

There are three types of immunohaemolytic anaemias, which are listed in Table 15.24.

Pathogenesis (Fig. 15.40)

Warm Antibody Type This is the most common form of immunohaemolytic anaemia; about half of the cases are idiopathic, whereas the other causes are listed in Table 15.24. Most common antibodies associated with this type of haemolysis are **IgG** and, in some cases, IgA. The mechanism of red cell destruction in this type of haemolytic anaemia is **opsonization** of red cells by IgG, followed by the phagocytic removal of antibody-bound portions of their membranes by splenic macrophages, resulting in the formation of **spherocytes** (Fig. 15.41). As in HS, the spherocytes are later sequestered and phagocytosed completely in the spleen, resulting in **extravascular haemolysis**. Moderate splenomegaly is seen in these cases.

Cold Agglutinin Type This subtype of immunohaemolytic anaemia is caused by **IgM** antibodies that bind to red cells with great affinity at low temperatures (0–4°C). The most common cause for cold agglutinin-induced haemolysis is **infection** by certain organisms like *Mycoplasma pneumoniae*, Epstein–Barr virus and cytomegalovirus; haemolysis associated with this type is generally self-limiting. Cold agglutinin immunohaemolytic anaemia is also seen

Table 15.24 Classification of Immunohaemolytic Anaemias and Their Causes, Types of Haemolysis and Features

Type of Immunohaemolytic Anaemia	Causes	Type of Haemolysis	Features
1. **Warm antibody type** IgG	1. **Primary** 2. **Secondary** A. Autoimmune disorders B. Drugs – penicillins, cephalosporins C. Lymphomas	Extravascular haemolysis at 37°C	Splenomegaly
2. **Cold antibody type** IgM	1. **Acute** Viral infections – *Mycoplasma pneumoniae*, Epstein–Barr virus, CMV, HIV 2. **Chronic** Lymphoid neoplasms	Extravascular haemolysis at less than 37°C with little intravascular haemolysis	Pallor, cyanosis, Raynaud phenomenon in the cooler parts of the body
3. **Cold haemolysin type – paroxysmal cold haemoglobinuria** IgG – Donath–Landsteiner antibody	Rare In children following viral infections	Intravascular haemolysis by IgG antibodies at less than 37°C	Substantial haemolysis, sometimes fatal

CMV, cytomegalovirus; HIV, human immunodeficiency virus.

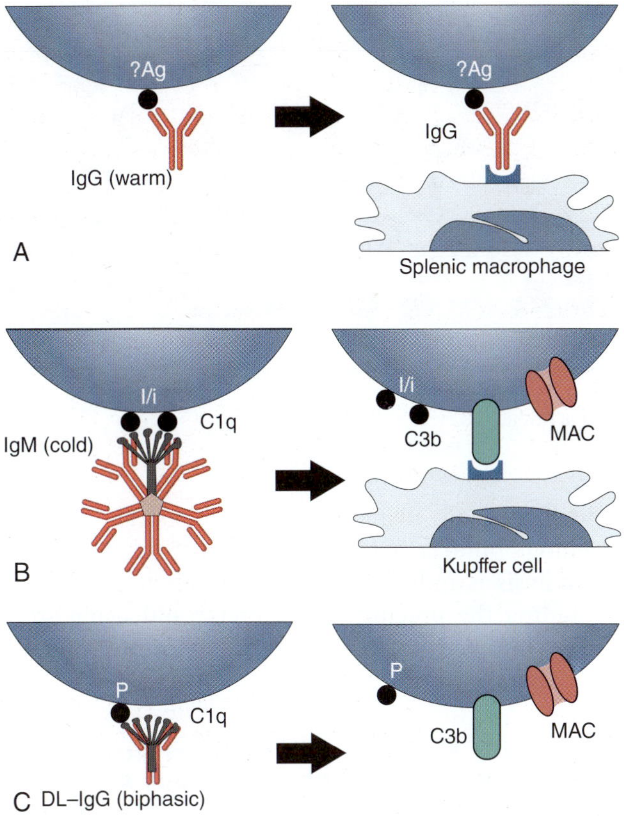

Fig. 15.40 Mechanism of haemolysis in warm autoimmune haemolytic anaemia (AIHA), cold AIHA and paroxysmal cold haemoglobinuria (PCH). (A) In warm reactive IgG AIHA, the red blood cell binds the autoantibody to a membrane-expressed cognate autoantigen and is trapped by spleen macrophages through Fc receptor interaction. (B) In cold reactive IgM AIHA, the I/i antigens on RBCs become covered with IgM class antibodies simultaneously fixing C1q whereupon the IgM leaves the cell at a higher temperature leaving opsonizing complement (C3b) and membrane attack complex (MAC) back on the cell. Thereafter, RBCs are trapped by liver macrophages (Kupffer cells) through complement receptor interaction. (C) In PCH, the biphasic Donath–Landsteiner IgG interacts with P antigen–carrying RBCs at cold temperature, fixes complement and leaves the cell surface at a warm temperature. Thereafter, complement-dependent haemolysis is triggered mainly through MAC perforation. (*Source:* From Stella T. Chou and Alan D. Schreiber. Autoimmune Hemolytic Anemia. Nathan and Oski's Hematology and Oncology of Infancy and Childhood. 8th edition. Elsevier 2015.)

in association with B-cell neoplasms, in which the haemolysis tends to be chronic.

Binding of IgM to RBCs occurs in the peripheries, such as fingers and toes where the temperature of the vascular bed is comparatively lower. This causes complement fixation and aggregation of RBCs (Fig. 15.40B), resulting in vascular obstruction causing cyanosis and Raynaud phenomenon. But before the bound complement can cause haemolysis, IgM detaches from RBCs in the circulation. However, the small quantity of C3b bound on it acts as an opsonin, leading to the removal of these cells by macrophages of the liver, spleen and bone marrow, producing haemolysis of variable severity. The predominant haemolysis in this type is extravascular, with the liver being the most common site.

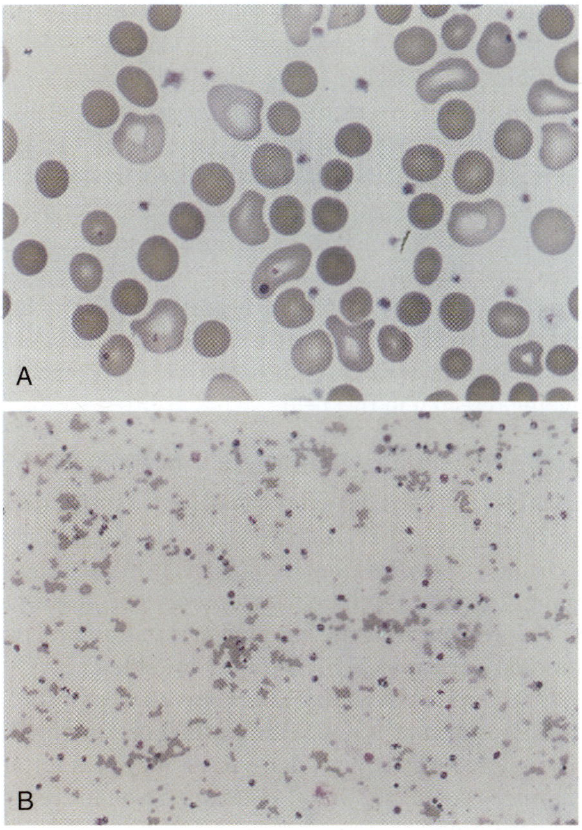

Fig. 15.41 Peripheral blood smear showing spherocytes in warm autoimmune haemolytic anaemia (AIHA) (A) and clumping of red blood cells (RBCs) in cold AIHA (B). (*Source:* From Stella T. Chou and Alan D. Schreiber. Autoimmune Hemolytic Anemia. Nathan and Oski's Hematology and Oncology of Infancy and Childhood. 8th edition. Elsevier 2015.)

Cold Haemolysin Type This group of antibodies is responsible for the rare entity called '**paroxysmal cold haemoglobinuria**'. The antibody responsible for this type of haemolysis is **IgG,** which binds to the P blood group antigen on the red cell surface at low temperatures of the extremities. This binding is followed by complement-mediated lysis of red cells when the blood circulates to warmer central parts of the body, resulting in intravascular haemolysis. The antibody that requires exposure to cold and warm temperatures for activation is called Donath–Landsteiner antibody. Cold haemolysin type is most often seen in children following viral infections. Generally, the haemolysis in this condition is self-limited.

Management

Investigations **Direct Coombs test:** The patient's red cells are mixed with sera containing antibodies that are specific for human immunoglobulin and complement. If the red cells are coated with immunoglobulin or complement, attachment of antibodies directed against them causes visible clumping. The test is explained in greater detail in Chapter 18.

The specific test used to identify Donath–Landsteiner antibody is Ham test.

Treatment Treating the underlying cause is often curative. Recent studies have shed light on the molecular mechanisms underlying AIHA, revealing the involvement of various pathways in its pathogenesis. This enhanced understanding has paved the way for targeted therapies, offering more effective and personalized treatment options. For instance, rituximab, an anti-CD20 monoclonal antibody, has emerged as a promising treatment for AIHA, particularly in cases resistant to conventional therapies like corticosteroids. These developments highlight the evolving landscape of treatment for immunohaemolytic anaemias and underscore the importance of ongoing research in this field.

Microangiopathic Haemolytic Anaemia PA 16.4

MAHA is a group of disorders characterized by the formation of microthrombi in small blood vessels, leading to mechanical haemolysis and thrombocytopenia. Prominent among these are thrombotic thrombocytopenic purpura (TTP) and atypical haemolytic uraemic syndrome (aHUS). Common causes of MAHA are listed in Table 15.25.

The common thread that runs between these disorders is a **microvascular lesion with luminal narrowing.** Red cells undergo mechanical injury when they pass through such narrowed blood vessels with the resultant **red cell fragmentation**.

Morphology

The hallmark finding is the presence of **schistocytes** (fragmented red cells), Burr cells, helmet cells and triangle cells in the peripheral smear apart from other common features of intravascular haemolysis (Fig. 15.42).

Treating the underlying disorder is the primary modality of treatment.

March haemoglobinuria

March haemoglobinuria is a rare haemolytic disorder usually observed in young males following marching or running on hard surfaces for a prolonged period. Traumatic destruction of red cells occurs within the vessels of the feet. The common complaint is passing reddish brown urine following physical exertion. Haemoglobinuria is transient in most cases, and the haemolysis is mild without causing obvious anaemia. Curtailing the precipitating exercise and using shoes with reinforced soles are helpful in preventing the haemolytic episodes.

Table 15.25 Causes of Microangiopathic Haemolytic Anaemia

Thrombotic thrombocytopenic purpura (TTP)
Haemolytic uraemic syndrome
Malignant hypertension
Disseminated intravascular coagulation (DIC)
Cardiac prostheses
Vasculitis associated with systemic lupus erythematosus (SLE)
Severe infections
Eclampsia

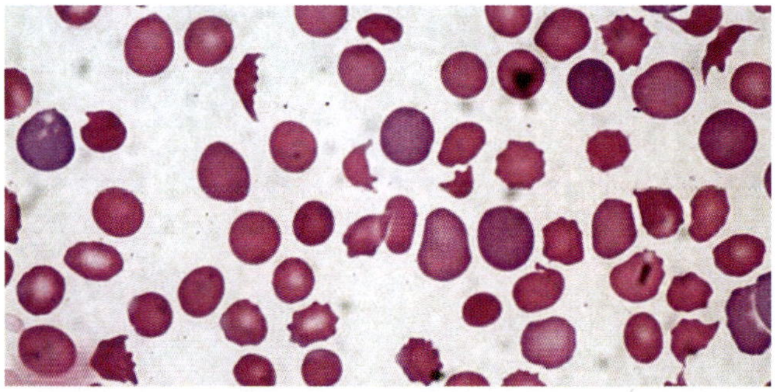

Fig. 15.42 Peripheral blood smear of microangiopathic haemolytic anaemia showing the presence of schistocytes. *(Source:* From Shiva Kumar R. Mukkamalla. Microangiopathic Hemolytic Anemia. Ferri's Clinical Advisor 2021. Elsevier 2021.)

Haemolytic Anaemia Due to Direct Action of Physical, Chemical and Infectious Agents PA 16.4

Haemolytic anaemia caused by physical, chemical and infectious agents represents a diverse group of disorders. These anaemias are induced by factors such as mechanical trauma to RBCs, exposure to certain chemicals or toxins, and infections. The pathophysiology involves the direct destruction or alteration of RBC membranes, leading to premature haemolysis.

Causes include extensive burns, chemicals agents like arsenic chloride and distilled water, and infectious agents like *Plasmodium* species and *Clostridium welchii.*

Haemolysis in malaria

In malaria due to *Plasmodium* species other than *P. falciparum*, the anaemia is generally mild. The mechanisms leading to anaemia are as follows:

- Excessive destruction of parasitized RBCs in the spleen
- Suppression of erythropoiesis by the inflammatory cytokines
- Suppression of erythropoietin production
- Shunting of iron from erythroblasts to stores

Haemolysis in *falciparum* malaria

Acute intravascular haemolysis, also called 'black water fever', occurs due to *P. falciparum* and is clinically characterized by fever, extreme fatigue and blackish discolouration of urine due to haemoglobinuria (and hence the name 'black water fever'). This is seen in patients with chronic malaria undergoing irregular treatment with quinine. Diagnosis is based on the demonstration of the parasite in blood films or detection of antigens by immunochromatography or by the quantitative buffy coat (QBC) method.

Haemolysis associated with clostridial infection

C. welchii sepsis is usually associated with septic abortion and commonly causes marked intravascular haemolysis with a poor prognosis. This organism releases lecithinase enzyme that acts on red cell membranes to form lysolecithins that have a strong haemolytic tendency.

Recent advancements have significantly improved our understanding and treatment of these conditions.

LABORATORY APPROACH TO A CASE OF ANAEMIA

PA 13.4

As discussed in the preceding sections, anaemia is not a primary disease but a manifestation of varied disorders and hence needs a complete workup before initiating treatment. Complete history taking and physical examination are equally important before laboratory approach to anaemia. Here, we discuss the laboratory approach to anaemia (Flowchart 15.1).

Investigations required for the approach:

- Complete blood cell count
- Peripheral smear study
- Reticulocyte count
- Serum LDH
- Serum bilirubin
- Serum iron studies
- Serum vitamin B_{12} levels
- Serum folic acid levels
- Haemoglobin electrophoresis
- Bone marrow examination
- Bone marrow – Pearl's Prussian blue staining
- Tests performed for specific anaemia
  - Osmotic fragility test – HS
  - NADPH assay – G6PD deficiency
  - Sickling test – sickle cell anaemia
  - NESTROFT test – thalassaemia
  - Flow cytometry – PNH
- Genetic studies in confirmation and genetic counselling

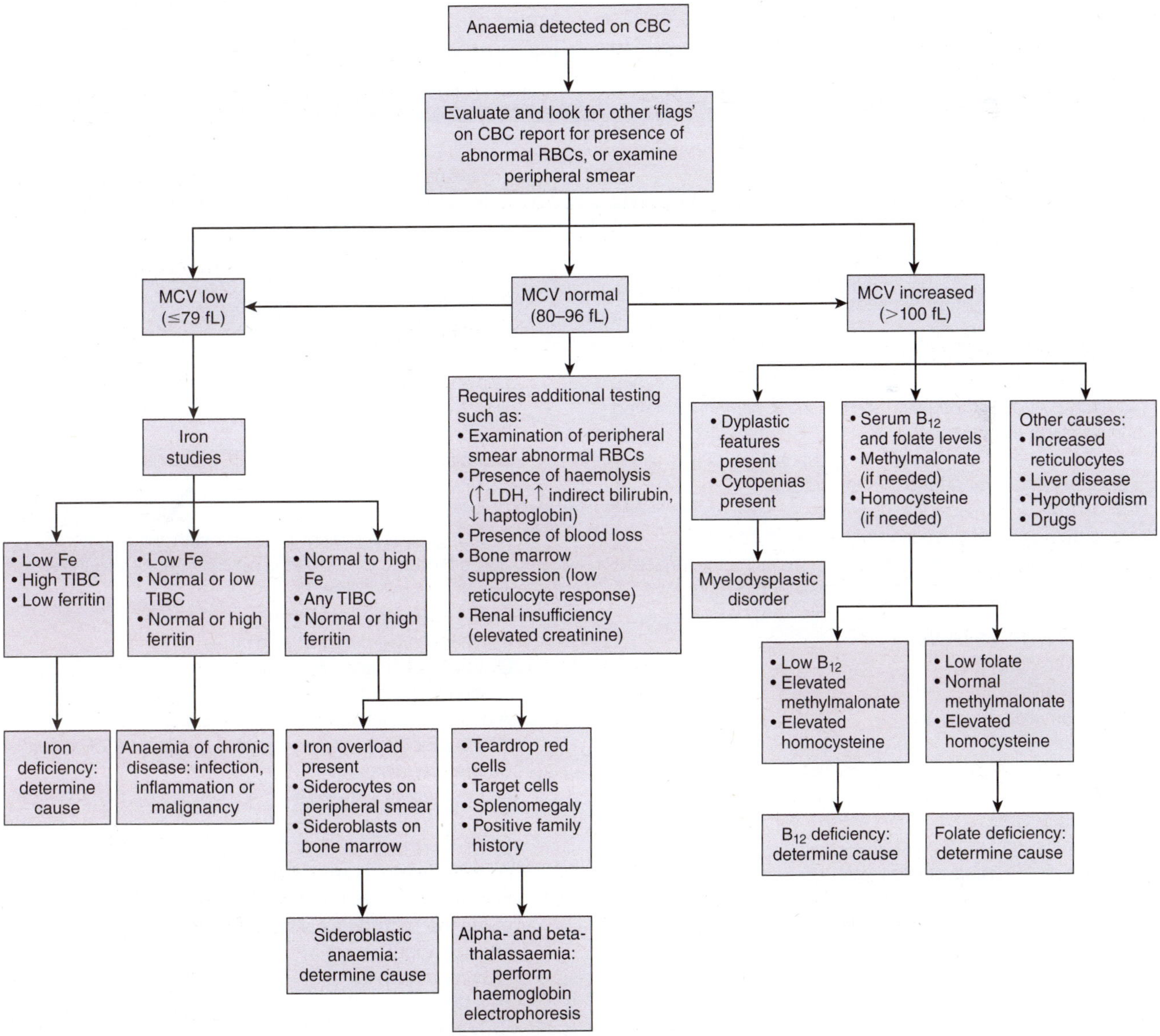

Flowchart 15.1 The laboratory approach to a case of anaemia. CBC, complete blood count; Fe, iron; LDH, lactate dehydrogenase; MCV, mean corpuscular volume; RBCs, red blood cells; TIBC, total iron-binding capacity (transferrin).

Table 15.26 Classification of Polycythaemia

Type	Subtype	Common diseases
Absolute polycythaemia		
1. **Primary**		Polycythaemia vera
2. **Secondary**	Compensatory	Lung and heart disease High-altitude sickness
	Paraneoplastic	Erythropoietin-secreting tumours
Relative polycythaemia	Haemoconcentration	Dehydration

POLYCYTHAEMIA

Polycythaemia, also known as polyglobulia, is a disease state with an abnormally high red cell count and/or haemoglobin. It can be **absolute** polycythaemia, with an increase in red cell production, or **relative** polycythaemia, due to haemoconcentration that occurs in dehydration (Table 15.26). Absolute polycythaemia can be due to **primary or secondary** causes. Primary polycythaemia is due to intrinsic abnormality of red cell progenitors. The most common cause of primary polycythaemia is polycythaemia vera due to mutations that result in erythropoietin-independent proliferation of red cell progenitors. It is discussed in detail in Chapter 16. Secondary polycythaemia is due to a compensatory increase in erythropoietin secretion. Hence, the erythropoietin levels are low or normal in primary polycythaemia and elevated in secondary polycythaemia cases. Polycythaemia that occurs due to stress is called **Gaisbock syndrome**.

Polycythaemia can cause complications due to **hyperviscosity of the blood**, thrombosis and bleeding and hence needs treatment. Emergency treatment is by phlebotomy and, depending on the underlying condition, it can be continued on a regular basis. Treating the underlying cause is the definitive treatment.

SELF-ASSESSMENT

Multiple Choice Questions

1. A 40-year-old patient presents with jaundice, dark urine and anaemia. The direct Coombs test is negative. Which condition is most likely?
   A. Autoimmune haemolytic anaemia
   B. Paroxysmal nocturnal haemoglobinuria
   C. Sickle cell anaemia
   D. Iron-deficiency anaemia
2. A patient with chronic kidney disease develops anaemia. Which pathophysiological mechanism is primarily involved in this type of anaemia?
   A. Decreased erythropoietin production
   B. Iron deficiency due to dietary factors
   C. Vitamin B_{12} deficiency
   D. Autoimmune destruction of red blood cells
3. A patient presents with a microcytic, hypochromic anaemia and a history of chronic gastrointestinal bleeding. What is the most likely cause of this anaemia?
   A. Vitamin B_{12} deficiency
   B. Folate deficiency
   C. Iron deficiency
   D. Haemolytic process
4. In a patient with suspected megaloblastic anaemia, which laboratory finding is most indicative of vitamin B_{12} deficiency rather than of folate deficiency?
   A. Macrocytosis
   B. Hypersegmented neutrophils
   C. Elevated homocysteine levels
   D. Elevated methylmalonic acid levels
5. A patient with anaemia and rheumatoid arthritis is most likely to have which type of anaemia?
   A. Anaemia of chronic disease
   B. Iron-deficiency anaemia
   C. Aplastic anaemia
   D. Haemolytic anaemia
6. A patient is diagnosed with anaemia and has a reticulocyte count of 0.5%. What does this suggest about the anaemia's aetiology?
   A. Haemorrhagic anaemia
   B. Haemolytic anaemia
   C. Anaemia of chronic disease
   D. Aplastic anaemia
7. A patient presents with anaemia, fatigue and a lemon-yellow skin complexion. Laboratory tests reveal macrocytic red cells. Which of the following deficiencies is most likely?
   A. Iron
   B. Folate
   C. Vitamin B_{12}
   D. Vitamin C
8. A young female patient presents with fatigue, headache and a high MCV. Her diet is predominantly vegan. Which anaemia is most likely?
   A. Iron-deficiency anaemia
   B. Vitamin B_{12}–deficiency anaemia
   C. Folate-deficiency anaemia
   D. Anaemia of chronic disease
9. A patient with known liver disease presents with anaemia. Which laboratory finding is most suggestive of anaemia due to liver disease?
   A. Low reticulocyte count
   B. Macrocytosis
   C. Microcytosis
   D. Normocytic, normochromic cells
10. In a patient with suspected drug-induced anaemia, which of the following drugs is most commonly associated with this condition?
    A. Acetaminophen
    B. Ibuprofen
    C. Methotrexate
    D. Lisinopril

11. A patient with a history of gastric bypass surgery presents with anaemia and neurological symptoms. Which type of anaemia is most likely?
    A. Iron-deficiency anaemia
    B. Anaemia of chronic inflammation
    C. Vitamin B_{12}–deficiency anaemia
    D. Folate-deficiency anaemia
12. A patient with systemic lupus erythematosus (SLE) presents with anaemia and a positive direct Coombs test. What type of anaemia is most likely?
    A. Autoimmune haemolytic anaemia
    B. Anaemia of chronic disease
    C. Iron-deficiency anaemia
    D. Aplastic anaemia
13. A patient with chronic obstructive pulmonary disease (COPD) develops anaemia. Which type of anaemia is commonly associated with COPD?
    A. Iron-deficiency anaemia
    B. Anaemia of chronic disease
    C. Aplastic anaemia
    D. Haemolytic anaemia
14. A patient with known HIV infection presents with macrocytic anaemia and low reticulocyte count. Which drug is likely contributing to this anaemia?
    A. Zidovudine
    B. Lamivudine
    C. Efavirenz
    D. Ritonavir
15. A patient is diagnosed with haemolytic anaemia. Laboratory findings show increased unconjugated bilirubin and low haptoglobin levels. Which additional test is most useful for confirming the diagnosis?
    A. Bone marrow biopsy
    B. Peripheral blood smear
    C. Urine examination
    D. Iron studies
16. A patient with a history of alcoholism presents with anaemia and a mean corpuscular volume (MCV) of 110 fL. What is the most likely cause of this anaemia?
    A. Iron deficiency
    B. Protein deficiency
    C. Vitamin B_{12} deficiency
    D. Direct alcohol toxicity on bone marrow
17. In a patient with microcytic anaemia, which finding differentiates thalassaemia from iron-deficiency anaemia?
    A. High ferritin levels
    B. Low reticulocyte count
    C. Elevated red blood cell count
    D. Elevated serum iron
18. A patient with a prosthetic heart valve develops anaemia with schistocytes on peripheral smear. What is the most likely diagnosis?
    A. Iron-deficiency anaemia
    B. Microangiopathic haemolytic anaemia
    C. Aplastic anaemia
    D. Megaloblastic anaemia
19. A patient presents with severe anaemia, jaundice and elevated lactate dehydrogenase (LDH). What type of haemolysis is most likely?
    A. Extravascular haemolysis
    B. Intravascular haemolysis
    C. Autoimmune haemolysis
    D. Drug-induced haemolysis
20. A patient with anaemia has a bone marrow biopsy showing increased cellularity and erythroid hyperplasia. What does this indicate about the anaemia's pathophysiology?
    A. It is likely due to a production problem.
    B. It is likely due to a destruction problem.
    C. It suggests an iron absorption issue.
    D. It indicates a vitamin deficiency.
21. In a patient with anaemia and elevated serum ferritin, which condition is most unlikely?
    A. Iron-deficiency anaemia
    B. Anaemia of chronic disease
    C. Hemochromatosis
    D. Sideroblastic anaemia
22. A patient with renal failure on erythropoietin therapy develops hypertension and a high haemoglobin level. What complication is this indicative of?
    A. Erythropoietin resistance
    B. Erythropoietin overdose
    C. Secondary polycythaemia
    D. Hyperviscosity syndrome
23. A patient with anaemia shows a low serum erythropoietin level. Which condition is this finding most consistent with?
    A. Anaemia of chronic disease
    B. Renal anaemia
    C. Haemolytic anaemia
    D. Iron-deficiency anaemia
24. A patient with anaemia has a high red cell distribution width (RDW) but normal MCV. What type of anaemia is this indicative of?
    A. Iron-deficiency anaemia
    B. Anaemia of chronic disease
    C. Sideroblastic anaemia
    D. Combined deficiency (iron and vitamin B_{12})
25. A patient with a history of intestinal resection presents with anaemia and neurological symptoms. Which type of anaemia is most likely?
    A. Iron-deficiency anaemia
    B. Anaemia of chronic inflammation
    C. Vitamin B_{12}–deficiency anaemia
    D. Folate-deficiency anaemia

Answers

1. (B); 2. (A); 3. (C); 4. (D); 5. (A); 6. (D); 7. (C); 8. (B); 9. (B); 10. (C); 11. (C); 12. (A); 13. (B); 14. (A); 15. (B); 16. (B); 17. (A); 18. (B); 19. (B); 20. (B); 21. (B); 22. (B); 23. (B); 24. (D); 25. (C)

Self-Assessment Questions

1. A 35-year-old man presented to casualty with acute blood loss following a road traffic accident. On examination, he had pallor. Explore the changes at the level of blood counts with respect to blood loss.
2. A 10-year-old child presented to the paediatrics outpatient department (OPD) with chief complaints being yellowish discolouration of the skin, abdominal distension, easy fatigability and loss of appetite. On examination, the child was anaemic and jaundiced with moderate splenomegaly.
   Laboratory investigations: Hb 6.5 g/dL, PCV 14%, bilirubin 6.5 mg/dL, indirect 5.3 mg/dL, reticulocyte count 8%
3. A 10-year-old child presented to the paediatrics OPD with chief complaints of yellowish discolouration of the skin, abdominal distension, easy fatigability and loss of appetite. A history of similar episodes was reported in one of the

parents. On examination, the child was anaemic and jaundiced with moderate splenomegaly.

Laboratory investigations: Hb 6.5 g/dL, PCV 14%, MCV 56 fL, MCH 16 pg, MCHC 40 g/dL, platelet count 175,000/mL, bilirubin 6.5 mg/dL, indirect 5.3 mg/dL, reticulocyte count 8%. Peripheral smear showed the presence of microspherocytes.

4. A 32-year-old African man who recently returned from a trip overseas was diagnosed with malaria due to *Plasmodium vivax*. After 4 days of therapy with primaquine, he developed fever, low back pain and dark urine.

   Laboratory investigations: Hb 6.5 g/dL, PCV 14%, reticulocyte count 10% (corrected). Peripheral smear showed the presence of bite cells, spherocytes, nucleated red cells and polychromatophilic red cells.

5. A 6-year-old child presented to the paediatrics OPD with chief complaints of painful episodes in hands and feet and easy fatigability. Family history was negative for similar episodes. On examination, the child was found to be anaemic and jaundiced with bone tenderness.

   Laboratory investigations: Hb 6.5 g/dL, PCV 14%, MCV 83 fL, MCH 28 pg, platelet count 275,000/mL, bilirubin 6.5 mg/dL, indirect 5.3 mg/dL, reticulocyte count 8%. Peripheral smear showed the presence of normocytic normochromic anaemia, sickle-shaped cells, nucleated red cells and polychromatophilic red cells.

6. A 5-year-old child presented with complaints of growth retardation, abdominal distension, easy fatigability and a history of two transfusions in the past. On examination, the child was short statured with frontal bossing and prominent cheekbones, pallor+, splenomegaly+ and bone tenderness+.

   Laboratory investigations: Hb 6.5 g/dL, PCV 14%, RBC count 5.6 million/mL, MCV 56 fL, MCH 16 pg, RDW 12, platelet count 375,000/mL, reticulocyte count 10% (corrected), Mentzer index 10 (<13). Peripheral smear showed microcytic hypochromic anaemia, target cells, nucleated red cells and polychromatophilic red cells.

7. A 45-year-old man presented with features of deep vein thrombosis. He also gave a history of passing red/brown-coloured urine early in the morning. On examination, he was anaemic with multiple purpuric spots.

   Laboratory investigations: Hb 8.5 g/dL, PCV 19%, MCV 69 fL, MCH 19 pg, total count 2000 cells/mm^3, platelet count 75,000/mL. Peripheral smear showed microcytic hypochromic anaemia. Screening test for autohaemolysis was positive. Flow cytometry was performed and results were awaited.

8. A 35-year-old woman presented with complaints of acute-onset fatigue and high-coloured urine. She gave a history of hospitalization for pneumonia a couple of weeks ago. On examination, she was anaemic.

   Laboratory investigations: Hb 6.5 g/dL, reticulocyte count 6.5% (corrected). Peripheral smear showed irregular clumping of RBCs, normoblasts and polychromatophilic red cells.

9. A 35-year-old woman presented with complaints of easy fatigability. She also had a history of excessive menstrual loss for the past 2 years. On examination, she was anaemic.

   Laboratory investigations: Hb 6.5 g/dL; MCV 65 fL; MCH 20 pg; RDW 19.5; reticulocyte count <0.5% (corrected); serum iron, ferritin and transferrin saturation low; serum TIBC elevated. Peripheral smear showed microcytic hypochromic RBCs with marked anisopoikilocytosis including pencil cells and target cells.

10. A 35-year-old alcoholic man presented with complaints of numbness, loss of position and vibration sense and easy fatigability. He also had a history of frequent episodes of oral ulcers and diarrhoea. On examination, he was anaemic and had a beefy red tongue.

    Laboratory investigations: Hb 6.5 g/dL; MCV 110 fL; MCH 34 pg; RDW 19.5; reticulocyte count <0.5% (corrected); serum iron, ferritin and transferrin saturation high; serum vitamin B_{12} markedly reduced.

11. A 35-year-old woman who had a known history of rheumatoid arthritis on irregular treatment presented with recent-onset easy fatigability. On examination, she was found to be anaemic.

    Laboratory investigations: Hb 6.5 g/dL, MCV 66 fL, MCH 20 pg, reticulocyte count <0.5% (corrected), serum iron and TIBC reduced, serum ferritin high, serum hepcidin high, serum erythropoietin low. Peripheral smear showed microcytic hypochromic anaemia.

12. A 40-year-old man who was receiving treatment with alkylating agents for non-Hodgkin lymphoma presented with easy fatigability, recurrent infections and frequent bleeding episodes. On examination, he was anaemic with multiple purpuric spots all over the body. The spleen was not palpable. Bone marrow aspiration was attempted, but the yield was nil.

    Laboratory investigations: Hb 6.5 g/dL, MCV 86 fL, MCH 28 pg, total count 2000 cells/mm^3, platelet count 15,000/mm^3, reticulocyte count <0.5% (corrected). Peripheral smear showed pancytopenia with normocytic normochromic anaemia.

Key

1. Acute blood loss changes
2. Extravascular haemolytic anaemia
3. Hereditary spherocytosis
4. G6PD deficiency
5. Sickle cell anaemia
6. Thalassaemia major
7. PNH
8. Cold AIHA
9. Iron-deficiency anaemia
10. Megaloblastic anaemia due to vitamin B_{12} deficiency
11. Anaemia of chronic disease
12. Aplastic anaemia

Topics for Self-Directed Learning

1. Congenital dyserythropoietic anaemia
2. Basophilic stippling of red blood cells
3. Hereditary persistence of fetal haemoglobin
4. Anaemia in chronic renal failure
5. Stem cell disorders
6. Different erythrocyte morphology and their associated disorders
7. Sideroblastic anaemia
8. NESTROFT test
9. Hereditary persistence of fetal haemoglobin
10. HbSC disease
11. Osmotic fragility test
12. Embryonic haemoglobins

MIND MAPS

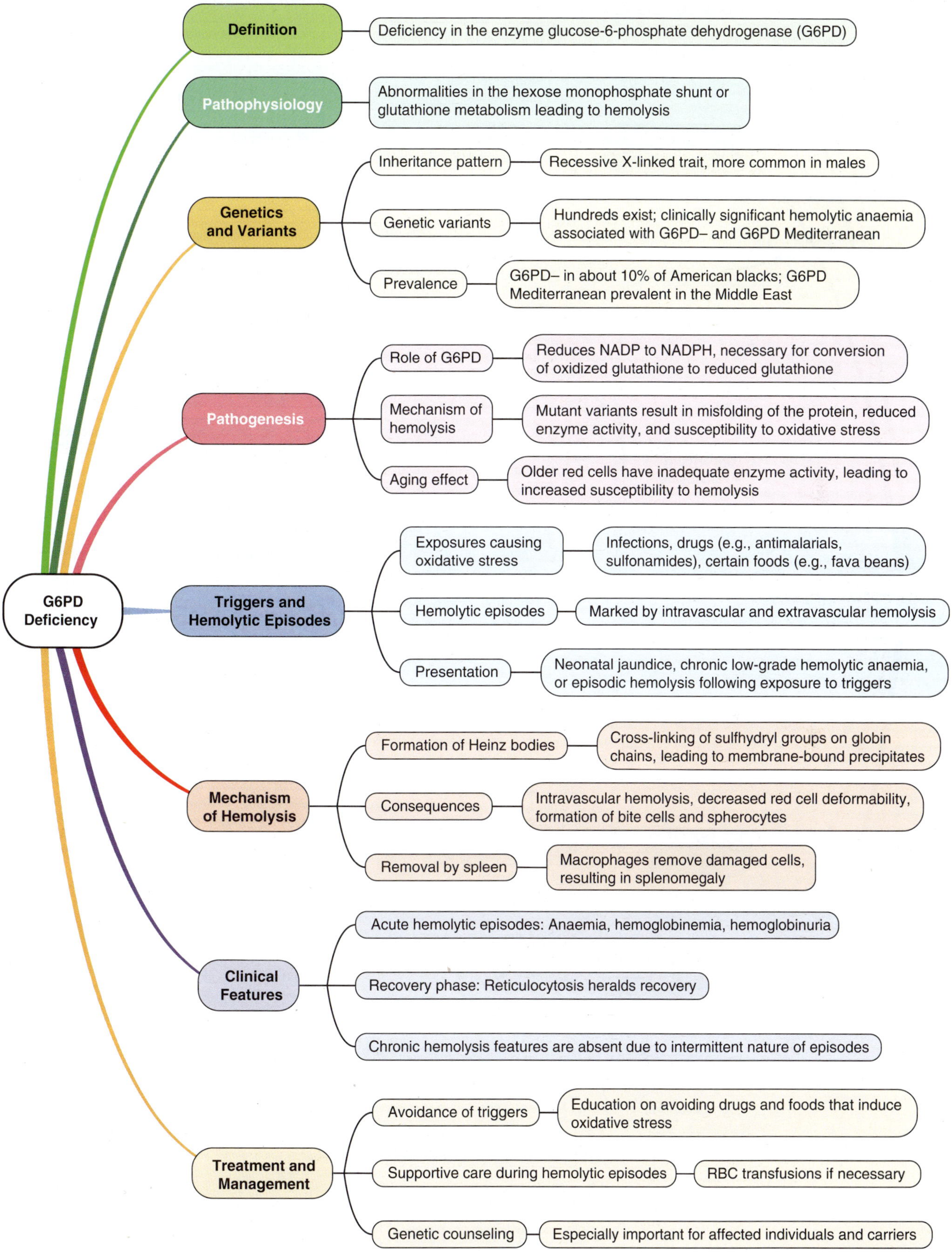
G6PD Deficiency
Definition
Deficiency in the enzyme glucose-6-phosphate dehydrogenase (G6PD)
Pathophysiology
Abnormalities in the hexose monophosphate shunt or glutathione metabolism leading to hemolysis
Genetics and Variants
Inheritance pattern
Recessive X-linked trait, more common in males
Genetic variants
Hundreds exist; clinically significant hemolytic anaemia associated with G6PD– and G6PD Mediterranean
Prevalence
G6PD– in about 10% of American blacks; G6PD Mediterranean prevalent in the Middle East
Pathogenesis
Role of G6PD
Reduces NADP to NADPH, necessary for conversion of oxidized glutathione to reduced glutathione
Mechanism of hemolysis
Mutant variants result in misfolding of the protein, reduced enzyme activity, and susceptibility to oxidative stress
Aging effect
Older red cells have inadequate enzyme activity, leading to increased susceptibility to hemolysis
Triggers and Hemolytic Episodes
Exposures causing oxidative stress
Infections, drugs (e.g., antimalarials, sulfonamides), certain foods (e.g., fava beans)
Hemolytic episodes
Marked by intravascular and extravascular hemolysis
Presentation
Neonatal jaundice, chronic low-grade hemolytic anaemia, or episodic hemolysis following exposure to triggers
Mechanism of Hemolysis
Formation of Heinz bodies
Cross-linking of sulfhydryl groups on globin chains, leading to membrane-bound precipitates
Consequences
Intravascular hemolysis, decreased red cell deformability, formation of bite cells and spherocytes
Removal by spleen
Macrophages remove damaged cells, resulting in splenomegaly
Clinical Features
Acute hemolytic episodes: Anaemia, hemoglobinemia, hemoglobinuria
Recovery phase: Reticulocytosis heralds recovery
Chronic hemolysis features are absent due to intermittent nature of episodes
Treatment and Management
Avoidance of triggers
Education on avoiding drugs and foods that induce oxidative stress
Supportive care during hemolytic episodes
RBC transfusions if necessary
Genetic counseling
Especially important for affected individuals and carriers

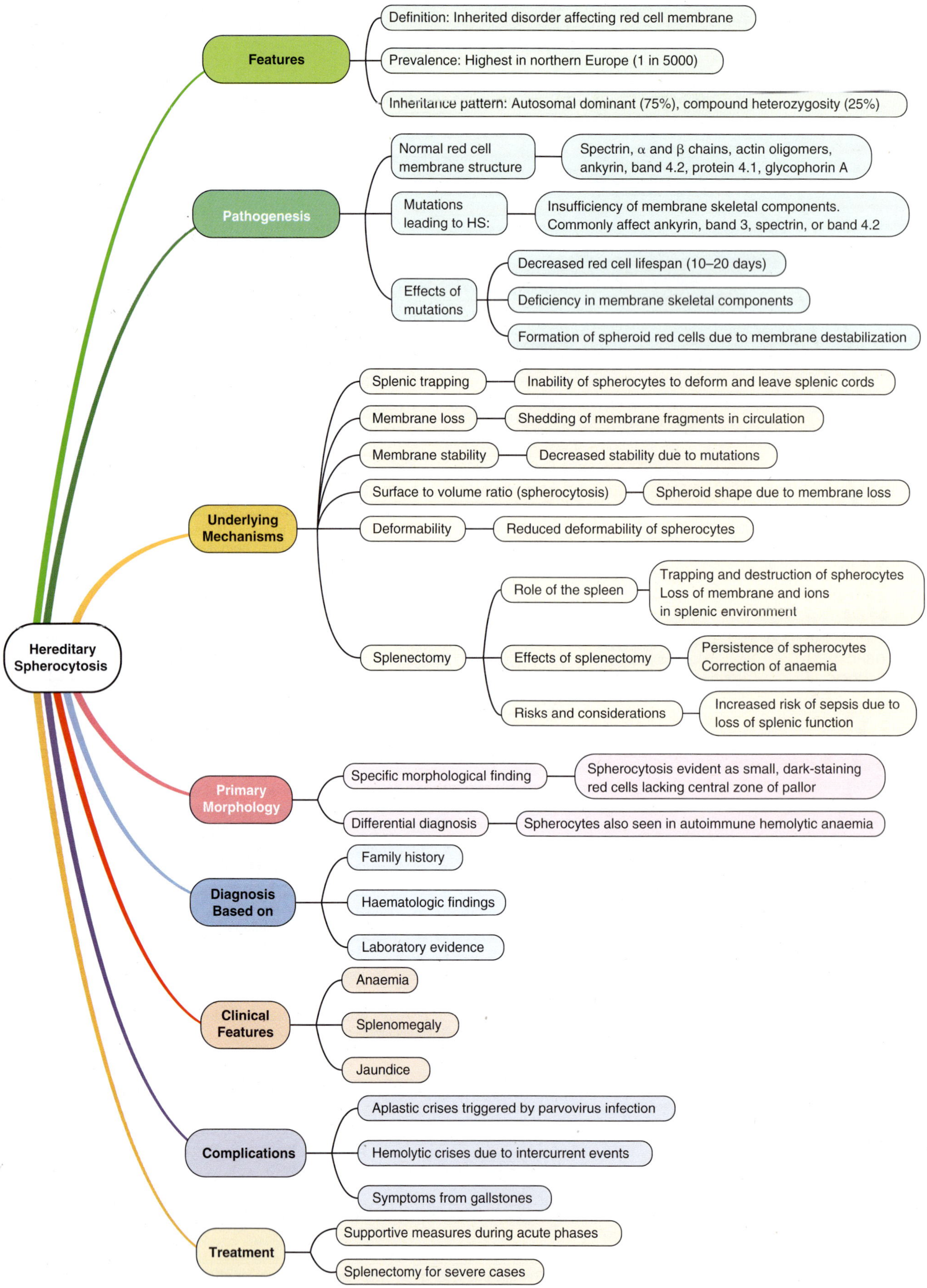
Hereditary Spherocytosis
Features
Definition: Inherited disorder affecting red cell membrane
Prevalence: Highest in northern Europe (1 in 5000)
Inheritance pattern: Autosomal dominant (75%), compound heterozygosity (25%)
Pathogenesis
Normal red cell membrane structure
Spectrin, α and β chains, actin oligomers, ankyrin, band 4.2, protein 4.1, glycophorin A
Mutations leading to HS:
Insufficiency of membrane skeletal components. Commonly affect ankyrin, band 3, spectrin, or band 4.2
Effects of mutations
Decreased red cell lifespan (10–20 days)
Deficiency in membrane skeletal components
Formation of spheroid red cells due to membrane destabilization
Underlying Mechanisms
Splenic trapping
Inability of spherocytes to deform and leave splenic cords
Membrane loss
Shedding of membrane fragments in circulation
Membrane stability
Decreased stability due to mutations
Surface to volume ratio (spherocytosis)
Spheroid shape due to membrane loss
Deformability
Reduced deformability of spherocytes
Splenectomy
Role of the spleen
Trapping and destruction of spherocytes
Loss of membrane and ions in splenic environment
Effects of splenectomy
Persistence of spherocytes
Correction of anaemia
Risks and considerations
Increased risk of sepsis due to loss of splenic function
Primary Morphology
Specific morphological finding
Spherocytosis evident as small, dark-staining red cells lacking central zone of pallor
Differential diagnosis
Spherocytes also seen in autoimmune hemolytic anaemia
Diagnosis Based on
Family history
Haematologic findings
Laboratory evidence
Clinical Features
Anaemia
Splenomegaly
Jaundice
Complications
Aplastic crises triggered by parvovirus infection
Hemolytic crises due to intercurrent events
Symptoms from gallstones
Treatment
Supportive measures during acute phases
Splenectomy for severe cases

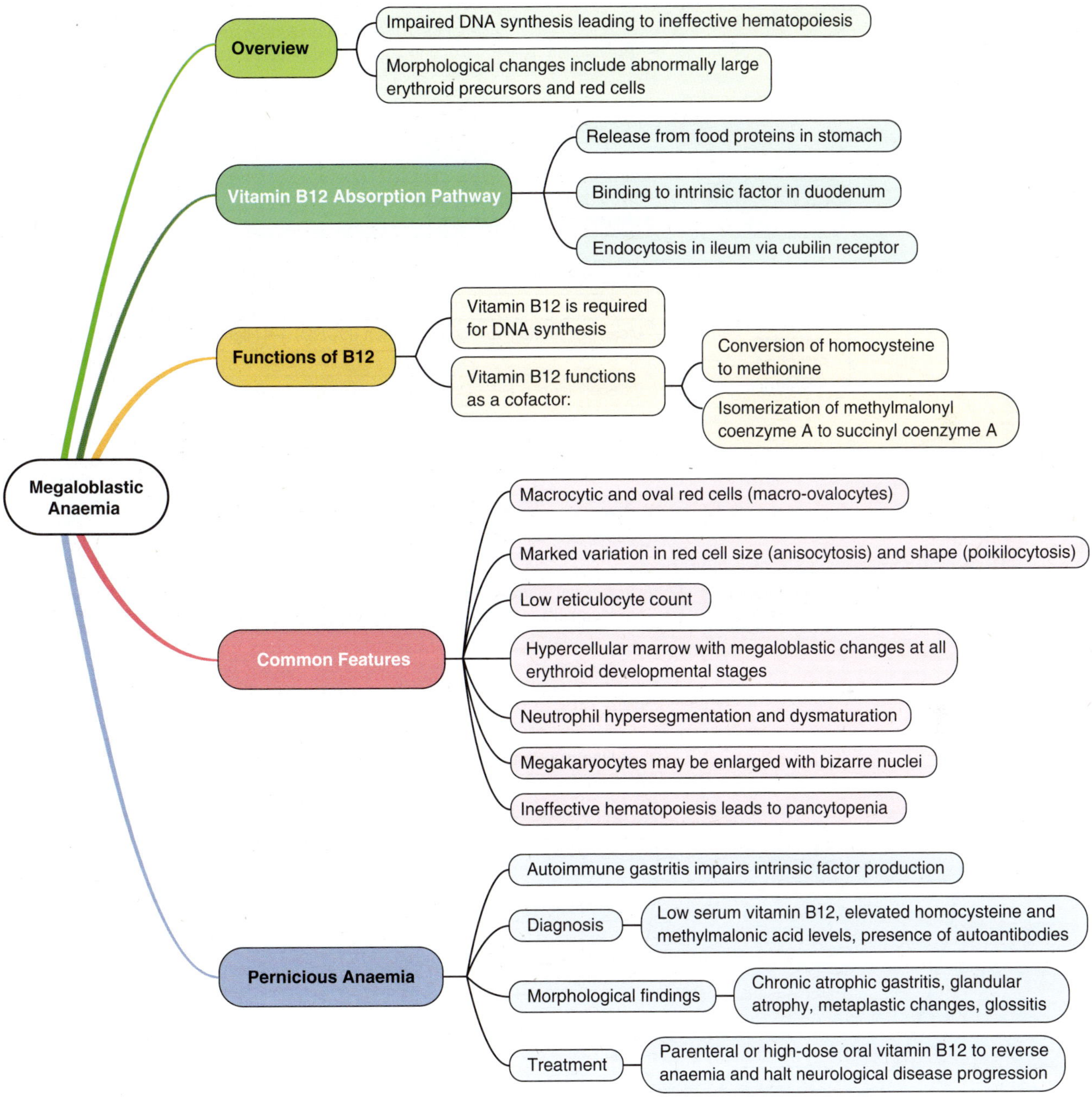
Megaloblastic Anaemia
Overview
Impaired DNA synthesis leading to ineffective hematopoiesis
Morphological changes include abnormally large erythroid precursors and red cells
Vitamin B12 Absorption Pathway
Release from food proteins in stomach
Binding to intrinsic factor in duodenum
Endocytosis in ileum via cubilin receptor
Functions of B12
Vitamin B12 is required for DNA synthesis
Vitamin B12 functions as a cofactor:
Conversion of homocysteine to methionine
Isomerization of methylmalonyl coenzyme A to succinyl coenzyme A
Common Features
Macrocytic and oval red cells (macro-ovalocytes)
Marked variation in red cell size (anisocytosis) and shape (poikilocytosis)
Low reticulocyte count
Hypercellular marrow with megaloblastic changes at all erythroid developmental stages
Neutrophil hypersegmentation and dysmaturation
Megakaryocytes may be enlarged with bizarre nuclei
Ineffective hematopoiesis leads to pancytopenia
Pernicious Anaemia
Autoimmune gastritis impairs intrinsic factor production
Diagnosis
Low serum vitamin B12, elevated homocysteine and methylmalonic acid levels, presence of autoantibodies
Morphological findings
Chronic atrophic gastritis, glandular atrophy, metaplastic changes, glossitis
Treatment
Parenteral or high-dose oral vitamin B12 to reverse anaemia and halt neurological disease progression

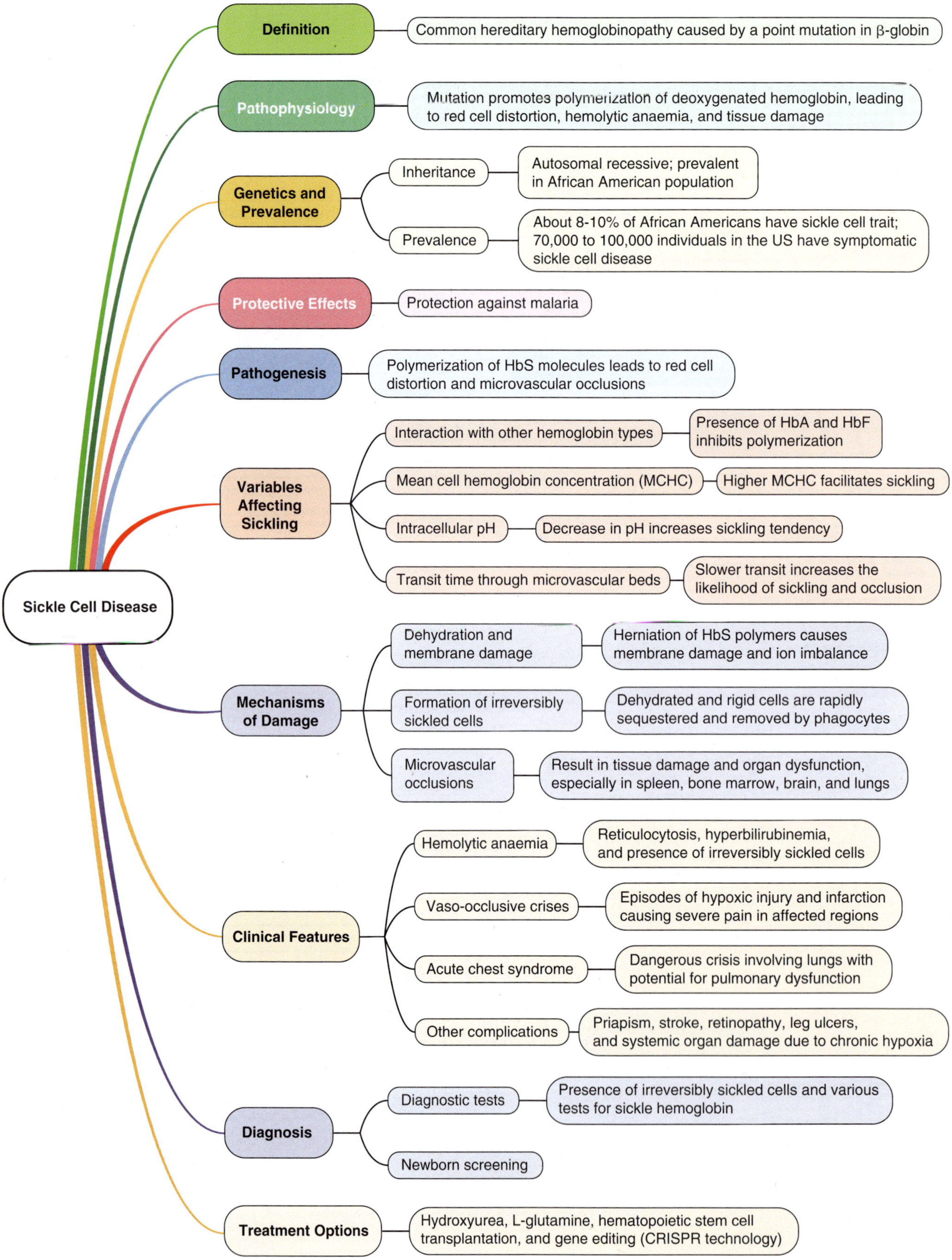
Sickle Cell Disease
Definition
Common hereditary hemoglobinopathy caused by a point mutation in β-globin
Pathophysiology
Mutation promotes polymerization of deoxygenated hemoglobin, leading to red cell distortion, hemolytic anaemia, and tissue damage
Genetics and Prevalence
Inheritance
Autosomal recessive; prevalent in African American population
Prevalence
About 8-10% of African Americans have sickle cell trait; 70,000 to 100,000 individuals in the US have symptomatic sickle cell disease
Protective Effects
Protection against malaria
Pathogenesis
Polymerization of HbS molecules leads to red cell distortion and microvascular occlusions
Variables Affecting Sickling
Interaction with other hemoglobin types
Presence of HbA and HbF inhibits polymerization
Mean cell hemoglobin concentration (MCHC)
Higher MCHC facilitates sickling
Intracellular pH
Decrease in pH increases sickling tendency
Transit time through microvascular beds
Slower transit increases the likelihood of sickling and occlusion
Mechanisms of Damage
Dehydration and membrane damage
Herniation of HbS polymers causes membrane damage and ion imbalance
Formation of irreversibly sickled cells
Dehydrated and rigid cells are rapidly sequestered and removed by phagocytes
Microvascular occlusions
Result in tissue damage and organ dysfunction, especially in spleen, bone marrow, brain, and lungs
Clinical Features
Hemolytic anaemia
Reticulocytosis, hyperbilirubinemia, and presence of irreversibly sickled cells
Vaso-occlusive crises
Episodes of hypoxic injury and infarction causing severe pain in affected regions
Acute chest syndrome
Dangerous crisis involving lungs with potential for pulmonary dysfunction
Other complications
Priapism, stroke, retinopathy, leg ulcers, and systemic organ damage due to chronic hypoxia
Diagnosis
Diagnostic tests
Presence of irreversibly sickled cells and various tests for sickle hemoglobin
Newborn screening
Treatment Options
Hydroxyurea, L-glutamine, hematopoietic stem cell transplantation, and gene editing (CRISPR technology)

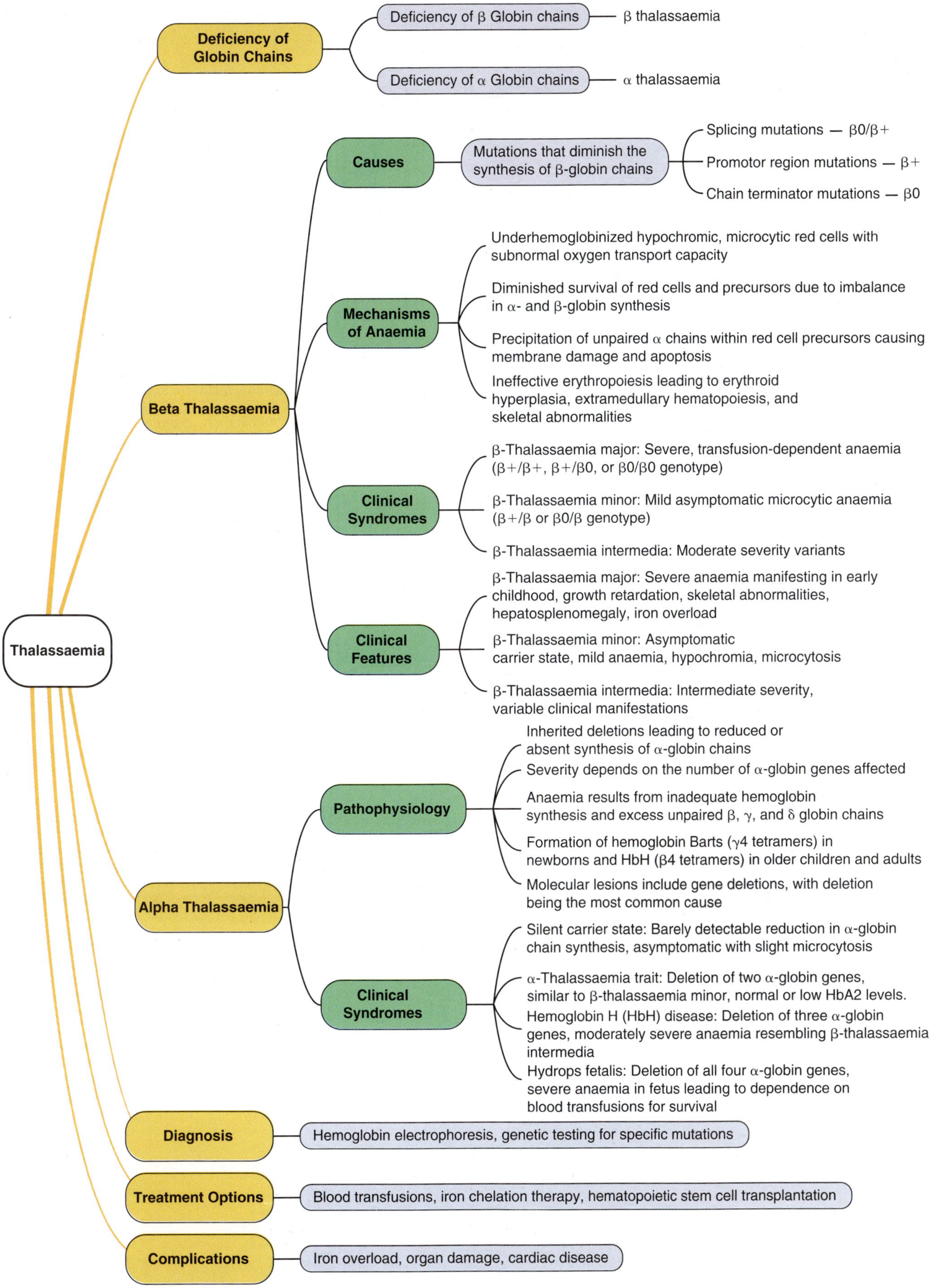
Thalassaemia
Deficiency of Globin Chains
Deficiency of β Globin chains
β thalassaemia
Deficiency of α Globin chains
α thalassaemia
Beta Thalassaemia
Causes
Mutations that diminish the synthesis of β-globin chains
Splicing mutations — β0/β+
Promotor region mutations — β+
Chain terminator mutations — β0
Mechanisms of Anaemia
Underhemoglobinized hypochromic, microcytic red cells with subnormal oxygen transport capacity
Diminished survival of red cells and precursors due to imbalance in α- and β-globin synthesis
Precipitation of unpaired α chains within red cell precursors causing membrane damage and apoptosis
Ineffective erythropoiesis leading to erythroid hyperplasia, extramedullary hematopoiesis, and skeletal abnormalities
Clinical Syndromes
β-Thalassaemia major: Severe, transfusion-dependent anaemia (β+/β+, β+/β0, or β0/β0 genotype)
β-Thalassaemia minor: Mild asymptomatic microcytic anaemia (β+/β or β0/β genotype)
β-Thalassaemia intermedia: Moderate severity variants
Clinical Features
β-Thalassaemia major: Severe anaemia manifesting in early childhood, growth retardation, skeletal abnormalities, hepatosplenomegaly, iron overload
β-Thalassaemia minor: Asymptomatic carrier state, mild anaemia, hypochromia, microcytosis
β-Thalassaemia intermedia: Intermediate severity, variable clinical manifestations
Alpha Thalassaemia
Pathophysiology
Inherited deletions leading to reduced or absent synthesis of α-globin chains
Severity depends on the number of α-globin genes affected
Anaemia results from inadequate hemoglobin synthesis and excess unpaired β, γ, and δ globin chains
Formation of hemoglobin Barts (γ4 tetramers) in newborns and HbH (β4 tetramers) in older children and adults
Molecular lesions include gene deletions, with deletion being the most common cause
Clinical Syndromes
Silent carrier state: Barely detectable reduction in α-globin chain synthesis, asymptomatic with slight microcytosis
α-Thalassaemia trait: Deletion of two α-globin genes, similar to β-thalassaemia minor, normal or low HbA2 levels.
Hemoglobin H (HbH) disease: Deletion of three α-globin genes, moderately severe anaemia resembling β-thalassaemia intermedia
Hydrops fetalis: Deletion of all four α-globin genes, severe anaemia in fetus leading to dependence on blood transfusions for survival
Diagnosis
Hemoglobin electrophoresis, genetic testing for specific mutations
Treatment Options
Blood transfusions, iron chelation therapy, hematopoietic stem cell transplantation
Complications
Iron overload, organ damage, cardiac disease

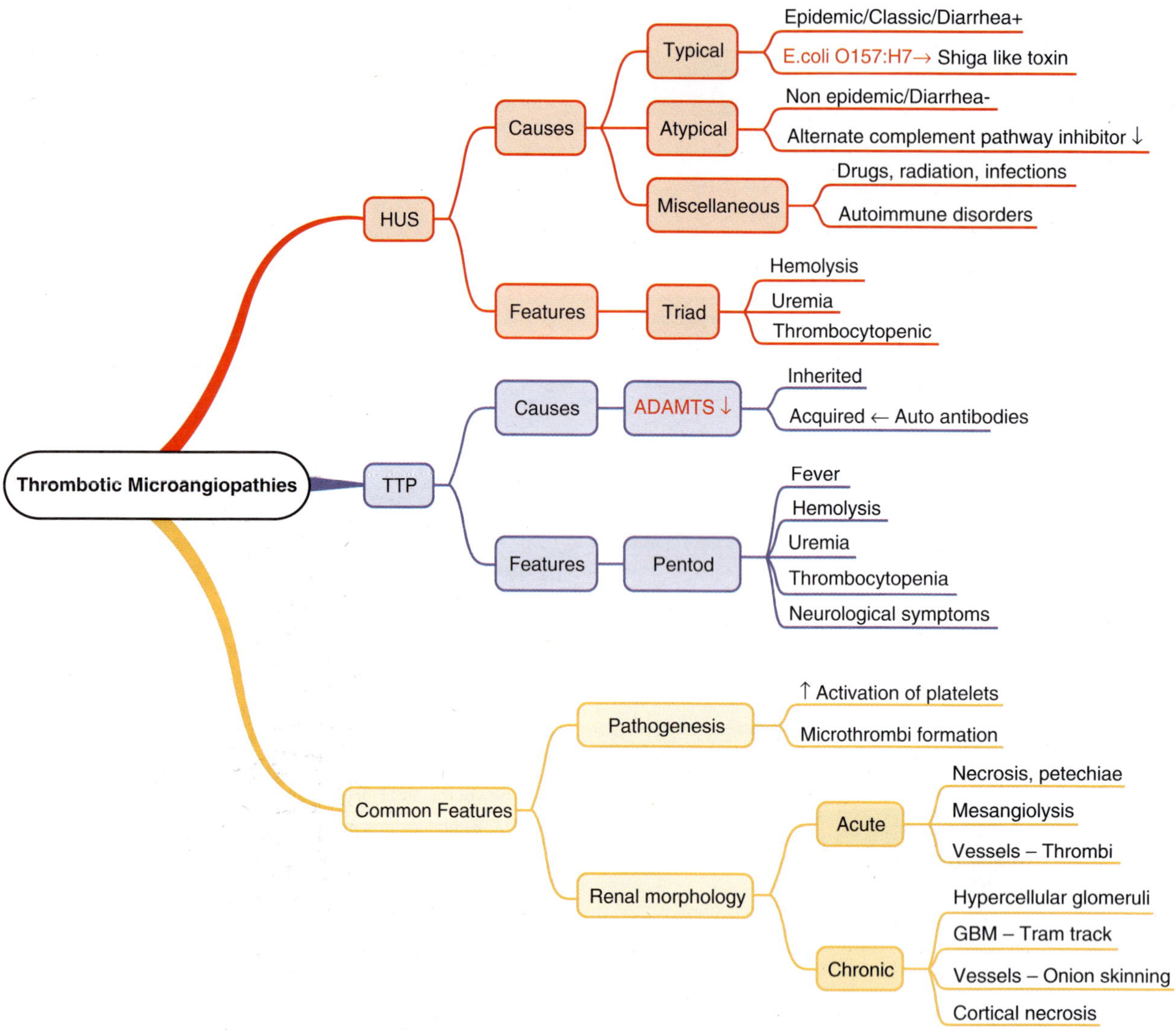
Thrombotic Microangiopathies
HUS
Causes
Typical
Epidemic/Classic/Diarrhea+
E.coli O157:H7→ Shiga like toxin
Atypical
Non epidemic/Diarrhea-
Alternate complement pathway inhibitor ↓
Miscellaneous
Drugs, radiation, infections
Autoimmune disorders
Features
Triad
Hemolysis
Uremia
Thrombocytopenic
TTP
Causes
ADAMTS ↓
Inherited
Acquired ← Auto antibodies
Features
Pentod
Fever
Hemolysis
Uremia
Thrombocytopenia
Neurological symptoms
Common Features
Pathogenesis
↑ Activation of platelets
Microthrombi formation
Renal morphology
Acute
Necrosis, petechiae
Mesangiolysis
Vessels – Thrombi
Chronic
Hypercellular glomeruli
GBM – Tram track
Vessels – Onion skinning
Cortical necrosis

Disorders of White Blood Cells, Lymph Nodes, Spleen and Thymus

16

Rajeswari Kathiah

PA 18.1 Enumerate and describe the causes of leucocytosis, **leucopenia, lymphocytosis and leukaemoid reactions**.

PA 18.2 Describe the aetiology, genetics, pathogenesis, classification, features and haematological features of **acute and chronic leukaemias**.

PA 19.1 Enumerate the causes and describe the differentiating features of **lymphadenopathy**.

PA 19.4 Describe and discuss the pathogenesis, pathology and the differentiating features of **Hodgkin and non-Hodgkin lymphomas**.

PA 19.6 Enumerate and differentiate the causes of **splenomegaly**.

CHAPTER OUTLINE

INTRODUCTION

Disorders of white blood cells (WBCs) can be broadly classified into two categories – the more common non-neoplastic diseases and the more dangerous neoplastic WBC disorders. Non-neoplastic disorders of WBCs are very common in humans and are encountered in daily practice, with manifestations ranging from simple to life-threatening infections. Functional abnormalities of WBCs, also called qualitative disorders of WBCs, are not so common, yet need to be identified with a high degree of clinical suspicion and managed appropriately. Non-neoplastic lymph node enlargement is one of the most common manifestations of a wide variety of underlying diseases and hence a complete knowledge of the causes, investigations and patterns is essential.

I. WHITE BLOOD CELLS AND LYMPH NODES

NON-NEOPLASTIC DISORDERS OF WHITE BLOOD CELLS

Non-neoplastic disorders of WBCs are almost always quantitative (numerical excess or deficiency of WBCs). Qualitative disorders refer to the structural and functional disorders of WBCs which may seldom accompany quantitative disorders. The clinically significant qualitative disorders are discussed in Chapter 3. Here, we discuss the quantitative disorders and few morphological abnormalities of WBCs.

A. **Non-neoplastic quantitative disorders of WBCs:**

1. **Leucocytosis:** It is a condition in which the number of circulating leucocytes is higher than normal. Leucocytosis is often synonymous with neutrophilia (which refers to the increase in the number of neutrophils). Leucocytosis can also result from inflammation or neoplasms or other causes as listed in Table 16.1.
2. **Leucopenia:** It is a decrease in the number of circulating leucocytes below the lower limit of normal.
3. **Leukaemoid reaction:** Leukaemoid reaction is characterized by a markedly increased WBC count with shift to left (increase in the number of immature cells in the neutrophil series) in peripheral blood in response to physiological stress or infection. Because of the presence of immature cells, it often mimics leukaemia, especially chronic myeloid leukaemia.
4. **Leucoerythroblastic reaction:** Leucoerythroblastic reaction refers to the presence of immature cells in the neutrophil series (granulocyte left shift) along with immature red blood cells (RBCs) and normoblasts in the peripheral blood.

LEUCOCYTOSIS PA 18.1

Because neutrophilia and lymphocytosis are very common entities, they are discussed in detail here; the causes for eosinophilia, monocytosis and basophilia are listed in Table 16.2.

Neutrophilia

Neutrophilia refers to an absolute increase in the neutrophil count above 7500 cells/mm^3. The most common manifestation of leucocytosis is neutrophilia; hence, the terms are used synonymously as mentioned earlier. The most common cause of neutrophilia is bacterial infections, especially pyogenic infections (Table 16.3). Of note,

Table 16.1 Leucocytosis and the Reference Values in Adults

Terms	Criteria
Leucocytosis	Total leucocyte count > 11,000/mm^3
Neutrophilia	Absolute neutrophil count > 7500/mm^3
Lymphocytosis	Absolute lymphocyte count > 4000/mm^3
Eosinophilia	Absolute eosinophil count > 600/mm^3
Monocytosis	Absolute monocyte count > 1000/mm^3
Basophilia	Absolute basophil count > 100/mm^3

Table 16.2 Causes of Increased WBC Counts

Type of Leucocytosis	Subcategories	Common Causes
Eosinophilia	Allergic diseases	Asthma Urticaria Rhinitis Drug reactions Type 1 hypersensitivity reactions Collagen vascular disorders
	Parasitic infestations	Filariasis Trichinosis Strongyloidiasis Toxocariasis Echinococcosis
	Dermatological disorders	Eczema Dermatitis herpetiformis Bullous pemphigoid
	Lung disorders	Loffler syndrome Tropical eosinophilia
	Haematological disorders	Myeloproliferative neoplasms Hodgkin disease Eosinophilic leukaemia
	Hypereosinophilic syndrome	
Monocytosis	Infections	Tuberculosis Brucellosis Kala-azar Malaria Typhoid Bacterial endocarditis
	Haematological malignancies	AML – M4 AML – M5 Chronic myelomonocytic leukaemia Myeloproliferative neoplasms Myelodysplastic syndromes Hodgkin disease
	Others	SLE RA Sarcoidosis
Basophilia		Myeloproliferative disorders Basophilic leukaemia IgE-mediated allergic disorders; inflammatory bowel disease Hypothyroidism

AML, acute myeloid leukaemia; RA, rheumatoid arthritis; SLE, systemic lupus erythematosus.

Table 16.3 Common Causes of Neutrophilia

Infectious causes:
- Acute bacterial infections by pyogenic organisms – abscess
- Appendicitis
- Osteomyelitis

Noninfectious causes:
- Tissue injury
- Burns
- Haemorrhage
- Haemolysis
- Acute myocardial infarction
- Gout
- Rheumatic fever
- Acute glomerulonephritis
- Asplenia
- Haematological malignancies
- Transient myeloproliferative disorder seen in Down syndrome
- Drugs – corticosteroids, lithium, etc.

neutrophilia is not always pathological and can also be seen in physiological conditions such as in newborn, pregnancy, following exercise and stress.

Morphology

In conditions of severe infections, following changes are commonly seen in the peripheral smear apart from neutrophilic leucocytosis (Fig. 16.1):

- Shift to left
- Toxic granules
- Döhle bodies
- Cytoplasmic vacuoles

Shift to left: Also referred to as left shift or blood shift is an increase in the number of immature leucocytes in the peripheral blood, especially the neutrophil band cells. The standard definition of a left shift is an absolute band form count of more than 700/mm^3. It is believed that cytokines, interleukin (IL)-1 and TNF accelerate the release of cells from the postmitotic reserve pool in the bone marrow, resulting in the increased number of immature cells in the peripheral blood. This systemic effect of inflammation often follows the course of active infection and other severe illnesses like hypoxia and shock.

Toxic granules (Fig. 16.2): Toxic granulation refers to dark coarse granules found in the cytoplasm of granulocytes, particularly neutrophils, in patients with inflammatory conditions. These granules are composed of peroxidase and acid hydrolase enzymes. Toxic granules are similar to the azurophilic granules that are found in immature granulocytes like promyelocytes but are usually not seen in the mature forms. Toxic granulation thus represents abnormal maturation of neutrophils. In a rare syndrome called Alder–Reilly syndrome, the neutrophils possess dark staining granules which may be confused with toxic granulation.

Döhle bodies (Fig. 16.3): Döhle bodies are light blue-grey, oval, basophilic inclusions of neutrophils which are thought to be remnants of the rough endoplasmic reticulum. These are often seen in conjunction with toxic granulation and are associated with burns, infection, trauma, etc. Their presence in mature and immature neutrophils on a blood smear can be normal if they are present only in small numbers.

Toxic vacuoles (Fig. 16.2): Toxic vacuolation is the presence of vacuoles in the cytoplasm of neutrophils as a response to infections or inflammatory conditions. The formation of toxic vacuoles represents increased phagocytic activity which is stimulated by the release of cytokines in response to inflammation or injury. It is often seen in bacterial infections, liver failure and alcohol toxicity. This finding when accompanied by toxic granules and shift to left is an indication of sepsis.

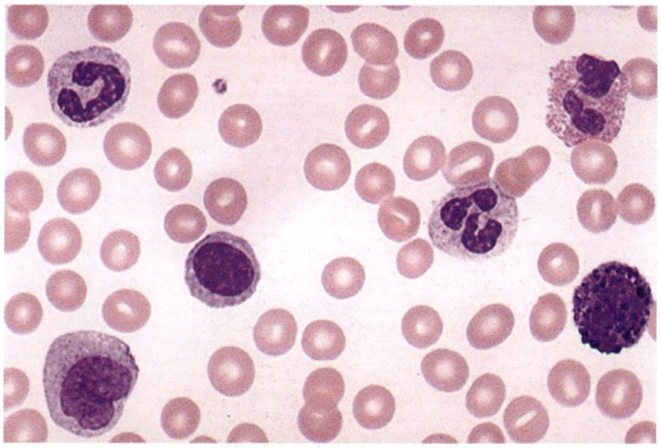

Fig. 16.1 Peripheral smear with normal WBCs shows a mature lymphocyte, neutrophils, eosinophil, basophil and monocyte. (*Source:* From Edward C. Klatt, Robbins and Cotran Atlas of Pathology. Elsevier. 2020.)

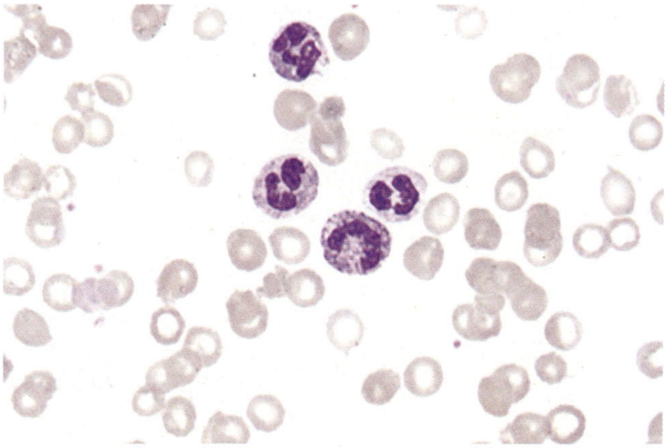

Fig. 16.2 Peripheral smear with toxic granules and cytoplasmic vacuoles in neutrophils. (*Source:* From Nancy S. Rosenthal. Hematopathology. Elsevier. 2017.)

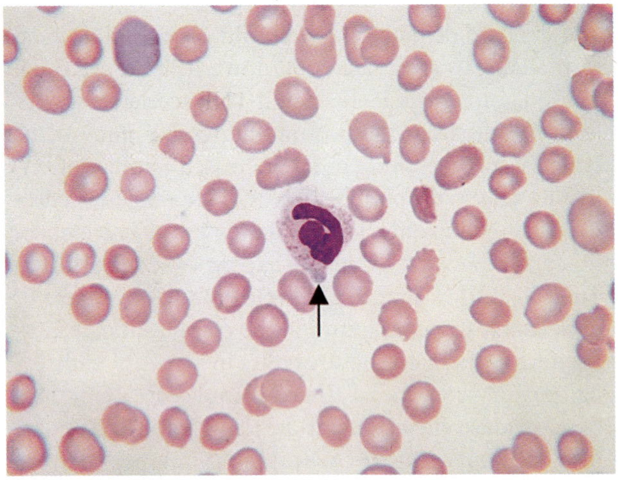

Fig. 16.3 Peripheral smear with Döhle bodies, a pale blue–grey amorphous inclusion near the cell membrane of the neutrophil. (*Source:* From Barbara J. Bain. Goldman-Cecil Medicine, 2-volume Set. Elsevier. 2020.)

Lymphocytosis **PA 18.1**

Lymphocytosis refers to the condition where there is an increase in absolute lymphocyte count beyond the normal range. Of note, physiological relative lymphocyte predominance (LP) exists in children younger than 12 years and elderly individuals older than 60 years. Lymphocytosis accompanies monocytosis in many disorders associated with chronic immunological stimulation. The commonest cause of lymphocytosis is viral infections; all other causes are listed in Table 16.4.

Lymphocytosis due to underlying haematological malignancies is important to detect and hence examination of the peripheral smear, and if necessary, bone marrow is indicated.

Table 16.4 Causes of Lymphocytosis

Category	Causes
Infections	
Viral	Infectious mononucleosis Cytomegalovirus infection Hepatitis Mumps Varicella
Bacterial	Tuberculosis Pertussis
Protozoal	Toxoplasmosis
Haematological malignancies	ALL CLL Prolymphocytic leukaemia Leukaemic phase of NHL
Stress lymphocytosis	Acute cardiovascular collapse Trauma Major surgery
Others	Monoclonal B-cell lymphocytosis Chronic infections Postvaccination Autoimmune disorders Postsplenectomy

ALL, acute lymphoblastic leukaemia; CLL, chronic lymphocytic leukaemia; NHL, non-Hodgkin lymphoma.

LEUCOPENIA **PA 18.1**

Reduction in total leucocyte count below the lower limit of normal is referred to as leucopenia. Leucopenia places individuals at an increased risk of infections, some of which can be fatal. Two common forms of leucopenia include neutropenia and lymphopenia. The causes of these two entities are listed in Table 16.5.

Neutropenia

Neutropenia is the reduction in the total number of neutrophils in the peripheral blood below the normal value ($<2000/mm^3$). Absolute neutrophil count above $1000/mm^3$ is generally considered adequate for phagocytic functions of neutrophils. Based on the neutrophil count, neutropenia is divided into three categories – mild, moderate and severe, as shown in Table 16.6 along with the risk of infection for each grade.

Agranulocytosis

Agranulocytosis refers to a clinically significant reduction in neutrophils (<500 cells/mm^3). Patients with agranulocytosis are susceptible to recurrent bacterial and fungal infections. Most common cause of agranulocytosis is drug toxicity, and the most common drugs being alkylating agents, antimetabolites, chloramphenicol, etc.

Symptoms and signs include malaise, chills and fever, followed by weakness and fatigue. Infections are often life-threatening and may cause death within hours to days. Treatment includes broad-spectrum antibiotics. G-CSF, a growth factor that stimulates the production of granulocytes from marrow precursors, is used especially in cases that follow myelosuppressive chemotherapy.

Lymphopenia

Lymphopenia, also called lymphocytopenia, is the condition in which patients present with abnormally low levels of lymphocytes. Lymphocytopenia can be T or B or NK (natural killer) lymphocytopenia.

Lymphocytopenia when severe is associated with a high risk of deadly infections by commensals and low-risk pathogens. Hence, regular monitoring of CD4 count by flow cytometry is essential. This is discussed in detail in Chapter 6.

LEUKAEMOID REACTION **PA 18.1**

Leukaemoid reaction is characterized by markedly increased WBC count, with shift to left as evidenced in the

Table 16.5 Common Causes of Neutropenia and Lymphopenia

Type of Leucopenia	Subcategory	Causes
Neutropenia	Infections	Miliary tuberculosis HIV infection Infectious mononucleosis Sepsis
	Drugs	Antimicrobials Analgesics Antithyroid drugs Cytotoxic drugs Phenytoin
	Immunological	Felty syndrome SLE
	Ineffective haematopoiesis	Megaloblastic anaemia
	Sequestration	Hypersplenism
	Bone marrow diseases	Aplastic anaemia Leukaemias Myeloproliferative neoplasms; myelodysplastic syndromes Space-occupying lesions of the marrow Lymphoma
	Miscellaneous	Cyclic neutropenia
		Kostman syndrome
		Chronic familial neutropenia
		Fanconi anaemia
Lymphopenia	T lymphocytopenia	HIV infection Chemotherapy Aplastic anaemia Irradiation
	B lymphocytopenia	High-dose steroids Aplastic anaemia Irradiation
	NK lymphocytopenia	Very rare

NK, natural killer; SLE, systemic lupus erythematosus.

Table 16.6 Grades of Neutropenia

Grade	Absolute Neutrophil Count	Risk of Infection
Mild	1000–1500/mm^3	No increased risk
Moderate	500–1000/mm^3	Mild risk
Severe	<500/mm^3	High risk

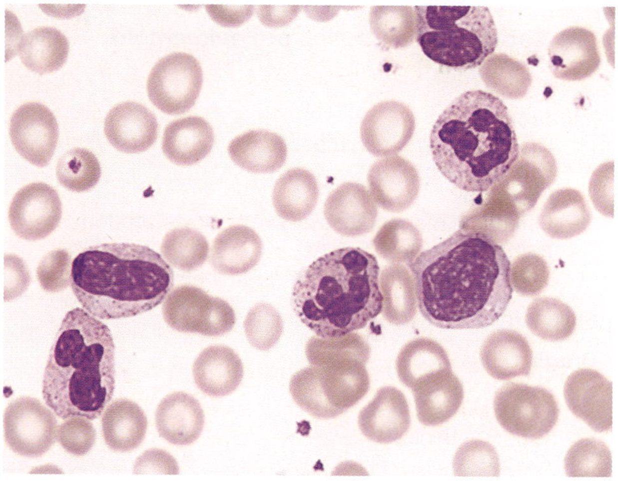

Fig. 16.4 Peripheral smear morphology of leukaemoid reaction. Left-shifted neutrophilic series with neutrophils, bands and myelocytes. The neutrophils also show coarse toxic granulation. (*Source:* From Neerja Vajpayee, Susan S. Graham, Sylva Bem. Henry's Clinical Diagnosis and Management by Laboratory Methods. Elsevier. 2017.)

peripheral blood picture due to nonleukaemic causes. Conventionally, leucocytosis exceeding 50,000/mm^3 with a significant increase in early neutrophil precursors is referred to as a leukaemoid reaction. Lymphocytic leukaemoid reaction can also occur following tuberculosis and pertussis. The peripheral blood smear may show myelocytes, metamyelocytes, promyelocytes and rarely myeloblasts (Fig. 16.4). Because of the presence of immature precursors, the peripheral blood picture may be confused with leukaemia. Leukaemoid reactions are most commonly caused by serious infections; the other causes are listed in Table 16.7.

In general, leukaemoid reactions are benign and are not life-threatening by themselves, although they are often a response to a notable disease state. However, it is important to differentiate myeloid leukaemoid reaction from chronic myeloid leukaemia, owing to their similar blood counts. The common differences between the two are listed in Table 16.8.

LEUCOERYTHROBLASTIC REACTION

Leucoerythroblastic reaction is defined by the presence of immature myeloid cells and nucleated RBCs in the peripheral blood. This is secondary to extramedullary haematopoiesis that disrupts the bone marrow–blood barrier, resulting in the release of premature cells into blood. Total leucocyte count may be normal or increased. Leucoerythroblastic picture is seen in a wide variety of settings which are listed in Table 16.9.

Peripheral blood smear morphology of leucoerythroblastic picture is discussed in Chapter 15. It is emphasized that leucoerythroblastic picture is not a disease per se but a manifestation of the underlying illness. Hence,

Table 16.7 Causes of Leukaemoid Reaction

Infections
- *Clostridium difficile* infection
- Tuberculosis
- Pertussis
- Infectious mononucleosis (lymphocyte predominant)
- Visceral larva migrans (eosinophil predominant)

Severe haemorrhage and haemolysis

Drugs
- Sulpha drugs
- Dapsone
- Glucocorticoids
- G-CSF
- All-*trans* retinoic acid

Ethylene glycol intoxication

Diabetic ketoacidosis

Organ necrosis
- Hepatic necrosis
- Ischaemic colitis

Asplenia

As a feature of trisomy 21

Paraneoplastic syndrome

Table 16.8 Differences Between Leukaemoid Reaction and Chronic Myeloid Leukaemia

Feature	Leukaemoid Reaction	Chronic Myeloid Leukaemia
Total leucocyte count	25,000–1 lakh/mm^3	≥1 lakh/mm^3
Differential count	Dominant cells – neutrophils Myeloblasts ≤5% Basophils – normal	All maturation stages Myeloblasts >5% Basophilia +
Toxic features	Toxic granules + Döhle bodies[a] +	Absent
NAP[b] score	Elevated	Reduced
Philadelphia chromosome	Absent	Present
Clonality	Polyclonal	Monoclonal
Massive splenomegaly	Absent	Present
Organ infiltration	Absent	May be present

[a]Döhle bodies: neutrophilic inclusion due to dilation of endoplasmic reticulum in sepsis and severe infections.
[b]NAP – neutrophil alkaline phosphatase activity tested by the stain.

Table 16.9 Causes of Leucoerythroblastic Blood Picture

Category	Causes
Infections	Miliary tuberculosis Sepsis
Bone marrow metastases	Carcinoma lung Carcinoma breast Carcinoma prostate Carcinoma of the GI tract Carcinoma thyroid Renal cell carcinoma
Haematological disorders	Myelofibrosis Severe haemolysis Lymphoma Myeloma
Storage disorders	Gaucher disease Niemann–Pick disease

GI, gastrointestinal.

investigations should be directed to find the predisposing cause, which needs be treated appropriately for reversal of the peripheral blood changes. Bone marrow examination may be required in most cases to arrive at a diagnosis.

MORPHOLOGICAL ABNORMALITIES OF WHITE BLOOD CELLS

Few inherited morphological abnormalities of WBCs need mention here. Many of them are associated with functional deficiency of neutrophils, while a few function normally.

1. **Pelger–Huët anomaly:** This is an autosomal dominant disorder in which the granulocytes are devoid of nuclear segmentation. Granulocyte nuclei may be rod-like, round or rarely may contain two segments. Though morphologically abnormal, these granulocytes function normally. Pelger–Huët-like cells called pseudo-Pelger–Huët cells are seen in acquired conditions like myelodysplastic syndromes (MDSs), acute myeloid leukaemia (AML) and myeloproliferative neoplasms (MPNs).
2. **Alder–Reilly anomaly:** This inherited disorder of granulocytes is characterized by the presence of abnormally large, darkly staining granules resembling toxic granules in the cytoplasm of neutrophils and monocytes. This abnormality is commonly seen in mucopolysaccharidoses such as Hurler and Hunter syndrome.
3. **May–Hegglin anomaly:** This uncommon disorder with autosomal dominant inheritance is characterized by a triad of thrombocytopenia, giant platelets

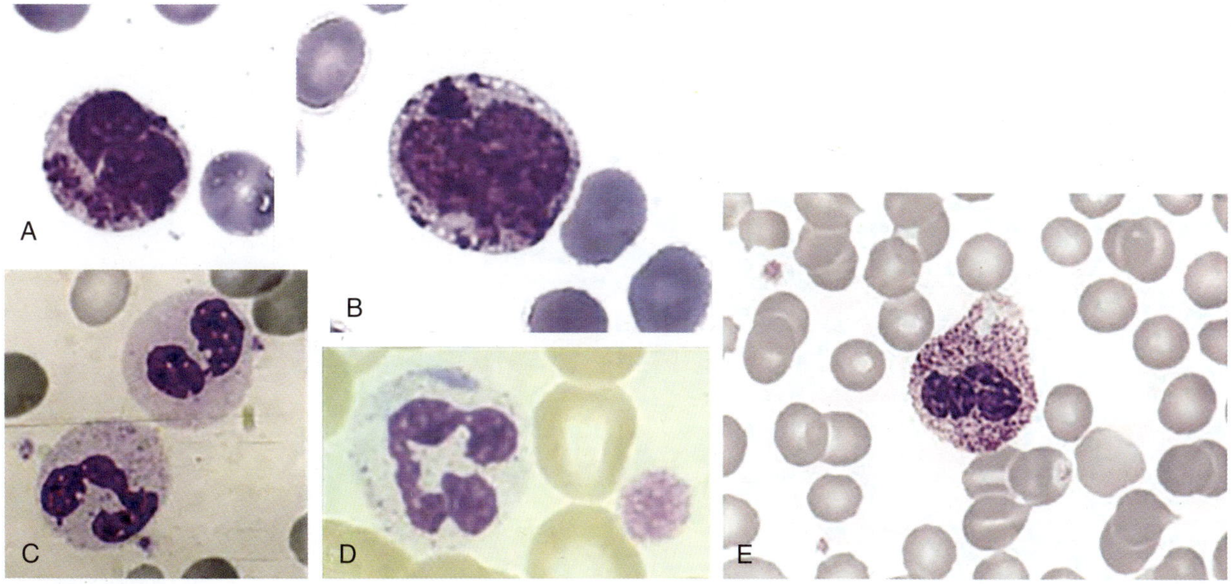

Fig. 16.5 (A and B) Peripheral blood smear of a patient with the Chediak–Higashi syndrome showing giant granules within the neutrophil series. (C) Peripheral blood neutrophil (up) showing the Pelger–Hu®t anomaly (bilobed nucleus). (D) May–Hegglin anomaly: giant platelet (left), neutrophil with greyish-blue cytoplasmic inclusion (right). (E) Smear in Alder–Reilly anomaly showing neutrophils with metachromatic granules. (*Source:* From G Zini. Blood and Bone Marrow Pathology. Elsevier. 2011. From Robert E. Hutchison, Katherine I. Schexneider. Henry's Clinical Diagnosis and Management by Laboratory Methods. Elsevier. 2017.)

and inclusions within granulocytes. The inclusions resemble Döhle bodies.

4. **Chediak–Higashi syndrome** (Fig. 16.5): The syndrome is explained in detail in Chapter 3. WBCs in this disorder are characterized by the presence of multiple giant cytoplasmic granules within the neutrophils and platelets.

NON-NEOPLASTIC DISORDERS OF LYMPH NODES

Lymphocytes originate from the stem cells in the bone marrow and differentiate in the central lymphoid organs, B cells in the bone marrow and T cells in the thymus. These further migrate and circulate through the blood and under the influence of cytokines and chemokines, home in to secondary lymphoid organs like lymph nodes, spleen, tonsils, adenoids and Peyer's patches. Lymph nodes are small, ovoid nodules normally ranging in size from a few millimetres to 2 cm. The primary function of lymph nodes is to filter out microorganisms and abnormal cells that have collected in the lymph. Lymph nodes are distributed in clusters along the course of lymphatic vessels located throughout the body. Lymph nodes are the most widely distributed and easily accessible lymphoid tissue examined frequently for diagnostic purposes.

LYMPHADENITIS PA 19.1

Lymphadenitis refers to the inflammation or enlargement of a lymph node. Lymph node enlargement is a common manifestation in a wide variety of diseases and may serve as the foreground for subsequent clinical investigation of diseases of the reticuloendothelial system or regional infection. Most of the cases represent a benign response to localized or systemic infection. Antigenic stimulation leads to the enlargement of primary follicles, with pale staining germinal centres resulting in the formation of secondary follicles. Paracortical T-cell region also can undergo hyperplastic changes. The extent and pattern of the morphological changes are dependent on the initiating stimulus and the intensity of the response.

B-cell region of lymph nodes (Fig. 16.6): cortical follicles (superficial)
T-cell region of lymph nodes (Fig. 16.6): paracortex (deeper)

The group of affected lymph nodes is purely dependent on the region drained by the lymph nodes normally. The onset and course of lymphadenitis can be acute, subacute or chronic.

Types of Lymphadenitis

Acute Nonspecific Lymphadenitis Acute nonspecific lymphadenitis most often results because of microbial infections of the regions drained by the nodes.

Example: acute mesenteric lymphadenitis due to acute appendicitis.

Morphology *(Fig. 16.7)*

The nodes are enlarged, engorged and grey–red. Microscopically, salient features include prominent, large, reactive germinal centres with numerous mitotic figures, macrophages engulfing particulate debris (tingible body

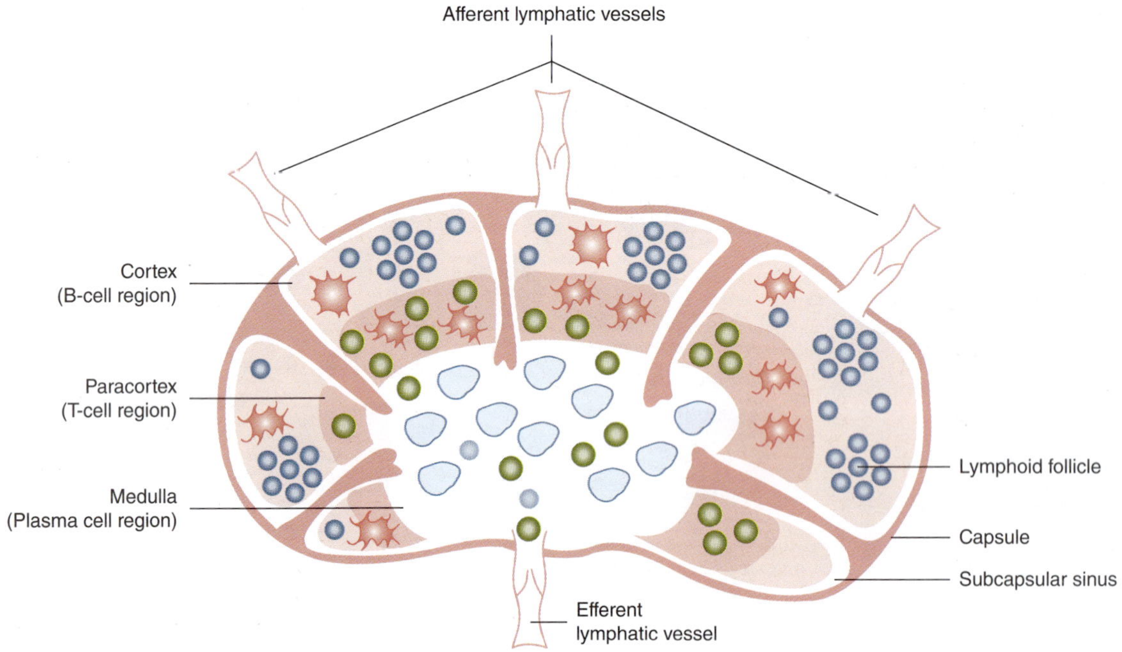

Fig. 16.6 Diagrammatic representation of B-cell (blue circles) and T-cell (green circles) regions of lymph nodes. (*Source:* From Randolph H. Stewart. Small Animal Critical Care Medicine. Elsevier. 2015.)

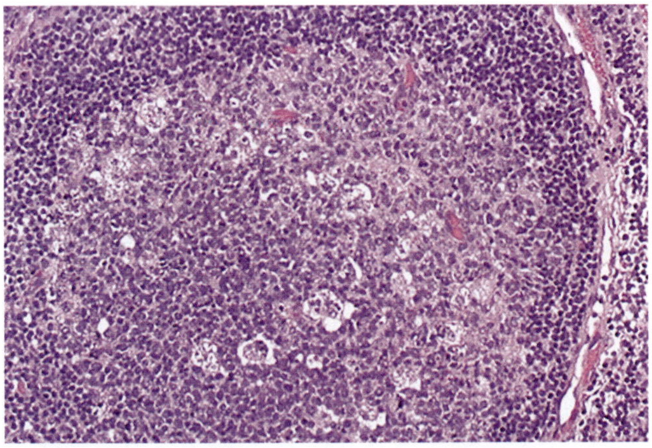

Fig. 16.7 Microscopy of acute nonspecific lymphadenitis showing a large follicle and germinal centre containing 'tingible body' macrophages. (*Source:* https://webpath.med.utah.edu/HEMEHTML/HEME120.html)

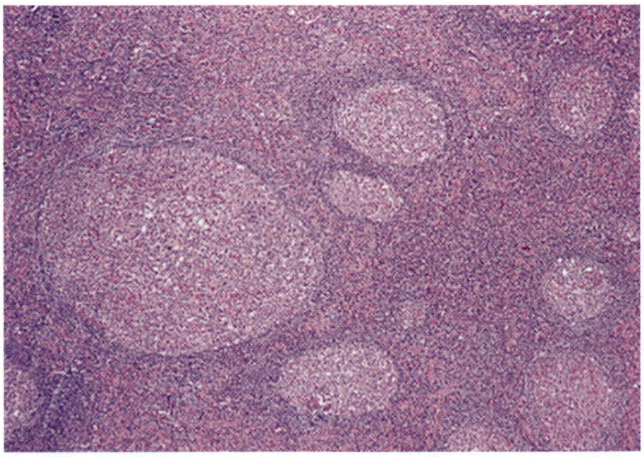

Fig. 16.8 Microscopy of follicular hyperplasia of chronic nonspecific lymphadenitis. (*Source:* From Daniel A. Arber. Rosai and Ackerman's Surgical Pathology-2 Volume Set. Elsevier. 2018.)

macrophages) and endothelial hyperplasia of the sinuses. With pyogenic organisms, the centres of the follicles may undergo necrosis with prominent neutrophilic infiltrate.

Clinical Features Nodes are usually enlarged and tender on palpation. With extensive suppurative inflammation, abscess with a draining sinus tract may follow.

Chronic Nonspecific Lymphadenitis Chronic antigenic stimulation produces several morphological patterns of reaction described below:

A. **Follicular hyperplasia:** This pattern is seen with stimuli that activate humoral immune responses. Morphologically, it is characterized by the prominence of secondary follicles surrounded by a collar of mantle zone (Fig. 16.8).
B. **Paracortical hyperplasia:** This pattern is seen with stimuli that trigger T-cell–mediated immune responses. T-cell region is filled with immunoblasts, with hypertrophied endothelial cells lining the sinusoids.
C. **Sinus histiocytosis:** This pattern is nonspecific and may be seen as a reaction of malignancy, commonly in carcinoma of breast. There is an increase in the number and size of cells that line lymphatic sinusoids, increased macrophages and markedly hypertrophic endothelial cells of the lymphatics (Fig. 16.9).

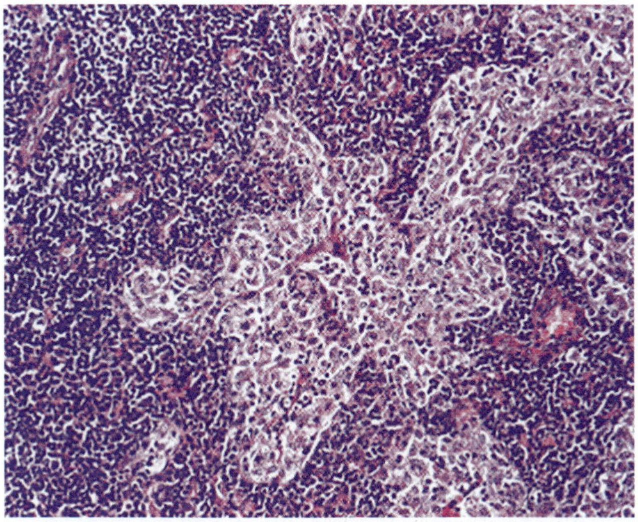

Fig. 16.9 Microscopy of sinus hyperplasia showing the presence of histiocytes and sinus lining cells in chronic nonspecific lymphadenitis. (*Source:* From Daniel A. Arber. Rosai and Ackerman's Surgical Pathology-2 Volume Set. Elsevier. 2018.)

Lymph nodes affected by chronic lymphadenitis are enlarged and nontender. Common group of lymph nodes affected are axillary and inguinal.

Haemophagocytic Lymphohistiocytosis Haemophagocytic lymphohistiocytosis (HLH), an uncommon disorder, also called **macrophage activation syndrome**, is characterized by systemic inflammation, cytopenias and shock-like picture due to hyperactive $CD8^+$ cells. This disorder is due to a highly stimulated, but ineffective, immune response to antigens which results in life-threatening cytokine storm and inflammatory reaction.

Types

- **Familial** form is a progressive disease that affects young children.
- **Acquired** form that affects older children and adults is associated with immunodeficiency and may be triggered by infectious agents, malignant neoplasms and graft versus host disease.

Pathogenesis The pathological hallmark of this disease is the excessive uncontrolled proliferation of activated macrophages and histiocytes, which phagocytose RBCs, WBCs and platelets, leading to the clinical symptoms of pancytopenia. A genetic defect in CD8 and NK cells enable them to perform their cytolytic activity in an excessive and prolonged manner when they cling on the pathogen-activating macrophages which go about functioning continuously. These activated macrophages are nonmalignant and not clonal in contrast to the malignant counterpart, Langerhans cell histiocytosis (LCH). The spleen, lymph nodes, bone marrow, liver, skin and membranes that surround the brain and spinal cord are the preferred sites of involvement.

Following are the factors involved in the pathogenesis of HLH:

- Failure of NK cells to induce apoptosis of the target cell, remove the antigenic stimulus and terminate the inflammatory response
- Accentuated Th1 response that leads to high levels of TNF-α and TNF-γ, causing pancytopenia
- Hepatosplenomegaly due to organ infiltration by activated lymphocytes and histiocytes
- Fever induced by IL-1 and IL-6

Morphology

Bone marrow examination is important in establishing the diagnosis (Fig. 16.10). Alternatively, spleen, lymph node or skin can be biopsied. The hallmark finding is the presence of macrophages phagocytosing RBCs, WBCs, platelets and precursors.

Clinical Features Clinical features include a sudden onset of systemic inflammatory response syndrome (SIRS), with symptoms including high unremitting fevers, malaise, rash, jaundice and myalgia, along with accompanying cytopenias, hepatosplenomegaly and generalized lymphadenopathy.

Laboratory Features Laboratory findings include hypofibrinogenaemia, markedly elevated ferritin and soluble IL-2 receptor, hypertriglyceridaemia, elevated transaminases and elevated lactate dehydrogenase (LDH).

Course and Prognosis The disease is uniformly fatal if left untreated. For acquired types, immediate treatment of the underlying predisposing condition is coupled with chemotherapy as treatment. Stem cell transplantation offers cure in familial forms.

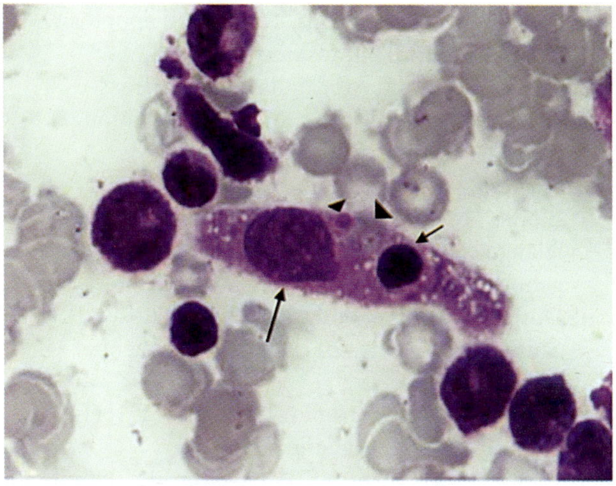

Fig. 16.10 Morphology of bone marrow aspiration in haemophagocytic syndrome. A macrophage with engulfed nucleated cell (arrow), RBC (small arrow) and platelet (arrowhead). (*Source:* From Pandiarajan Vignesh et al. The Journal of Allergy and Clinical Immunology: In Practice. Elsevier 2021.)

NEOPLASTIC PROLIFERATIONS OF WHITE BLOOD CELLS

Neoplastic disorders are the most important diseases of WBCs. These are of the following types:

- Lymphoid neoplasms
- Myeloid neoplasms
- Histiocytoses

Lymphoid neoplasms: This group includes neoplastic proliferations of B, T and NK cells. In many subtypes of these disorders, the neoplastic cell closely resembles a particular stage of lymphocyte maturation.

Myeloid neoplasms: This group includes neoplastic proliferations of myeloid progenitors. Further categorization of the group is discussed in the subsequent sections.

Histiocytoses: This is an uncommon group of neoplastic proliferation of macrophages and dendritic cells. LCH is a spectrum of neoplastic disorders due to the proliferation of immature dendritic cells.

Let us briefly discuss the aetiological factors involved in the development of WBC neoplasms before discussing the individual disorders.

AETIOLOGICAL AND PATHOGENETIC FACTORS IN WHITE BLOOD CELL NEOPLASIA: AN OVERVIEW

In most cases of leukaemias and lymphomas, aetiological factors are difficult to be established. Following are the aetiological factors associated with the genesis of lymphomas and leukaemias:

A. **Chromosomal abnormalities:**
Mutations causing white cell neoplasia fall under the following three categories:
  - Progrowth mutations – increased cell division, Warburg effect. Example: tyrosine kinase mutation, MYC translocation.
  - Prosurvival mutations – decreased apoptosis. Example: BCL2 translocation.
  - Transcription factor mutations – increased self-renewal. Example: MLL translocation, PML-RARA fusion.

B. **Inherited genetic factors:**
  - Bloom syndrome, Fanconi anaemia and ataxia–telangiectasia are preleukaemic conditions due to genomic instability.
  - Down syndrome and neurofibromatosis 1 (NF1) cause increased risk of childhood leukaemia.

C. **Viruses:**
  - Human T-lymphotropic virus type I (HTLV-I) – adult T-cell lymphoma/leukaemia
  - Epstein–Barr virus (EBV) – Burkitt lymphoma, Hodgkin lymphoma, NK-cell lymphoma
  - Kaposi sarcoma–associated herpesvirus (KSHV) – unusual B-cell lymphoma with malignant pleural effusion as presentation

D. **Chronic inflammation:**
  - *Helicobacter pylori* infection – gastric B-cell lymphoma
  - Gluten-sensitive enteropathy – T-cell lymphoma

E. **Iatrogenic factors:**
  - Ionizing radiation and chemotherapeutic drugs can induce mutations.

F. **Smoking:**
  - Due to benzene in tobacco smoke

Each of these factors is discussed in greater detail in Chapters 7 and 9.

LYMPHOID NEOPLASMS (FIG. 16.11)

Lymphoid neoplasms are categorized into peripheral and precursor B- and T-cell neoplasms. Let us understand a few fundamental terms before discussing the diseases.

White cell neoplasms are named leukaemia or lymphoma depending on their tissue distribution of disease at presentation.

Leukaemia: Neoplasms with a widespread involvement of bone marrow and (but not always) peripheral blood

Lymphoma: Neoplastic proliferation that presents as discrete tissue masses

The line of demarcation between leukaemias and lymphomas is often blurred as lymphomas may have leukaemic presentation and leukaemias may have lymphomatous presentation as the disease progresses.

The large group of lymphomas is broadly divided into two categories – **Hodgkin lymphoma (HL)** with its five subcategories and the larger group **non-Hodgkin lymphomas** (NHLs).

Neoplastic proliferation of plasma cells is a spectrum of disorders referred to as **plasma cell neoplasms** (also a category of NHL) which arise from the bone marrow with an infrequent involvement of lymph nodes or peripheral blood.

The clinical features of lymphoid neoplasms are determined by anatomic location of the disease. Most cases of NHL and all the cases of HL present as enlarged, nontender lymph nodes. The remaining cases of NHLs present with symptoms due to extranodal site involvement such as stomach, brain and skin.

Leukaemias, on the other hand, present with signs and symptoms of suppression of normal haematopoiesis due to the proliferating neoplastic cells.

Multiple myeloma, the most common plasma cell neoplasm, presents with bone pain and fractures due to lytic bone lesions.

Other specific features are discussed under individual diseases.

Current World Health Organization (WHO) classification of lymphoid neoplasms:

1. Precursor B-cell neoplasms – neoplasms of immature B cells
2. Peripheral B-cell neoplasms – neoplasms of mature B cells

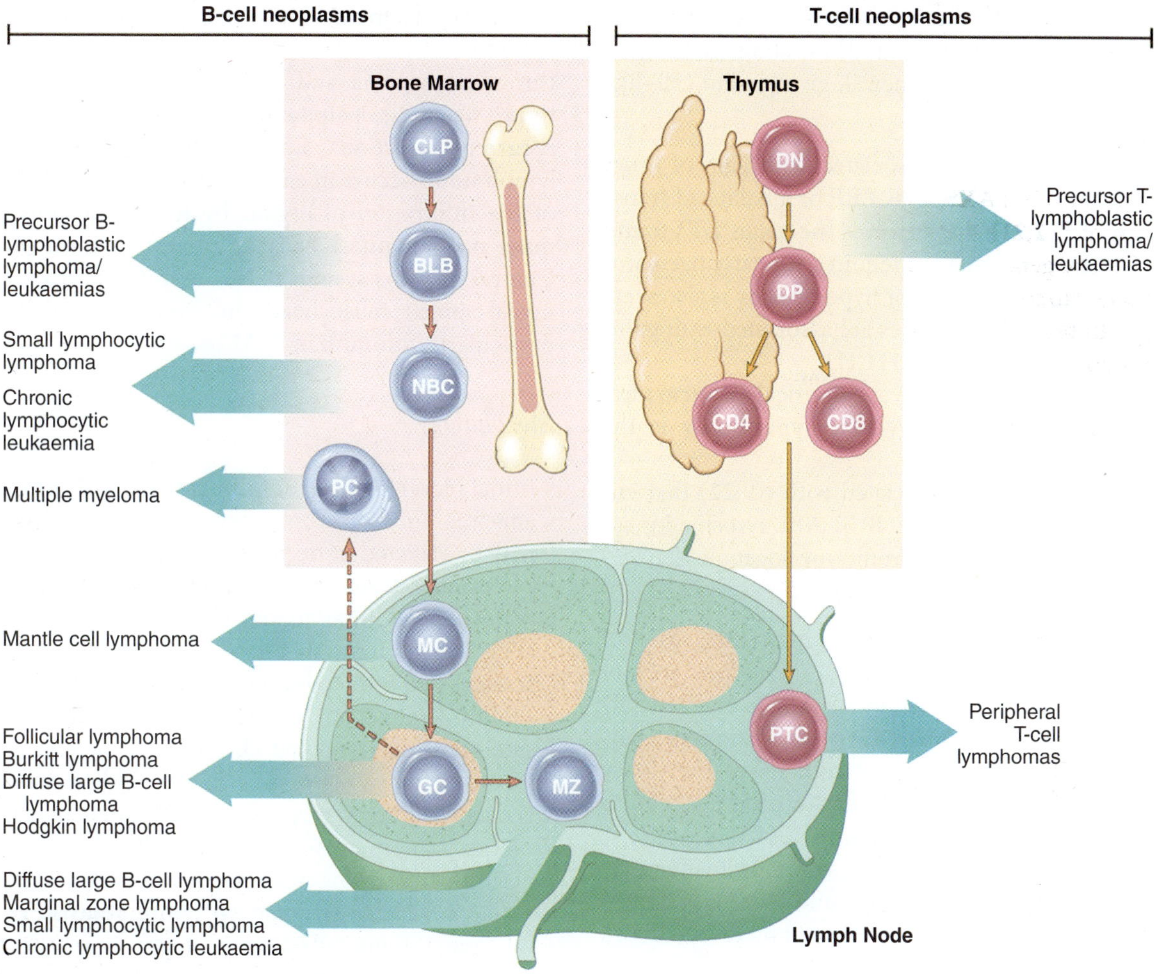

Fig. 16.11 Origin of lymphoid neoplasms. (*Source:* From Karen M. Frank, Alexander J. McAdam. Robbins & Cotran Pathologic Basis of Disease. Elsevier. 2021.)

3. Precursor T-cell neoplasms – neoplasms of immature T cells
4. Peripheral T- and NK-cell neoplasms – neoplasms of mature T and NK cells
5. Hodgkin lymphoma – neoplasms of Reed–Sternberg cell and its variants

All the lymphoid neoplasms share some common features, which are as follows:

- As we already know, the lymph node normally harbours a polyclonal population of immune cell subsets. Lymphoid neoplasms are characterized by monoclonal derivatives of the transformed cell that possess the same antigen receptor proteins.
- Histopathological examination of lymph nodes or the affected sites is a prerequisite for diagnosis.
- In total, 85%–90% of lymphoid neoplasms are of B-cell origin, with the remainder being T cell; NK-cell neoplasms are very rare.
- Antigen receptor gene rearrangement generally precedes transformation of lymphoid cells; hence, all the derivatives of the malignant progenitor share the same antigen receptor gene configuration and sequence and synthesize identical antigen receptor such as immunoglobulins or T-cell receptors.
- Lymphoid neoplasms are often associated with immune abnormalities.
- Neoplastic B and T lymphocytes recapitulate the behaviour of their normal counterparts.

Precursor B- and T-Cell Neoplasms **PA 18.2**

Acute Lymphoblastic Leukaemia/Lymphoma Acute lymphoblastic leukaemia (ALL)/lymphomas are neoplastic proliferations of immature B (pre-B) or T (pre-T) cells which are referred to as lymphoblasts. Close to 85% of ALLs are B-ALLs and the remaining are T-ALLs. Typically, B-ALLs manifest as leukaemias and T-ALLs as thymic lymphomas. Uncommonly, B-ALLs can present as lymphoma and T-cell ALLs with leukaemic picture. Because of their morphological similarities, B- and T-ALLs are discussed together here.

Pathogenesis Most of the genetic abnormalities associated with ALL cause dysregulation of expression and function of transcription factors involved in the development of T and B lymphocytes. The following genetic changes seen with ALLs act by disturbing the differentiation of lymphoid precursors and arresting maturation leading to accelerated self-renewal, giving stem cell–like properties to the altered cells:

- **B-ALL:** Most cases are associated with gain-of-function mutation of **PAX5, E2F, EBF** or a balanced translocation of **(12;21)** that involves the genes **ETV6 and RUNX1**, the genes that are required for early haematopoietic precursors. Hyper- or hypodiploidy is also seen.
- **T-ALL:** In total, 70% of cases are associated with gain-of-function mutation of **NOTCH1**.
- In total, 90% of ALLs have numerical or structural chromosomal changes of which **hyperploidy** is the most common.
- A fraction of ALLs is associated with **t(9;22)** that encodes a constitutively active BCR-ABL tyrosine kinase which is different from chronic myelogenous leukaemia (CML) (discussed in detail later).

As discussed in Chapter 7, malignancy is the result of multistep genetic damage and single mutations are not sufficient to produce ALL. Although ALL is a genetically simple tumour when compared with solid tumours, additional mutations like those that confer tyrosine kinase activity and RAS signalling that act to promote cellular growth are associated in the genesis of ALL.

Clinical Features ALL is the most common malignancy of children younger than 15 years, and there is a significant difference in the age group affected by B- and T-cell ALLs.

85% ALL – B cell – leukaemias, peak incidence at 3 years
15% ALL – T cell – lymphomas, peak incidence at adolescence
Less frequently, ALLs affect adults.

As the name suggests, these have an abrupt stormy onset within days to few weeks. The most common presenting features result from the disrupted haematopoiesis due to replacement of the marrow by malignant cells. Symptoms result from varying degrees of anaemia, thrombocytopenia and neutropenia, which include fatigue, weakness, palpitations, pallor, gum bleeding and recurrent infections. Enlargement of liver, spleen and lymph node occurs in early course of the disease because of the infiltration of organs by leukaemic cells. Scrotal mass may manifest because of testicular involvement. Central nervous system (CNS) manifestations and meningeal spread cause headache, vomiting and dizziness, particularly common in T-ALLs.

Morphology

Initial blood investigations in patients with ALL reveal anaemia and/or thrombocytopenia. The WBC count may be elevated or decreased or seldom even normal.

Peripheral smear examination reflects the blood counts in addition to the presence of lymphoblasts (Fig. 16.12). Both B- and T-ALL tumour cells have scant basophilic agranular cytoplasm with nuclei slightly larger than mature lymphocytes having delicate and finely stippled chromatin. Nucleoli may be inconspicuous to two per cell. The nuclear membrane is deeply subdivided, giving a convoluted appearance.

The bone marrow study that follows reveals a hypercellular marrow, with the normal elements being replaced with closely packed **lymphoblasts**. The mitotic rate is high, reflecting the aggressive nature of the tumour cells. In solid tumours, the tumour cells are admixed with tingible body macrophages that serve to remove the apoptotic cells, giving the **'starry sky'** appearance. Mediastinal thymic masses of T-ALL are often associated with lymphadenopathy and splenomegaly.

The morphology of lymphoblasts and myeloblasts is sometimes difficult to differentiate on smear exami-

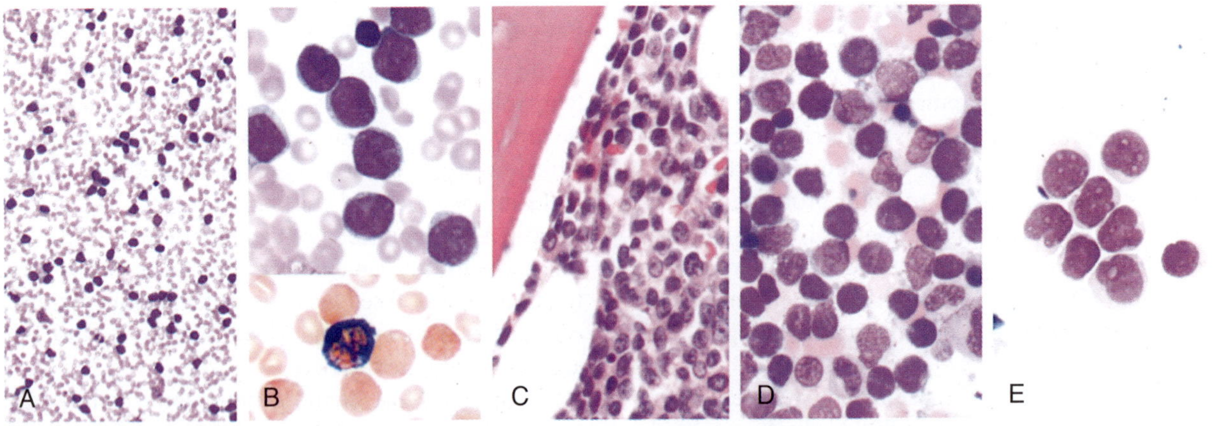

Fig. 16.12 Peripheral smear, bone marrow aspirate and CSF findings in ALL. (A) Increased white cell count with (B) increased lymphoblasts in (C) and lower insert showing negative MPO stain (positive stain is seen in neutrophil). (D) Increased cellularity of bone marrow. (E) Higher resolution of bone marrow demonstrates increased lymphoblasts. (*Source:* From Todd F. Roberts. Ferri's Clinical Advisor 2021. Elsevier. 2021.)

nation, but it is extremely essential to diagnose the two leukaemias as their treatment protocols are distinct. The features of lymphoblasts are compared with myeloblasts under the section 'acute myeloid leukaemia'.

Cytochemistry: In addition, lymphoblasts are PAS^+, whereas myeloid blasts are negative for PAS.

Immunophenotyping:

Pre-B- and pre-T-ALL – terminal deoxy-nucleotidyl transferase **(Tdt)** + (immature lymphoid marker)
B-ALL – B-cell markers + namely, CD19 and CD20
T-ALL – T-cell markers + namely, CD3 and CD7
CD marker profile of different cell lineages, leukaemias and lymphomas by immunophenotyping and flow cytometry is listed in the Table 16.15.

Clinical Features

Course and prognosis Many factors are associated with the clinical outcome of ALL and are listed in the following table:

Favourable Prognostic Factors	Unfavourable Prognostic Factors
2–10 years	<2 years
Low WBC count	Adults
Hyperdiploidy	Adolescents
Trisomy of chromosomes 4, 7, 10	Peripheral blast count >10,000
t(12;21)	Residual disease after therapy

ALLs are aggressive tumours with rapid disease progression and prove fatal. But with aggressive therapy, more than 95% of children acquire a complete remission and 75%–80% are cured, whereas the cure rate among adults is only about 35%–40%. Individuals with t(9;22) are effectively treated with BCR-ABL kinase along with combination chemotherapy. Patients labelled as 'cured' require long-term follow-up for early detection of minimal residual disease, which if present is predictive of a worse outcome.

Peripheral B-Cell Neoplasms **PA 19.4**

Lymphomas Lymphomas are a large and heterogeneous group of malignant neoplasms which originate primarily from lymph nodes or other lymphoid tissues. These are divided into two major types:

- HL
- NHL

Histogenesis A majority of HLs arise from the mature B lymphocyte at the germinal centre stage of differentiation, whereas NHLs arise from B or T lymphocytes (Table 16.10).

Clinical Features In NHL, involvement of multiple peripheral lymph nodes, extranodal disease, noncontiguous dissemination to distant organs and bone marrow involvement are more common. In contrast, HL is usually limited to a single axial lymph node region (mostly cervical), spreads in a contiguous manner and bone marrow involvement is rare. HL occurs predominantly in young adults, whereas NHL shows the increasing incidence with age.

Because of significant differences in the pathogenesis, management and prognosis, HL and NHL need to be diagnosed promptly.

Table 16.10 Differences Between Hodgkin and Non-Hodgkin Lymphomas

Feature	Hodgkin Lymphoma	Non-Hodgkin lymphoma
Age group	Usually young adults are affected	Incidence increases with age
Cell or origin	B lymphocyte	B or T lymphocyte
Lymph node involvement	Localized to a single axial group of nodes	Involvement of multiple peripheral nodes
Nature of spread	Orderly spread by contiguity	Noncontiguous spread
Mesenteric nodes and Waldeyer ring involvement	Rare involvement of mesenteric nodes and Waldeyer ring	Common involvement of mesenteric nodes and Waldeyer ring
Extranodal involvement	Extranodal presentation – rare	Extranodal presentation – common

Hodgkin Lymphoma

HL, formerly Hodgkin disease, was named after Thomas Hodgkin, who was first to describe abnormalities in the lymphatic system in 1832. However, Hodgkin did note that the earliest description of the disease may have been given by Marcello Malpighi in 1666.

HL is a group of lymphoid neoplasms that differ from NHL in many aspects. It is one of the most common malignancies of young adults and adolescents and is a potentially curable lymphoma in most cases. It is also the first human cancer to be successfully treated with radiation therapy and chemotherapy.

Epidemiology The incidence of HL is higher in males than in females. The sex predilection is most prominent in children, with 85% of cases affecting boys. The incidence of HL varies with age, with a clear bimodal distribution that is consistent across most countries. The initial peak is in young adults (15–34 years); HL is the most commonly diagnosed malignancy in teens aged 15–19 years. The second peak is in older adults (>55 years). There is also a significant difference in subtype based on age, with nodular sclerosing HL occurring in young adults and mixed cellularity (MC) HL commonly affecting the older age group.

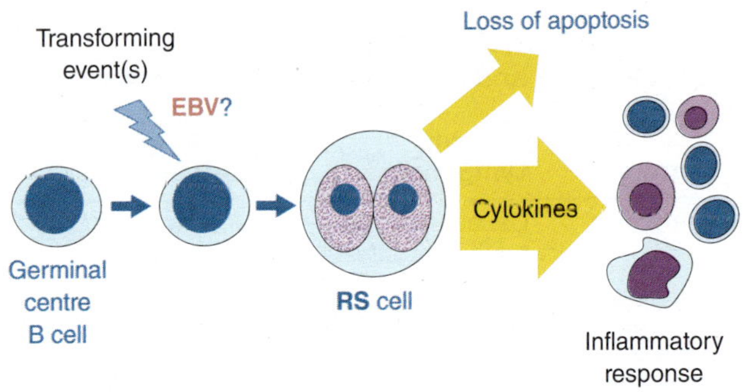

Fig. 16.13 Role of EBV in the pathogenesis of Hodgkin lymphoma.

Aetiology The exact aetiological factors for HL are not yet clearly known. Up to 30% of cases of classical Hodgkin lymphoma (CHL) may be positive for EBV proteins, highlighting the role of EBV in the genesis of HL (Fig. 16.13). The incidence of EBV positivity varies with subtype, and its association is stated in Table 16.11.

Genetic predisposition is an important risk factor in the development of HL. Around 1% of patients with HL have a family history of the disease, and siblings of an affected individual have three- to sevenfold increased risk of developing HL.

HIV-positive patients also have a higher incidence of HL compared with the general population. However, HL is not considered an AIDS-defining neoplasm.

Pathogenesis Activation of the transcription factor ***NF-κB*** is a common event in classic Hodgkin lymphoma (CHL), which can occur because of **EBV** infection with the resultant ***LMP1*** expression by EBV-infected cells. EBV-encoded proteins play a major role in the metamorphosis of B cells into RS cells.

The excessive accumulation of reactive cells in the background in tissues involved in CHL is because of the effect of a variety of cytokines, chemokines and other factors released by RS cells (e.g. IL-5, IL-10, M-CSF, eotaxin).

After recruitment, the reactive cells release factors that support the growth and survival of RS cells and also modify the reactive cell response.

Classification WHO classifies HL into five subtypes:

- Nodular sclerosis (NS)
- MC
- Lymphocyte rich (LR)
- Lymphocyte depletion (LD)
- LP

Table 16.11 Characteristic Features of Individual Subtypes of Hodgkin Lymphoma

Feature	Nodular Sclerosis	Mixed Cellularity	Lymphocyte Rich	Lymphocyte Depletion	Nodular Lymphocyte Predominance
Incidence	65%–70%	20%–25%	Uncommon	Uncommon	Uncommon
Age group	Young adults	Biphasic Young and older adults	Older adults	Older adults HIV-positive patients	Young adults
Sex predominance	M = F	M > F	M > F	M > F	M > F
Histopathological findings	Lymph nodes are divided into circumscribed nodules by deposition of collagen bands	Frequent mononuclear and classical RS cells in a background rich in reactive cells	Predominantly reactive lymphocytes with frequent mononuclear and classical RS cells	Paucity of lymphocytes with abundant RS cells	Nodular infiltrate of small lymphocytes and macrophages with rare classical RS cells
Type of RS cell	***Lacunar cells***	***Mononuclear and classical RS cells***	***Mononuclear and classical RS cells***	***Mummified RS cells***	***L&H type/popcorn cell***
Common stage of presentation	Stage I/II	Commonly presents in stage III/IV Constitutional symptoms +	–	Advanced stage of presentation with constitutional symptoms	–
EBV association	No	70%	40%	>90%	No
Immunophenotype	$CD15^+$, $CD30^+$	$CD15^+$, $CD30^+$	$CD15^+$, $CD30^+$	$CD15^+$, $CD30^+$	$CD20^+$, $BCL6^+$
Prognosis	Excellent	Very good	Very good to excellent	Worst	Excellent

EBV, Epstein–Barr virus; F, female; M, male.

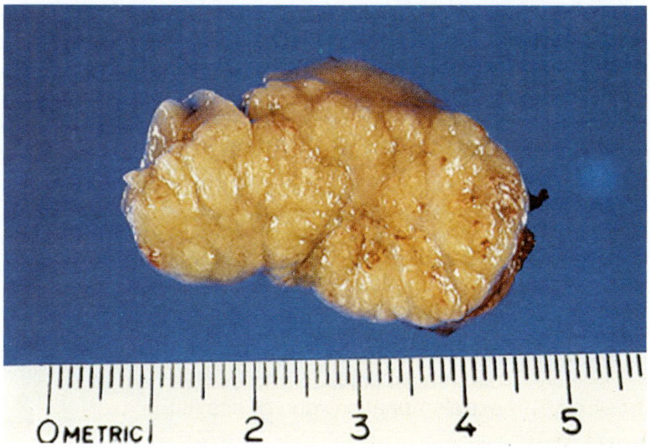

Fig. 16.14 Morphology of lymph node in Hodgkin lymphoma; gross – shows nodularity and sclerosis. (*Source:* From Daniel A. Arber. Rosai and Ackerman's Surgical Pathology-2 Volume Set. Elsevier. 2018.)

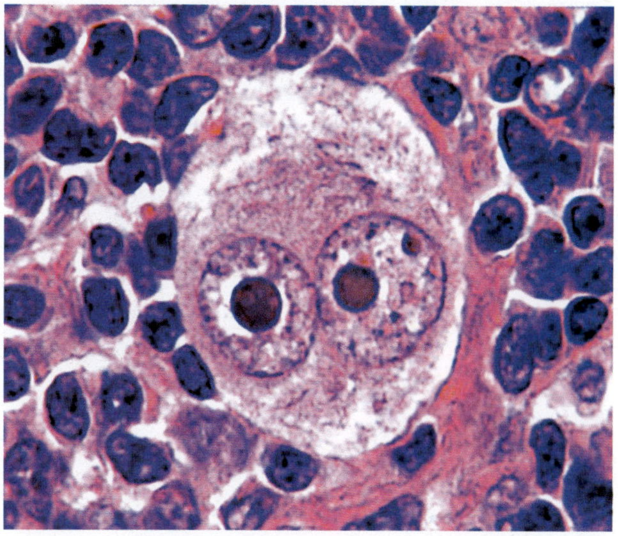

Fig. 16.15 Morphology of Hodgkin lymphoma with RS cells, high power, microscopy. (*Source:* From Daniel A. Arber. Rosai and Ackerman's Surgical Pathology-2 Volume Set. Elsevier. 2018.)

The first four subtypes have RS cells with similar immunophenotype and hence classified as ***classical*** forms of HL and the last subtype, LP, is termed ***nonclassical***.

Morphology (Fig. 16.14)

Enlarged lymph nodes are sampled for histopathological examination, and a careful search for the classical ***Reed–Sternberg cells***, which if found, prompts the diagnosis of HL. These RS cells are usually fewer in number and are often dispersed in a background of reactive inflammatory cells. RS cells are ***giant cells*** with a 45-μm diameter, multiple nuclei or single nuclei with multiple lobes, each with a large inclusion like a nucleolus of size of a small lymphocyte, 5–7 μm.

Many morphological types of RS cells exist (RS cell variants) and may be associated with the different types of HL.

Variants of RS cell:

- **Mononuclear variant:** RS cells with single nuclei
- **Lacunar variant:** RS cells with nuclei sitting inside a lacuna
- **Lymphohistiocytic variant:** RS cells with polypoid nuclei and inconspicuous nucleoli
- **Mummified variant:** RS cells that undergo pyknosis and cell death

Of note, RS-like cells are seen in NHLs, infectious mononucleosis and solid cancers.

Nodular Sclerosis (Fig. 16.15) This is the most common type of HL, constituting 65%–70% of cases. It is characterized by the presence of lacunar variant RS cells and the hallmark presence of lymphoid nodules surrounded by collagen bands that give the nodular appearance to the involved lymph nodes. Diagnostic RS cells are sparse and scattered against a background of polymorphous inflammatory infiltrate reactive T cells, eosinophils, plasma cells and macrophages.

Mixed Cellularity (Fig. 16.16) This type of HL constitutes 20%–25% of cases. Lymph nodes involved are diffusely effaced because of heterogeneous cellular infiltrate including T cells, eosinophils, plasma cells and macrophages along with RS cells. Classical RS cells and mononuclear RS cells are usually abundant.

Lymphocyte Rich This is an uncommon type of CHL in which reactive lymphocytes are the predominant cell type. In a majority of cases, nodes affected are diffusely effaced with vague nodularity because of the presence of residual follicles. This type is characterized by the presence of frequent mononuclear and diagnostic RS cells (Fig. 16.17).

Lymphocyte Depletion This is the least common type of HL, accounting for less than 5% of cases. This type is characterized by lack of lymphocytes coupled with relative abundance of classical or pleomorphic RS cells.

Nodular Lymphocyte Predominance This uncommon type of HL accounts for 5% of cases. Lymph nodes affected are effaced by nodular infiltrate of small lymphocytes admixed with macrophages. Classical RS cells are not easily seen, whereas L&H variant of RS cells, also called popcorn RS cells, are seen. Background contains B-cell follicles, reactive B cells and follicular dendritic cells along with scant eosinophils and plasma cells.

Following the establishment of morphological diagnosis of HL, the extent of the disease needs to be determined for treatment protocols. Staging of HL is done according to the Ann Arbor staging system, which has four stages, principally on the basis of lymph node involvement (Table 16.12).

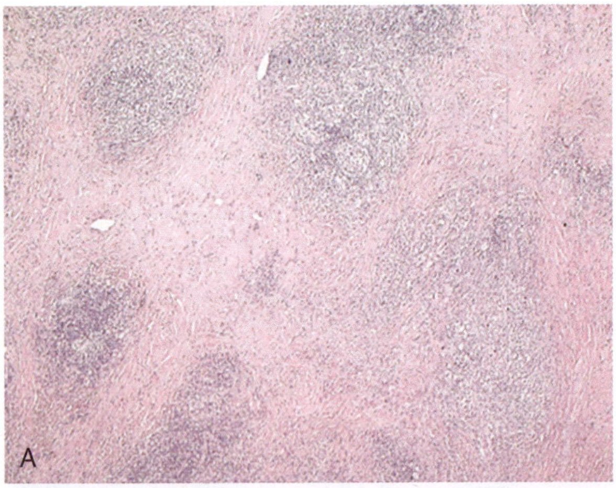

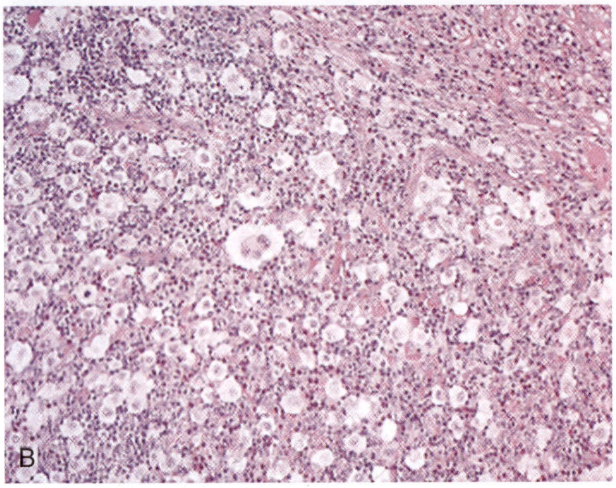

Fig. 16.16 Microscopy of lymph node in nodular sclerosis Hodgkin lymphoma. (A) Nodular sclerosis CHL. Cellular nodules are separated by concentric bands of mature collagen. (B) Close-up of cellular nodule shows numerous lacunar cells with clear cytoplasm intermingled with lymphocytes, neutrophils and eosinophils, with collagen bands rimming the nodule. (*Source:* From Jorge J. Castillo, Ann S. LaCasce. Ferri's Clinical Advisor 2021. Elsevier. 2021.)

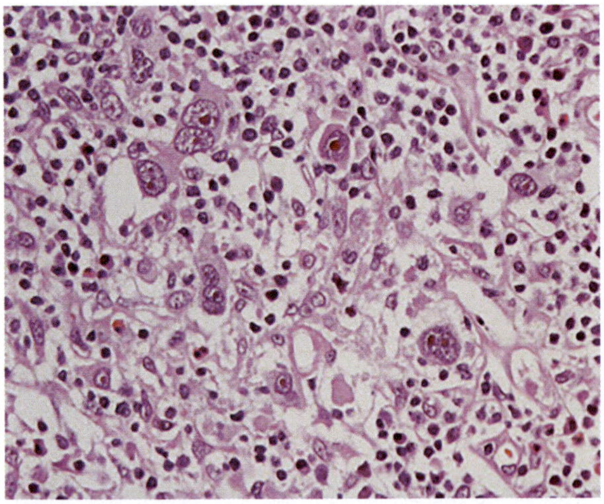

Fig. 16.17 Microscopy of lymph node in a mixed cellularity Hodgkin lymphoma shows typical HRS cells in a mixed cellular infiltrate, with lymphocytes, macrophages and eosinophils are visible. (*Source:* From Patricia A. Thistlethwaite, Jonathan R. Gower, Moises Hernandez, Yu Zhang, Andrew C. Picel, Anne C. Roberts. The Journal of Thoracic and Cardiovascular Surgery. Elsevier. 2018.)

Table 16.12 Clinical Staging of Hodgkin and Non-Hodgkin Lymphomas: Ann Arbor Staging System

Stage	Distribution of Disease
I	Single lymph node region (I)/single extralymphatic organ or site (IE)
II	Two or more lymph nodes on the same side of the diaphragm (II)/localized involvement of an extralymphatic organ or site (IIE)
III	Lymph nodes on both the sides of the diaphragm (III)/localized involvement of an extralymphatic organ or site (IIIE)
IV	Disseminated involvement of extranodal site(s)
A – absence of B symptoms	
B – fever, night sweats, loss of appetite and weight (>10% of body weight)	

Clinical Features Most commonly, patients present with painless lymphadenopathy and the disease spreads in an orderly fashion from nodes to spleen, liver and, rarely, bone marrow. Patients are commonly anaemic, which may be because of anaemia of chronic disease or bone marrow involvement.

Constitutional symptoms like unexplained weight loss of more than 10% of the total body weight within 6 months, unexplained fever or drenching night sweats are present in 40% of patients; collectively, these are known as 'B symptoms'.

Intermittent fever manifests in at least one-third of cases, and uncommonly, the classic Pel–Ebstein fever is observed, which is characterized by a high fever for 1–2 weeks, followed by an afebrile period of 1–2 weeks.

Chest pain, cough, shortness of breath or a combination of these may be present because of a large mediastinal mass or lung involvement, and haemoptysis occurs rarely. Pain at sites of nodal disease, precipitated by drinking alcohol, occurs in less than 10% of patients but is specific for HL.

Tumour stage is more important than the histological type from treatment perspective.

Laboratory Investigations Complete blood cell (CBC) count in patients with HL reveals anaemia, lymphopenia, neutrophilia and eosinophilia. Platelet counts are variable. Erythrocyte sedimentation rate (ESR) may be elevated and is commonly associated with poor prognosis. Serum LDH level may be elevated and is a marker of tumour burden. Test for HIV is important in the workup of HL because antiretroviral therapy can improve disease outcomes in HIV-positive patients. Screening for hepatitis B and C should also be considered because of their association with HL.

Treatment and Prognosis Treatment of HL is tailored to the type, stage and assessment of the risk of resistant disease. General treatment modalities include radiation therapy, induction chemotherapy, salvage chemotherapy and haematopoietic stem cell transplantation. Choice of treatment focuses on tailoring therapy to each patient according to age, risk of short-term and long-term toxicity and risk of relapse.

The cure rate of patients with stages I/IIA is close to 90% and even in patients with advanced disease (stages IVA and IVB), the disease-free survival at 5 years is 60%–70%.

The incidence of second malignancies that follow genotoxic drugs has come down with the use of newer safer drugs. Anti-CD30 antibodies provide excellent responses in patients with disease that failed to respond to conventional chemotherapy.

Non-Hodgkin Lymphomas

NHL is a group of disorders that include many clinicopathological subtypes, each with distinct epidemiologies, aetiologies, morphological, immunophenotypic, genetic and clinical features and responses to therapy. With respect to prognosis, NHLs can be divided into two groups – indolent and aggressive.

Classification of Non-Hodgkin Lymphoma (Table 16.13) Some of the common lymphomas are discussed in the subsequent sections.

Chronic Lymphocytic Leukaemia and Small Lymphocytic Lymphoma Both the chronic lymphocytic leukaemia (CLL) and small lymphocytic lymphoma (SLL) belong to the same spectrum, as they differ only in the presence of peripheral blood lymphocytosis, which is a common occurrence in CLL patients, whereas SLL patients present with lymphadenopathy and splenomegaly predominantly.

Table 16.13 Categorization of Common Lymphomas According to Their Biological Behaviour

Category	Lymphoma
Indolent	Follicular lymphoma Marginal zone lymphoma Extranodal marginal zone B-cell lymphoma (MALT lymphoma) Chronic lymphocytic leukaemia/small lymphocytic lymphoma Lymphoplasmacytic lymphoma Waldenström macroglobulinaemia
Aggressive	Diffuse large B-cell lymphoma Mantle cell lymphoma Burkitt lymphoma Precursor T-cell lymphoblastic lymphoma Peripheral T-cell lymphoma Lymphoblastic lymphoma Primary CNS lymphoma AIDS-associated lymphoma

CLL is the most common adult leukaemia in the western world, with a median age of 60 years and 2:1 male predominance. The disease is characterized by the accumulation of functionally incompetent lymphocytes.

Pathogenesis CLL arises from B cells that have been arrested during the B-cell differentiation pathway, intermediate between pre-B and mature B cells. An abnormal karyotype is associated with the majority of patients with CLL. The most common genetic abnormality is **deletion of 13q,** which occurs in more than 50% of patients. Most common genetic abnormality is *deletion 13q14.3.* Individuals with this abnormality have a relatively benign disease that usually manifests as stable or slowly progressive isolated lymphocytosis.

The presence of trisomy 12, which is observed in about 15% of CLL patients, is associated with atypical morphology and progressive disease. Deletion in the short arm of chromosome 17 has been associated with rapid progression, short remission and decreased overall survival. TP53 mutation is associated with extensive lymph node involvement, aggressive disease and shorter survival.

The growth of CLL/SLL is largely confined to ***proliferation centres***, where the tumour cells receive critical cues from the tumour microenvironment. Stromal cells in proliferation centres express factors that stimulate NF-κB which, in turn, promotes the proliferation and survival of tumour cells. These signals are transduced by B-cell tyrosine kinase (BTK), a finding that has helped in the development of targeted therapy for patients with CLL.

Morphology

The diagnosis of CLL depends on finding a total leucocyte count that is usually above 50,000 cells/mm^3, with more than 80% of cells being lymphocytes. Anaemia is commonly manifested. A low total count is seen with SLL in the presence of bone marrow infiltration. CLL should be considered if the absolute lymphocyte count is more than 5000/mm^3 in the absence of any other underlying cause. Platelet count may be normal or decreased, and thrombocytopenia becomes severe with progressive involvement of bone marrow by the tumour.

Peripheral blood smear (Fig. 16.18): In almost all the patients, more than 90% of neoplastic cells are small and mature looking lymphocytes with high N:C, scant cytoplasm and dense clumped chromatin with inconspicuous nucleoli. Smudge cells, also called basket cells, which are produced during spreading of blood film because of the fragility of lymphocytes, are characteristic feature of CLL.

A subset of CLL cases may have prominence of prolymphocytes (>10% but <55%), which are

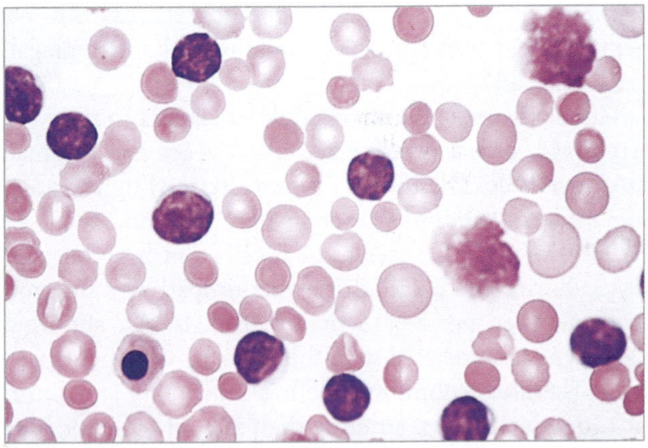

Fig. 16.18 Peripheral smear picture in CLL showing many mature lymphocytes. A few lymphocytes show disrupted cell membrane because of smearing process (smudge cells). Few spherocytes are seen, which is because of the coexistent haemolytic anaemia. (*Source:* From Karen M. Frank, Alexander J. McAdam. Robbins & Cotran Pathologic Basis of Disease. Elsevier. 2021.)

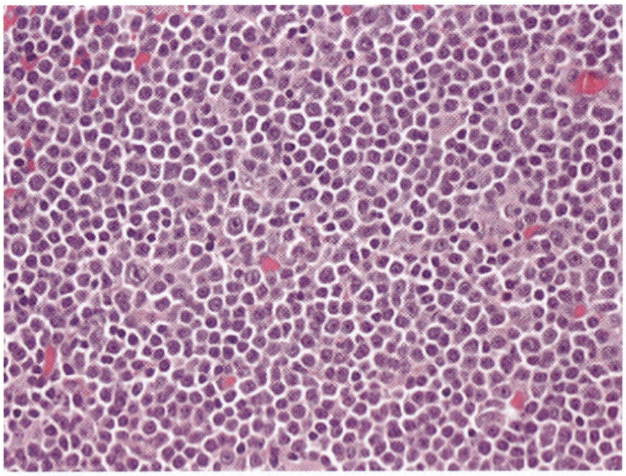

Fig. 16.19 Lymph node morphology in SLL shows alternating dark and light zones. The light zones comprise proliferation centres formed by prolymphocytes and paraimmunoblasts, whereas the smaller neoplastic CLL cells form the outer rim of dark zones. (*Source:* From Kedar V. Inamdar, Carlos E. Bueso-Ramos. Annals of Diagnostic Pathology. Elsevier. 2007.)

slightly larger than mature lymphocytes and have open chromatin and prominent or inconspicuous nucleoli. This category is designated as **CLL/PLL**.

Nucleated red cells and polychromatophilic RBCs are seen with the development of autoimmune haemolytic anaemia.

Bone marrow: Bone marrow can have any of the four patterns of involvement – interstitial infiltrates or aggregates:

- Interstitial
- Nodular
- Diffuse
- Mixed

Assessment of the pattern of infiltration of neoplastic cells in bone marrow has prognostic importance as a diffuse pattern is associated with aggressive disease and worse prognosis and a nodular pattern is associated with a favourable prognosis.

Lymph node: Lymph node architecture is diffusely effaced with an infiltrate predominantly of small lymphocytes admixed with a variable number of larger activated cells which gather to form proliferation centres. **Proliferation centres**, when seen, are pathognomonic of CLL/SLL.

Infiltrates are also seen in the white and red pulp of spleen and hepatic portal tracts (Fig. 16.19).

Immunophenotype

- Pan-B markers – CD19, $CD20^+$
- Special diagnostic markers – ***CD23 and*** $CD5^+$

Clinical Features Most patients with CLL are asymptomatic at diagnosis. Nonspecific symptoms like fatigue, loss of appetite and weight are the most common presentation. Generalized lymphadenopathy and splenomegaly are seen in half of the patients. Anaemia is due to replacement of marrow by the tumour, hypersplenism and autoimmune haemolysis. Hypogammaglobulinaemia due to disruption of normal immune function is the cause of recurrent infections. Paradoxically, 10%–15% of patients develop anaemia and thrombocytopenia because of autoantibodies against platelets and red cells, respectively.

Prognostic Factors The clinical course is highly variable, and the clinical stage is the most important indicator of prognosis. Binet and Rai staging systems are shown in Table 16.14. Apart from that, the following factors are associated with poor prognosis:

- Deletion of 11q and 17p
- Lack of somatic hypermutation

Table 16.14 Binet and Rai Staging System for Chronic Lymphocytic Leukaemia

Stage	Clinical Features
Binet:	
• A	Less than three areas of lymphadenopathy[a]
• B	More than three areas of lymphadenopathy[a]
• C	Anaemia (<10 g/dL) ± thrombocytopenia (<100 × 10^9/L)
Rai:	
• 0	Lymphocytosis in peripheral blood marrow only
• I/II	Lymphadenopathy[a] ± hepatosplenomegaly
• III/IV	Anaemia (<11 g/dL) ± thrombocytopenia (<100 × 10^9/L)

[a]Nodal areas: cervical, axillary, inguinal, spleen and liver.

- Expression of ZAP-70
- Presence of NOTCH1 mutation

Prognosis and Management Generally, the disease has an indolent course. Course and prognosis are extremely variable and depend on the clinical stage. In approximately 5%–10% of patients, CLL transforms to a more aggressive diffuse B-cell lymphoma, which is also referred to as **Richter syndrome**, due to acquisition of additional mutations. This stage is characterized by a rapidly enlarging mass in the spleen or lymph node.

Symptomatic patients are usually treated with gentle chemotherapy and immunotherapy. For young patients, haematopoietic stem cell transplantation is offered as the treatment of choice. BTK inhibitors are novel agents used with promising results.

Follicular Lymphoma Follicular lymphoma is the most common indolent NHL in the Western world, affecting middle-aged men and women equally, with the incidence increasing with age. Approximately 20% of NHLs diagnosed in the Western world are follicular lymphomas.

Aetiology Follicular lymphoma has an unknown aetiology. Family history is important as first-degree relatives are at high risk. Environmental factors like exposure to pesticides and herbicides are associated with the development of follicular lymphoma.

Pathogenesis Follicular lymphomas arise from germinal centre B cells and are strongly associated with the hallmark **t(14;18)** translocation. This translocation results in the overexpression of **BCL2,** which has antiapoptotic effect, helping the neoplastic cells to survive longer. Normal germinal centres contain plenty of B cells undergoing apoptotic cell death, whereas follicular lymphoma is strikingly devoid of apoptotic cells. In approximately 90% of cases, **MLL** gene is mutated, which leads to epigenetic changes. Especially in the early phase of the disease, the lymphoma cells grow within a network of reactive follicular dendritic cells, macrophages and T cells which influence the tumour growth and the response to therapy. Like their normal counterparts, follicular lymphoma cells have ongoing somatic hypermutation, which may promote transformation by causing point mutations or chromosomal aberrations.

Morphology

In a patient with suspected follicular lymphoma, peripheral blood findings are subtle, with 20% of patients showing lymphocytosis up to 20,000 cells/mm^3.

Lymph nodes: On histopathological examination (Fig. 16.20), lymph nodes show partial or complete effacement of architecture with similar sized neoplastic follicles, which are nonpolarized and lack mantle zones with the absence of tingible body macrophages in contrast to normal follicles and reactive hyperplastic follicles. Nodular or nodular and diffuse pattern with centrocytes (small cleaved cells) and centroblasts (larger cells with open chromatin, prominent nucleoli and moderate cytoplasm) is present with infrequent mitoses. The proportion of centroblasts defines the grade (Fig. 16.21).

Following lymph node biopsy and definitive diagnosis of follicular lymphoma, bone marrow studies are conducted to assess the extent of involvement. Bone marrow may show focal or extensive involvement. The tumours cells commonly aggregate as follicles in the paratrabecular region.

Spleen: White pulp of the spleen may be involved.
Liver: Portal tracts of the liver may be involved.

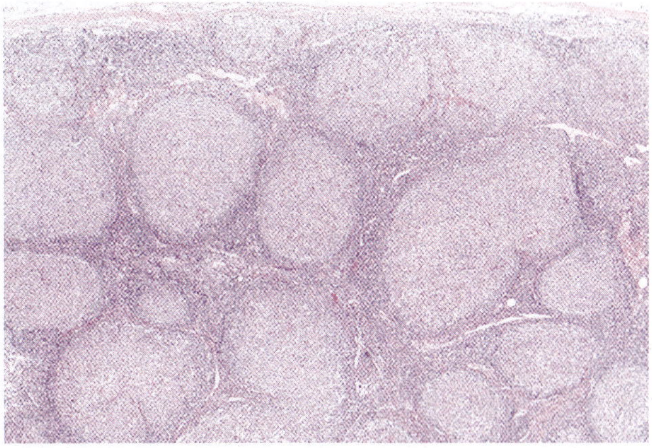

Fig. 16.20 Morphology of lymph node in follicular lymphoma, Low power – shows uniform-sized nodules distributed throughout the lymph node. (*Source:* From Rebecca L. King, Paul J. Kurtin. Hematopathology. Elsevier. 2018.)

Clinical Features Most patients present with painless generalized lymphadenopathy. Rare involvement of extranodal sites like the gastrointestinal tract and CNS can be observed. Fever, fatigue and weight loss are indicators of advanced disease.

Immunophenotyping

B-cell markers: CD19$^+$, CD20$^+$, CD10$^+$, Ig$^+$, BCL6$^+$
Special marker: ***BCL2***$^+$

Treatment and Prognosis Follicular lymphoma is an indolent disease with a chronic relapsing course. Low-dose chemotherapy and immunotherapy with anti-CD20 or localized radiotherapy are the usual treatment modalities. Roughly, 20%–30% of patients with follicular lymphoma worsen with transformation to aggressive diffuse large B-cell lymphoma (DLBCL), or Richter syndrome, which is associated with worse prognosis. Uncommonly, because of acquisition of MYC translocation, Burkitt-like lymphoma evolves. The median survival is less than 1 year after such transformations.

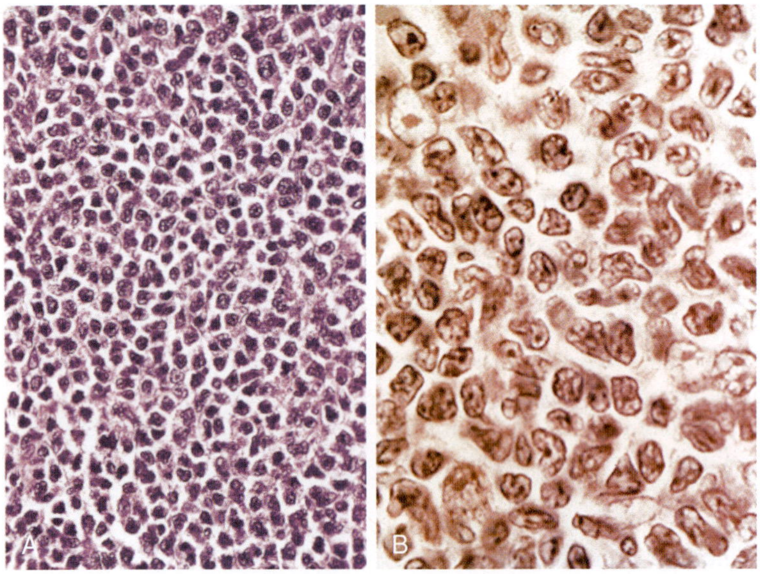

Fig. 16.21 Morphology of lymph node in follicular lymphoma; high power – shows homogeneous population of cells (A) which have cleaved nuclei (B). (*Source:* From Daniel A. Arber. Rosai and Ackerman's Surgical Pathology-2 Volume Set. Elsevier. 2018.)

Diffuse Large B-Cell Lymphoma DLBCL is the most common NHL which accounts for up to one-third of the lymphomas worldwide. It is also the NHL with worst prognosis. This lymphoma commonly affects men older than 60 years, whereas young adults and children are not spared. DLBCL is clinically and biologically heterogeneous and aggressive and includes two major subtypes. It may arise de novo, also called primary (common), or due to progression/transformation of a less aggressive NHL, referred to as secondary. One-third of cases arise from the transformation of follicular lymphoma.

Most common genetic abnormality: **BCL6** dysregulation and overexpression

Other genetic abnormalities: BCL2 or MYC overexpression

Special Subtypes

1. ***Immunodeficiency-associated large B-cell lymphoma*** – in HIV-positive patients and transplant recipients
2. ***Primary effusion lymphoma*** – strong association with KSHV/HHV-8 infection

Morphology

Morphologically, DLBCLs are characterized by diffuse growth pattern, mixed population of small and large cell sizes (usually 5 times normal lymphocytes) and enlarged vesicular nuclei with prominent nucleoli. Individual cells may have centroblastic, immunoblastic or plasmacytic morphology. Proliferation index is always high.
Immunophenotyping B-cell markers: $CD19^+$, $CD20^+$, $CD10^+$, Ig^+, $BCL6^+$

Clinical Features Diffuse large-cell lymphomas have a rapid growth rate and present as masses infiltrating tissues or obstructing organs. Most common presentation is a rapidly enlarging nodal or extranodal mass. These are fast-growing tumours with rapid fatality. At least half of the patients present in the advanced stage at the time of diagnosis.

The disease is uniformly fatal if untreated. Treatment with intense chemotherapy and adjuvant anti-CD20 improves the outcome.

Burkitt Lymphoma Burkitt lymphoma is characterized by rapidly proliferating tumour cells because of **MYC** overexpression. It is also the fastest growing tumour in humans. Burkitt lymphoma is named after Denis Parsons Burkitt, the Irish surgeon who first described the disease in 1958 while working in Africa. It is a lymphoma that predominantly affects children, whereas adults are involved rarely but with worse prognosis.

There are three clinical types of Burkitt lymphoma.

1. ***African or endemic type***: This type commonly affects the malaria endemic regions of the world, Africa, Brazil, etc. EBV association is seen in every patient of Burkitt lymphoma. Chronic malaria is believed to reduce resistance to EBV, allowing it to enter and proliferate. The disease characteristically involves the jaw or other facial bone (Fig. 16.22), distal ileum, caecum, ovaries or kidneys.
2. ***Sporadic or nonendemic*** or non-African type: This is the most common variant in malaria nonendemic regions of the world. It has predilection for abdominal viscera, especially the ileocaecal region. Only 15%–20% of cases are infected with EBV.
3. ***Immunodeficiency type in HIV patients:*** This variant is usually associated with HIV infection or in the setting of posttransplant patients who are taking

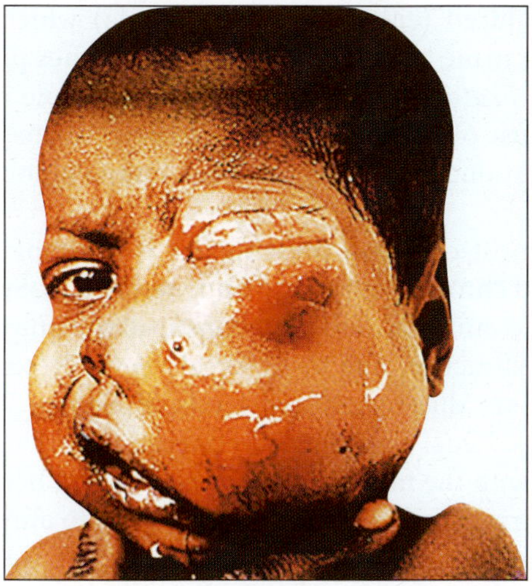

Fig. 16.22 African Burkitt lymphoma of mandible. (*Source:* From Ramya Kollipara, Stephen K. Tyring. Tropical Dermatology. Elsevier. 2017.)

immunosuppressive drugs. Burkitt lymphoma can be one of the diseases associated with the initial manifestation of AIDS. Twenty-five per cent of this variant is infected with EBV.

Pathogenesis All forms are strongly associated with ***MYC*** translocation and overexpression due to **t(8;14),** t(2;8) and t(8;22). The role of MYC in lymphomagenesis is explained in Chapter 7.

Morphology

Morphology of the affected organ shows diffuse effacement of architecture, with sheets of intermediate-size cells having high mitotic and apoptotic activities. Phagocytosis of the apoptotic cells by the macrophages gives the characteristic starry ***sky pattern*** (Fig. 16.23), which is the classical feature of Burkitt lymphoma.

Immunophenotyping B-cell markers: $CD19^+$, $CD20^+$, $CD10^+$, Ig^+, **$BCL6^+$**

Ki67 labelling index 100% (Ki67 is a proliferation marker; its level is high in most malignant tumours and exceptionally high [100%] in Burkitt lymphoma and is the hallmark diagnostic feature).

Course and Prognosis Burkitt lymphoma is a very aggressive tumour owing to its high proliferation index but responds well to chemotherapy. The results of chemotherapy depend on the time of diagnosis. Cure rate is high in children and young adults, whereas in adults, the prognosis is more guarded.

Plasma Cell Dyscrasias and Related Disorders

Plasma cell dyscrasias is the term used to describe the group of disorders characterized by neoplastic monoclonal proliferation of plasma cells, causing increased production of single homogeneous immunoglobulin.

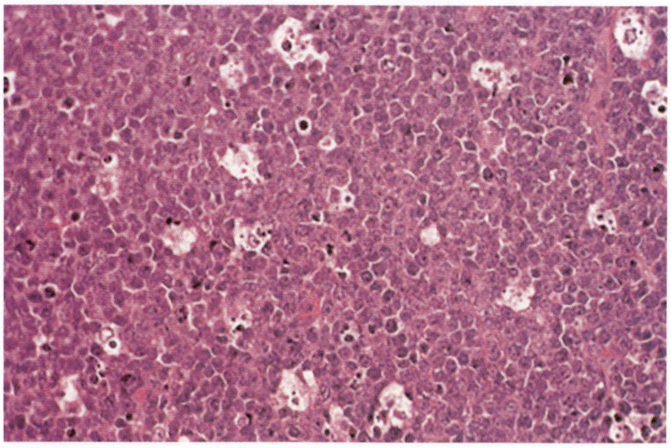

Fig. 16.23 Microscopy of Burkitt lymphoma lymph node showing a starry sky pattern. (*Source:* From Daniel A. Arber. Rosai and Ackerman's Surgical Pathology-2 Volume Set. Elsevier. 2018.)

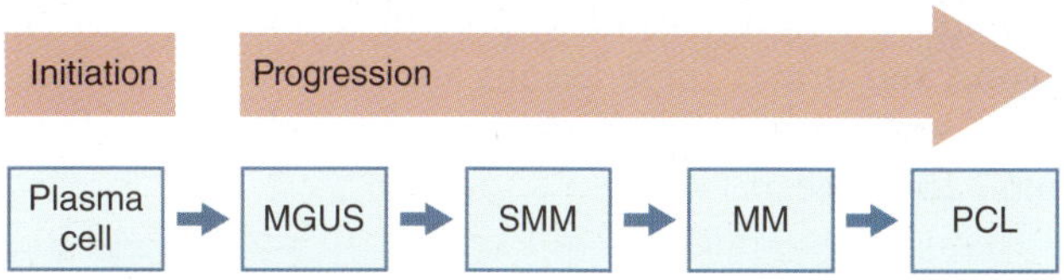

Fig. 16.24 Spectrum of plasma cell dyscrasias. MGUS, monoclonal gammopathy of undetermined significance; MM, multiple myeloma; PCL, plasma cell leukaemia; SMM, Smoldering multiple myeloma.

The clinicopathological entities in the spectrum are as follows (Fig. 16.24):

- MGUS – monoclonal gammopathy of undetermined significance
- Smouldering myeloma
- Plasmacytoma
- Multiple myeloma
- Waldenström macroglobulinaemia
- Heavy-chain disease
- Primary amyloidosis

Monoclonal Gammopathy of Undetermined Significance
This is the early stage of myeloma and the most common plasma cell dyscrasia. Almost all cases of multiple myeloma are preceded by an asymptomatic state called MGUS. Patients with MGUS are asymptomatic, with serum and urine Ig levels less than those in patients with myeloma. One per cent of such patients develop symptomatic myeloma every year. Regular assessment of serum M component levels and Bence Jones proteinuria is essential to identify early progression to multiple myeloma.

Serum and urine electrophoresis cut-offs for the diagnosis of MGUS are as follows:

- ***Serum: <3 g/dL of Ig***
- ***Urine: <6 mg/dL of Ig***

Smouldering Myeloma Smouldering myeloma marks a disease state between MGUS and multiple myeloma. The marrow plasma cells range between 10% and 30%, with serum and Ig levels similar to multiple myeloma but without symptoms.

Serum and urine electrophoresis cut-offs for the diagnosis of smouldering myeloma are as follows:

- ***Serum: >3 g/dL of Ig***
- ***Urine: >6 mg/dL of Ig***

The most defining criterion for differentiating smouldering myeloma from multiple myeloma is the absence of symptoms.

Solitary Myeloma/Plasmacytoma Solitary myeloma or plasmacytoma is an uncommon disorder characterized by solitary lesions of bone or soft tissue commonly involving the lungs, oropharynx or nasal sinuses. This disorder has modest elevations of M protein (explained later) in blood and urine. These lesions are cured by local resection, without which they progress to multiple myeloma after 10–20 years.

Multiple Myeloma Multiple myeloma is a plasma cell neoplasm characterized by the formation of multifocal tumour masses composed of plasma cells at multiple locations in the skeletal system, leading to multiple lytic bone lesions, hypercalcaemia, renal failure and acquired immune abnormalities due to suppression of normal immunoglobulin production.

Pathogenesis A common and early genetic abnormality noted in multiple myeloma is **t(11;14)**. MGUS carries the same genetic abnormality like multiple myeloma; with acquisition of additional genetic changes that involve RAS, p16 or MYC, it undergoes secondary changes in the bone marrow microenvironment and progresses to multiple myeloma.

Deletion of 17p is associated with worse prognosis, and **MYC overexpression** is associated with transformation to plasma cell leukaemia.

Increasing evidence suggests that the bone marrow microenvironment of tumour cells plays a pivotal role in the pathogenesis of multiple myeloma. Growth and survival of myeloma cells are dependent on **IL-6**, which is secreted by the tumour cells and also by the stromal cells. Elevated serum IL-6 levels are associated with active disease and poor outcome and are measures to assess prognosis.

Myeloma-derived **MIP-1α** upregulates RANKL expression by bone marrow stromal cells, which, in turn, activate osteoclasts which are the major mechanism for osteolytic bone lesions and the resultant hypercalcaemia and bone fractures. The downstream events of RANKL expression in bones is explained in Chapter 30.

Neoplastic plasma cells secrete monoclonal immunoglobulins which are referred to as **M component**. Apart from complete immunoglobulins, excess light chains are also produced (either kappa or lambda) which are excreted in urine and referred to as **Bence Jones protein**.

Clinical Features Clinical features of multiple myeloma are because of proliferation of neoplastic plasma cells and excess production of monoclonal immunoglobulins by them.

The most common presentation is pathological fractures and chronic pain due to bone resorption. Symptoms include confusion, lethargy, constipation, polyuria and renal dysfunction due to hypercalcaemia. Recurrent infections are due to reduced levels of normal immunoglobulins. Renal failure may be precipitated due to many factors, with the most important cause being Bence Jones proteinuria. There may be symptoms due to amyloidosis, which could exacerbate renal failure. Apart from these, there can be symptoms due to hyperviscosity (less often than Waldenström macroglobulinaemia) and also symptoms due to anaemia, leucopenia and thrombocytopenia.

Laboratory Investigations Laboratory investigations reveal anaemia, leucopenia and thrombocytopenia. Renal function tests may be abnormal with the onset of renal failure.

Morphology

Multiple myeloma most often present as lytic **bone lesions** (Fig. 16.25), especially involving axial skeleton (vertebral column, ribs, skull, pelvis, femur, clavicle and scapula) that appear radiologically as ***punched-out defects*** measuring up to 4 cm in diameter and grossly as soft red gelatinous masses. Such lesions begin in the medullary cavity, erode cancellous bone and destroy the bone cortex.

Peripheral blood smear examination: Rouleaux formation occurs because of high levels of circulating immunoglobulin, causing red cells to adhere to each other. Rarely, tumour cells may be seen in the peripheral blood with transformation to **plasma cell leukaemia.**

Bone marrow (Fig. 16.26): The important criterion is to detect a hypercellular marrow with more than ***30% plasma cells***, which may have completely replaced the normal haematopoietic elements. Neoplastic plasma cells may resemble normal appearing plasma cells or plasma blasts or other cytological variants like **Mott cells** (cells with multiple grape-like cytoplasmic inclusions), **flame cells** (cells with fiery red cytoplasm) or cells with inclusions like **fibrils, crystalline rods and globules** (Fig. 16.27).

Intracytoplasmic globular inclusions are referred to as **Russell bodies**, and intranuclear globular inclusions within the neoplastic plasma cells are referred to as **Dutcher bodies** (Fig. 16.28).

Immunophenotype Plasma cells are positive for ***CD138 (also known as syndecan-1) and CD56.***

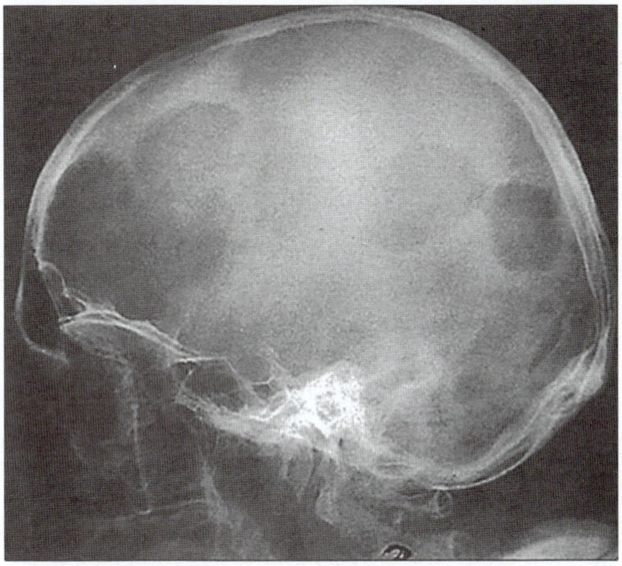

Fig. 16.25 X-ray picture of the skull with lytic lesions in multiple myeloma. (*Source:* From Michael Murphy, Rajeev Srivastava, Kevin Deans. Clinical Biochemistry. Elsevier. 2019.)

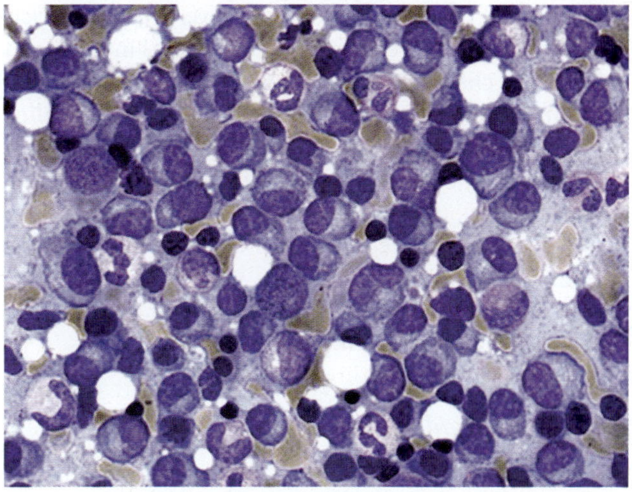

Fig. 16.26 Bone marrow morphology in multiple myeloma. (*Source:* From Olga Pozdnyakova. High-Yield Hematopathology. Elsevier. 2013.)

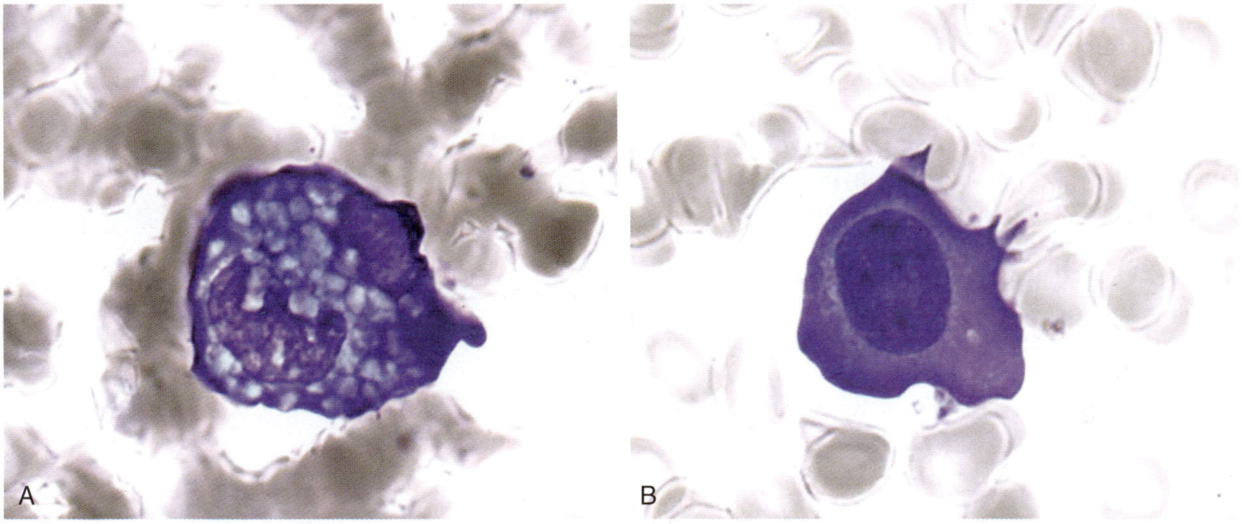

Fig. 16.27 (A) Mott cells and (B) flame cells seen in multiple myeloma, microscopy. (*Source:* From Olga Pozdnyakova. High-Yield Hematopathology. Elsevier. 2013.)

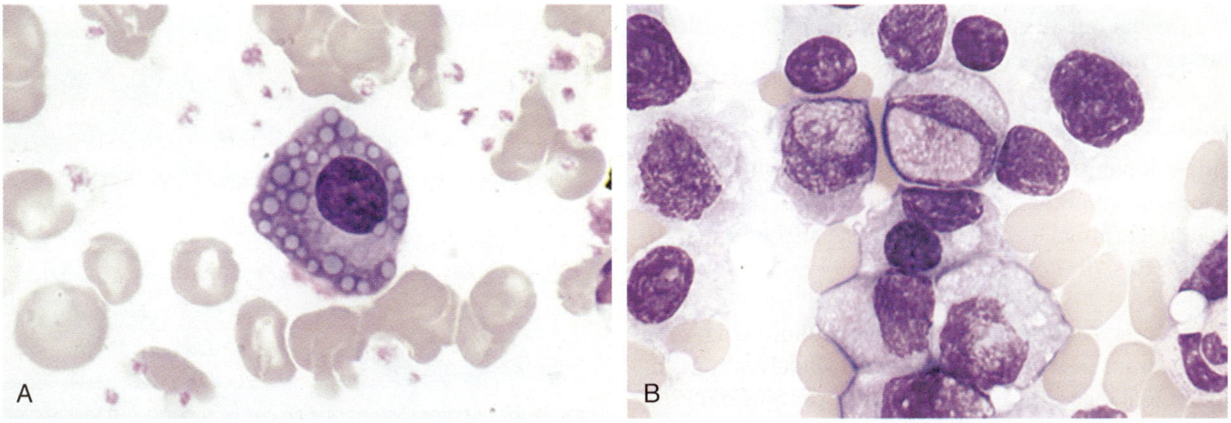

Fig. 16.28 Russell bodies (A) and Dutcher bodies (B) seen in multiple myeloma, microscopy. (*Source:* From Robert W. McKenna, Steven H. Kroft, Michael A. Linden. Hematopathology. Elsevier. 2017.)

Almost all the cases of multiple myeloma are associated with elevated levels of immunoglobulins in the blood and/or light chains. Most common monoclonal immunoglobulin is ***IgG***, followed by IgA. Other immunoglobulins are rare. Serum and urine electrophoresis is the commonly performed investigation which reveals the presence of monoclonal immunoglobulin, which is referred to as M protein. It is seen as spikes in the electrophoresis screen.

The usual levels and the criteria for M protein in multiple myeloma are as follows:

- ***Serum: >3 g/dL of Ig***
- ***Urine: >6 mg/dL of Ig***

Excessive production of M proteins usually of the IgA or IgG3 type results in hyperviscosity syndrome.

One per cent of myelomas are nonsecretory with no M component and need extensive workup.

Prognosis Patients with multiple bone lesions without treatment may survive less than a year.

- *Proteasome inhibitors* are bringing hope to patients with myeloma.
- Thalidomides inhibit myeloma cells.
- Biphosphonates help by inhibiting bone resorption.

Waldenström Macroglobulinaemia Waldenström macroglobulinaemia, also referred to as **hyperviscosity syndrome**, is due to elevated levels of ***IgM*** *and is* seen in association with lymphoplasmacytic lymphoma, where the B cells are differentiated into mature plasma cells.

All cases are associated with ***MYD88 mutations*** which activate ***NF-κB*** and signals involved in the B-cell receptor complex. Unlike multiple myeloma, this disorder is not associated with complications due to secretion of free light chains.

Patients present with nonspecific symptoms like fatigue, weakness, loss of weight and appetite. Lymphadenopathy, hepatomegaly and splenomegaly are seen in at least 50% of cases. Coombs test can reveal the presence of cold agglutinins causing autoimmune haemolytic anaemia. Prominent symptoms of *hyperviscosity syndrome* include visual impairment, neurological problems, bleeding and cryoglobulinaemia.

Mantle Cell Lymphoma

Mantle cell lymphoma is an uncommon lymphoma, with tumour cells resembling normal mantle zone B cells that surround germinal centres. It usually affects males in their fifth to sixth decades of life.

Pathogenesis Almost all mantle cell lymphomas have the hallmark translocation **t(11;14)**, which involves translocation of IgH locus on chromosome 11, resulting in ***cyclin D1*** overexpression. This translocation is detected in about 70% of cases by conventional karyotyping, and in the remaining cases fluorescent in situ hybridization (FISH) is helpful in detecting the genetic abnormality. Cyclin D1 acts by promoting the cells from G1 to S phase in the cell cycle.

Morphology

Lymph node enlargement is the predominant presentation with an infrequent involvement of extranodal sites and peripheral blood. Occasionally, mucosal involvement of the gut with polyp-like lesions referred to as *lymphomatoid polyposis* is seen.

Lymph node: There is effacement of architecture with expansion of the mantle zone with a nodular arrangement of homogeneous small cells with cleaved nuclei (Fig. 16.29). As the disease advances, the germinal centres become effaced, with obliteration of lymph node architecture.

A blastic variant, demonstrating numerous medium-to-large blast-like cells, has been reported.

Immunophenotyping B-cell markers: $CD19^+$, $CD20^+$, Ig^+

Special markers: ***CD5+ and cyclin D1+***

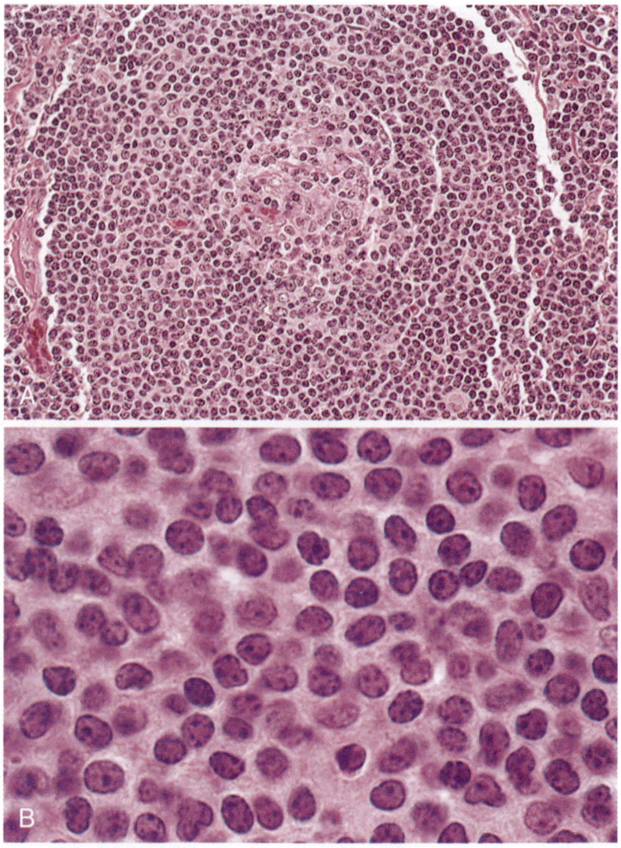

Fig. 16.29 Microscopy of Mantle cell lymphoma: (A) low power and (B) high power. (*Source:* From Olga Pozdnyakova. High-Yield Hematopathology. Elsevier. 2013.)

Clinical Features The most common presentation is painless lymphadenopathy and nonspecific symptoms.

Some patients present with symptoms due to the involvement of the spleen and gut. The lymphoma as such has poor prognosis but with ***blastoid transformation***, it has poorer prognosis with rapid fatality.

Patients are treated with chemotherapy, with less than one-third of patients achieving complete response. Haematopoietic stem cell transplantation is indicated in young patients and suitable candidates in whom it offers cure.

Marginal Zone Lymphoma

Marginal zone lymphoma is a group of B-cell lymphomas that arise in lymph nodes, spleen and extranodal sites. These extranodal tumours were previously found to be arising from mucosal sites and were referred to as mucosa-associated lymphoid tumours – **'MALTomas'**.

They represent an intermediate stage between reactive lymphoid hyperplasia and lymphomas.

Characteristics Characteristic features of extranodal marginal zone lymphomas are as follows:

- Commonly seen in tissues affected by chronic inflammatory/infectious/autoimmune disorders. Example: salivary gland in Sjögren syndrome, thyroid in Hashimoto thyroiditis and gastric mucosa in *H. pylori* infection.
- These remain localized for prolonged periods and spread only late in their disease course.
- If the inciting agent (e.g. *H. pylori*) is removed, these lymphomas may regress.

The disease begins as polyclonal immune reaction which develops to full-blown lymphoma by acquiring additional mutations like ***t(11;18)***, (14;18) or (1;14). Treating the primary cause of inflammation such as *H. pylori* in gastric MALTomas before the progression of polyclonal to monoclonal activation is beneficial and halts the neoplastic process.

All these translocations upregulate the expression of **BCL10** or ***MALT1*** protein, which, in turn, activates NF-κB which promotes growth and survival of B cells. With additional clonal evolution, metastatic spread and transformation to DLBCL occur.

Morphology of marginal cell lymphoma is discussed in Chapter 21.

Hairy Cell Leukaemia

Hairy cell leukaemia (HCL) is a rare B-cell neoplasm which predominantly affects middle-aged white men characterized by pancytopenia and splenomegaly and the presence of hairy cells in bone marrow and peripheral blood.

Pathogenesis More than 90% of cases of HCL are associated with activating point mutations of the serine/threonine kinase **BRAF**, which promotes growth by activating the MAPK pathway. The specific mutation of a valine to glutamate substitution at residue 600 is also associated with melanomas and LCH.

Clinical Features The clinical picture is dominated by the features because of infiltration of the bone marrow, liver and spleen. Splenomegaly is the most common manifestation. Hepatomegaly is less common, with lymphadenopathy being rare. Symptoms due to pancytopenia are common with anaemia, frequent infections and bleeding. Patients may also have an increased incidence of mycobacterial infections due to ***monocytopenia***.

Morphology

Peripheral smear (Fig. 16.30): This neoplasm derives its name owing to the presence of fine hair-like projections on the tumour cells. As evidenced by peripheral blood smear examination, hairy cells have round, oblong or reniform nuclei and moderate amounts of pale blue cytoplasm with thread- or bleb-like extensions that are best seen under a phase-contrast microscope.
Bone marrow (Fig. 16.31): Bone marrow though cellular, peripheral blood pancytopenia and dry tap are observed owing to the presence of delicate reticulin fibres enmeshing the cells. Hence, bone marrow biopsy is essential for diagnosis. On histopathological examination, the tumour cells show a perinuclear halo due to formalin fixation along with prominent cell borders, thereby exhibiting the classical *'fried egg appearance'*.
Spleen: Red pulp is densely infiltrated, resulting in the obliteration and atrophy of white pulp and a beefy gross appearance.
Cytochemistry: HCL cells show positivity with tartrate-resistant acid phosphatase (TRAP) enzyme.

Immunophenotyping
B-cell markers: $CD19^+$, $CD20^+$, surface Ig^+
Special markers: ***$CD11c^+$, $CD25^+$, $CD103^+$, $annexin^+$***

Treatment and Prognosis HCL has an indolent course which responds to gentle chemotherapy. Unlike most other lymphomas, single-agent therapy is common and usually successful. Purine analogues and interferons cause complete remission. BRAF inhibitors produce excellent results in cases that have failed conventional chemotherapy.

Non-Hodgkin Lymphomas: Peripheral T- and NK-Cell Neoplasms

Peripheral T-Cell and NK-Cell Lymphoma Peripheral T-cell tumours are a heterogeneous group of neoplasms that account for 5%–10% of NHLs. NK-cell tumours are very rare and are listed here.

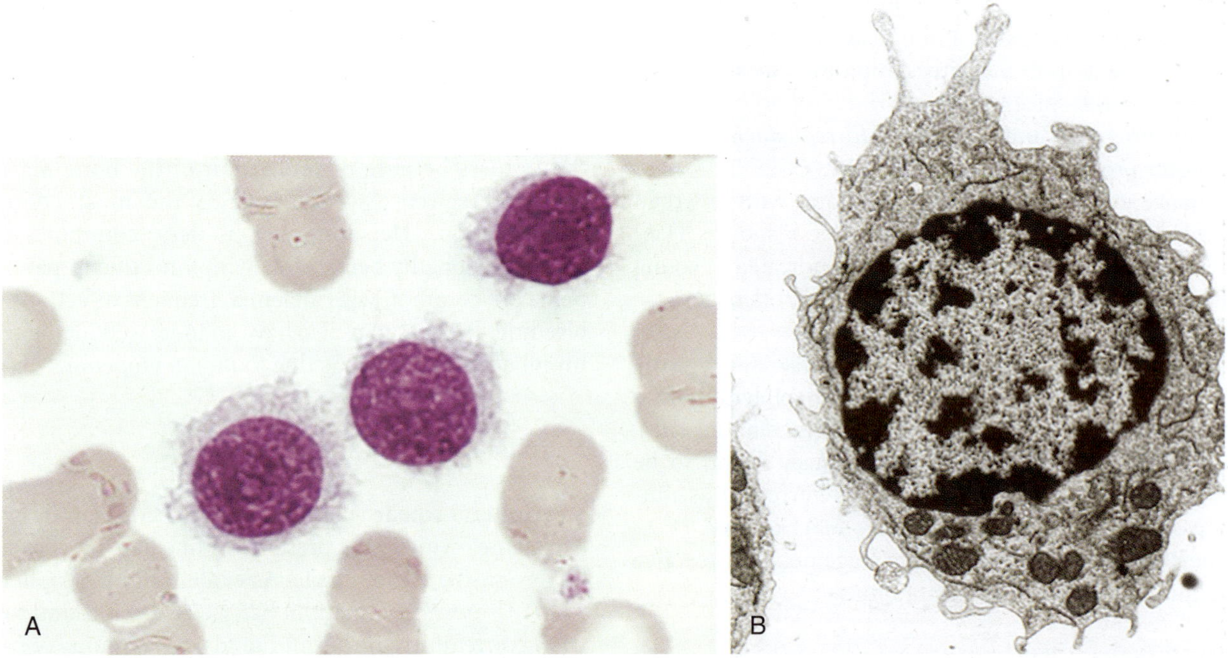

Fig. 16.30 Peripheral smear morphology in hairy cell leukaemia (A) and an electron micrograph of hairy cell (B). (*Source:* From Claire Dearden. Best Practice & Research Clinical Haematology. Elsevier. 2015.)

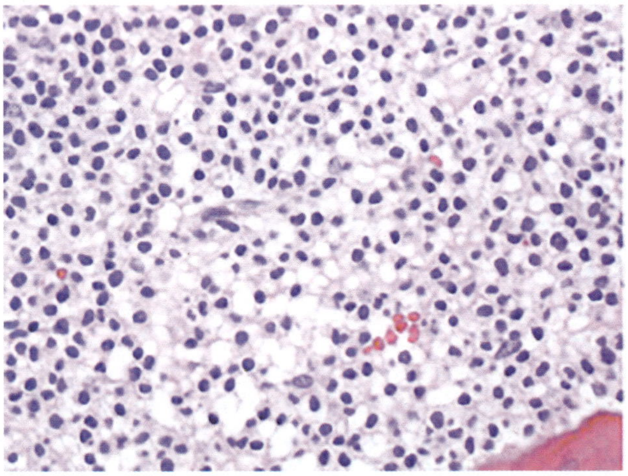

Fig. 16.31 Bone marrow morphology in hairy cell leukaemia shows hypercellularity with nuclei of hairy cells widely separated by abundant cytoplasm, giving a characteristic 'fried egg' appearance. (*Source:* From Rahul R. Naik, Alan Saven. Mayo Clinic Proceedings. Elsevier. 2012.)

Lymphomas under this category are as follows:

1. Peripheral T-cell lymphoma, unspecified
   This lymphoma arises from $CD4^+$ memory T cells and does not meet criteria for other T-cell lymphomas in the current WHO classification. It is also called Lennert lymphoma, and has an aggressive clinical course. Lymph node shows paracortical or diffuse infiltrate composed of medium- to large-sized cells with occasional Reed–Sternberg-like cells and clear cells.
2. Anaplastic large cell lymphoma
   It is a peripheral T-cell lymphoma composed of hallmark cells with kidney-shaped/horseshoe-shaped highly pleomorphic nucleus. The cells are strongly positive for CD30 with or without anaplastic lymphoma kinase (ALK) rearrangement. It presents with aggressive clinical course.
3. Adult T-cell leukaemia/lymphoma
   It is associated with early exposure to human T-lymphotropic virus-1 (HTLV-1) in endemic areas of Southwestern Japan, Caribbean basin, Africa and Middle East. ATCL arises after a long latency period and is more common in males. It manifests as exfoliative skin lesions, lymphadenopathy and hepatosplenomegaly. The tumour is composed of highly pleomorphic small- to medium-sized lymphoid cells positive for CD2, CD3, CD4 and CCR4.
4. Mycosis fungoides/Sezary syndrome
   Also known as cutaneous T-cell lymphoma, this is the neoplasm of $CD4^+$ T cells in the skin. Clinical manifestations occur in three phases – erythrodermic rash, plaque and tumour phase. Histologically, the tumour cells have cerebriform nuclei with marked nuclear membrane indentations. Presence of circulating tumour cells and generalized exfoliative erythroderma is called Sezary syndrome. Early phase has good prognosis. Plaque and tumour phases have 1–3 year survival.
5. Large granular lymphocytic leukaemia
   It is a chronic cytotoxic T-cell neoplasm with indolent course. It is associated with pancytopenia and autoimmune disorders. It shows a characteristic intrasinusoidal involvement in bone marrow, liver and spleen, and 50% cases show STAT3/STAT5b mutation.
6. Extranodal NK-/T-cell lymphoma
   It is also known as angiocentric T-cell lymphoma owing to its angiotropic and angiodestructive nature. It is

associated with EBV, and it is most common in Latin America and East Asia. Majority of patients show ulceration of nasal mucosa, infiltration by neoplastic lymphoid cells and necrosis.

Most tumours in this category are very aggressive with poor outcomes.

Common translocations and markers in lymphoid neoplasms are listed in Tables 16.15, 16.16 and 16.27.

Peripheral TANK neoplasms:

Peripheral T- and NK-cell neoplasms refer to the neoplasms of mature T cells and NK (natural killer) cells. These are a subset of lymphoid neoplasms, which generally share several common features.

Lymphoid neoplasms typically originate from a monoclonal derivative of a transformed cell, meaning the neoplastic cells are clones of a single cell type that possess the same antigen receptor proteins. This is in contrast to the normal polyclonal population of immune cell subsets found in lymph nodes.

For diagnosing these neoplasms, histopathological examination of lymph nodes or the affected sites is essential.

A significant majority of lymphoid neoplasms (approximately 85%–90%) are of B-cell origin. T-cell neoplasms form a smaller proportion, and NK-cell neoplasms are considered very rare.

Peripheral T- and NK-cell neoplasms are therefore a distinct group within lymphoid neoplasms, characterized by their cellular origin and specific monoclonal nature.

MYELOID NEOPLASMS

PA 18.2

Myeloid neoplasms are composite category of tumours originating from the haematopoietic stem cells in the marrow with a less frequent involvement of secondary haematopoietic organs. These generally present with symptoms due to altered haematopoiesis and are categorized into the following groups:

- AMLs
- MDSs
- MPNs
- MDS/MPN
- Myeloid/lymphoid neoplasms with rearrangement of PDGFRA, PDGFRB or FGFR1 or with PCM1-JAK2

Here, we discuss AML, MDS and MPNs in detail in the following sections.

Acute Myeloid Leukaemia

AML is a group of clonal neoplastic proliferation of haematopoietic precursor cells caused by acquired oncogenic mutations that result in the accumulation of excessive myeloblasts and other immature myeloid cells in the marrow. AML is genotypically and phenotypically extremely heterogeneous.

Epidemiology AML is more commonly diagnosed in developed countries and is more common among whites. Though AML affects persons of all age groups, the prevalence of AML increases with age and the median age of onset

Table 16.15 Important Translocations and Markers in Common Lymphoid Neoplasms

Leukaemia/Lymphoma	Common Genetic Abnormality	Immunophenotyping	Special Marker
B-cell ALL/lymphoma	t(12;21)	B-cell markers depending on the stage of maturation $CD10^{+}/-$	
T-cell ALL/lymphoma	NOTCH1 mutations	T-cell markers depending on the stage of maturation	
Burkitt lymphoma	t(8;14)	B-cell markers $CD10^{+}/-$	$BCL6^{+}$
Diffuse large B-cell lymphoma	Rearrangements involving BCL6, BCL2 or MYC	B-cell markers	
Follicular lymphoma	t(14;18)	B-cell markers $CD10^{+}/-$	$BCL2^{+}$
Extranodal marginal zone lymphoma	t(11;18)	B-cell markers	$MALT1^{+}$
Mantle cell lymphoma	t(11;14)	B-cell markers $CD10^{+}/-$	$CD5^{+}$ Cyclin $D1^{+}$
Hairy cell leukaemia	BRAF mutations	CD11c, CD25, CD103	$Annexin^{+}$ $TRAP^{+}$
Multiple myeloma	t(11;14)	Plasma cell markers	
CLL/SLL	Trisomy 12, deletion 11q, 13q, 17p	B-cell markers	CD5 and $CD23^{+}$

ALL, acute lymphoblastic leukaemia; CLL, chronic lymphocytic leukaemia; SLL, small lymphocytic lymphoma.

Table 16.16 Role of CD Markers in Leukaemia/Lymphomas

CD Marker	Marker For
Primary Stem Cell Marker	
CD34	Pluripotent HSCs and mast cells
Common Leucocyte Marker	
CD45[a]	All leucocytes
T-Cell Associated	
CD1	Langerhans cells
CD3[a]	Mature T cells
CD4[a]	Helper T cells
CD5	T cells
CD8[a]	Cytotoxic T cells
B-Cell Associated	
CD10[a]	B-cell marker, CALLA
CD19[a]	Pan-B marker
CD20	B-cell marker
CD21	Receptor for EBV
CD23	B-cell marker
CD79a[a]	Pan-B marker
Primary Monocyte or Macrophage Associated	
CD11c	Granulocytes, monocytes, macrophages; also in hairy cell leukaemia
CD13[a]	Monocytes and granulocytes
CD14[a]	Monocytes
CD15[a]	Granulocytes and Reed–Sternberg cells
CD33[a]	Myeloid progenitors and monocytes
CD64	Mature myeloid cells
Primary NK-Cell Associated	
CD16[a]	NK cells
CD56[a]	NK cells and neoplastic plasma cells
Primary Plasma Cell Associated	
CD38	Normal and neoplastic plasma cells
CD138[a]	Normal and neoplastic plasma cells
CD56	Neoplastic plasma cells
Activation Marker	
CD30[a]	Activated B cells, T cells and monocytes, Reed–Sternberg cells
Histiocytic Marker	
CD68	Histiocytes

EBV, Epstein–Barr virus; HSC, haematopoietic stem cell; NK, natural killer.
[a]High-yield markers.

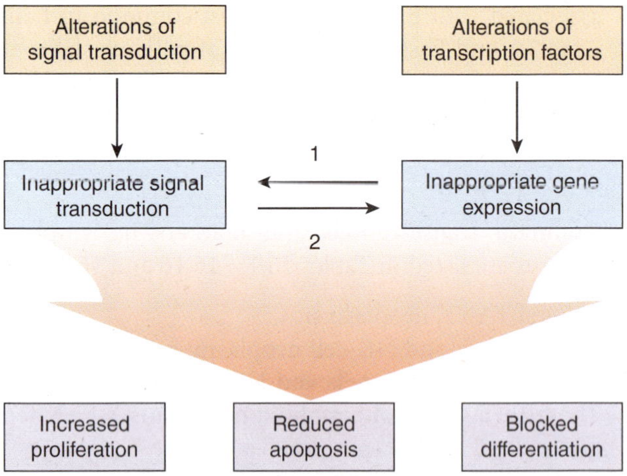

Fig. 16.32 Pathogenesis of AML.

is approximately 70 years. AML is more common in men than in women, especially in older patients. The likely explanation is that MDS is more common in men, and advanced MDS frequently evolves into AML. Some researchers have proposed that the higher prevalence of AML in men may be related to occupational exposure to carcinogens.

Pathogenesis (Fig. 16.32) Several factors have been implicated in the causation of AML.

- Environmental exposures to toxins and chemicals
- Drugs like alkylating agents used for cytotoxic chemotherapy and topoisomerase II inhibitors
- Viruses like HTLV-I are associated with adult T-cell leukaemia/lymphoma (ATLL)
- Antecedent haematological disorders like MDS (especially the type with excess blast) and MPNs
- Congenital disorders – Bloom syndrome, Down syndrome, congenital neutropenia, Fanconi anaemia and neurofibromatosis
- Familial syndromes
  - Germline mutations in the gene *AML1* (*RUNX1*, *CBFA2*) occur in the familial platelet disorder with predisposition for AML, an autosomal dominant disorder characterized by moderate thrombocytopenia, a defect in platelet function and a propensity to develop AML.
  - Mutation of *CEBPA* was described in a family with three members affected by AML.

However, most patients who present with de novo AML have no identifiable risk factor.

Classification Two staging systems are commonly used for AMLs:

- The French–American–British (FAB) system is based on morphology to define specific immunotypes.
- The World Health Organization (WHO) classification is based on chromosome translocations and evidence of dysplasia.

Table 16.17 WHO Classification of AML, 2016

Class	Prognosis	Morphology/Comments
I. **AML with recurrent genetic aberrations**		
1. AML with t(8;21)	Favourable	Myelocytic maturation with Auer rods
2. AML with inversion 16	Favourable	Myelomonocytic maturation with abnormal eosinophilic precursors with basophilic granules
3. AML with t(15;17) APL with PML-RARA	Intermediate	Numerous Auer rods, often in bundles (inconspicuous in microgranular variants), a high incidence of disseminated intravascular coagulation (DIC)
4. AML with t(11q23;v)	Poor	Monocytic differentiation
5. AML with normal cytogenetics and mutated NPM	Favourable	IHC for NPM+
II. **AML with MDS-like features**		
1. With prior MDS	Poor	Diagnosis based on clinical history
2. With multilineage dysplasia	Poor	Cells with dysplastic features like MDS
3. With MDS-like cytogenetics	Poor	Associated with 5q−7q− and 20q− aberrations
III. **AML therapy related**	Very poor	Following alkylator therapy or radiotherapy: >2–8 years latency period, MDS-like cytogenetics + Following topoisomerase II inhibitor n1–3 years latency period, MLL translocation +
IV. **AML, not otherwise specified** – intermediate prognosis		
1. Minimally differentiated		Myeloperoxidase (MPO) negative, blasts positive for myeloid antigens by flow cytometry
2. Without maturation		>3% blasts positive for MPO
3. With myelocytic maturation		Full range of myelocytic maturation
4. With myelomonocytic maturation		Myelocytic and monocytic maturation
5. With monocytic maturation		Nonspecific esterase-positive monoblasts and promonocytes predominance in marrow
6. With erythroid maturation		A. Erythroid myeloid subtype: >50% dysplastic erythroid precursors + >20% myeloblasts
		B. Pure erythroid subtype: >80% erythroid precursors without myeloblasts
7. With megakaryocytic maturation		Megakaryoblasts predominate in the marrow which are positive for GPIIb/IIIa, vWF Commonly associated with marrow fibrosis Most common AML in Down syndrome
V. **Myeloid sarcoma**		
VI. **Myeloid proliferations related to Down syndrome** • Transient abnormal myelopoiesis (TAM) • Myeloid leukaemia associated with Down syndrome		
VII. **Blastic plasmacytoid dendritic cell neoplasm**		
VIII. **Acute leukaemias of ambiguous lineage** • Acute undifferentiated leukaemia • Mixed phenotype acute leukaemia (MPAL) with t(9;22) (q34.1;q11.2); BCR-ABL1 MPAL with t(v;11q23.3); KMT2A rearranged • MPAL, B/myeloid, NOS • MPAL, T/myeloid, NOS		

WHO Classification of Acute Myeloid Leukaemia, 2016 *(Table 16.17)*

i. AML with recurrent genetic aberrations
ii. AML with MDS-related changes
iii. AML, therapy related
iv. AML, not otherwise specified
v. Myeloid sarcoma
vi. Myeloid proliferations related to Down syndrome

Genetics of Acute Myeloid Leukaemia The underlying pathogenesis causing AML is most likely the result of maturational arrest of bone marrow cells in the earliest stages of development. The mechanism of this arrest is under study, but in most cases, it involves the activation or inactivation of genes through chromosomal translocations and other genetic and/or epigenetic changes.

This developmental arrest results in two processes.

- First, the production of normal blood cells markedly decreases, leading to varying degrees of anaemia, thrombocytopenia and neutropenia.
- Second, the rapid proliferation of the myeloblasts, along with a reduction in their ability to undergo apoptotic cell death, results in their accumulation in the bone marrow, blood, spleen and liver.

Following are the genetic abnormalities commonly associated with AML:

- Many of the recurrent genetic aberrations disrupt the genes coding for transcription factors required for myeloid differentiation, e.g. t(8;21) and inv(16).
- Some genetic abnormalities result in activation of transcription factors, e.g. **t(15;17)**. The translocation creates a fusion gene that encodes a chimeric protein consisting of ***RAR***α fused to PML. This fusion protein interferes with the terminal differentiation of granulocytes, an effect that can be overcome by treatment with either **all-trans retinoic acid or arsenic trioxide**.
- In addition to this translocation, activating mutations in **FLT3**, a receptor tyrosine kinase that transmits signals mimicking normal growth factor signalling and thereby increasing cellular proliferation and survival. The significant number of AMLs is also because of epigenetic changes.
- **Clinical features**

  Symptoms of **bone marrow failure** because of suppression of normal haematopoiesis such as fatigue, fever, recurrent spontaneous bleeding due to anaemia, neutropenia and thrombocytopenia are very common. **Bleeding** can be superficial, deep or internal and can be fatal too. Procoagulants and fibrinolytic factors released by blasts in AML make bleeding a serious manifestation in AML when compared with ALL.

  Signs and symptoms because of **tissue infiltration** leading to splenomegaly, hepatomegaly and lymphadenopathy are fewer when compared with ALL. AML with monocytic differentiation tends to infiltrate tissues in the form of ***leukaemia cutis*** (skin infiltration) (Fig. 16.33) and gingival bleeding.

Laboratory Investigations The main purpose of laboratory investigations in a case of leukaemia is to confirm the diagnosis and more importantly to identify the specific lineage involved and its subtype.

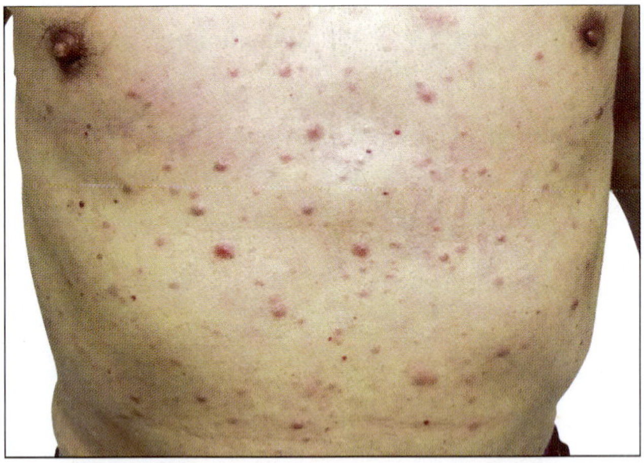

Fig. 16.33 Leukaemia cutis in AML, clinical picture. (*Source:* From https://www.msdmanuals.com/en-au/home/blood-disorders/leukemias/acute-myeloid-leukemia-aml)

Morphology

1. **Peripheral blood count** of blasts is highly variable, with values reaching more than 1 lakh/mm^3 commonly but under 10,000/mm^3 in 50% of patients. In such conditions of pancytopenia, a bone marrow examination is required to diagnose and confirm leukaemia.
2. **Peripheral smear** examination in these patients reveal the presence of myeloblasts and according to the recent WHO system, more than 20% blasts in the peripheral blood or bone marrow are necessary to diagnose AML. In subleukaemic leukaemia, the total count is normal or low but blasts are present in the peripheral blood whereas in aleukaemic leukaemia, blasts are not seen in the peripheral blood. Irrespective of the peripheral blood count, blasts are demonstrable in the bone marrow.
3. **Bone marrow** in AML contains more than 20% myeloid blasts. There may be more than one type of blast belonging to the myeloid series, which include myeloblast, monoblast or an erythroblast or blasts with hybrid features in the bone marrow. Myeloblasts (Fig. 16.34) have delicate nuclear chromatin and up to four nucleoli, more voluminous cytoplasm than lymphoblasts and cytoplasm often containing fine, azurophilic granules, which are MPO-positive. These cytochemical stains also help in differentiating them from lymphoblasts that are MPO-negative. Monoblasts have folded or lobulated nuclei lacking granules and stain cytochemically with nonspecific esterase positive. The morphological features of myeloblasts and lymphoblasts are shown in Table 16.18.
4. **Cytochemical staining** (Fig. 16.35): The nature and pattern of cytochemical staining are helpful in differentiating the different types of blasts and are shown in Table 16.19.

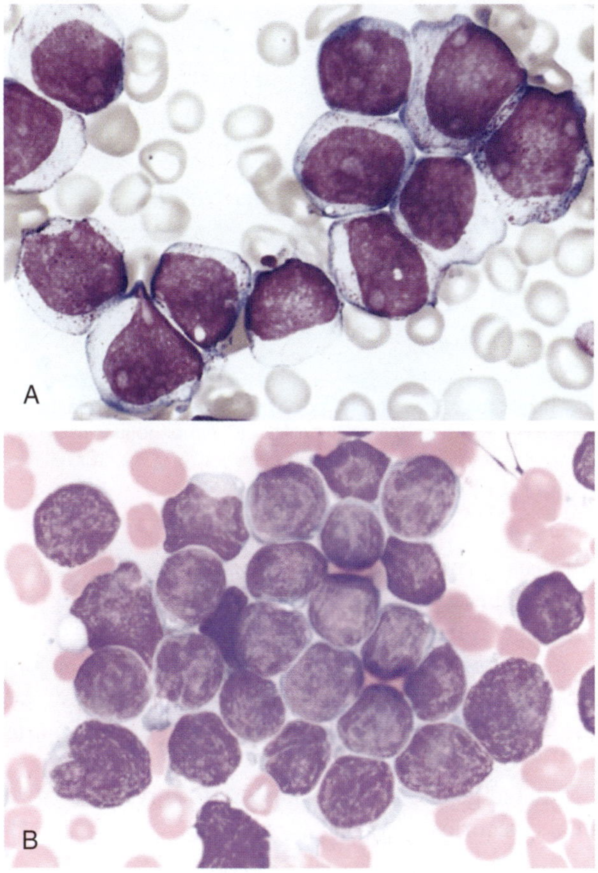

Fig. 16.34 Morphology of myeloblasts (A), which shows delicate nuclear chromatin, prominent nucleoli and fine azurophilic granules in the cytoplasm, and lymphoblasts (B), which shows blasts with small- to medium-sized round nuclei, scant cytoplasm, slightly condensed nuclear chromatin and indistinct nucleoli. (*Source:* From Karen M. Frank, Alexander J. McAdam. Robbins & Cotran Pathologic Basis of Disease. Elsevier. 2021.)

Table 16.18 Features of Myeloblast and Lymphoblast

Feature	Myeloblast	Lymphoblast
Cell size	Larger	Smaller
Volume of cytoplasm	Moderate	Scant
Auer rods	Present or absent	Absent
Chromatin	Delicate	Coarse
Nucleoli	One to four prominent	Inconspicuous to 2

5. **Immunophenotyping:** Myeloid-specific antigens are positive in AML and differentiate it from lymphoblasts. These are shown in Table 16.20.
6. **Cytogenetics:** Cytogenetics has a key role to play in the diagnosis and management of AML by detecting the karyotypic abnormalities. The cytogenetic abnormalities associated with different types of AML have been discussed earlier.
7. **Molecular genetic studies:** Molecular genetic tests like Southern blot analysis, polymerase chain reaction (PCR) and FISH are used in the diagnosis of specific types through identification of unique fusion genes formed because of genetic rearrangements, early detection of minimal residual disease and relapse, identification of lineage of leukaemic cells and detection of clonality.

Chloroma Chloroma is also known as ***myeloblastoma*** or ***granulocytic sarcoma.*** It is a haematopoietic stem cell tumour in which myeloblasts lodge themselves and proliferate at extramedullary sites, most commonly skin of the orbital and periorbital tissues. It is most commonly associated with **AML-M2**. It can also be seen in association with myelodysplastic and myeloproliferative syndromes.

Others Hyperleucocytosis characterized by a very high total count, usually more than 1 lakh, is associated with an increase in blood viscosity and leads to slowing down of blood circulation with headache, neurological symptoms, visual changes and respiratory distress.

AML subtypes like AML M3 are associated with DIC because of release of procoagulant substances from leukaemic cells.

Prognosis AML is a difficult disease to treat. Only 15%–30% of patients remain free of disease for 5 years. The outcome is different for different molecular subtypes. With the introduction of targeted therapy using all-trans retinoic acid and arsenic salts, AMLs with t(15;17) have the best prognosis and an 80% cure rate.

Myelodysplastic Syndromes

MDS is a heterogeneous group of acquired clonal stem cell disorders affecting elderly individuals. This group of disorders has in common the features of maturation defects associated with ineffective haematopoiesis along with a high risk of AML transformation. MDS is typically characterized by replacement of marrow progenitors with a transformed stem cell that retains the capacity to differentiate but does so in an ineffective and disordered fashion. These abnormal cells stay within the marrow, resulting in peripheral blood cytopenias.

Types of Myelodysplastic Syndrome

1. Primary MDS
2. Secondary MDS
   - t-MDS: Follows 2–8 years after genotoxic drug or radiation therapy
   - Exposure to chemicals like benzene and organic solvents

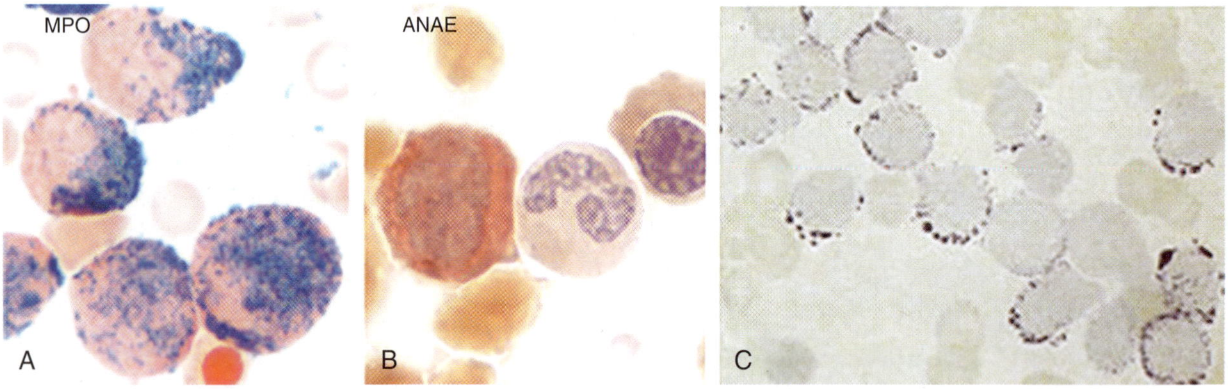

Fig. 16.35 Cytochemical reactions in acute leukaemia. (A) Myeloblasts show myeloperoxidase (MPO) positivity, while (B) monoblasts show nonspecific esterase positivity (compare left-side cell orange colour with unstained neutrophil on the right). In ALL, (C) lymphoblasts show block positivity with periodic acid–Schiff stain (PAS). (*Source:* From Stefan Faderl, Hagop M. Kantarjian. Hematology. Elsevier. 2018. (A–C) From A Porwit, M-C Béné. Blood and Bone Marrow Pathology. Elsevier. 2011.)

Table 16.19 Role of Special Stains in Acute Leukaemia

Type of Blast	Cytochemical Stain
Lymphoblast	PAS – block-like or dot-like positivity
Myeloblast	Myeloperoxidase positivity
Monoblast	Nonspecific esterase positivity
Erythroblast	PAS – diffuse positivity

Table 16.20 Lineage-Specific Cell Antigens of Acute Leukaemias

Lineage	Antigens
Myeloid	CD13, CD33, MPO, CD117, CD41, CD61, glycophorin A, CD14, CD15, CD36, lysozyme
B lymphoid	CD19, CD20, CD22, CD79a, surface Ig, cytoplasmic Ig, CD38
T lymphoid	CD2, CD3, CD5, CD7

- Genetic predisposition – Down syndrome, Fanconi anaemia, NF1

Both the forms of MDS have the risk of transformation to AML, but the frequency is high with t-MDS.

MDS is commonly associated with cytogenetic abnormalities; hence, cytogenetics is essential in the workup.

Pathogenesis

Pathogenesis of MDS is poorly understood. Evolution of MDS appears to be a multistep process. The initiating event is a somatic mutation of the stem cells, resulting in the formation of structurally and functionally defective haematopoietic cells with a shortened survival rate. Increased cellular proliferation coupled with enhanced apoptosis forms the basis for ineffective erythropoiesis and peripheral cytopenias. The MDS clone has growth advantage over the normal haematopoietic cells so that it expands slowly and suppresses normal haematopoiesis. MDS can present with varying degrees of single or multiple cytopenias including neutropenia, anaemia and thrombocytopenia.

Mutated genes can be grouped into three major functional categories.

- Epigenetic factors
- RNA splicing factors
- Transcription factors

The common chromosomal anomalies seen in both types of MDS are monosomies 5 and 7; deletions of 5q, 7q and 20q; and trisomy 8.

The MDS clone is unstable, and new genetic insults can accumulate over the original clone and initiate neoplastic transformation to AML.

Classification of Myelodysplastic Syndrome The FAB classification was recommended initially and was later modified by WHO (Table 16.21), which includes the percentage of blasts in the bone marrow, cytopenias, ring sideroblasts and dysplastic changes to differentiate the subtypes of MDS.

Clinical Features Median age of patients is generally 70 years. The development of MDS may be preceded a few years by an unexplained macrocytic anaemia with no evidence of megaloblastic anaemia and a mild thrombocytopenia or neutropenia. Clinical symptoms that should prompt a workup for MDS are low peripheral blood counts, usually from anaemia, thrombocytopenia or neutropenia.

MDS is usually discovered incidentally, but in half of the cases there may be symptoms because of ***pancytopenia***. Symptoms such as fatigue and malaise result from anaemia, recurrent infections due to leucopenia and bleeding manifestations due to thrombocytopenia.

Table 16.21 Recent WHO Classification[a] of MDS, 2016

MDS Type	Blast %	Dysplasia	Cytopenias	Others
MDS with single-lineage dysplasia (MDS-SLD)	<5	Dysplasia in ≥10% of one-cell line	One or two blood cytopenias	
MDS with multilineage dysplasia (MDS-MLD)	<5%	Dysplasia in ≥10% of cells in two or more haematopoietic lineages	One to three blood cytopenias	<15% ring sideroblasts
MDS with ring sideroblasts (MDS-RS)	0		Anaemia	≥15% of erythroid precursors with ring sideroblasts
MDS with isolated del(5q)	<5%	Unilineage erythroid dysplasia	Anaemia Thrombocytopenia +/−	Isolated del(5q)
MDS with excess blasts (MDS-EB)	EB 1 – 5%–9% – marrow or 2%–4% blasts in blood EB 2 – 10%–19% blasts in bone marrow or 5%–19% blasts in blood	Zero to three dysplastic bone marrow lineages	One to three blood cytopenias	
Unclassifiable MDS	<5	Single-lineage dysplasia or no dysplasia	+	Characteristic MDS cytogenetics

MDS, myelodysplastic syndrome.
[a]The WHO classification also includes a provisional category of refractory cytopenia of childhood, with cytopenias and <2% blasts in peripheral blood and dysplasia in one to three lineages and <5% blasts in bone marrow.

Worst prognosis is seen in patients with higher blast counts, more severe cytopenias and the presence of multiple clonal chromosomal abnormalities. Patients often die owing to complications of thrombocytopenia and neutropenia. In t-MDS, symptoms are more severe with rapid progression to AML.

Laboratory Findings Significant changes are noted in blood counts and morphology of patients with MDS. The peripheral blood count may show a single cytopenia (anaemia, thrombocytopenia or neutropenia) in the early phase or bicytopenia (two deficient cell lineages) or pancytopenia (three deficient cell lineages) in later stages. Cytopenias vary in degree from mild to severe.

Morphology

Marrow is usually hypercellular but can be normocellular or even hypocellular in a small fraction of patients. The most characteristic finding is ***dysplasia*** of the haematopoietic cells. The dysplastic features noted are as follows (Fig. 16.36):

1. **Erythroid lineage:** Dysplastic changes in RBC lineage (dyserythropoiesis) are characteristic, as well as ring sideroblasts, nuclear budding abnormalities, megaloblastoid maturation, nuclear cytoplasmic asynchrony and macro-ovalocytes in peripheral blood in the absence of vitamin B_{12} deficiency.
2. **Myeloid lineage:** Toxic granules, decreased secondary granules, Döhle bodies and pseudo-Pelger–Heut anomaly (hypolobated neutrophils) are present. Myeloblasts are increased but less than 19% in marrow and less than 10% in peripheral blood. The cut-off is 19%, as a blast count more than that would prompt a diagnosis of AML.
3. **Megakaryocytic lineage:** Pawn ball megakaryocytes (megakaryocytes with a single lobe or multiple separate lobes) in marrow, giant platelets in peripheral blood and micromegakaryocytes (dwarf forms) with poor nuclei lobulation are also commonly seen.

Treatment The standard care for patients with MDS is supportive therapy, which includes transfusion of blood components that are deficient and treatment of infections. The patients are followed up closely for the early diagnosis of AML transformation.

The more aggressive forms of therapy, such as stem cell transplantation and aggressive chemotherapy, are reserved for younger and fit patients with a high-risk disease.

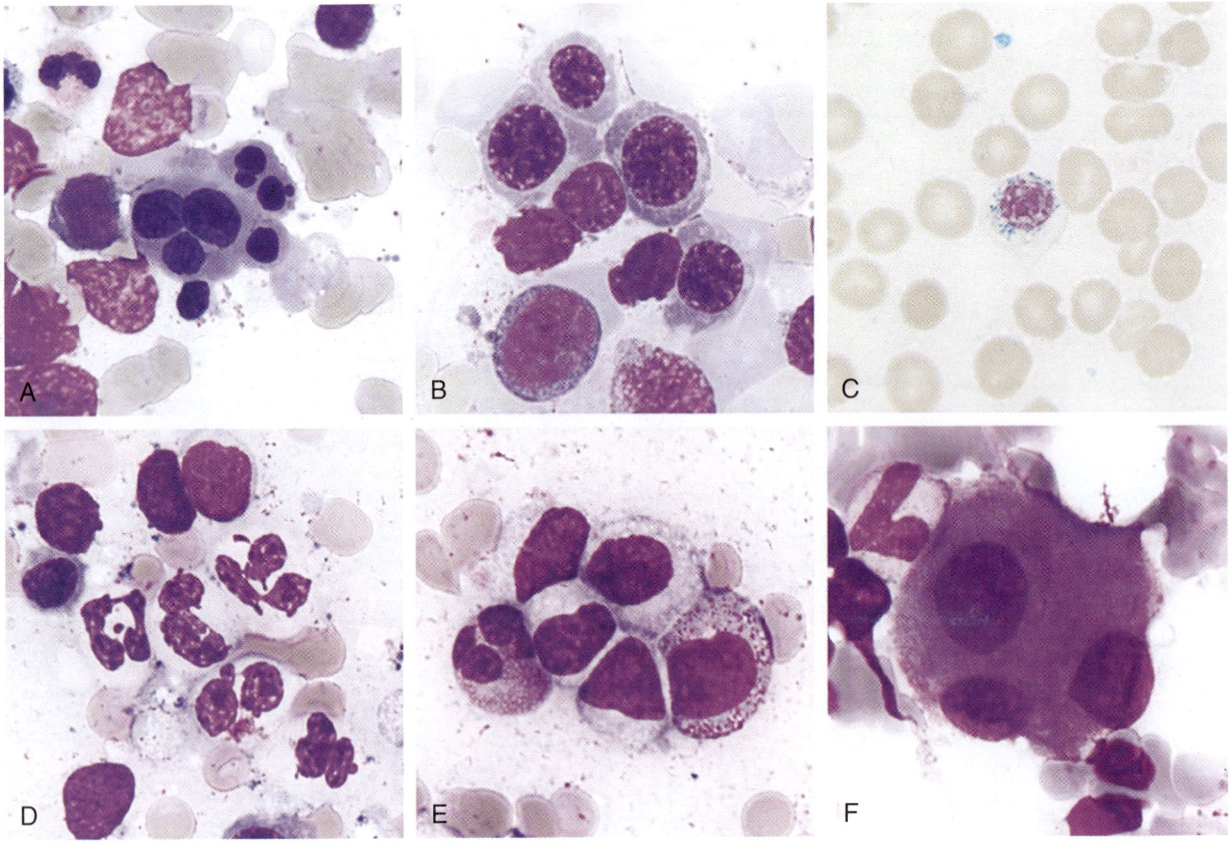

Fig. 16.36 MDS bone marrow smear. (A) Multinucleated erythroid precursor. (B) Megaloblastoid maturation of erythroid precursors with 'open' nuclear chromatin. (C) Ring sideroblast (Perl's Prussian blue stain). (D) Hypogranular neutrophils. (E) Pseudo-Pelger–Huët anomaly (hypolobated neutrophil). (F) Abnormal nuclear lobation in a megakaryocyte – a 'pawn ball' cell with three separated nuclei/nuclear lobes. (*Source:* From David P. Steensma, Richard M. Stone. Goldman-Cecil Medicine, 2-volume Set. Elsevier. 2020)

Myeloproliferative Neoplasms

MPNs are a group of haematopoietic stem cell disorders that are characterized by proliferation of one or more haematopoietic cell lines in the peripheral blood, distinct from acute leukaemia.

The characteristic features of this group of disorders are as follows:

- Clonal haematopoietic stem cell proliferations are present.
- Increased proliferative drive in the marrow is seen.
- One cell line predominates in each disorder.
- Maturation of cells is increased in number and is relatively normal.
- Extramedullary haematopoiesis because of homing of stem cells to secondary haematopoietic organs leads to splenomegaly and hepatomegaly.
- There is close relationship between different disorders with overlapping clinical features, interconversions and progression to AML.
- Transformation to spent phase is characterized by marrow fibrosis and peripheral blood cytopenias.

MPNs are generally distinguished from both MDS and MDS/MPN by the absence of monocytosis and morphological dysplasia, which include dyserythropoiesis and dysgranulopoiesis.

Classification The classification of MPNs is based on which cell line is most affected along with the patient's history, genetic findings and laboratory findings. There are seven subcategories in this group as listed by the latest WHO classification in 2016, and are given in Table 16.22.

Of note, mastocytosis, which was earlier included in this group, is no longer classified under the MPN category and is placed in its own disease category.

MPNs should be distinguished from each other as the treatment approach for each is different.

Pathogenesis CML is characterized by the presence of a hallmark chromosomal abnormality BCR-ABL translocation, also known as the Philadelphia chromosome. MPNs

Table 16.22 WHO Classification of Myeloproliferative Neoplasms, 2016

Chronic myeloid leukaemia (CML)
Polycythaemia vera (PV)
Primary myelofibrosis (PMF)
Essential thrombocythaemia (ET)
Chronic neutrophilic leukaemia (CNL)
Chronic eosinophilic leukaemia, not otherwise specified (CEL-NOS)
MPN, unclassifiable (MPN-U)

Table 16.23 Tyrosine Kinase and Other Mutations in Myeloproliferative Disorders

Disorder	Mutation
Chronic myelogenous leukaemia	BCR-ABL fusion gene
Polycythaemia vera	JAK2 point mutation
Essential thrombocythaemia	JAK2 point mutation MPL point mutation
Primary myelofibrosis	JAK2 point mutation MPL point mutation
Chronic neutrophilic leukaemia	CSF3R (nontyrosine kinase mutation)
Chronic eosinophilic leukaemia, not otherwise specified	Trisomy 8 (nontyrosine kinase mutation)

in which this abnormality is absent are known collectively as Philadelphia chromosome–negative MPNs, and the three most common forms of these are **primary myelofibrosis (PMF), polycythaemia vera (PV) and essential thrombocythaemia (ET)**. The BCR-ABL–negative MPNs are also called **classic MPNs**.

At the molecular level, all disorders of MPNs are due to **mutated tyrosine kinases** or other abnormalities in the signalling pathways resulting in growth factor independence (Table 16.23). Genetics of CML is discussed under its pathogenesis.

Genetics of a classic MPN is in large part elucidated. Somatic mutations are essential for clonal expansion of haematopoietic stem cells in MPNs.

The MPN-restricted mutations, including those in *JAK2*, calreticulin (*CALR*) and myeloproliferative leukaemia virus (*MPL*), abnormally activate the cytokine receptor/JAK2 pathway and their downstream effectors, more particularly the STATs. The most common mutation, *JAK2*V617F, activates the three main myeloid cytokine receptors, which include erythropoietin receptor, granulocyte colony–stimulating factor receptor, and MPL, whereas *CALR* or *MPL* mutants are restricted to MPL activation. This explains why *JAK2*V617F is associated with PV, ET and PMF, whereas *CALR* and *MPL* mutants are found in ET and PMF. Mutations in epigenetic regulators are involved in disease initiation and may precede the acquisition of *JAK2*V617F. Other mutations in epigenetic regulators also play a role in disease initiation and disease progression. Tyrosine kinase mutations do not impair differentiation but increase the production of one or more mature blood elements.

Individual disorders are discussed in detail in the following sections.

Chronic Myelogenous Leukaemia PA 18.2

CML, also known as chronic myeloid leukaemia, is an MPN, characterized by increased proliferation of the granulocytic cell line without the loss of their capacity to differentiate. Consequently, the peripheral blood cell count shows an increased number of granulocytes and their immature precursors, including occasional blasts. CML accounts for 20% of all leukaemias affecting adults.

Pathogenesis CML is characterized by a cytogenetic aberration consisting of a reciprocal translocation between the long arms of chromosomes 22 and 9 – ***t(9;22) (q34;q11)***. The translocation results in a shortened chromosome 22, an observation first described by Nowell and Hungerford who subsequently named it the Philadelphia (Ph1) chromosome after the city of discovery.

This translocation relocates an oncogene called *ABL* from the long arm of chromosome 9 to a specific breakpoint cluster region (*BCR*) in the long arm of chromosome 22. The *ABL* oncogene encodes a tyrosine protein kinase. The resulting ***BCR-ABL*** fusion gene (Fig. 16.37) encodes a chimeric protein with strong tyrosine kinase activity (210 kDa), which can be detected by FISH or PCR.

The expression of BCR-ABL tyrosine kinase leads to the development of CML phenotype through processes that are not yet fully understood, probably by inducing signals through progrowth and prosurvival pathways.

The presence of *BCR-ABL* rearrangement is the hallmark of CML, although this rearrangement has also been associated with other diseases. It is considered diagnostic when present in a patient with typical clinical manifestations of CML. The initiating factor of CML is still unknown, but exposure to ionizing radiation and benzene has been implicated.

Course of the Disease The disease is slowly progressive with three phases. The three phases of chronic myelogenous

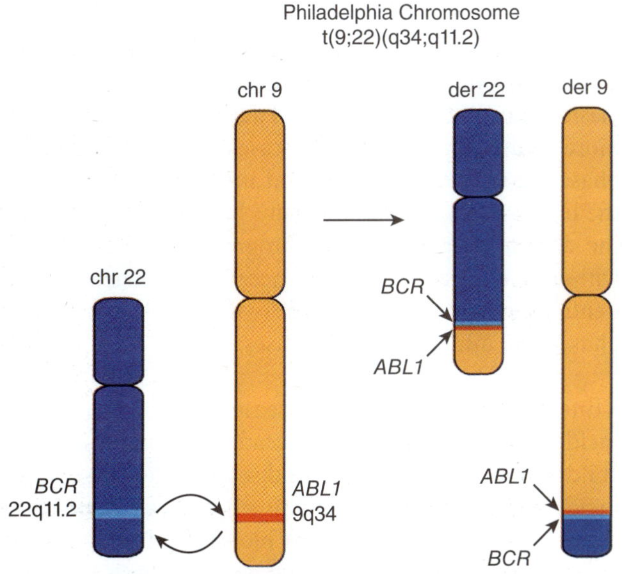

Fig. 16.37 BCR-ABL fusion in CML results from the reciprocal translocation of a portion of the ABL1 gene on chromosome 9 at band q34 to the region of the BCR gene on chromosome 22 at band q11.2. (*Source:* From Ritesh Rathore. Ferri's Clinical Advisor 2021. Elsevier. 2021.)

Table 16.24 Phases of CML

Phase of CML	WHO Definition
Chronic/classical/ stable phase	• Blasts <10% in peripheral blood and bone marrow
Accelerated phase	• Blasts 10%–19% of WBCs in peripheral and/or nucleated bone marrow cells • Peripheral blood myeloblasts and promyelocytes combined ≥30% • Peripheral blood basophils ≥20% • Persistent thrombocytopenia (<100 × 10^9/L) unrelated to therapy or persistent thrombocytosis (>1000 × 10^9/L) unresponsive to therapy • Increasing WBC counts and spleen size unresponsive to therapy • Additional clonal cytogenetic abnormalities in Philadelphia chromosome–positive cells
Blast crisis	• Blasts ≥20% of peripheral blood WBCs or nucleated bone marrow cells • Extramedullary blast proliferation • Large foci or clusters of blasts on bone marrow biopsy

CML, chronic myelogenous leukaemia; WBC, white blood cell.

leukaemia, as defined by WHO, are **classical, accelerated and blastic crisis** (Table 16.24).

After a variable period, the classical or chronic or stable phase progresses to ***accelerated phase*** with progressing anaemia, thrombocytopenia, increasing basophilia along with additional clonal cytogenetic abnormalities. In a majority of the patients, within 6–12 months, the accelerated phase terminates in a picture resembling acute leukaemia – ***blast crisis***, characterized by 20% or more of blasts, clinical deterioration and additional mutations. In more than two-thirds of the cases, the blasts in crisis phase are of myeloid origin and in the remaining cases, the blasts are of lymphoid origin. In about 30% of cases, the chronic phase suddenly progresses to blastic crisis without a clinically noticeable accelerated phase and patients present in the blastic crisis without the preceding phases in a minor fraction of cases.

Clinical Features CML is a disease of adults with a peak incidence in fifth and sixth decades but can also affect children and young adults. The disease is often discovered incidentally in its chronic phase when an elevated WBC count is revealed by a routine blood count or when an enlarged spleen is found during general physical examination.

The onset is insidious with nonspecific symptoms due to anaemia and hypermetabolism such as fatigability, weakness, excessive sweating, weight loss and anorexia. Sometimes, the first symptom may be abdominal discomfort due to splenomegaly.

In some patients who present in the accelerated phase of the disease (skipping the chronic phase), bleeding, petechiae and ecchymosis may be the dominant symptoms. In these situations, fever is usually associated with infections. Bone pain and fever, as well as an increase in bone marrow fibrosis, are indicators of the blast phase.

At the time of diagnosis, prognostic factors associated with a shorter duration of survival are older age, massive hepatosplenomegaly, an increased percentage of blasts, an increased number of basophils and marrow fibrosis.

Laboratory Findings In general, total leucocyte count is proportionate with size of the spleen, basophilia, blast percentage and degree of anaemia. Total leucocyte count is moderately to markedly increased and is usually above 100,000/mm^3.

Morphology (Fig. 16.38)

Peripheral smear: Anaemia is present in almost all patients at the time of diagnosis and is usually mild to moderate and normocytic and normochromic. Few normoblasts are seen in the peripheral smear along with an elevated WBC count with **shift to left of myeloid series**. Blast count is variable depending on the phase of the disease. Basophilia and eosinophilia are strikingly prominent. Platelet count is usually increased.

Marrow: Markedly **cellular marrow** with a myeloid to erythroid ratio of 10:1 to 50:1. Myeloid series show the predominance of maturing granulocytic precursors, **basophilia and eosinophilia**. **Megakaryocytes are also increased**, which may show dysplastic features. Erythroid progenitors are normal or may be decreased. A characteristic finding is the presence of scattered macrophages with wrinkled blue–green cytoplasm called **'sea blue histiocytes'.**

Spleen is markedly enlarged and congested because of extramedullary haematopoiesis.

Bone marrow aspiration is not crucial for the diagnosis of CML, whereas it is indicated for the following reasons:

1. To confirm or exclude blastic phase
2. Cytogenetic analysis for Philadelphia chromosome
3. Assessment of myelofibrosis

Cytogenetic analysis for the presence of Philadelphia chromosome, which if present, can be performed in all the cell lineages in more than 95% of cases. Even in cases that do not reveal the genetic abnormality, the translocation is cryptic and is revealed by FISH, Southern blot technique and PCR. Additional cytogenetic abnormalities are seen in accelerated and blastic crisis phases.

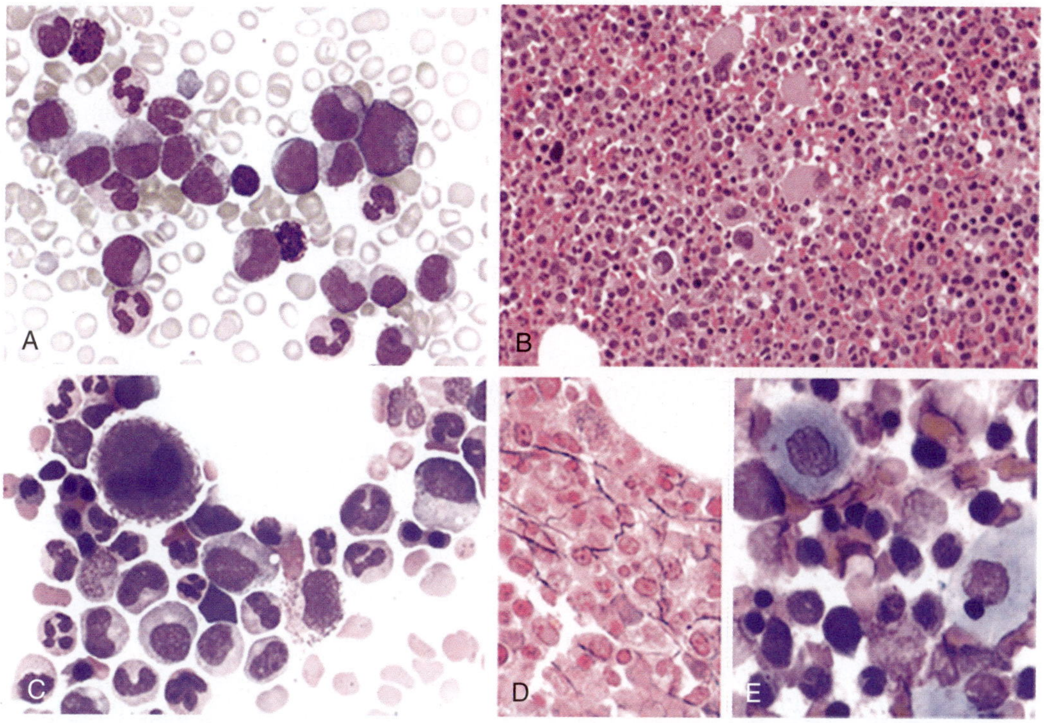

Fig. 16.38 CML. (A) Peripheral smear showing marked leucocytosis due to a granulocytic proliferation of all stages with particularly increased myelocytes and absolute basophilia. (B) Bone core biopsy illustrating markedly hypercellular marrow because of granulocytic proliferation and increased small hypolobated megakaryocytes. (C) Bone marrow aspirate showing the same granulocytic proliferation and small, 'dwarf' megakaryocytes. Mild fibrosis as seen on reticulin stain (D) and pseudo-Gaucher cells (E). (*Source:* From Ravi Bhatia. Hematology. Elsevier. 2018.)

Treatment CML was the first malignant disease to be associated with a chromosomal abnormality and the first malignant disease for which targeted molecular therapy became available as the treatment of choice. Imatinib mesylate, a potent and specific inhibitor of tyrosine kinase, became available in 1998 and is still the standard first-line treatment of newly diagnosed chronic-phase CML. Treatment with **BCR-ABL inhibitors** offers remission in more than 90% of patients.

In some patients, the emergence of resistance to BCR-ABL drugs is a major threat to the patients. In patients developing resistance or intolerance to the drug, the second line of drugs like hydroxyurea or α-interferon is tried with reduced efficacy.

For the accelerated phase, dasatinib or nilotinib are recommended for treatment. For the blast phase, tyrosine kinase inhibitor therapy either alone or in combination with chemotherapy, followed by allogeneic haematopoietic transplantation, is recommended.

Polycythaemia Vera

PV, also referred to as polycythaemia rubra vera, is an MPN characterized by **trilineage hyperplasia** (granulocytic, erythroid and megakaryocytic) in bone marrow with a predominant involvement of the erythroid series. The signs and symptoms are predominantly because of an increase in RBCs – erythrocytosis. It is essential to differentiate PCV from relative and absolute polycythaemia, as the treatment is completely different for all these conditions.

Pathogenesis This myeloproliferative disorder is associated with ***JAK2*** mutations. It has been found that mutation in tyrosine kinase *JAK2*V617F occurs in 95% of cases and a mutation in exon 12 occurs in another 4% of cases of PV. The *JAK2* mutation also occurs in a significant number of patients with PMF and ET. When both the copies of JAK2 are mutated, which happens in 25%–30% cases, the signals and proliferative drive by JAK2 are stronger.

JAK2 point mutation activates the JAK/STAT pathway which normally gets activated by many growth factors, mainly erythropoietin. In PCV, due to constitutively active JAK2, the red cell precursors are independent of erythropoietin. Hence, **the level of erythropoietin is consistently low**, which differentiates PCV from other causes of polycythaemia. The increase in blood viscosity due to an increase in haematocrit along with thrombocytosis results in frequent episodes of bleeding and thrombosis.

There are two phases of PV:

- **Proliferative or polycythaemic or cellular phase** characterized by proliferation of erythroid cells
- **'Spent' or postpolycythaemic phase** characterized by myelofibrosis and cytopenias

Progression to AML occurs in a significant proportion of patients.

Criteria for Polycythaemia Vera Diagnosis of PV requires the presence of either all three major criteria or the first two major criteria and one minor criterion.

Major Criteria

- Haemoglobin >16.5 g/dL or haematocrit >49% in men
- Haemoglobin >16 g/dL or haematocrit >48% in women
- Bone marrow biopsy: hypercellularity with trilineage proliferation and pleomorphic mature megakaryocytes
- Presence of *JAK2* or *JAK2* exon 12 mutation

Minor Criteria

- Subnormal serum erythropoietin level

Clinical Features PCV is an uncommon disease affecting males of 50–60 years of age. The disease is insidious in onset. There is an increase in total blood volume, but the increase in haematocrit is the major cause of symptoms. These factors result in abnormal blood flow, especially on the venous side, with patients being plethoric and cyanotic. Headache, dizziness, hypertension and gastric ulcers are also common symptoms. Pruritus due to histamine release from basophils and gout due to hyperuricaemia resulting from high cell turnover are also common.

High blood volume, altered blood flow and platelet function result in bleeding and thrombotic episodes. Chronic bleeding may result in iron deficiency, offering some relief from the complications by bringing down haematocrit.

Laboratory Features

Morphology

Peripheral smear (Fig. 16.39)

The RBC count, haemoglobin concentration and haematocrit are raised. Initially, red cells are normocytic and normochromic, with progression to spent phase (myelofibrosis), anisopoikilocytosis, teardrop cells and nucleated red cells (leucoerythroblastic blood picture).

There is mild to moderate leucocytosis, with shift to left up to the myelocyte stage. Basophils, eosinophils

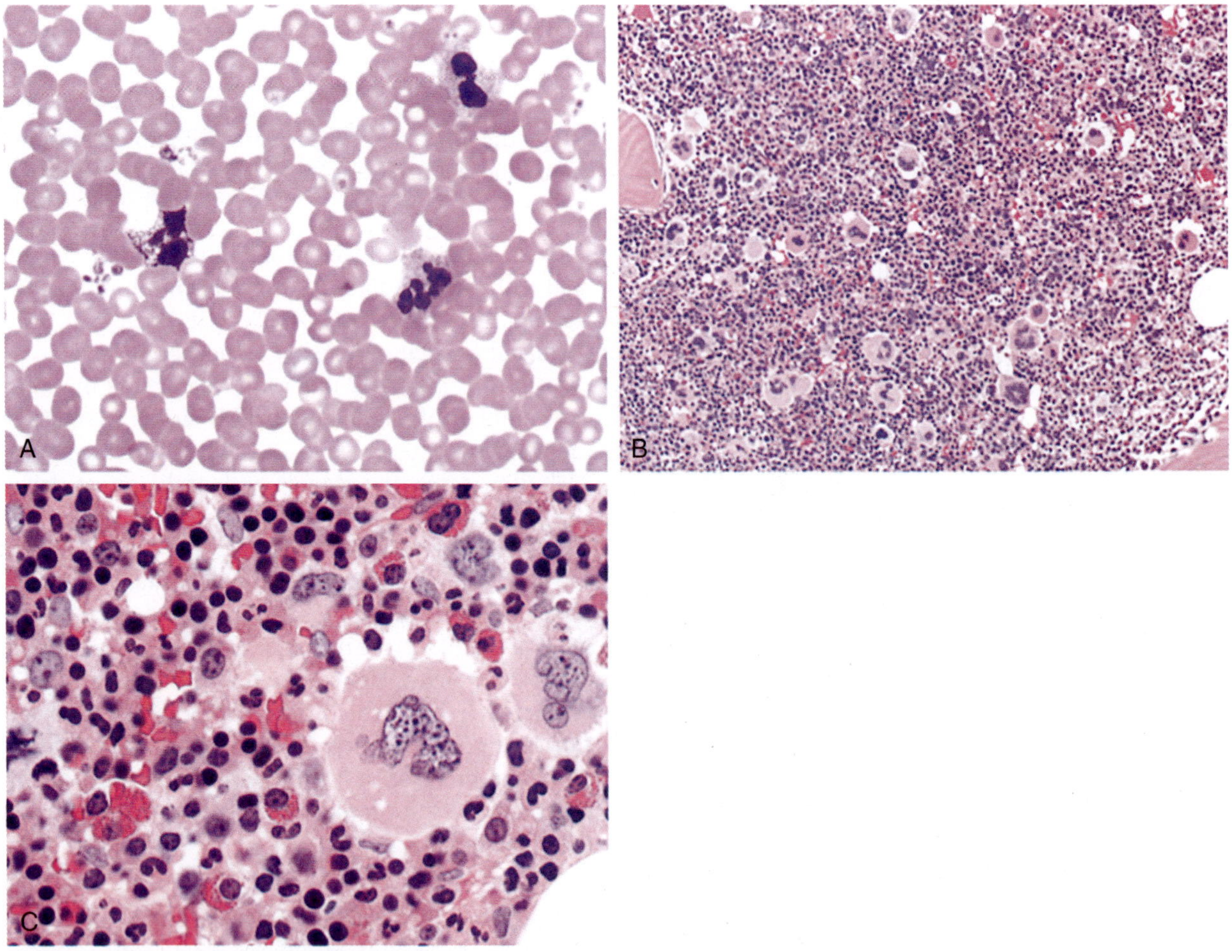

Fig. 16.39 Peripheral smear and bone marrow in polycythaemia vera. (A) Peripheral blood is characterized by mild neutrophilia and occasional basophils. (B) Bone marrow biopsy reveals hypercellularity. (C) Closer inspection shows panmyelosis. The megakaryocytes are variable in size but are not highly atypical or bizarre. (*Source:* From James W. Vardiman. Hematopathology. Elsevier. 2017.)

and monocytes are often increased. Platelet count is increased in 50% of patients and is usually more than 500,000/mm^3. Giant platelets are commonly seen.

Bone marrow

Marrow is hypercellular because of trilineage proliferation in the cellular phase, with 10% of cases with an increase in marrow reticulin fibres. Later, in the spent phase, the marrow is hypocellular because of marrow fibrosis.

Organomegaly is a common finding, which in the beginning is mild because of congestion and progresses to marked and massive because of extramedullary haematopoiesis in the spent phase.

Treatment Without treatment, the median survival of patients with PV is 18 months. Bleeding and thrombosis are common causes of death in untreated patients.

With simple phlebotomy, life can be extended up to 10 years by bringing down the haematocrit levels. In total, 15%–20% of patients after an average period of 10 years will progress to the spent phase because of the development of ***obliterative marrow fibrosis.***

Transformation to AML occurs in 1%–5% of patients.

Essential Thrombocytosis

Essential thrombocytosis (ET), also referred to as primary thrombocythaemia, is a chronic myeloproliferative disorder characterized by the neoplastic proliferation of megakaryocytes and an elevated platelet count in the peripheral blood.

Pathogenesis ET is associated with activating point mutations in ***JAK2*** (50%) or ***MPL*** (5%–10%), receptor tyrosine kinases, which are normally activated by thrombopoietin. The remaining cases are positive for ***calreticulin*** mutation, which also acts by activating JAK/STAT pathway. Constitutive JAK2 or MPL makes the megakaryocytes independent of their growth factor thrombopoietin.

Causes of reactive thrombocytosis should be ruled out in all cases of ET, especially in those without tyrosine kinase mutations.

Diagnostic Criteria Diagnosis requires meeting all four major criteria or first three major criteria and one minor criterion.

Major Criteria

- Platelet count is more than 450,000/mm^3.
- Bone marrow shows megakaryocytic proliferation with an increased number of enlarged mature megakaryocytes with hyperlobulated nuclei. No significant left shift of neutrophil granulopoiesis or erythropoiesis and a very rarely minor increase in reticulin fibres occur.
- Not meeting WHO criteria for BCR-ABL + CML, PV, PMF, MDS or other myeloid neoplasms.
- Presence of JAK2, CALR or MPL mutation.

Minor Criteria These include the presence of a clonal marker (e.g. abnormal karyotype) or the absence of evidence for reactive thrombocytosis.

Clinical Features ET is an uncommon disease of older adults with an indolent clinical course. Neoplastic platelets are qualitatively abnormal and dysfunctional, resulting in recurrent bleeding and thrombotic episodes. One characteristic symptom is ***erythromelalgia***, a throbbing and burning sensation of hands and feet caused by the occlusion of small arterioles by platelet aggregates.

Morphology

Peripheral smear (Fig. 16.40) shows an increase in platelets with abnormally large platelets, often accompanied by mild leucocytosis.

Marrow cellularity is only mildly increased with a marked increase in megakaryocytes, including abnormally large ones (Fig. 16.41). Delicate reticulin fibrils are often present without overt fibrosis.

Mild organomegaly due to modest extramedullary haematopoiesis is a common finding.

Progression to the spent phase and AML transformation is uncommon.

Treatment Median survival with treatment is 10–15 years. Treatment consists of gentle chemotherapy that suppresses thrombopoiesis. Addition of low-dose aspirin may be helpful in the presence of thrombosis. Causes of death include thrombosis, haemorrhage and AML transformation.

Primary Myelofibrosis

PMF is also called by other names such as chronic idiopathic myelofibrosis, myelofibrosis/sclerosis with myeloid metaplasia, agnogenic myeloid metaplasia, megakaryocytic

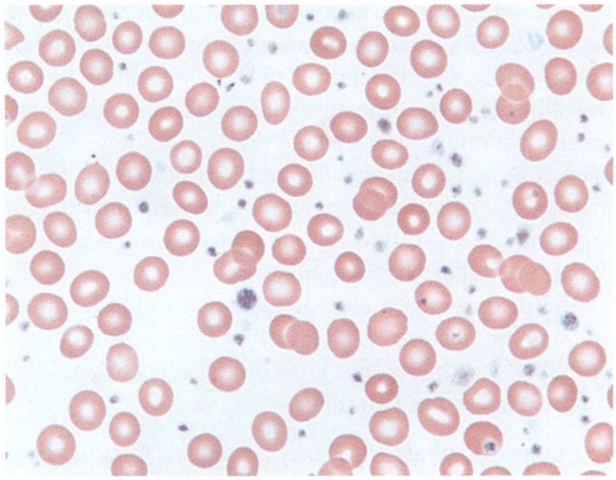

Fig. 16.40 Peripheral smear morphology in ET. (*Source:* From Marina Kremyanskaya, Vesna Najfeld, Bruce Petersen, Julie Teruya-Feldstein. Atlas of Diagnostic Hematology. Elsevier. 2021.)

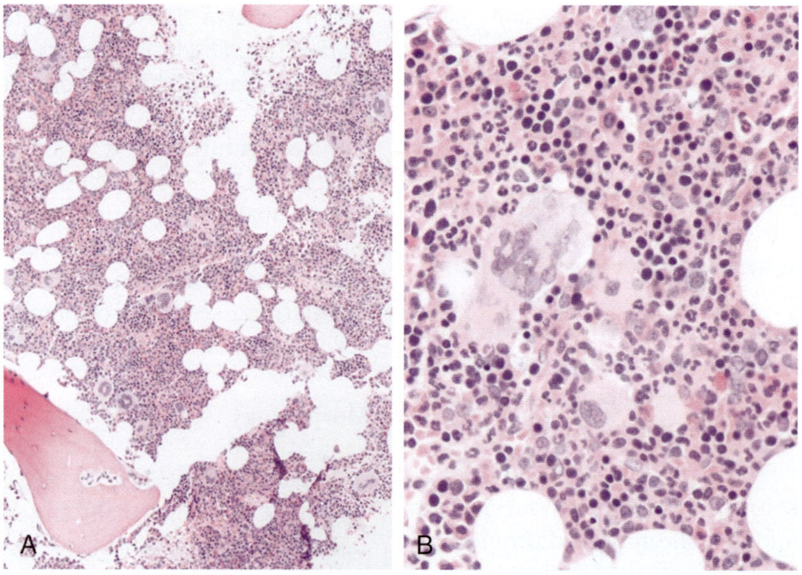

Fig. 16.41 Bone marrow morphology in ET. (A) Mildly hypercellular marrow with an isolated increase in megakaryocytes. (B) Megakaryocytes include hyperlobulated forms with staghorn morphology. (*Source:* From Marina Kremyanskaya, Vesna Najfeld, Bruce Petersen, Julie Teruya-Feldstein. Atlas of Diagnostic Hematology. Elsevier. 2021.)

myelosclerosis, idiopathic myelofibrosis and myelofibrosis with myeloid metaplasia.

PMF is an MPN that is characterized by trilineage proliferation with the predominance of granulocytic and megakaryocytic lineage and the development of ***obliterative marrow fibrosis*** with suppression of bone marrow haematopoiesis, leading to cytopenias and extensive extramedullary haematopoiesis. Bone marrow fibrosis is the result of stimulation of fibroblastic proliferation and synthesis of collagen.

The disorder shows a stepwise evolution from an initial prefibrotic/early stage to an overt fibrotic stage.

Pathogenesis ***JAK2*** mutations are associated in 50%–60% of cases, whereas a small subset (<1%) follows mutations in calreticulin. These mutations primarily cause megakaryocyte proliferation which release undue amounts of fibrogenic factors like platelet-derived growth factor ***(PDGF)***, basic fibroblast growth factor ***(bFGF)*** and transforming growth factor β (***TGF***-β), resulting in marrow fibrosis. The extensive marrow fibrosis eventually causes marrow failure by suppressing the bone marrow haematopoiesis. This is followed by displacement of haematopoietic elements from marrow to secondary haematopoietic organs, resulting in ***marked organomegaly*** due to extramedullary haematopoiesis.

This disorder resembles the spent phase of PCV and ET, and it is still unclear whether PMF is truly a distinct entity or PCV/ET with rapid progression to the spent phase.

The disease has two phases:

1. **Prefibrotic phase:** It usually presents with thrombocytosis. There are no blasts/borderline anaemia/borderline splenomegaly/borderline increased LDH. Misdiagnosis of ET is likely if the marrow is not completely examined.
2. **Overt phase:** It is characterized by thrombocytopenia, leucoerythroblastosis, anaemia, splenomegaly, increased LDH and increased myeloblasts (<20%). Transformation to AML occurs in approximately 5%–20% of cases at a median of 3 years after the diagnosis of the overt phase.

Diagnostic Criteria (for Prefibrotic Phase)

Major Criteria

- Megakaryocytic proliferation and atypia without reticulin fibrosis along with increased age-adjusted bone marrow hypercellularity, granulocytic proliferation and decreased erythropoiesis
- Not meeting the WHO criteria for *BCR-ABL1* + CML, PV, ET, MDS or other myeloid neoplasm
- Presence of *JAK2, CALR, or MPL* mutation or in the absence of these mutations, the presence of another clonal marker or the absence of minor reactive BM reticulin fibrosis

Minor Criteria

- Presence of one or more of the following, confirmed in two consecutive determinations:
  - Anaemia not attributed to a comorbid condition
  - Leucocytosis 11×10^9/L or more
  - Palpable splenomegaly
  - LDH level above the upper limit of the institutional reference range

Diagnosis requires all three major criteria and at least one minor criterion.

Clinical Features PMF is a disease of individuals older than 60 years. Anaemia and splenomegaly are common presentations. Fatigue, weight loss, night sweats, gout due to increased metabolism and high cell turnover are common.

The peripheral blood findings are nonspecific; hence, bone marrow biopsy is essential for diagnosis.

Morphology

In the initial phase of the disease, marrow is hypercellular with an increase in all the three cell lineages, a feature similar to PCV. **Megakaryocytes are large, dysplastic** and abnormally clustered, whereas erythroid and granulocytic precursors appear morphologically normal. At this stage, there is minimal fibrosis and the peripheral blood may show leucocytosis and thrombocytosis. As the disease progresses, the marrow becomes more fibrotic and hypocellular. Severe architectural distortion characterized by clusters of **atypical megakaryocytes** and the presence of haematopoietic elements within dilated sinusoids set in because of extensive fibrosis. In the advanced stage of the disease, marrow space gets converted to bone, a state called **'osteosclerosis'**.

This spent phase is characterized by marked splenomegaly and hepatomegaly due to extensive extramedullary haematopoiesis.

Peripheral smear (Fig. 16.42) reflects marrow fibrosis with the presence of normoblasts and precursors of granulocytes, a picture called ***'leucoerythroblastosis'***. Often seen are ***teardrop-shaped red cells*** (dacryocytes), which are damaged by the extremely fibrotic marrow during the release process. Peripheral smear also shows the presence of abnormally large platelets and basophilia.

Treatment Thrombocytosis could be managed with hydroxyurea and other palliative measures. Patients with milder disease may still be treated with supportive measures. Ruxolitinib, a *JAK1/JAK2* inhibitor, is the first chemotherapeutic agent to be approved for the treatment of myelofibrosis. Patients with refractory splenomegaly may be candidates for splenectomy. Patients with severe form of the disease with overt fibrosis should be considered for haematopoietic stem cell transplantation.

Chronic Neutrophilic Leukaemia

Chronic neutrophilic leukaemia (CNL) is an MPN characterized by clonal proliferation of mature neutrophils and is usually associated with activating mutations of the gene, encoding for the receptor for granulocyte colony–stimulating factor, also known as colony-stimulating factor (*CSF3R*). *CSF3R* mutations are specific to WHO-defined CNL. Diagnosis of CNL requires exclusion of other causes of neutrophilia such as infections and inflammatory

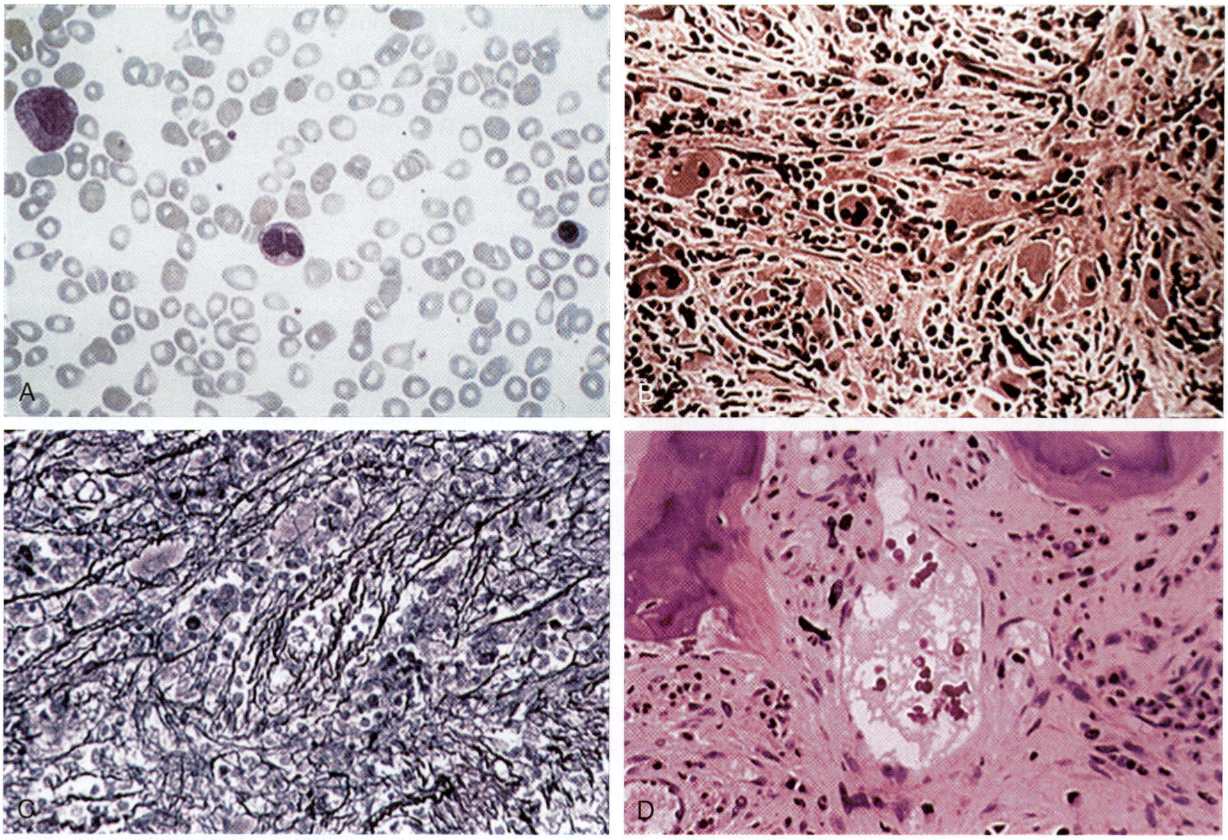

Fig. 16.42 Peripheral smear and bone marrow in PMF peripheral blood smear. (A) Leucoerythroblastic picture and teardrop cells, bone marrow showing fibrosis (B and C), and osteosclerosis and sinusoidal haematopoiesis (D) in primary myelofibrosis. (*Source:* From Ayalew Tefferi. Abeloff's Clinical Oncology. Elsevier. 2020.)

processes, metastatic cancer and plasma cell neoplasms with secondary neutrophilia. Mature-appearing neutrophilia also occurs in other myeloid malignancies, including atypical CML, *BCR-ABL1*-negative and chronic myelomonocytic leukaemia.

Diagnostic criteria for CNL are designed to exclude the possibilities of secondary and clonal neutrophilia associated with myeloid malignancies other than CNL.

Criteria for the diagnosis are as follows:

- Leucocytosis ($\geq 25 \times 10^9$/L), 80% or more segmented/band neutrophils
- Less than 10% of immature myeloid cells, less than 1% of circulating blasts
- Absence of dysgranulopoiesis or monocytosis (monocyte count $<1 \times 10^9$/L)

In clinical practice, the presence of a membrane proximal *CSF3R* mutation in a patient with neutrophilic granulocytosis should be sufficient for the diagnosis of CNL, regardless of the degree of leucocytosis.

Chronic Eosinophilic Leukaemia, Not Otherwise Specified

Chronic eosinophilic leukaemia, not otherwise specified (CEL-NOS) is an MPN with clonal eosinophilia.

Diagnostic Criteria

- Absolute eosinophil count 1.5×10^9/L or more in the peripheral blood with
- The presence of myeloblast excess (either >2% in the peripheral blood or 5%–19% in the bone marrow)
    - or
- Presence of a clonal cytogenetic abnormality

Cytogenetic abnormalities in CEL-NOS include trisomy 8 (the most frequent), t(10;11) (p14;q21) and t(7;12) (q11;p11).

Unlike the cases associated with *PDGFRA/B*-rearranged myeloid/lymphoid neoplasms with eosinophilia, imatinib therapy is ineffective in CEL-NOS.

The WHO MPN subcategory of MPN-U includes MPN-like neoplasms that cannot be clearly classified as one of the other six subcategories of MPNs described earlier. Patients with MPN-U might present with otherwise unexplained thrombosis, especially splanchnic vein thrombosis associated with a normal blood count.

LANGERHANS CELL HISTIOCYTOSIS

LCH is a complex disorder characterized by the proliferation of Langerhans cells. It can manifest in various forms, ranging from isolated bone lesions to multisystem involvement. Recent advancements have refined the understanding of LCH pathogenesis, emphasizing its potential roots in immune dysregulation rather than as a purely neoplastic process.

Pathogenesis

More than 50% of LCH cases are associated with valine to glutamate substitution at residue 600 in **BRAF**. In the remaining cases, mutations of TP53, RAS and MET are detected. LCH has varied presentations primarily because of homing of Langerhans cells which is due to an aberrant expression of chemokine receptors. Normal Langerhans cells express CCR6, whereas neoplastic Langerhans cells express **CCR6 and CCR7**. This permits the neoplastic cells to migrate into tissues that express the relevant chemokines – CCL20 (a ligand for CCR6) in the skin and bone and CCL19 and CCL21 (ligands for CCR7) in lymphoid organs.

LCH presents as several clinicopathological entities:

1. **Multifocal multisystem LCH, Letterer–Siwe disease**: Patients are usually younger than 2 years, but the occurrence in adults is not uncommon. The disease is characterized by ***systemic proliferation of Langerhans cells***, with cutaneous lesions over the trunk and scalp, resembling seborrhoeic eruptions, as a dominant clinical picture. Hepatosplenomegaly, lymphadenopathy, lung lesions and osteolytic bone lesions are also seen in most of the patients. Anaemia, thrombocytopenia and recurrent infections result because of extensive marrow infiltration. The course is fatal without intense chemotherapy, which would help 50% of the patients to survive up to 5 years.
2. **Unifocal and multifocal unisystem LCH (eosinophilic granuloma):**
   This type of LCH arises within the medullary cavities of bones, most commonly the calvarium, ribs and femur. Uncommonly, the lesions also arise from skin, lungs or stomach. This disease can be of two types depending on the distribution of the disease.
   a. **Unifocal:** Most common system affected is the skeletal system, which can be asymptomatic or may present with bone pain, tenderness, mass or pathological fracture. This type is indolent and may heal spontaneously or be cured by local excision or irradiation.
   b. **Multifocal unisystem:** This type usually presents with multiple erosive bony masses with expansion into the adjacent soft tissues; it commonly affects young children.
   c. **Hand–Schüller–Christian triad:** It is a subtype of multifocal unisystem LCH and a combination of calvarial bone defects and diabetes insipidus due to the involvement of posterior pituitary stalk of the hypothalamus and exophthalmos.
3. **Pulmonary LCH:**
   Pulmonary LCH, primarily seen in smokers, is a unique category of the disease characterized by reactive proliferation of Langerhans cells. It is notable for its potential to regress spontaneously on smoking cessation. Recent clinical studies have

highlighted the efficacy of targeted therapies in managing cases unresponsive to lifestyle modifications, emphasizing the importance of early diagnosis and personalized treatment plans.

Morphology

Irrespective of the clinical picture, the proliferating Langerhans cells have abundant, often vacuolated cytoplasm and vesicular nuclei containing grooves or folds. Langerhans cells possess their characteristic ***Birbeck granules*** (Fig. 16.43), which are seen only by electron microscopy. Under the electron microscope, these appear as ***'tennis racket'*** because of their pentalaminar tubules with a dilated terminal end. Eosinophilic granuloma subtype of LCH has a prominence of eosinophilic infiltrate along with the classical Langerhans cells and lymphocytes, plasma cells and neutrophils.

Immunophenotyping

Langerhans cells are positive for ***langerin (CD207), CD1a***, HLA-DR and S100.

Treatment

Unifocal bone lesions can be cured with surgical curettage. Since spontaneous resolution occurs in some cases, stable and asymptomatic lesions can be closely followed without intervention. Disseminated disease and progressive or recurrent bone lesions are treated with chemotherapy and/or steroids. The widespread organ involvement is associated with a poor outcome.

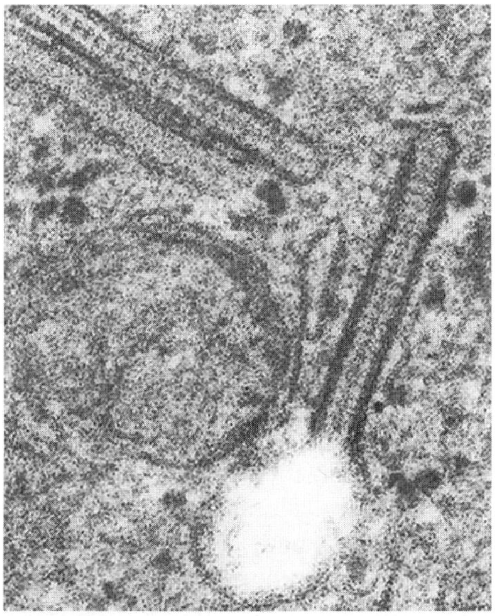

Fig. 16.43 Electron microscopy appearance of Langerhans cells displaying Birbeck granules with tennis racket appearance. (*Source:* From Barbara Young, Geraldine O'Dowd, Phillip Woodford. Wheater's Functional Histology. Elsevier. 2014.)

APPROACH TO A CASE OF ACUTE LEUKAEMIA/LYMPHOMA

Acute leukaemia, whether paediatric or adult, requires a meticulous approach for accurate diagnosis and effective treatment planning. Key steps in the diagnostic process include:

1. **History:** Recording any familial incidence of leukaemia/lymphoma and past exposure to genotoxic agents.
2. **Complaints:** Check for fatigue, recurrent infections in the recent past, bleeding episodes, dragging sensation in the abdomen (splenomegaly), headache, vomiting or nerve palsies (meningeal involvement), loss of appetite and weight and night sweats (hypermetabolic state).
   Clinical and laboratory evaluation: This includes a complete blood count, peripheral smear examination, and bone marrow analysis. Immunophenotyping, crucial for determining the leukaemia lineage, has advanced significantly, with newer markers aiding in more precise classification.
3. **Clinical examination:** Examine pallor, purpura/petechiae, splenomegaly, hepatomegaly, lymphadenopathy, sternal tenderness, nerve palsies and scrotal mass (testicular involvement in ALL).
4. **CBC:** This includes anaemia, leucocytosis/leucopenia or normal WBC count and thrombocytopenia.
5. **Peripheral smear examination:** Look for the presence of blasts, anaemia, thrombocytopenia and other additional findings (e.g. smudge cells in CLL).
6. **Buffy coat preparation:** Examine the smear for the presence of blasts in subleukaemic and aleukaemic leukaemias.
7. **ESR:** ESR is elevated in multiple myeloma.
8. **Bone marrow examination:** This is the most important test to check for cellularity and the predominant lineage and stage of differentiation. Check other lineages as well – erythroid and megakaryocytic. Calculate the exact percentage of blasts (20% blast is the cut-off for acute leukaemia) and additional findings (e.g. sea blue histiocytes in CML).
9. **Cytochemistry:** The cytochemical pattern of leukaemias is discussed.
10. **Immunophenotyping:** This is done to identify the lineage of the abnormal cells along with their stage of differentiation. Immunohistochemistry and flow cytometry are the techniques used for immunophenotyping.
11. **Cytogenetics:** This is done to detect the genetic abnormalities of leukaemias and lymphomas and to design the treatment (e.g. presence of BCR-ABL fusion directs treatment with BCR-ABL inhibitor).
12. **Bone marrow trephine biopsy:** This is done to confirm marrow involvement in lymphomas and to study the pattern of infiltration in lymphomas.

A case of lymphoma also should be approached in a similar manner, with the only exception being the biopsy of the affected site (lymph node/spleen/CNS/stomach) has to be sampled and examined.

II. SPLEEN

The spleen, a critical organ in immune function and blood filtration, can be involved in a variety of pathological conditions. Splenomegaly is a common manifestation in various systemic, hematopoietic and metabolic disorders. Advances in imaging techniques have improved the diagnostic accuracy for splenic diseases, and understanding the spleen's role in systemic diseases has become increasingly important in comprehensive patient management.

Before discussing diseases of the spleen, let us review the basic anatomy and physiology of the spleen briefly for a better understanding.

ANATOMY

The spleen is located in the upper left quadrant of the abdomen under the cover of the diaphragm and the rib cage and therefore cannot be normally palpated on clinical examination, except when it is enlarged. It is an intraperitoneal organ that is completely surrounded by peritoneum except at the splenic hilum.

The structure of spleen is organized into two areas – white pulp and red pulp. The white pulp consists of Malpighian or splenic follicles that are collections of lymphocytes around centrally located arterioles. Periarteriolar lymphocytes are mainly T lymphocytes.

Adjacent to this is the area of B lymphocytes which exhibit prominent germinal centres on antigenic stimulation.

Red pulp is made up of anastomosing cords and vascular sinuses. The splenic cords are made up of a network of macrophages. The vascular sinuses are lined by a discontinuous layer of endothelial cells to permit blood cells to traverse between sinusoids and cords.

The majority of the blood supply from the splenic artery passes from the smaller branches and arterioles into the capillaries and then into the splenic veins. A small fraction of the capillary blood passes slowly into the splenic cords; the blood from the cords then enters the sinuses through narrow slits between endothelial cells and then passes into the veins.

PHYSIOLOGY

Spleen is a natural filter for blood and a site of immune responses to antigens. A normal spleen weighs about ***150 g***. The spleen has four major functions:

- Phagocytosis of blood cells and particulate matter
- Antibody production
- Haematopoiesis in the fetus and a site for extramedullary haematopoiesis
- Sequestration of formed elements of blood

Spleen plays a pivotal role in the removal of unwanted elements from the blood. As the blood passes slowly through the splenic cords, macrophages recognize and phagocytose microorganisms and defective or damaged red cells occurring in various physiological and pathological conditions. Splenic macrophages also remove inclusions such as Howell–Jolly bodies or Heinz bodies from red cells. Spleen plays a role in both B-cell–mediated (humoral) and T-cell–mediated immune responses.

Spleen also functions as a site of haematopoiesis during fetal life. In some disorders such as thalassaemia major and myelofibrosis, extramedullary haematopoiesis may get reestablished in the spleen.

SPLENOMEGALY PA 19.6

The spleen is involved in all systemic inflammation, generalized haematopoietic disorders and many other metabolic disorders. In each of these disorders, the spleen undergoes enlargement (splenomegaly), which is the predominant manifestation of these disorders (Table 16.25).

When significantly enlarged, the spleen causes a dragging sensation in the left upper quadrant. Morphology of spleen in congestive splenomegaly is discussed in Chapter 4.

Classification of splenomegaly according to its weight:

Mild splenomegaly: Spleen weight less than 500 g
Moderate splenomegaly: Spleen weight 500–1000 g
Massive splenomegaly (Table 16.26; Figs 16.44 and 16.45): Spleen weight more than 1000 g

Hypersplenism

The clinical syndrome of hypersplenism does not definitively manifest with splenomegaly. The diagnostic criteria for hypersplenism are as follows:

- Splenic enlargement
- Peripheral blood cytopenias
- Normal or hypercellular marrow with a normal maturation pattern
- Normalization of blood parameters following splenectomy

Cytopenia results because of increased sequestration and phagocytosis of formed elements of blood by the abnormally functioning spleen. Normally, about one-third of total platelets in the body are pooled in the spleen and an enlarged spleen can sequester a large number of platelets to induce thrombocytopenia. A massively enlarged spleen can also trap and retain a considerable proportion of red cells and granulocytes to cause anaemia and neutropenia, respectively.

Table 16.25 Disorders Associated With Splenomegaly

Category	Common Causes
Infections	Infectious mononucleosis Tuberculosis Typhoid fever Malaria Brucellosis Cytomegalovirus Syphilis Kala-azar Histoplasmosis Subacute bacterial endocarditis
Congestive states related to portal hypertension	Cirrhosis of the liver Portal or splenic vein thrombosis Cardiac failure
Lymphohaematogenous disorders	Hodgkin lymphoma Non-Hodgkin lymphoma Multiple myeloma Myeloproliferative disorders
Haemolytic anaemias	Thalassaemia major Hereditary spherocytosis
Immunologic – inflammatory conditions	Rheumatoid arthritis Systemic lupus erythematosus
Storage diseases	Gaucher disease Niemann–Pick disease Mucopolysaccharidosis
Miscellaneous conditions	Amyloidosis Cysts Primary neoplasms Secondary neoplasms

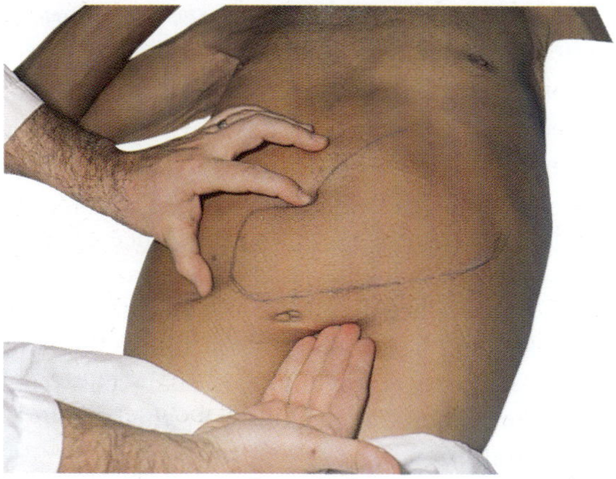

Fig. 16.44 Clinical picture of massive splenomegaly in a patient with CML. Note the splenic notch. (*Source:* From Mark H. Swartz. Textbook of Physical Diagnosis. Elsevier. 2021.)

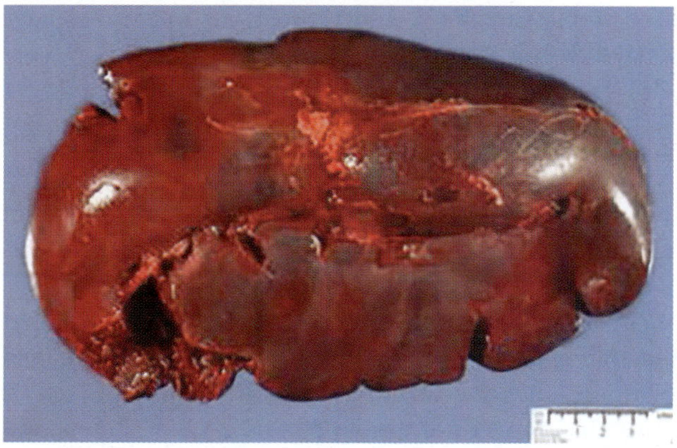

Fig. 16.45 Gross picture of a splenectomy specimen with massive splenomegaly in a patient with hereditary spherocytosis. (*Source:* From Sandra L. Hagen-Ansert. Textbook of Diagnostic Sonography. Elsevier. 2018.)

Table 16.26 Causes of Massive Splenomegaly

Chronic myeloid leukaemia
Myeloid metaplasia
Polycythaemia vera
Essential thrombocythaemia
Hairy cell leukaemia
β-Thalassaemia major
Indolent lymphomas
Kala-azar
Malaria
Gaucher disease

Tropical Splenomegaly

Tropical splenomegaly, also called hyper-reactive malarial syndrome (HMS), is prevalent in the regions endemic to malaria. Patients with HMS have high levels of antibody against *Plasmodium* species. Chronic antigenic stimulation is a key factor in the development of HMS. Though the exact mechanism is still unclear, evidence suggests that repeated or prolonged exposure to malaria elicits an exaggerated stimulation of polyclonal B lymphocytes, leading to an excessive and partially controlled production of polyclonal IgM.

Patients present with low-grade fever and massive splenomegaly. High levels of antimalarial antibodies are present in the blood along with elevated levels of IL-10 and IFN-γ.

Effective malarial chemoprophylaxis and eradication measures have been associated with regression of splenomegaly, correction of anaemia, lymphocytosis and fall in serum IgM levels. However, withdrawal of chemoprophylaxis in patients from malaria endemic regions has been associated with relapse.

III. THYMUS

Thymus is a derivative of third and fourth pharyngeal pouches which weighs around 10–35 g at birth, 20–50 g at puberty and 5–15 g in adults. In the presence of severe infection or HIV infection, it undergoes premature involution in children and young adults.

Thymus, when fully developed, is composed of two fused, well-encapsulated lobes which are divided into many lobules by the fibrous extensions from the capsule.

Histology of thymus reveals the presence of cortical, peripheral thymic epithelial cells and immature T lymphocytes. The epithelial cells in the medulla are compactly packed and have spindle shape unlike the polygonal shape of cortical thymic epithelial cells. Hassall corpuscles are whorls of medullary epithelial cells with hallmark keratinized cores.

Thymus plays a major role in cell-mediated immunity, which is discussed in greater detail in Chapter 6.

Developmental disorders like thymic hypoplasia or aplasia – as a part of DiGeorge syndrome, have also been discussed in Chapter 6. Apart from this, thymus can have isolated thymic cysts or thymic hyperplasia.

THYMOMAS

Thymus can give rise to many neoplasms such as germ cell tumours, lymphomas and carcinoids. Here, we discuss the pathology of thymomas.

Thymoma is a group of neoplasms that arise from thymic epithelial cells. WHO in the year 2015 has classified thymomas into the categories given in Table 16.27.

Because the clinical utility of this system is questionable, a simpler system that includes the surgical stage and the presence or absence of overt cytological features of malignancy is preferred. In this system, there are three subtypes:

1. Benign and noninvasive tumours
2. Invasive thymomas – cytologically benign tumours but locally invasive
3. Thymic carcinoma – cytologically malignant tumours

Morphology

Thymomas are grossly lobulated, firm, grey–white masses that may grow up to 20 cm in size. Most of these masses are encapsulated, but up to one-fourth of the tumours penetrate the capsule. Areas of necrosis and calcification may be present.

Noninvasive Thymomas

These are composed of medullary type or a mixture of medullary and cortical type epithelial cells. There is sparse infiltrate of thymocytes, whereas the mixed thymomas have dense infiltrate of thymocytes.

Invasive Thymomas

By definition, invasive thymomas have capsular penetration. The epithelial cells are more of cortical type admixed with numerous thymocytes. Generally, the cells are bland, and in rare cases with atypia, the tendency for aggressive behaviour is higher.

Thymic Carcinoma

These tumours are fleshy and grossly invasive. The most common histopathological type is squamous cell carcinoma, followed by lymphoepithelioma which is associated with EBV infection.

Clinical Course and Prognosis

Thymomas usually occur in adults older than 40 years and commonly manifest as an anterior superior mediastinal mass and with symptoms related to pressure on mediastinal structures. Around 30%–45% of tumours come to clinical attention during the workup of myasthenia gravis or pure red cell aplasia or Graves disease or pernicious anaemia.

Minimally invasive thymomas following a complete excision yield good prognosis, whereas the prognosis of widely invasive type and thymic carcinoma is guarded.

Table 16.27 WHO Classification of Thymomas, 2015

Type	Subtypes	Histological Features
Type A		Homogeneous population of neoplastic epithelial cells with spindle/oval shape, no nuclear atypia and accompanied by few or no non-neoplastic lymphocytes
Type AB		Mixed thymoma; tumours in which foci having the features of type A thymoma are mixed with foci rich in lymphocytes; the segregation of the two patterns can be sharp or indistinct
Type B	Type B1	Lymphocyte rich; resembles normal functional thymus by combining large expanses having normal thymic cortical areas with those resembling thymic medulla
	Type B2	Cortical; neoplastic epithelial component appears as scattered plump cells with vesicular nuclei, distinct nucleoli; heavy population of lymphocytes and perivascular spaces are common
	Type B3	Epithelial cells with round/polygonal shape and mild atypia, mixed with a minor component of lymphocytes; foci of squamous metaplasia and perivascular spaces common
Type C		Thymic carcinoma

SELF-ASSESSMENT

Multiple Choice Questions

1. Which of the following is not a cause of leucocytosis?
   A. Bacterial infections
   B. Viral infections
   C. Bone marrow disorders
   D. Increased physical exercise
2. What is the most common genetic abnormality in chronic lymphocytic leukaemia (CLL)?
   A. t(9;22)
   B. Deletion of 13q
   C. t(11;14)
   D. t(12;21)
3. Which lymphoma is associated with Reed–Sternberg cells?
   A. Non-Hodgkin lymphoma
   B. Hodgkin lymphoma
   C. Burkitt lymphoma
   D. Mantle cell lymphoma
4. What is the primary feature differentiating Hodgkin from non-Hodgkin lymphomas?
   A. Presence of B symptoms
   B. Involvement of lymph nodes
   C. Specific immunophenotyping
   D. Pattern of spread and distribution
5. What condition is characterized by an abnormal proliferation of immature white blood cells?
   A. Leukaemia
   B. Lymphoma
   C. Thrombocytopenia
   D. Anaemia
6. Which of the following is not a characteristic of acute myeloid leukaemia (AML)?
   A. Presence of Auer rods
   B. Origin from myeloid progenitor cells
   C. Expression of T-cell markers
   D. Increased myeloblasts in bone marrow
7. What is the primary cause of splenomegaly in myeloproliferative disorders?
   A. Lymphoid hyperplasia
   B. Extramedullary haematopoiesis
   C. Viral infection
   D. Congestion of splenic sinusoids
8. Which chromosome translocation is most commonly associated with Burkitt lymphoma?
   A. t(8;14)
   B. t(9;22)
   C. t(11;14)
   D. t(14;18)
9. What distinguishes a leukemoid reaction from chronic myeloid leukaemia?
   A. Presence of Philadelphia chromosome
   B. Elevated leucocyte alkaline phosphatase (LAP) score
   C. Lower white blood cell count
   D. Presence of lymphoblasts
10. Which of the following is not typically seen in neutrophilia?
    A. Toxic granulation
    B. Döhle bodies
    C. Cytoplasmic vacuoles
    D. Hypersegmented neutrophils
11. What factor is not associated with the development of lymphomas and leukaemias?
    A. Viral infections
    B. Radiation exposure
    C. Genetic predisposition
    D. Elevated blood glucose levels
12. In what condition are Reed–Sternberg cell variants commonly found?
    A. Follicular lymphoma
    B. Hodgkin lymphoma
    C. Chronic lymphocytic leukaemia
    D. Acute lymphoblastic leukaemia
13. Which of the following is not a feature of chronic lymphocytic leukaemia (CLL)?
    A. Increased number of mature lymphocytes
    B. Presence of smudge cells
    C. High levels of myeloblasts
    D. Lymphadenopathy
14. What is the primary distinguishing feature of acute lymphoblastic leukaemia (ALL)?
    A. Presence of Reed–Sternberg cells
    B. Predominance of immature lymphoid cells
    C. Increase in myeloblasts
    D. Proliferation of mature B cells
15. What characterizes marginal zone lymphomas?
    A. Rapidly dividing immature lymphocytes
    B. Association with chronic inflammatory disorders
    C. Predominance of Reed–Sternberg cells
    D. High incidence of bone marrow involvement
16. Which of the following is not a characteristic feature of multiple myeloma?
    A. Bence Jones proteinuria
    B. Lytic bone lesions
    C. Increased red blood cell count
    D. Hypercalcaemia
17. Which of the following is a distinguishing feature of non-Hodgkin lymphoma compared to Hodgkin lymphoma?
    A. Presence of B symptoms
    B. Painless lymphadenopathy
    C. More frequent extranodal involvement
    D. Reed–Sternberg cells
18. Which of the following is not a common cause of lymphadenopathy?
    A. Infections
    B. Autoimmune disorders
    C. Metabolic disorders
    D. Haematological malignancies
19. Which of the following conditions is characterized by the proliferation of plasma cells in the bone marrow?
    A. Lymphoma
    B. Myeloma
    C. Leukaemia
    D. Agranulocytosis
20. Which of the following is not typically associated with myeloproliferative neoplasms?
    A. Polycythaemia vera
    B. Chronic myelogenous leukaemia
    C. Hairy cell leukaemia
    D. Primary myelofibrosis

21. What is the hallmark of Waldenström macroglobulinaemia?
    A. Increased IgG levels
    B. High levels of IgM
    C. Presence of Reed–Sternberg cells
    D. Increased IgA levels
22. Which of the following is not a typical feature of acute lymphoblastic leukaemia (ALL)?
    A. High levels of myeloblasts
    B. Presence of lymphoblasts
    C. Rapid onset of symptoms
    D. Common in children
23. Which of the following is not a common finding in Hodgkin lymphoma?
    A. Bimodal age distribution
    B. Association with Epstein–Barr virus
    C. Presence of myeloblasts
    D. Lymph node enlargement
24. Which of the following is not a typical feature of chronic neutrophilic leukaemia?
    A. Elevated neutrophil count
    B. Presence of Philadelphia chromosome
    C. Splenomegaly
    D. Hypersegmented neutrophils
25. What distinguishes a leucoerythroblastic reaction?
    A. Presence of immature RBCs and WBCs in peripheral blood
    B. High levels of lymphoblasts
    C. Markedly increased WBC count
    D. Specific chromosome translocations

Answers

1. (D); 2. (B); 3. (B); 4. (D); 5. (A); 6. (C); 7. (B); 8. (A); 9. (B); 10. (D); 11. (D); 12. (B); 13. (C); 14. (B); 15. (B); 16. (C); 17. (C); 18. (C); 19. (B); 20. (C); 21. (B); 22. (A); 23. (C); 24. (D); 25. (A)

Self-Assessment Questions

1. A 16-year-old male patient presented to the emergency outpatient department (OPD) with signs and symptoms of acute appendicitis. Describe the peripheral smear findings expected in this patient.
2. A 25-year-old woman presented to the emergency OPD with complaints of generalized urticarial rashes following sulpha drug ingestion. Describe the CBC findings expected in this patient.
3. A 35-year-old patient presented with right molar caries tooth and right submandibular lymph node enlargement. Describe the histopathological features of the lymph node.
4. A 3-year-old child was brought with complaints of lethargy, recurrent infections and loss of appetite and weight since last 2 months. On clinical examination, it was found that the child was anaemic with purpuric spots over the body. There was also sternal tenderness. The paediatrician suspected leukaemia. What is your provisional diagnosis? Describe the peripheral smear and bone marrow findings.
5. A 55-year-old man presented with extreme fatigue, bleeding gums, and loss of weight and appetite. On examination, he was found to be anaemic with purpuric spots and splenomegaly. What is your probable diagnosis? Describe the peripheral smear and bone marrow findings.
6. A 26-year-old man presented with painless enlargement of cervical lymph node since past 6 months. He also complained of pain over the nodes following consumption of alcohol. What is your provisional diagnosis? Discuss the pathogenesis, types, morphological features and immunophenotyping of the disease.
7. A 2-year-old child was brought with acute intestinal obstruction, which was found to be due to ileocaecal mass. The mass was excised and submitted for histopathological examination. Microscopy revealed effacement of architecture with intermediate-size lymphoid cells interspersed with tingible body macrophages. What is your diagnosis? Discuss the aetiopathogenesis, morphology and immunophenotyping of the disease.
8. A 40-year-old male patient came with complaints of dragging sensation on the left side of the abdomen with loss of appetite and weight since past 6 months. His total leucocyte count was above 1 lakh/mm^3. What is your provisional diagnosis? Discuss the pathogenesis, peripheral smear and bone marrow morphology and cytogenetics of the disease.
9. Discuss the role of CD markers in leukaemia/lymphoma.
10. Discuss the role of special stains in leukaemias.
11. Differentiate between Hodgkin and non-Hodgkin lymphomas.
12. Discuss the causes of splenomegaly with fever.

Answers

1. Neutrophilia with reactive changes
2. Eosinophilia
3. Acute nonspecific lymphadenitis
4. Acute lymphoblastic leukaemia
5. AML – M5
6. Hodgkin lymphoma
7. Burkitt lymphoma
8. CML

Topics for Self-Directed Learning

1. FAB classification of ALL
2. BCR-ABL in ALL
3. Role of flow cytometry in leukaemias and lymphomas
4. Pathogenesis and features of peripheral T-cell lymphomas
5. Causes and morphology of splenic infarct
6. Heavy-chain disease
7. Mediterranean lymphoma
8. Role of molecular genetics in acute leukaemias
9. Peripheral smear findings in infectious mononucleosis
10. Lymphomas with leukaemia transformation
11. Haematogones
12. Minimal residual disease in leukaemias
13. Differentiate blast crisis phase of CML from AML
14. Criteria for complete remission in acute leukaemias following therapy
15. List the haematopoietic stem cell disorders

MIND MAPS

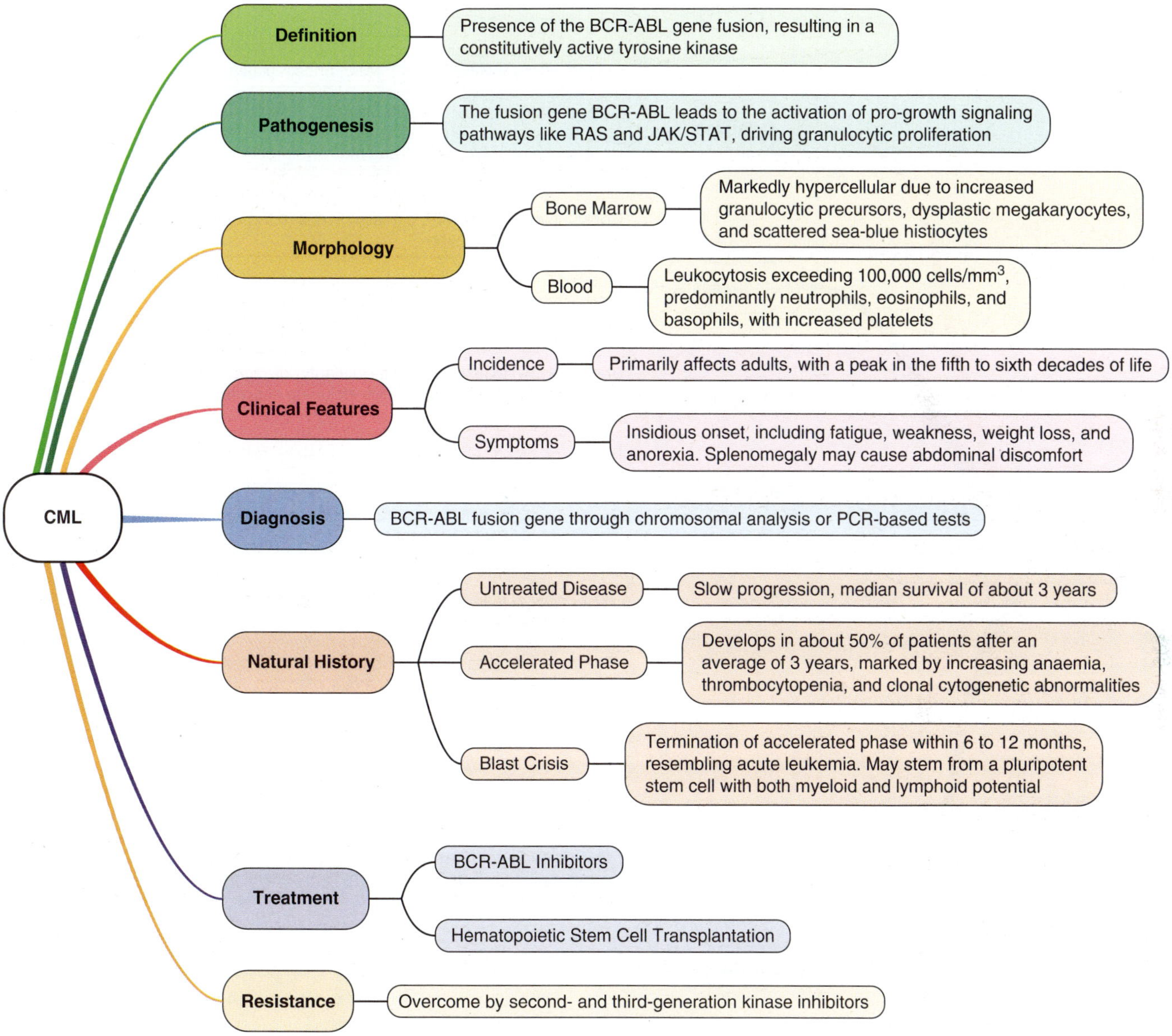
CML
Definition
Presence of the BCR-ABL gene fusion, resulting in a constitutively active tyrosine kinase
Pathogenesis
The fusion gene BCR-ABL leads to the activation of pro-growth signaling pathways like RAS and JAK/STAT, driving granulocytic proliferation
Morphology
Bone Marrow
Markedly hypercellular due to increased granulocytic precursors, dysplastic megakaryocytes, and scattered sea-blue histiocytes
Blood
Leukocytosis exceeding 100,000 cells/mm^3, predominantly neutrophils, eosinophils, and basophils, with increased platelets
Clinical Features
Incidence
Primarily affects adults, with a peak in the fifth to sixth decades of life
Symptoms
Insidious onset, including fatigue, weakness, weight loss, and anorexia. Splenomegaly may cause abdominal discomfort
Diagnosis
BCR-ABL fusion gene through chromosomal analysis or PCR-based tests
Natural History
Untreated Disease
Slow progression, median survival of about 3 years
Accelerated Phase
Develops in about 50% of patients after an average of 3 years, marked by increasing anaemia, thrombocytopenia, and clonal cytogenetic abnormalities
Blast Crisis
Termination of accelerated phase within 6 to 12 months, resembling acute leukemia. May stem from a pluripotent stem cell with both myeloid and lymphoid potential
Treatment
BCR-ABL Inhibitors
Hematopoietic Stem Cell Transplantation
Resistance
Overcome by second- and third-generation kinase inhibitors

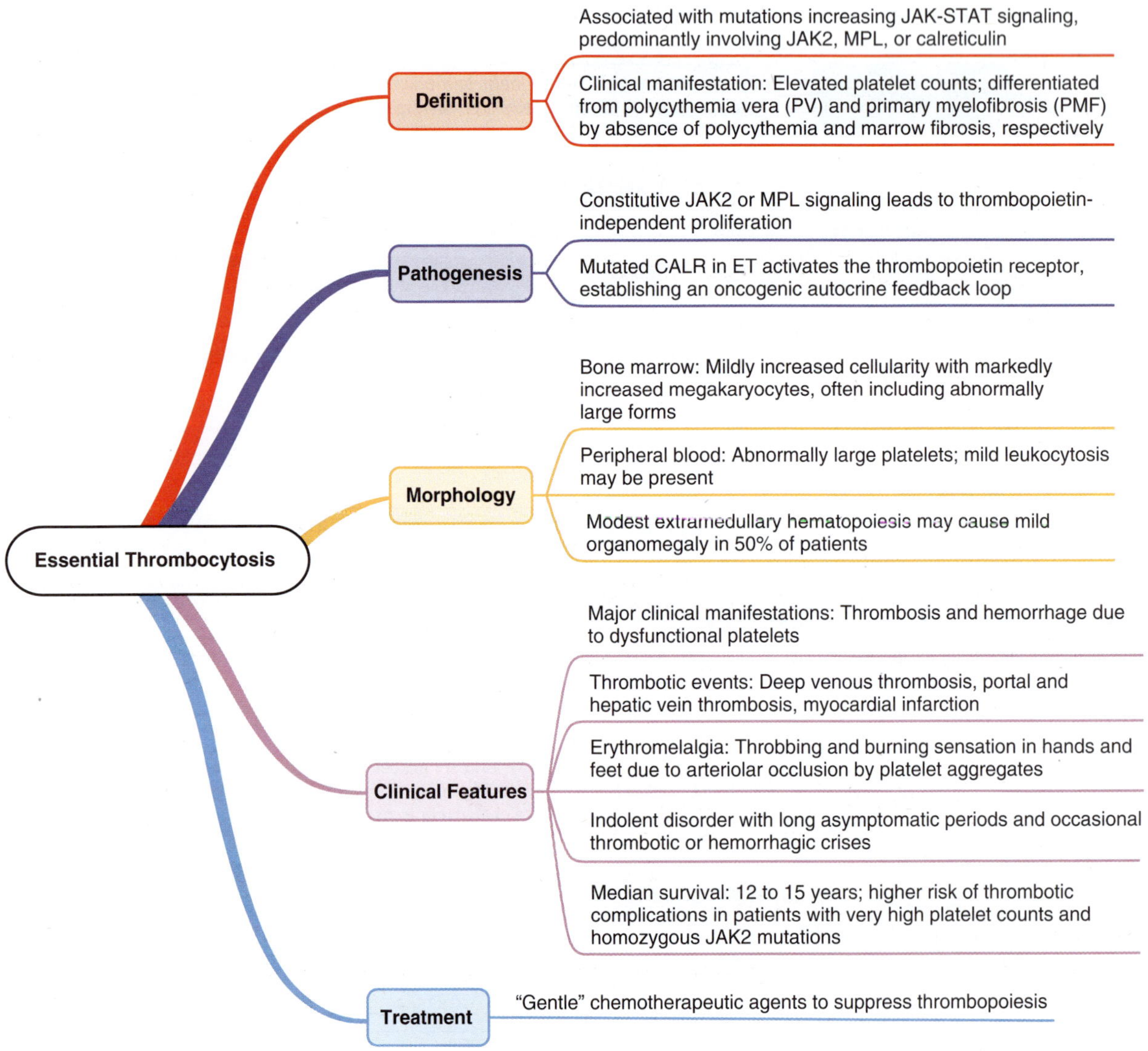
Essential Thrombocytosis
Definition
Associated with mutations increasing JAK-STAT signaling, predominantly involving JAK2, MPL, or calreticulin
Clinical manifestation: Elevated platelet counts; differentiated from polycythemia vera (PV) and primary myelofibrosis (PMF) by absence of polycythemia and marrow fibrosis, respectively
Pathogenesis
Constitutive JAK2 or MPL signaling leads to thrombopoietin-independent proliferation
Mutated CALR in ET activates the thrombopoietin receptor, establishing an oncogenic autocrine feedback loop
Morphology
Bone marrow: Mildly increased cellularity with markedly increased megakaryocytes, often including abnormally large forms
Peripheral blood: Abnormally large platelets; mild leukocytosis may be present
Modest extramedullary hematopoiesis may cause mild organomegaly in 50% of patients
Clinical Features
Major clinical manifestations: Thrombosis and hemorrhage due to dysfunctional platelets
Thrombotic events: Deep venous thrombosis, portal and hepatic vein thrombosis, myocardial infarction
Erythromelalgia: Throbbing and burning sensation in hands and feet due to arteriolar occlusion by platelet aggregates
Indolent disorder with long asymptomatic periods and occasional thrombotic or hemorrhagic crises
Median survival: 12 to 15 years; higher risk of thrombotic complications in patients with very high platelet counts and homozygous JAK2 mutations
Treatment
"Gentle" chemotherapeutic agents to suppress thrombopoiesis

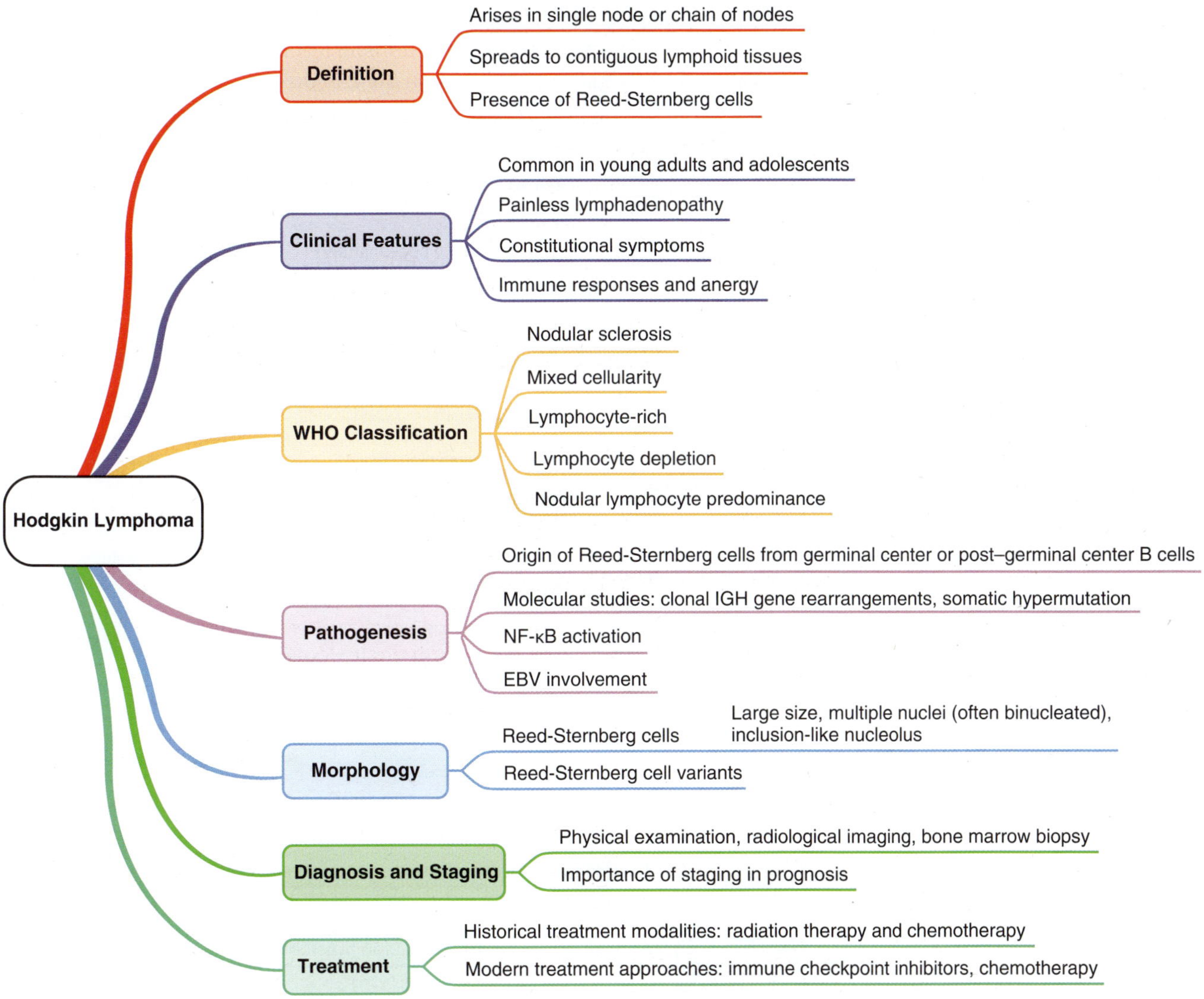
Hodgkin Lymphoma
Definition
Arises in single node or chain of nodes
Spreads to contiguous lymphoid tissues
Presence of Reed-Sternberg cells
Clinical Features
Common in young adults and adolescents
Painless lymphadenopathy
Constitutional symptoms
Immune responses and anergy
WHO Classification
Nodular sclerosis
Mixed cellularity
Lymphocyte-rich
Lymphocyte depletion
Nodular lymphocyte predominance
Pathogenesis
Origin of Reed-Sternberg cells from germinal center or post–germinal center B cells
Molecular studies: clonal IGH gene rearrangements, somatic hypermutation
NF-κB activation
EBV involvement
Morphology
Reed-Sternberg cells
Large size, multiple nuclei (often binucleated), inclusion-like nucleolus
Reed-Sternberg cell variants
Diagnosis and Staging
Physical examination, radiological imaging, bone marrow biopsy
Importance of staging in prognosis
Treatment
Historical treatment modalities: radiation therapy and chemotherapy
Modern treatment approaches: immune checkpoint inhibitors, chemotherapy

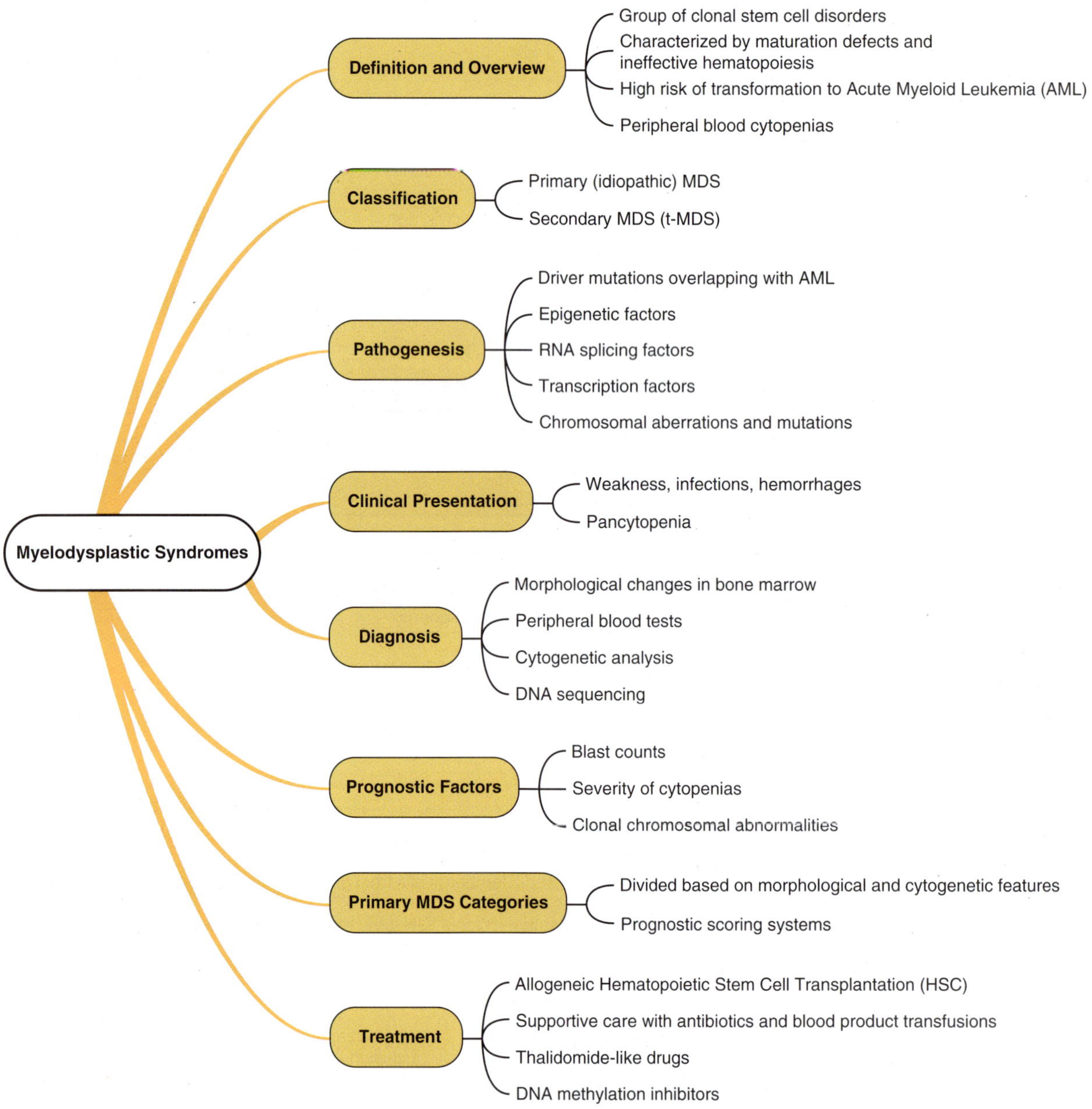

Myelodysplastic Syndromes
Definition and Overview
Group of clonal stem cell disorders
Characterized by maturation defects and ineffective hematopoiesis
High risk of transformation to Acute Myeloid Leukemia (AML)
Peripheral blood cytopenias
Classification
Primary (idiopathic) MDS
Secondary MDS (t-MDS)
Pathogenesis
Driver mutations overlapping with AML
Epigenetic factors
RNA splicing factors
Transcription factors
Chromosomal aberrations and mutations
Clinical Presentation
Weakness, infections, hemorrhages
Pancytopenia
Diagnosis
Morphological changes in bone marrow
Peripheral blood tests
Cytogenetic analysis
DNA sequencing
Prognostic Factors
Blast counts
Severity of cytopenias
Clonal chromosomal abnormalities
Primary MDS Categories
Divided based on morphological and cytogenetic features
Prognostic scoring systems
Treatment
Allogeneic Hematopoietic Stem Cell Transplantation (HSC)
Supportive care with antibiotics and blood product transfusions
Thalidomide-like drugs
DNA methylation inhibitors

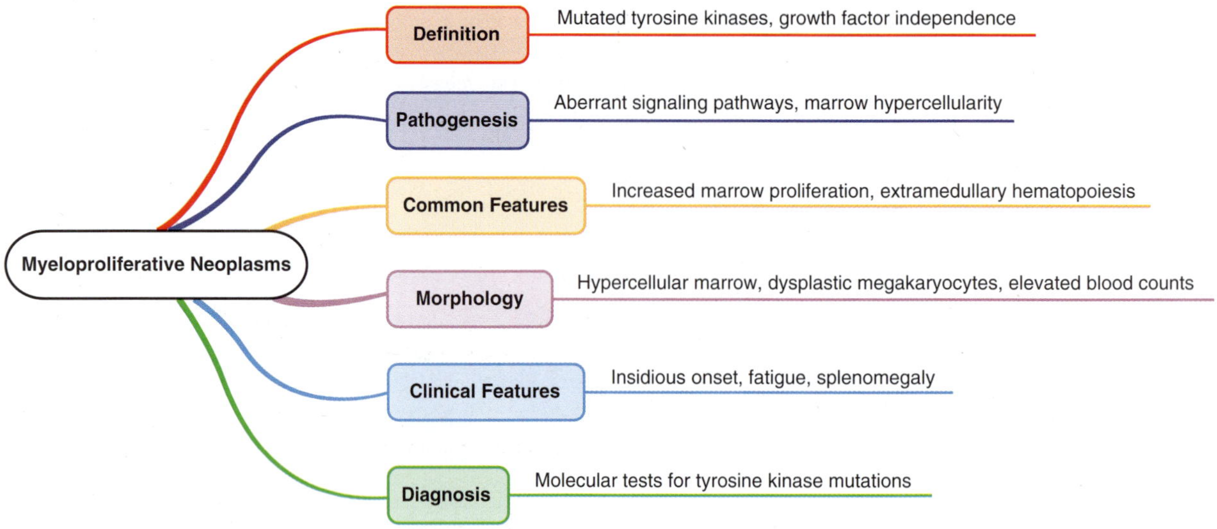

Myeloproliferative Neoplasms
Definition
Mutated tyrosine kinases, growth factor independence
Pathogenesis
Aberrant signaling pathways, marrow hypercellularity
Common Features
Increased marrow proliferation, extramedullary hematopoiesis
Morphology
Hypercellular marrow, dysplastic megakaryocytes, elevated blood counts
Clinical Features
Insidious onset, fatigue, splenomegaly
Diagnosis
Molecular tests for tyrosine kinase mutations

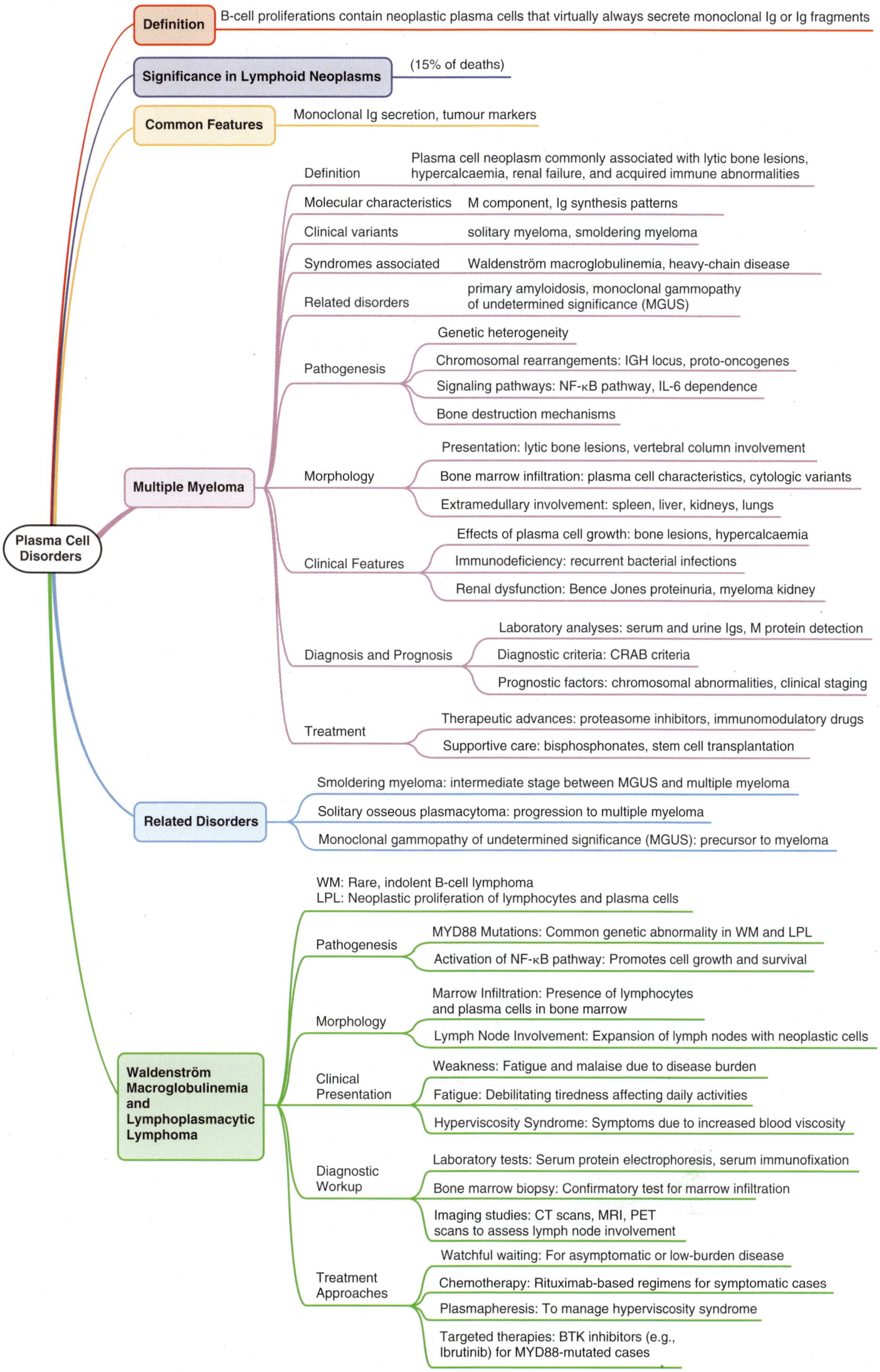
Plasma Cell Disorders
Definition
B-cell proliferations contain neoplastic plasma cells that virtually always secrete monoclonal Ig or Ig fragments
Significance in Lymphoid Neoplasms
(15% of deaths)
Common Features
Monoclonal Ig secretion, tumour markers
Multiple Myeloma
Definition
Plasma cell neoplasm commonly associated with lytic bone lesions, hypercalcaemia, renal failure, and acquired immune abnormalities
Molecular characteristics
M component, Ig synthesis patterns
Clinical variants
solitary myeloma, smoldering myeloma
Syndromes associated
Waldenström macroglobulinemia, heavy-chain disease
Related disorders
primary amyloidosis, monoclonal gammopathy of undetermined significance (MGUS)
Pathogenesis
Genetic heterogeneity
Chromosomal rearrangements: IGH locus, proto-oncogenes
Signaling pathways: NF-κB pathway, IL-6 dependence
Bone destruction mechanisms
Morphology
Presentation: lytic bone lesions, vertebral column involvement
Bone marrow infiltration: plasma cell characteristics, cytologic variants
Extramedullary involvement: spleen, liver, kidneys, lungs
Clinical Features
Effects of plasma cell growth: bone lesions, hypercalcaemia
Immunodeficiency: recurrent bacterial infections
Renal dysfunction: Bence Jones proteinuria, myeloma kidney
Diagnosis and Prognosis
Laboratory analyses: serum and urine Igs, M protein detection
Diagnostic criteria: CRAB criteria
Prognostic factors: chromosomal abnormalities, clinical staging
Treatment
Therapeutic advances: proteasome inhibitors, immunomodulatory drugs
Supportive care: bisphosphonates, stem cell transplantation
Related Disorders
Smoldering myeloma: intermediate stage between MGUS and multiple myeloma
Solitary osseous plasmacytoma: progression to multiple myeloma
Monoclonal gammopathy of undetermined significance (MGUS): precursor to myeloma
Waldenström Macroglobulinemia and Lymphoplasmacytic Lymphoma
WM: Rare, indolent B-cell lymphoma
LPL: Neoplastic proliferation of lymphocytes and plasma cells
Pathogenesis
MYD88 Mutations: Common genetic abnormality in WM and LPL
Activation of NF-κB pathway: Promotes cell growth and survival
Morphology
Marrow Infiltration: Presence of lymphocytes and plasma cells in bone marrow
Lymph Node Involvement: Expansion of lymph nodes with neoplastic cells
Clinical Presentation
Weakness: Fatigue and malaise due to disease burden
Fatigue: Debilitating tiredness affecting daily activities
Hyperviscosity Syndrome: Symptoms due to increased blood viscosity
Diagnostic Workup
Laboratory tests: Serum protein electrophoresis, serum immunofixation
Bone marrow biopsy: Confirmatory test for marrow infiltration
Imaging studies: CT scans, MRI, PET scans to assess lymph node involvement
Treatment Approaches
Watchful waiting: For asymptomatic or low-burden disease
Chemotherapy: Rituximab-based regimens for symptomatic cases
Plasmapheresis: To manage hyperviscosity syndrome
Targeted therapies: BTK inhibitors (e.g., Ibrutinib) for MYD88-mutated cases

Polycythemia Vera (PCV)

- **Definition**
  - Characterized by increased marrow production of red cells, granulocytes, and platelets (panmyelosis).
  - Predominantly manifests as polycythemia, contributing to clinical symptoms.
- **Pathogenesis**
  - Transformed progenitor cells exhibit decreased reliance on erythropoietin due to JAK2 mutations, leading to constitutive activation of the JAK/STAT pathway.
  - Elevated hematocrit causes increased blood viscosity and sludging, predisposing to thrombosis and bleeding.
  - Over 97% of cases associated with JAK2 mutation (valine-to-phenylalanine substitution at residue 617).
- **Morphology**
  - Marrow hypercellularity with subtle increase in red cell progenitors, granulocytic precursors, and megakaryocytes.
  - Moderate to marked reticulin fibrosis in about 10% of cases.
  - Late-stage characterized by extensive marrow fibrosis and extramedullary hematopoiesis, leading to organomegaly.
- **Clinical Features**
  - Incidence: 1 to 3 per 100,000 per year, usually in late middle age.
  - Symptoms: Plethora, cyanosis, headache, dizziness, hypertension, gastrointestinal symptoms, intense pruritus, peptic ulceration, hyperuricemia, and gout.
  - Complications: Increased risk of bleeding and thrombotic events, including deep venous thrombosis, myocardial infarction, stroke, and Budd-Chiari syndrome.
- **Diagnosis**
  - Elevated hemoglobin (>16 g/dL) and hematocrit (>55%), with white cell count (12,000 to 50,000 cells/mm³) and platelet count (>500,000 platelets/mm³).
  - Morphologic abnormalities and functional defects in platelets.
  - Thrombotic complications may precede typical hematologic findings.
- **Treatment**
  - Phlebotomy: Maintains red cell mass at normal levels, extending median survival to about 10 years.
  - JAK2 Inhibitors: Used mainly in patients with significant splenomegaly, although current efficacy is limited.
  - Progression to "spent phase" resembling primary myelofibrosis may occur in 15% to 20% of patients after an average of 10 years.
- **Transformation**
  - About 2% of patients transform to acute myeloid leukemia (AML), often lacking JAK2 mutations.
  - Transformation to acute lymphoblastic leukemia (ALL) is rare, consistent with myeloid progenitor origin.

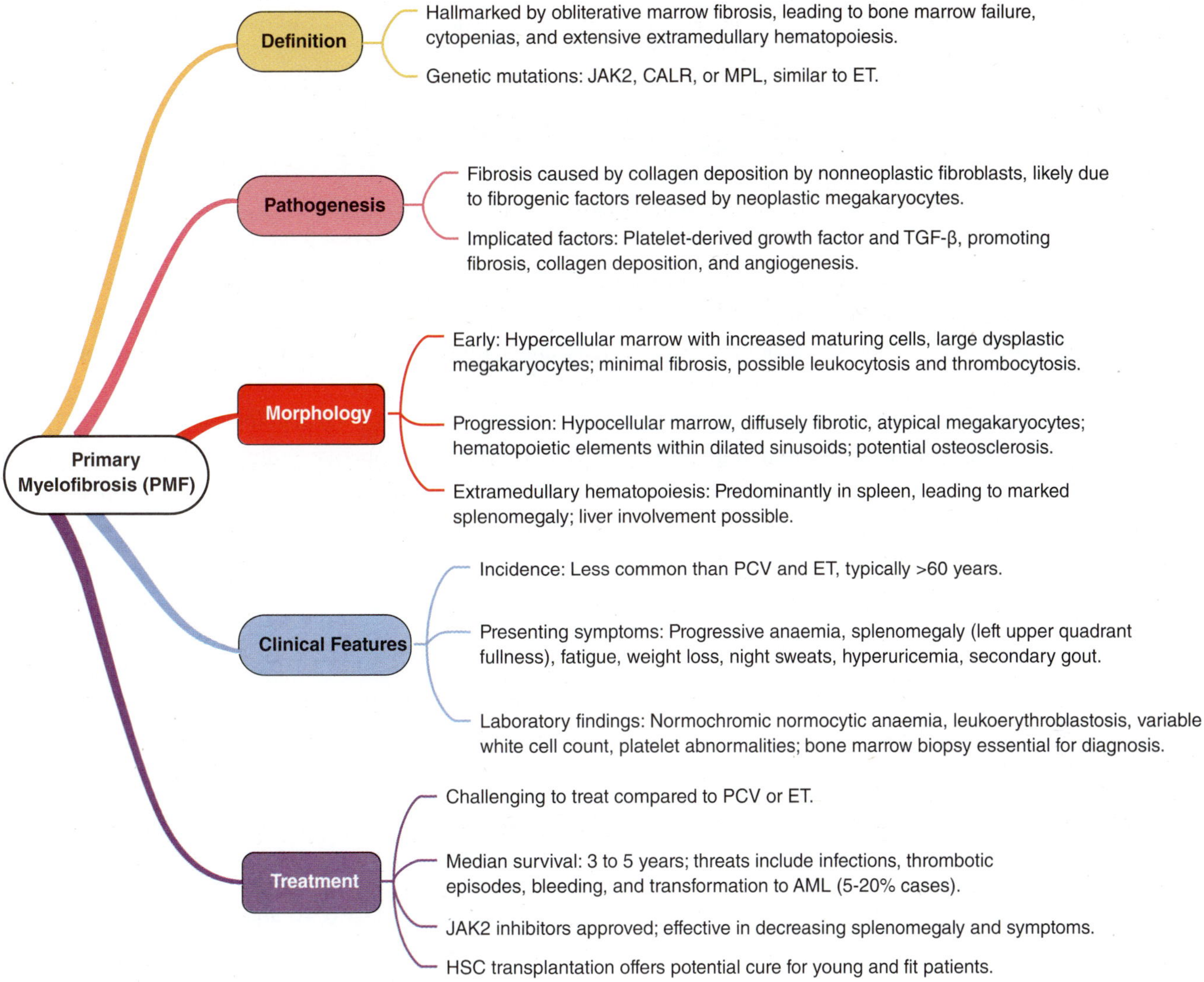
Primary Myelofibrosis (PMF)
Definition
Hallmarked by obliterative marrow fibrosis, leading to bone marrow failure, cytopenias, and extensive extramedullary hematopoiesis.
Genetic mutations: JAK2, CALR, or MPL, similar to ET.
Pathogenesis
Fibrosis caused by collagen deposition by nonneoplastic fibroblasts, likely due to fibrogenic factors released by neoplastic megakaryocytes.
Implicated factors: Platelet-derived growth factor and TGF-β, promoting fibrosis, collagen deposition, and angiogenesis.
Morphology
Early: Hypercellular marrow with increased maturing cells, large dysplastic megakaryocytes; minimal fibrosis, possible leukocytosis and thrombocytosis.
Progression: Hypocellular marrow, diffusely fibrotic, atypical megakaryocytes; hematopoietic elements within dilated sinusoids; potential osteosclerosis.
Extramedullary hematopoiesis: Predominantly in spleen, leading to marked splenomegaly; liver involvement possible.
Clinical Features
Incidence: Less common than PCV and ET, typically >60 years.
Presenting symptoms: Progressive anaemia, splenomegaly (left upper quadrant fullness), fatigue, weight loss, night sweats, hyperuricemia, secondary gout.
Laboratory findings: Normochromic normocytic anaemia, leukoerythroblastosis, variable white cell count, platelet abnormalities; bone marrow biopsy essential for diagnosis.
Treatment
Challenging to treat compared to PCV or ET.
Median survival: 3 to 5 years; threats include infections, thrombotic episodes, bleeding, and transformation to AML (5-20% cases).
JAK2 inhibitors approved; effective in decreasing splenomegaly and symptoms.
HSC transplantation offers potential cure for young and fit patients.

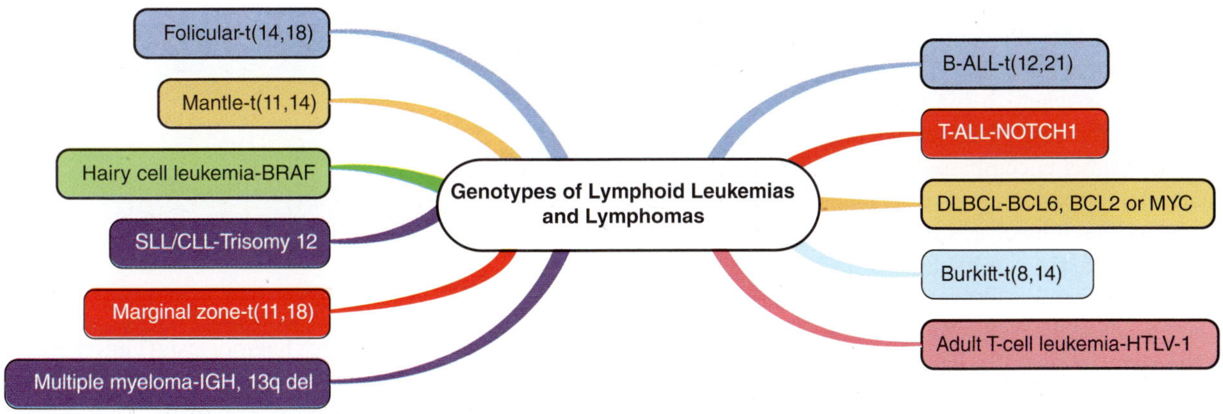
Genotypes of Lymphoid Leukemias and Lymphomas
Folicular-t(14,18)
Mantle-t(11,14)
Hairy cell leukemia-BRAF
SLL/CLL-Trisomy 12
Marginal zone-t(11,18)
Multiple myeloma-IGH, 13q del
B-ALL-t(12,21)
T-ALL-NOTCH1
DLBCL-BCL6, BCL2 or MYC
Burkitt-t(8,14)
Adult T-cell leukemia-HTLV-1

17 Bleeding Disorders

Rajeswari Kathiah

PA 21.1 Describe normal **haemostasis.**

PA 21.2 Classify and describe the aetiology, pathogenesis and pathology of **vascular and platelet disorders including immune thrombocytopenic purpura and haemophilias.**

PA 21.3 **Differentiate platelet from clotting disorders** based on the clinical and haematological features.

PA 21.4 Define and describe **disseminated intravascular coagulation**, its laboratory findings and diagnosis.

PA 21.5 Define and describe disseminated intravascular coagulation, its laboratory findings and diagnosis of **vitamin K deficiency**.

CHAPTER OUTLINE

REVIEW OF HAEMOSTASIS PA 21.1

Haemostasis is a critically controlled physiological process, essential for stopping bleeding at injury sites while preserving circulation elsewhere. It is a natural bodily response to vascular injury, forming a haemostatic plug to enable vessel repair. Haemostasis encompasses blood maintenance in a fluid state, clot formation upon vessel injury, and clot dissolution posthealing. It involves structures and factors such as blood vessels, platelets, clotting factors, and fibrinolytic factors, going through stages like vasoconstriction, primary and secondary haemostatic plug formation, and clot dissolution.

All the steps involved in haemostasis are discussed in detail in Chapter 4, and here we discuss the salient features of haemostasis with respect to bleeding.

Haemostasis involves the following features:

- Existence of blood in the fluid state
- Ability to form clot when the vessel is injured
- Dissolution of the clot when healing is complete

Structures and factors involved in the maintenance of haemostasis:

- Blood vessels
- Platelets
- Clotting factors
- Fibrinolytic factors

The steps involved in haemostasis:

1. A brief period of vasoconstriction
2. Primary haemostatic plug formation by platelets
3. Secondary haemostatic plug formation by clotting factors
4. Clot dissolution by fibrinolytic factors

The basic tests done to check haemostasis (Flowchart 17.1):

- Bleeding time (BT)
- Clotting time (CT)
- Prothrombin time (PT)
- Activated partial thromboplastin time (aPTT)

Special tests done to check haemostasis:

- Thrombin time (TT)
- Individual factor assay

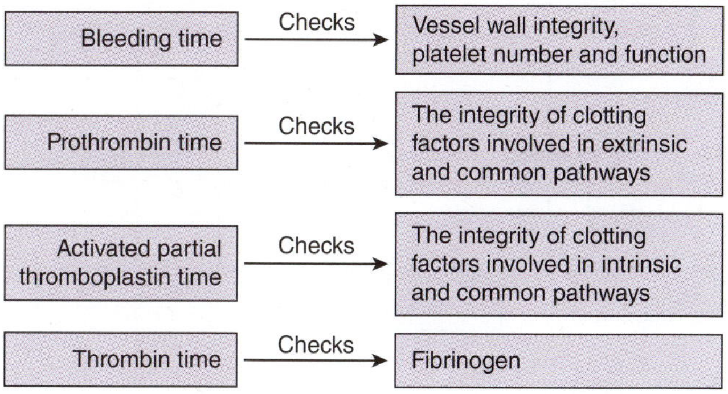

Flowchart 17.1 Basic tests for haemostasis.

- Platelet function tests
- Ristocetin cofactor (RCo) assay

TESTS DONE FOR ASSESSMENT OF HAEMOSTASIS (TABLE 17.1)

Before discussing the basic and specialized tests for assessing haemostasis, it is stressed that complete blood cell count and peripheral smear examination should be done in all the cases.

BT: This is a simple test in which a standard incision is made on the forearm and the time taken for the incision to stop bleeding is noted. The outcome of the test is dependent on capillary function quantity and quality of platelets.

Normal BT: 3–8 minutes

Table 17.1 Tests for Haemostasis – An Overview

Laboratory Test	Factor/Function Measured	Common Associated Disorders
Platelet count	Quantification of platelets	Thrombocytopenia/thrombocytosis
Bleeding time	Platelet number and function Vascular integrity	Quantitative platelet disorders Qualitative platelet disorders von Willebrand disease Collagen vascular disorders Acquired vascular disorders
Prothrombin time	Integrity of extrinsic and common pathways (factors I, II, V, VII, X)	DIC Liver disease Lupus anticoagulant Vitamin K deficiency Oral anticoagulants
Partial thromboplastin time	Integrity of intrinsic and common pathways (factors I, II, V, VIII, IX, X, XI, XII)	DIC Liver disease Lupus anticoagulant Vitamin K deficiency Heparin therapy
Thrombin time	Integrity of common pathway	DIC Afibrinogenaemia Hypo-/dysfibrinogenaemia Heparin therapy
Mixing studies	Checks whether the prolongation of PT or aPTT gets corrected after mixing with normal plasma	Factor deficiency Presence of inhibitors
Individual factor assay	Pathway in which the factor plays a role	Related disorders
Platelet function tests	Integrity of primary haemostatic plug formation by platelets	Platelet function disorders
Flow cytometry	Detection of surface glycoproteins on platelets	Bernard–Soulier syndrome Glanzmann thrombasthenia
Ristocetin cofactor assay	von Willebrand factor	von Willebrand disease
Fibrinogen **Fibrin degradation products**	Integrity of fibrinolysis	DIC Pulmonary embolism Deep vein thrombosis Recent myocardial infarction
D-dimer assay	Detection of cross-linked fibrin D-dimers Checks the formation of both thrombin and plasmin	More specific than FDP for DIC

aPTT, activated partial thromboplastin time; DIC, disseminated intravascular coagulation; FDP, fibrin degradation product; PT, prothrombin time.

CT: It is the time required for a sample of blood to coagulate under standard conditions. The integrity of the clotting cascade and the fibrinolytic system is on check with this parameter. CT is of limited value as it is insensitive and nonspecific and has been withdrawn from most of the laboratories.

Normal CT: 4–10 minutes

PT: It is useful in the evaluation of the extrinsic and common pathways of coagulation. In this test, tissue thromboplastin, which normally triggers the extrinsic pathway, and calcium are added to the sample and the time taken for the clot formation is measured.

Normal PT: 10–14 seconds

aPTT: This test is effective in assessing the factors involved in the intrinsic and common pathways. To perform the test, calcium, phospholipid and a surface activator such as kaolin are added to initiate the clotting cascade.

Normal aPTT: 30–40 seconds

TT: This test measures the time taken for a blood sample containing anticoagulant to clot after adding excess of thrombin.

Normal TT: 12–14 seconds

von Willebrand factor (vWF):RCo assay: This test measures the concentration and functional activity of vWF. Platelet aggregation to vWF in the presence of ristocetin is proportionate to the haemostatically active fraction of vWF. In this test, ristocetin and formalin-fixed platelets are added to the patient's platelet-poor plasma and the ability of the sample to passively agglutinate is checked. Formalin-fixed extrinsic platelets cannot secrete vWF and thus only the activity of the intrinsic vWF is tested.

Mixing studies: This test is done if there is isolated prolongation of PT or aPTT to determine whether it is because of factor deficiency or presence of inhibitor. In this test, PT or aPTT is repeated after using 50:50 mixtures of normal and the patient's plasma and it is noted whether normalization of the previously abnormal test occurs or not. In factor deficiency, following this mixing, the abnormal test results normalize. In the presence of inhibitors, the result depends on the type of inhibitors. Inhibitors may be immediate acting or delayed acting. With immediate-acting inhibitor, the test result becomes normal after mixing. With delayed-acting inhibitor, PT or aPTT becomes normal immediately after mixing but becomes prolonged after 1–2 hours of incubation at 37°C. If clotting factor deficiency is suspected, then individual factor assays need to be carried out.

Fibrin degradation products (FDPs): These are fragments formed by proteolytic digestion of fibrinogen or fibrin by the action of plasmin.

Normal: less than 10 μg/mL (conventional units) or less than 10 mg/L. An FDP level of more than 40 mg/mL is considered critical, indicating that there may be an underlying clotting disorder.

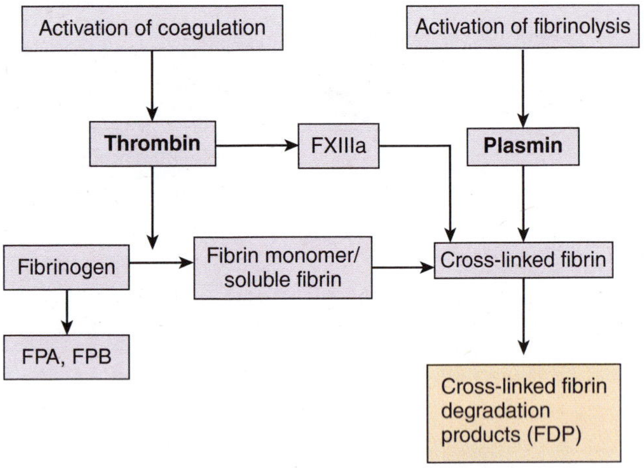

Flowchart 17.2 Generation of D-dimer.

D-dimer assay: D-dimer is the degradation product of cross-linked fibrin (by factor XIII). It reflects ongoing activation of the clotting cascade (Flowchart 17.2).

Normal: less than 250 ng/mL or less than 0.4 μg/mL.

BLEEDING DISORDERS

Bleeding disorders, or haemorrhagic diathesis, are a group of diseases resulting from defective haemostasis, leading to abnormal bleeding. These disorders can manifest as spontaneous skin or mucosal haemorrhages (e.g. petechiae, purpura, ecchymosis), or bleeding posttrauma or surgery. The causes are multifactorial, including vessel wall, platelet, clotting factors and fibrinolytic defects.

Causes of bleeding disorders can be grouped into the following categories:

- **Bleeding due to vessel wall abnormalities**
- **Bleeding due to platelet abnormalities**
- **Bleeding due to clotting factors abnormalities**
- **Bleeding due to fibrinolytic defects**

DISORDERS DUE TO VESSEL WALL ABNORMALITY PA 21.2

Bleeding due to vessel wall abnormalities comprises a heterogeneous group of disorders that clinically resemble bleeding due to platelet abnormalities. Abnormalities in the vessel wall can lead to bleeding due to damage to the capillary endothelium, defects in the subendothelial matrix, or problems with the extravascular connective tissue, such as weakened collagen observed in conditions like scurvy (Fig. 17.2). The disorders can be inherited or acquired (Table 17.2).

Inherited vascular bleeding disorders are caused by either vascular malformations or disorders of connective tissue, whereas acquired disorders have multiple causes such as increase in vessel wall fragility, decreased collagen and vasculitis.

Vascular bleeding disorders are characterized by easy bruising, petechiae, ecchymosis, mucosal bleeding and

Table 17.2 Inherited and Acquired Vascular Causes of Bleeding

Inherited Vascular Bleeding Disorders	Acquired Vascular Bleeding Disorders
Disorders of connective tissue matrix, e.g. Ehlers–Danlos syndrome, pseudoxanthoma elasticum Hereditary haemorrhagic telangiectasia	Henoch–Schönlein purpura Scurvy Drug reactions Vessel wall infections, e.g. meningococcal infection Steroid purpura Senile purpura Cryoglobulinaemia Devil's pinches – simple easy bruising

spontaneous bleeding from small vessels. Bleeding is usually mild (Fig. 17.1) but can be prominent as in scurvy or Henoch–Schönlein purpura (Fig. 17.3). Tests of haemostasis are usually normal except for mild **prolongation of BT**. Because the clinical features and the tests for haemostasis resemble platelet disorders, extensive clinical examination and extended laboratory testing are needed to differentiate the vascular bleeding disorders from platelet disorders, as the treatment of these two conditions are different.

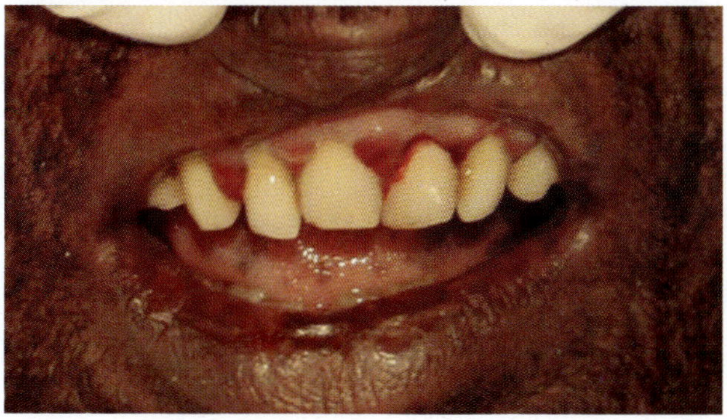

Fig. 17.1 Gum bleeding in vitamin C: clinical picture. (*Source:* From Stuart Ralston, Ian Penman, Mark Strachan, Richard Hobson. Davidson's Principles and Practice of Medicine. Elsevier. 2020)

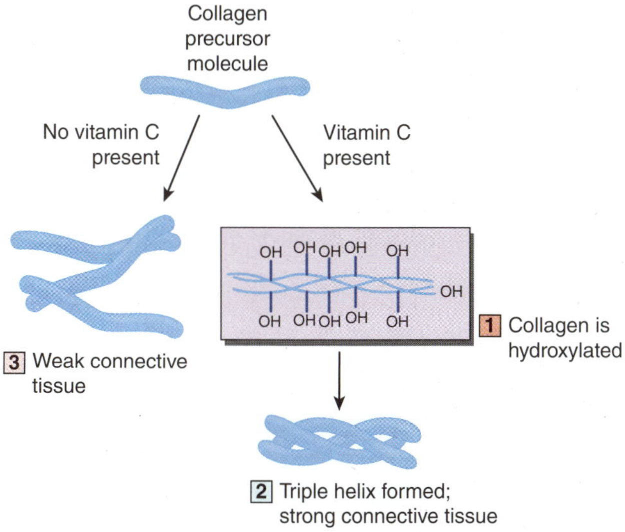

Fig. 17.2 Role of vitamin C in cross-linking of collagen. (*Source:* https://twitter.com/drjkahn/status/1005460799660478464)

DISORDERS DUE TO PLATELET ABNORMALITY

Platelets are crucial in haemostasis, transforming from discs to spiny spheres upon activation. They contain α- and dense granules, releasing proaggregatory materials like ADP and synthesizing thromboxane A2 (listed in Table 17.3) crucial for haemostatic plug consolidation. Platelet disorders, characterized by superficial bleeding and prolonged BT, are distinct from clotting factor deficiencies and require specific management approaches.

Once activated, platelets recruit additional platelets to the growing haemostatic plug by two major mechanisms – release of proaggregatory materials like ADP by their degranulation and synthesis of thromboxane A2 from arachidonic acid. All these act to consolidate the initial haemostatic plug by augmenting the participation of

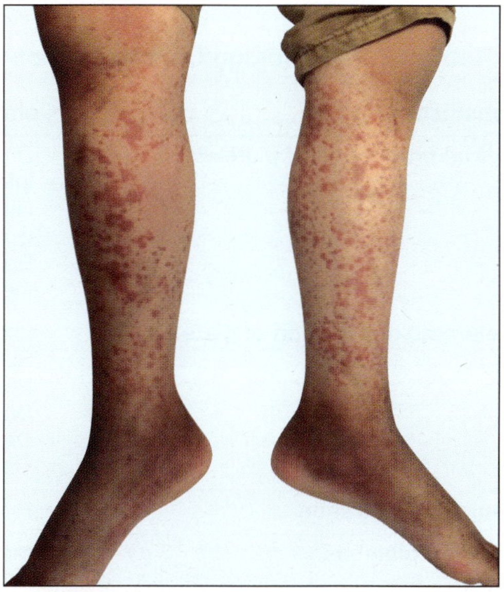

Fig. 17.3 Henoch– Schönlein purpura, clinical picture. (*Source:* From IgA vasculitis (Henoch–Schönlein purpura). Elsevier Point of Care. 2021.)

Table 17.3 Contents of α- and Dense Granules of Platelets

α-Granules	Dense Granules
PDGF	ADP
TGFβ	ATP
Platelet factor 4	Ionized calcium
IGF 1	Serotonin
von Willebrand factor	Histamine
Thrombospondin	
Fibrinogen	
Fibronectin	
Factor 5	

other platelets. In addition to this, when platelets are activated, negatively charged phospholipids move from the inner to the outer leaflet of the membrane bilayer. This provides the negative surface required for the action of enzymes and cofactors for the coagulation system, resulting in the formation of secondary haemostatic plug.

Platelet disorders lead to defects in primary haemostasis and cause signs and symptoms that are different from those of clotting factor deficiency. Platelet disorders are characterized by **superficial bleeding,** petechiae and purpura and are associated with **prolonged BT.**

Platelet disorders can be quantitative or qualitative and can be inherited or acquired.

QUANTITATIVE PLATELET DISORDERS, THROMBOCYTOPENIA PA 21.2

Thrombocytopenia, defined as a platelet count below the normal range (<150,000 cells/mm^3), leads to defective primary haemostatic plug formation. It can stem from various immunological or nonimmunological causes. Conversely, thrombocytosis (platelet count above the normal range) may also present with functional platelet abnormalities and is associated with myeloproliferative disorders, discussed in Chapter 16.

Immunological or nonimmunological causes of thrombocytopenia can be diagnosed with routine haematology, bone marrow aspiration cytology and platelet-specific tests (Table 17.4).

Thrombocytosis, which is defined as the elevation in the platelet count above the upper limit of normal reference range (>450,000 cells/mm^3), may also be associated with platelet functional abnormalities and is discussed under myeloproliferative disorders in Chapter 16.

Some common causes of thrombocytopenia are discussed here.

IMMUNE THROMBOCYTOPENIC PURPURA

Immune thrombocytopenic purpura (ITP) is an autoantibody-mediated disease marked by peripheral platelet destruction. Life span of platelets is reduced markedly to less than 1 hour against the normal life span of 7–10 days. Based on the duration of the disease, ITP can be classified into acute and chronic forms. The aetiology of the two forms is discrete.

Acute Immune Thrombocytopenic Purpura Acute ITP is commonly a disease of childhood, with no sex predilection. Children may develop ITP at any age, but the peak incidence is noted around 1–6 years of age. ITP usually precipitates itself following 1–2 weeks of viral illness, because of the formation of antiplatelet antibodies for presumably unknown reasons. The disease is self-limited and requires only supportive treatment.

Chronic Immune Thrombocytopenic Purpura Chronic ITP is more commonly a disease of adulthood and has a

Table 17.4 Common Causes of Thrombocytopenia

Mechanism	Common Causes
Impaired production of platelets	• Drugs: alcohol, thiazides, cytotoxic drugs • Infections: HIV, measles • Nutritional deficiencies: vitamin B_{12}, folate deficiency • Bone marrow failure: aplastic anaemia • Bone marrow infiltration: leukaemia, metastasis, granulomatous disease • Ineffective haematopoiesis: myelodysplastic syndromes
Accelerated destruction of platelets	• Immune thrombocytopenic purpura • SLE • Posttransfusion autoimmune destruction • Drugs: heparin, quinidine • Disseminated intravascular coagulation • Thrombotic microangiopathies
Splenic sequestration	• Hypersplenism
Dilution of platelets	• Massive transfusion of old stored blood

SLE, systemic lupus erythematosus.

higher predilection for females. The disease is insidious in onset but persists chronically. Chronic ITP can be primary (idiopathic) or secondary, and the secondary causes are listed as follows:

Causes of secondary chronic ITP:

- Physiological states like pregnancy
- Autoimmune disorders like systemic lupus erythematosus (SLE), antiphospholipid antibody syndrome
- Chronic infections like hepatitis C, HIV infection and *Helicobacter pylori* infection
- Drugs like heparin, quinine, quinidine, nonsteroidal anti-inflammatory drugs (NSAIDs) and anticonvulsants
- Certain malignancies like chronic lymphocytic leukaemia (CLL) and other lymphoproliferative diseases

***Pathogenesis** (Fig. 17.4)* Pathogenesis of both the forms, acute and chronic ITP, is the same and discussed together. The platelets are destroyed by opsonization by antiplatelet antibodies which then undergo splenic sequestration and destruction. This results in shortened life span of platelets and a compensatory increase in the number of megakaryocytes in marrow. The antiplatelet antibodies are directed against platelet glycoprotein **GPIIb/IIIa or GPIb/IX**

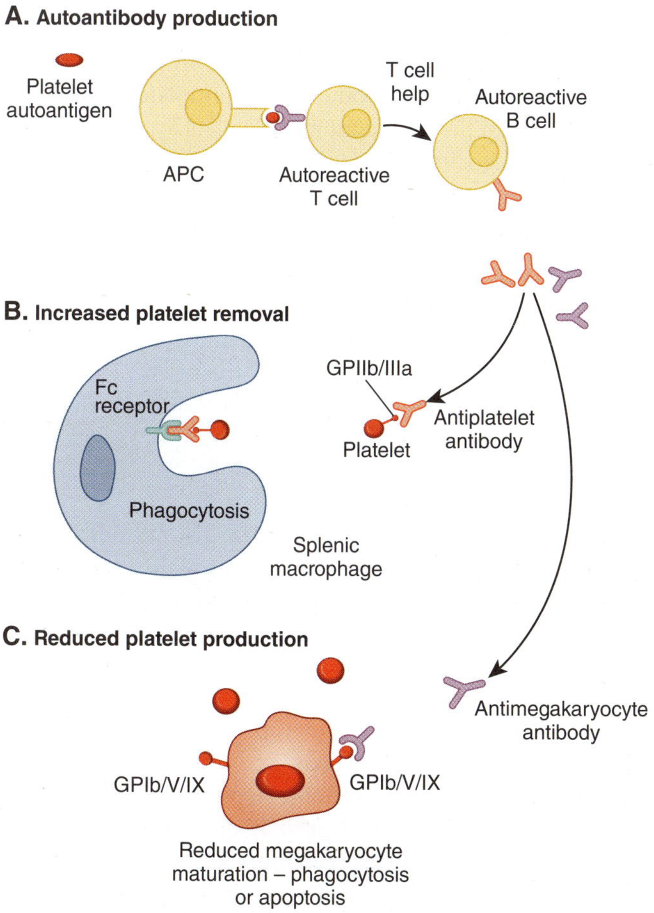

Fig. 17.4 Pathogenesis of ITP. (*Source:* From Wei A, Jackson SP. Boosting Platelet Production. Nat Med. 2008;14(9):917–918.)

complexes. In few cases, the antibodies against GPV, GPIa/IIa or GPIV have also been reported.

Role of Spleen in Immune Thrombocytopenic Purpura Spleen is the site of autoantibody production and is also the site of phagocytosis of the opsonized platelets. The slow passage of platelets through the splenic sinusoids, with a high local concentration of antibodies, and the presence of Fc-γ receptors on splenic macrophages make the spleen a unique site of platelet destruction.

Clinical Features ITP manifests as easy bruising (purpura) or as extravasated blood from capillaries into the skin and mucous membranes (petechiae). Patients also have an increased bleeding tendency. Despite the destruction of platelets by splenic macrophages, the spleen is normally not enlarged. In fact, an enlarged spleen should lead to a search for other possible causes for the thrombocytopenia as *splenomegaly excludes the diagnosis of ITP.*

Laboratory Findings and Morphology

ITP can be suspected based on the clinical findings. Morphological changes in peripheral blood, bone marrow and spleen are reported, but none of them are specific. Hence, *ITP is a diagnosis of exclusion.*

Platelet count: This is moderate to markedly reduced.

Peripheral smear (Fig. 17.5): Reduced platelets, with many being abnormally large giant platelets, are present. Smear may also show the presence of reactive/atypical lymphocytes, reflecting a recent viral illness in acute ITP.

Bone marrow: This may be normal or show increased megakaryocytes, with abnormal morphology such as large, nonlobulated single nuclei, cytoplasmic granules and cytoplasmic vacuoles.

Spleen (Fig. 17.6): Spleen is of normal size, with enlargement of follicles and congestion of sinusoids.

Serology: The presence of antiplatelet antibodies can be demonstrated on the surface of platelets or in the serum of patients.

Tests for haemostasis: BT is prolonged, whereas all the other tests are normal.

Course and Management

Acute Immune Thrombocytopenic Purpura (ITP) Patients usually spontaneously recover within 6 months. Intracranial haemorrhage might complicate the clinical course in a minority of the cases, when the platelet count drops below 10,000/μL, and half of those may be fatal. Steroids are required to control or prevent the bleeding episodes in such cases. Unfortunately, in a small percentage of children, the disease is not self-limited and progresses to chronic ITP.

Chronic Immune Thrombocytopenic Purpura (ITP) All patients respond to steroids, but most cases relapse. Patients with moderate thrombocytopenia usually need

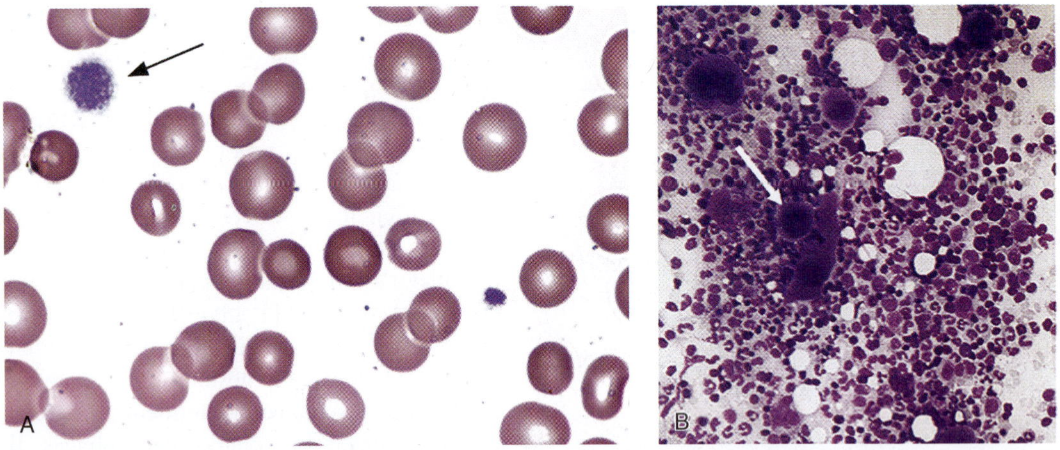

Fig. 17.5 Peripheral smear and bone marrow findings in ITP. (A) Blood smear shows large platelets. (B) Bone marrow aspirate shows increased numbers of megakaryocytes, with several being hypolobated and immature. (*Source:* From J. Paul Scott, Veronica H. Flood. Nelson Textbook of Pediatrics, 2-Volume Set. Elsevier. 2020.)

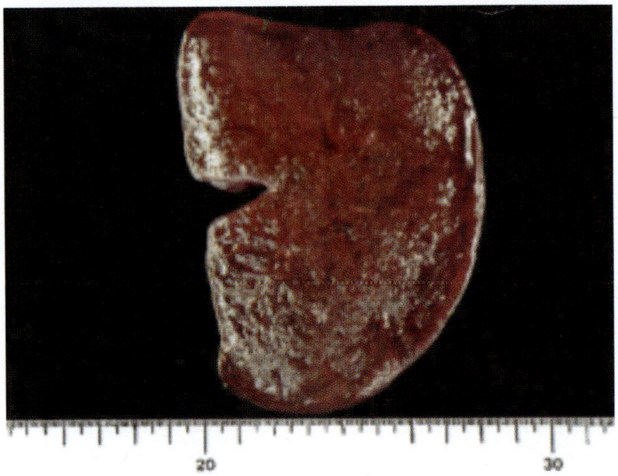

Fig. 17.6 Morphology of spleen in ITP. (*Source:* From Min Ju Kim, Kyoung Won Kim. Abdominal Imaging. Elsevier. 2017.)

only close follow-up and have a spontaneous recovery over a period of a year. Splenectomy may be indicated in patients with severe thrombocytopenia, but complications of splenectomy persist.

Immunomodulatory agents such as anti-CD20 may be beneficial in patients who fail to respond to splenectomy or in whom splenectomy is contraindicated.

Treatment with thrombopoietin mimetics is also effective by stimulating the production of platelets and improving the count.

HIV-Associated Thrombocytopenia Thrombocytopenia is one of the most common haematological manifestations in HIV-infected patients. Although often asymptomatic, the thrombocytopenia may be associated with a variety of bleeding abnormalities. Megakaryocytes are easy targets for HIV because these possess CD4 and CXCR4 receptors on their cell surfaces which serve as attachment sites for the virus, enabling it to enter and infect the cells. Low platelet count is further augmented by peripheral destruction of platelets.

The following is the list of mechanisms causing low platelet count in HIV infection:

- HIV-infected megakaryocytes undergo premature death by apoptosis.
- HIV infection suppresses platelet production in the marrow.
- B-cell hyperplasia and dysregulation in HIV infection result in the production of antiplatelet antibodies and in the destruction of platelets by opsonization and phagocytosis.
- Immune complex deposition (mechanisms discussed in Chapter 6) on platelets causes accelerated destruction.

HIV-associated thrombocytopenia responds well to zidovudine or antiretroviral combination therapy. Steroids, intravenous immunoglobulin and splenectomy are considered as secondary choices of treatment. Decisively, thrombocytopenia in HIV-infected patients may be treated with pharmacological stimulation of megakaryocytopoiesis.

Drug-Induced Thrombocytopenia Thrombocytopenia is a recognized side effect of treatment with a wide range of drugs. Though most cases of drug-induced thrombocytopenia are mild, some are complicated by life-threatening bleeding symptoms.

Heparin-Induced Thrombocytopenia Heparin is widely used for thromboprophylaxis and treatment of many medical and surgical conditions. Heparin-induced thrombocytopenia (HIT) is a potentially devastating immune-mediated adverse drug reaction. It is caused by the emergence of antibodies that activate platelets in the presence of unfractionated heparin. It is technically the most common cause of drug-induced thrombocytopenia, but the reduction in platelets is rarely sufficient to induce bleeding. However, thrombosis caused by the activation of platelets may affect various organs and lead to significant morbidity and mortality if unrecognized.

HIT has a unique pathogenesis and may present in two distinct forms: types I and II.

HIT type I, also called **nonimmune** heparin-associated thrombocytopenia, affects 10% of patients, usually within the first 48–72 hours of heparin administration. It is characterized by mild and transient thrombocytopenia without an increased risk of thrombosis. It is a nonimmunological response to heparin caused by the direct interaction between heparin and the circulating platelets, resulting in platelet clumping and sequestration. No diagnostic test is required to diagnose HIT type I, and most cases resolve spontaneously after discontinuation of heparin or even while receiving heparin.

HIT type II, also simply referred to as HIT, is caused by the formation of antibodies that activate platelets following administration of heparin. The principal antigen is a complex of heparin and platelet factor 4 (PF4), a tiny positively charged molecule found in the α-granules of platelets with uncertain function. Binding of heparin with PF4 induces a conformational change and the complex becomes immunogenic, resulting in the generation of antibodies against heparin–PF4 complex (HIT antibodies). The antibody interaction with the antigen forms heparin–PF4–IgG complex. This complex then activates platelets through its Fc receptors, resulting in the release of prothrombotic platelet-derived microparticles, leading to intravascular thrombosis, platelet consumption and thrombocytopenia.

Up to 8% of patients receiving heparin are at risk of developing HIT antibodies, but only 1%–5% of patients receiving heparin will progress to develop HIT with thrombocytopenia and one-third of those with thrombocytopenia develop thrombosis. This risk is much lesser with the administration of low-molecular-weight heparin.

THROMBOTIC MICROANGIOPATHIES

TMAs are characterized by thrombi formation in small vessels because of excessive platelet activation triggered by endothelial injury. This category includes diseases like haemolytic uraemic syndrome (HUS), thrombotic thrombocytopenic purpura (TTP), atypical haemolytic uraemic syndrome (aHUS), disseminated intravascular coagulation (DIC), malignant hypertension and antiphospholipid antibody syndrome.

The classical TMAs, HUS and TTP, are described here.

Though both the diseases are characterized by the presence of microvascular thrombi, microangiopathic haemolytic anaemia and multiorgan dysfunction, their aetiopathogenesis are different and hence discussed separately.

Haemolytic Uraemic Syndrome HUS commonly affects children, whereas adults, if affected, have worse outcomes. This disorder is characterized by the triad of haemolytic anaemia, uraemia and thrombocytopenia. Initial symptoms include bloody diarrhoea, fever, vomiting and fatigue. Thrombocytopenia and renal symptoms become prominent as the diarrhoea improves.

Aetiopathogenesis Most cases that occur following infectious diarrhoea are caused by a specific type of ***Escherichia coli called O157:H7***. Other bacteria such as *Streptococcus pneumoniae*, *Shigella* or *Salmonella* can also precipitate the disease, though uncommonly. The underlying mechanism involves the release of Shiga-like toxin by the bacteria into the systemic circulation. The toxin causes endothelial cell damage, especially in the microcirculation, and commonly affects the glomerulus. The damaged endothelial cells release cytokines that promote vasoconstriction and platelet microthrombus formation at the site of damage. The glomerular filtration rate decreases because of the end-organ damage caused by the microthrombi, resulting in uraemia. The red blood cells (RBCs) get mechanically destroyed when they pass through the platelet microthrombi, in the microcirculation, resulting in haemolytic anaemia. Thrombocytopenia occurs because of the consumption of platelets in the microthrombi.

Clinical features Bloody diarrhoea lasting about 5–10 days precedes the onset of symptoms. The classical symptoms are because of the following triad:

- Thrombocytopenia: mucosal bleeding, petechiae and purpura
- Microangiopathic haemolytic anaemia: fatigue, dyspnoea, pallor and jaundice
- Uraemia: haematuria, oliguria and anuria

Morphology

Morphological features of HUS and TTP are similar. Peripheral smear shows the presence of **schistocytes** (up to 10% of RBCs) along with the other features of haemolytic anaemia (Fig. 17.7).

Treatment involves supportive care and may include haemodialysis, steroids, blood transfusions or plasmapheresis. Many patients recover completely, whereas up to 25% acquire renal problems, which in less than 5% of patients become fatal.

Atypical Haemolytic Uremic Syndrome This uncommon disorder with poor outcome is a variant of HUS and is caused by uncontrolled complement activation by the alternate pathway along with the formation of microvascular thrombi. This dysregulation is due to mutations in the genes that encode complement regulatory proteins, **factor H, factor I, complement 3, factor B,** thrombomodulin or the presence of anti-FH antibody, resulting in unwarranted activation of the complement system.

aHUS presents at any age and is of acute onset in 20% of cases. The disease is precipitated by pregnancy, viral

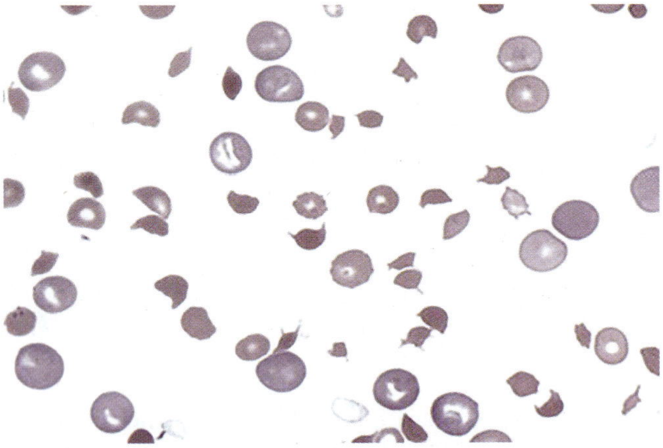

Fig. 17.7 Peripheral smear picture of HUS and TTP. Peripheral blood smear shows numerous schistocytes, red blood cell fragments and polychromatophilic RBCs. Platelets are absent. (*Source:* From Elizabeth A. Morgan. High-Yield Hematopathology. Elsevier. 2013.)

illness and sepsis. It presents as a systemic disorder; extrarenal features are seen in 25% of cases, and a catastrophic presentation with multiorgan involvement occurs in 5% of patients.

Therapy of aHUS is supportive, with attention to management of acute kidney injury and systemic complications.

Thrombotic Thrombocytopenic Purpura TTP is a type of thrombotic microangiopathy which is characterized by the systemic deposition of platelet thrombi, with an abundance of vWF in the microcirculation. This is caused by the deficiency of **ADAMTS13** (**A D**isintegrin **A**nd **M**etalloproteinase with **T**hrombo**S**pondin type 1 motif, member **13**) in the circulation. The deficiency of the enzyme may be congenital or due to antibodies inhibiting its activity.

Pathogenesis *(Fig. 17.8)* ADAMTS13 is a metalloprotease, also called vWF-cleaving protease, and is primarily

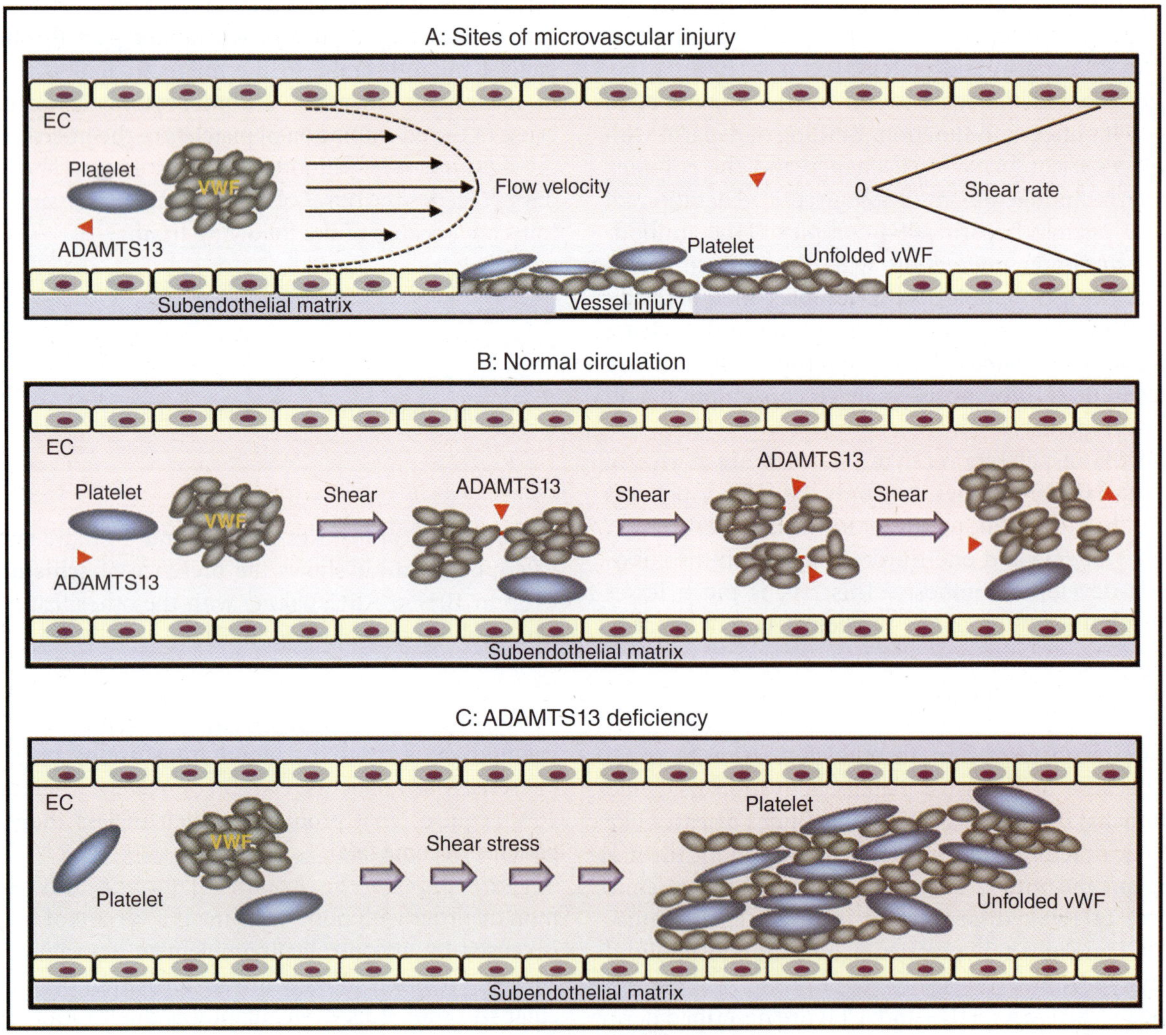

Fig. 17.8 Pathogenesis of microvascular thrombosis in thrombotic thrombocytopenic purpura. (A) At sites of vessel injury, von Willebrand factor binds to the exposed subendothelial collagen and becomes rapidly unfolded and activated by the shear stress. It provides the substrate for platelet adhesion. (B) In the circulation, von Willebrand factor is intermittently and partially unfolded by shear stress and gets cleaved by ADAMTS13, a plasma metalloprotease. This prevents thrombus extension. (C) Without proteolysis by ADAMTS13, von Willebrand factor is gradually unfolded and activated by shear stress, leading to von Willebrand factor–platelet aggregation and intravascular thrombosis. ADAMTS13, a disintegrin and metalloprotease with thrombospondin repeat, member 13; EC, endothelial cell; VWF, von Willebrand factor. (*Source:* From Han-Mou Tsai. The American Journal of Medicine. Elsevier. 2013.)

synthesized in the liver. The function of ADAMTS13 is to cleave von Willebrand multimers into smaller proteins and prevent them from triggering platelet aggregation. The deficiency of ADAMTS13 leaves the hyperadhesive vWF unchecked under high shear stress in the microcirculation, resulting in the formation of excessive and unwanted platelet thrombi. The deficiency is caused by inherited mutations of its gene, because of autoantibodies against ADAMTS13 or less commonly because of acquired inactivating mutations of ADAMTS13.

Clinical Features The classical symptoms are because of the following pentad:

- Fever
- Thrombocytopenia: mucosal bleeding, petechiae and purpura
- Microangiopathic haemolytic anaemia: fatigue, dyspnoea, pallor and jaundice
- Uraemia: haematuria, oliguria and anuria
- Neurological symptoms

TTP is an important differential diagnosis in patients presenting with microangiopathic haemolytic anaemia and thrombocytopenia. Early diagnosis of TTP is crucial, as untreated ITP can be fatal. More than 80% of patients are treated with plasma exchange, which removes the autoantibodies against TTP and replenishes uninhibited, functional ADAMTS13 enzyme from the donor plasma. The introduction of caplacizumab, an innovative anti-vWF nanobody, has revolutionized the treatment of TTP. Caplacizumab rapidly inhibits the interaction between ultra-large vWF multimers and platelets, effectively reducing the formation of microthrombi. This therapeutic advancement has demonstrated a significant reduction in morbidity and mortality in TTP patients, marking a substantial progress in the management of TTP.

QUALITATIVE PLATELET DISORDERS

Abnormal Bleeding due to Platelet Functional Disorders

Qualitative platelet disorders, either inherited or acquired, lead to varied bleeding episodes, diagnosed by history, physical examination, and prolonged BT in the presence of normal platelet counts. Disorders include adhesion, aggregation, storage pool, release reaction and signal transduction abnormalities.

The diseases are classified as disorders of the following events (Table 17.5):

- Adhesion
- Aggregation
- Storage pool
- Platelet release reaction
- Signal transduction

Bernard–Soulier syndrome (BSS) and Glanzmann thrombasthenia (GT), though very rare diseases, have given clear insights into platelet functions and are discussed as follows (Fig. 17.9).

Bernard–Soulier Syndrome BSS is a rare autosomal recessive bleeding disorder caused by the qualitative or quantitative defect of platelet glycoprotein complex **GPIb/V/IX**, which is the receptor complex for vWF. The presence of GPIb on platelets is essential for the normal adhesion of platelets to the subendothelial collagen. Patients with BSS may present with mild to severe bleeding tendency.

In BSS, BT is prolonged, with normal or low platelet counts, increased mean platelet volume (MPV) and more specifically enlarged platelets (giant platelets) in the peripheral smear.

Glanzmann Thrombasthenia GT is a rare inherited bleeding disorder caused by the deficiency of the platelet glycoprotein GPIIb/IIIa complex. Platelets do not aggregate to any aggregating agents except ristocetin.

Table 17.5 Common Causes of Qualitative Platelets Defects

Category of the Disorder	Common Inherited Causes	Common Acquired Causes
Defective adhesion	von Willebrand disease Bernard–Soulier syndrome	Myeloproliferative disorders
Defective aggregation	Glanzmann thrombasthenia Congenital afibrinogenaemia	Lymphoproliferative disorders
Storage pool disorders	Hermansky–Pudlak syndrome Wiskott–Aldrich syndrome Chediak–Higashi syndrome	Multiple myeloma Chronic liver disease Cardiopulmonary bypass
Granule and secretory defects	Storage pool disease Quebec platelet disorder	Uraemia Aspirin and NSAIDs
Signal transduction defects	G protein defects Thromboxane synthesis defects Cytoskeleton defects	

NSAID, nonsteroidal anti-inflammatory drug.

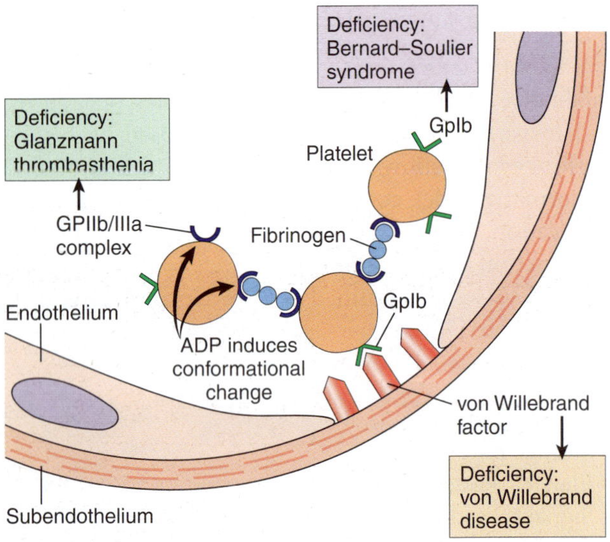

Fig. 17.9 Pathogenesis of Bernard–Soulier syndrome and Glanzmann thrombasthenia. (*Source:* From Peter Pytel, Douglas C. Anthony. Robbins & Cotran Pathologic Basis of Disease. Elsevier. 2021.)

GT is associated with normal platelet count and size, but the BT is prolonged. Platelet function studies highlight the abnormality at the level of aggregation.

Thrombocytopenia is a common event we come across every day and its evaluation is shown in Flowchart 17.3.

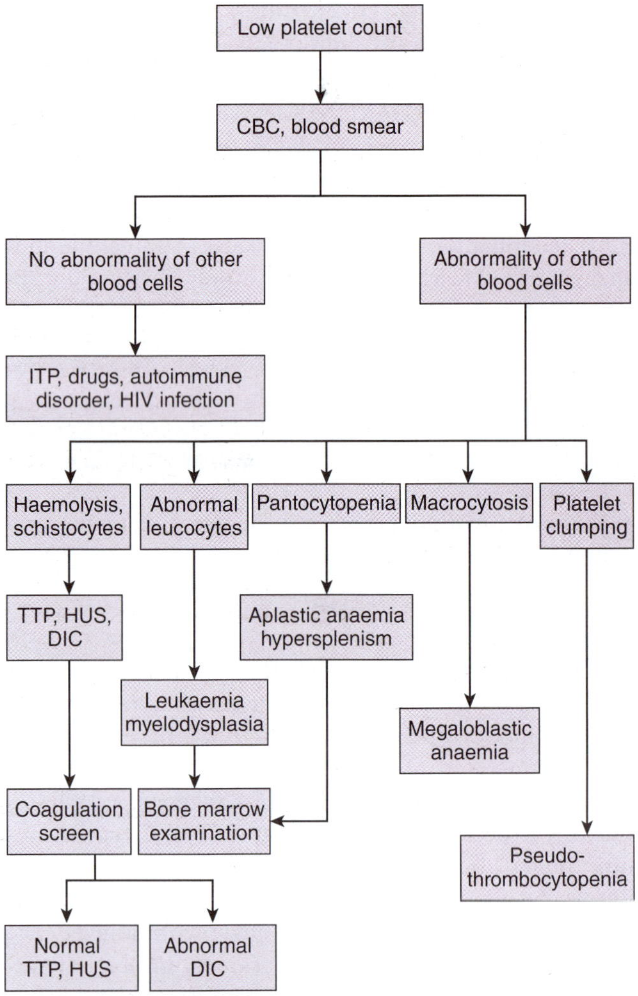

Flowchart 17.3 Laboratory approach to a case of thrombotic thrombocytopenia purpura.

BLEEDING DISORDERS DUE TO DEFECTS IN CLOTTING FACTORS

Haemophilia A

PA 21.2

Haemophilia A, also called factor VIII deficiency, is the most common congenital bleeding disorder associated with life-threatening complications.

Genetics It is inherited as an X-linked recessive trait, thus affecting males and homozygous females. Haemophilia A has been called a 'Royal disease' because the haemophilia gene, acquired as a spontaneous mutation by Queen Victoria, the Queen of England in the 18th century, was passed on to her descendants, affecting members of the Royal family.

The disease is caused by the mutations in factor VIII, an important factor in the coagulation cascade. The gene factor for factor VIII is a large gene located on a fragile region of the X chromosome. The most common mutation associated with severe haemophilia is inversion **of intron 22** and less commonly involves point mutations. In about 25%–30% of the patients, no family history can be detected, indicating new mutations as the cause of the disease. It is characterized by mild, moderate or severe bleeding episodes.

Pathogenesis Factor VIII is a plasma protein produced by the liver which circulates in the blood bound to its carrier protein, vWF. vWF stabilizes factor VIII and maintains its half-life at 8–12 hours, whereas the half-life of unbound factor VIII is only 2.4 hours.

Clinical Features Clinical severity is dependent on the level of factor VIII activity and can be divided into three categories:

1. **Mild:** >5% activity, >0.05 IU/mL, incidence 30%–40%
2. **Moderate:** 1%–5% activity, 0.01–0.05 IU/mL, incidence 10%
3. **Severe:** <1% activity, <0.01 IU/mL, incidence 50%

Bleeding may vary from posttraumatic or postoperative to spontaneous, depending on the severity of factor VIII deficiency. Spontaneous bleeding in haemophiliac patients takes the form of haemarthroses, bleeding into the major joints. Recurrent haemarthroses lead to progressive deformities that could result in crippling. Deep bleeding into muscles and the central nervous system may also occur. Superficial bleeding in the form of petechiae that are commonly seen in cases with platelet disorders is characteristically absent.

Laboratory Tests

- Platelet count – normal
- BT – normal
- PT – normal
- PTT – prolonged
- Factor VIII–specific assay – levels reduced

Introduction of recombinant factor VIII has been a breakthrough in the management of haemophilia A. Up until a decade ago, haemophiliac patients were treated with unscreened plasma-derived factor VIII, following which many of them contracted HIV infection. Nowadays, haemophiliac patients are treated with recombinant factor VIII infusions, which eliminates the risk of HIV transmission but about 15% of such patients develop antibodies against factor VIII, which is a therapeutic challenge.

Haemophilia B, Factor IX Deficiency, Christmas Disease PA 21.2

Haemophilia B, a bleeding disorder that clinically resembles haemophilia A, is due to the deficiency of factor IX that functions along with factor VIII to activate factor X in the coagulation cascade. This disease is also transmitted as an X-linked recessive trait with variable clinical severity. Laboratory tests are similar to haemophilia A, except for the normal levels of factor VIII and reduced factor IX in factor-specific assays. Patients are treated with recombinant factor IX.

von Willebrand Disease

von Willebrand disease (vWD) is the most common inherited bleeding disorder. It is a clinically heterogeneous haemorrhagic disorder caused by the deficiency or dysfunction of vWF. Unlike haemophilia, vWD affects both males and females equally, but the disease may be more pronounced in females because of menstrual blood loss.

The disease is named after the Finnish doctor, Erik von Willebrand, who was the first to describe inherited bleeding disorder in the families in Aland Islands. Though he could not identify the actual cause for the disease, he distinguished it from haemophilia and other bleeding disorders.

Role of von Willebrand Factor in Haemostasis (Fig. 17.10)

vWF is a large glycoprotein that circulates in the blood at low concentration. The gene for vWF is located on chromosome 12. vWF exists as a series of multimers varying in molecular weights. The building blocks of the multimers are dimers, held together by disulphide bonds.

When the need for its activity arises, it is released from the Weibel–Palade bodies in the endothelial cells and α-granules of platelets, where it is normally stored. Two major functions of vWF that help to maintain haemostasis are as follows:

1. vWF mediates the adhesion of platelets to the subendothelial collagen as a first step in primary haemostatic plug formation.
2. It binds and stabilizes factor VIII, prolonging its half-life.

Role of vWF in platelet adhesion is described in Chapter 4. Its role in stabilizing factor VIII is described here.

The main function of vWF is to bind noncovalently with the inactive factor VIII in circulation. In its unbound form, factor VIII rapidly degrades because of the degradative effects of protein C. vWF factor when bound to factor VIII stabilizes it in the circulation and localizes factor VIII to sites of platelet plug and subsequent clot formation.

Classification of von Willebrand Disease vWD is classified into types 1, 2 and 3 with primary and secondary classification as shown in (Table 17.6).

Acquired von Willebrand Disease This is a rare disorder that results from the development of **antibodies to vWF.** This disorder may arise in a variety of settings including lymphoproliferative, myeloproliferative cardiovascular

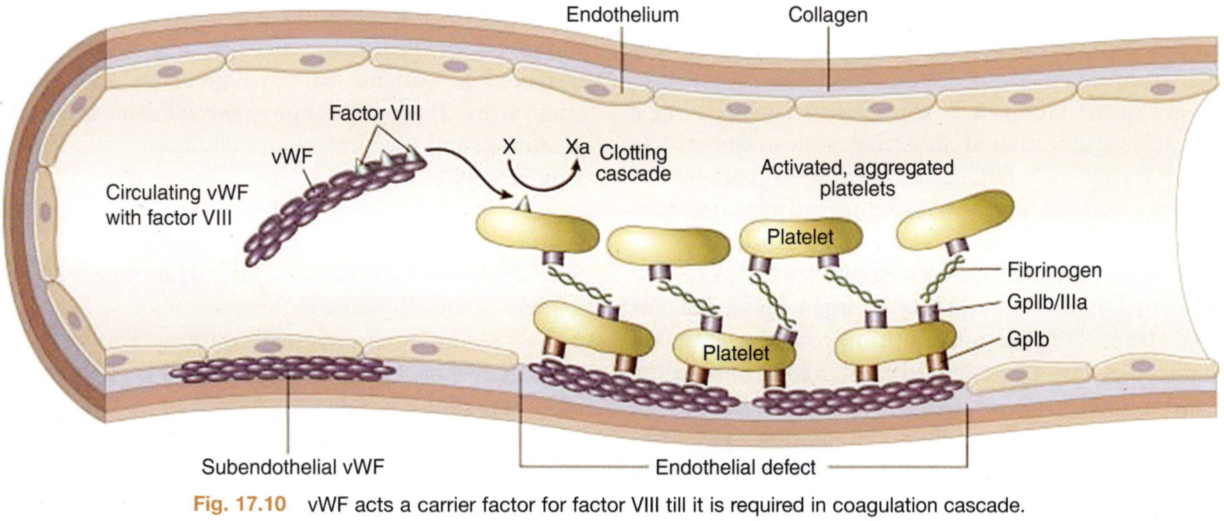

Fig. 17.10 vWF acts a carrier factor for factor VIII till it is required in coagulation cascade.

Table 17.6 von Willebrand Disease Types

Classification	Types	Defect
Primary classification	Type 1	Partial quantitative deficiency of vWF
	Type 2	Qualitative vWF defects
	Type 3	Complete quantitative deficiency of vWF
Secondary classification of type 2	Type 2A	Decreased vWF-dependent platelet adhesion without large multimers
	Type 2B	Increased affinity for platelet GPIb
	Type 2M	Decreased vWF-dependent platelet adhesion with large multimers
	Type 2N	Markedly decreased binding affinity for factor VIII

vWF, von Willebrand factor.

and autoimmune diseases and typically alleviates with the treatment of the underlying disease.

Laboratory findings

- Platelet count: normal
- BT: prolonged
- PT: normal
- aPTT: prolonged
- Ristocetin cofactor levels: reduced
- vWF-specific assay: reduced

For most affected individuals, vWD is a mild and docile and clinically severe haemorrhage manifests only as a result of trauma or invasive procedures. In vWD types II and III, bleeding may be severe and potentially life-threatening.

Levels of vWF normally increase with age.

The main treatment of patients with vWD is dependent on the type, clinical manifestation and severity of the disease is treated with desmopressin, recombinant vWF or vWF/factor VIII concentrates.

DISSEMINATED INTRAVASCULAR COAGULATION PA 21.4

DIC is a complex, acquired medical syndrome, which results from an aberrant activation of the coagulation pathways in the blood. It is not a disease in itself but a secondary complication arising from various underlying medical conditions. DIC is marked by a paradoxical occurrence of both excessive clotting and bleeding tendencies within the body. This condition can lead to the widespread formation of microthrombi, which can disrupt normal blood flow and lead to organ dysfunction or failure. Hence, DIC is a **consumption coagulopathy** that is characterized by a paradoxical combination of bleeding and thrombosis. The symptoms of DIC are often those of the underlying inciting condition. In addition, symptoms of thrombosis, embolism, organ dysfunction or bleeding may be present.

AETIOLOGY AND PREVALENCE

DIC is typically a secondary condition, arising as a complication from a range of clinical scenarios. It is estimated that around 1% of patients in hospital settings might develop DIC during their stay. Conditions like Gram-negative sepsis and adult respiratory distress syndrome (ARDS) are particularly prone to leading to DIC, with up to 20% of these patients developing this complication.

ACUTE VERSUS CHRONIC DISSEMINATED INTRAVASCULAR COAGULATION

DIC can manifest in two forms: acute and chronic.

Acute DIC: This form is usually triggered by a sudden exposure of the bloodstream to procoagulants, such as tissue factor or tissue thromboplastin, often found in conditions like sepsis or trauma. This leads to a rapid and overwhelming activation of the coagulation cascade, causing a severe consumption coagulopathy that can lead to life-threatening haemorrhages.

Chronic DIC: In contrast, chronic DIC is a more compensated form of the condition, where there is continuous or intermittent exposure to procoagulants. This form is often observed in patients with malignancies or large aortic aneurysms. The compensatory mechanisms are not overwhelmed, and the clinical and laboratory manifestations may be subtle.

Pathogenesis (Fig. 17.11 and Flowchart 17.4)

Several diseases, as listed in Table 17.7, may lead to DIC via one of the following pathways:

1. Systemic inflammatory response: This leads to the activation of cytokines, which then trigger the coagulation cascade.
2. Release of procoagulant material: The presence of procoagulant material in the circulation can lead to coagulation activation.

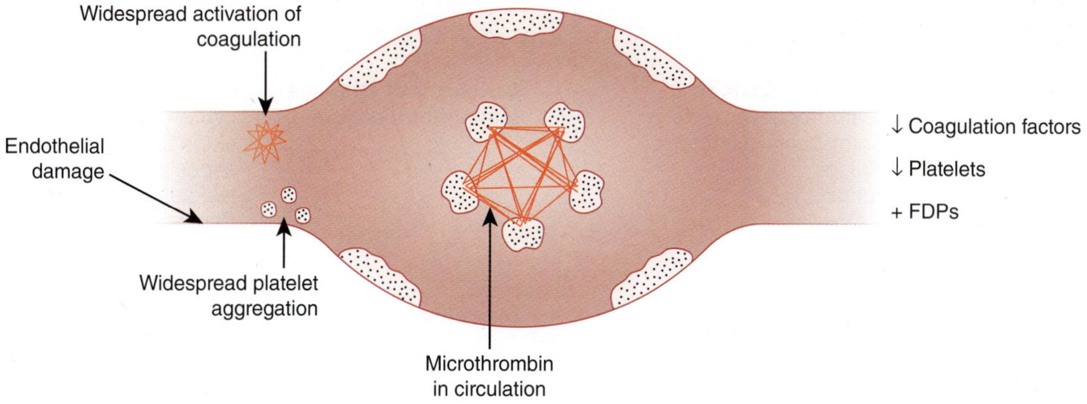

Fig. 17.11 Microthrombin formation in circulation in DIC.

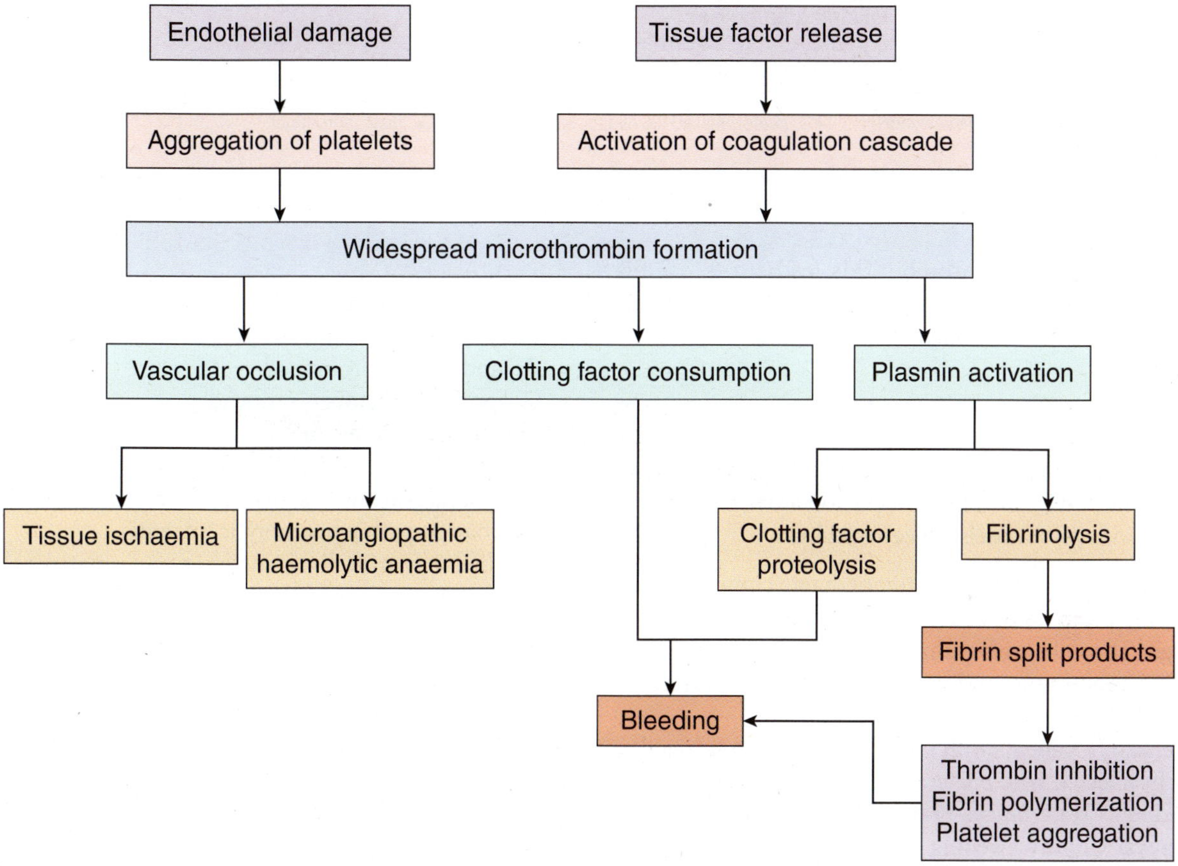

Flowchart 17.4 Pathogenesis of DIC.

The core mechanisms involved in DIC include:

- Increased thrombin generation: Predominantly mediated by the extrinsic pathway of coagulation, leading to widespread thrombin formation.
- Suppression of anticoagulant pathways: Key components like antithrombin, protein C, and protein S levels are reduced, exacerbating the situation.
- Impaired fibrinolytic pathways: Initially, there is an increase in fibrinolytic activity, followed by a suppression, mainly because of an increase in plasminogen activator inhibitor-1 (PAI-1).
- Activation of inflammatory pathways: The interaction between coagulation and inflammation is complex, with inflammation triggering coagulation, and the resultant thrombin exacerbating inflammatory activities.

Clinical Consequences The consequences of DIC are primarily twofold:

a. Consumption coagulopathy: This involves the consumption of clotting factors and platelets, leading to haemorrhagic diathesis.

Table 17.7 List of Diseases Commonly Associated With DIC

Category of Disease	Common Causes	Category of Disease	Common Causes
Sepsis	Gram-negative bacteria Gram-positive bacteria Viruses Fungi Protozoa Rickettsiae	**Malignant tumours**	Lymphoproliferative and myeloproliferative malignancies, especially acute promyelocytic leukaemia Pancreatic carcinoma Mucin-secreting carcinomas of the GI tract and ovary
Tissue injury	Burns Trauma[a] Snake envenomation	**Miscellaneous**	Pancreatitis Fat embolism Near drowning Acute haemolytic transfusion reaction ARDS Aortic aneurysm Prosthetic devices
Obstetric complications	Abruptio placentae Retained dead fetus Preeclampsia Eclampsia Septic abortion Amniotic fluid embolism Acute peripartum haemorrhage Acute fatty liver of pregnancy		

ARDS, adult respiratory distress syndrome; DIC, disseminated intravascular coagulation; GI, gastrointestinal.
[a]Especially neurotrauma.

b. Formation of microthrombi: This leads to ischaemia and failure of multiple organs, and is also responsible for microangiopathic haemolytic anaemia.

Morphology

Although any organ can be affected, the organs commonly affected by thrombus occlusion are brain, heart, lungs, kidneys, adrenals, spleen and liver.

Brain: Microinfarcts with haemorrhagic complication that may progress to neurological sequelae.
Lungs: Thrombi with pulmonary oedema, fibrin and hyaline membrane and resemble clinical manifestations of ARDS.
Adrenals: In patients with meningococcaemia, adrenals may be affected with bilateral massive haemorrhage, referred to as Waterhouse–Friderichsen syndrome.
Kidneys: Cloudy swelling of renal tubular epithelial cells in mild cases to bilateral renal cortical necrosis in severe cases.

Clinical Features Patients present with the symptoms of the underlying disease process. In acute DIC, onset is abrupt and fulminant, whereas in chronic DIC, onset is insidious. In cases due to obstetric complications, the disorder tends to be reversible if appropriately managed. Symptoms depend on the systems affected. In addition, there is typical bleeding in the form of petechiae, purpura and ecchymosis and bleeding through gingiva and mucosa. In chronic DIC, thrombotic complications dominate.

Laboratory Findings

- Haemoglobin – reduced
- Platelet count – reduced, not less than 30,000/mm^3
- PT and PTT – prolonged
- Coagulation factors – reduced
- Fibrinogen – reduced
- D-dimer and other FDPs – elevated
- Peripheral smear – schistocytes are seen because of microangiopathic haemolytic anaemia
- Cardiac enzymes, liver enzymes and creatinine – elevated in multiorgan failure

PT, aPTT, fibrinogen, platelet count and antithrombin levels should be serially monitored.

Treatment Treatment strategies focus on managing the underlying disease and replacing consumed coagulation factors and platelets.

Maintaining fibrinogen levels and replacing consumed coagulation factors and platelets are critical. Treatment may include transfusions of cryoprecipitate, fresh frozen plasma, and platelets, along with heparinization in cases with thrombosis.

The prognosis of DIC varies widely and is mainly dependent on the underlying cause of the syndrome.

VITAMIN K DEFICIENCY PA 21.5

Vitamin K is an essential, lipid-soluble vitamin that plays a major role in the production of coagulation factors. It is present in green leafy vegetables and oils such as olive, soybean, cottonseed and canola oils. There are three main types of vitamin K: K1, which is derived from plants; K2, which is derived from intestinal flora; and K3, which is synthetic and used for treatment.

Role of vitamin K in haemostasis:

1. Vitamin K is required for the synthesis of four clotting factors in the liver: **factors II, VII, IX and X.** Vitamin K acts as a cofactor for the γ-glutamyl carboxylase enzyme. γ-Carboxylation of these factors is essential for them to bind to ionic calcium in haemostasis (Fig. 17.12).
2. It is essential for the production of two anticoagulant factors: **protein C and protein S.**
3. It is required for the γ-carboxylation of osteocalcin, which is required for bone matrix synthesis.

Vitamin K deficiency can affect patients of any age but most often affects infants, especially preterm infants because of their sterile gut and absence of microbiota, which is normally the chief source of vitamin K. The common causes of vitamin K deficiency are chronic illness, malnutrition, chronic alcoholism, intestinal resection, chronic parenteral nutrition, malabsorption syndromes, cholestatic disease, inflammatory bowel disease and various drugs.

Clinical Features

The clinical findings of vitamin K deficiency are evident only if **hypoprothrombinaemia** is present. Bleeding is the predominant symptom, which is often evident in posttraumatic cases but can present spontaneously as well. Easy bruising is a typical finding.

Complications associated with vitamin K deficiency vary according to the age of onset. In newborns, it causes haemorrhagic disease of newborn, resulting in intracranial bleeding. Because vitamin K is required for bone matrix synthesis, osteoporosis is also associated with vitamin K deficiency.

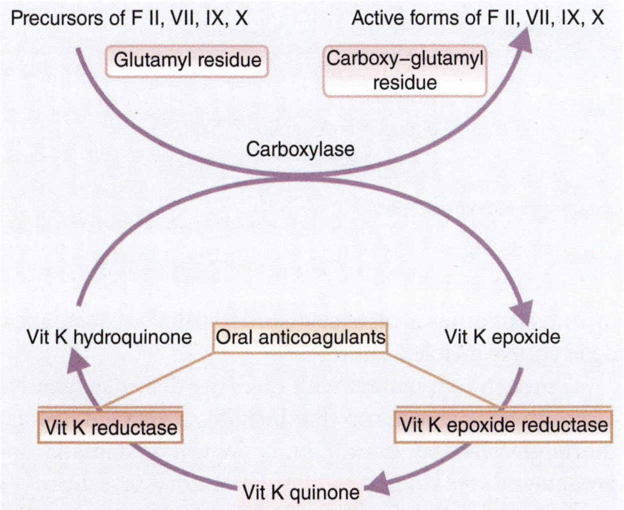

Fig. 17.12 Vitamin K–dependent γ-carboxylation of clotting factors and the mechanism of action of oral anticoagulants.

Laboratory Investigations

- BT – normal
- PT – prolonged
- aPTT – prolonged
- Serum vitamin K – reduced
- Des-γ-carboxy prothrombin (DCP) – elevated

Though vitamin K–dependent factors take part in the intrinsic, extrinsic and common pathways, factor VII of the extrinsic pathway has the shortest half-life, making prolonged PT an early marker of vitamin K deficiency. A clearly prolonged PT (INR > 3.5) along with normal levels of fibrinogen and platelet count is highly suggestive of vitamin K deficiency–related bleeding. Levels of specific vitamin K–dependent factors (factors II, VII, IX, X) are required for confirmation of the diagnosis.

The reduced levels of the factors are rapidly corrected with the parenteral administration of vitamin K.

PLATELET VERSUS CLOTTING DISORDERS (TABLE 17.8) PA 21.3

There are significant differences in history and clinical features of bleeding due to platelet or vascular disorders and disorders of coagulation which help in choosing the right battery of investigations.

APPROACH TO A PATIENT WITH BLEEDING DISORDER (FLOWCHART 17.5)

Diagnosing a bleeding disorder involves a detailed history, thorough physical examination, and laboratory investigations to determine the nature of the bleeding and to guide management. It is crucial to differentiate between platelet disorders and coagulation defects to plan appropriate treatments.

Careful History Taking

The following definitive points must be noted in history taking:

- Bleeding from childhood or recent onset?
- Bleeding – superficial or deep?
- Past history of transfusion, minor or major surgeries?
- Menstrual history in females
- Drug history
- Family history of bleeding disorder
- Easy bruising or posttraumatic bleeding?

Clinical Examination

A careful clinical examination is a must to establish the diagnosis of a bleeding disorder.

The purpose of clinical examination is to assess the site and severity of the bleeding. Often a complete history taking and careful physical examination will help to identify

Table 17.8 Differences Between Platelet and Clotting Factor Disorders

Feature	Platelet or Vessel Wall Disorder	Coagulation Disorder
Positive family history	Rare (except in vWD and hereditary haemorrhagic telangiectasia)	Common
Sex of the patient	Presentations are relatively more common in females	Up to 90% of inherited forms occur in males
Petechiae	Characteristic	Rare
Superficial ecchymosis	Small and multiple ones are characteristic	Large and solitary ones are characteristic
Deep dissecting haematomas	Rare	Characteristic
Haemarthrosis	Rare	Characteristic
Delayed bleeding (recurrence of bleeding from the same site, hours or days following injury)	Rare	Common
Bleeding from superficial cuts	Often profuse	Minimal and persistent

vWD, von Willebrand disease.

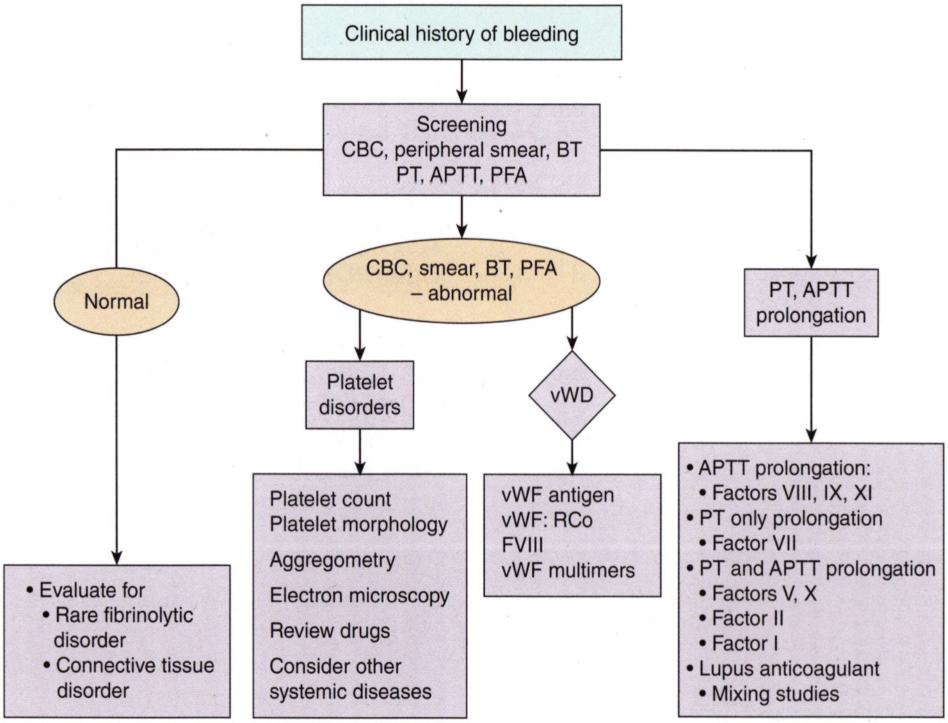

Flowchart 17.5 Approach to a case of bleeding disorder.

the haemostatic disorder with at least 90% accuracy. It should enable categorization of the disorder as inherited or acquired and the possibility of a systemic illness.

Laboratory Assessment

Careful and complete clinical examination allows the selection of appropriate plan for laboratory investigation. For every phase of haemostasis, screening tests that help in differentiating a platelet disorder from a coagulation defect are available (Table 17.9).

Approach to a patient with bleeding disorder requires a comprehensive workup that includes a detailed history, thorough physical examination, logical systematic approach and discriminate use of laboratory investigations to arrive at the diagnosis, to assess the severity and to plan the management.

Table 17.9 Commonly Done Tests for Haemostasis and the Common Disorders Associated With Their Abnormalities

Test	Probable Clinical Conditions
Prolongation of PT	Factor VIII deficiency Early oral anticoagulation therapy
Prolongation of aPTT	Deficiency of factors involved in the intrinsic or common pathway, von Willebrand disease Lupus anticoagulant
Prolongation of PT and aPTT	Deficiency of factors involved in the common pathway Oral anticoagulants Vitamin K deficiency Liver disease
Prolongation of PT, aPTT and TT	Fibrinogen deficiency Dysfibrinogenaemia Liver disease Heparin
Prolongation of BT with abnormal platelet function tests	Platelet function defects von Willebrand disease

aPTT, activated partial thromboplastin time; BT, bleeding time; PT, prothrombin time; TT, thrombin time.

SELF-ASSESSMENT

Multiple Choice Questions

1. What is the normal range for prothrombin time (PT)?
   A. 4–10 minutes
   B. 10–14 seconds
   C. 30–40 seconds
   D. 12–14 seconds
2. Which of the following is a characteristic feature of immune thrombocytopenic purpura (ITP)?
   A. Enlarged spleen
   B. Increased bleeding tendency
   C. Normal platelet count
   D. Shortened clotting time
3. Vitamin K is essential for the synthesis of which clotting factors?
   A. II, V, VIII and X
   B. II, VII, IX and X
   C. I, II, III and IV
   D. V, VII, IX and XII
4. Which of the following factors is deficient in haemophilia A?
   A. Factor VIII
   B. Factor IX
   C. Factor XI
   D. Factor V
5. Activated partial thromboplastin time (aPTT) tests the function of which pathways?
   A. Extrinsic and common
   B. Intrinsic and extrinsic
   C. Intrinsic and common
   D. Common pathway only
6. What is the primary cause of thrombocytopenia in HIV-infected patients?
   A. Immune complex deposition
   B. Decreased platelet production in marrow
   C. Premature death of megakaryocytes
   D. All of the above
7. Heparin-induced thrombocytopenia (HIT) type II is characterized by
   A. Mild thrombocytopenia without increased risk of thrombosis
   B. Antibodies against heparin–platelet factor 4 complex
   C. Transient thrombocytopenia resolving with continued heparin use
   D. Only occurs with low-molecular-weight heparin
8. Which of the following is not a typical feature of disseminated intravascular coagulation (DIC)?
   A. Formation of microthrombi
   B. Elevated fibrinogen levels
   C. Consumption of clotting factors
   D. Haemorrhagic manifestations
9. Bernard–Soulier syndrome is caused by a defect in which platelet glycoprotein complex?
   A. GPIIb/IIIa
   B. GPIb/V/IX
   C. GPIa/IIa
   D. GPV
10. What is the primary defect in Glanzmann thrombasthenia?
    A. Platelet aggregation
    B. Platelet adhesion
    C. Platelet release reaction
    D. Platelet signal transduction
11. Atypical haemolytic uraemic syndrome (aHUS) is caused by
    A. Bacterial toxins
    B. Uncontrolled complement activation
    C. ADAMTS13 deficiency
    D. Antibodies against vWF
12. What is the hallmark of thrombotic thrombocytopenic purpura (TTP)?
    A. Deficiency of ADAMTS13
    B. Increased platelet count
    C. High levels of factor VIII
    D. Prolonged bleeding time
13. Which factor is involved in both coagulation and bone matrix synthesis?
    A. Factor V
    B. Factor X
    C. Vitamin K
    D. Protein C
14. What is the most common cause of haemolytic uraemic syndrome in children?
    A. *Streptococcus pneumoniae*
    B. *Escherichia coli* O157:H7
    C. HIV infection
    D. Heparin administration
15. Chronic DIC is often observed in patients with
    A. Sepsis
    B. Malignancies
    C. Haemophilia
    D. Vitamin K deficiency
16. What distinguishes acute ITP from chronic ITP?
    A. Platelet count
    B. Duration of disease

C. Size of spleen
D. Age of onset

17. Which statement about von Willebrand disease is true?
A. Affects only males
B. Causes prolonged prothrombin time
C. Characterized by deficiency or dysfunction of vWF
D. Associated with high levels of factor VIII

18. In DIC, what is the significance of elevated D-dimer levels?
A. Indicates reduced platelet count
B. Suggests increased thrombin generation
C. Reflects ongoing activation of the clotting cascade
D. Signifies elevated fibrinogen levels

19. Which of the following is not a feature of qualitative platelet disorders?
A. Prolonged bleeding time
B. Normal platelet count
C. Elevated PT
D. Abnormal platelet function

20. The main treatment for severe cases of von Willebrand disease is
A. Heparin
B. Fresh frozen plasma
C. Desmopressin
D. Vitamin K

21. Which test is used to diagnose vitamin K deficiency–related bleeding?
A. Bleeding time
B. DCP assay
C. Prothrombin time
D. Activated partial thromboplastin time

22. What is the primary role of thrombin time (TT) in diagnostic testing?
A. Assessing platelet function
B. Measuring fibrinolytic activity
C. Evaluating extrinsic pathway of coagulation
D. Determining the time for clot formation after thrombin addition

23. In thrombotic microangiopathies, the damage to the endothelial cells results in
A. Decreased platelet activation
B. Formation of microthrombi
C. Elevated factor VIII levels
D. Reduced ADAMTS13 activity

24. Which of the following is a common clinical feature of platelet disorders?
A. Deep muscle bleeding
B. Petechiae and purpura
C. Haemarthroses
D. Prolonged clotting time

25. Which of the following is not a common cause of acquired vitamin K deficiency?
A. Chronic illness
B. High intake of green leafy vegetables
C. Chronic alcoholism
D. Intestinal resection

Answers

1. (B); 2. (B); 3. (B); 4. (A); 5. (C); 6. (D); 7. (B); 8. (B); 9. (B); 10. (A); 11. (B); 12. (A); 13. (C); 14. (B); 15. (B); 16. (B); 17. (C); 18. (C); 19. (C); 20. (C); 21. (C); 22. (D); 23. (B); 24. (B); 25. (B)

Self-Assessment Questions

1. A 5-year-old child was brought with the complaints of purpuric spots all over the body. There was also a history of fever 1 week ago. What do you think as the most common cause? Which test for haemostasis would be abnormal?
2. A 45-year-old man was taking warfarin as prophylaxis against pulmonary thromboembolism due to deep vein thrombosis. Which test for haemostasis would be abnormal?
3. A 52-year-old man who has completed his jail tenure of 12 years and got released presented with gum bleeding and purpuric spots. What do you think as the most common cause? Which test for haemostasis would be abnormal?
4. An 18-year-old man with a frequent history of deep bleeds into the muscles was investigated. His BT and PT were normal with PTT prolongation. What is your provisional diagnosis?
5. A 27-year-old woman developed DIC following septic abortion. What haemostatic abnormalities you expect in this patient?
6. A 9-year-old boy was brought with multiple purpuric spots. There was no history of fever in the recent past. On examination, he was found to be otherwise normal appearing. His platelet count, PT and aPTT were normal. BT was prolonged, and peripheral smear showed the presence of giant platelets. What is your provisional diagnosis? What tests would you like to perform?
7. A 25-year-old man was investigated for preoperative checkup. Following are his laboratory findings: platelet count normal; BT, aPTT prolonged with normal PT. What is your provisional diagnosis? What tests would you like to do?
8. A 35-year-old man met with road traffic accident and suffered heavy blood loss for which he underwent massive transfusion. One week later, his laboratory parameters are as follows: BT, PT and aPTT prolongation. What is your provisional diagnosis?

Answers

1. Acute ITP, bleeding time prolongation
2. PT and aPTT prolongation
3. Scurvy, BT prolongation
4. Haemophilia
5. BT, PT, aPTT, TT prolongation, FDP and D-dimer elevation
6. Bernard–Soulier syndrome, platelet functional studies
7. von Willebrand disease, vWF assay
8. Hypofibrinogenaemia following massive transfusion

Topics for Self-Directed Learning

1. Mechanical purpura
2. Osler–Rendu–Weber syndrome
3. Causes of giant platelets
4. Posttransfusion purpura
5. Pseudothrombocytopenia
6. Grey platelet syndrome
7. Genotype analysis of haemophilia
8. Inherited disorders of fibrinogen
9. Acquired inhibitors of coagulation
10. Lupus anticoagulant
11. International normalized ratio (INR)
12. Massive blood transfusion and bleeding
13. Oral anticoagulants

MIND MAPS

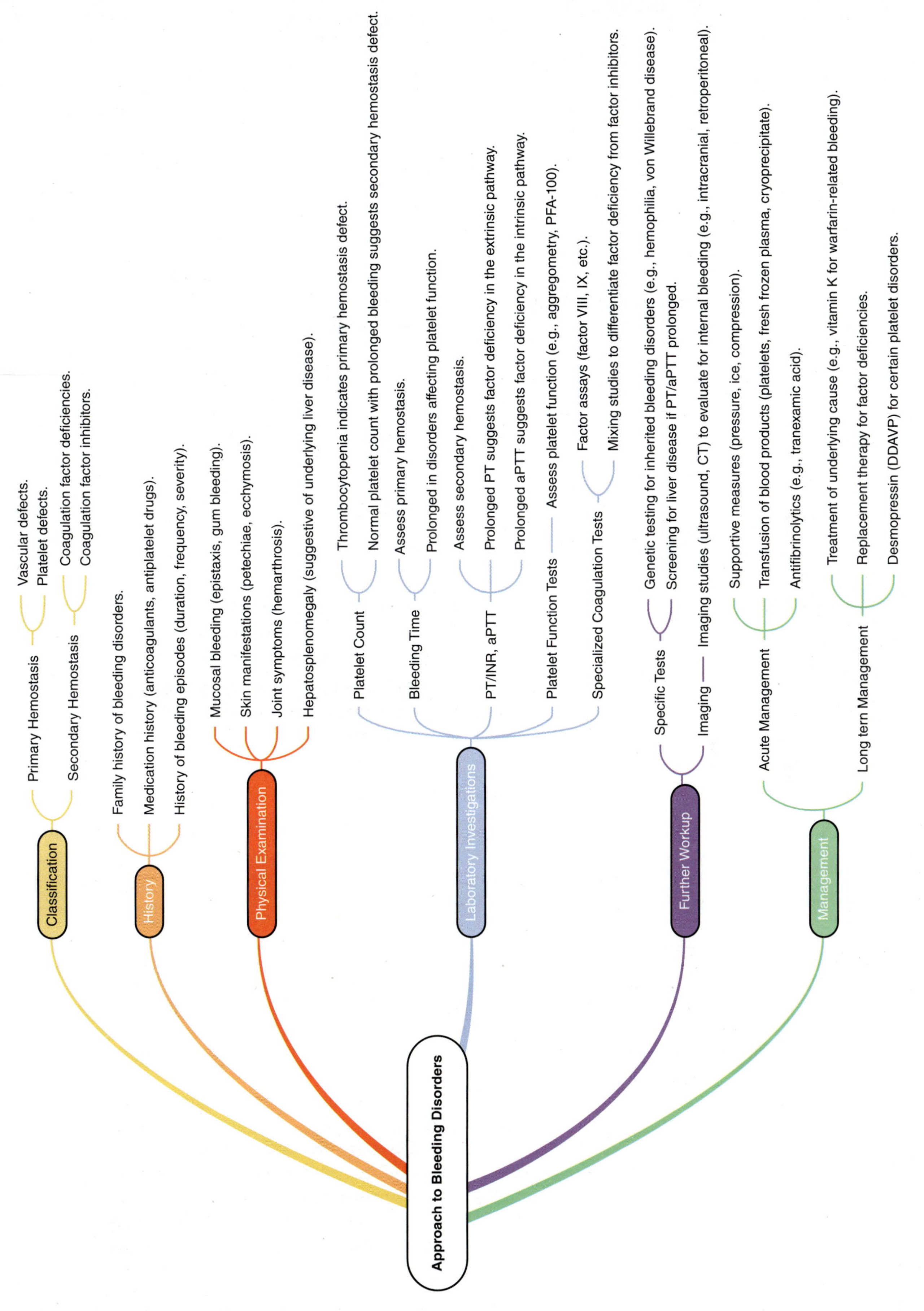
Approach to Bleeding Disorders
Classification
Primary Hemostasis
Vascular defects.
Platelet defects.
Secondary Hemostasis
Coagulation factor deficiencies.
Coagulation factor inhibitors.
History
Family history of bleeding disorders.
Medication history (anticoagulants, antiplatelet drugs).
History of bleeding episodes (duration, frequency, severity).
Physical Examination
Mucosal bleeding (epistaxis, gum bleeding).
Skin manifestations (petechiae, ecchymosis).
Joint symptoms (hemarthrosis).
Hepatosplenomegaly (suggestive of underlying liver disease).
Laboratory Investigations
Platelet Count
Thrombocytopenia indicates primary hemostasis defect.
Normal platelet count with prolonged bleeding suggests secondary hemostasis defect.
Bleeding Time
Assess primary hemostasis.
Prolonged in disorders affecting platelet function.
PT/INR, aPTT
Assess secondary hemostasis.
Prolonged PT suggests factor deficiency in the extrinsic pathway.
Prolonged aPTT suggests factor deficiency in the intrinsic pathway.
Platelet Function Tests
Assess platelet function (e.g., aggregometry, PFA-100).
Specialized Coagulation Tests
Factor assays (factor VIII, IX, etc.).
Mixing studies to differentiate factor deficiency from factor inhibitors.
Further Workup
Specific Tests
Genetic testing for inherited bleeding disorders (e.g., hemophilia, von Willebrand disease).
Screening for liver disease if PT/aPTT prolonged.
Imaging
Imaging studies (ultrasound, CT) to evaluate for internal bleeding (e.g., intracranial, retroperitoneal).
Management
Acute Management
Supportive measures (pressure, ice, compression).
Transfusion of blood products (platelets, fresh frozen plasma, cryoprecipitate).
Antifibrinolytics (e.g., tranexamic acid).
Long tern Management
Treatment of underlying cause (e.g., vitamin K for warfarin-related bleeding).
Replacement therapy for factor deficiencies.
Desmopressin (DDAVP) for certain platelet disorders.

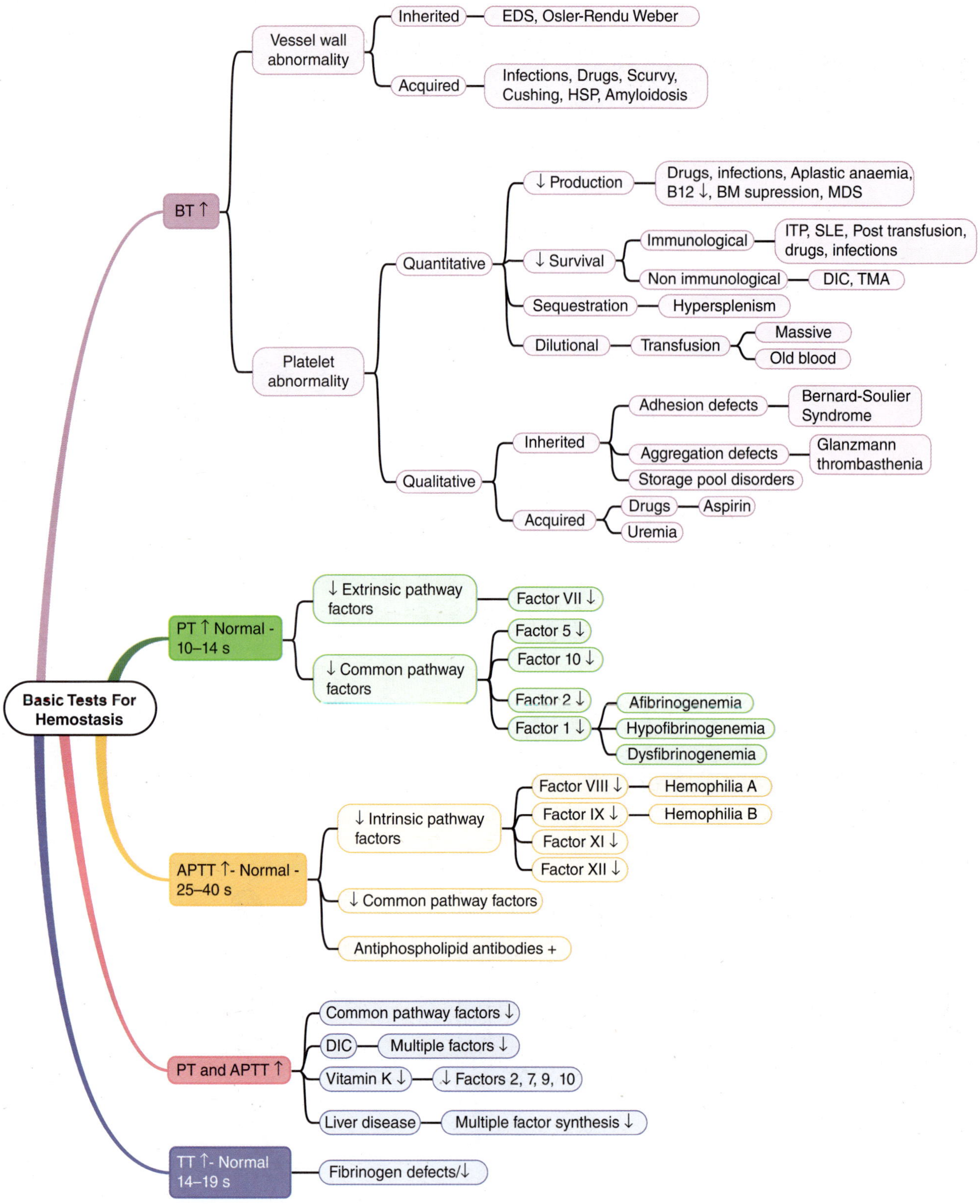
Basic Tests For Hemostasis
BT ↑
Vessel wall abnormality
Inherited
EDS, Osler-Rendu Weber
Acquired
Infections, Drugs, Scurvy, Cushing, HSP, Amyloidosis
Platelet abnormality
Quantitative
↓ Production
Drugs, infections, Aplastic anaemia, B12 ↓, BM supression, MDS
↓ Survival
Immunological
ITP, SLE, Post transfusion, drugs, infections
Non immunological
DIC, TMA
Sequestration
Hypersplenism
Dilutional
Transfusion
Massive
Old blood
Qualitative
Inherited
Adhesion defects
Bernard-Soulier Syndrome
Aggregation defects
Glanzmann thrombasthenia
Storage pool disorders
Acquired
Drugs
Aspirin
Uremia
PT ↑ Normal - 10–14 s
↓ Extrinsic pathway factors
Factor VII ↓
↓ Common pathway factors
Factor 5 ↓
Factor 10 ↓
Factor 2 ↓
Factor 1 ↓
Afibrinogenemia
Hypofibrinogenemia
Dysfibrinogenemia
APTT ↑- Normal - 25–40 s
↓ Intrinsic pathway factors
Factor VIII ↓
Hemophilia A
Factor IX ↓
Hemophilia B
Factor XI ↓
Factor XII ↓
↓ Common pathway factors
Antiphospholipid antibodies +
PT and APTT ↑
Common pathway factors ↓
DIC
Multiple factors ↓
Vitamin K ↓
↓ Factors 2, 7, 9, 10
Liver disease
Multiple factor synthesis ↓
TT ↑- Normal 14–19 s
Fibrinogen defects/↓

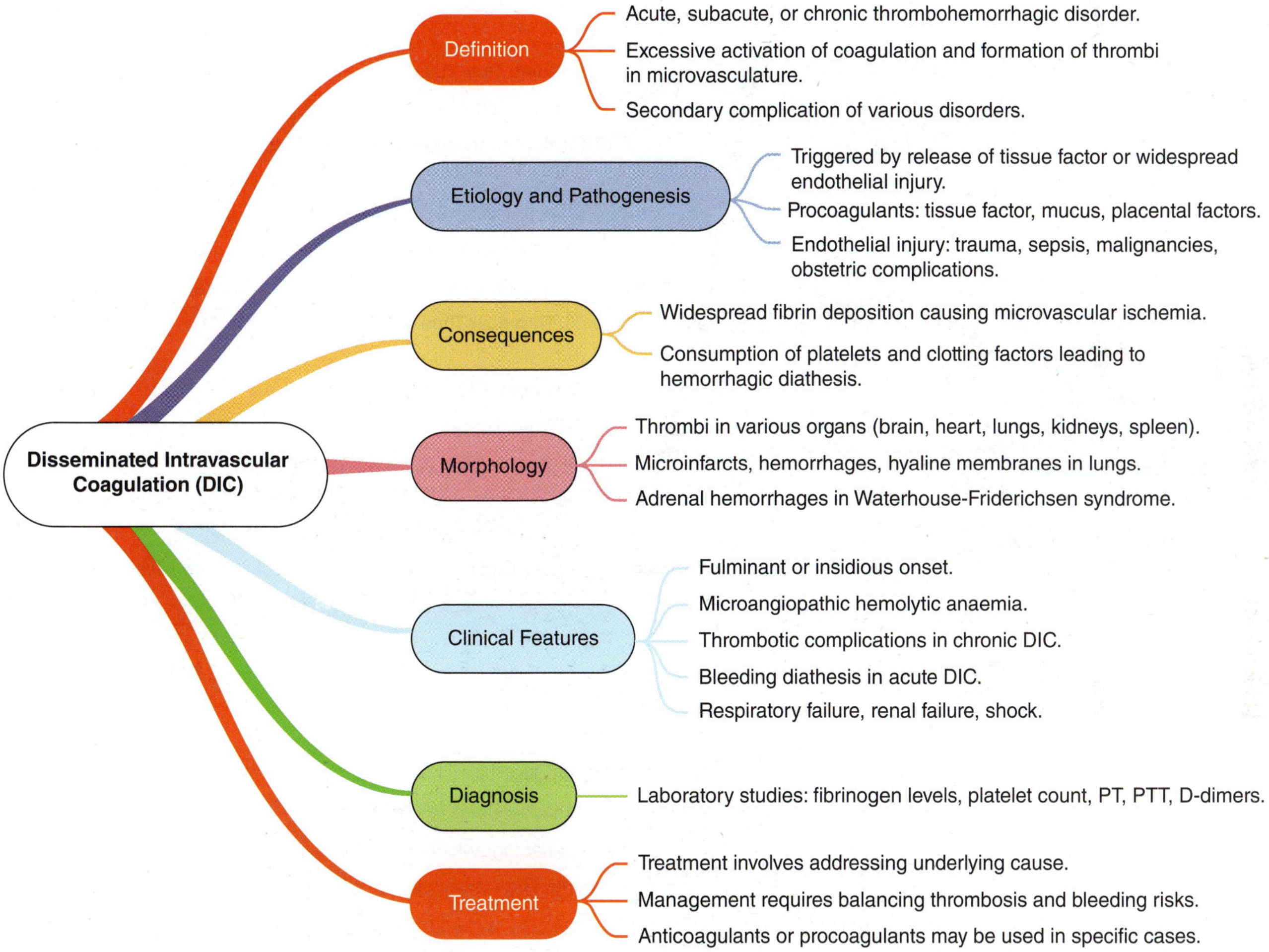
Disseminated Intravascular Coagulation (DIC)
Definition
Acute, subacute, or chronic thrombohemorrhagic disorder.
Excessive activation of coagulation and formation of thrombi in microvasculature.
Secondary complication of various disorders.
Etiology and Pathogenesis
Triggered by release of tissue factor or widespread endothelial injury.
Procoagulants: tissue factor, mucus, placental factors.
Endothelial injury: trauma, sepsis, malignancies, obstetric complications.
Consequences
Widespread fibrin deposition causing microvascular ischemia.
Consumption of platelets and clotting factors leading to hemorrhagic diathesis.
Morphology
Thrombi in various organs (brain, heart, lungs, kidneys, spleen).
Microinfarcts, hemorrhages, hyaline membranes in lungs.
Adrenal hemorrhages in Waterhouse-Friderichsen syndrome.
Clinical Features
Fulminant or insidious onset.
Microangiopathic hemolytic anaemia.
Thrombotic complications in chronic DIC.
Bleeding diathesis in acute DIC.
Respiratory failure, renal failure, shock.
Diagnosis
Laboratory studies: fibrinogen levels, platelet count, PT, PTT, D-dimers.
Treatment
Treatment involves addressing underlying cause.
Management requires balancing thrombosis and bleeding risks.
Anticoagulants or procoagulants may be used in specific cases.

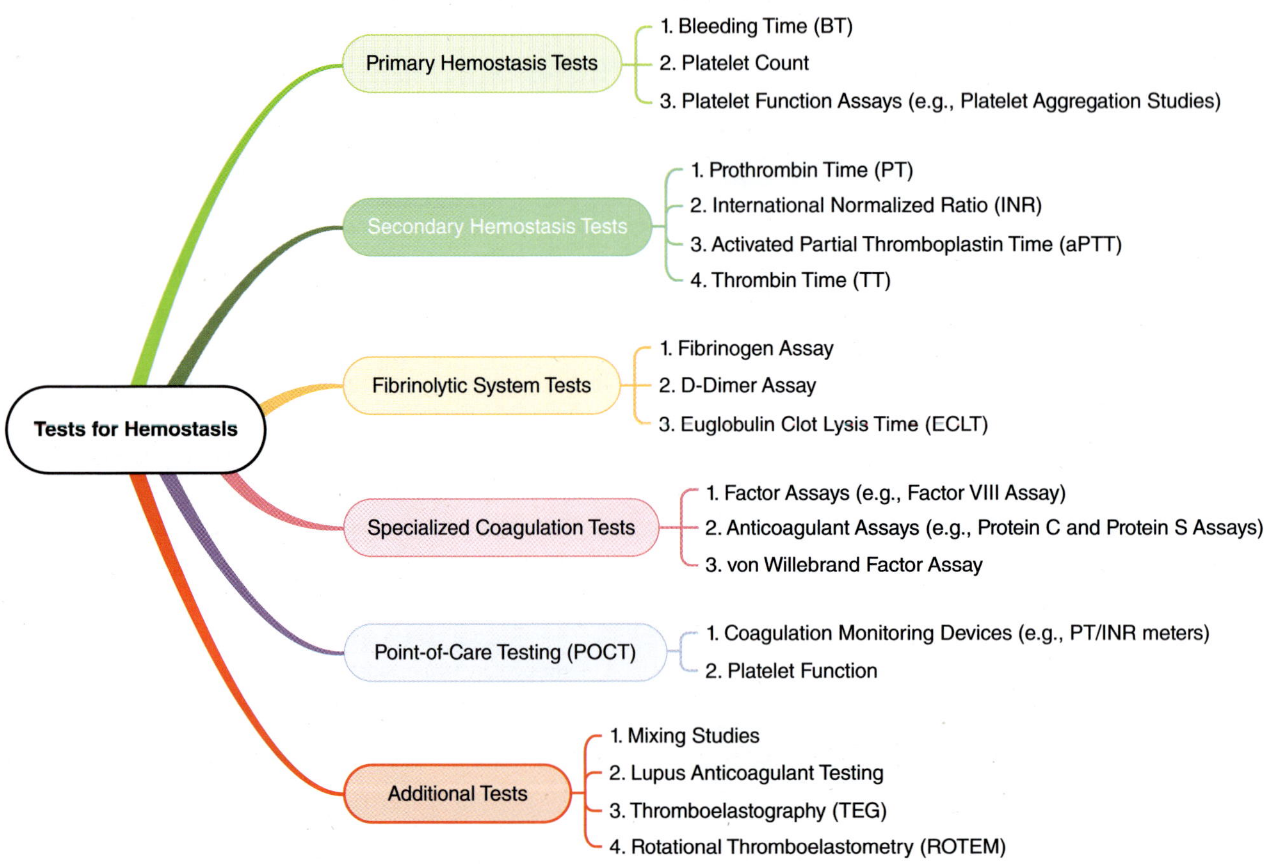
Tests for Hemostasis
Primary Hemostasis Tests
1. Bleeding Time (BT)
2. Platelet Count
3. Platelet Function Assays (e.g., Platelet Aggregation Studies)
Secondary Hemostasis Tests
1. Prothrombin Time (PT)
2. International Normalized Ratio (INR)
3. Activated Partial Thromboplastin Time (aPTT)
4. Thrombin Time (TT)
Fibrinolytic System Tests
1. Fibrinogen Assay
2. D-Dimer Assay
3. Euglobulin Clot Lysis Time (ECLT)
Specialized Coagulation Tests
1. Factor Assays (e.g., Factor VIII Assay)
2. Anticoagulant Assays (e.g., Protein C and Protein S Assays)
3. von Willebrand Factor Assay
Point-of-Care Testing (POCT)
1. Coagulation Monitoring Devices (e.g., PT/INR meters)
2. Platelet Function
Additional Tests
1. Mixing Studies
2. Lupus Anticoagulant Testing
3. Thromboelastography (TEG)
4. Rotational Thromboelastometry (ROTEM)

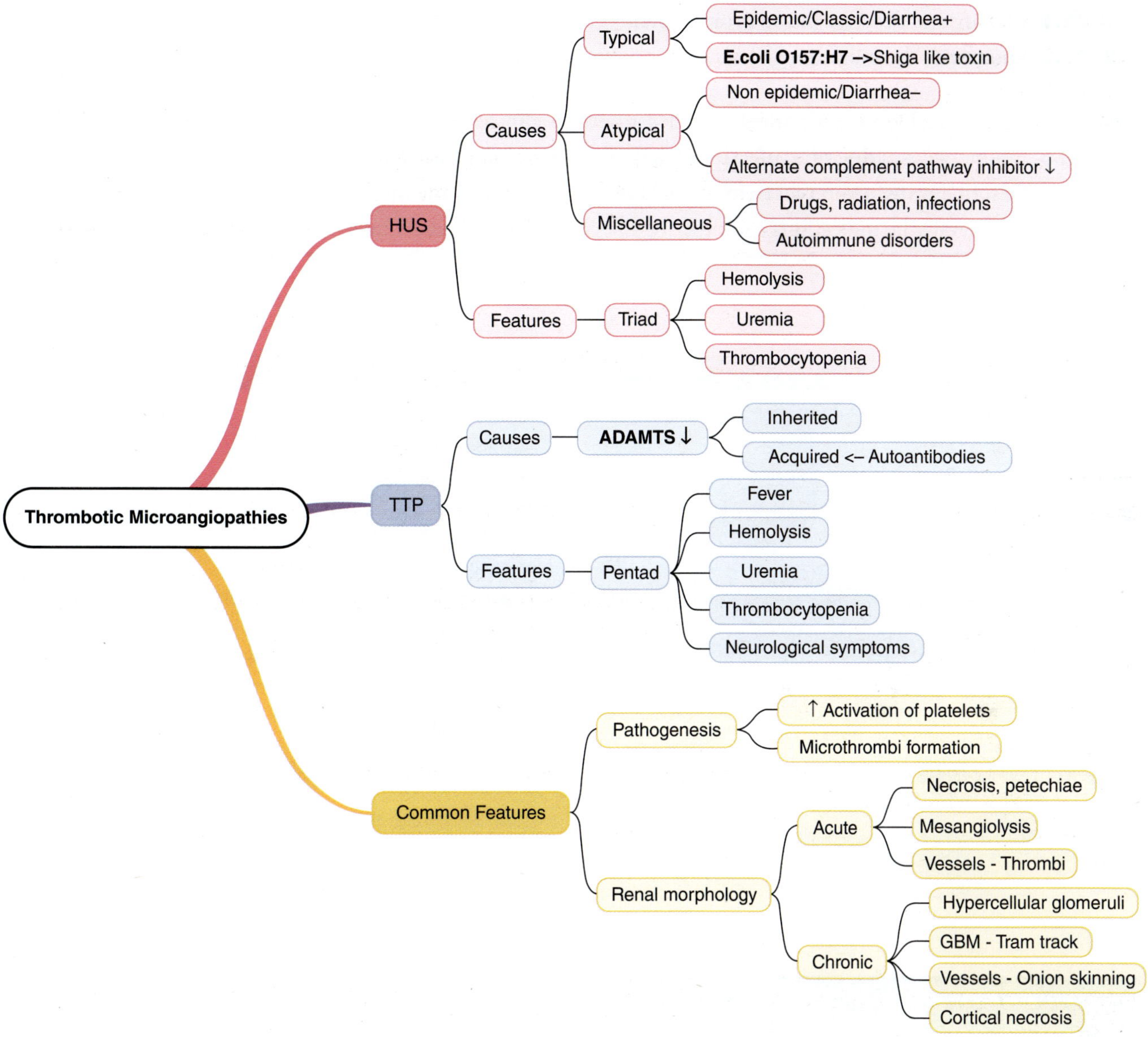
Thrombotic Microangiopathies
HUS
Causes
Typical
Epidemic/Classic/Diarrhea+
E.coli O157:H7 –>Shiga like toxin
Atypical
Non epidemic/Diarrhea–
Alternate complement pathway inhibitor ↓
Miscellaneous
Drugs, radiation, infections
Autoimmune disorders
Features
Triad
Hemolysis
Uremia
Thrombocytopenia
TTP
Causes
ADAMTS ↓
Inherited
Acquired <– Autoantibodies
Features
Pentad
Fever
Hemolysis
Uremia
Thrombocytopenia
Neurological symptoms
Common Features
Pathogenesis
↑ Activation of platelets
Microthrombi formation
Renal morphology
Acute
Necrosis, petechiae
Mesangiolysis
Vessels - Thrombi
Chronic
Hypercellular glomeruli
GBM - Tram track
Vessels - Onion skinning
Cortical necrosis

18 Transfusion Medicine

A Sivaramakrishnan

PA 22.1 Classify and describe **blood group systems** (ABO and RH).

PA 22.2 Enumerate the indications, describe the principles and enumerate and demonstrate the steps of **compatibility testing**.

PA 22.4 Enumerate **blood components** and describe their clinical uses.

PA 22.5 Enumerate and describe **infections transmitted by blood transfusion**.

PA 22.6 Describe **transfusion reactions** and enumerate the steps in the investigation of a transfusion reaction.

PA 22.7 Enumerate the indications and describe the principles and procedures of **autologous transfusion**.

CHAPTER OUTLINE

INTRODUCTION TO TRANSFUSION MEDICINE

Transfusion medicine is the branch of medicine that encompasses all the aspects of transfusion of blood and blood products. It includes collection of blood from the nonremunerated voluntary blood donors, component preparation and appropriate storage in cold chain, transfusion-transmissible infection (TTI) screening, pretransfusion compatibility tests, management and monitoring of clinical transfusion practices, therapeutic apheresis and stem cell harvest for clinical applications. To ensure the safety of blood and blood products, strict quality procedures and quality assurance systems must be in place, covering all the aspects of the transfusion chain, from donor selection to the outcome of transfusion.

BLOOD GROUP SYSTEMS (TABLE 18.1) PA 22.1

Blood group antigens (blood groups) are components of the red cell membrane and are **immunogenic**. Chemically, these are either glycolipids or glycoproteins. The polysaccharide component is responsible for the specificity, and

Table 18.1 Common Blood Group Systems in Practice

No.	System Name	System Symbol	Gene Name(s)	Number of Antigens	Chromosomal Location
001	ABO	ABO	*ABO*	4	9q34.2
002	MNS	MNS	*GYPA, GYPB, (GYPE)*	49	4q31.21
003	P1PK	P1PK	*A4GALT*	3	22q13.2
004	Rh	RH	*RHD, RHCE*	55	1p36.11
005	Lutheran	LU	*BCAM*	25	19q13.2
006	Kell	KEL	*KEL*	36	7q33
007	Lewis	LE	*FUT3*	6	19p13.3
008	Duffy	FY	*ACKR1*	5	1q21–q22
009	Kidd	JK	*SLC14A1*	3	18q11–q12

the amino acid fraction determines the antigenicity. Blood group substances are also secreted in saliva. These substances possess specificity but are not antigenic; however, in combination with another protein, these can evoke an immune response.

The locus for ABO blood group is present on **chromosome 9q34.2** and that of the Rh system on chromosome **1p36.11**.

There are currently 45 recognized blood group systems containing 360 red cell antigens (July 2023). Blood group antigens play an important role in clinical transfusion practice. Incompatibility between donor and recipient blood can lead to serious outcomes such as haemolytic transfusion reactions (HTRs).

ABO BLOOD GROUP SYSTEM

ABO genes contain multiple alleles which are located on the long arm of chromosome 9. The four major alleles are A1, A2, B and O. O is a 'silent' gene or 'amorph' and produces no gene product. The A and B genes are codominant, while O is recessive. The H gene is the base for the formation of A and B antigenicity. The H gene without alteration results in O group because of lack of A and B antigenicity.

The H gene and its allele h are present at a separate locus from the ABO genes and are independent. **The H gene produces an enzyme L-fucosyltransferase**, which is responsible for transfer of the specific sugar fucose to the precursor carbohydrate chains to form the H antigen. The H antigen forms the substrate for A and B enzymes. The h allele is an amorph. Homozygous hh is extremely rare and results in the production of the **Bombay phenotype**, which is characterized by the absence of the H antigen.

ABO ANTIGENS (FIG. 18.1)

The ABO blood group genes do not code directly for specific antigens; instead, these code for specific enzyme transferases, namely ***N*-acetylgalactosaminyltransferase and D-galactosyltransferase**. These enzymes, in turn, transfer the immunogenic sugars *N*-acetylgalactosamine and D-galactose, respectively, to the H substance to confer A and B specificity.

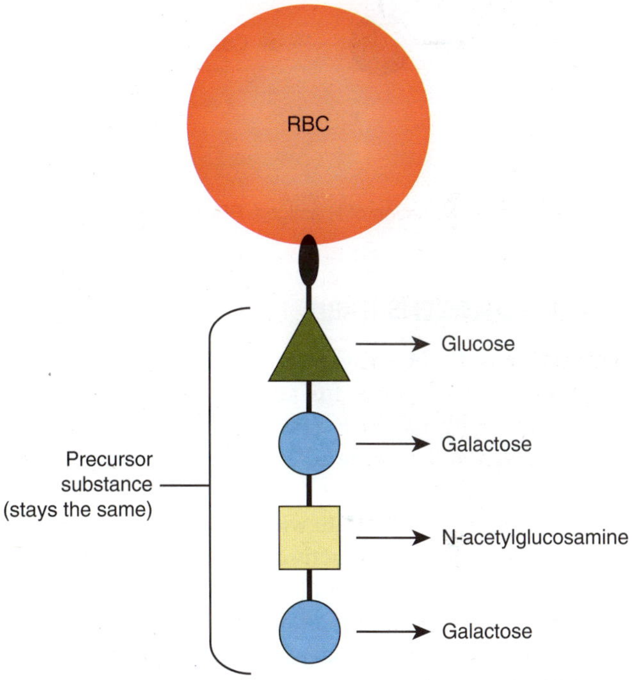

Fig. 18.1 Formation of precursor substance. RBC, red blood cell.

Formation of the H antigen (Fig. 18.2)

- The H antigen is the base upon which the A and B antigens are built.
- *A* and *B* genes code for the enzymes that add an immunodominant sugar to the H antigen.
- **Immunodominant sugars** are present at the terminal ends of the chains and confer the ABO antigen specificity.

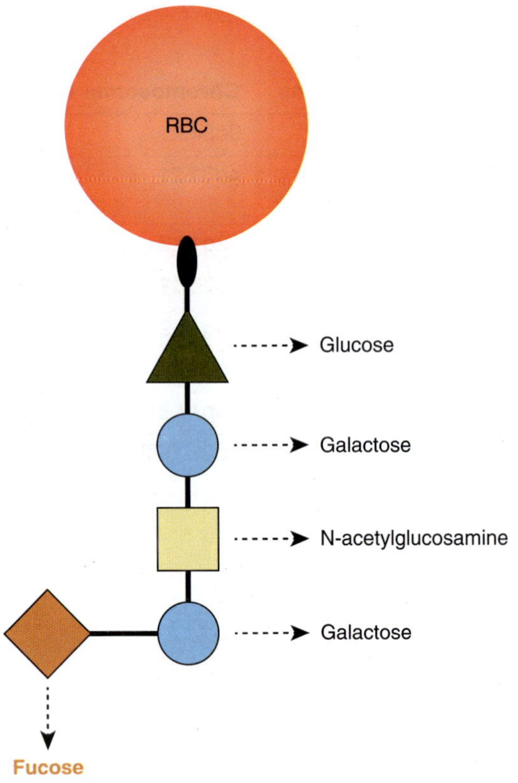

Fig. 18.2 Formation of H antigen. RBC, red blood cell.

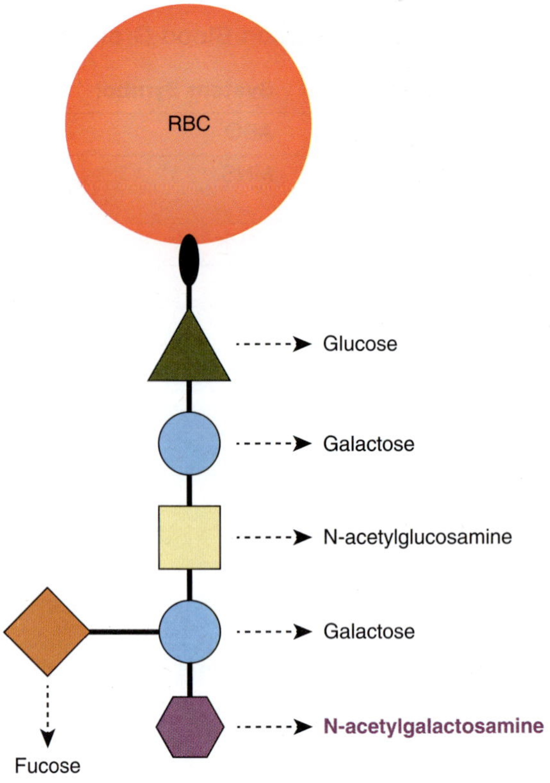

Fig 18.3 Formation of A antigen. RBC, red blood cell.

A AND B ANTIGENS (TABLE 18.2)

Formation of the A antigen (Fig. 18.3)

- The '*A*' gene codes for an enzyme *N*-acetylgalactosaminyltransferase (transferase) that adds ***N-acetylgalactosamine*** to the terminal sugar of the H antigen.
- Precursor carbohydrate with attached fucose (H antigen) + ***N-acetylgalactosamine*** → **A antigen**.

Formation of the B antigen (Fig. 18.4)

- The '*B*' gene codes for an enzyme D-galactosyltransferase that adds **D-galactose** to the terminal sugar of the H antigen.
- Precursor carbohydrate with attached fucose (H antigen) + **D-galactose** → **B antigen**.

Subgroups

- ABO subgroups differ in the amount of antigens present on the red blood cell (RBC) membrane.
- Subgroups have fewer antigens.
- Subgroups are the result of less effective enzymes. These are not very efficient in converting the H antigen to A or B antigen (fewer antigens are present on the RBC).
- **Subgroups of A are more common than subgroups of B.**

Subgroups of A

The two principal subgroups of A are A_1 and A_2.

- Both react strongly with reagent anti-A.
- To distinguish A_1 from A_2 red cells, the lectin *Dolichos biflorus* is used (anti-A_1).
- Eighty per cent of group A or AB individuals are subgroup A_1.
- Twenty per cent are A_2 and A_2B.

ABO ANTIBODIES

ABO is the most important system in transfusion practice because of the invariable presence of naturally occurring anti-A and anti-B antibodies (antibodies) in persons

Table 18.2 Enzymes, Immunodominant Sugars and Antigens of Blood Group Genes

Gene	Glucosyltransferase	Immunodominant Sugar	Antigen
H	L-fucosyltransferase	L-fucose	H
A	*N*-acetylgalactosaminyltransferase	*N*-acetyl-D-galactosamine	A
B	D-galactosyltransferase	D-galactose	B

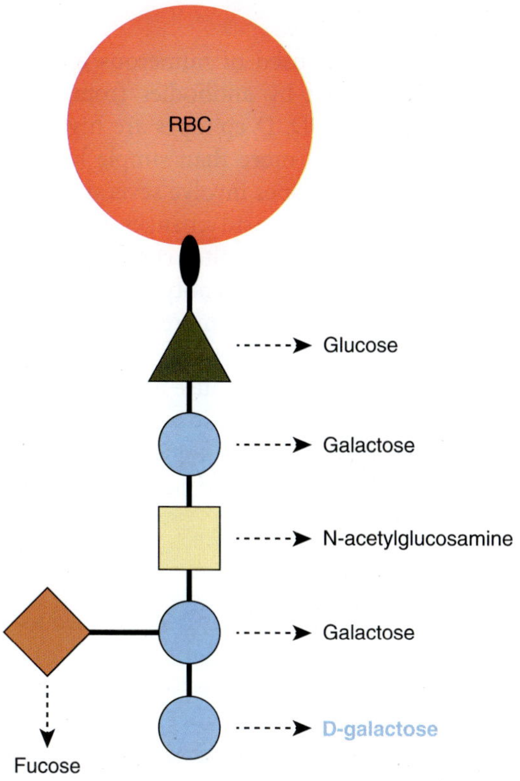

Fig. 18.4 Formation of B antigen. RBC, red blood cell.

Table 18.3 ABO Antigens and Their Corresponding Antibodies

Genotype	Blood Group (Phenotype)	Antigen on RBCs	Antibody in Plasma/Serum
AO/AA	A	A	Anti-B
BO/BB	B	B	Anti-A
AB	AB	AB	None
OO	O	H	Anti-A, anti-B
hh	Bombay blood group	None	Anti-H, anti-A, anti-B

RBC, red blood cell.

lacking the corresponding antigen. Group A individuals have anti-B antibodies in plasma, whereas group B individuals have anti-A agglutinin. Group O individuals have both anti-A and anti-B antibodies (Table 18.3) because of lack of antigens.

ABO antibodies are of two types – **naturally occurring and immune**. Naturally occurring antibodies are found in all individuals lacking the corresponding antigen and do not require the obvious exposure to an immunogen to be formed. They are **IgM** in nature. Many plants, animals and bacteria possess antigens that have A-, B- and H-like specificity. Exposure to these is believed to result in the production of naturally occurring IgM antibodies.

Immune antibodies in the ABO system are mostly produced after immunization as a result of either pregnancy or transfusion. These are **IgG** in nature.

Anti-A and anti-B are usually not produced by infants till 3–6 months of age. By 5–10 years of age, the antibodies reach a maximum titre which gradually declines thereafter. The antibodies found in the serum of infants at birth are mostly of maternal origin; therefore, only grouping based on antigens is recommended in newborns.

Anti-A is found in group B and group O individuals and reacts strongly with A_1 and A_2 cells. Anti-B is found in group A and O individuals. Anti-A and anti-B are found in group O individuals.

Anti-A_1 is found in 1%–8% of A_2 and 22%–35% of A_2B individuals. It is usually active at room temperature or below and is rarely clinically significant, except if it reacts at 37°C. Anti-H in Bombay blood group individuals reacts over a wide thermal range (between 4°C and 37°C) and may cause severe HTRs.

Landsteiner's Rule

If an antigen (Ag) is present on a patient's RBCs, the corresponding antibody (Ab) will NOT be present in the patient's plasma under 'normal conditions'.

BOMBAY BLOOD GROUP (h/h or O_h)

The Bombay blood group (H-deficient phenotype) was discovered in 1952 by Bhende et al. It is characterized by the absence of A, B and H antigens on red cells and in the body secretions and is expressed as phenotype 'Oh' because of inheritance of the *hh* gene. The h gene is an amorph and results in little or no production of L-fucosyltransferase and causes lack of the H antigen, resulting in **RBCs with no H, A or B antigen** (patient types as O).

The sera of these individuals show the presence of anti-A, anti-B and anti-H and react with O group cells which express the H antigen. These individuals possess normal ABO and secretor genes; however, the A, B and H antigens are not expressed because of the absence of the H gene. During blood grouping using RBCs, Bombay RBCs are not agglutinated with anti-A, anti-B or anti-H (no antigens present).

Bombay serum has strong anti-A, anti-B and anti-H, agglutinating all ABO blood groups. The lectin of *Ulex europaeus* has anti-H activity and can be used to detect the H antigen.

SECRETOR STATUS

The ability to secrete A, B and H substances is determined by the presence of a **secretor gene Se** in either the homozygous SeSe state or the heterozygous Sese state. This is inherited independently of the ABO and Hh genes. Eighty per cent of the population comprises secretors and 20% nonsecretors (sese) of A, B and H antigens.

A, B and H antigens are not only present on the red cells but also widely distributed throughout the body tissues except in the central nervous system. All individuals possessing the secretor gene (SeSe or Sese) secrete these antigens in all body fluids **except the cerebrospinal fluid.**

Rh BLOOD GROUP SYSTEM

After the ABO system, the Rh blood group system is the most important in clinical practice. The majority of Rh-negative individuals transfused with Rh-positive blood produce immune Rh antibodies. Rh antibodies are an important cause of haemolytic disease of the newborn (HDN) and can cause HTRs.

Of more than 50 described antigens, only 5 Rh antigens are common. These antigens are protein products of a complex system of three closely related genes present on chromosome 1. Three alleles *D/d*, *C/c* and *E/e* are inherited as a single unit (haplotype), and the d allele is amorphic.

Nomenclature

The **Fisher–Race** (DCE) nomenclature is adequate for description and understanding of clinically important problems. Rh antigens (D, C/c and E/e) are the products of corresponding genes. The D antigen is highly immunogenic and is more clinically important than the other Rh antigens.

Phenotype and Genotype in the Rh System

Phenotype denotes the expression of antigens on the RBCs. Genotype denotes the gene combination in a particular individual. Five antisera are routinely used to detect the phenotype. The phenotype thus detected gives the probable genotyping. Prediction of the possible genotype can be made from the known frequencies of the Rh genotype in the population.

Most D-negative (Rh-negative) phenotypes are the result of complete deletion of the *RHD* gene. Exposure to RhD in a D-negative individual often results in the production of anti-D. The immunogenicity of a protein is correlated with the degree of foreignness to the host, and the large number of amino acid differences explains why exposure to RhD can result in a potent immune response.

Antigens

The D antigen is the most immunogenic Rh antigen, followed by c and E antigens. Routine donor and patient typing tests only for D. Testing for other common Rh antigens is performed primarily to resolve or confirm antibody identification, with the exception that some sickle cell transfusion programmes (because of frequent transfusion requirements) perform Rh typing before transfusion to match patients and donors for D, C and E (in addition to the Kell antigen) to reduce alloimmunization.

D Antigen

The D antigen is composed of numerous epitopes that were originally defined by antibodies from D-positive people who made anti-D. D epitopes are highly conformational and consist of more than simple linear amino acid residues. Many epitopes involve several of the extracellular loops, and amino acid changes in intracellular regions of the protein can also alter D epitopes.

Most D-positive red cell phenotypes have a conventional RhD protein. However, more than 100 different RHD alleles that encode proteins with amino acid changes have been reported. These can cause numerous variations in the expression of D and include weak D, partial D and Del phenotypes. Red cells with some form of altered D expression are often encountered in routine transfusion practice.

Weak D (Formerly DU)

Weak D red cells have historically been defined as having a reduced amount of the D antigen, requiring an indirect antiglobulin test (IAT) for detection. The number of samples classified as weak D, however, depends on the characteristics of the typing reagents, which have changed over the years. Weak D expression results primarily from single-nucleotide mutations in RHD, which encodes amino acid changes predicted to be located intracellularly, or in the transmembrane regions of RhD, rather than on the outer surface of the red cell.

1. If transfused with Du blood, an individual who has anti-D antibodies (through previous sensitization by transfusion or pregnancy) is likely to develop severe haemolysis.
2. A sensitized Rh-negative mother having anti-D antibodies can produce haemolytic disease of the fetus and newborn (HDFN) in a Du-positive fetus.

D-Negative (Rh-Negative)

The D-negative phenotype is prevalent in White population (15%–17%), less likely in African black population (3%–5%) and rare in Asians (<0.1%). The D-negative phenotype has ascended multiple times, as evidenced by the different mutations responsible for lack of D expression in various ethnic groups. In most whites, it results from deletion of the entire RHD gene.

Rh Antibodies

Most Rh antibodies are IgG, although some sera may have an IgM component. Typically, Rh antibodies do not activate complement. As a result, in transfusion reactions involving Rh antibodies, haemolysis is primarily extravascular rather than intravascular. Unlike ABO antibodies that are natural, Rh antibodies are induced on exposure and almost always caused by red cell immunization from pregnancy or transfusion and usually persist for many years.

Most Rh antibodies should be considered as having the potential to cause clinically significant HDFN and transfusion reactions. Anti-c, clinically the most important Rh antibody after anti-D, may cause severe HDFN. Anti-C, anti-E and anti-e do not often cause HDFN and when they do, it is usually mild. If serum antibody levels fall below detectable levels, subsequent exposure to the antigen characteristically produces a rapid secondary immune response. The reactivity of Rh antibodies in the laboratory can be enhanced by enzyme treatment of the test red cells and most react optimally at 37°C.

PRETRANSFUSION COMPATIBILITY TESTS PA 22.2

PURPOSE

Pretransfusion compatibility tests are crucial to select blood components that do not cause transfusion reaction to the recipient and have acceptable survival in vivo. Pretransfusion compatibility tests confirm ABO compatibility between the component and the recipient. It detects almost all clinically significant unexpected antibodies and ensures that only compatible blood and blood components are transfused to the patient.

STEPS INVOLVED

- ABO/Rh blood group typing
- Compatibility test
- Antibody detection/identification

1. **ABO/Rh blood group typing**
   - In the ABO typing, the forward and reverse typing MUST match.
   - In the Rh typing, a negative control must be included.
   - Both of these tests indicate what type of blood should be given.

   Cell grouping (forward grouping)
   - It tests the patient's red cells with known anti-A and anti-B to determine the antigen expressed.

   Serum grouping (reverse grouping)
   - It tests the patient's serum with known A and B cells to determine the presence of antibody.
2. **Antibody detection/identification**
   - The antibody screen detects the presence of any unexpected antibodies in the patient's (recipient's) serum.
   - If antibodies are detected, it should be identified using panel cells.
   - If an antibody is present, units negative for the corresponding antigen must be selected for transfusion.
3. **Crossmatch**

   Purpose
   - Prevent transfusion reactions
   - Increase in vivo survival of red cells
   - Double-check for ABO errors
   - Another method of detecting antibodies

   Compatibility test method types
   - Manual tube technique (IS and IAT)
   - Gel technology
   - Electronic (computerized) crossmatch
   - Red cell affinity column technology (ReACT)
   - Solid-phase adherence assays (SPAA)

   Two types of crossmatch (Table 18.4)
   1. **Major crossmatch** (Fig. 18.5)
   2. **Minor crossmatch** (Fig. 18.6)

   Crossmatch technique consists of three phases
   1. Immediate spin or saline phase
   2. 37°C incubation phase
   3. Anti-human globulin (AHG) phase

Table 18.4 Major and Minor Crossmatches

Method	Major Crossmatch	Minor Crossmatch
Requirement	1. Recipient's serum 2. Donor's red cells	1. Donor's serum 2. Recipient's red cells
Aim	To detect compatibility of IgM/IgG antibody in the patient's serum against antigens on the donor's red cells	To detect compatibility of IgM/IgG antibody(ies) in the donor's serum against antigens on the recipient's red cells
Immediate spin or saline phase	1. Label the tube for each donor sample to be tested. 2. Put two drops of the patient's serum in a labelled tube. 3. Add one drop of 2%–5% saline suspended red cells of the donor. 4. Mix and incubate for 5–10 min (spin method). 5. Centrifuge at 1000 rpm for 1 min.	1. Label the tube. 2. Put two drops of the donor's serum in a labelled tube. 3. Add one drop of 2%–5% saline suspended red cells of the patient. 4. Mix and incubate for 5–10 min. 5. Centrifuge at 1000 rpm for 1 min.
Observation Inference	Agglutination and haemolysis Presence of agglutination and haemolysis indicates incompatibility	Agglutination and haemolysis Presence of agglutination and haemolysis indicates incompatibility

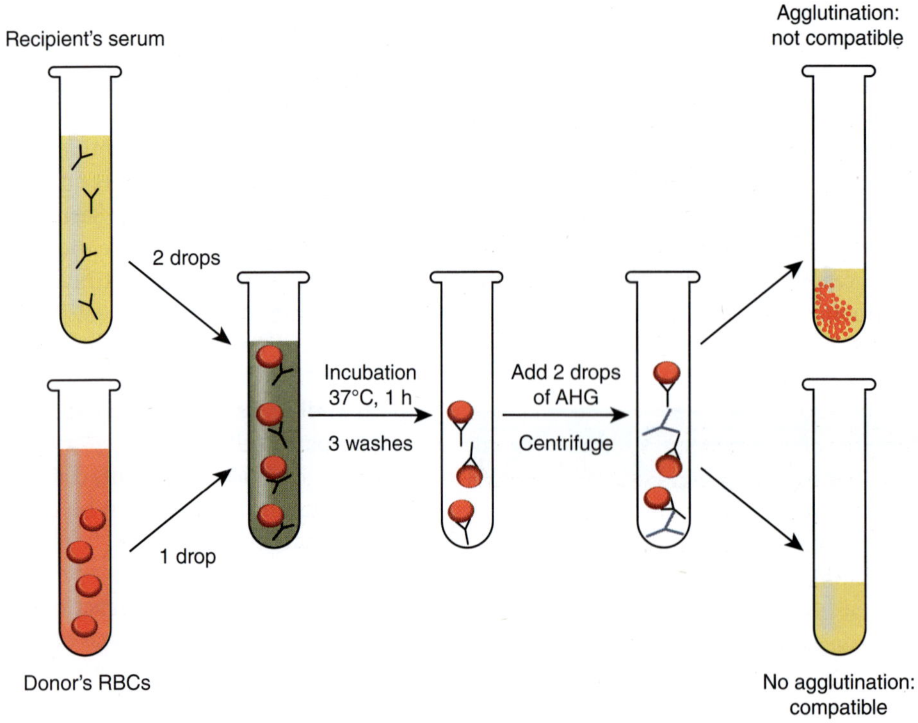

Fig. 18.5 Major crossmatch. AHG, anti-human globulin; RBCs, red blood cells.

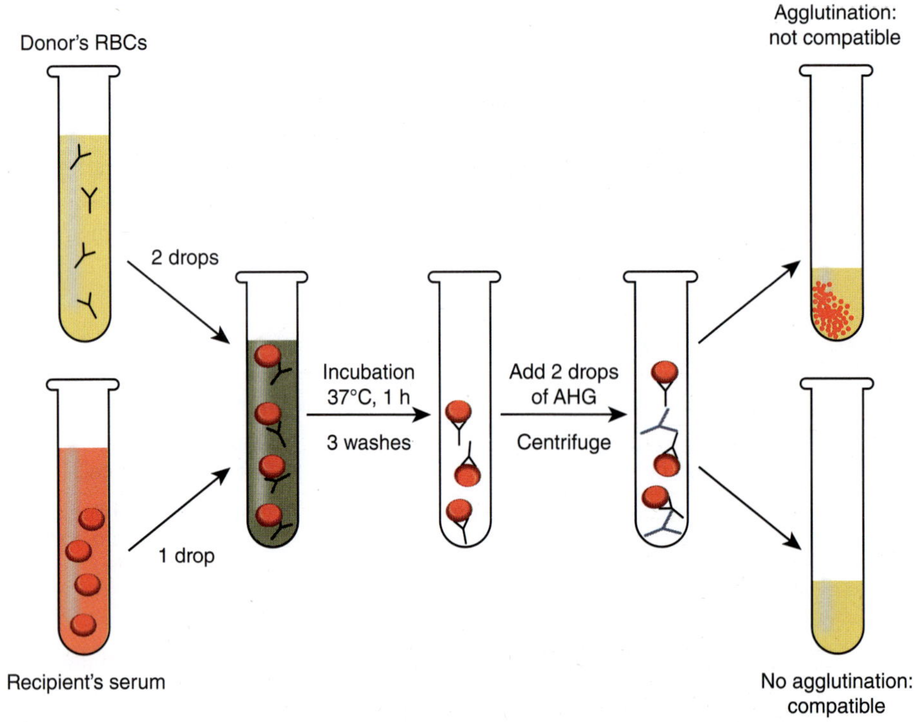

Fig. 18.6 Minor crossmatch. AHG, anti-human globulin; RBCs, red blood cells.

Saline technique
- Saline technique is designed to detect compatibility of IgM antibody(ies) in the donor's serum against antigens on the recipient's red cells.
- Label the tube. Put two drops of the donor's serum in a labelled tube. Add one drop of 2%–5% saline suspended red cells of the patient.
- Mix and incubate for 5–10 minutes. Centrifuge at 1000 rpm for 1 minute.
- Read the result; observe for haemolysis and agglutination. Agglutination or haemolysis indicates a positive result (incompatible).

Interpretation
- Saline technique is inadequate as a complete compatibility test because it is inadequate to detect clinically significant IgG antibodies.

37°C incubation and AHG phase test
- Indirect antiglobulin test (IAT) is the most important and widely used serological procedure to test the IgG compatibility between the donor and the patient. The majority of clinically significant antibodies are IgG and are detected by the AHG test.
- For major crossmatch, put two drops of the patient's serum in a labelled tube and add one drop of 2%–5% saline suspended red cells of the donor. In case of a minor crossmatch, put two drops of the donor serum in a labelled tube and add one drop of 2%–5% saline suspended red cells of the patient.
- Incubate for 30–60 minutes at 37°C.
- Centrifuge at 1000 rpm for 1 minute; check for haemolysis/agglutination.
- If there is no haemolysis/agglutination, wash the cells 3 times with normal saline and proceed to the next phase.

Anti-human globulin test
- Add two drops of polyspecific AHG serum to the washed cells.
- Centrifuge at 1000 rpm for 1 minute.

Interpretation
- Haemolysis or agglutination at any stage indicates incompatibility.

BLOOD COMPONENTS (CELLULAR AND PLASMA) AND PLASMA DERIVATIVES (FRACTIONS) PA 22.4

INTRODUCTION

Transfusion of blood and its components has undergone technological advancement, and its use is increasing. The practice of whole blood transfusion has largely been replaced by component therapy. The separation of blood into its various components has made it very economical as blood donated from a single donor can be utilized for many recipients at the same time by dividing it into its components, such as red cells concentrates, fresh frozen plasma (FFP), cryoprecipitates and platelet concentrates. Only the most appropriate blood component should be ordered and transfused. Awareness on the storage temperature and shelf life of components of blood products is essential for their effective storage and appropriate usage (Table 18.5).

OVERVIEW

Cellular components
- Packed red blood cell (PRBC) concentrate
- Platelet concentrate (random donor platelet)

Plasma components
- Fresh frozen plasma
- Cryoprecipitate
- Cryo-poor plasma

Apheresis products
- Erythrocytopheresis
- Plasmapheresis
- Plateletpheresis (single-donor platelet)
- Granulocytes apheresis

Plasma derivatives
- Albumin 5% and 25%
- Plasma protein fractions
- Factor VIII concentrate
- Immunoglobulins
- Fibrinogen
- Other coagulation factors

Table 18.5 Storage Temperature and Shelf Life of Blood Components

Component	Storage Temperature	Shelf Life	Compatibility
Packed red cells	2–6°C	30 days – without SAGM additive	ABO, Rh, crossmatch
Fresh frozen plasma	−30°C	1 year	ABO
Cryodeficient plasma	−30°C	5 years	ABO
Platelet Concentrate	22–24°C	5 days	ABO
Cryoprecipitate	−30°C	1 year	Any group

Whole blood

Whole blood contains 450 ± 45 or 350 ± 35 mL of donor blood plus anticoagulant solution. CPDA-1 is the commonly used anticoagulant for whole blood collection. Whole blood has a haematocrit value of 30%–40%. Stored whole blood has no functional platelets and coagulation factors.

RBC concentrates (packed red blood cells)

RBCs (packed red cells) are prepared by removing most of the plasma from a unit of whole blood.

Platelet concentrate can be prepared from the following:

1. Random donor platelet (prepared from 450-mL whole blood): It is prepared from a 450-mL whole blood bag kept at room temperature (20–22°C) **within 6–8 hours of collection.**
2. Single-donor platelet prepared by apheresis.

Precaution and storage: **The pH should never fall below 6.** A decline in pH causes the following:

- Change in the shape of platelets from disc to sphere
- Pseudopod formation
- Release of platelet granules which results in nonfunctional platelets

Agitation during storage helps exchange of gases, maintenance of pH and reduction in the formation of platelet aggregates. An agitator (flatbed) with 1- to 1.5-inch strokes at 70 cycles per minutes at 20–24°C gives good results.

Fresh Frozen Plasma

FFP is plasma obtained from a single donor either by normal donation or by plasmapheresis and rapidly frozen within 6–8 hours of collection. It contains **all coagulation factors** and thus great care must be taken during collection of blood, freezing and thawing to preserve their activity.

Cryoprecipitate

Cryoprecipitates are precipitated proteins of plasma, obtained from a single unit of fresh plasma (,200 mL) by rapid freezing within 6 hours of collection. It is rich in **factor VIII, von Willebrand factor (vWF), fibrinogen (factor XIII)** and fibronectin.

Cryoprecipitate-Poor Plasma

It is a by-product of cryoprecipitate preparation. It lacks labile clotting factors V and VIII and fibrinogen. It contains adequate levels of the **stable clotting factors II, VII, IX and X**. It is frozen and stored at −20°C or at a lower temperature for 5 years.

Granulocyte Concentrate

Granulocytes can be stored at 20–24°C, but these should be used as early as possible and not later than 24 hours. In the case of a single donor (apheresis), unit granulocyte count should be $1 \times 10^{10}/\mu L$.

Irradiation

Gamma irradiation in doses of 2500 cGy is given to blood units to prevent graft-versus-host disease (GVHD). Irradiation can damage the red cell membranes and increase the rate of potassium loss to approximately 1.5 mEq/day; however, once infused, the red cells have normal in vivo survival.

Leucocyte-reduced blood components

Leucocytes in blood components can cause the following:

- Nonhaemolytic febrile transfusion reaction (NHFTR)
- Human leucocyte antigen (HLA) alloimmunization
- Transmission of leukotropic viruses (cytomegalovirus [CMV], Epstein–Barr virus [EBV] and human T-lymphotropic virus type 1 [HTLV-1])
- Transfusion-related GVHD
- Transfusion-related acute lung injury (TRALI)
- Transfusion-related immunosuppression

Reducing the leucocytes content to less than 5×10^8 in 1 unit of RBCs prevents most of the NHFTRs. For other complications such as preventing transmission of CMV or alloimmunization to HLA antigens, leucocyte content must be reduced to less than 5×10^6 in a unit of packed red cells.

CLINICAL INDICATIONS OF BLOOD AND BLOOD COMPONENTS

1. **Whole blood**

   A 450-mL whole blood donation contains the following:

   - 450 mL of donor blood
   - 63 mL of anticoagulant preservative solution
   - Haemoglobin approximately 12 g/mL
   - Haematocrit 35%–45%
   - No functional platelets
   - No labile coagulation factors (V and VIII)

   Clinical indications – whole blood

   - Red cell replacement in acute blood loss with hypovolaemia
   - Exchange transfusion
   - Patients requiring red cell transfusions where red cell concentrates or suspensions are not available
   - Must be ABO and RhD compatible with the recipient

2. **Packed red cells (RBCs)**

   - These are used to increase oxygen-carrying capacity in bleeding patients who have surgical anaemia and nonpharmacologically treatable chronic anaemia.
   - If the patient's haemoglobin is more than 10 g/dL, transfusion of RBCs is most likely not required unless the patient is bleeding.
   - If the patient's haemoglobin is 7–10 g/dL, transfusion is only indicated if the patient is bleeding or symptomatic.
   - If the patient's haemoglobin is less than 7 g/dL, transfusion is most likely warranted.

3. **FFP**
   - Preoperative or bleeding patients requiring replacement of multiple coagulation factors (e.g. severe liver disease, disseminated intravascular coagulation [DIC])
   - To correct oral anticoagulant overdose
   - In a patient undergoing massive transfusion with coagulation deficiency
   - Thrombotic thrombocytopenic purpura (TTP)
   - Management of patients with selected coagulation factor deficiency
   - Management of patients with selected plasma protein such as C1 inhibitor deficiency
4. **Platelets**
   Adults
   a. Nonbleeding patients with failure of platelet production
      a. Platelet count less than 10,000/μL
      b. Invasive procedure with platelet count less than 50,000/mL
   b. Bleeding patients
      a. DIC with platelet count less than 50,000/μL
      b. Massive transfusion and platelet count less than 50,000/μL
      c. Active bleeding and platelet count less than 20,000/μL
      d. Diffuse bleeding following cardiopulmonary bypass and platelet count not available or less than 100,000/μL
      e. Platelet function defect
      f. Relative contraindications include patients with TTP, heparin-induced thrombocytopenia (HIT) and posttransfusion purpura (PTP)
5. **Cryoprecipitate**
   - Hypofibrinogenaemia (<80 mg/dL)
   - Consumptive coagulopathy (DIC)
   - Dysfibrinogenaemia
   - Afibrinogenaemia
   - Factor VIII deficiency (haemophilia A)
   - von Willebrand disease with bleeding or anticipated haemostatic challenge, i.e. surgery, biopsy or invasive procedure
6. **Cryo-poor plasma**
   This is primarily used for TTP to correct clotting factor deficiency except fibrinogen, factor VIII, factor XIII and vWF deficiency.

TRANSFUSION REACTIONS — PA 22.6

INTRODUCTION

Transfusion of blood and blood components is usually a safe procedure; however, untoward effects of transfusion can occur frequently. A transfusion reaction is defined as any untoward event which occurs during or after transfusion of blood or blood components.

As the blood or blood components transfused contain antigens and antibodies, transfusion reactions may occur because of incompatibility of antigens and antibodies to red cells, leucocytes, platelets or plasma proteins. These may vary from mild reactions to life-threatening complications.

TYPES OF TRANSFUSION REACTIONS (TABLE 18.6)

Transfusion reactions can be immune or nonimmune in nature. Both may be immediate or delayed. In the former, destruction of red cells begins during transfusion while the delayed reactions begin only days or weeks after there has been an immune response provoked by the transfusion.

IMMUNE MEDIATED TRANSFUSION REACTION

Immunological reactions are caused by red cell, leucocytes or platelet incompatibility or reaction to plasma components.

Haemolytic Transfusion Reactions

An HTR is the occurrence of abnormal destruction of red cells following transfusion. Most of these are due to red cell incompatibility. These reactions may be immediate/delayed and intravascular/extravascular.

Table 18.6 Adverse Effects of Transfusion

Immune-Mediated Transfusion Reactions		Nonimmune-Mediated Transfusion Reactions
Immediate	**Delayed**	
Immediate haemolytic transfusion reaction (IHTR) Febrile nonhaemolytic transfusion reaction (FNHTR) Anaphylaxis and anaphylactic reactions Transfusion-related acute lung injury (TRALI)	Delayed haemolytic transfusion reaction (DHTR) Alloimmunization Posttransfusion purpura (PTP) Transfusion-associated graft-versus-host disease (TA-GVHD) Immunosuppression	Bacterial contamination Transfusion-associated circulatory overload (TACO) Physical or chemical RBC damage Depletion and dilution of coagulation factors and platelets Iron overload Air embolism

RBC, red blood cell.

Intravascular reactions are characterized by destruction of red cells within the bloodstream with liberation of haemoglobin into the plasma. Extravascular haemolysis is characterized by phagocytosis of red cells by macrophages of the reticuloendothelial system. Acute haemolysis, both intravascular and extravascular, is of major clinical significance.

Immediate Haemolytic Reactions

An HTR refers to the occurrence of signs and symptoms of increased red cell destruction after transfusion. These reactions occur during transfusion or within few hours of transfusion.

Causes

1. Transfusion of ABO incompatible red cells is the commonest cause of these reactions as anti-A and anti-B are strongly haemolytic. Other non-ABO antibodies that may cause haemolysis are Kell, Kidd, Duffy, anti-Lewis, anti-P, anti-H, etc.
2. Accidental heating/freezing of blood may lead to lysis of red cells.
3. Injection of intravenous fluids other than normal saline into the circulation leads to damage of red cells.
4. Contact of red cells with 5% dextrose in vitro is one of the causes.
5. Red cell abnormality in a patient or donor may precipitate haemolysis after transfusion, e.g. G6PD deficiency and paroxysmal nocturnal haemoglobinuria (PNH).

Most ABO incompatible transfusions are because of failure to identify the patient correctly. Unconsciousness in a patient further increases the risk of transfusion of ABO incompatible blood, as there may be no signs and symptoms to call attention to the mismatched transfusion.

Administration of ABO incompatible blood can be because of the following:

1. Clerical errors
   a. Incorrect labelling on the
      - Blood bag
      - Pilot tubes
      - Recipient's sample
      - Request form
   b. Misidentification of the patient at the time of collection of the sample or transfusion of blood
   c. Mix-up of samples at the time of collection
2. Technical errors
   a. Error in blood grouping of donor and recipient samples
   b. Error in compatibility testing
      - Faulty technique
      - Weak antibodies not detected by routine tests
3. Destruction of recipient red cells by donor antibodies. This occurs because of the unselective use of group O blood, which may contain potent anti-A and anti-B.

Pathogenesis

Events following transfusion of incompatible red cells, e.g. Transfusion of B-positive blood to O-positive patient (recipient) results in antigen-antibody. Antigen–antibody complex formation on the incompatible red cells (anti-B antibody in the patient plasma combines with the B antigen on the transfused B-positive red cells). When the reciepient has preformed antibodies in their blood this results in acute intravascular hemolysis.

Clinical Features

Symptoms

- Chills
- Flushes
- Chest or back pain
- Sweating, nausea, vomiting
- Pain at the infusion site
- Restlessness
- Abdominal discomfort

Signs

- Fever with rigors
- Hypotension
- Tachycardia
- Haemoglobinuria
- Dyspnoea
- Oliguria
- Tachypnoea
- Anuria
- Pallor
- Cyanosis
- Shock and DIC

Any febrile transfusion reaction must be considered and managed as an immediate HTR until and unless proved otherwise.

Laboratory Evaluation of Suspected Haemolytic Reaction

The workup at the transfusion centre of a suspected transfusion reaction includes the following:

1. Check all the records to ensure that the correct unit of blood was transfused to the right patient. This includes the following:
   Patient details
   - Blood requisition form
   - Compatibility report
   - Labels

   Till the time a clerical error is ruled out, stop issue of all blood units from the centre, as it may lead to issue of another mismatched blood because of mix-up of samples or other clerical errors.
2. The following samples must be immediately sent to the laboratory and blood bank:
   - Posttransfusion sample in a plain vial (5 mL)
   - Posttransfusion sample in an EDTA vial (3 mL)
   - Blood bag along with transfusion set
   - Urine (posttransfusion) first sample

- Coagulation profile-citrated blood sample
- Blood cultures from the blood bag and the patient

The pretransfusion sample should be preserved in the laboratory for 7 days.

Investigation For evaluation of a patient with haemolytic reaction, the investigation may be divided into three parts:

1. Investigation for evidence of increased red cell destruction
2. Investigation for identification of cause of haemolysis
3. Investigation to follow up of a patient with proven haemolysis

Tests for Evidence of Increased Red Cell Destruction

1. Centrifuge the posttransfusion blood sample and examine the supernatant plasma. Compare this with the pretransfusion sample. A pink or red colour in the posttransfusion sample indicates haemolysis and the presence of free haemoglobin.
2. Perform a direct antiglobulin test (DAT) on the posttransfusion sample. A positive test indicates immune haemolysis. A negative DAT with haemoglobinaemia suggests a nonimmune haemolysis, e.g. due to mechanical trauma or thermal damage.
3. Reticulocyte count is raised in patients with haemolysis.
4. Obtain pre- and posthaemoglobin values.
5. Perform serum unconjugated bilirubin estimation.

Tests to Establish the Cause of Haemolysis

a. Repeat ABO and Rh grouping on the pre- and posttransfusion samples and from the bag. If blood group of the pre- and posttransfusion samples does not agree, it may be because of an error in patient identification, drawing or grouping of blood.
   If the donor sample is not of the same group as indicated on the bag, an error in labelling or grouping and also in the compatibility testing should be suspected.
b. Repeat the compatibility testing on the pre- and posttransfusion samples with a sample of blood from the bag.
   - If both the samples show incompatibility, there was an error in the pretransfusion testing. The donor sample may have been incorrectly labelled or the crossmatch reaction was incorrectly read as negative.
   - If the incompatibility is seen only with the posttransfusion sample, an anamnestic response should be suspected.
   - If both crossmatches are compatible and there is a strong suspicion of haemolysis, further tests are required.
c. Perform an antibody screening on the pre- and posttransfusion samples. If an antibody is detected, it should be identified using further tests. An antibody present only in the posttransfusion sample may be because of the following:
   - Anamnestic response (e.g. anti-Kidd and anti-Duffy antibodies)
   - Passively acquired antibody from donor plasma
d. Examine a stained peripheral blood film for spherocytes and crenated cells, the presence of which favours a diagnosis of immune haemolysis.

Tests for Nonimmune Haemolysis

1. Examine the bag for discolouration or clots. Take specimens from the bag for bacterial and fungal cultures and also for Gram staining.
2. Examine the plasma in the bag for the presence of free haemoglobin. If present, it indicates improper storage of the unit of blood, overheating or overcooling, injection of drugs or hypotonic solutions. The presence of free haemoglobin in the administration tubing suggests that the same tube was used for administration of dextrose/other solutions.
3. The possibility of mechanical/osmotic haemolysis should also be borne in mind.

Tests Done to Follow Up a Patient With Proven Haemolysis

1. Serum unconjugated bilirubin levels.
2. Plasma haemoglobin levels.
3. Serum haptoglobins: The level in the posttransfusion sample must be compared with that in the pretransfusion sample as the normal range is very wide.
4. Examine the posttransfusion urine sample for free haemoglobin. This is done in a freshly collected sample of urine. In the event of delay in evaluation of a haemolytic reaction, the urine may be tested for haemosiderin. The presence of intact red cells indicates haemorrhage and not haemolysis.
5. Perform a coagulation screen (prothrombin time [PT], activated partial thromboplastin time aPTT, thrombin time [TT]) and platelet count to check for DIC.
6. Monitor blood urea and serum creatinine to assess renal function.

Consequences of Haemolytic Transfusion Reaction

- Disseminated intravascular coagulation
- Renal failure due to haemoglobinaemia caused by intravascular haemolysis

Management of Acute Haemolytic Transfusion Reaction At the first suspicion of a haemolytic reaction, the following steps have to be undertaken:

1. Immediately stop the transfusion.
2. Maintain a patent intravenous line.
3. Ensure diuresis (diuretics, dopamine).
4. Provide cardiorespiratory support.
5. Maintain blood pressure, heart rate and adequate airway.
6. Check the patient's identification to see whether the patient received the intended unit of blood.
7. Report the reaction immediately to the transfusion centre.
8. Send samples to the blood bank for further testing.
9. Monitor blood urea and creatinine levels.

10. Perform a complete coagulation screen to rule out DIC.
11. Check any other patient receiving transfusion at the same time to prevent mortality associated with incompatible transfusion.

Delayed Haemolytic Transfusion Reaction

- These reactions occur days or weeks after the blood is transfused.
- The initial level of antibody in the recipient is low but the transfusion provokes an anamnestic response.
- The antibody titre rises rapidly thereafter with resulting haemolysis.
- Secondary immune response may occur because of previous pregnancy or transfusion.

Clinical Features The time course of a delayed haemolytic transfusion reaction (DHTR) is variable, ranging from an abrupt haemolytic episode to gradual destruction of red cells with little evidence of haemolysis. Maximal rate of destruction is 4–13 days after transfusion.

- Jaundice occurs 5–7 days after transfusion.
- Haemoglobinuria is not uncommon and is seen with antibodies of different specificities.
- DHTRs may occasionally be followed by renal failure.

Laboratory Features

1. A fall in haemoglobin levels not attributed to any other cause is noted.
2. There is an appearance of a new alloantibody.
3. Spherocytosis is observed in blood films which may be the only indicator.
4. DAT is positive. The test becomes positive a few days after transfusion and remains positive until all incompatible cells have been eliminated. With these features, a diagnosis of autoimmune haemolytic anaemia [AIHA] may be made, especially if the significance of a previous transfusion is not realized.
5. Antibody detection: The antibody responsible for the reaction may be detected by preparing an eluate (plasma contains antibody which is separated from the incompatible red cells) from the patient's red cells.

The antibody is detected 4–7 days after transfusion and peaks after 10–15 days.

Sensitive antibody detection techniques in pretransfusion testing may prevent DHTRs.

Nonhaemolytic Immune Transfusion Reactions

Nonhaemolytic immune transfusion reactions (NHTRs) are associated with an immunological reaction between antibodies in the patient's plasma and other antigenic constituents, e.g. platelets and leucocytes in donor blood.

Nonhaemolytic Febrile Transfusion Reaction

NHFTR is suspected when a temperature rise of 1°C or more occurs during or after the transfusion and no other cause could be found.

These are thought to be due to an immunological reaction against one or more of the transfused cellular or plasma components, usually leucocytes, though plasma proteins or platelets may be involved.

These reactions are more common in patients receiving multiple transfusions or in multiparous women. Endogenous pyrogens released during the antigen–antibody interaction stimulate the thermoregulatory centre to produce fever.

Clinical Manifestations

1. Fever and chills shortly after the start of transfusion or even after the transfusion is over. Temperature rise may be mild to severe.
2. Nausea, vomiting.
3. Hypotension and shock.

Management These reactions should be prevented. If mild, the reaction may be managed by slowing of the infusion and using antipyretics. Severe reactions, however, require active intervention. The reactions are often self-limiting. Leucocyte-reduced red cell concentrates should ideally be used in patients at risk. These may be prepared by filtration or centrifugation.

Filtration is the most frequently used technique to achieve leucodepletion. Third-generation in-line leucocyte filters, which remove 99.9% of white cells, are now available.

Allergic Transfusion Reactions

Allergic reactions occur most commonly because of infusion of plasma proteins. The severity of the reactions is variable and not necessarily dose-related.

a. Mild allergic reaction: urticaria
   This is a commonly encountered reaction characterized by a localized swelling of the superficial layers of the skin. The lesions are pruritic, raised, erythematous, sharply demarcated and transient.
   The reactions are due to allergy to a product in the donor plasma. IgE in the recipient reacts with antigens on the donor cells. The release of histamine causes the typical clinical features. The reactions are managed by administration of antihistamines. After the reaction has subsided, transfusion may be continued at a slow rate as the reaction is not likely to recur.
b. Severe allergic reaction: anaphylactoid reaction
   This is a rare and severe reaction. The symptoms of shock and unconsciousness may occur with transfusion of a few millilitres of blood.

Pathogenesis It occurs in IgA-deficient (IgA <1 mg/mL) patients who have developed anti-IgA after previous transfusion or pregnancy. The antibodies can fix complement. On reexposure to minute amounts of IgA, these patients develop anaphylactoid reaction. The incident of IgA deficiency is 1:1000.

Clinical features of the reaction are as follows:

- Cough
- Respiratory distress
- Bronchospasm
- Nausea, vomiting, abdominal cramps and diarrhoea
- Circulatory collapse
- Hypotension and shock

Diagnosis Diagnosis can be made by demonstration of antibody to IgA; however, this is not done in most laboratories. The absence of serum IgA may be demonstrated by immunodiffusion.

Management
1. Stop the transfusion.
2. Treat hypotension with fluids.
3. Give epinephrine injection (0.5 mg) subcutaneously if the patient is in shock.
4. Steroids (100–200 mg of hydrocortisone) are useful.

Prevention
1. Sensitized patients should be given blood and blood products deficient in IgA.
2. If red cells are required, deglycerolized and washed red cells may be used.
3. Transfusion should be given at a slow rate.

Because IgA-deficient donors may be difficult to find, autologous blood may be used.

Transfusion-Related Acute Lung Injury or Noncardiogenic Pulmonary Oedema

It is a rare reaction in which the recipient develops pulmonary oedema without a change in cardiac pressure. The proposed pathogenetic mechanisms are as follows:

a. Reaction between donor antileucocyte antibodies and recipient leucocytes forms aggregates. The aggregates are trapped in the pulmonary circulation with a change in vascular permeability.
b. Activation of complement C3a and C5a with release of histamine produces leucocyte aggregates. Pulmonary leucostasis causes microvascular occlusion, capillary leakage and pulmonary oedema.
c. Complement-activated granulocytes produce oxygen radicals which damage pulmonary endothelial cells and lead to increased vascular permeability and oedema.

Clinical Features
- Acute respiratory distress
- Fever with chills
- Cyanosis
- Hypotension

X-ray chest: Pulmonary infiltrates in the hilar region

Management
1. Stop the transfusion.
2. Provide respiratory support.
3. Give steroids.

Prevention Washed red cells may be used. Multiparous women and multitransfused patients should not be used as plasma donors, as their serum may have high titres of leucoagglutinating antibodies.

Graft-Versus-Host Disease

GVHD is a rare complication of transfusion that occurs in severely immunosuppressed individuals such as patients receiving chemotherapy/radiotherapy. Patients with lymphopenia and bone marrow transplant recipients are at risk, as also are neonates, especially those who receive exchange transfusion.

Pathogenesis The donor lymphocytes engraft and multiply in the recipient. The engrafted cells react with the host tissues to cause the clinical manifestations. The donor lymphocytes are not destroyed as the host is immunocompromised.

Clinical Features

- Fever
- Diffuse erythematous rash
- Diarrhoea
- Bone marrow suppression
- Infection

Prognosis The reaction is fatal in 90% of cases.

Prevention The use of irradiated blood and blood products can prevent GVHD. A radiation dose of 1500–5000 rad for 10 minutes renders 85%–95% of lymphocytes incapable of replication. Gamma irradiators are commercially available which can be used for irradiation of blood bags.

Posttransfusion Purpura

In this condition, marked thrombocytopenia develops 5–10 days after transfusion. It is found more often in multiparous women. In some patients, platelet-specific alloantibodies have been found (anti-PLA1). The antibody destroys not only the transfused platelets but also the patient's own platelets which are PLA1-negative. Thrombocytopenia is severe but self-limiting.

Platelet transfusions are not beneficial and if treatment is required, therapeutic plasmapheresis is suggested. Intravenous immunoglobulins have a proven role in the management of these patients.

Alloimmunization

Blood transfusion exposes a patient to several foreign antigens. If the recipient does not possess these antigens, antibodies are formed against them days, weeks or months after the transfusion. Alloimmunization may occur to red cell, white cell or platelet antigens as well as to plasma proteins.

Immunomodulation

Transfusion of blood is associated with changes in immune function. The effect is obvious in multitransfused patients. There is decreased lymphocyte responsiveness to phytohaemagglutinin and in a mixed lymphocyte culture, with pooled normal lymphocytes as stimulator cells. A reduced helper to suppressor ratio and decreased activity of natural killer (NK) cells are also observed.

Tumour Recurrence

Transfusion of blood has a detrimental effect on the outcome of cancer surgery. The difference in tumour-free survival in transfused and nontransfused patients is statistically significant, and the rate of recurrence in the latter group is lower.

Allograft Recipients

Transfusion also increases the survival of allografts by this immunosuppressive effect.

Infection

Transfusion is implicated in decreasing resistance to infection with viruses and bacteria. There is a highly significant association of transfusion with an increased incidence of postoperative infections.

In contrast, all these effects are not observed with the use of autologous blood.

NONIMMUNE REACTIONS

Bacterial Contamination of Blood

Bacterial contamination of blood may occur because of incorrect phlebotomy, improper handling during component preparations or improper storage. With strict adherence to appropriate protocols for phlebotomy and adequate equipment for storage being available, this is fortunately a rare complication.

Clinical Features

The symptoms are severe and occur because of endotoxin produced by Gram-negative bacteria. The patient may experience the following:

- High-grade fever
- Nausea, vomiting
- Diarrhoea
- Abdominal cramps
- Haemoglobinuria
- Shock
- DIC and renal failure

Management

1. Stop the transfusion immediately.
2. Examine the bag for discolouration/clots/colour of the blood and plasma/interface of cells and plasma.
3. Send blood from the blood bag, tubing and the recipient (posttransfusion) for culture at 4°C, 22°C and 37°C. Cultures must be done for bacteria (aerobic and anaerobic) and fungi.
4. Keep intravenous line patent.
5. Give broad-spectrum antibiotics, steroids and dopamine to manage shock.

Prevention

1. Maintain strict aseptic precautions during phlebotomy.
2. Store blood under adequate storage conditions.
3. Maintain aseptic precautions during component preparation.
4. Maintain the donor room area clean.
5. Send the reagents used for cleaning the venipuncture site for bacteriological examination at periodic intervals to check for contamination.

CIRCULATORY OVERLOAD

Patients with a compromised cardiopulmonary function may not tolerate a rapid increase in blood volume and develop hypervolaemia. This is specially seen in infants and elderly patients.

Clinical Features

During the transfusion, the patient may develop the following:

- Sudden severe headache
- Tachycardia
- Dyspnoea
- Cough
- Cyanosis
- Orthopnoea

Management

1. Stop the infusion immediately.
2. Place the patient in a sitting position.
3. Give diuretics.
4. Give oxygen, if required.

Prevention

1. Slow infusion to be given to patients at risk (1 mL/kg/h).
2. Give diuretics before starting the transfusion.

IRON OVERLOAD

Each unit of red cells contains 200 mg of iron. Patients who are on long-term transfusion therapy, such as those with thalassaemia, accumulate iron and develop organ dysfunction because of deposition of iron. Treatment is achieved by chelating agents such as desferrioxamine or newer compounds such as oral iron chelator L1.

TRANSFUSION-TRANSMISSIBLE INFECTIONS

These diseases are transmissible by blood transfusion and can cause morbidity and mortality in the recipients.

Common TTIs are discussed in the following section.

As large volumes of blood or blood components are given to patients during transfusion therapy, even a blood unit with a low viral load may cause infection in the recipient.

SUMMARY

Transfusion of blood is frequently associated with adverse reactions, which may be divided into immunological or nonimmunological. Acute intravascular haemolytic reactions are associated with high mortality. These result most often because of ABO incompatibility. As human error is the most common cause of these reactions, all efforts should be made to prevent such errors. All reactions should be adequately evaluated and recorded. The hospital transfusion committee should look into the causes of transfusion reactions and take steps to prevent these reactions.

TRANSFUSION-TRANSMISSIBLE INFECTIONS PA 22.5

INTRODUCTION

Major life-threatening complications due to blood transfusion are rare, and human error remains a common factor in many situations. The prominent hazard of blood transfusion is the risk of transmission of blood-borne infections. Understanding the infectious agents which are endemic in a particular region is important in implementing strategies to prevent the transmission of these infections. Provision of safe blood is of utmost importance, and its responsibility lies generally with the blood transfusion service.

The infections transmitted through blood can be divided into the following:

a. **Exogenous**
   Exogenous infections are those which are introduced into a blood unit from an external source.
b. **Endogenous**
   Endogenous infections are those which are transmitted from the donor's blood to the recipient.
   The infectious agents known to be transmitted through blood can be as follows:

1. Viruses
2. Bacteria
3. Protozoa

Viruses transmissible by blood transfusion
- Cytomegalovirus
- Epstein–Barr virus
- HTLV-1
- HTLV-2
- Herpes virus (HSV-1 and HSV-2)
- Hepatitis B virus
- Hepatitis delta virus (HDV)
- Hepatitis A virus (HAV)
- Hepatitis C
- Human immunodeficiency virus (HIV-1 and HIV-2)
- Serum parvovirus (B-19)

Bacteria transmissible by blood transfusion
- *Treponema pallidum* (syphilis)
- *Brucella abortus*
- *Yersinia enterocolitica*
- *Salmonella*

Parasites transmissible by blood transfusion
- *Plasmodium* species (malaria)
- *Trypanosoma cruzi* (Chagas disease)
- *Toxoplasma gondii* (mostly in immunosuppressed patients)
- *Leishmania donovani*
- Microfilariae
- *Babesia microti*

AUTOLOGOUS BLOOD DONATION PA 22.7

Autologous donation means blood and blood components collected from an individual and planned exclusively for subsequent autologous transfusion to that same individual. The advantages and disadvantages of autologous blood donation are given in Table 18.7.

Table 18.7 Advantages and Disadvantages of Autologous Blood Donation

Advantages of ABD	Disadvantages of ABD
Prevents TTI	Risk of bacterial contamination
No alloimmunization	Administrative error, e.g. ABO mismatch
Avoidance of transfusion reactions	Costlier
Avoidance of immunosuppression	More wastage
Conservation of blood resources	Perioperative anaemia
Patient satisfaction	Complex, especially in children

ABD, autologous blood donation; TTI, transfusion-transmissible infection.

Types of autologous blood donation

1. **Preoperative autologous donation**
   Donor weight ≥50 kg, then 450 mL collection
   Donor weight <50 kg
   (Volume collected = Donor weight in kg/50 × 450 mL)
   Haemoglobin ≥11 g%, haematocrit ≥33%
   Storage
   2–8°C
   Indications
   - Major orthopaedic procedures
   - Vascular surgery
   - Cardiac/thoracic surgeries
   - Radical prostatectomy
   - Neurosurgical procedures
2. **Acute normovolaemic haemodilution**
   Definition
   Removal of whole blood from a patient and restoring the circulating blood volume with an acellular fluid shortly before an anticipated significant surgical blood loss.
   - Performed immediately before or after induction of anaesthesia
   - Collection in standard blood bags containing anti-coagulant – ACD, CPDA, CPD/SAGM
3. **Intra- and postoperative blood recovery or blood salvage**
   Recovery of blood from surgical drains, followed by reinfusion after processing through a microaggregate filter. Upper limit of blood volume that can be reinfused: 1400 mL. If blood not used within 6 hours, then it is discarded. Practiced commonly in the following:
   - Cardiac surgeries
   - Orthopaedic surgery
   - Neurosurgery

Autologous transfusion should be considered as part of an approach for minimizing the risk associated with transfusion for patients having surgery, where blood loss is anticipated. All transfusions, whether allogeneic or autologous blood, carry a risk. Planning and appropriate treatment in advance of or during surgery may reduce transfusion requirements. Before transfusing a patient, always think twice whether it is necessary and if it can be avoided by using any alternative.

SELF-ASSESSMENT

Multiple Choice Questions

1. Which blood group is considered the universal donor for red blood cells?
   A. A
   B. B
   C. AB
   D. O
2. What is the most common cause of haemolytic transfusion reactions?
   A. Blood group incompatibility
   B. Donor blood contamination
   C. Patient's immune response
   D. Storage issues
3. Which component is typically transfused to treat haemophilia?
   A. Red blood cells
   B. Platelets
   C. Fresh frozen plasma
   D. Cryoprecipitate
4. What is the primary risk of a transfusion in a patient with a history of multiple transfusions?
   A. Infection
   B. Haemolysis
   C. Allergic reaction
   D. Alloimmunization
5. In a patient with cold agglutinin disease requiring transfusion, the best approach is
   A. Prewarming the blood products
   B. Using leukoreduced red cells
   C. Administering only AB plasma
   D. Avoiding transfusion altogether
6. A patient with paroxysmal nocturnal haemoglobinuria (PNH) is most at risk of which transfusion complication?
   A. Anaphylactic reaction
   B. Alloimmunization
   C. Iron overload
   D. Haemolysis
7. Which genetic mutation is most significantly associated with transfusion-related acute lung injury (TRALI)?
   A. HLA-DR
   B. HNA-3a
   C. ABO
   D. RHD
8. In a transfusion setting, the Bombay phenotype presents a challenge because:
   A. It is resistant to most anticoagulants
   B. It lacks A, B and H antigens on red cells
   C. It causes spontaneous agglutination of donor cells
   D. It is associated with recurrent febrile reactions
9. Massive transfusion protocol in trauma patients ideally requires a ratio of:
   A. 1:1:1 of RBCs, plasma and platelets
   B. 2:1:1 of RBCs, plasma and platelets
   C. 1:2:1 of RBCs, plasma and platelets
   D. 1:1:2 of RBCs, plasma and platelets
10. The most appropriate test to diagnose delayed haemolytic transfusion reaction (DHTR) is
    A. Direct antiglobulin test (DAT)
    B. Indirect antiglobulin test (IAT)
    C. Elution
    D. Haptoglobin levels
11. In a patient with sickle cell disease, the best transfusion strategy to prevent stroke is
    A. Chronic simple transfusions
    B. Exchange transfusion
    C. Periodic leukoreduced transfusions
    D. Transfusion only during crises
12. The primary mechanism of transfusion-associated graft-versus-host disease (TA-GVHD) is
    A. Donor T-cells attacking host tissues
    B. Host immune response against donor cells

C. ABO incompatibility
D. HLA alloimmunization

13. Which pathogen is not typically screened for in standard blood donations in the United States?
A. HIV
B. Hepatitis C
C. Babesia
D. Hepatitis B

14. 'TACO' (transfusion-associated circulatory overload) is best managed initially by:
A. Diuretics
B. Steroids
C. Antihistamines
D. Stopping the transfusion and sit the patient upright

15. In a patient with a history of anti-Jka antibody, which of the following blood types should be avoided?
A. Jka-positive
B. Kell-positive
C. Duffy-negative
D. MNS-positive

16. Which anticoagulant is preferred in a patient with heparin-induced thrombocytopenia requiring apheresis?
A. Heparin
B. Citrate
C. Warfarin
D. Argatroban

17. The most effective method to prevent transfusion-related Zika virus transmission is
A. NAT (nucleic acid testing)
B. Pathogen reduction technology
C. Donor travel history screening
D. Quarantining blood products

18. In platelet refractoriness, the first step should be:
A. Administering HLA-matched platelets
B. Checking for antiplatelet antibodies
C. Increasing the dose of platelets
D. Switching to apheresis platelets

19. The primary concern with transfusing 'old' red blood cells (close to expiration) is
A. Increased risk of bacterial contamination
B. Decreased oxygen-carrying capacity
C. Risk of alloimmunization
D. Potassium leakage leading to hyperkalaemia

20. The Rh-null phenotype is clinically significant due to
A. High risk of haemolytic disease of the fetus and newborn
B. Severe transfusion reactions with standard RhD-negative blood
C. Its extreme rarity and associated haematologic abnormalities
D. Lack of compatibility with most blood donors

Answers

1. (D); 2. (A); 3. (D); 4. (D); 5. (A); 6. (D); 7. (B); 8. (B); 9. (A); 10. (A); 11. (B); 12. (A); 13. (C); 14. (D); 15. (A); 16. (B); 17. (A); 18. (B); 19. (D); 20. (C)

Self-Assessment Questions

1. A patient with type B blood urgently needs a transfusion but type B blood is not available. Which alternative blood type can you safely transfuse?
2. During a transfusion, a patient develops a fever and chills. What is the most likely cause and how should it be managed?
3. A pregnant woman with O-negative blood is due for delivery. What prophylactic treatment should be considered to prevent haemolytic disease of the newborn?
4. A patient receiving a transfusion suddenly shows signs of back pain and dark urine. What is the likely complication and immediate action required?
5. In a trauma patient requiring massive transfusion, what are the key components to include in the transfusion protocol for balanced resuscitation?
6. A patient with a known history of anti-Kell antibodies needs a transfusion. What specific testing or blood type is required for safe transfusion?
7. For a patient undergoing chemotherapy, what transfusion considerations are important to prevent complications?
8. A patient with thalassaemia major requires regular transfusions. What long-term complication should be monitored and how is it managed?
9. During a transfusion, a patient complains of difficulty breathing and shows signs of hypotension. What is the likely cause and first line of treatment?
10. A patient with a history of multiple transfusions presents with elevated ferritin levels. What condition should be suspected and what are the management strategies?

Answers

1. Type O blood can be safely transfused as it is compatible with type B blood.
2. The patient is likely experiencing a febrile nonhaemolytic transfusion reaction. Management includes stopping the transfusion, administering antipyretics and evaluating for other causes.
3. Administration of Rh immune globulin (Rho(D) immune globulin) is recommended to prevent haemolytic disease of the newborn.
4. This is indicative of an acute haemolytic transfusion reaction. Immediate action includes stopping the transfusion and initiating supportive care.
5. The protocol should include a balanced ratio of red blood cells, plasma and platelets, often in a 1:1:1 ratio.
6. Transfusion with Kell-negative blood is required to avoid an immune reaction.
7. Transfusion of leukoreduced and irradiated blood products is important to minimize the risk of complications.
8. Iron overload is a common complication, managed with regular chelation therapy.
9. This could be a sign of a transfusion-related acute lung injury (TRALI). Immediate management includes stopping the transfusion and providing respiratory support.
10. The condition is likely transfusional haemosiderosis. Management strategies include iron chelation therapy and minimizing future transfusions.

Scenario-Based Questions

1. A 38-year-old man who met with an accident was shifted to the operation theatre as he needed urgent surgery. Two units of packed cell units were reserved and transfused postoperatively because of heavy blood loss. The patient complained of chest pain and breathlessness 20 minutes after starting the transfusion of the first unit of packed cells. He also had temperature of 101°F, chills, rigor and tachycardia.
   What is your provisional diagnosis? How would you like to investigate and manage the situation?
2. Design a protocol for pretransfusion testing.
3. Write a protocol for workup of transfusion reactions.
4. Describe ABO blood group antigens and their formation and structure.
5. Describe the Rh blood group system.
6. List blood components and their uses.
7. Discuss the adverse effects of blood transfusion.
8. List the transfusion-transmissible infections.
9. Enumerate and discuss the types of autologous blood transfusion.

Topics for Self-Directed Learning

1. Other blood group systems and their significance
2. Haemovigilance
3. Weak, partial and elevated D
4. Donor selection criteria
5. Donor deferral
6. Weak D/partial D Rh antigen types and their clinical significance
7. Apheresis technique

MIND MAPS

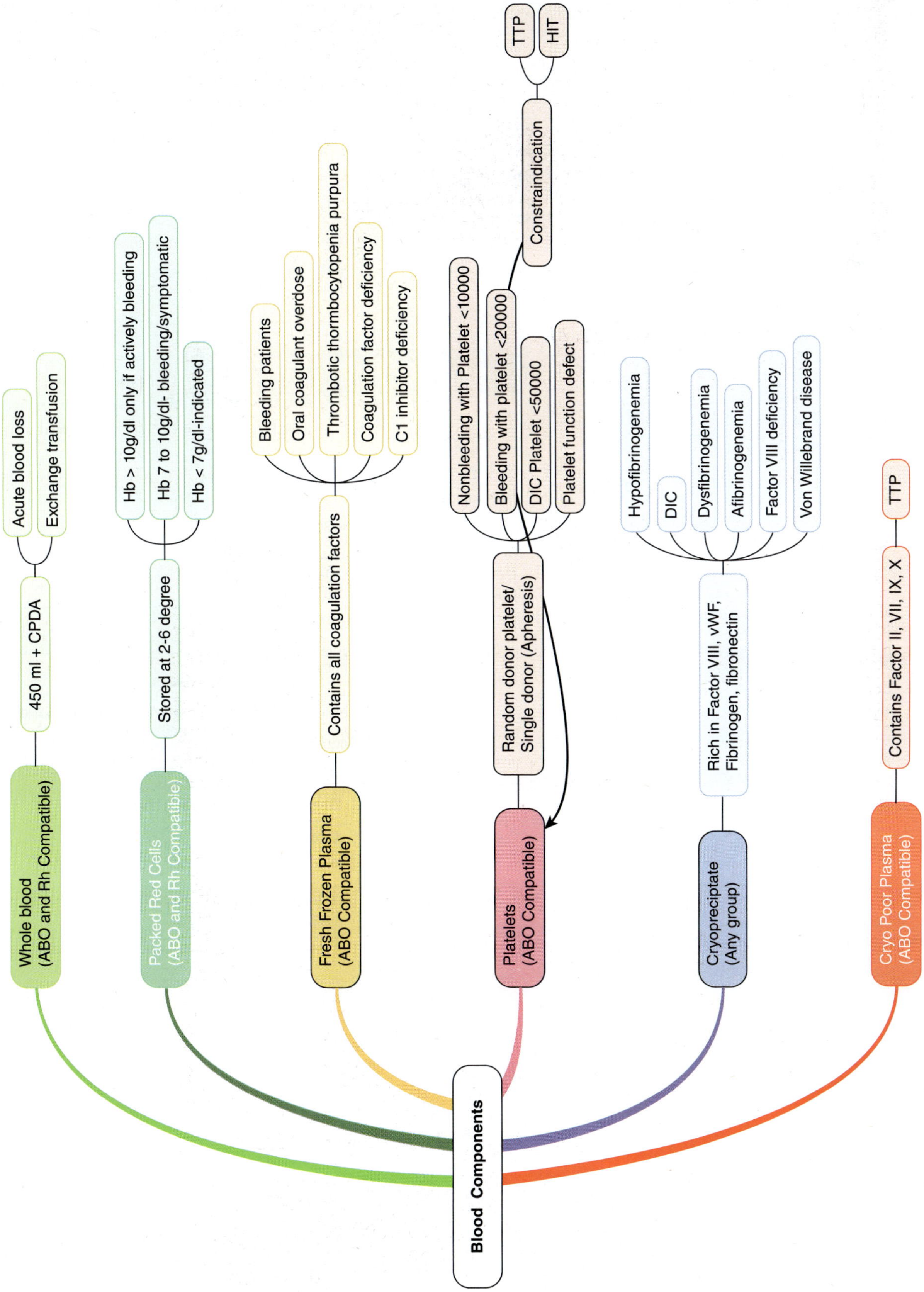
Blood Components
Whole blood (ABO and Rh Compatible)
450 ml + CPDA
Acute blood loss
Exchange transfusion
Packed Red Cells (ABO and Rh Compatible)
Stored at 2-6 degree
Hb > 10g/dl only if actively bleeding
Hb 7 to 10g/dl- bleeding/symptomatic
Hb < 7g/dl-indicated
Fresh Frozen Plasma (ABO Compatible)
Contains all coagulation factors
Bleeding patients
Oral coagulant overdose
Thrombotic thrombocytopenia purpura
Coagulation factor deficiency
C1 inhibitor deficiency
Platelets (ABO Compatible)
Random donor platelet/ Single donor (Apheresis)
Nonbleeding with Platelet <10000
Bleeding with platelet <20000
DIC Platelet <50000
Platelet function defect
Constraindication
TTP
HIT
Cryoprecipitate (Any group)
Rich in Factor VIII, vWF, Fibrinogen, fibronectin
Hypofibrinogenemia
DIC
Dysfibrinogenemia
Afibrinogenemia
Factor VIII deficiency
Von Willebrand disease
Cryo Poor Plasma (ABO Compatible)
Contains Factor II, VII, IX, X
TTP

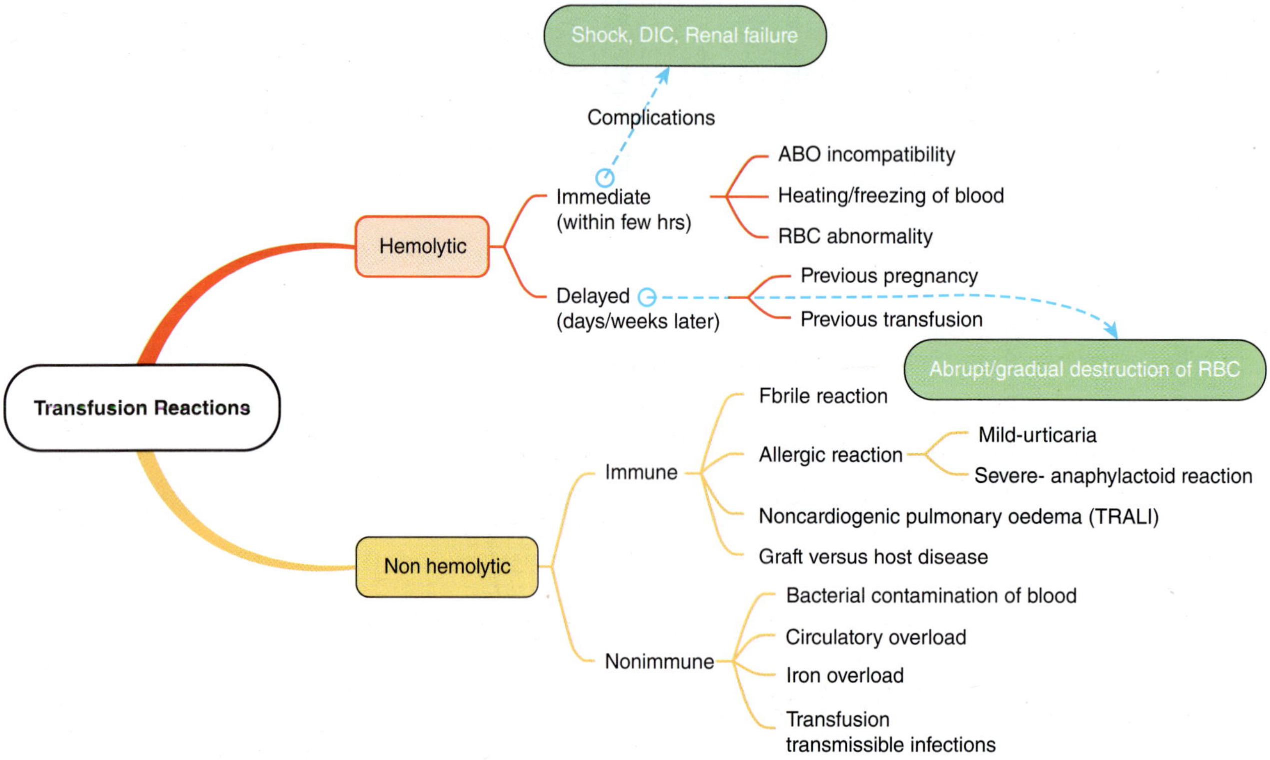
Shock, DIC, Renal failure
Complications
ABO incompatibility
Immediate
(within few hrs)
Heating/freezing of blood
Hemolytic
RBC abnormality
Previous pregnancy
Delayed
(days/weeks later)
Previous transfusion
Abrupt/gradual destruction of RBC
Transfusion Reactions
Fbrile reaction
Allergic reaction
Mild-urticaria
Severe- anaphylactoid reaction
Immune
Noncardiogenic pulmonary oedema (TRALI)
Graft versus host disease
Non hemolytic
Bacterial contamination of blood
Circulatory overload
Nonimmune
Iron overload
Transfusion
transmissible infections

The Lungs 19

V Eswari

PA 26.1 Define and describe the aetiology, types, pathogenesis, stages, morphology and complications of **pneumonia**.

PA 26.2 Describe the aetiology, gross and microscopic appearance, and complications of **lung abscess**.

PA 26.3 Define and describe the aetiology, types, pathogenesis, stages, morphology, complications and evaluation of **obstructive airway disease (OAD) and bronchiectasis**.

PA 26.4 Define and describe the aetiology, types, pathogenesis, stages, morphology, microscopic appearance and complications of **tuberculosis**.

PA 26.5 Define and describe the aetiology, types, exposure, environmental influence, pathogenesis, stages, morphology, microscopic appearance and complications of **occupational lung diseases**.

PA 26.6 Define and describe the aetiology, types, exposure, genetics, environmental influence, pathogenesis, stages, morphology, microscopic appearance, metastases and complications of **tumours of the lung and pleura**.

PA 26.7 Define and describe the aetiology, types, exposure, genetics, environmental influence, pathogenesis, morphology, microscopic appearance and complications of **mesothelioma**.

CHAPTER OUTLINE

INTRODUCTION

The lungs, the major organs of the respiratory system, function primarily to provide oxygen to the tissues for cellular respiration, remove the waste product carbon dioxide and help in maintaining acid–base balance. We begin with a brief review of the basic anatomy, histology and physiology of the lungs before delving into the pathology.

ANATOMY AND HISTOLOGY

Anatomy (Fig. 19.1)

The respiratory system develops as an outgrowth (laryngotracheal diverticulum) from the ventral wall of the foregut at the end of the third week of gestation. The distal end of the diverticulum dilates to form the lung bud that divides to form two primary bronchial buds. The bronchial buds divide and redivide to form the bronchial tree. The right main bronchus gives rise to three secondary bronchi, and the left main bronchus forms two secondary bronchi. During further development, secondary bronchi divide repeatedly, giving rise to progressively smaller airways termed bronchioles. Additional branching of the bronchioles leads to terminal bronchioles. The **right main bronchus is more vertical** and directly in line with the trachea. Hence, aspirations are more common on the right than on the left.

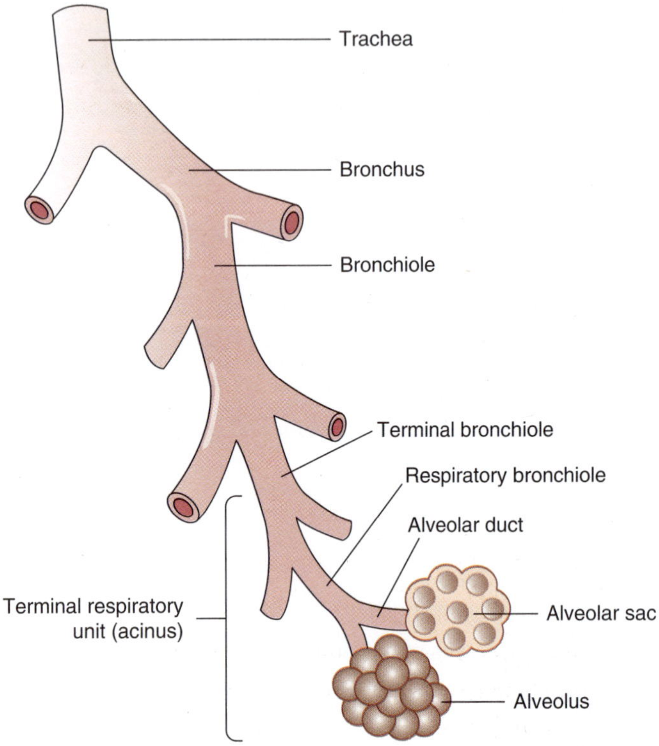

Fig. 19.1 Anatomy of lungs. (*Source:* From Paul Bass, Susan Burroughs, Norman Carr, Claire Way. Master Medicine: General and Systematic Pathology. Elsevier. 2009.)

The part of the lung distal to a terminal bronchiole is called an acinus, which is composed of respiratory bronchiole, alveolar duct and alveolar sac. A cluster of three to five terminal bronchioles, each with its appended acinus, is referred to as pulmonary lobule. The lungs have **dual blood supply** – oxygenated blood from bronchial arteries and venous blood from pulmonary arteries. These are also rich in intercommunicating lymphatics on the surface.

Histology

The entire respiratory tree including the larynx, trachea, bronchi and bronchioles is lined by pseudostratified ciliated columnar epithelium and contains goblet cells. They secrete mucus that serves as the first line of defence against incoming environmental pathogens. Cilia move the mucus-bound particulate up and away for expulsion from the body. The bronchial mucosa also contains **neuroendocrine cells** (NECs) that release factors such as serotonin, calcitonin and gastrin-releasing peptide (bombesin).

The trachea, bronchi and their bronchioles possess cartilage, smooth muscles and mucous glands in their walls. **Bronchioles have smooth muscles but lack cartilage** and submucosal glands.

Alveolar walls and septae have the following features:

Alveolar epithelium is a continuous layer made up of two types of cells:

- **Type 1 pneumocytes**, also known as membranous pneumocytes, make up 95% of the alveolar surface. These are flat and plate-like.
- **Type 2 pneumocytes** or granular pneumocytes extend into the alveoli and are covered by microvilli. They secrete surfactant, a phospholipoprotein that prevents the collapse of the lung, and are involved in the repair of alveolar epithelium.

Capillary endothelium forms the anastomotic capillaries in the alveolar walls.

The capillary basement membrane separates the capillary endothelium from the alveolar lining of the epithelial cells.

Alveolar macrophages are mononuclear phagocytes found in the **alveoli** of the lungs. They ingest small inhaled particles, assisting in the degradation, clearance and presentation of the antigen to adaptive immune cells.

The pores of Kohn are the sites of alveolar communications and are present between the adjacent alveolar walls that allow the passage of bacteria and exudate.

CONGENITAL ANOMALIES

Congenital anomalies of the lungs are rare, and the relatively common ones are described as follows:

Pulmonary hypoplasia

Pulmonary hypoplasia is characterized by the defective development of both the lungs and is caused by abnormalities that compress the lung or impede normal lung expansion in utero (congenital diaphragmatic hernia, oligohydramnios).

Bronchogenic cysts

This type of anomaly arises because of anomalous budding of the tracheobronchial tree and is commonly found in the mediastinum, behind the carina and in the lung parenchyma.

It is a unilocular cyst lined by the respiratory epithelium (cuboidal or columnar ciliated epithelium). The wall is made up of tissues like those of the normal bronchial tree, including cartilage, elastic tissues, mucous glands and smooth muscle. These do not usually communicate with the bronchial tree. This may be an incidental finding or can present as an obstruction or infection.

Pulmonary sequestration

Pulmonary sequestration, also referred to as accessory lung, is a rare congenital abnormality that is characterized by the presence of a nonfunctional lung tissue that, by definition, lacks any connection to the airway system and has abnormal blood supply derived from the aorta and its branches and not the pulmonary artery.

Types (Fig. 19.2)

Extralobar sequestration is most commonly seen in infants as abnormal mediastinal masses, and may be associated with other congenital abnormalities.

Intralobar sequestration is found within the lungs typically observed in older children and associated with recurrent infections.

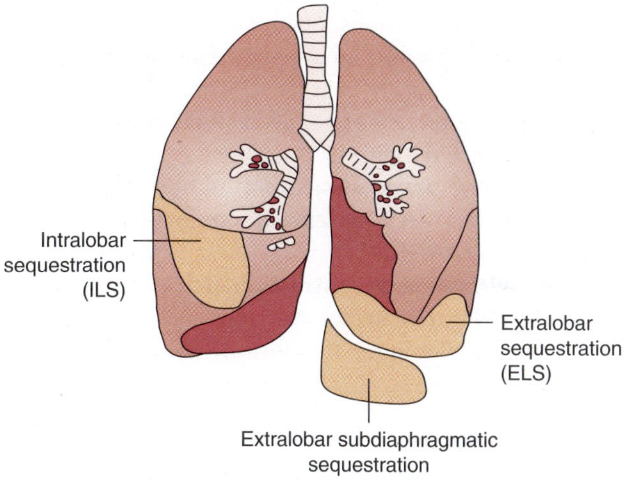

Fig. 19.2 Schematic representation of intralobar and extralobar pulmonary sequestrations. (*Source:* Reproduced from Classification of pulmonary sequestration | Radiology Case | Radiopaedia.org.)

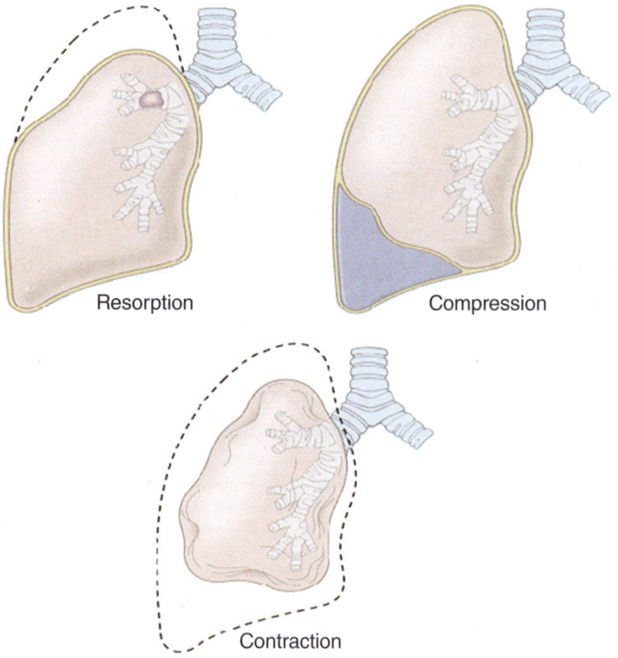

Fig. 19.3 Different types of acquired atelectasis. Dashed lines indicate normal lung volume. (*Source:* From Vinay Kumar, Abul K Abbas, Jon C Aster. Robbins Basic Pathology. Elsevier. 2018.)

ATELECTASIS

The word 'atelectasis' is derived from two Greek words *atelez* (meaning imperfect) and *ectasis* (meaning expansion). Atelectasis can be defined as a partial or completely reversible collapse of the small airways leading to impaired gas exchange, which may be acquired or inherited.

Acquired atelectasis: Collapse of the previously inflated lungs

Inherited or neonatal atelectasis: Incomplete expansion of the lungs

Types of acquired atelectasis (Fig. 19.3)

Obstructive atelectasis, also referred to as resorption atelectasis, is caused by a partial or complete obstruction of the airway most commonly due to mucus plugs and rarely by tumour fragments and foreign bodies. Air in the alveoli distal to the obstruction is reabsorbed, causing alveolar collapse. As a result, lung volume is diminished and the **mediastinum shifts towards the atelectatic lung.**

Nonobstructive atelectasis is of many types:

- **Compression atelectasis:** It occurs secondary to increased pressure exerted on the lungs, causing the alveoli to collapse. It is frequently encountered

in pleural effusions, pneumothorax or haemothorax. Compressed lung tissue cannot expand and is therefore poorly ventilated. Compression pushes the lung, resulting in a mediastinal shift away from the affected lung.
- **Adhesive atelectasis:** It occurs due to surfactant deficiency seen in acute respiratory distress syndrome (ARDS).
- **Cicatrization or contraction atelectasis:** It occurs due to parenchymal scarring, e.g. fibrosing diseases of the lung. This form of atelectasis is irreversible.

Clinical Features

Patients may present with dyspnoea, tachypnoea, absent breath sounds, cough with sputum production and diminished chest expansion.

PULMONARY OEDEMA

Pulmonary oedema results from accumulation of fluid in the air spaces and lung parenchyma, leading to impaired gas exchange and respiratory failure.

PATHOPHYSIOLOGY

The passive exchange of water between the capillary microcirculation and the interstitial fluid is largely determined by the hydrostatic pressure and oncotic pressure of these two compartments.

Oedema arises due to an imbalance between the hydrostatic pressure and the oncotic pressure.

The classification of pulmonary oedema is based on the underlying cause:

- Cardiogenic
- Noncardiogenic

Pulmonary oedema is also classified on the basis of the mechanism involved and is shown in Table 19.1.

Morphology

Gross The lungs are heavy and wet. Oedema first develops in the **basal regions** (greater hydrostatic pressure in the dependent areas). **Fibrosis and thickening** of the affected areas result in a gross, brown and firm appearance called **brown induration.**

Microscopy Microscopically, the alveolar spaces are predominantly filled with pale-staining eosinophilic material, which also occupies the perivascular interstitial spaces, resulting in the widening of the alveolar septa (Fig. 19.4). Within the alveolar septae and alveolar spaces, characteristic **heart failure cells** are seen. These cells are formed when extravasated red blood cells (RBCs) break down, releasing haemoglobin, which is then ingested by alveolar macrophages. The haemoglobin inside the macrophages is then converted into fine granules of golden brown haemosiderin.

Clinical Features

Patients with pulmonary oedema commonly experience dyspnoea due to impaired diffusion of oxygen into the pulmonary capillaries. **Orthopnoea** and **paroxysmal nocturnal dyspnoea** occur due to increased venous return to the already congested heart and lungs, especially when the patient lies in the supine position. **Rusty sputum** may occur due to rupture of the pulmonary capillaries. Wheezing may be due to peribronchial oedema.

ACUTE LUNG INJURY AND ACUTE RESPIRATORY DISTRESS SYNDROME

Acute lung injury (ALI) or ARDS is a state of **acute diffuse alveolar damage** characterized by **increased capillary**

Table 19.1 List of Causes of Pulmonary Oedema on the Basis of the Mechanism

Category	Mechanism of Pulmonary Oedema
Noninflammatory or haemodynamic oedema	• Increased hydrostatic pressure (e.g. congestive heart failure) • Decreased oncotic pressure (e.g. nephrotic syndrome, liver disease, protein-losing enteropathies, hypoalbuminaemia) • Lymphatic obstruction (e.g. carcinomatosis)
Inflammatory or microvascular injury	• Injury to pulmonary capillaries or alveolar lining cells • Adult respiratory distress syndrome, trauma, pneumonia, sepsis, near drowning, inhalation of gases (high concentration of oxygen, smoke), drugs like bleomycin and amphotericin
High altitude	• Owing to hypoxic pulmonary vasoconstriction and increase in the pulmonary artery pressure
Neurogenic oedema	• Spinal cord injury, subarachnoid haemorrhage (SAH), traumatic brain injury (TBI), intracranial haemorrhage, status epilepticus, meningitis and subdural haemorrhage

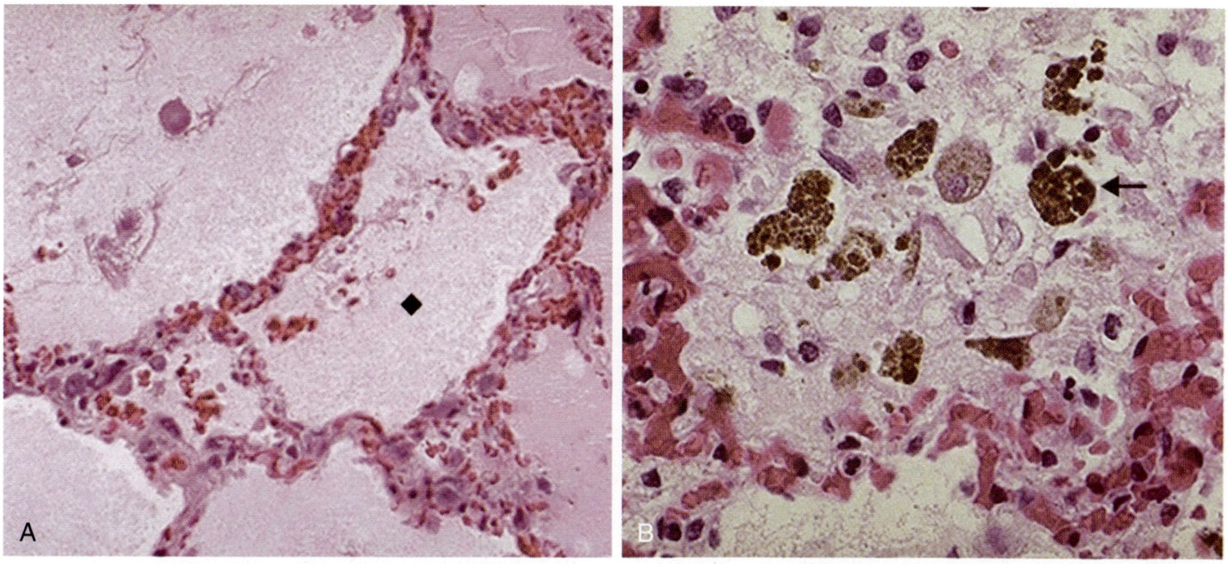

Fig. 19.4 Microscopy of pulmonary oedema. (A) The alveoli are filled with pink material (mark) and the alveolar capillaries in the septal walls are congested. (B) Alveolar spaces show haemosiderin-laden macrophages ('heart failure cells') containing brown cytoplasmic haemosiderin granules due to breakdown of RBCs (arrow). (*Source:* From Edward C Klatt. Robbins and Cotran Atlas of Pathology. Elsevier. 2021.)

permeability, pulmonary oedema and refractory hypoxaemia.

This syndrome is also referred to by the following names:

Adult hyaline membrane disease
Shock lung
Noncardiogenic pulmonary oedema

Table 19.2 lists the conditions that lead to ALI. Its features are as follows:

- Acute onset of severe hypoxaemia
- Signs of respiratory distress (dyspnoea, tachypnoea)
- Diffuse bilateral infiltrates in the chest X-ray
- No evidence of left atrial hypertension

PATHOPHYSIOLOGY

There are three phases of the disease (Fig. 19.5 and Flowchart 19.1):

1. Exudative/inflammatory
2. Proliferative
3. Fibrotic

The course of each phase and the overall progression of the disease are variable.

Exudative phase or inflammatory phase

This marks the initial phase. Injury to the alveolar epithelium triggers activation of alveolar macrophages recruiting neutrophils and circulating macrophages to the pulmonary sites of injury. These cells elaborate proteases, reactive oxygen species, eicosanoids, phospholipids and cytokines perpetuating inflammatory responses. Inflammatory cytokines, such as IL-1β, tumour necrosis factor alpha (TNF-α), IL-6 and IL-8, are

Table 19.2 List of Conditions Associated with Acute Respiratory Distress Syndrome

Category of the Disease	Common Causes
Infections	Sepsis[a] Diffuse pulmonary infections caused by viruses, *Mycoplasma*, pneumocystis pneumonia and miliary tuberculosis[a] Gastric aspiration[a]
Physical injury	Mechanical trauma including head injury[a] Near drowning Pulmonary contusions Fractures with fat embolism Burns
Chemical injury	Heroin overdose Methadone overdose Barbiturate overdose Acetylsalicylic acid overdoses
Inhalational irritants	Oxygen toxicity Smoke
Haematological diseases	Disseminated intravascular coagulation Transfusion-related acute lung injury (TRALI)
Pancreatitis	
Cardiopulmonary bypass	
Uraemia	
Hypersensitivity reactions	
Drugs	

[a] Most common causes.

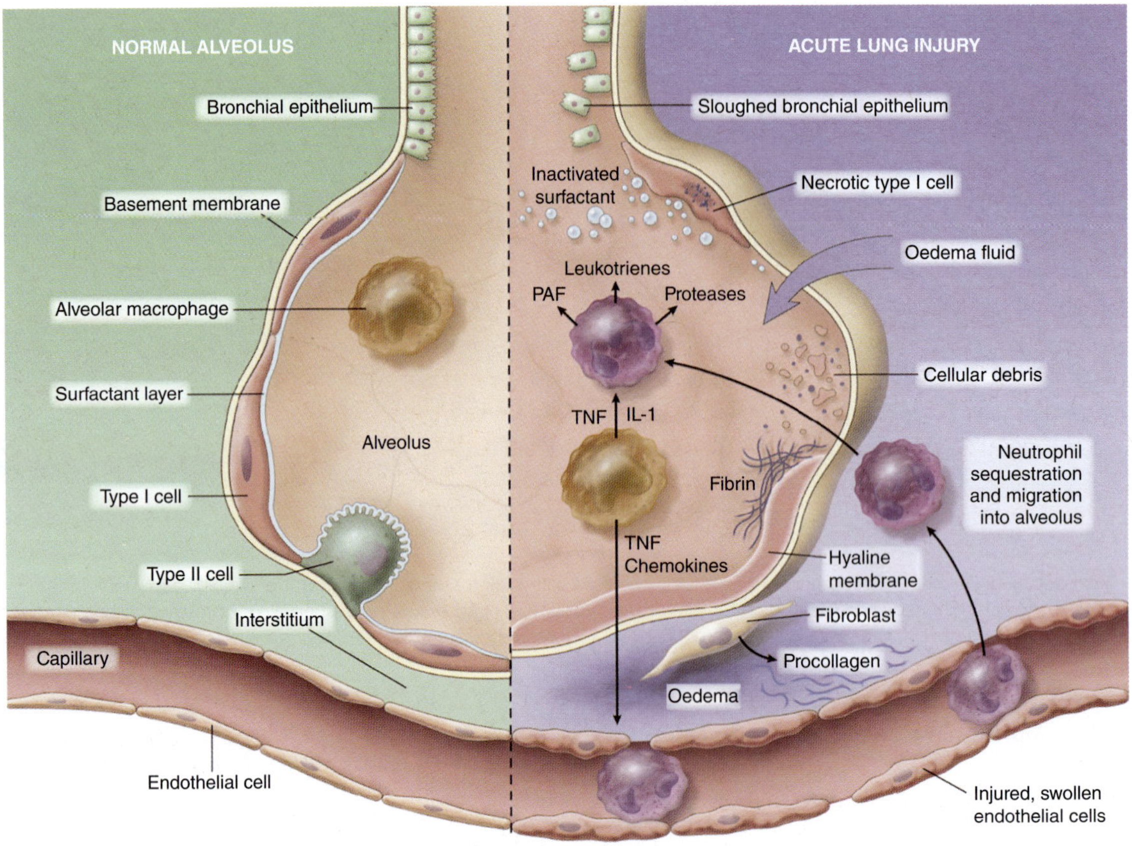

Fig. 19.5 Pathogenesis of ARDS. To the left is the normal alveolus and to the right is the injured alveolus in the early phase of acute lung injury. Neutrophils are sequestered in the pulmonary microvasculature (due to IL-1, IL-8 and TNF) and then migrate into the alveolus where they are activated. Leukotrienes, proteases, oxidants and platelet-activating factor (PAF) released by activated neutrophils contribute to local tissue damage, accumulation of oedema fluid, surfactant inactivation and hyaline membrane formation. TNF, tumour necrosis factor. (*Source:* From Vinay Kumar, Abul K Abbas, Jon C Aster. Robbins Basic Pathology. Elsevier. 2018.)

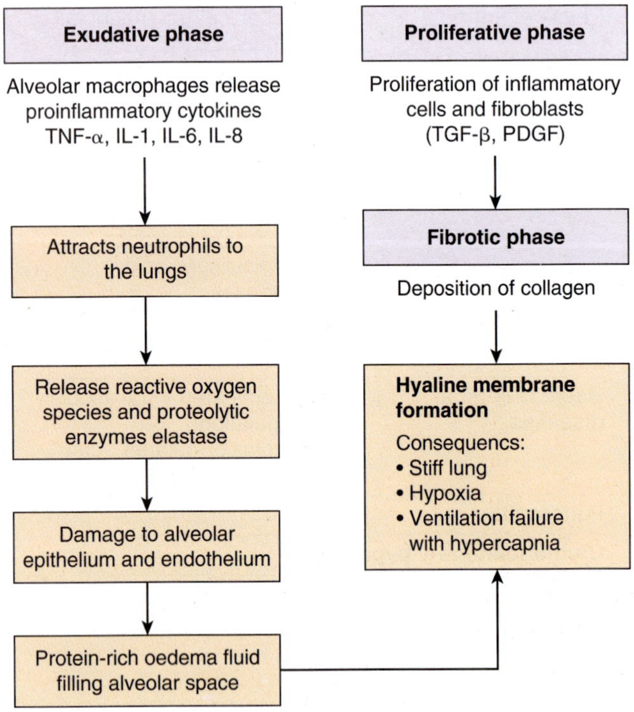

Flowchart 19.1 Pathogenesis of ARDS. TGF-β, transforming growth factor-β.

elevated in both bronchoalveolar lavage (BAL) fluid and circulating plasma in ARDS patients. Neutrophils also contribute to injury in the lung endothelium. Disruption of the epithelial–endothelial barrier leads to intra-alveolar and extra-alveolar flooding with protein-rich oedematous fluid. Type I alveolar epithelial cells undergo irreversible damage and are replaced by the deposition of proteins, fibrin and cellular debris forming hyaline membranes. In addition, injury to type II alveolar cells results in alveolar collapse.

Proliferative phase

Type II alveolar cells proliferate resulting in the regeneration of some epithelial cells. Fibrogenic cytokines such as transforming growth factor-β (TGF-β) and platelet-derived growth factor (PDGF) stimulate fibroblast proliferation. This leads to the formation of cellular junctions which in turn promote the expression of aquaporin and ion channels. These components play a crucial role in the reabsorption of fluid.

Fibrotic phase

Collagen deposition occurs in alveolar, vascular and interstitial beds. Though not seen in all patients, it is associated with increased mortality.

Morphology

Gross The lungs are heavy, firm, red and boggy.

Microscopy **Diffuse alveolar damage** is the characteristic histological manifestation of ARDS. Microscopically, alternate areas of collapsed and dilated alveoli lined by eosinophilic **hyaline membranes can be appreciated** (Fig. 19.6), which is the hallmark feature of the disease. The membrane is composed of fibrin admixed with cell debris derived from necrotic alveolar cells. Interstitial and intra-alveolar oedema, congestion and intra-alveolar haemorrhages with collection of neutrophils inside the capillaries are also seen. In the organizing stage, there is proliferation of type II pneumocytes, marked thickening of the alveolar septa due to collagen deposition and intra-alveolar fibrosis due to organization of fibrin-rich exudate.

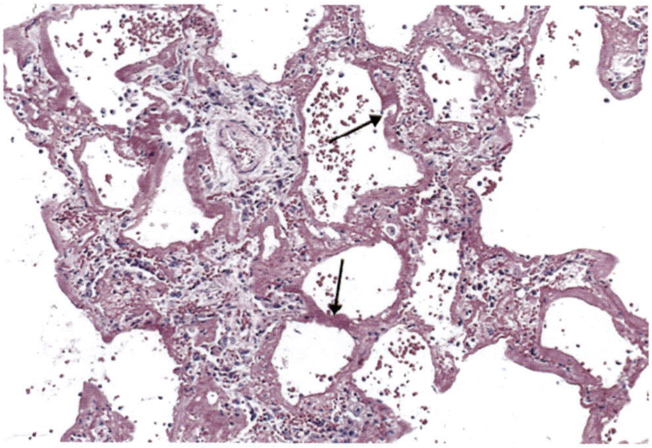

Fig. 19.6 Hyaline membrane lining the distended alveolar duct (arrowhead). (*Source:* From Vinay Kumar, Abul K Abbas, Jon C Aster. Robbins Basic Pathology. Elsevier. 2018.)

Clinical Features

The clinical symptoms may vary in intensity depending on the cause and severity, as well as the presence of underlying heart or lung disease.

Severe dyspnoea, tachypnoea, cyanosis, hypoxaemia, tiredness and drowsiness are seen. Fever and productive cough may be seen in infective aetiology. It may lead to respiratory failure.

Prognosis

Even with optimal therapy, the mortality rate is 60%. Patients who recover have normal pulmonary function with some residual diffusion defect. Advanced age, bacteraemia and multiorgan dysfunction are the predictors of a poor prognosis.

OBSTRUCTIVE AND RESTRICTIVE LUNG DISEASES (TABLE 19.3)

Obstructive lung diseases are characterized by a decrease in airflow due to increased resistance from partial or complete airway obstructions at any level. These obstructions can be either due to narrowing of the airway lumen or due to decrease in the elastic recoil of the surrounding pulmonary parenchyma, which has the effect of reducing the calibre of the lumen. Other causes of obstruction include tumours, aspirated foreign bodies, asthma, emphysema, chronic bronchitis, cystic fibrosis and bronchiolitis.

Restrictive lung diseases (RLDs) are characterized by reduced expansion of the lung parenchyma. The restriction may be either intrinsic to the lung or caused by external compression of the lung parenchyma as in severe scoliosis, chest wall tumours and expansion of the pleural space due to the presence of fluid or air.

Table 19.3 Differences Between Obstructive and Restrictive Lung Diseases

	Obstructive Lung Disease	Restrictive Lung Diseases
Definition	Increased resistance to airflow secondary to obstruction of airways	Reduced ability of the lung parenchyma to expand during inhalation resulting in decreased lung volume
Pulmonary function tests	FEV_1/FVC decreased	Decreased TLC:VC
Examples	Chronic obstructive airway diseases • Chronic bronchitis • Emphysema Bronchiectasis Asthma	Chest wall disorders Morbid obesity Kyphoscoliosis Polio Interstitial/infiltrative disease ARDS Pneumoconiosis

ARDS, acute respiratory distress syndrome; FEV_1, forced expiratory volume in 1 second; FVC, forced vital capacity; TLC, total lung capacity; VC, vital capacity.

OBSTRUCTIVE PULMONARY DISEASES

PA 26.3

Obstructive pulmonary diseases include **chronic bronchitis, emphysema, bronchial asthma and bronchiectasis**. Emphysema and chronic bronchitis are grouped together as chronic obstructive pulmonary disease (**COPD**).

COPD is a preventable and treatable disease characterized by airflow limitation that is not fully reversible. It is a heterogeneous lung condition characterized by chronic respiratory symptoms (dyspnoea, cough, sputum production and/or exacerbations) due to abnormalities of the airways (bronchitis, bronchiolitis) and/or alveoli (emphysema) that cause persistent, often progressive, airflow obstruction (Global Initiative for Chronic Obstructive Lung Disease, 2023).

Diagnostic criteria: In the appropriate clinical context, the presence of non-fully reversible airflow limitation (i.e. forced expiratory volume in 1 second [FEV_1]/forced vital capacity [FVC] <0.7 post-bronchodilation) measured by spirometry confirms the diagnosis of COPD (Global Initiative for Chronic Obstructive Lung Disease, 2023) (Table 19.4).

EMPHYSEMA

Emphysema is defined as an abnormal, **permanent enlargement of the air spaces distal to the terminal bronchiole** (respiratory bronchioles, alveolar duct and alveoli), with destruction of the walls and **without fibrosis**. Compensatory overinflation differs from emphysema by the absence of destruction of the alveolar walls.

Pathogenesis (Fig. 19.7)

Cigarette smoke and other toxic particles activate the macrophages in the respiratory tract and release neutrophil chemotactic factors such as IL-8, leukotriene B_4 and TNF. These cells further release proteases of different classes (elastase, matrix metalloproteinase). Neutrophil elastase induces apoptosis of small airways and alveolar epithelial cells by the intrinsic pathway, also known as the mitochondrial pathway, and destruction of elastin fibre in the lung parenchyma. A protease inhibitor, α_1-antitrypsin, plays a key role in controlling protease activities. Thus, a balance between protease and antiprotease is very important for the maintenance of the normal structure and function of the airway (Table 19.5).

Protease–antiprotease imbalance is a critical factor in the development of emphysema because the protease-mediated degradation of elastin is often irreversible.

Table 19.4 Differences Between Obstructive and Restrictive Patterns in Pulmonary Function Tests

Variables	Obstructive Pattern	Restrictive Pattern
Total lung capacity (TLC)	Increased	Decreased
Forced expiratory volume in 1 second (FEV_1)	Decreased	Decreased
Forced vital capacity (FVC)	Normal or slightly decreased	Decreased
FEV_1/FVC	Decreased	Normal
Functional residual capacity (FRC)	Increased	Decreased
Residual volume (RV)	Increased	Decreased

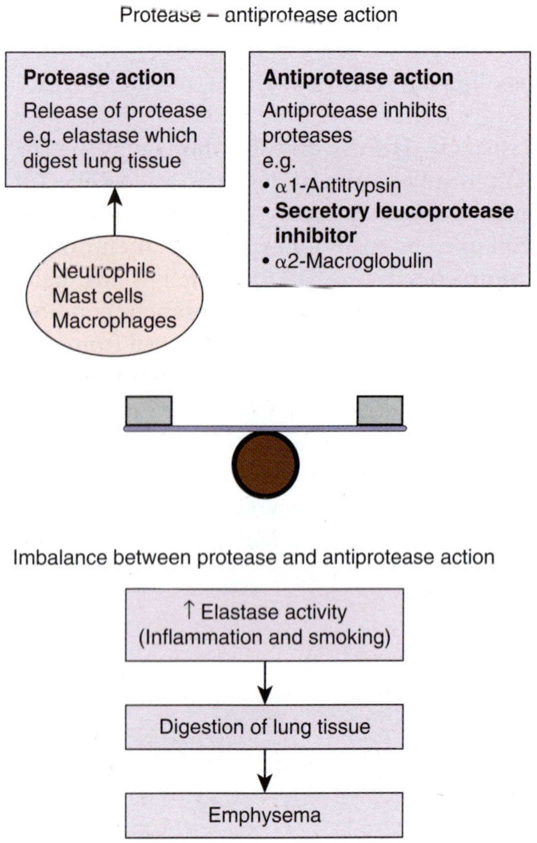

Fig. 19.7 Pathogenesis of emphysema.

Table 19.5 List of Proteases and Antiproteases in Emphysema

Proteases	Antiproteases
Serine proteases Neutrophil elastase Cathepsin G Proteinase 3	**α_1-Antitrypsin** Secretory leucoprotease inhibitor
Cysteine proteinases	Cystatins
Matrix metalloproteinase	Matrix metalloproteinase inhibitor

Factors contributing to this imbalance include the following:

- Low levels of α_1-antitrypsin
- Insufficient production of α_1-antitrypsin due to genetic defects
- Inactivation of α_1-antitrypsin by smoking-induced oxidants

SERPINA1 (serine protease inhibitor) gene located in the long arm of chromosome 14 encodes for the protein α_1-antitrypsin, which protects the body from neutrophil elastase. Mutations in the *SERPINA1* gene can cause either deficiency of α_1-antitrypsin or an abnormal form of the protein that cannot control neutrophil elastase. Environmental factors, such as exposure to tobacco smoke, chemicals and dust, have an impact on the severity of α_1-antitrypsin deficiency.

The most common allele of the *SERPINA1* gene, called M, produces normal levels of α_1-antitrypsin. Most people have two copies of the M allele (MM) in each cell. Other alleles of the *SERPINA1* gene lead to reduced levels of α_1-antitrypsin. For example, the S allele produces moderately low levels of this protein and the Z allele produces very little α_1-antitrypsin. Individuals with two copies of the Z allele (ZZ) in each cell are likely to have α_1-antitrypsin deficiency. Those with the SZ combination have an increased risk of developing lung diseases (such as emphysema), particularly if they smoke. Owing to destruction of the structural components that support small airways, the respiratory bronchioles collapse during expiration, leading to functional airflow obstruction.

Oxidative stress plays an amplifying mechanism. Oxidants are generated by cigarette smoke, other inhaled particles and inflammatory cells. These produce more inflammation and tissue damage by activation of inflammatory genes, inactivation of antiproteases, stimulation of mucus secretion and stimulation of increased plasma exudation.

Types of Emphysema

The following are the **types of emphysema** on the basis of anatomical distribution of septal damage (Fig. 19.8):

- **Centriacinar (centrilobular)**
  - This form of emphysema is most common and frequently seen in smokers often in association with chronic bronchitis.
- The central or the **proximal part** of the acinus formed by the respiratory bronchiole is damaged, with relative sparing of the distal alveoli. Thus, normal and emphysematous air spaces exist within the same acinus and lobule. The lesions are more common and severe in the apical segments of the **upper lobes**.
- **Panacinar (panlobular)**
  - There is a uniform enlargement of the acinus from the respiratory bronchiole to the distal alveoli. The entire acinus is damaged because all alveoli in the acinus are equally dilated. It tends to occur in the **lower zones and at the bases**. This type of emphysema is associated with **α1-antitrypsin** deficiency, an autosomal codominant disorder.
- **Distal acinar (paraseptal) emphysema**
  - In this type of emphysema, only the **distal part** of the acinus is involved. It occurs **adjacent to the lobular septa and pleura**, near areas of fibrosis, scarring or atelectasis, and is more severe in the upper half of the lungs.
  - Extension to the pleura causes spontaneous pneumothorax.
- **Irregular emphysema**
  - The acinus is irregularly involved and is always accompanied by **scarring**.
  - It is associated with bullae or apical blebs.

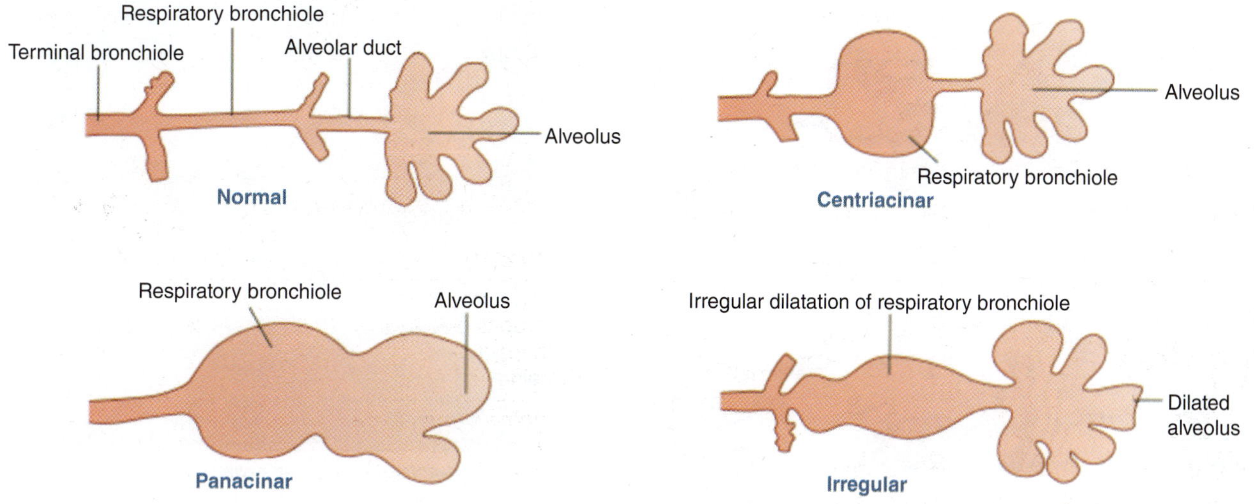

Fig. 19.8 Types of emphysema.

Morphology

Gross

The lungs are overinflated, spongy and enlarged, with the cut surface showing large distended alveoli (Fig. 19.9). Panacinar emphysema results in voluminous lungs; in contrast, centriacinar emphysema leads to less voluminous lungs with the upper two-thirds of the lung being more severely affected. Bullae are usually located in the lung apices and subpleurally but can occur anywhere in the emphysematous lung.

Microscopy

There is a marked enlargement of the air spaces with destruction of alveolar septa without fibrosis (Fig. 19.10). The alveolar capillaries are decreased. In the advanced stage, adjacent alveoli fuse to form large bullae that compress the nearby respiratory bronchioles and vasculature of the lung.

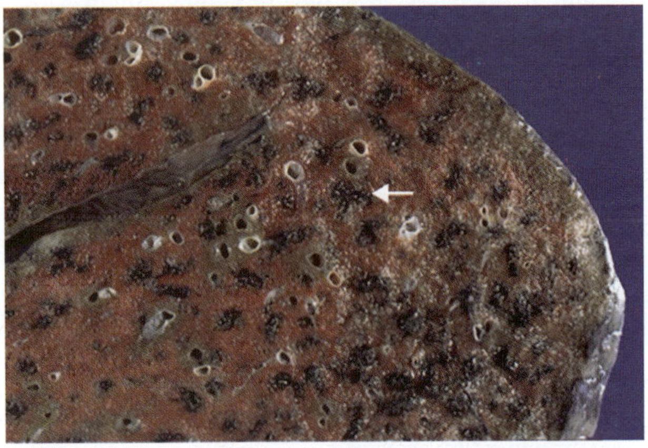

Fig. 19.9 Gross morphology of pulmonary centrilobular emphysema. The central lobular loss of lung tissue with black anthracotic pigmentation (←). (*Source:* From Edward C Klatt. Robbins and Cotran Atlas of Pathology. Elsevier. 2021.)

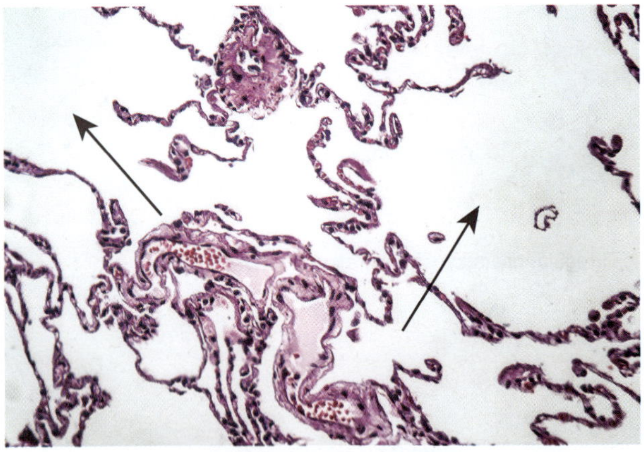

Fig. 19.10 Microscopy of lung emphysema showing enlargement of air spaces in lung tissue and destruction of alveolar septa.

Clinical Features

Patients present with dyspnoea with prolonged expiration, and they generally breathe through pursed lips. It may be associated with cough, wheezing and weight loss. Patients with emphysema are referred to as **pink puffers** (patients overventilate but remain well oxygenated, with normal saturation).

Complications

- Coronary artery disease
- Respiratory failure
- Cor pulmonale
- Massive collapse of the lungs (due to pneumonia)

Other Forms of Emphysema

- **Compensatory hyperinflation**
  Hyperexpansion of the residual lung parenchyma occurs following surgical removal of a diseased lobe or lung.
- **Obstructive overinflation**
  This condition can result from congenital lobar overinflation (hypoplasia of bronchial cartilage) or obstruction secondary to tumours or foreign bodies. Expansion of the lung occurs due to air trapping.
  Overinflation is due to the following:
  Air entering during inspiration, with the outflow being prevented during expiration
  Air entering through collaterals (pores of Kohn)
- **Bullous emphysema** (Fig. 19.11)
  - Large bullae (>1 cm in diameter) or subpleural blebs can occur in any form of emphysema. These are more commonly seen in irregular emphysema.
  - Occasionally, rupture of the bullae may give rise to pneumothorax.

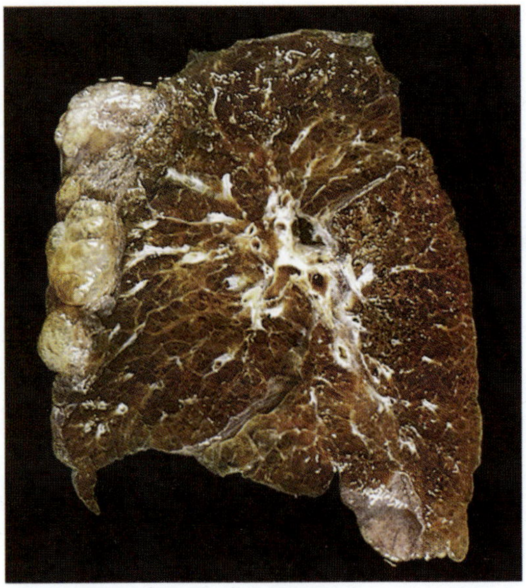

Fig. 19.11 Gross morphology of bullous emphysema with large subpleural bullae. (*Source:* From Vinay Kumar, Abul K Abbas, Jon C Aster. Robbins Basic Pathology. Elsevier. 2018.)

- **Interstitial emphysema (mediastinal emphysema)**
  This refers to the entry of air into the connective tissue stroma of the lung, mediastinum or subcutaneous tissue. Common causes include alveolar tear and fractured ribs. Entry of air into subcutaneous tissue produces crepitation over the chest.

CHRONIC BRONCHITIS

It is a clinical condition defined as persistent chronic cough with expectoration for at least 3 months per year for 2 consecutive years in the absence of any other identifiable cause.

Aetiology

Causes

Cigarette smoke	Active and passive inhalation
Inhalation of irritants	Environmental pollutants like dust, smog, industrial pollutants, toxic chemicals
Repeated exposure to infections	Viral infections – influenza types A and B Bacterial infections due to *Staphylococcus, Streptococcus* and *Mycoplasma pneumoniae*
Associated respiratory diseases	Asthma, cystic fibrosis and bronchiectasis

Pathogenesis

The normal inflammatory response of the respiratory tract to chronic irritants such as cigarette smoke is increased in COPD. The inflammation is further amplified by oxidative stress and excess of proteinases in the lung.

Inflammation, fibrosis and luminal exudates result in small airway obstruction, which correlates clinically with reduction in FEV_1 and the FEV_1:FVC ratio. Air gets trapped into the lungs during expiration, resulting in hyperinflation that reduces inspiratory capacity such that functional residual capacity increases, particularly during exercise, and this results in dyspnoea and limitation of exercise capacity.

Mucus hypersecretion, which is clinically responsible for productive cough in chronic bronchitis, is due to increased number of goblet cells and enlarged submucosal glands that occur as a response to chronic airway irritation by cigarette smoke and other noxious agents (Flowchart 19.2).

Mild to moderate pulmonary hypertension in COPD is due to hypoxic vasoconstriction of small pulmonary arteries, resulting in structural changes that include intimal hyperplasia and later smooth muscle hypertrophy/hyperplasia.

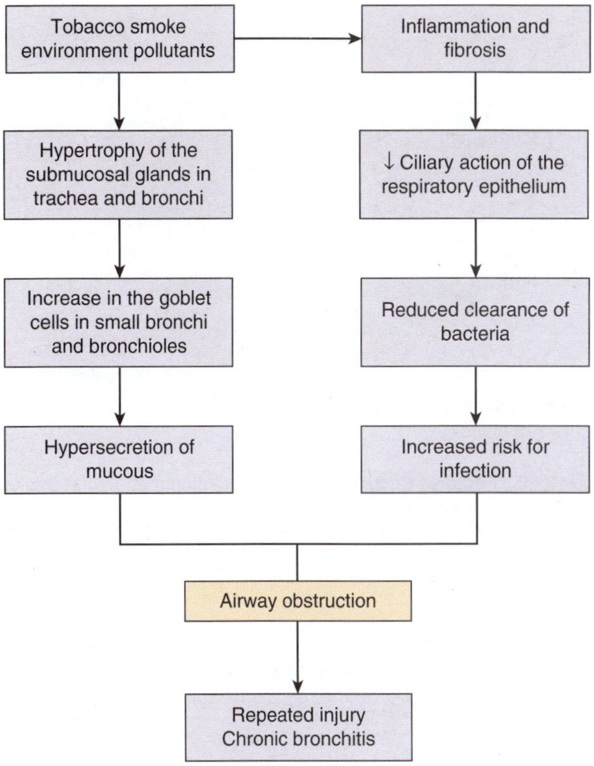

Flowchart 19.2 Pathogenesis of chronic bronchitis.

Morphology

Gross Boggy mucosa of the large airways is seen with excess mucous or mucopurulent secretions filling the bronchi and bronchioles (Fig. 19.12).

Microscopy Early changes show hypersecretion of mucus in large airways, with hypertrophy of submucosal glands in the trachea and bronchi (Fig. 19.13). Later, there is an increase in the goblet cells with mild chronic inflammation of the airways. In the submucosa, mucosal glands occupy an increasing proportion of the bronchial wall that is measured by the Reid index.

Reid Index

It is the ratio of thickness of mucous glands to the thickness of the wall between the epithelium and the cartilage. The normal Reid index is 0.4 but it is increased in chronic bronchitis.

The bronchial epithelium may show squamous metaplasia and dysplasia.

Reid index calculation: The percentage of bronchial wall thickness occupied by mucosal gland tissue is the Reid index (Fig. 19.14).

Clinical Features

These include chronic cough, dyspnoea, hypoxaemia, hypercapnia and cyanosis (**blue bloaters**).

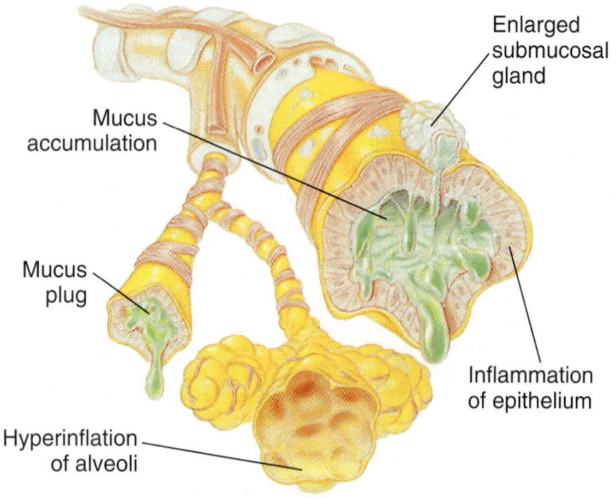

Fig. 19.12 Features of chronic bronchitis. Inflammation and thickening of mucous membrane with accumulation of mucus and pus in the airways leads to obstruction.

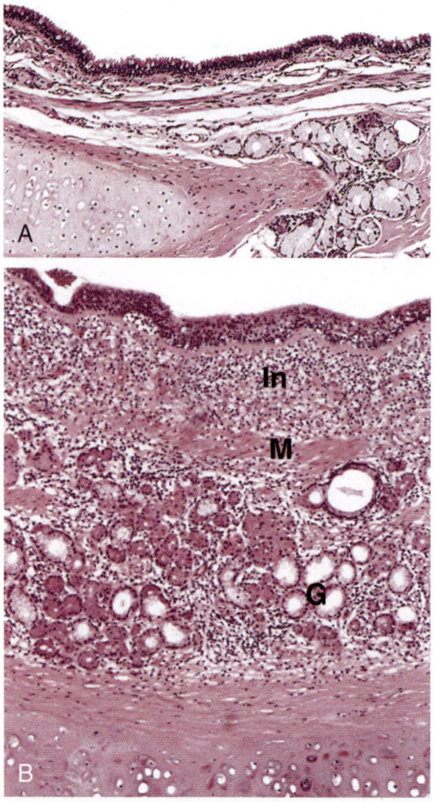

Fig. 19.13 (A) Normal bronchial wall. (B) Bronchial wall in chronic bronchitis – the chronic inflammatory infiltrate in the submucosa (In), hypertrophy of the mucosal smooth muscle (M) and hyperplasia of the mucosal glands (G) contribute to the increased thickness of the bronchial wall. (*Source:* From Geraldine O'Dowd, Sarah Bell, Sylvia Wright. Wheater's Pathology: A Text, Atlas, and Review of Histopathology. Elsevier. 2020.)

Facts 'Pink puffers' and 'blue bloaters' are older terms to describe the phenotype in emphysema and chronic bronchitis, respectively.

Emphysema: Pink puffer is a thin cachectic individual who experiences shortness of breath. He/she has a

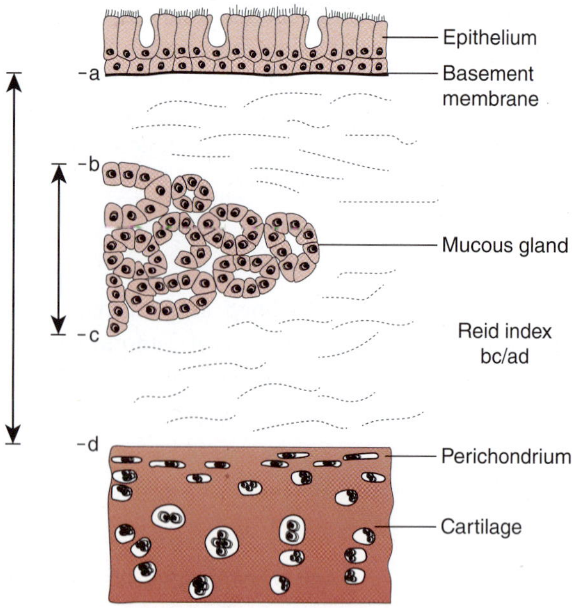

Fig. 19.14 Reid index calculation.

ventilation–perfusion defect, in which the alveoli and airways collapse during expiration, resulting in air trapping. Pursed lip breathing is beneficial in maintaining positive end-expiratory pressure, which helps keep the airways open. The person also has decreased lung compliance, which leads to increased work of breathing and dyspnoea.

Chronic bronchitis: Blue bloater is a large oedematous person with cyanosis. Airway obstruction leads to hypoxia, ventilation–perfusion mismatch, secondary pulmonary vasoconstriction leading to pulmonary hypertension and cor pulmonale. Hypoxaemia causes cyanosis.

Bronchial Asthma

Asthma is defined as a chronic inflammatory disease of the airways caused by an **increased responsiveness of the tracheobronchial tree** to a variety of stimuli and characterized by **episodic airway obstruction** due to narrowing of the airways that are relieved spontaneously or by therapy.

Types

i. Atopic Asthma

- The **most common type** of asthma is due to IgE-mediated (type I) hypersensitivity reaction.
- It usually begins in childhood and is triggered by environmental allergens (dusts, pollution and immune activation).
- A positive family history of asthma is common.
- Skin test with allergen results in wheal and flare reaction immediately.
- There is an increased serum IgE level.
- The presence of IgE antibodies specific for individual allergens can be detected by the radioallergosorbent test (RAST).

ii. Nonatopic Asthma

- Respiratory infection due to **viruses** is a common trigger.
- No allergen sensitization is indicated.
- A positive family history is less common.
- Negative skin test is reported.
- There is a low threshold of vagal receptors.

iii. Drug-Induced Asthma

A number of drugs are known to cause asthma, e.g. aspirin.

Drugs act by inhibiting the cyclooxygenase pathway of arachidonic acid metabolism, leading to a decreased production of prostaglandin E_2, which normally inhibits the enzymes involved in the generation of leukotrienes.

iv. Exercise-Induced Asthma

The increased ventilation during exercise results in increased osmolality in airway lining fluid. This triggers surface mast cells to release mediators such as leukotriene D_4, resulting in bronchoconstriction.

v. Occupational Asthma

It is triggered by fumes, organic and chemical dusts and gases in the workplace. Once the patient is sensitized to the trigger, a very low-dose exposure can induce the attack. These may be categorized as follows:

High-molecular-weight pollutants: These are compounds that trigger an IgE-dependent response. The effects are immediate or soon after exposure, e.g. flour and latex.

Low-molecular-weight pollutants: These compounds develop a complex immune response after repeated and long-term exposure, e.g. isocyanates and wood dusts.

Pathogenesis

Asthma is a chronic inflammatory disorder of the airways characterized by involvement of multiple inflammatory cells and mediators that contribute to distinct clinical and pathophysiological changes.

Inhaled allergen causes the release of cytokines IL-4 and IL-5 from the T helper type 2 (T_H2) cells.

IL-4 and IL-5 favour the production of IgE antibodies and recruitment of eosinophils, respectively. On re-exposure to the antigen, an immediate reaction occurs due to cross-linking of IgE bound to IgE receptors on the mast cells. Preformed chemical mediators are released from the mast cells that initiate the immediate reactions.

Leucocytes recruited to the site of injury release additional mediators that mediate late-phase reactions.

Airway Inflammation in Asthma (Table 19.6) Inflammation affects all the airways including upper respiratory pathways but is more pronounced in medium-sized airways.

Atopic asthma is characterized by immediate- and late-phase reactions.

Early or Immediate-Phase Reactions The early phase reactions in asthma are characterized by the release of several factors that lead to bronchospasm and other associated events like increased mucus production, increased vascular permeability and vasodilation. These factors include leukotrienes (C4, D4 and E4), acetylcholine (due to parasympathetic stimulation), histamine, prostaglandin D_2 and platelet-activating factor. These reactions occur within minutes and are commonly referred to as the early asthmatic response (Table 19.7).

Table 19.6 Inflammatory Cells in the Airways of Bronchial Asthma

Cells	Actions
Mucosal mast cells	Mast cells are activated by allergens through immunoglobulin E (IgE) receptor and release histamine, cysteinyl leukotrienes and prostaglandin D_2 on activation, producing bronchoconstriction
T lymphocytes	Present in increased numbers in asthmatic airways, T lymphocytes release the following specific cytokines: Interleukin IL-4 (stimulates the production of IgE) IL-5 (recruits eosinophils) IL-13 (stimulates bronchial submucosal glands to produce mucus secretion) Increased T_H2 cell activity may be due to a reduction in the regulatory T cells that normally inhibit T_H2 cells Increases in T_H17 cells are also seen that recruit neutrophils
Eosinophils	Release major basic proteins and eosinophilic cationic protein that damages airway epithelial cells
Dendritic cells	Antigen-presenting cells respond to the allergens from the airway surface and migrate to regional lymph nodes, interact with regulatory T cells to stimulate production of T_H2 cells from naive T cells
Macrophages	Release inflammatory mediators and cytokines that amplify the inflammatory response, especially in severe asthma
Neutrophils	Increased in the airways and sputum of patients with severe asthma and in smoking asthmatic patients

T_H2, T helper type 2.

Table 19.7 Mediators and Their Effects in Bronchial Asthma

Mediators	Effects
Leukotrienes C_4, D_4, E_4	Bronchoconstriction, increased vascular permeability and increased mucus secretion
Acetylcholine	Bronchoconstriction
Histamine	Bronchoconstriction
Prostaglandin D_2	Bronchoconstriction and vasodilatation
Platelet-activating factor	Platelet aggregation and release of serotonin

Late-Phase Reactions The late asthmatic response is delayed by hours. It is caused by a multitude of inflammatory cells, of which the T cells play an important role by producing cytokines that maintain and intensify the local inflammatory response.

Recruitment of leucocytes – neutrophils, eosinophils and macrophages – results in epithelial damage.

Understanding the concept of early and late-phase asthma is important in the treatment of asthma. Different therapies may be more effective at different points in the disease process. β_2-Agonists stabilize mast cells and are likely to be most effective in the early asthma response. Corticosteroids and leukotriene antagonists, with their anti-inflammatory effects, are more effective in the late asthmatic response.

Genetic Susceptibility

Polymorphism in the IL-13 gene has the strongest association with asthma or allergic disease.

Polymorphism in the gene encoding ADAM 33, a metalloproteinase, causes an increased proliferation of bronchial smooth muscle cells and fibroblasts, contributing to bronchial hyperreactivity and subepithelial fibrosis.

Environmental Factors

There is an increased prevalence of asthma in Western countries. This is due to exposure to airborne pollutants that initiate T_H2 response. An increase in the prevalence of allergic diseases in children could be explained by hygiene hypothesis, which presents the assumption that a reduced exposure to microorganisms leads to a disordered regulation of the immune system. Allergic diseases can be prevented by infection in early childhood transmitted by unhygienic contact with older siblings or acquired prenatally. Currently, the chances of cross-infection have been greatly reduced because of declining family size, improved household amenities and high standards of personal cleanliness. This may have resulted in the widespread expression of atopic disease.

Airborne allergens and viral respiratory infections have emerged as the most important factors in the development, persistence and, possibly, severity of asthma.

Airway remodelling involves an activation of many of the structural cells, with consequent permanent changes in the airway that increase airflow obstruction and airway responsiveness and render the patient less responsive to therapy.

Morphology

Gross The lungs are distended by overinflation. Bronchi and bronchioles are filled with thick mucus plugs.

Microscopy The sputum or BAL contains **eosinophils, Charcot–Leyden crystals** (crystalloids of eosinophil protein galectin-10), **Curschmann spirals** (Fig. 19.15) (mucus plugs containing degenerated epithelium) and **Creola bodies** (three-dimensional clusters of ciliated columnar cells sloughed from bronchial mucosa).

Histological features of airway remodelling are as follows (Fig. 19.16):

- Thickening of airway walls
- Deposition of fibrous tissue in the subepithelium
- Hypertrophy and hyperplasia of the bronchial smooth muscle and mucous glands
- Increased airway vascularity

Clinical Features

- Chest tightness
- Dyspnoea
- Wheezing
- Cough

Complications

- Superimposed infections
- Chronic bronchitis
- Pulmonary emphysema

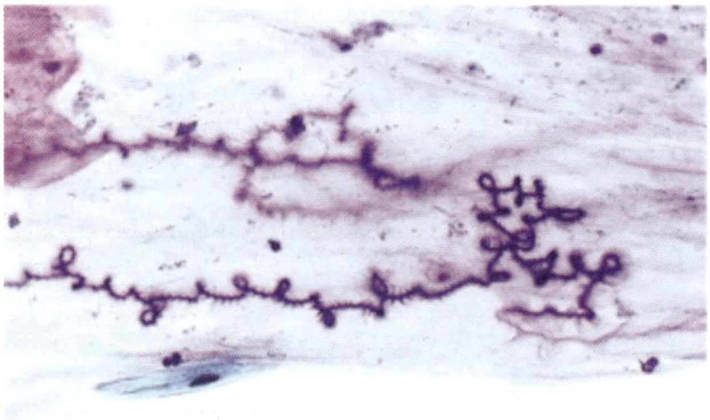

Fig. 19.15 Curschmann spirals on sputum cytology – inspissated mucous cast of the bronchioles. (*Source:* From Olivia McKinney, Isabel Woodman. Crash Course Pathology. Elsevier. 2019.)

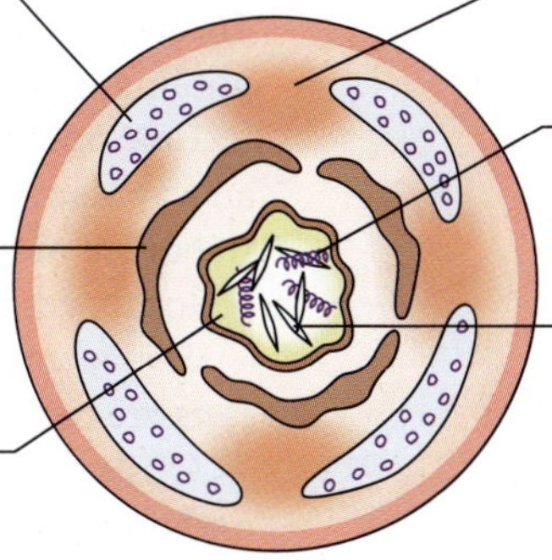

Fig. 19.16 Diagrammatic representation of the airway changes in asthma. (*Source:* Reproduced from Olivia McKinney, Isabel Woodman. Crash Course Pathology. Elsevier. 2019.)

- Bronchial asthma, which can progress to **status asthmaticus**, a prolonged and severe bout of bronchial asthma lasting for days and often responding poorly to therapy (in some cases, it can be life-threatening resulting in death)

BRONCHIECTASIS PA 26.3

Bronchiectasis refers to abnormal, **permanent dilation of the bronchi and bronchioles** with destruction of smooth muscle and elastic tissue. These present as obstructive lung disease with chronic productive cough, recurrent infections and progressive lung damage.

Predisposing Conditions (Table 19.8)

Kartagener Syndrome Kartagener syndrome is an autosomal recessive disorder with a genetic defect in the dynein gene.

Features of this syndrome are as follows:

- Bronchiectasis
- Situs inversus
- Sinusitis
- Infertility in males

It is characterized by ultrastructural changes in the microtubules causing **immobility of cilia** of the respiratory epithelium and sperms.

Allergic Bronchopulmonary Aspergillosis It occurs in patients with asthma and cystic fibrosis owing to mucus plug formation.

It is a hypersensitivity reaction to the fungus *Aspergillus fumigatus*, with activation of T_H2 cells. There is intense airway inflammation with eosinophils, high serum IgE levels and serum antibodies to *Aspergillus*.

Table 19.8 Aetiology of Bronchiectasis

Category	Examples
Obstruction of single bronchus	Tumour Foreign body Lymph node Airway compression
Obstructive airway disease	COPD Asthma α_1-Antitrypsin deficiency
Defects of mucociliary clearance	Cystic fibrosis Kartagener syndrome Primary ciliary dyskinesia
Immunodeficiency	Primary – hypogammaglobulinaemias Secondary – bone marrow transplantation, AIDS, malignancy
Fungal allergy	Allergic bronchopulmonary aspergillosis (ABPA)
Fibrosis	Postradiation Sarcoidosis
Postinfectious	Pneumonia Pertussis Mycobacterial infections Viral infections – measles, adenovirus influenza
Damage to the airways	Inhalational injury Gastro-oesophageal disease
Connective tissue diseases	Rheumatoid arthritis Sjögren syndrome
Idiopathic	

COPD, chronic obstructive pulmonary disease.

Morphological Classification of Bronchiectasis (Fig. 19.17)

Cylindrical (fusiform): This is the commonest form that involves the airways from 6th to 10th generations. The bronchi have uniform calibre. These do not taper and have parallel walls.

Varicose: This is relatively uncommon with a beaded appearance due to dilated bronchi having interspersed sites of narrowing.

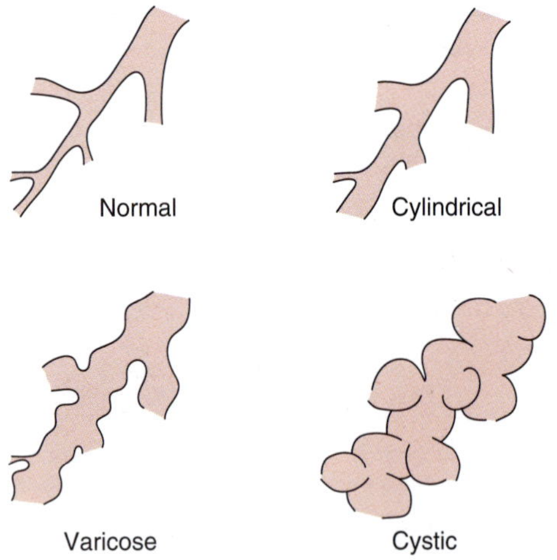

Fig. 19.17 Morphological types of bronchiectasis.

Saccular: This is the most severe form that occurs in proximal bronchi. Dilation ends in large cysts, saccules or grape-like clusters.

Pathogenesis (Flowchart 19.3)

The most widely known model for the development of bronchiectasis is Cole's 'vicious cycle hypothesis'. Microbial colonization initiates and perpetuates airway inflammation. Inflammatory cells such as neutrophils, lymphocytes and macrophages accumulate within the bronchial lumen. Neutrophils alter the function of the cilial epithelium, leading to changes in cilial beat frequency and mucous gland hypersecretion. This leads to impaired mucociliary clearance. The loss of mucociliary transport renders the airways susceptible to microbial colonization. The microbial infection triggers a cycle of chronic inflammation resulting in the release of inflammatory mediators.

Neutrophils play a key role in the tissue damage by releasing inflammatory cytokines, elastases and matrix metalloproteinases that destroy the bronchial elastin and other supporting lung structures, leading to permanent dilation of the bronchi.

The airway walls become thickened due to oedema or fibrosis. In proximal airways, the bronchi and bronchioles are dilated, with a reduction in supportive structure. These changes in airway structure further contribute to pooling of mucus, and the self-perpetuating cycle of infection and inflammation, which promotes progressive airway damage and recurrent infections. Depending on the cause of bronchiectasis, the extent of the disease may be localized, focal or diffuse.

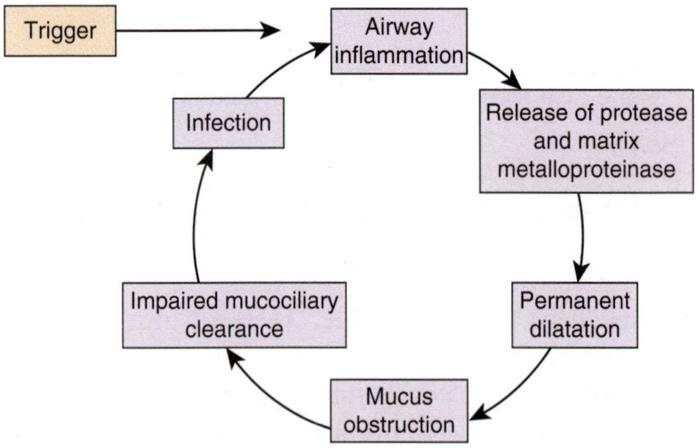

Flowchart 19.3 Pathogenesis of bronchiectasis.

Two factors required for the development of bronchiectasis are persistent infection and a defect in host defence.

Obstruction leads to an impaired clearing mechanism and predisposes to infection. Infection leads to inflammation with necrosis, fibrosis and eventually dilation of bronchi.

Morphology

Gross Bronchiectasis affects **lower lobes and** is **bilateral** in most cases. It is most severe in distal bronchi and bronchioles. Localized single segment is affected in obstructive aetiology.

The cut surface of the lungs shows cystically dilated airways – **honeycomb appearance.** The airways are dilated four times the normal size. The dilated bronchi and bronchioles can be traced to the pleural surface (Fig. 19.18). Lung parenchyma is reduced and fibrotic.

Microscopy The bronchial epithelium shows ulceration, whereas the bronchial wall displays infiltration by acute and chronic inflammatory cells, with destruction of muscle and elastic tissue that later show fibrotic replacement. The pleura in the affected areas shows fibrosis.

Clinical Features

- Chronic cough with foul-smelling sputum (due to anaerobic infection), which is the hallmark of this disease
- Haemoptysis (due to necrosis of the bronchial wall and bronchial vessel erosion)
- Sputum production, which varies with posture and is maximum within 2 hours of waking up (stagnation of sputum during sleep)
- Dyspnoea (airway obstruction)
- Secondary bacterial infection, which is frequent due to excessive bronchial secretion – *Haemophilus influenzae, Streptococcus, Pseudomonas aeruginosa* and various anaerobic organisms

Complications

- Lung abscess
- Pulmonary fibrosis
- Clubbing of fingers
- Brain abscess, amyloidosis and cor pulmonale, which are rare due to effective antibiotic treatment and physical therapy

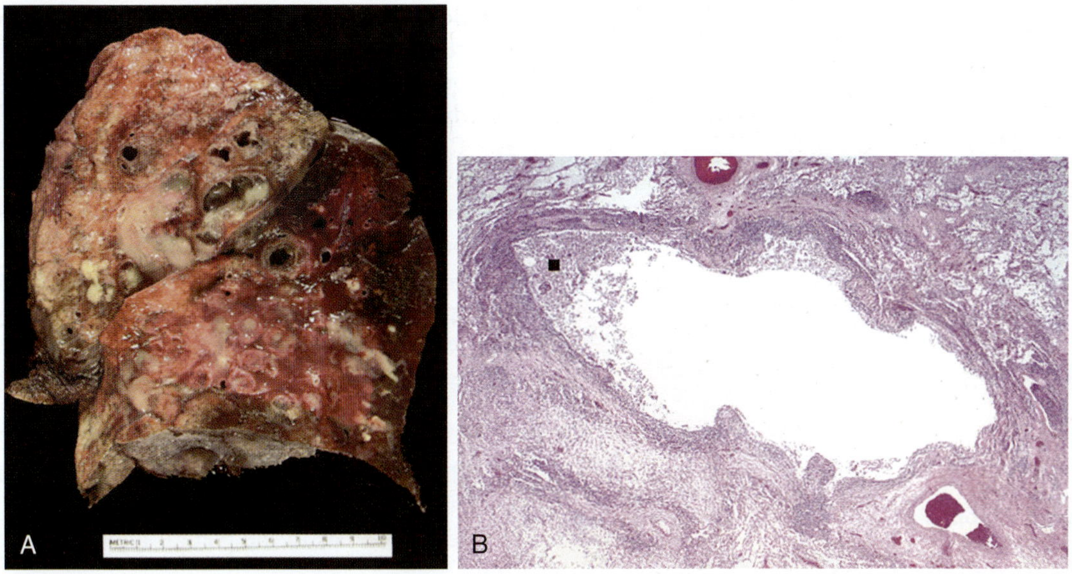

Fig. 19.18 (A) Gross morphology of bronchiectasis. (B) Permanent dilation of peripheral bronchi filled with purulent mucus and extending into subpleural regions. (*Source:* From Vinay Kumar, Abul K Abbas, Jon C Aster. Robbins Basic Pathology. Elsevier. 2018.)

Special Conditions

- Bronchiectasis with the predominant involvement of **upper lung fields is seen in cystic fibrosis.**
- Bronchiectasis with the predominant involvement of **lower lung fields is seen characteristically in chronic recurrent aspiration.**
- Bronchiectasis with the predominant involvement of **mid lung fields is seen in atypical mycobacterial infection and allergic bronchopulmonary aspergillosis.**

RESTRICTIVE LUNG DISEASES

RLDs are chronic, diffuse, interstitial lung diseases (ILDs) usually affecting the most peripheral and delicate interstitium of the alveolar walls. The predisposing factors are given in Table 19.9.

Pulmonary interstitium is composed of basement membranes of alveolar epithelial cells, capillary endothelial cells and the tissues between them, mostly made up of collagen elastic fibres, fibroblasts and mononuclear cells.

Hallmark features of RLDs

Hypoxia (damage to alveolar epithelium and pulmonary vessels hindering gas exchange) and **stiff lungs** (the lungs cannot expand easily) are the hallmark features of RLDs. Patients with ILD present with dyspnoea, tachypnoea, end-inspiratory crackles and cyanosis without wheeze.

Chest X-ray findings

Diffuse infiltration by small nodules, ground glass appearance and irregular lines are some of the findings.

Pulmonary function tests

These show restricted filling of the lung, decreased total lung capacity (TLC) and decreased FVC; FEV_1:FVC ratio is normal (Table 19.4).

Table 19.9 Causes of Restrictive Lung Diseases

Chronic Interstitial and Infiltrative Diseases of Lung
Chest wall abnormalities
• Kyphoscoliosis
• Ankylosing spondylitis
• Poliomyelitis
• Severe obesity
• Pleural diseases

Progression of the disease

The end stage of all the diseases in this category is diffuse interstitial pulmonary fibrosis leading to the following complications:

- Secondary pulmonary hypertension
- Cor pulmonale
- Respiratory failure

Categories of chronic RLDs

RLDs are categorized on the basis of the pathogenesis as given in Table 19.10.

FIBROSING LUNG DISEASES

Pulmonary fibrosis is the end stage of several diffuse parenchymal lung diseases characterized by excessive matrix deposition and destruction of the lung architecture leading to respiratory insufficiency.

Repeated subclinical injuries lead to epithelial damage and destruction of the alveolar–capillary basement membrane. This initiates the infiltration of fibrotic cells and the activation of (myo) fibroblasts. In pulmonary fibrosis, the normal resolution of inflammatory and mesenchymal cells through apoptosis and phagocytosis is dysregulated.

Table 19.10 Major Categories of Chronic Interstitial Lung Disease

Category	Common diseases
Fibrosing	Pneumoconiosis Idiopathic pulmonary fibrosis Associated with collagen vascular diseases Therapy related
Granulomatous	Sarcoidosis Hypersensitivity pneumonitis
Smoking related	Desquamative interstitial pneumonia Respiratory bronchiolitis–associated interstitial lung disease
Pulmonary eosinophilia	
Others	Langerhans cell histiocytosis Pulmonary alveolar proteinosis

PNEUMOCONIOSIS PA 26.5

Pneumoconiosis is a group of fibrosing pulmonary diseases caused by inhalation of mineral dusts, organic and inorganic particles, chemical fumes and vapours. It develops gradually over several decades following exposure to mineral dust (Table 19.11). The pathogenesis of fibrosis is through the release of fibrogenic chemical mediators.

Pathogenesis The severity of the disease depends on the following factors:

i) **Amount of dust retained in the lung**, which is determined by the following:
   a) Concentration of dusts in the air
   b) Duration of exposure
   c) Clearance mechanisms
ii) **Size, shape and buoyancy of particles:** Particles of size 10^5 μm are most dangerous, because the particles may reach and settle in the small airways and air sacs.

Table 19.11 List of Mineral Dust Pneumoconiosis

Mineral dust	Diseases
Coal	Anthracosis
Silica	Silicosis
Asbestos	Asbestosis
Beryllium	Berylliosis
Iron oxide	Siderosis
Barium sulphate	Baritosis
Tin oxide	Stannosis

iii) **Solubility and toxicity of the particles:** Small particles with highly soluble injurious substances may produce rapid lung damage. Larger particles resist dissolution, persist for many years and evoke fibrosis.
iv) **Concomitant tobacco smoking**
   Not all individuals exposed to inhaled dust develop lung pathology. This suggests that there is a genetic predisposition to develop disease.
   Several studies have proposed a genetic component (polymorphism in TNF-α). An understanding of interaction between genetic and environmental factors is crucial in identifying high-risk individuals.

Coal-Worker's Pneumoconiosis This disease is caused by inhalation of carbon dust from coal mines. The carbon pigment (anthracotic pigment) accumulates in macrophages, as well as in the pleural lymphatics and interstitium.

Course of the Disease The disease can manifest in different types and varying degrees of severity.

1. Asymptomatic Anthracosis It is the accumulation of carbon pigment–laden alveolar macrophages in the connective tissue along the lymphatics or in lymphoid tissue along the bronchi or in the hilum of the lung without a perceptible cellular reaction.

2. Simple Coal-Worker's Pneumoconiosis It is characterized by coal macules (1–2 mm in diameter) and coal nodules in the upper lobes and upper zones of the lower lobe with little pulmonary dysfunction. The coal macule consists of dust-laden macrophages with a small amount of collagen fibres arranged in a delicate network. The macules and nodules are seen adjacent to respiratory bronchioles. Alveolar dilation leads to centrilobular emphysema.

3. Complicated Coal-Worker's Pneumoconiosis (Black Lung Disease) It is characterized by progressive massive fibrosis that takes many years to develop. Black scars 2–10 cm in diameter are seen in the lung parenchyma. On microscopic examination, the scars consist of dense collagen and pigment, with the centre of the lesions being necrotic due to ischaemia. The walls of the respiratory bronchioles and blood vessels are thickened.

4. Caplan Syndrome This syndrome was first described in coal workers and is associated with rheumatoid arthritis and coal-worker's pneumoconiosis. The lungs show round, firm nodules with central cavitation, necrosis and calcification. These nodules show fibrinoid necrosis surrounded by palisading mononuclear cells and fibroblasts.

Clinical Features Individuals suffering from simple coal-worker's pneumoconiosis usually have chronic cough and dyspnoea on exertion. With progressive massive fibrosis, increasing respiratory distress, chest tightness, chronic cough with black sputum, pulmonary hypertension and cor pulmonale develop.

Silicosis (Knife Grinder's Disease) It is an occupational lung disease that majorly affects individuals working in construction units, mining, nonmetallic mineral products, pottery and glass industry.

It is caused due to prolonged exposure to silicon dioxide (silica).

Pathogenesis Silica exists in two forms – crystalline form and amorphous form (Flowchart 19.4).

Morphology

Gross Pale black silicotic nodules are seen in the upper zones of the lungs and hilar lymph nodes (Fig. 19.19). With progression of the disease, the nodules coalesce to form collagenous scars with central cavitation due to ischaemia. Lymph nodes show calcification. Chest X-rays of these patients reveal nodular lesions with characteristic eggshell calcifications.

Microscopy Coalescent collagenous nodules (fibrotic nodules) are seen in the upper lobes that may progress to massive fibrosis (Fig. 19.20). Birefringent silica particles can be seen with polarized light.

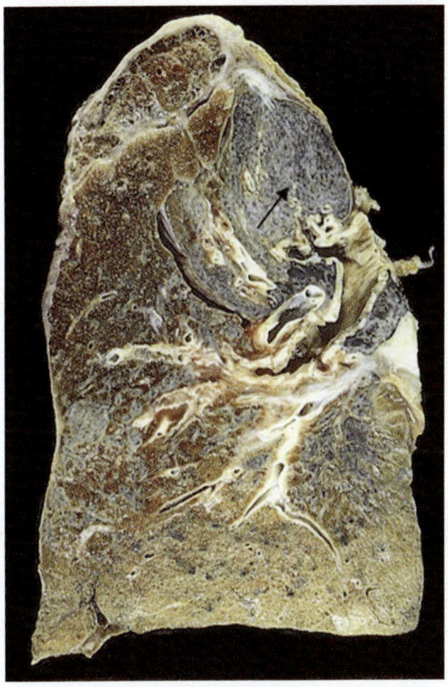

Fig. 19.19 Gross morphology of silicosis lung – scarring of the upper lobe of the lung (black arrow) into a small dark mass with pleural thickening. (*Source:* From Vinay Kumar, Abul K Abbas, Jon C Aster. Robbins Basic Pathology. Elsevier. 2018.)

Clinical Features The onset of silicosis may be slow and insidious (10–30 years after exposure), accelerated (within 10 years) or rapid (within weeks after intense exposure to fine dust rich in silica). The affected individuals develop shortness of breath on exertion, persistent cough, fatigue and tachypnoea.

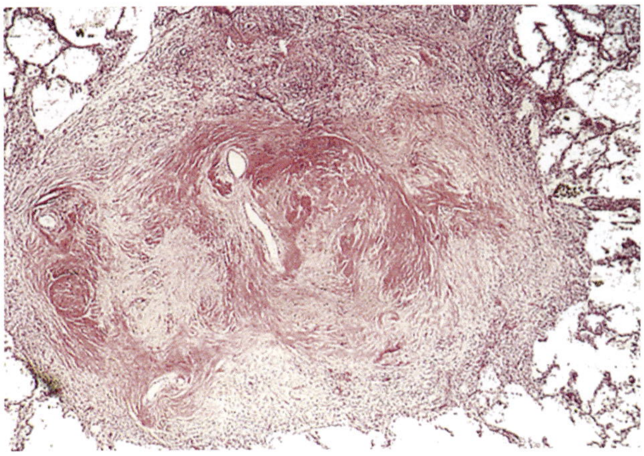

Fig. 19.20 Microscopic picture of silicosis lung – coalescent collagenous silicotic nodules. (*Source:* From Simon S Cross. Underwood's Pathology. Elsevier. 2019.)

Complications

- An increased susceptibility to tuberculosis (TB) (due to inhibition of phagocytic activity of macrophages by silica)

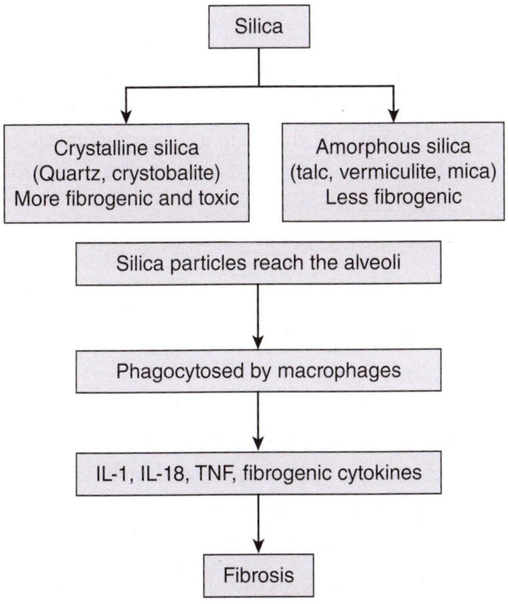

Flowchart 19.4 Pathogenesis of silicosis.

- Caplan syndrome
- Cor pulmonale
- Increased predisposition to lung cancer

Asbestosis Asbestosis is a condition caused by members of the family of crystalline hydrated silicates.

Asbestos occurs in the following two forms:

Serpentine (the most common form is chrysotile) consists of curved and flexible fibres that get impacted in the upper respiratory pathways and are removed by mucociliary clearance.

Amphibole (crocidolite, tremolite and amosite) pathogenic than serpentine forms.

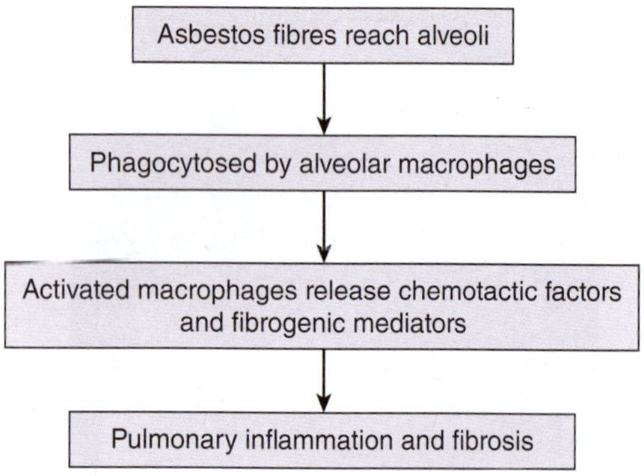

Flowchart 19.5 Pathogenesis of asbestosis.

Table 19.12 Asbestos-related Diseases

Lung	Parenchymal interstitial fibrosis (asbestosis), lung carcinoma
Pleura	Localized pleural plaques
	Diffuse pleural fibrosis
	Recurrent pleural effusions
	Mesotheliomas
Other malignancies	Laryngeal carcinoma
	Ovarian carcinoma
	Colon carcinoma

Pathogenesis (Flowchart 19.5) Asbestos fibres reach the alveoli easily and penetrate the alveolar epithelial cells, leading to diffuse interstitial disease (Table 19.12).

Morphology

Diffuse interstitial fibrosis with the characteristic asbestos bodies is the hallmark feature of asbestosis (Fig. 19.21).

These asbestos bodies are morphologically fusiform or beaded bodies, are golden brown in colour and consist of asbestos fibres coated with an iron-containing proteinaceous material (Fig. 19.22).

In addition, ferruginous bodies representing organic or inorganic fibres coated with complexes of iron and glycoprotein can be seen. Fibrosis begins around respiratory bronchioles and alveolar ducts and then extends to involve alveolar sacs and alveoli. The fibrous tissue distorts the lung architecture, producing enlarged air spaces enclosed by a thick fibrous wall (**honeycomb lung**). Asbestosis begins in the lower lobes and extends subpleurally, gradually involving the middle and upper lobes over time. The fibrous scarring may trap pulmonary arteries and arterioles, producing pulmonary hypertension.

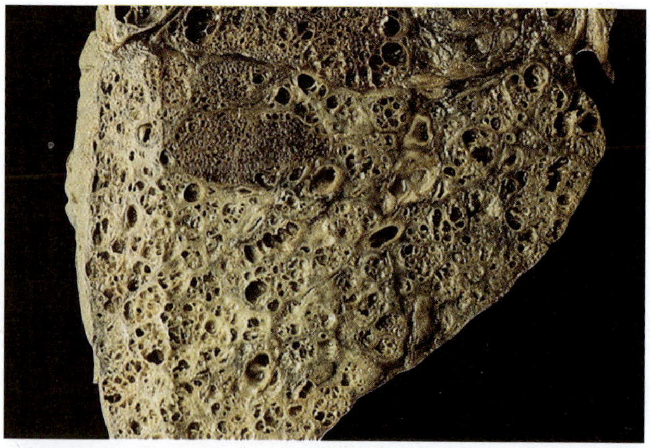

Fig. 19.21 Asbestosis lung. Gross – fibrosis has resulted in the formation of honeycomb lung. (*Source:* From Simon S Cross. Underwood's Pathology. Elsevier. 2019.)

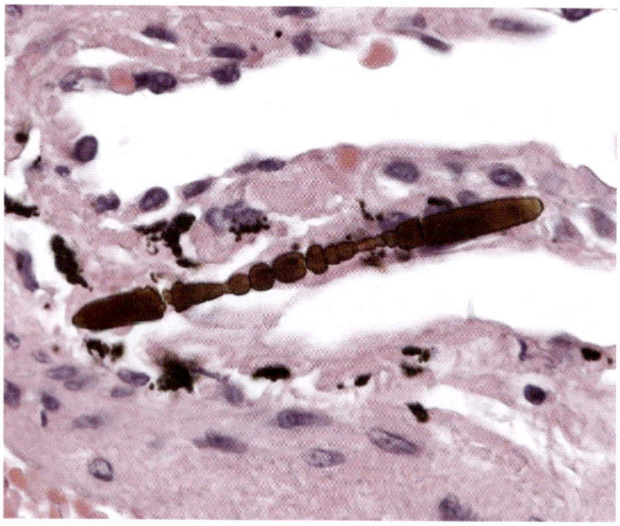

Fig. 19.22 Asbestosis lung. High-power view showing a brown-beaded appearance of asbestos bodies. (*Source:* From Geraldine O'Dowd, Sarah Bell, Sylvia Wright. Wheater's Pathology: A Text, Atlas, and Review of Histopathology. Elsevier. 2020.)

Parietal pleural plaques (Fig. 19.23) (acellular type I collagen deposition) occur in a symmetrical distribution involving the domes of the diaphragm and the posterolateral chest wall.

Fibrous adhesions may occur on visceral pleura.

Lung cancer: It is the most common tumour in an asbestos-exposed individual.

Malignant mesothelioma

- It is a rare and highly malignant neoplasm with 90% of the cases being associated with asbestos exposure.
- It typically presents with recurrent pleural effusion, dyspnoea and chest pain with a poor prognosis.

Clinical Features It has a slow, insidious onset with dyspnoea and cough (appearing 10–20 years after exposure)

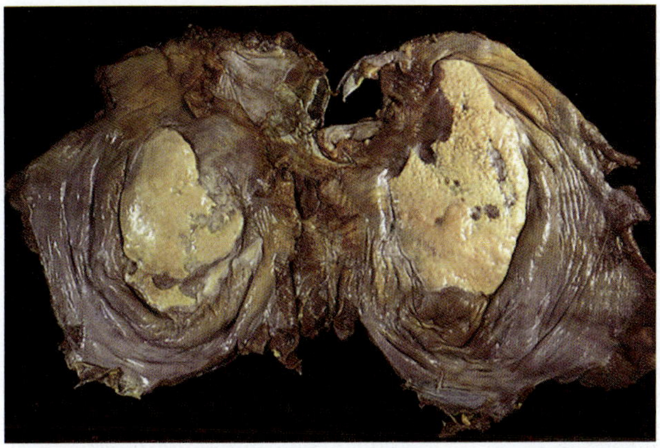

Fig. 19.23 Asbestos-related pleural plaques – large fibrocalcific plaques seen on the pleural surface of the diaphragm. (*Source:* From Vinay Kumar, Abul K Abbas, Jon C Aster. Robbins Basic Pathology. Elsevier. 2018.)

progressing to respiratory failure, cor pulmonale and eventually death.

Berylliosis Berylliosis is caused by a heavy exposure to beryllium and its salts. Beryllium is used in nuclear and aerospace industries and electronic equipment.

Two forms of berylliosis can occur:

Acute form occurs in people who are unusually sensitive to beryllium and its salts.

Pulmonary reaction

- Acute exudative chemical pneumonitis
- Alveoli filled with protein-rich fluid with the formation of hyaline membrane

Chronic form occurs after a delay of more than 20 years.

It is a cell-mediated hypersensitivity reaction with noncaseating epithelioid granulomas and seen diffusely scattered in the lung parenchyma.

Other Fibrosing Lung Diseases

Idiopathic Pulmonary Fibrosis (Usual Interstitial Pneumonia) It refers to a clinicopathological syndrome of unknown aetiology that causes progressive interstitial fibrosis and respiratory failure. Histologically, idiopathic pulmonary fibrosis is named **usual interstitial pneumonia (UIP)**, which shares features with asbestosis, hypersensitivity pneumonia and connective tissue diseases.

Pathogenesis Both genetic factors and environmental factors are implicated.

Genetic factors

Telomerase mutations

Telomerase is an enzyme that prevents cellular ageing by maintaining the length of telomeres at the ends of the chromosomes. Mutations of the telomerase produce telomere shortening in alveolar epithelial cells.

Surfactant mutations

Mutations in the surfactant genes create folding defects in the affected proteins. This leads to activation of the unfolded protein response, making the alveolar epithelial cells more sensitive to environmental factors.

Abnormal mucin

Increased secretion of an abnormal mucin MUC5B predisposes to alveolar injury.

Environmental factors Smoking, occupational exposure to chemicals, exposure to environmental toxins and irritants lead to epithelial injury, release of fibrogenic factors and an increased production of collagen and fibrosis.

Morphology

The pathological hallmark is temporal heterogeneity (in which different lung foci show patchy interstitial fibrosis in different stages of disease). Computed tomography (CT) of the lung shows fibrosis initially seen in subpleural patches but eventually results in diffuse fibrosis with end-stage 'honeycomb' lung.

Clinical Features Insidious onset is with progressive dyspnoea and cough. Hypoxaemia, cyanosis and clubbing occur late in the course of the disease. The course of the disease is variable with a poor prognosis.

Nonspecific Interstitial Pneumonia It may be idiopathic or associated with connective tissue diseases. Histologically, it shows both a cellular pattern and a fibrosing pattern. In the cellular pattern, there is chronic interstitial inflammation containing lymphocytes and plasma cells in uniform or patchy distribution. The fibrosing pattern consists of diffuse or patchy interstitial fibrosis in the same stage of development.

Clinical Features Patients usually present with dyspnoea and cough. Diagnostic features on CT scan are bilateral, symmetrical and predominantly lower-lobe opacities. These patients have a much better prognosis than those with UIP.

Cryptogenic Organizing Pneumonia (Bronchiolitis Obliterans Organizing Pneumonia) It is a disease of unknown aetiology. Patients present with cough and dyspnoea. Chest X-rays show subpleural and peribronchial consolidation.

Microscopically, it is characterized by **Masson bodies** (Fig. 19.24) – polypoidal plugs of loose connective tissue in the alveoli, alveolar ducts and bronchioles. Lung architecture is normal. There is no interstitial fibrosis or honeycomb lung.

Treatment is with steroids. It is important to note that organizing pneumonia with intra-alveolar fibrosis may occur secondary to a wide variety of lung injuries such as viral and bacterial pneumonias, toxin inhalation, connective tissue diseases and graft-versus-host disease in bone marrow transplant recipients. The course and prognosis depend on the type and severity of the underlying disorder.

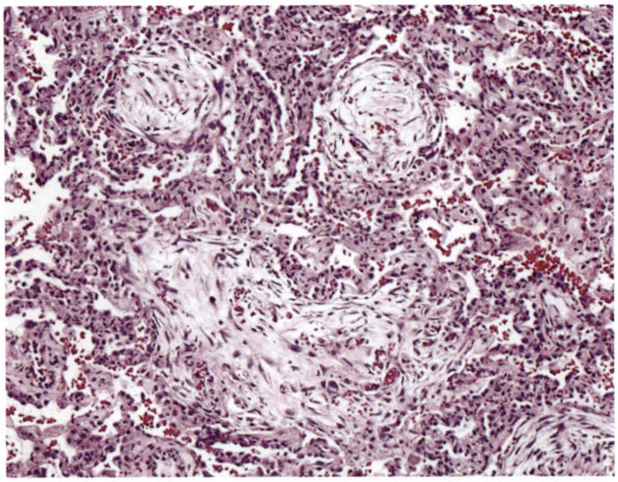

Fig. 19.24 Microscopy – Masson bodies (balls of fibroblast) in the alveolar spaces of cryptogenic organizing pneumonia. (*Source:* From Vinay Kumar, Abul K Abbas, Jon C Aster. Robbins Basic Pathology. Elsevier. 2018.)

Lung Involvement in Autoimmune Diseases

There is involvement of the lungs in autoimmune diseases (Table 19.13).

GRANULOMATOUS DISEASES (TABLE 19.14)

Granulomatous lung diseases refer to a wide spectrum of pathologies with variable clinical manifestations and outcomes but share a common feature of the presence of granulomas in the lung. It can be due to infectious and noninfectious diseases.

Sarcoidosis

It is a systemic granulomatous disease of unknown aetiology. It usually affects females more than males aged between 20 and 60 years. The most common presentation is bilateral hilar lymphadenopathy, and the involvement of the lungs is seen in about 90% of cases.

Table 19.13 Involvement of Lung in Autoimmune Diseases

Autoimmune Diseases	Pulmonary Diseases
Rheumatoid arthritis	Lungs are involved in 30%–40% of cases Chronic pleuritis with or without effusion Diffuse interstitial fibrosis Intrapulmonary nodules Follicular bronchiolitis Pulmonary hypertension
Systemic sclerosis	Diffuse interstitial fibrosis and pleural involvement
Systemic lupus erythematosus	Pneumonitis, pleurisy and pleural effusions

Table 19.14 List of Granulomatous Diseases of the Lungs

Category	Examples
Infectious lung disease	Tuberculosis and nontuberculous mycobacteriosis *Cryptococcus, Coccidioides, Histoplasma, Blastomyces and Aspergillus*
Noninfectious lung disease	Sarcoidosis Hypersensitivity pneumonitis Drugs Berylliosis Granulomatosis with polyangiitis Rheumatoid nodule Pulmonary Langerhans cell histiocytosis

Pathogenesis Disordered immune regulation, genetic factors and environmental factors contribute to the development of this disease.

Immunological Abnormalities Cell-mediated immune response occurs to an unidentified antigen.

- Pathogenic involvement of CD4 – T_H cells can lead to their accumulation in the alveoli and interstitium resulting in an elevated CD4:CD8 ratio.
- Increased level of the T_H1 cytokines – IL-2 responsible for T-cell expansion and interferon gamma (γ-IFN) cause macrophage activation.
- Increase in IL-8, TNF and Macrophage Inflammatory Protein (MIP)-1α leads to recruitment of T cells and monocytes aiding in the formation of granulomas. **TNF is a marker of disease activity in bronchoalveolar fluid (BAF)**.
- Anergy to common skin test antigens for *Candida* and TB purified protein derivative is seen.
- Polyclonal hypergammaglobulinaemia may also be seen.
- **Genetic factors:** Association of the disease with HLA-A1 and HLA-B8 is seen.

Morphology

Involved tissues show noncaseating granulomas (Fig. 19.25) composed of a collection of epithelioid macrophages and multinucleated giant cells surrounded by fibroblasts. Granulomas also contain **Schaumann bodies**, which are laminated concretions of calcium and proteins, and **asteroid bodies** – stellate inclusion in giant cells. These are seen in 60% of the granulomas but are not specific for sarcoidosis (Fig. 19.26).

Lung Small nodules (noncaseating granulomas) are predominantly seen in the upper lobes with bilateral hilar lymphadenopathy. Special stains should be used to exclude them because granulomas can also be caused by infectious diseases. The stains include acid-fast bacillus

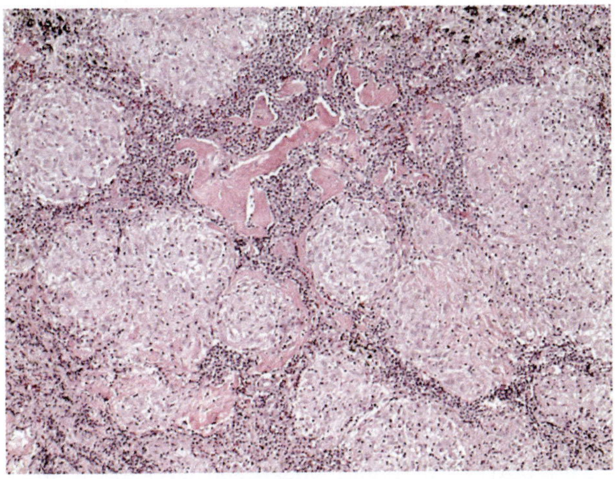

Fig. 19.25 Sarcoidosis – characteristic noncaseating granulomas. (*Source:* From Cancer Therapy Adviser, Imaging Sarcoidosis, 2017.)

(AFB) stain to rule out *mycobacteria* and Gomori methenamine silver (GMS) stain to rule out fungi. Granulomas are replaced by diffuse interstitial fibrosis in 5%–15% of cases.

Skin Erythema nodosum, maculopapular lesions and painless subcutaneous nodules are seen in one-fourth of cases.

Eye Iritis, iridocyclitis (unilateral or bilateral), corneal opacities, glaucoma, loss of vision and involvement of the posterior uveal tract may be seen. Ocular lesions are frequently accompanied by inflammation in the lacrimal glands with suppression of lacrimation (sicca syndrome).

Bone Phalangeal bones of the hands and feet are involved with small circumscribed resorption of the bone in the marrow cavity.

Other organs involved are the spleen, liver, parotid glands, muscle (sarcoid myositis), heart, brain (neurosarcoidosis seen in 5%–15% of cases) and pituitary glands.

Clinical Features The most common presentation is respiratory symptoms or abnormalities discovered on chest X-rays.

Bilateral hilar lymphadenopathy with lung mottling is a typical chest X-ray feature. Chest X-rays and CT scan of the chest are likely to show involvement of the disease process. Lung function tests show a restrictive pattern of defect.

Symptoms include fatigue, fever, night sweats, weight loss or respiratory abnormalities such as cough and dyspnoea.

Sarcoid macrophages are responsible for 1α-hydroxylation of vitamin D, with resultant 1,25-$(OH)_2$-vitamin D_3. This results in hypercalcaemia and hypercalciuria. Levels of angiotensin-converting enzyme (ACE) are elevated in sarcoidosis. Although ACE levels are not of diagnostic value, these may be useful in monitoring the progression of disease.

Course About 65%–70% of affected patients recover with minimal or no residual manifestation in the lung.

Hypersensitivity Pneumonitis **PA 26.5**

It is a spectrum of immunologically mediated interstitial lung disorders secondary to inhaled organic antigens (Table 19.15). It is also known as extrinsic allergic alveolitis because it damages the alveolar walls.

Pathogenesis It is due to type III and IV hypersensitivity reactions to an extrinsic antigen. In the acute phase of the disease, which occurs 4–6 hours after antigen exposure in a previously sensitized host, type III hypersensitivity reaction (immune complex) occurs. With continuous exposure, the disease enters a chronic phase, which is represented by type IV hypersensitivity reaction. Granulomas and interstitial fibrosis occur in the chronic phase.

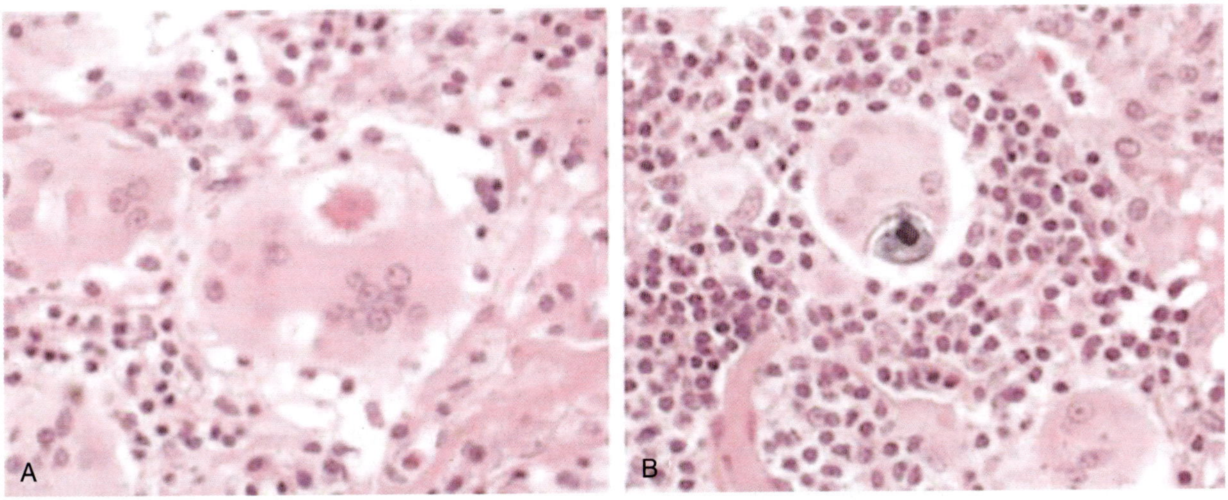

Fig. 19.26 Microscopy – sarcoidosis. Multinucleated giants cells with cytoplasmic inclusions. (A) Asteroid bodies. (B) Schaumann bodies.

Table 19.15 Inhaled Organic Antigens with Their Syndromes

Antigens	Syndromes
Mould hay	Farmer's lung
Bagasse (sugarcane)	Bagassosis
Cotton flex hemp	Byssinosis
Bird droppings	Bird fancier's or pigeon breeder's lung
Mushroom compost dust	Mushroom worker's lung
Malt dust	Malt worker's lung
Mouldy maple bark	Maple bark disease
Thermophilic bacteria (water reservoir)	Air conditioner or humidifier lung

Morphology

The histological changes are seen in bronchioles and include interstitial pneumonitis consisting of lymphocytes, macrophages, plasma cells, noncaseating granulomas, interstitial fibrosis and obliterative bronchiolitis.

Clinical Features Patients present with fever, cough and dyspnoea. Symptoms occur 4–6 hours after exposure and may last for 12 hours to several days. Chronic form of the disease leads to progressive respiratory failure.

SMOKING-RELATED INTERSTITIAL DISEASES

Smoking is associated not only with obstructive diseases but also with interstitial diseases. It is related to the development of several ILDs including desquamative interstitial pneumonia (DIP), respiratory bronchiolitis–associated interstitial lung disease (RBILD) and pulmonary Langerhans cell histiocytosis (PLCH).

A. **DIP**
It is commonly seen in smokers. Hallmarks of this disease are accumulation of plenty of macrophages with cytoplasmic brown pigment (**smoker's macrophages**) in the alveolar spaces and thickened alveolar septa. The term 'desquamative' came from the misconception that intra-alveolar macrophages were desquamated epithelial cells. Fibrosis is minimal and alveolar architecture is preserved. The average age of onset is 40 years, with cough and dyspnoea as the main complaints. It has a much better prognosis than UIP, with 10-year survival at 70%–100%; pathological changes regress following smoking cessation.

B. **RBILD**
RBILD is a common histological lesion in smokers. Pigmented intraluminal macrophages (smoker's macrophages) are seen in the first- and second-order bronchioles with peribronchial fibrosis. Symptoms are mild with a gradual onset of cough and dyspnoea. Cessation of smoking results in clinical improvement.

PULMONARY EOSINOPHILIA

Pulmonary eosinophilia is a collection of diseases characterized by similar morphology of eosinophil infiltration in the pulmonary interstitium and in the alveolar spaces and similar clinical scenarios with a prompt response to corticosteroids. It includes several entities, which are mentioned as follows:

- **Acute eosinophilic pneumonia with respiratory failure** Acute onset of dyspnoea, cough and fever follow with a rapid progression to respiratory distress. Chest X-rays show bilateral diffuse opacities. Blood eosinophils are usually normal but occasionally elevated (generally <500/mm^3). BAL fluid shows eosinophils greater than 25%. Histology shows eosinophils and diffuse alveolar damage.
  - **Löffler syndrome** is characterized by mild respiratory symptoms:
    - Peripheral blood eosinophilia
    - Transient migratory pulmonary infiltrates
    - Self-limiting
    - Associated with hypersensitivity to *Ascaris lumbricoides*
  - **Secondary chronic pulmonary eosinophilia** occurs secondary to adverse drug reactions; infection with fungi, bacteria and helminths; allergic bronchopulmonary aspergillosis; asthma; and vasculitis.
  - **Idiopathic chronic eosinophilic pneumonia** is characterized by focal areas of consolidation in the periphery of the lungs. Prominent interstitial and intra-alveolar lymphocytic and eosinophilic infiltrates are seen in peripheral lung fields. Patients present with fever, cough, night sweats, dyspnoea and weight loss. The condition is a diagnosis of exclusion.

PULMONARY LANGERHANS CELL HISTIOCYTOSIS (PAP)

It is a rare histiocytic disorder affecting exclusively the lungs of smokers. It is a form of ILD characterized by nodules composed of a heterogeneous cell population including cells that exhibit the phenotype of Langerhans cells, eosinophils, neutrophils, macrophages and osteoclastic type of giant cells. Langerhans cells are dendritic cells with grooved nuclei and function as antigen-presenting cells. The cells express S100, CD1a and CD207 (langerin) and contain intracytoplasmic Birbeck granules.

Recently, BRAF mutations are seen in PLCH, suggesting clonal proliferation. Cessation of smoking gives better results.

PULMONARY ALVEOLAR PROTEINOSIS

It is a rare disease characterized by a bilateral, patchy, asymmetric lung involvement with opacification on chest

X-rays. There is accumulation of surfactant in the alveolar and bronchiolar spaces due to macrophage dysfunction. It may be congenital, secondary or autoimmune.

Autoimmune PAP (also called acquired): It is due to autoantibody that inhibits the activity of granulocyte–macrophage colony-stimulating factor (GM-CSF), thereby impairing macrophage clearance of pulmonary surfactant.

Secondary PAP: It is associated with haematopoietic disorders, malignancies, immunodeficiency disorders, lysinuric protein intolerance and acute silicosis. These conditions affect macrophage function, leading to inadequate clearance of the surfactant from alveolar spaces.

Congenital PAP: It arises due to mutation in any of the following: ATP-binding cassette protein member 3 (ABCA3), surfactant protein C, surfactant protein B, GM-CSF or GM-CSF receptors.

Morphology

The lungs are enlarged and heavy; fluid exudes out on the cut section.

Microscopy reveals intra-alveolar accumulation of dense, granular, eosinophilic material containing lipid and Periodic Acid Schiff (PAS)-positive material (Fig. 19.27).

Clinical Features

Progressive dyspnoea, cyanosis and respiratory insufficiency may occur.

DISEASES OF PULMONARY BLOOD VESSELS

The two main types of pulmonary vascular disease are pulmonary embolism and pulmonary hypertension.

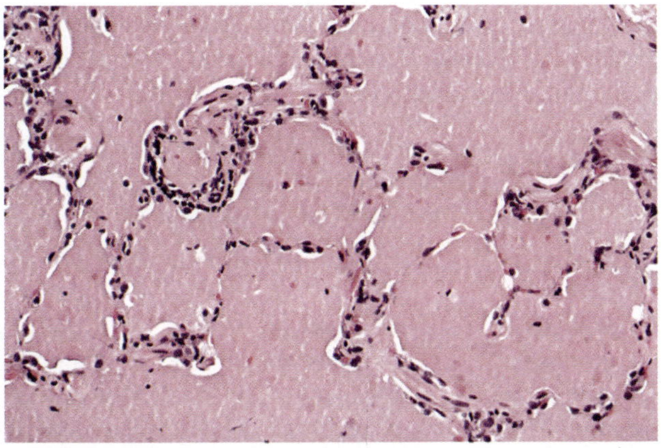

Fig. 19.27 Microscopic picture of pulmonary alveolar proteinosis. Alveoli are filled with dense granular protein lipid material. (*Source:* From Vinay Kumar, Abul K Abbas, Jon C Aster. Robbins Basic Pathology. Elsevier. 2018.)

Table 19.16 Risk Factors for Pulmonary Embolism

Hospitalized or bedridden patients
Cardiac disease
Malignancy
Hip fracture
Hypercoagulable states • Primary (factor V Leiden mutation, antiphospholipid antibody syndrome, prothrombin mutation) • Secondary (obesity, oral contraceptive use) • Indwelling central venous line – nidus for right atrial thrombi and can embolize to lungs • Small bone marrow emboli during cardiopulmonary resuscitation efforts

PULMONARY EMBOLISM

Pulmonary embolism is a blockage in one of the pulmonary arteries in the lungs. Pulmonary emboli result from a thrombus or blood clot, amniotic fluid, fat or air. Pulmonary embolism is a common and highly lethal condition and the leading cause of death in bedridden patients (Table 19.16).

Aetiology

Embolism originates from deep vein thrombosis (DVT) of the proximal veins of lower limbs – popliteal, femoral and iliac veins (>95% of cases).

The effects of pulmonary embolism depend on the size of the occluded vessel, nature of emboli and cardiovascular status.

A large embolus can get impacted at the bifurcation of the main pulmonary artery, forming a **saddle embolus**.

More commonly, multiple emboli or fragmented parts of a large embolus affect the lower lobes of the lungs.

Paradoxical embolism is the passage of an embolus from the right side of the heart into the left side of the heart through septal defects.

In patients with adequate cardiovascular function, blood supply to the lung is maintained by bronchial circulation despite pulmonary vascular obstruction. In such a situation, only pulmonary haemorrhage occurs. Pulmonary infarction occurs when there is an inadequate bronchial circulation, as in patients with heart or lung disease.

Pathogenesis

Hemodynamic effects

- Pulmonary embolism results in an increase in pulmonary vascular resistance because of mechanical obstruction by the embolus and vasoconstriction due to thromboxane A_2 and serotonin released from platelets.
- This results in an increase in the right ventricular afterload, dilation of the right ventricle and subsequent right-side heart failure. The elevated pulmonary

vascular resistance causes a decrease in the left ventricular preload and results in systemic hypotension.

Abnormalities in gas exchange

Pulmonary embolism increases dead space ventilation. The alveolar ventilation exceeds pulmonary capillary blood flow, contributing to ventilation–perfusion mismatch and hypoxaemia.

Morphology

Gross Pulmonary infarcts are haemorrhagic, raised red-blue wedge-shaped infarcts, with the apex pointing towards the hilus of the lung (Fig. 19.28). An occluded vessel is usually identified near the apex of the infarct. Pleural surface shows fibrous exudate. Fibrous replacement begins at the margin and eventually the infarct is converted into a scar.

Microscopy Haemorrhagic areas microscopically show red-blue areas of ischaemic necrosis of the alveolar walls, bronchioles and vessels.

Septic infarcts can occur if the infarct is caused by infected embolism. Neutrophilic inflammatory reaction is seen in the infarct.

Facts

Pulmonary infarcts are typically wedge shaped, with the apex of the wedge near the hilum and the base reaching the pleural surface. This pattern reflects the specific geographic region supplied by the branch of the pulmonary artery.

Clinical Features

Clinical features vary depending on the size of the embolus and the ability of the right ventricle to respond to increased afterload. Most of the pulmonary emboli (60%–80%) are small and clinically silent. Massive pulmonary embolism may present as cardiovascular collapse or even cardiac arrest. A diagnosis of pulmonary embolism should be considered in patients presenting with severe dyspnoea. Key physical findings are those of clinical shock: the patient is cold, clammy and hypotensive and the jugular venous pressure is elevated. Embolic obstruction of the small end arteriolar pulmonary branches can cause pulmonary infarction.

Patients present with dyspnoea, tachypnoea, fever, chest pain, cough, haemoptysis and pleural rub (due to fibrinous pleuritis). Embolic obstruction of medium-sized arteries may result in pulmonary haemorrhage. Only 10% of emboli cause infarction because the lung is supported by dual blood supply (pulmonary circulation and bronchial artery circulation), and three-fourths of the infarcts affect the lower lobes. In more than half of the cases, infarcts are multiple.

Multiple small emboli may lead to pulmonary hypertension and chronic cor pulmonale (Flowchart 19.6).

Risk of recurrence is high with pulmonary embolism.

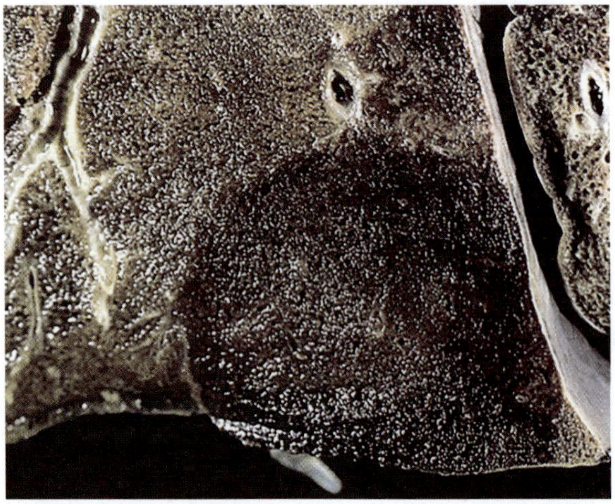

Fig. 19.28 Gross morphology of a small wedge-shaped haemorrhagic pulmonary infarct. (*Source:* From Vinay Kumar, Abul K Abbas, Jon C Aster. Robbins Basic Pathology. Elsevier. 2018.)

Investigations and Management

- An elevated D-dimer in the presence of symptoms is suggestive of pulmonary embolism.
- Ventilation–perfusion scan identifies areas of the lung with good ventilation but poor perfusion (V/Q mismatch).
- A spiral CT angiography of the lungs can detect pulmonary embolism by showing filling defects in the pulmonary arteries.
- X-rays of the chest show a wedge-shaped infarct 12–36 hours after the occurrence of embolism.
- Treatment is focused on stabilizing the clot with anticoagulation and to reduce extension of the clot, as well as looking for potential underlying causes.

PULMONARY HYPERTENSION

Pulmonary hypertension is defined as mean pulmonary arterial pressure greater than 20 mm Hg at rest, measured by right-side heart catheterization. Normally, pulmonary arterial circulation is a low-pressure high-flow system with much lower blood pressure than systemic blood pressure. WHO has classified pulmonary arterial hypertension into five groups (Table 19.17).

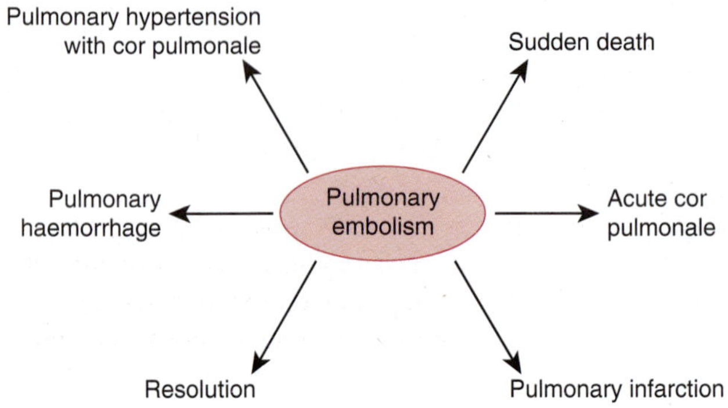

Flowchart 19.6 Consequences of pulmonary embolism.

Table 19.17 WHO Classification of Causes of Pulmonary Arterial Hypertension

Group 1: Pulmonary arterial hypertension
Increase in pulmonary vascular resistance
- 1.1. Idiopathic
- 1.2. Heritable
  (Inactivating germ line mutations in the gene encoding bone morphogenetic protein receptor 2 [BMPR2] are found in 75% of the familial cases of pulmonary hypertension)
- 1.3. Drug and toxin induced
- 1.4. Connective tissue diseases
- 1.5. HIV infection
- 1.6. Congenital heart disease
- 1.7. Portal hypertension

Group 2: Pulmonary hypertension due to left-sided heart disease
Increase in left atrial and pulmonary venous pressure
- 2.1. Left ventricular systolic and diastolic dysfunction
- 2.2. Valvular heart disease

Group 3: Pulmonary hypertension due to lung diseases and/or hypoxia
Increased pulmonary resistance to blood flow
- 3.1. COPD
- 3.2. Interstitial lung disease
- 3.3. Sleep apnoea

Group 4: Chronic thromboembolic pulmonary hypertension
Decreased functional cross-sectional area of pulmonary vascular bed

Group 5: Pulmonary hypertension with unclear or multifactorial mechanisms

COPD, chronic obstructive pulmonary disease.
(*Source:* Malik Bisserier et al. Targeting epigenetic mechanisms as an emerging therapeutic strategy in pulmonary hypertension disease. Fig. 2, January 2020, Vascular Biology 2(1):R17-R34.)

Morphology

Morphological changes are seen from the main pulmonary arteries down to the arterioles. **Medial hypertrophy** of the pulmonary muscular and elastic arteries as well as concentric and eccentric **intimal fibrosis** is observed (Fig. 19.29). Capillary tuft or plexiform arrangement of capillaries is seen in idiopathic and familial pulmonary hypertension, in human immunodeficiency virus (HIV) infection and in congenital heart disease with left-to-right shunt. Atheromatous deposit in large vessels is also seen.

The presenting features are dyspnoea, fatigue and anginal chest pain. Over time, respiratory distress, cyanosis and right ventricular hypertrophy appear. Decompensated cor pulmonale, often with superimposed thromboembolism and pneumonia, is the cause of death. Idiopathic pulmonary hypertension occurs in women 20–40 years of age and is associated with a poor prognosis.

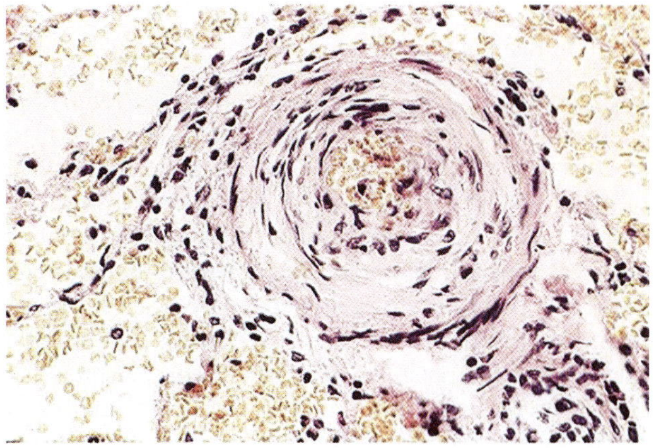

Fig. 19.29 Vascular changes in pulmonary hypertension. Medial hypertrophy of a pulmonary vessel. (*Source:* From Vinay Kumar, Abul K Abbas, Jon C Aster. Robbins Basic Pathology. Elsevier. 2018.)

TUBERCULOSIS PA 26.4

TB is a chronic, communicable, airborne bacterial disease caused by members of the *Mycobacterium tuberculosis* complex, which includes tubercle bacilli (*M. tuberculosis*), *M. bovis, M. africanum, M. microti, M. canettii, M. caprae* and *M. pinnipedii.* It usually affects the lungs but can affect any tissue or organ in the body.

Worldwide, TB is the leading cause of death from a single infectious agent. Globally, 7.5 million people were diagnosed and notified and about 1.3 million people died from TB in 2022 (*Global Tuberculosis Report*).

MYCOBACTERIA

- These are small, slender (4 μm), rod-shaped bacilli that are nonmotile and strict aerobes. (These therefore multiply better in pulmonary tissue, particularly at the apex, where oxygen concentration is higher than in the deeper organs.) Their cell envelope is composed of three macromolecules – peptidoglycan, arabinogalactan and mycolic acid – which are covalently linked to each other, and lipoarabinomannan (LAM), a lipopolysaccharide, anchoring to the plasma membrane.
- The cell wall component gives mycobacteria their characteristic staining properties. The organism stains weakly positive with Gram stain. The mycolic acid structure confers the ability to resist destaining by acid alcohol, after being stained by certain aniline dyes, leading to the term 'AFB'.
- The generation time of the bacillus is approximately 12–18 hours, so cultures must be incubated for 3–6 weeks at 37°C until proliferation becomes microscopically visible. The bacillus can withstand weak disinfectant and survive in a dry state for weeks.
- The bacteria can be demonstrated by the following methods:
  1. Ziehl–Neelsen staining
  2. Fluorescent dye method

3. Culture in Löwenstein–Jensen (LJ) media
4. Guinea pig inoculation

TRANSMISSION OF TUBERCULOSIS

M. tuberculosis bacilli are carried in airborne particles, called droplet nuclei, of 1- to 5-μm diameter. Infectious droplet nuclei are generated when persons having pulmonary or laryngeal TB disease cough, sneeze, shout or sing. These tiny particles remain suspended in the air for several hours. *M. tuberculosis* is transmitted through the air, **not** by surface contact. Transmission occurs when a person inhales droplet nuclei containing *M. tuberculosis*, and the droplet nuclei traverse the mouth or nasal passages, upper respiratory tract and bronchi to reach the alveoli of the lungs.

Other modes of transmission are **ingestion, inoculation and transplacental transmission**.

Pathogenesis

The outcome of infection in a previously unexposed, immunocompetent person depends on the development of antimycobacterial T-cell-mediated immunity (Fig. 19.30). These T cells control the host response to the bacteria that helps in protection, and results in development of pathological lesions such as caseating granulomas and cavitation. The steps in the infection process are as follows:

- **Entry into macrophages:** *M. tuberculosis* enters macrophages by phagocytosis, mediated by several receptors on the phagocyte such as mannose-binding lectin and CR3.
- **Replication in macrophages:** *M. tuberculosis* blocks the formation of the phagolysosome by inhibiting both $Ca^{2}+$ signals and the recruitment and assembly of the proteins that mediate phagosome–lysosome fusion. This allows bacteria to replicate unchecked within the vesicle, protected from the microbicidal action of the lysosomes. Thus, during the earliest stage of primary TB (<3 weeks) in the nonsensitized individual, bacteria proliferate in the pulmonary alveolar macrophages and air spaces, resulting in bacteraemia and seeding of multiple sites. The infected individuals generally remain asymptomatic or have mild flu-like symptoms. Multiple pathogen-associated molecular patterns of *M. tuberculosis*, including lipoproteins and glycolipids, are recognized by innate immune receptors, including toll-like receptors (TLRs) such as TLR2.
- **T_H1** response: About 3 weeks after infection, T_H1 cell gets differentiated (with the help of IL-12, which is produced by antigen-presenting cells) to become bactericidal due to exposure to mycobacterial antigens that enter draining lymph nodes.
- **T_H1**-mediated macrophage activation and killing of bacteria: T_H1 cells, both in lymph nodes and in the lung, produce **IFN-γ**, the critical mediator that enables macrophages to contain the *M. tuberculosis* infection.
    - IFN-γ stimulates maturation of the phagolysosome in infected macrophages, exposing the bacteria to a lethal acidic, oxidizing environment.
    - Second, IFN-γ stimulates expression of inducible nitric oxide synthase, which produces nitric oxide

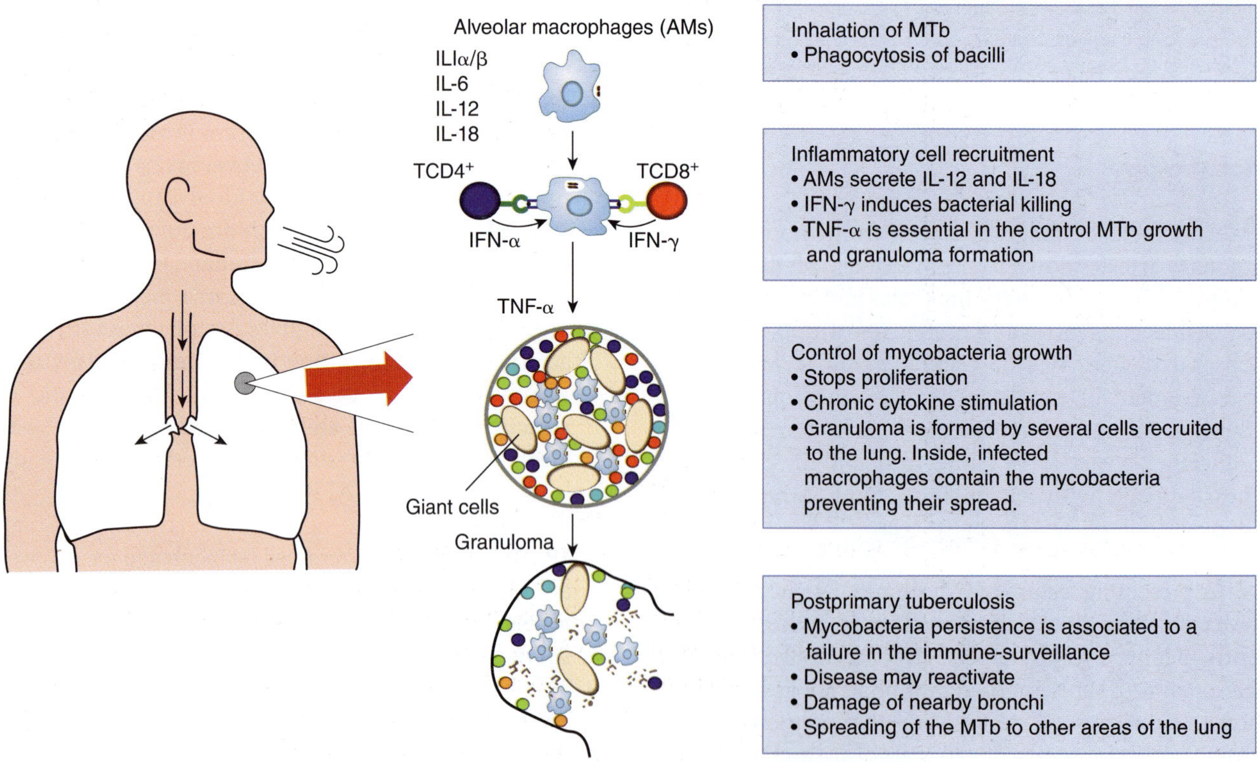

Fig. 19.30 Pathogenesis of *Mycobacterium tuberculosis*.

(NO). NO combines with other oxidants to create reactive nitrogen intermediates, which appear to be particularly important for killing of *Mycobacterium*.
- Third, IFN-γ mobilizes antimicrobial peptides (defensins) against the bacteria.
- Finally, IFN-γ stimulates autophagy, a process that sequesters and destroys damaged organelles along with intracellular bacteria such as *M. tuberculosis*.

- **Granulomatous inflammation and tissue damage:** T_H1 response orchestrates the formation of **granulomas and caseous necrosis**. Macrophages activated by IFN-γ differentiate into the 'epithelioid histiocytes' that aggregate to form granulomas; some epithelioid cells may fuse to form giant cells. In many people, this response halts the infection before significant tissue destruction or illness occurs. In other people, the infection progresses due to advanced age or immunosuppression and the ongoing immune response results in caseation necrosis. Activated macrophages also secrete TNF and chemokines, which promote recruitment of more monocytes.
- **Host susceptibility to disease:** People with genetic deficiencies in the IL-12 and IFN-γ pathways, including STAT1, a signal transducer for IFN-γ, are vulnerable to severe mycobacterial infections. The disease states that increase the risk of infection include diabetes mellitus, Hodgkin lymphoma, chronic lung disease (particularly silicosis), chronic renal failure, malnutrition, alcoholism, immunosuppression, HIV infection, drug abuse and smoking.
- **Immunological state in active TB:** Reactivation of latent infection occurring only in some individuals can be explained by the upregulation of IFN-responsive genes in the neutrophils of these individuals. This leads to an exaggerated response to IFN-1 and IFN-2 by the neutrophils, making IFN response an important cause of the disease process. The expression of these genes correlates with the severity of lung damage and is also shown to decrease following antitubercular treatment.

In summary, T_H1 cells are the important cells that help to protect us from TB by activating the macrophages to destroy the bacilli. But these also act as the main cause for tissue destruction. Reactivation of latent infection and reinfection is often associated with a greater level of tissue necrosis due to faster mobilization of the immune system. It is also important to realize that decrease in T-cell response indicates loss of resistance to the organism by the host body.

Primary pulmonary TB (PTB) is often seen in children following the primary exposure, whereas secondary PTB is common in adults following reactivation of the primary lesion. These lesions may resolve or progress to progressive PTB or miliary TB depending on the host immunity.

Intestinal TB contracted by the drinking of contaminated milk is common in countries where bovine TB is present and milk is not pasteurized. It can present as circumferential ulcerations that may lead to strictures in the small intestine (ileocecal region predominantly) and ascites.

Types of Tuberculosis

- Primary PTB
- Secondary TB
- Progressive PTB
- Miliary TB
- Extrapulmonary TB

Primary Pulmonary Tuberculosis

Primary TB is the infection in an individual who has not been previously infected or immunized. The common sites of primary infection are the lungs, hilar lymph nodes, tonsils, cervical lymph nodes, small intestine and mesenteric lymph nodes, with the lungs being the most common site.

Following inhalation of infected droplet nuclei, the bacilli localize in the distal air spaces of the lower part of the upper lobe and the upper part of the lower lobe, close to the pleura. After 2–8 weeks, a 1- to 1.5-cm area of grey-white inflammation with consolidation develops. This is known as **Ghon focus**.

The combination of parenchymal lung lesion (Ghon focus) with hilar lymph node enlargement is known as the **Ghon complex or primary complex** (Fig. 19.31).

Morphology

The characteristic lesion is a caseating granuloma, a localized lesion in the tissue consisting of a central area of caseous necrosis surrounded by epithelioid macrophages, lymphocytes and Langhans giant cells. Caseating granulomas may enlarge and progress but rarely reach more than 3 cm in diameter (Fig. 19.32). These may undergo calcification and heal with fibrosis and scarring.

Facts Virchow described caseous necrosis as 'fatty metamorphosis' because of abundant lipid and foamy macrophages. Caseation is a process of coagulation necrosis in which lipid-rich cells disintegrate and are converted into a homogeneous, structureless mass devoid of blood vessels.

Fate of Primary Tuberculosis

- **No progression:** Lesions heal by fibrosis and may also undergo calcification (detected in chest X-rays as the Ranke complex) in 95% of cases.
  A few viable bacilli may remain in these areas and go into a dormant state as long as the person's immune system remains active.
- **Progressive primary TB:** It occurs in malnourished children, the elderly and immunosuppressed individuals.

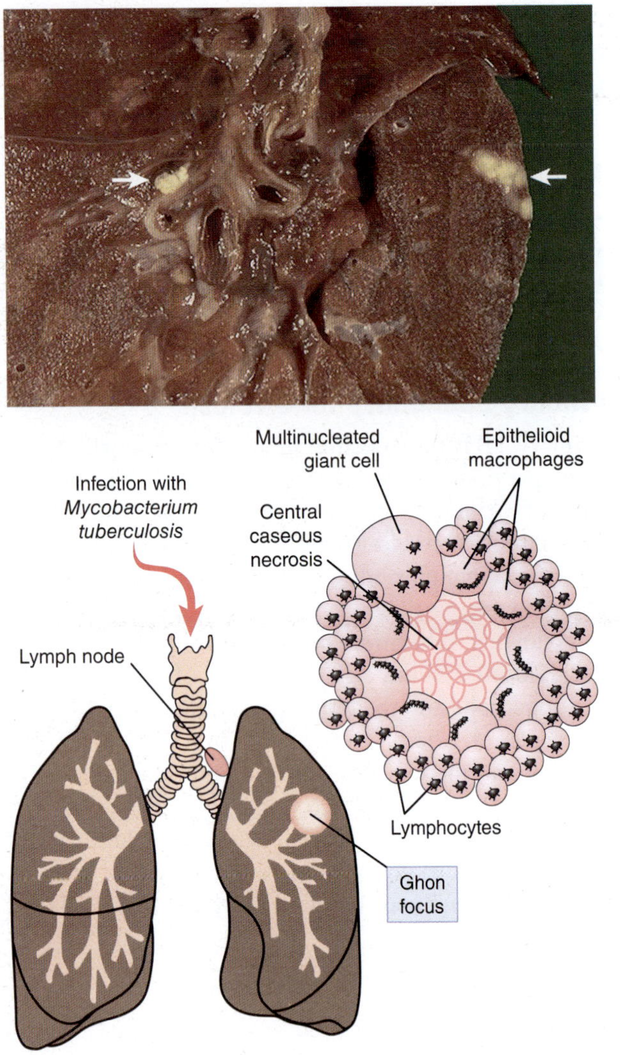

Fig. 19.31 Ghon complex in primary tuberculosis. A small yellow granuloma seen in subpleural (arrow) and hilar lymph node (arrow) next to bronchus.

Primary focus continues to grow and caseous material is disseminated to other parts of the lungs, causing lower- and middle-lobe consolidation, pleural involvement with effusion, empyema and hilar lymph node enlargement. Direct spread leads to erosion into the bronchial tree, producing foci of infection in other parts of the lungs.

Laryngeal TB may occur due to coughed infected sputum and intestinal TB due to swallowing of the infected sputum.

- **Primary miliary TB:** Bacilli may enter circulation through erosion of the blood vessel and disseminate to other parts of the body.
- **Progressive secondary TB:** This is due to reactivation of healed primary TB lesions.

Secondary Tuberculosis (Post-primary Tuberculosis)

It arises in a previously sensitized host, commonly due to reactivation of latent infection when the immune system is depressed, but may also occur due to exogenous reinfection. It progresses slowly and occurs in 10%–15% of patients.

Morphology

Classically, it involves the apical and posterior segments of the upper lobe of one or both the lungs. Regional lymph nodes are less commonly involved. **Cavity formation is common**. The apical lesion in secondary TB without lymph node involvement is known as the **Assman focus**. Such foci are circumscribed grey-white-yellow with central caseation and peripheral fibrosis.

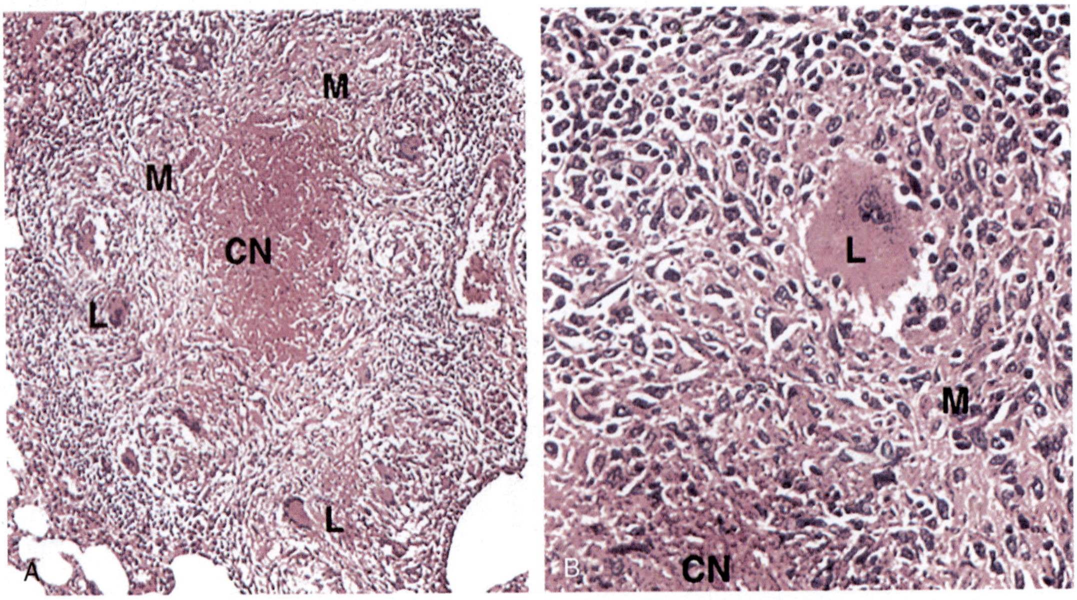

Fig. 19.32 Morphology of early pulmonary tuberculosis. (A) Early tubercle (medium power). (B) Early tubercle (high power) – caseous necrosis (CN) in the centre of the tubercle surrounded by a zone of epithelioid macrophages (M) with Langhans giant cells (L).

Facts Patients with cavitary lesions are highly infectious (100 million bacilli in a cavity of size of 2 cm) and are always smear positive because of high oxygen tension in the cavity that favours bacterial growth.

Fate of Secondary Tuberculosis

- **No progression:** Heals with fibrous scarring and calcification
- **Progressive secondary pulmonary TB**
- **Fibrocaseous TB**

  The central caseous necrosis either may break into a bronchus (open fibrocaseous TB) or can remain as a soft caseous lesion without breaking into bronchus or bronchiole, producing a noncavitary lesion.

  Grossly, the tuberculous cavity is spherical with a thick fibrous wall. The cavity is lined by a yellow caseous necrotic material, and the lumen is traversed by thrombosed blood vessels. There may be thickening of the overlying pleura. Microscopically, the wall and lumen of the cavity show caseous necrosis with dystrophic calcification and fibrosis.

  Complications of fibrocaseous TB

  Aneurysm of the patent arteries traversing the cavity (produces haemoptysis)
  Bronchopleural fistula (extension into the pleura)
  Tuberculous empyema (deposition of caseous material on the pleural surface)
  Thickened pleura (adhesions of the parietal pleura)
- **Tuberculous caseous pneumonia:** Exudative reaction with oedema, fibrin, polymorphs and macrophages
- **Miliary TB**

Progressive Pulmonary Tuberculosis

This is common in adults and immunocompromised hosts. The apical lesion of secondary TB may involve the adjacent lung parenchyma and erode into the bronchi, resulting in discharge of the necrotic material into the bronchi, leaving behind an empty cavity, and into the blood vessels resulting in haemoptysis. With adequate treatment, the cavity may heal with **fibrosis** (Fig. 19.33). But when treatment is inadequate or if the individual is immunocompromised, the bacilli may spread to other organs of the body through lymphatic channels and the bloodstream. This type of spread is known as miliary TB. The complications of progressive PTB include pleural effusions, tuberculous empyema and obliterative fibrous pleuritic.

Miliary Tuberculosis

Miliary TB refers to the presence of multiple small 2-mm-sized lesions (millet-like) with yellow-white consolidation (Fig. 19.34). They may be pulmonary (within the lung) or extrapulmonary in location. This type of dissemination may be seen following primary or secondary TB and represents 1%–3% of cases. Microscopically, the lesions are surrounded by macrophages and form granulomas.

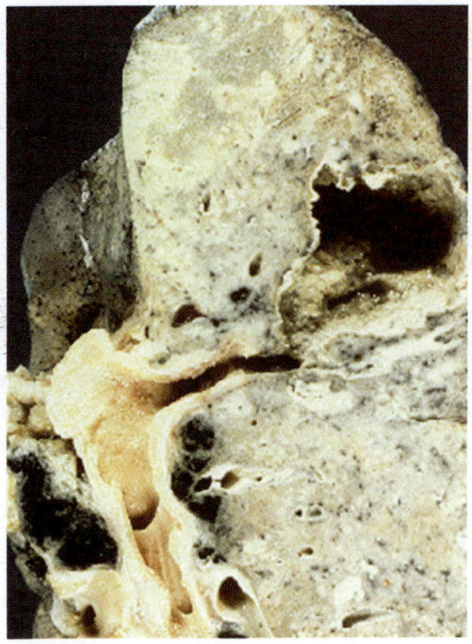

Fig. 19.33 Cavitating pulmonary tuberculosis – large cavity, which empties into an airway, apical consolidation and necrotic nodules. (*Source:* From Carol F. Farver, Jaishree Jagirdar, Pulmonary Pathology, Elsevier 2018.)

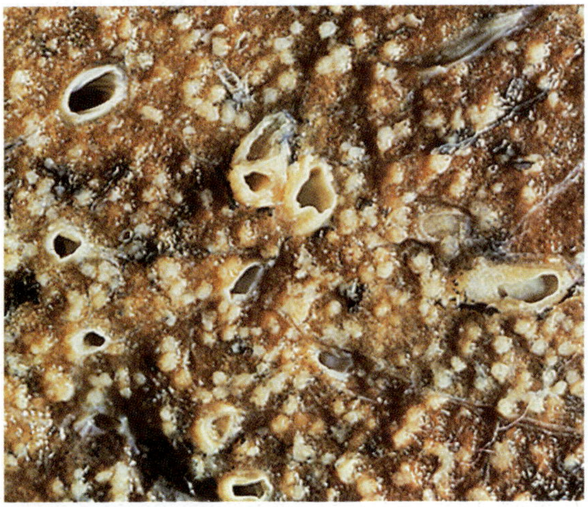

Fig. 19.34 Gross – miliary tuberculosis of the lung showing multiple grey-white granulomas. (*Source:* From Simon S Cross. Underwood's Pathology. Elsevier. 2019.)

Pulmonary Miliary Tuberculosis This occurs when the bacteria leaving the lung through the lymphatics circulate and reach other areas of the lungs (Fig. 19.35). This condition is rare but serious. 'Miliary' refers to the radiograph appearance of the lesions resembling millet seeds scattered throughout the lung. It is most common in severely immunocompromised persons. Up to 25% of patients with miliary TB have meningeal involvement.

Systemic Miliary Tuberculosis It occurs when bacteria disseminate through the systemic arterial system and spread to various organs.

It can involve any organ but is most prominent in the liver, bone marrow, spleen, fallopian tubes, meninges, kidney and epididymis.

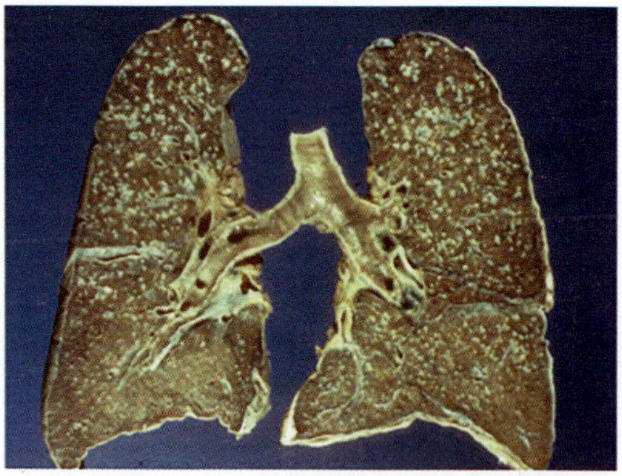

Fig. 19.35 Miliary tuberculosis. Innumerable millet-sized nodules are seen in the lung. (*Source:* From Richard L. Kradin, Eugene J. Mark. Diagnostic Pathology of Infectious Disease. Elsevier. 2018.)

Extrapulmonary Tuberculosis

Tuberculous lymphadenitis: Extrapulmonary TB occurs commonly due to hematogenous dissemination when the infection in the lungs results in the erosion of the alveolar epithelial cells with spread of infection into the pulmonary vein. The bacteria then reach the left side of the heart and through systemic circulation infect extrapulmonary organs and circulate back into the lungs. Once infected, the cell-mediated immune response is activated and granuloma formation occurs.

It is a common presentation of TB infection.

It is common in children and HIV-infected patients.

Cervical nodes are more frequently involved.

Single or multiple enlarged, matted, painless nodes are seen (scrofula).

Tuberculous meningitis

It is most common in children younger than 2 years and in HIV-infected individuals.

TB of bone and joints

Arthritis: Chronic monoarthritis with joint destruction occurs.

TB spine (Pott disease): It affects thoracic and lumbar vertebrae and disc resulting in destruction and deformation of the spine. Paraspinal 'cold' abscesses in these patients may track along tissue planes and present as an abdominal or pelvic mass.

Genitourinary TB

Renal involvement

It may present with dysuria, urinary frequency, nocturia, urgency, back and flank pain, abdominal pain and haematuria.

Genital TB

In women, tuberculous salpingitis and endometritis occur and most commonly present with irregular menstrual bleeding and sterility.

Adrenal TB

Spread of TB to the adrenals is usually bilateral, and both the adrenals are markedly enlarged. Destruction of the cortex leads to Addison disease.

Abdominal TB

It presents as circumferential ulcerations with stricture of the small intestine (ileocecal) and ascites.

TB of pleural and pericardial cavities

Cutaneous TB

Facts Patients with extrapulmonary TB are typically **not** infectious unless they have the following:

- Pulmonary disease along with extrapulmonary disease
- Extrapulmonary disease located in the oral cavity or in the larynx

TB pleural effusions may have underlying PTB that is masked on the chest radiograph due to the lung compression caused by the effusion fluid. These patients should be considered infectious until PTB is ruled out.

Clinical Features Systemic features like fever, night sweats, loss of appetite, weight loss (due to release of IL-1 and TNF by macrophages), chest pain and fatigue are common. Local symptoms of pulmonary infection – cough, haemoptysis and dyspnoea – are the usual presenting features.

Laboratory Diagnosis The diagnosis of pulmonary disease is based on the following:

1. The history, physical examination findings and radiographic findings of consolidation or cavitation seen in the apices of the lungs may lead to the diagnosis, but tubercle bacilli must be demonstrated for confirmation.
2. Acid-fast smears and cultures of the sputum of patients suspected of having TB should be performed. Culture on solid agar media shows growth at 3–6 weeks, whereas culture in liquid media shows growth within 2 weeks. **BACTEC system** is an automated system used for the rapid detection of mycobacteria.
3. PCR amplification of *M. tuberculosis* DNA enables rapid diagnosis by identifying the presence of *M. tuberculosis* and is also useful to identify resistance to rifampicin.
4. **The tuberculin (purified protein derivative (PPD) or Mantoux) skin test** (Fig. 19.36) is based on the delayed-type hypersensitivity (T-cell-mediated) reaction caused by infection. About 2–4 weeks after infection, an intracutaneous injection of purified protein derivative of *M. tuberculosis* induces a visible and palpable induration that peaks in 48–72 hours. This test however does not differentiate between infection and active disease.
5. QuantiFERON-TB Gold (QFT) is a highly sensitive and specific simple blood test that aids in the detection of *M. tuberculosis*. It is an IFN-γ release assay, commonly known as an IGRA, and is an alternative to the tuberculin skin test. Although the results of this test are not affected by prior vaccination, it cannot differentiate between latent infection and active disease.
6. Fine needle aspiration cytology (FNAC) of lymph node may be performed in patients presenting with lymph

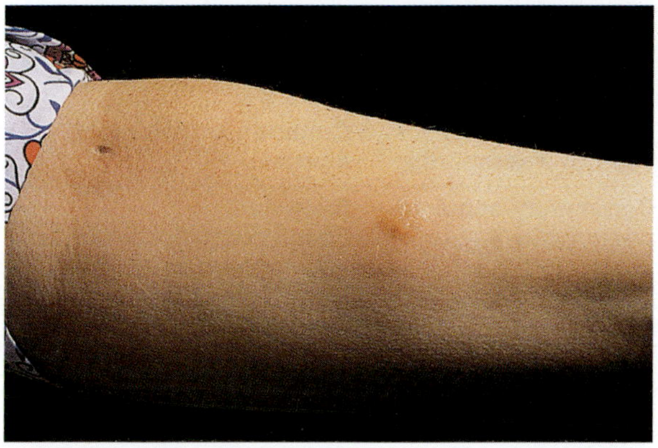

Fig. 19.36 A positive Mantoux test in a person previously immunized with the bacille Calmette–Guérin (BCG) vaccine. (*Source:* From Simon S Cross. Underwood's Pathology. Elsevier. 2019.)

node enlargement. Appearance of features suggestive of granuloma formation and demonstration of bacilli by AFB stain help in diagnosis.

Treatment Treatment of latent TB involves regimens with one or two antitubercular drugs, whereas active TB, particularly if it is a drug-resistant strain, will require a multidrug regimen. The most common medications used to treat TB are isoniazid, rifampin, ethambutol and pyrazinamide.

If the person has a drug-resistant TB, a combination of fluoroquinolones and injectable antibiotics, such as amikacin or capreomycin (Capastat), is used for 20–30 months.

Causes of Death in Tuberculosis

- Pulmonary haemorrhage
- Pulmonary insufficiency
- Sepsis due to disseminated TB
- Cor pulmonale
- Secondary amyloidosis

Tuberculosis and HIV The risk of TB increases by 2- to 5-fold in early HIV infection and by 20-fold in advanced HIV disease. In HIV-negative individuals, lymphadenitis tends to be unifocal and localized. In contrast, HIV-positive people almost always have multifocal disease, with systemic symptoms and involvement of either the pulmonary system or other organs by active TB. All stages of HIV infection are susceptible to TB. Depletion of CD4 T cells in HIV infection plays a major role in the increased risk of TB in HIV-infected individuals. TB can have a variety of presentations. In early HIV infection (relatively high CD4 cell count), TB presents as a reactivation pattern (upper lung zone infiltrates with cavities) as opposed to lower- and middle-zone infiltrates in advanced patients with low CD4 cell counts. The extent of immunodeficiency also determines the frequency of extrapulmonary TB, ranging from 10% to 15% in mild immunosuppression to more than 50% with severe immunodeficiency.

HIV-positive individuals have a high rate of sputum smear-negative disease because they are less likely to have cavitary lesions, anergy in the tuberculin skin test (absence of delayed-type hypersensitivity reaction) and the absence of characteristic granuloma formation in the tissues in the late stages of HIV infection.

PULMONARY INFECTIONS

The respiratory tract is the most common site of infection by pathogens because it is in direct contact with the physical environment and exposed to airborne organisms.

Upper respiratory tract infections such as common cold and pharyngitis are predominantly caused by viruses. Lower respiratory tract infections are caused by bacteria, virus, fungi and *Mycoplasma* organisms.

PNEUMONIA — PA 26.1

It is the infection of the lung parenchyma distal to the terminal bronchiole.

Pathogenesis

The microorganisms enter the lungs by one of the following four routes:

- Inhalation of microbes
- Aspiration of organisms
- Haematogenous spread from a distant focus
- Direct spread from an adjoining site of infection

Pneumonia can result whenever there is an impairment of local defence mechanisms and decrease in host systemic resistance.

Causes of impairment of local defence mechanisms are as follows:

a) **Loss or suppression of the cough reflex due to**
   - Coma
   - Anaesthesia
   - Neuromuscular disorders
   - Drugs

b) **Injury to the mucociliary apparatus**
   Impaired ciliary function
      Destruction of ciliated epithelium due to cigarette smoke and inhalation of corrosive gases
      Viral diseases
      Genetic defects of ciliary function – immotile, cilia syndrome

c) **Accumulation of secretions**
   Cystic fibrosis
   Bronchial obstruction

d) **Impaired phagocytic activity of alveolar macrophages due to**
   Alcohol

Tobacco smoke
Anoxia
O_2 intoxication
Pulmonary congestion and oedema

e) **Decrease in host systemic resistance**
- It can occur in defects of innate immunity (neutrophil and complement defects).
- It can occur in humoral immune deficiency (leading to an increased incidence of pyogenic infection).
- It can also occur in cell-mediated immune defects (an increased incidence of intracellular microbes like mycobacteria, herpes and organisms of low virulence).
- Germline mutation in MYD88 (adaptor for TLR) can lead to a decrease in host systemic resistance.
- Immunosuppressive agents lead to destructive pneumonia and leucopenia.

Classification of Pneumonia

On the basis of the anatomical part of the lung parenchyma involved, pneumonias are traditionally classified into three main types:

Lobar pneumonia

It is an acute bacterial infection involving a part of the lobe, the entire lobe or even two lobes of one or both the lungs. and typically does not affect bronchi. This condition may occur at any age but it is less common in infancy and in the late life. The most common organism causing lobar pneumonia is *Streptococcus pneumoniae* (>90%). Other organisms are *Staphylococcus aureus*, gram-negative bacteria such as *H. influenzae*, *Klebsiella pneumoniae*, *Pseudomonas*, *Proteus* and *Escherichia coli*.

Bronchopneumonia

It is characterized by patchy consolidation of the lung and involves terminal bronchioles. It tends to affect infants and the elderly as a secondary infection following viral infections. The common organisms are *S. pneumoniae*, *S. aureus*, *H. influenzae*, *Klebsiella* and *Pseudomonas*.

Interstitial pneumonia

It is characterized by inflammation of interstitial lung tissue. The inflammatory exudates are confined mostly to the alveolar interstitium. Alveolar exudate is not prominent. Consolidation is not a feature of this type of pneumonia. The most common organisms are viruses, especially respiratory syncytial virus (RSV), and *Mycoplasma*.

On the basis of clinical settings

Community-acquired pneumonia (CAP)
Healthcare-associated pneumonia
Hospital-acquired pneumonia
Ventilator-associated pneumonia (VAP)

On the basis of aetiology and pathogenesis (Table 19.18)

Table 19.18 Types of Pneumonia and Their Common Aetiological Agents

Type of Pneumonia	Common Aetiological Agents
Community-acquired pneumonia	**Bacteria** *Streptococcus pneumoniae* *Haemophilus influenzae* *Klebsiella pneumoniae* *Staphylococcus aureus* *Streptococcus pyogenes* *Pseudomonas aeruginosa*
Atypical pneumonia	Bacteria *Mycoplasma pneumoniae* Viruses Respiratory syncytial virus, influenza and parainfluenza virus, human metapneumovirus *Chlamydia* sp. *Coxiella burnetii*
Healthcare-associated pneumonia	Methicillin-resistant *S. aureus* *P. aeruginosa*
Hospital-acquired pneumonia	*S. aureus* S. pneumoniae Enterobacteriaceae *Pseudomonas*
Aspiration pneumonia	Anaerobic bacteria
Chronic pneumonia	**Bacteria** *Nocardia* *Actinomyces* Mycobacteria and atypical mycobacteria **Fungi** *Histoplasma capsulatum* *Blastomyces dermatitidis* *Coccidioides immitis*
Necrotizing pneumonia and lung abscess	Anaerobic bacteria *S. aureus* *S. pyogenes* *K. pneumoniae*
Pneumonia in the immunocompromised host	Cytomegalovirus *Pneumocystis jirovecii* *Mycobacterium avium* *Mycobacterium intracellulare* *Aspergillus* *Mucor* *Candida*

COMMUNITY-ACQUIRED PNEUMONIAS

CAP is defined as an acute infection of the lung parenchyma in a healthy person, acquired from the community in the absence of recent hospitalization or association with other healthcare facilities. It can be bacterial or viral in origin. In CAP, factors such as age, presence of coexisting illness, immunosuppression and splenic function influence the severity of pneumonia and increase the likelihood of certain organisms.

Table 19.19 Characteristic Features of Selective Community-Acquired Bacterial Pneumonias

Organism	Characteristic Features	Complications
Streptococcus* or *Pneumococcus	Most common cause of community-acquired acute pneumonia Seen in middle-aged, elderly or debilitated patients, those with cardiopulmonary disease and malnourished persons Produces rust-coloured sputum Diagnosis: Sputum Gram stain and blood culture Pneumococcal vaccine containing capsular polysaccharides is used in high-risk individuals, e.g. decreased and absent splenic function (sickle cell disease, postsplenectomy)	Empyema
Haemophilus influenzae	Pleomorphic, gram-negative organism, encapsulated and nonencapsulated forms seen Most common bacterial cause of acute exacerbations in COPD Pulmonary consolidation is lobular and patchy	In children, *H. influenzae* may follow a viral respiratory infection and has a high mortality rate Produces descending laryngotracheal bronchitis; small bronchi are plugged by dense fibrin-rich exudates producing airway obstruction
Staphylococcus aureus	Important cause of secondary bacterial pneumonia in children and adults following viral illness Important cause of hospital-acquired pneumonia Causes pneumonia in intravenous drug users	Associated with complications like lung abscess and empyema
Klebsiella pneumoniae	Gram negative Common in chronic alcoholic patients and diabetic patients Produces thick mucoid blood-tinged sputum (currant jelly sputum)	Lung abscess
Pseudomonas	Most commonly causes hospital-acquired infection Causes pneumonia in patients with cystic fibrosis, immunocompromised patients and neutropenic patients	Propensity to invade blood vessels
Legionella	Common in organ transplant recipients	

COPD, chronic obstructive pulmonary disease.

Morphology (Table 19.19)

Lobar Pneumonia In the preantibiotic era, lobar pneumonia was traditionally seen to evolve through four sequential but distinct stages described by Laennec.

Four stages of inflammatory responses are as follows (Figs 19.37 and 19.38):

1. **Stage of congestion (initial phase)**
   This phase lasts for 1–2 days.
   The lungs are red, heavy and boggy.
   Cut surface shows exudation of blood-stained frothy fluid.
   Dilation and congestion of the blood capillaries are seen in the alveolar walls. Pale eosinophilic oedematous fluid is present in the air spaces. Few neutrophils and numerous bacteria are present in the alveolar fluid.
2. **Stage of red hepatization (early consolidation)**
   This phase lasts for 2–4 days.
   The affected lobe is red, firm and airless with liver-like consistency. The red discoloration is caused by the extravasated red cells.
   The oedematous fluid is replaced by fibrin strands. Marked cellular exudates occur by neutrophils and RBCs.
3. **Stage of grey hepatization (late consolidation)**
   This phase lasts for 4–8 days.
   The affected lobe is greyish brown, firm and dry. The change in colour from red to grey begins at the hilum and spreads towards the periphery. Fibrinous pleurisy is prominent.
   The fibrin strands are dense and more numerous. There is progressive disintegration of red cells and neutrophils.
4. **Stage of resolution (final stage)**
   - Liquefaction of the solid fibrinous exudates occurs by enzymatic action. Granular and fragmented fibrin strands are seen in the alveolar spaces.

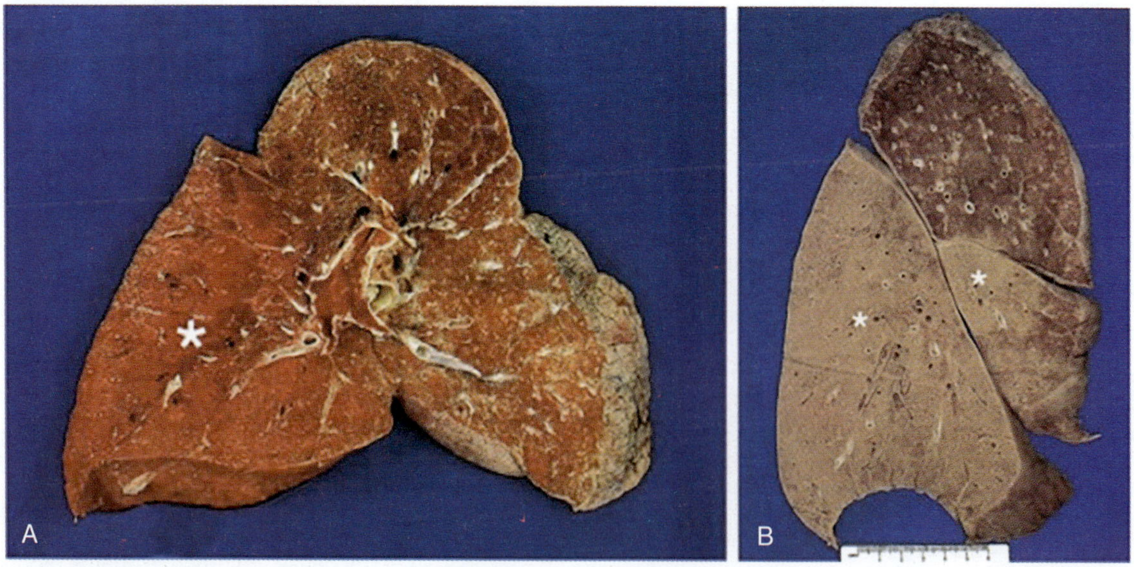

Fig. 19.37 Gross morphology of lobar pneumonia. (A) Red hepatization – the lower lobe (asterisk) is inflamed, consolidated and hyperaemic. (B) Grey hepatization – diffuse consolidation of the two lobes (asterisk). (*Source:* From Olivia McKinney, Isabel Woodman. Crash Course Pathology. Elsevier. 2019.)

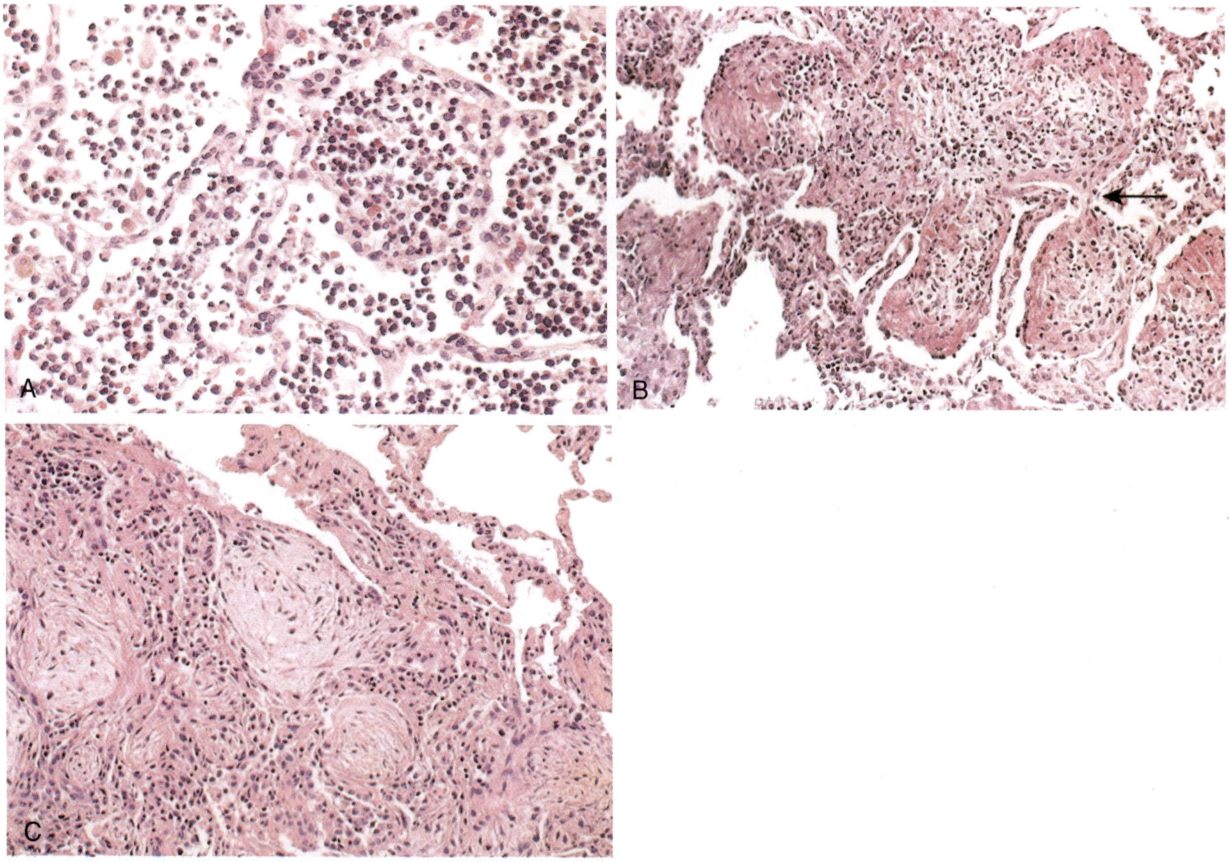

Fig. 19.38 Stages of pneumonia. (A) Red hepatization – note numerous intra-alveolar neutrophils with congested septal capillaries. (B) Grey hepatization shows fibrinosuppurative exudate in the alveoli. (C) Organizing pneumonia – exudates are converted into fibromyxoid masses rich in fibroblasts and macrophages. (*Source:* From Vinay Kumar, Abul K Abbas, Jon C Aster. Robbins Basic Pathology. Elsevier. 2018.)

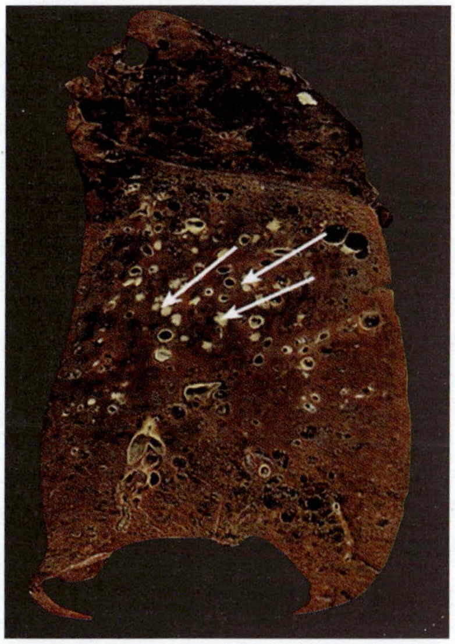

Fig. 19.39 Bronchopneumonia patchy consolidation and pus-filled bronchi (arrow) with upper-lobe emphysema. (*Source:* From Respiratory tract – Underwood's Pathology – Clinical Key Student.)

- Progressive removal of fluid as well as cellular exudates from the air spaces results in the restoration of normal lung parenchyma with aeration.
- The pleural reaction may also show resolution but may undergo organization, leading to fibrous obliteration of the pleural cavity.

Bronchopneumonia

Patchy areas of consolidation are seen in one or more lobes, frequently bilateral and involving the basal regions (lower zones), due to the tendency of the secretions to gravitate to the lower lobes (Fig. 19.39). Lesions are elevated, dry, granular, red or grey in colour and are often centred around a bronchiole. These patchy areas are best picked up by passing the fingertips on the cut surface.

Neutrophil-rich exudates filling the bronchi, bronchioles and adjacent alveolar spaces are seen.

Complications

Lobar pneumonia

The usual course of pneumonia is a complete resolution. Since the advent of antibiotics, complications are uncommon but still can occur in neglected cases and in patients with immunological defects. The complications are as follows:

- **Organization** (in about 3% of cases, resolution of the exudate does not occur but instead it gets organized; there is ingrowth of fibroblasts from the alveolar septa, resulting in fibrosed, airless leathery lung tissue)
- **Pleural effusion**
- **Abscess**
- **Empyema** (encysted pus in the pleural cavity occurs in less than 1% of the cases)
- **Metastatic infection** (bacteraemic dissemination to the heart and pericardium causes bacterial endocarditis, myocarditis and pericarditis and may also occur in the brain, kidney, spleen or joints)

Bronchopneumonia

Complete resolution is uncommon. There is some degree of destruction of the bronchioles, resulting in focal bronchiolar fibrosis that may eventually cause bronchiectasis.

Clinical Features

The symptoms of bacterial pneumonias are the sudden onset of fever with chills, cough with mucopurulent sputum and occasionally haemoptysis and pleuritic pain. The common physical findings are fever, tachycardia and tachypnoea; sometimes, cyanosis may occur if the patient is severely hypoxaemic and pleuritic friction rub when pleuritis is present. There is generally a marked neutrophilic leucocytosis. Blood cultures are positive in about 30% of cases. Chest radiograph may reveal consolidation.

COMMUNITY-ACQUIRED VIRAL PNEUMONIA (INTERSTITIAL PNEUMONIA, ATYPICAL PNEUMONIA)

It is marked by patchy inflammatory changes confined to interstitium of the lung without involving the air spaces. The term 'atypical' refers to lack of alveolar exudates, absence of physical findings such as consolidation, a moderate amount of sputum and a moderate elevation in the white cell count.

Aetiology

- Viruses
- RSV
- Influenza
- Adenoviruses
- Rhinoviruses
- Coxsackieviruses
- Cytomegalovirus
- *Mycoplasma pneumoniae*
- Psittacosis (*Chlamydia*)
- Q-fever (*Coxiella*)

Influenza Infections

Influenza viruses are enveloped RNA viruses. There are three types of influenza viruses – types A, B and C. Influenza A viruses are responsible for epidemic and pandemic outbreaks. These viruses have a segmented genome with eight strands of RNA. This property is responsible for the gene reassortment to occur among different subtypes of influenza, allowing a new subtype to form.

The virus contains three important envelope glycoproteins. These are haemagglutinin (HA) protein responsible for the viral entry into the cell, neuraminidase (NA) that facilitates the cell–cell spread of virus and matrix proteins that link the virus envelope with the virus core.

Antibody against HA is very protective and antibody against NA reduces the severity of the illness.

Influenza viruses escape from the body's immune system by **antigenic shifts** and **antigenic drift**.

Antigenic shift is seen only with influenza type A. It results from the replacement of HA with novel subtypes from other nonhuman influenza viruses. Introduction of new HA into the human virus is responsible for pandemics and millions of influenza-related deaths.

Antigenic drift results from the accumulation of mutations in the antibody-binding site in HA, NA or both. These mutations prevent antibodies formed against previous strains from being effective against the current strain, enabling spread throughout the partially immune population. Antigenic drift occurs in both type A and B viruses.

Pathogenesis The virus infection begins with the attachment of viral HA to sialic acid residues on the surface of the target host cells. In the lungs, the alveolar epithelial cells are the target cells for the virus. After attachment, the virus enters the host cell through receptor-mediated endocytosis. Viral RNA is released into the cytosol and travels into the nucleus of the infected cell and viral RNA is synthesized. NA facilitates the release of the daughter virions. Viral infection of alveolar epithelial cells inhibits their sodium channel, allowing transudate of the fluid and proteins into the alveolar spaces, and later leads to apoptosis of these cells.

Infected epithelial cells release inflammatory mediators. Activated neutrophils and macrophages eliminate the viral particles and the apoptotic bodies. The inflammatory by-products cause further injury to the airway. The increased risk of secondary bacterial infection may be due to delayed epithelial healing.

Severe Acute Respiratory Distress Syndrome

Severe acute respiratory syndrome (SARS) is a viral respiratory illness caused by a **coronavirus** called SARS-associated coronavirus (SARS-CoV). SARS was first reported in Asia in February 2003.

SARS-CoV-2 is the name given to the 2019 novel coronavirus. It is a new strain of coronavirus not previously identified in humans. WHO declared coronavirus disease 2019 (COVID-19) as the sixth public health emergency of international concern on 30 January 2020. Genetically, it is closely related to SARS-CoV-1. Infection is transmitted through respiratory droplets and surface contact, with a mean incubation period of 6 days. Symptoms of COVID-19 vary from being asymptomatic to having fever, cough, sore throat, general weakness, fatigue and muscular pain and, in the most severe cases, severe pneumonia, ARDS, sepsis and septic shock, all potentially leading to death. Clinical deterioration can occur rapidly, often during the second week of disease.

Morphology

All viral infections produce similar morphological changes. Upper respiratory infection is characterized by mucosal swelling and hyperaemia, submucosal mononuclear inflammatory infiltrate and excess mucous production leading to plugging of nasal chambers and Eustachian tubes.

Viral tonsillitis – follicular hyperplasia of the Waldeyer ring
Viral laryngotracheobronchitis and bronchiolitis

Lungs The lungs are heavy and congested and consolidation may be patchy or massive with the involvement of one or both the lungs.
Microscopy **Interstitial inflammation** involving the walls of the alveoli is seen with oedema of the alveolar walls. **Necrotizing bronchiolitis** with focal necrosis of the bronchiolar epithelium occurs, with mononuclear inflammatory infiltration in the walls.

Alveolar changes: Alveoli are usually free of exudates except in severe cases or in ARDS, in which cellular exudates are seen in alveoli and pink hyaline membrane lines the walls of alveoli. In the **organizing stage**, there is interstitial fibrosis obliterating the alveolar spaces.

Clinical Course It has a varied clinical course. Most cases present as severe upper respiratory infections or as chest colds, fever, headache and muscle pain. Later, dry nonproductive cough may develop due to tracheitis or bronchitis. Individuals who develop ALI develop profound dyspnoea and tachypnoea, followed by increasing cyanosis, hypoxaemia and respiratory failure. Chest radiographs may show patchy or diffuse consolidation.

Consequences

- Besides the two extremes – death and recovery – patients who survive acute episodes of ARDS may develop interstitial fibrosis and chronic pulmonary disease.

Complication

- Superimposed bacterial infection

HEALTHCARE-ASSOCIATED PNEUMONIA

Most common organisms isolated are methicillin-resistant *S. aureus* (MRSA) and *Pseudomonas*. The mortality rate is high with this type of pneumonia.

HOSPITAL-ACQUIRED PNEUMONIA

Pulmonary infections acquired during a hospital stay are called hospital-acquired pneumonia.

Risk factors

- Severe underlying disease
- Immunosuppression

- Prolonged antibiotic therapy
- Intravascular catheter and mechanical ventilators

Most common organisms

S. aureus

S. pneumoniae

Enterobacteriaceae and *Pseudomonas*

VENTILATOR-ASSOCIATED PNEUMONIA

VAP is a type of hospital-acquired pneumonia that occurs more than 48 hours after endotracheal intubation. The most common pathogens are gram-negative bacilli, *S. aureus* and antibiotic-resistant organisms.

ASPIRATION PNEUMONIA

Aspiration of gastric contents, foreign body and infected material from the oral cavity causes aspiration pneumonia (Table 19.20).

Histological: In chemical pneumonitis, haemorrhagic pulmonary oedema occurs with the presence of particles in the bronchioles. Lung abscess is a common complication if the patient survives.

Hypostatic pneumonia

It is the collection of fluid in the dependent parts of the lungs as seen in bedridden patients. The accumulated fluid in the basal zone and the posterior part of the lungs gets infected by bacteria from the upper respiratory tract and bacterial pneumonia ensues.

Lipid pneumonia

It is a noninfective pneumonia. It is of two types:

Exogenous lipid pneumonia is caused by aspiration of oily materials.

Endogenous lipid pneumonia involves the endogenous origin of lipids that cause pneumonic consolidation; e.g. tissue destruction by tumour, TB and bronchiectasis.

Morphology

Gross: The right lung is more commonly affected. The cut surface appears golden yellow.

Microscopy shows foamy macrophages within alveolar spaces, granuloma with foreign body giant cells and cholesterol clefts.

CHRONIC PNEUMONIAS

It is a pulmonary parenchymal infection lasting for weeks to months. In an otherwise healthy individual, chronic pneumonias are caused by slow-growing organisms like tuberculous and nontuberculous *Mycobacterium*; fungi such as *Histoplasma*, *Blastomyces* and *Cryptococcus*; mixed aerobic and anaerobic bacterial infections; and actinomycosis. In immunocompromised patients, chronic pneumonia is caused by *Pneumocystis jirovecii*.

Table 19.20 Aetiological Factors for Aspiration Pneumonia

Unconsciousness
Alcoholism
Neurological disorders affecting swallowing
Drowning
Necrotic oropharyngeal tumours
Premature infants
Congenital tracheoesophageal fistula

FUNGAL PNEUMONIAS

Histoplasmosis

It is caused by ***Histoplasma capsulatum***, an intracellular pathogen found inside the phagocytes. Infection is acquired by inhalation of dust particles contaminated with bird droppings. Clinical and morphological lesions are like those in TB. Clinically, patients present with fever, night sweats and cough.

Primary pulmonary involvement is often latent and may produce coin lesion on chest X-rays. Chronic progressive secondary lung disease is seen in lung apices. Involvement of other sites like the mediastinum, adrenals, meninges and liver also occurs. A widely disseminated disease is seen in immunocompromised individuals. Pathogenesis following infection is mediated by γ-IFN produced by helper cells that activate macrophages to kill the intracellular yeast.

Morphology

Diagnosis is by demonstration of epithelioid granulomas with caseous necrosis and the presence of 3- to 5-μm yeast forms in the tissue and within macrophages (Fig. 19.40). Healed lesions undergo **fibrosis** and **concentric calcification** (tree bark lesions) (Fig. 19.41). In immunosuppressed individuals, a fulminant widespread form occurs without granulomas.

Blastomycosis

Blastomyces dermatitidis is a dimorphic fungus. It occurs in three clinical forms – pulmonary, disseminated and cutaneous forms. Pulmonary blastomycosis may present as lobar consolidation, multilobar infiltrates, perihilar involvement, multiple nodules and miliary seedlings. Upper lobes are commonly involved. These resolve spontaneously or progress to the chronic form. The clinical symptoms are sudden onset of fever, chills, headache, anorexia, weight loss and productive cough. Histologically, granulomas may be seen and diagnosis is confirmed by the demonstration of **rounded budding yeast with double-contoured wall and nuclei** (Fig. 19.42).

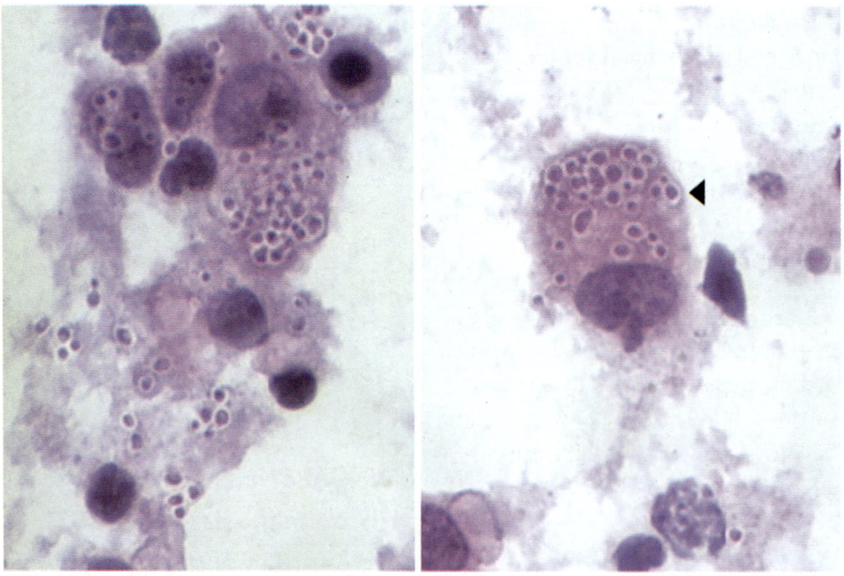

Fig. 19.40 Histoplasmosis of the lung. Microscopy – macrophages showing numerous small microorganisms with an artefactual clear zone around a central blue nucleus.

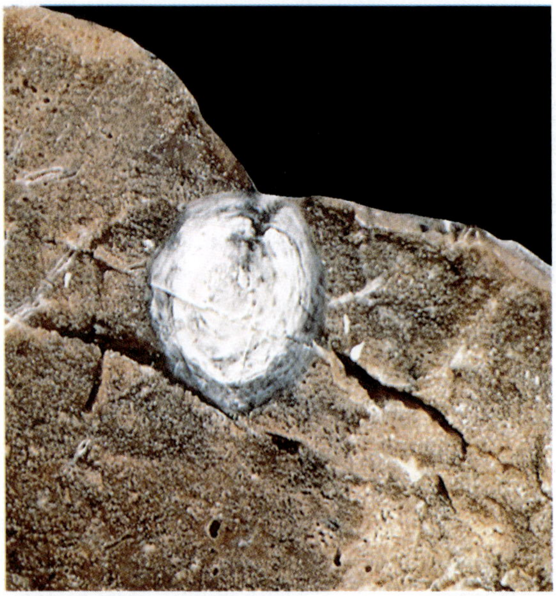

Fig. 19.41 Gross – histoplasmosis of the lung – laminated histoplasma granuloma of the lung. (*Source:* From Vinay Kumar, Abul K Abbas, Jon C Aster. Robbins Basic Pathology. Elsevier. 2018.)

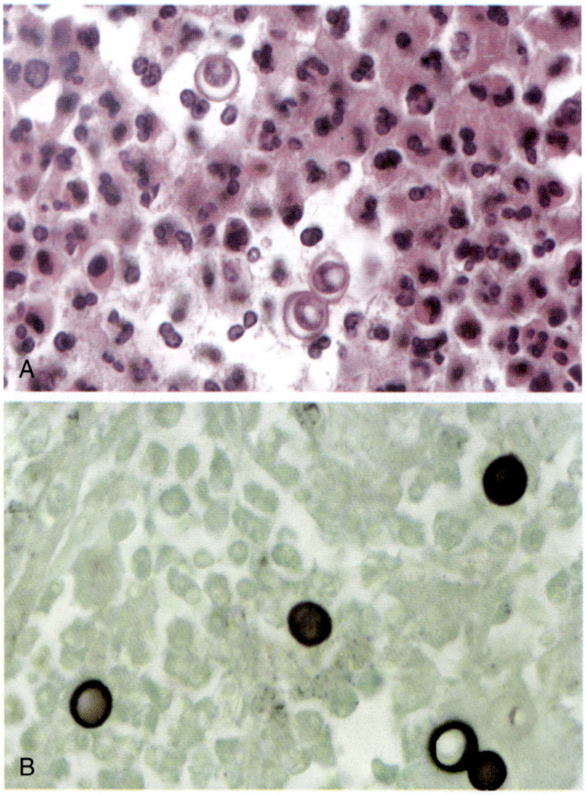

Fig. 19.42 Blastomycosis of the lung. (A) Round budding yeast forms with a thick wall and nuclei. (B) Silver stain. (*Source:* From The Lung – Robbins and Cotran Pathologic Basis of Disease – Clinical Key Student.)

Coccidioidomycosis

Coccidioides immitis is the causative organism. Primary and secondary lung lesions are similar to those in histoplasmosis. The inflammatory response to this infection can be granulomatous, pyogenic (when the host resistance is diminished or disease is widespread) or mixed. The San Joaquin Valley fever complex characterized by symptoms of fever, cough, pleuritic chest, pain, erythema nodosum or erythema multiforme is associated with this infection. To diagnose *Coccidioides*, the presence of **thick-walled nonbudding spherules with endospores inside macrophages or giant cells must be demonstrated**.

PNEUMONIA IN THE IMMUNOCOMPROMISED HOST

Pneumonia is the most common and serious complication in immunosuppressed individuals. Causes for immunosuppression may include diseases, immunosuppressive therapy, chemotherapy, irradiation and organ transplants. Immunocompromised patients may develop pneumonia due to the usual organisms, along with several other organisms that normally do not cause illness in healthy hosts. The common opportunistic infections are as follows:

Bacteria: *P. aeruginosa*, *Mycobacterium* sp., *Legionella pneumophila* and *Listeria*
Virus: Cytomegalovirus and herpesvirus
Fungi:– *P. jirovecii*, *Candida*, *Aspergillus*, *Cryptococcus*

P. jirovecii Pneumonia

Aside from *Pneumococcus*, *P. jirovecii* is the most common cause of pneumonia in AIDS patients. It is seen particularly when the CD4 count is less than 200/mm^3. It is also seen in individuals on immunosuppressive therapy.

Pulmonary Disease in HIV-Infected Patients

The respiratory symptoms are common complaints among HIV-infected individuals. The spectrum of pulmonary diseases in HIV-infected individuals includes HIV-related and non-HIV-related conditions (Table 19.21). Opportunistic infections caused by bacteria, viruses, fungi and parasites are prevalent in HIV-infected patients. The most frequent respiratory diagnoses in these patients **are upper respiratory tract infection, acute bronchitis** and **acute sinusitis.**

The development of specific type of pulmonary infections depends on the immune status of the patient as indicated by CD4 cell counts. Recurrent bacterial pneumonia and PTB are common when the CD4 cell counts are less than 400 cells/μL. Pneumocystis pneumonia (PCP) and disseminated TB are usually diagnosed when CD4 cell counts drop below 200 cells/μL. Disseminated *Mycobacterium avium* complex (MAC), fungal pneumonia and cytomegalovirus pneumonitis occur in patients with the most severe immunosuppression (CD4 cell counts less than 100 cells/μL).

Table 19.21 Spectrum of Respiratory Illness in HIV-Infected Patients

Category	Organisms
Bacteria	*Streptococcus pneumoniae* Haemophilus influenzae Gram-negative bacilli *Staphylococcus aureus* *Mycobacterium tuberculosis, Mycobacterium kansasii, Mycobacterium avium* complex
Fungi	*Pneumocystis jirovecii, Cryptococcus, Aspergillus, Coccidioides*
Virus	Cytomegalovirus, herpes simplex virus
Parasites	*Toxoplasma gondii, Strongyloides*
Neoplasms	Kaposi sarcoma, non-Hodgkin lymphoma

HIV, human immunodeficiency virus.

LUNG ABSCESS

PA 26.2

It is a local suppurative process within the lung characterized by necrosis of lung tissue.

Aetiology

Aspiration is the most common cause. The commonly isolated organisms include aerobic and anaerobic streptococci, *Staphylococcus* and gram-negative organisms.

Risk Factors

- Aspiration of infective material: This can occur in alcoholic patients and during anaesthesia, gingival and dental sepsis and coma (suppression of cough reflex).
- Preceding pneumonia: Lung abscesses following pneumonia are more often seen in pneumonia due to *Staphylococcus*, *Klebsiella* and fungal infections.
- Septic embolism: Infected emboli can arise from thrombophlebitis, infective endocarditis and intravenous drug abusers.
- Neoplasm: Postobstructive pneumonia can occur.
- Miscellaneous
  - Direct traumatic penetration of the lung, spread of infection from neighbouring organs and haematogenous seeding by pyogenic organisms

Primary Cryptogenic Abscess

When no cause is identified for the formation of abscess after excluding all the aforementioned causes, then it is called primary cryptogenic abscess.

Morphology

Gross Abscesses due to aspiration are more common on the right and are mostly single.

Multiple abscesses are found in the following conditions: post-pneumonia, bronchiectasis and septic emboli.

Abscesses range from few millimetres to large diameters. The cavity often contains exudate (Fig. 19.43).

Microscopy Suppurative destruction of the lung parenchyma occurs within the central area of cavitation. The cavity is initially surrounded by acute inflammation in the wall but later gets replaced by lymphocytes, plasma cells and macrophages. In more chronic cases, there is fibroblastic proliferation forming a fibrocollagenous wall. Continued infection leads to gangrene of the lung.

Clinical Features These include fever, cough with copious amount of foul-smelling purulent sputum and clubbing of the fingers and toes. It is always important to rule out an underlying malignancy that is present in 10%–15% of cases.

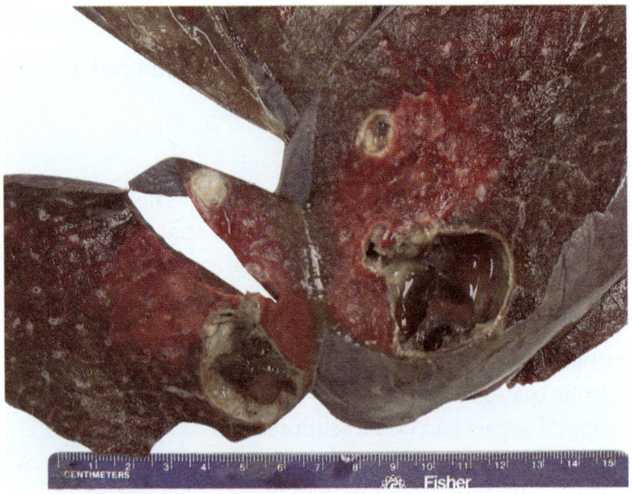

Fig. 19.43 Multifocal purulent lung abscesses seen in gross examination of lung.

Complications

These include extension into the pleural cavity, brain abscess and meningitis (due to septic emboli) and secondary amyloidosis (rare).

Table 19.22 Histological Classification of Malignant Epithelial Tumours of the Lung by WHO[a]

Squamous cell carcinoma
Adenocarcinoma Preinvasive lesion – atypical adenomatous hyperplasia and adenocarcinoma in situ (AIS) Minimally invasive adenocarcinoma Invasive adenocarcinoma (lepidic, papillary, acinar, micropapillary and solid) Invasive mucinous adenocarcinoma
Neuroendocrine tumours Small-cell carcinoma Large-cell neuroendocrine carcinoma Carcinoid tumours Preinvasive lesion – diffuse idiopathic neuroendocrine cell hyperplasia
Large-cell carcinoma
Adenosquamous carcinoma
Carcinoma with sarcomatoid type
Carcinoma of salivary gland type

[a] Simpler version.

TUMOURS PA 26.6

INTRODUCTION

Worldwide, the cancer burden is estimated to have risen to 18.1 million new cases and 9.6 million deaths. Lung, female breast and colorectal cancers are the leading types in terms of incidence. The most diagnosed cancer and the leading cause of cancer deaths in men and women include the lung cancer and the breast cancer, respectively. The increase in cancer burden is due to several factors like population growth, ageing and lifestyle changes in industrialized countries.

Table 19.23 Classification of Bronchogenic Carcinoma

Small-cell carcinoma (20%–25%)
Non-small-cell carcinoma (70%–75%) Squamous cell carcinoma Adenocarcinoma Large-cell carcinoma
Mixed (5%–10%)

LUNG CANCER

Lung cancer is the leading cause of cancer-related deaths. It occurs between the ages of 40 and 70 years, whereas only 2% of cases occur before 40 years of age. Among primary lung cancer, bronchogenic carcinoma is the most common form (95%). The classification of lung cancer is shown in Table 19.22.

For therapeutic purpose, bronchogenic carcinoma can be classified into three groups (Table 19.23).

Aetiological Factors

Smoking

- Most lung cancers are strongly associated with smoking. About 80% of lung cancers occur in active smokers or those who have stopped smoking recently.
- The risk in smokers who smoke more than 2 packs per day for 20 years is 60–70 times greater than in nonsmokers. Although cessation of smoking decreases the risk for lung cancer, it never returns to the nonsmoker level. Genetic changes can persist for many years in the bronchial epithelium of the smokers.
- The smoke from cigarette contains carcinogens like benzopyrene, 1,3-butadiene, polonium-210 and nicotine-derived nitrosoamino ketone, which lead to genetic mutations through DNA adduct formation. Adduct formation is caused by metabolic activation of these carcinogens by P450 cytochromes enzymes.

Industrial hazards: Industrial exposures such as asbestos, arsenic, chromium, uranium and nickel increase the risk of developing cancer.

Air pollution

Chronic exposure to air particulates in smog causes irritation, chronic inflammation and scarring, which increase the risk of lung cancers.

Table 19.24 Gene Mutations in Histological Types of Lung Carcinoma

Histological Type	Genes Associated
Squamous cell carcinoma	P53 mutations, loss of RB gene, loss of P16
Small-cell carcinoma	Amplification of MYC gene; loss of function involving TP53, RB, chromosome 3p deletion
Adenocarcinoma	K-ras mutation, EGFR mutation

Radiation

Long-term exposure to radon in uranium miners increases the risk of lung cancer. Radon gas is a product of uranium decay. It has the potential to ionize genetic material and cause genetic mutations that lead to lung cancer.

Molecular genetics (Table 19.24)

Lung cancers develop through a multistep process involving genetic and epigenetic alterations, with activation of growth-promoting pathways and inhibition of tumour suppressor genes. The histological subtypes of lung cancer are associated with distinctive molecular features.

Around 25% of lung cancers occur in nonsmokers. Cancers in nonsmokers are more likely to have epidermal growth factor receptor (EGFR) mutations.

Precursor Lesions

The following morphological types of precursor epithelial lesions are identified and the stages of progression are shown in Fig. 19.44:

- Squamous dysplasia and carcinoma in situ
- Atypical adenomatous hyperplasia
- Adenocarcinoma in situ
- Diffuse idiopathic pulmonary NEC hyperplasia

Squamous dysplasia (Fig. 19.45)

It is the precursor lesion of squamous cell carcinoma (SCC).

Epithelial changes associated with smoking include:

- Goblet cell hyperplasia
- Basal cell/reserve cell hyperplasia
- Squamous metaplasia
- Squamous dysplasia

Histologically, dysplasia exhibits the following features:

- Disordered squamous epithelium
- Loss of nuclear polarity
- Nuclear hyperchromasia and pleomorphism
- Mitotic figures

Dysplasia progresses through stages of mild, moderate and severe dysplasia. Carcinoma in situ is the immediate precursor of invasive SCC and has not yet penetrated the basement membrane.

Atypical adenomatous hyperplasia

It is characterized by the following features:

- Small lesions that are less than 5 mm in size

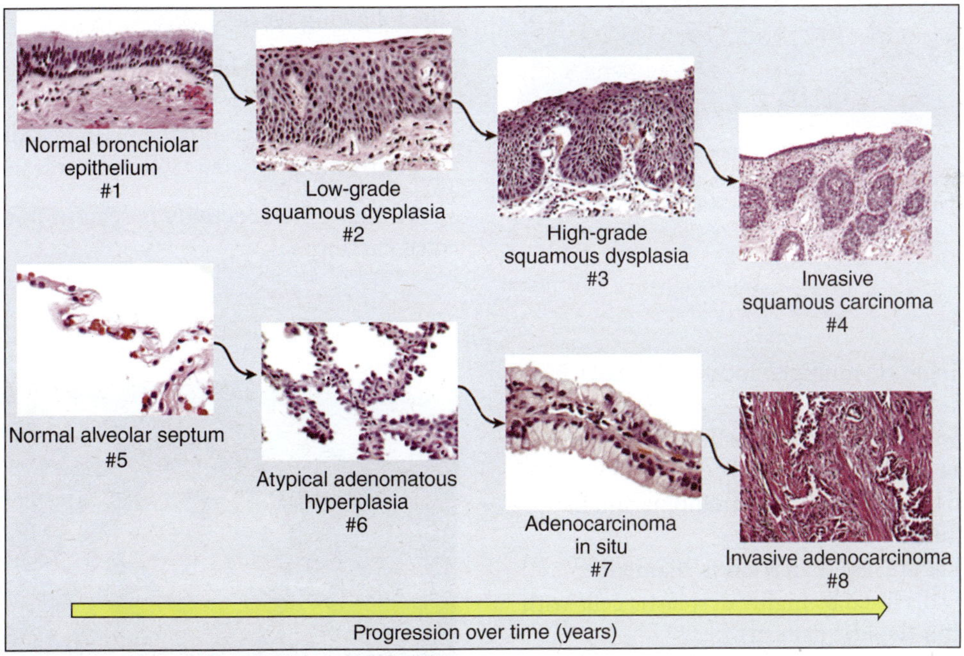

Fig. 19.44 Multistep carcinogenesis in the lung. Squamous cell carcinomas (SCCs) arise from the respiratory mucosa: (1) The earliest premalignant lesion is a low-grade squamous dysplasia; (2) the basaloid cells mature into large cells that become flat on the surface; (3) a high-grade squamous dysplasia with less distinct maturation, loss of polarity and cytological atypia; (4) invasive SCC with tumour cells infiltrating into the underlying stroma. Adenocarcinoma arise peripherally in alveoli and terminal bronchiole: (5) The precursor lesion is atypical adenomatous hyperplasia with a preserved alveolar architecture; (6) adenocarcinoma in situ; (7) dysplastic cells line the alveolar septae; and (8) invasive adenocarcinoma tumour cells spread beyond alveolar walls. (*Source:* From Lung Neoplasms, Primary – Ferri's Clinical Advisor 2021 – Clinical Key Student.)

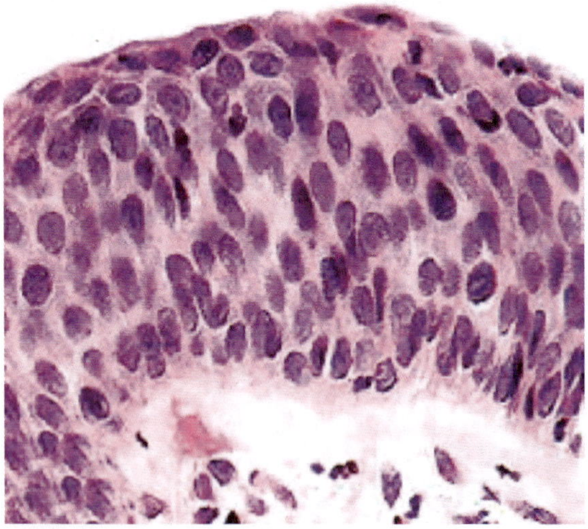

Fig. 19.45 Squamous dysplasia of the lung – characterized by loss of polarity, nuclear hyperchromasia and pleomorphism with mitotic figures. (*Source:* From Vinay Kumar, Abul K Abbas, Jon C Aster. Robbins Basic Pathology. Elsevier. 2018.)

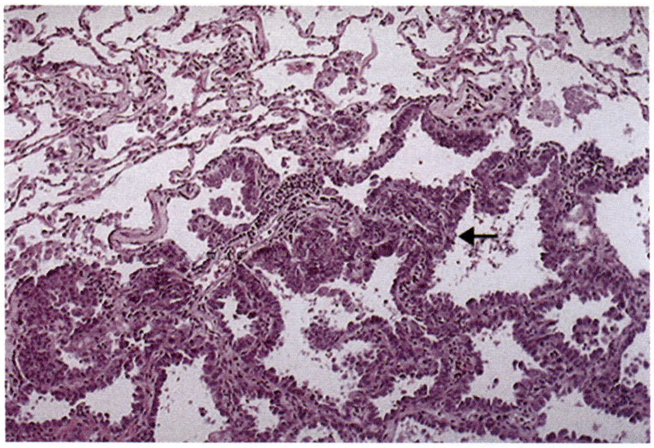

Fig. 19.46 Adenocarcinoma in situ of the lung previously known as bronchoalveolar carcinoma, with well-differentiated neoplastic columnar cells lining the alveolar septa (lepidic pattern). (*Source:* From Edward C Klatt. Robbins and Cotran Atlas of Pathology. Elsevier. 2021.)

- Can be single or multiple, located adjacent to or away from the tumour
- Alveolar walls lined by dysplastic pneumocytes

Adenocarcinoma in situ (Fig. 19.46)

It is also called bronchioalveolar carcinoma and has the following features:

- Lesions that are less than 3 cm in diameter
- Alveolar walls lined by highly dysplastic cells without invasion (lepidic pattern)

Adenocarcinoma in situ is classified into two types – mucinous and nonmucinous.

NEC hyperplasia

Normally, NECs are present as a single cell or in clusters in the respiratory epithelium. An increase in the number of these cells is called neuroendocrine hyperplasia.

Causes of NEC hyperplasia may be idiopathic (diffuse idiopathic NEC hyperplasia – precursor to neuroendocrine tumours) or inflammation/fibrosis.

Morphology

Lung carcinomas may be of the following types on the basis of location:

Central/hilar tumours are often associated with SCC.
Peripheral tumours are adenocarcinoma and large-cell carcinoma.

1. Squamous Cell Carcinoma

It is the most common type of lung cancer in India and mostly found in men. It is strongly associated with smoking. Well-characterized precursor lesions can be identified.

It presents as exophytic growth into the bronchial lumen, producing bronchial obstruction, atelectasis and infection. It may penetrate the wall of the bronchus, adjacent carina or mediastinum.

The cut surface is grey-white, firm and hard in consistency (Fig. 19.47). Large tumours have focal areas of necrosis or haemorrhage and may produce yellow or red mottling and softening. Necrotic focus may cavitate.

Histological features are like SCC elsewhere with keratinization and intercellular bridges. Keratinization may be in the form of squamous pearls or individual cells with abundant eosinophilic cytoplasm (Fig. 19.48B).

On the basis of the features, SCC are graded into the following types:

- Well-differentiated, with prominent and extensive keratinization
- Moderately differentiated, with keratinization seen
- Poorly differentiated, with keratinization rarely seen

A high mitotic activity is seen in poorly differentiated carcinomas.

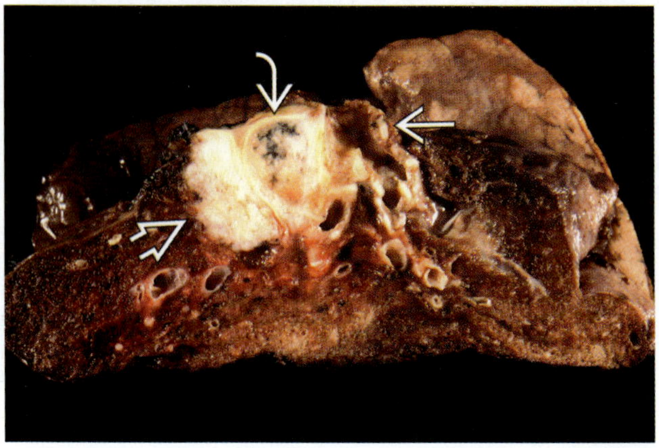

Fig. 19.47 Gross appearance of squamous cell carcinoma (SCC) of the lung shows a large, firm, tan-white tumour mass located adjacent to a large bronchus. Hilar lymph nodes are also involved by tumour.

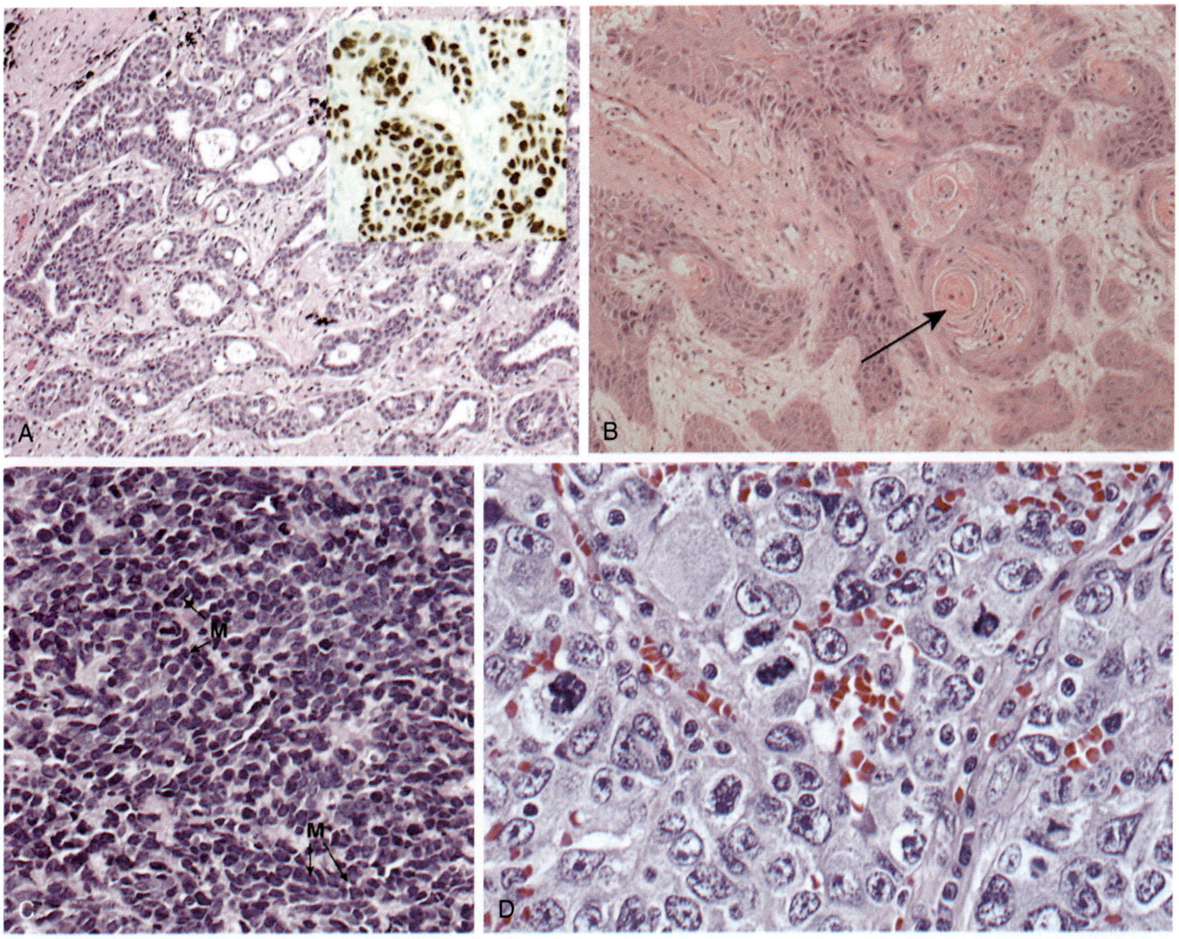

Fig. 19.48 Microscopy of carcinoma of lung. (A) Adenocarcinoma of the lung – tumour cells in acinar pattern; inset shows positivity for thyroid transcription factor-1. (B) Squamous cell carcinoma of the lung – well differentiated with keratin pearl formation (arrow). (C) Small-cell carcinoma of the lung – note the small basophilic cells with scant cytoplasm, a crushed nucleus and brisk mitotic activity (M). (D) Large-cell carcinoma – undifferentiated tumour cells with a large nucleus and prominent nucleoli. Note the numerous mitotic figures. (*Source:* From Gartner, Leslie P., Textbook of Histology, Elsevier 2021.)

2. Adenocarcinoma It is the most common type of lung cancer in women and in nonsmokers. Lesions are small and peripherally located (peripheral carcinomas) and are often associated with areas of scarring (scar carcinomas). These malignant epithelial tumours exhibit glandular differentiation and mucin production (Fig. 19.48A). Various growth patterns can be seen:

- Acinar
- Papillary, micropapillary
- Bronchioalveolar
- Solid

Microinvasive Adenocarcinoma These tumours (<3 cm) have a small invasive component (<5 mm) with a peripheral **lepidic growth pattern**. Mucinous adenocarcinoma spread aerogenously and can present as a single nodule, multiple nodules or entire lobe consolidation. Tumour cells elaborate thyroid transcription factor-1 (TTF-1, required for normal lung development).

3. Small-Cell Carcinoma These tumours are highly malignant and aggressive with strong association with smoking and affect both major bronchi and periphery of the lung. No preinvasive lesions are seen. The epithelial cells have the following features:

- Small size (these cells are smaller than small lymphocytes; are round, oval or spindle shaped, with ill-defined cell borders, scant cytoplasm and the nucleus exhibiting nuclear moulding; and contain fine granular nuclear chromatin [salt and pepper type] [Fig. 19.48C])
- High mitotic count
- **Azzopardi effect** (basophilic staining of the vascular walls due to encrustation by DNA from necrotic tumour cells)

Electron microscopy shows dense core of **neurosecretory granules**.

The tumour cells express neuroendocrine markers like **chromogranin, synaptophysin and CD57**. The tumour cells produce parathormone or parathyroid hormone (PTH)–like peptide (produce hypercalcaemia), suggesting that the tumour originates from neuroendocrine progenitor cells present in the respiratory epithelium. It is the most common bronchogenic carcinoma type associated with ectopic hormone production and paraneoplastic syndrome. This tumour is incurable by surgery but most responsive to radiotherapy and chemotherapy.

4. Large-Cell Carcinoma It is an undifferentiated malignant epithelial tumour. The tumour cells are large with moderate amount of cytoplasm and a large nucleus with prominent nucleoli (Fig. 19.48D). This tumour type is generally a diagnosis of exclusion and does not express any maker.

Variant: Large-cell neuroendocrine carcinoma – tumour cells are large with the expression of a neuroendocrine marker.

Tumour Spread The frequency of nodal involvement is greater than 50% involving hilar, bronchial, tracheal and mediastinal nodes. Cervical, supraclavicular and para-aortic nodes are also involved. Direct spread includes extension to the pleural surface, pleural cavity and pericardium. Haematogenous spread via blood vessels to the liver (30%–50%), adrenals (>50%), bones (20%), brain (20%) and opposite lungs may occur. On the basis of the size of the tumour and local invasion (T), nodal involvement (N) and distant metastasis status (M), the tumour is staged (Table 19.25).

Clinical Features Symptoms are quite variable and result from local effects, direct and distant metastasis and paraneoplastic syndromes. The most common symptoms are cough, haemoptysis, chest pain and weight loss. Apart from the above-mentioned symptoms, the tumour can cause various symptoms due to pressure on surrounding structures and secretion of various factors (Table 19.26).

Table 19.25 International Staging System for Lung Cancer

TX		Primary tumour cannot be assessed, or tumour proven by the presence of malignant cells in sputum or bronchial washings but not visualized by imaging or bronchoscopy
T0		No evidence of primary tumour
Tis		Carcinoma in situ
T1		Tumour 3 cm or less in the greatest dimension, surrounded by lung or visceral pleura, without bronchoscopic evidence of invasion more proximal than the lobar bronchus (i.e. not in the main bronchus)
	T1mi	Minimally invasive adenocarcinoma
	T1a	Tumour 1 cm or less in greatest dimension
	T1b	Tumour more than 1 cm but not more than 2 cm in greatest dimension
	T1c	Tumour more than 2 cm but not more than 3 cm in greatest dimension
T2		Tumour more than 3 cm but not more than 5 cm; or tumour with any of the following features: • Involves main bronchus regardless of distance to the carina, but without involving the carina • Invades visceral pleura • Associated with atelectasis or obstructive pneumonitis that extends to the hilar region, involving either part of the lung or the entire lung
	T2a	Tumour more than 3 cm but not more than 4 cm in greatest dimension
	T2b	Tumour more than 4 cm but not more than 5 cm in greatest dimension
T3		Tumour more than 5 cm but not more than 7 cm in greatest dimension or one that directly invades any of the following: chest wall (including superior sulcus tumours), phrenic nerve, parietal pericardium; or associated separate tumour nodule(s) in the same lobe as the primary
T4		Tumours more than 7 cm or one that invades any of the following: diaphragm, mediastinum, heart, great vessels, trachea, recurrent laryngeal nerve, oesophagus, vertebral body, carina; separate tumour nodule(s) in a different ipsilateral lobe to that of the primary
N = Regional lymph nodes		
NX		Regional lymph nodes cannot be assessed
N0		No regional lymph node metastasis
N1		Metastasis in ipsilateral peribronchial and/or ipsilateral hilar lymph nodes and intrapulmonary nodes, including involvement by direct extension
N2		Metastasis in ipsilateral mediastinal and/or subcarinal lymph node(s)
N3		Metastasis in contralateral mediastinal, contralateral hilar, ipsilateral or contralateral scalene or supraclavicular lymph node(s)
M = Distant metastasis		
M0		No distant metastasis
M1		Distant metastasis

Paraneoplastic Syndromes

Small-cell carcinomas are more commonly associated with ectopic hormone production.

The hormones produced by lung cancer are as follows:

- Adrenocorticotropic hormone (ACTH): Cushing syndrome
- Antidiuretic hormone (ADH): Hyponatraemia

Table 19.26 Local Effects Produced by the Lung Cancer

Clinical Features	Pathological Basis
Cough	Involvement of bronchial airways
Haemoptysis	Haemorrhage from the tumour
Chest pain	Tumour extension
Pneumonia, abscess, atelectasis	Obstruction
Pleural effusion	Invasion into pleura
Hoarseness	Recurrent laryngeal nerve
Dysphagia	Oesophageal invasion
Diaphragm paralysis	Phrenic nerve involvement
Rib destruction	Invasion into the chest wall
SVC syndrome	Compression of SVC
Horner syndrome	Invasion of cervical sympathetic plexus
Pericarditis, pericardial tamponade	Pericardial involvement

SVC, superior vena cava.

- PTH: Hypercalcaemia
- Calcitonin: Hypocalcaemia
- Gonadotropins: Gynaecomastia
- Serotonin: Carcinoid syndrome

Other systemic manifestations of lung cancer are as follows:

- Lambert–Eaton syndrome
  - Characterized by muscle weakness
  - Caused due to antibodies against neuronal calcium channels
- Peripheral neuropathy: Sensory
- Acanthosis nigricans
- Leukaemoid reaction
- Trousseau syndrome: Migratory thrombophlebitis
- Hypertrophic pulmonary osteoarthropathy: Clubbing of the fingers

Horner Syndrome

This syndrome is associated with apical lung cancers that invade the cervical sympathetic plexus. It presents with pain along the distribution of the ulnar nerve, anhidrosis, ptosis, miosis and enophthalmos on the same side as the lesion. These symptoms collectively define Horner syndrome. The tumours associated with this condition are Pancoast tumours.

Superior Vena Cava Syndrome

Compression or invasion of the superior vena cava, resulting in facial swelling and cyanosis along with dilation of the veins of the head, neck and upper extremities, is called superior vena cava syndrome.

NEUROENDOCRINE TUMOURS OF LUNG

It includes benign tumourlets, carcinoids, small-cell carcinoma and large-cell neuroendocrine carcinoma. Benign tumourlets are small hyperplastic nests of NECs seen in areas of chronic inflammation and scarring.

Carcinoid Tumours

These represent 1%–5% of all lung tumours occurring in the younger age group, younger than 40 years, with an equal sex incidence. It can occur in patients with multiple endocrine neoplasia. These have low-grade malignant potential with subclassification into typical and atypical carcinoids.

Morphology

Gross The location of the tumour may be central or peripheral. Central tumours grow as polypoidal mass projecting into the lumen of the bronchus with intact mucosa (Fig. 19.49). Peripheral tumours are solid and nodular. These can penetrate the bronchial wall and involve the peribronchial tissue producing collar button lesion.

Microscopy The tumour cells are arranged in an organoid, trabecular or palisading pattern, separated by fibrovascular septa. They have small, round, uniform nuclei with salt-and-pepper-type chromatin and a moderate amount of cytoplasm.

Features of Typical Carcinoids These are slow-growing indolent tumours with no necrosis and have mitotic counts less than 2 per 10 high-power fields (HPF). These do not metastasize and carry an excellent prognosis.

Features of Atypical Carcinoids Atypical carcinoids grow in a disorganized fashion with necrosis and lymphatic invasion. These have high nuclear pleomorphism, and mitotic counts between 2 and 10 mitoses per 10 HPF are seen. Metastasis to regional lymph nodes occurs at a rate between 5% and 10%, and the 5-year survival rate is 90%–95%. Immunohistochemistry (IHC) shows these cells to be positive for serotonin, chromogranin, neuron-specific enolase and other peptides. Electron microscopy shows dense-core neurosecretory granules.

Clinical Features The patients may present with cough and haemoptysis.

Complications

- Infections, bronchiectasis, emphysema and atelectasis due to intraluminal obstruction
- Carcinoid syndrome (5%–10% of cases) characterized by diarrhoea, flushing and cyanosis

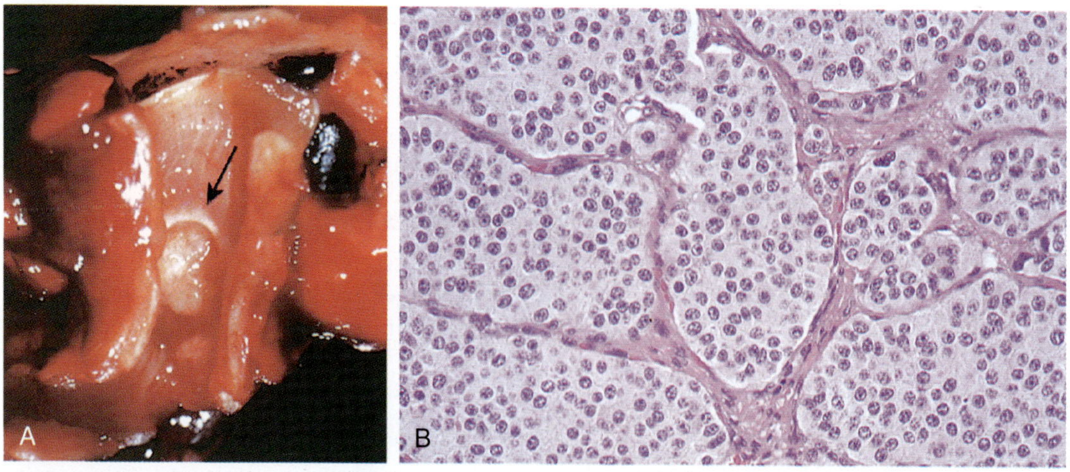

Fig. 19.49 (A) Gross picture of carcinoid showing a round, pale mass protruding into the bronchial lumen. (B) Microscopic picture of a carcinoid tumour – small round cells with uniform nuclei and a moderate amount of cytoplasm arranged in an organoid pattern. (*Source:* From Vinay Kumar, Abul K Abbas, Jon C Aster. Robbins Basic Pathology. Elsevier. 2018.)

METASTATIC TUMOURS

The lung is the most common site of metastatic tumours. These tumours have a much higher incidence than primary lung cancers. The primary ones may be carcinomas and sarcomas arising anywhere and spread via blood, through lymphatics or by direct continuity to the lungs.

Variable patterns of growth are seen. The most common pattern is multiple nodules scattered throughout the lungs, being more in the periphery. Other patterns like solitary nodule (cannon ball metastasis), endobronchial, pneumonic consolidation and pleural involvement are also seen (Figs 19.50 and 19.51).

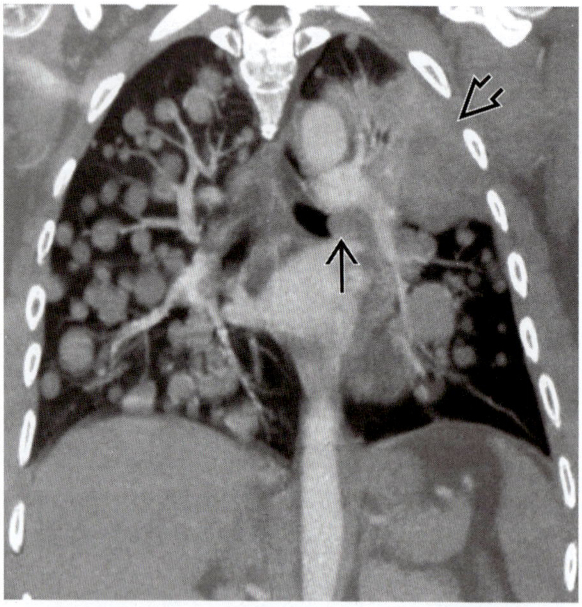

Fig. 19.50 Pulmonary metastases, gross – multiple grey-white nodules scattered throughout the lungs. (*Source:* From Vinay Kumar, Abul K Abbas, Jon C Aster. Robbins Basic Pathology. Elsevier. 2018.)

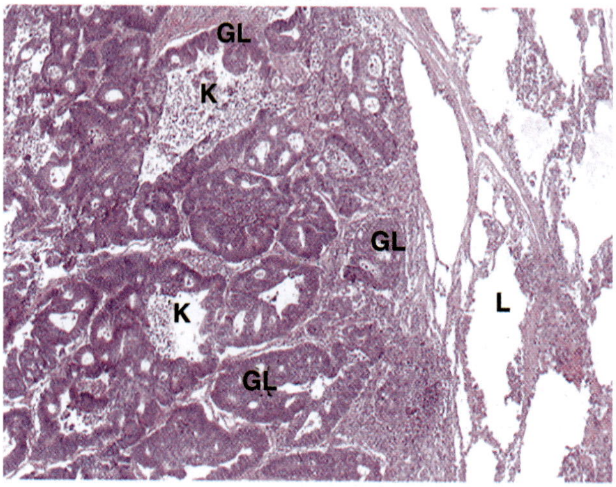

Fig. 19.51 Microscopic picture of pulmonary metastases – glands (GL) infiltrating the lung (L) tissue with the lumen containing dirty necrosis composed of karyorrhectic debris (K). (*Source:* From Respiratory System – Wheater's Pathology: A Text, Atlas, and Review of Histopathology – ClinicalKeyStudent.)

MISCELLANEOUS TUMOURS

Lymphangioleiomyomatosis

This is a pulmonary disease primarily affecting young women, and patients may present with dyspnoea, pneumothorax or chylous effusions.

Morphology

Gross: Cysts scattered diffusely throughout the lung with dilation of terminal air spaces, thickened interstitium and obstructed lymphatic vessels are seen.

Microscopy: It shows proliferation of epithelioid cells that express both markers of smooth muscle (actin) and melanocytes (HMB45).

Inflammatory Myofibroblastic Tumour

It is a rare tumour and more common in children. It may be asymptomatic or may present with fever, cough, chest pain and haemoptysis. Microscopically, proliferation of fibroblasts, myofibroblasts, lymphocytes and plasma cells is seen.

LUNG TRANSPLANTATION

Lung transplantation has become an accepted treatment option for end-stage pulmonary parenchymal and vascular disease. Selection of recipients and donors is important to decrease early graft failure. Mostly, single lung transplants are performed, although bilateral lungs and heart–lung transplants are also possible (Table 19.27).

CRITERIA FOR SELECTION OF LUNG TRANSPLANT RECIPIENTS

In 2014, the International Society for Heart and Lung Transplantation laid down the following criteria to be met for lung transplantation in adults with chronic end-stage lung disease:

High (>50%) risk of death from lung disease within 2 years if lung transplantation is not performed
High (>80%) likelihood of surviving at least 90 days after lung transplantation
High (>80%) likelihood of 5-year post-transplant survival from general medical perspective if there is adequate graft function

COMPLICATIONS OF LUNG TRANSPLANTS

- **Pulmonary infections**
  In the early weeks, bacterial infections are more common. Gram-negative bacteria, *S. aureus*, *Pseudomonas*, tuberculous and nontuberculous *Mycobacteria* species, *L. pneumophila* and *Listeria monocytogenes* are common. Viral infections with cytomegalovirus occur after 3–12 months. Fungi such as *Aspergillus* and *Candida* involve the anastomotic site and the lung.

Table 19.27 Indications for Lung Transplantation

• Non-neoplastic terminal lung diseases
• End-stage emphysema
• Idiopathic pulmonary fibrosis
• Cystic fibrosis
• Idiopathic primary pulmonary hypertension
• Bilateral lung transplant is performed when bilateral chronic infection is present (cystic fibrosis and bronchiectasis)

- **Rejection**
  Acute: It appears several weeks to months after surgery. It may present with fever, dyspnoea and cough with radiological infiltrates.
  Histological features of acute rejection include infiltration of small blood vessels and submucosa of the airways with lymphocytes, plasma cells, few eosinophils and neutrophils.
  Chronic rejection: It develops 3–5 years after transplantation and presents with cough and dyspnoea (due to pulmonary fibrosis).
  Histological features include bronchiolitis obliterans and fibrotic occlusion of the small airways, which may be partial or complete. In long-standing cases, bronchiectasis and pulmonary fibrosis may develop.
- **Complications such as anastomotic dehiscence and vascular thrombosis becoming rare** with improved surgical techniques
- **Malignancy:** Epstein–Barr virus (EBV)-associated B-cell lymphoma (rare)
- **Accelerated pulmonary arteriosclerosis**

Absolute contraindications for lung transplantation are as follows:
- Malignancy in the last 2 years
- Untreatable advanced dysfunction of another major organ system (e.g. heart, liver or kidney)
- Noncurable chronic extrapulmonary infection including chronic active viral hepatitis B, hepatitis C and HIV infection
- Significant chest wall or spinal deformity

PLEURA

The lungs are covered by a thin serous membrane – the visceral pleura – which is reflected onto the chest wall as parietal pleura at the hilum of each lung. The pleural cavity or the pleural space is the potential space between these two layers. Normally, a small amount of fluid (10–20 mL) is present in the pleural space that helps the layers to glide against each other.

Primary diseases of the pleura – neoplastic and non-neoplastic – are rare, and the pleura is usually involved secondarily by disease processes located elsewhere (e.g. bacterial pneumonia leading to empyema or lung carcinoma with metastases to the pleura) (Table 19.28).

PLEURAL EFFUSION

Pleural effusion is the collection of excess fluid in the pleural cavity. Normally, less than 15 mL of clear serous fluid lubricates the pleural surface.

Pleural effusion can be of the following types (Table 19.29):

A) Exudate or inflammatory
B) Transudate or noninflammatory

Table 19.28 Diseases of the Pleura

Category	Diseases
Non-neoplastic	Pleurisy Pleural effusion Pneumothorax Haemothorax
Neoplastic	Benign solitary fibrous tumour Malignant mesothelioma Secondaries

Table 19.29 Aetiopathogenesis of Pleural Effusion

Transudate effusion	**Alteration in hydrostatic or oncotic pressure** Congestive left heart failure Nephrotic syndrome Liver cirrhosis Hypoalbuminaemia
Exudate effusion	**Increased capillary permeability** Infections – pneumonia or tuberculosis Malignancy Inflammatory disorders like pancreatitis, lupus, rheumatoid arthritis, post–cardiac injury syndrome Chylothorax Asbestosis

For pleural fluid to accumulate, there must be an increase in hydrostatic pressure, decreased oncotic or pleural pressure, an increased microvascular permeability or impaired lymphatic drainage.

A) Inflammatory Effusion

Inflammation of the pleura with pleuritic chest pain is known as pleuritis or pleurisy.

Pleuritic chest pain is described as sharp pain aggravated by certain actions like taking deep breaths, coughing or sneezing. Infection or irritation causes inflammation and vascular congestion of the pleura.

Causes

- Infections
  - TB, pneumonia, abscess, bronchiectasis
- Infarction of the lung
- Systemic autoimmune diseases
- Metabolic (uraemia)
- Radiotherapy
- Neoplastic (haemorrhagic pleuritis)
- Rickettsial infections (haemorrhagic pleuritis)

The inflammation can resolve or may develop pleural effusions.

Depending on the character of exudates, it can be of the following types:

- Serous
- Fibrinous
- Serofibrinous
- Empyema
- Haemorrhagic pleuritis

Clinical Features Patients present with chest pain on breathing, and friction rub can be heard on auscultation. If the exudate is minimal, it resolves with complete resolution. Repeated attacks of pleurisy may result in organization, leading to fibrinous adhesion and obliteration of the pleural cavity. Haemorrhagic pleuritis differs from haemothorax in having inflammatory cells and exfoliated tumour cells.

Pyothorax: It involves effusion with a large number of neutrophils in the pleural cavity.

Causes

Infections of the pleura

Complication of bacterial pneumonia

Empyema Empyema is considered as a variant of pyothorax characterized by the accumulation of thick pus in the pleural cavity.

Causes

- Infections (most often associated with pneumonia due to *S. pneumoniae*, *S. aureus*, *H. influenzae*, group A *Streptococcus*, gram-negative organisms, TB and fungi)
- Rupture of a lung abscess into the pleural space
- Contamination introduced from trauma or thoracic surgery
- Extension of intra-abdominal abscesses

B) Noninflammatory Effusion

Hydrothorax It is the accumulation of noninflammatory serous fluid known as transudate effusion within the pleural space.

The fluid is typically clear and straw coloured and can be unilateral or bilateral depending on the underlying cause.

Causes

a) Increased hydrostatic pressure
b) Heart failure
c) Pulmonary oedema
d) Systemic oedema (renal failure and cirrhosis of the liver)

Haemothorax It refers to collection of blood within the pleural cavity.

Causes

a) Trauma to the chest wall or thoracic viscera
b) Rupture of aortic aneurysm

Chylothorax Accumulation of milky lipid-rich effusion is called chylothorax. It is caused due to rupture of the thoracic duct by trauma or obstruction of the thoracic duct by tumours.

PNEUMOTHORAX

Pneumothorax is defined as the collection of air in the pleural cavity from a ruptured bulla or penetrating injury to the chest leading to collapse of the lung.

Types

Spontaneous pneumothorax is defined as the spontaneously occurring presence of air in the pleural cavity in patients without a clinically apparent underlying lung disease. It occurs in young adults. It is of two types – **primary and secondary**.

Primary spontaneous pneumothorax occurs due to rupture of an emphysematous bulla or a subpleural bleb. It is typically seen in young adults. This condition usually resolves on its own as the air is absorbed by the body. However, in some cases, it can lead to the collapse of a portion of the lung, causing the trachea to shift towards the collapsed side.

Secondary spontaneous pneumothorax may develop as a complication of various underlying lung diseases, most commonly COPD and TB, but may also be seen in asthma, lung abscess, pulmonary infarcts, bronchogenic carcinoma and different forms of fibrotic and cystic lung diseases.

Traumatic pneumothorax is caused by penetrating injury to the chest wall.

Iatrogenic pneumothorax is caused by mechanical ventilation (which can lead to barotrauma due to high positive end-expiratory pressure), thoracocentesis and central venous catheter placement.

Tension Pneumothorax

Tension pneumothorax is a life-threatening large pneumothorax. The injured tissue acts as a valve flap, allowing air into the pleural space on inhalation but failing to release it during expiration, increasing the intrathoracic pressure. This eventually displaces mediastinal structures, which can interfere with venous return to the heart, causing cardiovascular collapse and shock.

Tension pneumothorax is a medical emergency and is treated with the insertion of a chest tube.

PLEURAL TUMOURS PA 26.6

Pleural tumours include benign, malignant and tumour-like lesions involving the pleura (Table 19.30). Malignant pleural neoplasms are more common than benign tumours.

Solitary Fibrous Tumour

It is a benign tumour that occurs in the pleura and less commonly in the lung. It is often attached to the pleural surface by a pedicle.

Table 19.30 Classification of Pleural Tumours

Primary	
	Benign – solitary fibrous tumour
	Malignant – malignant mesothelioma
Secondary	
	Primary from breast and lung

Morphology

Gross The tumour is solid, grey-white with a whorled appearance.

Microscopy The tumour is composed of spindle cells resembling fibroblasts interspersed between whorls of reticulin and collagen fibres. IHC is positive for CD34 and negative for keratin. Tumour size greater than 10 cm, presence of necrosis, nuclear pleomorphism and mitotic activity favour malignancy.

Malignant Mesothelioma PA 26.7

It is a rare aggressive malignant tumour that arises from mesothelial cells lining the body cavities (pleura, pericardium peritoneum) and tunica vaginalis.

Aetiology Asbestos exposure, with a long latent period of 25–45 years, is required for the development of a tumour. Average age of onset is 60 years.

Molecular genetics: Deletion of tumour suppressor gene CDKN2A/INK4a is seen in 80% of mesotheliomas.

Morphology

Gross Pleural mesotheliomas encase and compress the lung, extending into fissures and interlobar septa. The lung is ensheathed by thick, firm, white tumour tissue (Fig. 19.52).

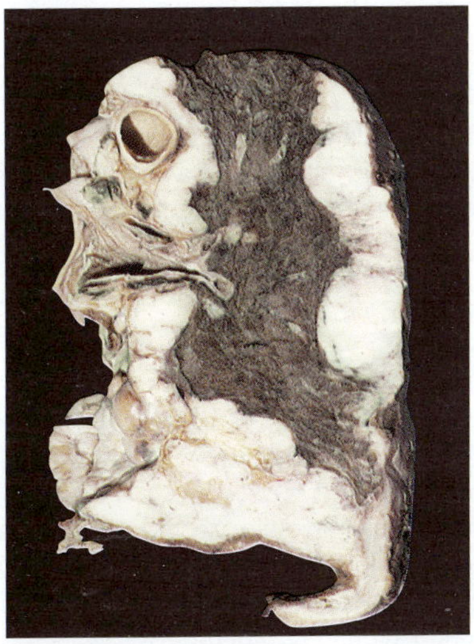

Fig. 19.52 Gross picture of malignant mesothelioma. Grey-white tumour encasing the lung. (*Source:* From Simon S Cross. Underwood's Pathology. Elsevier. 2019.)

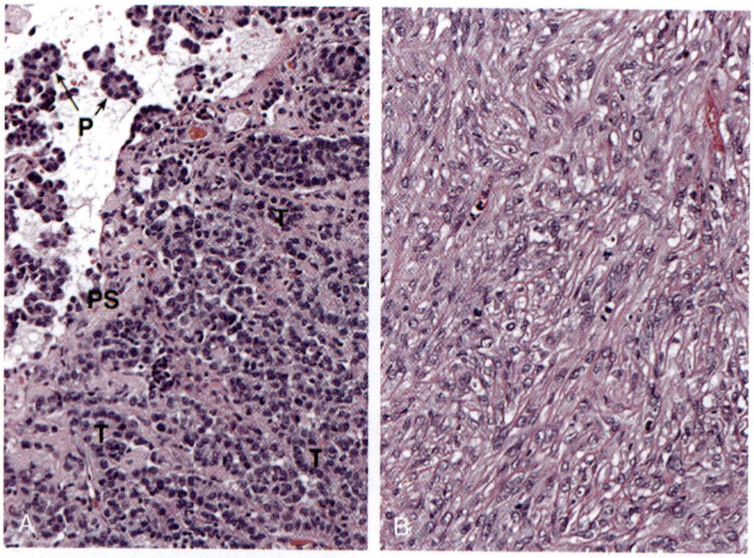

Fig. 19.53 Malignant mesothelioma of the pleura. (A) Epithelioid variant – the tumour is seen with a papillary architecture (P) on the pleural surface and also in glandular and tubular patterns. (B) Sarcomatoid variant – spindle cell type. (*Source:* From Geraldine O'Dowd et al. Wheater's Pathology: A Text, Atlas, and Review of Histopathology, 6th edition. Elsevier 2020.)

Microscopy The tumour may be of epithelioid type (60%), sarcomatoid type (20%) or mixed type (20%). The epithelioid component consists of tubular and papillary structures lined by cuboidal, columnar and flattened cells resembling adenocarcinoma, whereas the mesenchymal component consists of spindle cells resembling sarcoma. The biphasic type has both components (Fig. 19.53). The 2021 WHO classification system introduced a two-tier grading system (low grade and high grade) on the basis of nuclear atypia, mitosis and necrosis.

IHC: Mesotheliomas are positive for calretinin, cytokeratin 5 and 6 and Wilms tumour 1 (WT-1).

Clinical Presentation Patients may present with chest pain, dyspnoea, recurrent pleural effusions and pleural mass. Metastasis can occur to the lung parenchyma or mediastinal lymph nodes and to distant sites like the liver, bone and adrenals.

Prognosis Malignant mesothelioma has a poor prognosis, with 50% of patients succumbing to death within a year of diagnosis.

SELF-ASSESSMENT

Multiple Choice Questions

1. The most carcinogenic component of cigarette smoke is
   A. Nicotine
   B. Polycyclic hydrocarbons
   C. Cotinine
   D. All of the above
2. A 45-year-old male alcoholic was admitted with signs and symptoms of lung abscess. The most common mechanism of development of lung abscess in this patient would be ______.
   A. Antecedent primary lung infection
   B. Septic embolism
   C. Neoplasm
   D. Aspiration of infective material
3. A 55-year-old female patient was diagnosed with lung abscess. Which among the following histopathological features is expected in this patient?
   A. Neutrophilic infiltration in the interstitial septa
   B. Lymphocytic infiltration in the interstitial septa
   C. Suppurative destruction of the lung parenchyma within the central area of cavitation
   D. Neutrophilic infiltration of alveolar spaces
4. A 55-year-old female patient was diagnosed with lung abscess. Which among the following is expected as a complication in this patient?
   A. Secondary amyloidosis
   B. Brain abscess
   C. Empyema
   D. All of the above
5. A 49-year-old male, a chronic smoker, was admitted with signs and symptoms of emphysema. Which among the following types of emphysema is expected in this patient?
   A. Centriacinar
   B. Panacinar
   C. Distal acinar
   D. Irregular
6. ____________ is defined clinically as persistent cough with sputum production for at least 3 months in at least 2 consecutive years in the absence of any other identifiable cause.
   A. Emphysema
   B. Chronic bronchitis
   C. Bronchial asthma
   D. Bronchiectasis

7. The earliest change seen in chronic bronchitis is
   A. Narrowing of bronchioles
   B. Bronchiolitis obliterans
   C. Mucus hypersecretion
   D. Squamous metaplasia
8. Reid index is increased in
   A. Chronic bronchitis
   B. Emphysema
   C. Bronchiectasis
   D. Bronchial asthma
9. Which among the following findings is seen in the sputum or bronchoalveolar lavage specimen of patients with bronchial asthma?
   A. Eosinophilia
   B. Curschmann spirals
   C. Charcot–Leyden crystals
   D. All of the above
10. Which among the following features is not a part of 'airway remodelling' in bronchial asthma?
    A. Hypertrophy and/or hyperplasia of the bronchial wall muscle
    B. Sub–basement membrane fibrosis
    C. Increase in the size of the submucosal glands and number of airway goblet cells
    D. None of the above
11. Ghon complex is formed by
    A. Parenchymal lung lesion
    B. Lymph node
    C. Both of the above
    D. None of the above
12. A 35-year-old male was diagnosed with byssinosis, an occupational lung disorder. What was he probably exposed to in his workplace in your opinion?
    A. Sugarcane residue
    B. Tin oxide
    C. Cotton
    D. Bird droppings
13. A 48-year-old male works in a mining industry that involves asbestos fibres. On chronic exposure, which among the following diseases is he anticipated to develop?
    A. Mesothelioma
    B. Laryngeal carcinoma
    C. Colonic carcinoma
    D. All of the above
14. The most common manifestation of asbestos exposure is
    A. Diffuse pulmonary interstitial fibrosis
    B. Asbestos bodies
    C. Pleural plaques
    D. Mesothelioma
15. The most common type of lung carcinoma that affects nonsmokers is
    A. Adenocarcinoma
    B. Small-cell carcinoma
    C. Squamous cell carcinoma
    D. None of the above
16. The pulmonary lesion that is less than 3 cm in size and is composed entirely of dysplastic cells growing along preexisting alveolar septa is a feature of
    A. Atypical adenomatous hyperplasia
    B. Adenocarcinoma in situ
    C. Adenocarcinoma
    D. Squamous cell carcinoma
17. A 58-year-old male presented with persistent cough, chest pain, dyspnoea and weight loss. He was diagnosed as a case of bronchogenic carcinoma and his tumour was sampled. Electron microscopic examination revealed the presence of neurosecretory granules in the tumour cells. What is the histological type of lung carcinoma that the patient has?
    A. Squamous cell carcinoma
    B. Adenocarcinoma
    C. Bronchioloalveolar carcinoma
    D. Small-cell carcinoma
18. A 49-year-old male presented with cough, haemoptysis, diarrhoea, cutaneous flushing and cyanosis. On investigations, he was found to be having a 'collar button' lesion in the lung. What is the most likely diagnosis?
    A. Carcinoid tumour
    B. Silicosis
    C. Asbestosis
    D. All of the above
19. STAT6 is the marker for
    A. Small-cell carcinoma
    B. Solitary fibrous tumour
    C. Adenocarcinoma lung
    D. Squamous cell carcinoma of the lung
20. Which among the following markers is positive in mesothelioma?
    A. Cytokeratin 5/6
    B. WT1
    C. Calretinin
    D. All of the above

Answers

1. (B); 2. (D); 3. (C); 4. (D); 5. (A); 6. (B); 7. (C); 8. (A); 9. (D); 10. (D); 11. (C); 12. (C); 13. (D); 14. (C); 15. (A); 16. (B); 17. (D); 18. (A); 19. (B); 20. (D)

Self-Assessment Questions

1. A 45-year-old man suffering from liver cirrhosis died due to respiratory failure and his autopsy revealed diffuse changes in the lungs. What is the probable diagnosis? Describe the genetics, pathogenesis, morphological features and complications of the disease.
2. A 31-year-old woman presented with cough, dyspnoea, flushing, diarrhoea, hypotension and haematemesis for the past 6 months. Bronchial lesion was noted and investigated. What is your provisional diagnosis? Discuss the types, morphological features and histochemical and immunohistochemical markers of the disease.
3. A 59-year-old man, an asbestos factory worker for the past 30 years, presented with a lung mass. Investigations revealed a pleural-based mass, which was biopsied and examined. What is the most probable diagnosis? Discuss the aetiopathogenesis, morphological features, microscopic patterns, immunohistochemical markers and electron microscopic features of the tumour.
4. A 6-year-old boy accidentally inhaled a seed that got lodged into one of his bronchi. Chest X-rays showed the shift of the mediastinum towards the side of obstruction. What is the probable diagnosis? Discuss the aetiopathogenesis, types and morphological features of the disease.

5. A 48-year-old chronic smoker presented with chronic cough with expectoration for the past 4 months. He had similar episodes in the last 2 years. There was no other identifiable cause for his condition. Clinically, he was found to be dyspnoeic, cyanotic, hypoxic and hypercapnic. What is your probable diagnosis? Discuss the aetiopathogenesis, morphological features and complications of the disease.
6. A 65-year-old man with a 40-year history of tobacco use and a chronic productive cough for several years developed more severe dyspnoea and fever. He had an enlarged chest diameter and some mild blueness to the lips. A chest radiograph showed an enlarged heart and hyperlucent lung fields but no evidence of a pulmonary infiltrate. What is the most likely diagnosis? What is the most likely underlying mechanism associated with this disorder?
7. A 54-year-old man working in the mining industry for the past 32 years presented with a low-grade fever, cough with expectoration and loss of weight and appetite for the past 4 months. He also complained of breathlessness on exertion. X-rays of the lung revealed nodular lesions along with a cavitary lesion. There was also eggshell calcification noted in the lung parenchyma. What is your provisional diagnosis? Discuss the aetiopathogenesis, morphological features and complications of the disease.
8. A 35-year-old woman presented with complaints of shortness of breath and cough for the last 2 months. She also has had fatigue and mild subjective fever. Physical examination revealed several discrete subcutaneous nodules. No masses or organomegaly was found. A chest radiograph showed bilateral hilar lymphadenopathy but no lung or mediastinal masses. A biopsy of one of the skin nodules showed noncaseating granuloma. What are the diagnostic considerations? Discuss the pathogenesis and morphological features of the disease. What serum blood test can help confirm the diagnosis?
9. A 58-year-old male patient in the intensive care unit admitted for sepsis developed rapid-onset respiratory failure and died. Medicolegal autopsy was performed, and the microscopy of the lung tissue showed the presence of dilated alveoli lined by hyaline membrane. What is your diagnosis? Discuss the aetiopathogenesis and morphological features of the disease.
10. A 78-year-old man was brought to the emergency department. For the last several days, he has had fatigue, malaise, fever and a productive cough. A chest radiograph showed consolidation in the right lower lobe. A Gram stain of the sputum showed a predominance of gram-positive cocci in pairs and chains. What is the most likely diagnosis?

Answer Key

1. α_1-Antitrypsin deficiency – liver cirrhosis with panacinar emphysema
2. Carcinoid tumour
3. Mesothelioma
4. Atelectasis
5. Chronic bronchitis
6. Emphysema
7. Silicosis with pulmonary tuberculosis
8. Sarcoidosis
9. ARDS/ALI
10. Typical pneumonia

Topics for Self-Directed Learning

1. Differentiate between latent TB and active TB.
2. Differentiate between primary TB and secondary TB.
3. Differentiate between emphysema and chronic bronchitis.
4. Provide interpretation of pleural fluid in various diseases.
5. Describe the classification and pathophysiology of respiratory failure.
6. Provide interpretation of the pulmonary function test.
7. Describe mediastinal compartment anatomy and pathology.
8. Describe pulmonary haemorrhage syndromes.
9. Describe pathophysiology of obstructive sleep apnoea syndrome.
10. Describe clear cell tumour (sugar tumour) of the lung.

Head and Neck 20

Rajeswari Kathiah

PA 24.1 Describe the aetiology, pathogenesis, pathology and clinical features **of oral cancers.**

CHAPTER OUTLINE

Diseases of the head and neck range from simple infections to invasive malignancies. Common and histopathologically significant head and neck diseases are discussed under the following headings:

1. Oral cavity
2. Upper airway, which includes draining nodes, nasopharynx and larynx
3. Neck
4. Salivary glands

I. DISEASES OF THE ORAL CAVITY

Oral cavity includes many structures like teeth, gingiva, oral mucosa and connective tissue stroma. Though non-neoplastic lesions outnumber neoplastic lesions, oral cancer is the most common malignancy in low-socioeconomic countries like India, causing significant morbidity and mortality. Here, we describe some of the common non-neoplastic and neoplastic lesions of the oral cavity.

NON-NEOPLASTIC LESIONS

Two non-neoplastic lesions of the oral cavity deserve special mention and description here for their common incidence and morbidity they are associated with. The conditions are as follows:

- Aphthous ulcers
- Oral candidiasis

Aphthous Ulcers

Aphthous ulcers, also referred to as **recurrent aphthous stomatitis or canker sores**, are common lesions of the oral cavity that affect 50% of the population. These ulcers often present as recurrent, painful, superficial, mucosal ulceration of unknown aetiology. These are more often a familial disorder and have an association with immunological disorders like inflammatory bowel disease, coeliac disease, Behçet disease, autoinflammatory syndromes and immunodeficient states like HIV/AIDS. Patients present in early childhood or adolescence with recurrent, painful, small, round or ovoid ulcers. The margins are well-defined and erythematous, forming a halo and a central yellow or grey floor.

Morphology (Fig. 20.1)

The lesions are single or multifocal, superficial, hyperaemic, mucosal ulcerations covered by a thin exudate and rimmed by a narrow area of erythema.

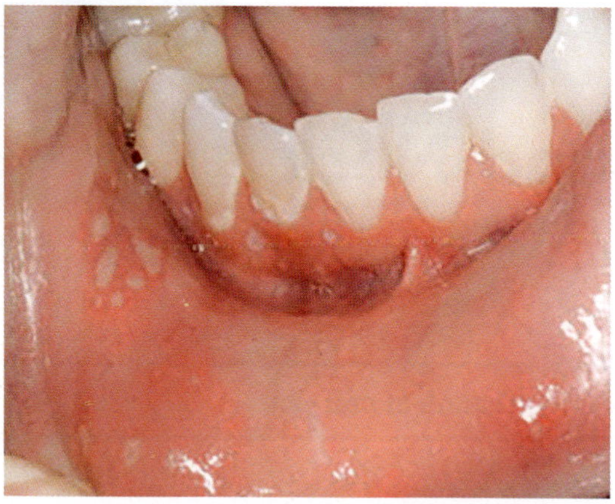

Fig. 20.1 Clinical picture of aphthous ulcer. (*Source:* From Nicholas Inman, Joshua Justice. Aphthous Ulcers. Elsevier 2022.)

The underlying submucosa shows inflammatory infiltrate that is composed of lymphocytes which are later replaced by polymorphs because of secondary bacterial infection.

Generally, the lesions resolve spontaneously in 7–10 days. However, in some cases, especially in immunocompromised patients, these lesions persist longer for many weeks and even months.

Oral Candidiasis

Oral candidiasis, also called **oral thrush**, is caused by the fungus *Candida albicans*, which is part of the normal oral microbiota in half of the population. It is the most common fungal infection of the oral cavity. The presence of *Candida* in mucosal surface is not considered to be a disease, but when *Candida* species become pathogenic and invade host tissues, oral candidiasis occurs. The most important factor in the transformation of oral commensal to pathogenic fungus is the immune status of the individual. Administration of broad-spectrum antibiotics, diabetes or AIDS can eliminate or alter the normal oral flora and predispose individuals to oral candidiasis.

Oral candidiasis can be present as primary or secondary forms (Table 20.1).

Table 20.1 Classification of Oral Candidiasis

Group	Forms
Primary candidiasis	Pseudomembranous Erythematous Hyperplastic plaque like, nodular *Candida*-associated lesions: denture-related stomatitis, angular stomatitis, etc.
Secondary candidiasis	Oral manifestations of systemic mucocutaneous candidiasis

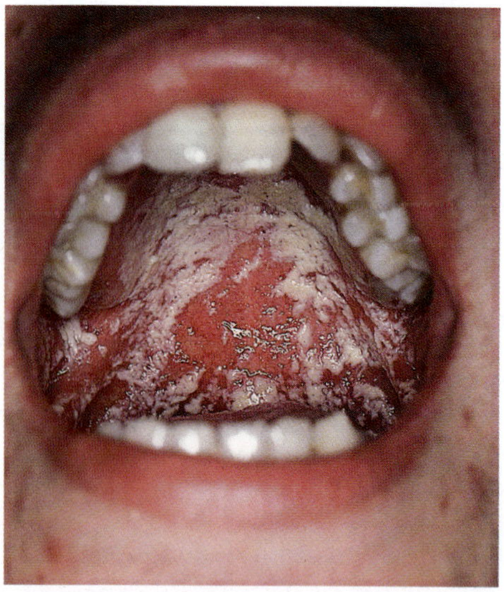

Fig. 20.2 Clinical picture of oral candidiasis affecting the dorsal tongue with the classical pseudomembrane. (*Source:* From Candidiasis. Elsevier Point of Care 2022.)

Morphology (Fig. 20.2)

Three main clinical presentations of candidiasis are **pseudomembranous, erythematous and hyperplastic**. The most common presentation is the pseudomembranous form and is referred to as **thrush**. It is characterized by individual patches of pseudomembranous white slough that can easily be scraped away to reveal the underlying erythematous base which may bleed. The pseudomembrane is made up of debris, fibrin and desquamated epithelium that has been invaded by the fungus. Fungus can be highlighted in tissue sections using stains like PAS.

The infection is generally confined to the superficial zone except in immunocompromised individuals in whom it may be deeply invasive.

Gold standard investigation is culture and sensitivity with identification of the organism.

Treatment includes antifungals and most importantly treatment of the predisposing factor.

PRECANCEROUS LESIONS

Precancerous lesions of oral mucosa, known as potentially malignant lesions in the recent years, comprise a group of diseases.

The common oral precancerous lesions are as follows:

- **Leucoplakia**
- **Erythroplakia**
- **Speckled leucoerythroplakia**
- **Oral submucous fibrosis (OSMF)**

For their close association, the first three lesions are discussed together, followed by OSMF.

Leucoplakia, Erythroplakia and Speckled Leucoerythroplakia

Leucoplakia is a firmly attached **white patch** on the mucous membrane which is associated with an increased risk of malignant transformation. The World Health Organization (WHO) defines leucoplakia as *'a white patch or plaque that cannot be scraped off and cannot be characterized clinically or pathologically as any other disease'*. Hence, this term is reserved for lesions that are present in the oral cavity for no apparent reason such as lichen planus or candidiasis. Because 5%–25% of such lesions are premalignant, all lesions should be considered precancerous until proven otherwise.

Leucoplakia is usually seen in people older than 40 years and is slightly more common in males. Causative factors include tobacco use, alcohol, ill-fitting dentures, chronic irritation and human papillomavirus (HPV) infection. Leucoplakia can occur anywhere in the oral cavity, but the most common site is gingival buccal sulcus and lesions on the floor of mouth are often dysplastic.

Proliferative verrucous leucoplakia, which is a form of verrucous leucoplakia, is characterized by multifocal presentation and has a strong potential for malignant transformation.

Erythroplakia, also called dysplastic erythroplakia, is a less common but more threatening condition. It is defined as *'a fiery red patch that cannot be characterized clinically or pathologically as any other definable disease'*. It is seen as red, velvety, eroded, flat or depressed area within the oral cavity.

Speckled leucoerythroplakia is an unusual form characterized by features intermediate between leucoplakia and erythroplakia. Such lesions often have *Candida* infection and have only 4% risk of malignant transformation. The risk is higher if the lesions are speckled or warty or located on the floor of the mouth or the ventral surface of tongue.

Morphology

Leucoplakia appears as solitary or multifocal white patches with sharp demarcation from the adjacent mucosa. At times, it appears as ridged verrucous plaques (Fig. 20.3).

On microscopic examination (Fig. 20.4), it may have features ranging from hyperkeratosis and acanthosis, with orderly maturation to frankly dysplastic changes which might blend with areas of carcinoma in situ.

Erythroplakia is usually associated with highly atypical epithelial changes with thin and atrophic epithelium and prominent vasculature. Atypical changes may range from severe dysplastic changes (Fig. 20.5) to carcinoma in situ or even microinvasion (Fig. 20.6).

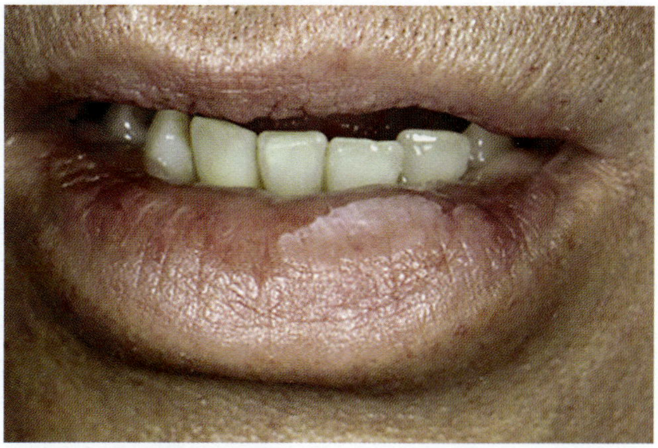

Fig. 20.3 Clinical picture microscopy of leucoplakia seen as thin white plaque over the lower lip. (*Source:* From James, Dinulos. Habif's Clinical Dermatology, 7e, Chapter 21. Elsevier 2021.)

Oral Submucous Fibrosis

OSMF is a chronic and potentially malignant lesion. It is seen commonly in Asians and affects both the sexes in their second and third decades of life. It is characterized by juxtaepithelial fibrosis of the oral cavity. The strongest risk factor for OSMF is chewing betel quid containing areca nut. Other factors like genetic and immunological predisposition also play a role in OSMF.

Patients present with burning sensation and/or intolerance to spicy food in the beginning which slowly progresses to fibrosis, causing difficulty in opening the mouth.

Clinical Stages OSMF is clinically divided into three stages, and the morphological features vary accordingly.

Stage 1: It represents erythema, vesicles, ulcers and melanotic pigmentation in the mucosa.

Stage 2: Rupture of vesicles and ulcers leading to fibrosis when they heal is the hallmark feature of this stage. Older lesions include vertical and circular palpable fibrous bands in the buccal mucosa and around the mouth or lips, resulting in marble-like appearance of the mucosa.

Stage 3: Leucoplakia is found in more than 25% of patients with OSMF.

Morphology

Microscopy (Fig. 20.7) Mucosal changes such as atrophy, pigment incontinence, ulceration with granulation tissue, hyperplastic changes, dysplasia and carcinoma may be seen in some cases.

Submucosal changes may include **fibrosis**, diffuse and chronic inflammatory infiltrate, atrophy of minor salivary glands, band-like infiltrate of inflammatory cells, oedema and congestion.

Despite the general accessibility of the oral cavity for physical examination, many malignancies are not diagnosed

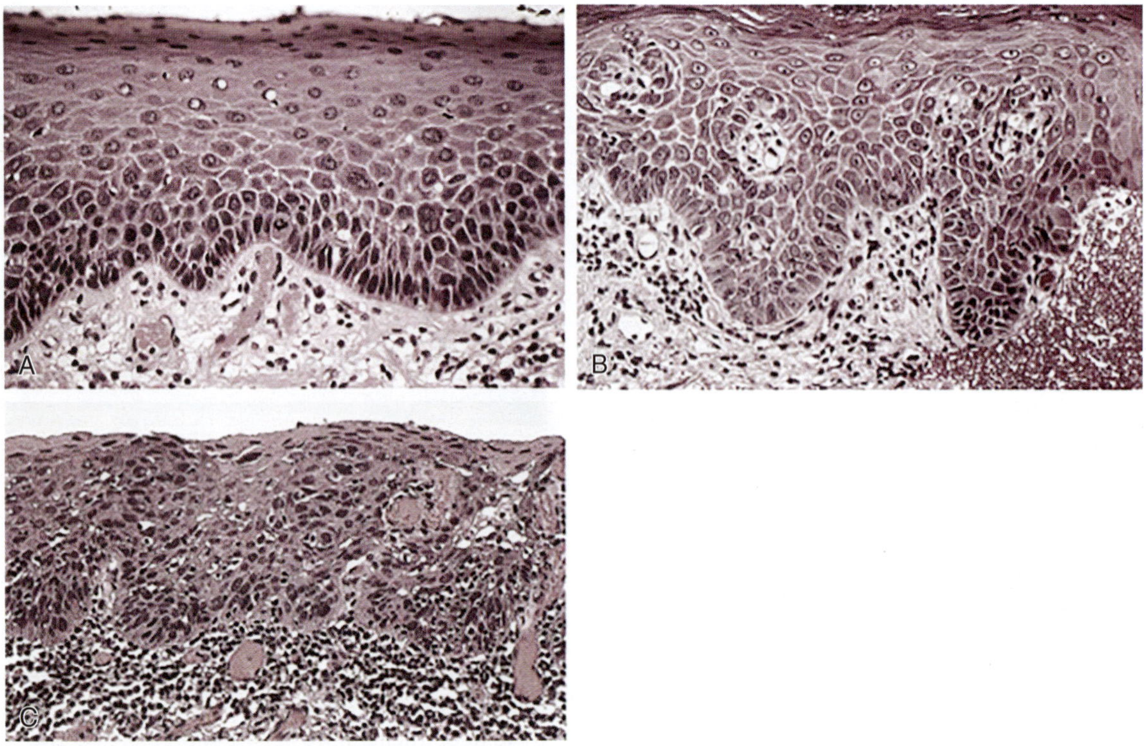

Fig. 20.4 (A–C) Microscopy of leucoplakia displaying a wide range of changes from mild to moderate to severe dysplasia. (*Source:* From James J. Sciubba. Cummings Otolaryngology. Elsevier 2021.)

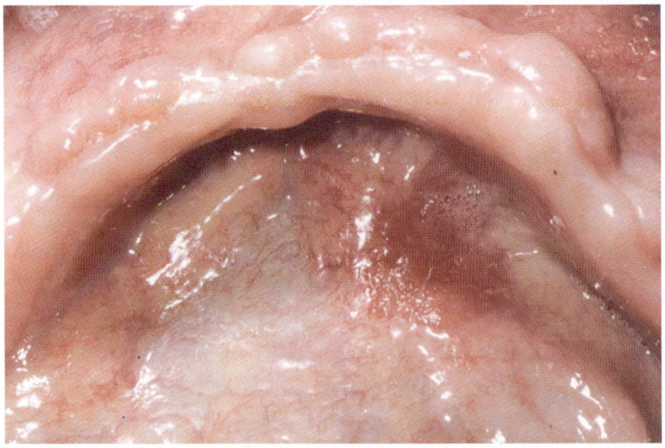

Fig. 20.5 Clinical picture of erythroplakia. (*Source:* From Edward E. Herschaft. Oral and Maxillofacial Pathology. Elsevier 2016.)

until late stages. In order to prevent malignant transformation of these precursor lesions, multiple screening and detection techniques have been developed. Early detection is of crucial importance as the survival rates markedly improve when the oral precancerous lesions are identified at an early stage.

MALIGNANT TUMOURS

Oral Squamous Cell Carcinoma PA 24.1

Oral squamous cell carcinoma (OSCC) represents 95% of all forms of head and neck malignancies, and over the last decade its incidence has increased by 50%. Squamous cell

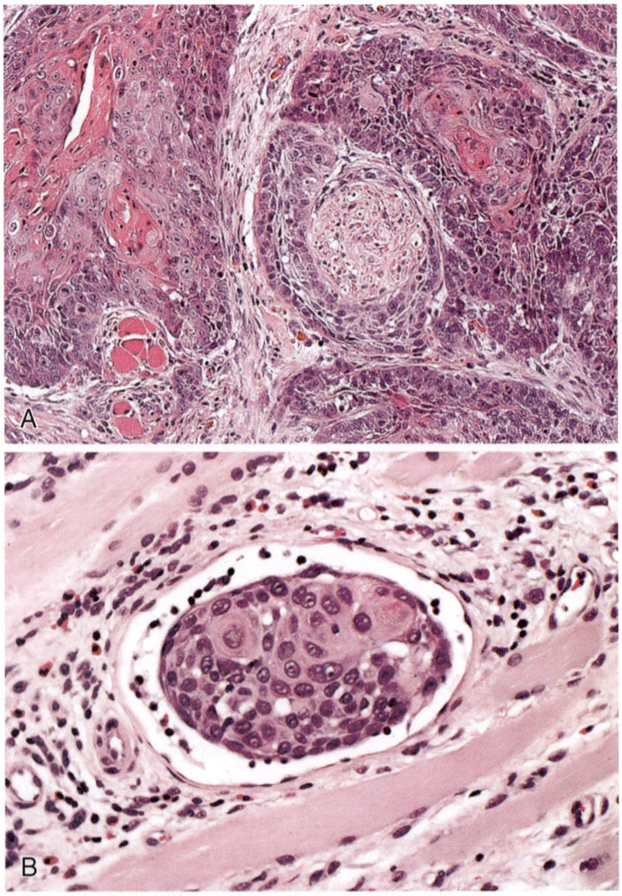

Fig. 20.6 (A and B) Microscopy of erythroplakia harbouring squamous cell carcinoma with a focus of vascular invasion. (*Source:* From Edward E. Herschaft. Oral and Maxillofacial Pathology. Elsevier 2016.)

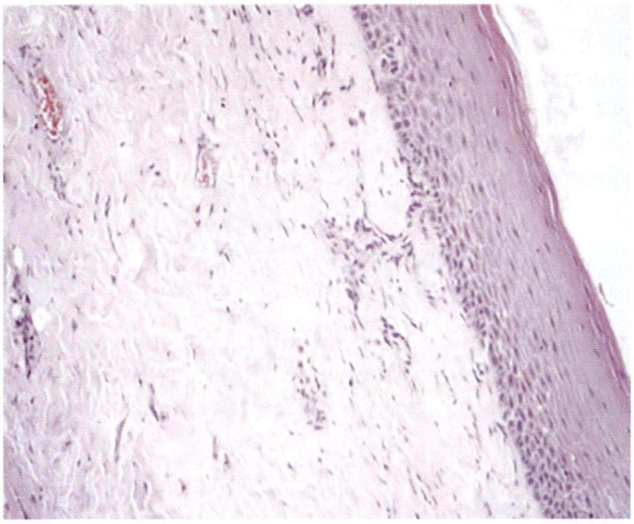

Fig. 20.7 Microscopy of oral submucous fibrosis characterized by juxtaposition of atrophic epithelium surfacing a subjacent fibrosis. (*Source:* From Usha Isaac, John S. Issac, and Noor Ahmed Khoso. Oral Surgery, Oral Medicine, Oral Pathology, Oral Radiology, and Endodontology, Volume 106, Issue 4. Elsevier 2008.)

carcinoma (SCC) of the head and neck region is the sixth most common malignancy in the world. It is also the most common malignancy in India affecting both men and women, accounting for 50%–70% of total cancer mortality.

Aetiological Factors Factors responsible for the development of OSCC include the following:

- Idiopathic
- Smoked tobacco
- Alcohol
- Betel nut and *paan* (betel leaf)
- Actinic radiation from sunlight
- HPV infection

Close to 75% of OSCCs, especially the ones involving the tonsils, base of tongue and pharynx, have strong association with oncogenic strains of **HPV** (Figs 20.8 and 20.9). In the recent years, the number of OSCC cases with HPV association has doubled and is predicted to increase exponentially in the year 2040.

One interesting fact about OSCC is its association with the development of **second primary tumours**, the incidence of which is up to 7% every year, the highest among all malignancies. The reason for such a high incidence of second primaries is the long-term exposure of the oral mucosa to the carcinogens. One school of thought is that the so-called second primaries are in fact **intraepithelial metastases**.

Survival rate is dependent on many factors. For example, patients with advanced tumour stage, multiple primaries and HPV negativity have worse prognosis when compared with early-stage, single primary and HPV-positive tumours. Hence, the most critical step in the management of OSCC is **early detection**.

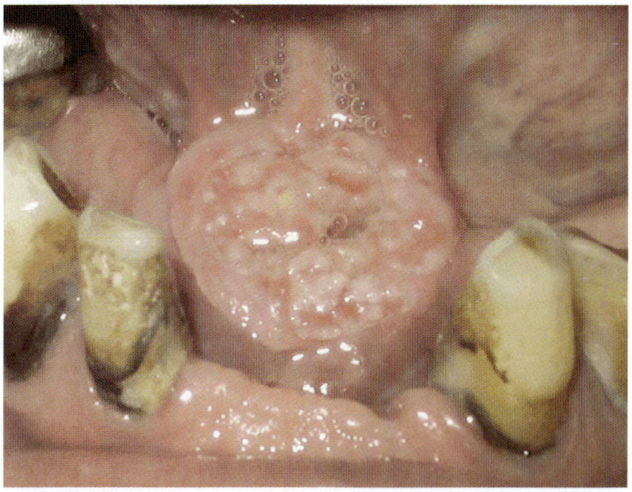

Fig. 20.8 Clinical picture of oral squamous cell carcinoma involving the floor of the mouth. (*Source:* From Silvana Canjau et al. Fluorescence influence on screening decisions for oral malignant lesions. Romanian Journal of Morphology and Embryology. 2018.)

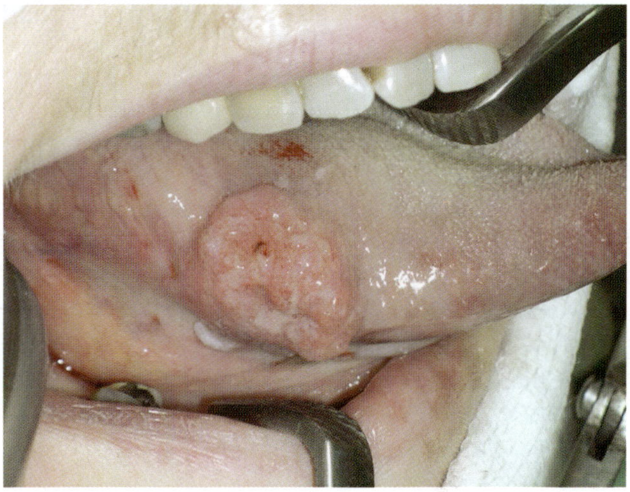

Fig. 20.9 Clinical picture of oral squamous cell carcinoma involving the lateral border of the tongue. (*Source:* From Sara Al-Mahozi, Zainab Salim, Nicholas J Malden, Crispian Scully and Victor Lopes. Tobacco habit-Associated oral disease and the negative effects on surgical outcomes. Dental Update. 2017.)

Molecular Pathology of Oral Squamous Cell Carcinoma

Oral carcinogenesis is a multistep process in which genetic changes lead to the disruption of the normal regulatory pathways that control basic cellular functions including cell division, differentiation, apoptosis and senescence. Evidence states that 6–10 genetic changes are required for the development of oral carcinogenesis. However, it should be noted that not all cases of dysplasia will progress to invasive malignancy and not all the OSCC cases will have a linear trend in development with a uniform timeline.

The most common gene mutated in OSCC is **TP53** and its associated genes like p63 and NOTCH1, whereas in

HPV-associated OSCC, the pathogenesis is similar to cervical cancer and includes the following:

- p16 overexpression
- Inactivation of p53 by E6
- Inactivation of Rb by E7

Morphology

OSCC predominantly affects anterior tongue, cheek, floor of mouth, retromolar area, gingiva or the buccal mucosa, tongue, lower lip and soft palate. In a typical case of SCC, invasive malignancy is preceded by the presence of premalignant lesions as described earlier and can have varied presentations.

In the beginning, the lesions appear as raised, firm, irregular pearly plaques or as irregular rough verrucous areas because of mucosal thickening and clinically mimic leucoplakia. Either of the patterns may have a background of leucoplakia or erythroplakia. Progression of these lesions is marked by the ulceration and formation of a protruding mass with irregular and indurated borders.

Microscopy (Fig. 20.10) Microscopically, the malignancies begin as dysplastic lesions which may not progress to carcinoma in situ before invading the underlying stroma, unlike carcinoma cervix, in which there is always a carcinoma in situ stage. The morphology of SCC ranges from well-differentiated keratinizing SCC to anaplastic or even sarcomatoid variants.

The tumours are widely infiltrative before giving rise to metastases. The pathway of spread depends on the site of primary lesion.

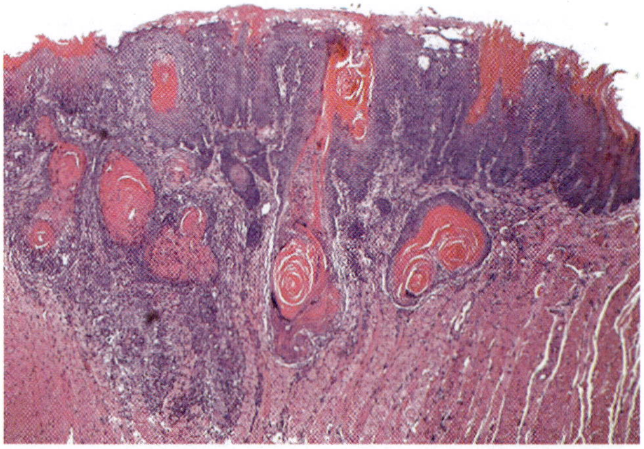

Fig. 20.10 Microscopy of oral squamous cell carcinoma characterized by nests and islands of malignant squamous cells invading the stroma. (*Source:* From Anthony Chang, Lora Hedrick Ellenson, Jonathan I. Epstein, Karen M. Frank, Matthew P. Frosch, Andrew Horvai, Aliya N. Husain, Zoltan G. Laszik, Alexander J. Lazar, Susan C. Lester, Mark W. Lingen, Tamara L. Lotan, Anirban Maitra, Alexander J. McAdam et al. Robbins Basic Pathology. Elsevier 2018.)

Cervical lymph nodes are the most common site of local metastasis, and the mediastinal lymph nodes are the most common site of distant metastasis. Lungs, liver and bones are affected in the due course.

Unfortunately, many patients present with such distant spread at the time of initial diagnosis.

II. DISEASES OF THE UPPER AIRWAYS

Upper airways include nose, pharynx and larynx. Infections and inflammations of these structures are most commonly encountered in daily practice, but most of them do not pose a threat to human lives.

NOSE

Nose is the most common site for inflammatory diseases like the common cold, which is more often due to viral infections but at times complicated by secondary bacterial infections.

Common inflammatory conditions affecting the nose are as follows:

- Infectious rhinitis
- Allergic rhinitis
- Nasal polyps
- Chronic rhinitis
- Sinusitis

Among these conditions, only nasal polyps require surgical excision if not responding to medical treatment and are submitted to histopathological examination.

Nasal Polyps

Nasal polyps are the result of repeated attacks of rhinitis, leading to the focal protrusions of nasal mucosa which can be up to 4 cm in length (Fig. 20.11). When the polyps are multiple, these can obstruct the airway and sinus drainage. Though most of the polyps show features pointing towards allergic aetiology, only less than 1% of patients have a history of allergy.

Morphology

On histological examination, nasal polyps consist of hyperplastic oedematous connective tissue with some seromucinous glands and inflammatory cells like neutrophils, eosinophils and plasma cells. In early stages, the surface is covered with normal respiratory epithelium, but later on, it undergoes metaplastic change to squamous epithelium because of constant irritation and inflammation (Fig. 20.12).

Necrotizing Lesions of the Upper Airways

Though not so common, necrotizing lesions of the upper airways are caused by varied diseases ranging from fungal

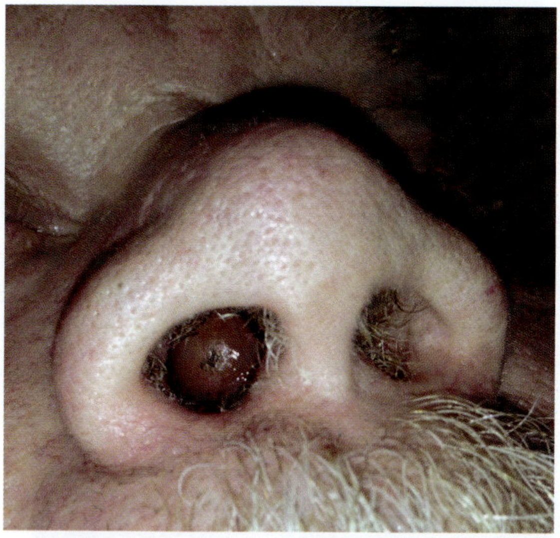

Fig. 20.11 Clinical picture of a nasal polyp. (*Source:* From Andrew H. Murr. Goldman-Cecil Medicine, 2-volume Set. Elsevier 2020.)

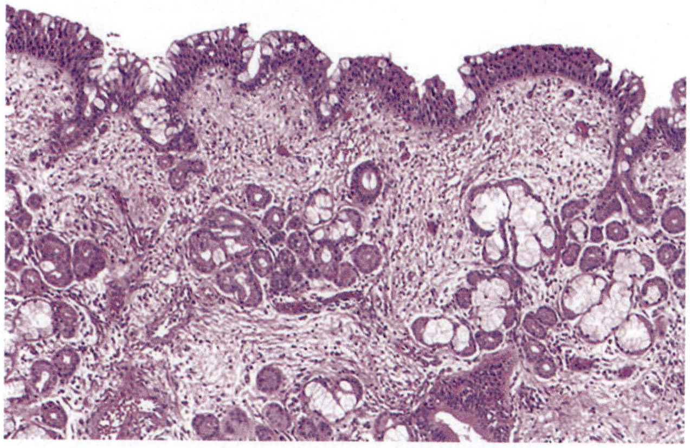

Fig. 20.12 Microscopy of nasal polyps characterized by focal squamous metaplastic change of the respiratory epithelium along with underlying loose oedematous stroma with hyperplastic mucous glands and inflammatory infiltrate. (*Source:* Seethala R.R., Pant H. (2010) Pathology of Nasal Polyps. In: Önerci T., Ferguson B. (eds) Nasal Polyposis. Springer, Berlin, Heidelberg.)

infections to aggressive malignancies. Following are the causes of necrotizing lesions of the upper airways:

a. **Invasive fungal infections** like mucormycosis in diabetics and immunocompromised individuals
b. Granulomatosis with polyangiitis, previously called Wegener granulomatosis
c. Churg–Strauss syndrome
d. Extranodal natural killer (NK)/T-cell lymphoma
e. Leishmaniasis
f. Syphilis
g. Tuberculosis
h. Leprosy
i. Rhinoscleroma
j. Cocaine-induced midline destructive disease
k. Idiopathic midline destructive disease

Any necrotizing lesions of the nose and upper airways need complete workup, as these are more often a manifestation of the underlying systemic disease.

NASOPHARYNX

Though the nasopharynx can be a site for varied pathologies, we restrict our discussion to nasopharyngeal carcinoma (NPC).

Tumours of the nose, sinuses and nasopharynx are as follows:

- Nasopharyngeal angiofibroma
- Sinonasal papilloma
- Olfactory neuroblastoma
- NUT midline carcinoma
- NPC

Nasopharyngeal Carcinoma

NPC is a rare tumour arising from the epithelium of nasopharynx. It accounts for 1% of all childhood malignancies.

The special features of NPC are as follows:

- **Distinctive geographical distribution** (common in some parts of Africa and the age group affected is different in different geographic locations)
- Strong association with **Epstein–Barr virus (EBV)**
- Close anatomic relationship to lymphoid tissue

Viral DNA studies in NPC have made it clear that EBV can infect epithelial cells and is associated with their malignant transformation. Apart from EBV infection, heredity, age and environmental factors are also implicated in the carcinogenesis. There is a high incidence of NPC within specific ethnic groups. The role of genes in the development of this tumour is supported by the presence of cytogenetic abnormalities, increased risk in patients with A2 HLA haplotype and the presence of affected first-degree relatives.

Environmental factors like diet rich in nitrosamines, smoking and chemical fumes also play an important role in the carcinogenesis of NPC.

WHO has classified NPC into the following three categories:

- **WHO 1: Well- to moderately differentiated** squamous or transitional cell carcinoma with keratin production
- **WHO 2: Nonkeratinizing carcinoma**
- **WHO 3: Undifferentiated carcinoma including lymphoepithelioma**

Morphology (Fig. 20.13)

On microscopic examination, NPC WHO 1, the keratinizing patterns, and WHO 2, the nonkeratinizing patterns, resemble the usual well-differentiated and poorly differentiated SCCs arising elsewhere. NPC WHO 3, the

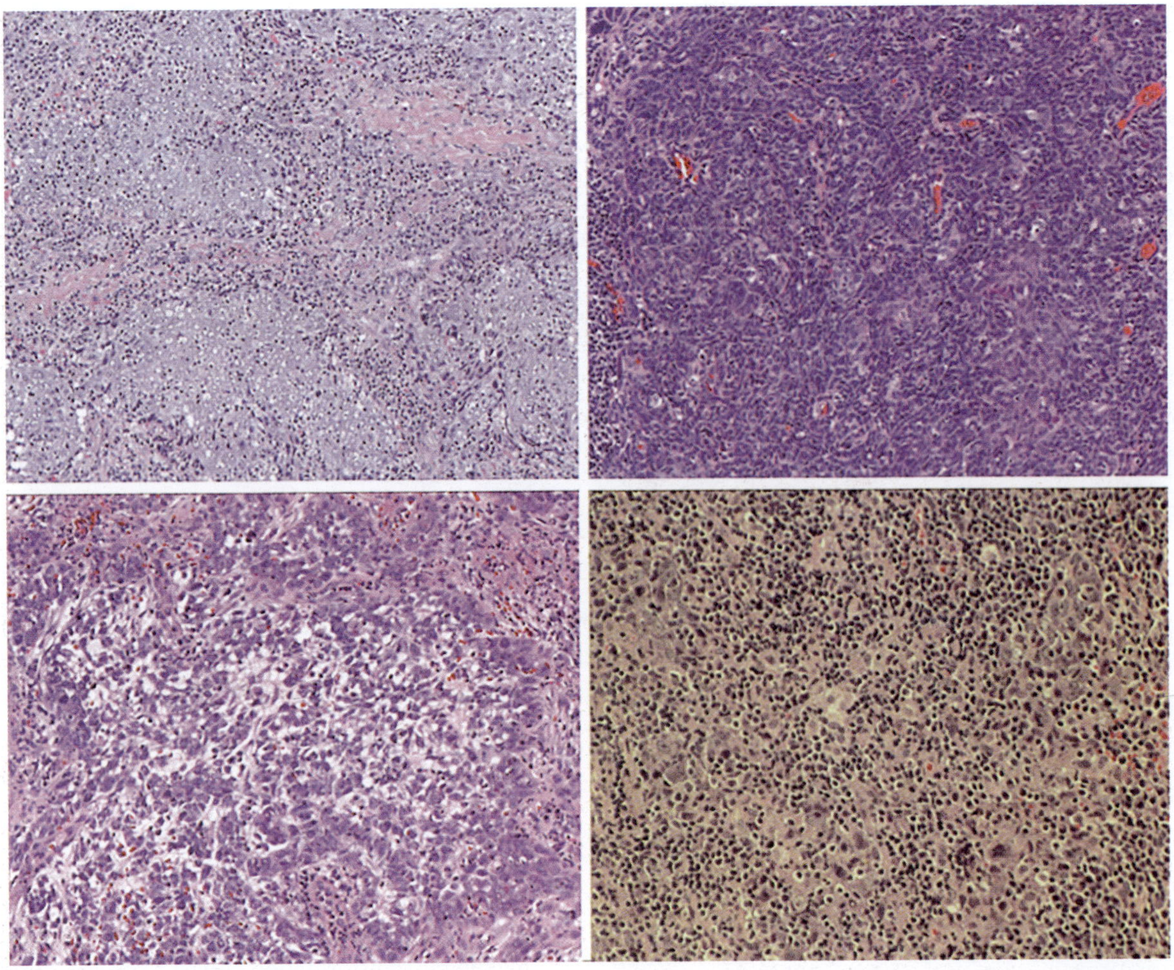

Fig. 20.13 Microscopy of nonkeratinizing nasopharyngeal carcinoma displaying syncytial architecture of epithelial cells arranged in islands and nests infiltrated with rich inflammatory infiltrate. (*Source:* From Lester D.R. Thompson. Diagnostic Immunohistochemistry. Elsevier 2019.)

undifferentiated carcinoma category, is composed of large epithelial cells with round to oval nuclei and prominent nucleoli and indistinct cell borders forming syncytium. Such syncytium of epithelial cells is admixed with non-neoplastic T lymphocytes. EBV genomes and EBV-encoded RNAs like EBER-1 and proteins like LMP-1 are identified by molecular techniques.

NPC rarely comes to medical attention before it has spread to regional lymph nodes. Enlargement and extension of the tumour lead to nasal obstruction, hearing defects, headache and cranial nerve palsies.

Radiotherapy is the treatment of choice. Nonkeratinizing variants have better prognosis with 5-year survival of 70%–98%, whereas the keratinizing variant has poorer prognosis with 5-year survival of 20%. This is attributed to the radiosensitive nature of the nonkeratinizing types when compared with keratinizing variant which is radio-resistant.

LARYNX

Most common diseases of larynx are inflammatory lesions, while tumours are uncommon.

Some of the relatively common lesions of larynx other than inflammatory diseases are listed as follows:

1. Vocal cord nodules and polyps
2. Squamous papilloma and papillomatosis
3. Laryngeal carcinoma

Vocal Cord Nodules and Polyps

Vocal cord nodules and polyps, also called **reactive nodules or polyps**, are seen in individuals who strain their vocal cords and those who smoke. These are also called '**singer's nodules**' because of their increased incidence in singers. These nodules and polyps are most often seen in adults. The nodules are bilateral (Fig. 20.14), whereas the polyps are unilateral.

Morphology

Reactive nodules are located on the true vocal cords and are small in size, up to few millimetres, smooth, rounded, sessile or pedunculated.

Histologically, they are covered by squamous epithelium (Fig. 20.15), which may become keratotic,

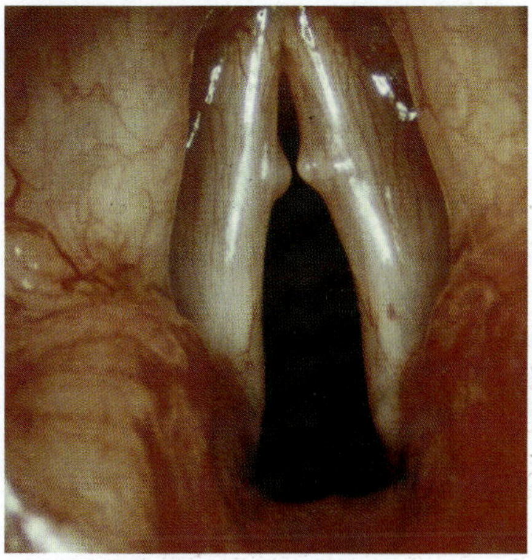

Fig. 20.14 Vocal nodules seen bilaterally in both cords.

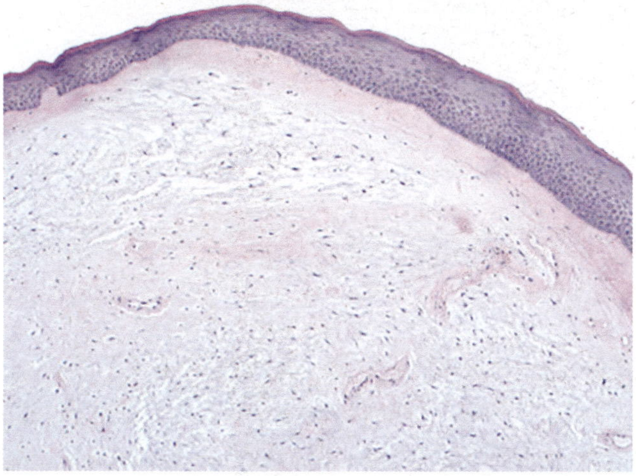

Fig. 20.15 Microscopy of laryngeal nodule displaying squamous epithelial lining and the underlying fibromyxoid stroma.

hyperplastic or even dysplastic. The central core of the nodule consists of loose myxoid stroma which may be vascular or fibrotic. Ulceration may be seen on the surface when there is impingement of opposing nodules.

These nodules and polyps are notoriously associated with voice change, leading to progressive hoarseness, but almost never turn malignant.

Squamous Papilloma and Papillomatosis

Squamous papillomas of larynx are benign tumours located on the true vocal cords. Clinically, these are seen as soft, raspberry-like growths that may grow up to 1 cm in diameter. On microscopic examination, these papillomas have finger-like projections, covered by stratified squamous epithelium enclosing the central fibrovascular core (Fig. 20.16). These may become ulcerated because of traumatic injury.

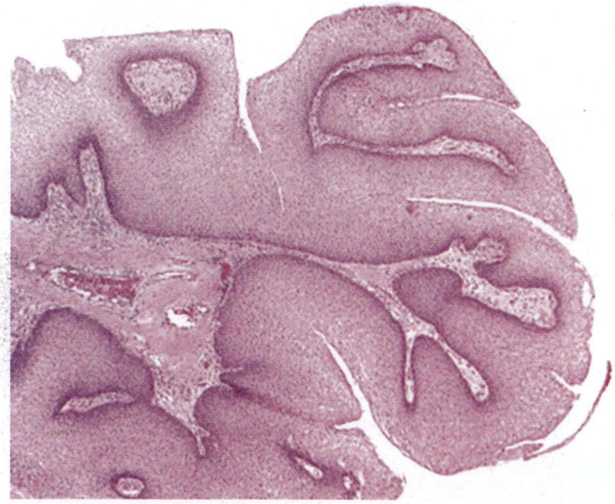

Fig. 20.16 Microscopy of laryngeal papilloma demonstrating the exophytic or papillary proliferation of squamous epithelium with central fibrovascular stroma; H&E, scanner view. (*Source:* From Ian O. Ellis, Andrew H.S. Lee, Sarah E. Pinder, Emad A. Rakha. Diagnostic Histopathology of Tumors, 2 Volume Set. Elsevier 2021.)

Laryngeal papillomatosis is a condition commonly seen in children and is characterized by the presence of multiple laryngeal papillomas. This condition is associated with **HPV type 6 and 11** infections. These papillomas generally regress spontaneously and do not turn malignant.

Laryngeal Carcinoma

Laryngeal cancers are typically SCCs with a significant cause of morbidity and mortality. A majority of the patients are men with a history of **smoking**, but cessation of smoking even up to the point of malignant transformation is helpful in reverting the epithelial changes. **Alcohol** consumption is a strong cofactor for smoking in the development of laryngeal carcinoma. Other risk factors include low-socioeconomic status, age older than 55 years, diet poor in nutrition and antioxidants, irradiation, asbestos exposure and HPV infection.

Hyperplasia–Dysplasia–Carcinoma Sequence of Laryngeal Carcinoma (Fig. 20.17) Before becoming frankly invasive, laryngeal carcinoma undergoes a spectrum of epithelial changes that range from hyperplasia, atypical hyperplasia, dysplasia and carcinoma in situ.

Not all cases of epithelial hyperplasia turn malignant. The risk is proportionate to the extent and grade of dysplasia, making histopathological examination crucial in the management of laryngeal growths.

Morphology

Gross The mucosal changes may be seen as smooth, white or erythematous focal thickenings to keratotic irregular verrucous or ulcerated lesions. These carcinomas may also have fungating appearance (Fig. 20.18).

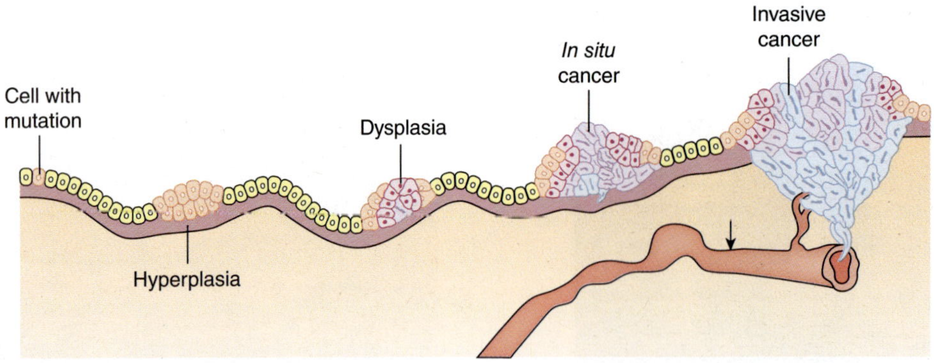

Fig. 20.17 Hyperplasia, dysplasia and carcinoma sequence model of laryngeal carcinoma. (*Source:* https://sphweb.bumc.bu.edu/otlt/mph-modules/ph/ph709_cancer/ph709_cancer_print.html)

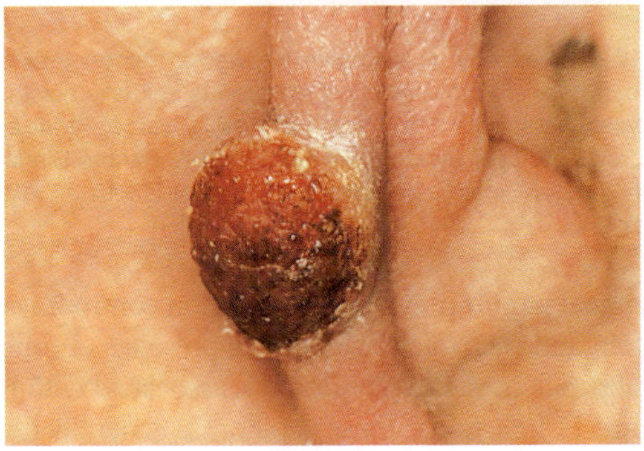

Fig. 20.18 Gross image of squamous cell carcinoma of the larynx.

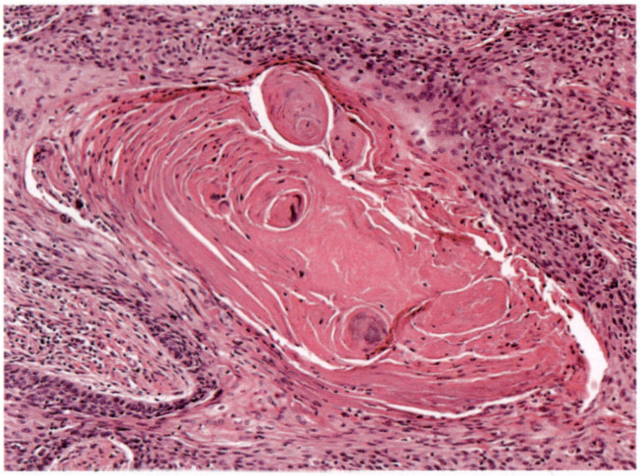

Fig. 20.19 Microscopy of laryngeal carcinoma characterized by the presence of nests of pleomorphic squamous cells infiltrating the stroma. Keratin pearls are seen; H&E, 100×. (*Source:* https://www.microscopyu.com/gallery-images/laryngeal-squamous-cell-carcinoma-at-10x-magnification)

More than 95% of laryngeal carcinomas are **SCCs**, and most of them arise from the true vocal cords, i.e. the glottis. Supraglottic cancers are less common, and subglottic cancers are the least common.

Laryngeal carcinomas are divided according to their location as follows:

a. **Glottic carcinoma**
b. **Supraglottic carcinoma**
c. **Subglottic carcinoma**
d. **Transglottic carcinoma**

The tumours limited to larynx are called intrinsic, and the ones that arise or extend outside the larynx are called extrinsic.

Microscopy (Fig. 20.19) Microscopically, the tumours look like the conventional SCCs that occur elsewhere. Areas of precancerous changes may be seen, and the degree of anaplasia is highly variable.

The clinical course of laryngeal cancer is dictated by its site of origin and its tendency to disseminate to the regional lymph nodes. Progressive continuous hoarseness, dysphagia, dyspnoea, dysphonia, cough and pain are the usual symptoms. Prognosis is dependent on the clinical staging. Early lesions may be treated with organ preservation techniques like laser surgery, microsurgery and radiotherapy. Advanced lesions require radical surgery along with chemotherapy and radiotherapy.

III. DISEASES OF THE NECK

Neck can be involved in many pathologies ranging from inflammatory to invasive malignancies. Here, we restrict our discussion to few common diseases.

THYROGLOSSAL DUCT CYST

Thyroglossal duct cyst is the most common congenital neck mass and the most common paediatric cystic neck anomaly. Thyroglossal duct is a transient epithelium-lined midline channel serving as the path of descent for the thyroid primordium from the foramen caecum. Foramen caecum is located at the junction of the anterior two-thirds and the posterior third of the tongue, beneath the thyroid cartilage where definitive thyroid development occurs.

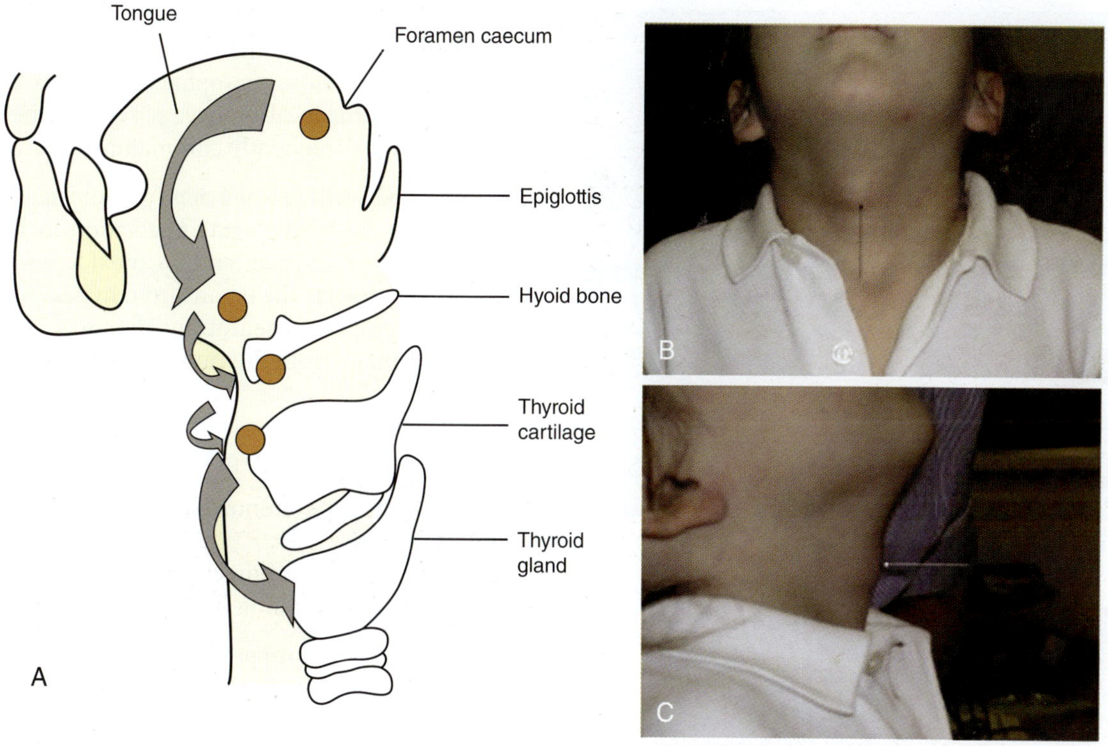

Fig. 20.20 (A) Illustration showing the migratory paths of thyroid gland and the sites of thyroglossal cyst. (B and C) Anterior and lateral views of a child with thyroglossal duct cyst. (*Source:* From Thyroglossal Duct Cyst. Elsevier Point of Care 2022.)

If a portion of the thyroglossal cyst persists, cystic lesions may arise following repeated cycles of infection and/or inflammation because it is lined by secretory epithelium. Cysts can arise anywhere along the course of the duct (Fig. 20.20).

Morphology

The cysts generally range in size from 1 to 4 cm in diameter and are lined by stratified squamous or pseudostratified ciliated columnar epithelium, with or without ectopic thyroid gland tissue and/or lymphoid tissue in the wall (Fig. 20.21). Occasionally, transitional lining is present. Accumulation of the secretions and debris causes enlargement of the cysts.

The cyst is treated by excision. Though malignant transformation is rare, it has been reported.

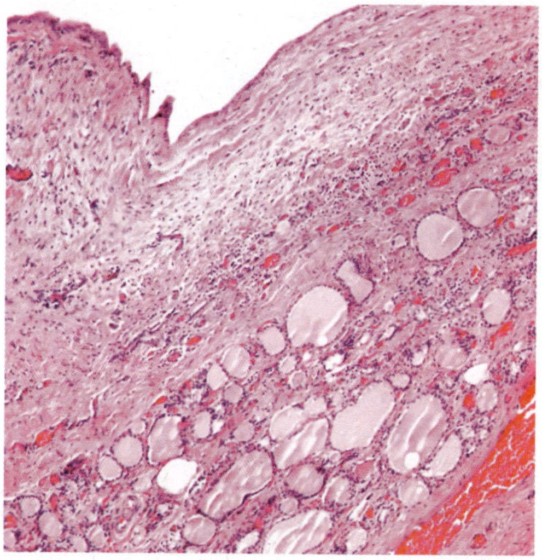

Fig. 20.21 Microscopy of thyroglossal duct cyst displaying a cyst with respiratory columnar epithelial lining, fibrous wall and benign thyroid tissue in the cyst wall. (*Source:* From Thyroglossal Duct Cyst. Elsevier Point of Care 2022.)

BRANCHIAL CYST

Branchial cysts are benign cysts located on the upper lateral aspect of the neck along the sternocleidomastoid muscle (Fig. 20.22). These are commonly seen in young individuals aged 20–40 years, and a majority of branchial cysts arise from second branchial arch remnants.

Morphology

These are well-circumscribed, slowly enlarging cysts ranging 2–5 cm in diameter. The cysts may contain watery or mucinous fluid or fluid with cellular debris made of desquamated cells. The cysts are lined by stratified squamous epithelium or pseudostratified columnar epithelium. Cyst wall usually contains collections of lymphoid tissue most often with germinal centres (Fig. 20.23).

These cysts can be treated by excision and rarely undergo malignant transformation.

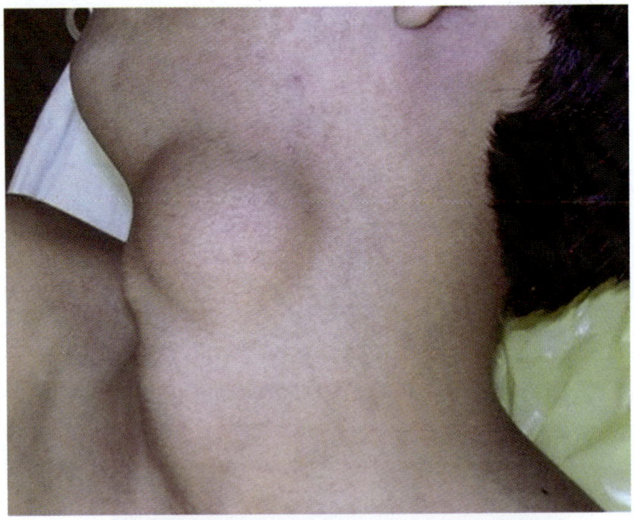

Fig. 20.22 Clinical picture of a branchial cyst.

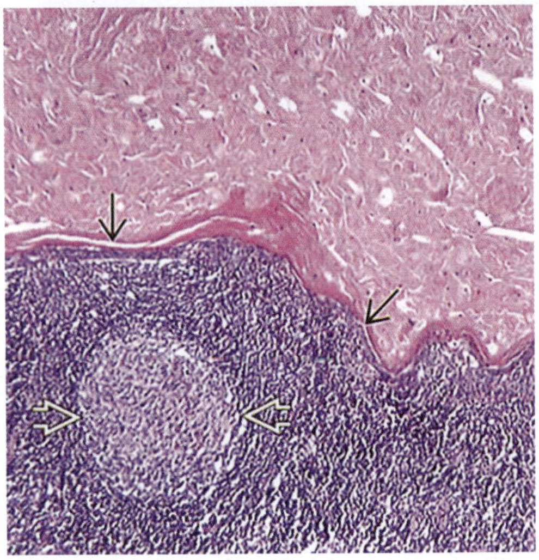

Fig. 20.23 Microscopy of branchial cyst with prominent lymphoid tissue in the wall. (*Source:* https://basicmedicalkey.com/branchial-cleft-cyst-3/)

PARAGANGLIOMA

Paragangliomas, also called **carotid body tumours**, are rare tumours that arise from paraganglia. Paraganglia are neuroendocrine cell clusters associated with the sympathetic and parasympathetic nervous systems. Because of the widespread location of paraganglia, paraganglioma can be seen in many locations. However, the most common location of paraganglioma is within the **adrenal medulla** (pheochromocytomas) and 70% of extra-adrenal paragangliomas arise in the head and neck regions.

There are two preferred locations of paraganglioma:

1. **Paravertebral paraganglia** – in organs of Zuckerkandl and bladder. In this location, tumours have sympathetic connections and are positive for chromaffin, a stain used for detection of catecholamines.
2. **In relationship to the great vessels of the head and neck** – from the aorticopulmonary chain including the carotid bodies, aortic bodies, jugulotympanic ganglia, ganglion nodosum of the vagus and clusters located in the oral cavity, nose, nasopharynx, larynx and orbit. Tumours in this location have parasympathetic innervation and are frequently chromaffin-negative.

Carotid body, which originates from the neural crest, is important in the body's acute adaptation to fluctuating concentrations of oxygen, carbon dioxide and pH. The carotid body protects the organs from hypoxic damage by releasing appropriate neurotransmitters. Carotid body tumours originate from the carotid body.

Pathogenesis

There are three different types of carotid body tumours:

1. Familial – most common; constitutes 85% of carotid body tumours
2. Sporadic – seen in younger patients
3. Hyperplastic – common in chronic hypoxia

The pathogenesis of paraganglioma is not completely understood. The mutation that is commonly seen in association with the tumour is the loss-of-function mutation of the genes encoding **succinate dehydrogenase** or SDH subunits or cofactors or proteins that are part of mitochondrial oxidative phosphorylation.

Morphology

Gross The carotid body tumour arises close to or enveloping the bifurcation of the common carotid artery and usually grows up to 6 cm in diameter. The tumour appears red–pink to brown in colour.

Microscopy (Fig. 20.24) Microscopic features of all paragangliomas are the same irrespective of their location. The tumour cells are arranged in their characteristic ***Zellballen pattern***, in which nests of round to oval chief cells are surrounded by delicate vascular septae. The supporting stromal cells in the periphery of the nests called sustentacular cells are typical. Individual tumour cells have abundant clear or granular cytoplasm and round to ovoid, occasionally vesicular nuclei. Pleomorphism and mitotic figures are not common findings. The chief cells are positive for neuroendocrine markers like synaptophysin, chromogranin, neuron-specific enolase, CD56 and CD57. The sustentacular cells are positive for S-100. The presence of neuroendocrine granules can be seen by electron microscopy.

Clinical Features

In general, carotid body tumours are painless, slow-growing masses in people aged between 40 and 60 years. These tumours are known for their recurrence following incomplete excision. These also metastasize to regional nodes and

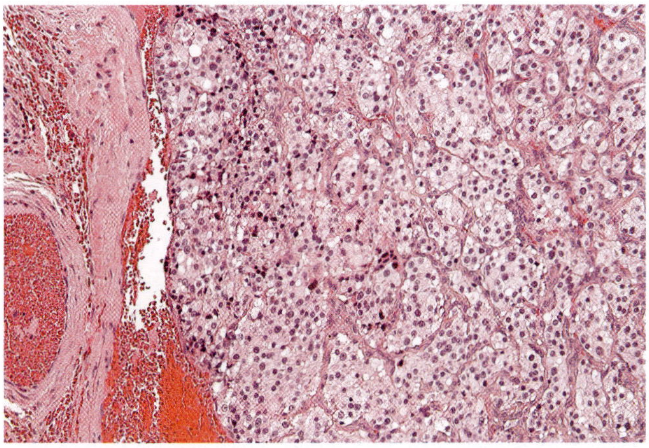

Fig. 20.24 Microscopy of paraganglioma. (*Source:* https://www.google.com/search?q=carotid+body+tumors+microscopy&rlz=1C1CHZL_enIN707IN710&source=lnms&tbm=isch&sa=X&ved=2ahUKEwju8cTKsfzsAhWOyzgGHU0vC6cQ_AUoAXoECA0QAw&biw=1366&bih=600#imgrc=589p2vdZGfZhuM)

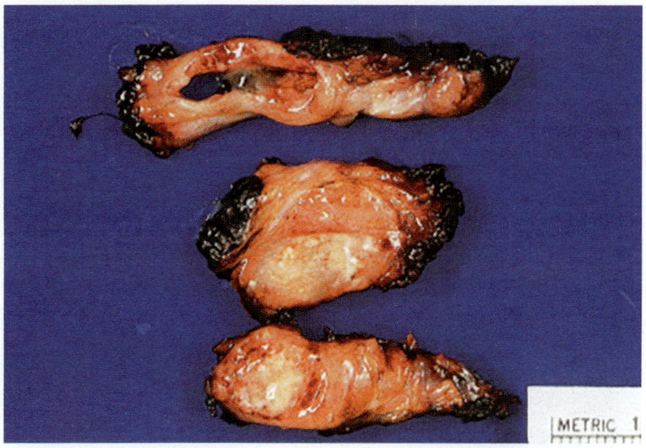

Fig. 20.25 Gross appearance of suppurative sialadenitis with pus formation. (*Source:* From Jonathan B. McHugh. Rosai and Ackerman's Surgical Pathology-2 Volume Set. Elsevier 2018.)

distant sites. Bitter facts are that there are no histological predictors of malignant behaviour and at least half of the tumours are fatal because of their locally infiltrative nature.

IV. DISEASES OF THE SALIVARY GLANDS

There are three major salivary glands, parotid, submandibular and sublingual, and numerous minor salivary glands widely distributed throughout the mucosa of the oral cavity. Salivary glands can be affected by inflammatory or neoplastic diseases, and few common ones are described here.

NON-NEOPLASTIC LESIONS

Sialadenitis

Sialadenitis is inflammation of salivary glands, usually the major salivary glands. The most commonly affected salivary gland is the parotid gland. The disease can be acute or chronic.

Sialadenitis may be triggered by trauma, viral or bacterial infection or autoimmune disease. Following are the predisposing factors for sialadenitis:

- Sialolithiasis
- Decreased salivary flow because of dehydration, post-surgical state and drugs
- Autoimmune disorders
- Viral infections; mumps is the most common cause of viral sialadenitis
- Bacterial infections like streptococcal and staphylococcal infections
- Poor oral hygiene
- Malnutrition

Acute suppurative sialadenitis is generally caused by *Staphylococcus aureus*, *Streptococcus* species and Gram-negative bacteria (Fig. 20.25). Acute sialadenitis may present itself as a red, painful and tender swelling. Histopathology shows infiltration of salivary glands by polymorphs. Once an abscess has formed, surgical drainage may be necessary.

Chronic sialadenitis is typically less painful and presents as a recurrent swelling usually after meals, without features of acute inflammation. Histopathology shows markedly hyperplastic lymphoid infiltrates with loss of salivary gland acini and infiltration of lymphocytes in the ducts.

Sialadenitis generally resolves with medications but, in some cases, may develop complications such as with the development of abscess and dental decay.

Sialolithiasis

Sialolithiasis is a common disease of the major salivary glands and is caused by the formation of sialoliths, which are calcified masses that develop in the intra- or extraglandular duct system. Sialoliths form as a result of mineralization of debris that has accumulated in the duct lumen. Nidus of formation is organic material such as bacteria, mucous and desquamated epithelial cells. Calcium salts are precipitated on the nidus because of supersaturation and deficit of crystallization inhibitors.

Morphology

Microscopic features are dilated ducts with squamous metaplasia or calculi, variable chronic inflammation with destruction of acini and fibrosis (Fig. 20.26).

Patients present with pain and swelling at mealtime, and in some cases there may be purulent ductal discharge. The usual diagnostic modalities are sialogram and ultrasonogram.

Treatment is surgical removal of calculus or gland. In recent years, disintegration of calculi with shock wave lithotripsy is used in the conservative management of sialolithiasis.

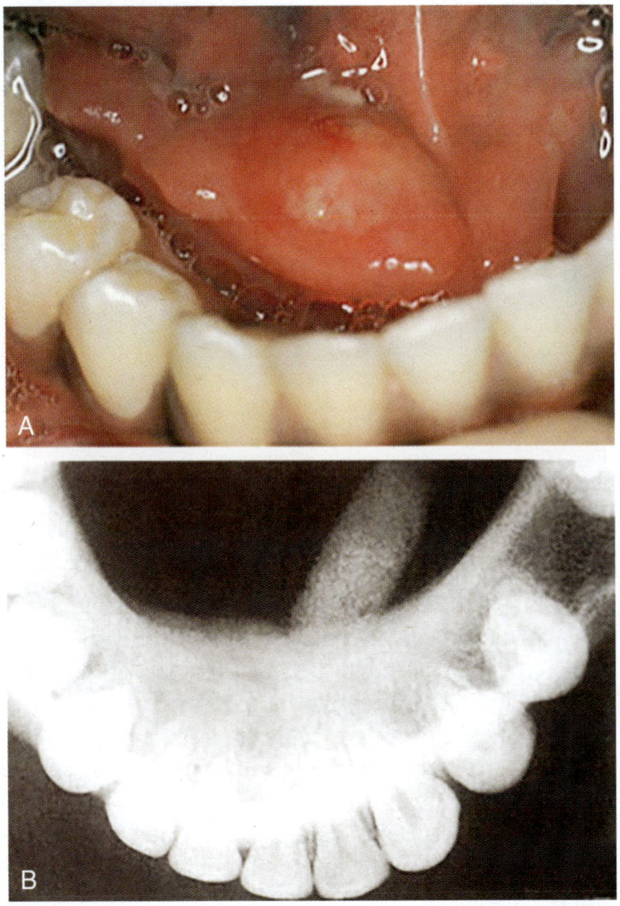

Fig. 20.26 Salivary calculus. (A) This sialolith obstructing a salivary duct is observed on the floor of the mouth. (B) A dental radiograph of the sublingual space reveals the size and location of the salivary calculus. (*Source:* From Brian Martin, Heather Baumhardt, Alene D'Alesio and Katelyn Woods. Zitelli and Davis' Atlas of Pediatric Physical Diagnosis. Elsevier 2018.)

Mucocoele

This is the most common pathology of the salivary glands and is a reactive process which occurs because of mucus extravasation. Common sites affected are lower lip, floor of the mouth and ventral tongue. Trauma to the salivary gland duct is the cause for mucus extravasation.

Morphology

Grossly, mucocoele is a nodular mass resembling gelatinous material.

Microscopic examination (Fig. 20.27) reveals the presence of pseudocyst cavity containing mucin, foamy histiocytes, neutrophils and granulation tissue along with obstructive changes in the salivary gland parenchyma.

Ranula: Ranula is the mucocoele located on the floor of mouth arising from the sublingual gland (Fig. 20.28).
Plunging ranula: This term is used if the mucin from an enlarged ranula dissects through the mylohyoid muscle to involve the cervical area.

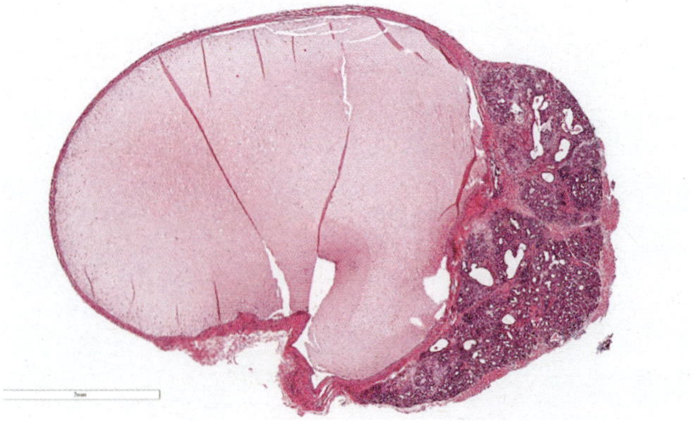

Fig. 20.27 Microscopy of mucocoele. Microscopy showing a fully excised mucocoele with extravasated mucin and the feeding minor salivary gland. (*Source:* From Nathan Lee, Tony Ng. Oral cavity & oropharynx: Salivary gland tumors & processes. PathologyOutlines.com, 2019-2022.)

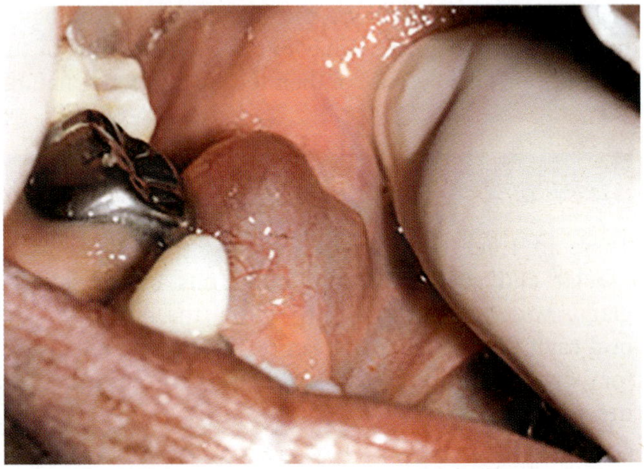

Fig. 20.28 Clinical picture of ranula seen as bluish fluctuant swelling on the floor of the mouth. (*Source:* From Brian Martin, Heather Baumhardt, Alene D'Alesio, Katelyn Woods. Zitelli and Davis' Atlas of Pediatric Physical Diagnosis. Elsevier 2018.)

NEOPLASMS

Though salivary glands have simple histology, they give rise to more than 30 histopathologically different neoplasms. A simpler version of classification of salivary gland neoplasms is given in Table 20.2.

A majority of the tumours arise from the parotid gland, and the remaining arise from the submandibular gland and only a small percentage of tumours affect sublingual glands and minor salivary glands. On the other hand, only less than 30% of parotid tumours are malignant whereas a majority of minor salivary gland tumours are malignant. Hence, it can be stressed that '*the likelihood of a salivary gland tumour being malignant is inversely proportionate to the size of the gland*'.

We restrict our discussion to common salivary gland neoplasms.

Table 20.2 WHO Classification of Salivary Gland Neoplasms, 2017[a]

Category of Tumours	Common Tumours
Benign	Pleomorphic adenoma Warthin tumour Oncocytoma Myoepithelioma Basal cell adenoma
Borderline	Sialoblastoma
Malignant	Mucoepidermoid carcinoma Acinic cell carcinoma Adenoid cystic carcinoma Secretory carcinoma Epithelial–myoepithelial carcinoma Polymorphous adenocarcinoma Carcinoma ex pleomorphic adenoma
Other epithelial lesions	
Soft-tissue lesions	
Haematolymphoid tumours	

[a]Simpler version of WHO classification, 2017.

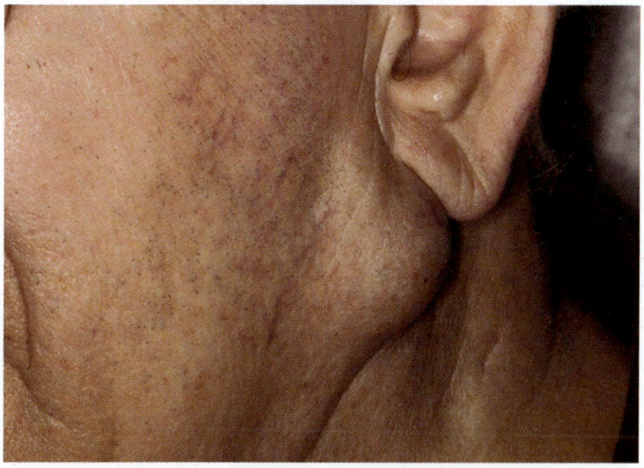

Fig. 20.29 Pleomorphic adenoma. Firm nodular mass of the left parotid gland lifting the earlobe at the angle of the mandible.

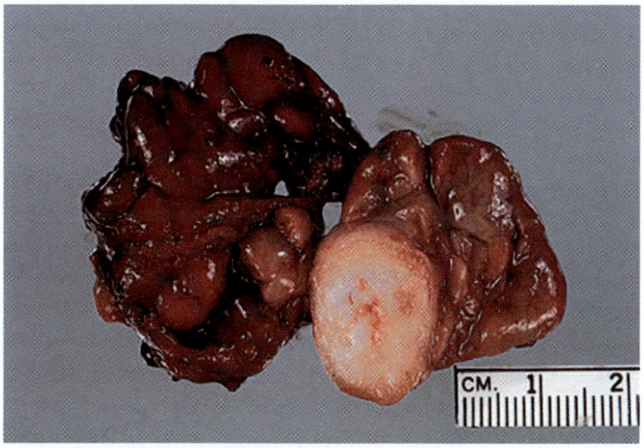

Fig. 20.30 Gross morphology of pleomorphic adenoma displaying a solid cut surface with a glistening appearance. (*Source:* From Jonathan B. McHugh. Rosai and Ackerman's Surgical Pathology-2 Volume Set. Elsevier 2018.)

Pleomorphic Adenoma

This is the most common benign neoplasm of the salivary glands and is also referred to as benign mixed tumour. It represents 45%–75% of all salivary gland tumours and 70%–80% of benign salivary gland tumours. This tumour affects superficial lobe of the parotid gland and is relatively uncommon in minor salivary glands. The exact aetiology of pleomorphic adenoma is unknown, but possible factors include radiation exposure and simian virus, SV40. Microscopically, pleomorphic adenoma has a highly variable appearance and hence the term 'pleomorphic'. It is composed of a mixture of ductal cells and myoepithelial cells, thereby showing differentiation towards epithelial and myoepithelial lineage.

Morphology

Gross Pleomorphic adenoma presents as a single, firm, mobile, well-circumscribed mass on gross examination (Fig. 20.29). Though these adenomas are encapsulated, there may be weak points in the capsule through which the tumour may protrude outside by forming pseudopods. This makes complete excision of the tumour difficult and also results in recurrences when simple enucleation of the tumour is attempted. Its colour may vary from whitish tan to grey to bluish, and its size may range from few millimetres to gigantic forms. The tumour may show bluish glistening areas because of the presence of cartilaginous tissue (Fig. 20.30). Degenerative and cystic changes may be seen on the cut surface. **Recurrent tumours tend to present as multiple nodules** of variable sizes.

Microscopy The prominent microscopic feature is the heterogeneity of tumours. The epithelial derivatives are ductal epithelial cells and myoepithelial cells arranged in ducts, acini, tubules, solid, cystic spaces, strands and sheets of cells (Fig. 20.31). These cells are set in a **chondromyxoid stromal** background containing islands of **cartilage** and even bone in rare cases. Usually, epithelial dysplasia or mitotic activity is not seen.

Pleomorphic adenoma usually presents as a slow-growing painless mass which may have been present for many years. Parotid tumours, in general, have the tendency to lift the ear lobe. Symptoms and signs depend on the location. With large tumours, patients present with facial nerve weakness. Pleomorphic adenoma in the deep

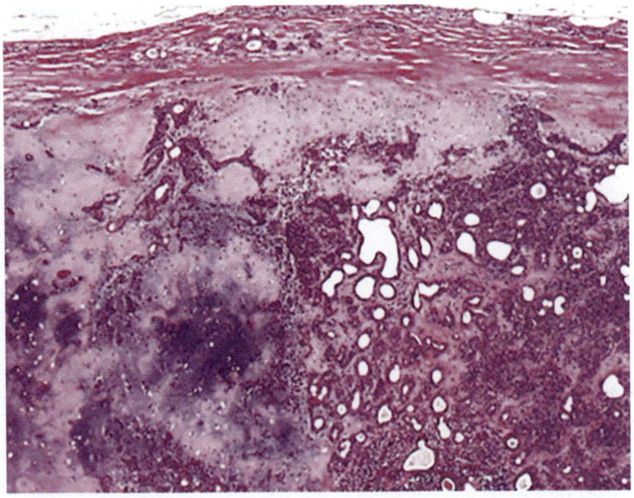

Fig. 20.31 Microscopy of pleomorphic adenoma showing biphasic components, epithelial and mesenchymal (cartilaginous stroma). (*Source:* From Jennifer R. Wang, Diana M. Bell, Ehab Y. Hanna. Cummings Otolaryngology. Elsevier 2021.)

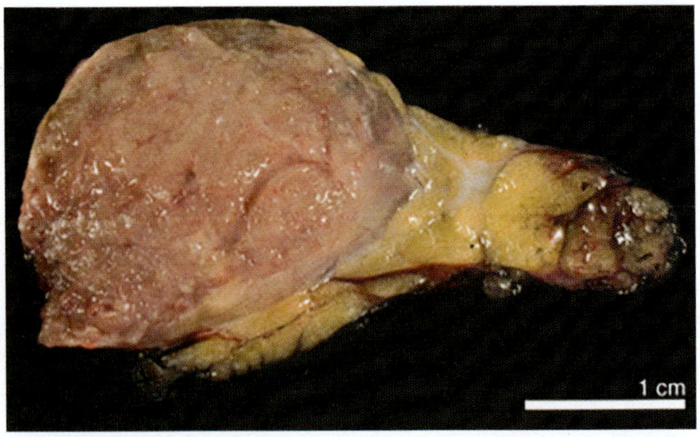

Fig. 20.32 Gross morphology of Warthin tumour. The presence of cystic spaces is characteristic of this tumour. (*Source:* From Jonathan B. McHugh. Rosai and Ackerman's Surgical Pathology-2 Volume Set. Elsevier 2018.)

lobe of the parotid gland may present as an oral retrotonsillar mass or parapharyngeal space tumour. Rapid enlargement of a tumour nodule should raise concern about the development of malignancy.

Carcinoma ex pleomorphic adenoma, also called malignant mixed tumour, is defined as a malignant neoplasm that develops in association with a benign primary or recurrent pleomorphic adenoma. The malignancy is usually an adenocarcinoma or an undifferentiated carcinoma. The tumour is highly infiltrative and tends to completely replace the pleomorphic adenoma at places. Occasionally, the entire lesion may be replaced, in which case, it would be difficult to justify the diagnosis.

Warthin Tumour

Warthin tumour, also referred to as 'papillary cystadenoma lymphomatosum', is a benign tumour and the second most common salivary gland neoplasm. This tumour almost always arises in the **parotid gland** and affects males more often than females. Around 10% of tumours are bilateral and 10% are multifocal. The tumour has a very strong association with **smoking**.

Morphology

***Gross** (Fig. 20.32)* Warthin tumours range in size from 2 to 5 cm. These are encapsulated and lobulated, with **multicystic** areas filled with mucinous or serous secretion. The overlying skin may be fixed, and the tumours may undergo haemorrhagic infarction, especially following fine-needle aspiration.

***Microscopy** (Fig. 20.33)* The hallmark feature of Warthin tumour is the presence of cystic spaces lined by a double layer of epithelial cells resting on a dense

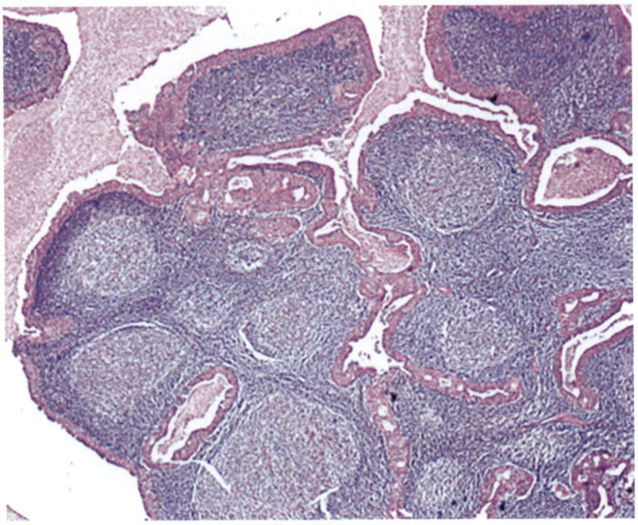

Fig. 20.33 Microscopic picture of Warthin tumour. (*Source:* From Jonathan B. McHugh. Rosai and Ackerman's Surgical Pathology-2 Volume Set. Elsevier 2018.)

lymphoid stroma containing variable germinal centres. The cystic spaces are narrowed by polypoid projections of lymphoepithelial elements. The double layer is distinctive; the upper layer is composed of palisading columnar cells with abundant, granular, eosinophilic cytoplasm, whereas the lower layer is composed of cuboidal to polygonal cells (Fig. 20.34). The upper-layer cells have numerous mitochondria and hence have the typical granular oncocytic appearance. There may be areas of squamous metaplasia.

Only 2% of Warthin tumours recur, and malignant transformation is very rare.

Mucoepidermoid Carcinoma

Mucoepidermoid carcinoma (MEC) is the most common malignant tumour of salivary glands and represents 15% of all salivary gland tumours. Parotid gland is the most

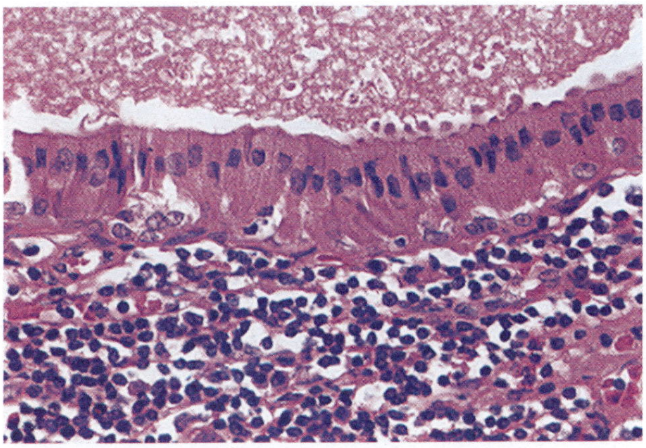

Fig. 20.34 Microscopic picture of Warthin tumour. High-power view of the lining of one of the cysts of Warthin tumour. The epithelium is tall and oxyphilic, with a discontinuous layer of small cells at the base. The stroma beneath contains a monotonous lymphocytic infiltrate. (*Source:* From Jonathan B. McHugh. Rosai and Ackerman's Surgical Pathology-2 Volume Set. Elsevier 2018.)

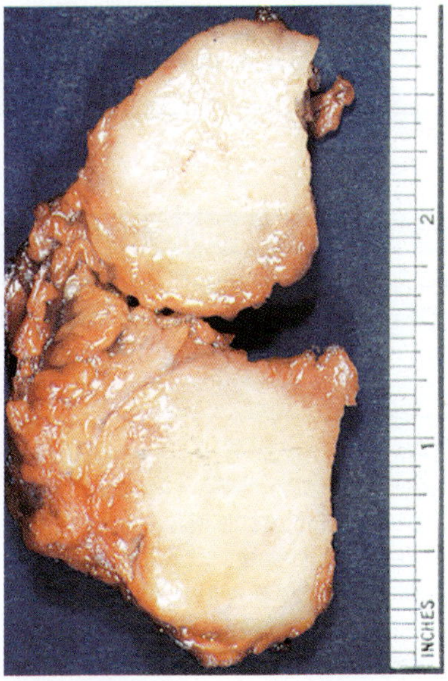

Fig. 20.35 Gross appearance of mucoepidermoid carcinoma. This particular tumour is entirely solid, without the cystic formations commonly seen in low-grade lesions. (*Source:* From Jonathan B. McHugh. Rosai and Ackerman's Surgical Pathology-2 Volume Set. Elsevier 2018.)

common site. In at least half of the cases, a balanced translocation t(11;19) (q21;13) resulting in the fusion of MECT1 and MAML2 genes, is believed to be the key factor in the tumorigenesis by activating NOTCH and cAMP-dependent signalling pathways.

Morphology

Gross (Fig. 20.35) MECs can grow up to 8 cm. Though these appear circumscribed, they lack well-defined capsule and have infiltrative borders. On the cut section, the tumours are grey–white and often contain microcystic spaces filled with mucin.

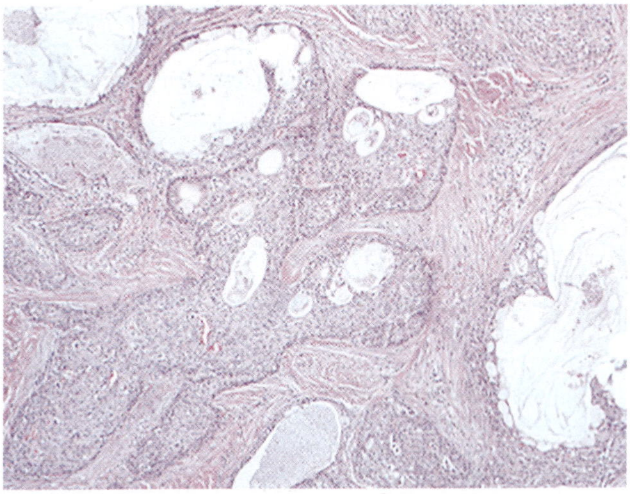

Fig. 20.36 Microscopic picture of low-grade mucoepidermoid carcinoma with predominant cystic areas. (*Source:* From Jonathan B. McHugh. Rosai and Ackerman's Surgical Pathology-2 Volume Set. Elsevier 2018.)

Microscopy The tumour is composed of cords, sheets, cystic spaces and clusters of mucous squamous, intermediate and clear cells, hence the name mucoepidermoid. The tumour cell appearance may range from bland to highly anaplastic. MECs are subclassified into low-, intermediate- and high-grade types.

Low grade: Mucinous and intermediate cells with bland nuclei form glandular spaces (Fig. 20.36).
High grade: Solid and infiltrative growth pattern of atypical epidermoid and intermediate cells is seen along with cytoplasmic clearing with a small number of mucinous cells. The intracystic component is less than 20%.

The course and prognosis of tumours depend on their grade. Low-grade tumours may invade local tissues, whereas high-grade tumours are widely invasive with distant spread and are associated with poorer prognosis. Other poor prognostic factors include male gender, older age, extraglandular extension, vascular invasion, presence of necrosis and a high mitotic rate.

Adenoid Cystic Carcinoma

Adenoid cystic carcinoma (ACC) is not a common tumour and is more often seen in minor salivary glands, especially the glands in the palate. The striking histopathological feature of the tumour is the presence of cribriform or adenoid cystic pattern. The characteristic clinical feature of the tumour is the high incidence of perineural invasion and spread. ACC also has a high incidence of recurrence and distance metastasis.

Acinic Cell Carcinoma

Acinic cell carcinoma is an uncommon malignancy of salivary gland, mainly affecting major salivary glands. It can be bilateral or multifocal. The characteristic histopathological finding is the presence of serous acinar cells with vacuolated cytoplasm, with little or no anaplasia and mitoses. The tumour has a less aggressive clinical course, with a very rare recurrence rate and a low incidence of metastasis. So, these are associated with good 5-year survival rates.

SELF-ASSESSMENT

Multiple Choice Questions

1. A 45-year-old male patient presents with a recently diagnosed OSCC at the base of the tongue. Biopsy results show HPV-positive status. Which of the following is most likely about his prognosis compared to HPV-negative OSCC patients?
   A. Poorer prognosis because of higher metastatic potential
   B. Similar prognosis with no significant difference
   C. Better prognosis and responsiveness to treatment
   D. Unpredictable prognosis because of variable genetic mutations
2. A 55-year-old woman with a history of tobacco use presents with a white patch on her buccal mucosa. Biopsy indicates dysplastic changes. This lesion is most likely:
   A. Leukoplakia
   B. Erythroplakia
   C. Lichen planus
   D. Candidiasis
3. In the study of OSCC, mutations in which gene are most commonly implicated in the pathogenesis of the disease?
   A. BRCA1
   B. KRAS
   C. TP53
   D. EGFR
4. A 60-year-old man presents with a 2-cm firm, painless solid mass in the parotid gland. Fine-needle aspiration cytology suggests a benign lesion. Which of the following is the most likely diagnosis?
   A. Warthin tumour
   B. Mucoepidermoid carcinoma
   C. Adenoid cystic carcinoma
   D. Pleomorphic adenoma
5. A patient with a long-standing history of leukoplakia develops a lesion on the lateral border of the tongue. The biopsy reveals invasive squamous cells. This finding indicates a transition from:
   A. Hyperkeratosis to OSCC
   B. Leukoplakia to OSCC
   C. Erythroplakia to OSCC
   D. Lichen planus to OSCC
6. A 50-year-old patient presents with a rapidly enlarging mass in the lower lip. Biopsy shows a mix of squamous, mucous and intermediate cells. This histological finding is characteristic of:
   A. Squamous cell carcinoma
   B. Mucoepidermoid carcinoma
   C. Adenoid cystic carcinoma
   D. Acinic cell carcinoma
7. A pathology report of a salivary gland tumour notes the presence of a t(11;19) translocation. This finding is most commonly associated with which of the following tumours?
   A. Warthin tumour
   B. Mucoepidermoid carcinoma
   C. Adenoid cystic carcinoma
   D. Pleomorphic adenoma
8. A patient diagnosed with OSCC shows a highly keratinized tumour with a well-differentiated pattern. This type of OSCC is most likely associated with:
   A. HPV infection
   B. Chronic alcohol abuse
   C. Sun exposure
   D. Genetic predisposition
9. In a patient with OSCC, which of the following is a strong indicator of poor prognosis?
   A. Presence of a well-differentiated tumour
   B. HPV-positive status
   C. Location on the floor of the mouth
   D. Early-stage diagnosis
10. A biopsy from a salivary gland tumour shows a cribriform pattern with perineural invasion. This pattern is characteristic of:
    A. Mucoepidermoid carcinoma
    B. Adenoid cystic carcinoma
    C. Acinic cell carcinoma
    D. Pleomorphic adenoma

Answers

1. (C); 2. (A); 3. (C); 4. (D); 5. (B); 6. (B); 7. (B); 8. (B); 9. (C); 10. (B)

Self-Assessment Questions

1. A 62-year-old man presented with complaints of a non-healing ulcer on the floor of the mouth for the past 6 months. He gave a history of tobacco chewing for the past 40 years. On examination, the ulcer was 2 × 1 cm in size and had an irregular border with heaped up margins. Cervical lymph nodes were enlarged, hard and fixed. What is your provisional diagnosis? Discuss the aetiopathogenesis and morphology of the disease.
2. A 32-year-old man presented with a painless white patch over the buccal mucosa. What is your provisional diagnosis? Discuss the pathology of the disease.
3. A 42-year-old man presented with a red, velvety, flat lesion in the oral cavity that could not be attributed to any pathology. What is your provisional diagnosis? Discuss the pathology of the disease.

Answers

1. Squamous cell carcinoma
2. Leukoplakia
3. Erythroplakia

Topics for Self-Directed Learning

1. Ameloblastoma
2. Odontogenic keratocyst
3. Haematolymphoid tumours of the oral cavity
4. Salivary duct carcinoma
5. WHO classification of salivary gland carcinoma
6. Epithelial–myoepithelial carcinoma
7. Actinomycosis of the head and neck region
8. Oral manifestations of HIV infection
9. Clinical manifestations of oral viral diseases
10. Inverted papilloma

The Gastrointestinal Tract

21

Gayathri Devi Thanigaimani

PA 24.2 Describe the aetiology, pathogenesis, pathology, microbiology, clinical and microscopic features of **peptic ulcer disease.**

PA 24.4 Describe the aetiology, pathogenesis and pathological features of **carcinoma of the stomach.**

PA 24.5 Describe the aetiology, pathogenesis and pathological features of **tuberculosis of the intestine.**

PA 24.6 Describe the aetiology, pathogenesis, and pathological and distinguishing features of **inflammatory bowel disease.**

PA 24.7 Describe the aetiology, pathogenesis, and pathological and distinguishing features of **carcinoma of the colon.**

CHAPTER OUTLINE

ANATOMY AND HISTOLOGY

The gastrointestinal (GI) tract is the alimentary canal that extends from the mouth at the upper end to the anus at the lower end. It is anatomically divided into oesophagus, stomach, small intestine and large intestine. The primary function of the GI tract includes food digestion, absorption of nutrients and expulsion of waste. These activities are carried out in conjunction with the accessory digestive organs such as pancreas, liver, salivary gland and gall bladder. Each part of the tract has unique anatomy and histology, and the pathology of disorders of each part is also different. Hence, these have different clinical presentations, enabling the clinician to evaluate the pathology.

BASIC PATTERN OF THE ALIMENTARY TRACT

The wall of the entire GI tract is lined by four layers, namely mucosa, submucosa, muscularis externa and serosa. The innermost layer is the mucosa, which is further subdivided into epithelium, lamina propria and muscularis mucosae. The submucosa consists of loose areolar tissue which fixes the mucosa onto the underlying muscle layer. It also contains lymphatic channels and blood vessels that branch into the mucosa and the muscularis. The muscularis externa, generally composed of smooth muscles, consists of an inner layer of circular muscle and an outer layer of longitudinal muscle. The layers are made up of smooth muscles and show some regional variations and thickening, forming sphincters. The outer serosa is the visceral peritoneum covering these structures.

The GI tract has a rich nerve supply in the form of two plexuses – the submucosal plexus of Meissner in the submucosa and the myenteric plexus of Auerbach, between the two layers of muscularis externa. The plexus contains both afferent and efferent neurons.

OESOPHAGUS

The oesophagus is a muscular tube, about **25 cm in length**, extending from the lower end of the pharynx at the level of C6 to the oesophagogastric junction at the level of T11. It passes through the superior and posterior mediastina and enters the abdomen by passing through the oesophageal hiatus in the diaphragm. For the sake of endoscopic evaluation, landmarks in the oesophagus are mentioned as the distance from the incisors.

Sphincters: The oesophagus has two important sphincters that aid in its function. The upper sphincter is an anatomical sphincter composed of the cricopharyngeus muscle. It is located at a distance of 18 cm from the incisor and helps in deglutition. The lower oesophageal sphincter (LES) functions as a physiological sphincter and is located just above the gastro-oesophageal junction. It plays a major role in preventing reflux of gastric contents into the oesophagus.

Histology: The wall of the oesophagus is composed of mucosa, submucosa and muscularis externa. Unlike other areas of the GI tract, the oesophagus is **not covered by serosa**. The oesophageal mucosa is lined by nonkeratinized stratified squamous epithelium. However, the distal end is replaced by columnar epithelium akin to the stomach, forming a squamocolumnar junction few centimetres above the oesophagogastric junction. The submucosa, in addition to loose connective tissue, has a few tubuloalveolar glands that secrete mucus. The muscularis externa of the oesophagus is the only part of the gut that is composed of striated muscle, especially in the proximal third, which facilitates the swallowing process.

STOMACH

The stomach is a J-shaped distensible muscular portion of the alimentary canal. The average capacity of the stomach is about 1.5–2 L in adults. It extends from the oesophagogastric junction above up to the pyloric junction below. It possesses an outer greater curvature and an inner lesser curvature. The stomach is divided into cardia, which is the junction of the oesophagus and the stomach; the fundus, which is the dome-shaped portion above the oesophageal junction; the body; and the pylorus (Fig. 21.1). The pyloric region is divided into pyloric antrum and pyloric canal. The circular muscle at the lower end of the stomach forms the pyloric sphincter which prevents regurgitation of duodenal contents into the stomach.

Histology (Fig. 21.2): The mucosa of the stomach is thrown into folds called ***rugae***. These rugae flatten when the stomach distends. The mucosa of the stomach is lined by mucus-secreting columnar epithelium. The unique feature of gastric mucosa is the presence of microscopic invaginations called *gastric pits* that contain gastric glands. The gastric glands that are present in the body contain predominantly chief cells that secrete the digestive enzymes, along with oxyntic or parietal cells that secrete

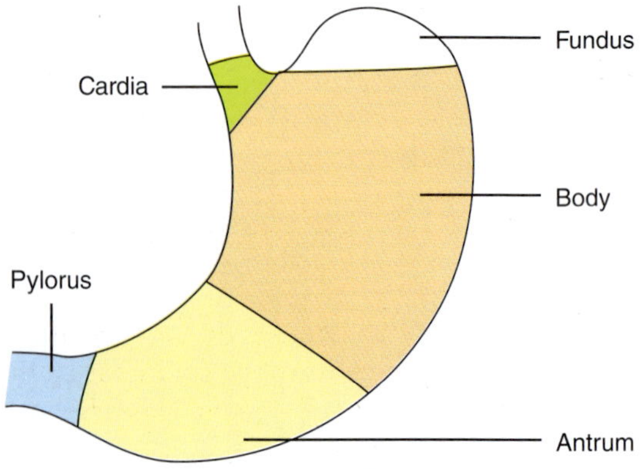

Fig. 21.1 Parts of the stomach.

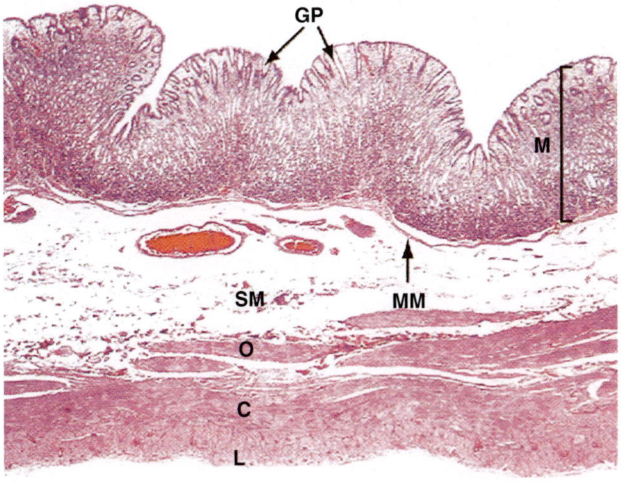

Fig. 21.2 Histology of the stomach. GP, gastric pits; M, mucosa; MM, muscularis mucosae; O, C and L, oblique, circular and longitudinal muscles; SM, submucosa. (*Source:* From Barbara Young, Geraldine O'Dowd and Phillip Woodford. Wheater's Functional Histology. 6th edition. Elsevier 2014.)

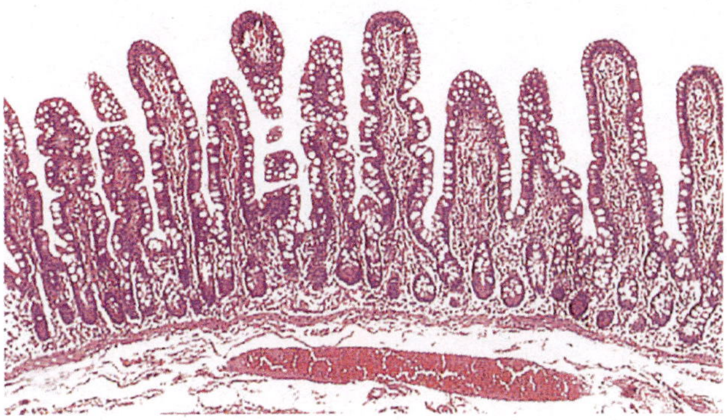

Fig. 21.3 Histology of the small intestine showing absorptive villi. (*Source:* From Barbara Young, Geraldine O'Dowd and Phillip Woodford. Wheater's Functional Histology. 6th edition. Elsevier 2014.)

hydrochloric acid and intrinsic factor and endocrine cells that secrete the hormone gastrin. The glands in the pylorus secrete mucus and gastrin.

SMALL INTESTINE

The small intestine is about 6 m in length and extends from the pyloric junction to the ileocaecal junction. It is marked by the duodenum above, which is the fixed part of the small intestine, and the jejunum and ileum below, which are the mobile portions.

The duodenum is about 25 cm in length and divided into four parts. The second part is particularly important because it contains the *ampulla of Vater* in which the pancreatic and biliary ducts open. The ileum and the jejunum are mobile and are attached to the mesentery. The upper two-thirds of the mobile portion is the jejunum, whereas the lower two-thirds is called the ileum. Most of the absorption takes place in the mucosal lining of the small intestine, so the lining is thrown into many folds and, unlike the fold of the stomach, these folds are permanent. The surface of these folds possesses *villi*, which are hair-shaped projections having blood and lymphatic channels running through their interiors. The villous surface accommodates many microvilli also, called *brush border cells*. Collectively, these intestinal folds, villi and microvilli increase the surface area of absorption. Further between the villi, the mucosal lining forms short invaginations called *crypts*.

Histology (Fig. 21.3): The mucosa of the small intestine is predominantly lined by absorptive columnar epithelium. Interspersed within these cells are mucus-secreting goblet cells and enzyme-secreting Paneth cells. Importantly, the invaginating crypts contain undifferentiated cells (stem cells) for ongoing replenishment of the epithelium. The duodenum is distinct in its structure from the jejunum and the ileum by the presence of mucus-secreting Brunner glands in the submucosa. Similarly, the ileum can be easily identified histologically by the presence of longitudinal aggregates of lymphoid follicles in the lamina propria along the antimesenteric border called *Peyer's patches.*

LARGE INTESTINE

The large intestine is about 1.5 m in length and extends from the ileocaecal junction to the anus. It is divided into caecum, ascending colon, transverse colon, descending colon, sigmoid colon, rectum and anal canal. Only the appendix, transverse colon and sigmoid colon are mobile, whereas the major part of the large intestine is fixed. The large intestine is identified grossly by the presence of *taeniae coli*, which are localized thickenings of the longitudinal muscle layer. There are three taeniae that converge at the base of the appendix and extend up to the rectosigmoid junction throughout the length of the colon. Their contractions facilitate peristaltic action of the large intestine, causing the appearance of haustrations and clefts on the surface of the colon. Running along the taeniae are small appendages that are peritoneum-lined protrusions of subserosal fat and are referred to as *appendices epiploicae.*

Near the ileocaecal junction, in the caecum, is located the vermiform *appendix*, which varies from 2 to 20 cm in length. It should be stressed here that the position of the appendix is variable and this is the commonest position. It is a true diverticulum with a narrow lumen that often gets obstructed, leading to acute appendicitis.

Histology: The mucosa of the large intestine has numerous *crypts* but is devoid of villi. The lining of the epithelium is majorly striated columnar epithelium that helps in absorption of water and electrolytes. The epithelium also contains numerous goblet cells for mucus secretion (Fig. 21.4). Occasional lymphoid follicles may be seen in the lamina propria. In the muscularis externa, the

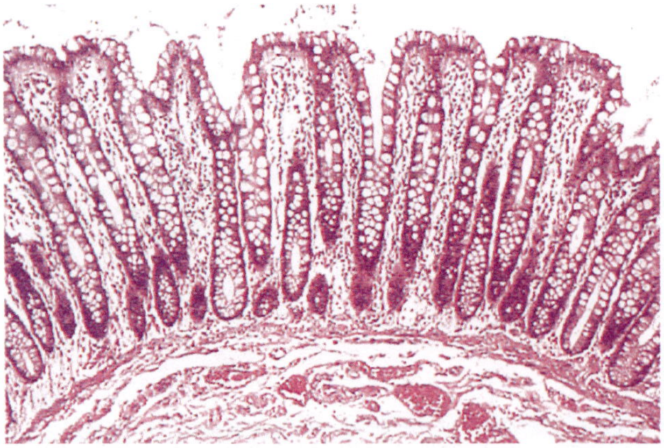

Fig. 21.4 Histology of the large intestine. Note the goblet cells. (*Source:* From Barbara Young, Geraldine O'Dowd and Phillip Woodford. Wheater's Functional Histology. 6th edition. Elsevier 2014.)

longitudinal muscle is thinned out due to aggregation of fibres in taeniae coli. The serosa layer is absent on the posterior side of the ascending and descending colon.

CONGENITAL ANOMALIES

ECTOPIA

Ectopia refers to the presence of normal tissues at abnormal locations other than the usual site. Ectopic tissue occurs at different sites in the GI tract. The common ectopic tissues in the GI tract are ectopic gastric mucosa and ectopic pancreatic mucosa.

1. **Ectopic gastric mucosa:** This may be seen in the oesophagus, small bowel or colon. The most frequent site is the upper third of the oesophagus where it is referred to as ***inlet patch***. The acid released from the ectopic tissue may cause oesophagitis, dysphagia, Barrett oesophagus and rarely adenocarcinoma. When it occurs in the intestines, it is called ***gastric heterotopia***. It may occasionally develop peptic ulcers and cause blood loss in stools.
2. **Ectopic pancreatic mucosa:** The favoured sites are the oesophagus and stomach. Although it is usually asymptomatic, it may be mistaken as invasive carcinoma when present in the deeper layers of the gastric wall.

MECKEL DIVERTICULUM

Diverticula are blind outpouchings that communicate with the bowel lumen. These are broadly classified into true diverticulum and false diverticulum. True diverticulum is lined by all anatomical layers, whereas false diverticulum is characterized by the absence of one or more layers. Meckel diverticulum is the most common true diverticulum that results due to failure of involution of the vitelline duct. It is commonly located on the antimesenteric side of the distal ileum.

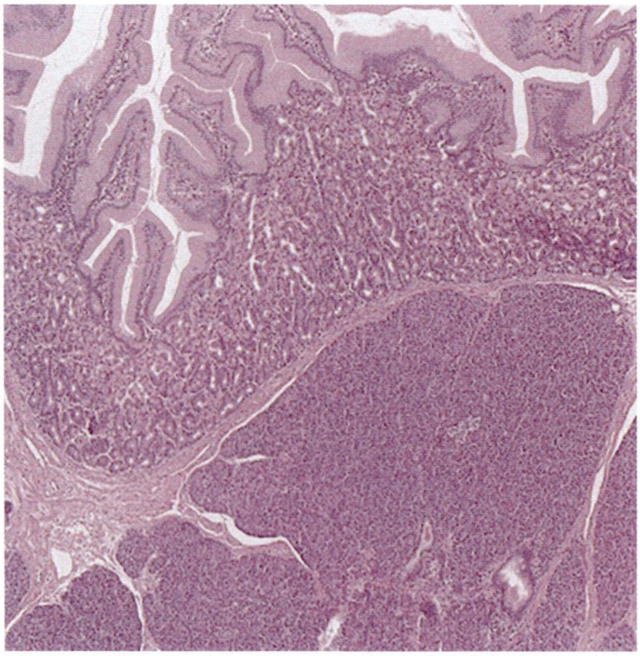

Fig. 21.5 Microscopy of Meckel diverticulum showing foci of gastric mucosa (right) and pancreatic tissue (left). (*Source:* Gastrointestinal and Liver Pathology: A Volume in the Series Foundations in Diagnostic Pathology, Third Edition: Amitabh Srivastava, Daniela S. Allende; Figure 16.1, Elsevier Inc., 2023.)

Meckel diverticulum is classically characterized by the '**rule of 2**':

- About 2% of the population is affected.
- It is usually found within 2 feet of the ileocaecal valve.
- It is 2-inch long.
- It is two times common in males.
- It presents with symptoms at 2 years of age (but is mostly asymptomatic).

Meckel diverticulum may occasionally contain **ectopic pancreatic or gastric tissue** (Fig. 21.5). Acid secreted by the gastric tissue can lead to peptic ulcers in the adjacent mucosa and occult bleeding that may mimic an acute appendicitis on the left side.

PYLORIC STENOSIS

Pyloric stenosis is caused by the obstruction of the gastric outlet due to hyperplasia of the muscularis propria in the pyloric region of the stomach. This muscular block is further aggravated by oedema and inflammation of the mucosa and submucosa of the pylorus. The aetiology of pyloric stenosis may be congenital or acquired. Congenital pyloric stenosis shows a multifactorial pattern of inheritance. It is more common in the first-born male child. Monozygotic twins have a 200-fold increased risk, whereas dizygotic twins and siblings have a 20-fold increased risk. Infants with Turner syndrome and trisomy 18 show a higher incidence, indicating a genetic basis for this condition.

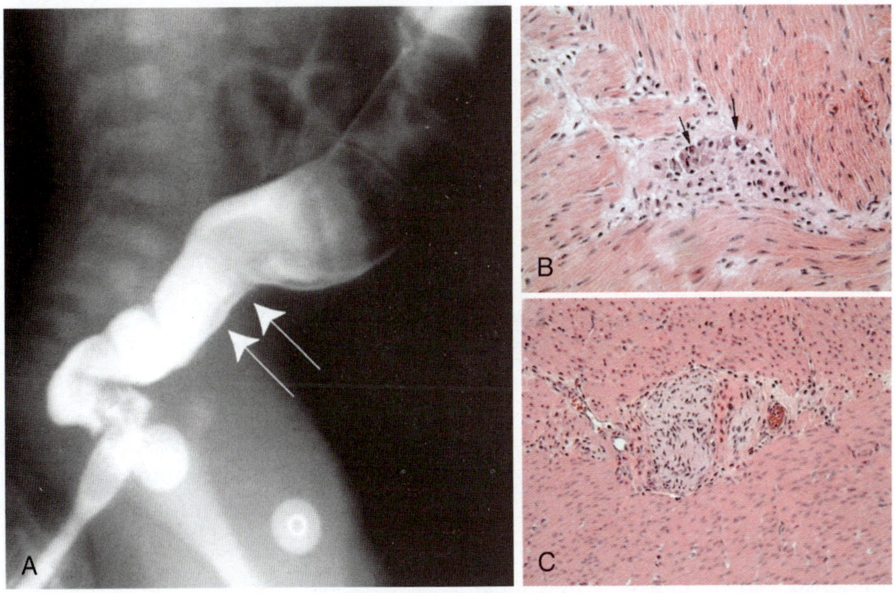

Fig. 21.6 Hirschsprung colon. (A) Barium enema study of a 3-month-old child showing narrowing of the distal colon, with the transition from dilated to narrowed colon demarcated by arrows. (B) Normal myenteric ganglion. Myenteric ganglion cells (arrows) are located normally in the plexus between the longitudinal and circular layers of the muscularis propria. (C) Aganglionic distal bowel of Hirschsprung disease showing hypertrophied nerve bundle. (*Source:* From Ada Hamosh, Roderick R. McInnes, Robert L. Nussbaum, Huntington F. Willard, Emily C. Lisi and Nara Sobreira. Clinical Case Studies Illustrating Genetic Principles. Thompson & Thompson Genetics in Medicine. 8th edition. Elsevier 2016.)

Infants usually present around the third to sixth weeks of life with regurgitation and nonbilious projectile vomiting immediately after feeding. Classical presenting findings include a 1- to 2-cm firm ovoid mass palpable on the right upper quadrant of the abdomen and visible peristalsis during and after feeding. The condition can be treated by surgery in which the hyperplastic muscles are split.

Acquired pyloric stenosis includes all conditions that cause gastric outlet obstruction such as scarring in peptic ulcers and carcinomas of the pylorus and pancreas.

HIRSCHSPRUNG DISEASE

Hirschsprung disease, also called **congenital aganglionic megacolon**, is an abnormal dilatation of a segment of the colon due to a distal functional obstruction. The lack of peristalsis in the affected segment is due to the *absence of parasympathetic ganglion cells* affecting both Auerbach and Meissner nerve plexuses. The neural crest cells that usually migrate to the rectum from the caecum either fail to migrate or die prematurely, leading to congenital aganglionosis.

The disease presents itself in about 1 in 5000 newborns, with an increased incidence in male children; about 10% of cases are seen in individuals with Down syndrome. The most common genetic defect associated with this condition is *loss-of-function mutation of RET* proto-oncogene.

Morphology

Gross: The aganglionic segment is normal or narrowed with dilation of the proximal normal intestine. The dilatation may be quite marked, occasionally leading to rupture and associated complications. The rectum is always involved along with a variable segment of the proximal intestine.

Microscopy: The involved segment shows the absence of ganglion cells and associated hypertrophied nerve bundles (Fig. 21.6). The absence of ganglion cells can be confirmed by immunohistochemistry for acetylcholinesterase enzyme. During surgery, the presence of ganglion cells should be confirmed in the proximal normal segment by frozen section to confirm the extent of resection.

Clinical Features

In the neonatal period, infants usually present with delay in passage of meconium, abdominal distension and bilious vomiting. Diagnosis can be confirmed by biopsy of the affected segment, which is usually taken at about 2 cm from the anal sphincter.

Treatment includes resection of the aganglionic segment and anastomosis. Acquired aganglionic megacolon is seen in *Trypanosoma cruzi* infection and Chagas disease.

OTHER ANOMALIES

Tracheo-oesophageal fistula is seen in about 1 in 800 newborns. Several anatomic variations exist. The most common type seen is type C, in which the upper segment of the oesophagus ends as a blind pouch (oesophageal atresia), with the distal segment communicating with the trachea as a tracheo-oesophageal fistula. Infants present in the newborn period with complaints of drooling of saliva and inability to accept feeds. Surgical correction of the deformity is usually done within the first few days of birth.

Imperforate anus is an inborn abnormality presenting as the most common form of intestinal atresia. It occurs due to failure of involution of the cloacal membrane. This malformation can be treated surgically and would require a lifetime follow-up.

Diaphragmatic hernia is the herniation of contents of the abdomen into the thoracic cavity. This causes pressure on the thoracic structures, which when marked can lead to pulmonary hypoplasia and respiratory failure.

OESOPHAGUS

ACHALASIA

Achalasia is characterized by a triad *of increased tone of LES, incomplete relaxation of LES and the absence of peristalsis of the oesophagus.*

Pathogenesis As mentioned earlier, LES is a functional sphincter that is controlled by a delicate balance between cholinergic and anticholinergic stimulations. Although the muscle thickness is the same as the rest of the oesophagus, it has a greater resting tone (Fig. 21.7). During swallowing, the relaxation of the sphincter is caused by the release of nitric oxide (NO) and vasoactive intestinal peptide (VIP) by the vagus nerve, which is an inhibitory neuron. Primary achalasia occurs due to the degeneration of the inhibitory neurons, extraoesophageal vagal nerve degeneration and degeneration of dorsal motor nucleus of the vagal nerve. Secondary causes of achalasia include Chagas disease, in which there is destruction of the myenteric plexus by *T. cruzi* infection. Other rare causes include diabetic autonomic neuropathy, amyloidosis, sarcoidosis and vagal dorsal motor nuclear lesions such as polio and tumour-related pseudoachalasia.

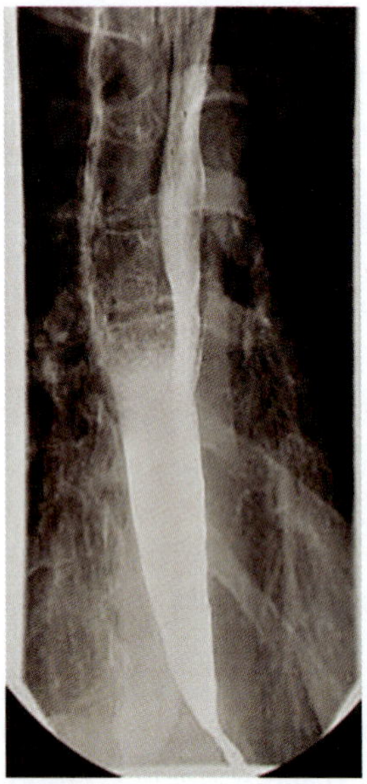

Fig. 21.7 Barium oesophagram in patients with achalasia demonstrating a dilated oesophagus and tapering of the distal oesophagus with the classical 'bird's beak' appearance. (*Source:* From Dawn L. Francis and David A. Katzka. Achalasia: Update on the Disease and Its Treatment. Gastroenterology. 2010;139:369–374.e2.)

Thus, the increased tone along with failure of relaxation of LES results in dysphagia. The lack of peristalsis also adds to the pathogenesis, causing dysphagia for liquids and solids. The condition also presents with regurgitation of food that is sometimes even a few days old, chest pain, hiccups and weight loss.

OESOPHAGITIS

Laceration and Perforation

Mallory–Weiss tear is a common cause of oesophageal laceration. It occurs due to forceful vomiting in which there is failure of relaxation of LES. The vigorous vomiting causes vertical tears in the cardiac gastric mucosa, which is usually **near the squamocolumnar junction** and in 10% of cases may extend into the oesophagus (Fig. 21.8). These

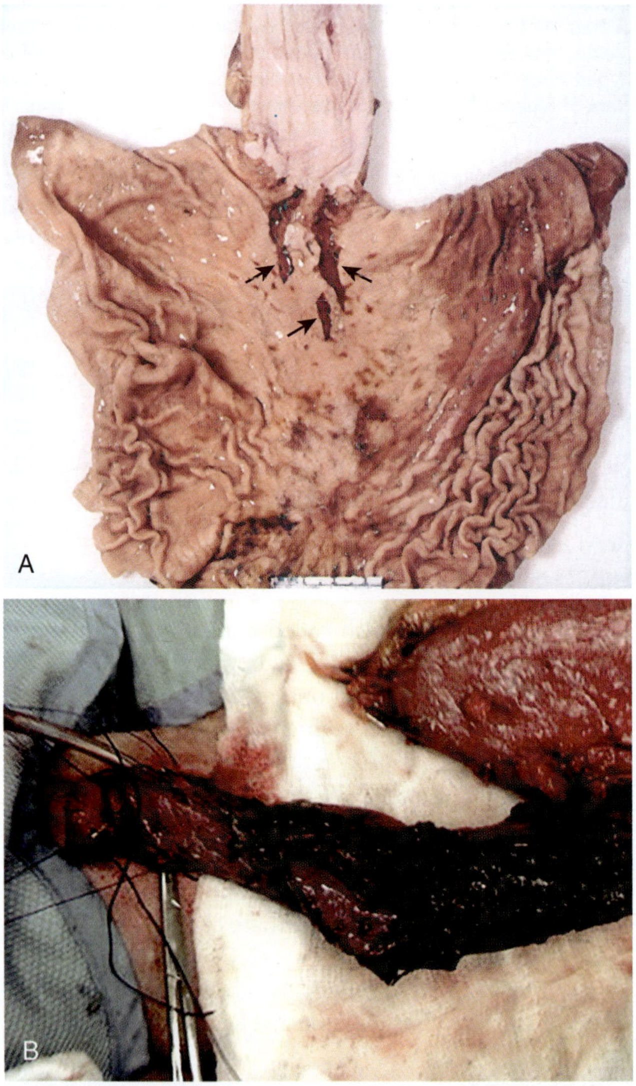

Fig. 21.8 Gross images of Mallory–Weiss tear – linear superficial tears at the oesophagogastric junction (A) and a longitudinal full-thickness tear in mid-oesophagus – Boerhaave syndrome (B). (*Source:* From Andrew J. Connolly, Walter E. Finkbeiner, Philip C. Ursell and Richard L. Davis. Atlas of Gross Autopsy Pathology. Autopsy Pathology: A Manual and Atlas. 3rd edition. Elsevier 2016.)

are **superficial tears** that present with haematemesis but heal spontaneously and rarely need intervention.

Boerhaave syndrome, on the contrary, is an oesophageal perforation due to forceful vomiting against a closed glottis (Fig. 21.8). The buildup of pressure is directly in the oesophagus, so it perforates at the weakest point, which is the **lower third**. The contents of the oesophagus are forced under pressure into the mediastinum, causing acute symptoms of chest pain and tachypnoea, mimicking a myocardial infarction. If left untreated, it can lead to serious consequences such as mediastinitis. Hence, **surgical intervention is required** for Boerhaave syndrome.

Chemical and Infectious Oesophagitis (Table 21.1)

Chemical oesophagitis causes damage to the squamous epithelium of the oesophagus, and the degree of damage depends on the quantity and concentration of the ingested agent. Alkalis cause more damage to the oesophagus with fibrosis due to their deeper penetration, whereas acids cause more damage to the stomach. The common complications associated with chemical- and radiation-induced oesophagitis are **fibrous scarring leading to stenosis**. Fungal and viral infections of the oesophagus are mostly seen only in immunocompromised patients or debilitated patients.

Endoscopy of patients with advanced candidiasis shows adherent grey–white pseudomembranes that contain aggregates of fungal pseudohyphae and inflammatory cells. Ulcers of herpes simplex virus (HSV) are punched out, whereas cytomegalovirus (CMV) ulcers are shallow with necrotic base. Biopsy in HSV ulcers should be taken from the margins to demonstrate viral inclusions in the nucleus, whereas biopsy in CMV ulcers should be taken from the base of the ulcer to demonstrate inclusions in the nucleus and cytoplasm.

Table 21.1 Causes of Chemical and Infectious Oesophagitis

Causes of chemical oesophagitis
Alcohol
Excessively hot fluids
Accidental ingestion of acids and alkalis
Acid and alkali ingestion in a suicide attempt
Dissolution of pills in the oesophagus
Chemotherapy induced
Radiotherapy induced
Causes of infectious oesophagitis
Immunocompetent patients
Herpes simplex virus infection
Immunosuppressed patients
Herpes simplex virus infection
Cytomegalovirus infection
Candidiasis (most common fungal infection)
Mucormycosis
Aspergillosis

Reflux Oesophagitis

Reflux oesophagitis is the inflammatory changes in the oesophagus induced by reflux of acidic gastric contents into the oesophagus commonly involving the lower end.

Pathogenesis The oesophagus lined by stratified squamous epithelium is sensitive to gastric acid–induced damage and hence has developed three levels of antireflux barriers to protect itself (Table 21.2). Failure of these barriers may result in acid from the stomach entering the oesophagus and damaging the squamous lining.

Morphology (Fig. 21.9)

In endoscopy, the earliest changes are oedema and redness. However, the reliable findings include easy bleeding, red streaks and erosions. Histological

Table 21.2 Levels of Antireflux Barriers in the Oesophagus and the Conditions Causing Failure of the Mechanisms

Levels	Mechanism	Causes of failure
Level 1	Intrinsic LES	Transient LES relaxation Food induced (chocolate, fat) Gastric distension (food, gas) Drug induced (barbiturates, morphine, diazepam, calcium channel blockers) Strain induced (coughing, bending) Hiatus hernia
Level 2	Oesophageal acid clearance by swallowing and secretions	Supine position Patients with oesophagitis Decreased salivation (sleep, smokers)
Level 3	Tissue resistance	Degradation of E-cadherin in cell junctions Bile acids in the reflux content

LES, lower oesophageal sphincter.

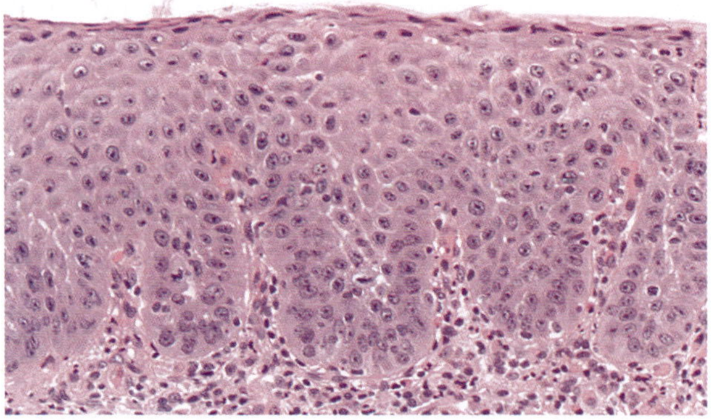

Fig. 21.9 Histology of reflux oesophagitis showing basal and suprabasal cell hyperplasia, elongation of the lamina propria papillae, lack of surface maturation with the presence of nucleated squamous cells at the surface of the epithelium and increased inflammation in the lamina propria. (*Source:* From Ana E. Bennett, John R. Goldblum and Robert D. Odze. Inflammatory Disorders of the Esophagus. Odze and Goldblum Surgical Pathology of the GI Tract, Liver, Biliary Tract and Pancreas. 3rd edition. Elsevier 2015.)

changes develop earlier than endoscopic changes. The sensitive findings are *basal cell hyperplasia* (>20% of epithelial thickness) and elongation of rete pegs, whereas the specific findings include the presence of *neutrophils and eosinophils* within the layers of squamous epithelium.

Clinical Features Gastro-oesophageal reflux disease (GERD) is common among patients in the older age group who present most commonly with heartburn and dysphagia. The symptoms tend to be worse after food intake, although the pH of the gastric contents tends to be higher postprandially than in an empty stomach. This is explained by the presence of an ***acid pocket*** in the upper end of the stomach that does not allow the pH increase after food intake. The severity of symptoms does not correlate with the histological changes seen in biopsy. The complications associated with GERD are *ulceration, haematemesis, strictures and Barrett oesophagus.*

OESOPHAGEAL VARICES

Oesophageal varices are abnormally dilated veins of portosystemic anastomosis located at the lower end of the oesophagus that tend to bleed and cause haematemesis.

Pathogenesis

The blood drained from the intestine by the portal circulation passes through the liver for first-pass metabolism before entering the caval system for drainage into the right heart. A block in this mechanism as seen in patients with cirrhosis results in opening up of alternate channels of drainage. One of the collateral channels includes the submucosal veins of the lower end of the oesophagus. These collateral channels are incapable of carrying large volumes of blood; hence, they dilate and may progressively leak or rupture, leading to life-threatening complications. Oesophageal varices are most commonly associated with alcoholic liver disease and hepatic schistosomiasis.

Morphology

The dilated veins are located beneath the oesophageal mucosa. The veins may not be visible during surgery because reduced pressure collapses them. In later stages, after rupture, the veins may be seen as ulcers or necrotic areas. Old ruptured veins may show venous thrombosis and inflammation.

Clinical Features

Patients with varices usually present with haematemesis when there is a bleed (Table 21.3). It is an emergency that needs to be managed medically with drugs to induce splanchnic vasoconstriction or by endoscopic sclerotherapy or surgical ligation. In spite of these measures, death occurs in 30% of patients and the rest tend to develop similar episodes in the future. Prophylactic treatment of high-risk patients with β-blockers may reduce the risk of bleeding.

BARRETT OESOPHAGUS

Barrett oesophagus is the *intestinal metaplasia of the distal oesophagus* as a consequence of GERD.

Pathogenesis

The stratified squamous epithelium of the oesophagus is sensitive to acidic gastric contents. Recurrent episodes of acid reflex damage the squamous epithelium and healing occurs by the metaplastic process. The stem cells of the oesophagus are reprogrammed to form columnar epithelium, and this increases the risk of malignant transformation in the distal oesophagus, leading to adenocarcinoma. Prolonged GERD and long-segment involvement are associated with an increased risk of dysplasia. Although adenocarcinoma of the oesophagus mostly arises from Barrett oesophagus, not all patients undergo malignant transformation.

Table 21.3 Causes of Haematemesis

Oesophageal Causes	Gastric Causes
Mallory–Weiss syndrome	Peptic ulcer
Oesophageal ulceration	Gastric cancer
Oesophageal varices	Gastric varices
GERD	Gastric angiodysplasia
Oesophageal cancer	

GERD, gastro-oesophageal reflux disease.

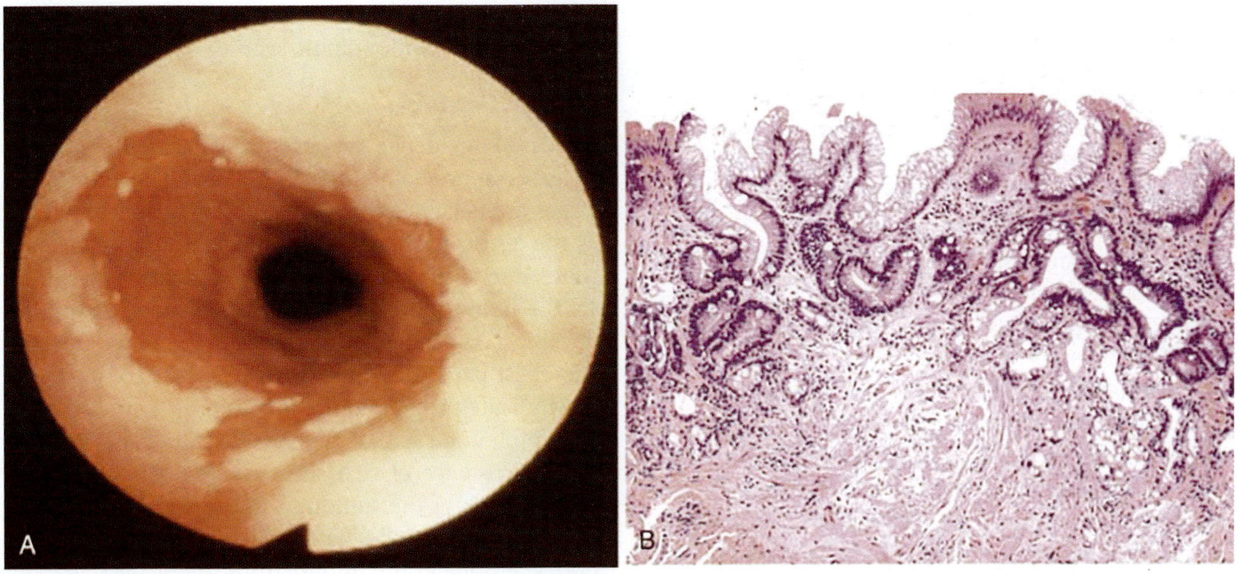

Fig. 21.10 Barrett oesophagus. (A) Tongues of gastric-appearing columnar mucosa extend proximal to the gastro-oesophageal junction. (B) Microscopy shows incomplete intestinal metaplasia, mucous columnar cells, scattered goblet cells and reactive changes in the base of the crypts. (*Source:* From Ana E. Bennett, John R. Goldblum and Robert D. Odze. Inflammatory Disorders of the Esophagus. Odze and Goldblum Surgical Pathology of the GI Tract, Liver, Biliary Tract and Pancreas. 3rd edition. Elsevier 2015.)

Morphology (Fig. 21.10)

Biopsy shows columnar epithelium replacing the squamous epithelium in the affected segment. The presence of *goblets cells*, denoting intestinal-type metaplasia, is diagnostic and essential to label the lesion a complete Barrett oesophagus. Goblets cells can be highlighted using special stains like Alcian blue or with immunohistochemical (IHC) markers like CK7 and CK20. Other cells such as gastric foveolar cells, though may be present, do not confirm the diagnosis. The biopsy of Barrett oesophagus is done not only to confirm the diagnosis but also to check for the presence of *dysplasia* (Fig. 21.11). If present, the severity needs to be assessed. Abnormal glandular architecture with budding, branching and nuclear features such as nuclear hyperchromatism, increased nuclear cytoplasmic ratio, clumping of chromatin and atypical mitosis are seen in both high-grade and low-grade lesions. However, the severity of morphological changes is much more in high-grade lesions with an increased risk of malignant transformation. Invasion of the lamina propria by dysplastic cells needs to be carefully looked for, because it defines transformation of dysplasia to intramucosal carcinoma.

Clinical Features

The criteria for the diagnosis of Barrett oesophagus include, first, the endoscopic confirmation of the columnar epithelium in the distal oesophagus above the oesophagogastric junction. This is usually seen as *tongue-like areas of red velvety mucosa* in the distal oesophagus, which otherwise has a pale glossy appearance in healthy tissue. The length of involvement has now helped to classify Barrett oesophagus *into long-segment, short-segment and ultra-short*-segment Barrett oesophagus. The second criterion is the biopsy finding of *metaplastic columnar epithelium* resembling the intestinal epithelium.

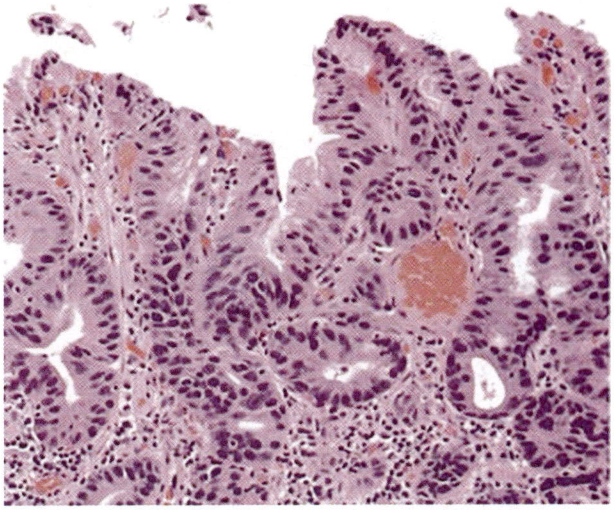

Fig. 21.11 High-grade dysplasia in a Barrett oesophagus showing a marked degree of nuclear pleomorphism, loss of polarity, increased N:C ratio and full-thickness stratification. (*Source:* From Ana E. Bennett, John R. Goldblum and Robert D. Odze. Inflammatory Disorders of the Esophagus. Odze and Goldblum Surgical Pathology of the GI Tract, Liver, Biliary Tract and Pancreas. 3rd edition. Elsevier 2015.)

Management of Barrett oesophagus depends on the presence of dysplastic changes. The treatment varies from simple follow-up with endoscopy and biopsy in low-grade lesions to surgical resection in multifocal high-grade lesions. Regular endoscopic follow-up helps to identify malignant transformation at an earlier stage and helps in better prognosis for the patient.

TUMOURS OF OESOPHAGUS

Tumours of the oesophagus include both benign and malignant tumours. The benign tumours comprise epithelial tumours like squamous papilloma and adenoma and mesenchymal tumours like leiomyoma, fibroma, lipoma, haemangioma and lymphangioma. The most common benign tumours among these are *leiomyoma*. The common malignant tumours of the oesophagus are *squamous cell carcinoma and adenocarcinoma.*

Oesophageal **squamous cell carcinoma** is the most common malignant tumour of the oesophagus worldwide. However, in developed Western countries, **adenocarcinomas** have become more common due to the increased incidence of associated risk factors (Table 21.4). Oesophageal carcinomas are more common in men and in Caucasians. The risk factors associated with squamous cell carcinoma and adenocarcinoma are different. The most common factors linked to oesophageal squamous cell carcinoma are tobacco use and excess alcohol consumption, whereas Barrett oesophagus with GERD increases the risk of adenocarcinoma.

Morphology

Diagnosis of oesophageal carcinomas requires endoscopy and biopsy. The most common site of squamous cell carcinoma is the middle third of the oesophagus, whereas adenocarcinoma usually involves the lower third because it is progressive of GERD. In the early stage, endoscopy shows normal mucosa or a plaque. As the lesion progresses, it may infiltrate into the wall, causing thickening and luminal narrowing, or it may form a protruding polypoidal mass.

Lesions diagnosed by screening endoscopies have a better prognosis than symptomatic lesions. The other investigations include barium contrast oesophagography and computed tomographic scan.

Table 21.4 Risk Factors for Oesophageal Carcinoma

Squamous Cell Carcinoma	Adenocarcinoma
Smoking	Barrett oesophagus
Alcohol (>140 g/week)	Obesity-associated GERD
Vitamin A, C and E deficiency	Tobacco use
Folic acid, zinc, selenium deficiency	Radiation exposure
Chronic thermal injury (hot liquids)	High fat content in food
Fungus-contaminated food	Higher socioeconomic status
Human papillomavirus infection	
Plummer–Vinson syndrome	
Achalasia	

GERD, gastro-oesophageal reflux disease.

Clinical Features

Increased incidence of oesophageal carcinoma in men suggests a protective effect of female hormones. Early stages are usually asymptomatic, and dysphagia develops as the lesion progresses. Dysphagia is first seen only for solids due to luminal obstruction and causes weight loss. As the lesion increases in size, dysphagia to liquids also develops. Anaemia, lymph node enlargement, odynophagia, chest pain and voice change are less commonly seen but indicate progression of the lesion.

Lymph node spread depends on the site of the primary lesion. Presence of rich submucosal lymphatics helps in early spread of the tumour. Lesions involving the upper third of the oesophagus tend to metastasize to cervical nodes, lesions in the middle third prefer mediastinal and paratracheal nodes, and those in the lower third involve the coeliac and gastric nodes.

SQUAMOUS CELL CARCINOMA

Pathogenesis

Tobacco smoking and excess alcohol intake increase the risk of squamous cell carcinoma by about fivefold each and, if present together, have a synergistic effect. Nutritional deficiencies increase the risk, whereas the intake of the antioxidant vitamins helps to counterbalance it. The risk associated with intake of hot liquids has not been conclusively proven, but intake of traditional fermented milk, *mursik*, in Kenya, which contains acetaldehyde, has been proven to be linked to squamous cell carcinoma. The genetic factors associated with this malignancy include amplification of **SOX2 and cyclin D1** and loss-of-function mutation in **TP53 and E-cadherin.**

Morphology

Gross: Squamous cell carcinoma is usually preceded by squamous dysplasia or carcinoma in situ, which progresses to a circumferential mass and often gets ulcerated (Fig. 21.12). Invasion into the submucosa and deeper layers can be seen on the cut section.

Microscopy: These carcinomas are usually moderate to well differentiated and composed of sheets of squamous epithelial cells with keratin pearl formation. The cells have pleomorphic hyperchromatic nuclei with an increased nuclear cytoplasmic ratio and atypical mitotic figures. These may also invade into the adjacent structures such as bronchi, aorta, pleura, pericardium, diaphragm and mediastinum.

ADENOCARCINOMA

Barrett oesophagus with metaplastic columnar epithelium is a fertile soil for the development of adenocarcinoma of

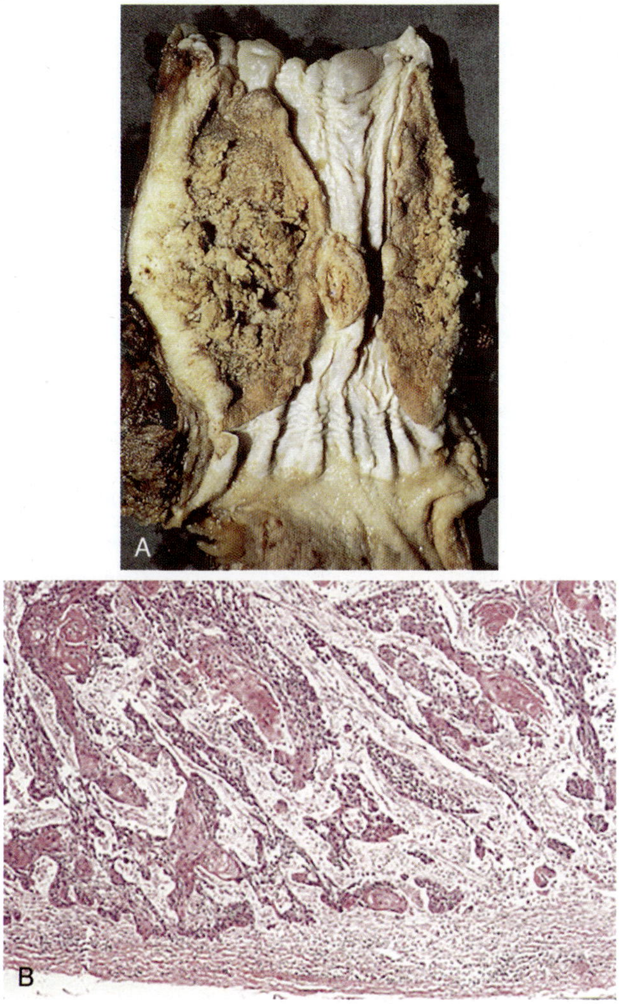

Fig. 21.12 Squamous cell carcinoma of the oesophagus, gross – showing ulcerative growth in mid-oesophagus (A) and microscopic appearance showing infiltrating islands of keratinizing squamous cells (B). (*Source:* From Fiona Campbell and Gregory Y. Lauwers. Tumors of the Esophagus and Stomach. Diagnostic Histopathology of Tumors. 5th Edition. Elsevier 2021.)

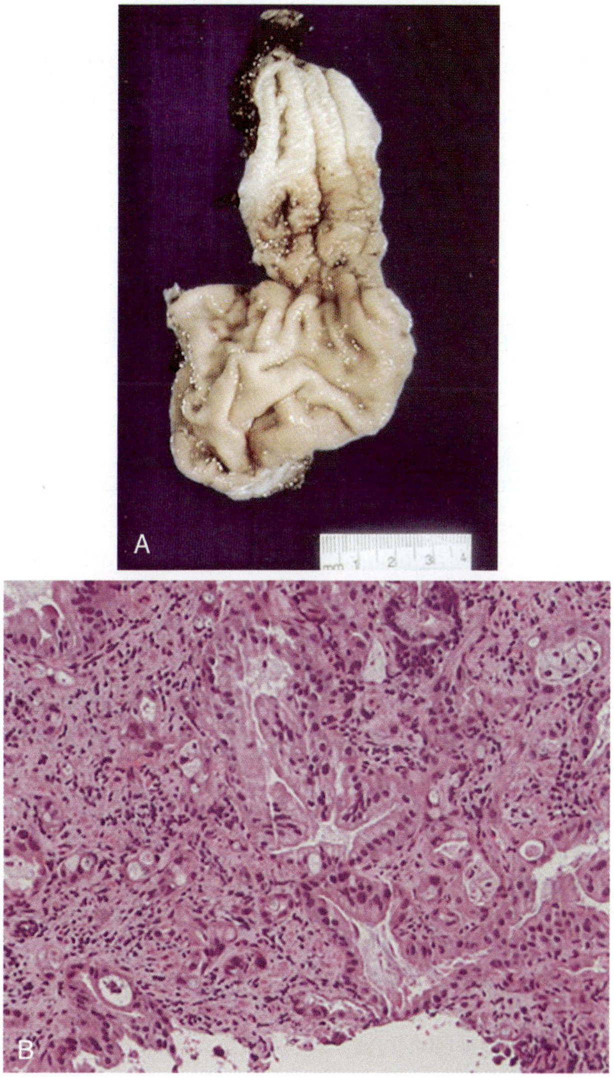

Fig. 21.13 Gross appearance of adenocarcinoma (A) showing an ulcerative lesion in the lower third of the oesophagus. Microscopy showing irregular, malignant glands with luminal mucin production involving oesophageal mucosa, with inflammatory stromal response (B). (*Source:* From Parakrama Chandrasoma, Yanling Ma and Evan E. Yung. Esophageal Mucosa in Health and Disease. Shackelford's Surgery of the Alimentary Tract. 8th edition. Elsevier 2019.)

the oesophagus. All factors that increase GERD are associated with an increased risk of adenocarcinoma. *Heliobacter pylori*, on the contrary, is protective because it reduces gastric acid secretion by causing atrophic gastritis and reduces the chances of developing adenocarcinoma. Statistics indicate that there is an increase in the incidence of adenocarcinoma worldwide by different mechanisms. A widespread increase in fatty food intake and treatment of *H. pylori* infection are some of the causes for an increase in the incidence of adenocarcinoma, especially in developed countries. The common chromosomal abnormalities associated with adenocarcinoma are **TP53** mutation and **p16/INK 4a downregulation**.

Morphology

Gross: Adenocarcinoma of the oesophagus most commonly occurs in the lower end of the oesophagus and may involve the upper end of gastric mucosa. The tumour is usually polypoidal, causing luminal obstruction (Fig. 21.13).

Microscopy: Intestinal-type glands are seen invading the underlying layers with often detectable adjacent areas of Barrett oesophagus. Occasionally, the tumour may be composed of diffusely infiltrating signet ring cells.

STOMACH

GASTROPATHY, ACUTE GASTRITIS AND ACTIVE GASTRITIS

Inflammation of gastric mucosa is called **gastritis**. When gastritis is associated with dense infiltration of the gastric

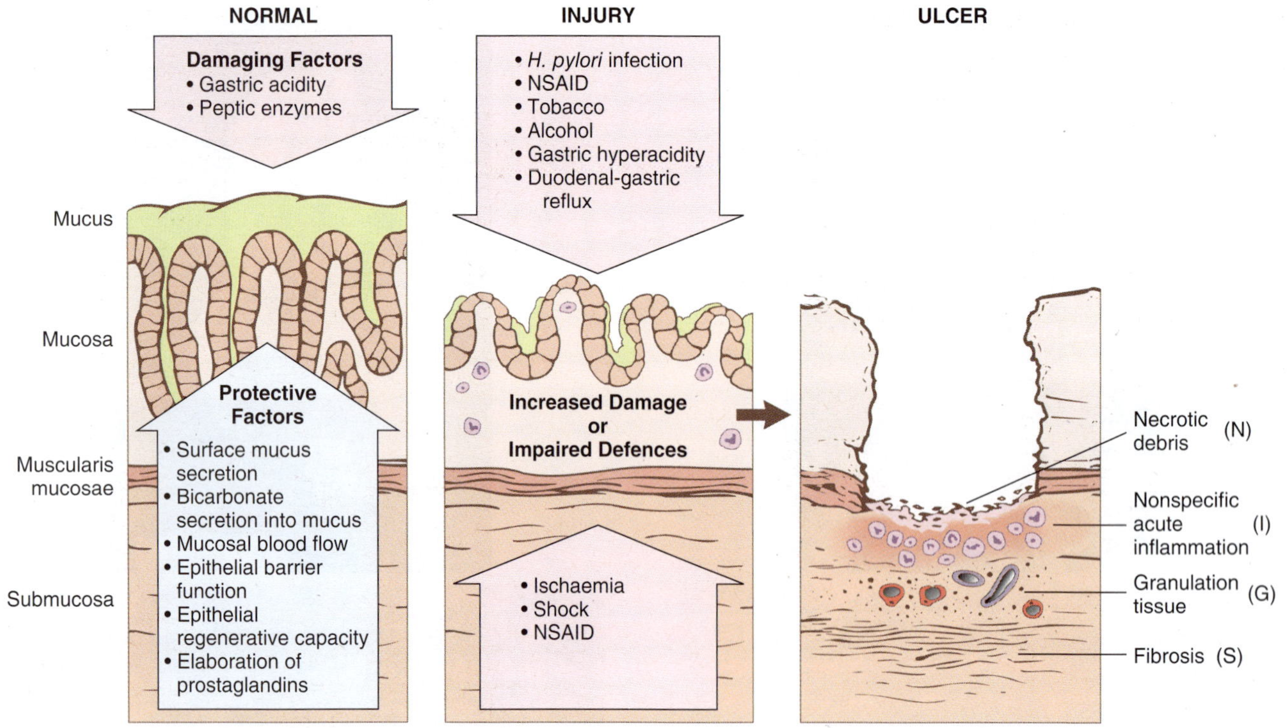

Fig. 21.14 Mechanism of gastric injury and protection. (*Source:* From Vinay Kumar, Abul K. Abbas and Jon C. Aster. Oral Cavities and Gastrointestinal Tract. Robbins Basic Pathology. 10th edition. Elsevier 2018.)

wall by neutrophils, it is termed **acute gastritis**, which is caused by invasive organisms. When the gastric mucosa shows neutrophils along with chronic inflammatory cell lymphocytes and plasma cells, it is termed **active gastritis** and this is much more a common entity than acute gastritis. When gastric injury or gastric dysfunction occurs with mucosa showing rare or absent inflammatory cells, it is termed **gastropathy**.

Protective mechanism of gastric mucosa (Fig. 21.14):

- The gastric foveolar cells secrete **mucus** that prevents food particles to come in contact with the epithelium.
- Below the mucus, there is a fluid layer containing **bicarbonate** secreted by the surface epithelial cells.
- Beneath the fluid layer, the **continuity of the gastric epithelium** acts as a barrier and prevents back diffusion of acid and digestive enzymes.
- To optimize the secretory and barrier functions, **surface foveolar cells** are completely replaced every 3–7 days.
- Furthermore, the acid secretion into the lumen is coupled with **alkaline bicarbonate secretion** into the mucosal capillaries, creating an alkaline tide.
- The acid that escapes all these defences and diffuses into lamina propria is washed by the **rich vasculature**.

Factors disrupting these defences:

- *Nonsteroidal anti-inflammatory drugs* (NSAIDs) that function by inhibiting cyclooxygenase (COX) enzyme-dependent prostaglandin synthesis (these prostaglandins are key elements in maintaining gastric mucus and bicarbonate production; nonselective COX inhibitors such as aspirin and ibuprofen cause more damage than selective COX-2 inhibitors such as celecoxib)
- *Urease-secreting H. pylori* infection and uraemic patients who have reduced bicarbonate secretion
- *Ageing* that causes reduced mucus and bicarbonate secretion
- *Altitude*-associated reduced oxygenation of tissues
- *Chemical-induced injury* as in acid–base ingestion, as well as excess alcohol consumption
- *Chemotherapy and radiotherapy*

Morphology

In patients with mild acute gastritis, biopsy shows an intact epithelium with oedema and vascular congestion of the lamina propria. Active gastritis is characterized by *corkscrew-type hyperplasia of foveolar cells*, epithelial proliferation and neutrophils in the epithelial layer. With the onset of severe gastritis, epithelial continuity is lost, forming erosions and leading to haemorrhage. The term **acute erosive haemorrhagic gastritis** is preferred when extensive areas of superficial erosion occur with concurrent haemorrhage.

Clinical Features

Acute gastritis and gastropathy present as epigastric pain. On the basis of the aetiology, some respond to antacids and proton pump inhibitors (PPIs), whereas others are refractory.

STRESS-RELATED MUCOSAL DISEASE

Stress-related mucosal diseases occur in patients under various clinical scenarios and have been given different names on the basis of their location and clinical association:

- **Stress ulcers** – seen in shock, severe trauma and stress
- **Curling ulcer** – occurs in the proximal duodenum in patients with severe trauma or burns
- **Cushing ulcer** – occurs in the stomach, duodenum and oesophagus in cases of increased intracranial pressure

Pathogenesis

Stress ulcers mostly occur due to *ischaemia of the gastric mucosa* as a result of splanchnic vasoconstriction seen in states of shock. This is aggravated by increased activity of inducible NO synthase and vasoconstriction by release of endothelin. Cushing ulcers are caused by increased gastric acid secretion due to *vagal nuclei stimulation* due to increased intracranial pressure.

Morphology

Stress-related ulcers are usually multiple and occur anywhere in the stomach unlike peptic ulcers that are solitary. The ulcers vary from shallow erosions to deep penetrating lesions. Acute ulcers are punched-out ulcers, with base containing acid-digested extravasated blood that appears brown to black. There may be associated inflammation involving all layers and localized serositis. Unlike peptic ulcers, these lack thickened blood vessels and scarring. These ulcers heal within days by complete re-epithelialization.

Clinical Features

Although stress-induced mucosal injury is seen in many patients admitted to the intensive care unit, significant bleeding requiring intervention is quite uncommon. Important strong risk factors for such bleeding include respiratory failure and coagulopathy, and these patients are benefitted by ulcer prophylaxis. Routine prophylaxis is not indicated for all patients because treatment of the underlying disorder satisfactorily improves the outcome.

CHRONIC GASTRITIS

Chronic gastritis refers to chronic inflammation of gastric mucosa characterized by infiltration of gastric mucosa by inflammatory cells in the lamina propria. It is classified into **chronic superficial gastritis and chronic atrophic gastritis** on the basis of the absence and presence of atrophy of gastric glandular epithelium, respectively.

Aetiology (Table 21.5)

There are various causes for chronic gastritis, the most common being *H. pylori* infection. Although the symptoms vary on the basis of aetiology, all forms of gastritis present with upper abdominal pain, nausea and occasional vomiting.

Table 21.5 Common Causes of Chronic Gastritis

H. pylori **(most common)**
Autoimmune (most common diffuse atrophic gastritis)
Radiation injury
Chronic bile reflux
Mechanical injury (nasogastric tube)
Crohn disease
Amyloidosis
Eosinophilic gastritis (commonly seen in soy protein allergy)
Lymphocytic gastritis (also called varioliform gastritis)
Granulomatous gastritis (associated with Crohn disease)

H. pylori Gastritis

H. pylori is the most common cause of chronic bacterial infection of the body. It causes chronic gastritis, peptic ulcer in the stomach and duodenum, gastric adenocarcinoma and gastric mucosa–associated lymphoma.

Organism *H. pylori* is a spiral-shaped bacillus that is capable of surviving in high acidic medium of the gastric mucosa by virtue of its motility and urease production. It is more common in developing countries, especially in people of low socioeconomic status due to overcrowding, poor sanitation and lack of hygiene. The mode of spread is from human to human by faecal–oral route.

Pathogenesis *H. pylori* is preferably located superficially just below the mucus layer where it creates a neutral pH using the urease enzyme. It strictly colonizes *only the gastric mucosa* and does not affect the areas of intestinal metaplasia. The bacterial factors that are responsible for virulence are as follows:

- Flagella – aids in motility
- Urease – converts urea to ammonia and increases local pH
- Adhesin – helps to adhere to host cells
- Toxins – Cag A causing multifocal atrophic gastritis

H. pylori infection can be antral colonization or colonization of the body and fundus. The former is more common, and patients more commonly develop peptic ulcer than adenocarcinoma (Flowchart 21.1).

Morphology (Fig. 21.15)

Distribution of *H. pylori* is irregular and as mentioned earlier is seen in the luminal surfaces of the mucosal cells. On endoscopy, the infected mucosa appears granular or nodular. Biopsy of the gastric antrum is more likely to yield a positive result, although two

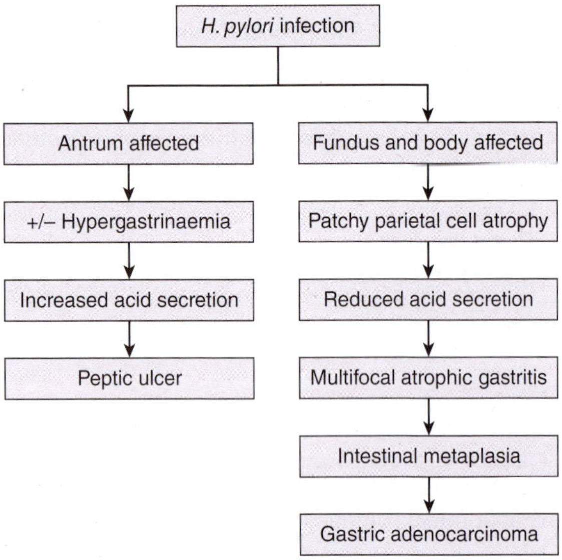

Flowchart 21.1 Pathogenesis of *H. pylori* infection based on site of colonization.

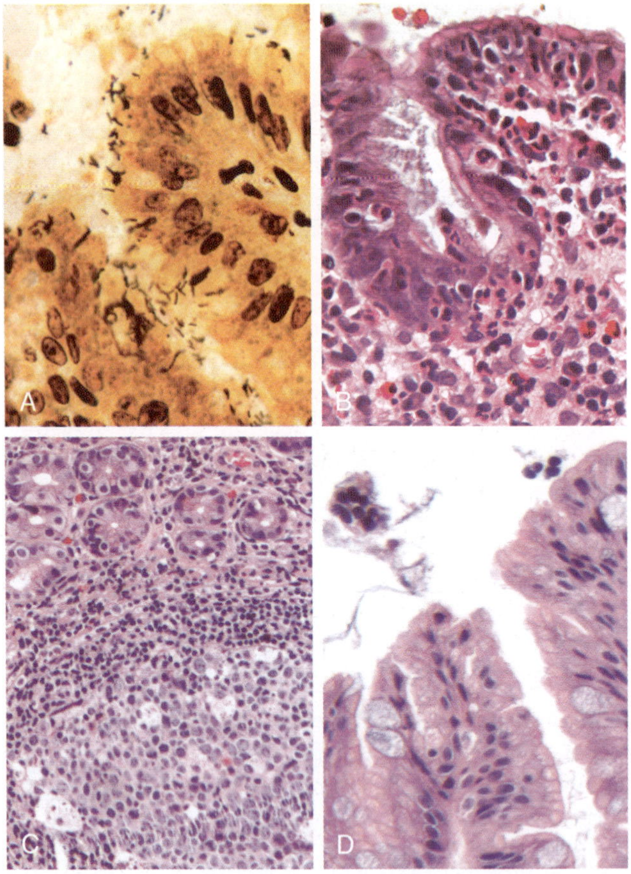

Fig. 21.15 Chronic gastritis. (A) Spiral-shaped *Helicobacter pylori* bacilli are evident in this Warthin–Starry silver stain. (B) Intraepithelial and lamina propria neutrophils are prominent. (C) Lymphoid aggregates with germinal centres and abundant subepithelial plasma cells within the superficial lamina propria are characteristic of *H. pylori* gastritis. (D) Intestinal metaplasia recognizable as the presence of goblet cells admixed with gastric foveolar epithelium. (*Source:* From Vinay Kumar, Abul K. Abbas and Jon C. Aster. Oral Cavities and Gastrointestinal Tract. Robbins Basic Pathology. 10th edition. Elsevier 2018.)

independent biopsy specimens from the antrum and corpus should be subjected to histopathology.

Microscopy: The classical findings include the following:

- Presence of neutrophils in the epithelial layer
- Pit abscesses (neutrophil accumulation in gastric pits)
- Plasma cells in the lamina propria
- Lymphoid aggregates, occasionally with a germinal centre

In due course, when atrophic gastritis sets in the oxyntic mucosa, the involvement is patchy with interspersed normal oxyntic cells unlike autoimmune gastritis that tends to be diffuse. Intestinal metaplasia if present poses risk of malignant transformation.

Clinical Features The gastritis associated with *H. pylori* infection is termed type B gastritis. It predominantly affects the antrum and leads to peptic ulcer disease (PUD). Occasionally, *H. pylori* may cause pangastritis and such patients are more prone to develop gastric carcinoma.

Laboratory Investigations iagnostic investigations in patients suspected of *H. pylori* gastritis include serology for *H. pylori* antibodies, urea breath test and faecal bacterial detection. Endoscopy and biopsy, though invasive, help to visualize the histological changes and assess risk of malignant transformation. The bacteria are best highlighted using silver stains like **Warthin–Starry and Steiner stains** and also using immunohistochemistry. The biopsy specimen can also be used for bacterial culture and PCR of bacterial DNA. Treatment includes antibiotics and PPIs. But eradication is difficult and reinfection is common.

Autoimmune Gastritis

Autoimmune gastritis is caused by immune-mediated *destruction of the parietal cells* of the gastric mucosa. It is referred to as type A gastritis and accounts for 10% of cases of chronic gastritis. The differences between *H. pylori* gastritis and autoimmune gastritis are listed in Table 21.6.

Pathogenesis Autoimmune gastritis is caused by CD4 cells that are directed against parietal cell components, resulting in the deficiency of intrinsic factor, but they may also destroy the adjacent chief cells.

The characteristic features are as follows:

- Presence of antibodies against parietal cells and intrinsic factor in serum
- Vitamin B_{12} deficiency
- Achlorhydria
- Antral endocrine cell hyperplasia
- Reduced levels of pepsinogen 1 in serum

Table 21.6 Differences between H. pylori and Autoimmune Gastritis

	H. pylori **Gastritis**	**Autoimmune Gastritis**
Also called	Type B gastritis	Type A gastritis
Location	Antrum	Body
Inflammatory infiltrate	Intraepithelial neutrophils, subepithelial plasma cells	Lymphocytes, macrophages
Location of inflammation	Predominantly superficial	Predominantly deep inflammation of the mucosa
Acid production	Increased to slightly decreased	Decreased
Gastrin	Normal	Increased
Serology	Antibodies to *H. pylori*	Antibodies to parietal cells
Sequelae	Peptic ulcer, adenocarcinoma, MALToma	Pernicious anaemia, adenocarcinoma, carcinoid
Associated with	Low socioeconomic status, poverty, rural residence	Thyroiditis, diabetes and other autoimmune disorders

MALT, mucosa-associated lymphoid tissue.

Clinical Features Autoimmune gastritis has a slow onset, and patients are symptomatic after two to three decades, usually around 60 years of age. It is more common in women and is often associated with other autoimmune disorders such as Hashimoto thyroiditis, type 1 diabetes mellitus, Addison disease and Graves disease. Vitamin B_{12} deficiency–associated anaemia in this condition is called **pernicious anaemia**, and it may be associated with other symptoms of vitamin B_{12} deficiency such as atrophic glossitis, beefy tongue, cerebral dysfunction and subacute combined degeneration of the spinal cord. The neurological symptoms are due to demyelination, axonal damage and neuronal death manifesting as peripheral neuropathy, including loss of position and vibration sense, sensory ataxia and limb weakness. These neuronal changes, unlike anaemia, cannot be reversed by correction of vitamin B_{12} deficiency. Another feature in these patients is iron-deficiency anaemia because gastric acid in the stomach is required for absorption of iron.

Morphology

Autoimmune gastritis shows diffuse damage of mucosa of the body and fundus in contrast to peptic ulcers in which involvement of the body, if present, is patchy. The antrum and cardia are not affected. The inflammatory infiltrate is mainly composed of lymphocytes and macrophages and is found deeper near the gastric glands. Areas of intestinal metaplasia with goblet cells may be seen. Such areas are at risk of developing adenocarcinoma, and the risk is greater than that in *H. pylori*–induced gastritis because it is associated with achlorhydria. Further changes related to vitamin B_{12} deficiency such as nuclear enlargement may be seen in the epithelial cells. Endocrine hyperplasia may be present and can be easily identified using immunostains for chromogranin.

Complications of Chronic Gastritis

The complications of chronic gastritis include peptic ulcer, mucosal atrophy with intestinalization, gastritis cystica, dysplasia and adenocarcinoma.

PEPTIC ULCER DISEASE PA 24.2

PUD is the chronic ulceration of gastric and duodenal mucosa. The major causes are *H. pylori infection, NSAIDs and cigarette smoking* (Fig. 21.16). Owing to reduction in *H. pylori* infection, PUD in the young population has reduced but its incidence in older patients has increased. The low-dose aspirin prescribed in older patients for cardiovascular benefits when combined with NSAIDs and cardiovascular diseases commonly prevalent in old age reduces gastric mucosal blood flow leading to this pattern.

Pathogenesis PUD generally occurs in patients with chronic gastritis. It is due to the imbalance between the factors that damage the gastric mucosa and the defence mechanisms. The sites of peptic ulcer are as follows:

- *Gastric antrum or duodenum*, which is the most common site, due to *H. pylori* infection of the antrum that causes increased gastric acid secretion
- *Gastric fundus and body* ulcers also caused by *H. pylori* infection or autoimmune gastritis (these lead to gastric atrophy and have lesser acid secretion and hence cannot damage the antrum and duodenum)
- *Ileum or Meckel diverticulum* due to ectopic gastric mucosa
- *Oesophagus* due to ectopic gastric mucosa or GERD

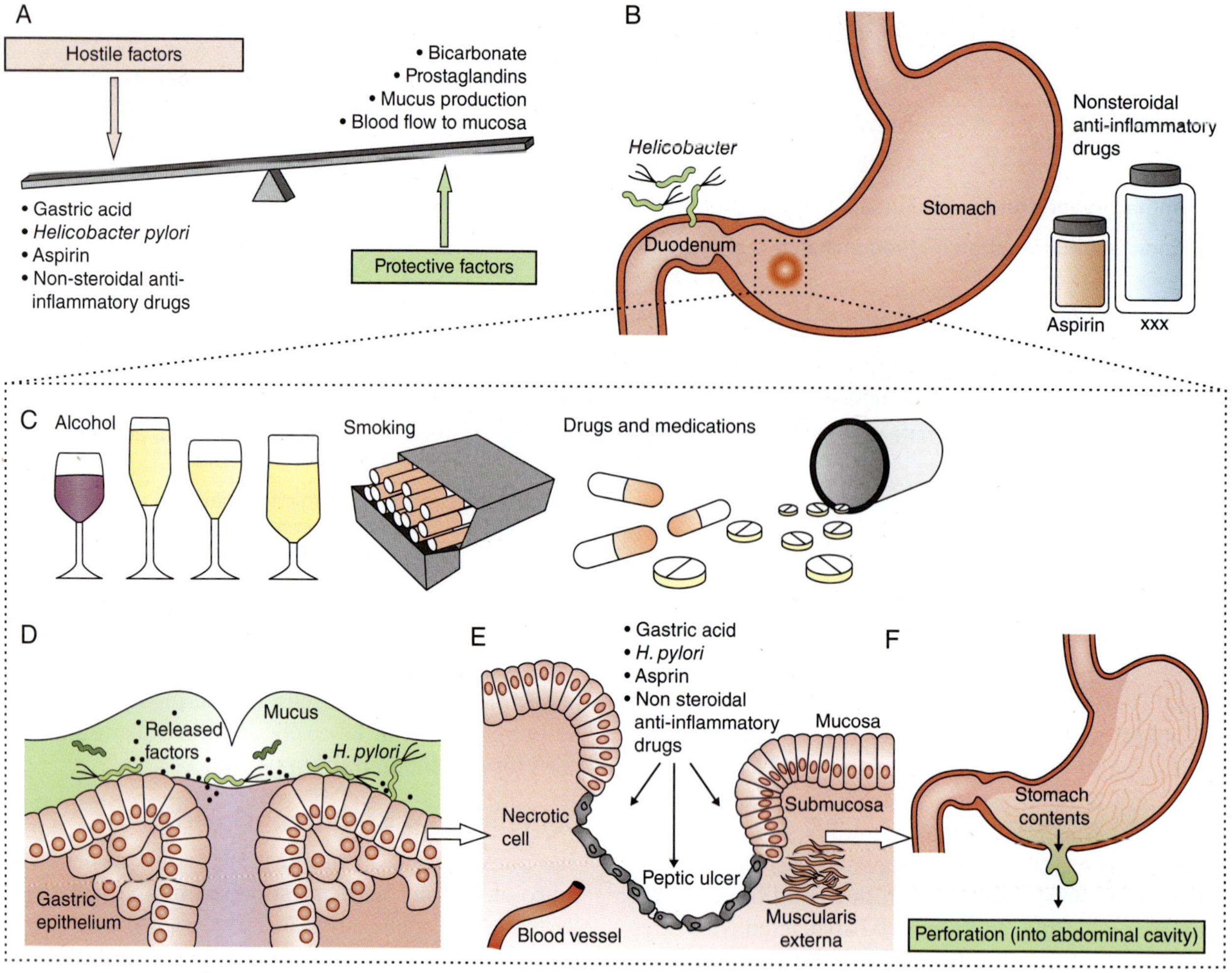

Fig. 21.16 (A–F) Factors leading to peptic ulcer development. (*Source:* From Jason W. Kempenich MD and Kenneth R. Sirinek MD, PhD. Acid Peptic Disease. The Surgical Clinics of North America. 2018;98:933-944.)

Morphology (Fig. 21.17)

The most common site is the proximal duodenum involving the anterior duodenal wall, followed by the lesser curvature of the stomach at the junction between the body and the antrum. These are mostly solitary, round to oval, punched-out ulcers. Chronic duodenal ulcers seldom become malignant, whereas gastric ulcers may turn malignant. Furthermore, benign gastric ulcers may mimic malignant ulcers, and vice versa (Table 21.7). Thus, every gastric ulcer should be considered malignant and subjected to histopathological examination to confirm the diagnosis.

Clinical Features Patients present with epigastric burning pain which usually occurs 1–3 hours after meal and is worse at night. The pain is generally relieved by alkali and is often associated with belching, bloating, nausea and vomiting. Some patients present late with complications that may sometimes be life threatening. Treatment includes removal of the offending agent and PPIs.

Complications (Table 21.8) The common complications associated with peptic ulcer are iron-deficiency anaemia, perforation, bleeding or gastric outlet obstruction.

HYPERTROPHIC GASTROPATHIES

These are diseases characterized by epithelial hyperplasia without inflammation leading to *giant cerebriform enlargement of gastric rugae.* Menetrier disease and Zollinger–Ellison syndrome (ZES) are the common examples of this pathology.

Menetrier Disease

It is a rare disorder associated with *diffuse hyperplasia of foveolar cells* of the gastric epithelium due to excess of transforming growth factor alpha (TGF-α).

Pathogenesis Menetrier disease has been shown to have a causative relationship with *H. pylori.* The foveolar cell hyperplasia is mainly seen in the body and fundus with sparing of gastric antrum. There is associated widening of the intercellular spaces, causing protein leakage and

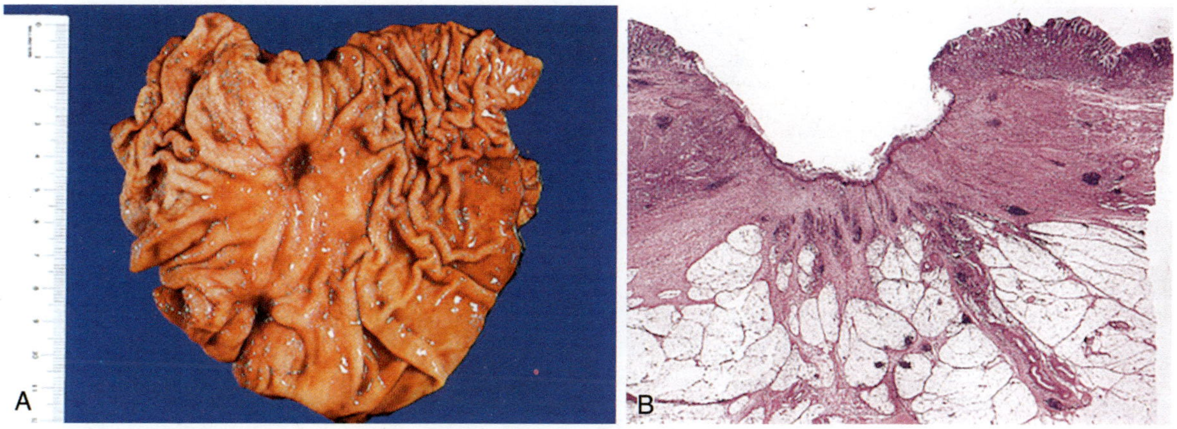

Fig. 21.17 (A) Gross appearance of a peptic ulcer with converging rugae. (B) Histology of the peptic ulcer showing overhanging mucosa on one edge and the sloping mucosa on the other with complete destruction of the external muscle layer. (*Source:* From John R. Goldblum. Stomach. Rosai and Ackerman's Surgical Pathology. 11th edition. Elsevier 2018.)

Table 21.7 Features of Benign Versus Malignant Ulcers

Peptic Ulcer	Malignant Ulcer
Punched-out ulcers	Large ulcers
Overhanging margins	Heaped-up margins
Depth – gastric muscularis propria	Necrotic base
Clean base due to peptic digestion of exudate	Malignant cells invading normal structures
Neutrophilic infiltrate with the underlying granulation tissue	
Scarring in the ulcer base forms radiating mucosal folds	

Table 21.8 Complications of Peptic Ulcers

Haemorrhage	Perforation	Obstruction
Most common (20% of patients)	Occurs in 5% of patients	Occurs in 2% of patients
Posterior wall ulcers	Anterior wall ulcers	Proximal duodenal ulcers
Owing to damage of blood vessels in the ulcer base	Erosion of the stomach wall	Scarring of ulcers during healing narrows the lumen

hypoproteinaemia. In addition, there is a reduction in parietal cells due to foveolar cell hyperplasia, resulting in hypochlorhydria or achlorhydria.

Morphology (Fig. 21.18)

Endoscopic view of the gastric lumen shows an increase in gastric rugosity in the body and fundus. Histologically, diffuse gastric foveolar cell hyperplasia imparts a *corkscrew-like appearance* of glands and occasional cystic dilation. Presence of intraepithelial lymphocytes may be seen. Hypoplasia of parietal cells and chief cells may be seen as patchy or diffuse glandular atrophy.

Clinical Features Menetrier disease usually presents with oedema and weight loss related to *hypoproteinaemia.* In children, it presents as a self-limiting disease following a respiratory infection. In adults, it is treated with anticholinergic drugs or octreotide and may be reversed by *H. pylori* eradication. TGF-α blocking agents are being tried now with promising results. Follow-up of patients is advised due to the increase in the *risk of adenocarcinoma* associated with this disease.

Zollinger–Ellison Syndrome

ZES is a state of *hypergastrinaemia* caused by gastrin-secreting tumours called *gastrinomas.* These are neuroendocrine tumours most commonly located in the duodenum and pancreas. The gastrin produced by these tumours stimulates acid secretion by the gastric mucosa, leading to hyperacidity.

Pathogenesis ZES may be sporadic in 80% of cases or associated with multiple endocrine neoplasia syndrome 1 (**MEN-1**). It can present as a constellation of symptoms that reflect the hypergastrinaemia associated with this disease. Common features of ZES include diarrhoea and multiple relapsing ulcers in atypical locations such as the distal duodenum and proximal jejunum (Flowchart 21.2).

Morphology

The gastric mucosa shows *doubling of oxyntic mucosa* with an associated increase in proliferation of mucus-secreting cells and endocrine cells in the gastric mucosa.

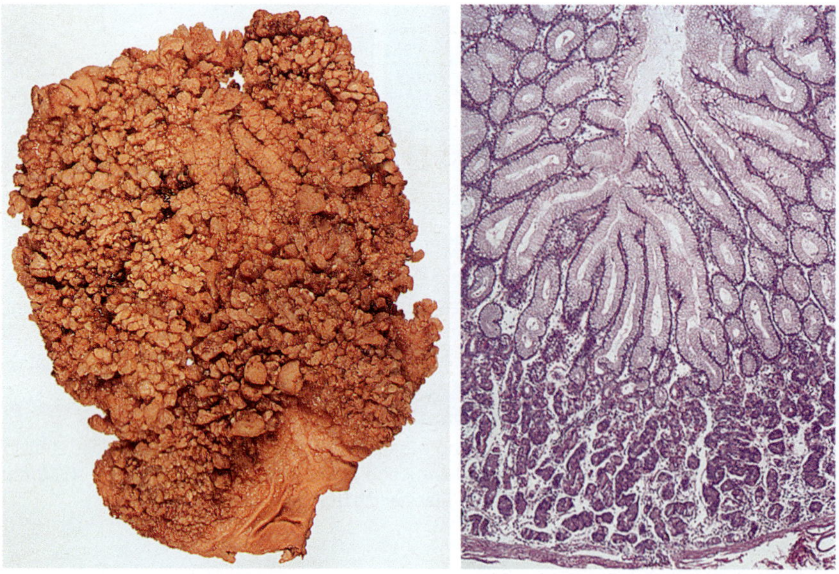

Fig. 21.18 Menetrier disease – gross appearance showing exuberant proliferative change (A) and microscopy showing marked hyperplasia of the foveolar epithelium along with atrophy of the underlying secretory mucosa (B). (*Source:* From John R. Goldblum. Stomach. Rosai and Ackerman's Surgical Pathology. 11th edition. Elsevier 2018.)

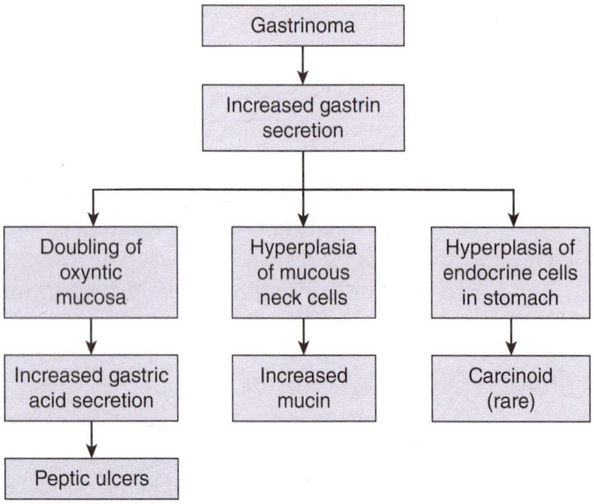

Flowchart 21.2 Common features of ZES.

Clinical Features Patients usually present with symptoms of peptic ulcer. Treatment aims at reduction of gastric acid secretion along with treatment of gastrinoma. Increased gastric acid secretion responds satisfactorily to PPIs and prevents gastric perforation. Sporadic gastrinomas are often solitary and occur in the pancreas but have a higher malignant potential. MEN-1-associated gastrinomas are multiple, located in the wall of the duodenum and have a low malignant potential. These tumours are detected by endoscopic ultrasonography and surgically managed.

GASTRIC POLYPS

Polyps or nodules are projections of the mucosa into the lumen of hollow organs above the level of surrounding mucosal lining. The polyps are detected in about 5% of endoscopies. Although hyperplastic polyps commonly exist, neoplasms of the stomach, both benign and malignant, can present as polyps.

Inflammatory and Hyperplastic Polyps

These constitute 75% of gastric polyps and are most common in the sixth decade of life. Chronic inflammation of the gastric mucosa causes injury, leading to reactive hyperplasia and polyp formation. Among the various causes of chronic inflammation, *H. pylori* is the most common cause, leading to polyps that may regress with bacterial eradication.

Inflammatory or hyperplastic polyps mostly occur as small (<1 cm in diameter), multiple, ovoid projections with a smooth surface or occasional superficial erosions. Microscopically, the polyps have dilated, elongated foveolar glands with oedematous lamina propria (Fig. 21.19). Polyps greater than 1.5 cm are surgically removed and subjected to histopathological examination to check for dysplastic changes.

Fundic Gland Polyps

Fundic gland polyps are formed due to *hyperplasia of parietal and chief cells.* The polyps occur sporadically in patients using PPIs or in patients with familial adenomatous polyposis (FAP). PPIs inhibit acid secretion, thereby stimulating gastrin secretion that causes growth of oxyntic glands. Patients usually present with nausea, vomiting and epigastric discomfort.

These polyps occur in the fundus or body as single/multiple well-circumscribed masses with smooth surface. Microscopically, the polyps are lined by parietal and chief cells (Fig. 21.20). Only FAP-associated polyps have malignant potential.

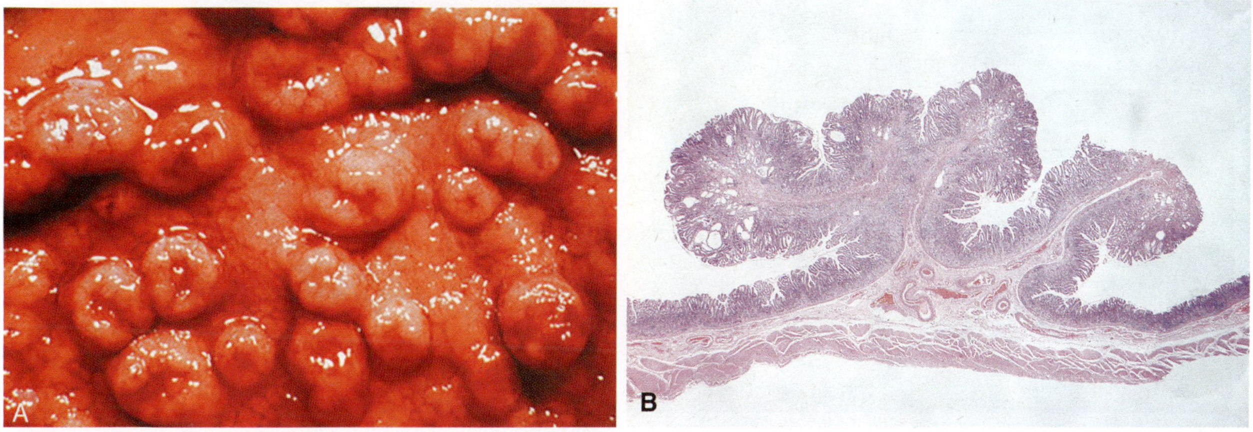

Fig. 21.19 Hyperplastic polyps, gross showing multiple polyps with central umbilication and microscopy. (*Source:* From John R. Goldblum. Stomach. Rosai and Ackerman's Surgical Pathology. 11th edition. Elsevier 2018.)

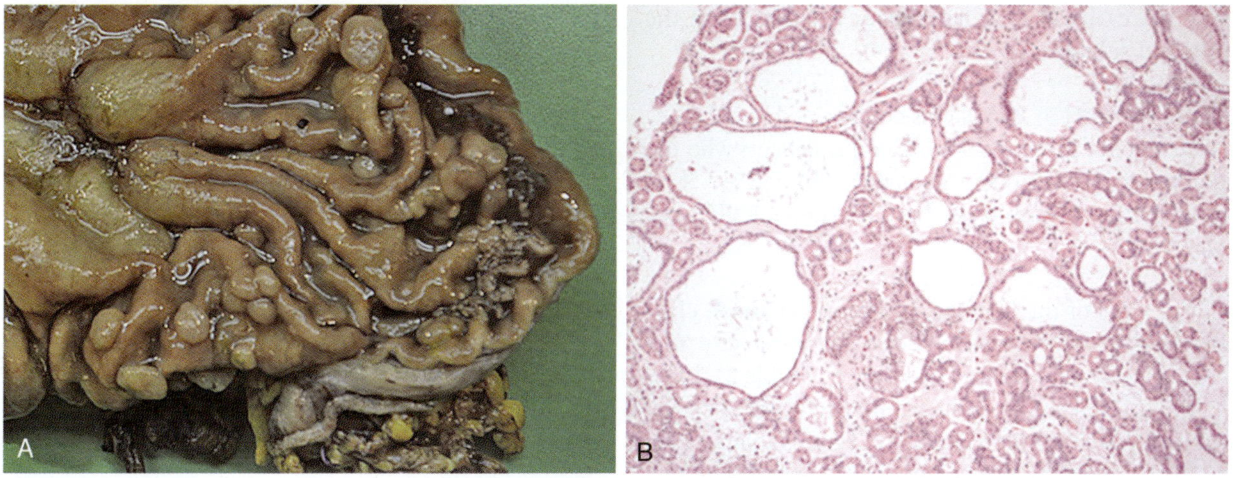

Fig. 21.20 Fundic polyps, gross (A) showing multiple fundic gland polyps and microscopy (B) showing cystically dilated glands lined by parietal and oxyntic cells. (*Source:* From Fiona Campbell and Gregory Y. Lauwers. Tumors of the Esophagus and Stomach. Diagnostic Histopathology of Tumors. 5th Edition. Elsevier 2021; Shoko Vos, Rachel S. van der Post and Lodewijk A.A. Brosens. Gastric Epithelial Polyps. Surgical Pathology Clinics 2020;13:431–452.)

GASTRIC TUMOURS

Gastric Adenoma

Gastric adenomas are polyps of the stomach showing *dysplastic changes* in the epithelium lining and glands. These are *premalignant* with a significant risk of transformation to invasive cancer. The adenomas constitute about 10% of gastric polyps and are common in males in their sixth decade of life. Their incidence is higher in patients with FAP. These usually arise in a setting of chronic gastritis with atrophy and intestinal metaplasia.

Morphology (Fig. 21.21)

Gastric adenomas occur as single lesions in the antrum, usually less than 2 cm, and lesions greater than 2 cm have a higher risk of malignant transformation. The columnar epithelium lining shows dysplastic changes that may be classified into low- and high-grade lesions. Glandular enlargement, pseudostratification, epithelial crowding and nuclear hyperchromasia are seen in both grades. High-grade lesions, in addition, show higher cytological atypia, glandular budding, gland-in-gland appearance and cribriform pattern.

Gastric Carcinoma

PA 24.4

Gastric adenocarcinoma is the most common cancer of the stomach, accounting for 90% of gastric malignancies. It is asymptomatic in many patients and does not present till late in the course of the disease, so it has a poor prognosis.

Epidemiology Gastric carcinoma shows a higher incidence in Japan, Chile, Costa Rica and Eastern Europe. Mass screening programmes in these areas help to identify

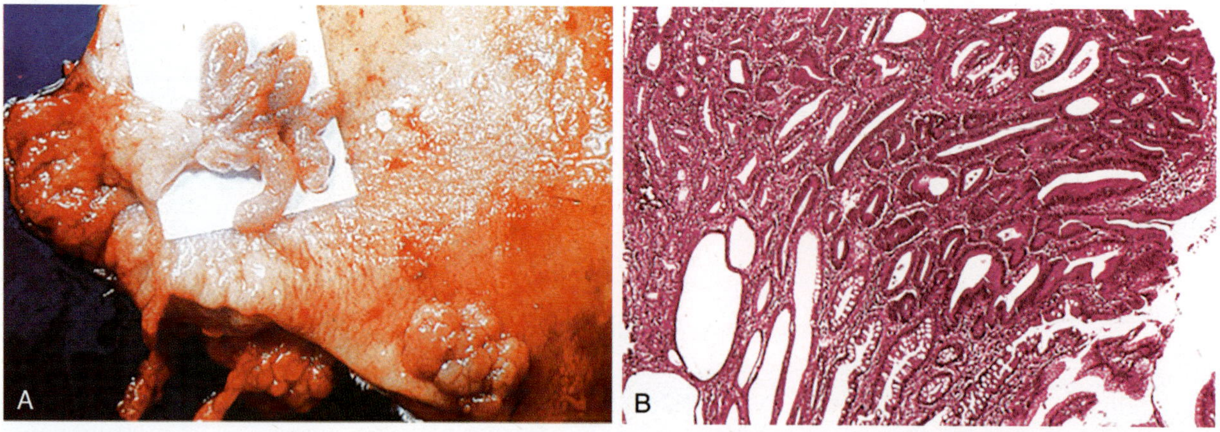

Fig. 21.21 Gastric adenomatous polyp, gross (A) showing a large polyp with finger-like projections and microscopy (B) showing crowding of glands. (*Source:* From John R. Goldblum. Stomach. Rosai and Ackerman's Surgical Pathology. 11th edition. Elsevier 2018.)

cases at an early stage when cancer involves only the mucosa and submucosa.

Aetiology (Table 21.9) *H. pylori* is documented to influence the occurrence of gastric adenocarcinoma. Patients who develop atrophic gastritis due to *H. pylori* infection are at an increased risk in comparison to those who develop PUD.

Classification

1. On the basis of the histological features, **Lauren classification** classifies gastric adenocarcinoma into two types – intestinal type and gastric type (Table 21.10).
2. On the basis of the location, adenocarcinoma is classified into **proximal type** and **distal type** (Table 21.11).
3. On the basis of the depth of invasion, gastric carcinoma can be classified into **early gastric cancer** and **advanced gastric cancer**. Gastric cancer involving only the mucosa and submucosa is called early gastric cancer, whereas the cancer showing invasion of the muscularis propria is denoted as advanced gastric cancer. The former is commonly diagnosed in Japan and has a better prognosis. The Japanese have further classified early gastric cancer as protruding, superficial or excavated (Fig. 21.22).

Table 21.9 Risk Factors for Gastric Carcinoma

- *H. pylori* infection
- Chronic atrophic gastritis
- Intestinal metaplasia
- Dysplasia
- Gastric adenoma
- Cigarette smoking
- Gastric surgery
- Genetic
- Family history of gastric cancer
- Familial adenomatous polyposis
- Hereditary nonpolyposis colorectal cancer
- Peutz–Jeghers syndrome
- Juvenile polyposis

Table 21.10 Intestinal Versus Diffuse Types of Gastric Carcinoma

Intestinal Type	Diffuse Type
• Decreasing incidence • Influenced by dietary and environmental factors • Old age • Composed of gland-like structures • Associated with mutation of the Wnt pathway, loss of function of APC gene and gain of function of β-catenin • Better prognosis	• Increasing incidence • Incidence same throughout the world • Young age • Composed of solitary signet ring cells • Associated with loss-of-function mutation of CDH1, which decreases expression of E-cadherin • Worse prognosis

Table 21.11 Proximal Versus Distal Types of Gastric Adenocarcinoma

Proximal Type	Distal Type
Involves the oesophago-gastric junction and gastric cardia	Involves the fundus, body and antrum
Location more prone to *H. pylori* infection, thus increased incidence	Location less prone to *H. pylori* infection, thus decreased prevalence

4. The **Borrmann classification** is based on the type of growth (Fig. 21.23):
   - Type I (polypoid)
   - Type II (fungating)
   - Type III (ulcerated)
   - Type IV (infiltrative)
5. **WHO classification, 2000**
   - Adenocarcinoma – intestinal type and diffuse type
   - Papillary adenocarcinoma
   - Tubular adenocarcinoma
   - Mucinous adenocarcinoma

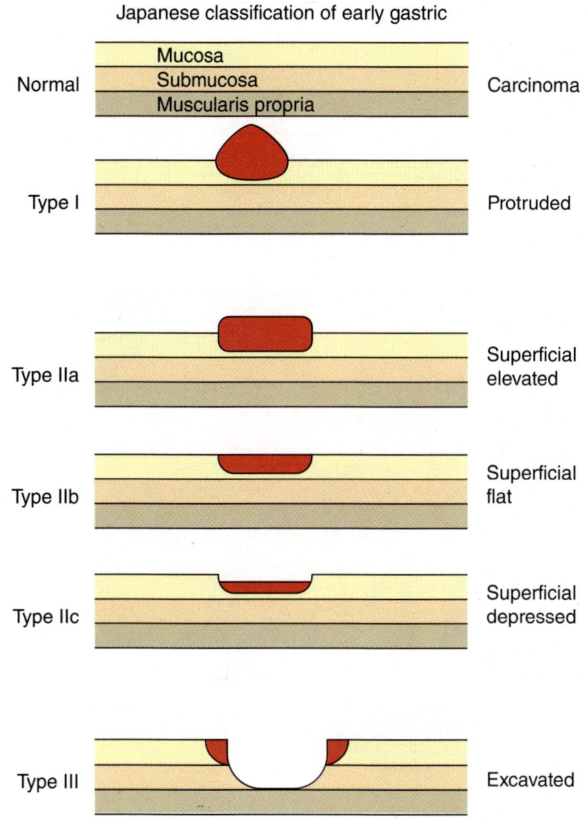

Fig. 21.22 Early gastric carcinoma, the Japanese classification.

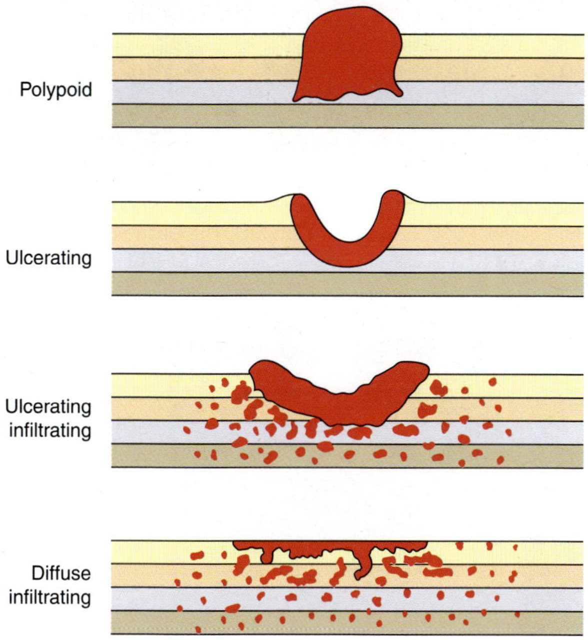

Fig. 21.23 Gastric carcinoma, the Borrmann classification.

- Signet ring cell carcinoma
- Adenosquamous carcinoma
- Squamous cell carcinoma
- Small cell carcinoma
- Undifferentiated carcinoma
- Others

Pathogenesis The development of gastric carcinoma follows multistep carcinogenesis. Normal gastric mucosa transforms into adenoma and later into carcinoma in a stepwise process as depicted in Flowchart 21.3. *H. pylori* has been classified as an important carcinogen involved in this process. Although it may cause both types of adenocarcinoma, the pathway to intestinal type is much better understood.

Morphology

The most common vulnerable sites of gastric carcinoma are the *gastric antrum and lesser curvature* than the greater curvature. On gross appearance, the tumour mass is made up of varying proportions of exophytic and endophytic components (Fig. 21.24).

- **Intestinal type** of tumours (Fig. 21.25) often forms bulky exophytic masses that may have an ulcerated surface. The ulcers have heaped-up margins and are microscopically composed of glandular structures lined by columnar neoplastic cells with apical mucin vacuoles.
- **The diffuse type** of tumours *infiltrates into the wall (endophytic)* of the stomach involving extensive areas. Occasionally, the entire gastric wall stiffens due to desmoplastic reaction. The extensive involvement of the stomach with loss of rugosity gives a leather bottle appearance, termed **linitis plastica**. Microscopically, due to loss of E-cadherin, the tumour is composed of dyscohesive **signet ring cells**, which have large mucin vacuoles pushing the nucleus to the periphery (Fig. 21.25). These cells are seen invading the mucosa and other layers singly or in small groups and may be mistaken for macrophages, making the diagnosis of the tumour difficult in punch biopsies.
- **Mucinous carcinoma** of the stomach grossly appears as a gelatinous soft mass. Microscopically, lakes of extracellular mucin with islands of floating neoplastic cells can be seen. This carcinoma has a better prognosis if not associated with any solid component.

Staging (Fig. 21.26) The important prognostic markers are *depth of invasion and nodal/distant metastasis* at the time of diagnosis. Hence, these markers have been used for staging of tumours by the tumour–nodes–metastasis (TNM) staging system. 'T' denotes the depth of invasion of tumour, 'N' refers to the presence or absence of nodal involvement and 'M' stands for metastatic status.

Clinical Features Intestinal-type gastric carcinoma is twice more common in males, with mean age being 55 years. These carcinomas arise from precursor lesions such as dysplasia and adenoma and are often seen in patients with atrophic gastritis and intestinal metaplasia.

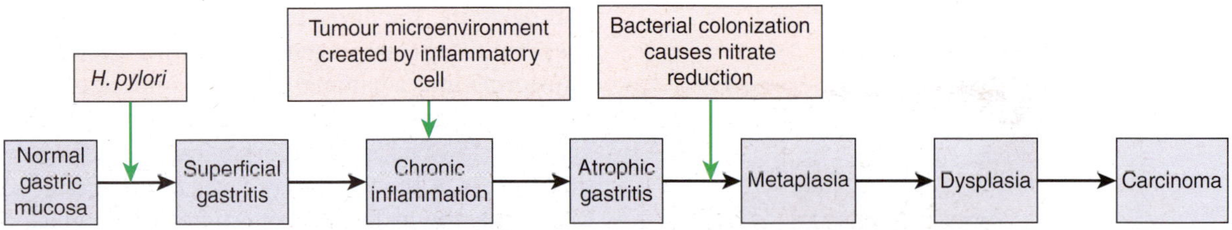

Flowchart 21.3 Adenoma–carcinoma sequence of gastric adenocarcinoma.

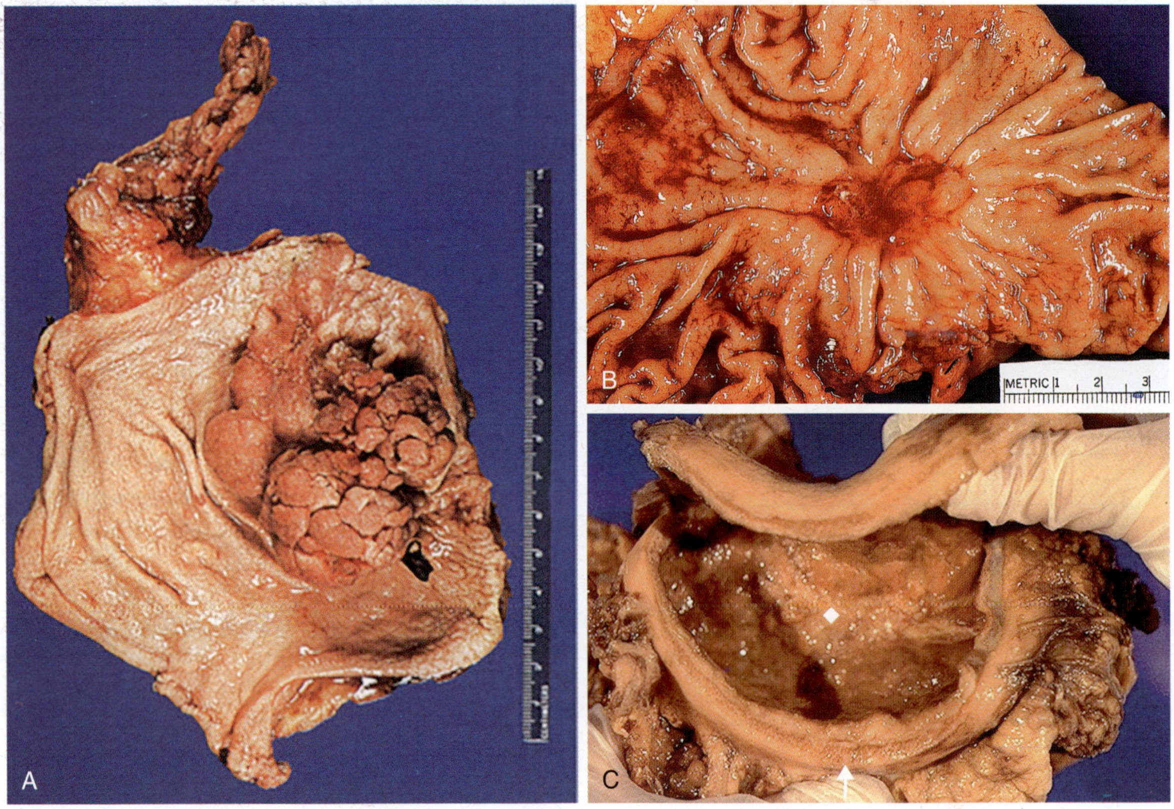

Fig. 21.24 Gastric carcinoma – gross appearance of polypoidal growth (A), ulcerative growth (B) and linitis plastica (C). (*Source:* From John R. Goldblum. Stomach. Rosai and Ackerman's Surgical Pathology. 11th edition. Elsevier 2018; Edward C. Klatt MD, The Gastrointestinal Tract. Robbins and Cotran Atlas of Pathology. 4th edition. Elsevier 2021.)

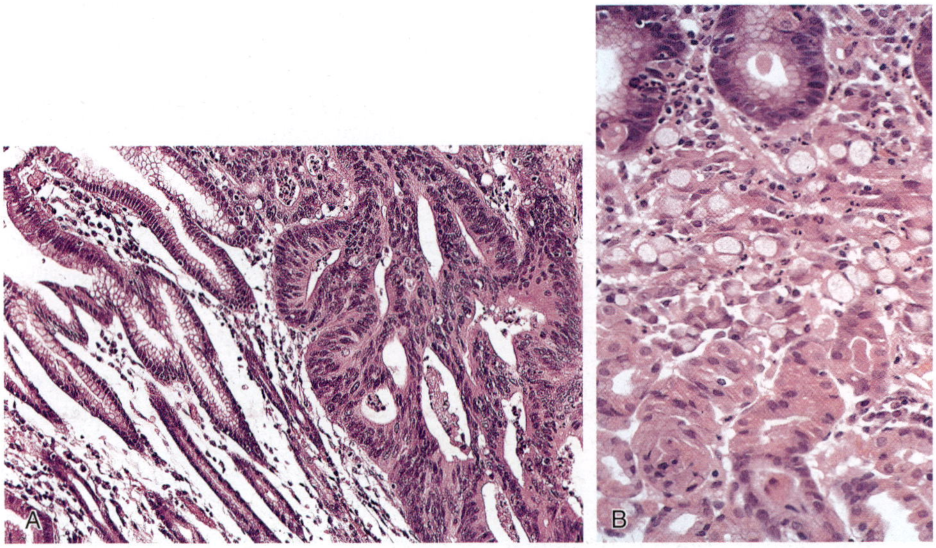

Fig. 21.25 Microscopic appearance of the intestinal type of gastric carcinoma (A) showing malignant glands, and diffuse type of gastric carcinoma (B) showing signet ring cells infiltrating the lamina propria. (*Source:* From John R. Goldblum. Stomach. Rosai and Ackerman's Surgical Pathology. 11th edition. Elsevier 2018; Fiona Campbell and Gregory Y. Lauwers. Tumors of the Esophagus and Stomach. Diagnostic Histopathology of Tumors. 5th edition. Elsevier 2021.)

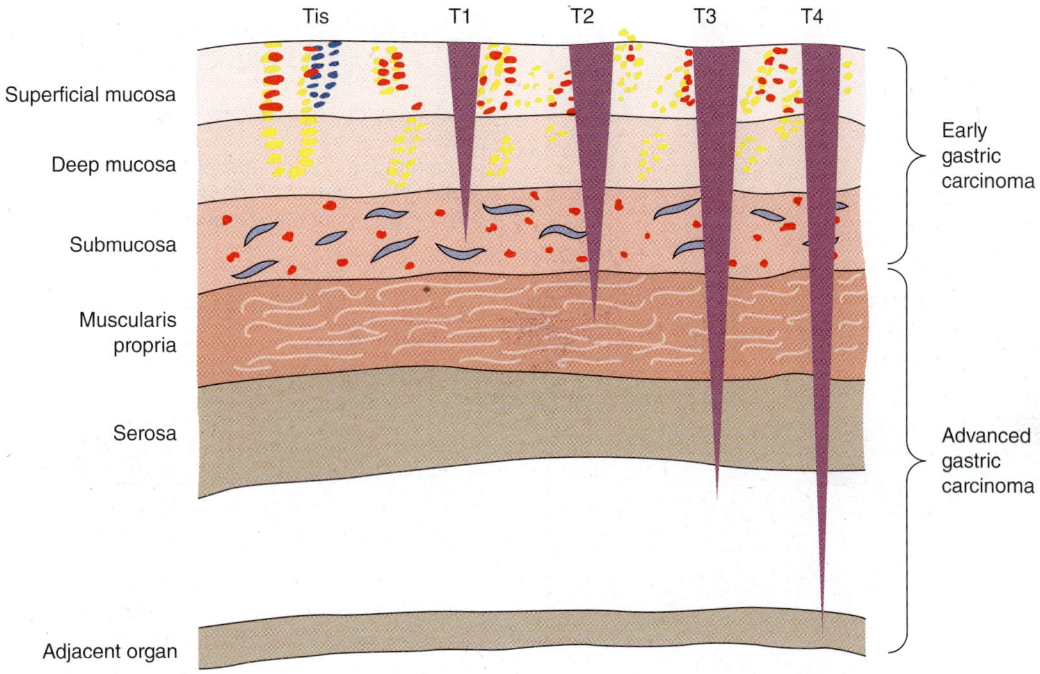

Fig. 21.26 In the TNM classification, T denotes depth of invasion; Tis designates carcinoma in situ, which is tumour cells confined to the epithelial lining of the stomach; T1 tumours are confined to the mucosa (T1a) and submucosa (T1b); T2 tumours invade the muscularis propria but not the serosa; T3 tumours penetrate the subserosal connective tissue without involving the visceral peritoneum or contiguous structures; and T4 tumours invade the serosa (visceral peritoneum) and may involve adjacent organs and tissues. TNM, tumour–nodes–metastasis.

The diffuse type of gastric carcinoma is not associated with any precursor lesions. The incidence of the intestinal-type gastric carcinoma has declined, whereas diffuse carcinoma is still stable in incidence. Patients often present with anaemia, asthenia and anorexia.

Dysphagia may be the presenting symptoms in tumours of the cardia or antrum due to mechanical obstruction. Some tumours present late with an epigastric lump or secondaries such as left supraclavicular node (**Virchow node**), ascites and umbilical nodule (**Sister Joseph nodule**).

Chemotherapy, followed by surgery, is recommended for patients without metastasis. The presence of metastasis is a poor prognostic marker and shifts the management towards chemotherapy and radiotherapy.

LYMPHOMA

The stomach is the most common site of extranodal lymphoma, especially Epstein–Barr virus (EBV)–associated lymphomas that are seen in transplant recipients who are taking oral immunosuppressants. The lymphomas of the stomach arise from mucosa-associated lymphoid tissue (MALT) and are hence called lymphomas of MALT or **MALToma**.

Pathogenesis

Most of the gastric lymphomas are **extranodal marginal zone lymphomas**. The pathogenesis is depicted in Flowchart 21.4.

H. pylori–induced inflammation causes activation of NF-κB, resulting in increased B-cell proliferation and survival. Patients with these lymphomas respond to *H. pylori* eradication treatment protocols with fewer chances of recurrences.

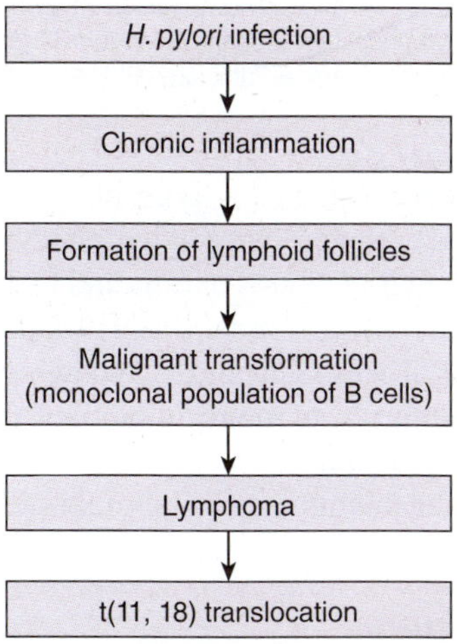

Flowchart 21.4 Pathogenesis of extranodal marginal zone lymphoma.

However, development of t(11,18) or any other MALToma-associated translocation makes the activation of NF-κB constitutive and such patients no longer respond to antibiotic treatment. Other indicators of nonresponse to antibiotic treatment are invasion into muscularis propria, nodal involvement, accumulation of additional mutations such as inactivation of p53 and transformation into more aggressive lymphomas such as **diffuse large B-cell lymphoma**.

Morphology (Fig. 21.27)

Microscopically, the MALTomas show diffuse infiltration of monoclonal lymphocytes into the lamina propria with the formation of lymphoid follicles, plasma

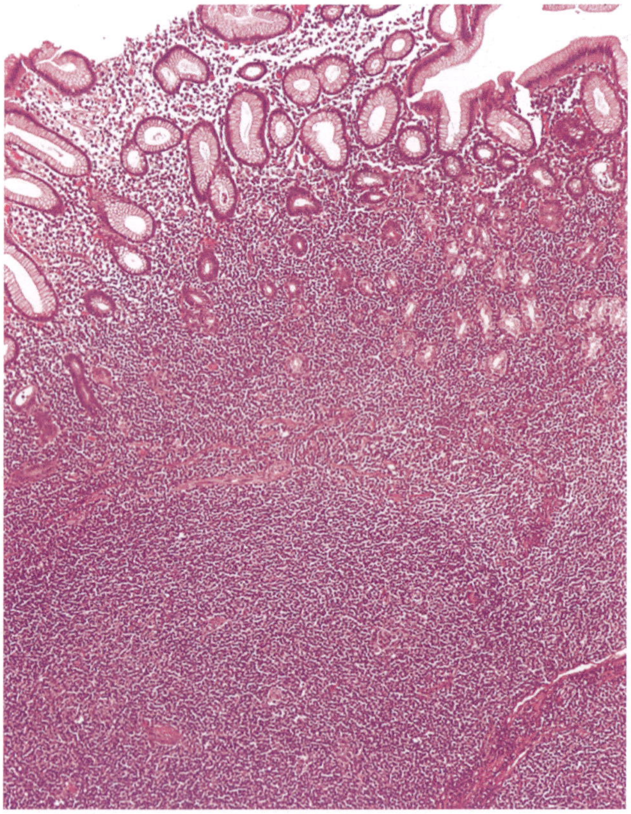

Fig. 21.27 Microscopic appearance of gastric lymphoma showing sheets of monotonous lymphocytes. (*Source:* From John R. Goldblum. Stomach. Rosai and Ackerman's Surgical Pathology. 11th edition. Elsevier 2018.)

cells and the diagnostic **lymphoepithelial lesion**, which refers to the presence of lymphocytes within the glands. The marker status of tumours includes positivity of mature B-cell markers CD19 and CD20, with markers for T cells CD5 and CD10 being negative. In addition, establishing monoclonality of the B cells using kappa or lambda chain of immunoglobulin or IgH gene rearrangements may be helpful in diagnosis.

Clinical Features

Patients commonly present with dyspepsia and epigastric pain or nonspecific symptoms. The investigation of choice for diagnosis is endoscopy with biopsy. However, these are often difficult to differentiate from *H. pylori* infection in gastric biopsies.

NEUROENDOCRINE TUMOURS

Neuroendocrine tumours originate from components of endocrine system scattered in the various parts of the body. The well differentiated tumours were formerly called carcinoids but this word is now restricted to ones located outside the GI tract. The most common site is the the GI tract, with the highest incidence in the small intestine. The next common site is the tracheobronchial tree and lungs. Neuroendocrine neoplasms are commonly associated with conditions that are listed in Table 21.12.

Table 21.12 Conditions Commonly Associated with Carcinoid

Endocrine cell hyperplasia
MEN-1
Autoimmune chronic atrophic gastritis
Zollinger–Ellison syndrome
Proton pump inhibitor therapy (rare)

MEN-1, multiple endocrine neoplasia syndrome 1.

Morphology

Macroscopically, these tumours are located either *submucosally or intramurally*. On the cut surface, the tumour is characteristically yellow or tan coloured and firm in consistency due to the intense desmoplastic reaction (Fig. 21.28). Microscopically, the well differentiated tumours are composed of islands, trabeculae, strands, glands or sheets of uniform cells with pink granular cytoplasm and stippled nucleus, salt and pepper pattern (Fig. 21.29). These usually do not exhibit pleomorphism, but poorly differentiated tumours may show the presence of anaplasia, high mitotic index and necrosis and are called neuroendocrine carcinoma. They exhibit TP53 and Rb mutations, and are further classified into small cell and large cell based on cell morphology.

Immunohistochemically, the neuroendocrine tumour cells express neuroendocrine markers such as **synaptophysin and chromogranin A**. Further neuroendocrine carcinomas show high Ki67 proliferative index expression.

Clinical Features

The incidence is highest in the sixth decade of life, but it may occur in any age, especially in the appendix. The clinical features of the tumour depend on the hormone it elaborates. Tumours producing gastrin cause peptic ulcer

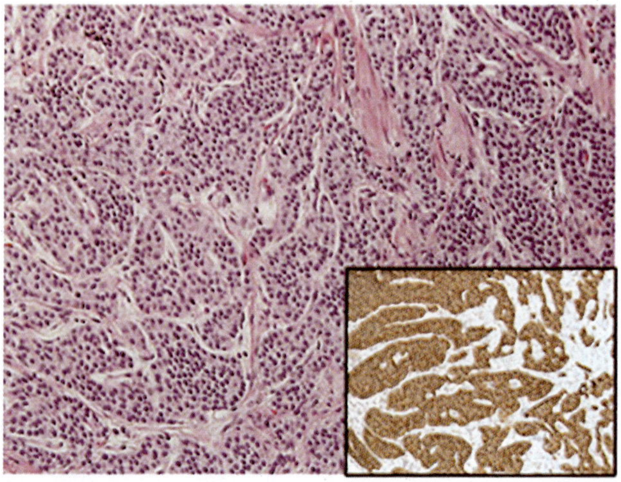

Fig. 21.28 Gastric carcinoid tumour – microscopy showing uniform round cells and IHC chromogranin stain positivity (inset). (*Source:* From Rathore, Bharti. Gastrinoma. Elsevier 2022.)

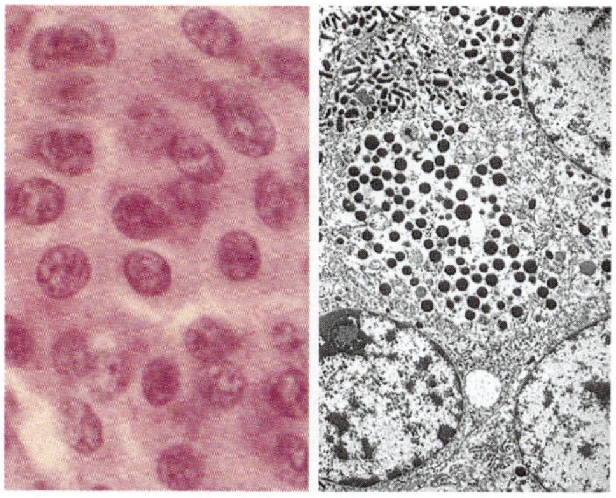

Fig. 21.29 High-power view showing salt and pepper chromatin in the nucleus of the cells, and electron microscopy shows cytoplasmic dense core neurosecretory granules. (Sodium Chloride. Drug information provided by Gold Standard. Elsevier.)

and ZES, whereas tumours of the small intestine elaborate vasoactive substances causing carcinoid syndrome. **Carcinoid syndrome** manifests as flushing, sweating, bronchospasm, abdominal colic pain and diarrhoea but is quite rare due to the inactivation of the released substances during the 'first-pass' metabolism in the liver. A sudden onset of carcinoid syndrome in patients with small intestinal carcinoid should warn the possibility of *liver metastasis*.

The behaviour of tumours and prognosis of the patient depend on the *location of the tumours*. Midgut carcinoids are more likely to be malignant, whereas appendiceal carcinoids are almost always benign.

The carcinoids are hence classified into foregut carcinoids, midgut carcinoids and hindgut carcinoids (Table 21.13).

Management of carcinoids depends on their grade and stage. Small carcinoids detected early may be resected endoscopically and followed up, whereas large carcinoids with invasion need open surgical resection and chemotherapy.

GASTROINTESTINAL STROMAL TUMOUR

GI stromal tumour (GIST) is the most common abdominal mesenchymal tumour. In the GI tract, the most common site is the stomach. Similarly, the most common mesenchymal tumour of the stomach is GIST, and it may be recalled here that the most common mesenchymal tumour of the oesophagus is leiomyoma. The tumour is postulated to originate from the interstitial *cells of Cajal* or the pacemaker cells of the muscularis propria. Precursors of GIST with low mitotic index are seen in about 20% of resected stomach samples, and these have a low risk of transformation to GIST. GIST is seen to peak around 60 years of age. An increased incidence is seen in neurofibromatosis 1 (NF1) and in children with Carney triad (gastric GIST, paraganglioma and pulmonary chondroma).

Pathogenesis

About 80% of the patients exhibit *gain-of-function mutation of receptors tyrosine kinase* (KIT), and about 8% show mutations of platelet-derived growth factor receptor α (PDGFRA). These may be sporadic or germline mutations and result in constitutively activated KIT or PDGFRA, causing tumour cell proliferation and survival. Although these mutations are the initiating steps in tumorigenesis, progression to overt GIST requires additional mutations.

Morphology

Macroscopically, the tumour is a large, solitary, solid, well-circumscribed mass protruding into the lumen and/or serosal surface. Mucosal ulceration may be seen. The cut surface shows a whorled appearance (Fig. 21.30). Microscopically, the tumour is classified on the basis of the type of cell – **spindle cell variant** composed of whorls of spindle cells or **epithelioid variant** when composed of epithelial-like cells (Fig. 21.31). The mitotic index is noted to help in prognosis. The most useful IHC marker is *KIT* seen in tumour cells.

Table 21.13 Features of Carcinoid According to its Location

Feature	Foregut Carcinoid	Midgut Carcinoid	Hindgut Carcinoid
Location	Oesophagus, stomach, proximal duodenum	Jejunum and ileum	Appendix and colorectum
Fraction of GI carcinoid	<20%	>40%	Appendix <25% Colorectum <25%
Symptoms	Gastritis, peptic ulcer, abdominal pain	Asymptomatic, obstruction, metastasis	Asymptomatic, abdominal pain, weight loss
Behaviour	Variable	Aggressive	Benign
Outcome	Good when associated with atrophic gastritis	Worse outcome, especially when associated with local invasion, necrosis and mitosis	Usually diagnosed early, thus have a good outcome

GI, gastrointestinal.

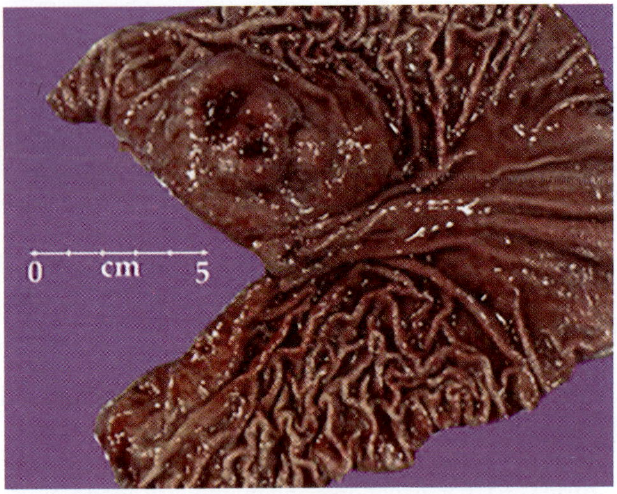

Fig. 21.30 Gross appearance of GIST as multiple submucous nodules. (*Source:* From Markku Miettinen, Jerzy Lasota, Gastroenterology Clinics of North America, Elsevier 2013.)

Clinical Features

GIST may be incidentally diagnosed during imaging or endoscopy or surgery. Occasionally, it presents with mucosal ulceration, causing bleeding and anaemia or mass effect. Management is by surgical excision of the tumour. The prognostic indicators are *tumour size, mitotic index and location*. Tumours less than 5 cm and having a low mitotic index metastasize or recur less commonly than mitotically active larger tumours. In addition, gastric GIST have a more favourable prognosis than intestinal GIST.

For surgically nonresectable tumours that have KIT or PDGFRA mutations, the drug of choice is the tyrosine kinase inhibitor – imatinib. In patients undergoing treatment, development of additional mutations leads to imatinib resistance.

SMALL INTESTINE AND COLON

Small intestine and colon are the important parts of the GI tract that help in absorption of nutrients and coherently interact with various antigens present in our food. The intestines also house a wide variety of bacteria that not only act as the beneficial flora but also make the gut a fertile soil for numerous infectious and inflammatory conditions.

MALABSORPTION AND DIARRHOEA

Malabsorption refers to defective absorption of nutrients such as fats, carbohydrates, proteins, vitamins, minerals, electrolytes and water. The hallmark of malabsorption is **steatorrhoea**, which is the passage of excess faecal fat which causes frothy, bulky, greasy, yellow-coloured stools that are difficult to flush.

Malabsorption results due to disturbance in one or more of the four phases of nutrient absorption.

The four phases of absorption are as follows:

1. **Intraluminal digestion** – breaking up of nutrients
2. **Terminal digestion** – done by brush border enzymes of the small intestine
3. **Transepithelial transport** – transport of nutrients by small intestinal epithelium
4. **Lymphatic transport** of absorbed lipids – forms the chyle

The symptoms of malabsorption overlap among the different phases, the most common being diarrhoea, flatus and abdominal pain. Malabsorption of vitamins can lead to various vitamin deficiencies and when chronic results in anaemia, weight loss and muscle wasting. Thus, the proper assessment by endoscopic evaluation with a small full-thickness mucosal biopsy is a must to determine the cause. Among the various causes of malabsorption, *coeliac disease is the most common* in India along with tropical sprue (Table 21.14).

Diarrhoea is defined as an increase in stool mass, frequency or fluidity, typically greater than 200 g/day. Painful, bloody, small-volume diarrhoea is called dysentery. The four types of diarrhoea are secretory, osmotic, malabsorptive and exudative diarrhoea (Table 21.15).

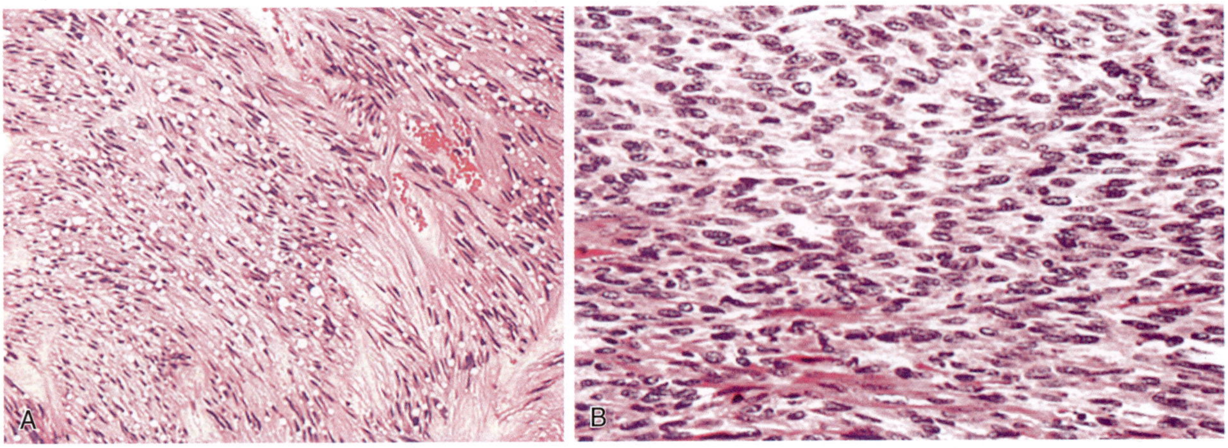

Fig. 21.31 Microscopy of GIST – (A) low grade showing perinuclear vacuoles and (B) high grade showing increased cellularity and absence of vacuoles. (*Source:* From John R. Goldblum. Stomach. Rosai and Ackerman's Surgical Pathology. 11th edition. Elsevier 2018.)

Table 21.14 Causes of Malabsorption

- Coeliac disease
- Environmental enteropathy
- Chronic pancreatitis
- Cystic fibrosis
- Primary bile acid malabsorption
- Carcinoid syndrome
- Autoimmune enteropathy
- Disaccharidase deficiency
- Whipple disease
- Abetalipoproteinaemia
- Viral, bacterial, parasitic gastroenteritis
- Inflammatory bowel disease

Having learnt an outline about malabsorption and diarrhoea, lets us now discuss a few common causes of malabsorption and their pathogenesis.

Cystic Fibrosis

Cystic fibrosis is caused by the absence of epithelial cystic fibrosis transmembrane conductance regulator (CFTR). It affects various organs, especially the lungs. The affected individuals have defective transport of chloride and bicarbonate ions, resulting in defective luminal hydration.

Affected individuals present with symptoms of malabsorption of fat and fat-soluble vitamins (Flowchart 21.5). This can, however, be corrected by pancreatic enzyme supplements.

Coeliac Disease

Coeliac disease or coeliac sprue is a **gluten-sensitive enteropathy** caused by an immune-mediated response to ingestion of food containing gluten in genetically predisposed individuals. The overall incidence is 0.6%–1% but varies in various regions on the basis of the diet and the genetic pattern.

Aetiology Coeliac disease is primarily the response to gluten present in wheat, barley and rye. Almost all individuals with coeliac disease have class II HLA-DQ2 or HLA-DQ8 allele, making it a critical influencing factor. The other contributing factors include polymorphisms of genes that regulate immunity and epithelial function.

Pathogenesis (Fig. 21.32) In individuals who are prone to coeliac disease, the response is triggered by ingestion of **gluten** in the diet. The gluten is broken down to **gliadin** by the luminal brush border enzymes. The gliadin further stimulates the production of IL-15 by the epithelial cells, thereby inducing the proliferation of CD8 cytotoxic lymphocytes within the epithelium. These cytotoxic lymphocytes express NKG2D, which acts as a receptor for MIC-A and destroys enterocytes that express MIC-A. The next phase of attack is due to the passage of the gliadin into the lamina propria through the CD8-damaged enterocytes. Here, the gliadin is deamidated by tissue *transglutaminase* and presented by HLA-DQ2 or HLA-DQ8 on antigen-presenting cells. This activates $CD4^+$ T cells to produce cytokines that cause tissue damage and induce plasma cells to produce various antibodies. These antibodies can be detected in sera of patients and are useful in diagnosis.

Noninvasive investigations in these patients include measurement of *IgA antibodies against tissue transglutaminase, IgA antiendomysial antibodies and IgG anti-tissue transglutaminase antibodies* (in patients with IgA deficiency). The absence of HLA-DQ2 and HLA-DQ8 can be tested for their high negative predictive values, but diagnosis cannot be confirmed by the presence of these alleles.

Morphology (Fig. 21.33)

Biopsy ideally should be taken from the second part of the duodenum or proximal jejunum. The histology findings include the following:

- Increased intraepithelial $CD8^+$ T lymphocytes
- Villous atrophy
- Crypt hyperplasia
- Loss of mucosal brush border
- Increased crypt mitotic rate
- Presence of plasma cells, eosinophils and mast cells in lamina propria

Among these, the first two findings are sensitive markers but not specific to coeliac disease. Hence, biopsy findings combined with serology help in making a specific diagnosis. On strict adherence to gluten-free diet, normal histology is restored in the mucosa in 6–24 months along with a decrease in titres of antibodies.

Table 21.15 Types of Diarrhoea

Type of Diarrhoea	Nature of Stool	Response to Fasting	Common Causes
Secretory diarrhoea	Isotonic stools	Persists on fasting	*Vibrio cholerae, Escherichia coli,* rotavirus infections
Osmotic diarrhoea	More concentrated than plasma	Relieved on fasting	Lactase deficiency
Malabsorptive diarrhoea	Associated with steatorrhoea	Relieved on fasting	Pancreatic insufficiency
Exudative diarrhoea	Purulent bloody stools	Persists on fasting	Inflammatory bowel disease, severe bacterial infections

Defective luminal hydration
↓
Thick secretions in pancreatic ducts
↓
Duct obstruction
↓
Chronic autodigestion of pancreas
↓
Pancreatic insufficiency
↓
Malabsorption

Flowchart 21.5 Pathogenesis of malabsorption in cystic fibrosis.

Clinical Features In adults, the common age of presentation is 30–60 years. It is more common in women than in men. It may present as follows:

- With typical symptoms of diarrhoea, abdominal bloating and fatigue
- Asymptomatic for long with the late presentation of anaemia and vitamin deficiency
- **Silent coeliac disease** with positive serology and villous atrophy but no symptoms
- **Latent coeliac disease** with positive serology but no villous atrophy

In children, males and females are equally affected at the time of introduction of gluten in the diet, between

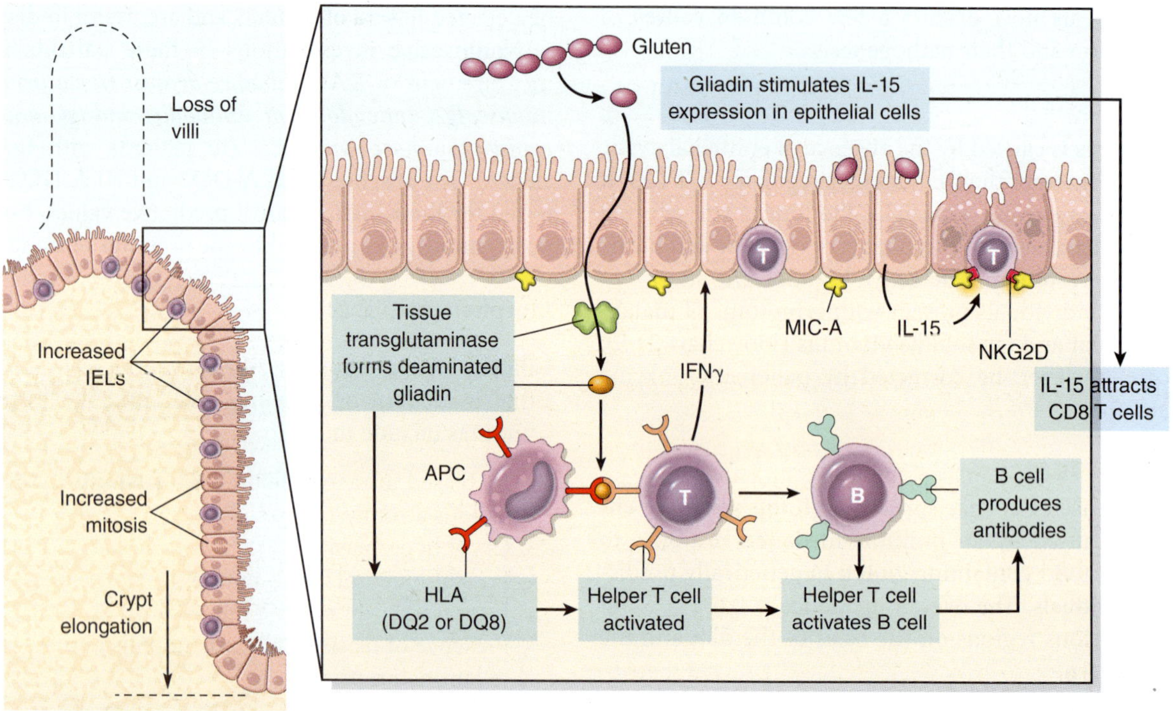

Fig. 21.32 Pathogenesis of coeliac disease showing the involvement of CD4 cells, CD8 cells and B cells. (*Source:* From Vinay Kumar, Abul K. Abbas and Jon C. Aster. The Gastrointestinal Tract. Robbins & Cotran Pathologic Basis of Disease. 10th edition. Elsevier 2021.)

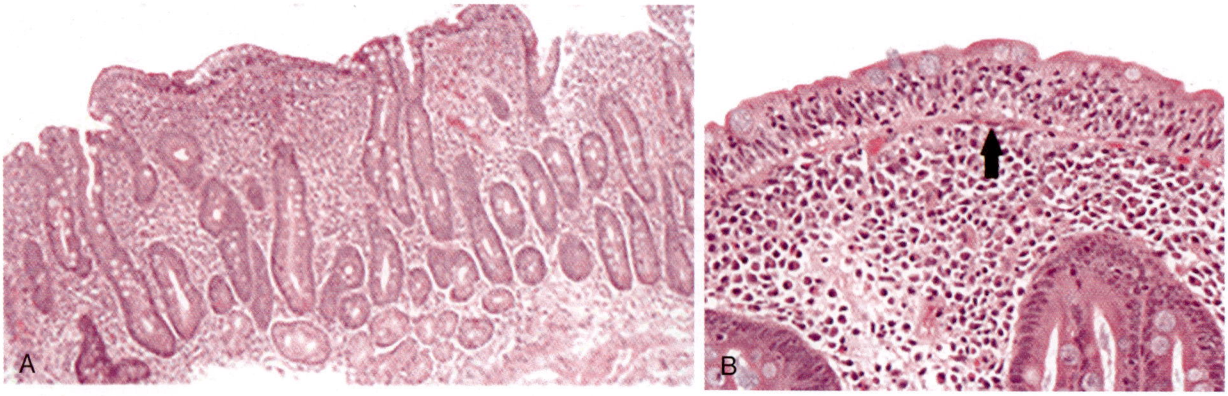

Fig. 21.33 Microscopic appearance of coeliac disease showing villous atrophy (A) and T cells in the epithelium with plasma cells in the lamina propria in a high-power view (B). (*Source:* From Stephen M. Lagana and Govind Bhagat. Biopsy Diagnosis of Celiac Disease. Gastroenterology Clinics of North America. 2019;48:39–51.)

6 and 24 months of age. The classical symptoms are irritability, abdominal distension, chronic diarrhoea, anorexia, failure to thrive, muscle wasting or weight loss. Some children may present late or have extraintestinal complaints such as joint pain, aphthous stomatitis, iron-deficiency anaemia, delayed puberty and short stature.

Other features of this disease include the presence of itchy blistering skin lesions, dermatitis herpetiformis, in about 10% of patients. The long-term complications include anaemia, female infertility, osteoporosis and cancers such as *enteropathy-associated T-cell lymphoma and small intestinal adenocarcinoma.* Strict adherence to gluten-free diet is the only mode of management available now that reduces symptoms and risk of long-term complications. However, relapse of symptoms when taking gluten-free diet may suggest *refractory sprue or development of cancer.*

Tropical Sprue

Tropical sprue, also called **environmental enteropathy or tropical enteropathy**, is a disorder encountered in developing countries with poor sanitation and bad hygiene. It is associated with chronic malabsorption, causing malnutrition and stunted growth. The defective mucosal immune response explains the high rates of oral vaccine failure in these regions. Intestinal biopsy findings are not specific and resemble those of severe coeliac disease. The aetiology is unknown, but possible causes are defective intestinal barrier function, chronic exposure to faecal pathogens and repeated bouts of diarrhoea within 2–3 years of birth. The deficiencies in these children are difficult to be corrected with oral diet or nutritional supplements, thereby affecting the physical and cognitive development. Globally, tropical sprue is considered to be one of the important causes of childhood death.

Lactase Deficiency

Lactase is a *disaccharidase enzyme* located in the apical brush border of epithelial cells of the small intestine. It converts the lactose present in the diet to glucose and galactose for absorption. The absence of lactase results in inability to absorb lactose that gets broken down by intestinal bacteria, releasing gas that causes bloating, abdominal pain, borborygmi, flatulence and explosive diarrhoea with frothy stools. Lactase deficiency is of two types:

- **Congenital lactase deficiency** is an autosomal recessive disorder. The affected infants present with symptoms on milk ingestion. Introduction of soy-based milk has helped in the management of these infants by relieving symptoms.
- **Acquired lactase deficiency** occurs following enteric viral or bacterial infections and usually resolves spontaneously. It is common in Afro-Americans and Native Americans.

The disorder usually manifests on intake of lactose-containing milk and milk products. Faecal pH and the presence of reducing sugar in stools help to diagnose this condition in suspected cases. *Biopsy is normal* because the disorder is biochemical with no associated histological changes.

Abetalipoproteinaemia

Abetalipoproteinaemia is a rare autosomal recessive disease in which the enterocytes are *unable to secrete triglyceride-rich lipoproteins.* The transfer of lipids to apolipoprotein B in the rough endoplasmic reticulum and production of triglyceride droplets in the smooth endoplasmic reticulum require microsomal triglyceride transfer protein (MTP). Without MTP, enterocytes cannot assemble or export lipoproteins. Hence, the lipids accumulate inside the enterocyte, causing vacuolization of small intestinal epithelial cells. This can be demonstrated by Oil Red O stain after a high-fat diet. Affected infants are unable to absorb fat and fat-soluble vitamins, resulting in steatorrhoea, diarrhoea and failure to thrive. The plasma lipoprotein levels show complete absence and peripheral smear shows *acanthocytic red cells* (burr cells).

INFECTIOUS ENTEROCOLITIS

Infection of the intestines is a very common problem encountered in developing and underdeveloped countries due to poor sanitation and hygiene. It may present with various symptoms such as diarrhoea, abdominal pain, dysentery, urgency, perianal discomfort or incontinence. It is one of the important causes of mortality among children. Enterocolitis may be caused by bacteria, virus or parasites. Among the various aetiological agents, enterotoxigenic *Escherichia coli, Vibrio cholerae* and enteric viruses (in paediatric cases) top the list (Table 21.16). The pathologically important infections are dealt with here in this chapter.

Table 21.16 Common Causes of Infectious Enterocolitis

Bacterial causes	Parasitic enterocolitis
Cholera	*Ascaris lumbricoides*
Shigellosis	*Strongyloides*
Enteric fever	*Necator duodenale* and
Clostridium difficile	*Ancylostoma duodenale*
Campylobacter jejuni	*Enterobius vermicularis*
Yersinia pestis	*Trichuris trichiura*
Escherichia coli	Schistosomiasis
Whipple disease	Intestinal cestodes
Mycobacterium species	*Entamoeba histolytica*
	Giardia lamblia
	Cryptosporidium
Viral causes	
Rotavirus	
Nova virus	
Adenovirus	

Salmonella Infection

Salmonella species are gram-negative bacilli within the family of Enterobacteriaceae. The two common types of clinical diseases in host humans include salmonellosis caused by *S. enteritidis* and typhoid caused by *S. enterica*.

Salmonellosis Salmonellosis is common in young adults and children due to ingestion of contaminated meat, especially when eaten raw or undercooked, eggs and milk. Vaccines are available for farm animals and humans, and newer vaccines have been found to give protection even in children. Infection spreads by the faeco-oral route, and the risk is higher among people with atrophic gastritis and those on acid-suppressive therapy.

Pathogenesis *Salmonella* causes damage to enterocytes in the following manner:

- **Virulence genes**, which enable it to transfer bacterial proteins into enterocytes and thereby gain entry into the enterocytes and grow there
- **Flagellin**, which activates TLR5 on host cells and activates host inflammatory response
- **Bacterial Lipopolysaccharides**, which activates TLR4
- Induces release of *hepoxilin A3* by epithelial cells that attract neutrophils, which potentiate mucosal damage

T-helper 1 and T-helper 17 cells are important for immunity against *Salmonella*, and individuals with defective T_H1 and T_H17 cells are at a high risk of disseminated salmonellosis. Diagnosis is established by stool culture.

Clinical Features The organism is shed in stools for several weeks even after resolution of symptoms. Thus, loose stools to profuse watery diarrhoea or dysentery and fever can bring salmonellosis into the differential. Most of the times, infection is self-limited, and the usage of antibiotics prolongs the carrier state or may cause relapse. Risk of extraintestinal complications is higher in patients with morbid conditions like malignancies, alcoholism, immunosuppression, cardiovascular dysfunction, haemolytic anaemia and sickle cell disease (probably due to immunity suppression).

Enteric Fever Typhoid fever or enteric fever is caused by *Salmonella enterica* whose two subtypes are *typhi* and *paratyphi*. In endemic countries, infection is due to *S. typhi*, whereas in travellers, *S. paratyphi* has been incriminated. In endemic areas like India, Mexico, Pakistan and Philippines, children and adolescents are mostly affected, and in developed countries, the only criterion is travel to an endemic country. Transmission occurs from person to person or via food and contaminated water. *S. typhi* or *S. paratyphi* often colonize the gall bladder and may cause gallstones and chronic carrier state.

Pathogenesis *S. typhi* bacilli invade the M cells of the small intestine and are taken by the macrophages to the mucosal lymphoid tissue. These are capable of disseminating through blood vessels and lymphatics that causes reactive hyperplasia of lymph nodes throughout the body and extraintestinal complications.

Clinical Features The common symptoms are anorexia, abdominal pain, bloating, nausea, vomiting and bloody diarrhoea. This is followed by a short asymptomatic phase and then progresses to develop bacteraemia and fever. Diagnosis by blood culture is positive only during the febrile phase. Antibiotic treatment can prevent disease progression. The patient may develop small erythematous maculopapular lesions, the **rose spots**, on the chest and abdomen. **Extraintestinal complications** include encephalopathy, meningitis, seizures, endocarditis, myocarditis, pneumonia and cholecystitis. *Salmonella* osteomyelitis is a unique complication seen in patients with sickle cell disease.

Morphology

Gross examination of the intestine shows *markedly enlarged Peyer's patches* in the terminal ileum up to 8 cm, producing plateau-like elevations and enlarged draining mesenteric lymph nodes. The ensuing mucosal damage causes *oval ulcers along the axis* of the ileum and occasional associated perforations (Fig. 21.34). Microscopy shows the enlarged Peyer's patches with acute and chronic inflammatory cell infiltration in the lamina propria.

The liver, bone marrow and lymph nodes show nodules called **typhoid nodules**, which are foci of parenchymal necrosis replaced by macrophage aggregates.

Pseudomembranous Colitis

Pseudomembranous colitis, also called **antibiotic-associated colitis**, is caused by ***Clostridium difficile***. This is the only organism that forms pseudomembrane on the intestinal mucosa and hence the name. Risk factors include old age, immunosuppression, hospitalization and antibiotic treatment. Although *C. difficile* colonization is common in hospitalized patients, not everyone develops this disease.

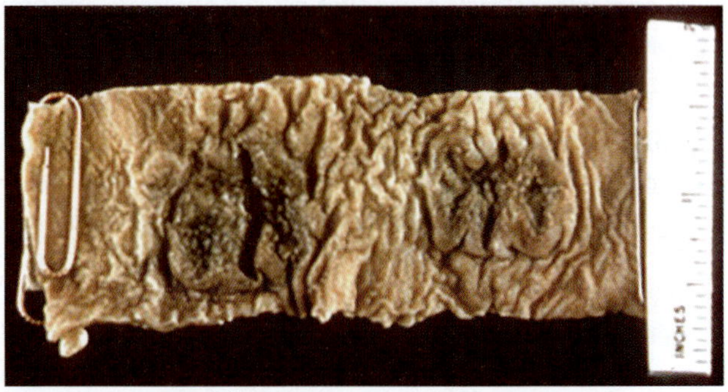

Fig. 21.34 Gross appearance of typhoid ulcers in the intestine. (*Source:* From Gregory Y. Lauwers, Mari Mino-Kendudson and Richard L. Kradin. Infections of the Gastrointestinal Tract. Diagnostic Pathology of Infectious Disease. 2nd edition. Elsevier 2018.)

Pathogenesis Frequent or prolonged use of antibiotics destroys the normal microbial flora, permitting the overgrowth of *C. difficile*. This condition is more common in those on immunosuppression therapy. The toxins (mainly toxin A and toxin B) released by *C. difficile* cause disruption of the epithelial cytoskeleton with loss of tight junction barrier, which further induces the release of cytokines and apoptosis.

Morphology

The important finding in this condition is the presence of **pseudomembrane** (Fig. 21.35). The infection first causes damage of the epithelium with neutrophilic infiltration of the lamina propria and thrombosis of capillaries. The crypts then get damaged and distended with mucopurulent exudate. These later erupt like a volcano, releasing the exudate on the surface, thereby forming the pseudomembrane. Hence, pseudomembrane is an adherent layer of inflammatory cells and debris at the sites of mucosal injury in the colon.

Clinical Features Symptoms of pseudomembranous colitis include fever, leucocytosis, abdominal pain, cramps, watery diarrhoea and dehydration. There may be hypoalbuminaemia due to protein loss. Stools may contain occult blood and leucocytes, but frank bloody diarrhoea is not seen. Diagnosis is by detection of *C. difficile* toxin in faeces and endoscopic biopsy. The condition responds well to metronidazole and vancomycin. However, in view of the emergence of antibiotic resistance, newer antibiotics and monoclonal antibodies against toxins A and B are being tried now.

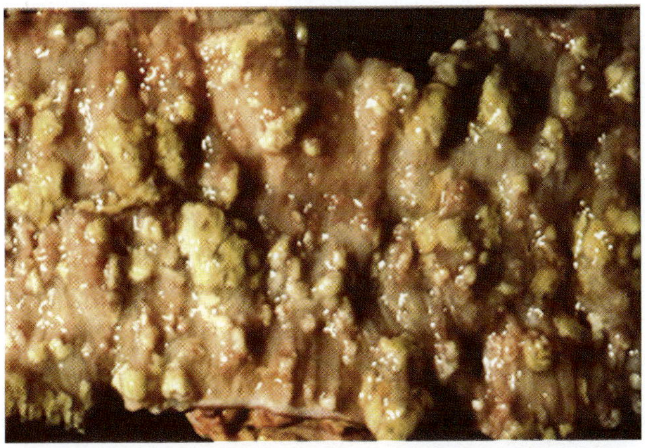

Fig. 21.35 Gross appearance of pseudomembranous colitis formed by coalescing, raised, adherent and yellow plaques that vary in size from 2 to 5 mm. (*Source:* From Ciarán P. Kelly and Sahil Khanna. Antibiotic-Associated Diarrhea and Clostridioides difficile Infection. Sleisenger and Fordtran's Gastrointestinal and Liver Disease. 11th edition. Elsevier 2021.)

Whipple Disease

Whipple disease is a rare disease first described as **intestinal lipodystrophy** by George Hoyt Whipple in 1907. It affects multiple organs, and patients present with extraintestinal manifestations months or years before malabsorption.

Pathogenesis Whipple disease is caused by the gram-positive actinomycete, *Tropheryma whipplei*. These organisms are engulfed by macrophages, and the macrophages accumulate in the lamina propria of the small intestine and in mesenteric lymph nodes. They cause obstruction in the lymphatics that absorb nutrients, especially fat. Thus, the malabsorption in Whipple disease is due to impairment in lymphatic transport.

Morphology

On endoscopic examination, the affected mucosa shows white or yellow plaques and a shaggy appearance of expanded villi. On microscopy, the lamina propria shows a dense accumulation of foamy macrophages containing periodic Schiff-positive, diastase-resistant granules (Fig. 21.36). These granules represent lysosomes laden with partially digested bacteria. These bacteria can be differentiated from intestinal tuberculosis causing *Mycobacterium tuberculosis* by acid-fast stains, because, unlike mycobacteria, they do not stain positive. Similar aggregation of bacteria-laden macrophages can be seen in mesenteric lymph nodes, synovial membranes of affected joints, cardiac valves, brain and other sites.

Clinical Features Whipple disease is common in Caucasian farmers who are exposed to soil or animals, with certain unidentified genetic factors playing a role in predisposition. The patients usually present with diarrhoea, weight loss and arthralgia. Extraintestinal symptoms include arthritis, arthralgia, fever, lymphadenopathy and neurological, cardiac or pulmonary disease.

Parasitic Enterocolitis

Parasitic enterocolitis, though not as common as bacterial or viral enterocolitis, causes a significant number of infections worldwide. About 20 parasites can be seen to infect the small intestine, but it is beyond the purview of this book. We discuss amoebiasis here due to the characteristic pathological changes it causes in the intestine.

Amoebiasis Amoebiasis is caused by *Entamoeba histolytica* and, like most other parasites, is transmitted by faeco-oral route. *E. histolytica* infection is quite prevalent in tropical countries with poor sanitation such as India, Mexico and Colombia and is an important cause of dysentery and liver abscess. The cysts of these parasites are

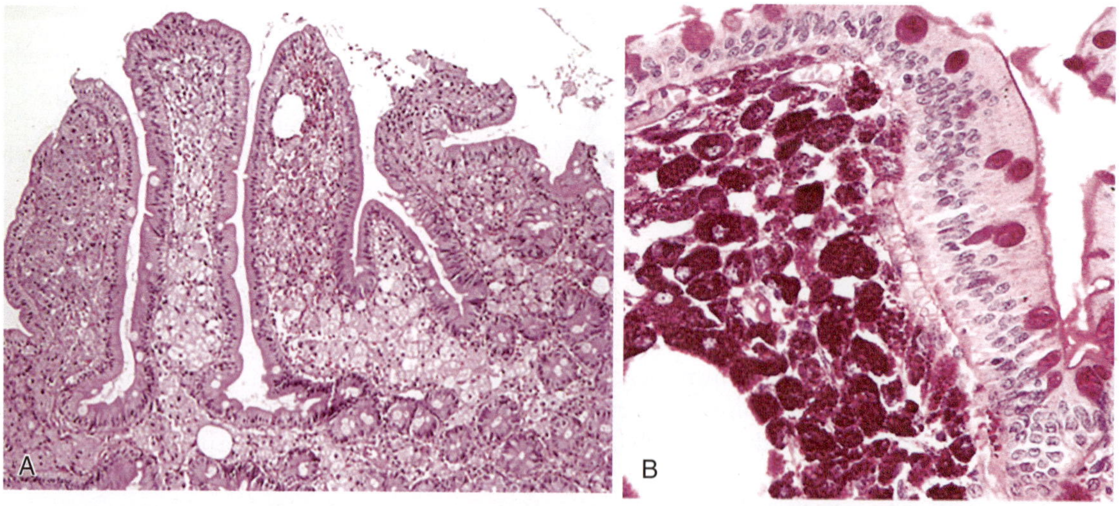

Fig. 21.36 Microscopic appearance of Whipple disease showing the lamina propria packed with histiocytes (A) and PAS stain demonstrating intracytoplasmic inclusions (B). (*Source:* From Laura W. Lamps. Small Bowel. Rosai and Ackerman's Surgical Pathology. 11th edition. Elsevier 2018; Robert E. Petras. Gastrointestinal System. In Differential Diagnosis in Surgical Pathology. Elsevier 2015.)

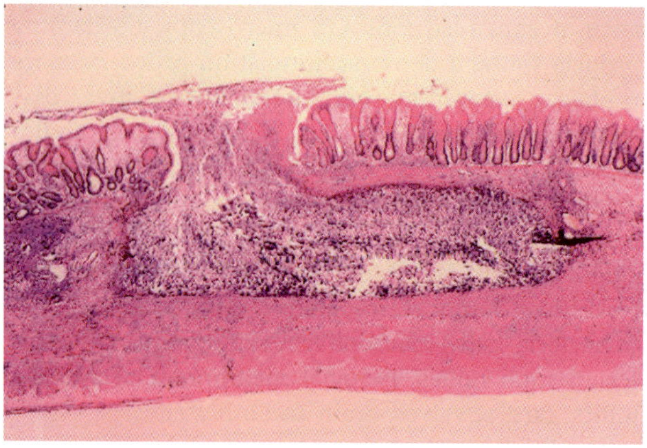

Fig. 21.37 Microscopic appearance showing flask-shaped mucosal ulceration with a widespread submucosal invasion. (*Source:* From Stanley SL. Amoebiasis. Lancet 2003; 361:1025–1034.)

resistant to gastric digestion and hence are able to reach the colon and colonize the epithelial surface. There they release trophozoites and amoebae that are capable of reproducing even in anaerobic conditions.

Morphology

Entamoeba colonizes the caecum and the ascending colon, but the sigmoid colon, rectum and appendix may also be involved. The pathogen invades the crypt and burrows laterally in the lamina propria, forming **flask-shaped ulcers** (narrow neck, broad base) (Fig. 21.37). Embolization to the liver through splanchnic vessels is seen in about 40% of patients who develop liver abscess. These abscesses are about 10 cm in diameter and contain **anchovy sauce pus** with shaggy lining surrounded by scanty inflammatory reaction. The abscesses persist longer and may spread the infection to the lungs and heart by direct extension and to the kidneys and brain through the bloodstream.

Clinical Features Amoebiasis usually presents with abdominal pain, bloody diarrhoea or weight loss. The occasional complications associated with significant mortality include *acute necrotizing colitis and megacolon*. The infection responds well to metronidazole, even for systemic diseases.

INTESTINAL TUBERCULOSIS PA 24.5

Tuberculosis of the small bowel is still a problem prevalent in countries where consumption of unpasteurized milk is common. The most common site of involvement is the *ileocaecal region*, which is the region of stasis, maximum rate of absorption, abundant lymphoid aggregates and close contact of bacilli with the mucosa. The jejunum and the colon are the next common sites. Tuberculosis resembles Crohn disease on both gross and microscopic examinations. It causes ulcers in the intestine that are *multiple and circumferential*. The muscularis externa is often damaged in these patients, and the presentation is mostly in the form of obstruction due to *strictures, adhesions or hyperplastic mural thickening*.

Patients usually present with abdominal pain, borborygmi or complications such as intestinal obstruction or less commonly with perforations. Investigations include imaging and barium studies that show many characteristic findings. Microscopically, the **tuberculous granulomas** are confluent granulomas with caseation necrosis in the centre and a peripheral rim of lymphocytes (Fig. 21.38). Acid-fast stains for the bacilli and PCR help to confirm the diagnosis whenever required. Early diagnosis prevents the

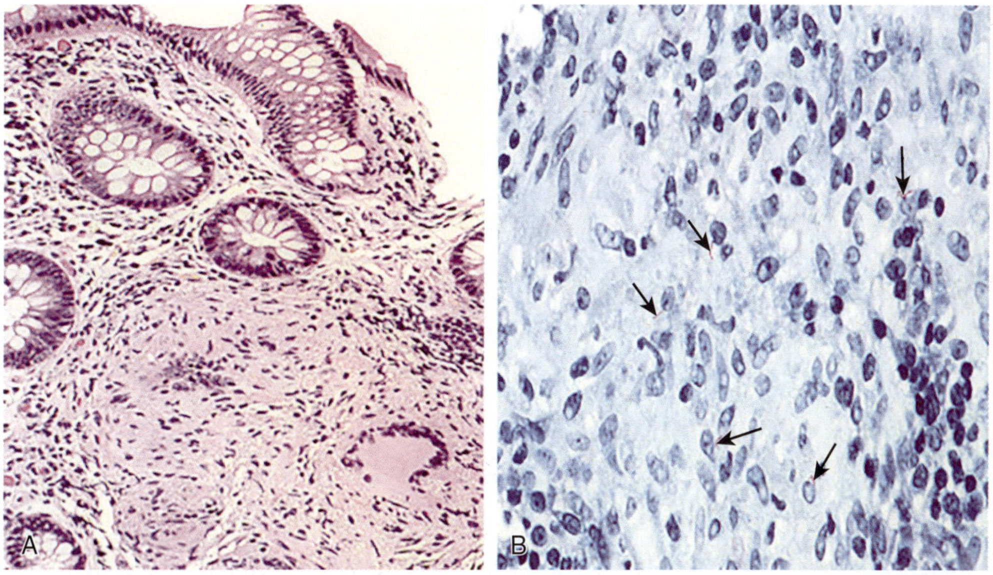

Fig. 21.38 Intestinal tuberculosis – microscopy (A) showing granulomas in the colonic mucosa and (B) Ziehl–Neelsen stain showing multiple red acid-fast bacilli. (*Source:* From Patrick L. Fitzgibbons. Histochemistry in the diagnosis of non-neoplastic gastrointestinal disorders. Seminars in Diagnostic Pathology. 2018;35:370–380.)

need for surgical intervention and shows better response to antitubercular therapy.

IRRITABLE BOWEL SYNDROME

Irritable bowel syndrome (IBS) is a disorder characterized by chronic, relapsing episodes of abdominal pain, bloating and changes in bowel habits. It is a diagnosis that depends purely on clinical symptoms and functional testing. IBS is actually a syndrome that includes multiple illnesses and is currently divided into several subtypes, as per successive revisions of the **Rome criteria**.

Pathogenesis

IBS is due to the influence of various factors, and the common theories include the following:

- **Dysregulated colonic contractions:** Decreased colonic contractions and transit rates cause *constipation-predominant IBS*, whereas increased colonic contractions and transit rates are associated with *diarrhoea-predominant IBS*.
- **Excess bile acid synthesis** or bile acid malabsorption is one of the causes of diarrhoea-predominant IBS because bile acids increase intestinal motility.
- **Defective brain–gut axis signalling** causes increased enteric sensory responses to GI stimuli.
- Onset of IBS is seen in some patients following infectious gastroenteritis, indicating that **change in gut microbiome** can trigger IBS. There may be some overlap in mechanisms underlying constipation-predominant and diarrhoea-predominant IBS. For example, single-nucleotide polymorphisms in immune mediators have been detected in both types.
- In some, **psychological stress and dietary changes** influence the onset of IBS.

Clinical Features

IBS is common in middle-aged women. The diagnosis is based on clinical criteria in which the individual has abdominal pain or discomfort that is relieved by defecation and change in stool frequency or form for at least 3 days per month for 3 months. The other causes of GI disorders such as infections and inflammation should be ruled out to make this diagnosis. Although IBS does not cause many complications, chronic pain and social issues may be a problem. Longer duration of symptoms reduces chances of improvement in patients.

IBS is not associated with serious long-term sequelae, but affected patients may undergo unnecessary abdominal surgery due to chronic pain and their ability to function socially may be compromised. The prognosis of IBS is most closely related to symptom duration, with a longer duration correlating with a reduced likelihood of improvement.

INFLAMMATORY BOWEL DISEASE PA 24.6

Inflammatory bowel disease (IBD) is a **chronic inflammatory condition** of the GI tract resulting from *inappropriate mucosal immune activation*. It comprises **ulcerative colitis** and **Crohn disease**. The major differences in these two conditions are the extent or site of involvement and the morphological expression of the disease (Fig. 21.39). Ulcerative colitis affects only the colon and involves only the mucosa and the submucosa, whereas Crohn disease

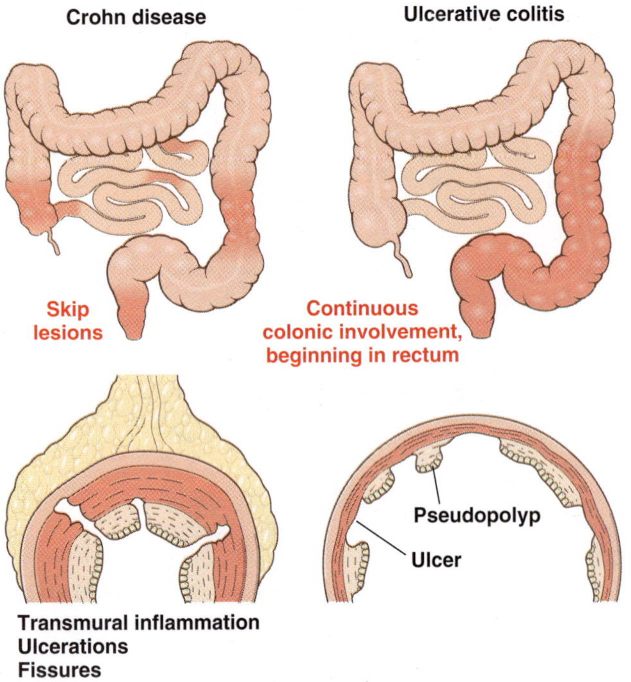

Fig. 21.39 Diagrammatic representation depicting the extent and depth of involvement of ulcerative colitis and Crohn disease. (*Source:* From Vinay Kumar, Abul K. Abbas and Jon C. Aster. The Gastrointestinal Tract. Robbins & Cotran Pathologic Basis of Disease. 10th edition. Elsevier 2021.)

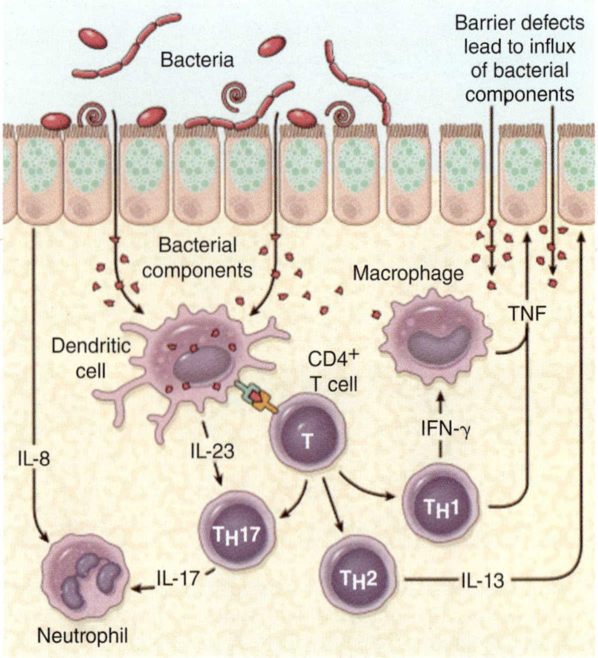

Fig. 21.40 Model of IBD pathogenesis.

may affect any part of the GI tract and involves all layers of the intestine (transmural).

Epidemiology

IBD usually affects the teens and those in early 20s, with ulcerative colitis being slightly common in females. It is noted to be more common in developed countries such as the United States and Europe compared with in the developing countries. The prevalence of helminth infection in the developing countries has shown to reduce the risk of IBD in animal models. But the recent trends of increases in IBD in Africa and Asia could be attributed to improvement in food storage and hygiene conditions and changes in food habits contributing to change in gut microbiome composition.

Pathogenesis (Fig. 21.40)

The important factors that play a combined role in causing IBD are genetic factors, alterations in host interactions with intestinal microbiota, intestinal epithelial dysfunction, aberrant mucosal immune responses and altered composition of the gut microbiome.

1. **Genetics**
   The concordance rate in monozygotic twins for Crohn disease is around 50%, whereas that for ulcerative colitis is only about 15%. This suggests that genetic factors are more dominant for Crohn disease than for ulcerative colitis.
   Genome-wide association studies have shown 160 genes associated with IBD, some of which are the same genes that are involved in the body's response to mycobacteria. Some of the genes strongly associated with Crohn disease include NOD2 (nucleotide oligomerization binding domain 2), ATG16L1 (autophagy-related 16-like) and IRGM (immunity-related GTPase M), but their exact role in the pathogenesis is yet to be identified.
2. **Mucosal immune responses**
   The role of mucosal immune responses in IBD is supported by the following observations:
   - T_H1 and T_H17 types of T-helper cells are activated in Crohn disease, and polymorphisms of IL-23 receptor of T_H17 reduce the risk of IBD.
   - Many proinflammatory cytokines such as TNF, IFN-γ and IL-13 and immunoregulatory molecules such as IL-10 and TGF-β are identified to be involved in the pathogenesis of IBD.
   - Thus, the role of deranged mucosal immune activation and defective immunoregulation has been shown to contribute to the development of IBD, making immunosuppressive drugs the mainstay in their treatment.
3. **Epithelial defects**
   Many epithelial defects have been described in IBD such as:
   - Patients with Crohn disease and their first-degree relatives have defects in the intestinal epithelial tight junction barrier function.
   - ECM1 polymorphisms, which increase the activity of matrix metalloproteinase-9, are noted in ulcerative colitis.

- HNFA polymorphisms, which are associated with maturity-onset diabetes (MODY), are also noted in patients with ulcerative colitis. MODY has already been proven to have reduced intestinal barrier function, thereby linking ulcerative colitis to the same.

4. **Microbiota**

   The link between microbiota and IBD is established from the following data:
   - Patients with Crohn disease having strictures, perforation and small bowel involvement show the presence of flagellin antibodies in their sera, whereas it is absent in patients with ulcerative colitis.
   - Clinical trials suggest that probiotic (or beneficial) bacteria or even faecal microbial transplants from healthy individuals may benefit IBD patients.

Morphology

The gross and microscopic findings in Crohn disease and ulcerative colitis are given in Table 21.17 and Figs 21.41 and 21.42.

Clinical Features

Crohn Disease Most patients present with intermittent attacks of relatively mild diarrhoea, fever and abdominal pain. Some may present with symptoms mimicking acute appendicitis or bowel perforation. The course of the disease has remissions and exacerbations. The triggers for disease reactivation include physical or emotional stress, specific dietary items and cigarette smoking.

Colonic disease may present as iron-deficiency anaemia, whereas extensive small bowel disease may present as hypoalbuminaemia due to protein loss, generalized nutrient malabsorption or vitamin B_{12} malabsorption. The common complications requiring surgical interventions include **fibrosing strictures**, especially of the terminal ileum, **fistulae** between loops of bowel and occasionally with the urinary bladder, vagina and abdominal or perianal skin, and **perforations**. Anti-TNF antibodies have created a big change in the management of Crohn disease.

Ulcerative Colitis Ulcerative colitis usually presents with attacks of bloody diarrhoea with stringy, mucoid material and lower abdominal pain that is temporarily relieved by defecation. The symptoms as in Crohn disease are remitting and relapsing. Most patients experience at least one relapse during the first 10 years, and about 30% require colectomy within the first 3 years. The factors that trigger ulcerative colitis include infectious enteritis, psychological stress and cessation of smoking; the latter is in contrast to Crohn disease, which is aggravated by smoking.

Extraintestinal Manifestations in Inflammatory Bowel Disease The common extraintestinal manifestations include *uveitis, migratory polyarthritis, sacroiliitis, ankylosing spondylitis, erythema nodosum and clubbing of the fingertips.* These overlap in Crohn disease and ulcerative colitis, but *pericholangitis and primary sclerosing cholangitis* occur with a higher frequency in ulcerative colitis than in Crohn disease. It should be noted that colectomy in patients with ulcerative colitis may help to relieve GI-related manifestations but extraintestinal manifestations still persist. Furthermore, the risk of *colonic adenocarcinoma* is increased in patients with long-standing IBD affecting the colon, especially in ulcerative colitis.

POLYPS

Polyps can occur in any part of the GI tract, but the most common site is the colorectum. The polyps initially start as flat elevations on the mucosa forming a sessile polyp (polyp that does not have a stalk) and progresses due to the proliferation of epithelial cells that exert a traction towards the lumen to form a pedunculated polyp. Polyps of the intestine are classified into non-neoplastic and neoplastic polyps.

Non-neoplastic Polyps

This category includes hyperplastic, inflammatory and hamartomatous polyps.

Hyperplastic Polyps

Hyperplastic polyps of the colon are benign polyps that present in the sixth or seventh decade of life. The decrease in the turnover of epithelial cells, and their delayed shedding, leads to 'piling up' of goblet cells and absorptive cells. These do not have malignant potential but should be distinguished from sessile serrated adenomas that have malignant potential. Occasionally, epithelial hyperplasia may occur as a response to an underlying malignancy, making it important to check for any adjacent mass while reporting a hyperplastic polyp.

These are commonly noted in the left colon as smooth nodular protrusions or sessile polyps on the crest of mucosal folds and are usually less than 5 mm in diameter. These polyps may be single or occasionally multiple. Microscopy shows elongated glands with infoldings, forming serrations, typically restricted to the upper third or less of the crypt. The glands are lined by mature goblet and absorptive cells.

Inflammatory Polyp

The polyp of **solitary rectal ulcer syndrome** comes under this category of inflammatory polyps. It is a single ulcerated or polypoid lesion occurring within 4–18 cm from the anal verge on the anterior rectal wall. It is due to *delayed relaxation of the anorectal sphincter* and is often associated with mucosal abrasions and ulcerations. It may

Table 21.17 Features of Crohn Disease Versus Ulcerative Colitis

Features	Crohn Disease	Ulcerative Colitis
Extent of involvement	**Any part of the GI tract**, mouth to anus	Colon and terminal end of the ileum (**backwash ileitis**)
Most common site	**Terminal ileum**, ileocaecal valve and caecum	Begins in the **rectum** and extends proximally
Type of involvement	Multiple, separate, sharply delineated areas of disease cause **skip lesions**	**Continuous** involvement
Depth of involvement	**Transmural**	**Superficial** – only mucosa and submucosa
Gross findings	**Aphthous ulcers** are the earliest lesions but may progress and coalesce into elongated **serpentine ulcers** oriented along the axis of the bowel	**Broad-based ulcers aligned along the long axis** of the colon
	Sparing of interspersed mucosa produces a coarsely textured **cobblestone appearance**	Isolated islands of regenerating mucosa may often bulge into the lumen to form **pseudopolyps** and their tips may fuse to create mucosal bridges
	Fissures that develop between mucosal folds may extend deeply to become **fistula tracts** or perforate	Flat and smooth mucosal surface without the normal folds due to **mucosal atrophy**
	Transmural oedema and inflammation along with submucosal fibrosis and muscularis propria hypertrophy may make the **intestinal wall thick and rubbery**	Mural thickening is not present and the serosal surface is normal; strictures are not seen
	Inflammation of the serosal surface due to transmural disease may cause mesenteric fat to get adherent to it (**creeping fat**)	Destruction of muscularis propria and neuronal plexus by inflammation causes **toxic megacolon**, which may perforate
Microscopy findings	**Crypt abscess** – clusters of neutrophils within a crypt	**Crypt abscess** – clusters of neutrophils within a crypt
	Crypt distortion and bizarre branching due to destruction and regeneration of crypts	**Crypt distortion and bizarre branching** due to destruction and regeneration of crypts
	Abrupt transition between ulcerated and adjacent normal mucosa and **microscopic skip areas**	Abrupt transition between ulcerated and adjacent normal mucosa but involvement is only in the mucosa and submucosa
	Epithelial cell metaplasia such as pseudopyloric metaplasia and Paneth cell metaplasia	**Epithelial cell metaplasia** such as pseudopyloric metaplasia
	Noncaseating granulomas are the hallmark of Crohn disease and are seen in the involved and/or uninvolved regions in any layer of the intestinal wall; however, the absence of granuloma does not rule out Crohn disease	**Absence of granuloma**
	Presence of **granulomas in mesenteric nodes** and skin	

GI, gastrointestinal.

get entrapped in the faecal stream and cause mucosal prolapse. The histological findings include epithelial hyperplasia, mixed inflammatory cell infiltrate and fibromuscular hyperplasia in the lamina propria.

Hamartomatous Polyps

These polyps occur sporadically or as a part of various syndromes, genetic or acquired. These are caused by germline mutations in proto-oncogenes or tumour suppressor genes and are associated with an increased risk of intestinal and extraintestinal malignancies.

Juvenile Polyps Juvenile polyps may be sporadic or syndromic and are due to malformations of the epithelium and lamina propria. These usually occur in young children, younger than 5 years. The most common site is the

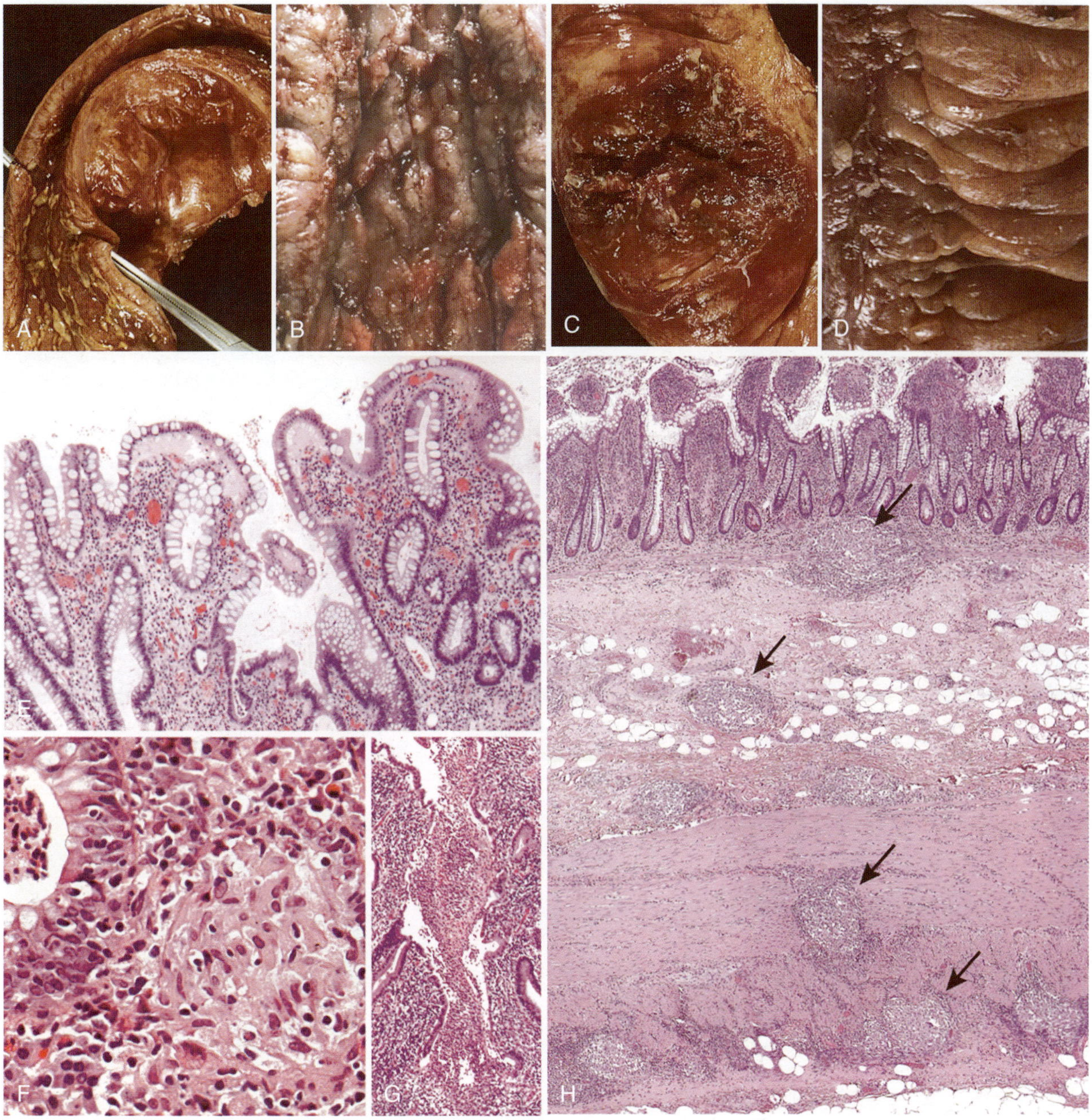

Fig. 21.41 Gross and microscopic features of Crohn disease. Gross: (A) Small intestinal stricture. (B) Linear mucosal ulcers, which impart a cobblestone appearance to the mucosa, and thickened intestinal wall. (C) Perforation and associated serositis. (D) Creeping fat. Microscopy: (E) Haphazard crypt organization results from repeated injury and regeneration. (F) Noncaseating granuloma. (G) Active Crohn disease with ulceration and purulent exudate. (H) Transmural Crohn disease with submucosal and serosal granulomas (arrows). (*Source:* From Vinay Kumar, Abul K. Abbas and Jon C. Aster. The Gastrointestinal Tract. Robbins & Cotran Pathologic Basis of Disease. 10th edition. Elsevier 2021.)

rectum, and the most common presentation is rectal bleeding. Occasionally, it may lead to complications such as intestinal obstruction or intussusception.

Sporadic juvenile polyps are usually solitary lesions in the rectosigmoid region with rare dysplastic changes and a very low risk of malignant transformation. These are the most common polyps in children and are also referred to as **retention polyps**. In contrast, individuals with the **autosomal dominant juvenile polyposis syndrome** have multiple polyps varying from 3 to as many as 100 hamartomatous polyps.

These polyps may cause severe haemorrhage due to ulceration and be associated with extraintestinal manifestations such as pulmonary arteriovenous malformations and other congenital malformations. The syndromic polyps may also undergo malignant transformation, with about 50% of patients developing colonic adenocarcinoma by 45 years of age. Juvenile polyps are proposed to be formed by mucosal hyperplasia and to be associated with mutations in genes involved in cellular growth. The one gene that has been identified to be involved is SMAD4 gene, with many more yet to be identified.

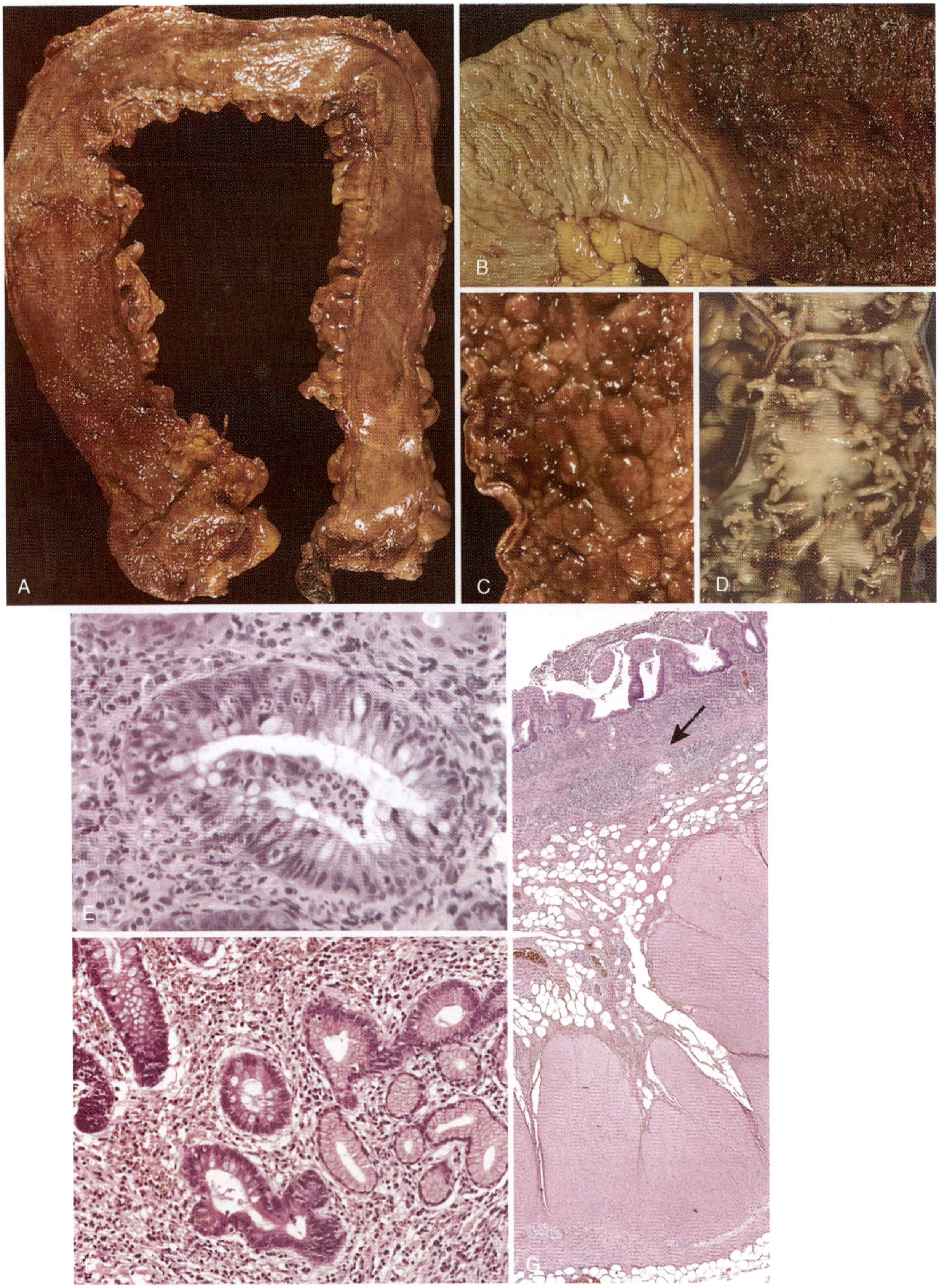

Fig. 21.42 Gross and microscopic features of ulcerative colitis. Gross: (A) Total colectomy with pancolitis showing active disease, with red granular mucosa in the caecum (left) and smooth, atrophic mucosa distally (right). (B) Sharp demarcation between active ulcerative colitis (right) and normal mucosa (left). (C) Inflammatory polyps. (D) Mucosal bridges that join inflammatory polyps. Microscopy: (E) Crypt abscess. (F) Pseudopyloric metaplasia (right). (G) Disease is limited to the mucosa (above the arrow). (*Source:* From Vinay Kumar, Abul K. Abbas and Jon C. Aster. The Gastrointestinal Tract. Robbins & Cotran Pathologic Basis of Disease. 10th edition. Elsevier 2021.)

Morphology

Sporadic and syndromic juvenile polyps have the same histology (Fig. 21.43). These polyps are less than 3 cm in diameter and typically pedunculated, smooth-surfaced and reddish lesions with characteristic cystic spaces apparent after sectioning. Histology shows dilated glands filled with mucin and inflammatory debris. The lamina propria is expanded with infiltration by mixed inflammatory cells.

Peutz–Jeghers Syndrome Peutz–Jeghers syndrome is an autosomal dominant syndrome that presents at a median age of 11 years. The features include multiple *GI hamartomatous polyps and mucocutaneous hyperpigmentation* seen as dark blue to brown macules on the lips, nostrils, buccal mucosa, palmar surfaces of the hands, genitalia and perianal region. These polyps should be distinguished from freckles that do not occur on mucosal surfaces. The importance of the diagnosis lies in the fact that these may initiate fatal **intussusception** and be associated with a markedly increased risk of several malignancies. The tumours to be screened for include sex cord tumours of the testes in children; gastric and small intestinal cancers in older children; and colon, pancreatic, breast, lung, ovarian and uterine cancers in adolescents and young adults.

Pathogenesis Individuals with this familial syndrome are born with a germline heterozygous loss-of-function mutation in the gene STK11. This means that these individuals are born with one normal allele and one defective allele, thereby heterozygous in nature. In sporadic Peutz–Jeghers syndrome, they may acquire the defective allele and become heterozygous. STK11 is a tumour suppressor gene, and loss of function of the heterozygous 'normal' copy of STK11 (second hit) results in malignant transformation.

Morphology (Fig. 21.44)

The sites of polyps in Peutz–Jeghers syndrome are the small intestine, stomach, colon, bladder and lungs in a decreasing order of frequency. The polyps are usually large, pedunculated and lobulated. Microscopically, the polyps contain an arborizing network of connective tissue, smooth muscle, lamina propria and glands lined by normal-appearing intestinal epithelium. The *branching appearance of muscularis mucosae* (smooth muscle) along with the lamina propria is a characteristic feature of polyps of Peutz–Jeghers syndrome that helps to differentiate it from other polyps.

Clinical Features Individuals present with multiple polyps in the small intestine, mucocutaneous hyperpigmentation and a positive family history. In patients who lack mucocutaneous pigmentation, STK11 mutations can help in the diagnosis, although it should be remembered that the absence of STK11 does not rule out Peutz–Jeghers syndrome.

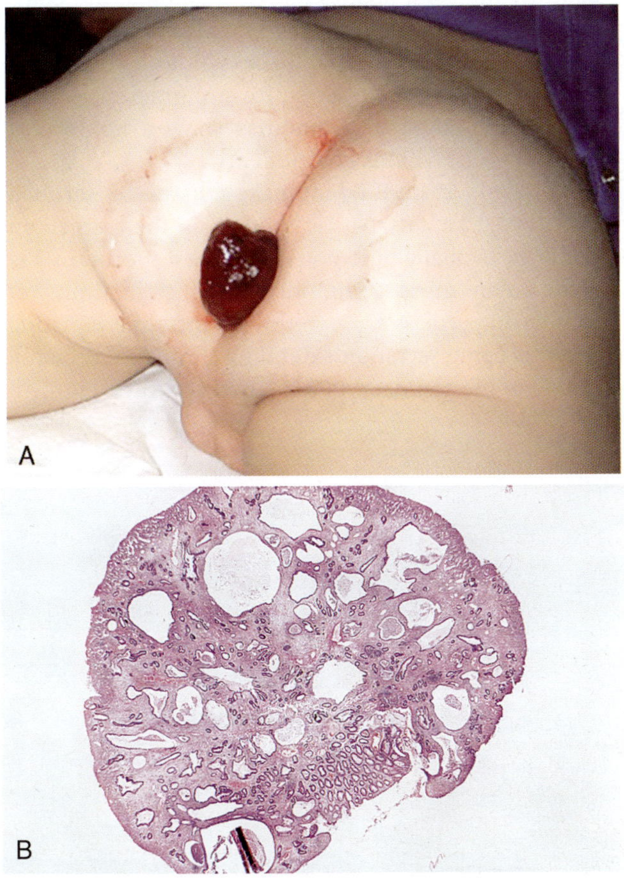

Fig. 21.43 Gross image (A) and microscopic appearance (B) of juvenile polyp showing cystically dilated glands and inflammatory cells in the oedematous lamina propria. (*Source:* From Sunil Shah, Elias Youssef, Maria Saccio and Barry Hahn. Juvenile Polyp. Journal of Emergency Medicine. 2011;41:e111–e112.)

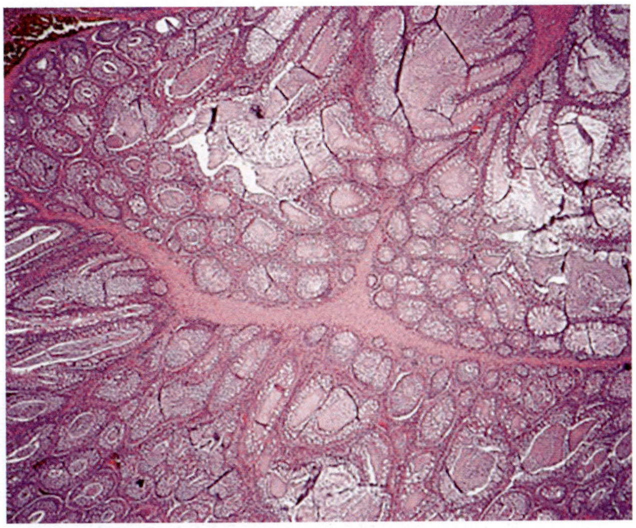

Fig. 21.44 Peutz–Jeghers polyp: branching muscle layer in the stalk derived from muscularis mucosae. (*Source:* From L.A.A. Brosens, M. Jansen, F.M. Giardiello and G.J.A. Offerhaus. Polyps of the small intestine. Diagnostic Histopathology. 2011;17:69–79.)

Neoplastic Polyps

Neoplastic lesions in the GI tract often produce mucosal protrusion or polyp. Such neoplasms include adenocarcinomas, neuroendocrine tumours, stromal tumours, lymphomas and metastatic cancers, but the most common neoplastic polyps are colonic adenomas.

Adenomas

Adenomas are the most common *precursors of colonic adenocarcinoma*. These are intraepithelial neoplasms that are common in Western countries among those who are older than 60 years and show a small male preponderance. The neoplasms present as solitary, sessile (Fig. 21.45) or pedunculated benign polyps, and the risk of malignant transformation depends on the *size of the polyp and the presence of high-grade dysplasia* on histological examination. Size less than 1 cm has a low risk of malignancy, and size greater than 4 cm has a 40% risk of malignant transformation. The incidence of adenomas is low in the Asian population but noted to increase due to changes in lifestyle and dietary habits. Surveillance of the at-risk population is by colonoscopy and polypectomy to reduce the incidence of colorectal adenocarcinoma.

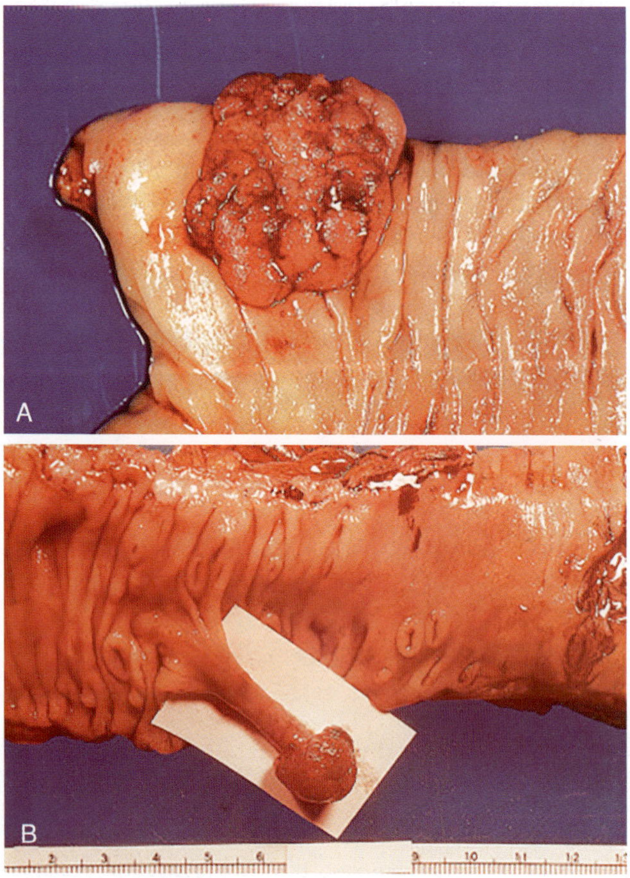

Fig. 21.45 Gross appearance of sessile adenoma (A) and pedunculated adenoma (B). (*Source:* From John R. Goldblum. Stomach. Rosai and Ackerman's Surgical Pathology. 11th edition. Elsevier 2018.)

Mostly, adenomas are clinically silent but large polyps may cause occult bleeding and anaemia and rare villous adenomas may cause hypoproteinaemic hypokalaemia by secreting large amounts of protein and potassium.

Morphology

The most important feature of adenoma is the presence of **epithelial dysplasia**. The adenomas are 0.3–10 cm in diameter and pedunculated or sessile polyps with velvety texture. Histologically, epithelial dysplasia is noted as nuclear hyperchromasia, elongation and stratification along with prominent nucleoli, eosinophilic cytoplasm and a reduction in the number of goblet cells. Pedunculated adenomas have fibromuscular stalks with prominent blood vessels. The stalk is usually covered by non-neoplastic epithelium, but dysplastic epithelium may be present.

Adenomas can be classified as **tubular, tubulovillous or villous** on the basis of their architecture. Tubular adenomas are common in the right colon, may be single or multiple, sessile or pedunculated, and are composed of glands with dysplastic changes (Fig. 21.46). These may lead to intussusception or changes in bowel habits. Villous adenomas are common in the rectosigmoid region and are usually single and sessile with papillary villous projections. These tend to encircle the entire circumference of the bowel. Tubulovillous adenomas show a mixture of glandular and villous components.

Sessile serrated adenomas are sessile serrated polyps that lack dysplastic changes in the epithelium but have a malignant potential. These occur in the right colon more commonly and histologically resemble hyperplastic polyps, with the differentiating features being serration extending throughout the full length of the gland, crypt dilatation and lateral growth (Fig. 21.47).

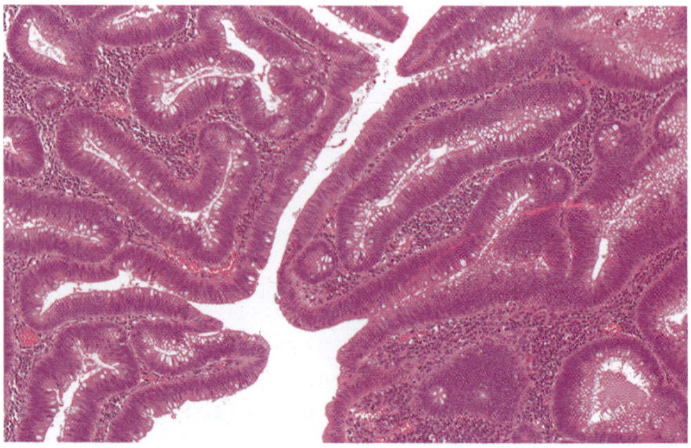

Fig. 21.46 Microscopic appearance of tubular adenoma with mild dysplasia. (*Source:* From John R. Goldblum. Large Bowel. Rosai and Ackerman's Surgical Pathology. 11th edition. Elsevier 2018.)

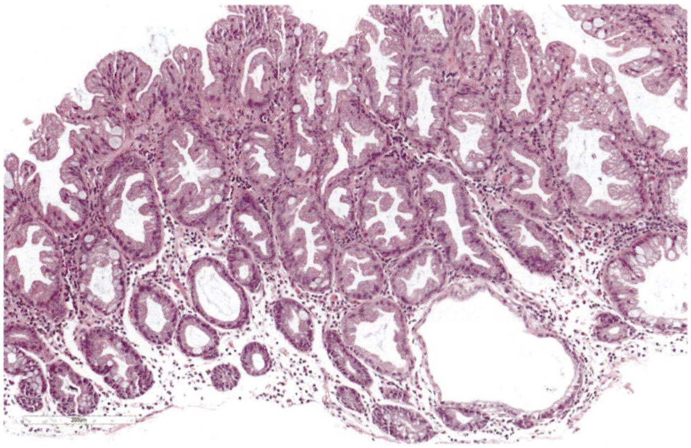

Fig. 21.47 Sessile serrated polyp showing full-length serration and cystic dilation of basal glands. (*Source:* From John R. Goldblum. Large Bowel. Rosai and Ackerman's Surgical Pathology. 11th edition. Elsevier 2018.)

Intramucosal carcinoma is diagnosed when dysplastic epithelial cells are seen invading the lamina propria or muscularis mucosae after crossing the basement membrane. The colonic mucosa does not have lymphatic drainage, so the presence of mucosal invasion does not confer metastatic potential to the tumour, making curative resection sufficient. But invasion beyond the muscularis mucosae or into the submucosal stalk of a pedunculated polyp transforms it into an invasive adenocarcinoma with a risk of metastasis. In such patients, the histological grade of the invasive component, the presence of vascular or lymphatic invasion and the distance of the invasive component from the margin of resection should be noted for planning further therapy.

Familial Polyp Syndromes

Familial adenomatous polyposis This is an autosomal dominant syndrome due to mutation of adenomatous polyposis coli gene, the **APC gene**, a negative regulator of the Wnt pathway. About 75% of cases are inherited, whereas 25% arise de novo. The individual usually presents with multiple adenomas that are about several thousands in the colorectal region. A minimum of 100 adenomas is required for diagnosis, and the adenomas, though numerous, are histologically similar to sporadic adenomas (Fig. 21.48). The *risk of malignant transformation in the colon is 100%* and so patients are offered prophylactic colectomy. However, the patient still carries a risk of malignancy in other parts of the GI tract, such as in adenomas near the ampulla of Vater or stomach. Extraintestinal manifestation includes *congenital hypertrophy of retinal epithelium,* which may be present at birth and used for early screening.

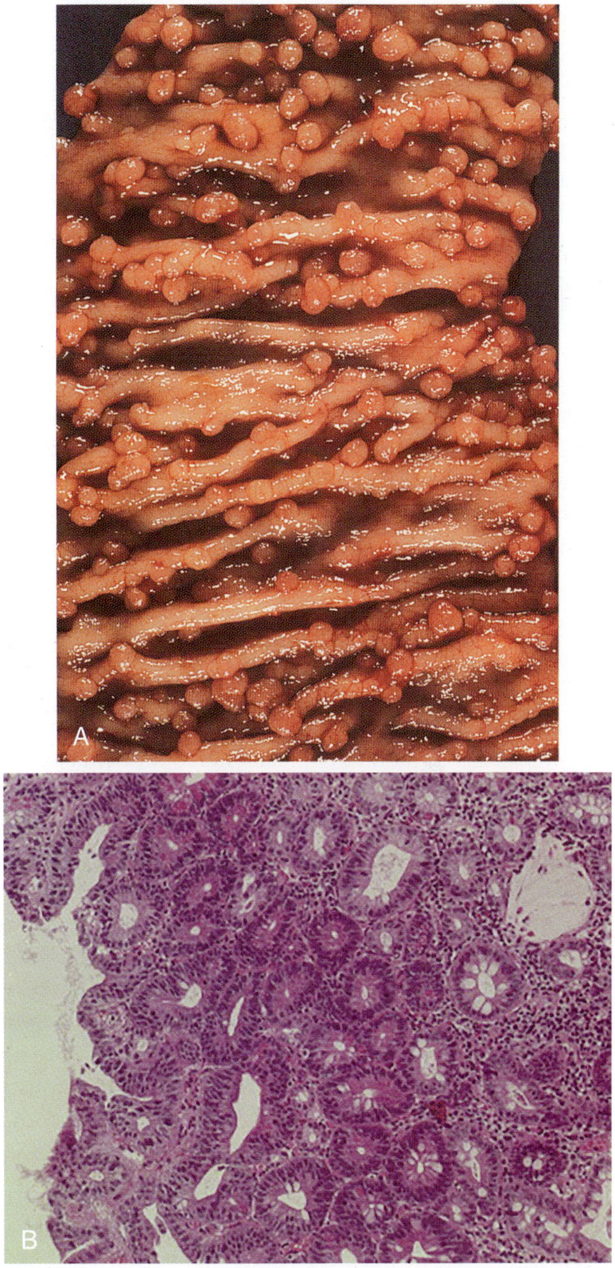

Fig. 21.48 Familial adenomatous polyposis, gross – showing the large bowel involved with innumerable small polyps (A) and microscopic appearance of FAP (B) showing a tubular adenoma resembling sporadic adenoma. (*Source:* From John R. Goldblum. Large Bowel. Rosai and Ackerman's Surgical Pathology. 11th edition. Elsevier 2018.)

Hereditary nonpolyposis colon carcinoma Hereditary nonpolyposis colon carcinoma (HNPCC) (**Lynch syndrome**) is the most common form of syndrome-associated colon cancer accounting for 2%–4% of colon cancers. It causes familial clustering of cancers at various sites such as the colorectum, endometrium, stomach, ovary, ureters, brain, small bowel, hepatobiliary tract, pancreas and skin. Cancers of the colon develop in these individuals at a younger age and are frequently located in the right colon. HNPCC is caused by inherited mutations in **MSH2 or MLH1** genes, which are responsible for repair of errors that occur during DNA replication. At birth, the individuals are heterozygous, with one mutant gene and one normal allele. The loss of second normal allele by mutation or epigenetic silencing leads to defects in mismatch repair, especially in areas containing short-repeat sequences called *microsatellites*. Thus, *failure in mismatch repair* and the resulting *microsatellite instability* are the basis of HNPCC.

ADENOCARCINOMA OF COLON PA 24.7

Adenocarcinoma of the colon is the most common GI malignancy worldwide. It is second in incidence among overall malignancies next to lung cancer. The incidence is the highest in North America, followed by other countries such as Europe, Australia, New Zealand and Japan, and low in countries such as South America, India and Africa. The incidence is high at 60–70 years of age.

Role of diet:

- **Low intake of dietary vegetable fibre:** This decreases stool bulk and alters the microbiota of the intestine. The altered microbial flora synthesizes toxic oxidative by-products, and these harmful chemicals remain in contact with colonic mucosa for a long duration due to the decreased stool bulk.
- **High intake of refined carbohydrates and fat:** High fat content in the diet increases hepatic synthesis of cholesterol and bile acids that get secreted into the intestine and get converted into carcinogens by intestinal bacteria.
- **Aspirin or other NSAIDs offer some degree of chemoprevention.** These drugs inhibit COX-2 enzyme that is necessary for the production of prostaglandin E_2, a mediator of epithelial proliferation after injury. About 90% of colorectal carcinomas and 40%–90% of adenomas highly express COX-2 and thereby, intake of these drugs may cause some degree of regression.

Pathogenesis

Development of colonic adenocarcinoma is due to a combination of molecular events that lead to the accumulation of mutations. In line with this, two pathways of development of colonic carcinoma are well studied – **the APC/β-catenin pathway and the microsatellite instability pathway**. The pathways differ in the genes involved but epigenetic events, which cause gene silencing, are the cause for progression in both pathways.

- **The APC/β-catenin pathway:**
  This pathway leads to the **classical adenoma–carcinoma sequence** (Fig. 21.49) seen in up to 80% of sporadic colon tumours. The loss of APC gene happens early in the course of the transformation, and both genes need to be deactivated for adenomas to develop. The mechanism of APC in cell proliferation is explained in Flowchart 21.6.
  Consequent to the loss of APC function, additional mutations occur and accumulate, promoting growth and transformation of adenoma to carcinoma. This includes mutations in KRAS, SMAD2, SMAD4 and TP53; in advanced stages, it also shows the expression of telomerase. Loss of function of tumour suppressor genes in this pathway is by chromosomal deletion, making **chromosomal instability** a hallmark of this pathway.
- **The microsatellite instability (MSI) pathway** (Fig. 21.50): Accumulation of microsatellite repeats occurs in patients with DNA mismatch repair defects. This condition is called **microsatellite instability** and the tumours are called **MSI high** or MSI-H tumours. The increased repeats may be located in coding or promoter regions of proteins involved in cell growth (such as type II TGF-β receptor) or apoptosis (such as BAX). This may lead to dysregulation of cell growth or inhibition of apoptosis, resulting in neoplastic transformation. This pathway of MSI has been found to be common in sessile serrated adenomas and associated cancers. These cancers often have prominent mucinous

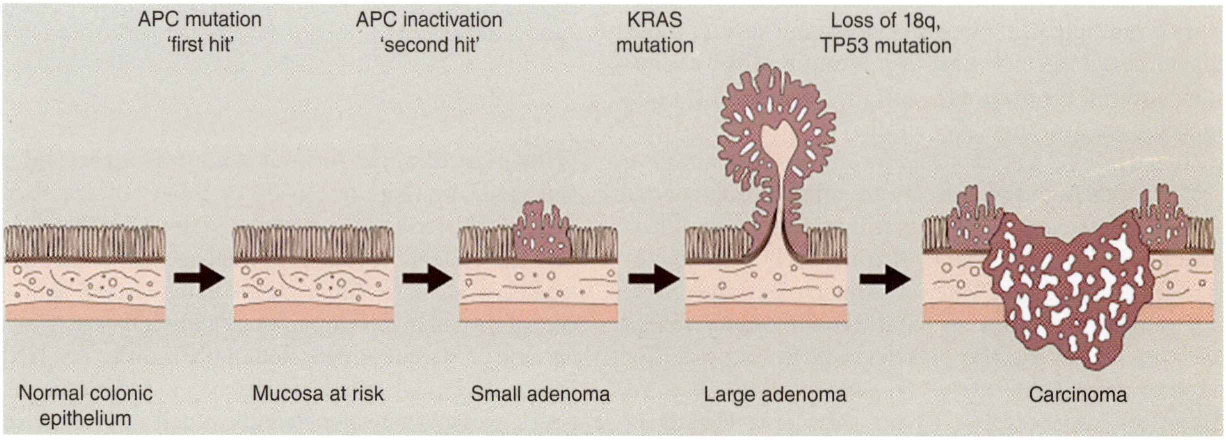

Fig. 21.49 Adenoma–carcinoma sequence of the APC/β-catenin pathway. (*Source:* From Clare Turnbull. Genomics in medicine. Medicine. 2018;46: 774–779.)

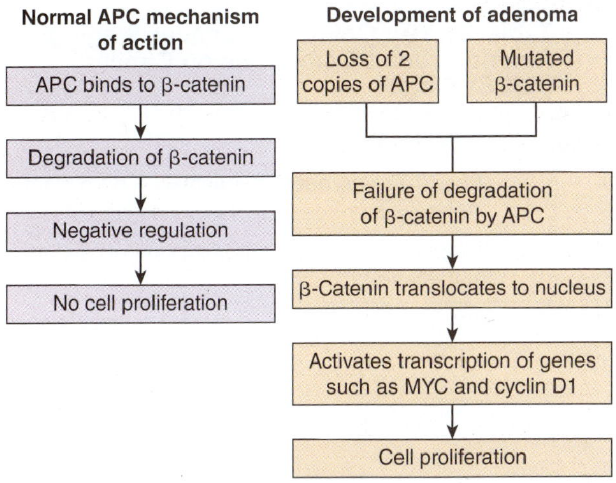

Flowchart 21.6 Mechanism of APC loss leading to adenoma.

differentiation and peritumoural lymphocytic infiltrates and are common in the right colon. Identifying patients with HNPCC is important for genetic counselling because of the elevated risk of a second malignancy of the colon or other organs and also because of the difference in prognosis and therapy.

Morphology

Adenocarcinoma of the colon may occur in any part of the colon and is usually detected late in the course of the disease. Tumours in the proximal colon, on the right side, are usually exophytic, polypoid masses that cause occult blood loss in stools and present as iron-deficiency anaemia. It has become a dictum that *old men or postmenopausal women presenting with iron-deficiency anaemia should be evaluated for GI malignancy.* In contrast, carcinomas in the distal colon, on the left side, tend to be circumferential lesions that produce 'napkin-ring' constrictions and luminal narrowing (Fig. 21.51). These commonly present with occult bleeding, changes in bowel habits, cramping and left lower-quadrant discomfort or even obstruction.

Microscopically, both right- and left-sided colonic adenocarcinomas are similar. These are composed of tall columnar dysplastic cells with invasion into the underlying stroma (Fig. 21.51). This invasion evokes a strong desmoplastic response, making the tumour firm in consistency. The tumours may show varying degrees of differentiation from glands to infiltrating sheets of cells. Some show abundant mucin secretion, making the tumour gelatinous, and such mucinous tumours are found to have a poorer prognosis. Occasionally, signet ring cell type of differentiation or neuroendocrine differentiation may be seen.

The two most important prognostic factors are *depth of invasion and the presence of lymph node metastases.* These factors were recognized by Dukes and Kirklin and form the core of the TNM classification (Tables 21.18 and 21.19). The T or tumour factor in the TNM classification gives importance to the depth of involvement, because it has been proved that invasion of the muscularis propria and beyond reduces survival. The N refers to nodal involvement and M to distant metastasis, the *liver being the most common site* except in rectal tumours, which do not drain by portal circulation. However, patients with a small number of metastases have better survival rates following resection of distant tumour nodules. The overall 5-year survival rates are similar in the United States, Europe, Japan and Australia at about 65%, whereas they are lower in countries such as China, India, the Philippines and Thailand at about 30%–42%.

TUMOURS OF THE ANAL CANAL

The anal canal can be divided into three parts on the basis of the epithelial lining – the upper zone lined by columnar rectal epithelium, the middle zone lined by transitional epithelium and the lower zone lined by stratified squamous epithelium. Hence, carcinomas of the anal canal may have a typical glandular pattern when arising from columnar epithelium, a basaloid pattern when derived from the basal layer of transitional epithelium or a squamous pattern when arising from squamous epithelium (Fig. 21.52). However, this differentiation is difficult and now proved to be unwarranted because they are histogenetically found to be **squamous carcinomas** showing varying patterns of differentiation. The most common site

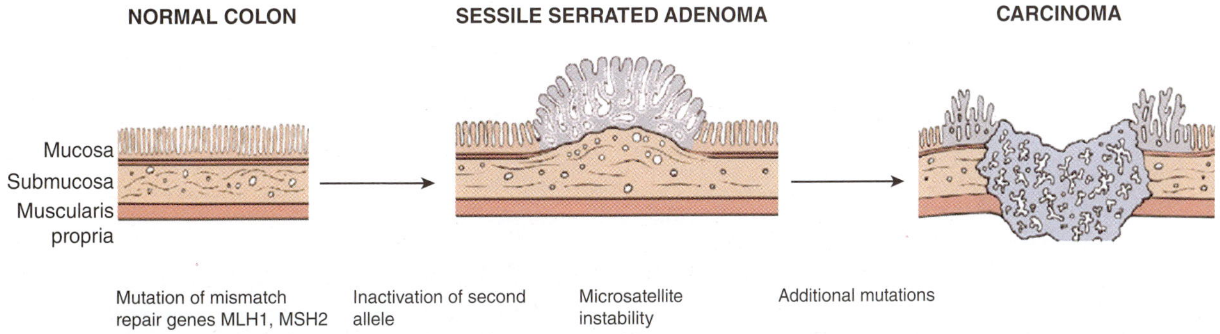

Fig. 21.50 Mechanism of the microsatellite instability pathway. (*Source:* From Vinay Kumar, Abul K. Abbas and Jon C. Aster. Oral Cavities and Gastrointestinal Tract. Robbins Basic Pathology. 10th edition. Elsevier 2018.)

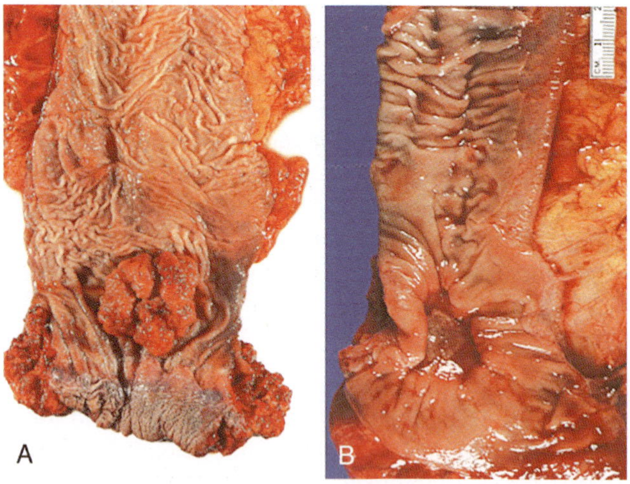

Fig. 21.51 Colonic adenocarcinoma, gross – showing proliferative growth (A) and penetrating ulcerative growth (B). (*Source:* From John R. Goldblum. Large Bowel. Rosai and Ackerman's Surgical Pathology. 11th edition. Elsevier 2018.)

Table 21.18 American Joint Committee on Cancer (AJCC) TNM Classification of Colorectal Carcinoma

Tumour	
Tis	Intraepithelial neoplasia
T1	Tumour invades submucosa
T2	Tumour invades into, but not through, muscularis propria
T3	Tumour invades through muscularis propria
T4	Tumour penetrates visceral peritoneum or invades adjacent organs
Regional lymph nodes	
NX	Lymph nodes cannot be assessed
N0	No regional lymph node metastasis
N1	Metastasis in one to three regional lymph nodes
N2	Metastasis in four or more regional lymph nodes
Distant metastasis	
MX	Distant metastasis cannot be assessed
M0	No distant metastasis
M1	Distant metastasis

TNM, tumour–nodes–metastasis.

is at the *pectinate line*, and the common presenting symptoms are bleeding, pain, mass and pruritus. The common risk factors include condyloma acuminatum, Crohn disease, lymphogranuloma venereum and human papillomavirus (HPV) infection, among which *condyloma acuminatum is considered as a precursor lesion.*

Table 21.19 Colorectal Cancer Staging: American Joint Committee on Cancer (AJCC) Stage[a]

Stage	TNM Finding
I	T1 or T2 + no nodal metastasis+ no distant metastasis
II	T3 or T4 + no nodal metastasis+ no distant metastasis
III	Any T + N1 or N2 + no distant metastasis
IV	Any T + any N + M1

TNM, tumour–nodes–metastasis.
[a]Simplified version.

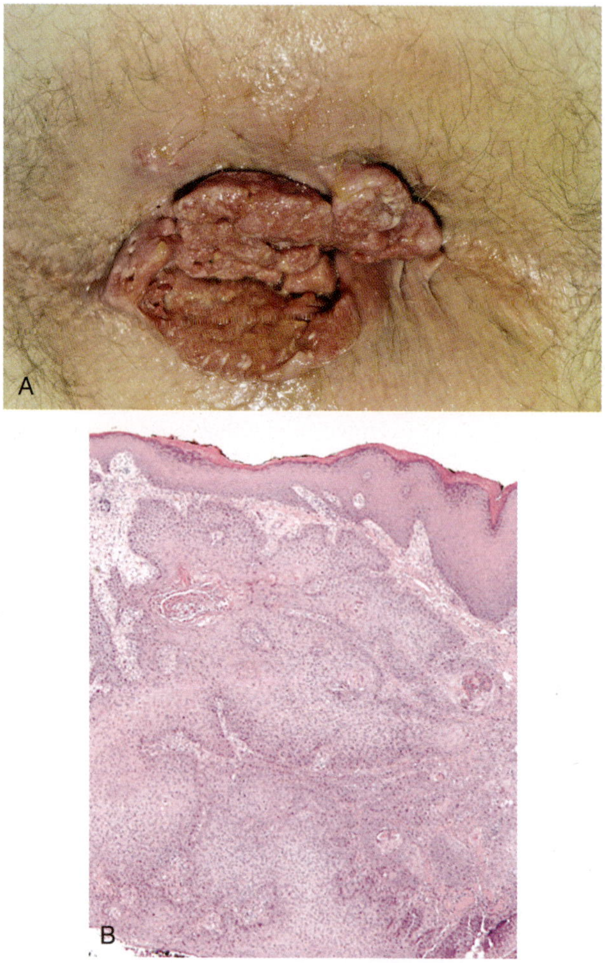

Fig. 21.52 Anal carcinoma, (A) gross – showing a proliferating mass in the anal canal and (B) microscopy showing invasive squamous cell carcinoma. (*Source:* From Cindy Kin and Andrew Shelton. Anal Malignancies. Colorectal Surgery. Saunders 2013.)

APPENDIX

The appendix is a **true diverticulum** of the caecum lined by all four layers of the intestine. Owing to its narrow lumen, it is prone to acute and chronic inflammation and may occasionally develop a mucocoele or tumour.

Acute Appendicitis

This is most common in adolescents and young adults, with a slight male preponderance. Symptomatically, it may mimic mesenteric lymphadenitis, acute salpingitis, ectopic pregnancy or Meckel diverticulum.

Pathogenesis The most common cause of acute appendicitis is luminal obstruction by a faecolith, gallstone, tumour or the intestinal worm *Enterobius vermicularis*. This may increase the intraluminal pressure, reducing the venous outflow, or may lead to stasis of luminal contents, promoting bacterial growth and inflammatory response.

Morphology

On gross appearance (Fig. 21.53), there is serosal congestion and dull granular erythematous serosa. The cut surface may show faecolith or ball of worms.

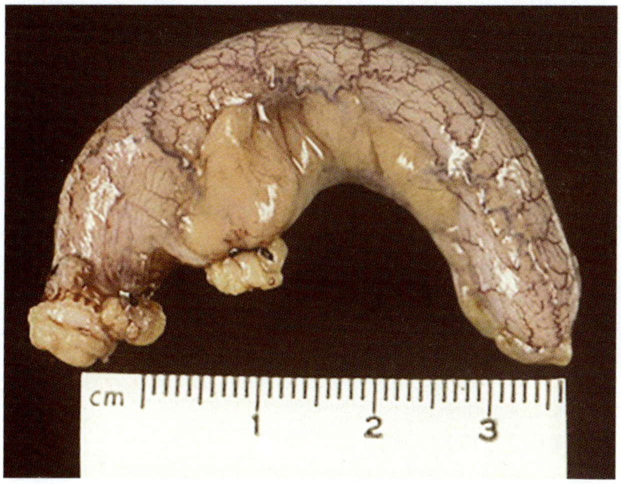

Fig. 21.53 Gross appearance of acute appendicitis. (*Source:* https://www.clinicalkey.com/#!/content/journal/1-s2.0-S1756231707001272?scrollTo=%231-s2.0-S1756231707001272-gr1.)

Microscopy shows mucosal ulceration, neutrophilic infiltration of muscularis propria (Fig. 21.54), which is a diagnostic criterion, and serosal congestion. A fibrinopurulent reaction on the serosa and focal abscesses in the wall may be seen in severe cases (**acute suppurative appendicitis**). When appendiceal blood supply gets compromised, large areas of haemorrhagic ulceration and gangrenous necrosis may develop, leading to **acute gangrenous appendicitis**, which may rupture and lead to suppurative peritonitis.

Clinical Features The patient is usually a child or young adult presenting with periumbilical pain that later localizes to the right lower quadrant, associated with nausea, vomiting, low-grade fever and neutrophilic leucocytosis. On examination, acute tenderness is noted at the McBurney point, which is two-thirds of the distance from the umbilicus to the right anterior superior iliac spine (**McBurney sign**). Late diagnosis may lead to periappendiceal abscess, gangrenous appendicitis, rupture and suppurative peritonitis. Other complications include pyelophlebitis, portal venous thrombosis, liver abscess and bacteraemia.

Tumours of the Appendix

- **Well-differentiated neuroendocrine tumour:** Also called **carcinoid**, this is the most common tumour of the appendix. It is usually located at the tip of the appendix and noticed as a bulbous swelling incidentally in resected specimens. It is about 2–3 cm and usually benign. Occasional local spread may be seen, but nodal and distant metastases are rare.
- **Benign adenomas and malignant adenocarcinomas:** These cause obstruction of the lumen and mimic acute appendicitis.
- **Mucocoele of the appendix:** The appendix is dilated, stretched and filled with mucin. It may be due to luminal obstruction, leading to the collection of inspissated

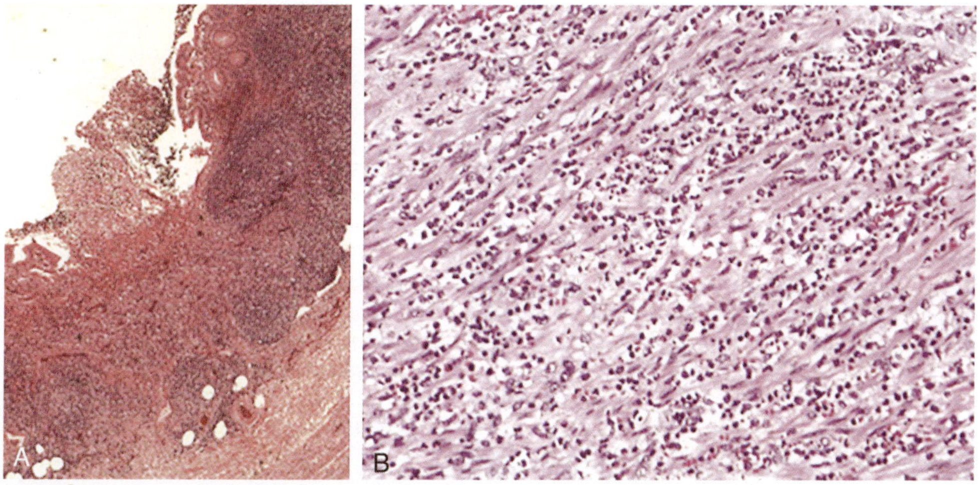

Fig. 21.54 Microscopy of early appendicitis with mucosal and submucosal acute inflammation and ulceration of the mucosa (A) and a high-power view showing neutrophilic infiltrate within the wall of the appendix (B).

mucin, or a consequence of **mucinous cystadenoma or mucinous cystadenocarcinoma**.

- **Mucinous cystadenocarcinoma:** This malignant neoplasm may spread to the peritoneum and cause **pseudomyxoma peritonei**, a condition in which the abdominal organs are coated with mucin secreted into the peritoneal cavity, creating marked adhesions between them (**frozen abdomen**).

SELF-ASSESSMENT

Multiple Choice Questions

1. A 45-year-old male presents with dysphagia and weight loss. Endoscopy shows a peptic stricture. What is the most likely cause?
   A. Oesophageal cancer
   B. Gastro-oesophageal reflux disease
   C. Achalasia
   D. Oesophageal varices
2. A 30-year-old female with a history of Crohn disease presents with abdominal pain and diarrhoea. Which is a common complication?
   A. Intestinal obstruction
   B. Peptic ulcer disease
   C. Gastrointestinal bleeding
   D. Hepatic encephalopathy
3. A patient with a history of alcohol abuse presents with haematemesis. What is the most likely diagnosis?
   A. Gastric ulcer
   B. Oesophageal varices
   C. Mallory–Weiss tear
   D. Gastritis
4. A 50-year-old man presents with jaundice, clay-coloured stools and dark urine. What is the most likely diagnosis?
   A. Hepatitis
   B. Cholecystitis
   C. Pancreatic cancer
   D. Haemochromatosis
5. A patient presents with severe abdominal pain radiating to the back, nausea and vomiting. Labs show elevated amylase and lipase. The most likely diagnosis is:
   A. Acute pancreatitis
   B. Cholecystitis
   C. Peptic ulcer disease
   D. Hepatic abscess
6. A 55-year-old male with a history of smoking and chronic GERD presents with progressive dysphagia. The most likely diagnosis is:
   A. Oesophageal spasm
   B. Oesophageal cancer
   C. Achalasia
   D. Zenker diverticulum
7. A patient with coeliac disease is most at risk of deficiency in which of the following?
   A. Vitamin B_{12}
   B. Vitamin D
   C. Iron
   D. All of the above
8. A 60-year-old male presents with painless jaundice. Which of the following is the most likely diagnosis?
   A. Acute hepatitis
   B. Pancreatic cancer
   C. Gallstones
   D. Alcoholic liver disease
9. A patient diagnosed with ulcerative colitis is at an increased risk for:
   A. Cholangiocarcinoma
   B. Colorectal cancer
   C. Pancreatic cancer
   D. Gastric cancer
10. A 40-year-old woman presents with recurrent right upper quadrant pain after meals. The most likely diagnosis is:
   A. Cholecystitis
   B. Hepatitis
   C. Pancreatitis
   D. Peptic ulcer disease
11. A patient with liver cirrhosis presents with ascites. Which of the following is the most likely cause?
   A. Portal hypertension
   B. Hepatic encephalopathy
   C. Spontaneous bacterial peritonitis
   D. Hepatocellular carcinoma
12. A 65-year-old male with a history of smoking presents with a change in bowel habits and rectal bleeding. What is the most likely diagnosis?
   A. Haemorrhoids
   B. Colorectal cancer
   C. Inflammatory bowel disease
   D. Diverticulitis
13. A patient presents with severe epigastric pain that improves with eating. The most likely diagnosis is:
   A. Gastric ulcer
   B. Duodenal ulcer
   C. Gastritis
   D. Pancreatitis
14. A patient with a history of NSAID use presents with epigastric pain and melena. The most likely diagnosis is:
   A. Gastric ulcer
   B. Duodenal ulcer
   C. Oesophageal varices
   D. Gastric cancer
15. A 70-year-old male presents with weight loss and a palpable mass in the right lower quadrant. The most likely diagnosis is:
   A. Appendicitis
   B. Colorectal cancer
   C. Diverticulitis
   D. Ileitis
16. A patient with a history of peptic ulcer disease now presents with acute abdominal pain and rigid abdomen. The most likely diagnosis is:
   A. Perforated ulcer
   B. Acute pancreatitis
   C. Cholecystitis
   D. Intestinal obstruction
17. A 50-year-old female with a long-standing history of heartburn now presents with Barrett oesophagus. This condition increases the risk of developing:
   A. Oesophageal varices
   B. Oesophageal adenocarcinoma
   C. Oesophageal squamous cell carcinoma
   D. Gastric cancer
18. A patient with a history of IBD presents with arthralgia and red, painful eyes. This is most likely indicative of:
   A. Rheumatoid arthritis
   B. Ankylosing spondylitis

C. Uveitis
D. Scleritis

19. A newborn presents with bilious vomiting and abdominal distension. The most likely diagnosis is:
    A. Pyloric stenosis
    B. Intussusception
    C. Hirschsprung disease
    D. Duodenal atresia
20. A patient presents with pruritus, fatigue and xanthelasma. Laboratory tests show elevated alkaline phosphatase. The most likely diagnosis is:
    A. Primary biliary cholangitis
    B. Hepatic cirrhosis
    C. Cholestasis of pregnancy
    D. Gallstones
21. A 35-year-old male with no significant medical history presents with acute epigastric pain and shock. CT scan shows pancreatic necrosis. What is the most likely complication?
    A. Pancreatic pseudocyst
    B. Haemorrhagic pancreatitis
    C. Chronic pancreatitis
    D. Pancreatic abscess
22. A 50-year-old female with a history of autoimmune hepatitis presents with progressive jaundice and ascites. A liver biopsy shows bridging fibrosis and regenerative nodules. The most likely diagnosis is:
    A. Acute hepatitis
    B. Primary sclerosing cholangitis
    C. Hepatocellular carcinoma
    D. Cirrhosis

Answers

1. (B); 2. (A); 3. (B); 4. (C); 5. (A); 6. (B); 7. (D); 8. (B); 9. (B); 10. (A); 11. (A); 12. (B); 13. (B); 14. (A); 15. (B); 16. (A); 17. (B); 18. (C); 19. (D); 20. (A); 21. (B); 22. (D)

Self-Assessment Questions

1. A neonate with a history of delayed passage of meconium had constipation, distension of the abdomen and failure to thrive. Rectal examination revealed an empty contracted rectum without faecal soiling. What is the diagnosis and pathogenesis and how will you confirm the diagnosis?
2. A 45-year-old obese chronic smoker with a severe feature of gastro-oesophageal reflux underwent upper GI endoscopy for evaluation. In the lower end of the oesophagus, endoscopy revealed proximal migration of squamocolumnar junction and smooth gastric mucosa. What is the likely diagnosis and histological finding?
3. A 70-year-old man who had progressively increasing dysphagia for the last 6 months accompanied by severe weight loss presented to the outpatient department. Examination revealed multiple enlarged lymph nodes in the neck. What is the diagnosis?
4. A 30-year-old highly strung nervous individual has burning type of pain lower down in the epigastrium, right of the midline, aggravated on an empty stomach and relieved on eating. The pain occasionally radiates to the back. What are the diagnosis, aetiology and complications?
5. A 65-year-old man whose blood group was A and who had a prolonged history of dyspepsia developed severe loss of appetite and weight loss recently. Of late, he felt ball-rolling movement in the stomach after food intake, followed by blood-stained vomitus. Examination revealed an epigastric mass and enlarged liver. What are the diagnosis, classification and morphological features?
6. A 50-year-old woman presented with chronic diarrhoea, abdominal bloating and fatigue. On questioning, she indicated that it worsened on eating biscuits and bread. Examination showed pallor and blistering lesions on the skin. What could be the cause for her symptoms?
7. A 28-year-old man admitted to intensive care and undergoing treatment of severe lower respiratory infection suddenly developed abdominal pain and watery diarrhoea. Stool examination showed leucocytes and occult blood. What are the diagnosis and recommended investigation?
8. A 30-year-old woman presented with recurrent attacks of bloody diarrhoea with stringy, mucoid material and lower abdominal pain that was temporarily relieved by defecation. She gave a history of a similar attack 2 years back for which she required hospitalization and treatment following which she was asymptomatic till 1 month back. On examination, aphthous ulcers were noted in the mouth, palpable mass in the right iliac fossa and a fistula in the anus. What are the diagnosis, pathogenesis and morphological findings possible?
9. A surgically resected tumour of the stomach was received in the histopathology department. The specimen showed a smooth intact mucosa and an underlying neoplasm composed of spindle-shaped cells with minimal pleomorphism. What are the diagnosis and mutations associated?
10. An elderly male patient developed intermittent colicky pain in the suprapubic area associated with altered bowel habits – episodes of constipation alternating with diarrhoea. A history of passing mucus with blood early in the morning was present. Examination revealed a vague mass in the left iliac fossa. What are the diagnosis and morphology of the lesion?

Answers

1. Hirschsprung disease
2. Barrett oesophagus
3. Oesophageal carcinoma
4. Gastric ulcer
5. Gastric adenocarcinoma
6. Coeliac disease
7. Pseudomembranous colitis
8. Inflammatory bowel disease
9. Gastrointestinal stromal tumour
10. Carcinoma of the colon

Topics for Self-Directed Learning

1. Tracheo-oesophageal fistula
2. Follow-up of patients with Barrett oesophagus
3. Pernicious anaemia
4. Ischaemic bowel disease
5. *E. coli* enterocolitis
6. Giardiasis
7. Intestinal manifestations of graft-versus-host disease
8. Sigmoid diverticulosis
9. Mucinous carcinoma of the stomach
10. Pseudomyxoma peritonei

MIND MAPS

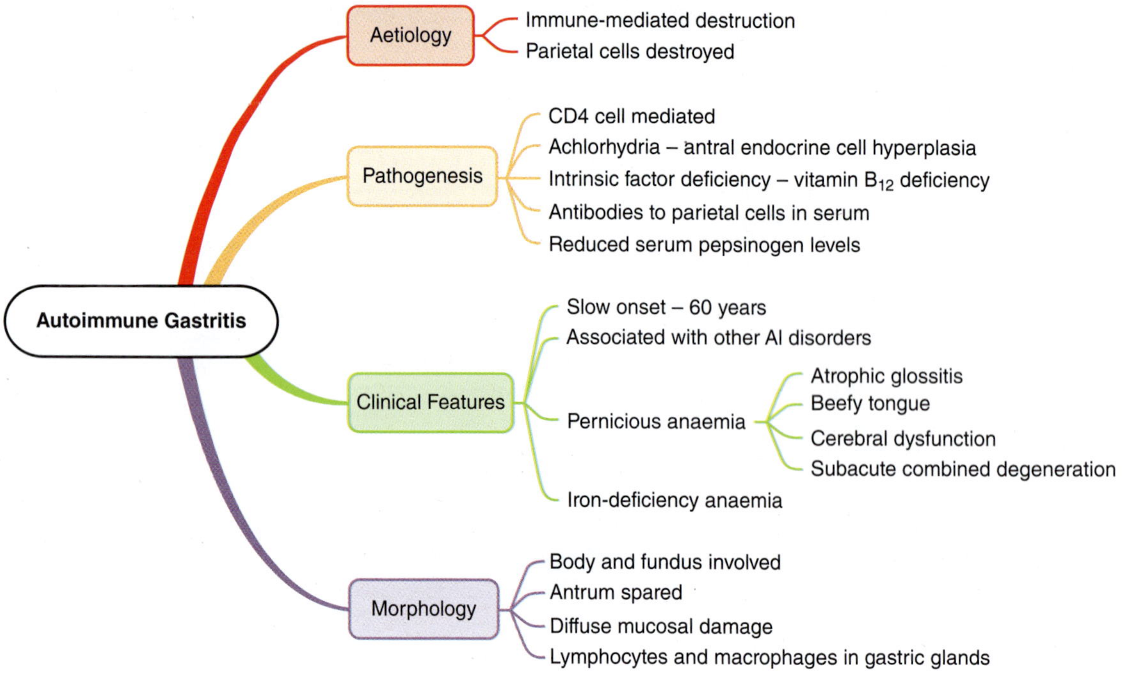
Autoimmune Gastritis
Aetiology
Immune-mediated destruction
Parietal cells destroyed
Pathogenesis
CD4 cell mediated
Achlorhydria – antral endocrine cell hyperplasia
Intrinsic factor deficiency – vitamin B_{12} deficiency
Antibodies to parietal cells in serum
Reduced serum pepsinogen levels
Clinical Features
Slow onset – 60 years
Associated with other AI disorders
Pernicious anaemia
Atrophic glossitis
Beefy tongue
Cerebral dysfunction
Subacute combined degeneration
Iron-deficiency anaemia
Morphology
Body and fundus involved
Antrum spared
Diffuse mucosal damage
Lymphocytes and macrophages in gastric glands

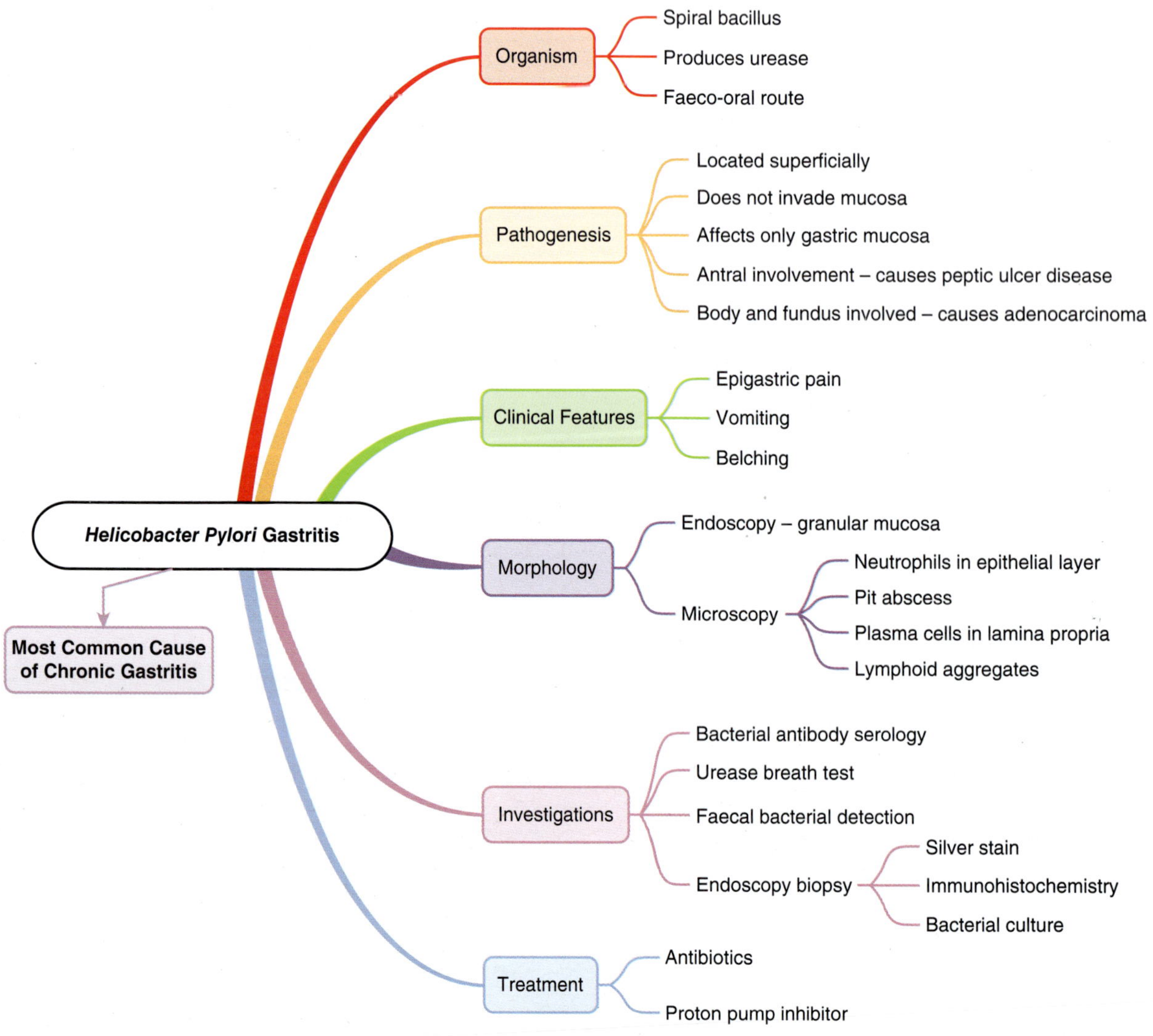
Helicobacter Pylori Gastritis
Most Common Cause of Chronic Gastritis
Organism
Spiral bacillus
Produces urease
Faeco-oral route
Pathogenesis
Located superficially
Does not invade mucosa
Affects only gastric mucosa
Antral involvement – causes peptic ulcer disease
Body and fundus involved – causes adenocarcinoma
Clinical Features
Epigastric pain
Vomiting
Belching
Morphology
Endoscopy – granular mucosa
Microscopy
Neutrophils in epithelial layer
Pit abscess
Plasma cells in lamina propria
Lymphoid aggregates
Investigations
Bacterial antibody serology
Urease breath test
Faecal bacterial detection
Endoscopy biopsy
Silver stain
Immunohistochemistry
Bacterial culture
Treatment
Antibiotics
Proton pump inhibitor

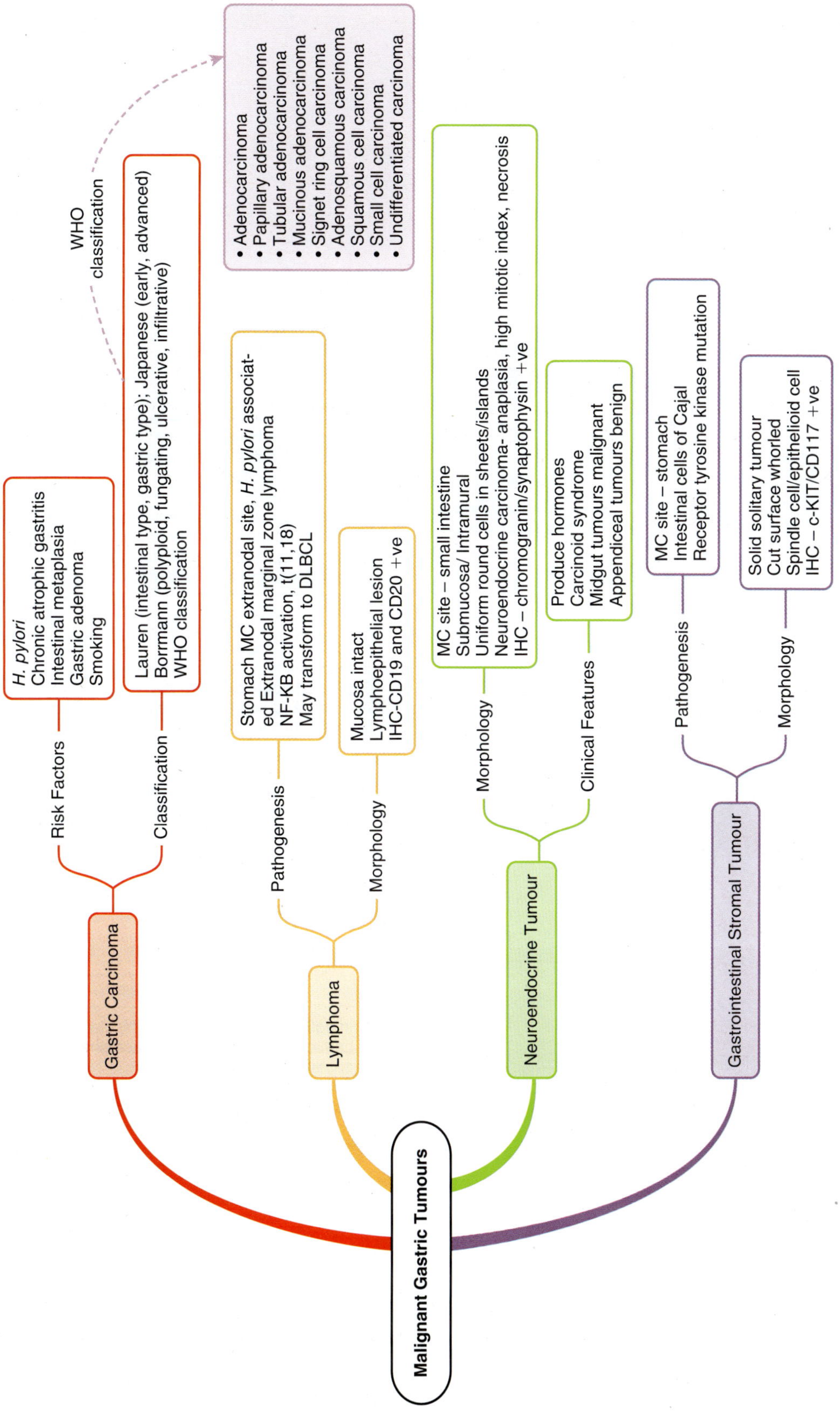
Malignant Gastric Tumours
Gastric Carcinoma
Risk Factors
H. pylori
Chronic atrophic gastritis
Intestinal metaplasia
Gastric adenoma
Smoking
Classification
Lauren (intestinal type, gastric type); Japanese (early, advanced)
Borrmann (polyploid, fungating, ulcerative, infiltrative)
WHO classification
WHO classification
• Adenocarcinoma
• Papillary adenocarcinoma
• Tubular adenocarcinoma
• Mucinous adenocarcinoma
• Signet ring cell carcinoma
• Adenosquamous carcinoma
• Squamous cell carcinoma
• Small cell carcinoma
• Undifferentiated carcinoma
Lymphoma
Pathogenesis
Stomach MC extranodal site, H. pylori associated Extranodal marginal zone lymphoma
NF-KB activation, t(11,18)
May transform to DLBCL
Morphology
Mucosa intact
Lymphoepithelial lesion
IHC-CD19 and CD20 +ve
Neuroendocrine Tumour
Morphology
MC site – small intestine
Submucosa/ Intramural
Uniform round cells in sheets/islands
Neuroendocrine carcinoma- anaplasia, high mitotic index, necrosis
IHC – chromogranin/synaptophysin +ve
Clinical Features
Produce hormones
Carcinoid syndrome
Midgut tumours malignant
Appendiceal tumours benign
Gastrointestinal Stromal Tumour
Pathogenesis
MC site – stomach
Intestinal cells of Cajal
Receptor tyrosine kinase mutation
Morphology
Solid solitary tumour
Cut surface whorled
Spindle cell/epithelioid cell
IHC – c-KIT/CD117 +ve

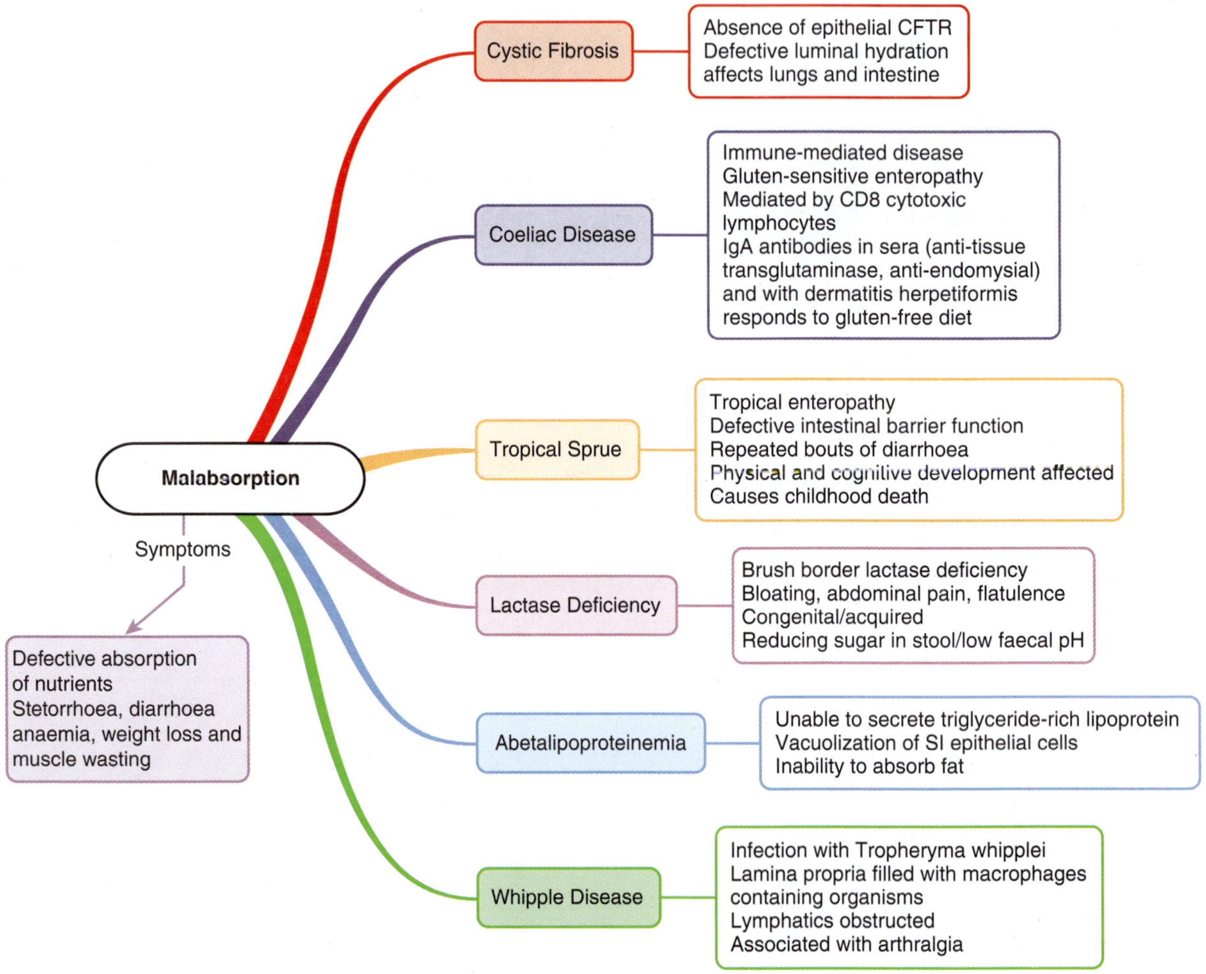

Malabsorption
Symptoms
Defective absorption of nutrients
Stetorrhoea, diarrhoea
anaemia, weight loss and muscle wasting
Cystic Fibrosis
Absence of epithelial CFTR
Defective luminal hydration
affects lungs and intestine
Coeliac Disease
Immune-mediated disease
Gluten-sensitive enteropathy
Mediated by CD8 cytotoxic lymphocytes
IgA antibodies in sera (anti-tissue transglutaminase, anti-endomysial)
and with dermatitis herpetiformis
responds to gluten-free diet
Tropical Sprue
Tropical enteropathy
Defective intestinal barrier function
Repeated bouts of diarrhoea
Physical and cognitive development affected
Causes childhood death
Lactase Deficiency
Brush border lactase deficiency
Bloating, abdominal pain, flatulence
Congenital/acquired
Reducing sugar in stool/low faecal pH
Abetalipoproteinemia
Unable to secrete triglyceride-rich lipoprotein
Vacuolization of SI epithelial cells
Inability to absorb fat
Whipple Disease
Infection with Tropheryma whipplei
Lamina propria filled with macrophages containing organisms
Lymphatics obstructed
Associated with arthralgia

Intestinal Polyps

- **Neoplastic Polyps**
  - Adenoma
    - Precursor of adenocarcinoma
    - Solitary sessile/pedunculated
    - Presence of epithelial dysplasia
    - Tubular/tubulovillous/villous
    - >4 cm, high-grade dysplasia – malignant risk high
  - Familial polyp syndromes
    - Familial adenomatous polyposis
      - APC gene mutation
      - >100 adenomas in colorectum
      - Risk of malignant transformation 100%
    - Hereditary nonpolyposis colon carcinoma
      - Lynch syndrome
      - MSH2/MLH1 gene mutation
      - Mismatch repair failure
      - Microsatellite instability
- **Non-neoplastic Polyps**
  - Hyperplastic polyps
    - Decrease in epithelial cell turnover
    - Delayed shedding
    - Piling up of goblet cells
    - Common in left colon
    - Serrations in upper third of crypt
  - Inflammatory polyp
    - Solitary rectal ulcer syndrome
    - Due to delayed relaxation of anorectal sphincter
    - May cause mucosal prolapse
  - Hamartomatous polyp
    - Germline mutations of proto-oncogenes/tumour suppressor genes
      - Juvenile polyps
        - Malformations of epithelium/lamina propria
        - Rectosigmoid region
        - Sporadic – low malignant potential
        - Syndromic – malignant risk
      - Peutz–Jeghers syndrome
        - Associated with mucocutaneous hyperpigmentation
        - Fatal intussusception
        - STK 11 gene mutation
        - Microscooy – arborizing muscle, lamina propria with glands

22 Liver and Gallbladder

K Meenakshisundaram, Indhu Kannan

PA 25.1 Describe bilirubin metabolism, enumerate the aetiology and pathogenesis of **jaundice**, and distinguish between direct and indirect hyperbilirubinaemias.

PA 25.2 Describe the pathophysiology and pathological changes seen in **hepatic failure** and their clinical manifestations, complications and consequences.

PA 25.3 Describe the aetiology and pathogenesis of **viral and toxic hepatitis**. Distinguish the causes of hepatitis on the basis of their clinical and laboratory features. Describe the pathology, complications and consequences of hepatitis.

PA 25.4 Describe the pathophysiology, pathology and progression of **alcoholic liver disease** including cirrhosis.

PA 25.5 Describe the aetiology, pathogenesis and complications of **portal hypertension**.

CHAPTER OUTLINE

INTRODUCTION

The liver is the largest visceral organ of the body and performs many vital functions that have an impact on all the body systems. It is the central organ for detoxification, metabolism, maintenance of homeostasis (production of coagulation factors), immunity, regulation of the endocrine system and vitamin storage. During prenatal development, the liver, in addition, aids in haematopoiesis. In the course of these essential functions, it is constantly exposed to a myriad of injurious agents, but fortunately, the liver has a remarkable functional reserve and regenerative capacity.

ANATOMY, HISTOLOGY AND FUNCTIONS OF THE LIVER

LIVER ANATOMY

The liver is a roughly triangular organ that resides predominantly in the right upper quadrant and extends across the abdominal cavity just inferior to the diaphragm, protected by the rib cage. An adult liver weighs 1400–1600 g, comprising approximately 2% of the total body weight. It measures about 10–12 cm vertically, 15–20 cm transversely and about 12–15 cm in thickness. Most of the liver is enclosed by a fibrous capsule, known as the Glisson capsule, which is further surrounded by the visceral peritoneum. A condensed extension of the peritoneum, the falciform ligament, divides the liver asymmetrically into two lobes - right and left - but, functionally, it is divided into eight segments with separate vascular supply and biliary drainage.

The liver has a unique dual blood supply, receiving approximately 60%–70% via the portal vein and the remainder via the hepatic artery. The portal vein brings to the liver blood containing absorbed nutrients along with contaminants such as drugs, toxins from food and by-products of blood cells recycling from the entire gastrointestinal (GI) tract, spleen and pancreas. The hepatic artery supplies oxygenated blood to the liver. Both the vessels enter the liver inferiorly at the porta hepatis, branch throughout the liver and empty their contents into the sinusoids. The sinusoids are designed with fenestrations to allow free access of the blood components to the hepatocytes for metabolic use. From here, the blood now devoid of metabolites is drained by the right, middle and left hepatic veins that empty into the inferior vena cava (IVC).

Liver Histology (Figs 22.1 and 22.2)

In histological terms, the liver is divided into repetitive hexagonal units called lobules. The best conceptualization of the liver architecture would be to understand it as the classical hepatic lobule that comprises a terminal hepatic venule (i.e. central vein) at the centre and portal tracts at the periphery. Each lobule is equipped with six portal tracts at each angle of the hexagon. The portal tract encloses a branch of the portal vein, a hepatic arteriole and the bile duct. Much of the lobule is occupied by the hepatocytes that are arranged in anastomosing cords of one- or two-cell thickness, radiating from the central vein. Hepatic acinus refers to the segment of liver tissue that is supplied by a single branch of the hepatic artery. Each hepatic acinus is divided into three zones:

Zone 1: It is the region that abuts the portal tract and receives the most oxygen-rich and toxin-rich blood.
Zone 2: It is the region between zone 1 and zone 3.
Zone 3: It is the region around the central vein that receives oxygen-poor and toxin-poor blood.

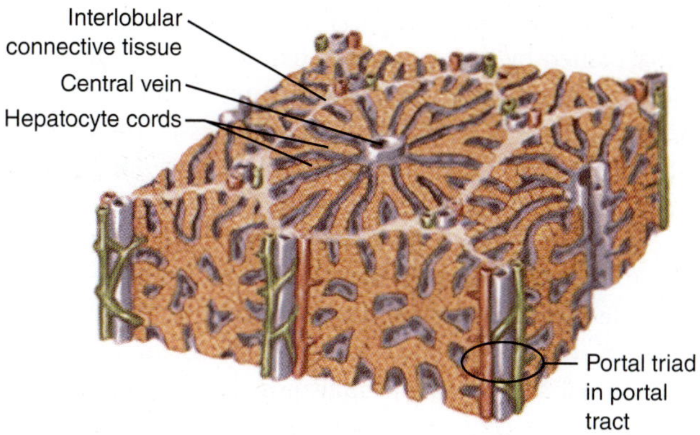

Fig. 22.1 The liver parenchyma is divided into hexagonal lobules, with a central vein **in the centre** and portal tracts in the periphery. (*Source:* From Dolores B. Njoku, Hovig V. Chitilian and Kate Kronish. Hepatic Physiology, Pathophysiology, and Anesthetic Considerations. Miller's Anesthesia. 9th edition. Elsevier 2020.)

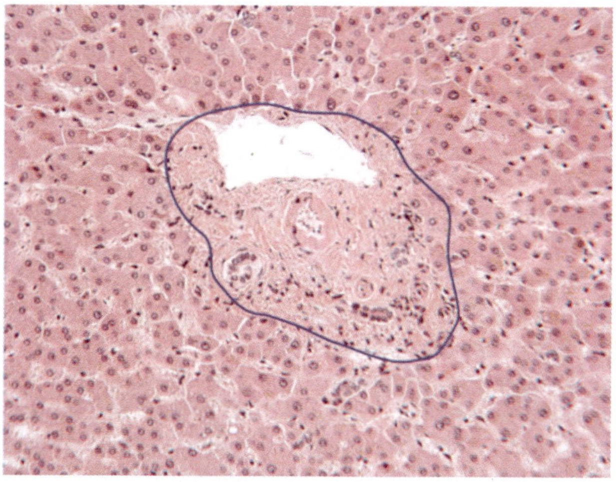

Fig. 22.2 Portal tract showing the thick-walled hepatic artery, bile duct and a large vessel with thin wall - portal vein. (*Source:* From Judith I. Wyatt and Beate Haugk. Liver, biliary system and pancreas. Underwood's Pathology. Seventh Edition. Elsevier 2019.)

Hepatic sinusoids run parallel to the hepatocyte cords and are lined by the specialized fenestrated endothelium. The perisinusoidal space between the endothelium and the hepatocytes is termed the 'space of Disse'. The hepatocytes extend their villi into the space of Disse for easy absorption of materials. The space of Disse also comprises fat-containing hepatic stellate cells, also called Ito cells, that function as vitamin A storage cells and play an important role in fibrogenesis in the disease state. Kupffer cells are liver resident macrophages that attach themselves to the luminal surface of the sinusoids and sometimes may extend into the space of Disse. Kupffer cells along with the lymphocytes within the liver parenchyma offer primary immune surveillance and perform phagocytic functions.

BILIARY TRACT

The biliary apparatus comprises the right and left hepatic ducts, common bile duct, cystic duct and gallbladder. The bile produced by the liver is transported through the innumerable bile canaliculi, which represent the smallest portions of the biliary tree. The canaliculi are located between the apical membranes of the adjacent hepatocytes and are sealed by tight junctions to prevent leakage. The canaliculi travel parallel to the sinusoids until they empty into the interlobular ductules (canals of Hering) at the edge of the lobules, which subsequently drain into the intrahepatic bile ductules within the portal tract. The ductules progressively join together to form larger ducts and eventually at the porta hepatis give rise to the right and left hepatic ducts. Slightly distal to the porta hepatis, the confluence of the right and left hepatic ducts delivers the common hepatic duct. The common hepatic duct is joined by the cystic duct from the gallbladder to form the common bile duct, which opens into the duodenum at the ampulla.

FUNCTIONS OF THE LIVER

This metabolically active organ is responsible for a staggering array of functions, and the most important ones are listed as follows:

- It interacts with the endocrine and GI systems and aids in digestion.
- It helps in the production and excretion of bile.
- It is involved in the metabolism of proteins, carbohydrates and lipids.
- The liver stores vitamins (mainly vitamins A, B_{12} and D), as well as iron and copper.
- It helps in detoxification of substances such as drugs and alcohol.
- The liver is responsible for bilirubin metabolism and conjugation.
- It helps in synthesis of many plasma proteins, such as albumin and clotting factors.

LIVER FUNCTION TESTS (TABLE 22.1)

Liver function tests (LFTs) are the measures of the concentration of proteins and enzymes produced by the liver or released by damaged hepatocytes. Most often, LFTs reflect the cause of hepatic injury rather than the functional capacity of the liver. Effectively, these tests can help in determining the hepatic or cholestatic origin of hepatic damage and the specific pattern of results often helps in organizing a differential diagnosis.

These tests and their interpretation with reference values are dealt with in Chapter 11.

Markers of hepatocellular injury	• ALT (alanine transaminase) (formerly glutamic pyruvic transaminase or SGPT) • AST (aspartate transaminase) (formerly glutamic oxaloacetic transaminase or SGOT)
Markers of cholestasis	• AP (alkaline phosphatase) • GGT (gamma-glutamyl transferase)
Markers of synthetic liver function	• Albumin • Prothrombin
Markers of liver excretory function	• Bilirubin, bile salts and bile pigment

Table 22.1 Liver Function Tests

Laboratory Test	Normal Range	Sources Other Than Liver
AST (aspartate aminotransferase)	<35 units/L	Cardiac and skeletal muscle
ALT (alanine aminotransferase)	<35 units/L	Skeletal muscle
GGTP (γ-glutamyl transpeptidase)	1–94 units/L	
Alkaline phosphatase	30–120 units/L	Bone
Total bilirubin	0.3–1.0 mg/dL	From haem breakdown
Direct bilirubin (conjugated)		
Total protein	6.0–8.3 g/dL	
Albumin	3.5–5.5 g/dL	
A/G ratio (albumin/globulin ratio)	>1	Total protein minus albumin = globulin
INR (based on prothrombin time)	0.9–1.1 (1)	

MECHANISMS OF INJURY AND REPAIR

The liver is vulnerable to a variety of disease processes, including infectious diseases, inflammatory conditions, metabolic disorders, toxic conditions, circulatory problems and neoplastic lesions. In general, symptoms of liver disease come into picture many years after the onset of injury because of its remarkable capacity of self-renewal and repair.

HEPATOCELLULAR INJURY

Liver cell injury can be triggered by any aetiology disturbing the normal homeostasis. The response to injury is reflected by the morphological changes in the hepatocytes and depends greatly on the type of insult and severity. The following is a brief list of the important cellular adaptive mechanisms adopted by the hepatocytes reflecting the impact of early liver damage:

- **Ballooning degeneration** (Fig. 22.3): Hepatocyte swelling (oedema) is a part of normal physiology with reference to regeneration and turnover. However, deranged cellular swelling is a feature of liver cell injury and is considered as a hallmark feature of alcoholic and nonalcoholic steatohepatitis (NASH). Hepatocytes with ballooning degeneration can be recognized as large cells with clear vacuolated cytoplasm and cellular oedema. These cells can also be seen in response to toxic and ischaemic injury causing ATP depletion.
- **Mallory–Denk bodies:** The ballooned hepatocytes often contain clumps of eosinophilic material, representing damaged intermediate filaments termed Mallory–Denk bodies. Apart from steatohepatitis (alcoholic and nonalcoholic), Mallory–Denk bodies accumulate in Wilson disease and cirrhosis, as well as in cholestatic conditions such as primary biliary sclerosis following exposure to certain drugs (e.g. amiodarone).

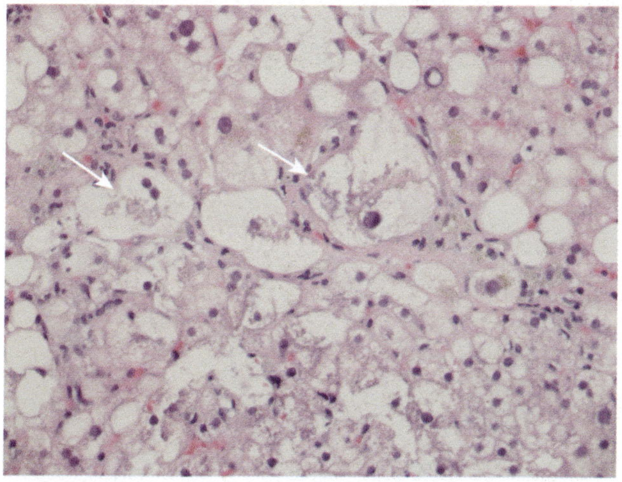

Fig. 22.3 Histopathological image of ballooning degeneration of hepatocytes with Mallory hyaline (arrows). (*Source:* From Kiyoko Oshima. Liver Histopathology. GI/Liver Secrets Plus. Saunders 2015.)

- **Steatosis** (Fig. 22.4): Accumulation of lipid droplets (LDs) within the hepatocyte is referred to as steatosis. It marks the most common and earliest response to alcohol-induced injury. Other common causes include hepatitis C infection and drugs such as corticosteroids and tetracyclines.
- **Cholestasis** (Fig. 22.5): It is defined as the stagnation of bile and bile products within the biliary tract due to obstructive or nonobstructive causes.

The aforementioned cellular changes may be viewed as reversible, but in the course of time, the threshold for compensation and recovery is exceeded and the hepatocytes undergo irreversible cell damage and die by necrosis or apoptosis. Necrosis is the predominant mode of death in conditions of extreme ATP depletion (as in ischaemic or hypoxic injury), toxin-related damage, most commonly acetaminophen induced, and oxidative stress. Loss of ATP results in loss of cellular membrane potentials and

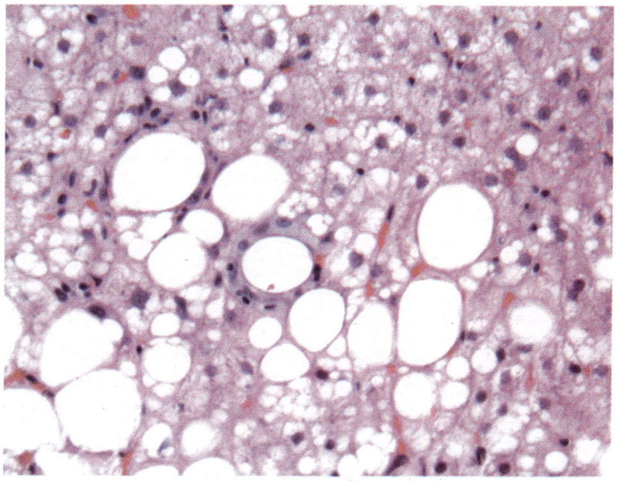

Fig. 22.4 Histopathological image showing steatosis surrounded by normal-appearing hepatocytes. (*Source:* From Elizabeth M. Brunt and Dina G. Tiniakos. Fatty Liver Disease. In Odze and Goldblum Surgical Pathology of the GI Tract, Liver, Biliary Tract and Pancreas. 3rd edition. Elsevier 2015.)

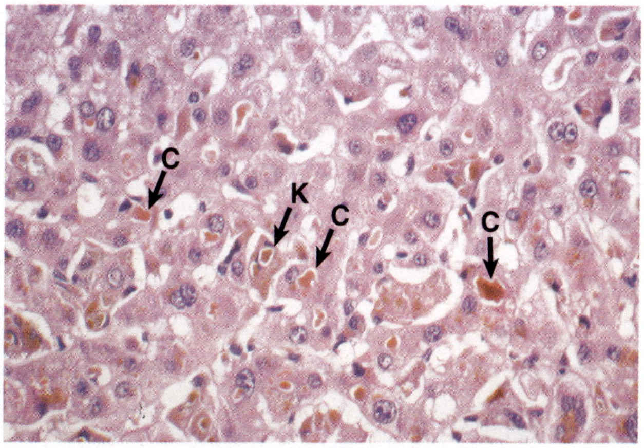

Fig. 22.5 Cholestasis characterized by inspissated bile within the bile canaliculi (C) (bile plugs) and within the Kupffer cells (K). (*Source:* From James H. Lewis. Liver Disease Caused by Anesthetics, Chemicals, Toxins, and Herbal and Dietary Supplements. In Sleisenger and Fordtran's Gastrointestinal and Liver Disease. 11th edition. Elsevier 2021.)

loss of function of channel/ion pumps, disturbing the calcium homeostasis. The resultant increase in the intracellular calcium and inflow of water causes plasma membrane rupture and release of cellular contents into the extracellular environment. This triggers an inflammatory response that further exacerbates tissue injury.

Several patterns of necrosis have been identified. ***Spotty or focal necrosis*** is the term used to describe necrosis of small clusters of hepatocytes accompanied by lymphocytes. ***Hepatocyte dropout/confluent necrosis*** refers to zones of hepatocyte death, most commonly zone 3 hepatocytes, especially in response to ischaemic insults. Severe forms of confluent necrosis can present as ***panacinar or submassive necrosis*** (necrosis of the entire lobule). When the necrosis spans over adjacent lobules in a portocentral or central–central pattern, it is called ***bridging necrosis*** (Fig. 22.6). The appearance of destroyed necrotic hepatocytes at the limiting plate or interphase between the parenchymal cells and the portal region is called ***piecemeal necrosis*** and the underlying condition interphase hepatitis (Fig. 22.7).

Apoptosis, as we already know from the previous chapters, is characterized by pyknosis, karyorrhexis and cellular fragmentation to form apoptotic bodies, which are quickly phagocytosed by the circulating Kupffer cells. Hepatocellular apoptosis is a regular feature of many liver diseases including viral hepatitis, autoimmune liver disease and alcohol- or drug-induced liver injury in which the infected or damaged cells are eliminated sensibly without spillage of contents into the external milieu.

In the liver, these apoptotic bodies are referred to as ***acidophil bodies*** (Fig. 22.8), identified as shrunken deeply

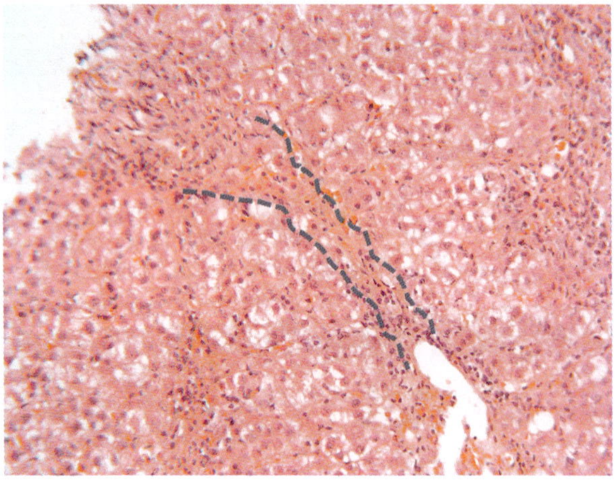

Fig. 22.6 Severe hepatitis with bridging necrosis. A confluent line of necrotic hepatocytes seen extending from the portal vein on the left to the central vein on the lower right – bridging necrosis. (*Source:* From Judith I. Wyatt and Beate Haugk. Liver, biliary system and pancreas. Underwood's Pathology. Seventh Edition. Elsevier 2019.)

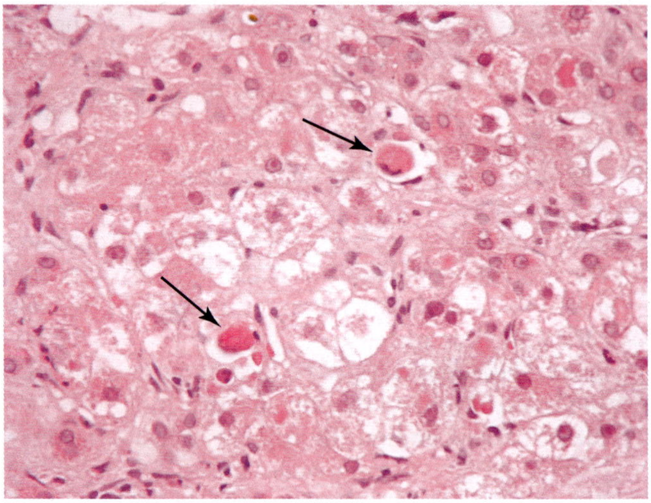

Fig. 22.8 Histopathological image showing acidophil bodies (marked with an arrow) within the sinusoids in a case of alcoholic steatohepatitis. (*Source:* From Yoh Zen, Kazuo Notsumata, Nobuyoshi Tanaka and Yasuni Nakanuma. Hepatic centrilobular zonal necrosis with positive antinuclear antibody: a unique subtype or early disease of autoimmune hepatitis? Human Pathology. 2007;38:1669-1675.)

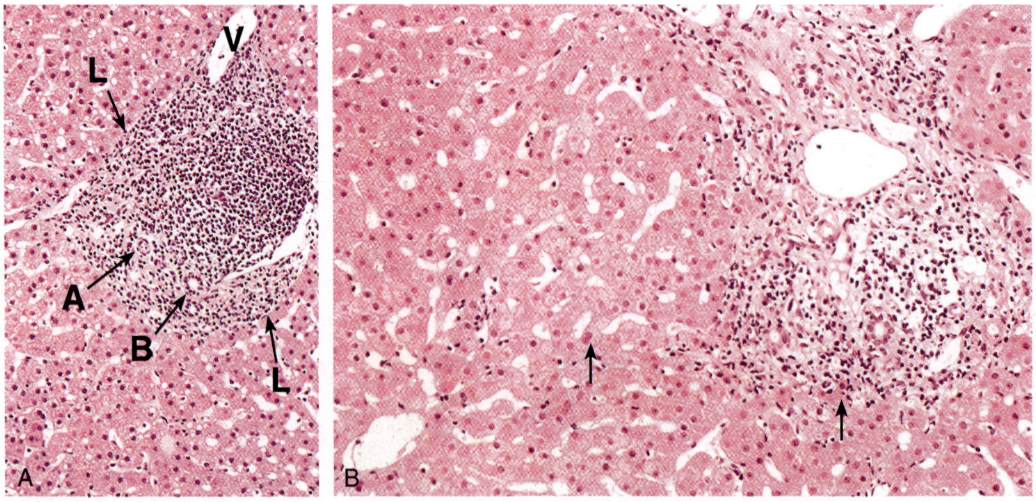

Fig. 22.7 (A) Portal tract is shown along with portal vein (V), bile duct (B) and hepatic artery (A), with inflammatory cells confined to the portal region. The periportal hepatocytes, called the limiting plate (L), are well preserved and show no necrosis. (B) Portal inflammatory cells seen spilling into the adjacent hepatic lobule causing hepatocyte necrosis – interface hepatitis. (*Source:* From Geraldine O'Dowd, Sarah Bell and Sylvia Wright. Liver and pancreaticobiliary system. In Wheater's Pathology: A Text, Atlas, and Review of Histopathology. 6th edition. Elsevier 2020.)

eosinophilic cells sometimes containing a small pyknotic nucleus. These apoptotic bodies were first described by scientist *William T. Councilman* in patients with yellow fever and were eponymously also known as *Councilman bodies*. Notably, physiological apoptosis, such as removal of senescent cells, and remodelling can also show the presence of acidophilic bodies.

REGENERATION

Liver regeneration is a process that is spontaneously activated following injury. Depending on the severity of the stimulus and the extent of cellular destruction, liver cell regeneration can be achieved by two cellular mechanisms: first, by compensatory hyperplasia and hypertrophy of the differentiated mature hepatocytes surrounding the destroyed cells, and, second, by the expansion and differentiation of the progenitor cells. As the bile ductules (canals of Hering) are the source of progenitor cells, bile ductular proliferation can be seen in the periportal region, an event known as bile ductular reaction. Another important event in regeneration is neoangiogenesis and vascular remodelling. Angiogenesis is the key step in chronic liver injury. The ongoing fibrosis and inflammation cause tissue hypoxia and the resultant generation of nitric oxide (NO), promoting vasodilatation. Vascular endothelial growth factor (VEGF) produced by the Kupffer cells, stellate cells and hepatocytes steps in next to activate the vascular buds. This is accompanied by enzymes (matrix metalloproteases [MMPs]) that clear the extracellular matrix (ECM) for new blood vessel formation.

FIBROSIS AND SCAR FORMATION PA 25.4

As mentioned earlier, regeneration aims at restoration of liver cell mass and is virtually beneficial in acute liver injury. The process is accompanied by appropriate inflammatory response and ECM remodelling. However, when the stimuli causing injury persist, the process of regeneration is exhausted, followed by fibrosis or scar formation. Thus, of note, fibrosis indicates chronic hepatitis. Activation of hepatic stellate cells is the central event in hepatic fibrosis. As already mentioned, hepatic stellate cells are quiescent (Fig. 22.9), nonparenchymal cells that function as vitamin A storage cells. On activation, these cells transform into fibrogenic myofibroblasts capable of producing type I and III collagen and fibronectin. Stellate cell activation is induced by Kupffer cells, which, after liver injury, produce large amounts of reactive oxygen species and fibrogenic cytokines – tumour necrosis factor alpha (TNF-α). Activated stellate cells produce cytokines such as TGF-β, PDGF, ET-1, and TNF and perpetuate their activation in an autocrine loop. Thus, hepatic stellate cells begin depositing elevated amounts of collagen and ECM material within the hepatic parenchyma, disturbing the normal cellular functions. In the space of Disse, ECM deposition causes blockade of the sinusoidal fenestrations, a process known as ***capillarization of sinusoids***, resulting in loss of protein exchange between the blood and hepatocytes, further deteriorating the liver function. Fibrosis initially sets in the periportal region, extending spikes of fibrous tissue into the lobules. Over time, periportal fibrosis may link the adjacent portal tracts or central vein forming

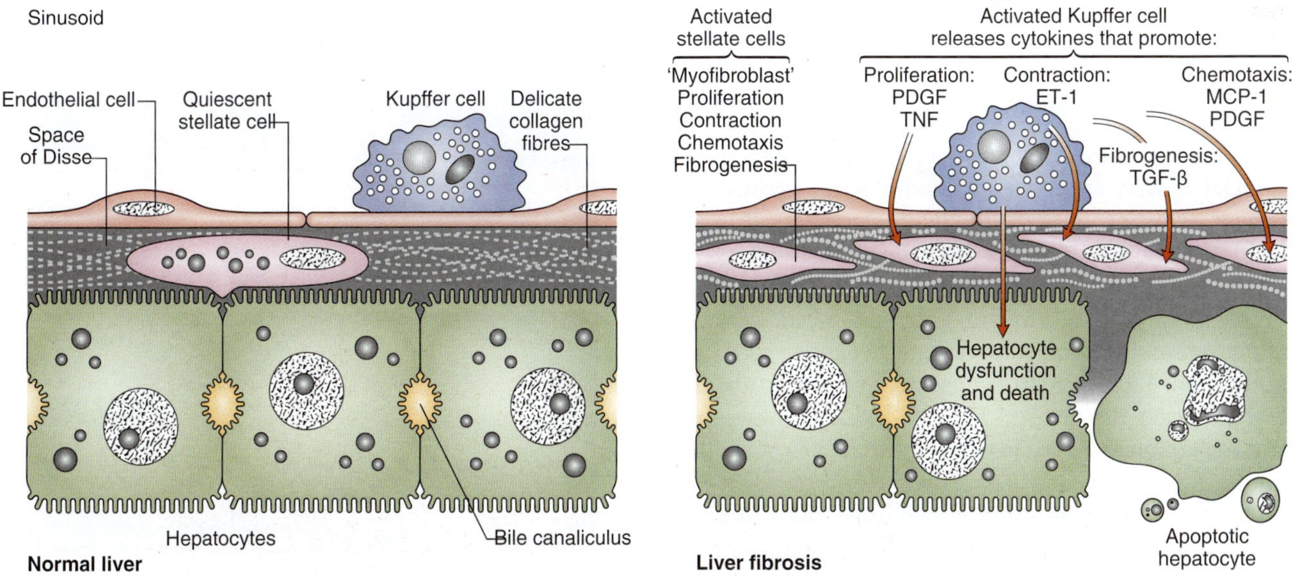

Fig. 22.9 On the left are the normal hepatocytes with quiescent stellate cells. In response to injury and inflammation, activated Kupffer cells, endothelial cells, hepatocytes and lymphocytes express cytokines that trigger the stellate cells into fibrogenesis. (*Source:* From James M. Crawford, Paulette Bioulac-Sage and Prodromos Hytiroglou. Structure, Function, and Responses to Injury. MacSween's Pathology of the Liver. 7th edition. Elsevier 2018.)

bridging fibrosis. Eventually, progressive hepatocyte loss and extensive fibrosis give rise to the condition of diffuse scarring, termed ***cirrhosis***.

Kupffer cells and macrophages release cytokines including TGF-β. These cytokines cause proliferation and activation of stellate cells, and also their chemotaxis to the site of injury. Fibrogenesis of the liver is stimulated, especially by TGF-β.

On the contrary, removal of stimuli, as in the reduction of viral load post-therapy or suppression of viral replication, can result in inactivation of stellate cells. Fibrolysis is attempted by the enzymes MMPs released by the hepatocytes causing partial absorption of the septae, resulting in incomplete septal cirrhosis. In the past, fibrosis was considered to be an obstinate process that would not reverse. Recent advances have brought out therapeutic measures that have achieved remission of relatively thin fibrous septa in patients with chronic hepatitis B virus (HBV)/hepatitis C virus (HCV) infection and autoimmune hepatitis. Future studies aim at antifibrotic therapies for other conditions like NASH and biliary disorders. Interestingly, although the fibrosis may regress, neovascularization imparts an irreversible architecture to the liver and may not regress.

LIVER FAILURE PA 25.2

Liver failure marks the most severe form of liver injury with a loss of 80%–90% of its functional capacity. Two forms of liver failure, acute liver failure and chronic liver failure, and a third form, acute-on-chronic liver failure, have being recently recognized. Acute liver failure is a result of sudden massive destruction of hepatocytes, whereas chronic liver failure is more insidious in onset. The prognosis is much worse for an acute liver failure.

ACUTE LIVER FAILURE

Acute liver failure is defined as an acute liver illness associated with encephalopathy and coagulopathy in a patient with no preexisting liver diseases, occurring within a period of 26 weeks since the onset of illness.

The two most common aetiological factors of acute liver injury include viral and drug-induced hepatitis. Other causes such as autoimmune hepatitis, neoplastic infiltration, Budd–Chiari syndrome, veno-occlusive diseases, Wilson disease and hypoxia-induced liver injury and malignancies have also been attributed to acute liver injury.

In the United States, more than 2000 cases of drug-induced acute liver failure are being reported annually, with more than 50% of cases caused by acetaminophen overdose. Although, theoretically, toxic ingestion of more than 150 mg/body weight can cause liver failure, recent reports suggest that even lower doses contribute to liver damage. Partly due to the easy over-the-counter availability of the drug, therapeutic misadventures are common with acetaminophen. In addition, intentional suicidal ingestion of the drug has been documented in 20% of reported cases. Fortunately, most patients with acetaminophen toxicity recover with early *N*-acetylcysteine therapy and supportive care.

Among viral infections, hepatitis A and hepatitis E are the prime causes of acute liver failure. Hepatitis B infection is another potential cause of acute liver failure, mostly in the Asian population. Other rare viral causes include cytomegalovirus, Epstein–Barr virus (EBV), parvovirus, adenovirus and HIV infections.

Morphology

Grossly, the liver is shrunken with loss of more than one-third of its weight. The morphological features of acute liver failure depend entirely on the severity and duration of the insult. Massive hepatic necrosis, referred to as fulminant hepatic necrosis in the past, is the most dreaded complication of acute liver failure (Fig. 22.10).

Microscopy reveals **extensive hepatocyte loss and collapse of the collagenous framework** at places. Debris, macrophages and variable inflammatory infiltrate can be seen in the portal regions and within the lobule. Consequences of acetaminophen overdoses are discussed in detail in the subsequent text. Although viral infections cause damage over months, morphologically, the liver shows evidence of regeneration, bile ductular reactions and scarring.

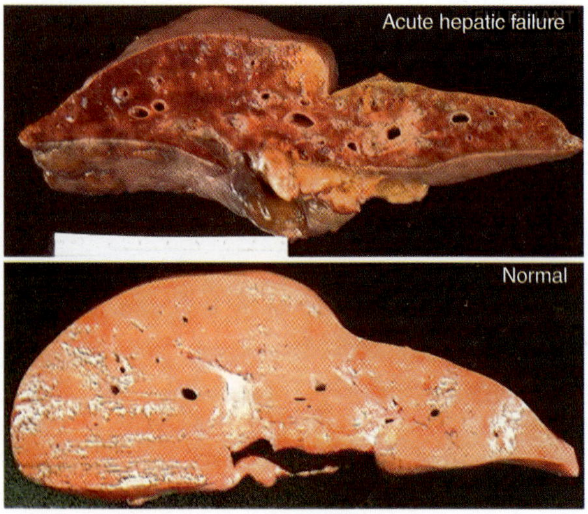

Fig. 22.10 In comparison with the normal liver, in conditions of acute hepatic failure, the liver macroscopically shows evidence of shrinkage, capsular wrinkling and areas of necrosis. (*Source:* From Brendan M. McGuire and Michael B. Fallon. Acute Liver Failure. Andreoli and Carpenter's Cecil Essentials of Medicine. 9th edition. Saunders 2016.)

Clinical Features

Manifestations of acute liver failure may range from simple constitutional symptoms as in nausea, vomiting, malaise and mild jaundice to life-threatening encephalopathy, severe hypotension or coagulation defects. High levels of serum transaminases in the blood can be noted during the initial phase due to liver enlargement, hepatocyte swelling and oedema. Over time, as the parenchyma is destroyed, the liver shrinks and transaminases drastically reduce. The clinical course typically follows that of multiple-organ failure. Some major manifestations of acute liver failure are briefly discussed as follows:

- ***Cholestasis:*** It can occur as a consequence of disturbed bile metabolism. Drug-induced cholestasis may be caused by direct injury to the bile duct or mitochondrial damage, as in acetaminophen toxicity. Retention of bile salts and bilirubin exposes the cells to the toxic effects of bile, further exacerbating the damage.
- ***Hepatic encephalopathy:*** It is a critical neurological manifestation of acute liver failure. Patients may present with mild drowsiness, disturbed consciousness, slow slurry speech along with increased severity, flapping tremors and deep coma. Prognosis is directly related to the grade of encephalopathy, thus warranting prompt diagnosis. The underlying pathogenesis of hepatic encephalopathy has been associated with elevated ammonia levels in acute hepatic failure. Normally, ammonia is excreted through the urea cycle that primarily takes place in the liver. In liver failure, an increased amount of ammonia in the circulating blood is capable of crossing the blood–brain barrier and causing profound effects on the brain cells. Exposure to ammonia causes an increased production of glutamine in the astrocytes. Glutamine being an osmolyte results in water influx and swelling, precipitating cerebral oedema and encephalopathy.
- ***Coagulopathy:*** As we already know, many clotting factors are produced by the liver. Thus, coagulation abnormality is an apparent sign of acute liver failure identified by increased prothrombin time and low levels of coagulation factors. In most patients, clinically significant spontaneous bleeding is uncommon; hence, correction by administration of fresh frozen plasma is not advocated because prothrombin time is an important prognostic marker similar to encephalopathy. Some patients may progress to present with disseminated intravascular coagulation.
- ***Portal hypertension:*** It is a more common manifestation of chronic liver failure (explained later). In acute liver failure, portal hypertension is mainly caused by the collapse of sinusoids, resulting in reduction of the intrahepatic vascular space. Ascites is the major clinical consequence of portal hypertension in liver failure.
- ***Hepatorenal syndrome:*** It is defined by the occurrence of acute renal failure in patients with acute liver failure with no history of renal dysfunction. Pathogenesis of hepatorenal syndrome is not completely understood but has been proposed to be initiated by portal hypertension–induced systemic vasodilation, resulting in hypovolaemia and diminished renal perfusion. However, renal dysfunction potentially reverses with improvement in hepatic function.

CHRONIC LIVER FAILURE AND CIRRHOSIS PA 25.4

Chronic liver failure is a resultant of a continuous process of inflammation, destruction, deterioration of liver function and regeneration of the liver parenchyma, progressing to the end stage, traditionally known as cirrhosis.

The most common cause of chronic hepatic failure worldwide is chronic viral hepatitis caused especially by hepatitis B or C infection. Similarly, autoimmune diseases, alcohol liver disease, genetic diseases and Budd–Chiari syndrome are included in the aetiological spectrum of chronic hepatic failure.

The term 'cirrhosis' was first defined by Laënnec in 1826. It is derived from the Greek word *scirrhous*, meaning tawny referring to the brown-yellow colour of the diseased liver at autopsy. Only about 100 years later, in 1930, the pathogenesis of the term was described as parenchymal destruction, regeneration and scarring. Since then, the term has been widely in use and has been accepted as a self-perpetuating irreversible process. ***Cryptogenic cirrhosis*** is the term applied to cirrhosis of uncertain aetiology.

Morphology

Grossly, the liver appears 'hob nailed', with **nodules** on the external surface as well as on the cut surface. The liver may be shrunken and is typically yellowish brown in colour, whereas other features depend on the underlying aetiology. Micronodular cirrhosis is the term used to define nodules less than 3 mm (Fig. 22.11). A classical example would be the end stage of alcohol-induced liver injury, referred to as Laënnec cirrhosis (explained later). In macronodular cirrhosis, the nodules are larger than 3 mm and are mostly a consequence of chronic viral hepatitis (Fig. 22.12).

Microscopically, cirrhosis is described as the **presence of fibrotic septa connecting portal tracts and the central vein or adjacent lobules**. These fibrous septa also dissect into the parenchyma, causing architectural distortion and encircle hepatocyte islands to form the characteristic nodules. The extent of fibrosis is often studied by the use of special stains that highlight collagen. A few nodules that may show features of regeneration are referred to as ***regenerative nodules*** and are not requisite for the diagnosis of cirrhosis. Finally, morphological features of regression that include the presence of thin incomplete scars and ductular reactions may be seen. Masson's trichrome stain is a special stain that is routinely used to demonstrate cirrhosis.

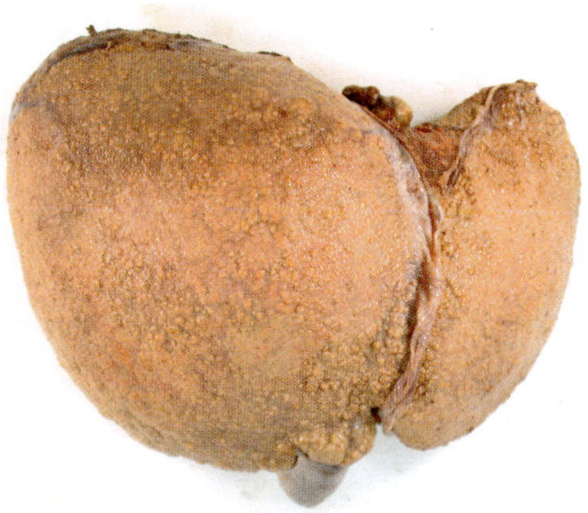

Fig. 22.11 Macroscopy of cirrhotic liver showing multiple tiny cirrhotic nodules (<3-mm diameter). (*Source:* From Judith I. Wyatt and Beate Haugk. Liver, biliary system and pancreas. Underwood's Pathology. Seventh Edition. Elsevier 2019.)

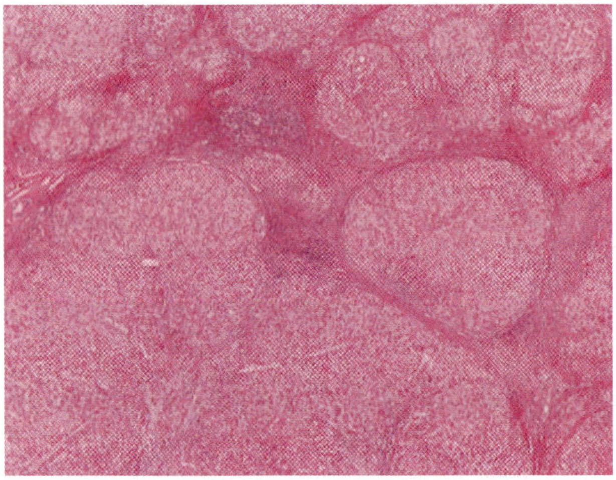

Fig. 22.12 Histopathological image showing mixed micronodular and macronodular cirrhosis in chronic hepatitis C infection. (*Source:* From Prodromos Hytiroglou. Hepatitis C. Practical Hepatic Pathology: A Diagnostic Approach. 2nd edition. Elsevier 2018.)

Clinical Features

Although a significant proportion of individuals with ongoing chronic liver failure present asymptomatically, some present with nonspecific symptoms such as anorexia, weight loss and fatigue. Apart from the jaundice, coagulopathy, encephalopathy and other symptoms related to hepatocyte dysfunction, as in acute hepatic failure, chronic liver failure causes impaired oestrogen metabolism leading to hyperoestrogenaemia and persistent cholestasis causing intense pruritus. Hyperoestrogenaemia-induced vasodilation produces spider angiomas of the skin characterized by a central pulsating arteriole with radiating small vessels. In males, the excess oestrogen can cause hypogonadism and gynaecomastia. Of note, 4%–12% of patients with cirrhosis, especially in the setting of portal hypertension, present with hepatopulmonary syndrome characterized by progressive insidious dyspnoea. Hypoxaemia is

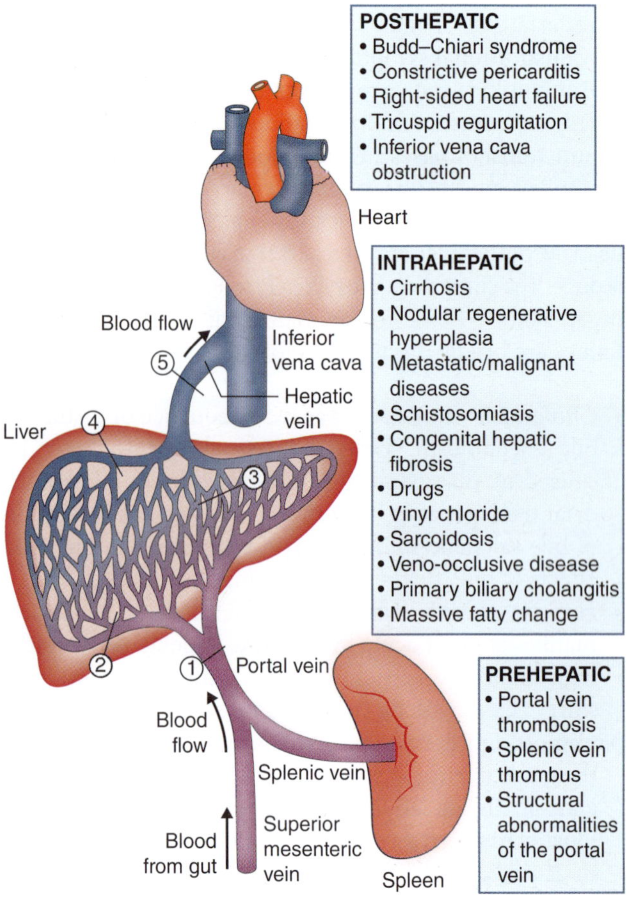

Fig. 22.13 Causes of portal hypertension.

probably caused by the right-to-left shunting of blood through the dilated vessels, causing ventilation–perfusion mismatch.

Three important dreaded complications that may develop in patients with chronic liver failure include portal hypertension, hepatocellular insufficiency and hepatocellular carcinoma (HCC).

Portal Hypertension **PA 25.5**

Portal hypertension is defined as a sustained increase in the portal venous pressure. The mechanisms causing portal hypertension revolve around the increase in vascular resistance due to obstruction of the portal circulation practically at any level. Hence, the causative factors can be conveniently categorized as prehepatic (due to narrowing of the portal vein or due to thrombosis of the portal vein), intrahepatic and posthepatic (due to heart failure, constrictive pericarditis and hepatic vein outflow tract obstruction [HVOTO]). The most common cause of portal hypertension is cirrhosis (intrahepatic) (Fig. 22.13).

The **pathophysiology** of portal hypertension (Flowchart 22.1) is multifactorial and complex. The logical explanations of the mechanisms underlying portal

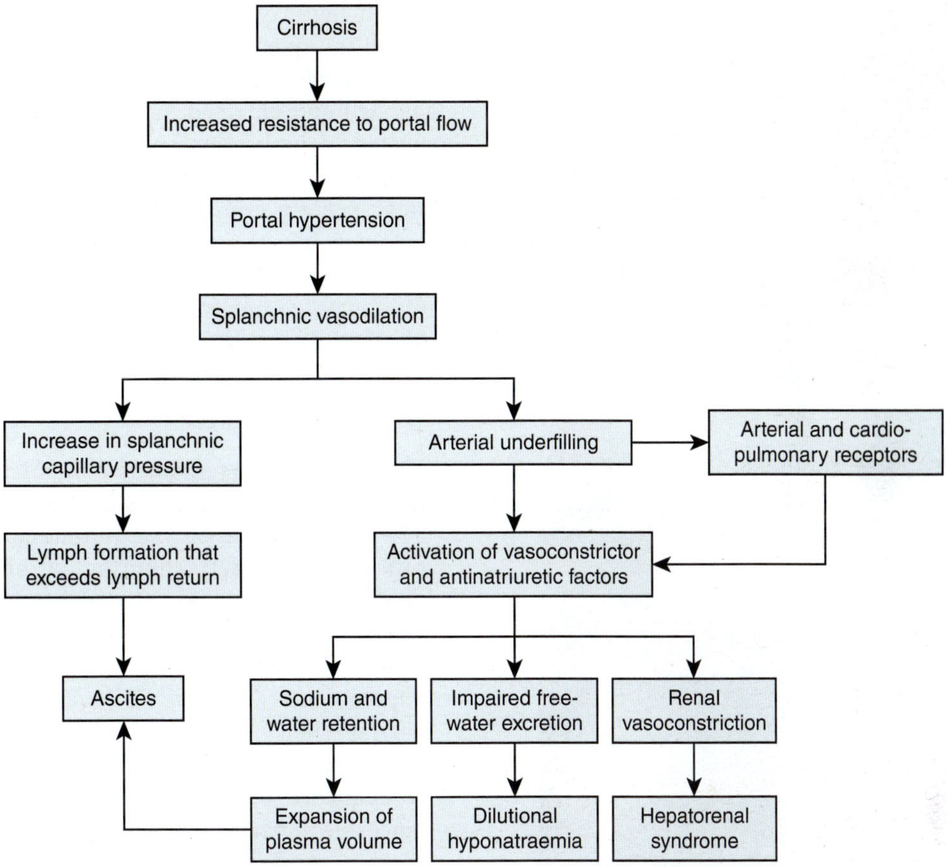

Flowchart 22.1 Pathophysiology of portal hypertension and ascites. (*Source:* From Tricia Brentjens, Paul David Weyker and Christopher A.J. Webb. Diseases of the Liver and Biliary Tract. Stoelting's Anesthesia and Co-Existing Disease. 7th edition. Elsevier 2018.)

hypertension could be in conditions such as cirrhosis, fibrotic nodules, trapping the small portal veins, obliterating them or causing external pressure in the process of parenchymal architectural distortion. The activated stellate cells in response to injury cause scarring of sinusoids. Further sinusoidal remodelling induces the release of vasoconstrictors like endothelin-1, and reduced availability of NO together contributes to narrowing of vessels. Increased resistance of blood flow through the portal circulation parallels arterial vasodilation, especially in the splanchnic circulation contributed by NO, VEGF and TNF. This worsens the condition by increasing the venous influx through the portal system. Progressively, mesenteric artery vasodilation augments system circulatory dysfunction, further reducing effective blood volume.

The major clinical manifestations of reduced effective blood volume due to portal hypertension include hepatic encephalopathy, ascites, portosystemic venous shunts and congestive splenomegaly.

Ascites (Flowchart 22.1) Ascites, excess accumulation of fluid in the peritoneal cavity, is a frequent manifestation of portal hypertension. In general, the fluid is serous with less protein content and scattered mesothelial cells and lymphocytes. In chronic cases, the fluid from the peritoneal cavity crosses the diaphragm through transdiaphragmatic lymphatics and may produce hydrothorax on the right side. The occurrence of ascites in cirrhosis and portal hypertension marks a poor prognosis. The pathogenesis of ascites can be attributed to the peripheral arterial vasodilation that reduces the cardiac output, eventually triggering the renin–angiotensin system. The resultant expansion of plasma volume paralleling with decreased albumin synthesis by the liver lowers the plasma oncotic pressure, forcing fluid accumulation within the peritoneal space causing ascites.

Portosystemic Shunts In portal hypertension, in an attempt to decompensate the pressure, the blood may be redirected through the portosystemic anastomoses (the anastomotic vessels between the systemic and the portal circulation). As these are thin vessels, when a large volume of blood passes through them for a prolonged period of time, the veins abnormally dilate and are thus referred to as varices. The most concerning among these are the oesophageal varices (Fig. 22.14), which may give rise to haematemesis and eventually result in death in 50% of patients. The major sites of these anastomoses include the rectum (manifesting as haemorrhoids), gastro-oesophageal junction (varices), the retroperitoneum and the abdominal wall (caput medusae – engorged vessels seen radiating from around the umbilicus) (Fig. 22.15).

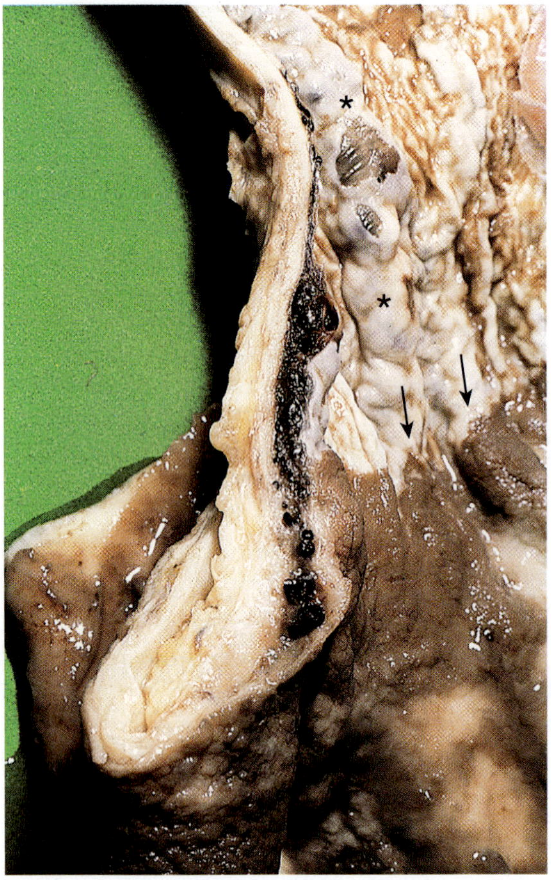

Fig. 22.14 Oesophageal varices – dilated, tortuous veins (marked with *) at the squamocolumnar junction (marked with an arrow) in a patient who died of cirrhosis. (*Source:* From Judith I. Wyatt and Beate Haugk. Liver, biliary system and pancreas. Underwood's Pathology. Seventh Edition. Elsevier 2019.)

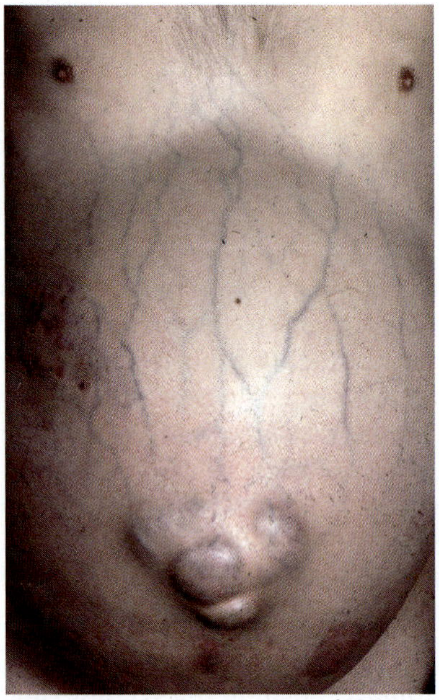

Fig. 22.15 Distended engorged paraumbilical veins in a patient with portal hypertension – caput medusae. (*Source:* From Ali W. Majeed and Ahmed Al-Mukhtar. Clinical investigation of hepatopancreatobiliary disease. Blumgart's Surgery of the Liver, Biliary Tract and Pancreas. 6th edition. Elsevier 2017.)

Splenomegaly Owing to the decreased blood flow through the splenic vein due to portal hypertension, the spleen unable to drain the blood within it becomes congested and enlarged. Congestive splenomegaly is an expected complication of portal hypertension. The spleen may enlarge to massive sizes as much as 1000 g. Pancytopenia is common among patients with massive splenomegaly.

Pulmonary Complications of Portal Hypertension Both cirrhosis and portal hypertension contribute to the development of pulmonary syndromes – portopulmonary hypertension and hepatopulmonary syndrome.

- Hepatopulmonary syndrome manifests in about 30% of patients with cirrhosis and portal hypertension. The vasodilation of the pulmonary capillary bed causes right-to-left shunting of blood, provoking ventilation–perfusion mismatch and eventually hypoxaemia. Patients suffer from dyspnoea and shortness of breath, especially in the upright position. Supplemental oxygen in such patients provides partial relief.
- Portopulmonary hypertension is hypothesized to be a consequence of increased pulmonary vascular resistance due to portal hypertension. The exact pathophysiological mechanism underlying this condition is yet to be properly understood. Unfortunately, in most patients, portopulmonary hypertension does not reverse even after liver transplantation.

ACUTE-ON-CHRONIC HEPATIC FAILURE

Acute-on-chronic liver failure refers to a condition in which a subgroup of stable cirrhotic patients suddenly develop organ failure, with more than 50% of cases labelled as having no identifiable precipitating event. Most relatable, patients with chronic hepatitis B infection superimposed with hepatitis D infection may experience an acute exacerbation. In the Western population, acute alcohol injury and bacterial infection prove to be common precipitating factors. In recent times, acute-on-chronic liver failure has drawn attention due to the significant morbidity and mortality it has caused. Treatment is directed towards the control of the precipitating factor, and the outlook in most patients is guarded.

HEPATITIS PA 25.3

Hepatitis refers to an inflammatory condition of the liver. Although the most common aetiology would be viral infection causing viral hepatitis, other conditions such as autoimmune hepatitis, drug-induced hepatitis and alcoholic hepatitis are well established.

INFECTIOUS HEPATITIS

Infectious hepatitis is by default thought to be caused by viruses, importantly by five heterotrophic viruses. The next discussion elaborates the illness commonly referred to as viral hepatitis.

Viral Hepatitis

Viral hepatitis is the term used to describe inflammation of the liver caused by viral infection. Worldwide, more than 32 million people are affected by viral hepatitis and are at a high risk of hepatic failure. Although many virus and infectious agents can be attributed to causing viral hepatitis, the term 'viral hepatitis' prioritizes the hepatotropic viruses A, B, C, D and E. The next segment discusses the pathological features unique to each type of virus responsible for infection.

Hepatitis A Virus Hepatitis A viral (HAV) particle was first demonstrated by Feiinstone et al. in the early 1970s. HAV infection is usually self-limited with no carrier state and is responsible for at least 20%–25% of clinical viral hepatitis cases in the developing countries.

Epidemiology HAV infection is highly contagious and spreads by the faeco-oral route and by ingestion of contaminated food and water. Shellfish-borne outbreaks of HAV infection due to consumption of undercooked or raw shellfish, oysters and clams are well known because they concentrate the virus from the seawater polluted with human sewage. Conditions that contribute to the propagation of infection among young children include crowded households and poor sanitization. However, with the advent of vaccination, hepatitis A infection has entered a declining phase.

Pathogenesis HAV is a small, nonenveloped, single-stranded, RNA-containing virus, approximately 27 nm in diameter, belonging to the family of picornavirus. On entry into the liver, the virus replicates within the hepatocytes and can also be demonstrated within the Kupffer cells. HAV is not directly cytopathic to the hepatocyte but triggers the host's immune response, the HAV-specific $CD8^{+}$ T lymphocytes and NK cells, causing destruction of the infected cells.

Clinical Features The incubation period of HAV ranges from 2 to 6 weeks. The prodromal phase is characterized by nonspecific symptoms such as fatigue and weight loss, whereas jaundice develops later. The virus is shed in the blood, bile and stools in the preicteric incubation period and declines after the onset of jaundice. IgM anti-HAV antibody appears in the serum with the initiation of symptoms and persists for 3–6 months. In the recovery phase of acute infection, IgG anti-HAV appears, offering lifelong immunity against HAV infection. The disease usually takes a benign clinical course, with complete recovery in most patients, and rarely may give rise to chronic cholestasis.

Hepatitis B Virus HBV is one of the most common infectious agents and is estimated that more than 350 million people are infected with hepatitis B worldwide. Clinical outcomes of the infection depend greatly on the patient's age, comorbid conditions and immune response. HBV-induced cirrhosis is considered to be the leading cause of liver transplant in China.

Epidemiology The high-prevalent regions of HBV infection include the Western Pacific Rim and Southeast Asia. The high carrier states in these endemic areas are sustained by vertical transmission from the mother to her child. Unlike HAV that spreads through the faeco-oral route, HBV does not spread through food or water. The virus is present in the blood, saliva and semen and spreads majorly by unprotected sex, contaminated needles and syringes and blood transfusion. Hence, routine screening for viral particles has been implemented vigorously before transfusion of blood products, virtually eliminating post-transfusion HBV infection.

With the advent of vaccination against HBV, much of the epidemiology is changing, with a significant decline in the prevalence, especially in the endemic regions.

Pathogenesis HBV is a hepatotropic DNA virus belonging to the Hepadnaviridae family. The virus particle (infectious virion), 'Dane particle' (Fig. 22.16), measures 42 nm and is a double-shelled structure consisting of an outer lipid envelope containing the hepatitis B surface antigen (HBsAg) and an inner nucleocapsid containing the hepatitis B core antigen (HBcAg) that surrounds the viral genome and the enzyme polymerase. The viral genome is composed of circular, partially double-stranded DNA with several open-reading frames, encoding the following proteins:

- ***HBsAg:*** These antigens were referred to as Australian antigens in the past after they were first discovered in Australia in the 1960s. The S gene codes for HBsAg, which is produced independently of the viral core. Although these antigens are secreted in large quantities into circulation, they are immunogenic but not infectious.
- ***HBcAg:*** The nucleocapsid core contains the core antigen (HBcAg) and another E antigen (HBeAg), both products of the C gene. The C gene also includes a

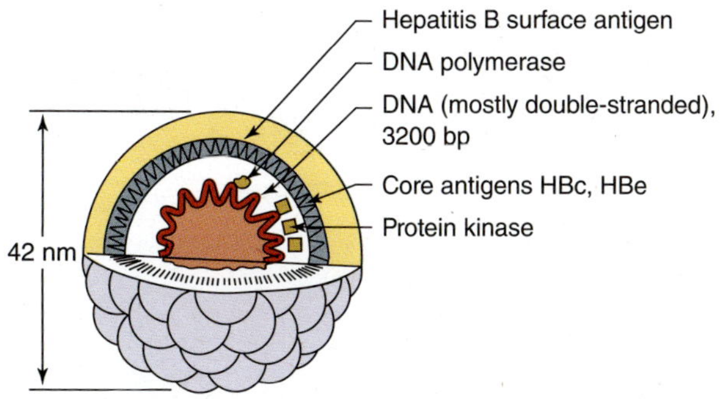

Fig. 22.16 HBV – Dane particle. (*Source:* From Hepatitis B. Elsevier Point of Care. 2021.)

precore and core regions. Although the core region of the C gene gives rise to the C antigen, translation of the entire C gene is required for the development of the E antigen. The important function of the C antigen is assembly of the complete virion.

- ***HBV polymerase:*** The P gene codes for the enzyme that carries out both DNA polymerase and reverse transcriptase activities.
- ***Hepatitis B X protein (HBx)***: The HBx antigen functions by activation of viral transcription and has been linked to the development of HCC in chronic HBV infection.

The virus attaches itself to the hepatocyte by binding of HBsAg to the bile salt transporter, sodium taurocholate cotransporting polypeptide (NTCP). The virus then uncoats and the viral DNA gains entry in the hepatocyte nucleus, following which viral replication takes place. The viral DNA is converted into a covalently closed circular DNA (cccDNA), which serves as a template for transcription of viral mRNA. Following translation, the nucleocapsid enveloping process takes place within the endoplasmic reticulum. The complete viral protein in then released into circulation. Some of the nucleocapsids are recycled to the nucleus to continue the cycle. The persistence of cccDNA makes it difficult for the clearance of viral particles even with intense antiviral therapy (Fig. 22.17).

HBV is not directly cytopathic, because it exists in a carrier state in which the individual is asymptomatic despite the viral load. CD8$^+$ T lymphocytes recognize the target viral antigens expressed by infected hepatocytes and the resulting immune attack is responsible for the destruction of hepatocytes as well as the clearance of the virion particles. Remarkably, the cytotoxic T lymphocytes also de-energize the virus replicative intermediates, preventing the spread of infection. In 90% of immunocompetent individuals, HBV infection resolves after an acute phase. A minority progress to chronic hepatitis probably due to the immune tolerance developed by the cytotoxic lymphocytes or the viral particles undergoing constant mutations that escape the immune surveillance.

Clinical Features (Flowchart 22.2) HBV has a prolonged incubation period of about 6 weeks to 6 months. Presenting

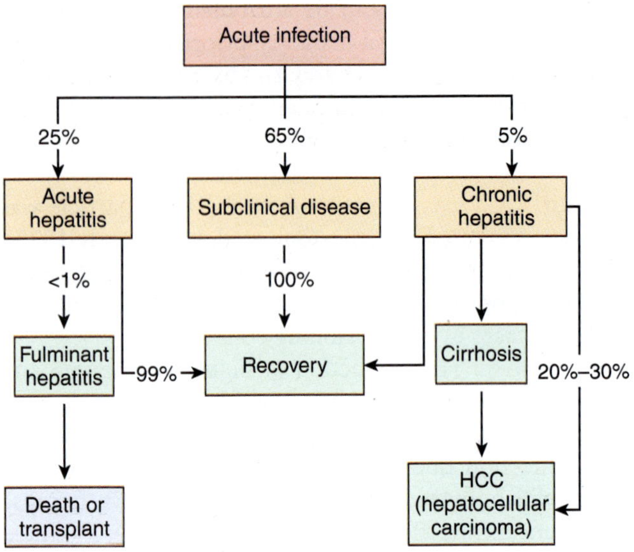

Flowchart 22.2 Clinical consequences of HBV infection. (*Source:* From Ryan M. Gill and Sanjay Kakar. Liver and Gallbladder. Robbins & Cotran Pathologic Basis of Disease. 10th edition. Elsevier 2021.)

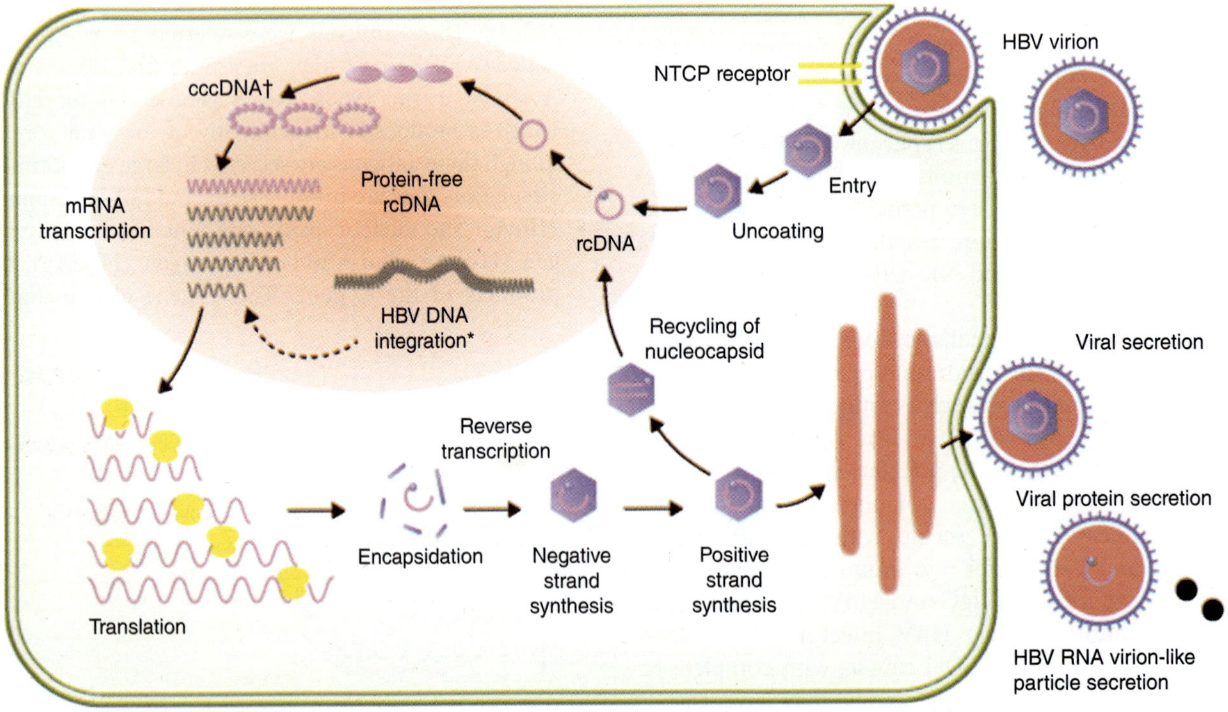

Fig. 22.17 Lifecycle of HBV. (*Source:* From Hepatitis B. Elsevier Point of Care. 2021.)

symptoms are similar to those of HAV infection but may be more severe. Serological tests and antigens levels in the blood are important determinants of the clinical course. The following are the immunological markers studied in HBV infection (Fig. 22.18):

- **HBsAg:** HBsAg is the first marker to appear in the blood in about 6 weeks postexposure and is an indicator of active ongoing infection. The levels gradually decline in 3–6 months during the recovery phase. However, persistent levels of HBsAg in the blood imply a carrier state.
- **Anti-HBs antibody:** Simultaneously or shortly after the disappearance of HBsAg, anti-HBs begins to rise, implying complete recovery and also offering a lifelong immunity. These antibodies may be of both IgM and IgG types. Patients who progress to chronic liver disease show an impaired production of anti-HBs antibodies.
- **HBeAg:** It can be detected in the serum for a transient period during acute illness. Anti-HBe replaces HBeAg soon after its disappearance. The seroconversion of HBeAg to anti-HBe is carefully monitored because it indicates waning of acute infection. Persistence of HBeAg beyond 10 weeks is indicative of the development of chronic disease or a carrier state.
- **HBcAg:** The core antigen is not seen in the blood of infected patients. Anti-HBc can however be detected and is a marker of prior HBV infection.
- **HBV DNA:** Detection by molecular hybridization is the most sensitive indictor of HBV infection.

As already mentioned, most patients experience an acute infection with complete resolution. The risk of progression

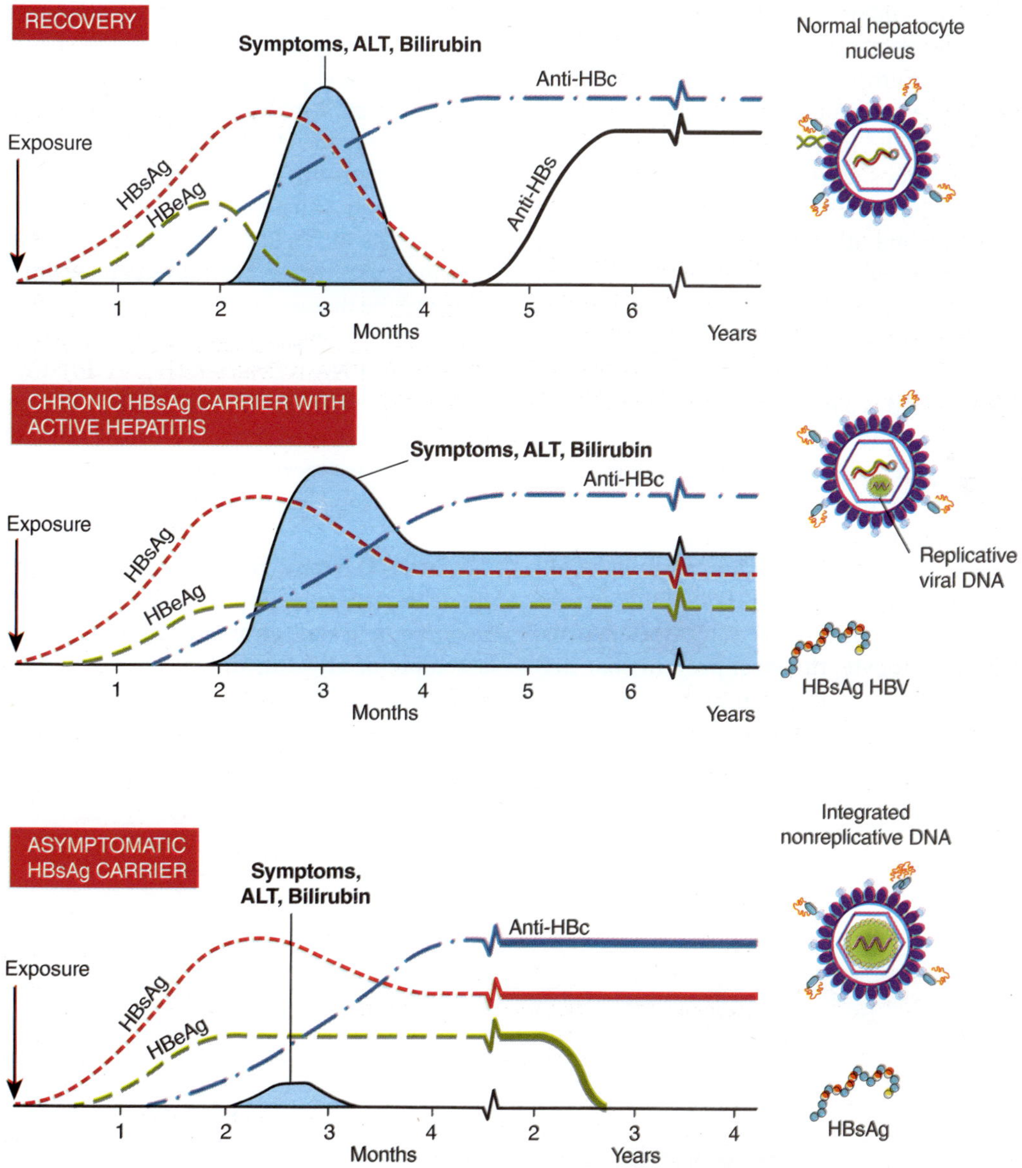

Fig. 22.18 Serological markers in events of HBV infection.

to chronicity depends greatly on the age of the patient and the duration of illness. About 5% of HBV-infected individuals develop chronic infection, of whom 20%–30% are capable of progressing to cirrhosis or carcinoma. In total, 90% of infants who acquire the disease through perinatal transmission move into a phase of chronic hepatitis and dreadfully HCC. In such patients, treatment with antiviral drugs and reverse transcriptase inhibitors can only slow down the process but not eliminate it.

Hepatitis C Virus HCV infection is one of the most common causes of chronic liver failure. Owing to its high risk of progression into cirrhosis, end-stage liver disease and HCC, HCV infection represents a formidable public heath challenge worldwide.

Epidemiology According to the World Health Organization (WHO), the estimated global prevalence of HCV infection is 2.2% of the general population. The geographic distribution of HCV infection indicates that the infection has been an endemic in many populations for centuries. A high seroprevalence is observed in North America and Western Europe; Egypt is rated as having the highest seroprevalence, with a reported rate of 22%.

Parenteral spread is the most effective means of viral transmission. Intravenous drug abuse, multiple sexual partners, needlestick injury with contaminated blood and perinatal transmission are other less efficient risk factors. Screening of donated blood for HCV antibodies has caused a drastic downfall in the incidence of new cases, especially in the United States.

Pathophysiology HCV is a small, enveloped, single-stranded RNA virus and is a member of the Flaviviridae family. The genome of HCV encodes many functional proteins, which include two envelope proteins (E1 and E2) and five core proteins (p7, NS2, NS3, NS5A and NS5B). The lifecycle of HCV begins with the binding of HCV to receptors, such as low-density lipoprotein receptor, on the hepatocyte surface. Following attachment, the particles are internalized by endocytosis. Once within the hepatocyte, the viral protein coat dissolves and the viral RNA is released into the cytoplasm. The viral RNA takes over the liver cell machinery, directing it to produce viral proteins. Many copies of HCV RNA are produced with the help of the polymerase enzyme within the membranous web of the endoplasmic reticulum. HCV core protein interaction with LDs is believed to be essential for the recruitment of other viral components involved in viral assembly. Finally, the viral proteins are assembled to form a complete virion particle. The immature virus buds migrate to the cell surface and are eventually released into the circulation.

In the recent years, the treatment of hepatitis C has been directed towards developing specific drug antagonists against the viral proteins. Direct-acting antivirals (DAAs) are recommended for therapy by WHO for patients with chronic HCV infection. DAA medications are by mechanisms NS3 protease inhibitors and NS5A and NS5B polymerase inhibitors.

Clinical Features (Flowchart 22.3) The incubation period for HCV is similar to that of HBV (6 weeks to 6 months). Within the first 1–2 weeks of infection, HCV RNA can be detected in the blood. Weeks later, anti-HCV antibodies begin to appear in the serum and persist through the chronic phase.

The clinical symptoms of HCV hepatitis are usually mild or asymptomatic. Complete recovery of the acute liver disease occurs in a very few infected individuals. Most patients enter a phase of chronic hepatitis, of which cirrhosis develops in 2%–24% of patients in about 10–30 years. Serum transaminases typically fluctuate during the chronic phase of the disease. Some patients may even show normal transaminase levels; thus, therapy needs to be initiated once HCV RNA is detected (Fig. 22.19). Comorbid conditions, older age group and alcohol use are risk factors involved in accelerating the progression of the disease. According to a recent survey, about 4% of patients with cirrhosis develop HCC every year.

Hepatitis D Virus Hepatitis D virus (HDV), also known as delta virus, is composed of a negative-stranded RNA genome and an envelope consisting of HBsAg. The assembly of HDV in the liver requires HBsAg, so HDV infection almost always occurs either simultaneously with HBV infection (coinfection) or follows HBV infection

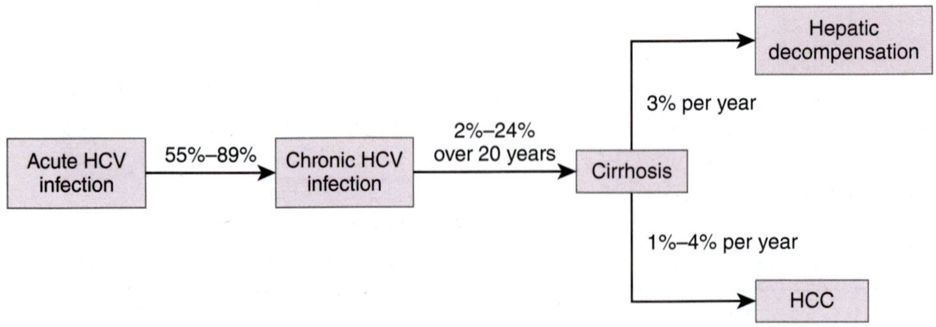

Flowchart 22.3 Clinical outcomes of HCV infection. (*Source:* From Jacinta A. Holmes and Raymond T. Chung. Hepatitis C. Sleisenger and Fordtran's Gastrointestinal and Liver Disease. 11th edition. Elsevier 2021.)

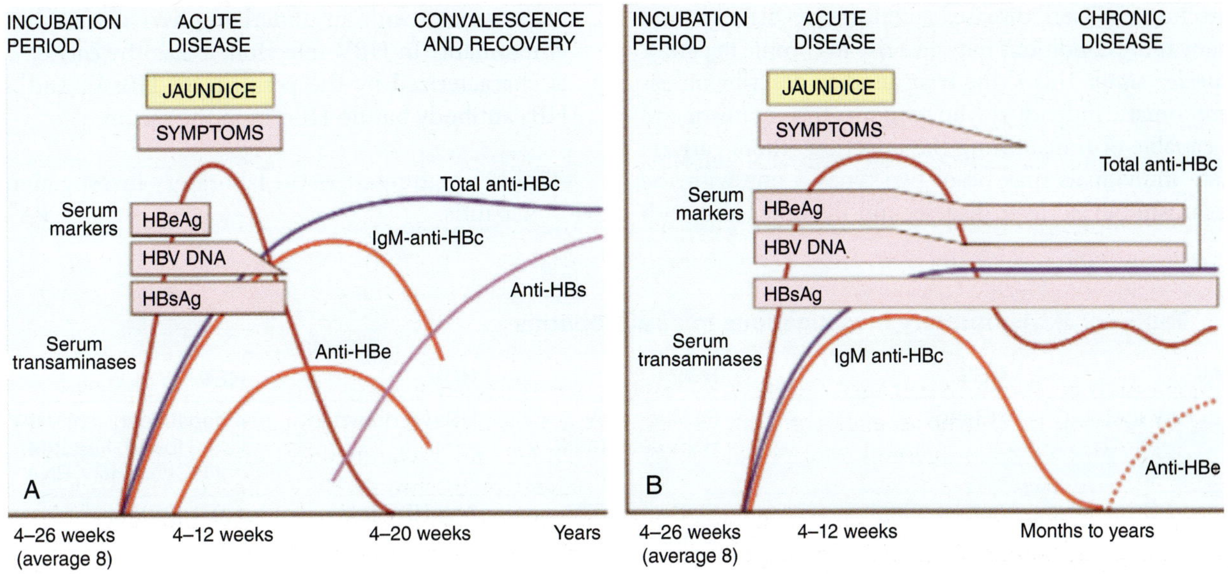

Fig. 22.19 Serological markers in acute and chronic HCV infections (*Source:* From Hepatitis B. Elsevier Point of Care. 2021.)

(superinfection). It is estimated that about 5% of individuals with HBV infection have coinfection with HDV. The disease transmission is similar to that of HBV and follows the parenteral route. HDV infection, especially in HBV carriers, typically increases the severity of disease and also the risk of progression to cirrhosis and HCC.

Hepatitis E Virus Like HAV, hepatitis E virus (HEV) is an acute, self-limited pathological agent. HEV-induced hepatitis accounts for at least half of the cases of acute viral hepatitis in young patients. Though self-limited, HEV infection in pregnancy is associated with high mortality.

Epidemiology Large epidemics of HEV outbreaks have been reported in India, Nepal and Mexico, mostly due to contamination of water supplies following heavy rains. HEV is also a potential zoonotic pathogen and can be transmitted via undercooked animal meat in developed countries. Parenteral and vertical transmission of the disease has also been recorded.

Pathogenesis HEV is an unenveloped, icosahedral, positive-stranded RNA virus, belonging to the Herpesviridae family. It does not cause direct cytopathic effects in the hepatocytes; the disease process rather stems from the host immune response.

Clinical Features The incubation period of HEV is about 4-5 weeks. Complete resolution of infection is possible within 2–4 weeks after the onset of illness. HEV particles are shed in the stool even before the evidence of clinical illness. During the illness phase, serum transaminases rise in the blood accompanied by elevated IgM anti-HEV. In the recovery phase, IgG anti-HEV antibodies can be detected.

In immunocompetent individuals, chronic disease and carrier states are almost obsolete. In immunocompromised patients, especially in those with HIV infection, chronic hepatitis is discernible.

Clinicopathological Syndromes of Viral Hepatitis

As we already know, both HAV and HEV infections are characterized by a self-limiting course and are not complicated by significant clinical sequelae. Thus, much focus is hurled over HBV and HCV pathogenesis and their disease processes, especially because HCV is modest in causing cirrhosis and HCC. The disease courses of viral hepatitis can be categorized as follows:

- ***Acute asymptomatic infection with recovery:*** These cases are incidentally detected, with the only evidence of ongoing infection being mildly elevated serum transaminases. With recovery, antiviral antibodies can be detected in the serum. This type of clinical course is most common with HAV and HBV infections that manifest as a subclinical disease.
- ***Acute symptomatic hepatitis*** **(acute viral hepatitis):** The most common manifestation of hepatotropic viruses includes acute hepatitis. The course of infection can be clinically classified into three phases. In the prodrome phase patients develop symptoms such as vomiting, headache, myalgia and photophobia. Some patients curiously present with altered olfaction and taste, particularly to coffee and cigarettes. This is followed by the icteric phase, which is characterized by jaundice and ecchymoses (due to reduced vitamin K levels). The final phase is the convalescence phase.
- ***Acute liver failure with massive to submissive hepatic necrosis:*** Globally, HAV and HEV are the most common causes of viral hepatitis causing acute liver failure.
- ***Chronic hepatitis:*** It is defined as symptomatic, biochemical or serological evidence of continuing or relapsing hepatic disease for more than 6 months. Apart from HBV and HCV infection, combined HBV and HDV

infection, Wilson disease, autoimmune diseases and many more conditions may give rise to chronic hepatitis.

- ***Carrier state:*** This is the term used to describe an asymptomatic individual who harbours the organism and is capable of transmitting the infection. These carrier-state individuals may be of two types – one with the organism but no liver disease, and the other also with the organism with an underlying liver disease but asymptomatic. In HBV infection, a 'healthy carrier state' is characterized by the presence of HBsAg and anti-HBs antibody but no HBeAg in the serum.

Table 22.2 summarizes the laboratory investigations in viral hepatitis. PA 25.6

Table 22.2 Laboratory Investigations in Viral Hepatitis

HAV	HBV	HCV	HDV	HEV
Anti HAV IgM +	HBsAg+	PCR for HCV RNA detected	HBsAg detected	if negative for anti-HAV igM, HbsAg, HBcIgM, antiHCV or HCV RNA
Blood PCR postive	Anti HBc IgM +;	ELISA for HCV anitbodies+	Anti HDV IgM+	Anti HEV IgM+
Acute HAV infection	PCR for HBV DNA+	Acute HCV infection	PCR for HDV RNA+	PCR for HEV RNA+
Anti-HAV IgG+	Acute HBV or flare up of chronic HBV	Anti HCV -; PCR negative	Acute HDV infection	Acute hepatitis E
Past infection (recovered)	Anti HBc IgG+; HBsAg+; HBeAg +; HBV DNA +/-	Chronic infection	Anti HDV IgG+	
	Chronic infection		Blood PCR negative	
	Anti HBc IgG+; HBsAg+; HBVDNA +/-; no symptoms/no deranged LFTs		Chronic infection	
	Chronic carrier state			

Morphology

The morphological spectrum of acute and chronic viral hepatitis has many features similar to those of autoimmune hepatitis, drug-induced hepatitis and Wilson disease (Fig. 22.20). Thus, it is of critical importance to evaluate the clinical history carefully.

Morphologically, the hallmark feature of acute viral hepatitis is the presence of **dead hepatocytes**. Grossly, the liver may appear shrunken, especially when associated with acute liver failure. Microscopically, widespread ballooning of hepatocytes with acidophilic bodies and focal spotty necrosis can be seen as in other causes of acute hepatitis. Mononuclear cells, mostly lymphocytes with variable plasma cells and eosinophils, would be seen infiltrating the portal region and constituting lobular inflammation. Areas of necrosis are often accompanied by scavenging macrophages to clear the cellular debris. Necrosis of hepatocytes may range from focal or confluent to panlobular or panacinar necrosis. Massive hepatic necrosis is a characteristic of liver failure.

Chronic viral hepatitis is defined by dense portal lymphocytic or lymphoplasmacytic inflammation and definitive fibrosis (Fig. 22.21). Often, the inflammatory cells can be seen breaching the limiting plate, causing interphase hepatitis and lobular hepatitis. As the severity increases, confluent necrosis may form bands of bridging necrosis connecting adjacent portal tracts. Progressive loss of periportal hepatocytes due to piecemeal necrosis results in deposition of collagen-causing fibrosis, progressing to periportal fibrosis and subsequently cirrhosis (Fig. 22.22). Features of bile ductular proliferation may be apparent in the portal region. In cases of HCV infection, lymphocyte aggregates or follicles are often present.

In HBV infection, the hepatocytes characteristically show '**ground glass appearance**' due to the accumulation of HBsAg within the cytoplasm (Fig. 22.23). HBsAg can be further demonstrated by immunostains to confirm the diagnosis. In HCV infection, focal steatosis in addition to focal bile duct injury can be a clue to diagnosis.

Although serological markers prompt the diagnosis of viral hepatitis, liver biopsy is preferred to assess the stage of fibrosis and the grade of inflammatory activity to plan treatment protocols.

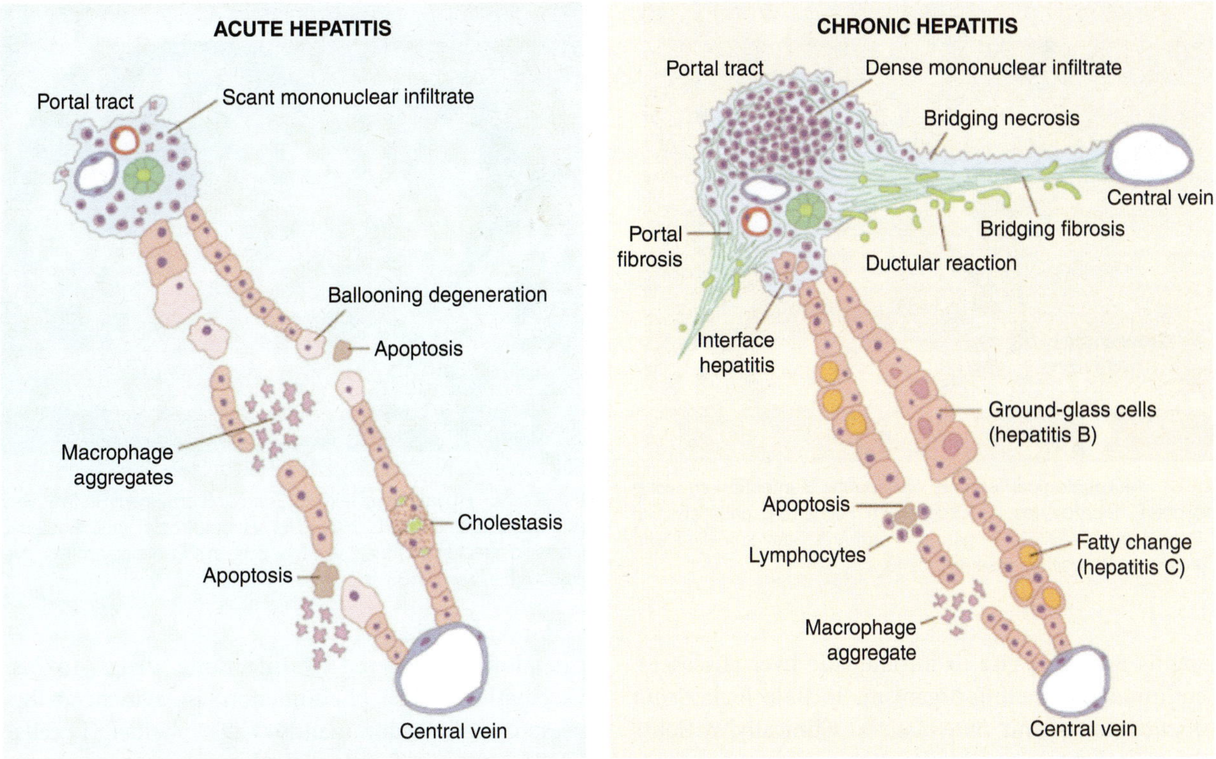

Fig. 22.20 Schematic representation of acute and chronic changes in viral hepatitis. (*Source:* From Vinay Kumar, Abul K. Abbas and Jon C. Aster. Liver and Gallbladder. Robbins Basic Pathology. 10th edition. Elsevier 2018.)

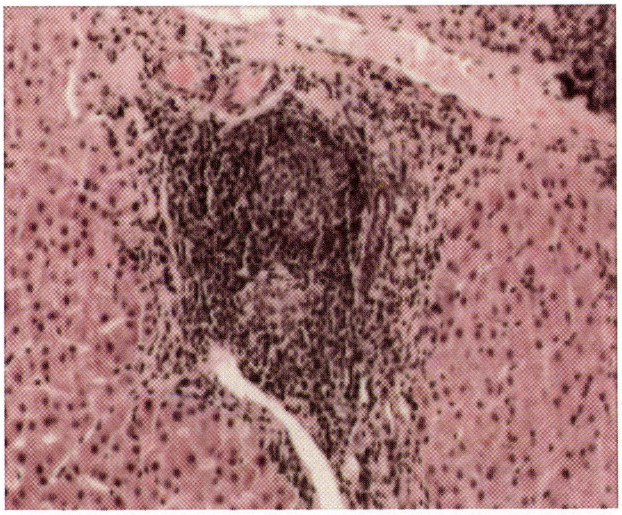

Fig. 22.21 Lymphoid follicle within the portal tract seen in a case of chronic HCV infection. Though not specific for HCV infection, findings of such complete follicles raise a high suspicion for HCV infection. (*Source:* From Neil D. Theise, Henry Charles Bodenheimer and Maria Guido. Viral Hepatitis. MacSween's Pathology of the Liver. 7th edition. Elsevier 2018.)

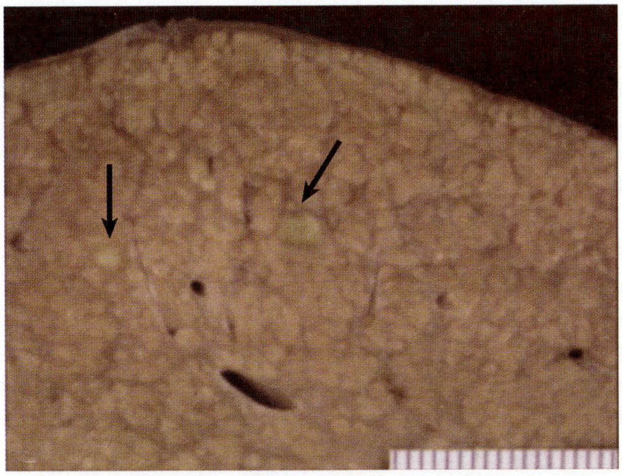

Fig. 22.22 Gross image of the liver showing micronodular cirrhosis caused by HCV infection. Note two nodules (arrows), which show microscopic evidence of hepatocellular carcinoma. (*Source:* From Neil D. Theise, Henry Charles Bodenheimer and Maria Guido. Viral Hepatitis. MacSween's Pathology of the Liver. 7th edition. Elsevier 2018.)

Nonviral Hepatitis

Other Infections and Infestations Apart from viral infection, the liver is also vulnerable to bacterial, parasitic and fungal infections. This could be a part of systemic or localized infection to the liver. Systemic infections can cause liver injury by direct invasion or indirectly through toxins and cytokines released by the organism. Typical examples include *Salmonella typhi* in typhoidal fever or *Staphylococcus aureus* in toxic shock syndrome.

Pyogenic cholangitis: Biliary obstruction causing cholestasis is profoundly linked to inviting bacterial infection and causing cholangitis. In serve infection, ascending

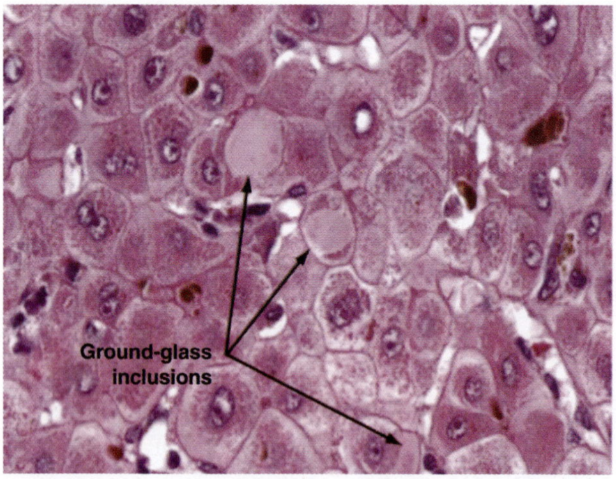

Fig. 22.23 Morphological features of hepatitis B infection showing ground-glass hepatocytes. (*Source:* From Harry L.A. Janssen and Scott Fung. Hepatitis B. Sleisenger and Fordtran's Gastrointestinal and Liver Disease. 11th edition. Elsevier 2021.)

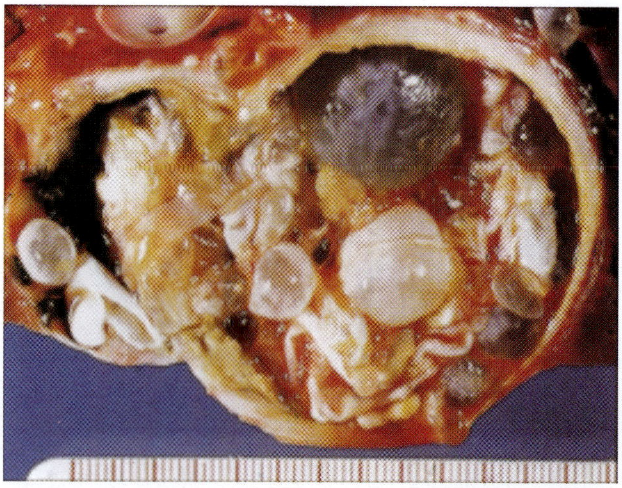

Fig. 22.24 Hydatid cyst – liver. (*Source:* From Sherif R. Zaki, Venancio A.F. Alves and Gillian L. Hale. Non-Hepatotropic Viral, Bacterial, and Parasitic Infections of the Liver. MacSween's Pathology of the Liver. 7th edition. Elsevier 2018.)

cholangitis may give rise to intrahepatic liver abscesses. The commonest infecting organisms include *Escherichia coli*, *Pseudomonas* and *Enterobacter*. Clinically, patients present with right upper-quadrant pain and fever, sometimes with hepatomegaly and jaundice. Ultrasonography (USG)–guided drainage of abscesses and appropriate antibiotic therapy are beneficial in most patients. In the setting of septicaemia, the liver typically shows features of bile ductular reaction along with cholestasis.

The liver is also frequently involved in disseminated infections such as amoebic liver abscess and hepatic tuberculosis. Histologically, typical granulomas may be present but the yield of acid-fast bacillus is generally low.

Parasitic infections of the liver are common only in highly endemic areas; thus, travel history needs to be carefully evaluated in such patients. *Entamoeba histolytica* infection, schistosomiasis and *Echinococcus* infection (Fig. 22.24) are some of the dominant parasitic infections of the liver. Liver fluke infections are common, especially in Southeast Asia, and serve as a potential risk factor in the development of cholangiocarcinoma (CCA).

AUTOIMMUNE HEPATITIS

Autoimmune hepatitis is a chronic inflammatory condition of the liver characterized by elevated levels of circulating autoantibodies and serum immunoglobulins.

Aetiopathogenesis

More than 70% of autoimmune hepatitis cases occur in women. The aetiopathogenesis underlying autoimmune hepatitis remains obscure. The current proposed theory suggests a failure of immune tolerance in genetically susceptible individuals. The resultant T-cell-mediated inflammation can also be triggered by infections, drugs, toxins and vaccination. This phenomenon is evidenced by the presence of predominantly $CD4^+$ helper T cells and $CD8^+$ cytotoxic T cells at the interphase.

Morphology

Histologically, autoimmune hepatitis has features similar to those of acute and chronic hepatitis. Characteristically, the inflammatory infiltrate is rich in **plasma cells** and may appear as clusters typically at the interphase (Fig. 22.25). Emperipolesis is another important feature that can be observed. Apparent necrosis of hepatocytes, depending on the severity of the illness, may present as confluent, panacinar or bridging necrosis. Interestingly, rosettes (Fig. 22.26), referring to clusters of hepatocytes surrounding dilated biliary canaliculi, can be appreciated.

Clinical Features Most patients present with nonspecific symptoms of fatigue, mild right upper-quadrant discomfort and anorexia. Very few patients may present with acute liver failure. Severe forms may present with hepatomegaly and jaundice.

Most of the histological features are less sensitive to rely on to make a diagnosis. Thus, the International Autoimmune Hepatitis Group has proposed simplified diagnostic criteria according to which patients can be classified as 'probable' or 'definite' (Table 22.3).

Two types of autoimmune hepatitis have been recognized on the basis of the autoantibodies in the serum. Table 22.4 compares the key features of type 1 and type 2 autoimmune hepatitis.

The severity and outcome of autoimmune hepatitis do not correlate with the levels of autoantibodies because of

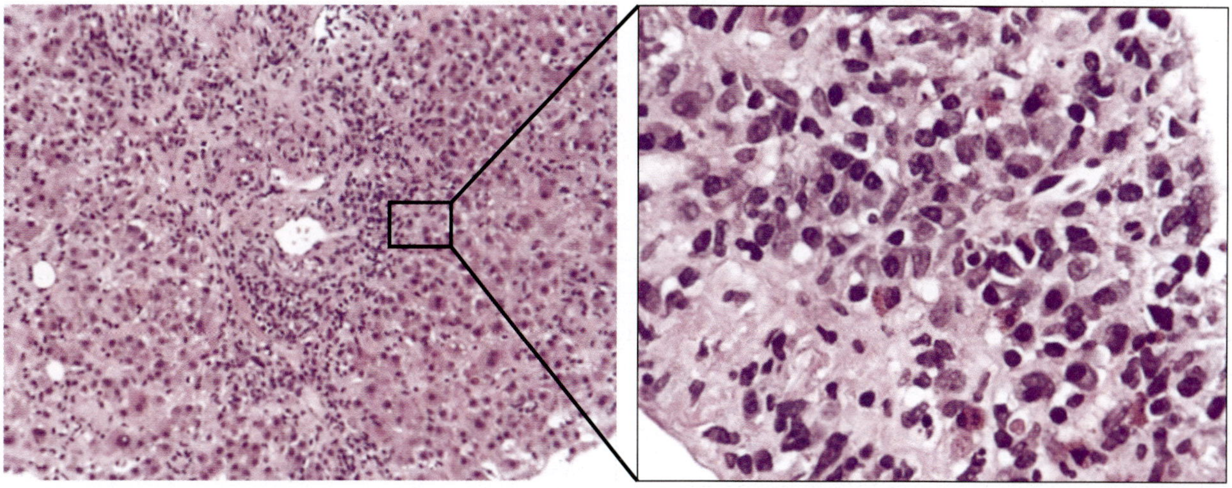

Fig. 22.25 Portal tract expanded with dense inflammatory infiltrate causing interface hepatitis. Inflammatory cells are predominantly plasma cells admixed with a few lymphocytes. (*Source:* From Cristina D. Cole and Romil Saxena. Autoimmune Hepatitis. Surgical Pathology Clinics. 2013;6:259–276.)

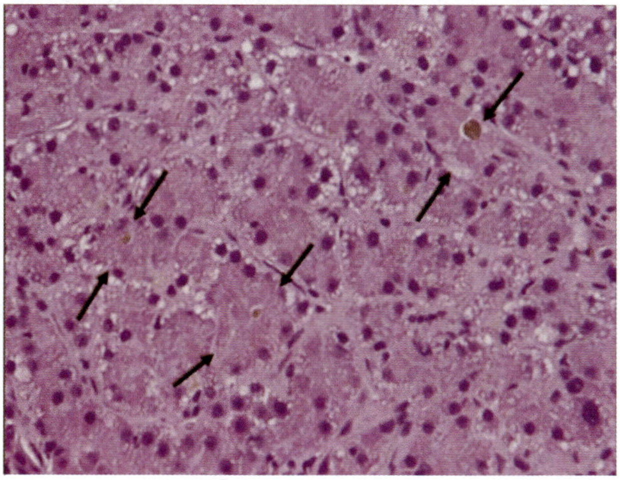

Fig. 22.26 Hepatocyte rosettes formed around sinusoids with bile plugs (arrows). (*Source:* From Cristina D. Cole and Romil Saxena. Autoimmune Hepatitis. Surgical Pathology Clinics. 2013;6:259–276.)

Table 22.3 Simplified Diagnostic Criteria Proposed by the International Autoimmune Hepatitis Group (2008)

		Points
Autoantibodies	ANA or ASMA or LKM >1:80	2
	ANA or ASMA or LKM >1:40	1
	SLA/LP positive (>20 units)	0
IgG (or gamma-globulins)	>1.10 times normal limit Upper normal limit	2 1
Liver histology	Typical for autoimmune hepatitis	2
	Compatible with autoimmune hepatitis	1
	Atypical for autoimmune hepatitis	0
Absence of viral hepatitis	Yes No	2 0

the existence of seronegative autoimmune hepatitis. Treatment options include immunosuppression with prednisone. Most patients show significant resolution within 1 year of therapy.

DRUG- AND TOXIN-INDUCED LIVER INJURY

Drug- or toxin-induced liver injury (DILI) is a heterogeneous adverse reaction to nearly any medication or xenobiotic compound that can cause liver disease. It is indeed the most common cause of acute liver failure in the United States. The liver is responsible for the metabolism of drugs and toxins, so it also bears the brunt of the toxin exposure. About 10% of patients may progress to chronic liver failure.

Pathogenesis

The smooth endoplasmic reticulum and enzymes such as cytochrome P450 and cytochrome reductase form the major drug-metabolizing machinery of the liver. These enzymes are predominant in the central zone, so necrosis of the perivenular hepatocytes is typical of drug-induced liver injury. The two mechanisms by which drugs cause liver injury are as follows:

a. **Dose-dependent or direct hepatotoxicity**, in which the drug effect is predictable in the exposed individual, a prototype example being acetaminophen toxicity.

Table 22.4 Key Differences Between Type 1 and Type 2 Autoimmune Hepatitis

Features	Type 1	Type 2
Approximate incidence	95%	5%
Autoantibodies detected	ANA (anti–smooth muscle antibody), ASMA (anti–smooth muscle actin)	Anti-liver/kidney microsomal antibody (LKM type 1)
Serum IgG levels	Elevated +++	+
Age group of patients	Young adults and the elderly	Children
Progression to cirrhosis	45%	80%
HLA association	HLA DR3/DR4	HLA DR3/DR7
Prognosis	Good	Poor, high relapse rates

Along with acetaminophen, its toxic metabolite *N*-acetyl-*p*-benzoquinone imine (NAPQI) produced by cytochrome P450 is responsible for hepatoxicity. Zone 3 hepatocytes are the first to respond to NAPQI in conditions of acetaminophen overdose. In addition, factors that accelerate cytochrome P450, especially alcohol, can exacerbate acetaminophen toxicity, thus cautioning the use of paracetamol as a hangover prophylactic.

b. **Idiosyncratic reactions** (hypersensitivity response) are more common and occur in an unpredictable fashion in a small fraction of the exposed population usually 1–3 months after exposure (Table 22.5). In these patients, injury usually reflects an unusual sensitivity or side effect, emphasizing the genetic and environmental influences, which include preexisting liver disease, female sex and ageing, and many more that play a role in individual susceptibility. The most common drug associated with idiosyncratic reactions is isoniazid; apart from isoniazid, many antimicrobials, anticonvulsants and nonsteroidal drugs are also implicated in similar reactions.

Table 22.5 Factors Implicated in the Pathogenesis of Idiosyncratic Drug Reactions

Environment	Drug	Host
• Tobacco • Alcohol • Diet • Other toxin exposure	• Duration • Lipophility • Chemical nature	• Age • Gender • Immune status • Preexisting diseases • Genetic variations • Metabolism

Morphology

DILI can trigger a whole spectrum of morphological changes in the liver that span from zonal necrosis to cholestatic pathologies, acute and chronic hepatitis and fatty liver. A few drugs show characteristic patterns such as acetaminophen that causes centrilobular necrosis, which may progress to panlobular necrosis at very high doses. Hepatocyte loss is accompanied by ballooning and variable fatty changes. Inflammation is usually sparse.

Idiosyncratic drug reactions more commonly present with features of acute hepatitis ranging from inflammation with necrosis to fatal massive hepatic cirrhosis. Typically, drug-induced hepatitis and associated liver enzyme elevation resolve with the cessation of the drug.

Cholestatic pathologies that include interlobular and intralobular bile duct injury are common among unpredictable responses to drugs such as oestrogen, androgens and sulphamethoxazole. Steatohepatitis pattern of injury can be observed among drugs like tamoxifen, amiodarone, tetracycline, valproic acid and methotrexate. Drugs such as azathioprine and oxaliplatin cause endothelial injury, leading to sinusoidal obstruction syndrome (older terminology – veno-occlusive disease) (Table 22.6).

Clinical Course

Clinicopathological features of DILI are highly nonspecific and overlap with those of viral and autoimmune hepatitis and thus must be considered in the differential diagnosis while evaluating liver diseases. Correlation between drug intake and onset of disease is of primary importance in the diagnosis of DILI. The diagnosis of idiosyncratic drug reactions is mostly made as a diagnosis of exclusion. Liver enzyme profile can help in recognizing a pattern of injury because we already know the following:

- Hepatocellular – if ALT is five or more times the normal value or the ALT/ALP ratio is more than 5
- Cholestatic – if ALP is two or more times the normal value and the ALT/ALP ratio is less than 2
- Mixed – if both ALP and ALT are increased with the ALT/ALP ratio is 2–5

FATTY LIVER DISEASE

The term 'fatty liver' was eponymously used to describe acute liver disease (ALD) in the past. It was subsequently recognized that steatosis is very common in a myriad of

Table 22.6 List of Drugs and Toxins Capable of Producing Hepatotoxicity and Their Pathological Changes

Pathological Changes	Agents
A. Acute liver disease	
1. *Zonal necrosis*	Carbon tetrachloride Acetaminophen Halothane
2. *Massive necrosis*	Halothane Acetaminophen Methyldopa
3. *Fatty change*	Tetracycline Salicylates Methotrexate Ethanol
4. *Hepatitis*	Methyldopa Isoniazid Halothane Ketoconazole
5. *Granuloma formation*	Sulphonamides Methyldopa Quinidine Allopurinol
6. *Cholestasis*	Sex hormones (including oral contraceptives) Chlorpromazine Nitrofurantoin
7. *Veno-occlusive disease*	Cytotoxic drugs
8. *Hepatic/portal vein thrombosis*	Oral contraceptives
B. Chronic liver disease	
1. *Fibrosis–cirrhosis*	Methotrexate
2. *Focal nodular hyperplasia*	Vinyl chloride Vitamin A Sex hormones
3. *Adenoma*	Sex hormones
4. *Hepatocellular carcinoma*	Sex hormones

conditions. It has now become apparent that steatosis and steatohepatitis can also be found in patients with type 2 diabetes and metabolic syndrome. This huge spectrum of diseases can be reasonably referred to as ***nonalcoholic fatty liver disease (NAFLD)***, considering steatosis as a part of ***nonalcoholic fatty liver (NAFL)*** and steatohepatitis associated with ***NASH***.

Both alcoholic fatty liver disease and NAFLD share many similarities and have been discussed together as given next.

ALCOHOLIC LIVER DISEASE PA 25.4

The harmful effects of excess alcohol (ethanol, ethyl alcohol) have been well known since many decades. ALD is the most frequent cause of liver disease in the Western countries. The three forms of ALD are as follows:

- Steatosis or fatty change
- Alcoholic hepatitis
- Cirrhosis

The progression greatly depends on the pattern of alcohol intake, whereas the type of alcoholic beverage makes little, if any, difference.

PATHOGENESIS (FLOWCHART 22.4)

Alcohol exposure and the development of cirrhosis follow a dose-dependent relationship. As much as 80 g of alcohol (six beers or 8 ounces of 80 proof liquor) consumed over a short period produces reversible fatty liver changes. However, in general, a daily intake of 30 g of undiluted alcohol or 80 g of alcohol for more than 10 years can cause severe liver disease. Apart from the amount of alcohol, other risk factors involved in the causation of ALD are listed as follows:

- Gender: Women have an increased susceptibility to develop ALD even with a much lower dose. Although the exact reasons are largely unknown, some evidence suggests that oestrogen may be an important pathogenic cofactor in causing liver disease.
- Ethnic and genetic factors: The rate of ethanol metabolism is genetically controlled. Genetic polymorphisms of alcohol dehydrogenase (ADH) and microsomal P450 oxidases have been significantly contributing to alcoholic liver damage. Among the different populations, cirrhosis rates are higher in the United States, with rates much higher among African Americans.
- Comorbid conditions: Other metabolism syndromes, malnutrition and HBV or HCV infections may accelerate disease progression.

The ethanol that is consumed is rapidly absorbed from the stomach and metabolized primarily in the liver. Within the hepatocytes, alcohol is oxidized to acetaldehyde and to acetate by the action of various enzymes, including ADH, cytochrome P450 and catalase. The oxidative pathway of alcohol generates excess NADH, causing an altered NADH/NAD ratio subsequently inhibiting fatty acid oxidation and promotion of lipogenesis.

In addition, alcohol is believed to cause increased permeability of the intestinal barrier, leading to release of lipopolysaccharide (LPS) derived from gut bacteria into portal circulation. LPS-stimulated Kupffer cells release cytokines and reactive oxygen species, causing hepatocyte damage and necrosis. Lipid accumulation also contributes to inflammation. Alcohol also impairs hepatic metabolism of methionine, causing increased homocysteine production that may induce endoplasmic stress response. Mitochondrial damage and cellular membrane damage may be produced by CYP2E1, a component of the cytochrome P450 system, which may also enhance

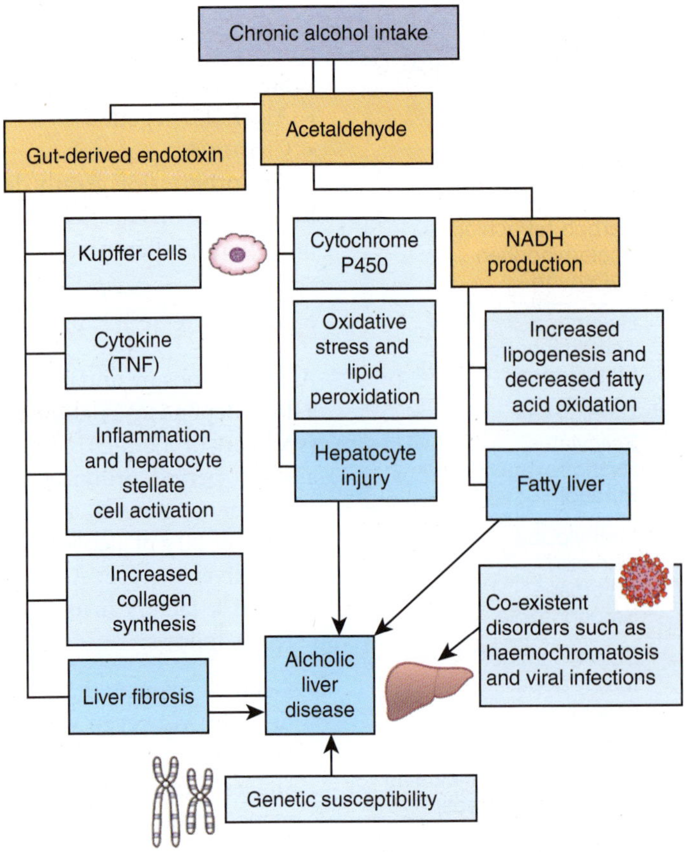

Flowchart 22.4 Pathogenesis of alcoholic liver disease.

the conversion of other drugs to toxic metabolites. Thus, ALD induces a maladaptive state in the liver that exacerbates all other stimuli, altering the homeostasis. The progression of this detrimental process eventually causes fibrosis and cirrhosis.

MORPHOLOGY

Grossly, the ***alcoholic fatty liver*** is enlarged (may weigh up to 4–6 kg) and is soft, greasy and yellowish (Fig. 22.27). Characteristic microscopic features include steatosis, which ranges from minute LDs within the cytoplasm of the hepatocytes, **microvesicular steatosis**, to large coalesced droplets filling up the entire cell, pushing the nucleus to the periphery and causing macrovesicular steatosis (Fig. 22.28), the latter being the predominant form in ALD.

Despite the conspicuous morphological changes, alcoholic fatty liver is reversible with cessation of alcohol intake.

In a small subset of patients, an acute form of alcohol-induced liver injury is precipitated by the consumption of bouts of alcohol over a long period of time. Repeated episodes of alcoholic hepatitis on the preexisting fatty liver disease are almost the forerunner of cirrhosis.

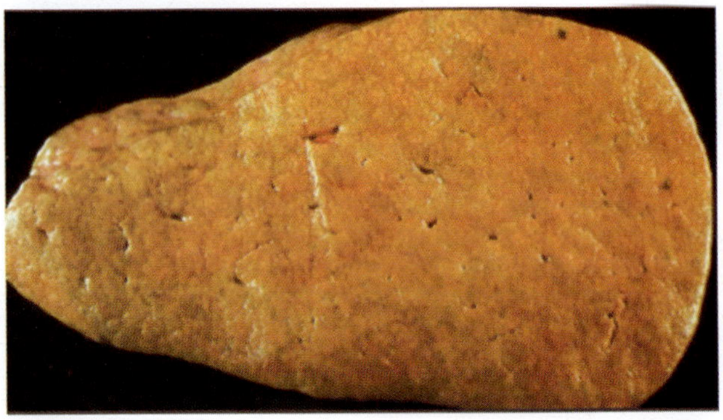

Fig. 22.27 Enlarged, pale yellow liver with micronodular cirrhosis in a patient with alcoholic liver disease. (*Source:* From Alcoholic Liver Disease. Elsevier Point of Care. 2021.)

Alcoholic hepatitis can be reliably diagnosed morphologically. The prominent features include the following:

- ***Ballooned hepatocytes*** (Fig. 22.29): These are enlarged, swollen hepatocytes with accumulation of fat, protein and water. In addition, there is accumulation of iron within hepatocytes. In some hepatocytes, cytokeratin intermediate filaments get accumulated and are known as **Mallory–Denk bodies.** These inclusion bodies are better visualized in destroyed and damaged hepatocytes where they appear as bright eosinophilic masses. Clusters of ballooned hepatocytes,

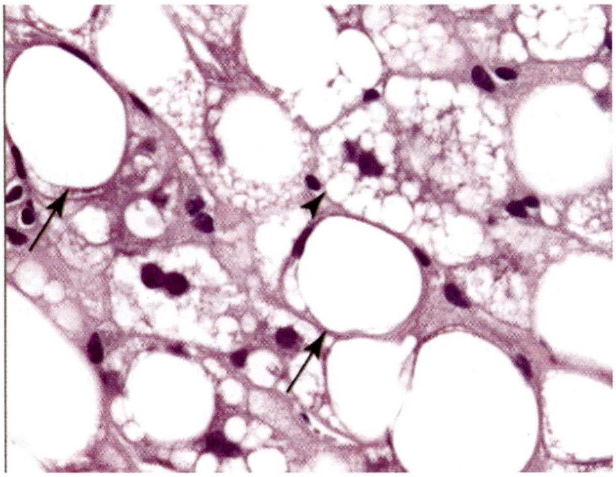

Fig. 22.28 Histopathological image showing microvesicular and macrovesicular steatosis. Microvesicular steatosis with a centralized nucleus (arrowhead). Macrovesicular steatosis with the nucleus pushed to the periphery (arrow). (*Source:* From Neil D. Theise and Romil Saxena. Algorithmic Approach to Diagnosis of Liver Disorders. Odze and Goldblum Surgical Pathology of the GI Tract, Liver, Biliary Tract and Pancreas. 3rd edition. Elsevier 2015.)

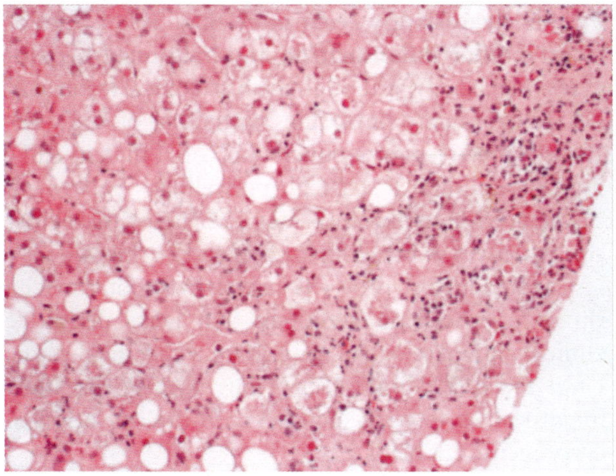

Fig. 22.29 Histopathological image of alcoholic steatohepatitis with evidence of steatosis, ballooning degeneration and Mallory hyaline. (*Source:* From Laura W. Lamps. Liver: Non-Neoplastic Diseases. Rosai and Ackerman's Surgical Pathology. 11th edition. Elsevier 2018.)

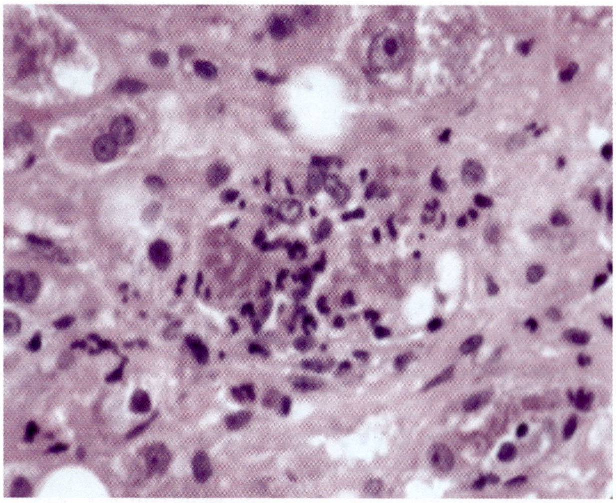

Fig. 22.30 Neutrophil aggregates around Mallory hyaline. (*Source:* From James M. Crawford. Histologic Findings in Alcoholic Liver Disease. Clinics in Liver Disease. 2012;16:699–716.)

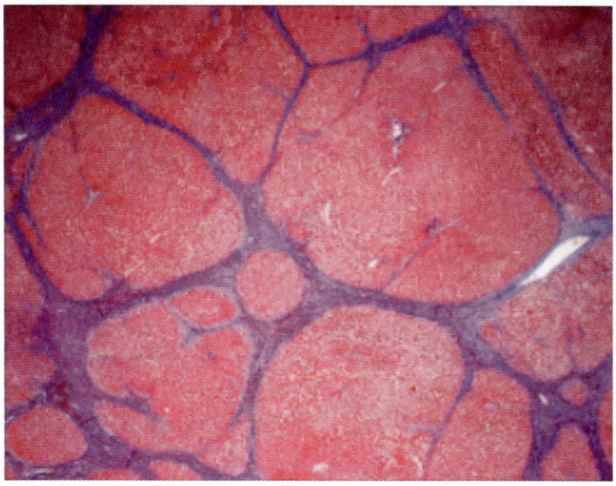

Fig. 22.31 Mixed micro- and macronodular cirrhosis in a patient with abstinence from alcohol over a long period of time. Stain – Masson's trichrome. (*Source:* From Lindsay Alpert and John Hart. The Pathology of Alcoholic Liver Disease. Clinics in Liver Disease. 2016;20:473–489.)

especially those with Mallory–Denk bodies, are often rimmed by neutrophils (Fig. 22.30). Typically, the liver architecture is not conspicuously damaged. Mallory hyaline and ballooned hepatocytes are not specific for alcoholic hepatitis but are essential for the diagnosis. They can also be seen in NASH, Wilson disease and other chronic cholestatic syndromes.

- ***Inflammation and necrosis:*** Neutrophil clusters are usually prominent around the ballooned hepatocytes, especially with Mallory hyaline. Lymphocytic infiltrates are common in the lobular and periportal regions along with an increase in the presence of macrophages. Necrosis is usually minimal and focal and, rarely, may progress to confluent necrosis.
- ***Fibrosis:*** **Perisinusoidal or pericellular fibrosis** begins usually in zone 3, producing a 'web-like' or 'chicken wire' appearance. This may progress to portal/periportal fibrosis, consequently bridging fibrosis and cirrhosis. Laënnec cirrhosis is the term applied to the micronodular cirrhosis occurring in ALD (Fig. 22.31). Even at this stage of early scarring, reversal of morphological changes is possible with cessation of alcohol intake. However, regression of full-blown alcoholic cirrhosis is extremely rare.

CLINICAL FEATURES

Patients with alcoholic hepatitis typically present with weight loss, anorexia, abdominal discomfort and, in some cases, tender hepatomegaly. Initially, mild elevation of serum bilirubin and AP levels is indicative of hepatic steatosis but elevated levels of serum transaminases and hyperbilirubinaemia are suggestive of alcoholic hepatitis. Importantly, serum ALT is raised to more than twice its normal level and a deranged AST/ALT ratio of 2:1 can be observed. This is particularly useful as in other chronic liver diseases, in which AST tends to be elevated.

Patients with alcoholic cirrhosis may, in addition, manifest neutrophilic leucocytosis, hypoprotinaemia with reversal of the albumin/globulin ratio and anaemia due to severe liver dysfunction; the overall consequences of alcoholic liver disease are elucidated in Flowchart 22.5. Although liver biopsy is not routinely indicated in these patients, biopsy may be required to rule out other causes of hepatic disease. Prognosis of early stage liver disease is favourable; however, 20% of cases may still progress to cirrhosis. Feared complications of alcoholic liver cirrhosis include recurrent infections, hepatorenal syndrome, hepatic coma, variceal bleed, hepatic encephalopathy and, rarely, HCC.

NONALCOHOLIC FATTY LIVER DISEASE

NAFLD is defined by the accumulation of fat in the liver (steatosis) in individuals with no history of alcohol ingestion or minimal quantities of alcohol intake and also in the absence of secondary causes such as Wilson disease, HCV infection and drugs. The acceptance level of daily alcohol intake, though not accurately defined, is less than 20 g per day in men and 10 g per day in women. Notably, trace fat deposits can also occur in the liver of healthy adults. Steatosis involving more than 5% hepatocytes may be considered pathological.

Pathogenesis

Steatosis and steatohepatitis form the spectrum of NAFLD. Though not fully understood, the pathogenesis of NAFLD is closely associated with type 2 diabetes mellitus and insulin resistance.

Increased calorie or rather inappropriate increase in calorie intake causes increase in free fatty acid (FFA) burden on the liver. Insulin resistance at the level of adipose tissue fails to supress lipolysis, further increasing the circulating FFAs. This coupled with de novo lipogenesis overtaxes the liver and brings about an accumulation of triglyceride LDs within the hepatocytes (steatosis). A small fraction of FFAs may be released as very low-density lipoprotein (VLDL). The lipotoxicity accelerates the synthesis of proinflammatory cytokines such as TNF-α by the adipocytes. Steatosis is also sensitive to oxidative stress, with a resultant damage to the mitochondria and plasma membrane consequently leading to cell death in the form of apoptosis or necrosis. Further release of cytokines TNF-α and TNF-β by the Kupffer cells causes activation of stellate cells and scarring.

Morphology

The important morphological features of NASH include **steatosis** involving more than 5% of hepatocytes, **lobular inflammation and ballooned hepatocytes** (Fig. 22.32). Although the histological features of NASH have many similarities with those of ALD, steatosis is much less pronounced in NASH than in ALD. Fibrosis follows the usual pericellular pattern of 'chicken wire' appearance (Fig. 22.33), with regular consequences of bridging fibrosis and cirrhosis.

Cryptogenic cirrhosis is the term applied to cirrhosis of uncertain aetiology that lacks definitive clinical and histological criteria for a specific disease. Until recently, NASH (burnt-out NASH) has been hypothesized to be associated with the causation of cryptogenic cirrhosis.

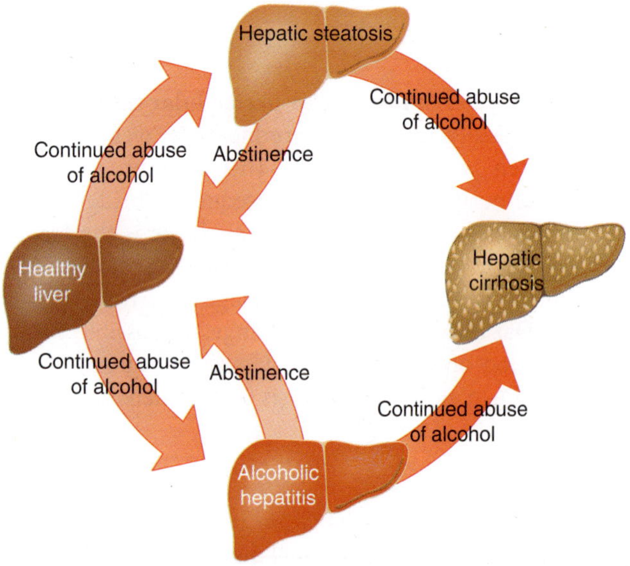

Flowchart 22.5 Consequences of alcohol abuse on the liver.

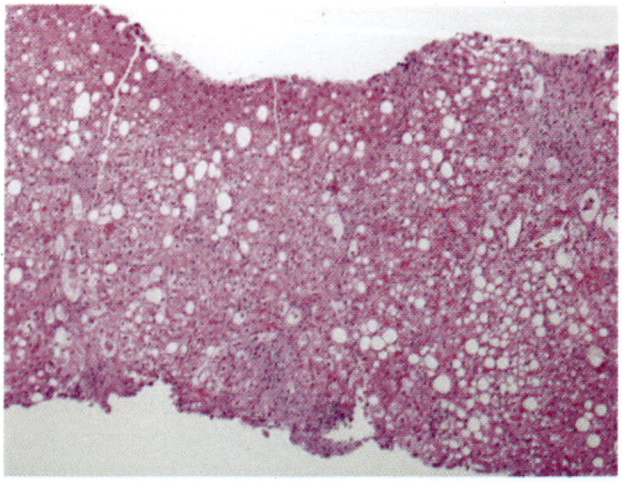

Fig. 22.32 NASH – mixed steatosis. (*Source:* From Gregory Thomas Brown and David E. Kleiner. Histopathology of nonalcoholic fatty liver disease and nonalcoholic steatohepatitis. Metabolism. 2016;65:1080–1086.)

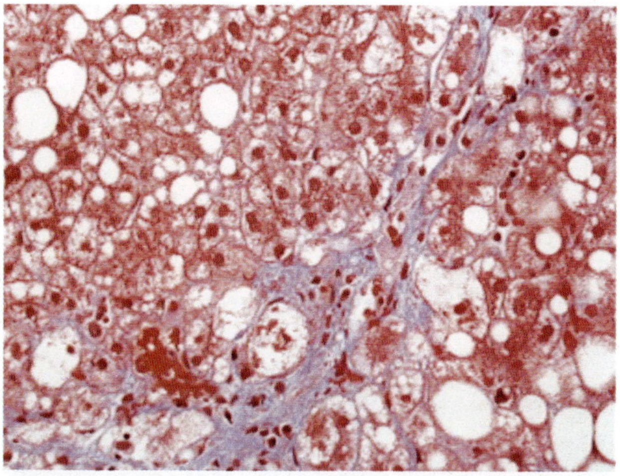

Fig. 22.33 Chicken wire pattern of fibrosis in NASH. (*Source:* From Gregory Thomas Brown and David E. Kleiner. Histopathology of nonalcoholic fatty liver disease and nonalcoholic steatohepatitis. Metabolism. 2016;65: 1080–1086.)

Clinical Features (Fig. 22.34)

Usually, asymptomatic individuals are insidiously diagnosed by radiological imaging. Serum liver enzymes may also show only a moderate increase. Liver biopsy is considered primarily to rule out other causes and to assess the severity and extent of fibrosis.

Treatment protocols are majorly directed towards correcting the underlying causes of obesity and insulin resistance.

The obesity epidemic has been increasingly involving the paediatric age group with ascending numbers of paediatric NAFLD cases and is a problem of demanding concern.

INHERITED LIVER DISEASES

Inherited liver diseases are a group of metabolic and genetic defects that typically cause early chronic liver involvement. In the next sections, we shall discuss the significant disorders – Wilson disease, α_1-antitrypsin deficiency and haemochromatosis.

HAEMOCHROMATOSIS (TABLE 22.7)

Haemochromatosis is characterized by iron overload due to excessive iron absorption. The most outward

Table 22.7 Aetiological Factors of Haemochromatosis

Hereditary haemochromatosis	Mutations of the HFE gene Mutations of the ferroportin (hepcidin gene) Congenital atransferrinaemia Aceruloplasminaemia
Secondary haemochromatosis (haemosiderosis)	Dietary iron overload Parenteral iron overload – blood transfusions Long-term haemodialysis Severe chronic haemolytic anaemias Chronic liver disease – HCV infection Alcoholic cirrhosis Porphyria cutanea tarda

HCV, hepatitis C virus.

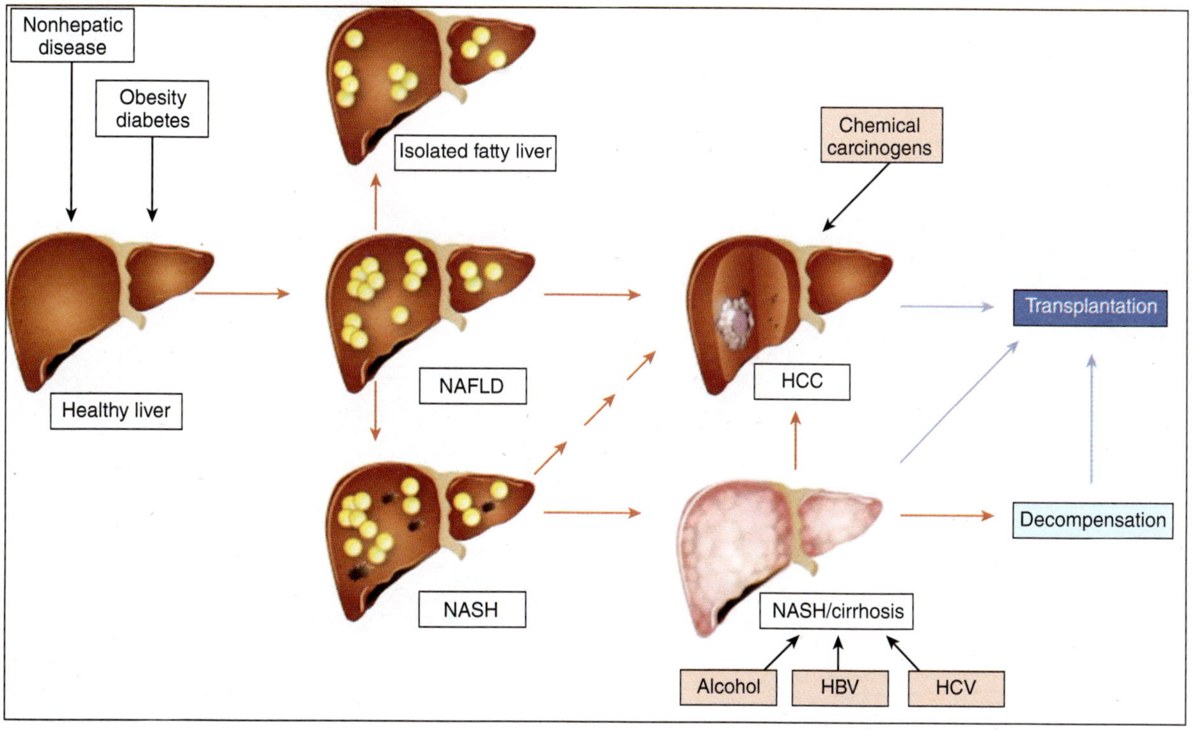

Fig. 22.34 Clinical outcomes and progress of NAFLD. (*Source:* From Diren Beyoğlu and Jeffrey R. Idle. The metabolomic window into hepatobiliary disease. Journal of Hepatology. 2013;59:842–858.)

manifestation of haemochromatosis is due to deposition of this excess iron within organs; the usually affected organs include the liver, pancreas, heart, joints and endocrine organs. Haemochromatosis due to inherited disorders can be classified as hereditary or primary haemochromatosis. Secondary haemochromatosis (haemosiderosis) is an acquired disorder resulting from parenteral administration of iron, most commonly in the form of blood transfusions.

Pathogenesis (Fig. 22.35) Iron levels are maintained by controlled mechanisms of regulation of iron absorption from the intestine. In haemochromatosis, this regulation is lost and there is an excess absorption of iron. The symptoms manifest when iron store is more than 20 g in the body. The iron that is deposited in the tissue is toxic to the liver because of the generation of free radicals and production of collagen from stellate cells; moreover, DNA damage predisposes to HCC.

Hepcidin, a peptide, is a negative regulator of iron absorption and is secreted by the liver. It binds to the iron efflux channel ferroportin and causes its internalization and proteolysis, preventing the release of iron stores from within the intestinal epithelial cells and macrophages. Thus, physiologically, hepcidin aims at lowering plasma iron levels. In hereditary forms of haemochromatosis, loss-of-function mutations of the HAMP gene that encodes for hepcidin cause iron overload. In addition, mutations involving the HFE gene producing a cysteine-to-tyrosine substitution at amino acid 282 (C282Y) are seen in about 70% of patients.

Morphology (Fig. 22.36)

The most important feature is deposition of haemosiderin in the parenchymal organs like the **liver, pancreas, myocardium, pituitary, adrenals, thyroid gland, joints and skin**. Long-standing cases show features of cirrhosis and fibrosis in the pancreas.

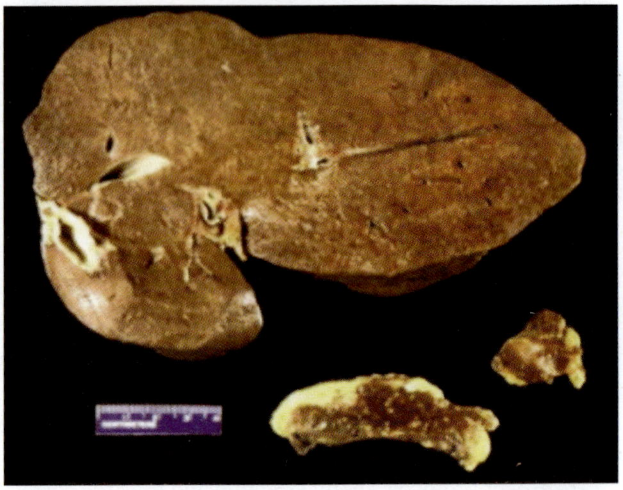

Fig. 22.36 Autopsy specimen of a patient who died of haemochromatosis. Note the rusty brown colour of the liver due to excessive iron deposition. (*Source:* From Hemochromatosis. Elsevier Point of Care. 2022.)

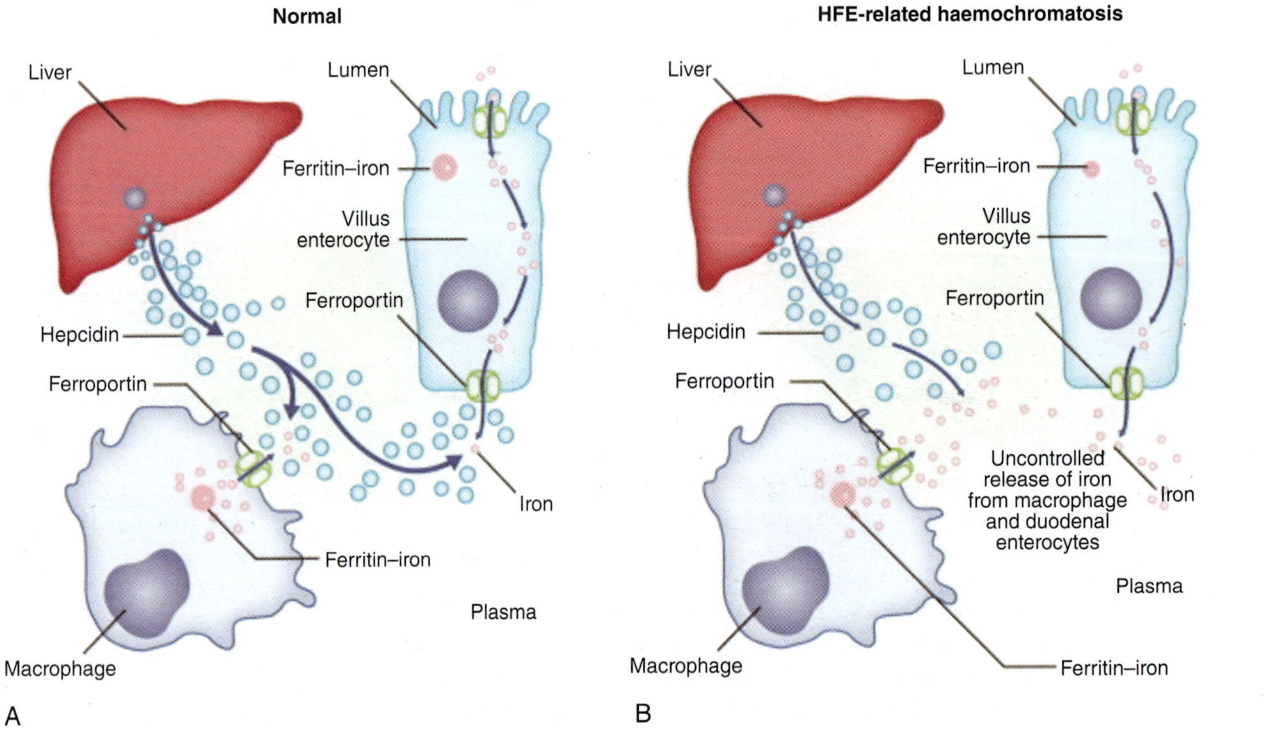

Fig. 22.35 (A) Normal iron metabolism. (B) Iron metabolism in haemochromatosis. (*Source:* From Paul C Adams Dr and James C Barton MD. Haemochromatosis. The Lancet. 2007;370:1855–1860.)

Grossly, the liver may appear slightly enlarged and brownish in colour. In the later course of the disease, a small shrunken liver with micronodular cirrhosis may be evident. Microscopically, haemosiderin appears as **golden brown pigment** in hepatocytes mostly in the periportal hepatocytes. Perls Prussian blue is the special stain for demonstration of haemosiderin, which stains the iron deposits blue (Fig. 22.37). Inflammation is characteristically absent. Iron being a potential toxin, long-term deposition leads to cirrhosis.

Normal iron content of liver tissue is 1 mg/g of dry weight. In haemochromatosis, the content rises to greater than 10 mg/g and an amount of more than 22 mg/g is associated with the development of fibrosis and cirrhosis.

The pancreas shows haemosiderin pigmentation concentration in the islet and acinar cells. Diffuse interstitial fibrosis may also be seen in long-standing cases.

Myocardium also shows haemosiderin deposits with delicate fibrosis in the interstitium.

In the skin, in addition to haemosiderin, an increase in melanin pigment is seen for unknown reasons. Haemosiderin deposition in the joint synovial linings may present as acute synovitis.

Clinical Features Haemochromatosis mostly presents in males as a clinically evident disease after 40 years of age. Common presenting signs and symptoms include hepatomegaly, skin pigmentation, diabetes, cardiac dysfunction and arthritis. Rarely, patients present with impotency. Hepatomegaly, skin pigmentation and diabetes comprise a classic triad seen in long-standing cases. Death may result from cirrhosis or cardiac failure. The risk of HCC is enormously increased in these patients.

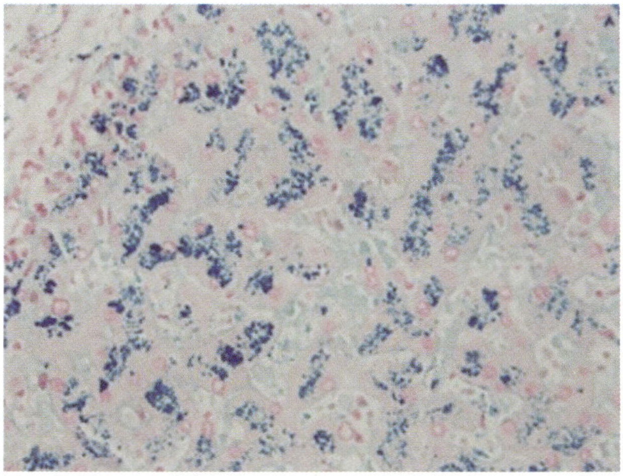

Fig. 22.37 Hepatocytes with enormous amounts of accumulated iron stains by Perls stain in haemochromatosis. (*Source:* From Kiyoko Oshima. Liver Histopathology. GI/Liver Secrets Plus. Saunders 2015.)

Haemochromatosis is mostly diagnosed before the liver undergoes irreversible damage because the patients present with early symptoms. DNA sequencing is essential to confirm the diagnosis. In addition, evaluation of the patient must include investigations to rule out secondary causes of haemochromatosis such as thalassaemia and myelodysplastic syndrome. Screening of all family members of a patient is routinely advocated to detect asymptomatic carriers. Regular phlebotomy can help in clearing the iron stores and delay the complications. Prognosis is usually favourable with prompt treatment.

WILSON DISEASE

Wilson disease is an autosomal recessive disorder characterized by reduced copper excretion in bile. This is commonly due to mutation of the ATP7B gene. The resultant excess copper accumulates in the liver, brain and eyes. The normal body copper level is 50–150 mg.

The copper that is absorbed from the gut is transported to the liver. In the liver, it is incorporated into ceruloplasmin and secreted in blood. Excess copper is transported through the bile to be excreted in the faeces. The ATP7B gene, located on chromosome 13, codes for a transmembrane enzyme that transports copper into bile. Loss-of-function mutations of this gene lead to a decrease in copper transport into bile and decrease incorporation and secretion of ceruloplasmin. Copper thus stagnates within the liver and induces profound toxicity. Hepatic injury is caused majorly by the reactive oxygen species generated by the Fenton reaction of copper. Consequently, the destroyed hepatocytes release the non-ceruloplasmin-bound copper that spills into the circulation to be deposited principally in the basal ganglia and the cornea. Predilection to these organs exists because the ATP7B and ATP7A genes are believed to be responsible for the entry and exit of copper at the blood–brain barrier and the choroid plexus epithelia.

Morphology

The liver may show varied morphological patterns including fatty change with necrosis and features of acute hepatitis or chronic hepatitis; in long-standing cases, cirrhosis may be observed. Liver biopsy in patients with Wilson disease most often shows features of chronic hepatitis that include moderate to severe portal inflammation, focal to confluent hepatocyte necrosis, steatohepatitis and perisinusoidal fibrosis. Copper can be demonstrated in the tissue by the use of **rhodamine** stain, and copper-associated protein is demonstrated by Orcein stain. Hepatic copper content of more than 250 μg/g dry weight is diagnostic (Fig. 22.38).

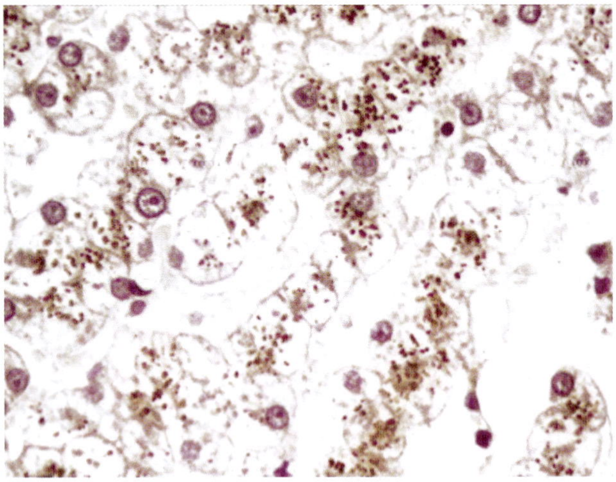

Fig. 22.38 Copper deposits identified as coarse, orange-brown pigment on rhodamine stain. (*Source:* From Neil D. Theise and Romil Saxena. Algorithmic Approach to Diagnosis of Liver Disorders. Odze and Goldblum Surgical Pathology of the GI Tract, Liver, Biliary Tract and Pancreas. 3rd edition. Elsevier 2015.)

Copper deposited in the basal ganglia of the brain often leads to brain atrophy. In the eye, deposition of copper in the Descemet membrane of the cornea is clinically seen as **Kayser–Fleischer rings**.

Clinical Features Wilson disease manifests between 6 and 40 years of age as a liver disease or Parkinson disease–like syndrome. Laboratory investigations reveal decreased serum ceruloplasmin levels, increased copper content in the liver and increased urinary excretion of copper.

Copper chelation therapy with D-penicillamine has shown significant improvement in many patients. Liver transplantation is the treatment of choice in cirrhotic patients.

α_1-ANTITRYPSIN DEFICIENCY

α_1-Antitrypsin deficiency is an autosomal recessive disorder characterized by very low levels of antitrypsin. This protein serves as a major inhibitor of proteases such as cathepsin G, proteinase 3 and neutrophil elastase. Thus, deficiency of the protein leads to the unchecked action of proteinases and causes many conditions, the most relatable being pulmonary emphysema due to unchecked neutrophil elastase activity.

α_1-Antitrypsin is produced by hepatocytes. The gene responsible for synthesis is located on chromosome 14 and many alleles are on record. PiMM is seen in more than 90% of individuals (Pi stands for protease inhibitor). PiS is a form in which there is a reduced level of this protein, and Pi null means no detectable protein in blood.

PiZ variants have less than 10% of normal of serum levels.

Pathogenesis

The disease-associated variant, PiZZ, is characterized by single amino acid substitution of lysine for glutamine at amino acid position 342. This abnormally misfolded protein accumulates within the hepatocyte, causing endoplasmic reticulum stress and mitochondrial dysfunction. This triggers cell death by apoptosis.

Morphology

The hallmark feature is the presence of **cytoplasmic eosinophilic globular inclusions** in hepatocytes (Fig. 22.39), which are highlighted with periodic acid–Schiff (PAS) stain. Mostly, these inclusions are seen in periportal hepatocytes but may progress to involve the central hepatocytes, especially in patients with PiZZ variant. However, the severity of the disease is not determined by the number of inclusions.

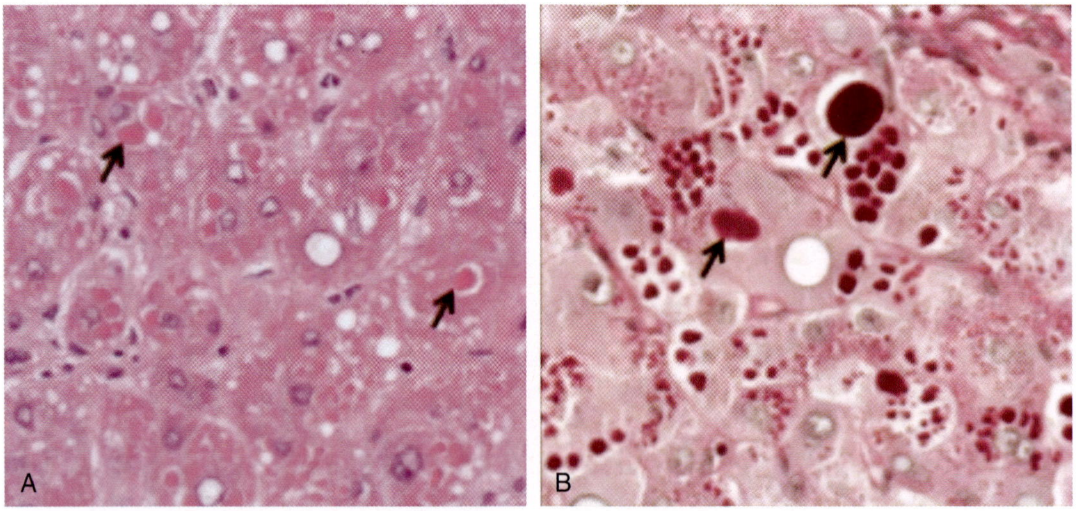

Fig. 22.39 Liver biopsy in a patient with α_1-antitrypsin deficiency showing cytoplasmic eosinophilic globular inclusions in hepatocytes (A, H&E; and B, PAS stain) marked with arrows. (*Source:* From Deniz Kuscuoglu, Sabina Janciauskiene, Karim Hamesch, Johannes Haybaeck, Christian Trautwein and Pavel Strnad. Liver – master and servant of serum proteome. Journal of Hepatology. 2018;69:512–524.)

Clinical Features

Unfortunately, most patients present with severe disease and rapid progression to cirrhosis. Liver transplant may be curative in most patients, but other organ manifestations of the deficiency persist.

CHOLESTATIC DISEASES

Bile is a physiological aqueous solution secreted by the liver. It is composed of mainly bile salts, phospholipids, conjugated bilirubin, electrolytes and water. Let us take an overview of the metabolism of bilirubin before delving into the depth of cholestatic diseases.

BILIRUBIN METABOLISM (FIG. 22.40) PA 25.1

Bilirubin is a toxic metabolite of haem degradation that is safely detoxified in the liver and excreted into the bile. Although 80% of the bilirubin is derived from the breakdown of senescent red blood cells (RBCs) in the spleen and also prematurely destroyed RBCs in the bone marrow, a smaller fraction originates from the turnover of haem-containing proteins present majorly in the liver and muscle, e.g. cytochrome P450 and myoglobin.

Bilirubin is generated by a two-stage reaction that occurs in the reticuloendothelial system, particularly the spleen, and partly by Kupffer cells of the liver. Within these cells, haem oxygenase catalyses the rate-limiting step in the breakdown of haem, which removes iron (which is transported to the marrow for recycling) from the haem, leaving a green pigment biliverdin. Biliverdin is then converted to bilirubin by biliverdin reductase and is released into the circulation. This type of bilirubin is referred to as indirect or unconjugated bilirubin. In the plasma, bilirubin travels bound to albumin because it is water insoluble but is lipophilic. In ideal conditions, no free (non–albumin bound) unconjugated bilirubin can be found in the plasma. In addition, albumin binding resists glomerular filtration, ensuring that no unconjugated bilirubin is excreted in the urine.

On reaching the liver, albumin detaches from the bilirubin at the level of the sinusoids. Hepatic uptake of unconjugated bilirubin is a passive process and is dependent on a concentration gradient. Within the hepatocytes, in the endoplasmic reticulum, the enzyme uridine diphosphate glucuronosyltransferase (UGT1A1) conjugates bilirubin with one or two molecules of glucuronic acid, rendering it nontoxic and water soluble for easy excretion. This conjugated bilirubin is transported through the bile canaliculi and excreted with the bile into the duodenum. While in the gut, the conjugated bilirubin is degraded by enzymes β-glucuronidases, produced by the gut microflora, to produce urobilinogen. Although most of the urobilinogen is excreted in the faeces in the form of stercobilinogen, a minor fraction is returned to the bile (enterohepatic circulation) and some of it is lost in the urine.

PATHOPHYSIOLOGY OF HYPERBILIRUBINAEMIA

Jaundice refers to the clinical manifestation of hyperbilirubinaemia. The normal serum levels of bilirubin are usually less than 1 mg/dL. As bilirubin levels rise in the body, it tends to deposit in tissues, particularly in those that are rich in elastin. The most sensitive indicator is yellow discolouration of the sclera, termed scleral icterus, which becomes evident when the plasma bilirubin levels cross 3 mg/dL.

In the past, the clinical jaundice was classified into prehepatic, hepatic and posthepatic types. Prehepatic jaundice was caused by the excess production of bilirubin, overtaking the liver's capacity to conjugate, thus resulting in predominantly unconjugated bilirubin. Intrahepatic causes include parenchymal liver diseases affecting the coagulation ability of the liver and interfering with the excretion of bilirubin. Thus, hepatic jaundice is characterized by

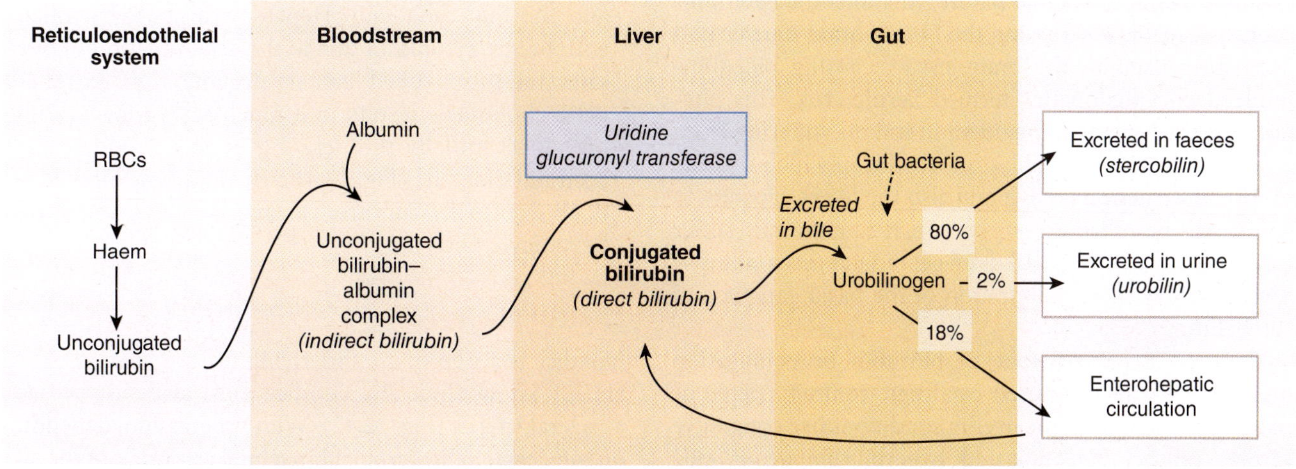

Fig. 22.40 Bilirubin metabolism.

Table 22.8 Aetiology of Unconjugated and Conjugated Hyperbilirubinaemias

Unconjugated Hyperbilirubinaemia	Conjugated Hyperbilirubinaemia
• **Excess production of bilirubin** • Haemolytic anaemias • Intra- and extravascular haemolysis • Dyserythropoiesis • **Decreased hepatic uptake** • Drugs • Sepsis • **Impaired bilirubin conjugation** • Genetic defects such as Crigler–Najjar syndrome and Gilbert syndrome • Physiological neonatal jaundice • Breast milk jaundice	• **Hereditary diseases** such as Dubin–Johnson syndrome, Rotor syndrome • **Acquired hepatocellular disease** – viral hepatitis, alcohol-induced injury, cirrhosis, Wilson disease, autoimmune • **Biliary obstruction** • Mechanical obstructions in the form of choledocholithiasis or strictures • Tumours – cholangiocarcinoma, carcinoma of the head of the pancreas • Extrahepatic biliary atresia • Cholangitis

elevated levels of unconjugated or conjugated bilirubin, sometimes both. Posthepatic jaundice, clearly obstructive jaundice due to mechanical obstruction of the extrahepatic biliary passage, is reflected by a rising dominant conjugated bilirubin level.

Hence, the categorization of jaundice on the basis of the predominant type of bilirubin present in the serum – unconjugated or conjugated – can be helpful in determining the aetiology. Table 22.8 elicits the mechanisms and aetiological factors underlying unconjugated and conjugated hyperbilirubinaemias.

Predominantly Unconjugated Hyperbilirubinaemia

Unconjugated hyperbilirubinaemia is commonly a resultant of an imbalance between the synthesis and the catabolism of bilirubin. Clinically, any condition leading to rapid destruction of RBCs and release of large quantities of bilirubin into the plasma can cause unconjugated hyperbilirubinaemia, the most apparent being haemolytic anaemia due to haemoglobinopathies, incompatible blood transfusions and malaria.

Although most of the bilirubin is bound to albumin, at very high concentrations, the unbound fraction rises. Owing to its lipid-soluble nature, this unconjugated bilirubin is capable of crossing the blood–brain barrier and depositing itself in the brain tissue, causing bilirubin-induced encephalopathy, termed kernicterus. This phenomenon is particularly evident in infants suffering from a severe form of erythroblastosis fetalis, in which the rate of RBC destruction is high and also the liver's capacity to conjugate the bilirubin is poor. Such infants may suffer from lifelong neurological damage; in fatal cases, autopsy reveals yellowish discolouration of the basal ganglia and cerebellum.

Reduced hepatic uptake of bilirubin or conjugation disturbances can be caused by drugs, contrast agents or reduced blood flow to the liver in conditions like congestive cardiac failure. Unconjugated hyperbilirubinaemia due to drugs such as rifampicin and novobiocin or contrast administration usually resolves within 48 hours of discontinuation.

Predominantly Conjugated Hyperbilirubinaemia

Conjugated hyperbilirubinaemia occurs mostly due to defective excretion of bilirubin, which may involve the microscopic bile ducts within the liver (intrahepatic cholestasis) or mechanical obstruction of the extrahepatic biliary passage (extrahepatic cholestasis). The conjugated bile is thus released or regurgitated back into the circulation to be excreted by the kidney, because it is water soluble, most often giving rise to tea- or cola-coloured urine. Apart from the rare hereditary diseases affecting bilirubin excretion, conditions causing inflammatory damage to the hepatocytes, especially viral hepatitis, ALDs and autoimmune diseases, cause increased concentrations of conjugated bilirubin.

Morphology

Theoretically, with obstruction to bile flow, liver biopsy in hyperbilirubinaemia reveals features of cholestasis. Intrahepatic cholestasis is characterized by greenish brown bile plugs occupying the hepatocytes and the bile canaliculi. Hepatocytes appear swollen with foamy cytoplasm due to the accumulation of bile salts, and this is called feathery degeneration. Extrahepatic cholestasis results in a much severe form, with bile ducts initially proliferating to accommodate the accumulating bile (Fig. 22.41). However, the bile canaliculi eventually rupture, causing bile leak and focal hepatocyte necrosis.

Clinical Features

Jaundice is a sign of an underlying disease process. As we already know, clinically, jaundice most evidently presents as scleral icterus (Fig. 22.42). With progression, depending on the degree of hyperbilirubinaemia, yellowing of the skin and mucous membrane may be noticeable. Other signs and

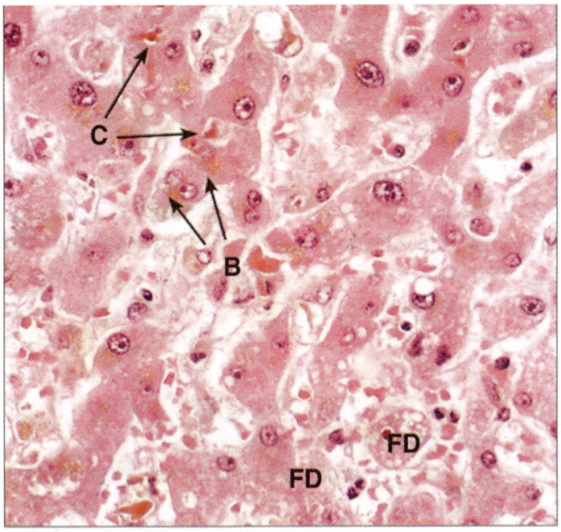

Fig. 22.41 A patient with gallstones causing extrahepatic biliary obstruction resulting in bile accumulation within the hepatocytes (B), canalicular cholestasis (C) and feathery degeneration of the hepatocytes with foamy cytoplasm (FD). (*Source:* From Olaya I. Brewer Gutierrez and Anthony N. Kalloo. Obstructive Jaundice: Endoscopic Therapy. In Current Surgical Therapy. 13th edition. Elsevier 2020.)

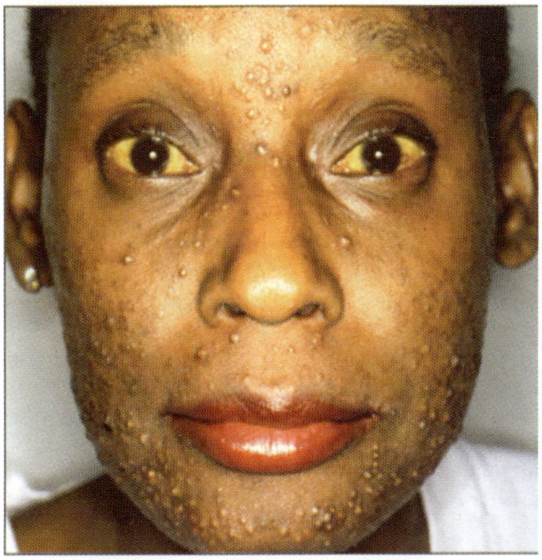

Fig. 22.42 A patient with clinically evident jaundice presenting with scleral icterus and eruptive xanthoma on the face. (*Source:* From James E. Fitzpatrick, Whitney A. High, W. Lamar Kyle. Urgent Care Dermatology: Symptom-Based Diagnosis. Elsevier. 2018.)

symptoms of cholestasis include fatigue, xanthoma and troublesome pruritus due to irritation of bile salts. Bile is necessary for fat absorption, so cholestasis can result in fat malabsorption and absorption of fat-soluble vitamins (A, D, E and K). Thus, patients manifest symptoms of their deficiencies, for instance, vitamin K inadequacy can cause bleeding tendencies, reflected by the increased prothrombin time.

LARGE BILE DUCT OBSTRUCTION

The most common cause of obstruction of large bile ducts includes choledocholithiasis – stones. Other causes include malignant neoplasms of the head of the pancreas, strictures due to previous surgery or ischaemia and primary sclerosing cholangitis (PSC; described later). In neonates, biliary atresia, cystic fibrosis and choledochal cysts are common causative factors of bile duct obstruction. The resultant cholestasis is reversible in the early pathogenetic stage, but persistence of obstruction can lead to chronic liver injury, fibrosis and, ultimately, cirrhosis, here referred to as ***biliary cirrhosis***. The accumulated bile invites bacterial infection, and most patients present with fever, chills and jaundice.

Morphology

The hallmark changes noted on liver biopsy include **cholestatic hepatocytes** with bile pigments within their cytoplasm. In areas of necrosis, the regurgitated bile pigments and bile plugs can be observed within the canaliculi. Apoptotic cells and bile ductular reaction may be prominent in the periportal region. ***Pericholangitis*** refers to the infiltrating neutrophils associated with ductules at the interface. In severe cases of bile duct obstruction, bile extravasates into the hepatic parenchyma to form bile lakes and bile infarcts (Fig. 22.43).

In advanced disease, swelling of the periportal hepatocytes (***feathery degeneration***) can be seen along with Mallory hyaline and bile pigment. Ultimately, fibrosis and cirrhosis set in (Fig. 22.44).

In cases of severe sepsis, canalicular cholestasis is accompanied by intense bile ductular proliferation at the interface – ductular or cholangiolar cholestasis.

NEONATAL JAUNDICE

Neonatal jaundice may be caused by both unconjugated and conjugated hyperbilirubinaemia. More than 75% of unconjugated hyperbilirubinaemia is physiological and is a mild and transient event. Newborns tend to have

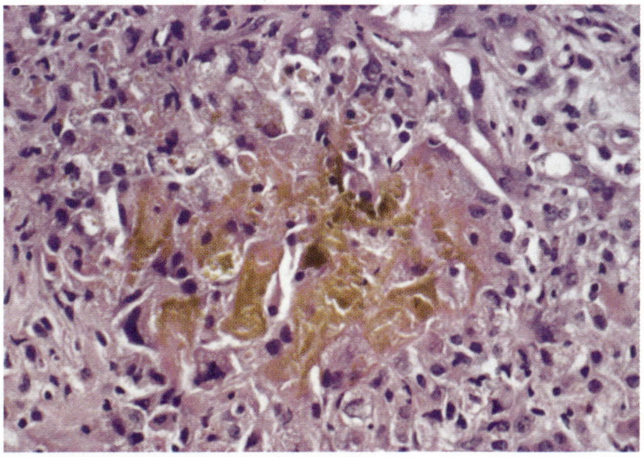

Fig. 22.43 In severe cases of bile duct obstruction, bile extravasates into the hepatic parenchyma to form bile lakes and bile infarcts. (*Source:* From Jay H. Lefkowitch. Scheuer's Liver Biopsy Interpretation. Elsevier. 2021.)

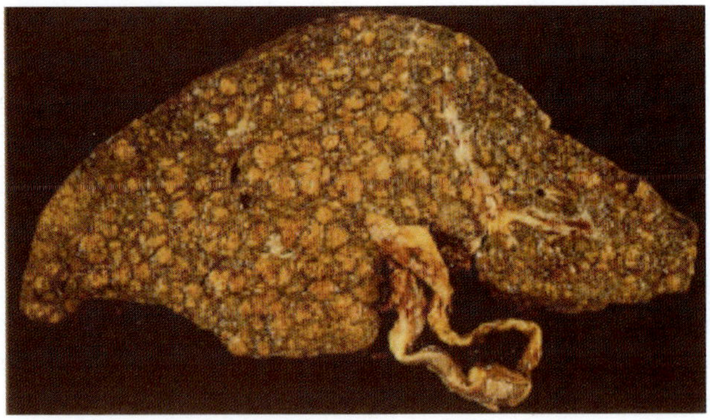

Fig. 22.44 A gross image of biliary cirrhosis of the liver. Note the greenish tinge due to cholestasis and micronodularity. (*Source:* From Christine Sempoux, Maria Guido, Romil Saxena. Practical Hepatic Pathology: a Diagnostic Approach. Elsevier. 2018.)

elevated bilirubin levels due to the greater production and faster breakdown of RBCs in their first few days of life. In addition, the newborn's immature liver is not capable to excreting the bilirubin as quickly as that of an adult. The accumulating unconjugated bilirubin manifests as physiological jaundice typically on days 2–4 of birth and resolves within 2 weeks. A few infants may require treatment with phototherapy (blue light), which converts the bilirubin into water-soluble isomers for easy excretion. Sometimes, physiological jaundice may be superimposed by breast milk jaundice, which presents much later at about 2 weeks of birth. The exact aetiology of breast milk jaundice has not been evaluated but has been postulated to be due to the presence of certain enzymes in breast milk that interfere with conjugation.

Notably, jaundice developing within the first 24 hours of birth is always pathological.

Pathological jaundice can be caused by both unconjugated and conjugated hyperbilirubinaemias (Table 22.9). Haemolytic anaemias due to hereditary causes (G6PD deficiency or pyruvate kinase deficiency), especially ABO/Rh incompatibilities, give rise to an exaggerated bilirubin production (>5 mg/dL per day). Other causes of neonatal hyperbilirubinaemia are listed in Table 22.8.

HEREDITARY NONHAEMOLYTIC HYPERBILIRUBINAEMIA

Inherited disorders of bilirubin metabolism majorly involve four syndromes, namely Gilbert, Crigler–Najjar, Dubin–Johnson and Rotor syndromes, among which the first two are characterized by unconjugated hyperbilirubinaemia and the other two by conjugated hyperbilirubinaemia. Except for Gilbert syndrome, which occurs in about 2%–10% of the general population, the other syndromes are extremely rare.

Table 22.10 elicits the inheritance patterns along with pathophysiological and other characterizations of these genetic disorders.

BILIARY ATRESIA

Biliary atresia is a congenital biliary disorder characterized by the partial or complete absence of the extrahepatic

Table 22.9 Neonatal Jaundice – Aetiology

Unconjugated Hyperbilirubinaemia	Conjugated Hyperbilirubinaemia
Physiological neonatal jaundice	Infections: TORCH, hepatitis A and B
Hereditary haemolytic diseases	Alagille syndrome
Infection or sepsis	Dubin–Johnson syndrome
Haematomas (following vacuum-assisted delivery)	Rotor syndrome
Haemolytic disease of the newborn	α_1-Antitrypsin deficiency
Crigler–Najjar syndrome	Cystic fibrosis
Gilbert syndrome	Idiopathic neonatal hepatitis
	Biliary atresia

Table 22.10 Types of Hereditary Hyperbilirubinaemia

Crigler–Najjar syndrome	Type 1 – autosomal recessive Absence of conjugating enzyme (UGT1A1) Type 2 – autosomal dominant Markedly reduced conjugating enzyme	Profound jaundice with severe unconjugated hyperbilirubinaemia High risk of kernicterus Life threatening, poor response to treatment Moderate unconjugated hyperbilirubinaemia Good prognosis
Gilbert syndrome	Autosomal dominant Decreased UGT activity	Mild unconjugated hyperbilirubinaemia Benign condition, excellent prognosis
Dubin–Johnson syndrome	Autosomal recessive Decreased hepatic excretion of bilirubin	Mild, nonpruritic jaundice Predominantly conjugated hyperbilirubinaemia Greenish black pigmented liver Benign condition, no treatment required
Rotor syndrome	Autosomal recessive Defective transport of bilirubin	Similar to Dubin–Johnson syndrome but no hepatic pigmentation

biliary tree. By incidence, it has contributed to a consistent 25%–30% of neonatal jaundice cases worldwide.

Aetiopathogenesis of biliary atresia is largely unknown. Contemporarily, biliary atresia is postulated as an idiopathic destructive fibroinflammatory process of the extrahepatic biliary tree, resulting in the complete replacement of bile ducts by fibrotic remnants or partial obstruction. Viral infections during the perinatal period, autoimmune reactions and genetic mutations have also been attributed as causative agents recently.

Two phenotypes of biliary atresia exist – the fetal and perinatal forms. The fetal form is less common and presents with defective morphogenesis of the extrahepatic biliary system at birth. The latter is characterized by normal-appearing bile ducts at birth, which later undergo sclerosis in the perinatal period.

Morphology

Grossly, the liver is enlarged, firm and **greenish black** due to cholestasis. The involved segments of the biliary system show features of distortion and narrowing and may be reduced to small atretic cords.

Histologically, the characteristic features seen on a liver biopsy include bile duct proliferation involving the portal tracts diffusely, portal oedema, ductular bile plugs and lobular neutrophilic inflammation. Progression of the disease leads to cirrhosis in untreated cases.

Clinical Features

Affected infants present with jaundice, dark-coloured urine, pale stools and hepatomegaly, and eventually develop biliary cirrhosis with portal hypertension and end-stage liver disease. If left untreated, death may follow within the first 2 years of age.

Surgical reconstruction by Kasai portoenterostomy, if performed within the first 2 months of life, yields a good prognosis. In the majority of cases, due to intrahepatic progression of the disease or late detection, surgery success rates fall drastically. In such patients, liver transplant is considered. Biliary atresia now constitutes the most common indication for liver transplant in the paediatric population.

Neonatal hepatitis has histological features similar to those of biliary atresia. Before considering surgery, it is important to confirm the diagnosis of biliary atresia by means of USG or HIDA scans with technetium-99m (^{99m}Tc). USG reveals an incomplete biliary tree. ^{99m}Tc is a dye that is usually excreted in the bile when injected. In cases of biliary atresia, there is a complete lack of the compound in the bile.

NONOBSTRUCTIVE NEONATAL CHOLESTASIS

This group of disorders can be categorized as follows:

- **Alagille syndrome:** This syndrome is responsible for 2%–6% of neonatal cholestasis. Most cases show mutations in the JAG1 gene and NOTCH 2 receptor, both of which are involved in the development of the biliary ducts. The typical diagnostic features include broad forehead, deep-set eyes, cardiac abnormalities, butterfly vertebrae and most importantly paucity of bile ducts.
- **Metabolic diseases:** Tyrosinaemia and galactosaemia may sometimes present with cholestasis.

AUTOIMMUNE CHOLANGIOPATHIES

Autoimmune cholangitis or autoimmune cholangiopathy is a chronic inflammation of the liver and a variant syndrome of autoimmune hepatitis. We now discuss two main autoimmune cholangiopathies – primary biliary cirrhosis and PSC.

PRIMARY BILIARY CHOLANGITIS

Primary biliary cholangitis (PBC) is an autoimmune disease characterized by nonsuppurative destruction of medium-sized intrahepatic bile ducts accompanied by portal inflammation and scarring, leading to cirrhosis.

The incidence is higher in females. Predominantly middle-aged individuals are affected, with a peak incidence in their fifth decade. Both genetic and environmental factors are involved in the development of this disease. It is insidious in onset, and the usual presentation is weakness and pruritus with hepatomegaly. Xanthelasmas of the eyelids, hyperpigmentation and arthropathy are also seen. Years later, signs and symptoms of cirrhosis with portal hypertension supervene.

Biochemically, an elevation in serum AP and cholesterol levels is always present. GGT is also elevated. Bilirubin is elevated when hepatic failure sets in. The characteristic feature of PBC is the presence of antimitochondrial antibodies.

Pathogenesis

PBC is an autoimmune disorder with antimitochondrial antibodies targeting E2 component of pyruvate dehydrogenase complex (PDC) (E2-PBC). The mechanism proposed is the aberrant expression of MHC class II molecules on bile duct epithelial cells and action of autoreactive T cells.

Morphology

PBC is a focal and variable disease, with different stages seen in different segments of the liver. **Small-duct biliary fibrosis and cirrhosis** are the characteristic features. Small ducts are infiltrated by lymphocytes and surrounded by macrophages and plasma cells forming

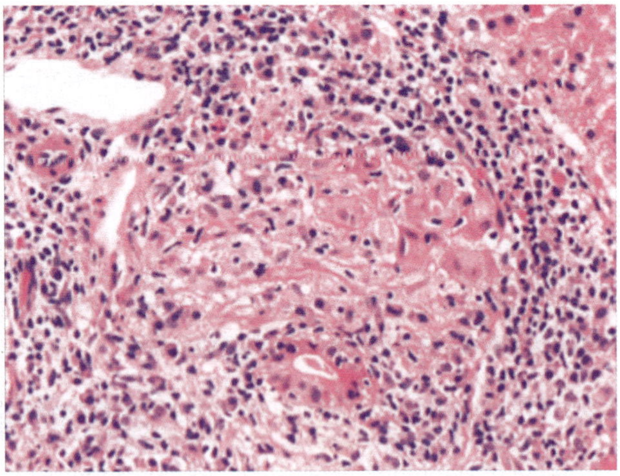

Fig. 22.45 Florid inflammation and a loose portal granuloma in a case of primary biliary cholangitis. (*Source:* From Jay H. Lefkowitch, Handbook of Liver Disease. Elsevier 2018.)

noncaseating granulomas (Fig. 22.45). The inflammatory cells gradually destroy the ducts, which undergo obstruction and secondary liver damage. Portal tracts proximally undergo bile ductular proliferation. Progressive obstruction leads to cholestasis. End stage shows scarring, fibrosis and cirrhosis.

Grossly, early stages show a normal liver but later on the liver gets a green colour due to bile stasis. Liver surface is smooth and glistening. End stage is characterized by fine nodularity due to fibrous bands resulting in micronodular cirrhosis.

Clinical Features

Insidious in onset, the patients present with fatigue, abdominal pruritus and discomfort. Skin pigmentation, xanthelasmas, steatorrhoea, and malabsorption-related osteomalacia and osteoporosis may be evident. Late stages present with jaundice and signs of portal hypertension such as variceal bleed.

The incidence of HCC is increased in patients with PBC. The major cause of death is liver failure, followed by massive GI bleed and infection. Other autoimmune disorders like Sjögren syndrome, systemic sclerosis, rheumatoid arthritis, Raynaud phenomenon and coeliac disease are also likely to be associated in certain individuals suffering from PBC. Treatment with ursodeoxycholic acid has been beneficial. The mechanism of action is not clear. End-stage liver disease requires transplantation.

PRIMARY SCLEROSING CHOLANGITIS

PSC is a fibrosing condition of intra- and extrahepatic bile ducts with dilation of uninvolved segments. The fibrosis is due to inflammation and it causes obstruction. This disease is very common between 20 and 40 years of age, with slight male predominance, and is commonly associated with inflammatory bowel disease, especially ulcerative colitis.

Pathogenesis

PSC is an inflammatory disorder caused by T cells active against gut antigens cross-reacting with bile duct antigens. In addition, numerous autoantibodies are detected in patients with PSC. These are anti–smooth muscle antibodies, antinuclear antibodies, rheumatoid factor and atypical p-ANCA, which also play a role in the inflammation. These cause fibrosis and strictures in the biliary tract.

Morphology

PSC is a **fibrosing cholangitis** of bile ducts, with lymphocytic infiltrate, progressive atrophy of the bile duct epithelium and obliteration of the lumen. The concentric periductal fibrosis around affected ducts (*'onion skin fibrosis'*) is followed by their disappearance, leaving behind a solid, cord-like fibrous scar (Fig. 22.46). In between areas of progressive stricture, bile ducts become ectatic and inflamed, presumably due to the result of downstream obstruction. As the disease progresses, the liver becomes markedly cholestatic, culminating in biliary cirrhosis much like that seen with primary and secondary biliary cirrhosis.

Clinical Features

Patients are usually asymptomatic with persistent elevated levels of serum AP. In addition, they present with fatigue, pruritus and jaundice. Severe disease results in weight loss, ascites and GI bleed. Risk of development of CCA is increased. The risk of development of pancreatitis and HCC is also increased.

Radiology shows a characteristic beading with contrast medium due to irregular strictures and dilations in the

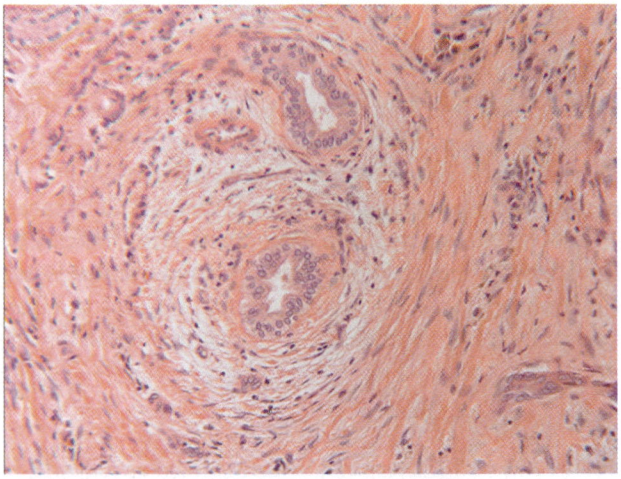

Fig. 22.46 Primary sclerosing cholangitis with characteristic lamellated periductal onion skin fibrosis accompanied by moderate inflammatory infiltrate. (*Source:* From Judith I. Wyatt, Beate Haugk. Underwood's Pathology: a Clinical Approach. Elsevier. 2019.)

biliary tree. Cholestyramine is the drug used in treatment, but in end-stage disease, transplant is the definitive treatment.

NODULES AND TUMOURS OF THE LIVER

Hepatic tumours and masses are a diverse group of disorders that include tumour-like masses and benign and malignant lesions. An overview of the common nodules and tumours encountered in the liver is provided next.

NON-NEOPLASTIC MASS LESIONS

Focal Nodular Hyperplasia

Focal nodular hyperplasia (FNH) is a benign, non-neoplastic condition of the liver arising in a noncirrhotic liver parenchyma. It is the second most common lesion occurring in the liver, next to haemangiomas.

Pathogenesis FNH is mostly considered as a reaction to focal injury, explicitly a preexisting vascular malformation, haemangioma or Budd–Chiari syndrome. In simple terms, FNH occurs in conditions that can alter the blood flow to the liver.

Morphology

Macroscopically, FNH can be described as a solitary, well-circumscribed, unencapsulated nodule located mostly in the **subcapsular location**. Most FNHs exhibit a **central stellate scar** (Fig. 22.47), the most recognizable gross feature that helps in differentiating them from other hepatic lesions, particularly hepatic adenomas.

Microscopically, the hepatic parenchyma is divided into nodules by the fibrous septa that radiate from the central scar. Bile ductular proliferation and inflammatory infiltrate are conspicuous, but interlobular bile ducts are typically absent. Hepatocytes within the nodules show a benign-looking nucleus and are arranged as one- to two-cell-thick plates. Immunohistochemical (IHC) staining with glutamine synthetase (GS) demonstrates a map-like pattern, useful in the diagnosis of FNHs (Fig. 22.48).

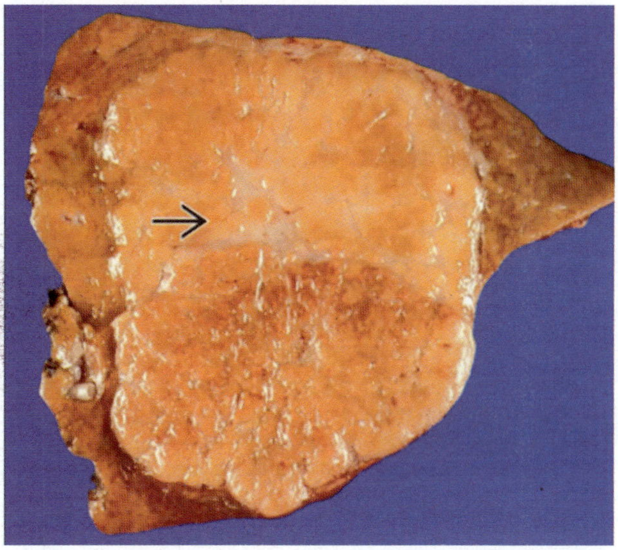

Fig. 22.47 Photomicrograph of a well-circumscribed nodule (FNH) with the central scar. FNH, focal nodular hyperplasia. (*Source:* From Michael P. Federle, Peter D. Poullos, Sidhartha R. Sinha. Imaging in Gastroenterology. Elsevier. 2018.)

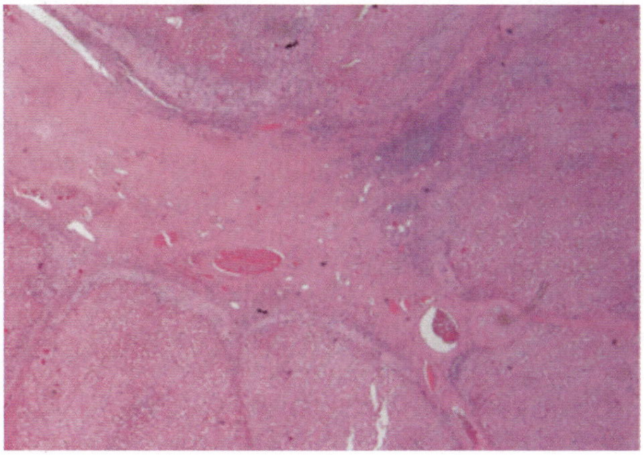

Fig. 22.48 Histomorphological features of FNH – thick fibrous septa separating nodules of hepatocytes. Note the absence of portal tracts. (*Source:* From Luiz Paulo Guido, Monica T. Garcia-Buitrago. Diagnostic Histopathology. Elsevier. 2021.)

Clinical Features FNH is mostly an incidental diagnosis because most patients are asymptomatic. The characteristic central scar is visible even on imaging. Patients mostly require only supportive treatment, and resection is considered only in large masses.

BENIGN NEOPLASMS

Cavernous Haemangiomas

The most common benign liver tumour is cavernous haemangioma. Macroscopically, it is less than 2 cm in diameter, discrete red-blue soft nodule located beneath the capsule. Microscopically, cavernous haemangiomas are composed of vascular channels surrounded by fibrous connective tissue (Fig. 22.49).

Hepatic Adenoma

Hepatic adenoma is a benign neoplasm arising from hepatocytes. Hepatic adenomas are also called liver cell adenomas and are mostly seen in young women who use oral contraceptives. The importance of recognizing these adenomas is that they may be mistaken for HCCs. Subcapsular adenomas can rupture and can cause fatal intraperitoneal haemorrhage.

Pathogenesis Three molecular subtypes of adenoma have been recognized in the recent history:

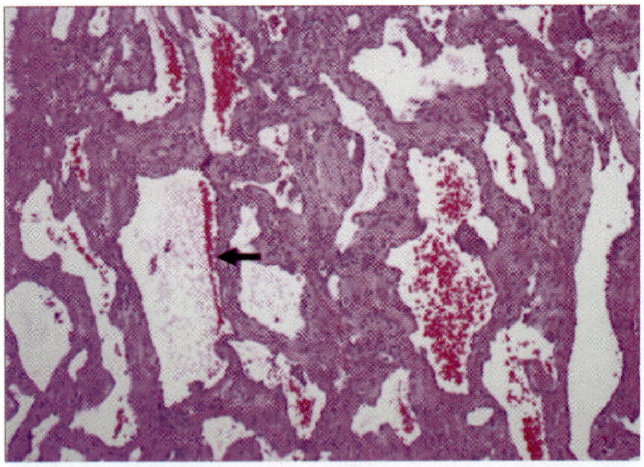

Fig. 22.49 Cavernous haemangioma of the liver, with thick-walled vascular channels intersecting the hepatic parenchyma. (*Source:* From Sudhakar K. Venkatesh, Vishal Chandan, Lewis R. Roberts. Liver Masses: A Clinical, Radiologic, and Pathologic Perspective. Clinical Gastroenterology and Hepatology. Elsevier. 2014.)

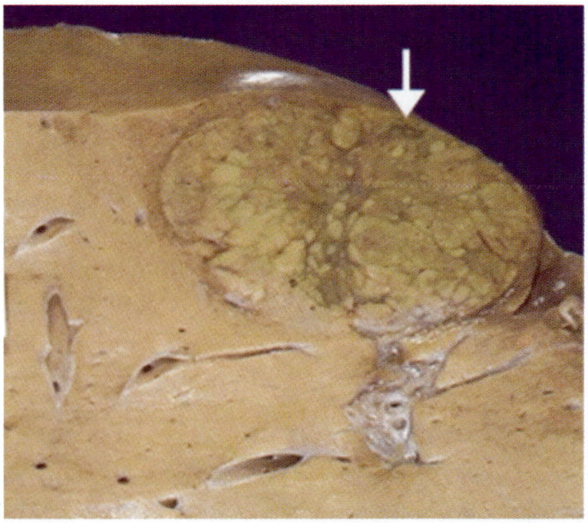

Fig. 22.50 Hepatic adenoma, gross features – characterized with a well-demarcated, tan-coloured solitary mass. (*Source:* From Edward C. Klatt. Robbins and Cotran Atlas of Pathology. Elsevier. 2020.)

- Hepatocyte nuclear factor for 1-alpha (HNF1α): Nearly all hepatic adenomas show loss-of-function mutations of HNF1α. This subtype is associated with a very minimal risk of malignant transformation and has a strong female predilection.
- Inflammatory hepatocellular adenoma: Activating mutations of gp130 resulting in the activation of JAK-STAT signalling is associated with this subtype. These adenomas are also more common in women. These tumours have a greater risk of malignant transformation.
- β-Catenin-activated hepatocellular adenoma: It is characterized by activating mutations in the β-catenin gene. These tumours are strongly associated with oral contraceptive use and bear the highest risk of malignant transformation.

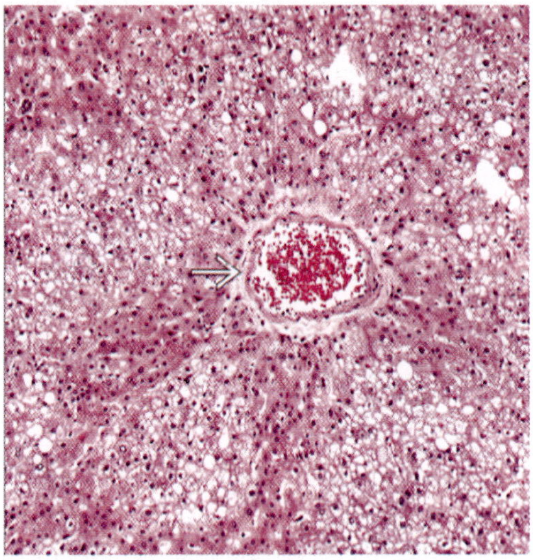

Fig. 22.51 Microscopically, hepatic adenoma features a thin-walled blood vessel (arrow), with surrounding tumour cells showing abundant steatosis or fatty changes. (*Source:* From Shefali Agrawal, Sheela Agarwal, Thomas Arnason, Sanjay Saini, Jacques Belghiti. Management of Hepatocellular Adenoma: Recent Advances. Clinical Gastroenterology and Hepatology. Elsevier. 2015.)

Morphology

Gross: Adenomas are usually solitary but can be multiple. Lesions are well demarcated, pale, yellow tan in colour and often bile-stained (Fig. 22.50). These nodules are mostly located below the capsule. Their size varies from 2 to 30 cm in diameter. These are well demarcated. Microscopically, these adenomas are composed of sheets and cords of cells resembling normal hepatocytes (Fig. 22.51). Although portal tracts are characteristically absent, fatty change is a usual finding in a particular type defined by *HNF1α* mutation. Two other molecular subtypes of hepatic adenoma include hepatic adenoma with β-catenin activation and an inflammatory hepatic adenoma characterized by upregulation of C-reactive protein.

Clinical Features Like FNHs, these tumours are also mostly detected insidiously. Mostly, cessation of oral contraceptive use is sufficient to prevent complications. Resection may be considered for tumours greater than 5 cm in diameter.

MALIGNANT TUMOURS

Both primary and secondary metastatic tumours are common in the liver. Primary carcinomas include HCCs (which arise from hepatocytes), CCAs (which arise from bile ducts), hepatoblastoma and angiosarcomas.

Angiosarcoma of the liver resembles that occurring elsewhere. The primary liver form is of interest because of its association with exposure to vinyl chloride, arsenic or Thorotrast essentially for several decades. Highly aggressive neoplasms metastasize widely.

Hepatoblastoma

It is the most common liver tumour in the paediatric population (younger than 3 years).

Hepatoblastomas show activation of WNT/β-catenin signalling pathway. These are also seen in association with familial adenomatous polyposis (FAP) syndrome, as well as with Beckwith–Wiedmann syndrome.

Morphology

Morphologically, two variants can be noted (Fig. 22.52). Epithelial type consists of fetal hepatocytes, embryonic hepatocytes or both, composed of primitive cells that are small polygonal cells forming acini, tubules or papillae. Mixed type is composed of epithelial and mesenchymal components in the form of primitive cartilage, osteoid or muscle.

Affected children mostly present with symptoms of liver failure. Close to 20% of the tumours metastasize at the time of their evaluation. However, patients respond well to treatment and the overall survival rate is 80%.

Hepatocellular Carcinoma

HCC is the third most frequent cause of cancer deaths worldwide. The development of carcinoma is strongly associated with chronic HBV and HCV infections. The incidence of HCCs is more in males.

Pathogenesis The predisposing factors for HCC include viral infections by hepatotropic viruses like HBV and HCV, alcoholism, NASH and contaminants. Other factors such as age, gender, chemicals, hormones and nutrition also play a role in the development of HCCs. An increased incidence is also seen in glycogen storage diseases, hereditary haemochromatosis, α_1-antitrypsin deficiency and tyrosinaemia.

Transmission of HBV from the mother to her infant increases the incidence 200-fold. Exposure to aflatoxin, from the fungus *Aspergillus flavus*, which is a contaminant of peanuts and grains, also increases the risk of cancer.

The main reason for the development in chronic viral infections is repeated cycles of cell death and regeneration that lead to inefficient DNA repair and accumulation of mutations. HBV integrates with the host cell genome and activates proto-oncogenes and transforms the cell. HBV X protein plays a major role in this transformation. These mutations result in preneoplastic changes known as hepatocyte dysplasia. This then progresses to HCC because of point mutations in genes like KRAS and p53 and expression receptors of hepatocyte growth factor such as c-MET. Activation of WNT or AKT pathways is also seen in many tumours.

Morphology

Grossly, HCC may be unifocal, multifocal or a diffusely infiltrative cancer. HCCs are paler but can have a greenish tinge due to bile secretion. One characteristic feature of HCC is the **invasion of vascular structures**, especially the portal vein (Fig. 22.53). The tumour may grow as a mass extending into IVC and even up to the right side of the heart. Satellite nodules may also be seen in the liver. The lungs may get involved by haematogenous spread, and lymphatic spread may involve the perihilar, peripancreatic and para-aortic nodes.

Microscopically, HCC can vary from being a well-differentiated to being an undifferentiated anaplastic tumour. Well-differentiated and moderately differentiated

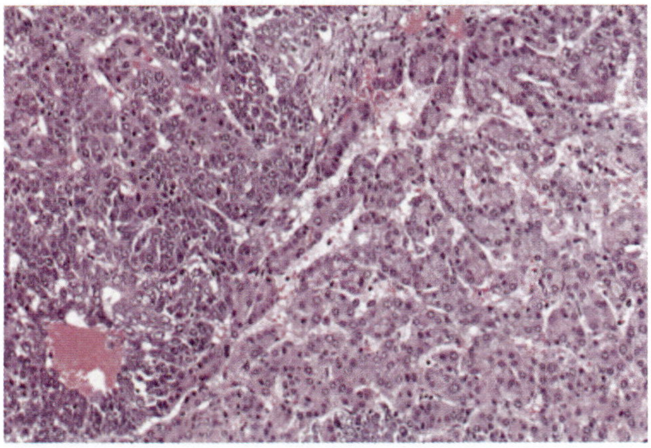

Fig. 22.52 Hepatoblastoma. Histomorphology showing a mixture of uniform cuboidal cells in the right (fetal cells) and darker cells with angulated hyperchromatic nuclei in the left (the embryonic cells). (*Source:* From Linda D. Ferrell, Sanjay Kakar. Diagnostic Histopathology of Tumors, 2 Volume Set. Elsevier. 2021.)

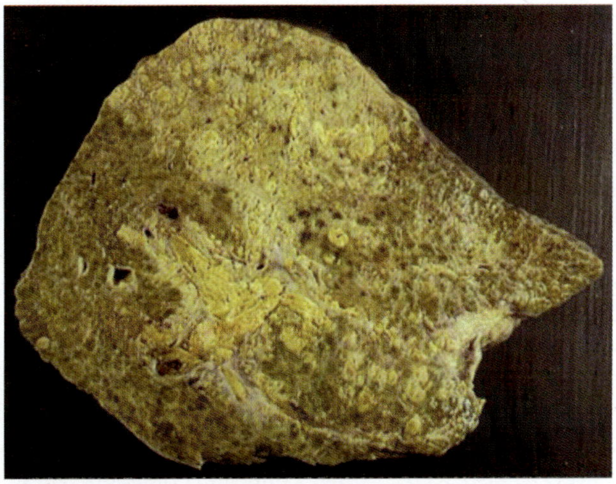

Fig. 22.53 Gross micrograph of hepatocellular carcinoma (diffusely infiltrative) arising out of a cirrhotic liver with cholestasis. Tumour shows venous invasion (left of the centre). (*Source:* From Linda D. Ferrell, Sanjay Kakar. Diagnostic Histopathology of Tumors, 2 Volume Set. Elsevier. 2021.)

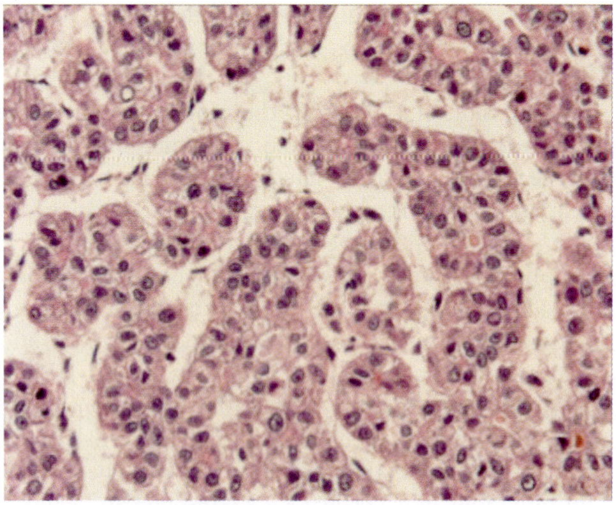

Fig. 22.54 Well-differentiated hepatocellular carcinoma with polygonal tumour cells arranged in cords and trabeculae. (*Source:* From Linda D. Ferrell, Sanjay Kakar. Diagnostic Histopathology of Tumors, 2 Volume Set. Elsevier. 2021.)

tumours show neoplastic cells arranged in trabeculae similar to normal liver cell plates but of more than three-cell-layer thickness (Fig. 22.54). Occasionally, the acinar pattern can be seen. Anaplastic tumours show pleomorphic cells with tumour giant cells and sometimes composed of undifferentiated cells resembling sarcoma.

Fibrolamellar carcinoma is a variant of HCC occurring in young adults with no sex predilection. The affected age group is 20–40 years. Prognosis is better in these patients because there is no underlying chronic liver disease. The cause of this variant is not known. Grossly, it presents as a single, large, hard tumour with fibrous bands. Microscopically, it is composed of polygonal cells with abundant cytoplasm having a round nucleus and prominent nucleoli. Cells are arranged in cords and nests, with intervening dense collagen bundles (Fig. 22.55).

Clinical Features Clinical manifestations of HCC are variable with upper abdominal pain, malaise, fatigue and weight loss. Sometimes, symptoms present as an abdominal mass or upper abdominal fullness. In few cases, the presentation may be fever, jaundice and GI bleed. Paraneoplastic syndromes are not infrequent with HCCs, especially in advanced stages. The most common manifestations include hypercholesterolaemia, hypoglycaemia and erythrocytosis.

The tumour marker of HCC is serum **α-fetoprotein**, which is increased in half of the patients. Elevation of this marker is also seen in other conditions like yolk sac tumours, cirrhosis, massive liver necrosis, chronic hepatitis, pregnancy, fetal death, anencephaly and spina bifida.

Causes of death in HCC include cachexia, massive bleeding in the GI tract, liver failure or rarely rupture of the tumour producing intraperitoneal haemorrhage. Surgery is the treatment of choice for small tumours. Radiofrequency ablation and chemoembolization may be required to shrink large tumours. The overall prognosis is poor.

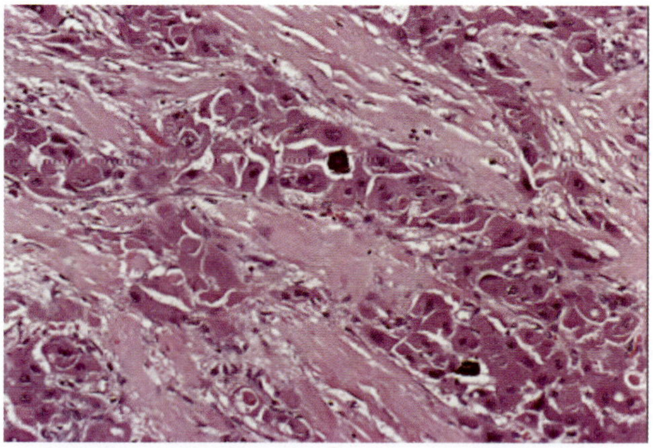

Fig. 22.55 Fibrolamellar carcinoma liver showing cords of tumour cells, with granular cytoplasm and macronucleoli in a background of dense collagenous stroma. (*Source:* From Linda D. Ferrell, Sanjay Kakar. Diagnostic Histopathology of Tumors, 2 Volume Set. Elsevier. 2021.)

Cholangiocarcinoma

CCA is the second most common primary malignant tumour of the liver, arising from the biliary tree. Risk factors for the development of CCA are PSC, congenital fibropolycystic diseases of the biliary system, HCV infection and exposure to Thorotrast. Infections of the biliary tract by liver flukes are also a major risk factor in the development of this cancer.

Pathogenesis Activation of the AKT signalling pathway is frequently encountered in CCAs. In addition, overexpression of antiapoptotic protein MCL-1, increased expression of KRAS and decreased expression of p53 are seen. Amplification of epidermal growth factor receptors and decreased expression of the cell-cycle regulator and tumour suppressor p16/ink4A are also proposed in the development of this malignancy.

Two forms of CCA – intrahepatic and extrahepatic – are noted, the former being more common. ***Klatskin tumours*** are those that arise in the perihilar zone. CCAs also arise near the ampulla of Vater where these are known as periampullary carcinomas. This subgroup also includes adenocarcinoma of the duodenum.

Prognosis is poor, and patients survive only 6 months postdiagnosis. Mostly, these tumours are identified due to biliary obstruction. Cholangitis and right upper-quadrant pain are also the presenting features in few cases.

Morphology

Extrahepatic tumours are usually small nodules within the bile duct, presenting as polyp or papillary lesions and sometimes as diffusely infiltrative lesions. Intrahepatic

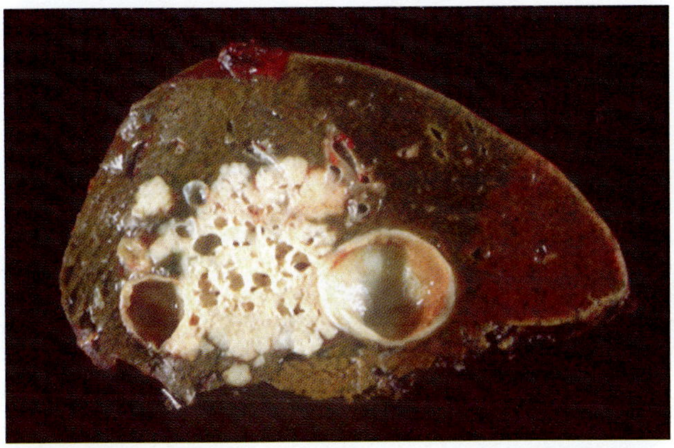

Fig. 22.56 Gross image of resected intrahepatic cholangiocarcinoma reveals a sclerotic, solid mass.

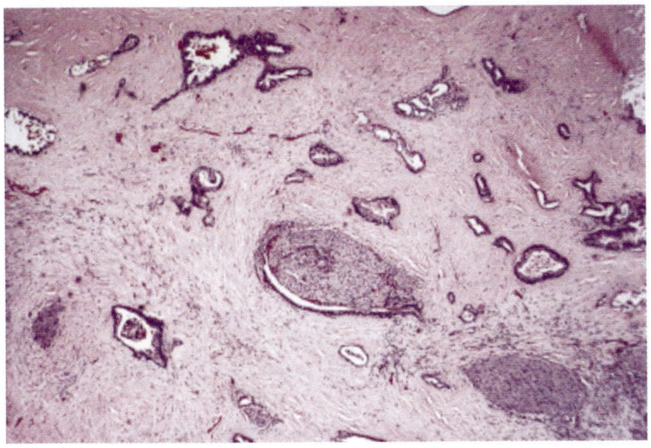

Fig. 22.57 Cholangiocarcinoma with marked desmoplastic stroma and perineural invasion. (*Source:* From Linda D. Ferrell, Sanjay Kakar. Diagnostic Histopathology of Tumors, 2 Volume Set. Elsevier. 2021.)

tumours can grow as tree-like masses in the liver when they grow along the portal tract or they can form nodules (Fig. 22.56).

Microscopically, these are adenocarcinomas with dense fibrous tissue. Differentiation can range from well-differentiated to moderately and poorly differentiated tumours. Well-differentiated tumours are composed of glandular structures lined by cuboidal to columnar cells. These tumours are markedly desmoplastic, producing dense fibrous tissue (Fig. 22.57). The tumours can spread via lymphatics and blood. Haematogenous spread occurs to the lungs, vertebra, adrenals and brain.

HCC and CCA may coexist in the same patient. These can be separate masses or collision tumours. Mixed tumours are also encountered in which there is a focus of hepatocellular differentiation in a CCA, and these tumours are believed to arise from the precursor cells that may differentiate into both hepatocytes and cholangiocytes.

METASTATIC TUMOURS

The liver is involved in metastatic tumours more commonly than in primary carcinomas. Most common primary sources are from the colon, breast, lung and pancreas. Leukaemias, melanomas and lymphomas may also involve the liver. The involved liver shows multiple nodules and gross hepatomegaly. Presentation includes jaundice and abnormal elevations of liver enzymes. The liver is very prone to metastatic tumour deposits, so the difficulty arises in differentiating a primary HCC from metastatic tumour cells with a similar morphology. In these situations, the use of IHC markers such as Hep par-1, which are specific markers for hepatocytes, can prove helpful.

GALLBLADDER

The gallbladder is a small sac that is located in a fossa on the inferior surface of the liver. The primary function of the gallbladder is to store the bile that is produced by the liver and release it when needed. About 1 L of bile is secreted by the liver every day. The bile that enters the gallbladder is concentrated by losing its water content by diffusion through the gallbladder wall. The adult gallbladder has a capacity of 50 mL.

CONGENITAL ANOMALIES

Congenital abnormalities of the gallbladder are rare, with most of them being virtually diagnosed with no clinical significance. Agenesis, meaning the complete absence of gallbladder, duplication and accessory bile ducts are among the few documented developmental abnormalities of the gallbladder. Bile duct abnormalities (Fig. 22.58) include chloledochal cysts, choledochal diverticula, choledochocoeles and Caroli disease (multiple intrahepatic dilations).

CHOLELITHIASIS

Cholelithiasis is the term applied to the presence of gallstones within the gallbladder or the extrahepatic biliary. A massive 700,000 cholecystectomies are being performed annually in the United States for gallstone disease alone. Though very common, the exact prevalence is low is some countries because most patients are asymptomatic.

Epidemiology

Gallstones are of two types – cholesterol stones and pigment stones. Cholesterol stones are composed of crystalline cholesterol monohydrate and are more common in the developed nations. Pigmented gallstones consist of bilirubin calcium salts. These arise mostly due to haemoglobinopathies and less commonly due to bacterial or parasitic infections.

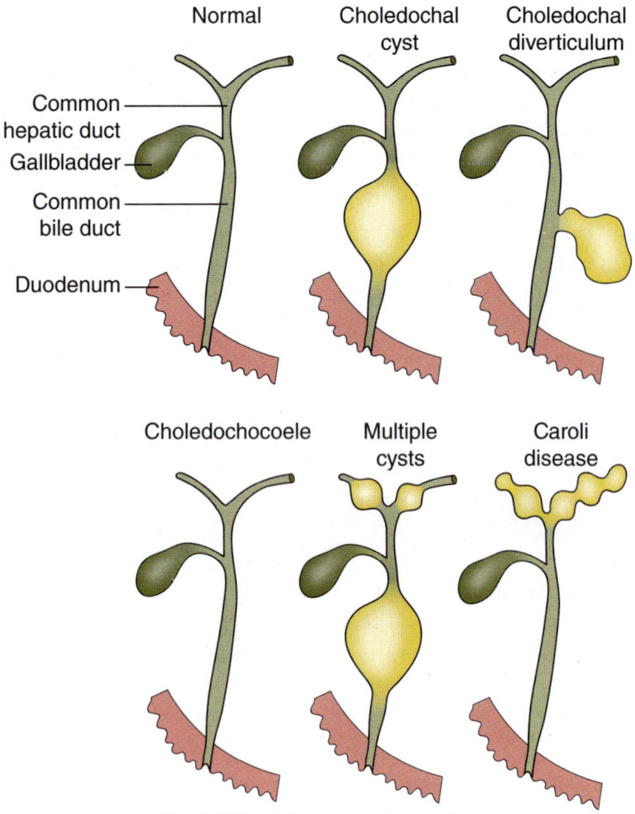

Fig. 22.58 Bile duct abnormalities.

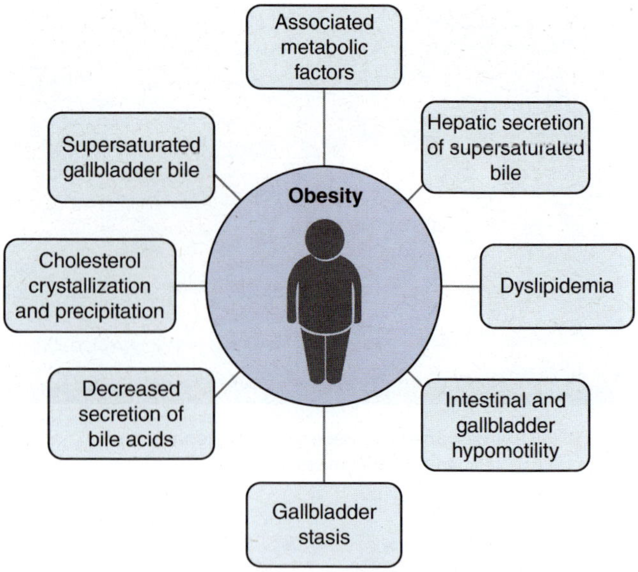

Fig. 22.59 Pathogenesis of gallstones.

Risk factors associated with cholelithiasis include the following:

- **Age and sex:** Gallstones are more common among the middle-aged and older individuals. Perimenopausal women are twice more affected with gallstone disease than men. Obesity and metabolic syndromes (diabetes, genetic hyperlipoproteinaemias) apparently hold a strong correlation with the occurrence of gallstone disease. Interestingly, moderate alcohol intake lowers biliary cholesterol concentration and decreases the risk of gallstones.
- **Environmental factors:** Rapid weight loss over a short period of time has been strongly associated with gallstone disease. Oral contraceptive use and women with several pregnancies record the highest incidence of cholesterol gallstones.

Pathogenesis (Fig. 22.59)

Cholesterol is insoluble in water. To be excreted in bile, cholesterol is converted into mixed micelles by the addition of bile acids and lecithin. When the concentration of cholesterol exceeds that of bile acids and lecithin, also referred to as **supersaturation of bile**, the unstable cholesterol aggregates to form cholesterol monohydrate crystals that later precipitate as cholesterol stones.

Pigmented stones are a resultant of chronic haemolysis in which large amounts of unconjugated bilirubin are produced, burdening the liver. The excess unconjugated bilirubin precipitates are calcium bilirubinate, generating pigmented gallstones. In addition, infections of the biliary tract by *E. coli*, *Ascaris lumbricoides* or liver flukes contribute to pigmented stone formation.

Morphology

Cholesterol stones are more common and may range from being 100% pure to containing 50% cholesterol. These stones appear hard, pale yellow in colour with a glistening cut surface. Usually, these occur as multiple stones with tight apposition to each other. Cholesterolosis is the term applied to the condition in which tiny cholesterol stones diffusely occupy the mucosa of the gallbladder.

Pigmented gallstones are brown-black in colour and range from tiny size to as much as 1.5 cm in diameter. These are soft and crumble easily.

Mixed gallstones are most common (80%) and contain an admixture of calcium salts, bile pigments and fatty acids. The cut surface shows a typical lamellated structure with alternating layers of dark pigment and pale white cholesterol (Figs 22.60 and 22.61).

Clinical Features

The majority of patients are asymptomatic throughout their lifetime. Some may experience symptoms typically after a heavy fatty meal as colicky pain in the right upper quadrant of the abdomen or in the epigastrium. Cholecystectomy is the treatment of choice.

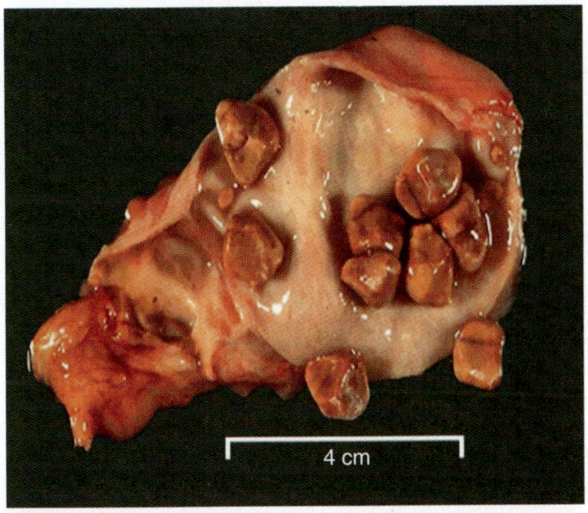

Fig. 22.60 Gross morphology of calculous cholelithiasis. (*Source:* From Edward C. Klatt. Robbins and Cotran Atlas of Pathology. Elsevier. 2020.)

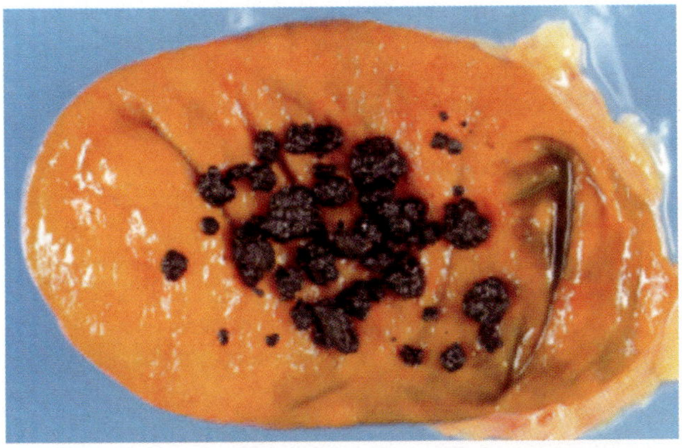

Fig. 22.61 Gross morphology of calculous cholelithiasis with pigmented gallstones. (*Source:* From Andrew J. Connolly, Walter E. Finkbeiner, Philip C. Ursell, Richard L. Davis. Autopsy Pathology: A Manual and Atlas. Elsevier. 2016.)

The most common complications of gallstones include acute cholecystitis, gallstone pancreatitis and gallstone ileus (which results from the perforation of the gallbladder by chronic gallstones and inflammation with consequent fistula formation). Rarely, carcinoma can supervene.

CHOLECYSTITIS

Cholecystitis or inflammation of the gallbladder can be acute or chronic and is almost always associated with gallstones. Acute cholecystitis is a medical emergency and is the most common indication for cholecystectomy.

Acute Cholecystitis

Acute cholecystitis is most commonly caused by obstruction of the neck of the gallbladder or the cystic duct by gallstone.

Pathogenesis A total of 90% of cases are linked to obstruction of the gallbladder outlet, whereas the remaining 10% (acalculous cholecystitis) are contributed by sepsis, trauma and infection. Obstruction of the cystic duct or gallbladder neck results in the release of phospholipase enzyme by the gallbladder epithelium. This enzyme hydrolyses the mucous coat over the epithelium, exposing it to the toxic action of bile salts. The resultant cellular damage invites inflammatory cells and its sequelae.

Morphology

Grossly, the gallbladder is congested, enlarged and oedematous and may show serosal haemorrhages. Gallstones are usually apparent.

Microscopically, the mucosa shows features of oedema, congestion, erosion and sparse neutrophilic infiltration.

Clinical symptoms of acute calculous include progressive upper-quadrant pain lasting more than 6 hours accompanied by fever, nausea and vomiting. The symptoms usually resolve within 24 hours. Acalculous cholecystitis usually presents with complaints of the underlying disorder. Complications of acute cholecystitis include empyema of the gallbladder, gangrenous cholecystitis, biliary peritonitis due to leak of bile into the peritoneum and cholecystoenteric fistula.

Chronic Cholecystitis

Chronic cholecystitis is the most common disease of the gallbladder. Repeated episodes of acute cholecystitis with persistent inflammation give rise to chronic cholecystitis.

Morphology

The gallbladder wall is thickened and fibrotic. Gallstones are usually found in the lumen. The mucosa may show ulcerations and sludge (fine calculus particles). Microscopically, the gallbladder wall shows diffuse chronic inflammation. Rokitansky–Aschoff sinuses, which are deep outpouchings of mucosa that extend into or even beyond the muscularis, may be seen, although not always apparent (Fig. 22.62). Long-standing inflammation may cause calcification of the gallbladder wall, giving rise to porcelain gallbladder (Fig. 22.63).

Clinical Features Most patients present with vague symptoms, whereas some may complain of pain in the right hypochondrium, which is typically episodic. USG examination can reveal the diagnosis. Cholecystectomy is the most sought-after method for solution.

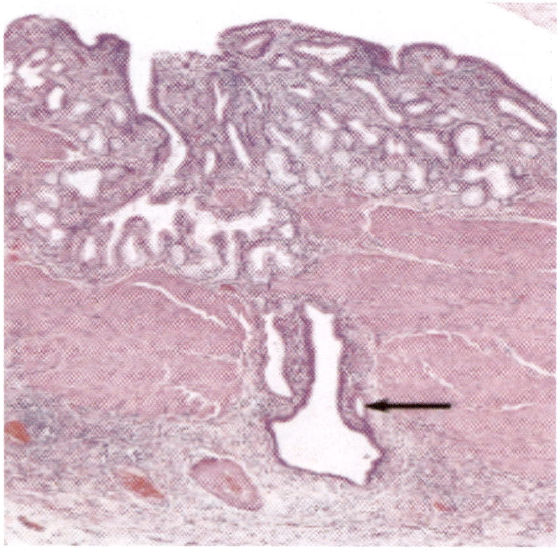

Fig. 22.62 Chronic cholecystitis. Microscopy reveals diffuse chronic inflammation with Rokitansky–Aschoff sinuses (arrow). (*Source:* From Judith I. Wyatt, Beate Haugk. Underwood's Pathology: a Clinical Approach. Elsevier. 2019.)

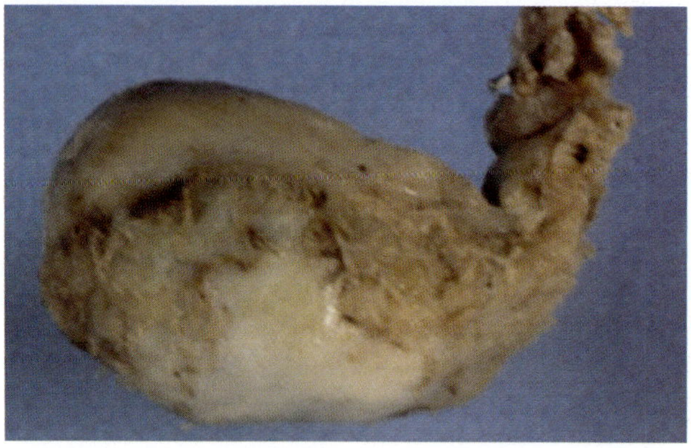

Fig. 22.63 Porcelain gallbladder – the entire wall of the gallbladder has been replaced by calcification. (*Source:* From Laura W. Lamps. Rosai and Ackerman's Surgical Pathology - 2 Volume Set. Elsevier. 2018.)

CARCINOMA OF THE GALLBLADDER

Adenocarcinoma of the gallbladder is not an uncommon tumour. With the ongoing trend in cholecystectomies, the incidence of gallbladder carcinoma has decreased. Adenocarcinoma may be detected incidentally in 2% of patients undergoing cholecystectomy. Aetiopathogenesis has been associated with cholelithiasis and chronic cholecystitis.

Morphology

Adenocarcinoma of the gallbladder more commonly occurs in the fundus. Grossly, the tumour presents as a discrete nodule or an infiltrative mass diffusely involving the bladder wall. Microscopically, the tumour is usually well differentiated with a characteristic desmoplastic stroma. Anaplastic and poorly differentiated tumours have also been reported. The tumours may progressively infiltrate the adjacent organs by peritoneal spread.

Clinical Features

Presenting symptoms are insidious and overlap with those of cholecystitis and cholelithiasis. Metastasis to the lungs and direct extension to the liver mark a poor prognosis. The overall 5-year survival rate is less than 3%. Adjuvant chemotherapy is often offered to such patients but is not definitively curative.

SELF-ASSESSMENT

Multiple Choice Questions

1. A 45-year-old male with a history of alcohol abuse presents with jaundice, ascites and spider angiomas. Liver biopsy shows micronodules. Which stage of alcoholic liver disease is most likely?
   A. Alcoholic steatohepatitis
   B. Alcoholic fatty liver
   C. Alcoholic cirrhosis
   D. Acute alcoholic hepatitis
2. A patient with chronic hepatitis C develops portal hypertension. Which of the following mechanisms is primarily responsible for this condition?
   A. Increased hepatic artery resistance
   B. Obstruction of hepatic venous outflow
   C. Sinusoidal fibrosis and increased intrahepatic resistance
   D. Splanchnic arterial vasodilation
3. A 50-year-old female presents with pruritus and fatigue. Laboratory tests show elevated alkaline phosphatase and positive antimitochondrial antibodies. Which condition is most likely?
   A. Primary sclerosing cholangitis
   B. Primary biliary cholangitis
   C. Alcoholic liver disease
   D. Nonalcoholic steatohepatitis
4. A patient with acute liver failure shows elevated serum ammonia and altered mental status. Which of the following complications is the patient most likely experiencing?
   A. Hepatic encephalopathy
   B. Spontaneous bacterial peritonitis
   C. Hepatorenal syndrome
   D. Portal hypertensive gastropathy
5. In a patient with haemochromatosis, which organ is typically NOT affected by excess iron deposition?
   A. Liver
   B. Pancreas
   C. Spleen
   D. Heart
6. A patient with viral hepatitis shows ground glass hepatocytes on biopsy. Which virus is most likely responsible?
   A. Hepatitis A virus
   B. Hepatitis B virus
   C. Hepatitis C virus
   D. Hepatitis E virus

7. A 35-year-old woman with no history of alcohol abuse has elevated liver enzymes and liver biopsy showing steatohepatitis. What is the most likely diagnosis?
   A. Alcoholic liver disease
   B. Nonalcoholic fatty liver disease (NAFLD)
   C. Acute viral hepatitis
   D. Autoimmune hepatitis
8. A patient with Budd–Chiari syndrome would show which of the following findings?
   A. Portal vein thrombosis
   B. Hepatic vein thrombosis
   C. Hepatic artery aneurysm
   D. Splenic vein thrombosis
9. A patient presents with Kayser–Fleischer rings and neurological symptoms. Which diagnostic test would be most confirmatory?
   A. Serum ceruloplasmin
   B. Liver function tests
   C. α-Fetoprotein
   D. Anti–smooth muscle antibody
10. In Wilson disease, which of the following substances accumulates in the liver due to defective excretion?
    A. Iron
    B. Copper
    C. α_1-Antitrypsin
    D. Bilirubin
11. A patient with chronic alcoholism develops ascites and hepatic encephalopathy. What is the most likely cause?
    A. Acute hepatitis
    B. Cirrhosis
    C. Hepatocellular carcinoma
    D. Cholelithiasis
12. A patient with jaundice has a liver biopsy showing bridging necrosis. Which condition is most likely?
    A. Alcoholic hepatitis
    B. Autoimmune hepatitis
    C. Drug-induced liver injury
    D. Viral hepatitis
13. In α_1-antitrypsin deficiency, which type of emphysema is typically seen?
    A. Centrilobular
    B. Panlobular
    C. Paraseptal
    D. Irregular
14. A patient with a history of intravenous drug use presents with jaundice and arthralgia. Hepatitis virus RNA is detected. What is the most likely diagnosis?
    A. Hepatitis C
    B. Hepatitis B
    C. Alcoholic hepatitis
    D. Autoimmune hepatitis
15. A patient with acute liver failure is found to have an overdose of a common analgesic. Which drug is most likely responsible?
    A. Aspirin
    B. Ibuprofen
    C. Paracetamol
    D. Naproxen
16. A 60-year-old patient presents with a history of progressive fatigue, skin hyperpigmentation and diabetes mellitus. Laboratory tests reveal elevated serum ferritin and transferrin saturation. Liver biopsy shows extensive iron deposition. Which condition is most likely?
    A. Wilson disease
    B. α_1-Antitrypsin deficiency
    C. Haemochromatosis
    D. Chronic viral hepatitis
17. A patient with a history of alcohol abuse presents with portal hypertension and splenomegaly. What is the most likely underlying pathology?
    A. Cirrhosis
    B. Acute hepatitis
    C. Cholangiocarcinoma
    D. Hepatic vein thrombosis
18. A patient with cirrhosis develops renal failure without other apparent causes. What is the most likely diagnosis?
    A. Acute tubular necrosis
    B. Glomerulonephritis
    C. Hepatorenal syndrome
    D. Diabetic nephropathy
19. In a patient with portal hypertension, which of the following is a common site for variceal bleeding?
    A. Oesophagus
    B. Stomach
    C. Duodenum
    D. Colon
20. A patient presents with high serum iron and transferrin saturation but normal ferritin levels. Which condition is this indicative of?
    A. Haemochromatosis
    B. Anaemia of chronic disease
    C. Iron-deficiency anaemia
    D. Thalassaemia

Answers

1. (C); 2. (C); 3. (B); 4. (A); 5. (C); 6. (B); 7. (B); 8. (B); 9. (A); 10. (B); 11. (B); 12. (D); 13. (B); 14. (A); 15. (C); 16. (C); 17. (A); 18. (C); 19. (A); 20. (A)

Scenario-Based Questions

1. A 26-year-old female patient was incidentally recognized as $HBsAg^+$ at the blood bank. Liver function tests performed revealed the following: albumin, 4 g/dL; AP, 109 units/L; AST/ALT, <1; and $HBsAg^+$, HBc IgG^+, $HBeAg^-$ and HBV DNA, <10 copies/mL. What is the likely diagnosis?
2. A 60-year-old male patient with a long history of alcoholism presented with right upper-quadrant pain and confused state of mind. Laboratory tests were as follows: bilirubin, 2 mg/dL; ALT, 63 IU/L; AST, 125/L; albumin, 31 g/L; AP, 248 IU/L; and PT, 20 seconds; blood counts showed thrombocytopenia. On examination, the patient was found to have grade II encephalopathy and palmar erythema. What is the probable diagnosis?
3. A 27-year-old woman presented with complaints of myalgia, nausea and vomiting. Her physical examination revealed slight yellowish discolouration of the sclera. There was no history of drug or alcohol intake in the recent months. On further questioning, she stated that she had lost her taste for coffee and cigarettes. Laboratory results showed a serum bilirubin level of 1.8 mg/dL and serum transaminases were slightly elevated. What diagnosis would you make of this patient?

4. A 5-year-old boy presented with complaints of body ache and mild fever. His physical examination revealed mild liver tenderness but no significant lymphadenopathy or organomegaly. Laboratory examination showed mildly elevated serum transaminases and bilirubin. He further stated that many of his friends at the day care he attended complained of similar symptoms. He recovered without incident. What is the most likely organism that could have caused infection in this boy?
5. A 50-year-old woman presented with fatigue and mild right upper-quadrant pain. Liver function tests performed revealed elevated AST and ALT levels. On follow-up for several months, serum transaminases remained elevated. Liver biopsy morphologically showed evidence of chronic inflammation at the interface, also destroying the surrounding hepatocytes. Further investigations revealed anti–smooth muscle antibodies and antinuclear antibodies to be present in the patient's serum. In addition, lupus erythematosus (LE) test was positive. What is the diagnosis of this patient?
6. What are the differential diagnoses of acute hepatitis?
7. Discuss the approach to a case of cirrhosis.
8. Discuss the approach to a case of jaundice.
9. What are the complications of gallstones?

Answers

1. Chronic HBV carrier state
2. Alcoholic hepatitis with liver failure
3. Acute viral hepatitis
4. Hepatitis A virus
5. Autoimmune hepatitis

Topics for Self-Directed Learning

1. Drug-induced liver injury in clinical practice
2. Targeted drug therapy in viral hepatitis
3. Special stains used in liver pathology
4. IHC markers in hepatobiliary tumours
5. IgG4-related diseases
6. Hepatic and biliary stem cell/progenitor niche reprogramming in disease and regeneration
7. Newer insights into the mechanisms of cholestasis

The Pancreas

23

Rajeswari Kathiah

PA 32.6 Describe the aetiology, pathogenesis, morphology, laboratory findings, morphological features, complications and metastases of **pancreatic cancer**.

CHAPTER OUTLINE

ANATOMY AND HISTOLOGY OF PANCREAS

The pancreas is an organ of the digestive system and the endocrine system. It is located in the abdomen, stretching from the inner curvature of the duodenum to the left upper abdomen near the hilum of the spleen, and functions as a gland. It is approximately 12–15 cm long, lobulated and salmon-coloured in appearance. Anatomically, the pancreas can be divided into **head, neck, body and tail**. Two ducts, the main pancreatic duct and a smaller accessory pancreatic duct, run through the body of the gland, joining the common bile duct near the ampulla of Vater. In most individuals, the main pancreatic duct joins the common bile duct just proximal to the papilla of Vater and the accessory duct drains into the duodenum through a separate minor papilla (Figs 23.1 and 23.2).

The **exocrine pancreas** accounts for 80%–85% of the organ and is composed of **acinar cells** that secrete digestive enzymes in the inactive proenzyme form. After secretion, these enzymes are transported by a group of ductules and ducts to the duodenum, where they are activated.

The **endocrine pancreas** constitutes only 1%–2% of the gland and is composed of 1 million clusters of **islets of Langerhans**, which are responsible for the secretion of endocrine hormones.

As mentioned earlier, the pancreas has both an endocrine function and a digestive exocrine function. As an endocrine gland, it acts mostly by regulating blood sugar levels by secreting hormones like **insulin, glucagon, somatostatin and pancreatic polypeptide**. As an exocrine gland, it acts by being a part of the digestive system, secreting pancreatic juice rich in **digestive enzymes** into the duodenum through the pancreatic duct. The pancreatic juice contains bicarbonate, which neutralizes the acid entering the duodenum from the gastric mucosa, and digestive enzymes, which breakdown carbohydrates, proteins and fats in the food.

CONGENITAL ANOMALIES

Although congenital anomalies and variations of the pancreas are often discovered as incidental findings, some of them may lead to unexplained clinical symptoms such as recurrent abdominal pain, nausea and vomiting. Such congenital anomalies of the pancreas are seen in approximately 10% of children and include pancreatic agenesis, hypoplasia, ectopia, pancreatic divisum and annular pancreas. Recognition of these anomalies is important as these may be surgically correctable causes of recurrent pancreatitis and gastric outlet obstruction.

The pancreas arises from the fusion of dorsal and ventral outpouchings of the foregut. During the development of the pancreas, which is a complex process, expansion of the duodenum causes the ventral bud to rotate and pass

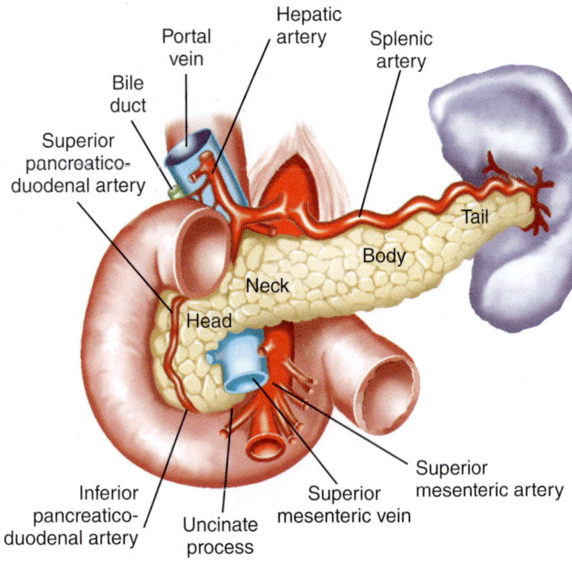

Fig. 23.1 Anatomy of the pancreas. (*Source:* From Megha S. Mehta, Bradley A. Barth and Sohail Z. Husain. Anatomy, Histology, Embryology, and Developmental Anomalies of the Pancreas. Sleisenger and Fordtran's Gastrointestinal and Liver Disease. 11th edition. Elsevier 2021.)

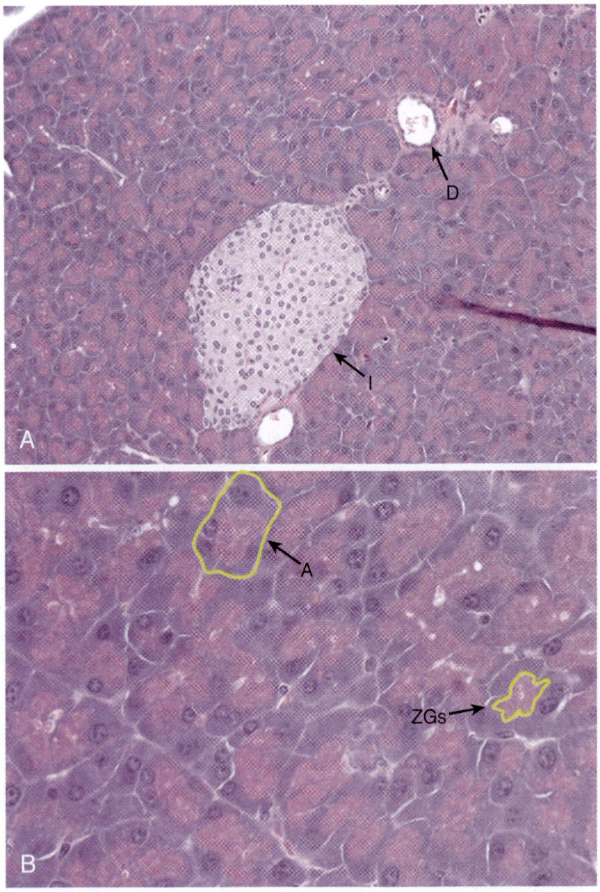

Fig. 23.2 Histology of the pancreas. (A) A low-power histological section of the pancreas showing a ductule (D) and an islet (I) (H&E). (B) A higher-power section showing numerous acini (A), which contain eosinophilic zymogen granules (ZGs). (*Source:* From Megha S. Mehta, Bradley A. Barth and Sohail Z. Husain. Anatomy, Histology, Embryology, and Developmental Anomalies of the Pancreas. Sleisenger and Fordtran's Gastrointestinal and Liver Disease. 11th edition. Elsevier 2021.)

behind the duodenum from right to left and fuse with the dorsal bud. This fusion of the dorsal and ventral pancreatic primordia is prone to incompleteness and imperfections, resulting in congenital variations and anomalies of the pancreas. The ventral bud forms the posterior head and the uncinate process, whereas the dorsal bud forms the anterior head, body and tail. Following this fusion, the ductal systems anastomose, a complicated process with a wide range of possible outcomes. The portion of the ventral duct between the dorsal–ventral fusion and the major papilla is termed the duct of Wirsung. The portion of the dorsal duct upstream to the dorsal–ventral fusion point is called the main pancreatic duct.

PANCREATIC DIVISUM

This is the most common congenital anomaly of the pancreas, with an incidence of 4%–14%. This results from the failure of fusion of the dorsal and the ventral ducts during development. Three variants have been described: type 1 or classical divisum, in which there is a complete failure of fusion; type 2, in which dorsal drainage is dominant in the absence of the main pancreatic duct; and type 3 or incomplete divisum, where a small communicating branch is present. In pancreatic divisum, the bulk of the pancreas drains into the duodenum through the small-sized minor papilla. Although most patients are asymptomatic, in some patients, this anomaly is associated with recurrent pancreatitis due to inadequate drainage of pancreatic secretions via the minor papilla.

ANNULAR PANCREAS (FIG. 23.3)

In this anomaly, the pancreas is present as a **band-like** or ring-like organ that completely encircles the second portion of the duodenum. This abnormal shape of the pancreas can be a cause of **duodenal obstruction**.

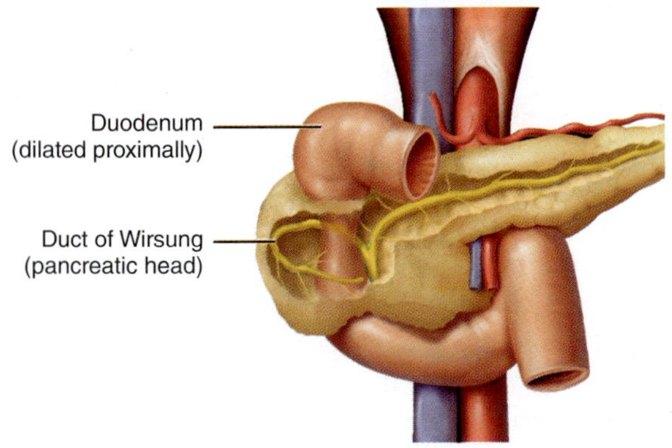

Fig. 23.3 Graphic shows the annular pancreas in which there is abnormal rotation and fusion of the ventral and dorsal pancreatic anlage resulting in a circumferential mass of pancreatic tissue that encircles and narrows the duodenum. The duct draining the pancreatic head encircles the second portion of the duodenum. This condition may remain asymptomatic or may result in obstruction of the duodenum, often in neonates.

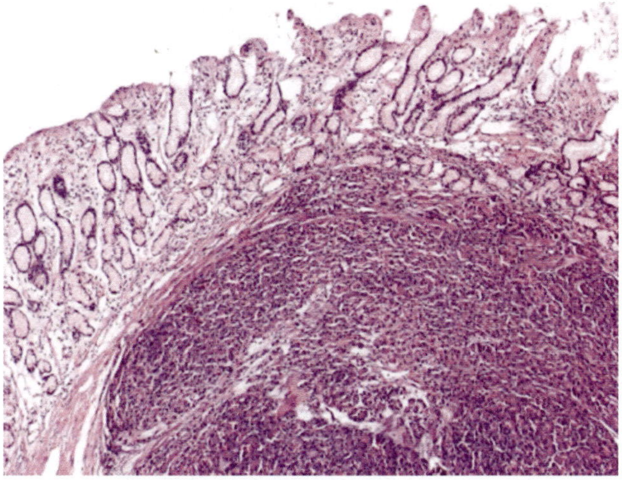

Fig. 23.4 Microscopy of the ectopic pancreas in gastric mucosa. (*Source:* https://pancreas.imedpub.com/heterotopic-pancreas-in-the-stomach-a-case-report-and-a-brief-review-of-the-literature.php?aid=1868)

ECTOPIC PANCREAS (FIG. 23.4)

Abnormal location of normal pancreatic tissue is termed as the ectopic pancreas and is found in 2% of routine autopsies. The common sites for ectopia are **stomach, duodenum, jejunum**, Meckel diverticulum and ileum. The pancreatic tissue in the ectopic site continues the secretory function. This anomaly is usually silent, but in a few cases, this may cause pain and mucosal bleeding.

AGENESIS

Complete failure of the development of pancreas is very rare. Some cases are due to inherited mutations of **PDX1**, a gene that is critically required for the development of the pancreas.

PANCREATITIS

Pancreatitis is the inflammation of the pancreatic parenchyma, which can be acute or chronic. Both forms are triggered by injuries to the pancreas, leading to autodigestion of the pancreas by its own enzymes.

In its normal state, the pancreas is protected from autodigestion by its own enzymes by the following mechanisms:

- Almost all the digestive enzymes of the pancreas are synthesized in the inactive proenzyme form and are packaged within secretory granules as zymogen granules.
- These proenzymes are activated by trypsin, which is produced and stored in the inactive form trypsinogen and activated by enteropeptidase in the duodenum. This maintains the intrapancreatic activation of proenzymes at a very minimal level.
- Acinar and ductal cells secrete trypsin inhibitors, such as serine protease inhibitor Kazal type 1 (SPINK1), which prevent intrapancreatic trypsin activity.

Table 23.1 Aetiological Factors for Acute Pancreatitis

Category	Common Causes
Metabolic	Alcoholism Hypercalcaemia Hyperlipoproteinaemia
Obstructive	Gallstones Trauma to the pancreas Iatrogenic injury to the pancreas
Genetic mutations	In the genes encoding trypsin, trypsin regulators and calcium regulators
Infections	Mumps
Acute ischaemia	Shock Thromboembolism Vasculitis
Drugs	Azathioprine Antiretroviral drugs Oestrogen

Pancreatitis is the result of the derangement of any or a combination of these protective mechanisms. Acute and chronic pancreatitis has different clinical and pathological presentations and is discussed in detail as follows.

ACUTE PANCREATITIS

Acute pancreatitis is a clinical condition characterized by a **reversible** parenchymal injury to the pancreas due to inflammation induced by varied aetiological factors. This is a relatively common condition in western countries, with a yearly incidence of 20 cases per 100,000 persons. The causes of acute pancreatitis are listed in Table 23.1, and the most common causes include **alcoholism** and **pancreatic duct obstruction** caused by biliary stone.

Pathogenesis (Fig. 23.5)

Pancreatitis is caused by inappropriate release and activation of pancreatic enzymes, which result in the destruction of pancreatic tissue and trigger an acute inflammatory reaction. Intrapancreatic activation of trypsin activates other proenzyme forms, such as prophospholipase and proelastase, which result in the digestion of fat and elastic fibres of the blood vessels, respectively. The kinin, coagulation and complement systems also get activated by the same trypsin mechanism. All these lead to inflammation, damage of blood vessel walls and small vessel thrombosis, which further aggravate acinar cell damage with the amplification of intrapancreatic activation of digestive enzymes.

The mechanisms leading to inappropriate intrapancreatic activation of pancreatic enzymes are as follows:

1. **Pancreatic duct obstruction** by gallstones or alcohol-associated concretions increases intraductal pressure, resulting in accumulation of the enzyme-rich interstitial

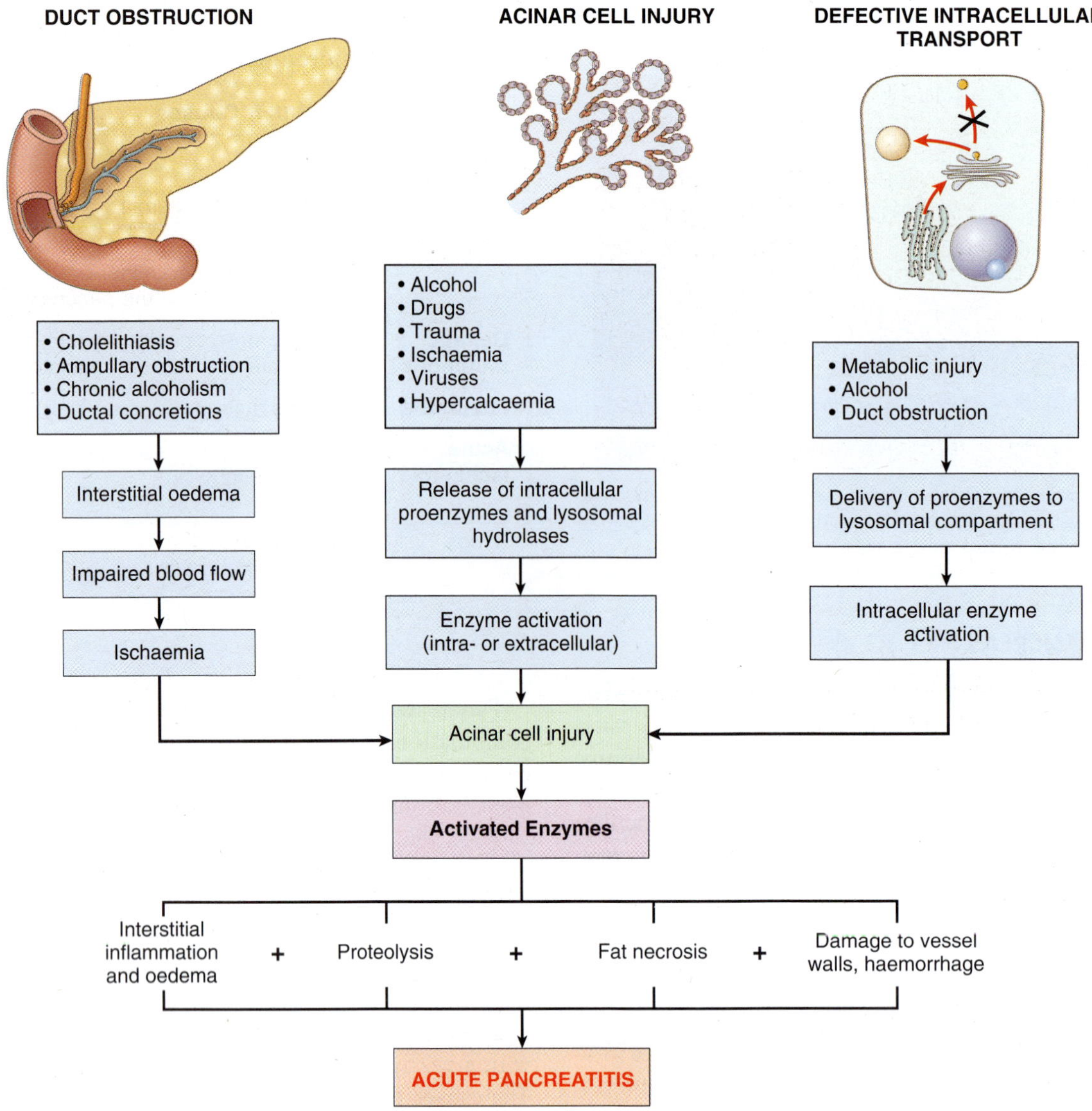

Fig. 23.5 Pathogenesis of acute pancreatitis. (*Source:* From Acute Pancreatitis. Elsevier Point of Care. 2022.)

fluid. This leads to fat necrosis that attracts neutrophils, which, in turn, release cytokines and cause interstitial oedema. This results in the impairment of blood flow and induces ischaemia, resulting in acinar cell injury.

2. **Acinar cell injury** caused by alcohol, drugs, trauma, ischaemia, infections and hypercalcaemia results in the premature release of proenzymes and lysosomal hydrolases within the pancreatic parenchyma.
3. **Defective intracellular transport of proenzymes** within the acinar cells occurs when the pancreatic proenzymes are inappropriately delivered to the intracellular compartment containing lysosomal hydrolases.

Role of Alcohol in Acute Pancreatitis

Alcohol can precipitate acute pancreatitis by any of the aforementioned mechanisms. The other mechanisms are as follows:

- Alcohol causes transient contraction of the sphincter of Oddi, and chronic alcoholism results in intraductal concretions by causing secretion of protein-rich pancreatic fluid.
- Alcohol is also directly toxic to pancreatic acinar cells.
- It also induces oxidative stress.

Hereditary Pancreatitis This entity is characterized by repeated attacks of acute severe pancreatitis that begins in the childhood, leading to chronic pancreatitis. The disease is due to genetic defects that increases or sustains the activity of trypsin. Three common genes that are mutated in hereditary pancreatitis are as follows:

1. PRSS1
2. SPINK1
3. CFTR

Most importantly, patients with hereditary pancreatitis are at a high risk of developing pancreatic carcinoma because of the association of chronic inflammation and malignancy.

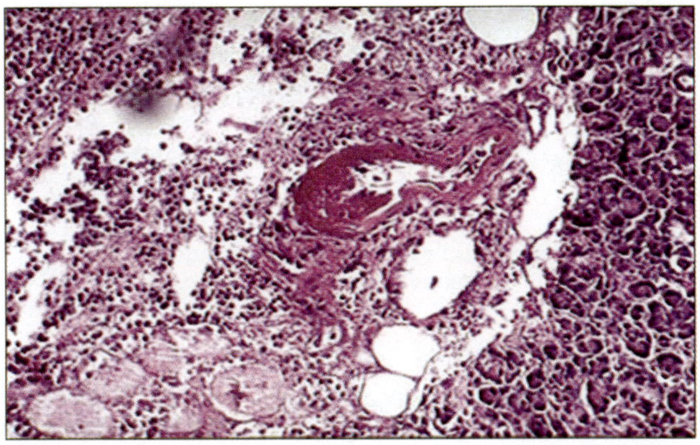

Fig. 23.6 Microscopy of acute severe pancreatitis with areas of inflammation and necrosis. A blood vessel within the necrotic area with fibrinoid necrosis is also seen. (*Source:* https://slideplayer.com/slide/9915942/)

Morphology (Fig. 23.6)

Morphology of acute pancreatitis varies from mild oedema to severe necrosis and haemorrhage depending on the severity of the inflammation. The fundamental changes are as follows:

- Acute inflammation
- Microvascular leakage and interstitial oedema
- Fat necrosis
- Parenchymal destruction
- Vessel wall damage and interstitial haemorrhage

The extent of each of these changes depends on the chronicity and severity of the disease. The pancreas is grossly swollen, indurated, oedematous, haemorrhagic or necrotic along with areas of fat necrosis. **Fat necrosis** is the result of lipase activity, and the released fatty acids combine with calcium to form insoluble salts which appear as yellow–white chalky areas.

There are many forms of acute pancreatitis, and the terminologies used for them are described as follows (Table 23.2):

- **Acute interstitial pancreatitis** – mild inflammation with oedema and fat necrosis
- **Acute necrotizing pancreatitis** – more severe form of inflammation with extensive necrosis which may be associated with haemorrhage
- **Haemorrhagic pancreatitis** – extensive parenchymal necrosis along with vast areas of haemorrhage
- **Biliary pancreatitis** – bile reflux through the common bile duct into the pancreatic duct due to abnormal junction between the two ducts
- **Infected pancreatic necrosis** – due to secondary infection of necrotic foci
- **Postoperative pancreatitis** – due to trauma of exploration of common bile duct, gastric resection surgeries, etc.

Table 23.2 Terminologies in Acute Pancreatitis[a]

Term	Definition
Acute pancreatitis	Acute inflammation of the pancreas with the variable involvement of peripancreatic tissues
Mild acute pancreatitis	Interstitial oedema of the pancreas; typically a benign clinical course with minimal organ dysfunction and full recovery
Moderately severe acute pancreatitis	Evidence of pancreatic necrosis with infectious complications and/or organ failure that resolves within 48 h of onset
Severe acute pancreatitis	Pancreatitis with associated organ failure that persists beyond 48-h duration
Acute fluid collection	Pancreatic or peripancreatic fluid, evident early in the course of disease; lacks wall/organization
Pancreatic pseudocyst	Collection of pancreatic juice contained within a capsule of fibrous tissue that arises after an episode of acute pancreatitis
Pancreatic necrosis	Diffuse or focal loss of viability of pancreatic parenchyma or peripancreatic fat
Pancreatic abscess	Localized collection of pus within pancreatic or peripancreatic tissue, containing little or no necrotic material

[a]Atlanta classification system for acute pancreatitis, 2012.
From Dave D. Paskar and John C. Marshall. Acute Pancreatitis. Critical Care Medicine: Principles of Diagnosis and Management in the Adult. 5th edition. Elsevier 2019.

Clinical Features

Acute abdominal pain is the predominant manifestation of acute pancreatitis. The pain is intense and constant and is localized to the upper back and left shoulder. The pain may be mild to excruciating, often accompanied by nausea, vomiting and loss of appetite. Severe acute pancreatitis is a medical emergency.

Laboratory Findings

Approximately 5% patients die during the first week, and the overall mortality varies from 20% in acute pancreatitis to 50% in haemorrhagic pancreatitis. A marked elevation in serum amylase and lipase levels is characteristic, and glycosuria is seen in some cases. Hypocalcaemia may be noted because of the precipitation of calcium soaps in fat necrosis. Imaging using computed tomography (CT) scan shows changes depicting inflammation and oedema of the pancreas and is an important investigation in patients suspected with acute pancreatitis.

Development of disseminated intravascular coagulation (DIC), adult respiratory distress syndrome (ARDS) and shock points towards the onset of systemic inflammatory response. The onset of systemic inflammatory response syndrome (SIRS) and acute tubular necrosis is a poor prognostic factor.

Management

'Resting' the pancreas by complete restriction of oral intake along with intravenous fluids and analgesics is the mainstay of treatment.

CHRONIC PANCREATITIS

Chronic pancreatitis is the chronic inflammation of pancreas characterized by irreversible destruction of the exocrine pancreas and fibrosis, which at a later stage progresses to the destruction of the endocrine pancreas.

Causes of Chronic Pancreatitis

- Chronic alcohol intake (the most common cause)
- Chronic pancreatic duct obstruction due to calculi or tumours
- Autoimmune pancreatitis
- Familial hereditary pancreatitis
- Nonalcoholic chronic tropical pancreatitis due to protein–calorie malnutrition
- Oxidative stress in idiopathic pancreatitis
- Secondary forms of autoimmune chronic pancreatitis associated with primary biliary cirrhosis and Sjögren syndrome
- Infections in immunocompromised patients

Pathogenesis

Chronic pancreatitis is mostly due to recurrent attacks of acute pancreatitis. This causes repeated episodes of perilobular fibrosis, duct distortion and altered pancreatic secretions, which eventually result in loss of pancreatic parenchyma and fibrosis. Injury to pancreatic tissue activates a complex interplay of growth factors, cytokines and chemokines, leading to the deposition of extracellular matrix and fibroblast proliferation that culminates into pancreatic fibrogenesis. This parenchymal damage and fibrosis is further aggravated by infiltration with inflammatory cells that release fibrogenic mediators such as **TGF-β and PDGF** (Fig. 23.7).

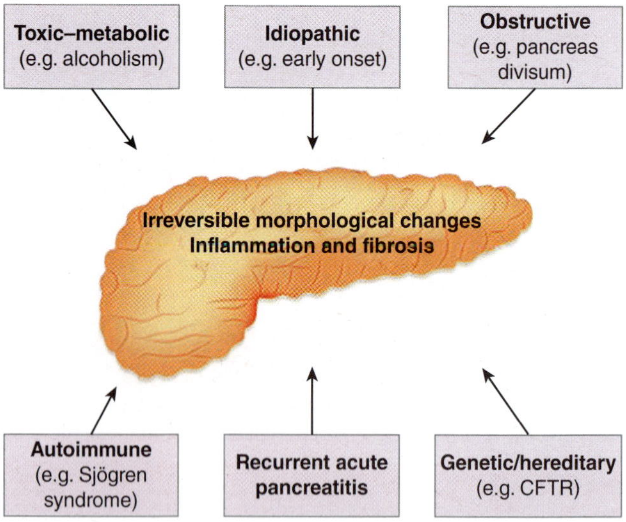

Fig. 23.7 Pathogenesis of chronic pancreatitis. (*Source:* From Giuseppe Orlando, Lorenzo Piemonti, Camillo Ricordi, et al. Transplantation, Bioengineering, and Regeneration of the Endocrine Pancreas, Volume 2, Elsevier Inc., 2020.)

Morphology (Fig. 23.8)

Characteristic morphological features of chronic pancreatitis are **fibrosis, atrophy and acinar loss** with pancreatic duct dilation. Grossly, the gland is hard and shrunken with dilated ducts. In the cases caused by alcoholism, intraluminal protein plugs and visible calcified concretions are commonly seen. In all these cases, there is a prominent chronic inflammatory infiltrate around the lobules and ducts. The lining epithelial cells of the ducts are atrophic or hyperplastic and may have areas of squamous metaplasia. Islets of Langerhans are usually spared and are lost at later stages. In autoimmune pancreatitis, there is prominent infiltration of IgG4-secreting plasma cells.

Clinical Features

Clinical manifestations are varied and characterized by recurrent episodes of acute pancreatitis. Diagnosis of chronic pancreatitis requires a high degree of suspicion. Abdominal pain is the most common presentation, and the presence of associated steatorrhoea and diabetes point in favour of this entity. During every attack, there is an elevation of **serum amylase** levels in early stages. CT scan and ultrasonography (USG) show the presence of pancreatic calcifications. Exocrine pancreatic insufficiency causes malabsorption and manifests in the form of oedema and weight loss.

Though the disease is not a life-threatening condition, the long-term prognosis is poor. The clinical presentation is complicated by the development of malabsorption and diabetes mellitus. In approximately 10% of patients, **pancreatic pseudocysts** develop and 40% of patients with hereditary pancreatitis have an increased risk of developing **pancreatic carcinoma**.

NON-NEOPLASTIC CYSTS OF THE PANCREAS

Cystic lesions of the pancreas is a group of pancreatic lesions with a characteristic cystic morphology. A majority of pancreatic cysts are non-neoplastic and can be classified into congenital cysts and pseudocysts. The common cystic lesions of the pancreas are listed in Table 23.3.

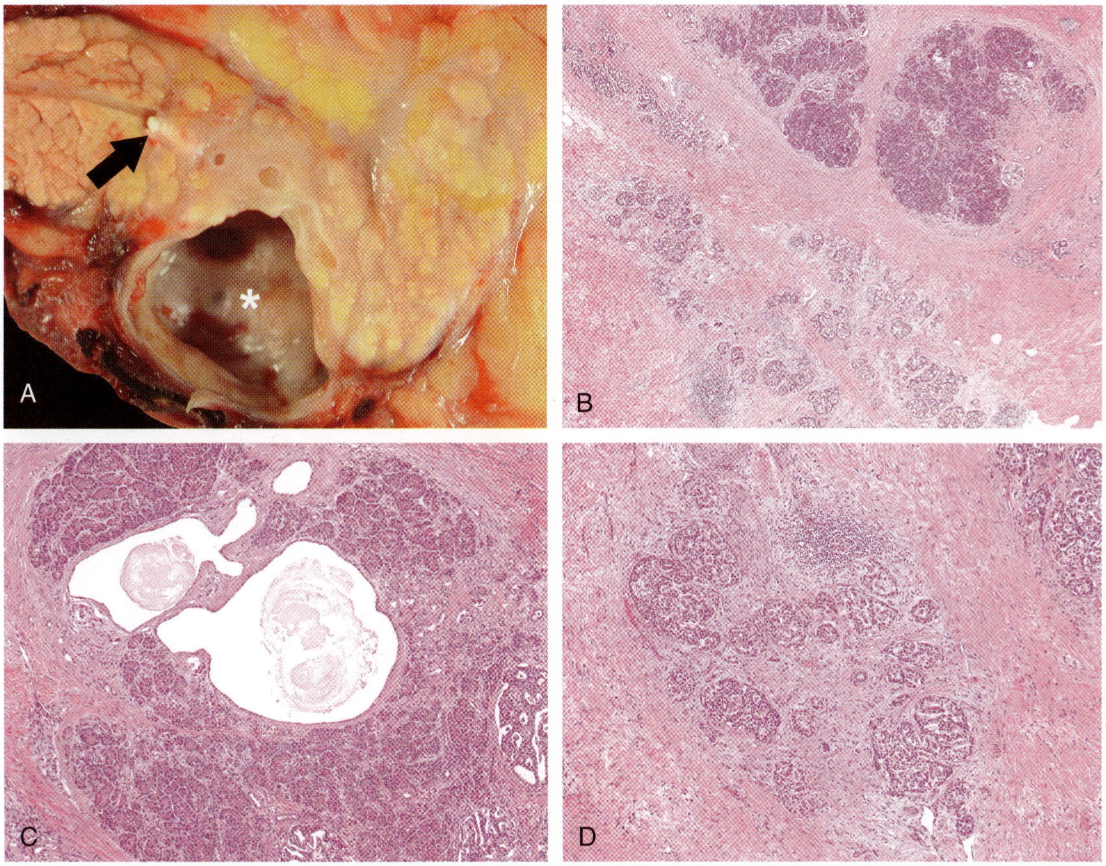

Fig. 23.8 (A) Although dependent on the aetiology (calculus, *black arrow*), the gross changes in obstructive chronic pancreatitis are confined to the pancreatic parenchyma distal to the obstruction. In addition, long-standing cases may develop retention cysts (*asterisk*). (B) Microscopically, pancreatic acinar, ductal and islet cell parenchyma are replaced by variable amounts of perilobular and interlobular fibrosis (H&E, original magnification ×40). (C) Because of the obstruction, normal concretions from the pancreatic ducts cannot exit the pancreas and result in ductal dilatation with intraluminal proteinaceous plugs (H&E, original magnification ×200). (D) As chronic pancreatitis continues, further fibrosis and parenchymal loss are identified with islets of Langerhans often found in aggregates (H&E, original magnification ×200). (*Source:* From Chronic Pancreatitis. Elsevier Point of Care. 2021.)

Table 23.3 Common Cystic Lesions of the Pancreas

Category	Common Examples
Non-neoplastic cysts	**Congenital cysts** • Sporadic • As a part of inherited syndromes • Autosomal dominant polycystic kidney disease • von Hippel–Lindau disease **Pseudocysts**
Neoplastic Cysts	
Benign	Serous cystic neoplasms
Precancerous	Intraductal papillary mucinous neoplasms Mucinous cystic neoplasms
Malignant	Solid pseudopapillary neoplasm Pancreatic serous cystadenocarcinoma Pancreatic mucinous cystadenocarcinoma

Here, we discuss the two common non-neoplastic cysts of the pancreas – congenital cysts and pseudocysts.

CONGENITAL CYSTS OF THE PANCREAS

True congenital cysts are extremely rare and pose a unique diagnostic and surgical challenge. These are thought to arise from the anomalous development of pancreatic ducts. Congenital cysts are generally asymptomatic and are discovered as incidental abdominal swellings but may become symptomatic when these cause pressure on adjacent organs.

Morphology

Congenital cysts range from 1 mm to 5 cm in diameter and are unilocular, thin-walled cysts. These cysts are lined by bland cuboidal cells and contain clear serous fluid.

As shown in Table 23.3, congenital cysts can be sporadic or a part of inherited syndromes like autosomal dominant polycystic kidney disease and von Hippel–Lindau disease.

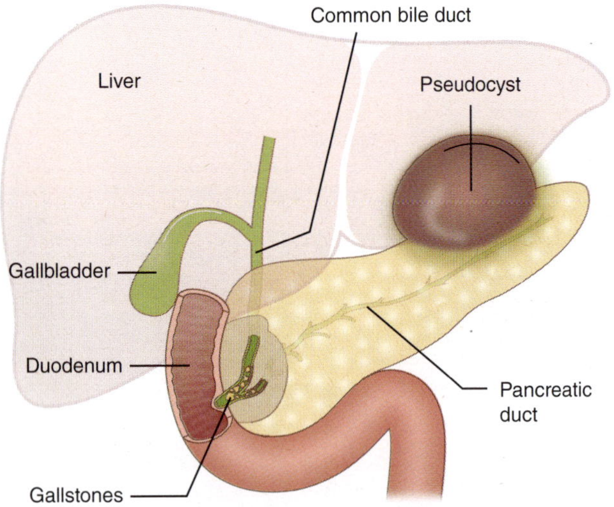

Fig. 23.9 Illustration of a pseudocyst of the pancreas.

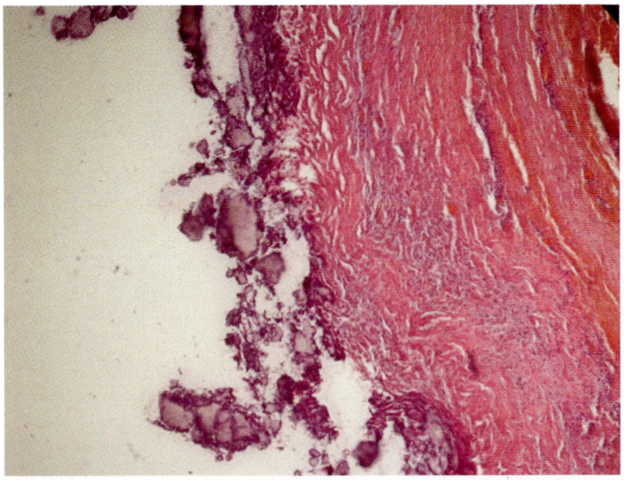

Fig. 23.10 Microscopy of pseudocyst of pancreas – note the absence of a lining epithelium, unlike true cysts. (*Source:* Courtesy of AFIP and PathologyOutlines.com)

The presence of congenital cysts of the pancreas should prompt workup to rule out associated inherited syndromes because of the morbidity and mortality of the associated lesions.

PANCREATIC PSEUDOCYSTS

Pancreatic pseudocysts account for the vast majority of cysts in the pancreas, which may be close to three-fourths of the cystic lesions of the pancreas. These commonly occur after an attack of acute pancreatitis in patients with chronic alcoholic pancreatitis. These may also occur as a result of **traumatic injury** to the pancreas.

Morphology (Figs 23.9 and 23.10)

Pancreatic pseudocyst is a circumscribed collection of fluid rich in pancreatic enzymes, blood and necrotic tissue usually communicating with the pancreatic ducts. It is typically located in the lesser sac of the omentum or retroperitoneum between the stomach and the transverse colon or between the stomach and the liver. Pseudocysts range from 2 to 30 cm in diameter. These are called pseudocysts because they do not have an epithelial lining, which is one of their characteristic features. The pseudocysts take up to 6 weeks to form following their predisposing condition.

Pancreatic pseudocysts present with abdominal discomfort and indigestion. Complications include infection, haemorrhage, compression, obstruction or rupture.

Diagnosis usually requires radiological investigations like CT and magnetic resonance cholangiopancreatography (MRCP).

Pancreatic pseudocysts can be managed conservatively with total parental nutrition. Surgical procedures like cystogastrostomy/cystojejunostomy/cystoduodenostomy are indicated if the cyst fails to resolve by 6 weeks following conservative management.

PANCREATIC NEOPLASMS

The pancreas gives rise to a large variety of distinct neoplasms which may be solid, cystic or intraductal. Pancreatic neoplasms recapitulate the various lines of differentiation present in the normal gland.

BENIGN AND LOW-GRADE CYSTIC NEOPLASMS

A majority of pancreatic cysts are non-neoplastic, whereas only 5%–15% of pancreatic cysts are neoplastic. Though invasive pancreatic malignancies can also present as cystic masses, here we restrict our discussion to benign, precancerous cystic neoplasms and low-grade malignant neoplasms of the pancreas.

- **Serous cystic neoplasms**
- **Mucinous cystic neoplasms**
- **Intraductal papillary mucinous neoplasms (IPMNs)**
- **Solid pseudopapillary neoplasm, papillary cystic neoplasm**

Serous Cystic Neoplasms (Serous Cystadenomas)

Serous cystadenomas are benign, focal cystic neoplasms which account for one-fourth of the cystic neoplasms of the pancreas and are commonly seen in the tail of the pancreas. It is more common in women and in those older than 50 years.

Morphology (Fig. 23.11)

The tumours are usually multicystic and characterized by the presence of tiny cysts of size with spongy appearance.

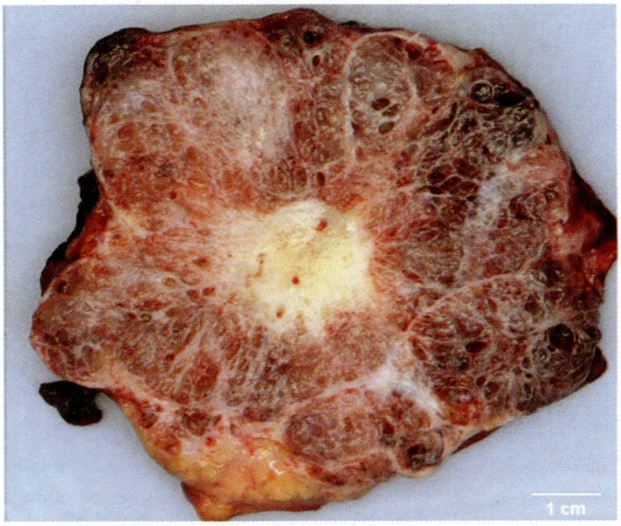

Fig. 23.11 Gross morphology of serous cystadenoma showing a well-circumscribed tumour with a characteristic spongy-appearing cut surface and a prominent central stellate scar. (*Source:* https://www.webpathology.com/image.asp?case=253&n=15)

The usual presentation is abdominal pain. The tumours are managed by surgical excision. The VHL gene is inactivated in most of these tumours.

Mucinous Cystic Neoplasms

Mucinous cystic neoplasms are **precursors to invasive carcinomas** and are malignant in approximately 25% of cases. These neoplasms mostly occur in women and are usually located in the tail of the pancreas as a painless slow-growing mass. The cyst wall is thin and may contain calcification in up to 15% of patients, which is the pathognomonic feature. The cavities rarely communicate with the pancreatic ducts. Features like irregularity of the walls, focal thickening, larger size of the cyst and solid regions within or outside the cyst are features indicative of malignancy. Endoscopic USG-guided fine-needle aspiration may be difficult as these cysts contain a thick viscous fluid which is an important clue for their diagnosis.

Morphology (Fig. 23.12)

Microscopically, the cyst wall is lined by columnar or cuboidal mucinous epithelial cells in approximately half of the cases, which is a diagnostic feature. The underlying stroma resembles ovarian stroma. This is pathognomonic and is helpful in differentiating this entity from an IPMN.

These lesions are associated with genetic mutations of TP53, KRAS and RNF43 and are generally excised owing to their high probability for malignant transformation.

Intraductal Papillary Mucinous Neoplasms

IPMNs are mucin-producing tumours which are usually seen in men older than 60 years.

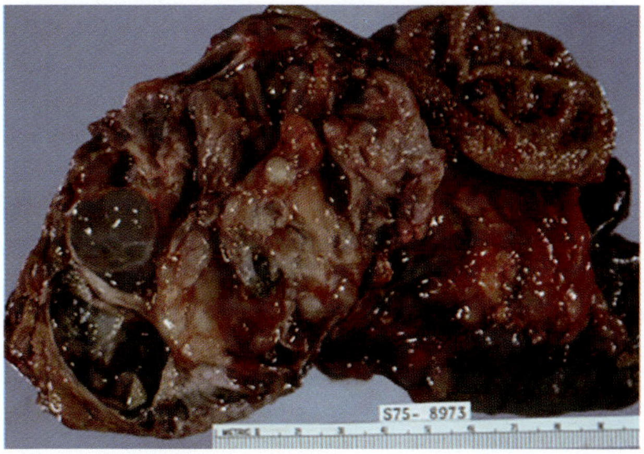

Fig. 23.12 Morphology of mucinous cystic neoplasms with the characteristic multilocular appearance with abundant mucin. (*Source:* From C. Robalo, J.O. Silva, J. Teixeira Oliveira, C. Silva, C. Branco, V. Simões, A. Canha, P. Soares, J. Daniel, D. Sousa Silva and J. Davide. Mucinous Cystadenoma of the Pancreas – A Case Series. HPB. 2021;23:S908-S909.)

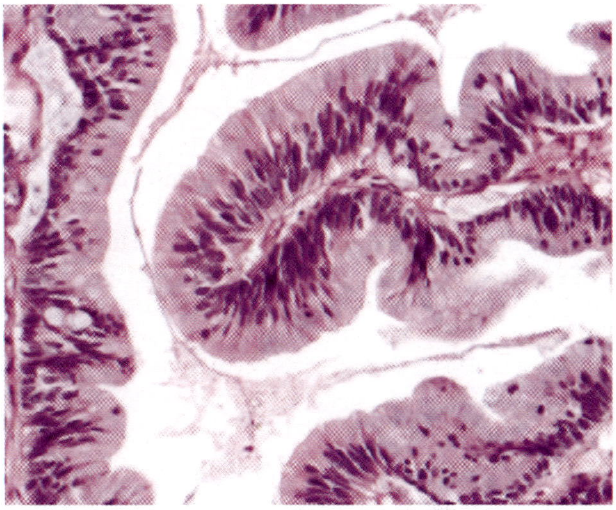

Fig. 23.13 Intraductal papillary mucinous neoplasms – microscopy (*Source:* https://pancreas.imedpub.com/obstructive-chronic-pancreatitis-andor-intraductal-papillary-mucinous-neoplasms-ipmns-a-21year-long-case-report.php?aid=2932)

Morphology (Fig. 23.13)

Unlike mucinous cystic neoplasms, IPMNs commonly involve the head of the pancreas and occupy part or whole length of the main pancreatic duct or side branches. Accordingly, IPMNs are divided into main duct type, branch duct type and mixed type. Most patients with an IPMN do not have invasive malignancy, and the progression of lesion is generally slower than mucinous cystadenomas.

Two classical features that help in differentiating IPMNs from mucinous cystic neoplasms are as follows:

a. Partial or diffuse dilatation of the main pancreatic duct
b. Absence of the dense ovarian stroma

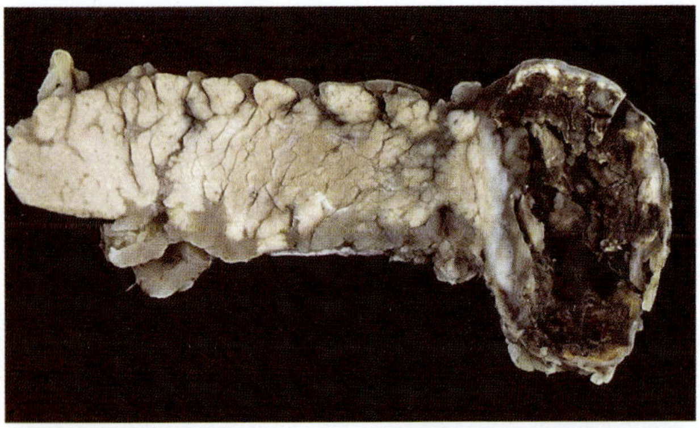

Fig. 23.14 Gross image of a solid pseudopapillary neoplasm of the pancreas with predominant areas of haemorrhagic necrosis. (*Source:* From Olca Basturk, Günter Klöppel and David S. Klimstra. Tumors of the Exocrine Pancreas. Diagnostic Histopathology of Tumors. 5th edition. Elsevier 2021.)

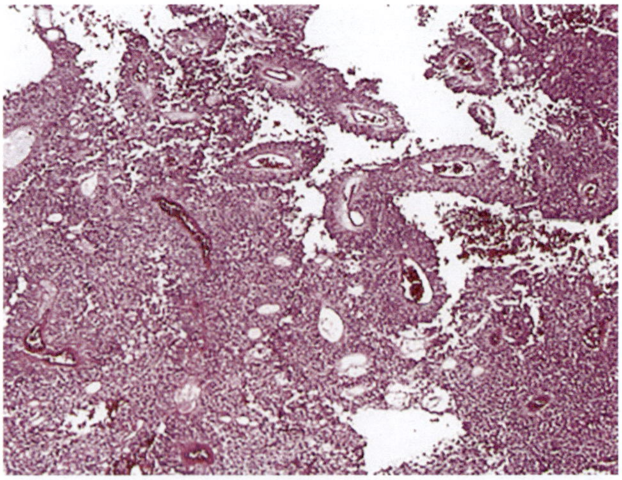

Fig. 23.15 Microscopy of solid pseudopapillary neoplasm consisting of sheets of cells and degenerative pseudopapillary structures. (*Source:* From Olca Basturk, Günter Klöppel and David S. Klimstra. Tumors of the Exocrine Pancreas. Diagnostic Histopathology of Tumors. 5th edition. Elsevier 2021.)

These lesions are associated with genetic mutations of **GNAS, KRAS, TP53, SMAD4 and RNF43**, and these lesions have to be excised to prevent malignant transformation.

Solid Pseudopapillary Neoplasm, Papillary Cystic Neoplasm

This locally invasive **low-grade malignant** pancreatic tumour is commonly seen in young females and is always noted in the tail or body of the pancreas. The tumours are grossly characterized by large, well-circumscribed lesions with solid and cystic areas filled with haemorrhagic debris (Fig. 23.14).

Morphology (Fig. 23.15)

Microscopically, the solid areas show the presence of branching papillae overlying a fibrovascular myxoid stroma while the cystic areas contain necrotic material in a haemorrhagic background.

Characteristically, the tumours are always associated with hyperactivation of the Wnt signalling pathway because of mutations of the β-catenin oncogene. Most patients can be cured by surgical excision with excellent prognosis.

PANCREATIC CARCINOMA PA 32.6

Pancreatic carcinoma is the 10th most common cancer in men and the 9th most common cancer in women, but it is the 4th leading cause of cancer deaths. It is a highly aggressive malignancy and responsible for 8% of all cancer-related deaths. Pancreatic carcinoma is estimated to become the second leading cause of cancer-related deaths by 2030.

Infiltrating ductal adenocarcinoma is by far the most common type of pancreatic malignancy, accounting for approximately 90% of all pancreatic malignant neoplasms. Hence, the terms 'pancreatic cancer' and 'pancreatic ductal adenocarcinoma' are used synonymously.

Precursors to Pancreatic Ductal Adenocarcinoma

Infiltrating pancreatic ductal carcinomas arise from precancerous lesions in small ducts of the pancreas called **'pancreatic intraepithelial neoplasia' (PanIN)** (Fig. 23.16). The disease progresses through several stages before becoming invasive. The sequence of PanIN to pancreatic carcinoma is strongly supported by the following observations (Fig. 23.17):

- PanIN is very often found in pancreatic parenchyma close to invasive carcinoma.
- PanIN precedes pancreatic carcinoma in experimental models.
- PanIN and pancreatic carcinoma share the same genetic and epigenetic changes.

Aetiological Factors

Pancreatic carcinoma can arise from the exocrine or endocrine pancreas, but 93% of carcinomas develop from the exocrine pancreas. Approximately **75%** of all pancreatic carcinomas occur within the **head or neck** of the pancreas, 15%–20% occur in the body of the pancreas and 5%–10% occur in the tail.

Pancreatic carcinoma primarily affects people aged 60–80 years. Following are the risk factors associated with pancreatic cancer:

- Tobacco smoking, the most common recognized risk factor
- Obesity and dietary factors because consumption of diet rich in fats is associated with greater risk
- Chronic pancreatitis; risk is higher in hereditary pancreatitis

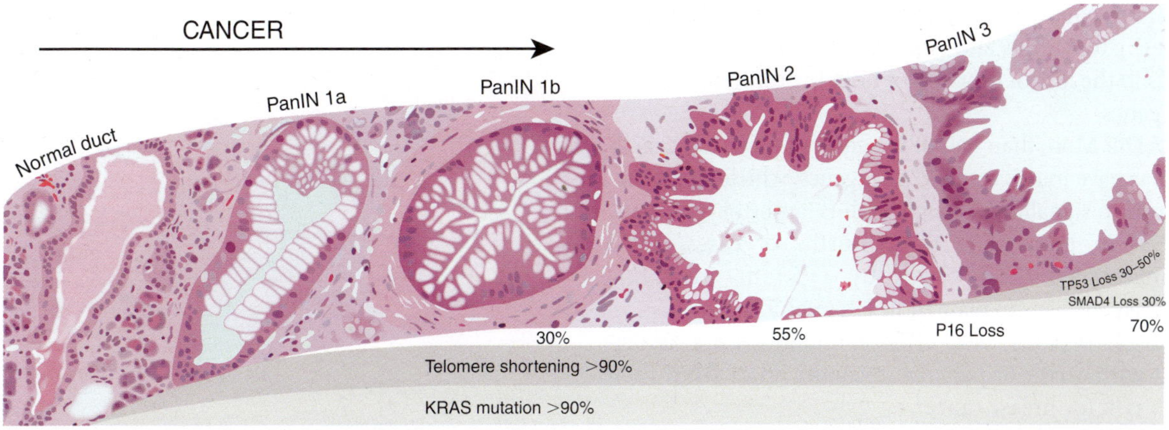

Fig. 23.16 Progression of normal pancreatic ducts through PanIN to invasive carcinoma. (*Source:* https://www.researchgate.net/figure/Pancreatic-cancer-develops-from-the-well-defined-precursor-lesions-pancreatic_fig2_303853276)

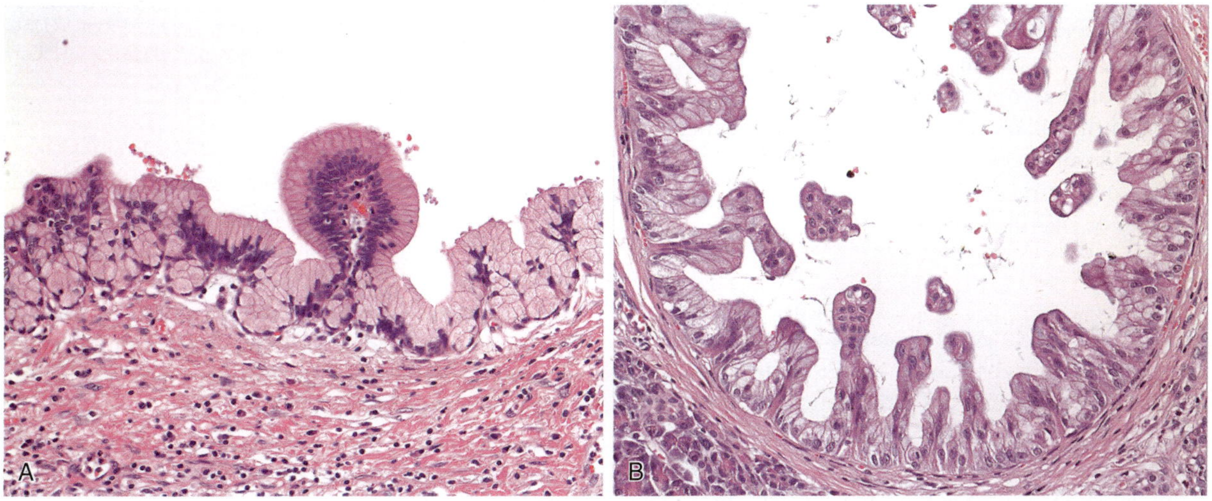

Fig. 23.17 (A and B) Microscopy of PanIN. (*Source:* From Olca Basturk, Günter Klöppel and David S. Klimstra. Tumors of the Exocrine Pancreas. Diagnostic Histopathology of Tumors. 5th edition. Elsevier 2021.)

- Alcohol consumption, especially when associated with chronic pancreatitis
- Family history of pancreatic cancer
- Genetic factors (described in the following section)
- Long-standing diabetes mellitus
- Race – black men have the highest incidence rate
- Inherited syndromes, listed in Table 23.4.

Pathogenesis

Molecular genetics of pancreatic adenocarcinoma have been studied in detail. Of these tumours, 80%–95% have activating mutations of the KRAS2 gene, 85%–100% have mutations in the CDKN2 gene, 50% have p53 mutations and 55% have mutations or homozygous deletion of the Smad4 gene. Some of these mutations are also seen in high-risk precursors of pancreatic cancer.

1. **KRAS:** The initial changes appear to be related to KRAS2 gene mutations and telomere shortening. KRAS is a small GTP-binding protein that is usually involved in signal transmission of growth factor receptors and activates many progrowth pathways.

Table 23.4 List of Inherited Syndromes Associated With Pancreatic Cancer

Syndrome	Genes Mutated
Hereditary breast and ovarian cancer syndrome	BRCA1 or BRCA2
Hereditary breast cancer	PALB2
Familial atypical multiple mole melanoma syndrome (FAMMM)	P16/CDKN2A
Familial pancreatitis	PRSS1
Lynch syndrome	MLH1 or MSH2
Peutz–Jeghers syndrome	STK11

2. **Telomere shortening:** A critical shortening of telomere length in precancerous lesions may predispose PanIN to progress to invasive carcinoma because of the progressive accumulation of genetic mutations.
3. **CDKN2A:** This is the most commonly mutated tumour suppressor gene in pancreatic cancers. Because this

complex codes for two important tumour suppressor genes, p16/INK4a and ARF, inactivation of CDKN2A leads to the loss of function of both the tumour suppressor genes.
4. **SMAD4:** More than half of the cases of pancreatic carcinomas have inactivated SMAD4 genes, which play a major role in signalling through TGF-β family of receptors.
5. **TP53:** In more than three-fourths of cases, TP53 is inactivated. Role played by TP53 in preventing tumorigenesis is explained in Chapter 7.
6. **BRCA2:** Persons with BRCA2 mutations are associated with a risk of pancreatic cancer apart from their high risk for breast cancer.

Apart from the aforementioned genes, there are many other mutations and genetic changes like DNA methylation abnormalities associated with the development of pancreatic carcinoma.

A majority of the carcinomas of pancreatic head cause obstruction of the common bile duct, resulting in the distension of the biliary tree and jaundice. The cancers of the body and tail do not cause obstruction and remain silent for a long time, leading to a larger size and advanced stage at the time of presentation.

Morphology

Gross (Fig. 23.18) In general, pancreatic cancers present as grey–white, stellate, hard and ill-defined masses. The two classical features of pancreatic cancer are its highly invasive nature and the tendency to evoke an intense desmoplastic response. Pancreatic carcinoma has the tendency to invade the adjacent structures like spleen, adrenals, colon, stomach and most notably nerves, blood vessels and the serosal surfaces.

Microscopy (Fig. 23.19) Most common histological type of pancreatic carcinoma is **ductal adenocarcinoma** in which the neoplastic cells are arranged in a glandular pattern. Less common histological types include giant cell carcinoma, adenosquamous carcinoma, microglandular adenocarcinoma, mucinous carcinoma, cystadenocarcinoma, papillary cystic carcinoma, acinar cystadenocarcinoma and acinar cell cystadenocarcinoma.

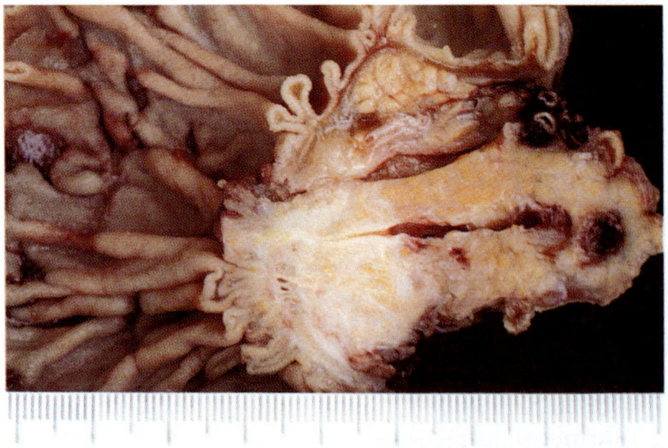

Fig. 23.18 Gross morphology of ductal adenocarcinoma in the head of the pancreas showing invasion of the ampulla and the duodenal wall and obstruction of the common bile duct and the pancreatic duct. (*Source:* From Olca Basturk, Günter Klöppel and David S. Klimstra. Tumors of the Exocrine Pancreas. Diagnostic Histopathology of Tumors. 5th edition. Elsevier 2021.)

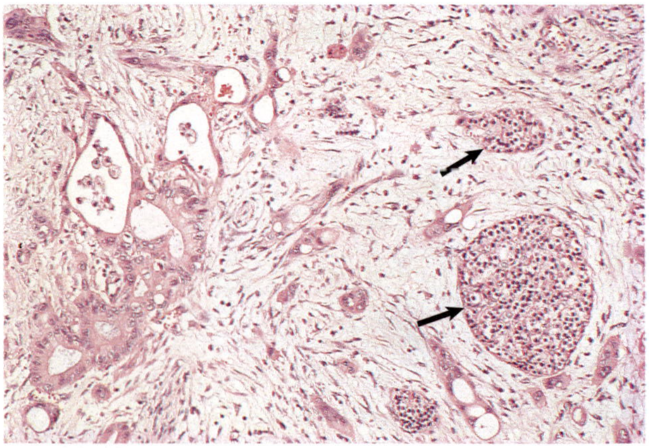

Fig. 23.19 Microscopic picture of pancreatic cancer showing the neoplastic glands with atypical nuclei invested by dense fibrous connective tissue, thus mimicking the texture of chronic pancreatitis when the gland is palpated during surgery. Islets of Langerhans (arrowed) survive at the edge of the tumour. (*Source:* From Judith I. Wyatt and Beate Haugk. Liver, biliary system and pancreas. Underwood's Pathology. Seventh Edition. Elsevier 2019.)

There are no histological differences between carcinomas of the head, body and tail of the pancreas. The vast majority of them are moderate to poorly differentiated adenocarcinomas with a highly infiltrative pattern and a severe desmoplastic response.

A common finding in these carcinomas is the presence of **perineural invasion**, which is the reason for the intense pain the patients commonly present with.

Clinical Features

Patients with pancreatic cancers are usually asymptomatic until the tumour invades the adjacent structures. A majority of patients present with a gradual onset of nonspecific symptoms like anorexia, malaise, nausea, fatigue and midepigastric or back pain, before presenting with relatively specific symptoms and signs mentioned as follows:

- Significant weight loss is a characteristic feature.
- Unrelenting nocturnal pain is a common complaint but usually a sign of advanced disease.
- Recent-onset diabetes mellitus can be a clue to the underlying disease.
- Painless obstructive jaundice and intense pruritus occur because of common bile duct obstruction in tumours of the head of the pancreas.
- Venous thrombosis and migratory thrombophlebitis (**Trousseau sign**) due to the release of platelet-activating

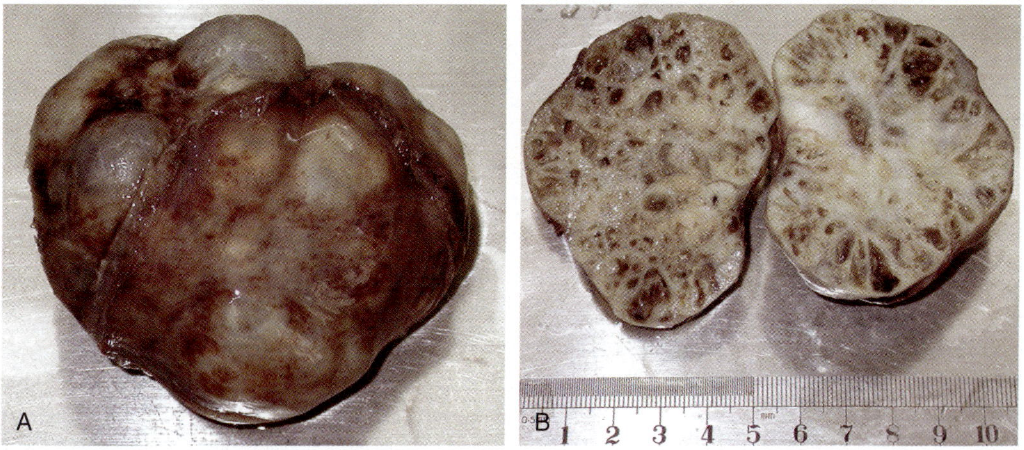

Fig. 23.20 (A and B) Gross morphology of pancreatoblastoma with a solid nodular growth pattern. (*Source:* From Bharti Rathore. Bone Tumor, Primary Malignant. Elsevier 2022.)

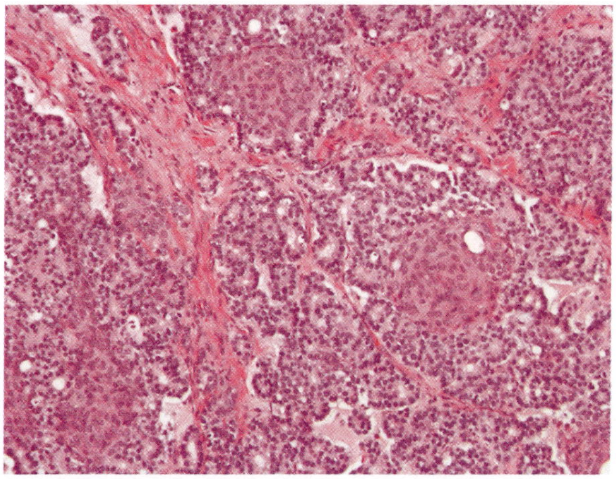

Fig. 23.21 Microscopy of pancreatoblastoma with a lobulated solid and acinar growth pattern and scattered squamoid corpuscles. (*Source:* From Olca Basturk, Günter Klöppel and David S. Klimstra. Tumors of the Exocrine Pancreas. Diagnostic Histopathology of Tumors. 5th edition. Elsevier 2021.)

factors and procoagulants from the tumour cells and necrotic cells may be the first symptom in some patients.
- Gallbladder may be palpable – **Courvoisier sign.**
- Ascites, abdominal mass, paraumbilical subcutaneous metastases (Sister Mary Joseph nodules), palpable nodules in the rectal pouch (Blumer shelf) and the palpable metastatic cervical nodes indicate an advanced incurable stage of the disease.

Radiological tests like CT scanning, transcutaneous USG, endoscopic USG, MRI, endoscopic retrograde cholangiopancreatography help in confirming the location of the cancer and the extent of invasion. Tumour markers such as **CA19-9** antigen and **CEA** are elevated in 75%–85% and 40%–45% of patients, respectively. Though they cannot be used to diagnose the disease, these markers can be used to monitor the disease activity and tumour response to treatment.

Course and Prognosis

In general, the course of pancreatic cancer is brief and rapidly progressive as most of the cases present in an advanced and widely invasive inoperable stage.

PANCREATOBLASTOMA

Pancreatoblastoma is the most common malignant pancreatic tumour in children. It is a rare malignant neoplasm of the pancreas affecting children between the ages of 5 and 15 years. Pancreatoblastoma arises from the epithelial exocrine cells of the pancreas. The tumour is grossly characterized by partial encapsulation and lobulation.

Morphology (Figs 23.20 and 23.21)

Microscopic findings are quite characteristic with the presence of a mixture of **acinar cells and squamoid corpuscles**.

It is a slow-growing tumour with a varied presentation and a better survival rate.

SELF-ASSESSMENT

Multiple Choice Questions

1. A 45-year-old male presents with severe epigastric pain radiating to the back and elevated serum amylase levels. A CT scan reveals pancreatic enlargement. Which of the following is the most likely diagnosis?
   A. Pancreatic carcinoma
   B. Chronic pancreatitis
   C. Acute pancreatitis
   D. Pancreatic pseudocyst
2. A patient with a history of heavy alcohol use presents with persistent abdominal pain and calcifications in the pancreas on imaging. Which of the following is the most likely diagnosis?
   A. Acute pancreatitis
   B. Chronic pancreatitis

C. Pancreatic adenocarcinoma
D. Pancreatic neuroendocrine tumour

3. A 55-year-old woman presents with jaundice, weight loss and a painless palpable gallbladder. Imaging shows a mass in the head of the pancreas. Which of the following is the most likely diagnosis?
   A. Chronic pancreatitis
   B. Pancreatic carcinoma
   C. Pancreatic pseudocyst
   D. Pancreatic serous cystadenoma
4. A patient presents with a cystic lesion in the pancreas, and EUS-FNA suggests a mucinous cyst. Which of the following is the most likely diagnosis?
   A. Serous cystadenoma
   B. Mucinous cystic neoplasm
   C. Intraductal papillary mucinous neoplasm (IPMN)
   D. Pancreatic pseudocyst
5. A 60-year-old patient presents with diabetes, skin rash and weight loss. Imaging reveals a lesion in the pancreas. Which of the following is the most likely diagnosis?
   A. Pancreatic adenocarcinoma
   B. Chronic pancreatitis
   C. Pancreatic neuroendocrine tumour
   D. Pancreatic pseudocyst
6. A biopsy from a pancreatic mass shows cells arranged in a trabecular pattern with amyloid deposits. This finding is indicative of:
   A. Pancreatic adenocarcinoma
   B. Chronic pancreatitis
   C. Pancreatic neuroendocrine tumour
   D. Pancreatic serous cystadenoma
7. A 50-year-old female presents with a history of multiple episodes of pancreatitis. Imaging reveals a calcified mass in the pancreatic duct. Which of the following is the most likely diagnosis?
   A. Chronic pancreatitis with pancreatic stones
   B. Pancreatic adenocarcinoma
   C. Intraductal papillary mucinous neoplasm (IPMN)
   D. Pancreatic serous cystadenoma
8. A patient presents with a solid pancreatic mass with well-defined borders on imaging. A biopsy reveals epithelial cells with clear cytoplasm. Which of the following is the most likely diagnosis?
   A. Pancreatic neuroendocrine tumour
   B. Pancreatic pseudocyst
   C. Pancreatic adenocarcinoma
   D. Solid pseudopapillary tumour
9. A patient presents with steatorrhea, diabetes mellitus and a history of recurrent abdominal pain. Which of the following is the most likely diagnosis?
   A. Acute pancreatitis
   B. Chronic pancreatitis
   C. Pancreatic pseudocyst
   D. Pancreatic adenocarcinoma
10. A patient with a pancreatic mass shows elevated serum levels of CA 19-9. This finding is most suggestive of:
   A. Pancreatic neuroendocrine tumour
   B. Chronic pancreatitis
   C. Pancreatic adenocarcinoma
   D. Intraductal papillary mucinous neoplasm (IPMN)

Answers

1. (C); 2. (B); 3. (B); 4. (B); 5. (C); 6. (C); 7. (A); 8. (D); 9. (B); 10. (C)

Scenario-Based Questions

1. A patient presents with abdominal pain, weight loss and jaundice. Imaging reveals a mass in the head of the pancreas and dilatation of the common bile duct.
   Discuss the differential diagnosis, necessary investigations to confirm the diagnosis and potential treatment options for this patient.
2. A 30-year-old woman with no significant medical history presents with recurrent episodes of severe abdominal pain radiating to the back. Laboratory tests reveal elevated serum lipase levels.
   Describe the likely diagnosis, the pathophysiology behind the symptoms, and the management approach, including both immediate and long-term strategies.
3. During a routine check-up, a 55-year-old man is found to have a cystic lesion in the pancreas on abdominal ultrasound. He is asymptomatic and has no history of pancreatitis.
   Explain the approach to differentiate between benign and malignant cystic lesions of the pancreas and the subsequent management plan for this patient.
4. A patient diagnosed with a pancreatic neoplasm has a biopsy revealing a well-differentiated tumour with a trabecular pattern and positive chromogranin A staining.
   Discuss the implications of these histopathological findings, including the type of tumour, prognosis and treatment options.
5. A 60-year-old patient with a history of chronic pancreatitis presents with steatorrhoea and new-onset diabetes mellitus.
   Explain the connection between the patient's chronic pancreatitis and their current symptoms, and outline a comprehensive management plan.

Topics for Self-Directed Learning

1. Compare and contrast the mediators involved in acute and chronic pancreatitis.
2. Describe involvement of the pancreas and other organs in IgG4 disease.
3. Describe involvement of the pancreas in von Hippel–Lindau disease.
4. Describe somatic molecular alterations in pancreatic carcinoma.

The Kidney

24

S Shanmugapriya, Gayathri Devi Thanigaimani

PA 28.1 Describe the **normal histology** of the kidney.

PA 28.2 Define, classify and distinguish the clinical syndromes and describe the aetiology, pathogenesis, pathology, morphology, clinical, laboratory and urinary findings, and complications of **renal failure**.

PA 28.3 Define and describe the aetiology, precipitating factors, pathogenesis, pathology, laboratory and urinary findings, progression and complications of **acute renal failure**.

PA 28.4 Define and describe the aetiology, precipitating factors, pathogenesis, pathology, laboratory urinary findings, progression and complications of **chronic renal failure**.

PA 28.5 Define and classify glomerular diseases. Enumerate and describe the aetiology, pathogenesis, mechanisms of glomerular injury, pathology, distinguishing features and clinical manifestations of **glomerulonephritis**.

PA 28.6 Define and classify glomerular diseases. Enumerate and describe the aetiology, pathogenesis, mechanisms of glomerular injury, pathology, distinguishing features and clinical manifestations of glomerulonephritis of **IgA nephropathy**.

PA 28.7 Enumerate and describe the findings in **glomerular manifestations of systemic disease**.

PA 28.8 Enumerate and classify **diseases affecting the tubular interstitium**.

PA 28.9 Define and describe the aetiology, pathogenesis, pathology, laboratory and urinary findings, progression and complications of **acute tubular necrosis**.

PA 28.10 Describe the aetiology, pathogenesis, pathology, laboratory findings, distinguishing features, progression and complications of **acute and chronic pyelonephritis and reflux nephropathy**.

PA 28.11 Define, classify and describe the aetiology, pathogenesis, pathology, laboratory and urinary findings, distinguishing features, progression and complications of **vascular diseases of the kidney**.

PA 28.12 Define, classify and describe the genetics, inheritance, aetiology, pathogenesis, pathology, laboratory and urinary findings, distinguishing features, progression and complications of **cystic diseases of the kidney**.

PA 28.13 Define, classify and describe the aetiology, pathogenesis, pathology, laboratory and urinary findings, distinguishing features, progression and complications of **renal stone disease and obstructive uropathy**.

PA 28.14 Classify and describe the aetiology, genetics, pathogenesis, pathology, presenting features, progression and spread of **renal tumours**.

PA 28.15 Describe the aetiology, genetics, pathogenesis, pathology, presenting features and progression of **thrombotic angiopathies**.

CHAPTER OUTLINE

INTRODUCTION AND BASICS

'And righteousness shall be the girdle of his loins, and faithfulness the girdle of his **reins**'. From time immemorial, the kidneys along with the heart have been the considered seats of conscience and reflection, which has several references as 'Reins' in the *Bible* and the *Talmud*.

The ancient Indian Ayurvedic system has considered the kidneys to be the key player of the cleansing system in the body and the colour of urine as the determinant of health and temperament of a person.

The kidneys are important organs of our body that help to purify our blood, filtering out toxic substances. Abnormalities in the renal function may occur in any age group due to several pathologies that are dealt with in this chapter.

For better understanding of the pathological disorders of the kidney, it is better to compartmentalize the different morphological zones of the kidney, which are as follows:

1. Glomerular compartment
2. Tubular compartment
3. Interstitium
4. Blood vessels

Primary disorders of the glomerulus are immune complex mediated, whereas disorders affecting the tubulointerstitial compartment are toxin induced or due to infectious agents. This will be a reflection of the manifestations of the disease that makes it easy to narrow down to a precise diagnosis.

ANATOMY (FIG. 24.1)

Each kidney is bean shaped weighing approximately 150 g in adults, which ranges from 125 to 175 g for men and 115 to 155 g for women.

The kidney is surrounded by four layers of fat and fascia, namely the renal capsule, perirenal fat, Gerota's fascia and pararenal fat – the outermost layer. The cut surface of the kidney shows differentiation into the cortex and the medulla. The medulla projects into the cortex in the form of conical-shaped renal pyramids; the tips of the pyramid are called papillae and terminate in the minor calyces; the minor calyces join to form major calyces. The major calyces finally drain the collected urine into the renal pelvis from which arise the ureters. The region of the kidney containing the pelvis of the ureter is called hilum. Apart from the ureter, the hilum also contains the renal artery, vein and lymphatics.

A **nephron** is the functional unit of the kidney. Each kidney contains approximately 1 million nephrons. The first part of the nephron is the **glomerulus** (renal corpuscle), which lies mainly in the renal cortex, followed by the **proximal convoluted tubule**, which also lies mainly in the renal cortex. This is followed by the loop of Henle, which is partly in the cortex and partly extends deep into the medulla. The loop of Henle is composed of a thin part and a thick part. This is followed by the distal convoluted tubule that lies in the renal medulla. Part of the **distal convoluted tubule** comes into contact with the hilum of the glomerulus and afferent arteriole. Cells in the hilum of the glomerulus and those in the distal convoluted tubule and afferent arteriole are modified to form the **juxtaglomerular apparatus**. The convoluted tubule ends into the collecting duct that lies partly in the cortex and partly in the medulla. In the medulla, collecting ducts descend in the pyramids and unite at the tips of the renal pyramid to form ducts of Bertini that discharge urine into the renal pelvis. The structure of a nephron includes glomeruli and tubules.

HISTOLOGY OF KIDNEY (FIG. 24.2) PA 28.1

The glomerulus consists of Bowman's capsule, Bowman's space and the glomerular capillary tuft (filtration unit). There are three types of cells that can be seen in the structure of the glomerulus – the epithelium, which is two layered, namely visceral epithelia (the **podocytes**) and the parietal epithelium that line Bowman's space;

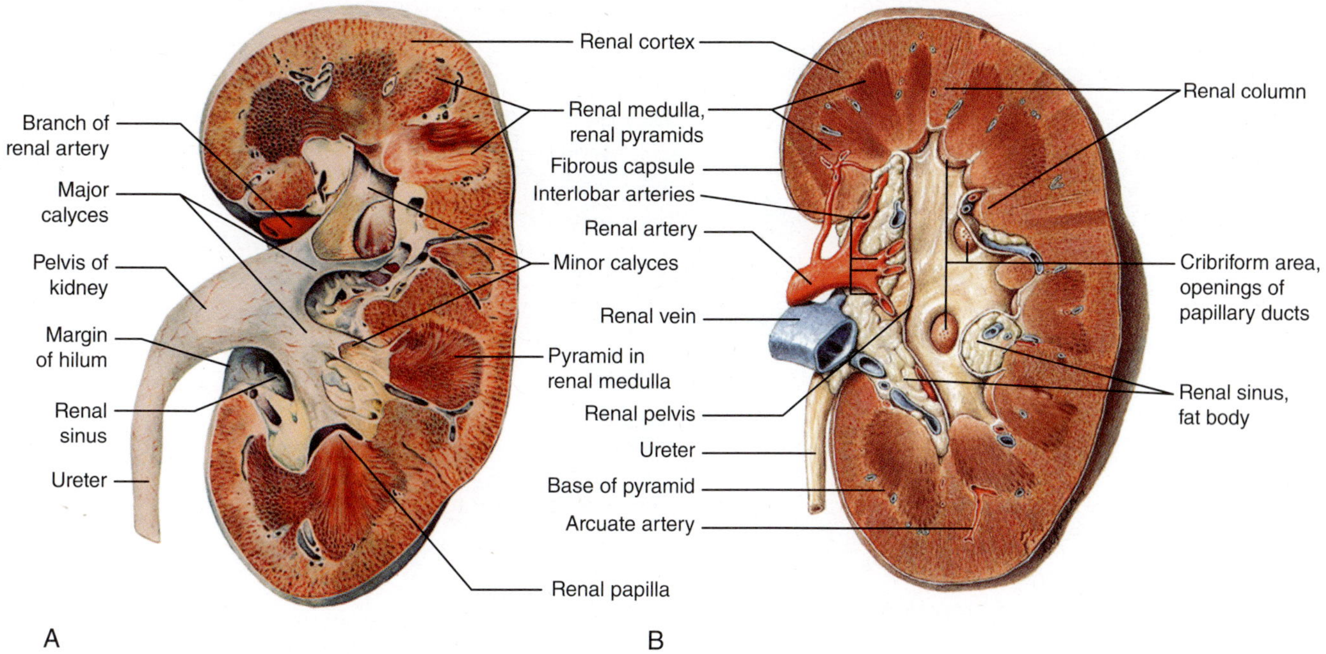

Fig. 24.1 (A and B) Anatomy of the kidney. (*Source:* From Acute Kidney Injury. Elsevier Point of Care. 2022.)

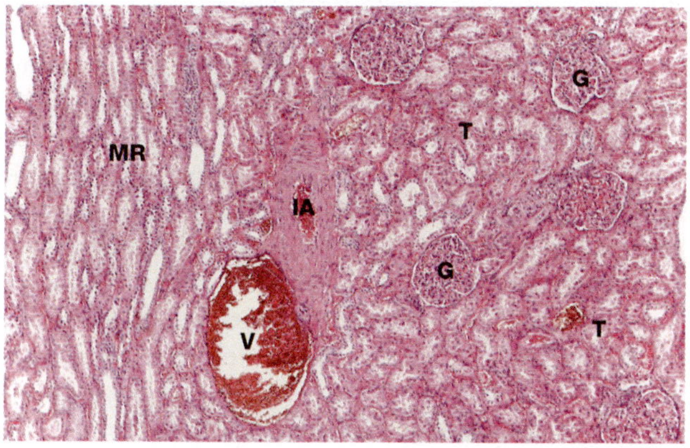

Fig. 24.2 Histology of renal cortex shows glomeruli with interspersed tubules. G, glomeruli; IA, interlobar artery; MR, medullary ray; T, tubules; V, vein. (*Source:* From Barbara Young BSc Med Sci (Hons), PhD, MB BChir, MRCP, FRCPA, Geraldine O'Dowd BSc (Hons), MBChB (Hons), FRCPath and Phillip Woodford MB BS, FRCPA. Urinary system. Wheater's Functional Histology. 6th edition. Elsevier 2014.)

the vascular endothelium of the capillaries; and the mesangial cells, which are mostly located near the vascular pole. The proximal tubules are lined by cuboidal cells that have abundant cytoplasm to the extent of obscuring the lumen. The distal convoluted tubules may be distinctly identified by the presence of lumen inside the tubules. The medulla comprises tubules forming a pyramidal arrangement that terminates into a transitional epithelium-lined urinary space called minor calyx. The cortical regions may be seen between the renal pyramids and are called renal columns.

The renal pelvis is lined by transitional epithelium. It extends downward as the ureter, which is also lined by transitional epithelium and is surrounded by muscular coat that helps in peristalsis.

BLOOD FLOW IN KIDNEY

The kidneys receive 25% of the cardiac output. The renal artery divides into the anterior and posterior branches that further divide several times to give rise to vessels in the order of interlobar arteries that courses through the lobes, divides into the arcuate artery at the corticomedullary junction and finally divides into the interlobular arteries and afferent arterioles. These then proceed to become efferent arterioles that, in turn, become the peritubular vascular network that finally unites to form the renal vein. The cortex is supplied by the peritubular vascular network, and the medulla is supplied by the vasa recta that arise from the efferent arteriole.

PHYSIOLOGY OF FILTRATION

The major components of the glomerular filtration apparatus are as follows (Fig. 24.3):

- **Endothelium:** The capillary endothelium is fenestrated, with fenestra being about 70–100 nm.
- **Glomerular basement membrane (GBM):** It is made up of a dense central layer (lamina densa) flanked on either side by thinner layers (lamina rara interna and lamina rara externa). GBM is composed of type IV

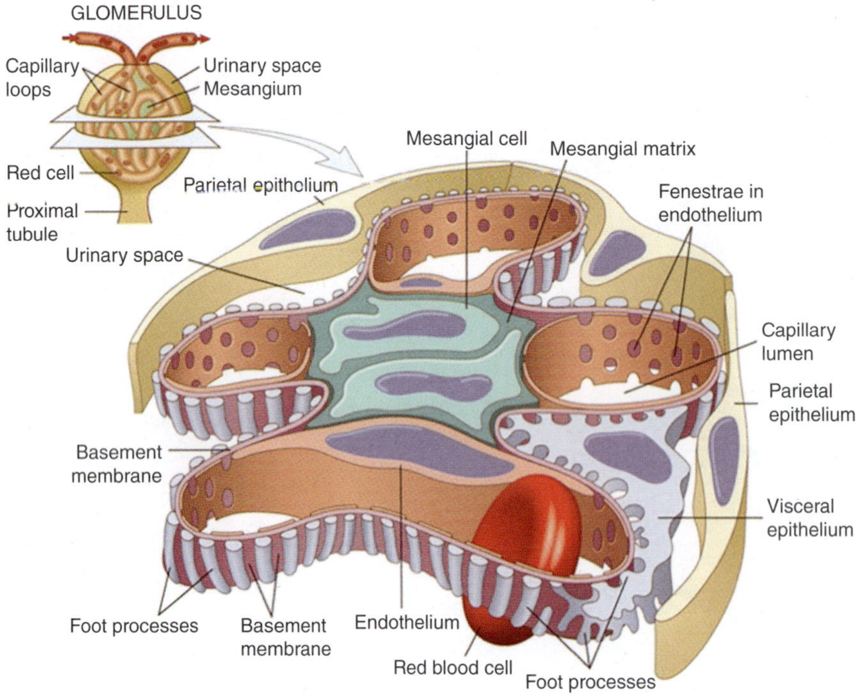

Fig. 24.3 Schematic representation of a glomerular lobe showing compartments of the glomerular lobe and their association with each other.

collagen (α1–α6 chains), laminin, proteoglycans, entactin, fibronectin and several other glycoproteins. The slit diaphragm of the visceral epithelium contains proteins such as nephrin, podocin and CD2-associated protein. Interspersed between the glomerular capillary tuft is the mesangial matrix.

- **Visceral epithelial cells:** Also called podocytes, these cells have interdigitating foot processes that are embedded on the rara externa of GBM, with a slit of 20–30 nm between adjacent foot processes forming the filtration slit.
- **Mesangial cells** are embedded in the mesangial matrix between the capillaries. In general, there are one to two mesangial cells per mesangial area. More than three cells per mesangial area will be considered as mesangial increase in cellularity.

The mechanism of filtration in the glomerular apparatus is based on the size and charge of the solute. Glomerular membranes are negatively charged due to heparan sulphate and allow only neutral and positively charged molecules to pass through. Charge-based barrier function is important in restricting the entry of albumin and other proteins into urine. The podocytes are the important factors maintaining the size-dependent glomerular filtration of the solute with the help of the filtration slits. Defects in the podocytes, which are generally termed 'podocytopathies', will lead to nephrotic syndrome.

RENAL FUNCTIONS

The kidneys play a major role in the normal functioning of the body. Excretion of metabolic waste products such as urea, creatinine and many drugs takes place through the kidney. The kidneys regulate **water and electrolyte balance**, thereby maintaining the total body water and plasma osmolarity. They play a major role in **regulating blood volume and blood pressure** through the renin–angiotensin system.

When stimulated, the juxtaglomerular granular cells secrete renin, which kick-starts a sequence of events that increase blood volume and cause vasoconstriction to maintain normal BP levels (discussed in Chapter 13).

Another important function of the kidneys is maintenance of **acid–base balance**. The proximal tubular epithelial cells secrete hydrogen ion and reabsorb bicarbonate ion, thereby increasing the alkali reserve of the body and preventing the development of metabolic acidosis. The kidneys also help in haematopoiesis by secreting EPO for regulating red blood cell (RBC) production. EPO secretion occurs in the interstitial fibroblasts of the kidneys.

The other function of the kidneys that needs mention is its **activation of vitamin D**. It converts 25-(OH) vitamin D into the active form, 1,25 dihydroxy-vitamin D, which not only is important for maintaining the bone mineralization and serum calcium levels but is also an important modulator of the immune, renal and cardiovascular systems.

CLINICAL MANIFESTATIONS OF RENAL DISEASE

Renal diseases involve the four fundamental morphological components of the kidney, causing the following:

- Glomerular diseases
- Tubular diseases

- Interstitial diseases
- Vascular diseases

Clinical manifestations of renal diseases give an important clue to the underlying pathology. Most of the renal pathologies usually present as one of the following clinical conditions:

Azotaemia

Azotaemia is defined as a condition associated with elevated blood urea nitrogen (BUN) and creatinine levels, which are caused by decreased glomerular filtration rate (GFR). The causes may be renal or extrarenal in origin. On the basis of the aetiology, azotaemia may be divided into prerenal azotaemia and postrenal azotaemia.

Prerenal azotaemia: It is mainly due to hypoperfusion of the kidney in the following conditions: hypotension, excessive fluid loss, shock, volume depletion, congestive heart failure (CHF) and cirrhosis.

Postrenal azotaemia: It is due to obstructed urine flow distal to the kidney such as in the case of urinary calculi and ureteric carcinoma.

Uraemia

Uraemia refers to the clinical presentation of azotaemia. It indicates the failure of renal excretory function. Apart from the elevated biochemical parameters, the patient may present with metabolic and endocrine alterations. Patients may exhibit secondary involvement of other organs such as the gastrointestinal (GI) tract (uraemic gastroenteritis), peripheral nerves (peripheral neuropathy) or heart (uraemic fibrinous pericarditis) due to elevated levels of toxic waste retained in the blood in patients with renal failure.

Nephritic syndrome

It is a glomerular disease that presents with a specific constellation of symptoms such as gross and microscopic haematuria showing diminished GFR, mild to moderate proteinuria and hypertension.

Nephrotic syndrome

It is a glomerular disease whose typical manifestations are heavy proteinuria (>3.5 g/day), hypoalbuminaemia, severe oedema, hyperlipidaemia and lipiduria.

Rapidly progressive renal failure (rapidly progressive glomerulonephritis [RPGN])

It is a glomerular condition in which there is a rapid decline of >50% of GFR within 3 months with the presence of crescents in at least 50% of the glomeruli.

Asymptomatic haematuria and proteinuria

These two are an early manifestation of minimal glomerular disease.

Acute kidney injury (AKI)

AKI, previously called acute renal failure, may occur in glomerular, tubular, interstitial and vascular injuries. It presents with a rapid decline in GFR within hours or days, presenting as oliguria, anuria and dysregulation of fluid and electrolytes leading to retention of urea and creatinine.

Chronic kidney disease (CKD)

Chronic renal disease, previously called chronic renal failure (CRF), refers to a diminished GFR of less than 60 mL/min/1.73 m^2 for the duration of 3 months and/or persistent albuminuria. It usually is a consequence in many chronic renal diseases and presents with symptoms of impairment or loss of renal functions such as uraemia, dehydration, oedema, hypokalaemia, metabolic acidosis, hyperphosphataemia, hypocalcaemia, anaemia, hypertension, CHF, nausea, vomiting, gastritis, colitis and oesophagitis, myopathy, neuropathy and dermatitis.

End-stage renal disease (ESRD)

It indicates the terminal stage of uraemia and is diagnosed by a GFR of less than 5% of normal.

Renal tubular defects

The disorders that primarily affect the tubular compartment are termed renal tubular defects. The common presentations of renal tubular defects are nocturia and metabolic acidosis. The common causes include familial nephrogenic diabetes, renal tubular acidosis, cystinuria, lead toxicity and nephronophthisis–medullary cystic disease.

Urinary tract obstruction

Obstruction of the urinary tract may lead to secondary infection causing bacteriuria or pyuria. The obstruction may be due to causes within the lumen or external pressure and may be at the level of the kidney, ureter, bladder or urethra.

Nephrolithiasis

It usually manifests as pain or haematuria.

Renal tumours

Renal tumours may present as haematuria, pain or a mass depending on the stage or may occasionally remain asymptomatic and present with atypical clinical presentation such as pyrexia of an unknown origin.

RENAL FAILURE PA 28.2

All renal diseases, irrespective of the aetiology, may evolve into major pathological syndromes –AKI or CKD. Let us review the definition and presentation of each before we move on to study the various causes and mechanisms of renal injury.

ACUTE KIDNEY INJURY PA 28.3

As the name indicates, it is a condition of rapid onset of renal dysfunction characterized by the development of oliguria or at times anuria leading to an increase in BUN and creatinine. The causes of AKI are classified as follows:

- **Prerenal causes:** These causes are due to hypoperfusion of the kidney, which may be a consequence of hypovolaemia or cardiac pump failure.

- **Intrarenal causes:** These causes are related to the various pathologies affecting the kidney such as vascular anomalies, glomerular damage, acute tubular necrosis due to ischaemia and toxin or tubulointerstitial nephritis.
- **Postrenal causes:** These may be due to obstruction at any level of the urinary tract due to calculi, tumour, external compression, etc.

Clinical Features

Clinical features may be specific to the aetiology of the renal failure:

- **Acute nephritis**–related causes may present with haematuria, oedema, mild hypertension and mild proteinuria. There may be associated fluid retention due to decreased GFR and increased salt and water reabsorption in distal nephron.
- **Tubular pathology**–related symptoms can be divided into three phases, each having its own presentation:
  - **Oliguric phase**
    It is characterized by urine output of less than 400 mL/day, which may last for up to 7–10 days. The patient presents with symptoms of azotaemia, metabolic acidosis, hyperkalaemia, hypernatremia and hypervolaemia. The specific gravity of urine in these patients is low.
  - **Diuretic phase**
    In this phase, there is an improvement in urinary output but due to the lack of secretion or reabsorption taking place in the tubules, the specific gravity of the urine is fixed and equal to the specific gravity of the ultrafiltrate of the glomeruli, which is 1.010.
  - **Recovery phase**
    In this phase, there is recovery of renal function.
- **Prerenal syndrome**
  This condition is seen in renal damage caused by ischaemia due to hypovolaemia or hypotension. The renal parameters – BUN and creatinine – are elevated and the patient presents with oliguria.
  AKI due to reduced renal perfusion and hypovolaemia is reversible to some extent by correction of the pathology leading to it, whereas renal failure caused by renal injury and damage may not respond well to treatment. Correction of the pathology leading to the acute renal shutdown should be initiated as early as possible for a better prognosis.

CHRONIC KIDNEY DISEASE PA 28.4

CKD, previously called CRF, is a condition characterized by progressive and irreversible decline in renal function leading to azotaemia, uraemia and metabolic acidosis. The aetiology may be classified on the basis of the pathogenesis as follows:

Disorders of the glomerular compartment
- Primary glomerular diseases
- Secondary diseases (diabetes, hypertension, autoimmune)

Table 24.1 Stages of Chronic Renal Failure

Stage	GFR	Clinical Presentation
Decreased renal reserve	50% normal	BUN and creatinine normal
Renal insufficiency	25% normal	BUN and creatinine elevated
Renal failure	10% normal	Uraemic symptoms
End-stage renal disease	5% normal	Renal and extrarenal symptoms

BUN, blood urea nitrogen; GFR, glomerular filtration rate.

Disorders of the tubulointerstitial pathology
- Vascular disorders
- Infections
- Drugs/toxins – acetaminophen, phenacetin, aspirin
- Obstructive uropathy

All these conditions are discussed in detail in the corresponding sections of the chapter.

Stages of Chronic Renal Failure

CRF is divided into four stages on the basis of GFR and are given in Table 24.1.

Clinical Features

The clinical features may be renal or extrarenal.

The **primary renal symptoms** are as follows:

- Metabolic acidosis, which produces Kussmaul breathing, hyperkalaemia and hypercalcaemia
- Hyperkalaemia, which may cause cardiac arrhythmia, weakness, nausea, diarrhoea and muscular irritability
- Retention of sodium and water that causes overload leading to CHF
- Hyperuricaemia that manifests as gout, joint stiffness and urate renal stones
- Azotaemia producing confusion, oedema and tachycardia

The **secondary extrarenal symptoms** due to renal failure are as follows:

- Anaemia – due to decrease in EPO production from the diseased kidney
- Uraemic frost – deposit of urea in sweat
- CHF due to volume overload
- GI bleed and irritation due to uraemia-induced platelet dysfunction and increased vascular malformations in these patients
- Osteomalacia due to decreased vitamin D from kidneys
- Osteitis fibrosa cystica due to elevated levels of parathormone, followed by low calcium levels

The basic principle of management is treatment of the underlying cause and renal replacement therapy in the form of dialysis or renal transplant for suitable patients.

Management of patients with CRF includes maintenance of BP and haemoglobin levels (greater than 10 g/dL), vitamin D supplements to reduce renal bone disease, maintenance of acid–base balance and correction of dyslipidaemia. Renal replacement in the form of dialysis may be required when the toxin levels in blood go high, and definitive management with renal transplant may be considered in suitable patients.

GLOMERULAR DISEASES PA 28.5

To understand the pathogenesis of glomerular diseases, it is important to understand the morphology of the glomerular filtration apparatus, which has been explained in the previous sections of this chapter.

Glomerular diseases are classified into primary glomerulopathies, systemic diseases and hereditary disorders (Table 24.2).

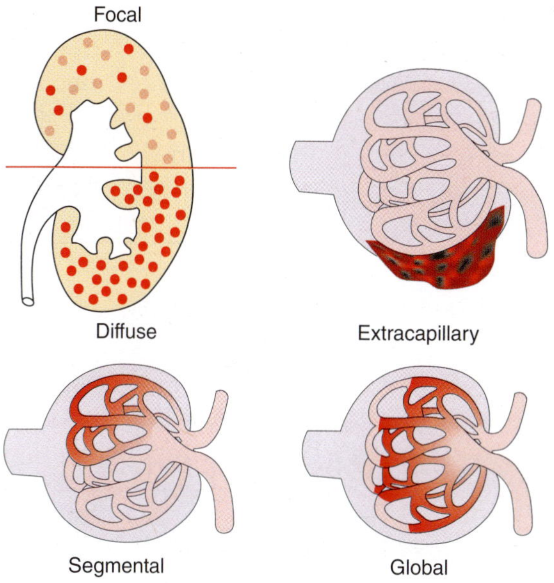

Fig. 24.4 Representation of the descriptive terms.

PATHOLOGICAL RESPONSES OF THE GLOMERULUS TO INJURY

Glomerular diseases do not follow the same pattern of involvement. On the basis of the nature and severity of the aetiology, they may show different patterns of distribution. Identifying the pattern may give a clue to the aetiology of the disease. On the basis of the distribution of the injury to the glomeruli, the terminologies used for description are explained as follows (Fig. 24.4):

- **Diffuse:** All glomeruli in the renal parenchyma are affected.
- **Focal:** A fraction of glomeruli is affected, whereas others are uninvolved.
- **Global:** Pathology involves the entire glomeruli.
- **Segmental:** Only a part of the glomeruli is involved, whereas the rest is functional.

Table 24.2 Glomerulopathies

1. **Primary glomerulopathies** Acute postinfectious glomerulonephritis Rapidly progressive glomerulonephritis Membranous nephropathy Minimal change disease Focal segmental glomerulosclerosis Membranoproliferative glomerulonephritis Dense deposit disease C3 glomerulonephritis IgA nephropathy Chronic glomerulonephritis
2. **Systemic disease with glomerular involvement** Systemic lupus erythematosus Diabetes mellitus Amyloidosis Goodpasture syndrome Microscopic polyarteritis Granulomatosis with polyangiitis Henoch–Schönlein purpura Bacterial endocarditis Secondary to multiple myeloma Thrombotic microangiopathy
3. **Hereditary disorders** Alport syndrome Thin basement membrane disease Fabry disease Podocyte/slit diaphragm protein mutations

Acute glomerular response to injury is characterized by proliferation of mesangial and endothelial cells. Furthermore, there may be infiltration of the glomeruli by leucocytes (neutrophils, monocytes and lymphocytes) leading to a hypercellular appearance of glomeruli. When the damage progresses, there may be a crescent formation by proliferation of epithelial cells that get bound to each other by fibrin that had leaked into Bowman's space from blood due to GBM injury.

Chronic glomerular response to injury includes basement membrane thickening, hyalinosis and sclerosis. GBM thickening may be due to immune complex deposition on the subendothelial side, on the subepithelial side or within the basement membrane, or amyloid, fibrin or cryoglobulin deposition, or an increased synthesis of basement membrane protein as in diabetic glomerulosclerosis or additional matrix synthesis as in membranoproliferative glomerulonephritis (MPGN). Hyalinosis of glomeruli may be due to capillary wall injury in the glomeruli, leading to exudation of plasma proteins. Sclerosis on the other side is due to excess deposition of extracellular matrix material in the mesangium and capillary wall and is an important finding in diabetic glomerulosclerosis.

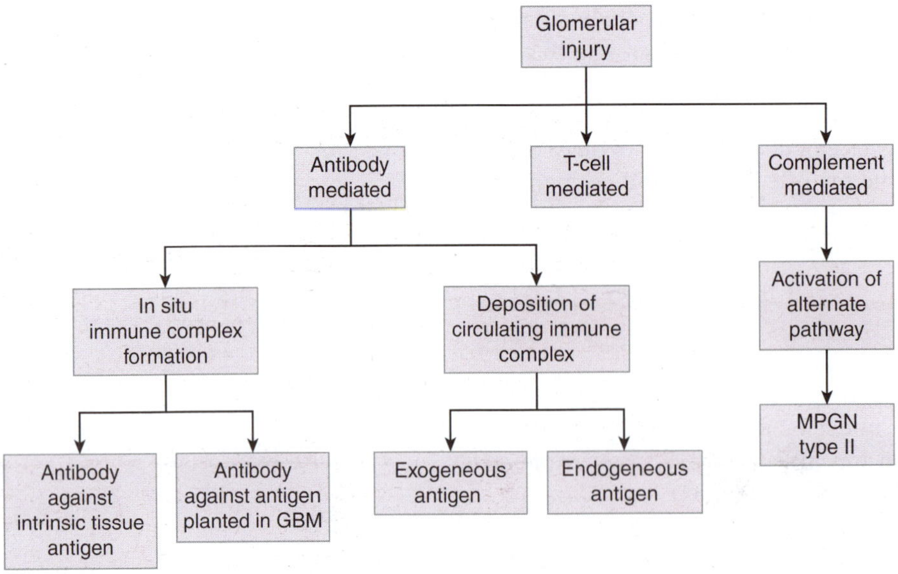

Flowchart 24.1 Pathogenesis of glomerular injury.

PATHOGENESIS OF GLOMERULAR INJURY (FLOWCHART 24.1)

Glomerular injury usually occurs due to the activity of the immune system. It may follow any one of the three pathways – antibody mediated, cell mediated or complement mediated, the former being the most common and discussed in detail next.

Antibody-Mediated Injury

Antibodies may form immune complexes in the glomerulus or may form immune complexes in circulation and get deposited in the glomeruli (Fig. 24.5).

In situ immune complex formation may occur due to the following two mechanisms:

- Immune complex formed by antibodies against **fixed intrinsic tissue antigen**
  The common intrinsic antigens are the NC1 domain of the α3 chain of type IV collagen seen in anti-GBM nephritis, which produce a characteristic diffuse linear staining by immunofluorescence, and podocyte antigen phospholipase receptor 2 (PLA2R) seen in membranous nephropathy (MN), which gives diffuse granular staining by immunofluorescence and mesangial antigens.
- Antibodies against the **planted antigen** that bind to the anionic component of GBM
  Exogenous antigens including infectious agent, drugs, bovine milk antigen and other cationic proteins and endogenous antigens such as DNA, nuclear proteins, immunoglobulins and IgA may get planted in GBM and trigger an immune response.

Circulating Immune Complex Deposition

This is a type 3 hypersensitivity reaction in which circulating immune complexes formed against exogenous or endogenous antigens may get deposited in the glomeruli in spite of having no immunological specificity to the glomerulus. The triggering antigens may be **endogenous** (DNA and tumour antigens that may be associated with systemic lupus erythematosus [SLE] or IgA nephropathy) or **exogenous** (streptococcal proteins, hepatitis B, hepatitis C, *Treponema pallidum* and *Plasmodium falciparum*). This localization of immune complexes occurs due to their physiochemical properties and haemodynamic factors along with molecular charge and the size of the reactant (Fig. 24.6).

Large circulating complexes are not nephritogenic because these are cleared by macrophages, but the small ones are prone to get filtered and trapped. **Cationic antigens** are capable of crossing the anionic GBM and hence the complexes may reside in the subepithelial side of GBM (between the outer surface of GBM and the podocytes). On the contrary, **anionic antigens** are unable to cross GBM and are trapped in the subendothelial side (between the endothelial cell and GBM). Lastly, antigens with **neutral charge** tend to accumulate in the mesangium.

The other determinant of this deposition is the duration of exposure. If the exposure of antigen is short-lived as in postinfectious glomerulonephritis (PIGN), the complexes are cleared by leucocytes, macrophages, mesangial cells and proteases. Exposure for a prolonged period of time as in SLE or hepatitis can lead to membranous or membranoproliferative glomerulonephritis type.

The **antigen–antibody complexes** deposited in the glomeruli lead to inflammatory reaction after activation of complement and cause injury. Immune complexes in the subendothelium have inflammatory pathology, but deposits in the subepithelium, such as in MN, have noninflammatory pathology. This immune complex

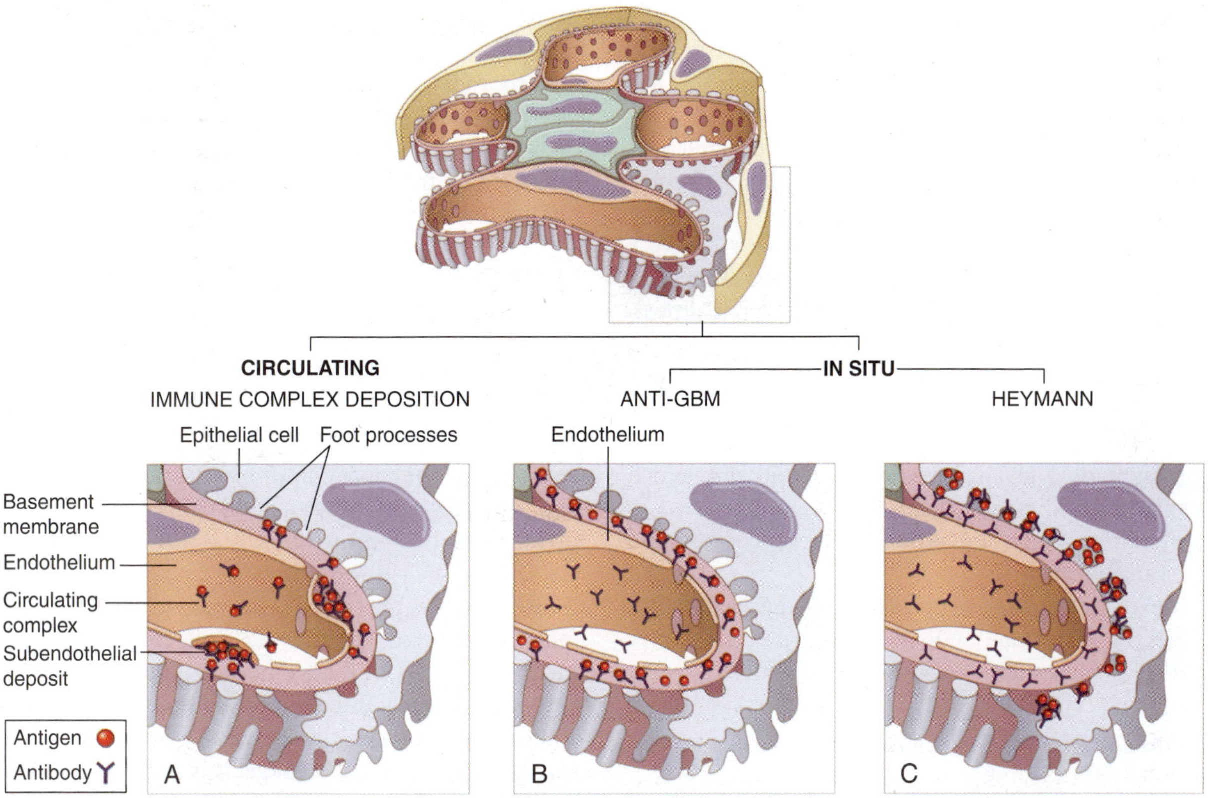

Fig. 24.5 Antibody-mediated glomerular injury. Deposition of circulating immune complex–mediated and in situ antigen mediated. (*Source:* Robbins & Cotran Pathologic Basis of Disease, 10e: South Asia Edition, Volume 2, 2nd ed.: Jon C. Aster, Vinay Kumar, Abul K. Abbas, Elsevier, 2020.)

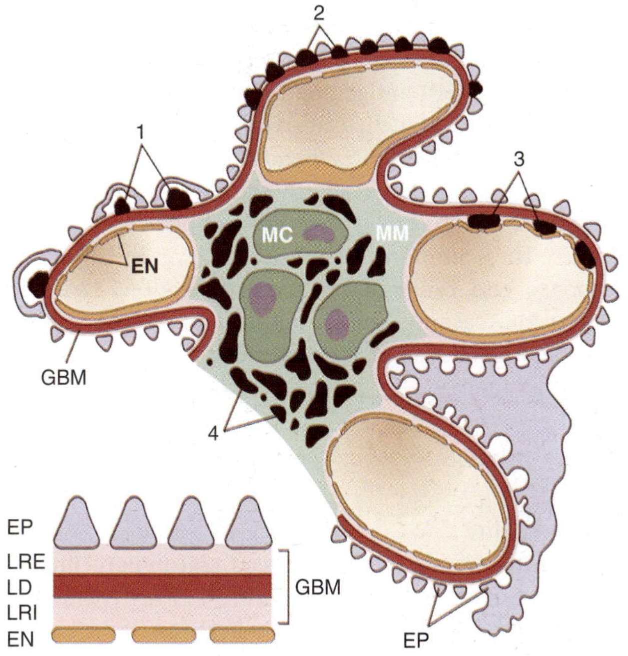

Fig. 24.6 Schematic representation of sites of immune complex deposition. Localization of immune complexes in the glomerulus: (1) subepithelial humps, as in acute glomerulonephritis; (2) membranous deposits, as in membranous nephropathy and Heymann nephritis; (3) subendothelial deposits, as in lupus nephritis and membranoproliferative glomerulonephritis; and (4) mesangial deposits, as in IgA nephropathy. EN, endothelium; EP, epithelium; GBM, glomerular basement membrane; LD, lamina densa; LRE, lamina rara externa; LRI, lamina rara interna; MC, mesangial cell; MM, mesangial matrix.

deposition is often associated with **proliferation of mesangial and endothelial cells**.

A specific pattern of damage is seen in some glomerular diseases such as **podocyte injury** in some primary and secondary glomerular diseases and **mutation** of nephrin and podocin of the slit diaphragm in hereditary nephrotic syndrome.

On the basis of these factors, the patterns of localization of immune complex in glomeruli are as follows:

- Subepithelial as in PIGN
- Epimembranous as in MN and Heymann nephritis
- Subendothelial as in lupus nephritis and MPGN
- Mesangial as in IgA nephropathy

Mediators of Glomerular Injury

After the deposition of immune complex in the glomeruli, there are a multitude of factors that cause damage to the glomeruli. These include the role of cells and soluble mediators.

a. **Cells**
   - Neutrophils and monocytes
     These activate complement (C5a) and release proteases that cause GBM lysis. The oxygen-derived free radicles produced by these cells cause damage to the surrounding cells, and the arachidonic acid metabolites produced reduce GFR.

- Macrophages and T lymphocytes
  The factors released by these cells include proteases, growth factors, eicosanoids and nitric oxide (NO).
- Platelets
  The platelets damage the glomeruli by causing vascular injury through the release of oxidants, chemokines, eicosanoids and growth factors.
- Mesangial cells
  These cells may be stimulated even in the absence of neutrophils to release eicosanoids, chemokines, growth factors, endothelin and reactive oxygen species.

b. **Soluble mediators**
- Complement, which does not require leucocytes for activation
- Eicosanoids, NO, angiotensin and endothelin, which cause haemodynamic changes
- Cytokines, which are produced by leucocytes and mesangial cells
- Growth factors such as platelet-derived growth factor (PDGF), FGF and VEGF
- Fibrin, which stimulates crescent formation

MECHANISM OF PROGRESSION IN GLOMERULAR DISEASES

When GFR reduces below 30%–50%, the progression to end-stage renal failure is inevitable. The two histological types seen in this stage are as follows:

a. **Glomerulosclerosis**
   This is an adaptive form of focal segmental glomerulosclerosis (FSGS) termed 'perihilar' variant. The kidney shows progressive hyalinosis and sclerosis involving the vascular pole (perihilar) of the glomeruli along with glomerulomegaly. This may be due to glomerular injury or nonglomerular pathology with associated proteinuria. The main factor involved in causing fibrosis is TGF-β.

b. **Tubulointerstitial fibrosis**
   This is a commonly seen component of acute and chronic glomerulonephritis (GN) and is characterized by tubular damage and interstitial inflammation. The tubular injury is mainly due to ischaemia of the tubules below the sclerosed glomeruli, inflammation of the surrounding interstitium and reduced blood flow in the peritubular vessels. The extent of tubular damage correlates with the renal function and the severity of glomerular damage. The tubular damage finally leads to activation of cytokines and growth factors leading to fibrosis.

We will now proceed to review the various types of glomerular injury, their pathogenesis, morphological changes and clinical features, a brief comparison of which is given in Table 24.3.

NEPHRITIC SYNDROME

Nephritic syndrome refers to inflammation of the glomeruli characterized by the symptom complex of oliguria, haematuria, mild proteinuria, hypertension and azotaemia. The proteinuria and the associated oedema are milder than those in nephrotic syndrome. These may be primary or associated with other diseases such as SLE. The causes of nephritic syndrome are listed in Table 24.4 and are discussed in the subsequent sections. In this chapter, we discuss the common causes of nephritic syndrome.

Postinfectious Glomerulonephritis

This group comprises GN occurring as a consequence of infection-induced immune complex deposition characterized by diffuse proliferation of cells within the glomerulus leading to hypercellularity along with influx of granulocytes (exudation) and hence called acute proliferative GN. The most common infection associated with this syndrome is streptococcal infection; hence, it is divided into two groups.

Acute Poststreptococcal Glomerulonephritis This is often considered as the classical immune complex–mediated disease of the glomerulus. It appears 1–4 weeks after streptococcal infection of the skin or pharynx, more commonly after skin infection. Although it may affect children and adults of any age, it is most frequently seen in children 6–10 years of age.

Aetiology and Pathogenesis Post-streptococcal GN is an immune complex–mediated disease caused by **group A β-haemolytic streptococci** types 12, 4 and 1 (nephritogenic strains) that constitutes 90% of the cases. The antigens have been identified to be streptococcal pyogenic exotoxin B (SpeB) antigen and streptococcal glyceraldehyde-3-phosphate dehydrogenase (GAPDH) that get initially deposited on the subendothelial side of the basement membrane that leads to the in situ formation of immune complexes following the binding of specific antibodies. These immune complexes elicit an inflammatory response and cause complement activation. Later, for unknown reasons, the immune complexes migrate to subepithelial side of the basement membrane and get deposited there.

Morphology (Fig. 24.7)

Light microscopy

Glomerulus

The glomeruli appear enlarged and **hypercellular**. The pathology is global and diffuse. The hypercellularity is mainly due to the proliferation of the endothelial and mesangial cells along infiltration of the glomeruli by leucocytes, mainly neutrophils and monocytes, leading to an exudative pattern of injury. Occasionally, there is extracapillary increase in cellularity (crescent), which signifies a poor prognosis. The capillary lumina are obliterated by the proliferating and infiltrating cells.

Table 24.3 Summary of Immune-Mediated Glomerular Diseases

Disease	Pathogenesis	LM	IF	EM
Membranous	In situ immune complex deposition (PLA2R antigen)	Capillary wall thickening	Capillary wall granular IgG and C3	Subepithelial deposits
IgA nephropathy	Abnormal IgA glycosylation	Mesangial hypercellularity	Mesangial dominant IgA (and some C3)	Mesangial deposits
Membranoproliferative glomerulonephritis (MPGN)	Immune complex deposition	Endocapillary hypercellularity, mesangial sclerosis, 'double contouring'	Capillary wall IgG (less IgM) and C3	Subendothelial deposits
C3 glomerulonephritis (C3GN)	Dysregulation of alternative pathway of complement	Variable features, but often similar to those of MPGN	Capillary wall dominant C3 (less or no Igs)	Variable, but subendothelial deposits
Dense deposit disease (DDD)	Dysregulation of alternative pathway of complement	Variable, but often similar to those of MPGN or mesangial cell hypercellularity	Capillary wall dominant C3 (less or no Igs)	Dense deposits in GBM
Postinfectious glomerulonephritis	Immune complex deposition, planted or circulating antigen	Endocapillary hypercellularity	Capillary wall IgG and C3	Subepithelial 'hump' deposits
Anti-GBM disease	Circulating anti-GBM antibodies (antigen is $\alpha 3$ chain of COL4)	Capillary wall necrosis and crescents	Capillary wall linear IgG and C3	No deposits, GBM ruptures
Pauci-immune glomerulonephritis	Antineutrophil cytoplasmic antibodies (ANCAs)	Capillary wall necrosis and crescents	No or sparse Ig/C3 staining	No or sparse deposits
Lupus nephritis (classes I–VI)	Immune complex deposition	Variable, class-dependent	'Full-house' staining for all Igs, C3 and C1q	Numerous deposits typically (location is class-dependent)

EM, electron microscopy; GBM, glomerular basement membrane; IF, immunofluorescence; LM, light microscopy; PLA2R, podocyte antigen phospholipase receptor 2.

Table 24.4 Causes of Nephritic Syndrome

1. Acute proliferative (postinfectious) glomerulonephritis
2. Rapidly progressive (crescentic) glomerulonephritis
3. IgA nephropathy (Berger disease)
4. Hereditary nephritis (Alport syndrome)
5. Membranoproliferative glomerulonephritis
6. Goodpasture syndrome
   Secondary to systemic diseases
   a. Systemic lupus erythematosus
   b. ANCA small-vessel vasculitides
   c. Infective endocarditis
   d. Cryoglobulinaemia
   e. Haemolytic uraemic syndrome
   f. Henoch–Schönlein purpura

ANCA, antineutrophil cytoplasmic antibody.

Tubulointerstitium

The tubules show red cell casts, and the interstitium is widened because of oedema and infiltration by mononuclear cells.

Immunofluorescence The biopsies taken within 2–3 weeks of the disease generally show diffuse, irregular, granular coarse deposits of IgG and C3 along the glomerular capillary wall and the mesangium (starry sky pattern). IgM is present in >50% of the cases. IgA and C1q are absent.

Electron Microscopy Amorphous, electron-dense immune complex deposits are commonly seen as subepithelial 'humps'. Electron-dense deposits may also be seen in the subendothelial side, in the mesangium and in the intramembranous site.

Clinical Course Children usually present with a sudden onset of malaise, fever, periorbital oedema, oliguria and haematuria producing smoky or **cola-coloured urine**. Urine examination reveals mild proteinuria and intact RBCs. There is mild to moderate hypertension. In adults, the presentation may be in the form of sudden onset of hypertension or oedema. Blood examination reveals elevated BUN and ASO (Anti-streptolysin O) titre and low

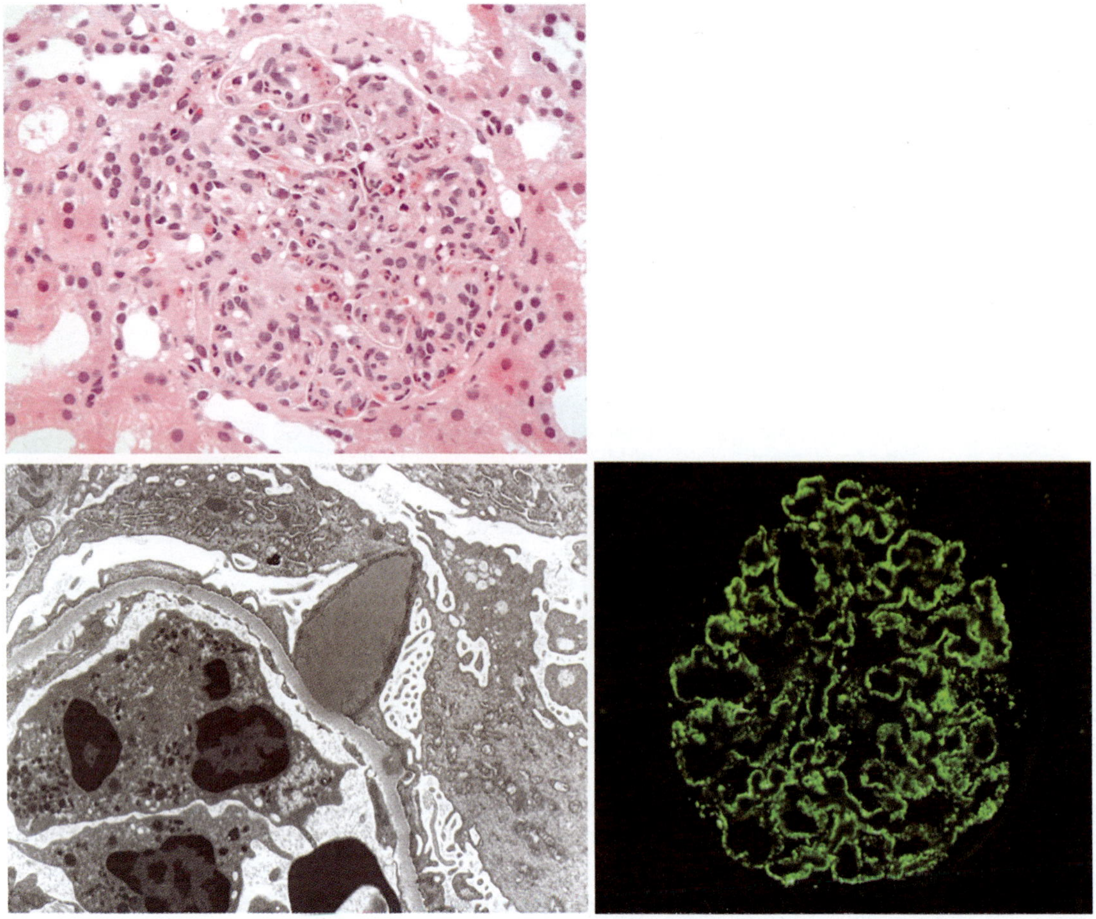

Fig. 24.7 Poststreptococcal glomerulonephritis – light microscopy, electron microscopy (EM) and immunofluorescence (IF). Light microscopy shows hypercellular glomerulus with endocapillary proliferation. EM shows subepithelial deposits of immune complexes. IF shows granular deposits. (*Source:* From Poststreptococcal Glomerulonephritis. Elsevier Point of Care. 2021.)

C3. The reduction in C3 complement levels may be attributed to the consumption of C3 in the glomeruli for the immune complex–associated complement activation.

Prognosis Prognosis is good in children. They require only supportive management to maintain water and sodium balance, and about 95% of children show complete recovery. Less than 1% of cases progress to RPGN and chronic GN. However, the disease is more likely to persist as haematuria, proteinuria and hypertension in about 40% of adults and in a proportion of them, it eventually leads to RPGN and chronic GN.

Nonstreptococcal Acute Glomerulonephritis This may be due to infection caused by various organisms such as:

- Bacteria: *Staphylococcus*, *Pneumococcus* infection
- Viruses: Hepatitis B, hepatitis C, mumps, measles, HIV infection, varicella
- Parasites: Malaria, toxoplasmosis

Among these, staphylococcal infection may produce IgA deposit rather than IgG immune complexes (IgA-dominant acute post-staphylococcal GN).

Rapidly Progressive Glomerulonephritis/ Crescentic Glomerulonephritis

RPGN is not a specific disease but rather a severe form of GN associated with severe glomerular damage and **crescent formation** in a majority of the glomeruli. It is the consequence of several glomerular pathologies that cause severe injury and is not due to any specific aetiology. The crescents are formed by proliferation of parietal epithelial cells along with the infiltrating monocytes and macrophages.

Aetiology and Pathogenesis RPGN is mostly an immune-mediated pathology. It can be classified into three types, the causes of which are listed in Table 24.5:

Type I RPGN: It is an **anti-GBM antibody**-mediated destruction of the glomeruli. The formation of antibodies is stimulated by viruses or exposure to hydrocarbons, and the antibodies are mainly directed against antigen located in the noncollagenous domain of $\alpha3$ chain of collagen type IV. This collagen is a component of GBM and the lung alveolar basement membrane, making them the target for antibodies. The patient hence presents with renal failure and pulmonary haemorrhage and it is called **Goodpasture**

Table 24.5 Causes of Rapidly Progressive Glomerulonephritis

Type I (anti-GBM antibody) Renal limited Goodpasture syndrome
Type II (immune complex) Idiopathic Postinfectious glomerulonephritis Lupus nephritis Henoch–Schönlein purpura IgA nephropathy Others
Type III (pauci-immune) ANCA-associated Idiopathic Granulomatosis with polyangiitis (formerly Wegener granulomatosis) Microscopic polyangiitis

ANCA, antineutrophil cytoplasmic antibody; GBM, glomerular basement membrane.

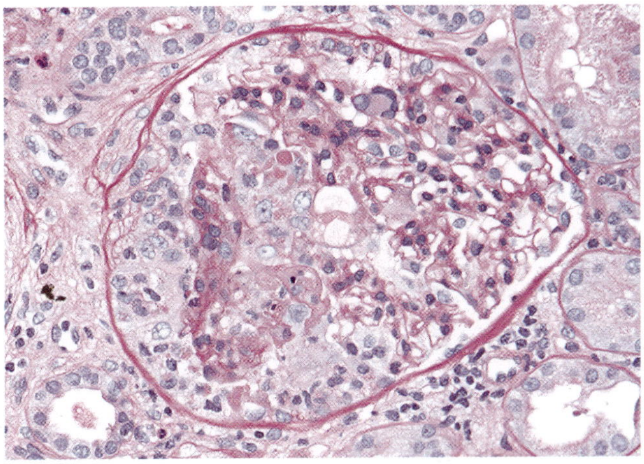

Fig. 24.8 Microscopy of crescentic glomerulonephritis. RPGN glomerulus showing cellular crescent compressing the capillary tuft. (*Source:* Neeraja Kambham. Kidney: Non-Neoplastic Diseases. Rosai and Ackerman's Surgical Pathology. 11th edition. Elsevier 2018.)

syndrome. The incidence is about 15%, and management is by plasmapheresis to remove the antibodies.

Type II RPGN: It is an immune complex–mediated destruction of the glomeruli. The immune complexes may be formed due to PIGN, lupus nephritis, Henoch–Schönlein purpura (HSP) and IgA nephropathy. The incidence is about 25%, and patients are not benefitted by plasmapheresis.

Type III RPGN: Also called **pauci-immune GN**, it encompasses the crescentic RPGNs that do not fall under the aforementioned two categories due to the absence of anti-GBM antibodies and immune complexes under electron microscopy and immunofluorescence. However, more than 90% of cases demonstrate antineutrophil cytoplasmic antibody (ANCA), either **c-ANCA** (anti-PR3 ANCA) or **p-ANCA** (anti-myeloperoxidase), in their blood. The aetiology is idiopathic or associated with systemic vasculitis (granulomatosis with polyangiitis and microscopic polyangiitis), but both are considered to be manifestations of small-vessel vasculitis, limited to the kidney in the former but systemic in the latter. Evidence of the role of ANCA in causing this disease is surfacing, so plasma exchange may be of help.

Morphology

On **gross** examination, the kidneys are enlarged with cortical petechial haemorrhages.

Light microscopy reveals the presence of **crescents** in the urinary space of the glomeruli which is a hallmark of RPGN (Fig. 24.8). The crescents are formed by proliferation of parietal cells, monocytes, macrophages and fibrin, often with the prominence of the fibrin strands between the cell layers, and more than 50% of glomeruli should have crescents for making the diagnosis. The crescents can be cellular, fibrocellular and fibrous crescents. On light microscopy, one important feature to differentiate between anti-GBM and pauci-immune GN is the type of crescents. The crescents in anti-GBM disease are temporally homogenous, whereas the crescents in pauci-immune GN are heterogenous. Segmental glomerular necrosis located adjacent to segments of glomeruli that do not show inflammation or proliferation is an important feature of pauci-immune type of RPGN. The tubules often show mild atrophy and the interstitium contains inflammatory cells. Restoration of normal glomerular architecture may occur with early aggressive therapy; else, often healing leads to scarring and glomerular sclerosis.

Immunofluorescence Immunofluorescence is performed in biopsies showing crescents under light microscopy for identification of the type of RPGN (Flowchart 24.2):

Type I RPGN (anti-GBM antibody): There are linear deposits of IgG along GBM along with more granular and discontinuous staining of C3 (Fig. 24.9).

Type II RPGN (immune complex): The staining pattern depends on the specific etiological cause of immune complex–mediated RPGN.

Type III RPGN (pauci-immune): There are few or no deposits.

Electron Microscopy Electron microscopy shows rupture of GBM.

Clinical Course Patients with RPGN usually present with haematuria, RBC casts, proteinuria, azotaemia and anaemia along with hypertension and oedema. In addition to these findings, patients with Goodpasture syndrome may have pulmonary haemorrhage with recurrent haemoptysis. Serum levels of anti-GBM, antinuclear antibody and

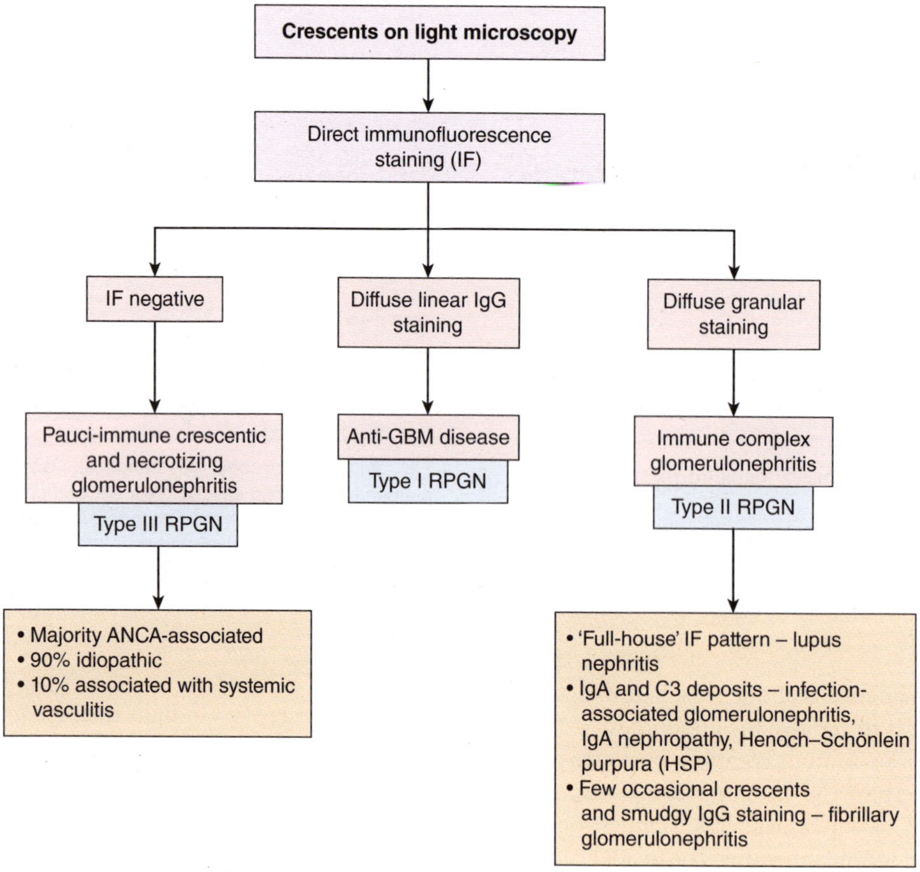

Flowchart 24.2 Approach to diagnosis – crescents in light microscopy.

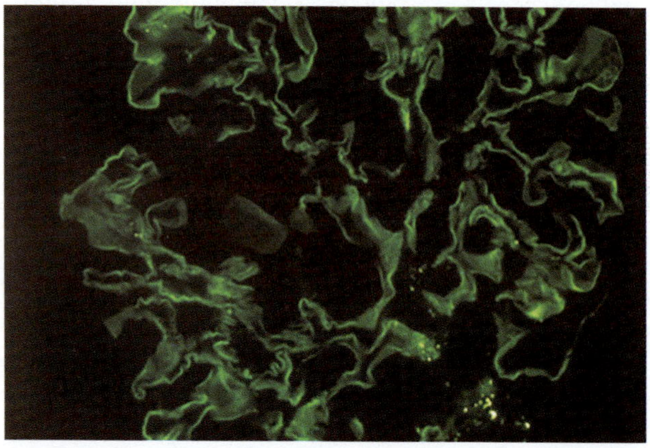

Fig. 24.9 Immunofluorescence in Goodpasture syndrome showing linear deposits of IgG directed against BM antigen. (*Source:* Neeraja Kambham. Kidney: Non-Neoplastic Diseases. Rosai and Ackerman's Surgical Pathology. 11th edition. Elsevier 2018.)

ANCA antibodies may help to identify the type of RPGN. It may lead to progressive renal involvement and oliguria.

Prognosis On early identification and aggressive treatment with plasmapheresis, cytotoxic agents and steroids, patients may show recovery. However, delay in diagnosis or treatment often leads to rapid loss of renal function and death from renal failure.

ISOLATED GLOMERULAR DISEASES

Although most glomerular pathologies manifest in the glomeruli, these may eventually involve the other structures and proceed to cause renal failure. But this group of diseases has manifestations only in the glomeruli without much involvement of the rest of the renal structures. Hence, these are called isolated glomerular diseases and have a better prognosis.

IgA Nephropathy (Berger Disease) PA 28.6

IgA nephropathy is the most common type of GN worldwide, especially among adults. It is characterized by the presence of mesangial IgA deposits and a clinical history of haematuria.

Aetiology and Pathogenesis (Fig. 24.10) Berger disease is mostly idiopathic and often follows respiratory or GI tract exposure to viruses, bacteria and food proteins. It presents 1–2 days following respiratory infection. Similar features may be seen in a variant of HSP and in secondary IgA nephropathy that follows extrarenal diseases like liver disease, coeliac disease, psoriasis, dermatitis herpetiformis, ankylosing spondylitis and inflammatory bowel disease.

The primary form of IgA nephropathy is due to an increase in the serum polymeric IgA levels and the

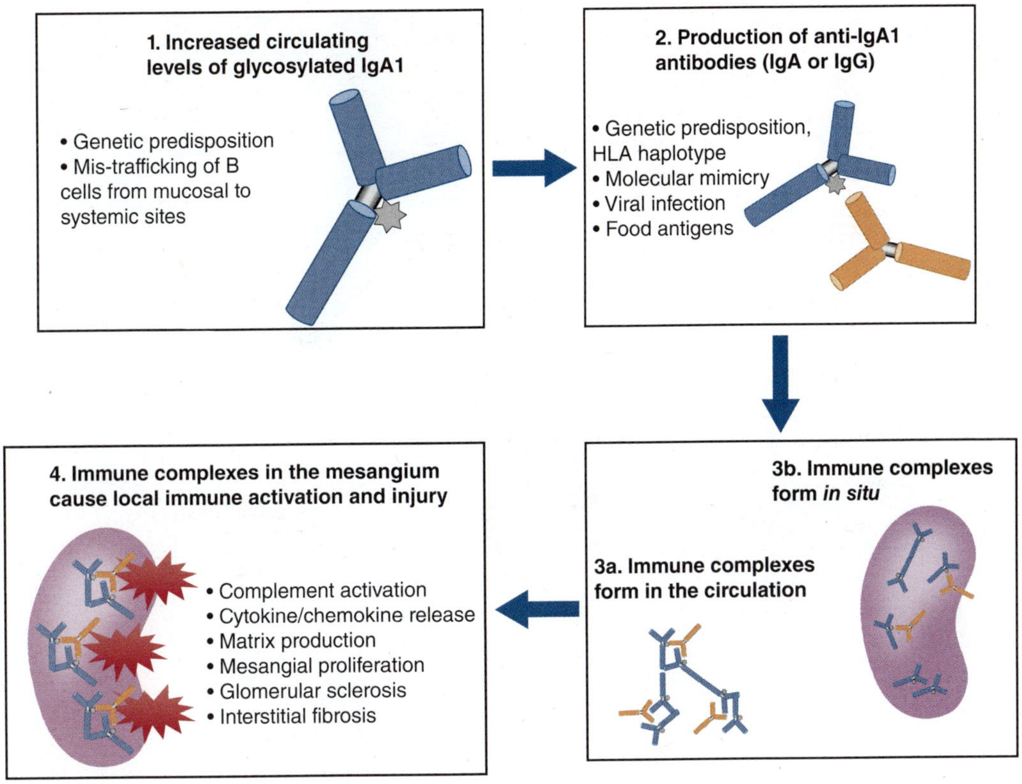

Fig. 24.10 Pathogenesis of IgA nephropathy.

formation of aberrant **glycosylated IgA** that triggers IgG autoantibody production. The glycosylated IgA may form immune complexes in circulation and get deposited in the mesangium or may get localized in the mesangium and trigger in situ immune complex formation. In both cases, the mesangium reacts by depositing more matrix and proliferation of mesangial cells. Ultimately, activation of complement by alternate pathway occurs, which is reflected by the absence of C4 and C1q and the presence of only C3 in the mesangium.

Morphology (Fig. 24.11)

Light Microscopy The glomeruli may show a normal morphology or may show mesangial widening due to increased matrix or hypercellularity or IgA deposition or a combination of these. The other specific findings include endocapillary proliferation in mesangioproliferative GN, segmental proliferation in focal proliferative GN or crescent formation in crescentic GN. Occasionally, healed glomeruli may show focal segmental sclerosis. The Oxford classification of IgA nephropathy, which is a histopathological classification, is currently in use for grading IgA nephropathy. The criteria taken into consideration include **mesangial hypercellularity (M), endocapillary hypercellularity (E), segmental glomerulosclerosis (S), tubular atrophy/interstitial fibrosis (T)** and the presence of crescents (C) – MEST-C score.

Immunofluorescence The dictum for a diagnosis of IgA nephropathy is the demonstration of dominant or codominant IgA in the mesangium. The staining pattern should be at least 1+ in intensity with predominant IgA1 deposits. C3 staining is seen in almost all the cases. There is minimal IgG and IgM staining with negative C1q on immunofluorescence. One unique feature on immunofluorescence is the increased staining of lambda over kappa.

Electron Microscopy On electron microscopy, there is immune complex–type electron-dense deposits in the mesangium and beneath the paramesangial GBM.

Clinical Course IgA nephropathy mostly affects older children and young adults (M > F). The common symptoms include gross haematuria following respiratory, urinary and GI tract infections. But in about 40% of cases, the symptoms may be recurrent microscopic haematuria with or without proteinuria. Only about 5%–10% of cases may progress to develop acute nephritic syndrome.

Prognosis IgA nephropathy tends to progress slowly, with progression to CRF seen in 15%–40% of cases over a 20-year period. Most children with HSP recover completely, but some children and adults may progress to renal failure, and recurrence is frequently noted in transplanted kidney.

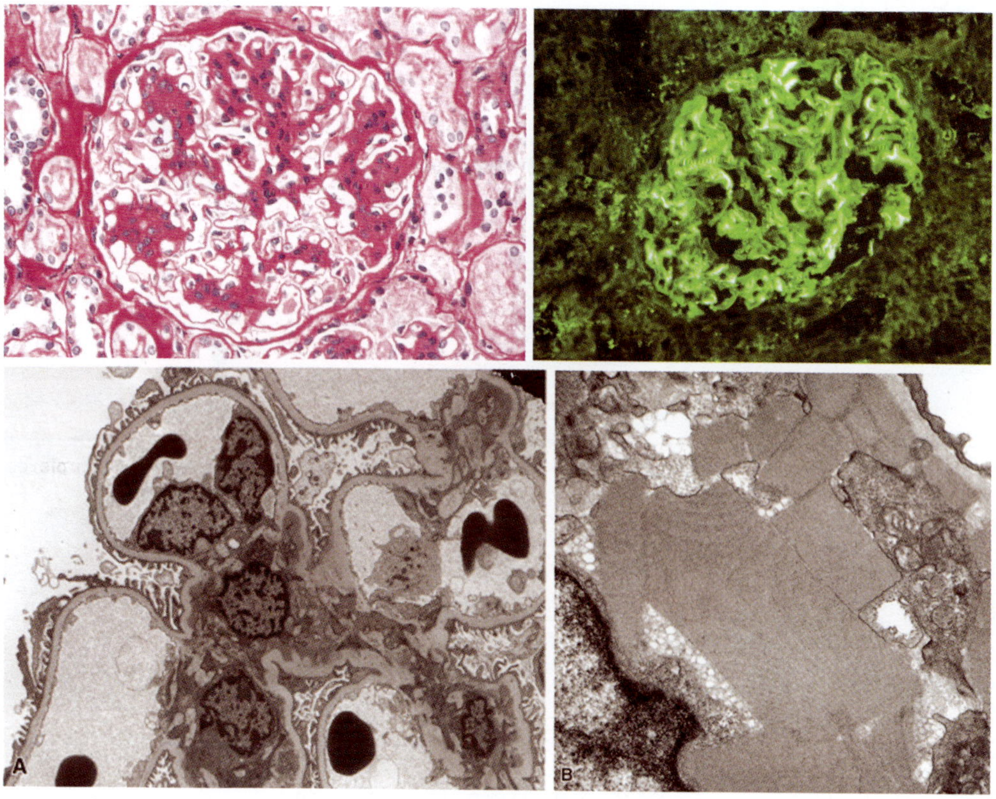

Fig. 24.11 Microscopy, immunofluorescence (IF) and electron microscopy (EM) of IgA nephropathy. Microscopy shows mesangial widening and hypercellularity IF shows mesangial IgA deposits. EM shows mesangial deposits and a lattice pattern of deposits at closer view. (*Source:* From Edgar Fischer, Lisa A. Cerilli and Donna J. Lager. Glomerular Diseases – Primary. Practical Renal Pathology. Saunders 2013.)

Hereditary Nephritis

Hereditary nephritis includes a cluster of heterogeneous familial renal diseases caused by mutations in collagen genes and commonly affects the glomeruli. The two important ones discussed here are Alport syndrome and thin basement membrane lesion (benign familial haematuria).

Alport Syndrome Alport syndrome is a syndrome of mutated collagen synthesis that leads to haematuria, nerve deafness and eye disorders such as lens dislocation, posterior cataracts and corneal dystrophy. Haematuria may progress to CRF due to a defect in collagen type IV, which is crucial for the integrity of GBM.

Aetiology and Pathogenesis It is a disorder caused by mutations in collagen genes that may exhibit different patterns of inheritance due to the presence of collagen genes in autosomes and X chromosome. X-linked pattern of inheritance is the common one that is associated with mutation in α5 chain of type IV collagen (COLA5) and is more common in men. Autosomal dominant and autosomal recessive patterns of inheritance are less common but show equal incidence in men and women.

Morphology

Light Microscopy In the early course of the disease, there is no significant change seen. However, in the later stages, there is the presence of FSGS that progresses to global sclerosis. In addition, there is *prominent interstitial foamy cell change* (nonspecific yet typically seen) along with tubular atrophy and interstitial fibrosis.

Immunohistochemistry/immunofluorescence Routine immunofluorescence may show nonspecific trapping of IgM.

Special immunofluorescence shows the absence of staining of GBM and tubular basement membrane (TBM) by antibodies to α3, α4 and α5 and the absence of staining by antibodies to α5 in skin biopsies.

Electron microscopy (Fig. 24.12) GBM and TBM show irregular foci of thickening and thinning with splitting and lamination of lamina densa of GBM, giving a **basket-weave appearance**.

Clinical Course The classical features include gross or microscopic haematuria with microscopic RBC casts. It usually affects individuals between 5 and 20 years of age and progresses to failure in males between 20 and 50 years

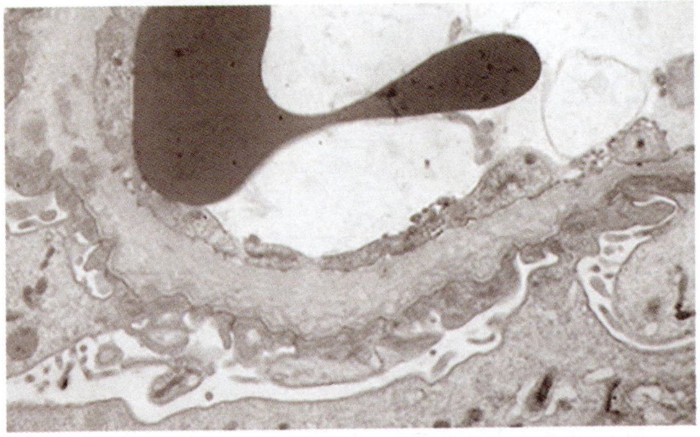

Fig. 24.12 Electron microscopy (EM) of Alport syndrome glomerulus. Basement membrane shows thickening and splitting of lamina densa into multiple strands (basket-weave appearance). (*Source:* From Michelle N. Rheault and Clifford E. Kashtan. Alport Syndrome and Other Familial Glomerular Syndromes. Comprehensive Clinical Nephrology. 6th edition. Elsevier 2019.)

of age. The associated symptoms may include nerve deafness and various eye disorders like lens dislocation and posterior cataract as discussed earlier.

Prognosis There is a progressive decline in renal function.

Thin Basement Membrane Nephropathy (Benign Familial Haematuria) This is an X-linked inheritance caused by mutation in α3 and α4 chains of type IV collagen. Occasional autosomal inheritance may also be seen. The disease runs a benign clinical course with haematuria and mild proteinuria. Electron microscopic examination reveals diffuse **thinning of GBM** between 150 and 225 nm (normal 300–400 nm). Prognosis is excellent with no progression.

NEPHROTIC SYNDROME

Nephrotic syndrome is a glomerular pathology that is caused by damage of the glomerular capillary walls resulting in increased permeability to plasma proteins. The main components of nephrotic syndrome include **massive proteinuria** (>3.5 g/day), hypoalbuminaemia (plasma albumin levels <3 g/dL), generalized oedema, hyperlipidaemia and lipiduria.

Pathophysiology

The mechanisms of development of symptoms of the nephrotic syndrome are interlinked and are explained in Flowchart 24.3.

Proteinuria that occurs in nephrotic syndrome depends on the severity of glomerular damage. Mild cases show highly selective proteinuria in which only low-molecular-weight proteins such as albumin are lost, whereas severe cases exhibit poorly selective proteinuria in which low- and high-molecular-weight proteins such as albumin and globulin are lost. The loss of the globulins (immunoglobulins) makes the patient vulnerable to infections, especially staphylococcal and pneumococcal infections. In addition, loss of anticoagulants such as antithrombin III leads to a hypercoagulable state, predisposing to the development of thrombotic and thromboembolic complications such as renal vein thrombosis.

Causes

Nephrotic syndrome may be due to the primary disease of the glomerulus or secondary to other systemic diseases. The causes for both are given in the following table, and few important ones are discussed in detail next:

Causes of Nephrotic Syndrome

a. **Primary glomerular diseases**	b. **Systemic diseases**
1. Minimal change disease	i. Diabetes mellitus
2. Membranous nephropathy	ii. Amyloidosis
3. Focal segmental glomerulonephritis	iii. Systemic lupus erythematosus
4. Membranoproliferative glomerulonephritis	iv. Drugs (NSAIDs, penicillamine, heroin)
	v. Infections (malaria, syphilis, hepatitis B and C, HIV infection)
	vi. Malignancy (carcinoma, lymphoma)
	vii. Bee sting allergy, hereditary nephritis

Membranous Nephropathy

MN, also called membranous glomerulopathy, causes nephrotic syndrome in young and middle-aged adults (aged 30–60 years). It is defined by the characteristic thickening of GBM due to immune complex deposition on the subepithelial side of the basement membrane.

Aetiology It can be either primary/idiopathic MN that constitutes 80% of the cases or secondary MN that is due to a variety of causes such as:

- Drugs (penicillamine, captopril, gold, mercury, NSAIDs)
- Tumours (carcinoma of the lung, colon and melanoma)
- SLE
- Infections (hepatitis B, hepatitis C, syphilis, schistosomiasis, malaria)

Pathogenesis MN is an immune complex–mediated disease in which the antibody formation is triggered against planted or endogenous antigens. The most common antibody in the primary form is directed against M type of phospholipase A2 receptor (PLA2R) antigen (70% of cases), whereas thrombospondin type 1 domain–containing 7A (THSD7A) constitutes the remainder of the primary MN. In secondary forms, a variety of newer antigens have been discovered that include nerve epidermal growth factor–like 1 (NELL-1) protein, EXT1/2 (exostosin 1/2) and semaphorin 3A, which are associated with specific secondary causes of secondary MN. The lesions **resemble Heymann nephritis** studied in rat models by inducing antibodies against podocyte antigens of rats.

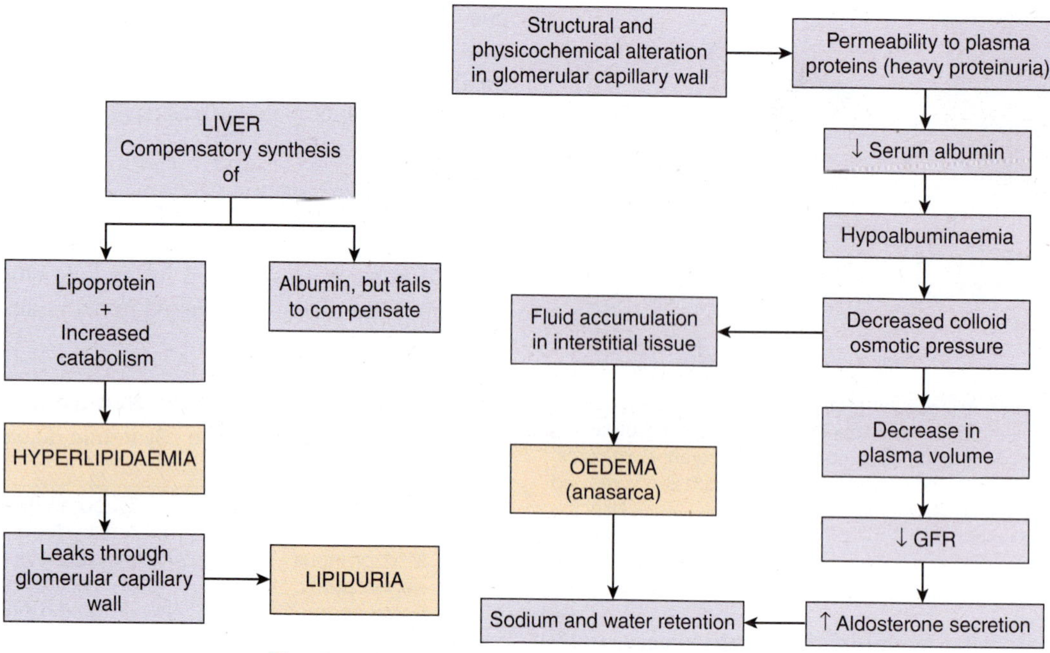

Flowchart 24.3 Pathophysiology of nephrotic syndrome.

The mechanism of glomerular insult in MN is by activation of complement by the subepithelial immune complex deposits, which in turn leads to direct attack on the glomerulus by C5–C9 (membrane attack complex) that causes the epithelial and mesangial cells to secrete proteases and oxidants, thereby damaging the glomerular capillary wall. It is because of the subepithelial localization of the immune complex deposits that there is absence of inflammatory cells in MN. IgG4, which is the predominant type of antibody deposited in MN, is a poor activator of classical complement pathway, which makes the pathway of complement activation an unsolved mystery.

Morphology

Light Microscopy The glomeruli appear normal in the early stage. Later, a diffuse uniform thickening of the glomerular capillary wall is seen in the well-developed stage. In untreated patients, the disease may evolve into a stage of segmental sclerosis or global sclerosis along with profound interstitial fibrosis and tubular atrophy.

Jones methenamine silver, a special stain, will reveal the subepithelial deposits as 'spikes' (Fig. 24.13).

Immunofluorescence On immunofluorescence, there are diffuse, granular, fine deposits of IgG and C3 in GBM. In addition, IgM and IgA may also be seen.

Electron microscopy (Fig. 24.14) Subepithelial deposits are noted in early stages, which later have a '**spike and dome**' appearance due to deposition of basement membrane material between the humps of subepithelial deposits. As the disease progresses, the deposits lose their electron density and appear as vacuolated **moth-eaten areas** within the thickened basement membrane.

Clinical Course Individuals present with full-blown nephrotic syndrome without antecedent illness. About 15% of patients present with non-nephrotic proteinuria (<3.5 g/24 h). Haematuria and mild hypertension may be present. Proteinuria is nonselective and nonresponsive to corticosteroids. Progression of the disease leads to increasing sclerosis of glomeruli as well as the tubulointerstitial compartment, resulting in renal insufficiency presenting as raised serum creatinine levels and hypertension.

Prognosis MN has a slow and indolent course with remission in 40% of cases. Although proteinuria is present in 60% of cases, only 40% progress to renal failure in 10–20 years. Unfortunately, recurrence has been noted in about 40% of cases of transplanted kidney. Antibodies to PLA2R and the other newer antigens (NELL-1, EXT1/2, semaphorin 3A) are now being used as routine markers for diagnosis, disease progression and response to treatment.

Podocytopathies

Podocytopathies are the specific group of glomerular disease characterized by proteinuria that is attributed to damage or dysfunction of podocytes.

This damage may be inherent to the podocyte itself due to genetic causes or from other extrinsic factors. The primary podocytopathies include:

1. Minimal change disease (MCD)
2. FSGS
3. Collapsing glomerulopathy
4. Diffuse mesangial sclerosis (DMS)

Pathogenesis The different morphological forms of podocytopathies are actually a reflection of the type

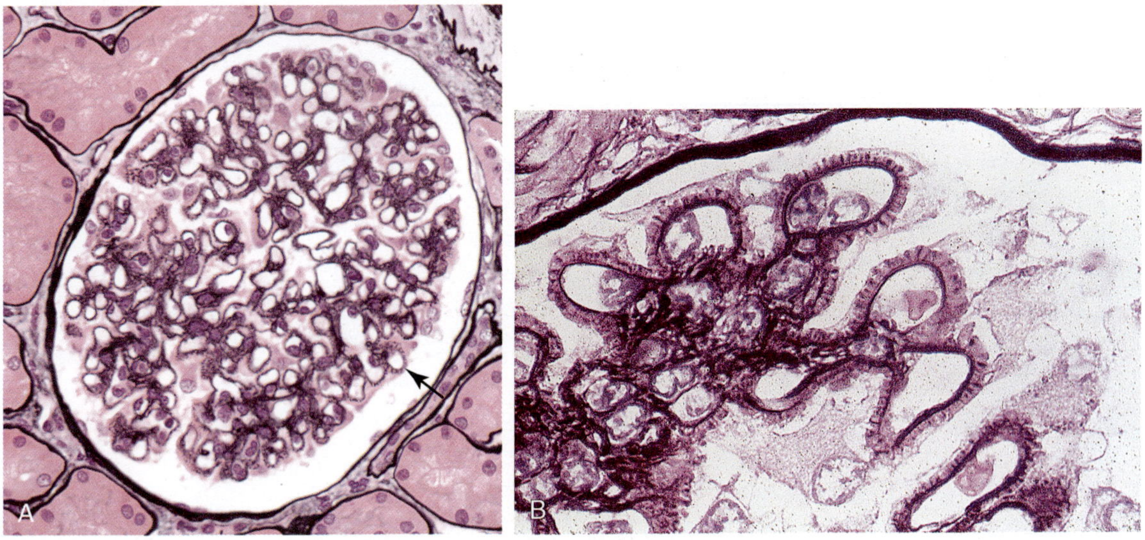

Fig. 24.13 (A) Silver stain showing thickened basement membrane (BM), and (B) a closer view showing a spike and dome pattern. (*Source:* From Anthony Chang and Zoltan G. Laszik. The Kidney. Robbins & Cotran Pathologic Basis of Disease. 10th edition. Elsevier 2021.)

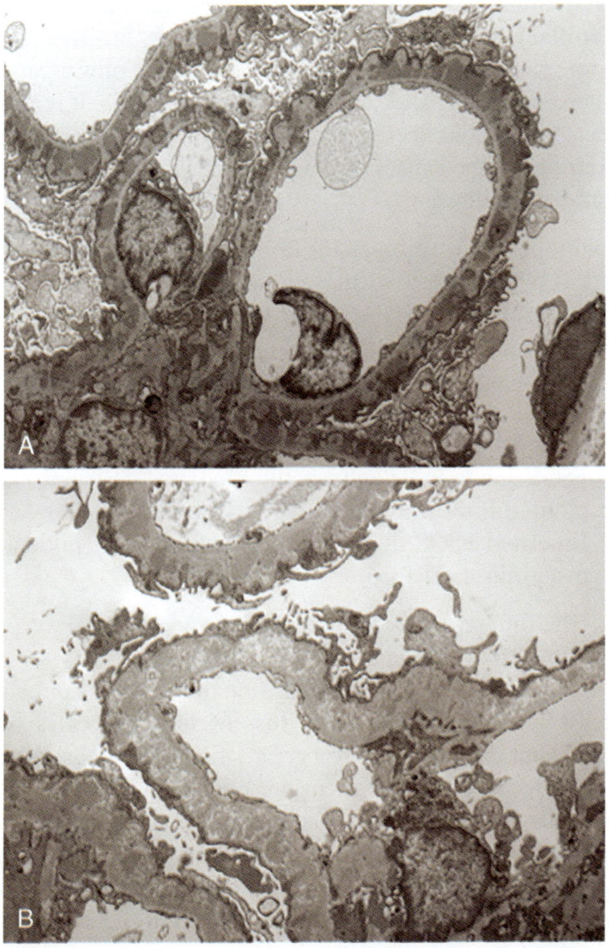

Fig. 24.14 Electron microscopy (EM) appearance of membranous nephropathy showing a spike and dome pattern (A) and thickened basement membrane (BM) with radiolucent vacuolated areas in advanced stages (B). (*Source:* From Edgar Fischer, Lisa A. Cerilli and Donna J. Lager. Glomerular Diseases – Primary. Practical Renal Pathology. Saunders 2013.)

of reparative response of the podocyte to a specific form of insult/injury (Flowchart 24.4).

Minimal Change Disease

MCD, also called **lipoid nephrosis**, is a benign disorder that frequently causes nephrotic syndrome in children aged 2–6 years. It is the most common cause of nephrotic syndrome in the paediatric age group. It is less common in adults. It is called MCD because the morphological changes are not visible by light microscopy and electron microscopic examination is required to confirm the diagnosis. The characteristic features are the occurrence of **selective proteinuria**, and an excellent response to steroids is seen in these patients.

Aetiology and Pathogenesis The disease is caused by immunological damage of the glomeruli. It usually follows respiratory infection or immunization and may be associated with atopic disorders. Hodgkin lymphoma, which is associated with T-cell defects, has also been found to be associated with MCD. Secondary MCD may also be due to NSAID use and may be associated with acute interstitial nephritis. The hypothesis is that proteinuria is the **podocyte injury** (podocytopathy) and associated **loss of charge barrier** in the filtration membrane of the glomeruli. The mechanism of protein leakage may be attributed to the following:

- Transcellular passage of proteins through the epithelial cells
- Passage through residual spaces between damaged foot processes
- Leakage through abnormal spaces that develop under the foot process that directly abuts the basement membrane
- Leakage through areas of detachment of epithelial cells from the basement membrane

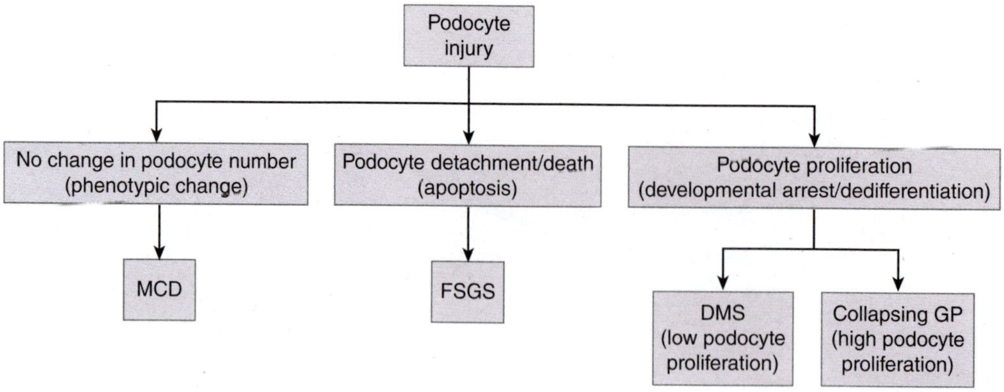

Flowchart 24.4 Podocyte injury.

Morphology

Light Microscopy As the name implies, the glomeruli appear normal. However, it is important that the tubular cells are filled with lipid and protein due to tubular reabsorption of lipoproteins that had been filtered by the glomeruli due to their defective filtration apparatus. These cells may be shed and appear in urine. Before signing out a report of MCD, it is important to analyse as many histopathological sections as possible so as to not miss any FSGS because it carries a worse clinical course and a bad prognosis.

Immunofluorescence Immunofluorescence shows absent immunoglobulin or complement deposits.

Electron microscopy (Fig. 24.15) This is the diagnostic investigation. It shows uniform and **diffuse effacement of foot process**, with an inability to visualize the slit diaphragms normally seen between the foot processes. This actually reflects the flattening, retraction and swelling of foot processes of the epithelial cells. This effacement of foot processes is also present in other conditions such as membranous glomerulopathy and diabetic nephropathy that are associated with proteinuria. Hence, the diagnosis of MCD can be made only if the effacement is associated with normal glomeruli by light microscopy and there are no electron-dense deposits on the basement membrane.

Clinical Course The children have a good renal function despite the massive proteinuria. There is no hypertension or haematuria. About 90% of children respond dramatically to corticosteroids and can become steroid dependent or steroid resistant. Even steroid-dependent children recover on reaching puberty. In adults, the response is slow and relapse may occur but long-term prognosis is good.

Prognosis Long-term prognosis is excellent in children. MCD never progresses to renal failure. If MCD progresses to renal failure, it is likely that the initial glomerular pathology was FSGS and not MCD.

Focal Segmental Glomerulosclerosis

FSGS is the most common cause of nephrotic syndrome worldwide in adults, accounting for about 20%–30% of cases, with a frequent occurrence in children. **It may be defined as a 'segmental solidification of the glomerular capillary tuft with accumulation of extracellular matrix, often with an adhesion (synechia) between the capillary tuft and Bowman's capsule'.**It involves only some glomeruli and even in those glomeruli, only a part is affected a part is affected, hence the name FSGS. It is associated with nonselective proteinuria.

Aetiology The causes of FSGS have helped in its classification as follows:

- Idiopathic or primary FSGS
- FSGS associated with HIV infection (HIV-associated nephropathy [HIVAN]) or heroin addiction (heroin nephropathy)
- Post–adaptive FSGS as a response to renal ablation, reflux nephropathy, renal agenesis or dysplasia, obesity, sickle cell disease or advanced hypertensive nephropathy
- FSGS due to IgA nephropathy-mediated destruction of glomeruli resulting in scarring (secondary FSGS)
- Inherited FSGS due to genetic mutations in podocin, α-actinin-4, TRPC6

The differences between primary and secondary types are given in Table 24.6.

Pathogenesis FSGS is a disease of the visceral epithelial cells (podocytes) that suffer **loss of foot processes** like MCD but differ from it by a greater frequency of haematuria, reduced GFR, hypertension, nonselective proteinuria, absence of response to steroids and greater chances of progression to chronic renal disease. Hyalinosis seen in the glomeruli is due to plasma protein/lipid entrapment that occurs due to the **hyperpermeability of GBM**. Genetic basis of FSGS may be due to one of the following mutations:

- Mutation in NPHS1 on chromosome 19q13 that encodes nephrin, a component of the slit diaphragm that controls the glomerular filtration process, gives rise to CNS of the Finnish type.

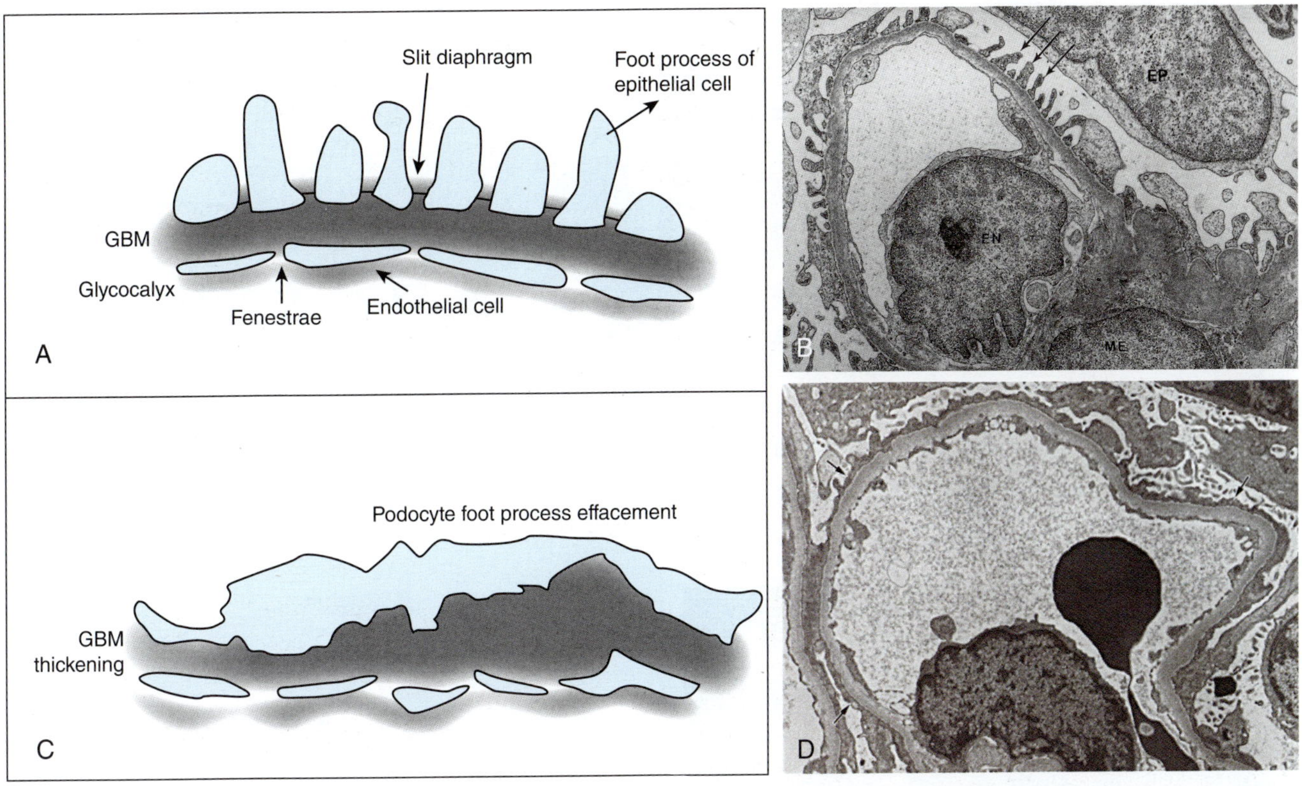

Fig. 24.15 Schematic representation and electron microscopy (EM) view of normal; arrows showing podocytes with foot process (A and B) versus effaced foot processes (C and D). (*Source:* From Neeraja Kambham. Kidney: Non-Neoplastic Diseases. Rosai and Ackerman's Surgical Pathology. 11th edition. Elsevier 2018.)

Table 24.6 Differences Between Idiopathic and Secondary Focal Segmental Glomerulosclerosis

Primary	Secondary
Abrupt in onset	Insidious
Normal-sized glomeruli, less parenchymal atrophy	Glomerular hypertrophy noted in unaffected glomeruli Loss of parenchyma with focal interstitial fibrosis and global glomerulosclerosis seen
Diffuse global podocyte foot process effacement	Segmental podocyte foot process effacement
No evidence of background renal damage	Evidence of the aetiology noted (IC, crescents, DM, Fabry disease, Alport syndrome, HTN)

DM, diabetes mellitus; HTN, hypertension; IC, immune complex.

- Mutation in NPHS2 on chromosome 1q25–q31 that encodes podocin, also a component of the slit diaphragm, gives rise to autosomal recessive steroid-resistant nephrotic syndrome.
- Mutation in α-actinin-4 gives rise to autosomal dominant FSGS, which has a higher tendency to cause renal insufficiency.

Morphology

Light Microscopy (Fig. 24.16) Primary FSGS involves the juxtamedullary glomeruli, with progression to cortical involvement as the disease evolves. There is sparing of glomeruli and involvement is seen partly in few glomeruli. In the sclerotic segments, capillary lumen may get occluded by hyalinosis. Extensive sampling is mandatory because the lesion may be missed due to insufficient glomeruli.

Collapsing glomerulopathy is the variant of FSGS characterized by segmental capillary tuft collapse (wrinkling and folding) in at least one glomerulus associated with podocyte hypertrophy and/or hyperplasia (pseudocrescent), seen in HIV infection, drug-induced toxicity and microvascular injury. The tubules show atrophy and interstitial fibrosis. It is characteristically associated with a poor prognosis.

Immunofluorescence (Fig. 24.17) Nonspecific entrapment of IgM and C3 deposits are seen in the sclerotic areas and mesangium.

Electron microscopy Diffuse effacement of foot processes is seen in the sclerotic and nonsclerotic areas.

Variants of FSGS Variants of FSGS are distinguished with the help of light microscopic features and are useful

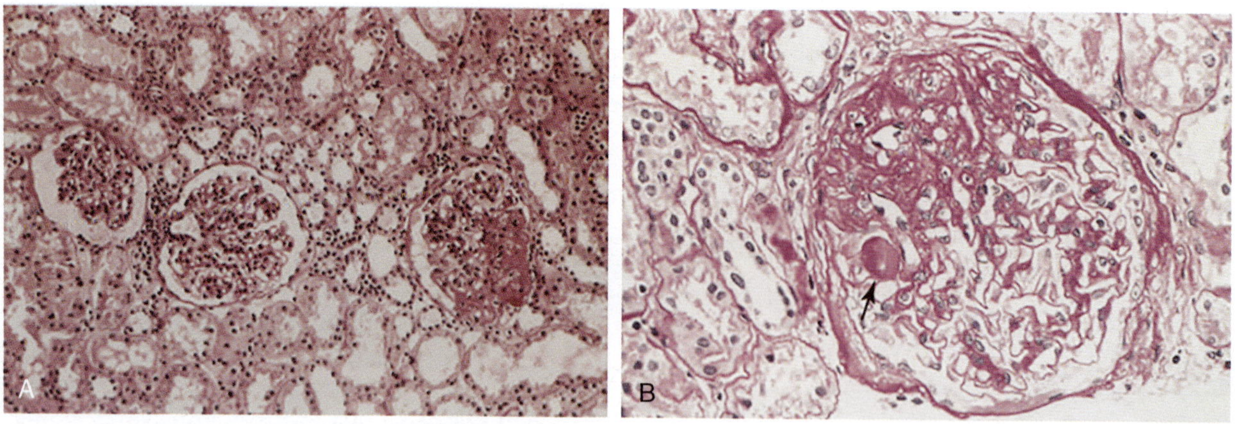

Fig. 24.16 Light microscopy (LM) of FSGS showing segmental sclerosis of one of the three glomeruli (A) with hyaline deposition evident at closer view (B). (ROBBINS)

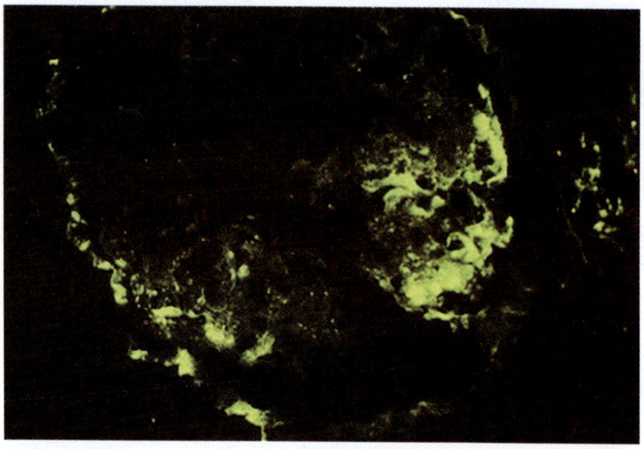

Fig. 24.17 Immunofluorescence (IF) showing segmental deposition of IgM in FSGS. (*Source:* From Neeraja Kambham. Kidney: Non-Neoplastic Diseases. Rosai and Ackerman's Surgical Pathology. 11th edition. Elsevier 2018.)

to predict response to therapy and prognosis. The collapsing variant has the highest chance of progression to ESRD.

Type	Features
Perihilar variant	Perihilar hyalinosis and sclerosis in at least 50% of glomeruli (secondary FSGS)
Tip variant	Segmental lesion with the expansion of glomerular tuft at the origin (tubular pole)
Collapsing variant	Collapse of tuft with visceral cell hyperplasia and hypertrophy in at least one glomerulus (Fig. 24.18)
Cellular variant	Segmental endocapillary hypercellularity
FSGS NOS (Not otherwise specified)	Lacks features of other variants

FSGS, focal segmental glomerulosclerosis.

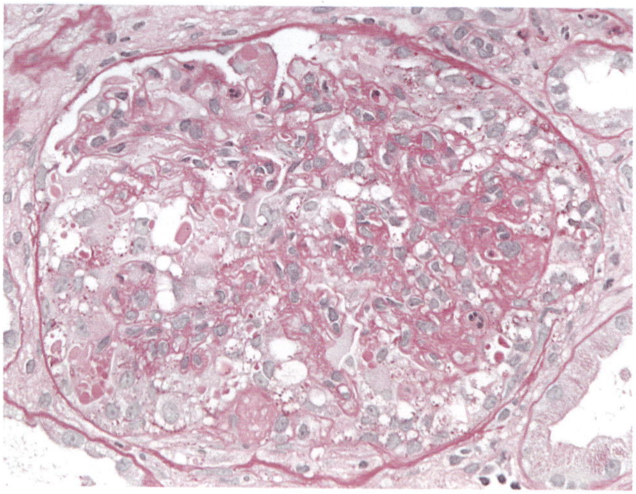

Fig. 24.18 Light microscopy (LM) of collapsing variant of focal segmental glomerulosclerosis showing obliteration of Bowman's space by podocyte proliferation and retraction of the basement membrane (BM) of glomeruli. (*Source:* From Neeraja Kambham. Kidney: Non-Neoplastic Diseases. Rosai and Ackerman's Surgical Pathology. 11th edition. Elsevier 2018.)

Clinical Course Both MCD and FSGS are podocytopathies. The incidence of haematuria and hypertension is more with FSGS and the response to steroids is poor.

Prognosis Children have a better prognosis than adults. The collapsing variant seen in HIV-infected patients has an unfavourable prognosis, whereas the tip variant has a better prognosis. Progression to ESRD in 10 years is seen in 50% of cases.

HIV-Associated Nephropathy

HIVAN is a classic triad of collapsing glomerulopathy type of FSGS, tubulointerstitial inflammation and microcystic tubular dilation. Microscopy shows cystically dilated glands filled with proteinaceous material along

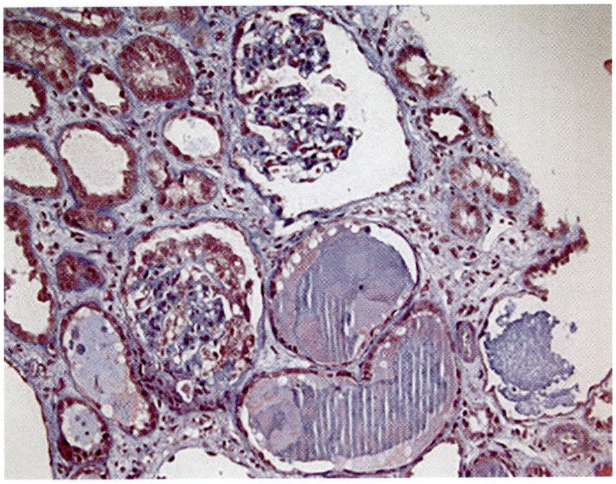

Fig. 24.19 Microscopy of HIV-associated nephropathy showing tubular dilation with casts and collapsing glomerulopathy. (*Source:* From Edgar Fischer, Lisa A. Cerilli and Donna J. Lager. Glomerular Diseases – Primary. Practical Renal Pathology. Saunders 2013.)

with fibrosis and inflammation (Fig. 24.19). Electron microscopy reveals tubuloreticular inclusion bodies that represent modified endoplasmic reticulum in the endothelium. The other HIV-associated renal lesions are as follows:

- Acute interstitial nephritis due to drugs or infection
- Thrombotic microangiopathy (TMA)
- PIGN

Diffuse Mesangial Sclerosis

DMS may be defined as an increase in mesangial matrix without mesangial cellular proliferation, leading to obliteration of glomerular capillaries and eventual glomerulosclerosis.

It is generally a histological finding in CNS or infantile nephrotic syndrome (INS). It can occur as an isolated histological finding or it can be syndromic and associated with Frasier syndrome (gonadoblastoma, CNS, pseudohermaphroditism) or Denys–Drash syndrome (Wilms tumour, CNS, pseudohermaphroditism). DMS carries a worse prognosis and is steroid resistant.

Membranoproliferative Glomerulonephritis

MPGN refers to a pattern of injury characterized by diffuse mesangial expansion due to endocapillary proliferation and increased mesangial matrix, and thickened capillary walls, often with a split 'tram-track' appearance.

MPGN, previously called mesangiocapillary GN, accounts for 5%–10% of cases of nephrotic syndrome in children and young adults. The presentation is a combination of nephrotic–nephritic picture. It is a morphological pattern evidenced in the glomeruli that may be a consequence of two different pathways of immune-mediated injury. Hence, MPGN is classified into type I (due to immune complex and complement deposition) and type II (due to complement activation that puts it under group C3 glomerulopathies).

Aetiology and Pathogenesis MPGN is an immune-mediated GN. It involves activation of classical and alternate complement pathways. The aetiology may be a primary damage to the glomeruli (primary or idiopathic MPGN) or secondary to other diseases (secondary MPGN). Idiopathic MPGN is an immune complex–mediated GN often due to planted antigens associated with hepatitis B/C and cryglobulinaemia, whereas secondary MPGN may be due to SLE, hepatitis B and C, HIV infection, schistosomiasis, endocarditis, α-antitrypsin deficiency and malignancies such as chronic lymphocytic leukaemia.

Two Types of MPGN (Flowchart 24.5) MPGN was earlier classified on the basis of the location of deposits as type I (mesangial and subendothelial deposits), type II (mesangial and intramembranous) and type III (subendothelial, intramembranous and subepithelial electron-dense deposits). But newer classification is based on the pathogenetic pathway and is given as follows:

1. Type I MPGN: This may be due to planted antigens stimulating immune complex formation in situ or deposition of circulating preformed immune complexes.
2. Type II MPGN: Also called C3 glomerulopathy, it includes C3 **glomerulonephritis** (C3GN) and dense deposit disease (DDD).
3. Type III MPGN of Anders and Burkholder: It is an immune complex–associated MPGN with no known causative factors (idiopathic).

C3GN and DDD

'By definition, both C3GN and DDD are defined as at least a two-level increase (2+) in fluorescence intensity of isolated C3 deposits compared with other immunoglobulins'.

DDD

The pathogenesis of DDD involves activation of alternate complement pathway (Fig. 24.20), which is evidenced by decreased C3 levels and factor B, decreased properdin and normal C1 and C4 levels. Normally, C3 convertase is labile and gets degraded spontaneously due to the action of factor H or I, but in DDD, an autoantibody, namely **C3 nephritic factor**, is formed that binds to C3 convertase and prevents inactivation. This leads to continuous C3 activation and hypocomplementaemia. The other mechanisms for hypocomplementaemia include decreased synthesis of C3 by the liver and mutation of factor H, factor I and membrane cofactor protein (MCP).

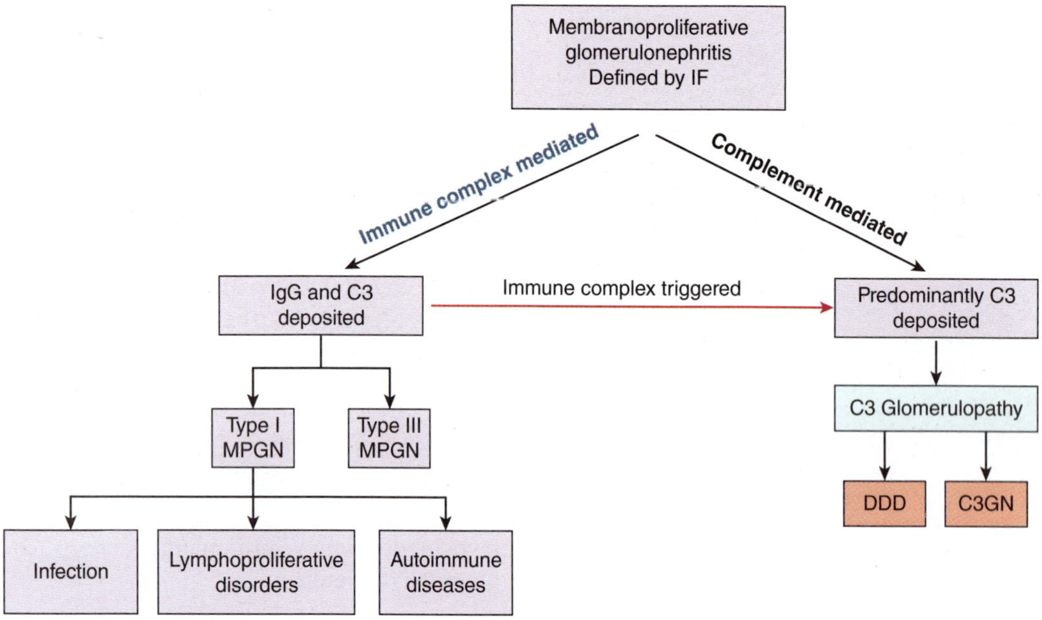

Flowchart 24.5 Classification of membranoproliferative glomerulonephritis.

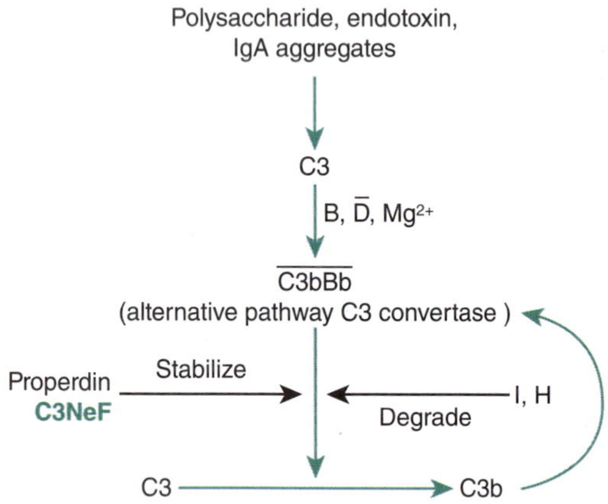

Fig. 24.20 Alternative complement pathway in dense deposit disease (type II MPGN).

Morphology

Light microscopy (Fig. 24.21)

Type I MPGN

Glomeruli are large and hypercellular, with lobular accentuation due to proliferation of endothelium, mesangium and leucocytes. There is interpositioning of the mesangial cell between the endothelium and GBM causing **duplication/splitting of GBM**, giving a '**tram-track**' appearance. Crescents may be present.

Type II MPGN DDD and C3GN

Although both these conditions were earlier stratified under the category of MPGN, the morphological patterns on light microscopy may show varying patterns like membranoproliferative pattern, mesangioproliferative pattern, exudative pattern or crescentic pattern of injury.

In addition, there is the presence of dense eosinophilic, refractile, ribbon-like thickening of GBM and tubules that are periodic acid–Schiff (PAS) positive in DDD.

Type III MPGN of Anders and Burkholder

The light microscopic features are similar to those of membranoproliferative GN type 1.

Immunofluorescence

In type I and type III MPGN, granular deposits of IgG, C3, C1q and C4 in GBM are present.

In DDD and other C3 glomerulopathies, granular/linear deposits of C3 are present in GBM on its either side and in the mesangium as **mesangial rings**. C3 deposits may also be present in TBM. As discussed earlier, the C3-dominant deposits should have a 2+ increase in the magnitude of the fluorescence compared with other immunoglobulins.

IgG, C1q and C4 are absent in C3 glomerulopathy, indicating the absence of classical pathway involvement.

Electron Microscopy (Fig. 24.22)

In type I MPGN, electron-dense deposits are present in the subendothelium.

In DDD, ribbon-like, homogeneous, electron-dense intramembranous deposits are present (lamina densa of GBM). Similar dense deposits may also be seen in the mesangium.

This deposit is characteristically absent in C3 glomerulopathy, thus differentiating it from DDD.

In type III MPGN, deposits are seen in the subendothelial, mesangial and intramembranous sites.

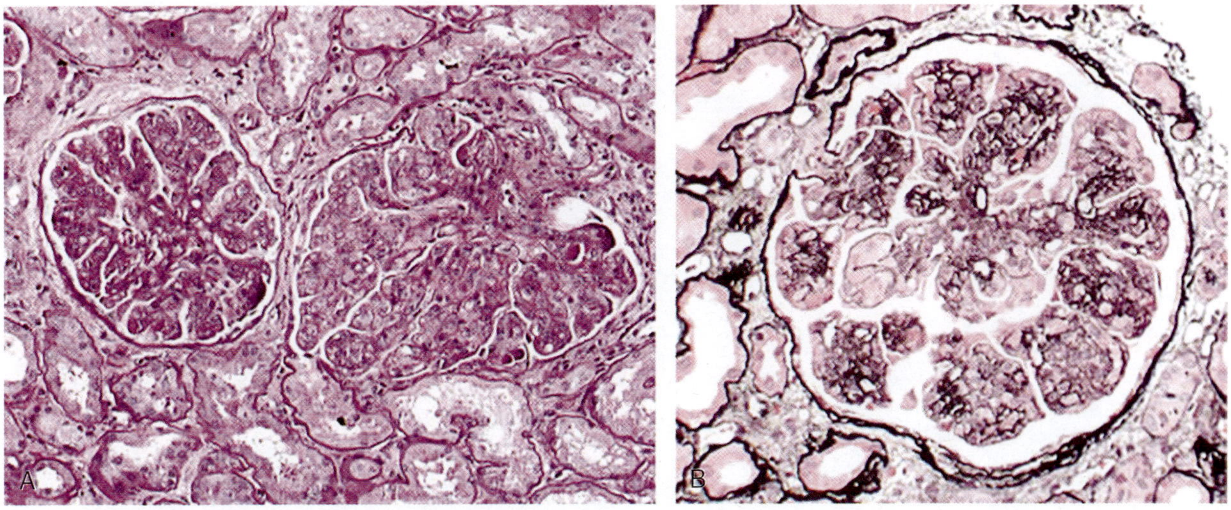

Fig. 24.21 MPGN light microscopy shows mesangial and endocapillary proliferation (A) and silver stain shows splitting of the basement membrane (tram-track appearance) (B). (*Source:* From Edgar Fischer, Lisa A. Cerilli and Donna J. Lager. Glomerular Diseases – Primary. Practical Renal Pathology. Saunders 2013.)

Clinical Course Primary MPGN is seen in young adults as mild proteinuria and haematuria. DDD occurs in younger individuals compared with C3 glomerulopathy. Treatment with steroids, immunosuppressive drugs and antiplatelet drugs is not proven to have any benefit.

Prognosis Prognosis is poor. Only few remissions occur spontaneously in either type.

- Some develop crescents and progress to RPGN.
- Forty per cent of patients progress to end stage renal disease (ESRD).
- Thirty per cent of patients develop renal insufficiency.
- Thirty per cent of patients have persistent nephrotic syndrome without renal failure.

In C3 glomerulopathy and DDD, if transplanted, 90% of transplant recipients have a risk of recurrence and progression to ESRD, and 50% develop renal failure.

GLOMERULAR LESIONS ASSOCIATED WITH SYSTEMIC DISEASES PA 28.7

Many systemic diseases such as infections, metabolic disorders and autoimmune diseases affect the kidneys directly and indirectly and produce lesions in the glomeruli. We shall study the diseases in detail in the respective chapters, but here we review their glomerular lesions briefly.

Lupus Nephritis

About 50% of patients with SLE have renal involvement. According to the current classification, glomerular diseases are grouped into six patterns (classes I–VI). Class I is the least common, and class IV, which shows **wire loop lesions** (Fig. 24.23), is the most common pattern. One class can evolve into another class over time.

An activity and a chronicity score are mandatory in cases of lupus nephritis. The activity score is based on proliferation, the presence of crescents, fibrinoid necrosis, neutrophilic infiltration, interstitial inflammation and subendothelial deposits (wire loop lesions). The chronicity score is based on the presence of fibrous crescents, glomerulosclerosis, interstitial fibrosis and tubular atrophy.
The various classes are divided on the basis of the features of lupus nephritis discussed in detail in Chapter 6 under Systemic Lupus Erythematosus.

Henoch Schonlein Purpura (HSP)

HSP is associated with purpuric skin lesions on the extensor surface of the arms, legs and buttocks, along with abdominal pain, intestinal bleeding, arthralgia and renal manifestations. The renal involvement may be in the form of the following:

- Gross and microscopic haematuria
- Nephritic syndrome
- Nephrotic syndrome
- RPGN

HSP commonly affects children between 3 and 8 years old and adults. Symptoms usually follow respiratory infection and atopy. Pathogenesis is due to deposition of predominant IgA deposits in the mesangium of the kidney as well as in the dermal vessels and the vessels of the GI tract. In addition, IgG and C3 may be present in the mesangium and vessels in the dermis and the GI tract. The disease course is variable and haematuria may recur. Prognosis is usually excellent in children but worse if associated with crescents.

Bacterial Endocarditis

Bacterial endocarditis may cause focal and segmental necrotizing GN or diffuse exudative and proliferative GN or show an MPGN pattern. Rarely, it may also lead to crescentic GN.

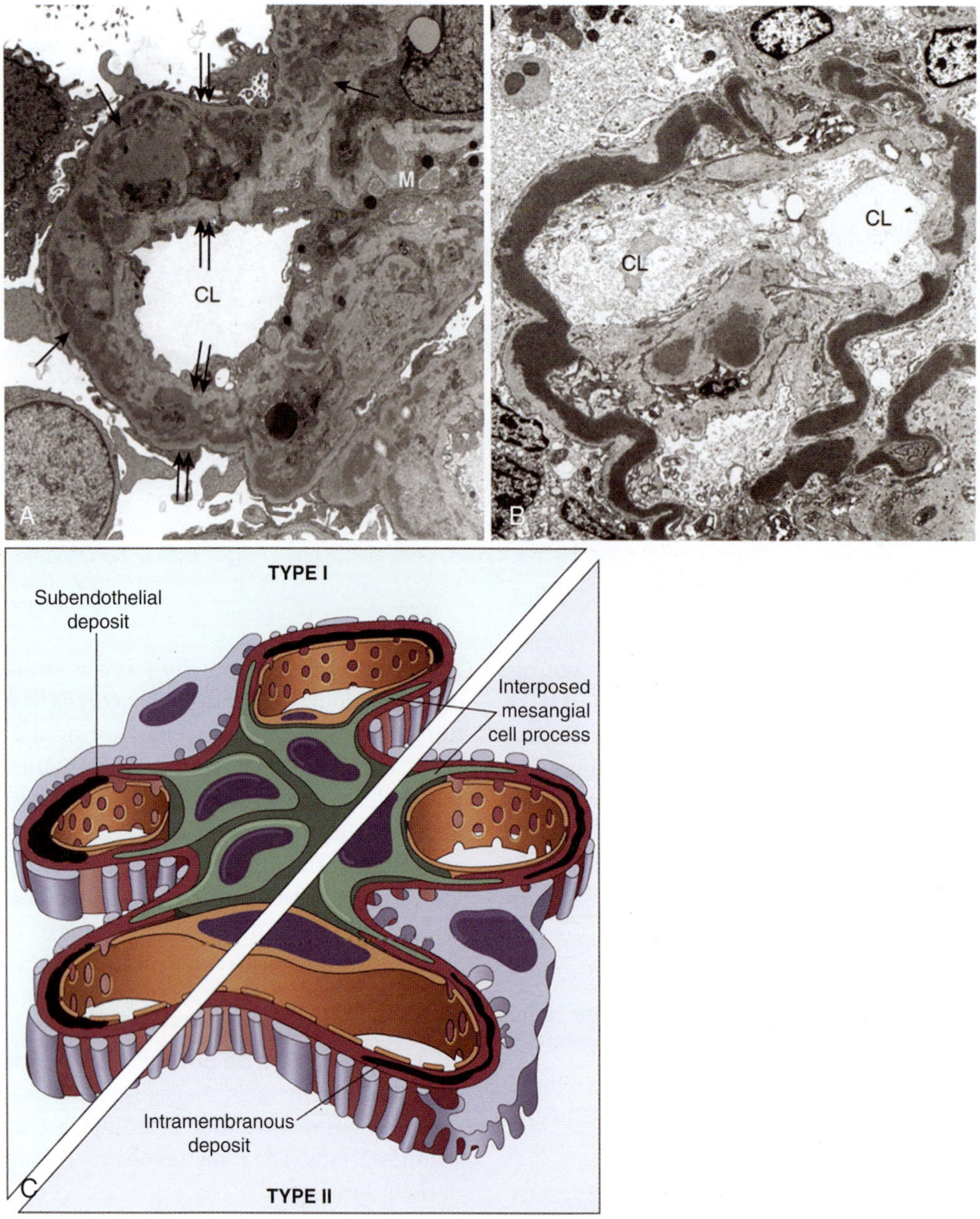

Fig. 24.22 Type I versus type II MPGN – schematic representation. Electron microscopy (A) shows deposits trapped between duplicated basement membrane, whereas (B) shows dense homogeneous intramembranous deposit, both exemplified by the schematic representation (C). MPGN, membranoproliferative glomerulonephritis. (*Source:* ([A], Courtesy Dr. Jolanta Kowalewska, Cedars-Sinai Medical Center, Los Angeles, Calif. [B and C] Robbins & Cotran Pathologic Basis of Disease, 10th ed.: Abul K. Abbas, Jon C. Aster, Vinay Kumar, Fig. 20.17, Elsevier Inc. 2021.)

Diabetic Nephropathy

The glomerular lesions in diabetic nephropathy include nodular glomerulosclerosis (**Kimmelstiel–Wilson disease**) that is pathognomonic of diabetic nephropathy, diffuse glomerulosclerosis and capillary basement membrane thickening. The renal vascular lesion is arteriolosclerosis, and the other manifestations are pyelonephritis and papillary necrosis. The topic will be dealt with in detail in Chapter 28.

Fibrillary GN

Fibrillary GN is a rare form of GN in which there is deposition of fibrillary Congo red negative amyloid-like deposits in the mesangium. The glomeruli show an MPGN pattern or mesangioproliferative changes in microscopy and the pathogenesis is unknown. On immunofluorescence, there is a specific pattern of ill-defined smudgy (nongranular) deposits of IgG and C3 in the mesangium and GBM. Electron microscopy shows fibrillary deposits of 15- to 30-nm diameter in the mesangium and GBM.

Other conditions that show glomerular lesions are Goodpasture syndrome, microscopic polyangiitis, granulomatosis with polyangiitis, essential mixed cryoglobulinaemia and amyloidosis.

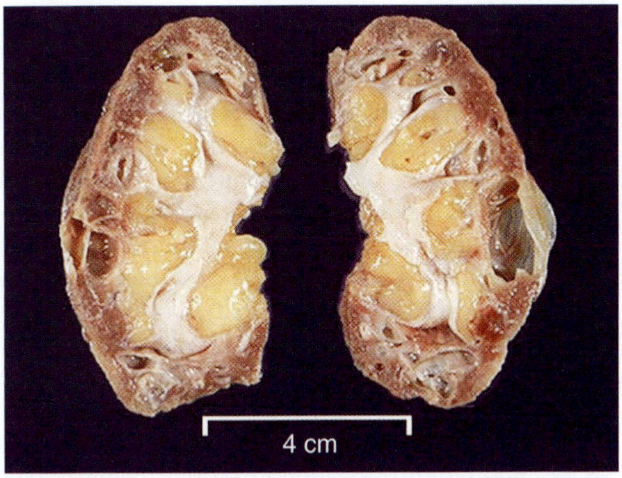

Fig. 24.23 Light microscopy showing wire loop lesions in lupus nephritis (PAS stain). (*Source:* From Neeraja Kambham. Kidney: Non-Neoplastic Diseases. Rosai and Ackerman's Surgical Pathology. 11th edition. Elsevier 2018.)

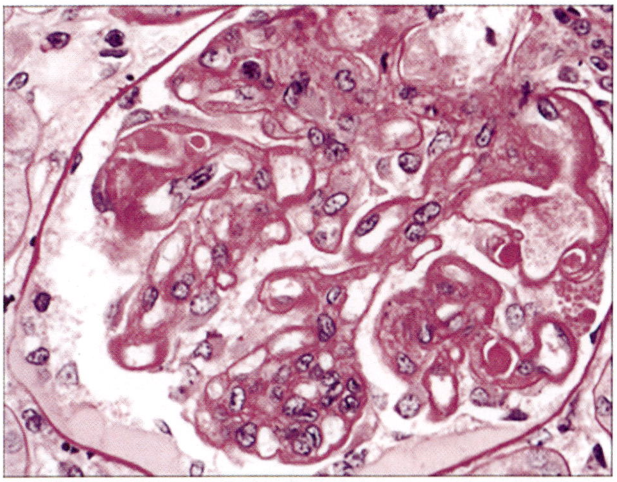

Fig. 24.24 Gross appearance of contracted kidney in chronic glomerulonephritis. (*Source:* From James W. Little DMD, MS, Craig S. Miller DMD, MS and Nelson L. Rhodus DMD, MPH. Chronic Kidney Disease and Dialysis. Little and Falace's Dental Management of the Medically Compromised Patient. 9th edition. Elsevier 2018.)

CHRONIC GLOMERULONEPHRITIS

Chronic GN refers to the end-stage glomerular disease that may be due to any kidney disease with a specific type of GN or can occur without any antecedent history of acute GN.

Aetiology and Pathogenesis

The glomerular diseases that may eventually lead to chronic GN are as follows:

- Membranous Nephropathy
- Membranoproliferative glomerulonephritis
- IgA nephropathy
- Focal segmental glomerulosclerosis
- Crescentic glomerulonephrtis
- PSGN, which is a rare cause, except in adults

Chronic GN in cases without a history of glomerular disease may be attributed to asymptomatic forms of GN that went undiagnosed.

Morphology

Gross (Fig. 24.24) The kidneys are **symmetrically contracted** with a diffusely **granular cortical surface**. The external surface appears red-brown. The cut surface shows thinned-out cortex with an increase in peripelvic fat.

Light Microscopy In early stages, the glomeruli show changes related to the primary glomerular disease. Later, the glomeruli are obliterated by the leaked-out plasma proteins, increased mesangial matrix, collagen and basement membrane–like material and finally get sclerosed. The tubules are atrophied. The interstitium shows lymphocytic infiltrate and fibrosis. The associated hypertension causes arterial and arteriolar scleroses.

Clinical Course

Chronic GN develops insidiously and slowly progresses to renal insufficiency. Patients may present with proteinuria, microscopic haematuria, hypertension and azotaemia. Later, proteinuria diminishes due to sclerosis-associated loss of glomerular filtration.

Prognosis

MPGN may cause uncontrolled hypertension leading to ESRD. After it develops, the primary involvement of the kidney compartment is difficult to analyse. Death may occur due to uraemia and electrolyte imbalance, if not treated by dialysis or transplantation.

APPROACH TO PATIENTS WITH GLOMERULAR DISEASES

Glomerular diseases may be classified into five broad categories on the basis of their clinical presentation or by histopathology. On the basis of clinical manifestations, the categories are nephrotic, nephritic, RPGN, chronic GN and isolated urinary abnormalities. Each category has a set of diagnostic features that are given in Table 24.7.

Diagnosis of these conditions is helped by an elaborate history, clinical examination, biochemical and serological evaluation and finally a renal biopsy.

- **Clinical history** helps to establish the nature of the disease, especially to differentiate whether the pathology is a **primary** renal disease or is **secondary** to a systemic disease. Glomerular diseases may be secondary to systemic autoimmune diseases, metabolic diseases such as diabetic mellitus, infections such as hepatitis and HIV infection, drug intake such as NSAIDs, and tumours such as Hodgkin lymphoma and colonic carcinoma.

Table 24.7 Categories of Glomerular Diseases and Their Manifestations

Syndromes	Manifestations
Nephritic syndrome	Haematuria, azotaemia, variable proteinuria, oliguria, oedema and hypertension
Rapidly progressive glomerulonephritis	Acute nephritis, proteinuria and acute renal failure
Nephrotic syndrome	>3.5 g/day proteinuria, hypoalbuminaemia, hyperlipidaemia, lipiduria
Chronic renal failure	Azotaemia → uraemia progressing for months to years
Isolated urinary abnormalities	Glomerular haematuria and/or subnephrotic proteinuria

- **Examination** of the patient helps to identify periorbital oedema, dependent oedema, evidence of streptococcal skin lesions and other signs of azotaemia. Signs of systemic disease such as SLE and uncontrolled diabetes must be identified. Measurement of BP helps to diagnose hypertension, which is an important manifestation of acute GN.
- **Urine analysis** is performed to check for proteinuria and haematuria.
- **Urine microscopy of sediments** helps to identify renal casts – RBC casts are seen in acute GN, whereas lipid casts are a feature of nephrotic syndrome. RBCs in urine can be attributed to glomerular pathology when microscopy shows dysmorphic RBCs and acanthocytes.
- A **24-hour urine examination** helps to identify **oliguria** and quantification of **proteinuria**. Normal protein loss in urine is less than 150 mg/day, and albumin contributes up to 20–30 mg. Increased protein excretion is a hallmark of glomerular disease. **Nephrotic range proteinuria** is defined as a urine protein excretion of more than 3.5 g/day, and proteinuria less than that quantity is labelled as **non-nephrotic proteinuria**. Proteinuria of less than 2 g/24 h in the absence of significant haematuria and other symptoms of nephritic syndrome is termed asymptomatic proteinuria and requires a close observation.
- **Urine protein-to-creatinine ratio** is a convenient alternative to 24-hour urine protein estimation because it is a random spot examination. A value of more than 3.5 indicates nephrotic range proteinuria.
- **Serum albumin** estimation helps to identify hypoalbuminaemia (>3.5 g/dL), which is a component of nephrotic syndrome presentation. Hypoalbuminaemia in nephrotic syndrome can be attributed to urinary losses of albumin, insufficient compensation by hepatic synthesis and increased albumin catabolism in the kidney in these patients.
- **Serology to identify infectious aetiology** and to evaluate the presence of autoimmune disorders may help in secondary glomerular diseases.
- **Renal imaging studies:** Newer imaging methods to evaluate glomerular function have been attempted with good success rates. These methods are especially useful in diseases with patchy renal involvement in which biopsies have the chances of missing the lesion. Dynamic contrast-enhanced (DCE) MRI and blood oxygen level–dependent (BOLD) MRI help in functional evaluation of the kidney.
- **Renal biopsy:** Renal biopsy helps to directly evaluate the renal parenchyma, confirm the diagnosis and perform ancillary tests such as immunofluorescence. This is an important investigation in various renal pathologies, so we shall review renal biopsy briefly here. The indications for renal biopsy include the following:
  - Unexplained renal failure
  - Acute nephritic syndrome
  - Nephrotic syndrome
  - Isolated non-nephrotic proteinuria
  - Isolated glomerular haematuria
  - Renal transplant rejection
  - Collagen tissue diseases such as SLE

The procedure is performed using a Tru-Cut needle under imaging guidance, and two cores of 1-cm length and 1.2-mm diameter are sent to the laboratory. The tissue is divided into three parts, one each for histopathology, electron microscopy and immunofluorescence. A **minimum of five glomeruli** should be seen to consider the biopsy as adequate (Fig. 24.25). In histopathology, a number of stains are used to evaluate the various components of the renal tissue and they are enlisted in Table 24.8.

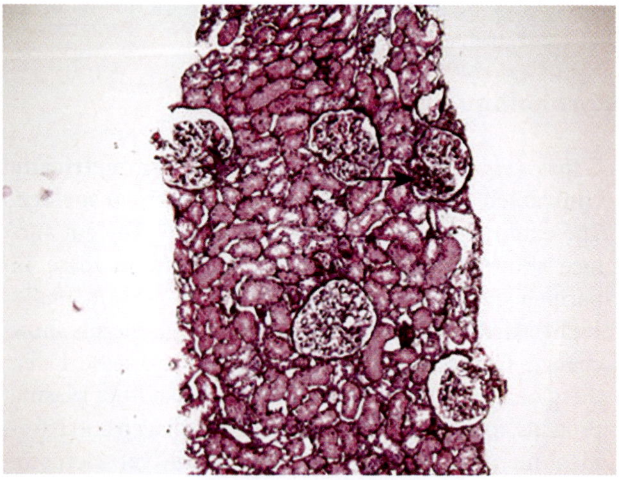

Fig. 24.25 Renal biopsy core showing five glomeruli (silver stain). (*Source:* From Edgar Fischer, Lisa A. Cerilli and Donna J. Lager. Glomerular Diseases – Primary. Practical Renal Pathology. Saunders 2013.)

Table 24.8 Stains Used in Histopathology Evaluation of Renal Biopsy

Stain	Utility
Haematoxylin and eosin stain (H and E)	General evaluation, cellular characteristics, type of inflammation
Periodic acid–Schiff stain	Glomerular cell number, basement membrane, mesangium, tubular basement membrane, hyaline (red colour)
Silver methenamine (Jones)	Basement details (black colour)
Masson's trichrome	Extracellular glomerular matrix and tubular basement membranes (blue or green)
Congo red	Amyloid
Von Kossa	Calcification
Acid fuchsin orange G	Protein deposition (immune complex)
Sirus red	Fibrosis

Immunofluorescence is performed on frozen sections of unfixed tissue. The commonly used markers include fluorescein-labelled antibodies against immunoglobulins (primarily IgG, IgM and IgA), complement components (primarily C3, C1q and C4), fibrin, and kappa and lambda light chains.

The tissue for electron microscopy is fixed in 2%–3% glutaraldehyde and processed. The electron microscopic examination helps to localize deposits, detect extremely small deposits and identify alterations of cellular and basement membrane structure.

All these investigations guide the clinician to make an appropriate diagnosis of the renal pathology and titrate the treatment to the patient.

TUBULAR AND INTERSTITIAL DISEASES

Diseases that affect the interstitium tend to affect the tubules also. Factors that affect the tubulointerstitial compartment may be divided into ischaemic/toxic and inflammatory causes.

ACUTE TUBULAR INJURY/NECROSIS PA 28.9

Acute tubular injury (ATI) is the most common cause of AKI with oliguria. It leads to AKI with or without necrosis of renal tubular epithelial cells. It may be caused by ischaemia or direct toxic injury. The damage to tubular epithelial cells results in decline of renal function, leading to decreased GFR and increased creatinine.

Aetiology

On the basis of the cause, ATI can be broadly classified into the following:

- **Ischaemic ATI:** The ischaemia due to decreased blood flow may be caused by the following:
  - Microscopic polyangiitis
  - Malignant hypertension
  - Haemolytic uraemic syndrome (HUS)
  - Thrombotic thrombocytopenic purpura (TTP)
  - Disseminated intravascular coagulation
  - Hypovolaemic shock
  - Mismatched blood transfusion
- **Nephrotoxic ATI:** This is caused by direct toxic injury due to the passage of the following toxins through the tubules:
  - Myoglobin
  - Haemoglobin
  - Monoclonal light chains
  - Bile
  - Drugs and heavy metals (CCl_4, mercury, gentamicin)
  - Radiocontrast dye

Pathogenesis (Flowchart 24.6)

Disturbances in blood flow

Compromise in blood flow to the kidney leads to haemodynamic alteration and affects glomerular filtration. The basis of the blood flow disturbance may be due to the following mechanisms:

- **Endothelial injury** → causes increase in endothelin and decrease in NO and prostaglandins synthesis → leads to intrarenal vasoconstriction → reduced blood flow → decreased oxygen delivery to the thick ascending limb and straight segment of the proximal tubule
- **Ischaemia** → leads to alteration in epithelial cell polarity → redistribution of Na^+–K^+-ATPase from the basolateral to the luminal surface of tubule epithelium → decreased proximal tubular reabsorption of sodium → causes increased sodium delivery to distal tubules → tubuloglomerular feedback triggered → renin–angiotensin system activated → eventually results in vasoconstriction

Tubule cell injury

Injury to the tubules is due to ischaemia and toxins (Fig. 24.26). The ischaemic tubular cells express cytokines and adhesion molecules and recruit leucocytes. The injured cells obstruct the lumen, decrease GFR and cause interstitial inflammation. The tubulointerstitial leak caused by the damage of tubular epithelium leads to interstitial oedema that further damages the tubules and decreases GFR further.

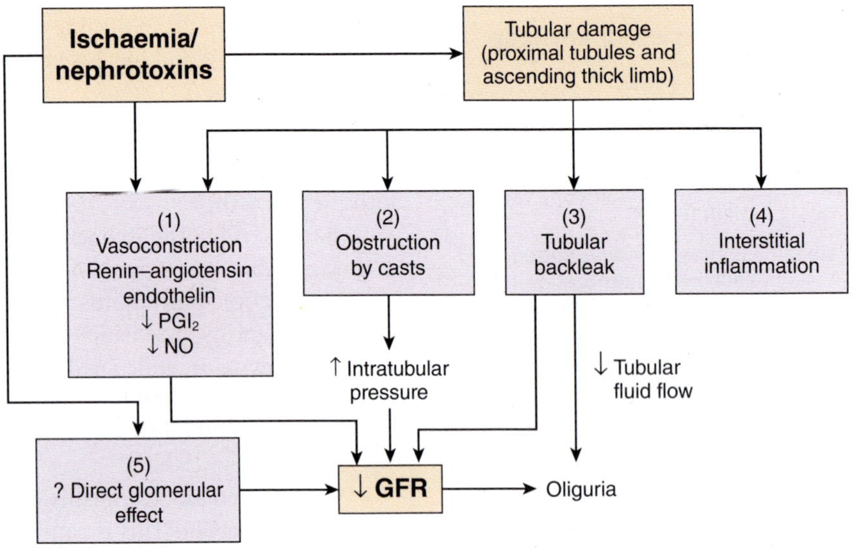

Flowchart 24.6 Pathogenesis of acute tubular injury.

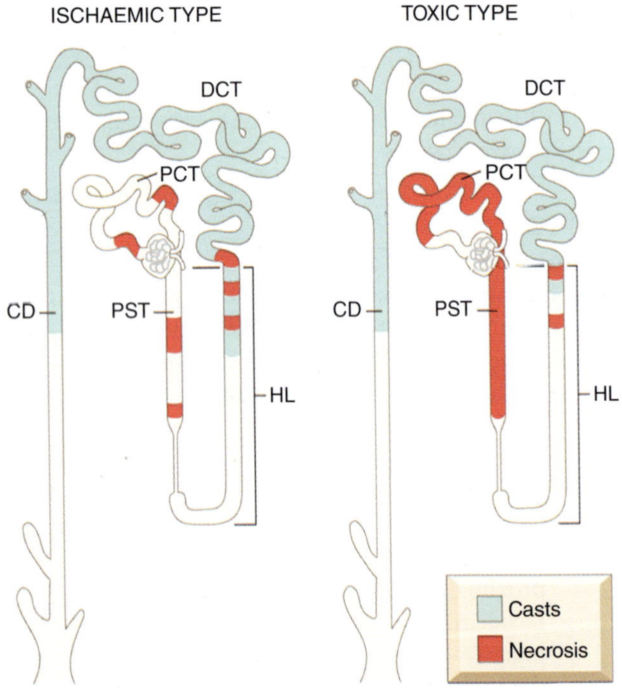

Fig. 24.26 Patterns of injury in ischaemic versus toxic acute tubular injury. In the ischaemic type, tubular necrosis is patchy; relatively short lengths of tubules are affected, and proximal straight tubule (PST) segments and ascending limbs of Henle's loop (HL) are most vulnerable. In toxic acute tubular injury, extensive necrosis is present along the proximal convoluted tubule (PCT) segments with many toxins (e.g. mercury), but necrosis of the distal tubule, particularly ascending HL, also occurs. In both types, lumens of the distal convoluted tubules (DCT) and collecting ducts (CD) contain casts.

Morphology

Light Microscopy (Fig. 24.27) **Ischaemic ATI** predominantly affects the straight portion of the proximal tubule and the ascending thick limb in the renal medulla as skip lesions. There is also associated rupture of the basement membrane (**tubulorrhexis**) and occlusion of the distal tubule and collecting duct by proteinaceous cast composed of Tamm–Horsfall protein, haemoglobin and plasma protein. The interstitium shows oedema and inflammatory cell infiltrate composed of neutrophils, lymphocytes and plasma cells. Evidence of regeneration of damaged epithelium may also be seen.

Toxic ATI changes are more evident in the proximal convoluted tubule in the form of necrosis, which is more prominent than in ischaemic aetiology. TBM is usually spared. Specific changes include the following:

- Mercuric chloride: Large acidophilic inclusions
- Carbon tetrachloride: Accumulation of neutral lipid in injured cells
- Ethylene glycol: Vacuolar degeneration of tubules and calcium oxalate crystals in the lumen

Clinical Course

Initiation phase: Patients usually presents with mild oliguria and increased BUN due to decreased GFR.

Maintenance phase: It is characterized by moderate oliguria, increased BUN and creatinine, hyperkalaemia, metabolic acidosis, uraemia and fluid overload.

Recovery phase: The urine output improves with return of BUN and creatinine to normal values along with development of hypokalaemia.

Prognosis

Prognosis depends on the severity and underlying disease. Ischaemic ATI has a better chance of recovery than toxic ATI. Preexisting renal disease with no supportive management progresses to ESRD.

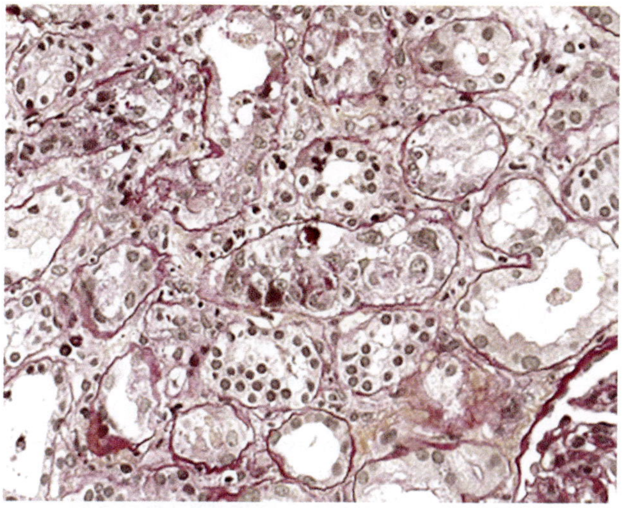

Fig. 24.27 Light microscopy of acute tubular injury showing dilated tubes with sloughing of tubular epithelium. (*Source:* From Ming Zhou, George J. Netto and Jonathan I. Epstein. Acute Tubular Necrosis. High-Yield Uropathology. Saunders 2012.)

Table 24.9 Causes of Tubulointerstitial Nephritis

Genetic
Ciliopathies
Nephronophthisis
ADTKD9 (autosomal dominant tubulointerstitial kidney disease)
Mitochondrionopathies
Crystal deposition and transport diseases
Infections
Acute pyelonephritis
Ascending infection
Haematogenous spread
Bacterial, fungal, viral, others
Chronic pyelonephritis
Nonobstructive (reflux associated)
Obstructive
Xanthogranulomatous
Malakoplakia
Obstructive uropathy
Hydronephrosis without infection
Reflux-associated nephropathy
Metabolic
Nephrocalcinosis
Acute phosphate nephropathy
Urate nephropathy
Secondary oxalosis
Immunological tubulointerstitial nephritis
Drug induced (antibiotics, diuretics, nonsteroidals)
Associated with systemic vasculitis
Lupus associated, Sjögren syndrome associated
Antitubular basement membrane disease
IgG4-related tubulointerstitial nephritis
Tubulointerstitial nephritis with uveitis
Toxic tubulointerstitial nephritis
Drug induced
Aminoglycosides
Cyclosporine
Lithium
Analgesics
Cisplatin
Heavy metal toxicity
Lead, mercury and others

TUBULOINTERSTITIAL NEPHRITIS PA 28.8

Renal diseases of this group are associated with inflammatory changes in tubules and interstitium, manifesting principally as azotaemia in patients. These may be primary or a consequence of a variety of renal diseases – glomerular, vascular, cystic and metabolic. In the primary form, the glomeruli are spared or affected late with the absence of nephritic or nephrotic syndrome. The defects in tubular function are manifested as an inability to concentrate urine (causing polyuria and nocturia), decreased excretion of acids, salt wasting and defects in tubular reabsorption.

Aetiology

The causes of tubulointerstitial nephritis are enlisted in Table 24.9.

Types

Acute tubulointerstitial nephritis develops rapidly in a short duration, and morphology shows interstitial oedema and leucocytic infiltration of the interstitium and tubules.

Chronic interstitial nephritis has an insidious onset, with the morphology of mononuclear infiltration of the interstitium and tubules along with interstitial fibrosis and tubular atrophy.

Pyelonephritis PA 28.10

Pyelonephritis is a disorder characterized by inflammation of the interstitium and tubules and renal pelvis. It often develops as a complication of urinary tract infection. It may be acute (which is more commonly due to bacterial infection affecting the lower urinary tract and ascending up to involve the kidney) or chronic (which apart from infection can be contributed by other factors such as vesicoureteric reflux and obstruction of the urinary tract).

Aetiology and Pathogenesis (Fig. 24.28) The following organisms are implicated in the aetiology:

- Gram-negative bacilli (*E. coli*, *Proteus*, *Klebsiella* and *Enterobacter*)
- Mycobacterial and fungal organisms
- Uncommon pathogens such as *Staphylococcus faecalis*
- Viruses like polyomavirus, adenovirus and cytomegalovirus in immunocompromised individuals

Ascending infection is the most common cause of pyelonephritis. Haematogenous infection due to septicaemia and endocarditis is less common and is mainly

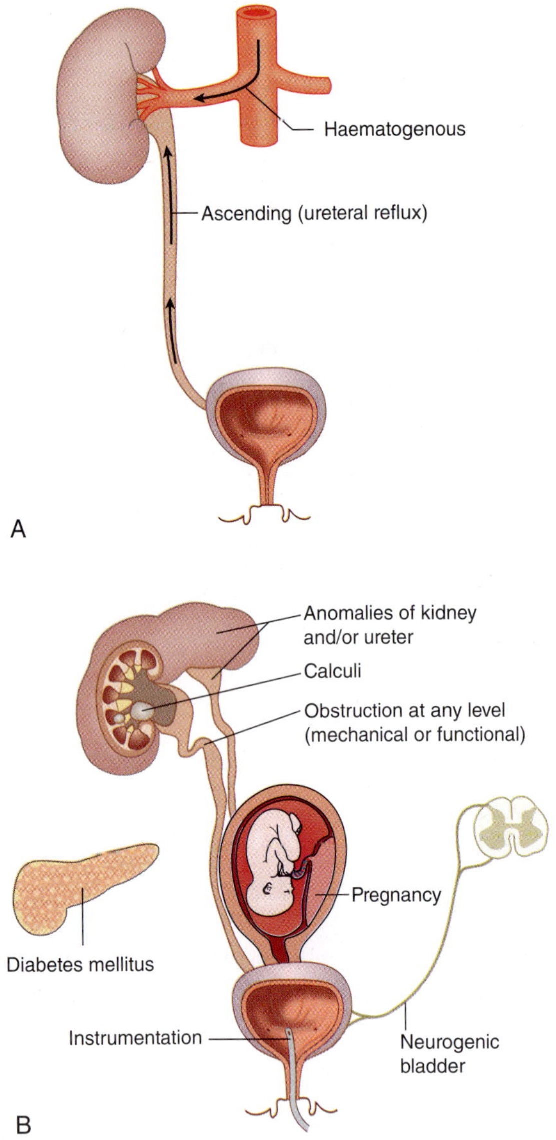

Fig. 24.28 Pathways of infection of renal tissue and predisposing factors. (*Source:* From L. Maximilian Buja and Gerhard R.F. Krueger. Kidneys, Ureters, and Urinary Bladder. Netter's Illustrated Human Pathology. 2nd edition. Saunders 2014.)

seen in debilitated and immunosuppressed patients. Ascending infection occurs in the following two steps:

- **Colonization of the distal urethra** and introitus occurs by coliform bacteria using their p-fimbriae (pili) or adhesins encoded by pyelonephritis-associated pili (pap) gene or in organisms that have fimbriae with renal tropism.
- **Movement of the organism** from the urethra to the kidney, which occurs more commonly in females due to a shorter urethra, hormonal changes and the absence of antibacterial protection offered by seminal fluid in males. The ascending infection is often seen in cases of instrumentation and catheterization of the bladder. The organism then ascends from the bladder to the kidneys due to the following:
  - **Urinary tract obstruction** due to prostatic hypertrophy, tumours or calculi or neurogenic bladder dysfunction and uterine prolapse, which lead to incomplete emptying of the bladder and stasis. This promotes multiplying of bacteria and favours spread of infection.
  - **Vesicoureteral reflux:** The main factor that promotes the movement of infection from the bladder to the kidney is the incompetence of the vesicoureteral valve. This may be due to short intravesical portion of the ureter or the infection itself weakening the ureteral contractility or acquired valve failure as in spinal cord injury.
  - **Intrarenal reflux:** The vesicoureteral reflux leads to infected urine reaching the renal pelvis. From the renal pelvis, it may enter the renal parenchyma through open ducts in the tip of concave papillae at the upper and lower poles of the kidney. These refluxes can be diagnosed by voiding cystourethrogram.

Acute Pyelonephritis

Acute pyelonephritis is the acute inflammation of the kidneys caused by viral or bacterial infection leading to suppuration. The method of spread of infection to the kidney may be through blood or an ascending infection through the ureters.

Morphology

Gross (Fig. 24.29) The cut surface of the kidney may show a discrete focal abscess or wedge-shaped abscess. ***Light Microscopy*** Examination reveals patchy interstitial suppurative inflammation and liquefactive necrosis. Intratubular aggregates of neutrophils may be seen that form WBC casts in urine. Neutrophilic tubulitis and tubular necrosis may be seen. Glomeruli are resistant in early stages but get affected in later stages.

Clinical Features Acute pyelonephritis is common in females younger than 40 years and in men older than 40 years who have increased chances of urinary stasis due to prostatic hypertrophy. It is often associated with precipitating factors such as pregnancy, urinary tract obstruction such as calculi, ureteric instrumentation, diabetes mellitus, vesicoureteric reflux and immunosuppression. Patients usually present with sudden onset of pain at the costovertebral angle along with fever and symptoms of bladder irritation such as dysuria, urgency and frequency.

Investigation and management

Urine examination reveals the presence of pus cells (**pyuria**) and urinary white cell casts, with casts indicating an upper urinary tract infection. Urine culture, however, helps to identify the causative organism and antibiotic sensitivity will help.

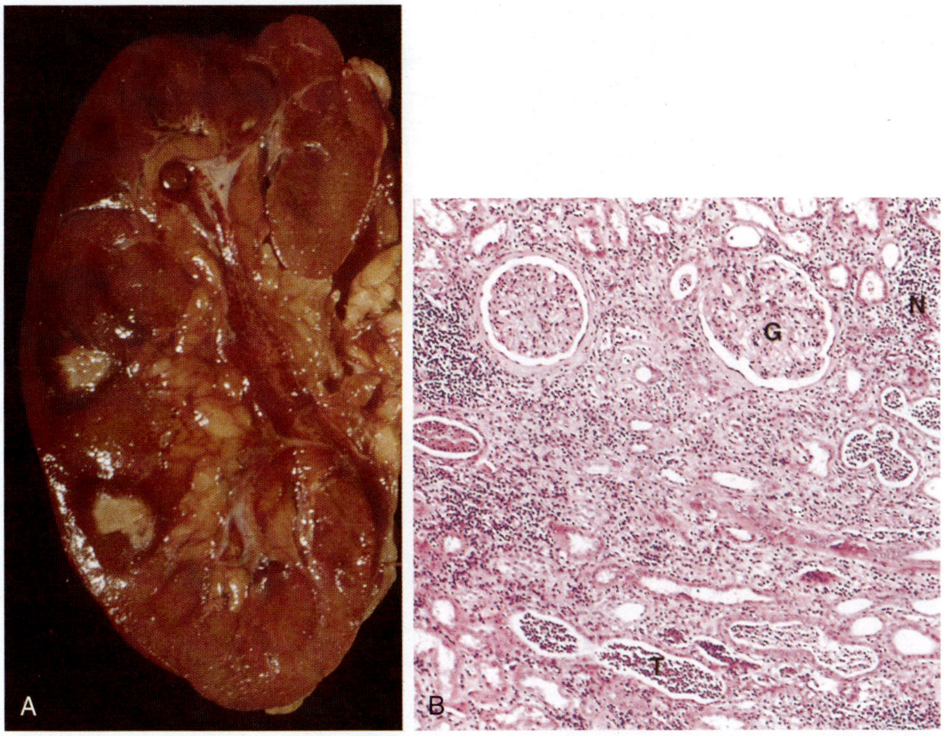

Fig. 24.29 Acute pyelonephritis – gross representation (A) shows abscesses in the form of yellowish streaks and blunting of calyces, and microscopy (B) shows neutrophilic infiltration in interstitium and collecting tubules, forming focal abscess. (*Source:* From Alton B. Farris and G. Petur Nielsen. Genitourinary Infectious Disease Pathology. Diagnostic Pathology of Infectious Disease. 2nd edition. Elsevier 2018; Geraldine O'Dowd, Sarah Bell and Sylvia Wright. Urinary system. Wheater's Pathology: A Text, Atlas, and Review of Histopathology. 6th edition. Elsevier 2020.)

Complications Complications include **papillary necrosis**, which is coagulative necrosis of distal two-thirds of the renal pyramid; **pyonephrosis**, which is pus filling the renal pelvis and calyces; and **perinephric abscess**, which is the extension of pus to the perinephric space (Fig. 24.30). Healing after the episode leads to scarring and deformation of the underlying calyx and pelvis, causing long-term consequences such as CRF.

Chronic Pyelonephritis

Chronic pyelonephritis is the chronic inflammation of the tubules and interstitium that causes scarring of calyces and pelvis. It can be of two types – **reflux nephropathy** (which is more common especially in children due to infection superimposed on vesicoureteric infection) and **chronic obstructive pyelonephritis** (which is precipitated by obstruction causing repeated bouts of inflammation).

Morphology

Gross (Fig. 24.31) The kidneys are asymmetrically and irregularly scarred. Reflux-associated changes include prominent scars at the poles and coarse discrete corticomedullary scars overlying blunted calyces.

Light Microscopy Microscopic changes include atrophy and hypertrophy of tubules with dilation and thyroidization (dilated tubules filled with secretions and casts). The interstitium shows chronic inflammatory cells and fibrosis in the cortex and medulla. The interlobular vessels show intimal sclerosis and hyaline arteriosclerosis. Glomerular changes include periglomerular fibrosis. A rare variant is chronic pyelonephritis or **xanthogranulomatous pyelonephritis** (Fig. 24.32) caused by obstruction with superimposed *Proteus* infection. Grossly, yellowish orange nodules mimic renal cell carcinoma (RCC) and hence are clinically important. Microscopy shows foamy macrophages, lymphocytes, plasma cells and neutrophils.

Clinical Features Clinical features include mild proteinuria, recurrent episodes of fever, back pain and pyuria. Patients may develop complications such as renal insufficiency due to failure to seek medical help early. Children develop symptoms of polyuria and nocturia due to hyposthenuria (inability to concentrate urine).

Prognosis Chronic pyelonephritis may progress to an adaptive form of secondary FSGS following the loss of renal mass or ESRD.

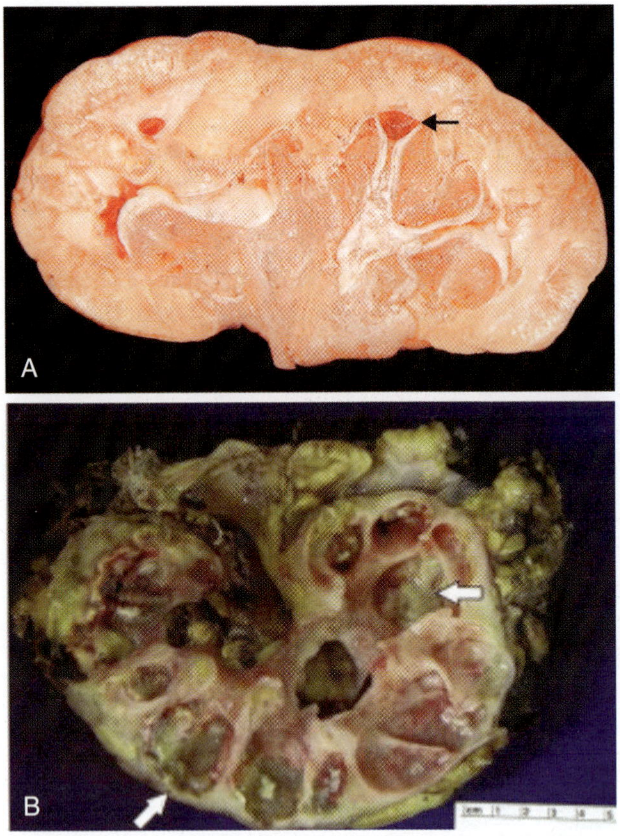

Fig. 24.30 Gross representation of papillary necrosis (A) and pyonephrosis (B). (*Source:* From Edward C. Klatt. The Kidneys. Robbins and Cotran Atlas of Pathology. 4th edition. Elsevier 2021; Nancy A. Hammond, Paul Nikolaidis and Frank H. Miller. Infectious and Inflammatory Diseases of the Kidney. Radiologic Clinics of North America. 2012;50:259–270)

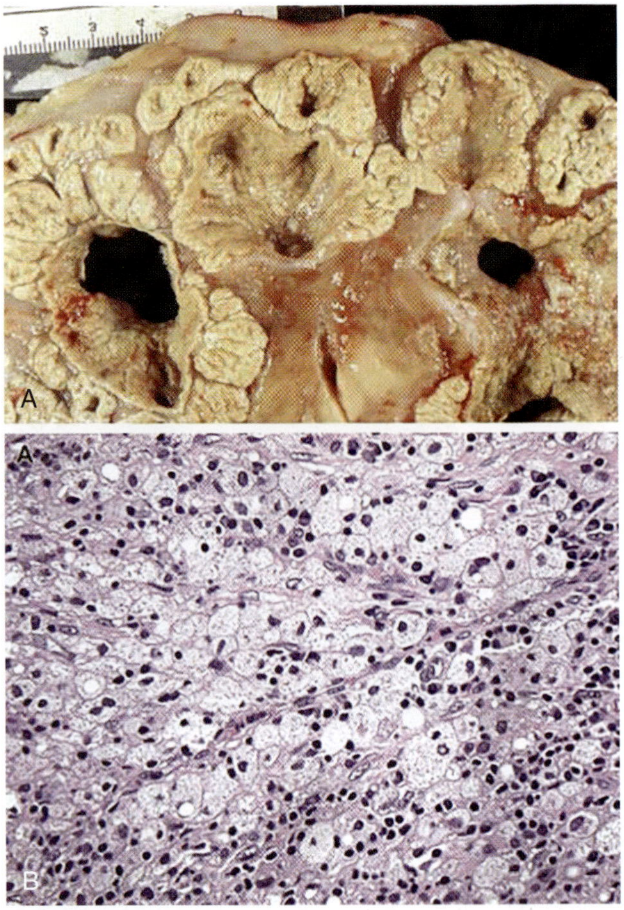

Fig. 24.32 Xanthogranulomatous pyelonephritis – (A) gross representation shows dilated pelvicalyceal system filled with yellowish debris, and (B) microscopy shows mixed inflammatory infiltrate and cholesterol clefts. (*Source:* Donna J. Lager, Neil A. Abrahams, Practical Renal Pathology, A Diagnostic Approach. © 2013 Elsevier Inc. From Glenn G. Fort. Renal Abscess. Elsevier 2022; Jean Hou and Leal C. Herlitz. Renal Infections. Surgical Pathology Clinics. 2014;7:389–408.)

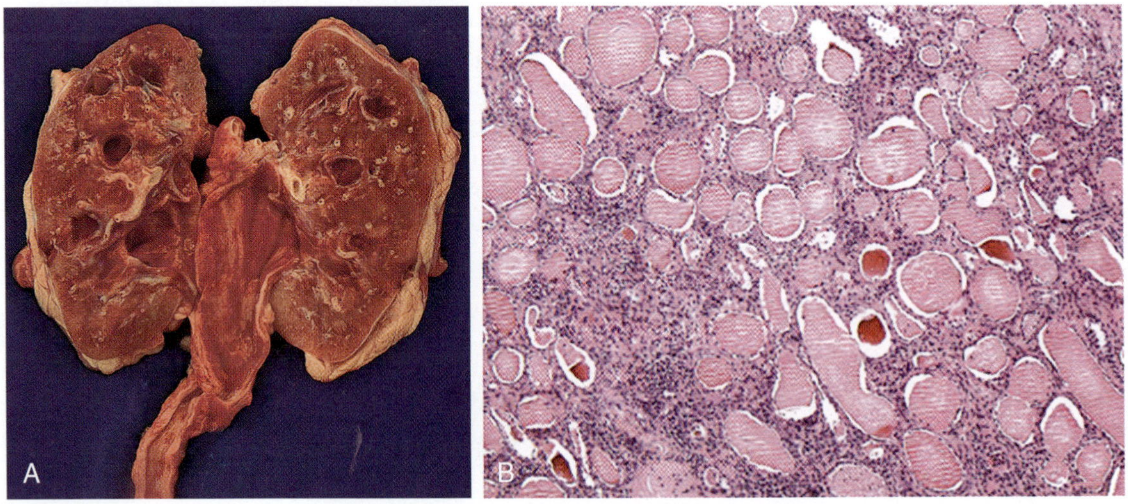

Fig. 24.31 Chronic pyelonephritis – gross representation (A) shows dilation of pelvicalyceal system and thinning of the cortex, and microscopy (B) shows thyroidization of tubules and inflammatory cell infiltration of the interstitium. (*Source:* From Andrew J. Connolly, Walter E. Finkbeiner, Philip C. Ursell and Richard L. Davis. Atlas of Gross Autopsy Pathology. Autopsy Pathology: A Manual and Atlas. 3rd edition. Elsevier 2016; Jean Hou and Leal C. Herlitz. Renal Infections. Surgical Pathology Clinics. 2014;7: 389–408.)

TUBULOINTERSTITIAL NEPHRITIS DUE TO DRUGS AND TOXINS

Drug- and toxin-induced tubulointerstitial nephritis is the second most common cause of AKI. The mechanism of injury may be a hypersensitivity reaction triggered as an immunological response or an ATI or chronic renal damage due to cumulative effect on the kidney.

Aetiology and Pathogenesis

The common cause for this type of renal injury is IgE- or T-cell-mediated immune reaction to the drugs such as:

- Penicillin
- Rifampicin
- Thiazides
- NSAIDs
- Allopurinol and cimetidine
- Phenacetin

Morphology

Light Microscopy Microscopic changes include tubulitis, interstitial oedema and infiltration by lymphocytes, macrophages, plasma cells, eosinophils and neutrophils, especially in the medulla where concentration of the drug is often high. Methicillin, thiazides and rifampicin cause non-necrotizing granuloma. NSAIDs cause MCD. In analgesic nephropathy, the papilla may show various stages of necrosis, calcification, fragmentation and sloughing.

Clinical Features

Drug-induced nephritis usually presents 15 days after drug intake along with fever, eosinophilia, rash, nephrotic syndrome, haematuria, leucocyturia and oliguria with raised serum creatinine levels. Papillary necrosis is another important feature that presents as gross haematuria and acute renal colic due to urinary tract obstruction. The other conditions that may cause papillary necrosis are sickle cell anaemia/trait, diabetes mellitus, urinary tract obstruction and renal tuberculosis.

Management

In about 30%–40% of cases, the causative agents are not identified and management is difficult. In known cases, withdrawal of the offending drug may reverse the changes, although it may take years in some cases or lead to permanent damage in some cases. Few cases have also been found to develop urothelial carcinoma of the renal pelvis. A few causes of drug/toxin induced tubulointerstitial nephritis need special mention below due to their common occurrence or different pathogenic mechanisms.

Analgesic Nephropathy

Analgesic nephropathy is a nephropathy caused by intake of NSAIDs. NSAIDs are one of the common drugs taken by the general population without medical consultation. The incidence of this condition can be reduced only by creating awareness about it among all classes of people. NSAIDs commonly used are nonselective cyclooxygenase (COX) inhibitors, function by inhibiting prostaglandin synthesis. The risk is also seen in selective COX-2 inhibitors, which spare the GI tract but still affect the kidney because COX-2 is expressed in the kidney in contrast to COX-1 that is expressed in the gastric mucosa. The renal syndromes associated with analgesic intake are as follows:

- AKI
- Acute hypersensitivity interstitial nephritis
- MCD
- MN

Light Chain Cast Nephropathy

Light chain nephropathy is caused by multiple myeloma and is called myeloma kidney.

Aetiology and Pathogenesis The factors that cause damage to the kidney in patients with myeloma are as follows:

- **Bence–Jones proteinuria and cast nephropathy:** Renal toxicity is due to Ig light chains that are filtered by the glomerulus called Bence–Jones proteins and tubular casts formed by these proteins and those secreted by the ascending limb of Henle called Tamm–Horsfall protein. These proteins are directly toxic to the epithelial cells or combine with urinary Tamm–Horsfall protein that can lead to obstruction of the tubular lumina, which is termed light chain cast nephropathy (LCCN).
- **Amyloidosis (AL type):** The light chains that are usually lambda light chains (λ) can cause similar damage leading to LCCN.
- **Light chain deposition** disease due to κ-subtype nonfibrillar light chain deposition occurs mainly in GBM and mesangium. In addition, similar deposits may be seen in the tubules, interstitium and blood vessels.
- **Hypercalcaemia and hyperuricaemia** are associated with bone destruction and high cell turnover.

Morphology

Tubules are dilated and appear obstructed by dense eosinophilic casts that appear laminated, fractured and surrounded by giant cells (Fig. 24.33). The casts may rupture the tubules and produce granulomatous reaction. The interstitium shows inflammatory cells and fibrosis. Light chains can be demonstrated by PAS stain to be deposited along the basement membrane of tubules. The presence of light chains can be confirmed by immunofluorescence with antibodies against kappa and lambda light chain of immunoglobulin to establish the clonality. The features of the associated conditions such as amyloidosis, light chain deposition disease, nephrocalcinosis and infection may be evident.

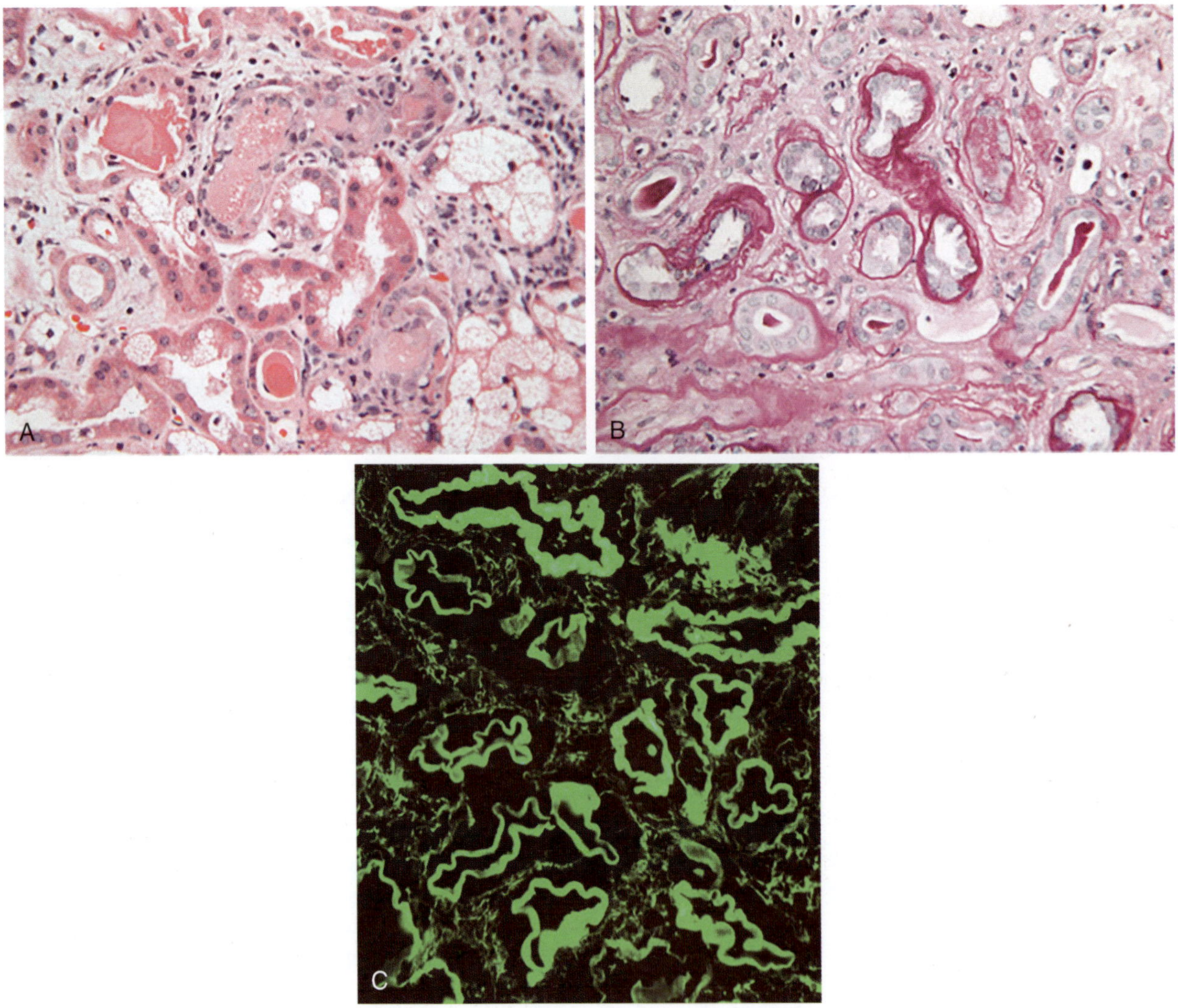

Fig. 24.33 (A) Myeloma kidney. Dilated tubules filled with eosinophilic hard casts, with giant cell reaction and inflammatory cell infiltrates. (B) Light chain deposition along tubular basement membrane (TBM) in PAS. (C) Light chain (kappa light chain) deposition along TBM. (*Source:* From Ashley B. Irish. Myeloma and the Kidney. Comprehensive Clinical Nephrology. 6th edition. Elsevier 2019.)

Clinical Features The patient may present with features of CKD or AKI. In 70% of cases of multiple myeloma, Bence–Jones proteinuria occurs resulting in this picture.

Bile cast nephropathy (cholaemic nephrosis)

The development of renal impairment in patients with severe or advanced liver disease in the form of bile casts in distal tubules causing tubular toxicity leading to AKI is termed bile cast nephropathy (cholaemic nephrosis). The serum bilirubin levels are markedly elevated.

The bile casts are yellowish green and can cause direct toxicity to the tubular epithelial cells or obstruction. They may be demonstrated by a special stain called Hall's stain.

Management involves treating the liver condition that will reverse the renal impairment.

VASCULAR DISEASES PA 28.11

Most renal disorders and systemic disorders may affect the blood vessels of the kidney. Among them, hypertension is a very important one because it may be both an aetiology and a consequence of renal damage. Here, we discuss some of the important vascular diseases of the kidney.

HYPERTENSIVE VASCULAR DISEASES

Systemic hypertension may affect the kidney and cause benign or malignant nephrosclerosis depending on the severity of hypertension.

Benign Nephrosclerosis

Nephrosclerosis is the sclerosis of renal arterioles and small arteries commonly seen in patients with hypertension. It may be both a cause and a consequence of nephrosclerosis. The pathology leads to ischaemic changes in the renal parenchyma. Severity of the lesions depends on the hypertension status and the presence of coexistent diabetes.

Pathogenesis The medial and intimal thickening seen in the blood vessels of these patients is due to haemodynamic changes associated with hypertension, ageing and genetic defects. The second important change is the hyalinization of arteriolar walls due to endothelial injury leading to plasma protein exudation and deposition of basement membrane matrix.

Morphology

Gross (Fig. 24.34) The kidneys appear normal or symmetrically reduced in size due to cortical scarring and shrinking. The cortical surface appears fine and granular, giving a grainy leather appearance.
Microscopy Hyaline arteriolosclerosis is the thickening of the wall of the arterioles and small arteries by hyalinization leading to narrowing of the lumen. This is accentuated by **fibroelastic hyperplasia** of the interlobular and arcuate arteries that is manifested by medial hypertrophy, duplication of the internal elastic lamina and increased myofibroblastic tissue in the intima. The vascular compromise by the vessel narrowing leads to tubular atrophy and interstitial fibrosis. The glomeruli show sclerosis, periglomerular fibrosis and collapse of GBM. The subcapsular scars represent sclerosed glomeruli and tubular dropout.

Prognosis Renal insufficiency occurs after prolonged shypertension.

Malignant Nephrosclerosis

This is a vascular disorder associated with malignant hypertension (BP >200/120 mm Hg) or accelerated hypertension. It is a medical emergency that requires antihypertensive therapy to prevent irreversible renal damage.

Aetiology and Pathogenesis Malignant hypertension may occur in normotensive individuals but is more common in patients with preexisting essential hypertension or hypertension caused by secondary causes or preexisting renal diseases such as GN or reflux nephropathy.

The vascular injury (Flowchart 24.7) starts off due to hypertension or vasculitis as endothelial injury and results in increased vascular permeability that leads to fibrinoid necrosis of arterioles and small arteries. This activates the platelets to form intravascular thrombosis and release of platelet factors, especially PDGF that triggers proliferation of medial smooth cells leading to hyperplastic arteriosclerosis. This is followed by activation of the renin–angiotensin system and elevated renin levels that worsen the intrarenal vasoconstriction through angiotensin II.

Morphology

Gross The size of the kidneys varies according to the duration of disease. The cortical surface has pinpoint haemorrhage, giving a **'flea-bitten'** appearance (Fig. 24.35).
Microscopy Microscopic changes include fibrinoid necrosis of arterioles seen as smudgy eosinophilic deposition, whereas the glomeruli show necrosis and microthrombi. The most important change is the hyperplastic arteriolitis seen due to proliferation of smooth muscle cells giving an **onion skin appearance** (Fig. 24.35).
Clinical Features Common presentation is with systolic pressure of more than 200 mm Hg and diastolic pressure of more than 120 mm Hg. Retinal examination may show papilloedema and retinal haemorrhage. The patient may develop proteinuria, microscopic and macroscopic haematuria due to renal damage, or headache and vomiting due to an increase in intracranial tension.

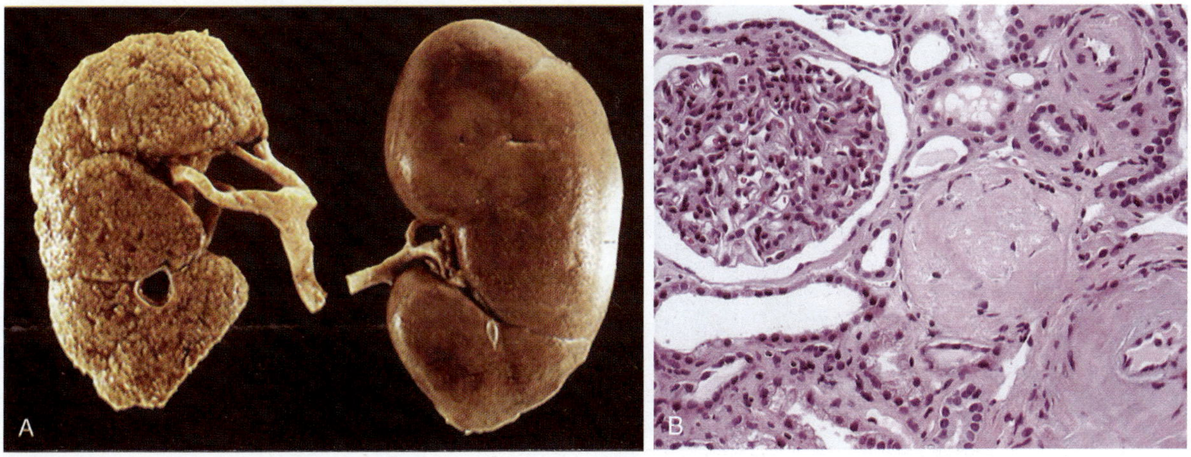

Fig. 24.34 Benign nephrosclerosis – gross representation (A) shows the granular contracted kidney on the left (contrast normal kidney on the right), and microscopy (B) shows sclerosed glomerulus in the centre and thick-walled artery on the lower right. (*Source:* From Stephen M. Bonsib. Nonneoplastic Diseases of the Kidney. Genitourinary Pathology: Foundations in Diagnostic Pathology. 2nd edition. Saunders 2015.)

RENAL ARTERY STENOSIS

Hypertension associated with unilateral renal artery stenosis accounts for about 2%–5% of cases of hypertension. It is unique in being a **surgically correctable cause of hypertension**, although complete normalization is not always possible. The cause for hypertension is ischaemia of the kidneys caused by the obstruction in the vessel. The causes for the renal artery obstruction may be attributed to atheroma seen in atherosclerosis of the vessels, leading to narrowing of the renal artery at the origin (M > F). Fibromuscular dysplasia is another important cause that involves the intima, media or adventitia (F > M). Ischaemia of the renal parenchyma triggers the juxtaglomerular apparatus to increase the secretion of renin that generates angiotensin II and leads to hypertension.

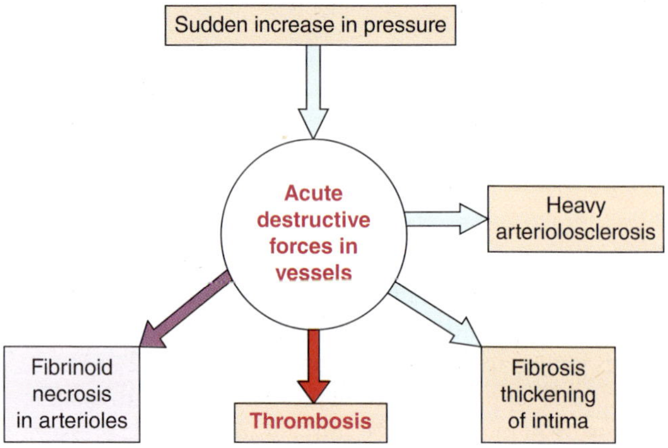

Flowchart 24.7 Mechanism of vascular damage in hypertension.

Morphology

The involved kidney is reduced in size. Microscopy shows crowded glomeruli, atrophied tubules and interstitium displaying fibrosis and inflammatory cell infiltration.

Clinical Features and Management

Renal artery stenosis is suspected in the early onset of hypertension in young patients, sudden worsening of hypertension in known cases of atherosclerosis, patients with malignant or unresponsive hypertension or those with sudden symptoms of azotaemia or gross discrepancy of more than 1.5 cm in the size of either kidney. Invasive angiography is the gold standard for diagnosis. Management is possible by stenting, balloon angioplasty or revascularization. It is aimed at lowering the BP, which may be successful in most cases of fibromuscular dysplasia by surgery, although medical management may also be attempted in cases of atherosclerosis.

THROMBOTIC MICROANGIOPATHIES PA 28.15

TMAs may be primary or secondary. Their causes are given in Table 24.10.

Aetiology and Pathogenesis

The main event in the pathogenesis of TMAs is endothelial injury with the formation of intravascular platelet microthrombi that lead to vascular compromise of the distal organs, platelet consumption-induced thrombocytopenia and intravascular haemolysis of RBCs. The events that lead to these changes are given next.

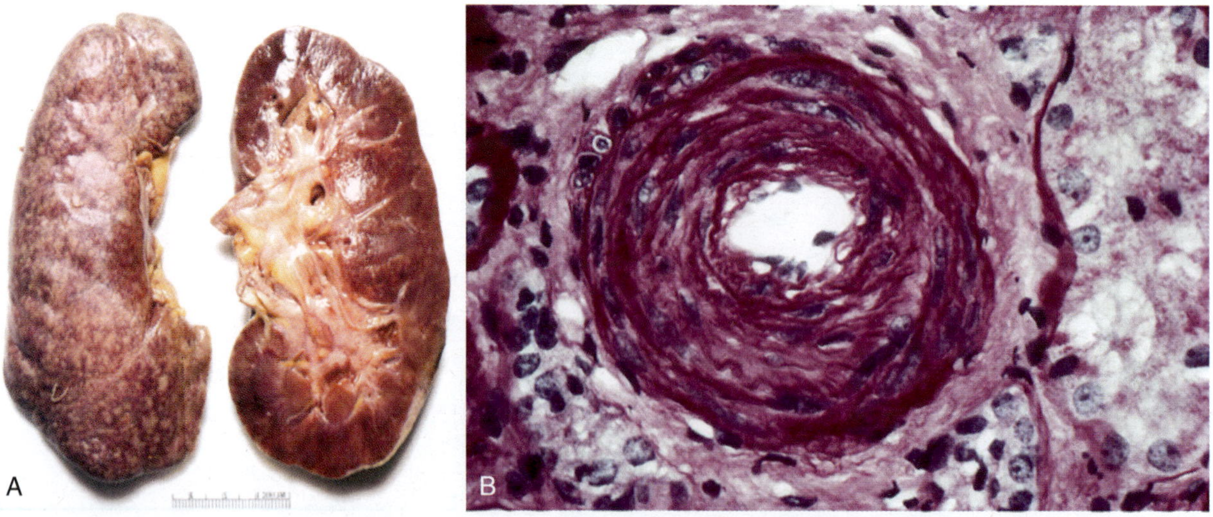

Fig. 24.35 Malignant nephrosclerosis – gross representation (A) shows the flea-bitten kidney, and microscopy (B) shows myointimal proliferation of artery (onion skin appearance). (*Source:* From Andrew J. Connolly, Walter E. Finkbeiner, Philip C. Ursell and Richard L. Davis. Atlas of Gross Autopsy Pathology. Autopsy Pathology: A Manual and Atlas. 3rd edition. Elsevier 2016.)

Table 24.10 Causes of Thrombotic Microangiopathy

Primary Causes
- Thrombotic thrombocytopenic purpura
- Haemolytic uraemic syndrome (HUS)
- Typical HUS
- Atypical HUS
- Drug mediated

Secondary Causes
- Malignant hypertension
- Scleroderma-associated thrombotic microangiopathy
- Pregnancy
- Chemotherapy
- Antiphospholipid antibodies
- Transplant rejection

Endothelial Injury Endothelial injury leads to activation of complement, platelet activation and thrombosis. Endothelin that is released causes vasoconstriction, whereas a decrease in prostaglandin I_2 and NO synthesis causes thrombosis in the glomerular capillaries, afferent arterioles and interlobular arteries.

Platelet Activation and Aggregation Various factors in HUS and TTP may lead to platelet activation and aggregation.

HUS is due to Shiga-like toxin, whereas atypical HUS is because of inhibitors of regulatory mediators of the complement pathway. The important cause attributed to TTP is the deficiency of ADAMTS13 due to acquired inhibitors, which causes increase in von Willebrand factor multimers that promote platelet aggregation. It can also be due to genetic causes due to deficiency of ADAMTS13.

Let us now review the pathogenesis of each subtype (Flowchart 24.8).

Typical Haemolytic Uraemic Syndrome

Typical HUS is a syndrome complex consisting of the triad of microangiopathy haemolytic anaemia, thrombocytopenia and acute renal damage. It is also called epidemic or **classical or diarrhoea-positive HUS**. The endothelial injury is caused by Shiga-like toxin produced by O157:H7 strain of *E. coli* or occasionally due to *Shigella dysenteriae*. It mainly affects children and older adults. Following an episode of influenza-like symptoms or diarrhoea, the patient develops haematemesis, melaena, severe oliguria, haematuria, microangiopathic haemolytic anaemia, thrombocytopenia and, in a few cases, prominent neurological changes. Hypertension may be present. The mechanism by which Shiga-like toxin causes this effect is based on the inflammatory changes it causes. The toxin causes an increased expression of leucocyte adhesion factor on endothelial cells leading to endothelial activation, increase in endothelin and decrease in NO synthesis, all contributing to endothelial apoptosis, platelet activation and vasoconstriction. On prompt management, recovery may occur but the renal damage caused by the syndrome may lead to a guarded prognosis in the long term.

Atypical Haemolytic Uraemic Syndrome

It is also called nonepidemic or diarrhoea-negative HUS. It is caused by inherited mutations of complementary regulatory proteins – factor H, factor I and CD46 – of the alternate pathway. It may be associated with antiphospholipid syndrome, complications of pregnancy and oral contraceptives, vascular disorders such as systemic sclerosis and malignant hypertension or chemotherapy/radiation. The prognosis is guarded because the underlying disorder is difficult to treat.

Thrombotic Thrombocytopenic Purpura

TTP is a pentad of fever, neurological symptoms, microangiopathic haemolytic anaemia, thrombocytopenia and

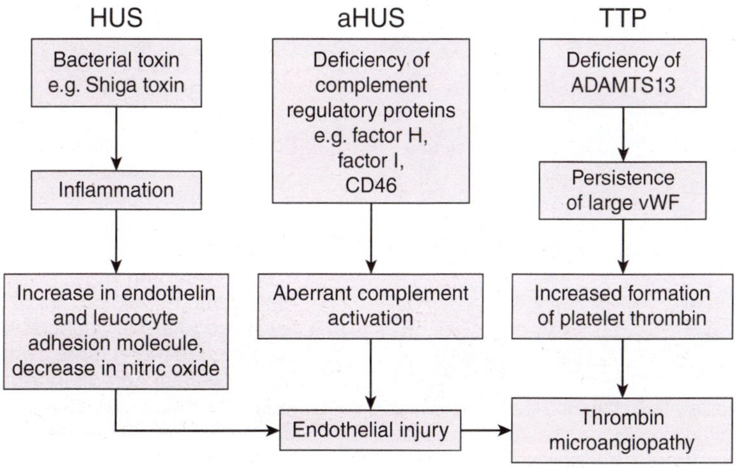

Flowchart 24.8 Pathogenesis of typical haemolytic uraemic syndrome (HUS) versus atypical haemolytic uraemic syndrome (aHUS) versus thrombotic thrombocytopenic purpura (TTP).

renal failure. It is associated with acquired or inherited deficiency of ADAMTS13. The most important cause for deficient ADAMTS13 activity is the formation of autoantibodies against it that are inhibitory in nature and manifest at age less than 40 years. The inherited cause is mostly inactivation of ADAMTS13 by mutations of its gene.

Morphology

The kidney shows patchy or diffuse cortical necrosis and subcapsular petechiae.

Microscopic examination shows capillaries occluded by thrombus and fibrinoid necrosis (Fig. 24.36).

The glomeruli are hypercellular with thickening and reduplication of the basement membrane of vessels giving an '**onion skin appearance**'. There may be associated mesangiolysis.

TTP is more common in women, and the most common cause of the clinical symptoms is the formation of widespread intravascular thrombi. Among the pentad of symptoms, **neurological symptoms predominate** in patients. Treatment with plasma exchange that removes autoantibodies is successful in treating 80% of patients.

Other renal vascular disorders are given as follows and description of these is out of scope of this book:

- Atherosclerotic ischaemic renal disease
- Atheroembolic renal disease
- Sickle cell nephropathy – affects sickle cell trait and fully blown sickle cell disease
- Diffuse cortical necrosis following abruptio placentae
- Renal infarcts

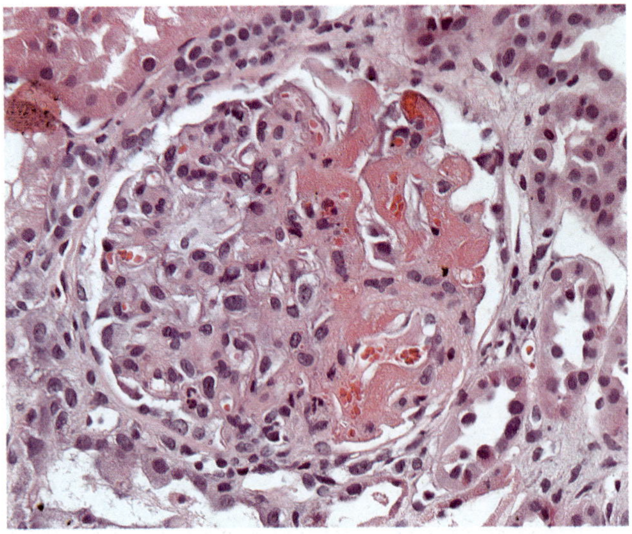

Fig. 24.36 Glomerulus with capillary fibrin thrombi, karyorrhexis and entrapped fragmented red blood cells in acute thrombotic microangiopathy. (*Source:* From Neeraja Kambham. Kidney: Non-Neoplastic Diseases. Rosai and Ackerman's Surgical Pathology. 11th edition. Elsevier 2018.)

CYSTIC DISEASES OF THE KIDNEY PA 28.12

Renal cystic diseases are a group of hereditary, developmental and acquired conditions that present with cystic lesions in the kidney. These often prove to be a diagnostic challenge for clinicians, radiologists and pathologists and may be confused with malignant tumours. The lesions that come under this category are listed in Table 24.11. However, we shall study the important ones in this chapter.

AUTOSOMAL DOMINANT (ADULT) POLYCYSTIC KIDNEY DISEASE

Autosomal dominant (adult) polycystic kidney disease (adult PKD) is a hereditary disorder, often presenting in adults, characterized by multiple cysts that expand and together destroy the renal parenchyma (Flowchart 24.9). The incidence is about 1 in 1000 live births. The development of this disorder, like the syndromes associated with tumour suppressor gene, requires inactivation of both the genes for the disorder to develop. Hence, on inheriting one mutated APKD gene, a second hit on the other normal allele leads to adult PKD. The involvement of kidneys is always bilateral.

Genetics and Pathogenesis

Adult PKD may be caused by a variety of mutations.

- Mutation in PKD1 that is located on chromosome 16p13.3 and encodes **polycystin-1**: It is expressed in tubular epithelial cells of the distal nephron. Individuals with this mutation have a risk of developing renal failure with increasing age, with the risk being 5% at 40 years of age and 95% at 70 years of age.
- Mutation in PKD2 that is located on chromosome 4q21 and encodes **polycystin-2**: It is expressed in tubular epithelium and also on some extrarenal tissue. The risk of renal failure is comparatively less and is

Table 24.11 Cystic Diseases of the Kidney

- Polycystic kidney disease
  - Autosomal dominant (adult) polycystic disease
  - Autosomal recessive (childhood) polycystic disease
- Medullary cystic disease
  - Medullary sponge kidney
  - Nephronophthisis
- Multicystic renal dysplasia
- Acquired (dialysis-associated) cystic disease
- Localized (simple) renal cysts
- Renal cysts in hereditary malformation syndromes (e.g. tuberous sclerosis)
- Glomerulocystic disease
- Extraparenchymal renal cysts (pyelocalyceal cysts, hilar lymphangitic cysts)

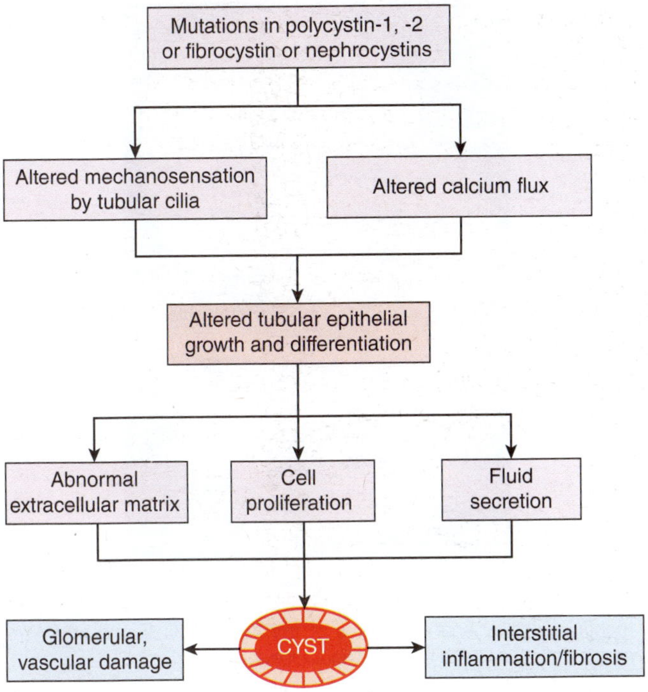

Flowchart 24.9 Mechanism of cyst formation in polycystic kidney disease.

about 5% at 50 years of age and increases to 45% at 70 years of age.

The hypothesis that is currently accepted in the pathogenesis of this disease is the presence of a defect in the cilia–centrosome complex of tubular epithelial cells. The cilia act as mechanosensor, detecting changes in the fluid flow within the lumen of the tubules. On the basis of the signals received by the sensor, the intracellular calcium levels are altered. Polycystin-1 and polycystin-2 are localized in the cilium and form the protein complex that regulates the intracellular calcium levels. Mutation in these proteins results in failure to form the polycystin complex or formation of aberrant complex, which fails to maintain the intracellular calcium levels optimally, thereby affecting the pathways that regulate cellular proliferation, apoptosis and secretory functions. This also affects the interaction of epithelial cells with extracellular matrix, leading to fibrosis and contributing to cyst formation. The bottom line is that **dysfunction of cilia** alters the ion flux and results in cyst formation. Following the formation of multiple cysts, the disease process that leads to **hypertension** is explained in Flowchart 24.10.

Morphology

Gross (Fig. 24.37) The involvement of the kidneys is bilateral, which become enlarged and heavy weighing up to 4 kg, with multiple cysts The external surface is bosselated replacing the entire kidney parenchyma. The cysts are found on the inner as well as on the outer surface of the kidneys. They can occur at any level of nephron and may be 4 cm in diameter. The cut surface shows cysts filled with serous or haemorrhagic fluid.

Microscopy The cyst may be lined by the epithelium of any part of the nephron depending on the origin. When Bowman's capsule is involved, the glomerular tuft may be seen compressed on one side.

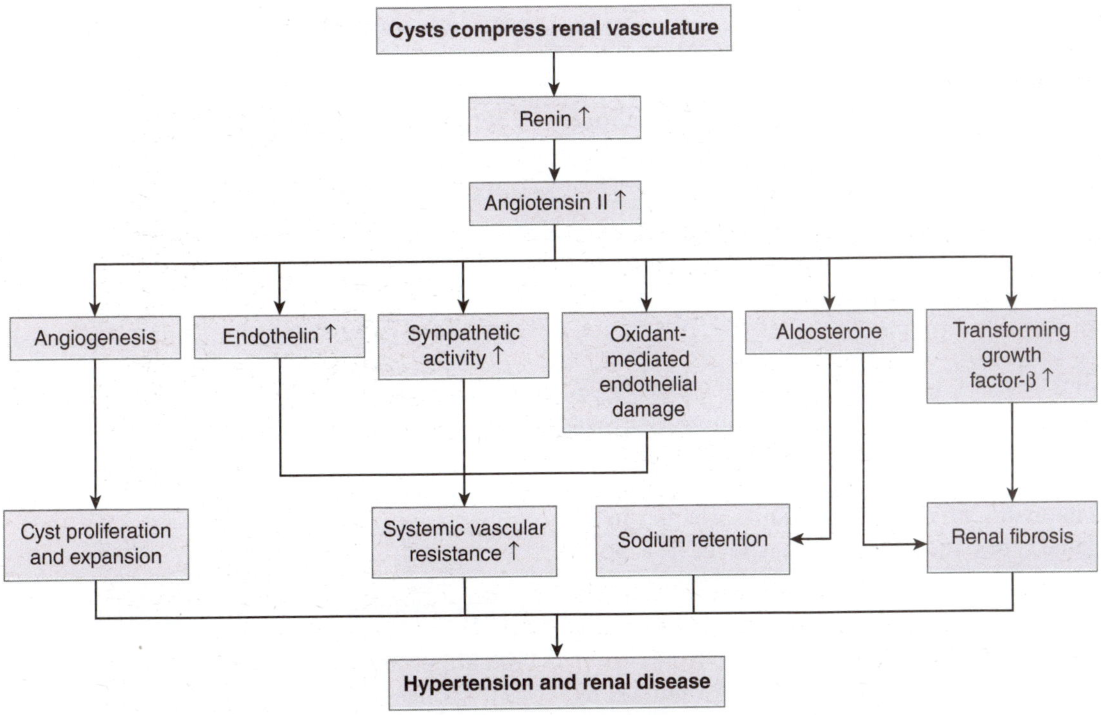

Flowchart 24.10 The disease process in adult polycystic kidney disease.

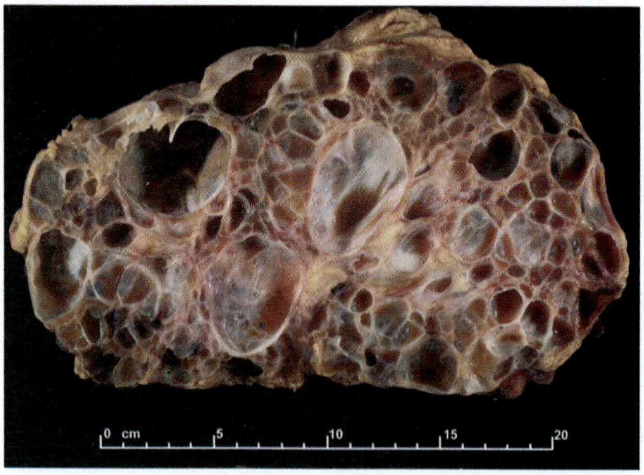

Fig. 24.37 Gross representation of adult polycystic kidney disease. (*Source:* From Ian S.D. Roberts. Kidney diseases. Underwood's Pathology. 7th edition. Elsevier 2019.)

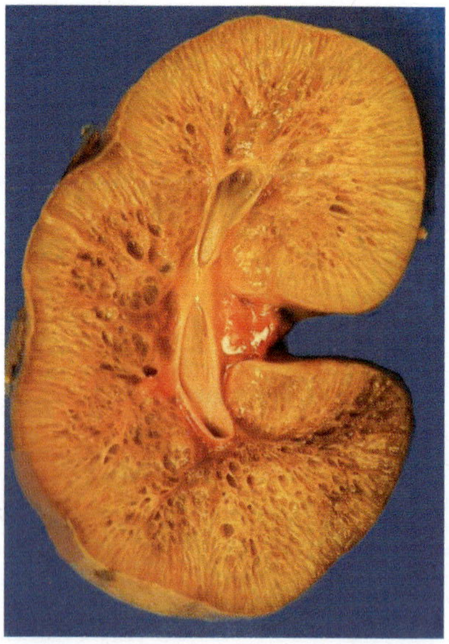

Fig. 24.38 Gross representation of childhood polycystic kidney disease. (*Source:* From Hsi-Yang Wu and Howard M. Snyder. Developmental and Positional Anomalies of the Kidneys. Holcomb and Ashcraft's Pediatric Surgery. 7th edition. Elsevier 2020.)

Clinical Features

Adult PKD produces symptoms after the fourth decade of life due to enlargement of the kidneys. The patients usually present with intermittent gross haematuria, proteinuria, polyuria and hypertension. The massively enlarged kidneys may produce **dragging sensation in the loin**, and cystic dilation may cause flank pain. Progression of the disease is accelerated in **sickle cell trait** in males. The other congenital lesions often associated with adult PKD are polycystic disease in the liver, spleen, pancreas and lungs. These may also have associated intracranial berry aneurysm which may cause death in up to 4%–10% of affected individuals and mitral valve prolapse may be seen in up to 25% of patients.

Prognosis

The disease has a protracted course, with patients progressing slowly to uraemic disease. The causes of death include coronary or hypertensive heart disease in about 40% of cases, infection in 25% of cases and ruptured berry aneurysm/intracerebral haemorrhage in 15% of cases.

AUTOSOMAL RECESSIVE (CHILDHOOD) POLYCYSTIC KIDNEY DISEASE

Autosomal recessive (childhood) PKD is an entity that is totally different from adult PKD. It is classified into four types on the basis of the timing of presentation and the presence of associated hepatic lesions. The categories are perinatal, neonatal, infantile and juvenile. The perinatal and neonatal types present at birth and have a poor prognosis.

Genetics and Pathogenesis

Autosomal recessive PKD is associated with mutations of **PKHD1 gene** in chromosome 6p21–23 that encodes **fibrocystin**, expressed in the adult and fetal kidney, liver and pancreas. Fibrocystin in the renal parenchyma is found in the cilia of tubular epithelial cells. It has been found to play a role in the differentiation of collecting ducts and biliary ducts. Hence, it has been implicated in the causation of renal and hepatic cysts.

Morphology

Gross (Fig. 24.38) The kidneys are enlarged with a smooth contour. The cut section reveals small cysts in the cortex and medulla, giving it a sponge-like appearance. The dilated channels appear to be arranged perpendicular to the cortical surface.

Microscopy The cysts are lined by cuboidal cells arising from dilated collecting tubules.

Prognosis

Affected infants succumb during infancy itself. If they survive beyond infancy, they eventually develop congenital hepatic fibrosis, characterized by periportal fibrosis and biliary ductular proliferation, which is the lesion of concern in older children with this disorder. They often develop portal hypertension and splenomegaly.

CYSTIC DISEASE OF RENAL MEDULLA

The important cystic diseases of the medulla are medullary sponge kidney, nephronophthisis and adult-onset medullary cystic disease.

Medullary Sponge Kidney

Medullary sponge kidney applies to the disorder characterized by **multiple cystic dilation** of the collecting ducts in the medulla. It is often an incidental finding in radiology in adults and may be associated with nephrolithiasis. The renal function is normal, and the microscopic examination shows these cysts to be lined by the cuboidal epithelium/transitional epithelium.

Nephronophthisis and Adult-Onset Medullary Cystic Disease

These cysts are found in the corticomedullary junction. Although the initial pathology is in the medulla, the damage to the cortical tubulointerstitium is the cause of the final renal dysfunction. It is of three types:

- Sporadic, nonfamilial
- Familial juvenile nephronophthisis – associated with blindness, cerebellar manifestations, mental retardation and liver fibrosis (children usually present with polyuria and polydipsia, reflecting the loss of concentrating ability of the kidney, sodium wasting and tubular acidosis)
- Renal–retinal dysplasia

Genetics and Pathogenesis Juvenile nephronophthisis has been found to be associated with mutation of about 16 genes (NPHP1–NPHP11; JBTS2, JBTS3, JBTS9 and JBTS11). Mutation in adult-onset medullary is found in MCKD1 and MCKD2 genes and is found to lead to end-stage kidney disease in adult life.

Morphology

The kidney is small and contracted. The cut surface shows multiple cysts concentrated around the **corticomedullary junction**. Microscopy shows the cysts to be lined by the cuboidal epithelium. The cortex shows tubular atrophy, thickened TBM and interstitial fibrosis with preserved glomeruli.

Clinical Features A positive family history with unexplained CRF in young adults should raise the suspicion of nephronophthisis.

MULTICYSTIC RENAL DYSPLASIA

Multicystic renal dysplasia is the most common cause of cystic renal disease in **infancy**. In this disorder, the kidneys are enlarged, irregular and cystic, with unilateral or bilateral involvement. The kidneys show the presence of multiple dilated noncommunicating cysts, immature collecting duct and undifferentiated mesenchyme, especially cartilage. These may be associated with ureteropelvic obstruction or ureteral agenesis. In unilateral cases, the opposite kidney functions normally, giving these patients a good prognosis following the removal of the affected kidney. Bilateral cases usually result in renal failure.

ACQUIRED (DIALYSIS-ASSOCIATED) CYSTIC DISEASE

Patients on long-term dialysis due to ESRD show multiple cortical and medullary cysts. The cysts contain clear fluid containing calcium oxalate crystals and are lined by the flattened epithelium. The cysts may bleed leading to haematuria and the patients show an increased risk of developing RCC.

Concluding the various cystic diseases of the kidney, a comparison of the gross appearances of the various cystic lesions is given in Fig. 24.39.

OBSTRUCTIVE UROPATHY (URINARY TRACT OBSTRUCTION) PA 28.13

Obstruction of the urinary tract is an important risk factor for infection and stone formation. Unrelieved obstruction may lead to hydronephrosis, which is associated with loss of renal parenchyma (obstructive uropathy) leading to renal failure. The obstruction may be sudden or insidious,

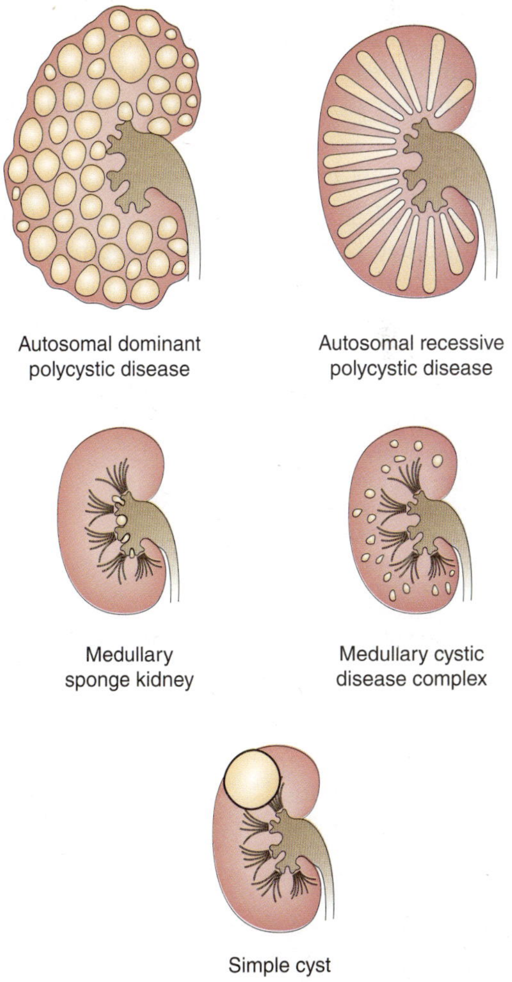

Fig. 24.39 Comparison of various cysts of the kidney.

unilateral or bilateral, extrinsic or intrinsic and partial or complete. The various causes are given in Table 24.12.

HYDRONEPHROSIS

Hydronephrosis is the **aseptic** dilatation of the renal pelvis and calyces due to loss of renal parenchyma as a consequence of urinary tract obstruction. This can be explained by the persistence of glomerular filtration even when there is complete obstruction of the urinary tract leading to diffusion of filtrate back into the interstitium and perirenal space. This causes dilatation of the renal pelvis and calyces, and the high pressure created in this region is transmitted through the collecting tubules to the cortex causing cortical atrophy and medullary vascular compression. All this leads to diminished blood flow in the medulla and a diminished concentrating ability of the tubules, which later progresses to interstitial fibrosis.

Morphology (Fig. 24.40)

The kidney is variably enlarged, on the basis of the severity and duration of the obstruction. The pelvis and calyces are dilated with associated interstitial inflammation even in the absence of infection. In chronic cases, there is cortical tubular atrophy and marked diffuse interstitial fibrosis. The apices of pyramids become cup shaped. In advanced cases, the kidney is converted into a thin-walled cystic structure with total parenchymal atrophy, loss of the pyramids and cortical thinning.

Clinical Features and Management

Symptoms of hydronephrosis are usually those of the underlying disorder. Distension of the renal capsule and the collecting system may cause pain in later stages.

Table 24.12 Causes of Urinary Tract Obstruction

- Congenital anomalies
- Posterior urethral valve
- Urethral stricture
- Meatal stenosis
- Bladder neck obstruction
- Severe vesicoureteric reflux
- Urinary calculi
- Benign prostatic hypertrophy
- Carcinoma of prostate, bladder, cervix, uterus and retroperitoneal lymphoma
- Inflammation
- Prostatitis
- Ureteritis
- Urethritis
- Retroperitoneal fibrosis
- Sloughed papilla, clot
- Pregnancy
- Cystocoele and prolapse
- Functional
- Spinal cord damage
- Diabetic nephropathy
- Dysfunctional bladder

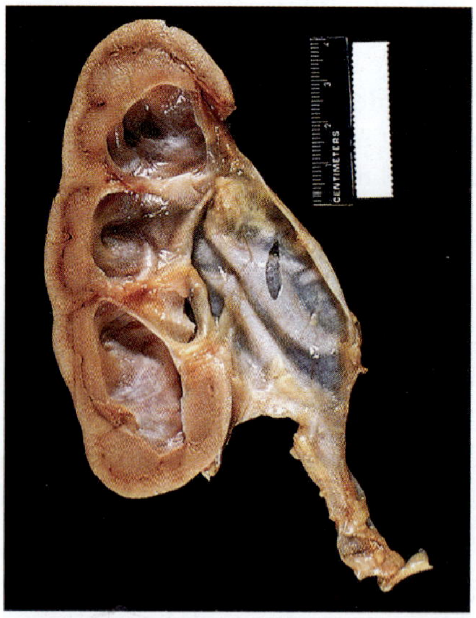

Fig. 24.40 Gross representation of hydronephrosis. (*Source:* From Natalija Kovacevic, David A. Leavitt. Hydronephrosis. Elsevier 2020.)

- **Unilateral obstruction** is usually asymptomatic. It may be an incidental finding on ultrasound scan. Relieving the obstruction may reverse the pathology in early stages.
- **Bilateral partial obstruction** disturbs the concentrating ability of the tubules, resulting in polyuria and nocturia. Distal tubular acidosis may develop later. The complications include secondary renal calculi, tubulointerstitial nephritis, scarring of the papilla and hypertension.
- **Bilateral complete obstruction** is a fatal condition unless this obstruction is relieved promptly. On removing the obstruction, postobstructive diuresis may develop, resulting in excessive loss of body water and sodium chloride.

UROLITHIASIS

Urolithiasis is a common problem worldwide, with an average incidence of 5%–10%. Men are more commonly affected than women, and the average age of presentation is between 20 and 30 years.

Aetiology and Pathogenesis

The common types of urinary stones and their incidence are as follows:

- Calcium oxalate and phosphate: 70%
- Triple stones or struvite stones (magnesium ammonium phosphate): 15%
- Uric acid stones: 5%–10%
- Cysteine stones: 1%–2%

The process of stone formation (Flowchart 24.11) is mainly attributed to **supersaturation** of the stone constituent in urine, leading to reduced solubility. The other factors that exaggerate the process include changes in urinary pH, decreased urinary volume, bacterial infection and deficiency of inhibitors of crystal formation (pyrophosphate, diphosphonate, citrate, glycosaminoglycans, osteopontin and nephrocalcin).

Clinical Features

Affected individuals may remain asymptomatic or present with renal colic, abdominal pain and haematuria. Obstruction of the urinary tract and thus the trauma caused may predispose to secondary urinary tract infection.

Calcium Oxalate Stones Calcium oxalate stones are radiopaque. **High pH** (alkaline) of urine favours calcium phosphate crystal formation. The common causes of calcium stones are as follows:

- Hypercalciuria without hypercalcaemia (50%) – due to absorptive hypercalciuria and renal hypercalciuria
- Hypercalcaemia with hypercalciuria (10%) – due to hyperparathyroidism, diffuse bone disease and sarcoidosis
- Hyperoxaluria (5%) – due to hereditary primary oxaluria (0.5%) or acquired intestinal overabsorption (4.5%)
- Hyperuricosuria (20%) with or without hypercalciuria – the uric acid acting as a nidus for calcium oxalate deposition
- Hypocitraturia associated with chronic diarrhoea
- Idiopathic (20%)

Magnesium Ammonium Phosphate (Struvite) Struvite stones are associated with *Proteus* infection and staphylococci (urea-splitting bacteria). This leads to an increase in the concentration of ammonia in urine and favours the precipitation of these stones. Urine contains mainly urea, so a large quantity of ammonia is generated, resulting in large **staghorn calculus** formation (Fig. 24.41).

Uric Acid Uric acid stones are radiolucent. **Low pH** favours uric acid crystal formation. The causes of uric acid stone formation are as follows:
- Hyperuricaemia (gout, leukaemia)
- Hyperuricosuria
- Idiopathic

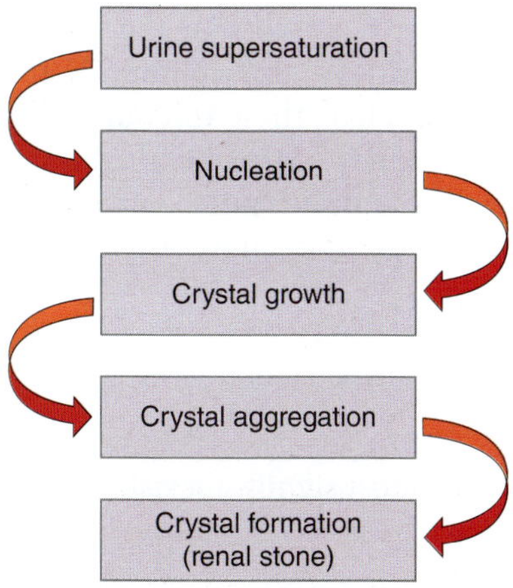

Flowchart 24.11 Formation of renal stones.

Cysteine Cysteine stone formation is due to a **genetic defect** in renal reabsorption of amino acid cysteine. Cysteine tends to crystallize in acidic urine.

Morphology

Renal calculi may be single or multiple but are usually unilateral. The calculi may be formed in the renal pelvis, where they are likely to be small with a smooth or an irregular surface, or in the urinary bladder. In some cases, progressive deposition of salts over the niche in the pelvis leads to the formation of branching structures that take the form of the renal pelvicalyceal system and are called staghorn calculi.

Management

Small stones may cause acute pain while they pass through the urinary tract along with urine. Some stones may cause urinary tract obstruction and either may require intervention in the form of induced diuresis to flush the stone out of the system or may require additional procedures to crush the stone to enable it to be flushed out. Rare complications associated with urolithiasis include obstruction leading to abscess formation, fistula formation and CRF.

NEOPLASMS OF THE KIDNEY PA 28.14

Neoplasms in the kidney, like any other site, may be benign or malignant. The latter is more clinically significant. The list of neoplasms is given in Table 24.13.

BENIGN NEOPLASMS

Renal Papillary Adenoma

Papillary adenomas are small adenomas arising from the renal tubules. These adenomas are asymptomatic and often have papillary architecture. These are often noticed in the cortex in autopsy as well-circumscribed nodules of less than 1.5 cm. Microscopy shows complex branching papillae or tubules and glands of cuboidal to hexagonal cells. These tumours are potentially malignant, with the risk of metastasis increasing with an increase in the size of tumours.

Angiomyolipoma

As the name indicates, these are tumours composed of blood vessels, muscle and fatty components derived from **perivascular epithelioid cells**. These occur in up to 50% of individuals with tuberous sclerosis. Their susceptibility to develop spontaneous haemorrhage makes them a clinically significant finding.

Oncocytoma

Oncocytoma is an epithelial cell neoplasm composed of cells with abundant mitochondria-rich eosinophilic

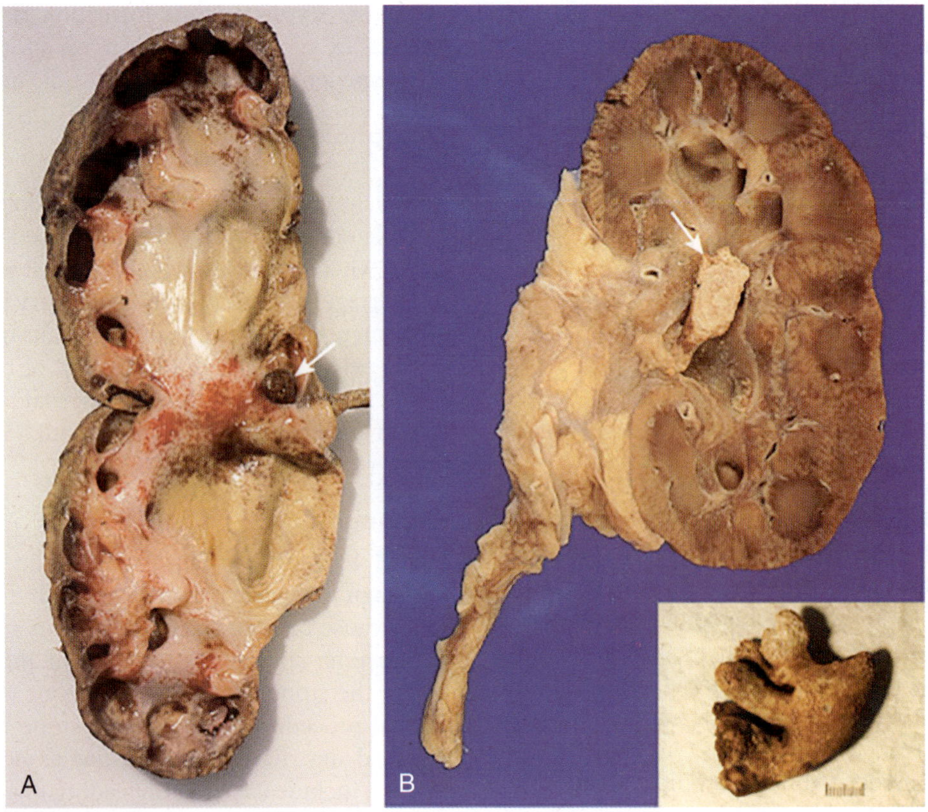

Fig. 24.41 Gross appearance of the kidney showing small round calculi (A) (white arrow) and staghorn calculi in renal pelvis (B) (white arrow). (*Source:* From Andrew J. Connolly, Walter E. Finkbeiner, Philip C. Ursell and Richard L. Davis. Atlas of Gross Autopsy Pathology. Autopsy Pathology: A Manual and Atlas. 3rd edition. Elsevier 2016.)

Table 24.13 Renal Neoplasms

Benign	Malignant
Epithelial	**Epithelial tumours**
Renal papillary adenoma	**Molecularly defined renal cell carcinoma**
Oncocytoma	FH-deficient RCC
Mesenchymal	**MET family of RCC**
Angiomyolipoma	TFE3-rearranged RCC (Xp11)
	TFEB-rearranged RCC t(6,11)
	TFEB-amplified RCC
	Renal cell carcinoma
	Clear cell carcinoma
	Papillary carcinoma
	Chromophobe carcinoma
	Collecting duct (Bellini duct) carcinoma
	Medullary carcinoma
	Mesenchymal tumours
	Sarcoma
	Sarcomatoid carcinoma
	Rhabdomyosarcoma
	Synovial sarcoma
	Leiomyosarcoma
	Angiosarcoma
	Haematolymphoid
	Lymphoma – Diffuse large B cell Lymphoma
	Plasmacytoma

FH, fumarate hydratase; RCC, renal cell carcinoma.

cytoplasm arising from the **intercalated cells of the collecting ducts**. The neoplasm appears as a well-circumscribed, nonencapsulated tumour that is homogeneous tan or mahogany brown with a central scar and is composed of large eosinophilic cells with benign nuclei containing prominent nucleoli. The abundant cytoplasm is ultrastructurally made up of abundant mitochondria.

Renal Cell Carcinoma

RCCs are tumours that arise from the epithelium of renal tubules. They constitute more than 90% of the malignancies that occur in the kidney in both sexes.

The tumour is twice as common in men than in women and usually presents in the sixth and seventh decades of life. Mostly, this tumour is sporadic, with only 4% being familial. These tumours may arise in any portion of the kidney but occur predominantly in the poles, especially the **upper pole**. Sarcomatoid and rhabdoid changes can occur in all types of RCC and make the prognosis poor.

Risk Factors The risk factors associated with RCC are as follows:

- Tobacco – the most significant risk factor
- Obesity
- Hypertension
- Oestrogen exposure

- Asbestos
- Petroleum products and heavy metals
- ESRD
- Acquired cystic disease
- Tuberous sclerosis

Associations With Renal Cell Carcinoma The syndromes associated with familial RCC are as follows:

- **Von Hippel–Lindau (VHL) syndrome:** VHL gene on chromosome 3p25 is involved in sporadic and familial clear cell RCC. Familial forms develop bilateral and multiple neoplasms.
- **Fumarate hydratase (FH)–deficient RCCs:** It was previously called 'hereditary leiomyomatosis and renal cell cancer syndrome'. This is an autosomal dominant disease that is associated with mutation of FH gene. Patients are prone to develop multiple cutaneous and uterine leiomyoma and high-grade papillary carcinoma that metastasize early.
- **MIT family of tumours:** It constitutes two types of genes – one is TFE3-rearranged RCCs (Xp11) and the other is TFEB-rearranged t(6,11) or amplified RCC. The most common morphological phenotype of these tumours is papillary pattern with TFEB amplified RCCs showing unique expression of melanocytic markers like MART1.
- **Birt–Hogg–Dubé syndrome:** This is also autosomal dominant in inheritance and is caused by mutation of BHD gene that expresses folliculin. The presentation is in the form of a group of lesions that include fibrofolliculoma, trichodiscoma, acrochordons, cysts in the lung and RCC.

Classification of Renal Cell Carcinoma RCCs are classified on the basis of the cytogenetic, genetic and histological features of the tumours.

- **Clear cell carcinoma:** Clear cell RCCs are the most common type of renal carcinoma accounting for up to 70%–80% of cases. These arise from **proximal tubular epithelium** of the nephrons. About 90% are sporadic, whereas the rest of them are familial. **Mutation of VHL** gene is involved in both sporadic and familial cases, and it may be associated with VHL syndrome also. Irrespective of the nature of origin, these tumours are associated with loss of VHL gene at **3p chromosome**. VHL gene acts a tumour suppressor gene. Hence, deletion of one gene plus hypermethylation-induced inactivation of second gene leads to complete loss of function of VHL gene and triggers the development of clear cell RCC. Inactivation of VHL gene leads to high levels of hypoxia-inducible factor 1 (HIF-1) even in the absence of hypoxaemia, which, in turn, triggers VEGF, insulin-like growth factor-1 (IGF-1) and other growth-promoting genes. The other mutations noted in this tumour include genes that regulate histone modification and control epigenetics.
- **Papillary carcinoma:** Papillary carcinomas account for up to 10%–15% of cases of RCCs. These may be familial or sporadic types but are not associated with 3p deletion. The chromosomal abnormalities associated with them include **trisomy 7 and 17 and loss of Y chromosome** in males. Chromosome 7 is mapped to MET that encodes tyrosine kinase receptor for hepatocyte growth factor, and mutation of MET is also seen in sporadic papillary carcinoma.
- **Chromophobe carcinoma:** These carcinomas account for up to 5% of cases of RCCs and are associated with multiple chromosome losses and hypodiploidy. These arise from intercalated cells of collecting ducts and have an excellent prognosis.
- **Multilocular cystic renal neoplasm:** These neoplasms are multicystic low-grade variant of clear cell RCCs, presenting in the middle-aged men more than in females. These have a minimal risk of recurrence and metastasis. Genetically, these are associated with **loss of 3p** like clear cell RCCs.
- **Collecting duct (Bellini duct) carcinoma:** This is a rare variant with an incidence of less than 1% of cases of RCCs. It arises from **collecting ducts in the medulla**, and although it may be associated with several chromosome losses, it does not have any specific mutations.

Morphology

Clear cell RCCs are solitary, unilateral lesions. These are variable in size and are found bulging out, distorting the renal surface, but are well defined and confined within the renal capsule, with the cut surface appearing yellow-grey and variegated in appearance with haemorrhage and necrosis (Fig. 24.42). Microscopically, these lesions are composed of solid, trabecular and tubular patterns with interspersed delicate branching blood vessels **(chicken wire blood vessels)**. The cells are round with clear/granular cytoplasm filled with glycogen and lipids. The lesions have a unique pattern of spread in that these may **invade the renal vein** and extend through the inferior vena cava up to the right side of the heart. On immunohistochemistry, these tumours show positivity for CA-IX (carbonic anhydrase IX) and CD10.

Papillary carcinomas are named so because of their papillary architecture. These are often multifocal and bilateral and arise from the **distal convoluted tubule**. The cut surface of the tumour is haemorrhagic and cystic. Microscopy shows papillary growth composed of a core containing interstitial foam cells and lined by cuboidal to columnar cells (Fig. 24.43). The stroma is scanty and vascularized. The presence of psammoma bodies is another notable feature of this variant. On immunohistochemistry, these tumours show positivity for cytokeratin-7 (CK-7) and α-methylacyl-CoA racemase (AMACR).

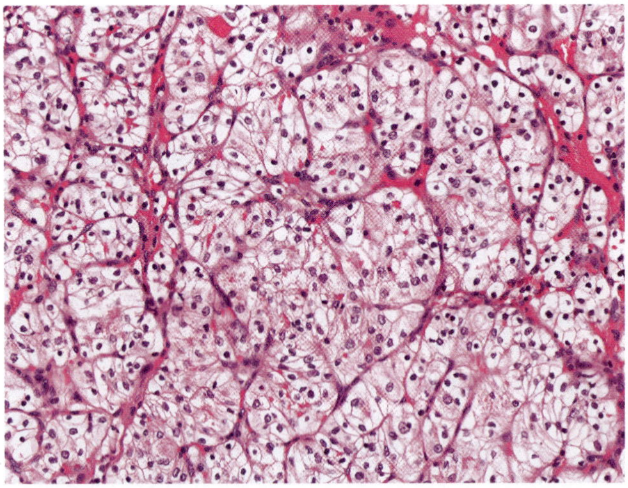

Fig. 24.42 Microscopy shows sheets of clear cells with thin delicate blood vessels – clear cell RCC. (*Source:* From Christopher D.M. Fletcher. Tumors of the Urinary Tract. Diagnostic Histopathology of Tumors. 5th edition. Elsevier 2021.)

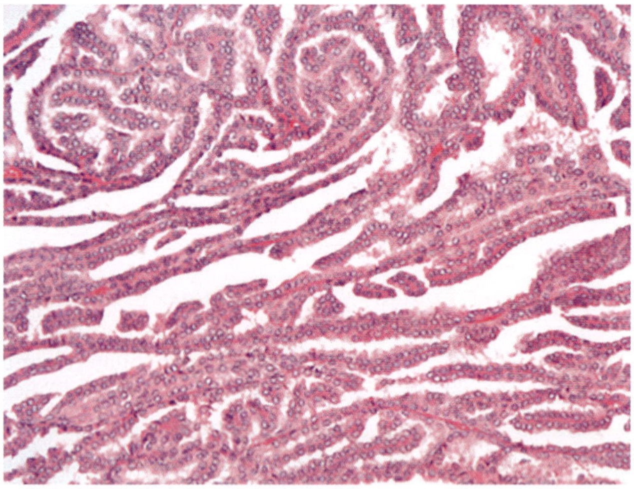

Fig. 24.43 Microscopy of papillary RCC showing branching papillae with a fibrovascular core lined by a single layer of cells. (*Source:* From Jesse K. McKenney. Kidney: Tumors and Tumorlike Conditions. Rosai and Ackerman's Surgical Pathology. 11th edition. Elsevier 2018.)

Chromophobe RCCs (Fig. 24.44) are tumours composed of cells with prominent cell membrane, eosinophilic cytoplasm with a wrinkled nucleus and **perinuclear halo** arranged as sheets around blood vessels. On immunohistochemistry, these tumours show positivity for c KIT (CD 117).

Multilocular cystic renal neoplasms are unilateral and composed of cysts of varying sizes filled with clear, serous or gelatinous fluid and no mural nodules. Microscopically, these neoplasms show cysts with septa composed of groups of clear cells similar to cells of clear cell RCCs.

In the collecting duct of Bellini carcinoma, the tumour is located in the medullary region. The malignant cells show hobnailing and are arranged in glands in fibrotic stroma.

Medullary carcinoma: It is similar to collecting duct carcinoma arising from the medulla. Morphologically, it shows glandular tissue in an adenoid cystic pattern within a desmoplastic stroma. These tumours show loss of integrase interactor-1 (INI-1). This tumour is seen at a greater frequency in patients with sickle cell trait.

The commonest grading system for RCC, especially clear cell and papillary RCC, is the Fuhrmann or International Society of Urological Pathology (ISUP) grading system (Table 24.14).

Rarely, sarcomas and haematolymphoid malignancies can occur in the kidney. The commonest sarcoma in the kidney is sarcomatoid carcinoma. Other tumours include synovial sarcoma, rhabdomyosarcoma, leiomyosarcoma and angiosarcoma.

Among the haematolymphoid malignancies, the commonest one is diffuse large B-cell lymphoma.

A summary of morphological features, IHC markers and molecular genetic changes of the variants of RCC is given in Fig. 24.45.

Clinical Features The triad of presenting symptoms in RCCs includes **costovertebral pain, palpable mass and intermittent haematuria**. Patients may sometimes be asymptomatic, with the tumour being noted incidentally, or present with nonspecific symptoms such as unexplained fever, malaise and weight loss when the tumour has attained large dimensions. In fact, at times, patients may present with symptoms of metastasis without any clinical feature related to the primary.

The tumour is also known for being notorious in producing **paraneoplastic syndromes** due to abnormal hormone production. The paraneoplastic symptoms associated with RCCs include polycythaemia, hypercalcaemia, hypertension, hepatic dysfunction, feminization, masculinization, eosinophilia, Cushing syndrome, amyloidosis and leukaemoid reaction.

Prognosis is not bad in cases diagnosed early by incidental radiological imaging, with the 5-year survival without distant metastasis being 95%. Unfortunately, due to its late presentation, metastasis is common in about 25% of cases; at the time of diagnosis itself, the most common site is the lungs, followed by bones, lymph node, liver, adrenals and brain in the descending order. The average 5-year survival rate is 70%, being further reduced to 60% in the presence of renal vein or perinephric invasion. Radical nephrectomy is the treatment of choice, but partial nephrectomy may be attempted with success in small

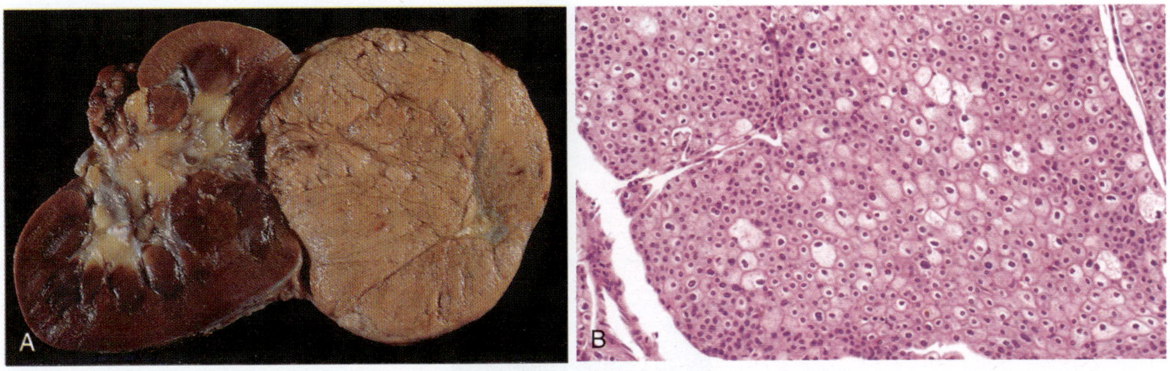

Fig. 24.44 (A) Grossly well-circumscribed brown tumour, and (B) microscopy showing perinuclear halo – chromophobe RCC. (*Source:* From Christopher D.M. Fletcher. Tumors of the Urinary Tract. Diagnostic Histopathology of Tumors. 5th edition. Elsevier 2021; Anthony Chang and Zoltan G. Laszik. The Kidney. Robbins & Cotran Pathologic Basis of Disease. 10th edition. Elsevier 2021.)

Table 24.14 Fuhrmann or International Society of Urological Pathology (ISUP) Grading System

Grade 1	Grade 2	Grade 3	Grade 4
Tumour cell nucleoli invisible or small and basophilic at 400× magnification	Tumour cell nucleoli conspicuous at 400× magnification and inconspicuous at 100× magnification	Tumour cell nucleoli eosinophilic and conspicuous at 100× magnification	Tumour cells show extreme nuclear pleomorphism and/or tumour giant cells and/or sarcomatoid and/or rhabdoid change

tumours less than 4 cm. Adjuvant therapy with tyrosine kinase and VEGF inhibitors may be helpful.

Urothelial Carcinoma of Renal Pelvis

These tumours make up 5%–10% cases of primary renal tumours. They arise from **renal pelvis urothelium** and range from benign papilloma to invasive urothelial carcinoma. These tumours may be detected early when small, due to **haematuria** that occurs when the tumour undergoes fragmentation. The location of the tumour may lead to urinary flow obstruction and cause **hydronephrosis**. They may be occasionally multiple, and about 50% may be associated with urothelial carcinoma of the bladder. These are also seen associated with Lynch syndrome and analgesic nephropathy. On gross examination (Fig. 24.46), urothelial tumours are solitary tumours but occasionally may be multiple, involving the pelvis, ureters and bladder. In 50% of cases, a preexisting or concomitant bladder urothelial tumour may be evident. Microscopically, these tumours resemble bladder urothelial carcinomas. Prognosis is good, with the 5-year survival rate ranging from 50%–100% in low-grade tumours to 10% in high-grade tumours.

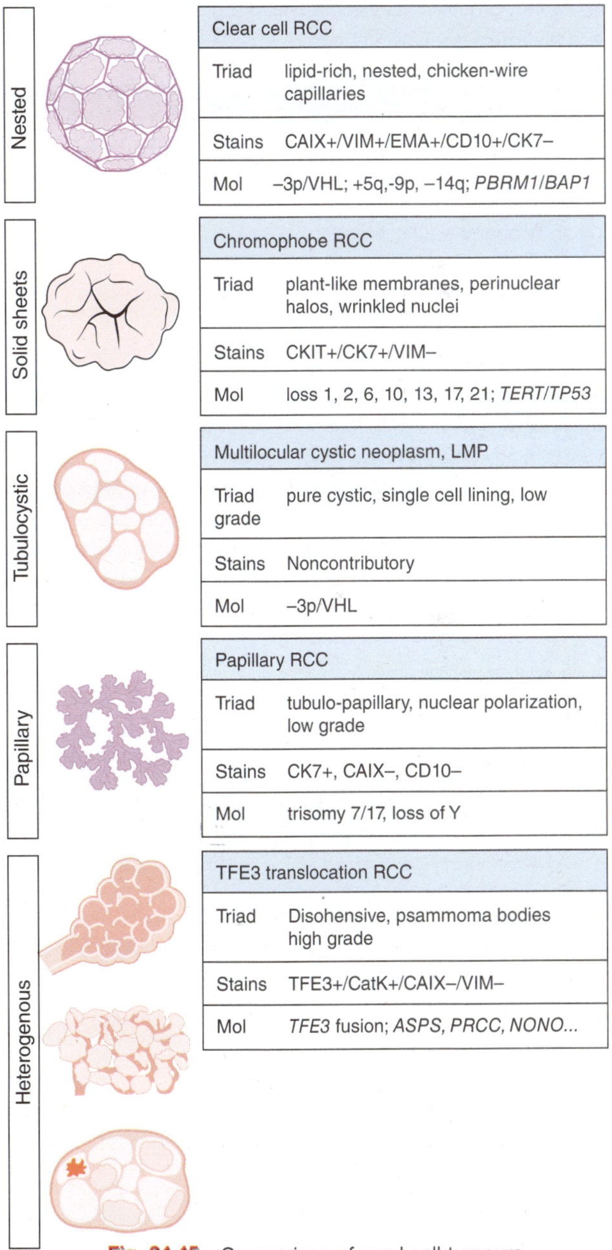

Fig. 24.45 Comparison of renal cell tumours.

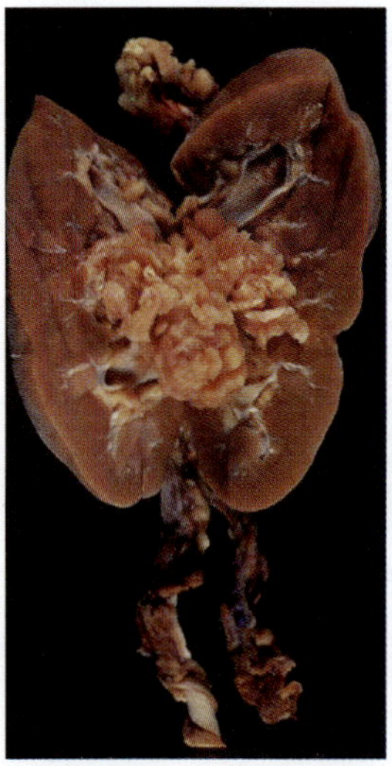

Fig. 24.46 Urothelial carcinoma occupying the renal pelvis. (*Source:* From Christopher D.M. Fletcher. Tumors of the Urinary Tract. Diagnostic Histopathology of Tumors. 5th edition. Elsevier 2021.)

SELF-ASSESSMENT

Multiple Choice Questions

1. Phagocytic cells of kidney are
   A. Visceral epithelial cells
   B. Parietal epithelial cells
   C. Mesangial cells
   D. All of the above
2. Acute kidney injury can result from damage to
   A. Interstitium
   B. Vessels
   C. Tubules
   D. Any of the above
3. A 25-year-old male was brought with signs and symptoms of rapidly declining renal function. He was investigated and renal biopsy was performed. Light microscopy showed the presence of cellular crescents, immunofluorescence highlighted linear IgG and C3, and electron microscopy showed no deposits. Which among the following mechanisms is implicated as a cause in this patient?
   A. Immune complex mediated
   B. Anti–GBM antibody mediated
   C. ANCA mediated
   D. Any of the above
4. Compared with nephritic syndrome, the feature that is not commonly seen in nephrotic syndrome is
   A. Proteinuria
   B. Haematuria
   C. Oedema
   D. None of the above
5. Electron microscopic finding of subepithelial humps in renal biopsy is the characteristic feature of
   A. Postinfectious glomerulonephritis
   B. Minimal change disease
   C. Membranoproliferative glomerulonephritis
   D. MPGN type I
6. Type III RPGN is
   A. Pauci-immune RPGN
   B. ANCA associated
   C. Negative for anti-GBM antibodies
   D. All of the above
7. PLA2R is the antigen implicated in the pathogenesis of
   A. Minimal change disease
   B. Membranous glomerulopathy
   C. IgA nephropathy
   D. Anti-GBM nephritis
8. Tram-track appearance of GBM in silver or PAS stain is a feature seen with
   A. MPGN
   B. PSGN
   C. FSGS
   D. Membranous nephropathy
9. A 22-year-old male patient presented with complaints of haematuria. He was investigated. Renal biopsy was performed that showed mesangial widening and immunofluorescence highlighted the presence of mesangial deposits of IgA and C3. Electron microscopy confirmed the presence of electron-dense deposits predominantly in the mesangium. What is your diagnosis in this patient?
   A. Type I MPGN
   B. Type II MPGN
   C. Beger disease
   D. None of the above
10. A 7-year-old male child presented with purpuric skin lesions, abdominal pain, intestinal bleeding and arthralgias along with renal abnormalities. Renal biopsy IF showed the presence of IgA deposits in the mesangium. What do you think is the diagnosis?
    A. Minimal change disease
    B. Henoch–Schönlein purpura
    C. Membranous nephropathy
    D. Any of the above
11. Tubulointerstitial disorders are distinguished clinically from the glomerular diseases by
    A. Absence of nephritic or nephrotic syndrome
    B. Salt wasting
    C. Metabolic acidosis
    D. All of the above

12. Which among the following conditions is a predisposing factor for the development of pyelonephritis?
    A. Urinary tract obstruction
    B. Stasis of urine
    C. Vesicoureteral reflux
    D. All of the above
13. The hallmark feature of acute pyelonephritis is
    A. Intratubular aggregates of neutrophils
    B. Neutrophilic tubulitis
    C. Tubular injury
    D. All of the above
14. The histopathological feature that differentiates chronic pyelonephritis from acute pyelonephritis is
    A. Tubulointerstitial inflammatory infiltrate with mononuclear cells
    B. Pelvicalyceal scarring
    C. Both of the above
    D. None of the above
15. Large multicystic kidneys associated with liver cysts and berry aneurysms are a feature of
    A. Adult polycystic kidney disease
    B. Childhood polycystic kidney disease
    C. Medullary sponge kidney
    D. Simple cysts
16. Which among the following syndromes is associated with the development of RCC?
    A. Hereditary papillary carcinoma
    B. Von Hippel–Lindau (VHL) syndrome
    C. Birt–Hogg–Dubé syndrome
    D. All of the above
17. Xp11 translocation carcinoma is associated with
    A. Papillary architecture
    B. Clear cells
    C. Overexpression of TFE3
    D. All of the above
18. A 65-year-old male was investigated for renal mass. Biopsy was performed that showed a malignant neoplasm composed of pale eosinophilic cells, with a perinuclear halo, arranged in solid sheets with a concentration of the largest cells around blood vessels. What is your diagnosis?
    A. Chromophobe renal carcinoma
    B. Clear cell carcinoma
    C. Papillary carcinoma
    D. Collecting duct carcinoma
19. Which among the following statements is false regarding RCC?
    A. The classic clinical features of renal cell carcinoma are costovertebral pain, palpable mass and haematuria.
    B. The most reliable clue is haematuria.
    C. It is locally invasive.
    D. RCC does not tend to metastasize widely
20. Medullary carcinoma is seen in patients with
    A. Diabetes
    B. Sickle cell trait
    C. Hypertension
    D. All of the above

Answers

1. (C); 2. (D); 3. (B); 4. (B); 5. (A); 6. (D); 7. (B); 8. (A); 9. (C); 10. (B); 11. (D); 12. (D); 13. (D); 14. (C); 15. (A); 16. (D); 17. (D); 18. (A); 19. (D); 20. (B)

Self-Assessment Questions

1. A 10-year-old boy presented to the paediatric outpatient department (OPD) with fever, malaise, nausea, oliguria and cola-coloured urine. He was treated for sore throat 1 week back. On examination, his blood pressure was 150/100 mm Hg. What is your diagnosis?
2. A 4-year-old boy presented to OPD with swelling of his legs and face over the past 1 week. On eliciting history, he reported that his urine was white coloured. His blood pressure was 110/70 mm Hg. What is your diagnosis?
3. A 23-year-old male patient presented with cough and haemoptysis to the medical OPD. He also gave a history of red-coloured urine for the past 15 days. His computed tomographic scan showed ground glass opacities of the lungs. Renal biopsy immunofluorescence showed linear deposits along the basement membrane. What is the diagnosis?
4. A 50-year-old male patient on the third postoperative day after gastrectomy developed severe oliguria. He was dyspnoeic and confused for the past 2 hours. On reviewing his notes, it was found that intravenous fluids were stopped 24 hours back but the patient did not take oral fluids due to nausea. What is the probable diagnosis?
5. A 45-year-old woman with a history of recurrent urinary infections developed fever and loin pain for the past 1 week. She gave a history of increased urine output over the past 2 days. Her blood pressure was elevated and imaging showed contracted kidneys. What is your diagnosis?
6. A 68-year-man presented to the emergency department with acute headache, nausea, vomiting and visual disturbance. His blood pressure was 200/120 mm Hg. His urine was red in colour, and his blood tests revealed elevated levels of renin. What is the diagnosis? What will be the gross appearance of kidneys?
7. A 30-year-old man presented with severe pain radiating from the loin to groin along with haematuria. There was severe pain in the costophrenic angle. He was a known case of acute leukaemia on chemotherapy. What is the likely cause of his symptoms?
8. A 45-year-old man presented with complaints of dragging sensation in the loin and haematuria. He also gave a history of recent-onset hypertension and had episodes of abdominal pain, followed by passing clots in urine. On ultrasound scan, the kidneys were grossly enlarged with multiple cysts. What is the gene responsible for this problem?
9. A known patient with sickle cell anaemia presented with complaints of abdominal pain and haematuria for the past 3 days. He had an episode of sickle cell crisis a few days back that evolved into localized flank pain now. What is the possible reason?
10. A 60-year-old man was being investigated for unexplained fever for the past 10 days. He gave a history of weight loss and loss of appetite for the past 1 month. Imaging showed a mass in the upper pole of the kidney. What is the possible diagnosis?

Answers

1. Poststreptococcal glomerulonephritis
2. Minimal change disease (nephrotic syndrome)
3. Goodpasture syndrome
4. Ischaemic acute kidney injury
5. Chronic pyelonephritis

6. Malignant hypertension – flea-bitten kidney
7. Urolithiasis – urate stone
8. Adult autosomal dominant polycystic kidney disease
9. Papillary necrosis
10. Renal cell carcinoma

Topics for Self-Directed Learning

1. Congenital anomalies of the kidney
2. Interpretation of renal biopsy
3. Role of immunofluorescence in renal biopsies
4. Pathologies in the transplanted kidney
5. Molecular diagnosis of tumours of the kidney
6. Amyloidosis of kidney
7. Light chain and heavy chain deposition disease of kidney
8. Renal diseases of pregnancy
9. Drug-induced renal damage

MIND MAPS

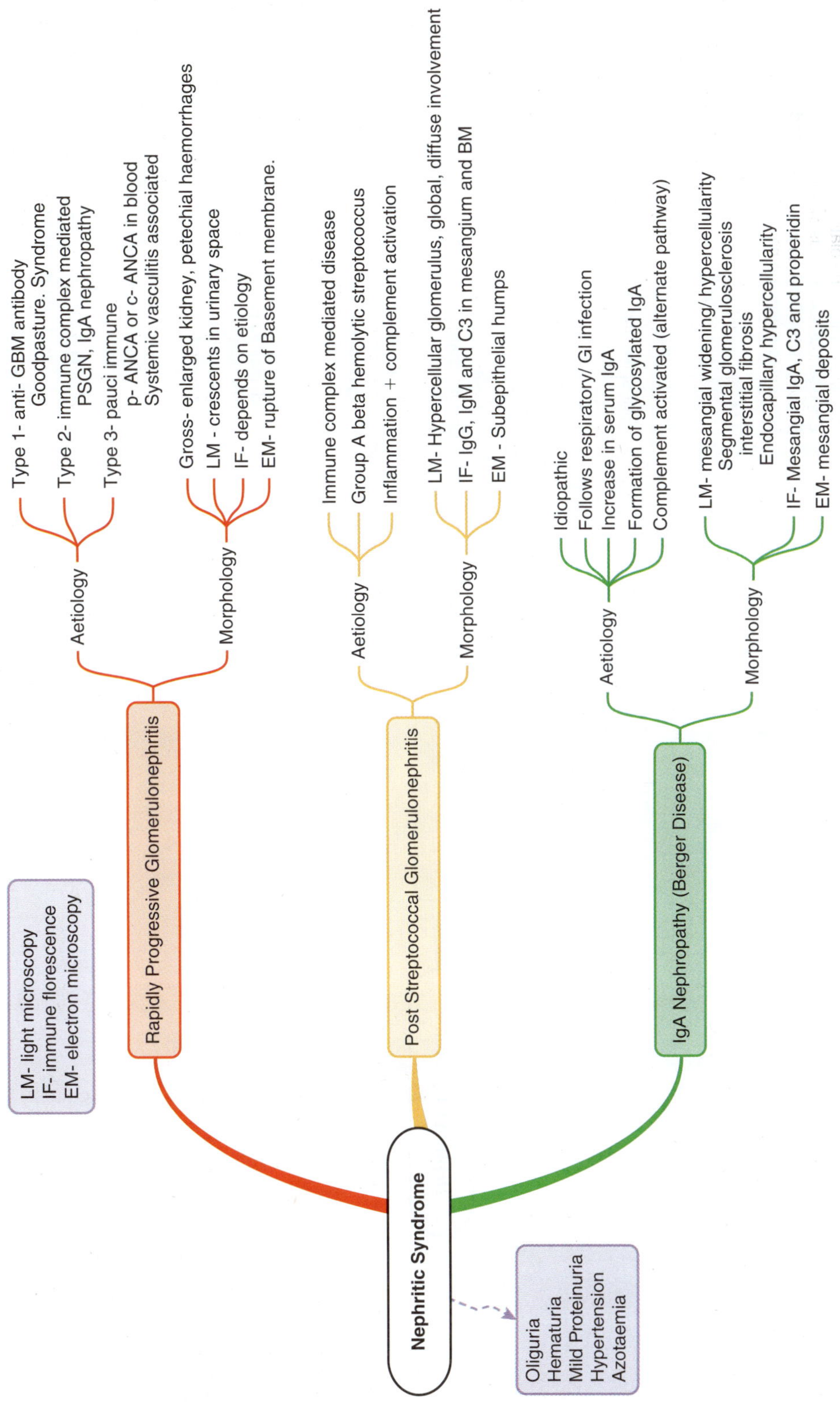
LM- light microscopy
IF- immune florescence
EM- electron microscopy
Nephritic Syndrome
Oliguria
Hematuria
Mild Proteinuria
Hypertension
Azotaemia
Rapidly Progressive Glomerulonephritis
Aetiology
Type 1- anti- GBM antibody
Goodpasture. Syndrome
Type 2- immune complex mediated
PSGN, IgA nephropathy
Type 3- pauci immune
p- ANCA or c- ANCA in blood
Systemic vasculitis associated
Morphology
Gross- enlarged kidney, petechial haemorrhages
LM - crescents in urinary space
IF- depends on etiology
EM- rupture of Basement membrane.
Post Streptococcal Glomerulonephritis
Aetiology
Immune complex mediated disease
Group A beta hemolytic streptococcus
Inflammation + complement activation
Morphology
LM- Hypercellular glomerulus, global, diffuse involvement
IF- IgG, IgM and C3 in mesangium and BM
EM - Subepithelial humps
IgA Nephropathy (Berger Disease)
Aetiology
Idiopathic
Follows respiratory/ GI infection
Increase in serum IgA
Formation of glycosylated IgA
Complement activated (alternate pathway)
Morphology
LM- mesangial widening/ hypercellularity
Segmental glomerulosclerosis
interstitial fibrosis
Endocapillary hypercellularity
IF- Mesangial IgA, C3 and properidin
EM- mesangial deposits

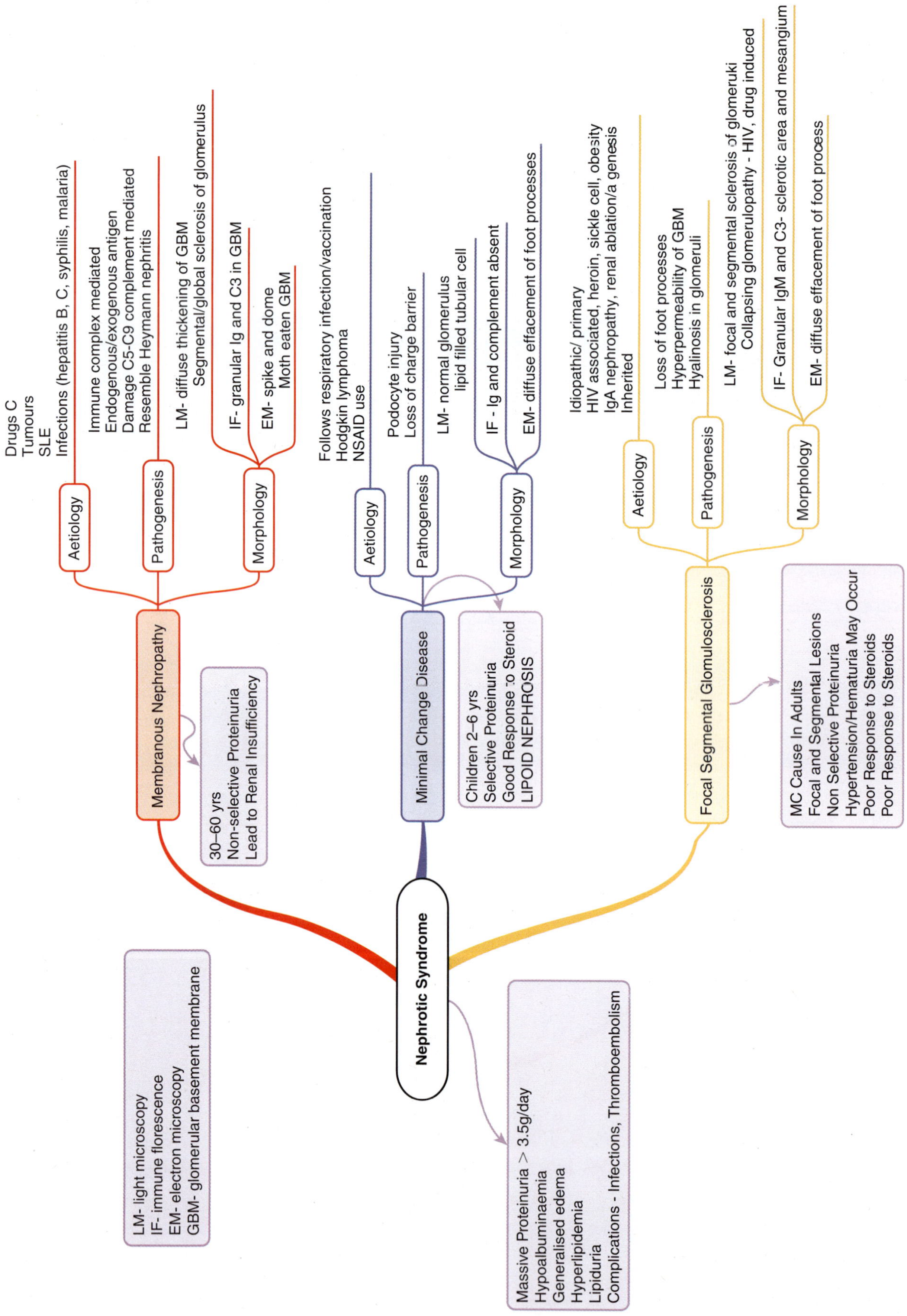
Nephrotic Syndrome
Membranous Nephropathy
Aetiology
Drugs C
Tumours
SLE
Infections (hepatitis B, C, syphilis, malaria)
Pathogenesis
Immune complex mediated
Endogenous/exogenous antigen
Damage C5-C9 complement mediated
Resemble Heymann nephritis
Morphology
LM- diffuse thickening of GBM
Segmental/global sclerosis of glomerulus
IF- granular Ig and C3 in GBM
EM- spike and dome
Moth eaten GBM
30–60 yrs
Non-selective Proteinuria
Lead to Renal Insufficiency
Minimal Change Disease
Aetiology
Follows respiratory infection/vaccination
Hodgkin lymphoma
NSAID use
Pathogenesis
Podocyte injury
Loss of charge barrier
Morphology
LM- normal glomerulus
lipid filled tubular cell
IF - Ig and complement absent
EM- diffuse effacement of foot processes
Children 2–6 yrs
Selective Proteinuria
Good Response to Steroid
LIPOID NEPHROSIS
Focal Segmental Glomulosclerosis
Aetiology
Idiopathic/ primary
HIV associated, heroin, sickle cell, obesity
IgA nephropathy, renal ablation/a genesis
Inherited
Pathogenesis
Loss of foot processes
Hyperpermeability of GBM
Hyalinosis in glomeruli
Morphology
LM- focal and segmental sclerosis of glomeruki
Collapsing glomerulopathy - HIV, drug induced
IF- Granular IgM and C3- sclerotic area and mesangium
EM- diffuse effacement of foot process
MC Cause In Adults
Focal and Segmental Lesions
Non Selective Proteinuria
Hypertension/Hematuria May Occur
Poor Response to Steroids
Poor Response to Steroids
LM- light microscopy
IF- immune florescence
EM- electron microscopy
GBM- glomerular basement membrane
Massive Proteinuria > 3.5g/day
Hypoalbuminaemia
Generalised edema
Hyperlipidemia
Lipiduria
Complications - Infections, Thromboembolism

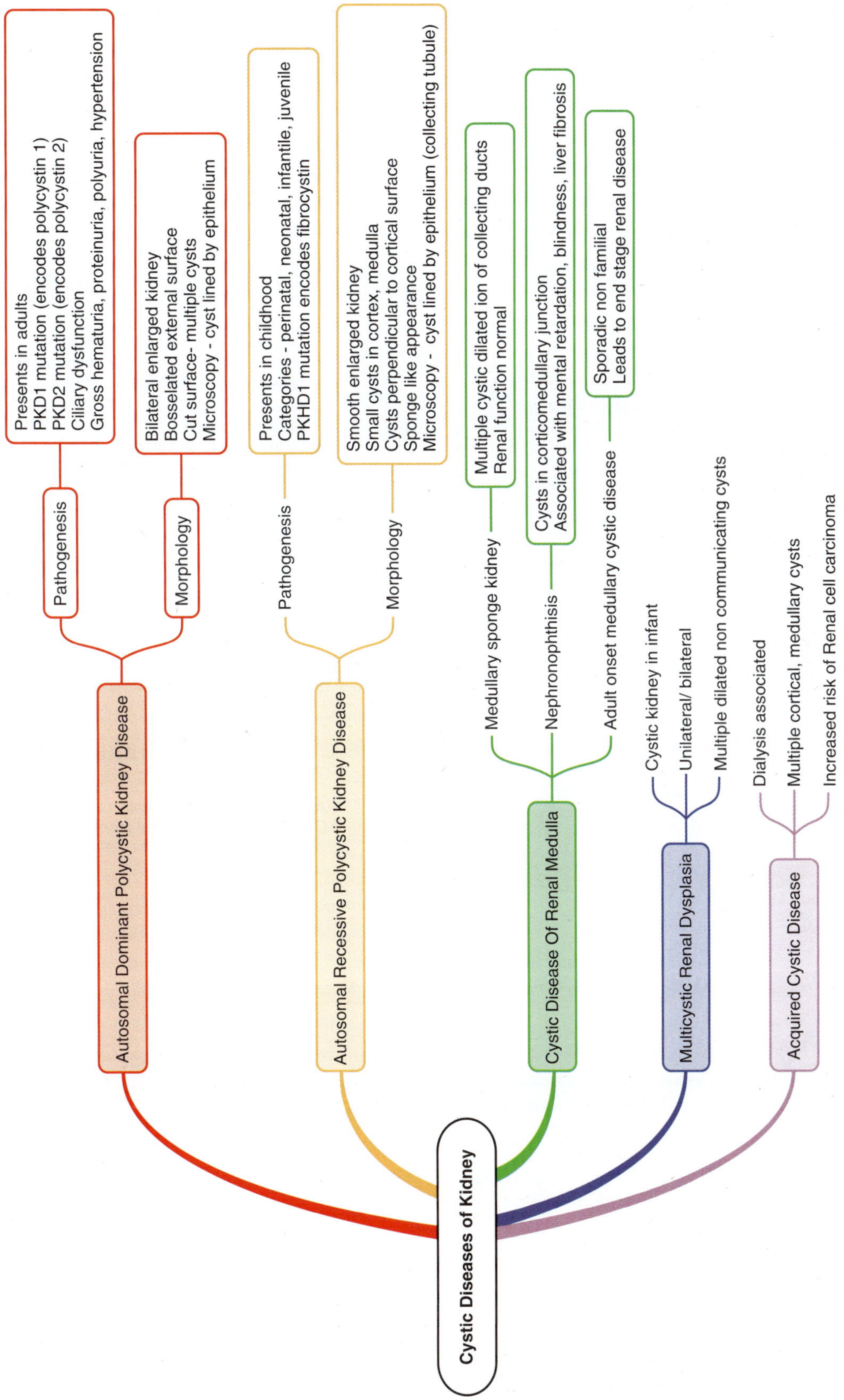
Cystic Diseases of Kidney
Autosomal Dominant Polycystic Kidney Disease
Pathogenesis
Presents in adults
PKD1 mutation (encodes polycystin 1)
PKD2 mutation (encodes polycystin 2)
Ciliary dysfunction
Gross hematuria, proteinuria, polyuria, hypertension
Morphology
Bilateral enlarged kidney
Bosselated external surface
Cut surface- multiple cysts
Microscopy - cyst lined by epithelium
Autosomal Recessive Polycystic Kidney Disease
Pathogenesis
Presents in childhood
Categories - perinatal, neonatal, infantile, juvenile
PKHD1 mutation encodes fibrocystin
Morphology
Smooth enlarged kidney
Small cysts in cortex, medulla
Cysts perpendicular to cortical surface
Sponge like appearance
Microscopy - cyst lined by epithelium (collecting tubule)
Cystic Disease Of Renal Medulla
Medullary sponge kidney
Multiple cystic dilated ion of collecting ducts
Renal function normal
Nephronophthisis
Cysts in corticomedullary junction
Associated with mental retardation, blindness, liver fibrosis
Adult onset medullary cystic disease
Sporadic non familial
Leads to end stage renal disease
Multicystic Renal Dysplasia
Cystic kidney in infant
Unilateral/ bilateral
Multiple dilated non communicating cysts
Acquired Cystic Disease
Dialysis associated
Multiple cortical, medullary cysts
Increased risk of Renal cell carcinoma

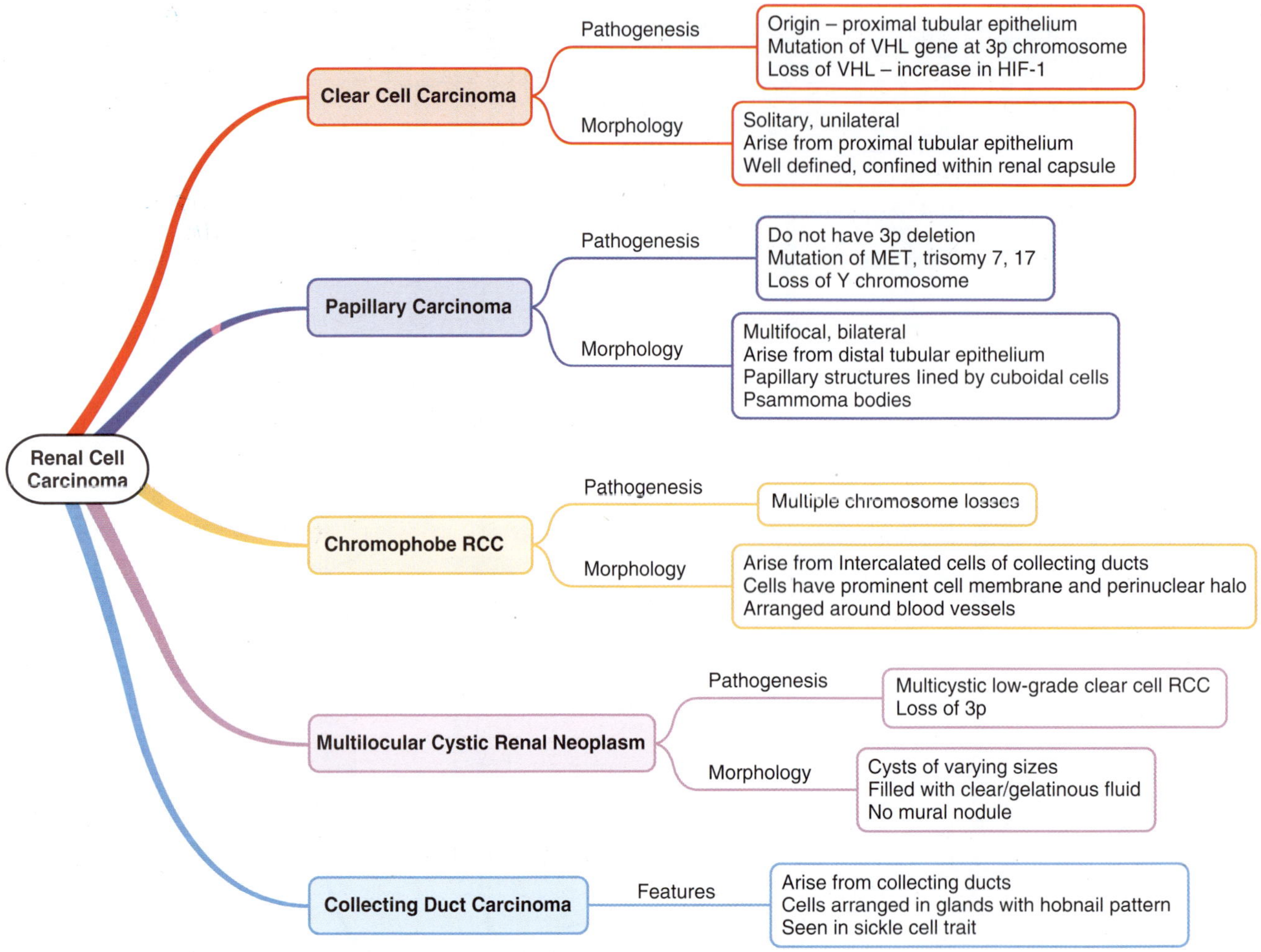
Renal Cell Carcinoma
Clear Cell Carcinoma
Pathogenesis
Origin – proximal tubular epithelium
Mutation of VHL gene at 3p chromosome
Loss of VHL – increase in HIF-1
Morphology
Solitary, unilateral
Arise from proximal tubular epithelium
Well defined, confined within renal capsule
Papillary Carcinoma
Pathogenesis
Do not have 3p deletion
Mutation of MET, trisomy 7, 17
Loss of Y chromosome
Morphology
Multifocal, bilateral
Arise from distal tubular epithelium
Papillary structures lined by cuboidal cells
Psammoma bodies
Chromophobe RCC
Pathogenesis
Multiple chromosome losses
Morphology
Arise from Intercalated cells of collecting ducts
Cells have prominent cell membrane and perinuclear halo
Arranged around blood vessels
Multilocular Cystic Renal Neoplasm
Pathogenesis
Multicystic low-grade clear cell RCC
Loss of 3p
Morphology
Cysts of varying sizes
Filled with clear/gelatinous fluid
No mural nodule
Collecting Duct Carcinoma
Features
Arise from collecting ducts
Cells arranged in glands with hobnail pattern
Seen in sickle cell trait

25 The Lower Urinary Tract and Male Genital System

Ramya Krishna

PA 29.1 Classify testicular tumours and describe the pathogenesis, pathology, presenting and distinguishing features, diagnostic tests, progression and spread of **testicular tumours.**

PA 29.2 Describe the pathogenesis, pathology, presenting and distinguishing features, diagnostic tests, progression and spread of **carcinoma of the penis.**

PA 29.3 Describe the pathogenesis, pathology, hormonal dependency, presenting and distinguishing features, urological findings and diagnostic tests of **benign prostatic hyperplasia.**

PA 29.4 Describe the pathogenesis, pathology, hormonal dependency, presenting and distinguishing features, diagnostic tests, progression and spread of **carcinoma of the prostate.**

PA 29.5 Describe the aetiology, pathogenesis, pathology and progression of **prostatitis.**

PA 28.16 Describe the aetiology, genetics, pathogenesis, pathology, presenting features and progression of **urothelial tumours.**

CHAPTER OUTLINE

I. LOWER URINARY TRACT

The lower urinary tract includes the **renal calyces, renal pelvis, ureters, urinary bladder and urethra**, which together aid in storage and excretion of urine. Let us briefly discuss the development, anatomy and histology before considering the pathological conditions of the lower urinary tract.

DEVELOPMENT, ANATOMY AND HISTOLOGY

DEVELOPMENT OF THE LOWER URINARY TRACT

The intermediate mesoderm and the primitive urogenital sinus together give rise to the urogenital system.

The **collecting system of the kidney** is derived from the **ureteric bud**, which arises from the distal part of the mesonephric duct. The ureteric bud grows cranially and dilates to form the ampulla. The ampulla divides repeatedly, of which the first three to five generations fuse to form the renal pelvis. The subsequent divisions form minor calyces and collecting tubules.

The **urinary bladder** develops from the proximal dilated part of the vesicourethral canal along with the proximal part of the allantois. The distal narrow part of the vesicourethral canal develops into the primitive urethra.

The **female urethra** is derived from the primitive urethra and the pelvic part of the urogenital sinus.

The **male urethra** comprises prostatic, membranous and penile segments, of which the prostatic urethra is derived from the primitive urethra and the pelvic part of the urogenital sinus, the membranous urethra is derived from the pelvic part of the urogenital sinus, and the penile urethra is derived from the phallic part of the urogenital sinus.

ANATOMY

The **renal pelvis** is a funnel-shaped proximal segment of the ureter. It originates in the kidney and is continuous with the ureter. The primary function of the renal pelvis is conduction of urine from the kidneys to the ureters.

The **ureters** are bilateral tubular structures, measuring about 25 cm in length, and serve as channels for the formed urine to reach the bladder.

The **urinary bladder** is a tetrahedral hollow viscus located within the pelvic cavity. Anatomically, it consists of an apex, a base and a neck. The urinary bladder is composed of two lateral walls, a posterior wall and a dome or superior wall. The trigone of the bladder is a triangular area on the posterior wall, with vertices formed by the two ureteric orifices and the internal urethral orifice.

The **female urethra** measures 2 inches in length, extending from the internal to the external urethral orifice. Owing to the short length of the urethra, women are more susceptible to infections like cystitis, which may ascend further via the ureter and manifest as pyelonephritis over a period of time.

The **male urethra** measures about 8 inches in length and opens at the end of the external urethral meatus. The urethra is divided into four segments, namely preprostatic urethra, prostatic urethra, membranous urethra and spongy or penile urethra.

HISTOLOGY

The urinary bladder and ureters histologically comprise four layers, namely the innermost mucosa, lamina propria, muscularis propria and the outermost adventitia or serosa. The mucosa is lined by **transitional epithelium, except for the distal urethra, which is lined by the non-keratinizing stratified squamous epithelium**. The transitional epithelium is stratified, comprising three to six layers of cells, and includes the basal cuboidal epithelium, the intermediate columnar epithelium and the surface epithelium containing specialized umbrella/dome cells that maintain impermeability, irrespective of the urinary solute concentration.

CONGENITAL ANOMALIES OF THE LOWER URINARY TRACT

The incidence of congenital anomalies of the kidneys and the urinary tract is approximately 4.2 per 10,000 live births. Although most of them have minimal clinical significance, certain anomalies can be severe enough to cause urinary obstruction or necessitate renal replacement therapy.

URETERS

Diverticula: These are saccular outpouchings from the wall of the ureters. Diverticula can be congenial or acquired. Congenital diverticulum is a true diverticulum that arises due to aberrant development of the ureteric bud, whereas acquired diverticulum is a pseudodiverticulum arising due to mechanical obstruction, calculi, iatrogenic causes, etc. These defects may be asymptomatic or may manifest in recurrent infections due to urinary stasis.

Ectopic ureter: In this condition, the ureter terminates into structures other than the urinary bladder such as the proximal urethra, seminal vesicle, vas deferens, fallopian tubes, uterus or vagina. Ectopic ureter is more common in women than in men.

Double/bifid ureters (Fig. 25.1): These are commonly associated with a double renal pelvis or with the anomalous development of a large kidney having a partially bifid pelvis, terminating in separate ureters. These double ureters pursue their independent course to the bladder but

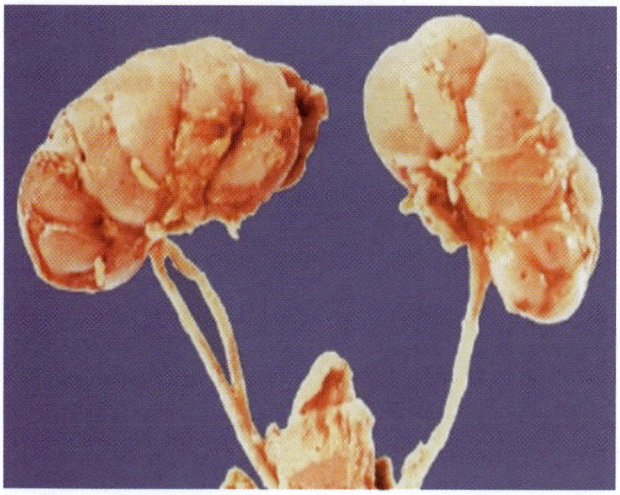

Fig. 25.1 Gross appearance of a bifid ureter. (*Source:* From Natalija Kovacevic, David A. Leavitt. Hydronephrosis. Elsevier 2022.)

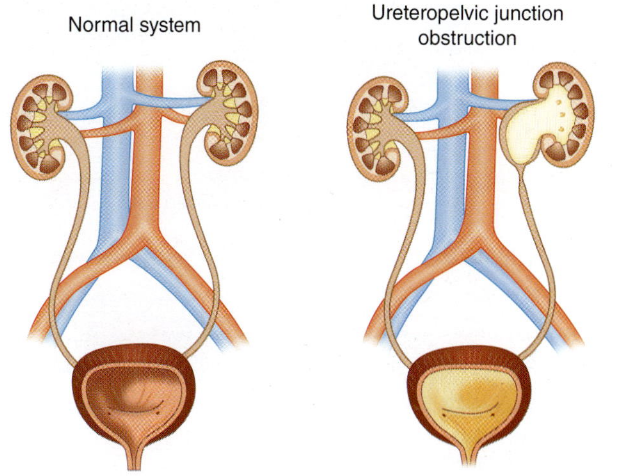

Fig. 25.2 Diagrammatic representation of ureteropelvic junction obstruction causing hydronephrosis on the left side.

drain through a single ureteric orifice. Bifid ureter is a relatively common incidental finding with no clinical significance.

Hydroureter: Dilation, elongation and tortuosity of the ureters can be congenital or acquired defects with an underlying neurogenic cause.

Ureteral agenesis: It is an extremely rare condition, occurring due to failure of development of the mesonephric diverticulum and is often associated with ipsilateral renal agenesis.

Ureteropelvic junction obstruction (Fig. 25.2): It is the most common cause of hydronephrosis in infants and children, with a slight male preponderance. Ureteropelvic junction obstruction usually presents unilaterally, although bilateral occurrences are not uncommon, accounting for 20% of the total cases. The underlying pathology has been ascribed to abnormal organization of smooth muscle bundles and excess deposition of stromal collagen between the smooth muscle bundles or can also be due to congenital extrinsic compression of the ureteropelvic junction by the renal vessels.

URINARY BLADDER

Vesicoureteral reflux (Fig. 25.3): It is defined as the retrograde regurgitation of urine from the urinary bladder up through the ureters into the kidney. It is the most common congenital anomaly, contributing to about 30% of the total cases of congenital urogenital anomalies. Long-standing vesicoureteral reflux often leads to recurrent renal infections and chronic pyelonephritis.

Diverticula (Fig. 25.4): These are pouch-like evaginations of the bladder wall, ranging from 1 to 10 cm in length. Diverticula can be congenital or acquired on the basis of the underlying aetiopathogenesis. Congenital diverticula occur due to failure of muscle development or bladder

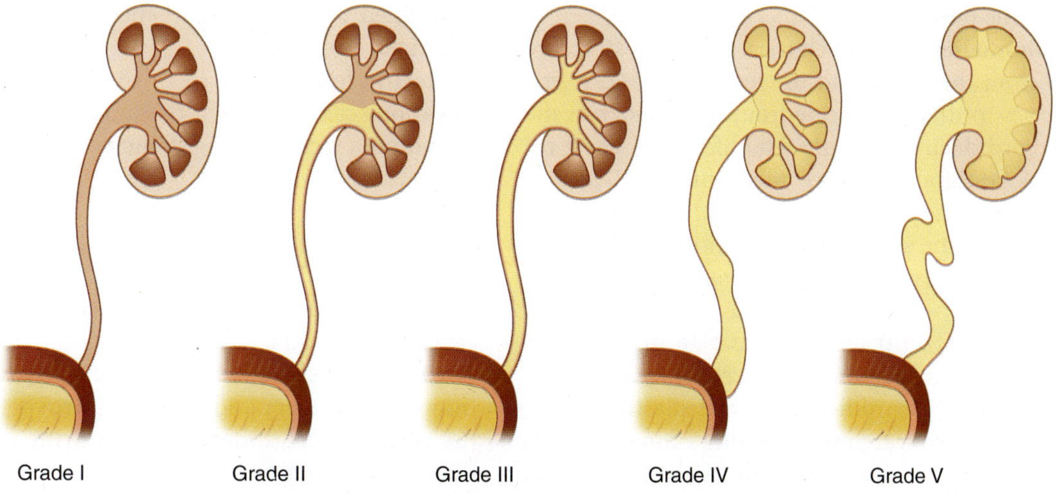

Fig. 25.3 Picture depicting the retrograde flow of urine in vesicoureteral reflux.

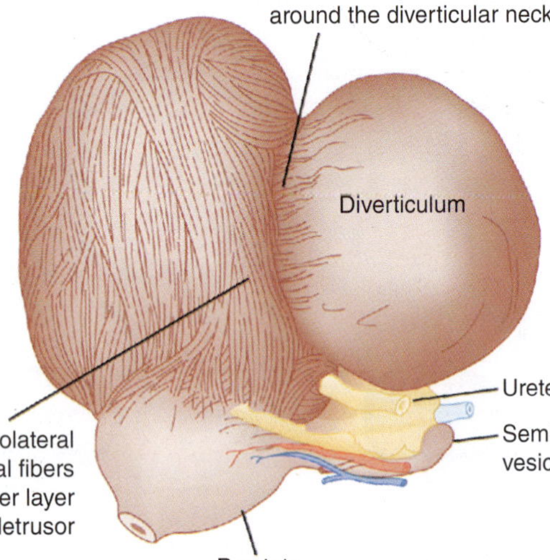

Fig. 25.4 Diagrammatic representation of bladder diverticulum. (*Source:* https://abdominalkey.com/bladder-and-female-urethral-diverticula/#s0010.)

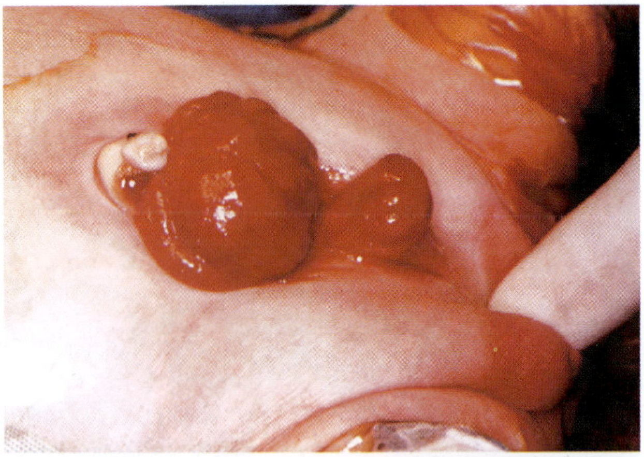

Fig. 25.5 Clinical picture of exstrophy of bladder. (*Source:* From George Jabboure Netto and Mahul B. Amin. The Lower Urinary Tract and Male Genital System. Robbins & Cotran Pathologic Basis of Disease. 10th edition. Elsevier 2021.)

outlet obstruction. Acquired diverticula are commonly associated with prostatic enlargement causing **urinary outflow obstruction** and marked bladder muscle hypertrophy. Diverticula are usually small and asymptomatic but occasionally may provoke clinical signs in response to urinary stasis, persistent infections, formation of calculi and vesicoureteric reflux due to their impingement on the ureter. They may rarely also give rise to urothelial carcinomas, which present only in advanced stage due to the poorly formed delicate muscular wall of the diverticulum.
Exstrophy of the bladder (Fig. 25.5): It is a developmental anomaly in which the **bladder mucosa is exposed to the exterior** through a defect in the anterior abdominal wall. The exposed mucosa of the bladder may undergo colonic glandular metaplasia or squamous metaplasia, which in due course can manifest in malignancies like squamous cell carcinoma, adenocarcinoma and rarely urothelial carcinoma. The bladder remnant is also at a higher risk for contracting **recurrent infections**, which can gradually ascend through the urinary tract and manifest in chronic pyelonephritis.
Urachal anomalies: The urachus is a tubular structure that runs from the bladder to the umbilicus, and it primarily serves to drain the urine from the bladder to the umbilical cord during the early fetal life. Later on, it remains as a **vestigial structure** measuring 3–10 cm in length, located in the preperitoneal pyramidal area formed by the bladder dome and obliterated umbilical arteries. It is usually obliterated after birth but, in rare instances, may remain patent anywhere in its course, manifesting in a fistulous urinary tract/patent urachus as a urachal cyst, umbilical sinus or vesicourachal diverticulum. The urachal cysts are lined by urothelium or metaplastic glandular epithelium. Adenocarcinomas arising from such cysts are not uncommon, accounting for 0.1%–0.3% of all bladder malignancies.

URETHRA

Rare congenital anomalies of the urethra include posterior urethral valves, congenital urethral stricture, megalourethra, urethral duplication, hypospadias, epispadias, anterior urethral valves and diverticula. A few of these conditions like epispadias and hypospadias are discussed under penis.

DISEASES OF THE URETERS

INFLAMMATION

Inflammation of the ureters is rarely associated with infections and is of limited clinical significance. It is of the following subtypes on the basis of the histomorphology:
Ureteritis cystica: Owing to chronic irritation, infections or inflammatory conditions, the mucosa of the ureters shows cysts of varying sizes, ranging from 1 to 5 mm, lined by normal urothelium and containing clear contents.
Ureteritis follicularis: In this condition, fine granular elevations can be seen in the mucosa due to aggregates of lymphocytes forming follicles in the subepithelial region.

OBSTRUCTIVE LESIONS OF URETER

Ureteric obstruction can be due to intrinsic or extrinsic causes (Table 25.1).

Ureteric obstruction manifests as **hydroureter** (dilation of the ureter) and **hydronephrosis** (distension of the renal calyces and pelvis with urine due to urinary outflow obstruction distal to the renal pelvis) and subsequently may lead to **pyelonephritis** on the basis of

Table 25.1 Causes of Ureteric Obstruction

Intrinsic Causes	Extrinsic Causes
Calculi: Renal in origin, usually small calculi (<5 mm) get impacted at any of the three anatomical sites of ureteral constriction	**Pregnancy:** Owing to relaxation of smooth muscles or pressure on ureters at pelvic brim due to the enlarging fundus
Strictures: Congenital/acquired	**Endometriosis:** As in the case of pelvic lesions associated with scarring
Blood clots: Massive haematuria due to renal calculi, tumours or papillary necrosis	**Tumours:** Carcinomas of the rectum, bladder, prostate, ovaries, uterus and cervix; lymphomas and sarcomas
Tumours: Urothelial carcinomas arising in ureters or benign tumours like papilloma/fibroepithelial polyps	**Periureteral inflammation:** Owing to salpingitis, diverticulitis, peritonitis or sclerosing retroperitoneal fibrosis
Neurogenic: Interruption of neural pathways to the bladder	

the duration and severity of obstruction. Unilateral obstruction occurs more likely due to conditions involving the proximal ureter, whereas bilateral obstruction is due to distal causes like nodular hyperplasia of the prostate.

Of all the causes, **sclerosing retroperitoneal fibrosis** requires special mention due to its association with group of **'IgG4-related diseases'**. Sclerosing retroperitoneal fibrosis is more common in males than in females, and it causes ureteral stenosis or obstruction. It is characterized by a proliferative inflammatory process with fibrosis, encasing the retroperitoneal structures, and manifests as **hydronephrosis**. The other organs involved in this disorder include the pancreas and salivary glands. Microscopic examination of the affected organ shows fibrous tissue with prominent lymphoid infiltrate, often with germinal centres, plasma cells producing IgG4 antibodies and eosinophils. Treatment primarily involves corticosteroids, but patients may eventually require ureteral stenting or ureterolysis due to the development of steroid resistance.

TUMOURS AND TUMOUR-LIKE CONDITIONS OF THE URETER

Primary ureteric tumours are rare and are classified into benign and malignant neoplasms. Benign tumours are usually small and are of mesenchymal in origin.

Fibroepithelial polyp is a tumour-like condition that presents as a small mass projecting into the lumen of the ureter, commonly in children. The polyp is primarily composed of loose vascularized connective tissue with an overlying normal urothelium.

Malignant tumours of the ureter are usually uncommon, affecting elderly individuals in their sixth or seventh decade of life. Uretic tumours are histologically being urothelial carcinomas in the majority of cases, similar to those arising from the renal pelvis and the bladder. These urothelial carcinomas of the ureter are at times multifocal or can occur concurrently with those of the urinary bladder or renal pelvis.

DISEASES OF THE URINARY BLADDER

INFLAMMATION (CYSTITIS)

Acute and chronic cystitis: Infections in the urinary bladder are commonly of bacterial origin; in untreated cases that lack timely intervention, they may ascend the urinary tract and manifest in pyelonephritis. Some of the most common organisms causing cystitis include *Escherichia coli*, *Proteus*, *Klebsiella*, *Enterobacter*, *Mycobacterium tuberculosis*, *Candida albicans*, *Cryptococcus* in immunosuppressed individuals, *Schistosoma haematobium*, adenovirus, *Chlamydia* and *Mycoplasma*. The predisposing factors for recurrent infections include bladder calculi, diabetes mellitus, instrumentation, urinary stasis due to prostatic enlargement and existing immunocompromised state. Owing to shorter urethras, women are at a higher risk for developing cystitis than men.

Morphology

Microscopy

Cystitis may show many of the following microscopic forms on the basis of the aetiology:

Cystitis due to infections: It shows acute or chronic nonspecific inflammation, mostly with neutrophilic infiltrate within the mucosa.

Chronic cystitis: Owing to persistence of bacterial infections, it shows mononuclear inflammatory infiltrate in the mucosa.

Haemorrhagic cystitis: It shows ulcerated surface urothelium with congested vasculature and extensive haemorrhage in lamina propria. A variable amount of cytological atypia in the epithelium may be observed in patients receiving cytotoxic antitumour drugs like cyclophosphamide.

Follicular cystitis: It is not associated with infections but shows lymphoid follicles in the mucosa and muscularis layers.

Eosinophilic cystitis: It shows submucosal eosinophilic infiltrate that is typically nonspecific and subacute. An underlying systemic allergic disorder has to be ruled out.

Radiation cystitis: Owing to irradiation of the bladder, it shows haemorrhage with fibrin, haemosiderin pigment deposition, acute-on-chronic inflammatory infiltrate with submucosal oedema and vascular ectasia.

Clinical Symptoms Associated With Cystitis

The common presenting symptoms of cystitis include an increased frequency of micturition, lower abdominal pain and dysuria. The other less commonly encountered symptoms include urge to urinate even after completion of voiding, haematuria and a low-grade fever.

Special Forms of Chronic Cystitis

Interstitial Cystitis (Chronic Pelvic Pain Syndrome) Frequently seen in women, it presents with clinical symptoms of cystitis. Cystoscopy, after luminal distension, shows fissures and punctate haemorrhages in the mucosa, mimicking low-grade bladder tumours. Although the aetiology remains unknown and management is empirical, microscopic examination shows increased mast cells within the mucosa and transmural fibrosis in advanced cases.

Malakoplakia It is a distinctive disorder involving the urinary bladder and other sites like the lungs, bones, kidneys, colon, prostate and epididymis due to acquired defects in phagocytic function. Commonly, it follows chronic bacterial infection by organisms like ***E. coli or Proteus***, especially in immunocompromised individuals.

Morphology

Gross: The bladder mucosa typically shows soft, **yellowish**, slightly elevated plaques of 3–4 cm in diameter.
Microscopy: The lamina propria shows large **foamy macrophages** with abundant granular cytoplasm, admixed with a few multinucleate giant cells and lymphocytes. The characteristic findings include the presence of laminated mineralized concretions due to calcium deposition in the lysosomes of macrophages, known as **Michaelis–Gutmann bodies** (Figs 25.6 and 25.7).
Special stain for calcium: von Kossa stain stains calcium deposit in black colour.
Immunohistochemistry: CD68 helps to label the macrophages.

Polypoid Cystitis It occurs due to injury to the bladder mucosa, most commonly due to indwelling catheters. Owing to marked submucosal oedema, the urothelium is thrown into broad polypoidal projections lined by normal transitional cells.

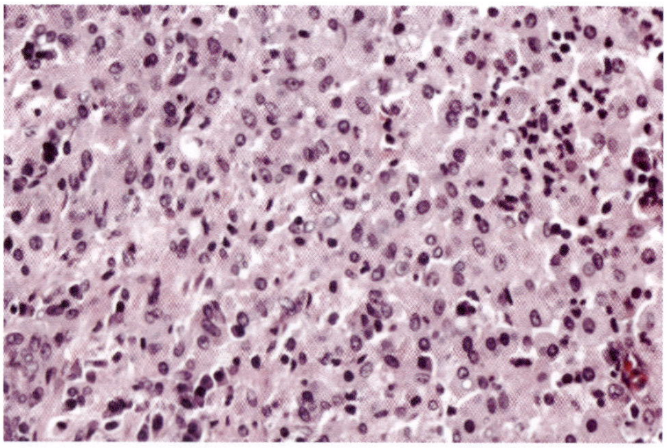

Fig. 25.6 Microscopy of malakoplakia of the urinary bladder – note the presence of sheets of macrophages. (*Source:* From Fang-Ming Deng and Jonathan Melamed. Nonneoplastic Diseases of the Urinary Bladder. Genitourinary Pathology: Foundations in Diagnostic Pathology. 2nd edition. Saunders 2015.)

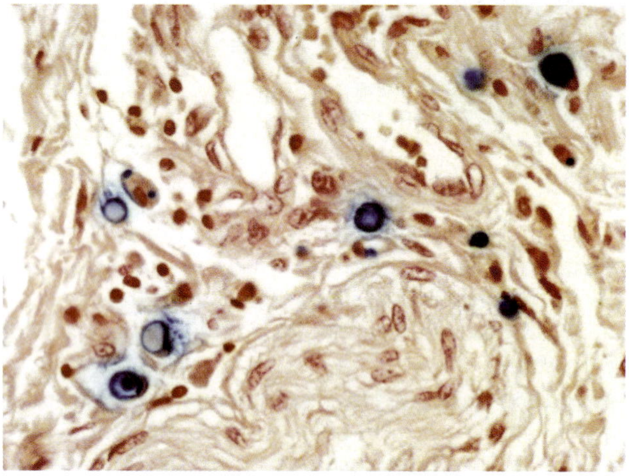

Fig. 25.7 Microscopy of malakoplakia – Perl's Prussian blue stain for iron highlighting the Michaelis–Gutmann bodies. (*Source:* From Fang-Ming Deng and Jonathan Melamed. Nonneoplastic Diseases of the Urinary Bladder. Genitourinary Pathology: Foundations in Diagnostic Pathology. 2nd edition. Saunders 2015.)

METAPLASTIC LESIONS OF THE URINARY BLADDER

Cystitis glandularis and cystitis cystica: These are common incidental lesions of the bladder in which the Von Brunn nests of urothelium grow inwards into the lamina propria. Either the epithelial cells in the centre of these nests undergo metaplastic change into cuboidal or columnar epithelium, which is referred to as **cystitis glandularis**, or the epithelium can retract in the centre, producing cyst-like spaces lined by flat urothelium, referred to as **cystitis cystica**. If these two changes coexist, the condition is called **cystitis cystica et glandularis.** In cystitis glandularis, the epithelium can occasionally show goblet cells, referred to as intestinal or colonic metaplasia.
Squamous metaplasia (Fig. 25.8): In response to chronic inflammation or injury, the urothelium gets replaced by stratified nonkeratinizing squamous epithelium because

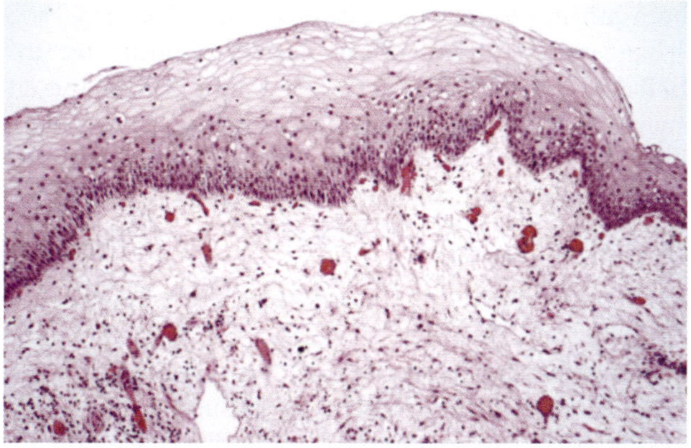

Fig. 25.8 Microscopy of squamous metaplasia in the urinary bladder. (*Source:* From Fang-Ming Deng and Jonathan Melamed. Nonneoplastic Diseases of the Urinary Bladder. Genitourinary Pathology: Foundations in Diagnostic Pathology. 2nd edition. Saunders 2015.)

the latter is more durable. Interestingly, glycogenated stratified squamous epithelium is a common finding at the trigone of the bladder in women of reproductive age. Trigonal squamous epithelium is a physiological variant occurring in response to hormonal stimuli unassociated with injury and should not be considered as a metaplastic change.

Nephrogenic adenoma: It is an uncommon lesion that occurs due to implantation of the shed renal tubular cells at the sites of discontinuous or injured urothelium. These lodged tubular cells are cuboidal and resume growth at the sites of injury in a papillary pattern. These lesions are usually small and can also infiltrate the underlying lamina propria and superficial detrusor muscle, mimicking malignancy.

OBSTRUCTIVE LESIONS

Similar to the ureter, obstruction of the urinary bladder outlet is of clinical significance due to its impact on the kidneys. Some of the common causes are given in Table 25.2 and Fig. 25.9.

Urinary bladder obstruction can be acute or chronic in onset. In cases of acute obstruction or in terminally ill patients with decreased micturition reflex mechanisms,

Table 25.2 Causes of Urinary Bladder Obstruction

- Nodular hyperplasia of the prostate in men
- Cystocoele of the bladder in women
- Urethral strictures – congenital/iatrogenic/inflammation induced
- Calculi
- Neurogenic bladder
- Tumours
- Blood clots
- Gravid uterus in pregnant women
- Foreign body in the urinary bladder
- Trauma with pelvic fracture

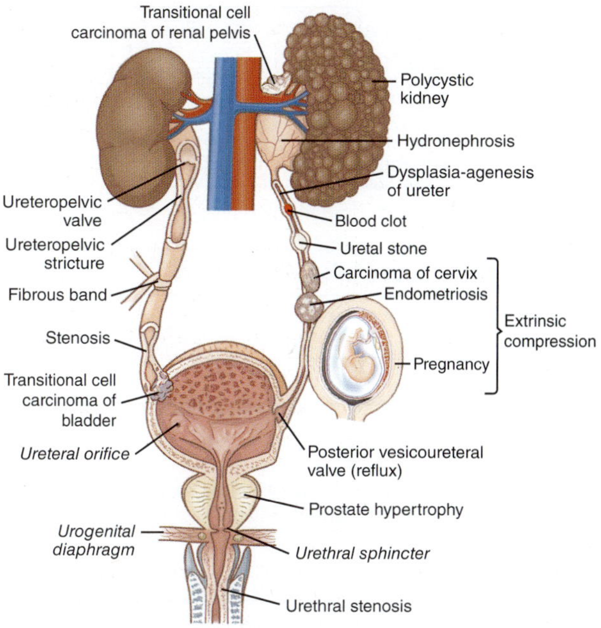

Fig. 25.9 Diagrammatic representation of lesions causing urinary tract obstruction. (*Source:* https://basicmedicalkey.com/wp-content/uploads/2016/09/B9780323088541000382_f38-01ab-9780323088541.jpg.)

Table 25.3 Common Mechanical Causes of Urinary Tract Obstruction

Ureter	Bladder Outlet	Urethra
Congenital		
Ureteropelvic junction narrowing or obstruction	Bladder neck obstruction	Posterior urethral valves
Ureterovesical junction narrowing or obstruction and reflux	Ureterocele	Anterior urethral valves
Ureterocele	Damage to S2–4	Stricture
Retrocaval ureter		Meatal stenosis
Vesicoureteral reflux (VUR)	VUR	Phimosis

the bladder may become extremely dilated, reaching up to the level of the pelvic brim or umbilicus, and the wall gets markedly thinned out with no trabeculations.

The common mechanical causes of urinary tract obstruction at all levels are listed in Table 25.3.

In chronic conditions, the bladder wall undergoes pathological changes gradually over a period of time and ultimately manifests in bilateral hydroureters and hydronephrosis if left untreated (Flowchart 25.1).

NEOPLASMS

Bladder tumours are the seventh most common tumours worldwide. As per the Indian Cancer Registry data, it is

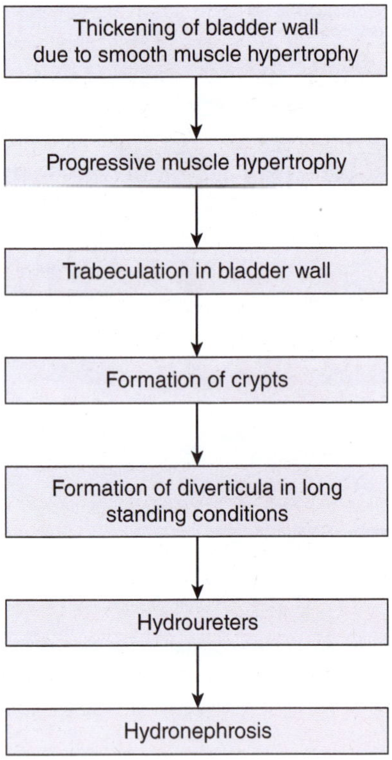

Flowchart 25.1 Series of events following the gradual onset of obstruction.

the ninth most common cancer accounting for 3.9% of all cancers. About **95% of the bladder tumours are urothelial in origin**, whereas the remaining 5% are mesenchymal in origin. These tumours may be located either in the upper urinary tract (renal pelvis and ureter) or in the lower urinary tract (bladder and proximal urethra).

Urothelial Tumours PA 28.16

Bladder urothelial tumours are more common, accounting for 90%–95% of the total cases, ranging from small benign lesions to aggressive multifocal carcinomas.

There exist two distinct precursor lesions that develop into invasive urothelial carcinomas, which include the more common **noninvasive papillary neoplasms** and the relatively less frequent **flat noninvasive urothelial carcinomas (carcinoma in situ [CIS])**. The WHO classification of urinary bladder tumours published in 2022 is given in Table 25.4.

Incidence and Aetiology Urothelial carcinomas show higher incidence rates in males than in females at a ratio of 3:1. These are more common in the elderly population with no significant familial transmission. Some of the important causative factors are as follows:

- **Cigarette smoking:** Smoking is the most important causative factor that increases the risk by three- to

Table 25.4 WHO Classification of Urinary Bladder Tumours (2022)

Histological Type	Benign Neoplasms	Noninvasive Neoplasms	Invasive Neoplasms
Urothelial tumours	Urothelial papilloma	Papillary urothelial neoplasm of low malignant potential (PUNLMP)	Infiltrating urothelial carcinoma (low grade/high grade)
	Inverted urothelial papilloma	Noninvasive papillary urothelial carcinoma, low grade Noninvasive papillary urothelial carcinoma, high grade Urothelial carcinoma in situ	
Squamous cell neoplasms	Squamous papilloma		Verrucous carcinoma Pure squamous cell carcinoma
Glandular neoplasms	Villous adenoma		Adenocarcinoma, NOS
Mesenchymal tumours	Leiomyoma		Leiomyosarcoma
	Haemangioma		Angiosarcoma
	Rhabdomyoma		Rhabdomyosarcoma
Rare malignant tumours	Urachal carcinoma, Diverticular carcinoma, Well-differentiated neuroendocrine tumour, small cell and large cell Carcinoma, malignant melanoma, lymphoma, Urethral accessory gland carcinoma, tumours of the Mullerian type		
Secondary tumours	From cervix, uterus, prostate and rectum		

(*Source:* WHO 2022 Update on the Classifications of Urinary Tract Neoplasms: George J. Netto. WHO Classification of the Urinary and Male Genital Tumours, 5th edition series, Page 5.)

sevenfold, depending on the duration and type of tobacco smoked. A majority of bladder carcinomas in men (50%–80%) are associated with the use of cigarettes. Cigars, pipes and smokeless tobacco are associated with a relatively smaller risk.

- **Industrial exposure to aryl amines:** Benzidine, 2-naphthylamine and related compounds are associated with an increased risk of developing bladder carcinomas. It usually manifests 15–40 years after the first exposure.
- **Drugs and dietary supplements:** Drugs like pioglitazone, used in the management of diabetes, and dietary supplements like aristolochic acid increase the risk of developing bladder tumours.
- ***S. haematobium infection:*** In endemic areas like Egypt and Sudan, it is an established risk. The ova of these trematodes are deposited in the bladder wall and incite a brisk chronic inflammatory response that induces progressive mucosal squamous metaplasia, dysplasia and rarely neoplasia. A majority of such neoplasms are squamous cell carcinomas, followed by urothelial carcinomas and adenocarcinomas.
- **Long-term exposure to analgesics and cyclophosphamide:** A prolonged exposure to analgesics manifests as analgesic nephropathy, whereas exposure to cyclophosphamide induces haemorrhagic cystitis and increases the risk of bladder carcinoma.
- **Irradiation:** Administered for pelvic malignancies, it increases the risk of urothelial carcinoma occurring several years after the initial exposure.

Pathogenesis Urothelial carcinomas are associated with several acquired genetic alterations (Table 25.5) that lead to the activation of growth factor receptor signalling pathways. Analysis of the genomes of precursor lesions and invasive urothelial carcinomas has shown two distinct molecular pathways of tumour progression (Fig. 25.10). The non-muscle-invasive papillary neoplasms often have gain-of-function mutations that increase signalling through growth factor receptor pathways, such as amplification of the FGFR3 tyrosine kinase receptor gene and activating mutations in the genes encoding RAS and PI3-kinase. These tumours have an increased tendency to recur but progression to muscle-invasive bladder carcinoma occurs in only about 20% of the cases. The majority of muscle-invasive bladder tumours develop by progression from 'flat' CIS. Although mutations that disrupt the function of p53 and RB genes are prevalent in all muscle-invasive cancers, these are observed much early in CIS than in noninvasive papillary neoplasms.

Morphology

Pathological features of some of the common urothelial tumours are described here.

Gross appearance

Urothelial tumours commonly present either as purely papillary neoplasms or as nodular/flat tumours arising commonly from the lateral or posterior wall of the bladder base. The papillary tumours range from 1 to 5 cm in diameter and at some instances may be multifocal.

Table 25.5 Genetic Alterations and Their Implications on Tumour Behaviour

Genetic Alterations Associated With Noninvasive Low-Grade Papillary Neoplasms	Genetic Alterations Associated With High-Grade Muscle Invasive Tumours
Gain-of-function mutation in FGFR3 Activating mutations in HRAS oncogene Loss of genetic material in chromosome 9	Loss-of-function mutation in TP53 and RB tumour suppressor genes

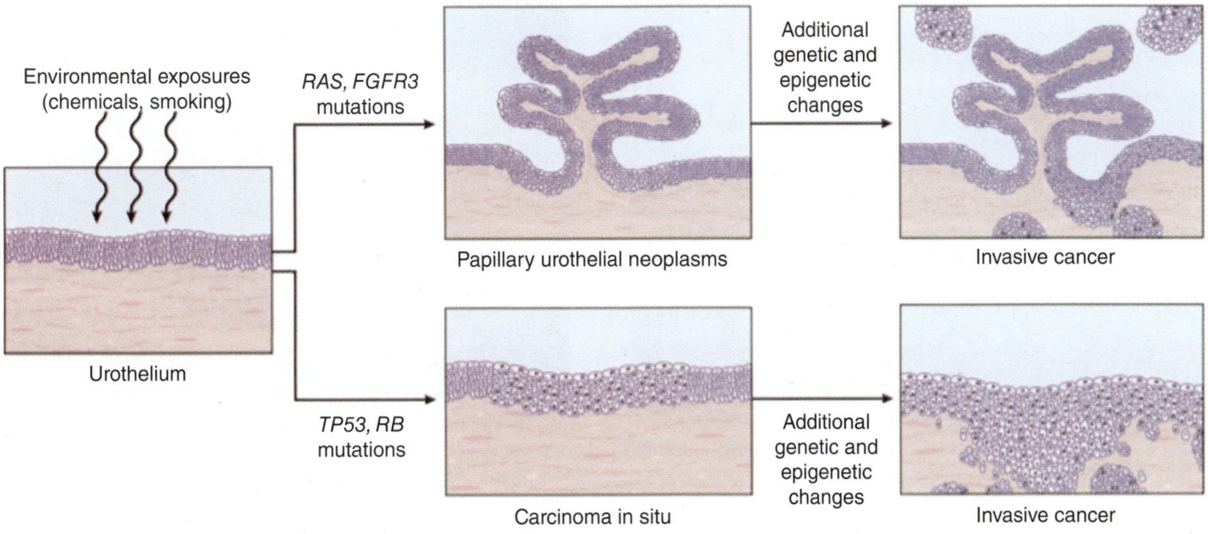

Fig. 25.10 Schematic picture of genetic alterations and their implications on tumour behaviour.

Urothelial papillomas

These are usually seen in young individuals as small delicate exophytic structures attached to the mucosa by a stalk. Microscopically, the individual finger-like papillae are lined by normal urothelium with central core of loose fibrovascular connective tissue. **Inverted papillomas** are those in which the growth extends downwards into the lamina propria as interanastomosing cords of cytologically bland urothelium (Fig. 25.11). Papillomas are generally benign lesions with rare instances of recurrence and progression.

Papillary urothelial neoplasm of low malignant potential (PUNLMP)

On cystoscopy, these tumours are larger than papillomas, mimicking low- or high-grade papillary carcinomas. These exhibit a histomorphology similar to that of papillomas but possess a **thicker urothelium**.

Low-grade noninvasive papillary urothelial carcinoma

These tumors have an orderly architectural appearance with mild loss of nuclear polarity and slight variation in nuclear size and shape. There are infrequent mitotic figures predominantly towards the base. These tumours have a tendency to recur and may also rarely invade but are not generally life-threatening.

High-grade noninvasive papillary urothelial carcinoma

These tumours show **architectural disarray and loss of polarity**. The individual cells contain pleomorphic hyperchromatic nuclei with several scattered mitotic figures, a few of them being atypical. On comparison with low-grade tumours, these tumours have a much higher incidence of progression to muscle-invasive bladder cancer and subsequent metastasis.

CIS

On cystoscopic examination, these lesions appear as areas of mucosal irregularity with hyperaemia or as areas of thickened wall without any evidence of intraluminal mass. These tumours are commonly multifocal and may extend to the ureters or urethra. The histomorphology of these tumours ranges from full-thickness dysplasia to scattered malignant cells exhibiting '**pagetoid**' spread within the urothelium. If unattended, 50%–75% of these tumours progress to invasive tumours.

Invasive urothelial carcinoma (Fig. 25.12)

Invasive urothelial carcinomas can be **low grade** or **high grade** on the basis of the cytomorphology and frequently exhibit squamous differentiation in variable proportions. A majority of these are high-grade tumours that show striking nuclear pleomorphism, hyperchromatic nuclei with irregular nuclear contours, sharp nuclear corners, numerous mitoses with atypical mitotic figures and moderate to abundant amount of cytoplasm (Fig. 25.13). The extent of invasion into the muscularis mucosae at the time of diagnosis determines the prognosis to a large extent. However, detrusor muscle invasion indicates a poor prognosis.

These tumours are well known for their morphological diversity, some of which include nested, large nested, microcystic, micropapillary, plasmacytoid, sarcomatoid, giant cell, lipid-rich and clear cell variants.

Immunohistochemical (IHC) markers for urothelial carcinoma

CK7, CK20, uroplakin, GATA3 and p63 are expected to be positive.

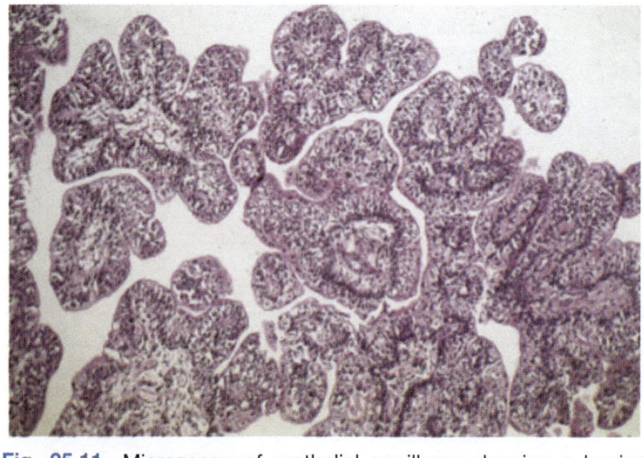

Fig. 25.11 Microscopy of urothelial papilloma showing a benign neoplasm composed of papillae lined by bland urothelium. (*Source:* From Christopher D.M. Fletcher. Tumours of the Urinary Tract. Diagnostic Histopathology of Tumours. 5th edition. Elsevier 2021.)

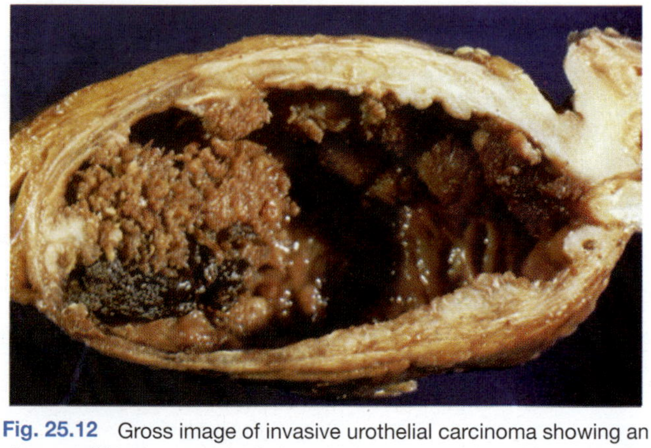

Fig. 25.12 Gross image of invasive urothelial carcinoma showing an ulceroproliferative, exophytic brownish tumour mass arising from the wall of the urinary bladder. (*Source:* From Christopher D.M. Fletcher. Tumours of the Urinary Tract. Diagnostic Histopathology of Tumours. 5th edition. Elsevier 2021.)

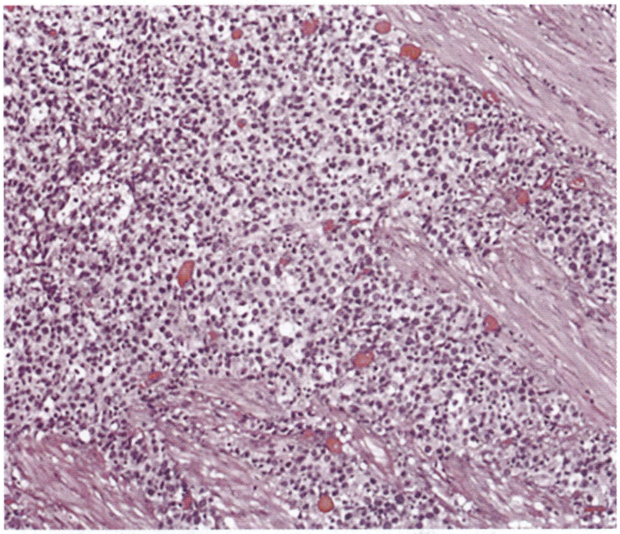

Fig. 25.13 Microscopy of invasive papillary urothelial carcinoma, high grade, showing pleomorphic tumour cells in sheets invading the muscularis mucosae. (*Source:* From Christopher D.M. Fletcher. Tumours of the Urinary Tract. Diagnostic Histopathology of Tumours. 5th edition. Elsevier 2021.)

Tumour progression and spread

The high-grade invasive tumours progressively invade the adjacent structures like the prostate, seminal vesicles, ureters, vagina, rectum and retroperitoneum. About 40% of these tumours metastasize to regional lymph nodes.

The extent of spread of these tumours at the time of diagnosis is the determining factor of the overall prognosis and hence staging of these tumours needs to be precise.

These tumours are further grouped under various categories on the basis of the tumour–node–metastasis (TNM) staging. The staging system and further stage grouping for urinary tract tumours arising from the renal pelvis and ureters and urethra in males and females are provided separately by WHO and American Joint Committee on Cancer (AJCC) (Table 25.6). These are suggested to be referred for further elaborate understanding.

Other Epithelial Tumours of the Bladder

Squamous cell carcinoma These account for 3%–7% of bladder tumours and are commonly associated with

Table 25.6 The TNM and AJCC Systems (2016) for Staging Bladder Tumours

Primary Tumour (T)	
Tx	Primary tumour cannot be assessed
T0	No evidence of primary tumour
Ta	Noninvasive papillary carcinoma
Tis	Carcinoma in situ: 'flat tumour'
T1	Tumour invades lamina propria
T2	Tumour invades muscularis propria
T2a	Tumour invades superficial muscularis propria (inner half)
T2b	Tumour invades deep muscularis propria (outer half)
T3	Tumour invades perivesical soft tissue
T3a	Microscopically
T3b	Macroscopically (extravesical mass)
T4	Tumour invades any of the following: prostate, uterus, vagina, pelvic wall, abdominal wall
T4a	Tumour invades the prostate, uterus or vagina
T4b	Tumour invades pelvic wall or abdominal wall
Regional Lymph Nodes (N)	
Nx	Regional lymph nodes cannot be assessed
N0	No regional lymph node metastasis
N1	Single regional lymph node metastasis in the true pelvis (perivesical, obturator, internal and external iliac or sacral lymph nodes)
N2	Multiple regional lymph node metastases in the true pelvis (perivesical, obturator, internal and external iliac or sacral lymph node metastasis)
N3	Lymph node metastasis to the common iliac lymph nodes

Continued

Table 25.6 The TNM and AJCC Systems (2016) for Staging Bladder Tumours—cont'd

Distant Metastasis (M)	
M0	No distant metastasis
M1	Distant metastasis
M1a	Distant metastasis limited to lymph nodes beyond the common iliac group of nodes
M1b	Non–lymph node distant metastases

AJCC, American Joint Committee on Cancer; TNM, tumour–node–metastasis.
(*Source: AJCC Cancer Staging Manual,* Eighth ed., Springer, New York, 2016.)

chronic irritation or infections like schistosomiasis. Mixed urothelial carcinomas with squamous differentiation are more common than pure squamous cell carcinomas of the bladder. These tumours are exophytic, fungating masses with surface ulceration. The extent of differentiation varies from well-differentiated keratinizing tumours to anaplastic forms with focal squamous differentiation.

Adenocarcinoma Primary adenocarcinomas of the bladder are rare and histologically similar to the adenocarcinomas occurring in other organs.

Clinical course These carcinomas present with symptoms of **painless haematuria** with an occasional increase in the frequency of micturition and dysuria. These tumours have a tendency to recur, with a higher histomorphological grade following excision of initial low-grade tumours. However, this depends on several variables like tumour size, grade, stage, unifocal or multifocal tumours, previous recurrence rates and presence of associated dysplasia or CIS in the adjacent mucosa.

Invasive urothelial carcinomas are associated with a 30% mortality rate once the tumour infiltrates lamina propria. In general, squamous cell carcinomas and adenocarcinomas of the bladder have a poorer prognosis than urothelial carcinomas. Early detection and adequate follow-up are the key for a better prognosis in these tumours.

Tumours detected at an early stage through cystoscopy and biopsy require subsequent follow-up and monitoring through repeated cystoscopy and cytological examination of urine. The **Paris system for urothelial neoplasia** is followed for cytological assessment of urine samples as a diagnostic tool and for routine follow-up of patients diagnosed with urothelial malignancies. The system is followed primarily to detect high-grade urothelial carcinoma by cytological examination of urine samples. Urine samples collected for cytological examination can also be used for detecting chromosomal abnormalities like aneuploidy of chromosomes 3, 7, 17 and 9p deletions by fluorescent in situ hybridization (FISH).

Management of bladder carcinomas depends largely on the clinical stage, grade and type of tumour. The treatment could be diagnostic **transurethral resection** for low-grade papillary tumours. Intravesical instillation of attenuated strain of ***Mycobacterium bovis* (BCG)** can be carried out in tumours exhibiting a higher tendency of recurrence such as high-grade noninvasive papillary tumours, noninvasive flat tumours with full-thickness dysplasia and multifocal tumours. The bacteria in BCG elicit local inflammatory reaction that aids in tumour destruction. **Radical cystectomy** is performed for tumours invading muscularis propria, CIS or high-grade papillary urothelial tumours resistant to BCG and CIS extending into prostatic urethra and ducts.

Malignant Mesenchymal Tumours (Sarcomas)

These rare tumours are large, fleshy, soft, grey-white and solid, protruding into the lumen and measuring around 10–15 cm in the greatest dimension. The most common sarcoma of the bladder in adults is **leiomyosarcoma**; in children or infants, it is embryonal rhabdomyosarcoma.

DISEASES OF THE URETHRA

INFLAMMATORY LESIONS

Urethritis is conventionally classified into **gonococcal and nongonococcal causes**. The organisms causing nongonococcal urethritis include *Chlamydia trachomatis* and *Mycoplasma*. In some instances, urethritis can be due to noninfectious agents as in reactive arthritis comprising a clinical triad of arthritis, conjunctivitis and urethritis.

Urethritis may be accompanied by cystitis in women and prostatitis in men. The pathological changes are similar to inflammation at other sites of the urinary tract. Urethritis itself is not a cause of clinical concern, but the subsequent implications on the kidneys require prompt attention.

TUMOURS AND TUMOUR-LIKE CONDITIONS

Urethral caruncle is an inflammation-induced tumour-like lesion which presents as a small reddish painful mass at the external urethral meatus of elderly women. It comprises inflammatory granulation tissue lined by friable but intact mucosa.

Benign tumours of the urethra include condylomas, inverted urothelial papilloma, squamous papillomas and urothelial papillomas.

Primary carcinomas of the urethra are rare; the tumours arising from the proximal urethra show urothelial differentiation and those from the distal urethra show squamous differentiation.

II. MALE GENITAL SYSTEM

The male genital system includes the penis, testis and epididymis, and prostate.

DEVELOPMENT, ANATOMY AND HISTOLOGY OF THE MALE GENITAL SYSTEM

DEVELOPMENT

The **external genitalia (penis)** develop from swellings that appear around the urogenital membrane.

The **testes** are derived from the coelomic epithelium covering the nephrogenic cord. Spermatozoa develop from primordial germ cells that arise in the region of the yolk sac. The **duct system** of the testis is derived from mesonephric tubules and the mesonephric duct.

The **prostate** develops embryologically from the buds arising from the caudal part of the vesicourethral canal and the pelvic part of the urogenital sinus

ANATOMY

The **penis** is the male sex organ and comprises the glans penis covered by prepuce, two columns of corpus cavernosum and a column of corpus spongiosum enclosing the penile urethra.

In the scrotum, the **testes** are paired organs, completely surrounded by double-layered tunica vaginalis – the outer parietal and the inner visceral layers. The visceral layer encloses the capsule of the testis, known as tunica albuginea. The tunica albuginea gives rise to numerous incomplete collagenous septae that divide the testis into about 250 testicular lobules. Within each lobule, there are one to four highly convoluted seminiferous tubules producing the spermatozoa. The seminiferous tubules converge upon the rete testis, from which 15–20 small ducts called the ductuli efferentes conduct spermatozoa to the extremely tortuous first part of the ductus deferens, which is the epididymis.

The adult **prostate gland** weighs about 10–15 g and is located at the neck of the urinary bladder in the pelvic cavity. The base of the prostate points superiorly towards the urinary bladder, and it encloses the prostatic urethra within. The prostate comprises five distinct lobes, which include an anterior lobe, a posterior lobe, a median lobe and two lateral lobes (Fig. 25.14). There is a partial capsule enclosing the posterior and lateral aspects of the prostate, but the anterior and apical surfaces are bounded by the anterior fibromuscular stroma. **McNeal's model** divides the gland into three zones, namely the central zone (base of the gland), peripheral zone (lateral aspect of the gland) and transition zone (periurethral region in the centre) for practical purposes.

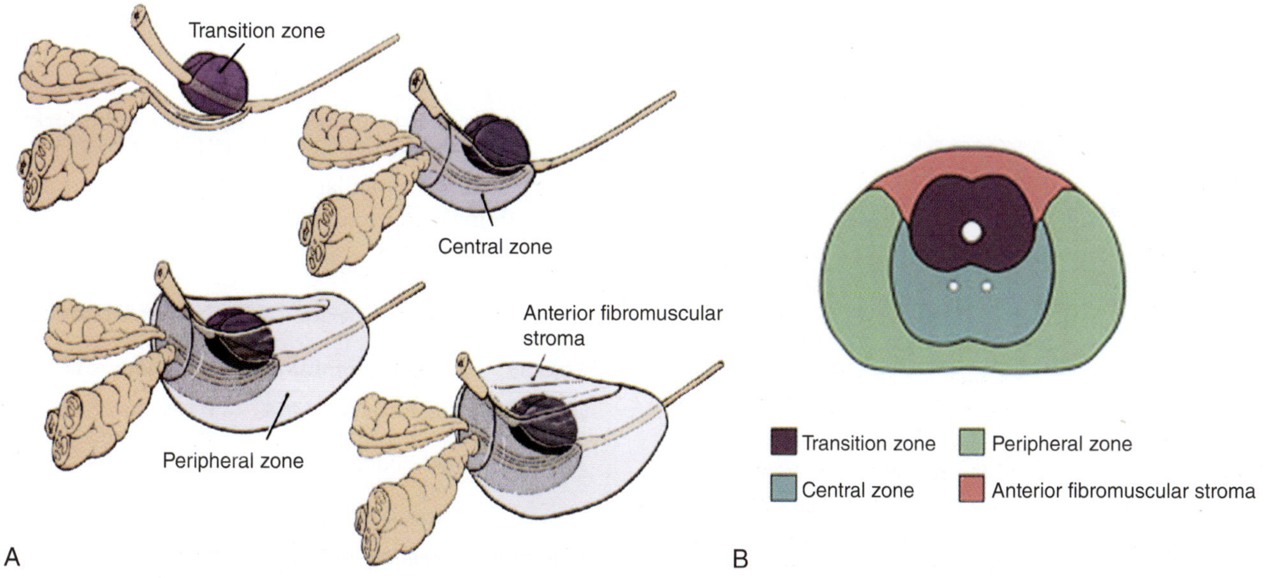

Fig. 25.14 Diagrammatic representation of zones of the prostate (A) and a cross-sectional representation (B). (*Source:* From Parviz K. Kavoussi. Surgical, Radiographic, and Endoscopic Anatomy of the Male Reproductive System. Campbell-Walsh-Wein Urology. 12th edition. Elsevier 2021; Joseph H. Yacoub and Aytekin Oto. MR Imaging of Prostate Zonal Anatomy. Radiologic Clinics of North America. 2018;56:197–209.)

HISTOLOGY

The **penis**, on cross-section, comprises three columns of erectile tissue – the two dorsal columns of corpora cavernosa and a single ventral column of corpora spongiosum through which the penile urethra runs. The penile urethra in adults is lined by columnar or pseudostratified columnar epithelium that gets gradually replaced by stratified nonkeratinizing squamous epithelium towards the tip of the penis.

The **testis** comprises convoluted seminiferous tubules demonstrating intraluminal spermatogenesis and spermiogenesis. The Sertoli cells can be seen within the tubules, amidst the germ cells. These Sertoli cells aid in nourishing the developing sperms and also secrete hormones like inhibin and anti-Müllerian hormone. The stroma interspersed between the seminiferous tubules is scant and contains Leydig cells that produce testosterone. The **epididymis** is a tubular structure lined by pseudostratified ciliated columnar epithelium and contains a thick muscularis layer. The final maturation of spermatozoa occurs in the epididymis.

The **prostate** consists of branched tubuloacinar glands embedded in a fibromuscular stroma. These tubuloacinar glands are lined by a bilayered epithelium that occasionally shows papillary invaginations (Fig. 25.15). The entire gland is divided into four unequal zones, namely the transition zone surrounding the prostatic urethra, the central zone surrounding the ejaculatory ducts, the peripheral zone accounting for 70% of the gland and the anterior fibromuscular stroma.

CONGENITAL ANOMALIES

PENIS

There are a few commonly encountered congenital anomalies of the penis.

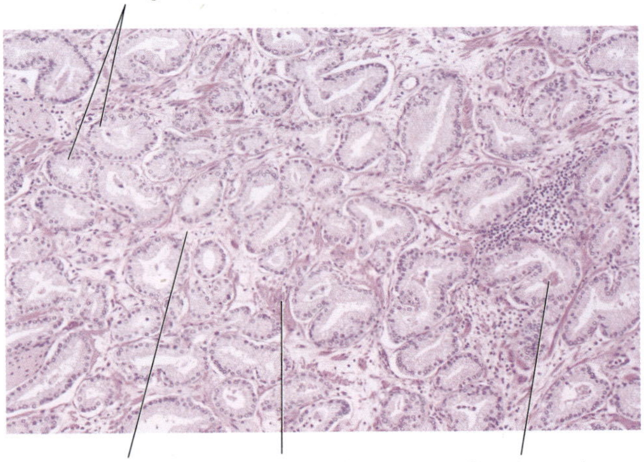

Fig. 25.15 The histology of the prostate gland.

Aphallia

Aphallia, also known as agenesis of the penis, is due to the failure of development of the genital tubercle during embryonic life.

Epispadias and Hypospadias

Hypospadias is the second most common congenital anomaly of male external genitalia, following cryptorchidism. In hypospadias, the urethra opens onto the **ventral surface of the penis** or scrotum. In epispadias, the urethra opens onto the **dorsal surface of the penis** and it is a relatively rare anomaly. These defects occur due to malformation of the urethral groove and the urethral canal. Epispadias and hypospadias draw clinical attention to consequences like ascending urinary tract infections due to a narrow orifice and infertility due to hampered physiological ejaculation and insemination.

Phimosis

The orifice of the prepuce is too small to permit normal retraction. Phimosis may present as a developmental anomaly or may result due to repeated infections causing scarring of the preputial ring. Consequently, persistent accumulation of secretions favours the development of infections and malignancy.

TESTIS AND EPIDIDYMIS

Congenital anomalies of the testis are extremely rare except for the undescended testes (**cryptorchidism**). The other rare anomalies include **anorchia** (absence of one or both testes) and **synorchism** (fusion of testes).

Cryptorchidism

It is defined as the complete or partial failure of the intra-abdominal testes to descend down into the scrotal sac. This condition is usually associated with testicular dysfunction and subsequent development of testicular malignancy. Cryptorchidism occurs in 1% of 1-year-old boys and may be accompanied by other genitourinary tract malformations like hypospadias (Table 25.7).

The phases of testicular descent are discussed briefly henceforth for better understanding.

Table 25.7 Phases of Testicular Descent

Phases	Transabdominal	Inguinoscrotal
Descent	The testis descends down from the mid-abdomen to the brim of the pelvis or lower abdomen	The testis descends through the inguinal canal into the scrotal sac
Hormone involved	Müllerian-inhibiting substance	Androgen-induced calcitonin gene–related peptide

Cryptorchidism is usually unilateral but can also be bilateral in 25% of the cases.

Morphology

Gross: The cryptorchid testis is small in size and firm in consistency due to the fibrotic changes.
Microscopy: Histological changes start by 2 years of age; tubular atrophy begins by 5–6 years of age and becomes advanced by puberty. It includes arrested germ cell maturation within the seminiferous tubules, dense hyalinization within the tubules and thickening of the basement membrane (Fig. 25.16). There is concomitant increase in interstitial stroma. Leydig cells appear prominent because these are spared. Germ cell neoplasia in situ (**GCNIS**) may be present in cryptorchid testes and can be a likely **precursor for subsequent germ cell tumours**.

Similar histological features may be seen in the contralateral testis in a patient with unilateral cryptorchidism, indicating that cryptorchidism is a marker of the underlying intrinsic defect in the development or functioning of the testis.

Clinical Features and Complications Cryptorchidism is usually asymptomatic, noticed only during clinical examination by the presence of an empty scrotal sac. The complications that the cryptorchid testis might be prone to include trauma, concomitant inguinal hernia and testicular carcinoma. Malignancy might also occur in the contralateral descended testis in unilateral cases, reinforcing the presence of a defective testicular development in association with malposition of the testis.

Management Orchiopexy is performed around 6–12 months of age, usually before the histological changes set in (by 2 years of age).

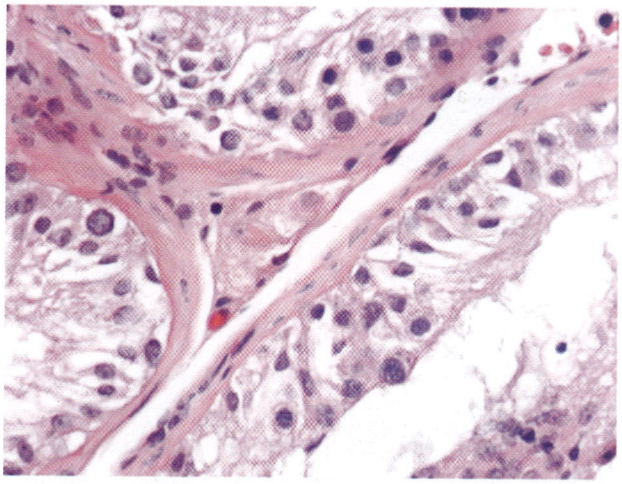

Fig. 25.16 Microscopy of the cryptorchid testis showing maturational arrest of spermatogonia. (*Source:* From Jesse K. McKenney. Testis and Testicular Adnexa. Rosai and Ackerman's Surgical Pathology. 11th edition. Elsevier 2018.)

PROSTATE

Congenital anomalies of the prostate are extremely rare and some of them include agenesis, hypoplasia, congenital prostatic cysts and ectopia. These are usually associated with underlying anomalies of other urogenital organs.

DISEASES OF THE PENIS

INFLAMMATORY LESIONS

Inflammation of the penis invariably involves the glans penis and the prepuce. The inciting agents may be specific organisms causing sexually transmitted diseases like syphilis, gonorrhoea, chancroid, granuloma inguinale and genital herpes (discussed in detail in Chapter 8) or may be nonspecific organisms like *C. albicans*, anaerobic bacteria, *Gardnerella* and pyogenic bacteria causing balanoposthitis. Most of these cases occur in uncircumscribed men with poor genital hygiene, leading to the accumulation of secretions, cellular debris, bacteria and sweat known as 'smegma'. The smegma acts as a local irritant and causes inflammatory scarring with subsequent phimosis.

TUMOURS

Tumours of the penis are generally rare, and the most common of these are carcinomas of the penis, followed by condyloma acuminatum. A few common benign lesions of the penis like condyloma acuminatum and Peyronie disease are explained briefly.

Condyloma Acuminatum

It is a benign wart caused by sexually transmitted **human papillomavirus (HPV)**. The strains of HPV associated with condyloma are type 6 and less commonly type 11 (discussed in greater detail in Chapter 26). These warts are seen on the perineum or external genitalia, mainly along the inner surface of prepuce and coronal sulcus (Fig. 25.17). Condylomas tend to recur but rarely undergo malignant transformation.

Morphology

Gross: It appears as single or multiple, tiny or large, pedunculated or sessile reddish papillary excrescences.
Microscopy: It shows hyperplastic papillary fronds lined by acanthotic stratified squamous epithelium with parakeratosis (Fig. 25.18). The epithelial cells show orderly maturation with no evidence of atypia or dysplasia. The characteristic feature of HPV infection to be noted is 'koilocytosis', seen as cytoplasmic vacuolation in mature squamous cells.

Peyronie Disease

Peyronie disease is a benign condition of unknown aetiology, resulting in the formation of fibrous bands in the

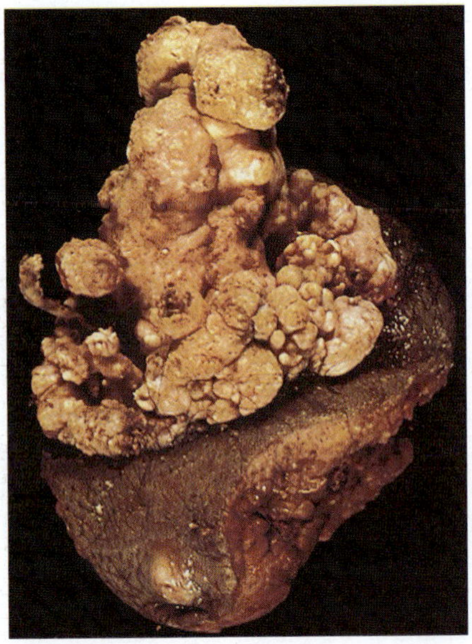

Fig. 25.17 Clinical picture of condyloma acuminatum showing an exophytic multinodular grey-brown tumour arising from the skin.

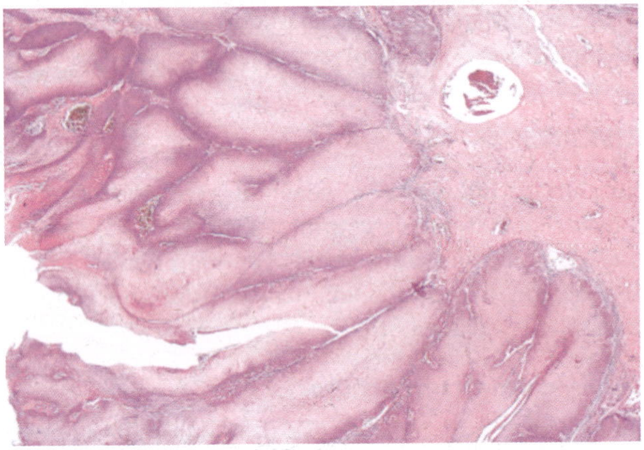

Fig. 25.18 Microscopy of condyloma acuminatum showing a hyperplastic papillary squamous epithelium with a noninvasive base. (*Source:* From Eduardo Calonje, Fiona Lewis, Chris Bunker, Diego Fernando Sánchez Martínez and Antonio L. Cubilla. Diseases of the anogenital skin. McKee's Pathology of the Skin. 5th edition. Elsevier 2020.)

corpus cavernosum of the penis. It leads to abnormal penile curvature and pain during intercourse.

Precursor Lesions and Invasive Malignancies

Penile carcinoma is an unusual malignancy with an incidence rate of 0.7–2.3 cases per 100,000 persons in India. Usually, squamous cell carcinomas are reported in a majority of cases. The precursor lesions for squamous cell carcinomas are described as penile intraepithelial neoplasia (PeIN) and exhibit features of intraepithelial squamous cell atypia.

Penile Intraepithelial Neoplasia Penile carcinomas show a bimodal pathway of carcinogenesis; hence, precursor lesions are broadly classified as follows:

- HPV related
- HPV unrelated

The term **PeIN** is the newer terminology to denote squamous intraepithelial lesion (SIL), which is also known as erythroplasia of Queyrat (lesion in the mucosal surface of the glans) and Bowen disease (lesion in the skin of the shaft of the penis). PeIN is further classified into two types:

- Differentiated/simplex (HPV unrelated)
- Undifferentiated (HPV related)

In the male external genitalia, two distinct pathological lesions display features of CIS, namely **Bowen disease** and **Bowenoid papulosis**. Both the conditions are strongly associated with infection by **high-risk HPV strain, type 16.**

Bowen Disease It is a premalignant condition involving the skin over the shaft of the penis and scrotum in men usually older than 35 years. The lesion grossly appears as a solitary thickened grey-white or velvety plaque (Fig. 25.19). Histological features include a hyperproliferative epidermis, with cells showing loss of polarity, dysplasia and occasional atypical mitotic figures (Fig. 25.20). The basement membrane at the dermoepidermal junction is intact with no evidence of infiltration of tumour cells. However, 10% of these patients can progress to develop squamous cell carcinoma after several years.

Bowenoid Papulosis It is also a premalignant condition but with almost negligible chances of progression to malignancy and with a tendency to regress spontaneously. The onset of Bowenoid papulosis is at a younger age than that in Bowen disease. These lesions are usually multiple, reddish brown and papular (Fig. 25.21). Microscopically, it is indistinguishable from Bowen disease.

Invasive Carcinoma PA 29.2 Squamous cell carcinomas of the penis are usually encountered in men aged 40–70 years,

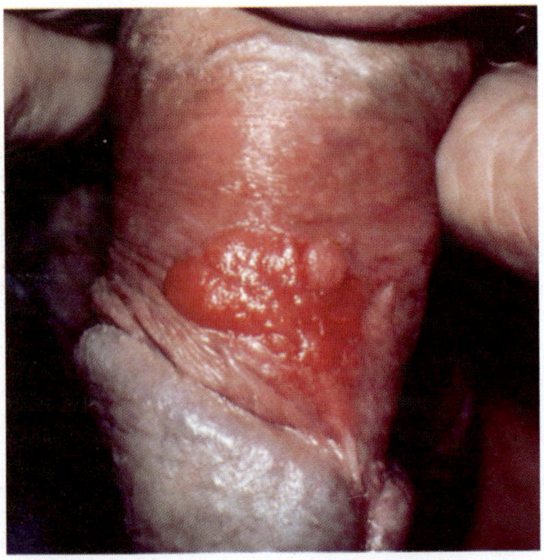

Fig. 25.19 Clinical picture of Bowen disease showing an erythematous flattened plaque involving the glans penis. (*Source:* From William D. James, Dirk M. Elston, James R. Treat, Misha A. Rosenbach and Isaac M. Neuhaus. Epidermal Nevi, Neoplasms, and Cysts. Andrews' Diseases of the Skin. 13th edition. Elsevier 2020.)

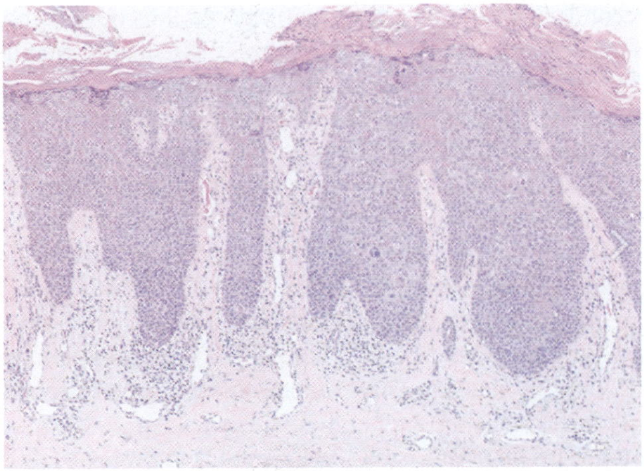

Fig. 25.20 Microscopy of Bowen disease showing epidermal hyperkeratosis and papillomatosis with full-thickness dysplasia. The papillary dermis shows mononuclear inflammatory cell infiltrate.

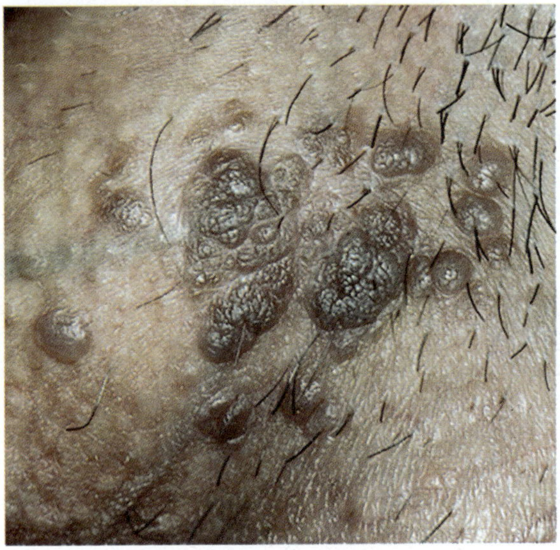

Fig. 25.21 Clinical picture of Bowenoid papulosis showing multiple elevated brownish papules on the skin.

accounting for 10%–20% of all malignancies in males. The common predisposing factors include poor genital hygiene and high-risk HPV infections, mainly type 16 and type 18. Cigarette smoking has also been associated with an increased risk of these tumours. Circumcision, which involves surgical removal of the foreskin, aids in maintaining good genital hygiene by limiting the accumulation of smegma and hence it serves as a protective measure in preventing carcinoma of the penis.

Presenting features: Penile tumours commonly present as discrete fungating exophytic masses or as an ulcer over the glans or prepuce. These are not usually associated with bleeding or pain, and patients may present with symptoms of urinary obstruction due to the tumour infiltrating the penile urethra.

Pathogenesis: There are two pathogenetic pathways associated with penile carcinomas, namely:

High-risk HPV-related pathogenesis: Disruption of RB protein/p16/p21 pathway (discussed in detail in Chapter 7) is observed similar to other HPV-related tumours of the cervix and head and neck carcinomas. In total, 30%–50% of these cases do not typically harbour TP53 mutation.

Non-HPV-related pathogenesis: It is further divided into two subgroups, one with TP53 mutation and the other with high chromosomal instability.

Classification of penile tumours on the basis of gross patterns of growth

- **Superficial spreading:** Tumours extend horizontally and are limited to the lamina propria or superficial corpus spongiosum only.
- **Vertical growth:** Tumours invade deeper structures by extending vertically and infiltrating the penile urethra. The surface of these tumours is usually ulcerated.
- **Verruciform:** These tumours are exophytic and papillomatous with variable extension into the deeper structures.
- **Multicentric tumours:** Two or more independent foci of carcinomas are noted.

Morphology

Gross: Penile tumours originate on the glans penis or along the inner surface of the prepuce, near the coronal sulcus. These may be **papillary or flat** tumours. The papillary tumours grow as exophytic fungating masses, whereas the flat lesions appear as areas of epithelial thickening with focal ulceration (Fig. 25.22).

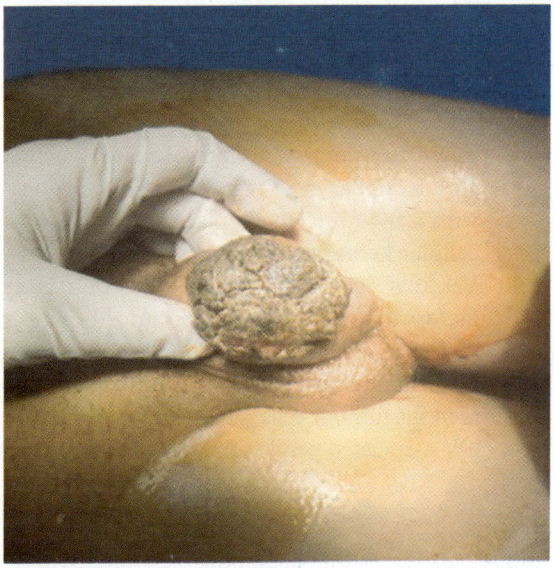

Fig. 25.22 Clinical picture of squamous cell carcinoma of the penis showing an exophytic grey-brown tumour mass with surface ulceration. (*Source:* From Yongrui Zhang, Runhui Tian, Zhanmeng zhu and Kaimin Guo. Giant squamous cell carcinoma of penis with rapid progression. Urology Case Reports. 2021;34:Article 101496.)

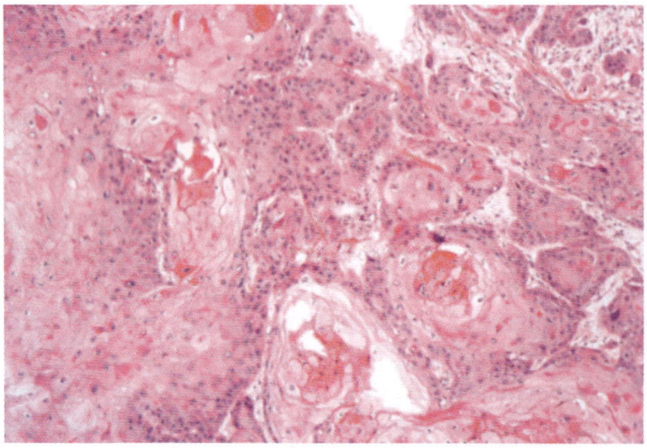

Fig. 25.23 Microscopy of squamous cell carcinoma of the penis showing tumour cells arranged in diffuse sheets and nests with prominent individual cell keratinization. (*Source:* From Eduardo Calonje, Fiona Lewis, Chris Bunker, Diego Fernando Sánchez Martínez and Antonio L. Cubilla. Diseases of the anogenital skin. McKee's Pathology of the Skin. 5th edition. Elsevier 2020.)

Microscopy: Both the papillary and flat tumours are squamous cell carcinomas demonstrating various degrees of differentiation, explained as follows (Fig. 25.23):

Well-differentiated squamous cell carcinoma (grade 1)

These tumours show malignant cells arranged in sheets with slightly enlarged nuclei and with abundant eosinophilic cytoplasm. Prominent intercellular bridges and individual cell keratinization can be observed.

Moderately differentiated squamous cell carcinoma (grade 2)

These tumours show more disorganized growth, comprising cells with high nucleocytoplasmic ratio, less evident individual cell keratinization and increased mitotic activity.

Poorly differentiated squamous cell carcinoma (grade 3)

These tumours show foci of solid sheets, nests and irregular aggregates of pleomorphic cells with a high nucleocytoplasmic ratio, no definite cellular keratinization and numerous mitoses.

Vascular invasion of tumour emboli is a vital factor that governs the prognosis and hence demands a careful search in all tumours.

Immunohistochemistry: IHC marker p53 is diffusely positive in the tumour cells. p16 positivity indicates high-risk HPV-associated penile squamous cell carcinomas.

Tumour progression: Squamous cell carcinomas of the penis are usually slow growing, although those arising within the glans, prepuce or coronal sulcus often spread early to the underlying structures like Buck's fascia. These carcinomas are usually painless until they undergo secondary ulceration with superimposed infection. Pathological assessment of these tumours is essential in staging the tumours according to their microscopic extent and depth of invasion. Nodal metastasis is very rare in tumours that invade only the lamina propria, whereas it is relatively common in the tumours that have invaded the urethra. Clinical assessment of regional lymph node involvement is inaccurate, because only 50% of enlarged inguinal nodes in patients with penile squamous cell carcinoma contain metastatic tumour deposit, with the rest showing only reactive lymphoid hyperplasia. Hence, pathological assessment of lymph nodes suggestive of harbouring tumour deposits becomes crucial in staging these tumours.

Staging: The penile carcinomas are staged on the basis of the extent of invasion of the tumour into the underlying structures with or without associated lymphovascular and perineural invasion. The lymph nodal spread is categorized on the basis of the number of ipsilateral or bilateral inguinal lymph nodes with metastatic deposits and presence of extranodal extension.

Treatment and prognosis: Carcinoma of the penis can be treated by local resection or partial/total penectomy, according to the size, location and histopathological type of the tumour. Local recurrence is extremely rare if the surgical margins are negative. Controversy still exists in the role of elective inguinal lymphadenectomy. Radiation therapy for penile tumours is contraindicated due to their high tendency of anaplastic transformation. The overall 5- and 10-year survival rates for squamous cell carcinoma of the penis are 77% and 71%, respectively. The prognosis depends on the following factors:

- **Tumour stage:** Higher the stage, poorer is the prognosis.
- **Microscopic type:** Verrucous and warty carcinomas have a better prognosis than basaloid or sarcomatoid carcinomas.
- **Microscopic grade:** Higher the grade, poorer is the prognosis.
- **Vascular invasion:** If present, it indicates a poor prognosis.
- **Marker p53 expression:** Overexpression is significantly associated with lymph node metastasis and hence a poorer prognosis.

Verrucous Carcinoma (Ackerman Tumour) Verrucous carcinoma is an exophytic variant of squamous cell carcinoma that is locally invasive, very well differentiated and very rarely metastasizing. It accounts for 2%–3% of penile squamous cell carcinomas.

Clinical features: These are long-standing tumours seen in the elderly population in their sixth or seventh decade of life and carry an excellent prognosis.

Morphology

Gross (Fig. 25.24): The tumour is an exophytic, papillomatous, grey-white irregular mass. The surface varies

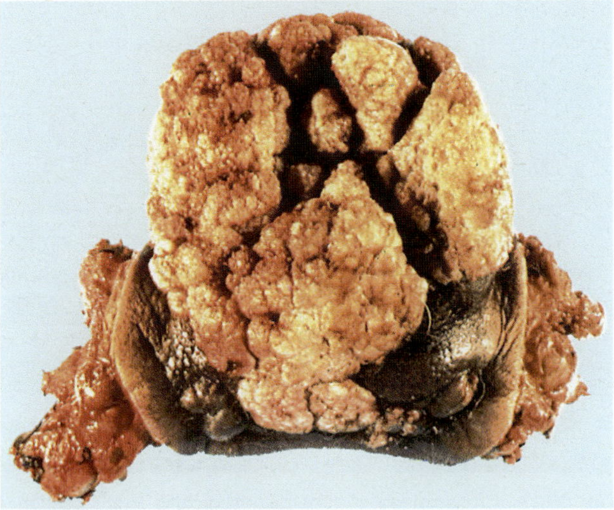

Fig. 25.24 Gross morphology of verrucous carcinoma of the penis – note that the large destructive, cauliflower-like mass has extensively replaced the penis. (*Source:* Courtesy of AFIP and PathologyOutlines.com, https://www.pathologyoutlines.com/topic/penscrotumpenisverr.html.)

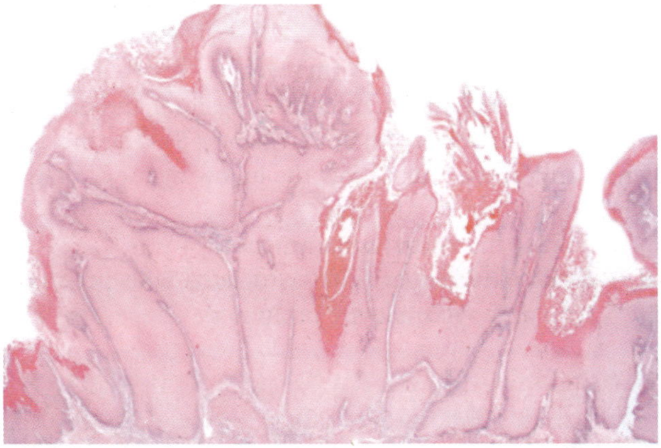

Fig. 25.25 Microscopy of verrucous carcinoma of the penis showing a cauliflower-like exophytic grey-white lesion arising from the skin over the glans penis. (*Source:* From Eduardo Calonje, Fiona Lewis, Chris Bunker, Diego Fernando Sánchez Martínez and Antonio L. Cubilla. Diseases of the anogenital skin. McKee's Pathology of the Skin. 5th edition. Elsevier 2020.)

from being fungating to macronodular. The cut surface shows serrated, papillary, grey-white appearance.
Microscopy (Fig. 25.25): Verrucous carcinoma is well-differentiated squamous cell carcinoma with a sharp delineation at the tumour–stromal junction. There is hyperorthokeratosis, papillomatosis and acanthosis. The tumour is broad based and pushes rather than infiltrates the subepithelial tissue. The nuclei are bland. Slight atypia may be seen at the basal cell layer.

DISEASES OF THE TESTIS AND EPIDIDYMIS

Distinct pathological conditions can be seen in the testis, of which tumours carry the utmost importance, followed by inflammatory conditions, testicular torsion and testicular atrophy.

TESTICULAR ATROPHY

Some causes of testicular atrophy are listed in Table 25.8.

Morphology (Fig. 25.26)

Gross: The testis is symmetrically small in size and firm in consistency.

Table 25.8 Causes of Testicular Atrophy

- Progressive atherosclerotic narrowing of blood vessels in elderly patients
- Chronic inflammatory orchitis
- Cryptorchidism
- Chronic malnutrition
- Irradiation
- Prolonged exposure to antiandrogens in the management of prostatic carcinoma
- Hypopituitarism
- Klinefelter syndrome

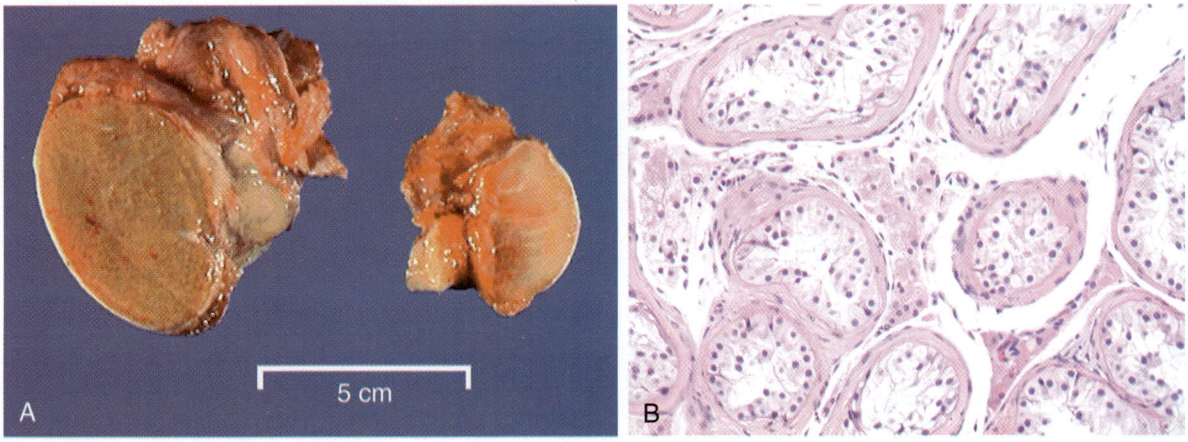

Fig. 25.26 (A) Gross image of the atrophic testis on the right side in comparison with the normal testis on the left. (B) Microscopy of the atrophic testis – note the presence of seminiferous tubules with Sertoli cells and the absence of spermatogenesis. In addition, note the presence of Leydig cell hyperplasia. (*Source:* From Edward C. Klatt. The Male Genital Tract. Robbins and Cotran Atlas of Pathology. 4th edition. Elsevier 2021.)

Microscopy: The testicular parenchyma shows arrested germ cell maturation within the seminiferous tubules, presence of dense hyalinization and thickening of the basement membrane. There is abundant interstitial stroma with prominent Leydig cells.

INFLAMMATORY LESIONS

These lesions of the testis and epididymis are further subdivided into nonspecific and specific inflammation on the basis of the aetiology.

Nonspecific Epididymitis and Orchitis

Epididymitis and subsequent orchitis commonly follow infections of the urinary tract, either through the vas deferens or through the lymphatics of the spermatic cord. The cause of epididymitis varies with age and can be classified as shown in Table 25.9.

Granulomatous Orchitis

Idiopathic granulomatous orchitis is seen in middle-aged men. It presents acutely as a tender testicular mass associated sometimes with fever. Histologically, it comprises granulomas restricted only to seminiferous tubules of the testis (Figs 25.27).

Specific Inflammation

The three specific inflammatory lesions of the testis and epididymis include gonorrhoea, tuberculosis and syphilis, of which the former two involve the epididymis first, whereas syphilis involves the testis first, followed by rest of the sites.

Gonorrhoea: This bacterial infection extends retrograde through the posterior urethra to the prostate, seminal vesicles, epididymis and testis. It can cause extensive destruction of the parenchyma, leading to abscess formation.
Mumps: Being a systemic viral infection, it may cause acute interstitial orchitis in 20%–30% of the infected postpubertal males.

Table 25.9 Causes of Epididymitis

	Age Group		
	Children	Younger Than 35 Years	Older Than 35 Years
Aetiology	Congenital genitourinary abnormality	Sexually transmitted infections	Common urinary tract pathogens
Organisms involved	Gram-negative rods	*Chlamydia trachomatis, Neisseria gonorrhoeae*	*Escherichia coli, Pseudomonas*

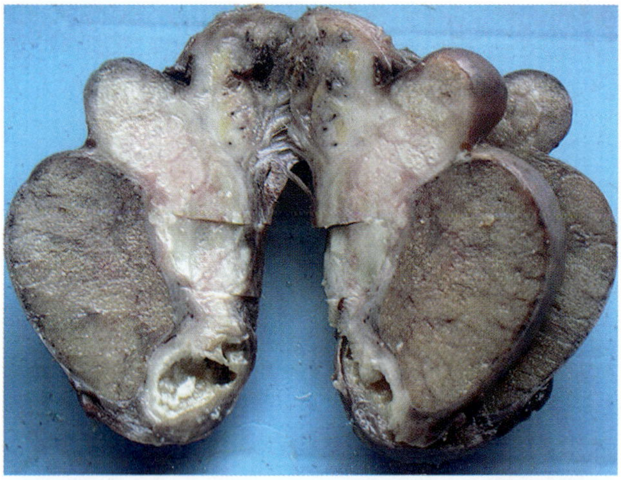

Fig. 25.27 Gross image of tuberculous orchitis – cut section of the orchidectomy specimen showing a lesion in the epididymis with fibrosis and caseous necrosis.

Tuberculosis: It begins at the epididymis and extends to the testis, producing caseating granulomatous inflammation.
Syphilis: It almost always involves the testis, and occasionally the epididymis, in both congenital and acquired syphilis (discussed in detail in Chapter 8). The morphological appearance may show the following:

(1) Production of gummas
(2) Diffuse interstitial inflammation
(3) Obliterative endarteritis associated with perivascular lymphoplasmacytic infiltrates

TESTICULAR TUMOURS PA 29.1

Testicular tumours are rare tumours with an incidence rate of less than 1 per 100,000 men in the Indian subcontinent and account for 1%–2% of all neoplasms in men globally. These are broadly classified into **germ cell tumours** and **sex cord–stromal tumours.** Germ cell tumours account for 95% of all testicular tumours, whereas 5% of cases are contributed by the sex cord–stromal tumours. The testicular tumours and their subcategories are listed in Table 25.10.

Germ Cell Tumours

These are aggressive tumours with a higher tendency to disseminate rapidly, whereas sex cord–stromal tumours are generally benign. Germ cell tumours are commonly seen in young individuals between 15 and 35 years of age. These are further subclassified into **seminoma** and **nonseminomatous tumours** (Table 25.11).

Predisposing factors: Both genetic and environment factors are found to play a crucial role in the pathogenesis of testicular tumours.
Environmental factors: Testicular germ cell tumours are associated with a spectrum of disorders known as

Table 25.10 Testicular Tumor Classification

Germ cell tumours derived from germ cell neoplasia *in situ*
- Noninvasive germ cell neoplasia
  - Germ cell neoplasia *in situ*
  - Gonadoblastoma
- Germinoma family of tumours
  - Seminoma
- Nonseminomatous germ cell tumours
  - Embryonal carcinoma
  - Yolk sac tumour, postpubertal-type
  - Choriocarcinoma
  - Teratoma, postpubertal type
  - Teratoma with somatic-type malignancy
  - Mixed germ cell tumours of the testis

Germ cell tumours unrelated to germ cell neoplasia *in situ*
- Spermatocytic tumour
- Teratoma, prepubertal type
- Yolk sac tumour, prepubertal type

Sex cord stromal tumours of testis
- Leydig cell tumour
- Sertoli cell tumours
- Granulosa cell tumours

Germ cell tumours in fibroma the coma group
- Mixed and other sex cord stromal tumours

Other tumours
- Testicular lymphoma

(*Source:* WHO Classification 2022.)

Table 25.11 Differences Between Seminoma and Nonseminomatous Germ Cell Tumours

Features	Seminoma	Nonseminomatous GCT
Clinical stage at presentation	Commonly in stage I	Commonly in stage II or III
Tumour behaviour	Grow slowly, hence remain confined to the testis for a longer duration	Grow rapidly, hence spread to distant sites occurs very early in the course of the disease
Route of metastatic spread	Lymphatic dissemination involving the iliac and para-aortic lymph nodes	Haematogenous dissemination, involving the lungs and liver and lymphatic route
Management	Radiotherapy is the preferred choice	Chemotherapy and surgery are preferred because they are less radiosensitive
Prognosis	Usually good	Poor

GCT, germ cell tumour.

'testicular dysgenesis syndrome' (TDS), the components of which include cryptorchidism, hypospadias and poor sperm quality. It has been observed that these conditions are more pronounced in individuals who were exposed to pesticides and nonsteroidal oestrogens in utero. The most common association however is with cryptorchidism, which is seen in approximately 10% of testicular germ cell tumours.

Genetic factors: There is a strong familial predisposition associated with the development of testicular germ cell tumours. The relative risk of these tumours is 4 times higher than normal in fathers and sons of affected patients and is 8–10 times higher in brothers. There are several genetic loci linked to an increased familial germ cell tumour risk, some of which are the genes encoding the ligand for the receptor tyrosine kinase KIT and BAK.

Differentiation in germ cell tumours: The seminomatous tumours are composed of cells that resemble primordial germ cells. The nonseminomatous tumours are composed of undifferentiated cells that resemble embryonic stem cells, as seen in embryonal carcinoma, and can also differentiate along other cell lineages, giving rise to yolk sac tumours, choriocarcinomas and teratomas.

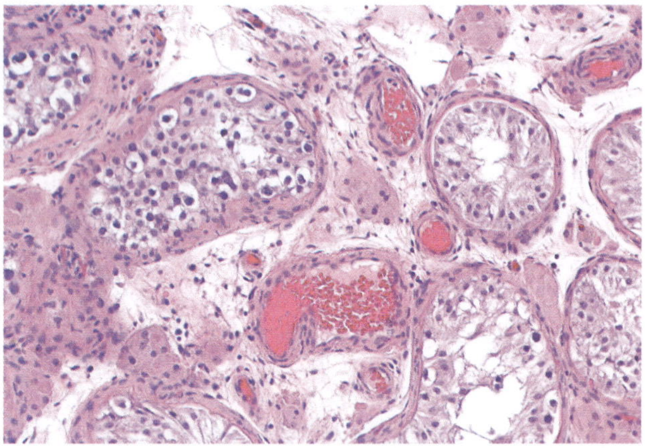

Fig. 25.28 Microscopy of ITGCN showing seminiferous tubules with a thickened basement membrane, lined by neoplastic cells that are large, round to polygonal with clear cytoplasm, coarse nuclear chromatin and prominent nucleoli. Two of the seven seminiferous tubules in the image show ITGCN, indicating that the involvement is patchy and not diffuse.

Pathogenesis Most testicular germ cell tumours, except for prepubertal yolk sac tumours, teratomas and spermatocytic tumour, arise from a preexisting precursor lesion called **intratubular germ cell neoplasia (ITGCN)**. ITGCN is presumed to arise in utero and stay dormant until puberty, after which it may give rise to any of the germ cell tumours.

ITGCN consists of **atypical primordial germ cells** with large nuclei and clear cytoplasm, which are about twice the size of normal germ cells (Fig. 25.28). These cells retain the expression of the transcription factors **OCT3/4** and **NANOG**, which are essential in maintaining pluripotent stem cells. There are some genetic alterations observed in ITGCN that are usually seen in germ cell tumours and include reduplication of the short arm of chromosome 12 in the form of an isochromosome i(12p) and activating mutations in the gene encoding KIT receptor tyrosine kinase. About 50% of individuals with ITGCN are found to develop invasive germ cell tumours within 5 years of diagnosis.

Clinical Features of Testicular Germ Cell Tumours Painless enlargement of the testis is the characteristic feature of germ cell tumours. Biopsy of a testicular neoplasm is associated with a risk of tumour spillage, so an open biopsy or radical orchidectomy is preferred. Testicular tumours spread through the lymphatic route and retroperitoneal para-aortic nodes are the first group of nodes to be involved, followed by the mediastinal and supraclavicular nodes. Haematogenous spread is primarily to the lungs, but it may also spread to the liver, brain and bones. Nonseminomatous germ cell tumours tend to metastasize earlier and more frequently through the haematogenous route.

Seminoma (classical or typical): Seminomas are the most common type of germ cell tumours with their peak incidence during the third decade of life. These arise from a preexisting ITGCN, which is also referred to as **GCNIS**. After puberty, these indolent GCNIS lesions give rise to seminomas. Similar to ITGCN, seminomas contain isochromosome 12p, express OCT3/4 and NANOG and some of these tumours also show KIT activating mutations.

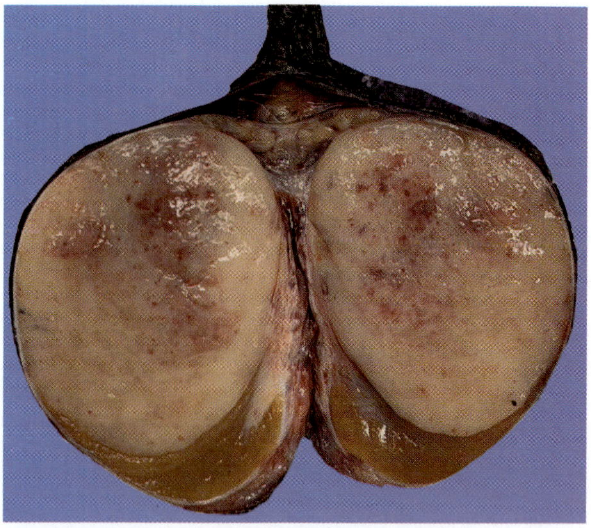

Fig. 25.29 Note the presence of a sharply demarcated, nodular pink tan tumour.

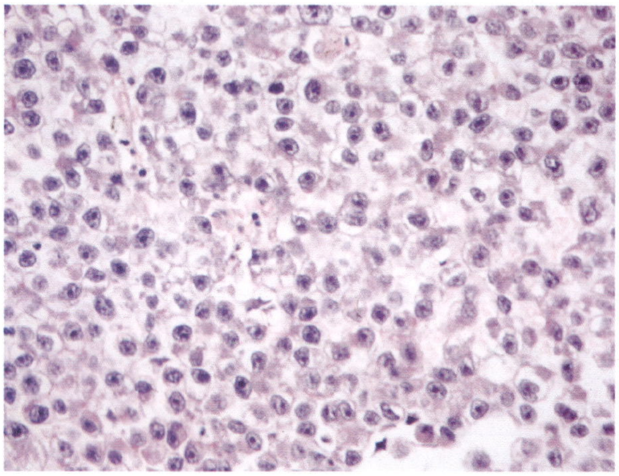

Fig. 25.30 Microscopy of classical seminoma displaying sheets of clear cells with lymphocytic infiltrate in the fibrous septa.

Morphology

Gross (Fig. 25.29): Seminomas produce bulky well-circumscribed masses often taking up the shape of the testis. On sectioning, these show a homogeneous, grey-white, lobulated cut surface devoid of haemorrhage or necrosis. These can extend to the epididymis, spermatic cord or rarely even the scrotal sac.

Microscopy (Fig. 25.30): Seminoma shows poorly demarcated lobules bordered by delicate fibrous septa and contains sheets of large uniform cells that are round to polyhedral in shape with a distinct cell membrane, clear cytoplasm and a large centrally placed nucleus with one or two conspicuous nucleoli. The fibrous septa show mild to moderate lymphocytic infiltrate. Mitoses are variable. The clear cytoplasm contains varying amounts of glycogen.

Variants

- **Anaplastic seminomas:** These show anaplastic features including frequent tumour giant cells and greater mitotic activity. However, anaplastic seminoma has an excellent prognosis similar to classical seminoma.
- **Seminomas with syncytiotrophoblasts:** These account for 15% of seminomas and show elevated levels of serum human chorionic gonadotropin (hCG).
- **Seminomas with granulomatous reaction:** These show ill-defined granulomas amidst the usual tumour cell population.

Immunohistochemistry: Seminoma cells stain positively for KIT, OCT4 and placental alkaline phosphatase (PLAP).

Spermatocytic tumor It is a distinctive, rare, slow-growing germ cell tumour commonly seen in elderly men. It accounts for 1%–2% of germ cell tumours. The affected individuals are generally older than 65 years. It is a slow-growing tumour with low metastatic potential, so the prognosis is excellent.

Morphology

Gross: These tumours have a soft, pale grey cut surface with occasional mucoid cysts.

Microscopy (Fig. 25.31): It shows three distinct intermixed cell populations:

- Medium-sized cells containing a round nucleus and eosinophilic cytoplasm (the most predominant)
- Smaller cells with a narrow rim of eosinophilic cytoplasm resembling secondary spermatocytes
- Uninucleate or multinucleate giant cells that are occasionally scattered

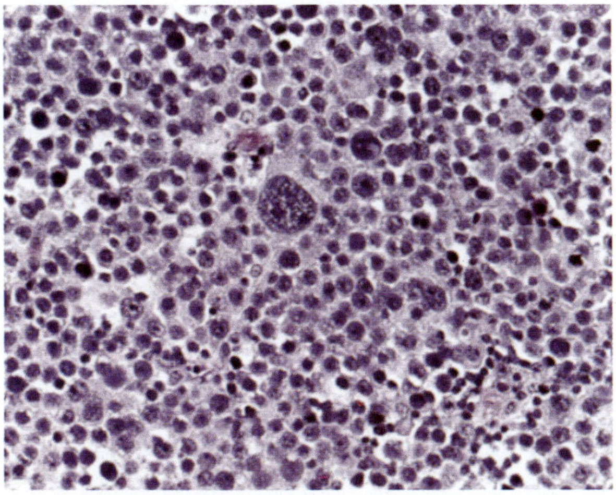

Fig. 25.31 Microscopy of spermatocytic tumor showing an admixture of small, medium-sized and large cells. (*Source:* From Ming Zhou, George J. Netto and Jonathan I. Epstein. Spermatocytic Seminoma. High-Yield Uropathology. Saunders 2012.)

Unlike typical seminomas, spermatocytic tumor lack lymphocytes, granulomas, syncytiotrophoblasts and extratesticular sites of origin, and are not associated with ITGCN.

Nonseminomatous Germ Cell Tumours

1. Embryonal Carcinoma

Embryonal carcinomas are aggressive tumours seen in individuals 20–30 years of age.

Morphology

Gross: Most primary tumours are smaller than seminomas and do not replace the entire testis, but extension through the tunica albuginea into the epididymis or cord is observed frequently. The cut surface of the tumour is often variegated, with interspersed foci of haemorrhage and necrosis and poorly demarcated at the margins.

Microscopy (Fig. 25.32): It shows primitive epithelial cells arranged in solid, pseudoglandular, alveolar, tubular or papillary patterns. Well-formed glands are absent. The neoplastic cells are large and anaplastic having hyperchromatic nuclei with prominent nucleoli. The cell borders are indistinct. Mitotic figures and tumour giant cells are seen frequently.

Immunohistochemistry: OCT 3/4 and PLAP, cytokeratin and CD30 stain positive on the tumour cells.

2. Yolk Sac Tumour (Endodermal Sinus Tumour) It is the most common testicular tumour in infants and children younger than 3 years. It usually carries a very good prognosis. In adults, the pure form of this tumour is rare but yolk sac elements may be frequently seen in combination with embryonal carcinoma.

Morphology

Gross: These are nonencapsulated tumours with a homogeneous, yellowish white, mucinous cut surface.

Microscopy (Fig. 25.33): It shows a reticular network of medium-sized cuboidal or flattened cells. Occasionally, papillary structures, solid cords of cells, tubules and glandular structures may be observed. In around

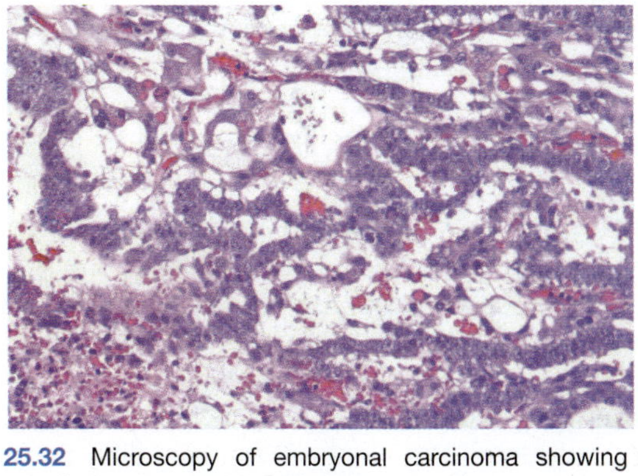

Fig. 25.32 Microscopy of embryonal carcinoma showing large tumour cells forming primitive tubules.

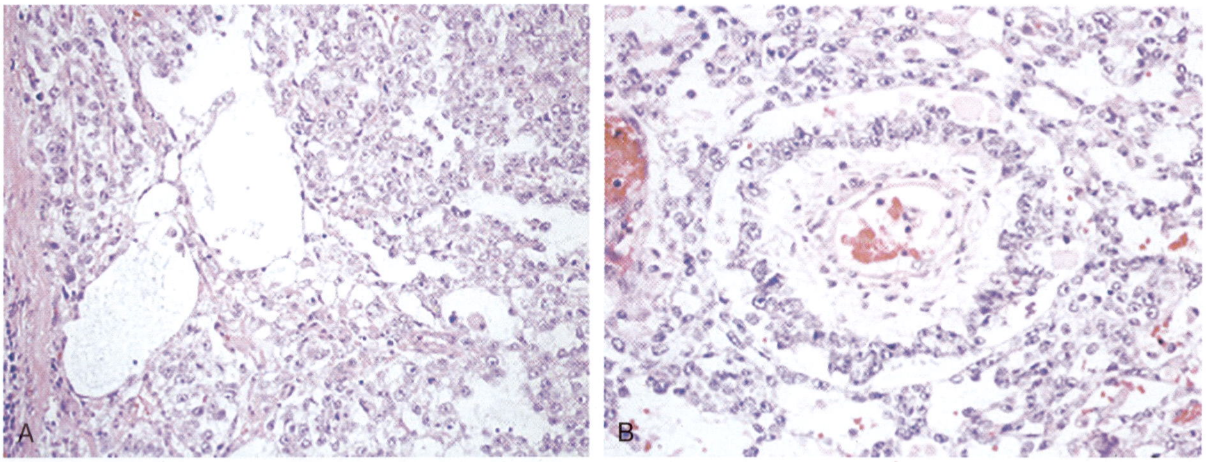

Fig. 25.33 Microscopy of yolk sac tumour showing (A) moderate nuclear atypia, a frequent reticular growth pattern and microcyst formation, and (B) the Schiller–Duval body. (*Source:* From Brooke E. Howitt and Daniel M. Berney. Tumours of the Testis. Surgical Pathology Clinics. 2015;8:687–716.)

50% of the tumours, **Schiller–Duval bodies** may be seen. These consist of a mesodermal core with a central capillary surrounded by visceral and parietal layers of cells resembling primitive glomeruli. Eosinophilic, **hyaline-like globules**, which are positive for α-fetoprotein (AFP), can be seen within the cytoplasm of some of the cells.

Immunohistochemistry: AFP and α_1-antitrypsin positivity is present.

3. Choriocarcinoma Choriocarcinoma is a highly malignant testicular tumour. It is commonly seen alongside other germ cell tumours and only rarely presents in its 'pure' form, constituting less than 1% of all germ cell tumours. These exhibit a peculiar tendency of being completely absent at the primary tumour site, whereas the lymph node concurrently harbours the metastatic tumour deposits and hence it is known as 'burnt-out' or **'vanishing tumour'**.

Morphology

Gross (Fig. 25.34): Choriocarcinomas often are felt as small palpable nodules with no definite testicular enlargement. Typically, these are small tumours, rarely measuring more than 5 cm in diameter, and show extensive areas of haemorrhage and necrosis with foci of cystic change.

Microscopy (Fig. 25.35): These tumours primarily contain two cell types – **syncytiotrophoblasts** and **cytotrophoblasts**. Syncytiotrophoblasts are large multinucleated cells with abundant eosinophilic vacuolated cytoplasm containing HCG. Cytotrophoblasts are polygonal cells with distinct cell borders, clear cytoplasm and a fairly uniform nucleus.

Immunohistochemistry: HCG positivity is present.

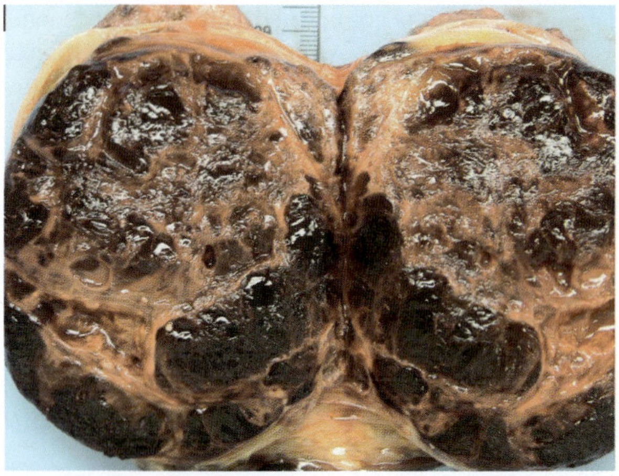

Fig. 25.34 Gross appearance of choriocarcinoma showing a well-circumscribed, grey-brown tumour with extensive areas of haemorrhage.

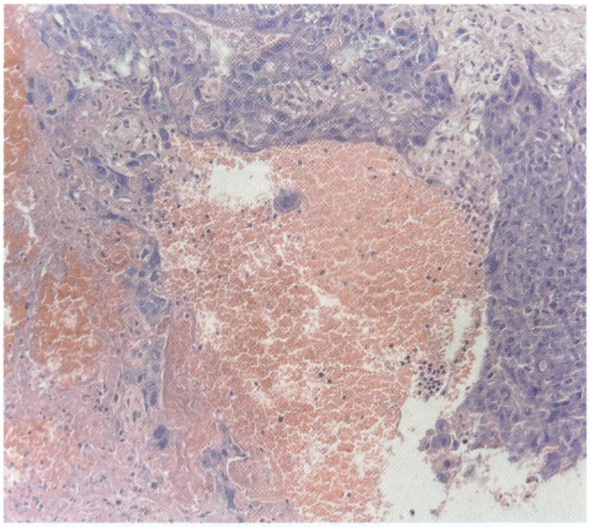

Fig. 25.35 **Microscopy of choriocarcinoma.** Classical **biphasic appearance** in a testicular **choriocarcinoma** consisting of **mononucleated cytotrophoblastic cells** with clear cytoplasm closely associated with and capped by **multinucleated syncytiotrophoblasts** with deeply eosinophilic cytoplasm.

4. Teratoma Teratoma is a germ cell tumour composed of several types of tissue representing the derivatives of one or more of the germinal layers (**endoderm, mesoderm and ectoderm**). It may be composed of exclusively well-differentiated mature tissue or may have an interspersed immature component. Teratoma may occur at any age from infancy to adult life. Pure forms of teratoma are common in infants and children. In adults, pure teratomas are rare, constituting only 2%–3% of germ cell tumours, whereas the incidence of teratomas mixed with other germ cell tumours is approximately 45%.

Morphology (Fig. 25.36)

Gross: Teratomas are usually large tumours, ranging from 5 to 10 cm in diameter, and showing a heterogeneous cut surface comprising grey-white solid and cystic areas, foci of bone, cartilaginous tissue, hair and even well-formed teeth with or without areas of haemorrhage and necrosis.
Microscopy: Teratomas show a heterogeneous admixture of tissue components comprising mainly the neural tissue, muscle bundles, islands of cartilage, strips of squamous epithelium, thyroid follicles, bronchial or bronchiolar epithelium and intestinal glands, all embedded in a fibrous or myxoid stroma.

Teratoma with malignant transformation: It is a rare condition in which the tissue components of teratoma may give rise to secondary tumours like squamous cell carcinoma, mucin-secreting adenocarcinoma, sarcoma or other tumours. The significance of recognizing a non-germ cell malignancy within a teratoma is that these secondary tumours are chemoresistant; hence, surgical resection is the mandatory choice for management.
Prognosis: Usually in children, differentiated mature teratomas have a benign course. in contrast, in postpubertal males, all teratomas, irrespective of morphology, are regarded as malignant tumours with metastatic potential.

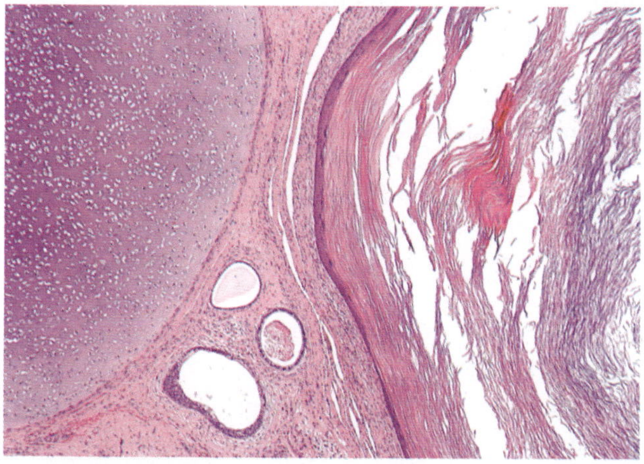

Fig. 25.36 Microscopy of teratoma showing cartilage on the left and stratified squamous epithelium with keratin flakes on the right.

5. Mixed Germ Cell Tumours About 60% of testicular tumours show two or more germ cell tumours coexisting with each other. The commonly encountered concoction includes teratoma and embryonal carcinoma with yolk sac tumour, seminoma with embryonal carcinoma and embryonal carcinoma with teratoma. The presence of more aggressive element indicates a poorer prognosis; hence, a through histopathological examination of the entire tumour becomes crucial in management and predicting the outcome.

For all testicular tumours, distant metastasis, if present, usually occurs within the first 2 years of treatment. Owing to their distinct biological behaviour and variable prognostic value, exact typing of germ cell tumours is essential.

Tumour Markers in Germ Cell Tumours of the Testis (Table 25.12) Germ cell tumours of the testes often secrete specific polypeptide hormones or enzymes, the elevated levels of which can be detected in the peripheral blood by sensitive assays.

Significance of evaluating biomarkers in testicular tumours is as follows:
- To categorize the testicular tumours
- In staging these tumours (persistently elevated HCG or AFP levels in postorchidectomy patients indicate stage II disease irrespective of lymph node status)
- To assess the tumour burden
- To monitor the response to therapy, subsequent follow-up for recurrence

Tumour progression and staging: The primary tumours are staged on the basis of their extent of spread into the adjacent structures and by the presence/absence of lymphovascular invasion. The metastatic deposits are initially seen in the retroperitoneal para-aortic nodes, followed by mediastinal and supraclavicular nodes. Haematogenous spread is primarily to the lungs and, rarely, the liver, brain or bones may also be involved. These tumours are also well known to show morphologies in the metastatic site that are different from those in the primary location, which is attributed to forward or backward differentiating capacity of the pluripotent stem cells. Hence, techniques

Table 25.12 Elevated Levels of Biomarkers in Specific Testicular Tumours

Marker	Indicative Tumours
β-HCG	Choriocarcinoma
AFP	Nonseminomatous GCT
PLAP	Seminoma, embryonal carcinoma
Lactate dehydrogenase	Denotes tumour burden

AFP, α-fetoprotein; GCT, germ cell tumour; HCG, human chorionic gonadotropin; PLAP, placental alkaline phosphatase.

like immunohistochemistry are required to ascertain the nature of the tumour.

Management of Testicular Germ Cell Tumours Germ cell tumours are assessed through scrotal ultrasound scan and an open or ultrasound-guided percutaneous testicular biopsy. However, radical orchidectomy remains the definitive management protocol for all testicular tumours along with pre- or postoperative chemotherapy and radiotherapy as and when indicated.

Sex Cord–Stromal Tumours

On the basis of their histogenesis and differentiation, sex cord–stromal tumours are further classified into Leydig cell tumours and Sertoli cell tumours.

Leydig Cell Tumours These tumours are commonly seen in individuals between 20 and 60 years of age. Leydig cell tumours present as testicular swelling or gynaecomastia in adults and sexual precocity in children. Tumours of Leydig cells are peculiar in a way that they may elaborate androgens, oestrogens and even corticosteroids occasionally.
Morphology (Fig. 25.37)

Gross: These tumours range in size from 1 to 5 cm and present as well-circumscribed nodules with a distinct homogeneous golden brown cut surface.
Microscopy: Leydig cells are large, round to polygonal cells with abundant granular eosinophilic cytoplasm containing lipid droplets, vacuoles, lipofuscin pigment and typical rod-shaped crystalloids of Reinke, seen in 25% of the tumours. These neoplastic Leydig cells are morphologically similar to the Leydig cells seen in normal testicular parenchyma. Although most of these tumours are benign, 10% of them may be malignant with a metastatic potential.

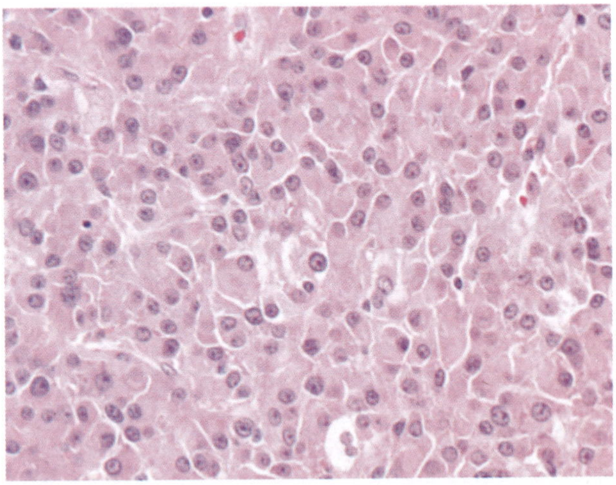

Fig. 25.37 Microscopy of Leydig cell tumour showing diffuse sheets of cells with definite cell borders, abundant eosinophilic cytoplasm, a round to oval nucleus and a prominent nucleolus. (*Source:* From Jesse K. McKenney. Testis and Testicular Adnexa. Rosai and Ackerman's Surgical Pathology. 11th edition. Elsevier 2018.)

Sertoli Cell Tumours Sertoli cell tumours are commonly seen in middle-aged men, presenting as a slowly enlarging mass in the testis. These are hormonally silent tumours.
Morphology

Gross: These tumours present as small, firm nodules measuring 2–4 cm in size with a homogeneous grey-white to tan-yellow cut surface.
Microscopy: The tumour cells are arranged in solid sheets, tubules, trabeculae or retiform pattern. The individual cells are uniformly round with oval or elongated nuclei and pale eosinophilic cytoplasm. There is no nuclear atypia or mitotic activity. Similar to Leydig cell tumours, these tumours are mostly benign, with an exception of 10% of them that may display a malignant potential.

Gonadoblastoma Gonadoblastomas are rare neoplasms arising in gonads with varying forms of testicular dysgenesis and comprise a mixture of germ cells and gonadal stromal elements. Rarely, the germ cell component turns malignant, giving rise to seminoma.

Morphology

Gross: These appear as yellow-tan nodules ranging from 1 to 8 cm in size with a gritty cut surface.
Microscopy: It shows irregular clusters of immature Sertoli cells surrounding the germ cells. The stroma shows large polygonal cells reminiscent of Leydig cells amidst areas of calcification.

Testicular Lymphoma Lymphomas of the testes can be primary or secondary tumours accounting for 5% of all testicular neoplasms. These are mostly aggressive non–Hodgkin lymphomas presenting in the advanced clinical stage and are generally encountered in men older than 60 years. The most common testicular lymphomas include diffuse large B-cell lymphoma, Burkitt lymphoma and Epstein-Bar Virus (EBV) positive extranodal natural killer (NK)/T cell lymphoma.
Morphology

Gross: These appear as tan-pink fleshy masses replacing the normal testicular parenchyma.
Microscopy (Fig. 25.38): The testicular parenchyma appears distorted and infiltrated by neoplastic lymphoid cells, splaying the intervening seminiferous tubules.

PARATESTICULAR TUMOURS

Paratesticular tumours can be benign or malignant masses arising from structures adjacent to the testis. The benign tumours include lipoma, leiomyoma, fibroma, haemangioma and the most common adenomatoid tumour,

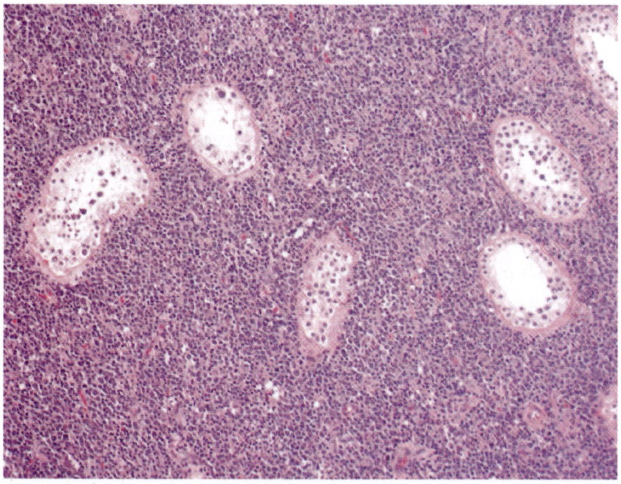

Fig. 25.38 Microscopy of testicular lymphoma. Note the destruction of tubules by the lymphoma cells.

which requires a brief mention. The most common malignant paratesticular tumour seen in children is rhabdomyosarcoma, whereas in adults, it is the liposarcoma. Paratesticular rhabdomyosarcoma is a rare malignancy arising from mesenchymal tissues of the spermatic cord, epididymis and testis. It will be discussed in detail along with its soft-tissue counterpart in Chapter 30.

Adenomatoid tumour of the testis: It is the benign tumour of mesothelial origin, presenting as a small, well-circumscribed, tan-white nodule in the upper pole of the epididymis. Microscopically, these tumours show tubules, cords and nests lined by cuboidal cells containing moderate to abundant amount of eosinophilic cytoplasm with several vacuoles and a bland nucleus.

PROSTATE

The three most common pathological conditions affecting the prostate, which merit an elaborate note, include inflammation, benign prostatic nodular hyperplasia and prostatic carcinoma. The benign prostatic hyperplasia (BPH) commonly involves the transition zone of the prostate, whereas adenocarcinoma involves the peripheral zone of the gland.

INFLAMMATION: PROSTATITIS PA 29.5

Prostatitis is divided into several categories, namely:

- Acute bacterial prostatitis
- Chronic bacterial prostatitis
- Chronic abacterial prostatitis
- Granulomatous prostatitis

Features of these four categories are listed and compared in Table 25.13.

Laboratory Diagnosis

Bacterial prostatitis: Culture of prostatic secretions should have bacterial counts 10 times higher than those of bladder or urethral cultures.

Chronic abacterial prostatitis: There should be more than 10 white blood cells per high-power field (WBC/HPF) in prostatic secretions and bacterial cultures are negative.

Table 25.13 Differences Between the Various Categories of Prostatitis

Factor	Acute Bacterial Prostatitis	Chronic Bacterial Prostatitis	Chronic Abacterial Prostatitis/Chronic Pelvic Pain Syndrome	Granulomatous Prostatitis
Organisms	*E. coli*, enterococci, staphylococci	*E. coli*, enterococci, staphylococci	Nil	*Mycobacterium tuberculosis*, BCG vaccine instillation, fungal infections in immunocompromised individuals
Mode of infection	Intraprostatic urine reflux, lymphohaematogenous route, iatrogenic	Recurrent urinary tract infections	No recurrent infections of urinary tract	Lymphohaematogenous route, local administration of BCG vaccine into the bladder
Clinical symptoms	Fever, chills, dysuria	Low back pain, dysuria, perineal and suprapubic discomfort	Low back pain, dysuria, perineal and suprapubic discomfort	Nonspecific
Confirmation	Urine culture positivity	Urine culture positivity and leucocytosis in urine	Urine culture negative and leucocytes >10/HPF	Biopsy showing necrotizing or non-necrotizing granulomas

HPF, high-power field.

Prostatitis should not be diagnosed on needle biopsy alone; it is a clinical diagnosis on the basis of quantitative bacterial cultures and microscopic examination of fractionated urine specimens and expressed prostatic secretions.

Morphology

Gross: In acute prostatitis, several tiny disseminated abscesses with large focal areas of necrosis and an overall congested gland are observed. Biopsy is not an indication for acute prostatitis, rather a contraindication due to the likelihood of sepsis. If these features are found as incidental findings on surgically resected specimens or core biopsies, these deserve a significant mention.

Microscopy (Fig. 25.39): It shows prostatic parenchyma with neutrophilic aggregates within the lumen of tubuloalveolar glands, as well as sheets of lymphocytes and macrophages in the stroma.

The diagnosis of acute or chronic prostatitis is usually made with the clinical and laboratory findings. Inflammatory changes seen in biopsies should be described as acute or chronic inflammation rather than prostatitis. These changes may be seen coexisting with adjacent benign nodular hyperplasia or adenocarcinoma of the prostate gland.

BENIGN PROSTATIC HYPERPLASIA (NODULAR HYPERPLASIA) PA 29.3

Nodular hyperplasia is the most common benign lesion of the prostate in men older than 50 years. The tendency of BPH to turn into malignancy over the years is absolutely negligible; hence, it is not a precancerous condition.

Aetiology and Pathogenesis

Three theories have been suggested for the development of BPH:

1. **Dihydrotestosterone (DHT) hypothesis:** DHT is formed in the prostate from testosterone through the action of an enzyme called type 2 5α-reductase. This enzyme is located almost entirely in the stromal cells and in a few basal cells of the prostate; hence, stromal cells are responsible for androgen-dependent prostatic growth. DHT binds to the nuclear androgen receptor (AR) present in both stromal and epithelial prostatic cells and stimulates the transcription of androgen-dependent genes, their growth factors and receptors like fibroblast growth factor (FGF) family and transforming growth factor (TGF)-β and thereby results in nodular hyperplasia of the prostate.
2. **Embryonic reawakening theory:** FGFs produced by stromal cells of the prostate are paracrine regulators of androgen-stimulated epithelial growth during the embryonic prostatic development. Some of these pathways may be reawakened in the adulthood, resulting in prostatic hyperplasia.
3. **Stem cell theory:** An increase in prostatic stem cell count or an increase in clonal expansion of preexisting stem cells results in prostatic hyperplasia.

Morphology

Gross (Fig. 25.40): An enlarged gland, weighing 60–100 g with fairly discrete nodules in the periurethral region, is the hallmark of BPH. These nodules can gradually obstruct the urethra in due course. The nodules that develop early are entirely stromal in origin, whereas the epithelial nodules arise later in the disease course. On sectioning, the nodules may be pinkish, soft, exuding milky white prostatic fluid when the glands form the major component or may be pale

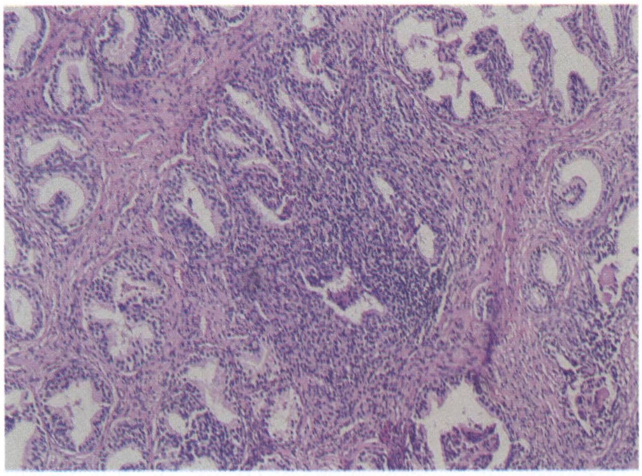

Fig. 25.39 Microscopy of prostatitis – numerous lymphocytes are seen in the stroma.

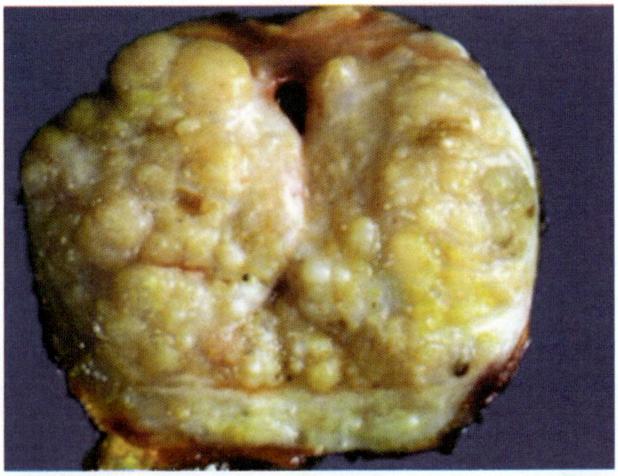

Fig. 25.40 Gross appearance of BPH. Note the nodular appearance of the enlarged gland.

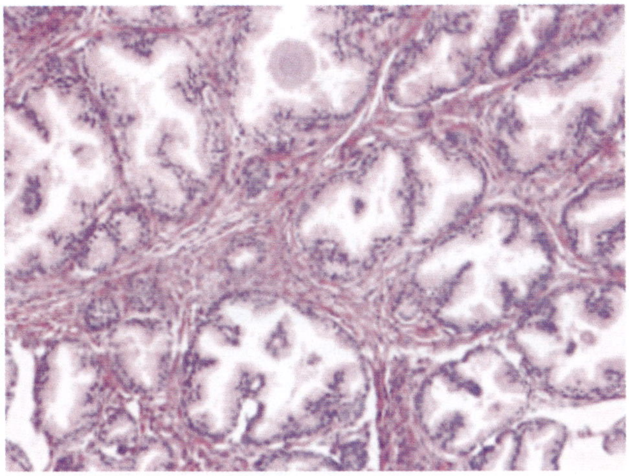

Fig. 25.41 Microscopy of BPH showing large cystically dilated glands lined by bilayered epithelium.

grey and tough due to the predominance of fibromuscular stroma.

Microscopy (Fig. 25.41): It shows several compactly arranged small to large cystically dilated glands lined by benign bilayered epithelium, comprising an inner columnar layer and an outer cuboidal or flattened epithelium. The stroma shows prominent fibromuscular hyperplasia.

Clinical Features

Urinary obstruction due to narrowing of the urethral orifice

Subsequent bladder hypertrophy and enlargement due to urinary retention

Residual urine acting as a nidus for repeated infections

Increased urinary frequency, incontinence, nocturia and dysuria

Investigations

- A urinary frequency and volume chart maintained to monitor the urine output and gauge the impedance to the urinary outflow due to nodular hyperplasia
- A routine urine examination to exclude urinary tract infection
- A postvoid bladder scan to assess the volume of urine retention occurring within the bladder
- Digital rectal examination (DRE) to evaluate the extent of prostatic enlargement and the lobes involved
- Prostate-specific antigen (PSA) levels to exclude any occult malignancy
- An ultrasound examination of the renal tract to assess for hydroureter or hydronephrosis due to the mechanical obstruction of urinary outflow and to measure the volume of the prostate gland
- Urodynamic studies and cystoscopic examination
- Prostatic biopsy showing features of BPH with no evidence of atypia or malignancy

Management

These lesions have almost no chance for malignant transformation and hence are managed conservatively.

1. **Mild BPH:** It is empirically managed by reducing the fluid intake before bedtime and by lowering the intake of alcohol and caffeine. The most commonly used and effective medical therapy for BPH includes α-blockers, which decrease the prostate smooth muscle tone by inhibiting the α_1-adrenergic receptors and **inhibitors of** 5α-reductase, which aids in shrinking the prostate by inhibiting the synthesis of DHT.
2. **Moderate to severe BPH:** Management includes several minimally invasive procedures like transurethral resection of the prostate (TURP), high-intensity focused ultrasound scan, laser therapy, transurethral microwave thermotherapy, transurethral electrovaporization and transurethral needle ablation using radiofrequency. All these procedures reduce the overall volume of the gland, which aids in relieving the symptoms.

PROSTATIC ADENOCARCINOMA PA 29.4

Prostatic tumours are primarily classified into epithelial and mesenchymal tumours. Adenocarcinoma of the prostate is the most common malignancy among men older than 50 years, with an annual incidence rate of 9–10/100,000 population according to the Indian Council of Medical Research (ICMR). It is the second most common cancer in men worldwide, with an average of 1.3 million cases every year. The incidence of these tumours is directly proportional to the advancing age among men. Both hereditary and environmental factors play a significant role in the pathogenesis of these tumours.

Genetic factors: The incidence of prostatic adenocarcinoma is the highest among American blacks and the lowest in the East Asian population. The disease has been found to manifest in familial clusters and in a hereditary form, supporting that genetic factors determine the disease onset and progression.

Environmental factors: High calorie intake, high body mass index (BMI), consumption of animal fat and certain toxins containing cadmium have been found to increase the risk, whereas intake of soy and other phytoestrogens, selenium, vitamin A, vitamin D and antioxidants is associated with a reduction in risk.

Prostatic carcinomas have a precursor lesion known as prostatic intraepithelial neoplasia (PIN), which is the forerunner of malignancy, which is detected incidentally on core needle biopsies or resected specimens of the prostate, either as solitary lesions or coexisting with invasive carcinomas (Fig. 25.42).

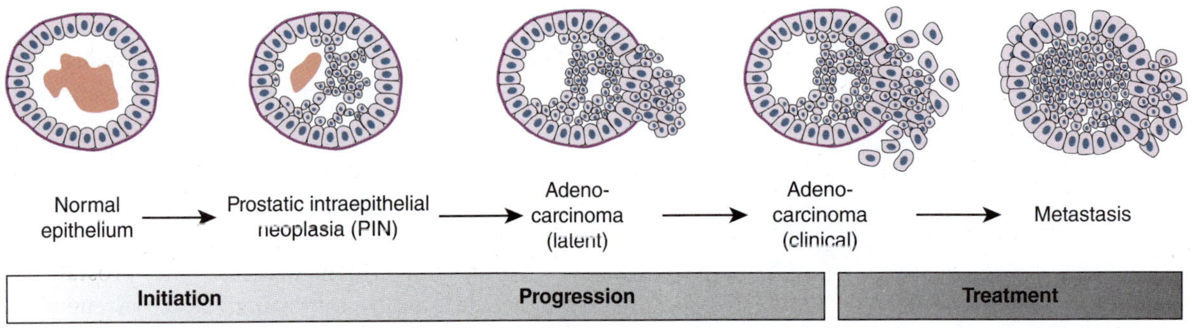

Fig. 25.42 Schematic picture depicting the progression of prostatic adenocarcinoma. (*Source:* Molecules 2022, 27, 5730, Fig. 1, page 8.)

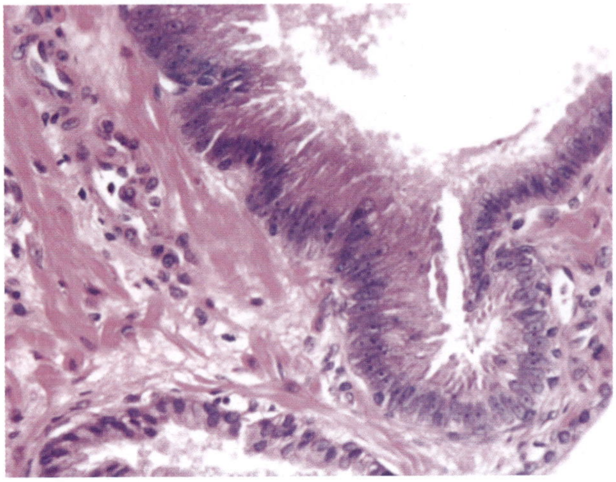

Fig. 25.43 Microscopy of PIN showing glands lined by atypical cells. (*Source:* From Jonathan I. Epstein. Pathology of Prostatic Neoplasia. Campbell-Walsh-Wein Urology. 12th edition. Elsevier 2021.)

Prostatic Intraepithelial Neoplasia

PIN consists of architecturally benign prostatic acini lined by cytologically atypical cells (Fig. 25.43). It is further subclassified into low-grade PIN (LG-PIN) and high-grade PIN (HG-PIN). In HG-PIN, mild architectural abnormality, nuclear atypia characterized by enlarged nuclei, hyperchromatism, overlapping nuclei with prominent nucleoli and amphophilic cytoplasm are observed.

Both PIN and adenocarcinoma of the prostate are typically seen in the peripheral zone of the prostate. PIN has been observed to be coexisting with invasive carcinoma frequently. It has been found that molecular changes found in invasive carcinomas, like rearrangements involving ETS genes, are also observed in PIN, gaining evidence that PIN could potentially be a precursor lesion for invasive carcinoma.

Aetiopathogenesis of Prostatic Adenocarcinoma Various factors play a role in the pathogenesis of prostatic carcinoma that include age, race, family history, hormonal levels and certain environmental factors. A positive family history increases the risk of developing prostatic carcinoma at an early age by several folds.

Androgens are found to play an important role in the pathogenesis of prostate cancer. The growth and survival of tumour cells of prostatic adenocarcinoma depend on the androgens, which bind to **AR** and induce the expression of progrowth and prosurvival genes. In normal individuals, there is a significant variation in the length of the CAG repeats, which affect the AR function. ARs with the shortest stretches of polyglutamine have the highest sensitivity, whereas those with the longest stretches have the least sensitivity to androgens. **Example:** African Americans have the shortest CAG repeats, exhibiting best prognosis, whereas Asians have the longest CAG repeat chains, indicating a poorer outcome.

However, most of the tumours eventually become resistant to androgen blockade. The tumour cells escape through a multitude of mechanisms like acquisition of hypersensitivity to low levels of androgen, ligand-independent AR activation, mutations in AR that permit it to be activated by nonandrogen ligands and other epigenetic changes that activate the alternative signalling pathways, which may bypass the need for AR itself.

The other genetic alterations are as follows:

- Germline mutations in tumour suppressor gene BRCA2
- TMPRSS2–ERG gene fusion
- Germline mutations in HOXB13, a gene encoding transcription factor that regulates prostatic development
- Genetic alterations like amplification of the 8q24 locus containing the MYC oncogene
- Deletion involving the PTEN tumour suppressor
- Deletion or mutation in TP53
- Deletion of the RB gene

The most common epigenetic alteration in prostate carcinoma is hypermethylation of the glutathione *S*-transferase (GSTP1) gene, which downregulates GSTP1 expression. The GSTP1 gene located on chromosome 11q13 plays a vital role in the pathway that prevents damage from a range of carcinogens.

The other genes silenced by epigenetic modifications in prostate carcinomas include several tumour suppressor genes like RB, CDKN2A, MLH1 and MSH2.

Morphology

Gross (Fig. 25.44): In the majority of cases, carcinoma of the prostate arises in the **peripheral zone** of the gland, especially in the posterior location. On sectioning, the tumour is firm and gritty with a grey-white cut surface. The local extension of tumour most commonly involves periprostatic tissue, seminal vesicles and base of the urinary bladder.

Microscopy (Fig. 25.45): A majority of the prostatic adenocarcinomas produce well-defined glandular patterns. The glands are typically smaller than benign glands and are lined by a single layer of uniform, bland-looking cuboidal or low columnar epithelium. These glands **lack the basal cell layer** and are more crowded without definitive branching or papillary invaginations. The individual tumour cells contain a large pleomorphic nucleus with one or more prominent nucleoli and pale to clear or amphophilic cytoplasm. Crystalloids, glomerulations and mucinous fibroplasia and **perineural invasion** are common findings in these tumours, whereas mitotic activity is usually insignificant.

Immunohistochemistry **p63 and HMW cytokeratin:** Labels the basal cell layer that is absent in adenocarcinoma.

α-Methyl acyl-coenzyme A-racemase (**AMACR**): Positive in tumour cells of adenocarcinoma

PSA: Positive in adenocarcinoma (it stains normal, benign and malignant prostatic glands, so it is not tumour specific; it can be used to identify prostatic cancer of occult primary origin)

NKX3.1, P501S (prostein): Newer antibodies for poorly differentiated prostatic adenocarcinoma

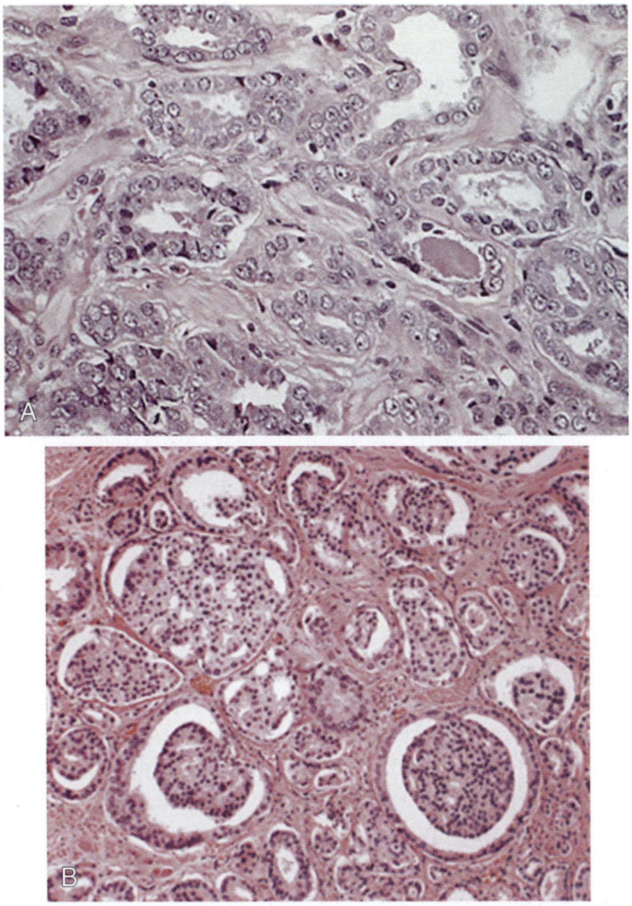

Fig. 25.45 Microscopy of prostatic adenocarcinoma showing glands lined by atypical cells that lack the basal layer (A) and glands with glomerulations (B). Glomeruloid structures are characterized by dilated glands containing an intraluminal proliferation of malignant epithelium, which is attached only to the one edge of the gland. (*Source:* From Christopher D.M. Fletcher. Tumours and Tumour-like Conditions of the Male Genital Tract. Diagnostic Histopathology of Tumours. 5th edition. Elsevier 2021.)

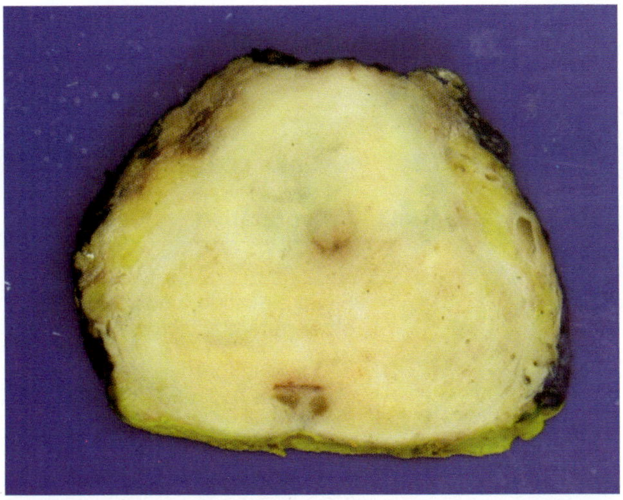

Fig. 25.44 Gross appearance of prostatic adenocarcinoma showing a grey-yellow, firm, poorly delimited tumour involving the prostate gland. (*Source:* https://www.pathologyoutlines.com/imgau/prostateprostaticCAgeneralZynger2.jpg.)

Novel Biomarkers of Significance The following novel biomarkers are assessed in the urine sample of male patients with prostatic carcinoma and are found to be elevated:

- Urine PCA3 level assessment
- Urine TMPRSS2–ERG fusion DNA level assessment

These novel markers enable us to detect and subsequently follow up patients with prostatic carcinomas by analysing their urine samples.

Clinical Features Prostatic adenocarcinomas are initially asymptomatic due to their posterior location. Only advanced tumours present with symptoms of increased frequency of micturition, dysuria, incomplete voiding of urine, erectile dysfunction or haematuria due to impingement of the tumour over the urethra. Rarely, in advanced cases, patients may present with bone pain due to metastatic deposits.

Grading and staging: Grading is of specific significance in prostatic carcinomas, because the grade and stage are the best prognostic predictors. Prostate carcinomas are graded according to the well-known Gleason system, which stratifies the tumour into five grades on the basis of the glandular patterns of differentiation, and these grades ultimately indicate the tumour prognosis.

Gleason grading system (Fig. 25.46)

The Gleason grading system may be used for assessing prostatic core needle biopsies and resected specimens of prostatic adenocarcinomas. The grades are assigned on the basis of the primary and secondary patterns of tumour, which represent the most widely observed patterns in a particular case. Grade 1 and 2 are not used for needle biopsy specimens; very rarely used in grading radical prostatectomy specimens. Addition of the primary and secondary grades gives the Gleason score, which denotes the overall tumour differentiation and thereby its prognosis.

Grade 1: These are single discrete, closely packed uniform round glands arranged in well-circumscribed nodules.

Grade 2: These are fairly circumscribed tumour nodules with less closely packed discrete glands minimally infiltrating the adjacent non-neoplastic prostatic stroma.

Grade 3: These are single discrete glands of varying sizes with irregularly separated, ragged and poorly defined edges infiltrating the stroma. The neighbouring glands are separated by at least a wisp of intervening stroma.

Grade 4: These include coalescent or fused glands in a cribriform pattern with the absence of intervening stroma.

Grade 5: These have solid sheets or nests of cells with no glandular differentiation.

Gleason scoring system: A majority of prostatic carcinomas exhibit more than one histological pattern, which are given a Gleason score by adding the primary (the predominant) and the secondary (the second predominant) patterns. The final Gleason score determines the biological behaviour of the tumour. A Gleason score of 2–6 indicates well-differentiated tumours with an excellent prognosis, whereas tumours with a score of 7 are moderately to poorly differentiated; those with a score of 8–10 are poorly or undifferentiated tumours exhibiting aggressive behaviour.

However, deficiencies in this Gleason system of reporting have impacted patient care and have prompted the need for grade grouping of these tumours on the basis of the overall Gleason score as follows:

Grade group 1: Gleason score less than or equal to 6
Grade group 2: Gleason score 3 + 4 = 7
Grade group 3: Gleason score 4 + 3 = 7
Grade group 4: Gleason score 8 (4 + 4/5 + 3/3 + 5)
Grade group 5: Gleason score 9 − 10

PSA in Prostatic Carcinoma

PSA is produced by the prostatic epithelium and is normally secreted in the semen. Normally, in men, only minute amounts of PSA circulate in the serum. Elevated blood levels of PSA occur commonly in malignancy (Table 25.14). However, elevated PSA levels are also observed in conditions like BPH, prostatitis, infarction of nodular hyperplasia, iatrogenic causes and ejaculation to an extent, leading an uncertainty in the interpretation of the results. In a majority of cases, a serum level of 4 ng/mL is considered as the cutoff between normal and abnormal levels.

PSA levels alone cannot precisely indicate a malignancy, so several other derivatives of PSA are used to delineate the benign changes from malignancy and include the following:

PSA density (Table 25.15): The ratio between serum PSA value and volume of the prostate gland is elevated in malignancy.

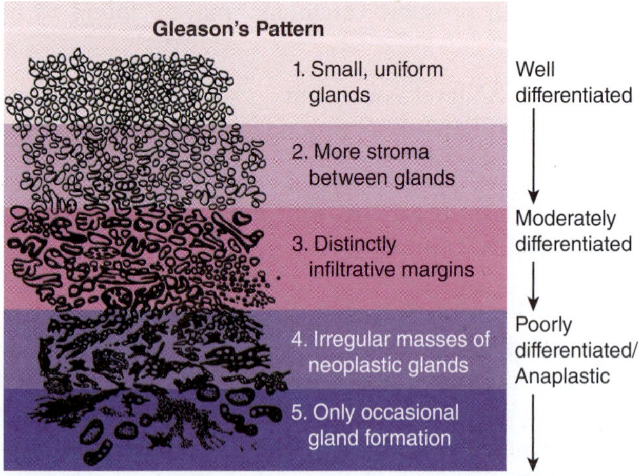

Fig. 25.46 (Schematic diagrams of the Gleason grading system. (*Source:* https://upload.wikimedia.org/wikipedia/commons/thumb/b/bc/Gleasonscore.jpg/290px-Gleasonscore.jpg)

Table 25.14 PSA Level and Its Significance

PSA Level (ng/mL)	Interpretation
0–2.5	Normal
2.6–4	Slight elevation, correlation with other potential factors is required
4.0–10	Suspicious for malignancy; 25% chance of having a prostatic carcinoma
>10	Highly suspicious of malignancy; 50% chance of having a prostatic carcinoma

PSA, prostate-specific antigen.

Table 25.15 Derivatives of PSA and Their Formulae

Parameter	Formula
PSA density	Serum PSA level: Volume of the prostate gland
PSA velocity	Rate of change in PSA value with time
Percentage of free PSA	([Free PSA]/[total PSA]) × 100

PSA, prostate-specific antigen.

Table 25.16 Age-Specific PSA Levels

Age Group (Years)	Upper Limit of PSA Level (ng/mL)
40–49	2.5
50–59	3.5
60–69	4.5
70–79	6.5

PSA, prostate-specific antigen.

PSA velocity: The rate of change in PSA value with time is high in men with prostatic carcinoma.

Age-specific reference ranges of PSA (Table 25.16): The upper age-specific PSA reference ranges are 2.5 ng/mL for men 40–49 years of age, 3.5 ng/mL for men 50–59 years of age, 4.5 ng/mL for men 60–69 years of age and 6.5 ng/mL for men 70–79 years of age.

Percentage of free PSA: The value ([Free PSA]/[total PSA]) × 100 is lower in men with prostatic adenocarcinoma. The immunoreactive PSA exists in two forms – a major fraction that is bound to α_1-antichymotrypsin and a minor free fraction. The minor free fraction is the parameter of interest, which is higher in benign prostatic diseases than in malignancy.

Tumour Progression Tumours detected incidentally at an early stage (clinically T1a) are found to be indolent when followed even up to 10 years (Table 25.17). However, advanced tumours spread through lymphatics to the obturator nodes and eventually to the para-aortic nodes. Haematogenous spread occurs chiefly to the bones of axial skeleton such as the vertebral column, pelvis, ribs, skull and sternum due to their rich capillary network in the marrow. These bony metastases are typically multiple and osteoblastic in nature. The presence of bony metastasis indicates a disseminated tumour and hence prognosis is usually guarded (Fig. 25.47).

Management Prostatic carcinomas are treated by surgery, radiation therapy and hormonal treatment. These

Table 25.17 Staging of Prostatic Adenocarcinoma (AJCC, 2016)

'T' Category
- T1: Clinically inapparent tumor not palpable not visible by imaging
- T2: Organ confined
- T3: Extraprostatic extension
- T3a: Extraprostatic extension (unilateral or bilateral) or microscopic invasion of the bladder neck
- T3b: Tumour invades seminal vesicles
- T4: Tumour is fixed or invades adjacent structures other than seminal vesicles such as external sphincter, rectum, bladder, levator muscles and/or pelvic wall

'N' Category
- N0: No positive regional nodes
- N1: Metastases in regional nodes

'M' Category
- M1: Distant metastasis

AJCC, American Joint Committee on Cancer.
(*Source:* American Joint Committee on Cancer (AJCC) tumor-node-metastasis (TNM) Staging Manual, 8th ed.)

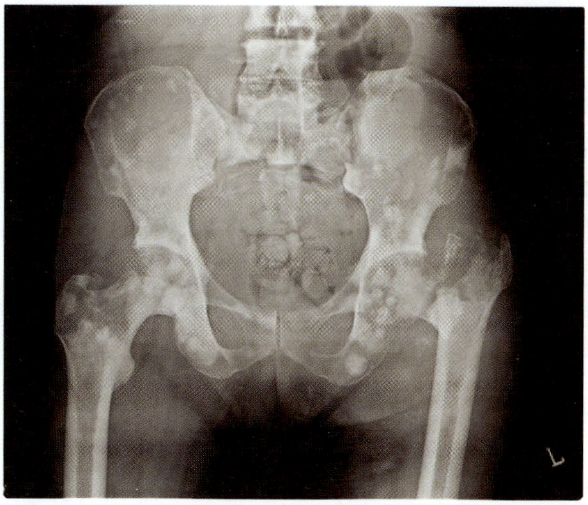

Fig. 25.47 Radiological appearance of bony metastasis in prostatic adenocarcinoma – multiple sclerotic lesions seen at the pelvic bones and proximal femora in a case of carcinoma of the prostate with a pathological fracture through the intertrochanteric plane.

tumours have a good overall survival rate, with an average life expectancy of 15 years in more than 90% of the patients. The present management of choice for clinically localized tumours is radical prostatectomy. The prognosis following radical prostatectomy is based on the pathological stage, margin status and Gleason grade. Alternative management for localized prostatic carcinomas is either external-beam radiation therapy or interstitial radiation therapy. Advanced metastatic carcinoma is treated by androgen deprivation therapy, which can be achieved either by administration of synthetic analogues of luteinizing hormone–releasing hormone (LHRH) or by orchidectomy. Although androgen deprivation therapy induces remissions, eventually, these tumours become resistant to testosterone withdrawal and this heralds the progression of disease and subsequent death.

OTHER TUMOURS

The less common epithelial tumours of the prostate are adenocarcinoma arising from prostatic ducts and adenosquamous and pure squamous cell carcinomas of the prostate. Tumours with abundant mucinous secretions are termed colloid carcinomas of the prostate. The most aggressive variant of prostatic carcinoma is small-cell/neuroendocrine carcinoma. The mesenchymal tumours of the prostate include rhabdomyosarcoma, angiosarcoma, leiomyoma and leiomyosarcoma. Lymphomas, although rare, are also encountered in the prostate.

SELF-ASSESSMENT

Scenario-Based MCQs

1. A 70-year-old male presents with nocturia, hesitancy and a decreased stream. Digital rectal examination reveals an enlarged, nontender prostate. The most likely diagnosis is
   A. Acute prostatitis
   B. Prostate cancer
   C. Benign prostatic hyperplasia
   D. Urethral stricture
2. A 55-year-old smoker presents with painless haematuria. Cystoscopy reveals a red, velvety area on the bladder wall. The most likely diagnosis is
   A. Acute cystitis
   B. Bladder cancer
   C. Urolithiasis
   D. Glomerulonephritis
3. A 25-year-old male experiences sudden-onset testicular pain. Physical examination reveals a high-riding testicle with a horizontal lie. The most likely diagnosis is
   A. Epididymitis
   B. Testicular torsion
   C. Orchitis
   D. Hydrocele
4. A patient presents with dysuria, frequency and urgency. Urinalysis shows pyuria. The most likely causative organism is
   A. *Escherichia coli*
   B. *Chlamydia trachomatis*
   C. *Mycoplasma genitalium*
   D. *Klebsiella pneumoniae*
5. A 40-year-old male presents with a palpable, painless mass in the testis. Serum markers show elevated AFP and hCG levels. The most likely diagnosis is
   A. Testicular torsion
   B. Varicocele
   C. Testicular tumour
   D. Epididymitis
6. A 65-year-old male with a history of diabetes mellitus presents with dysuria, fever and lower back pain. Urinalysis reveals pyuria and bacteriuria. The most likely diagnosis is
   A. Acute prostatitis
   B. Benign prostatic hyperplasia
   C. Bladder cancer
   D. Urethral stricture
7. A 30-year-old male presents with scrotal pain and swelling. Doppler ultrasound shows reduced blood flow to the testicle. The most immediate concern is
   A. Hydrocele
   B. Testicular cancer
   C. Testicular torsion
   D. Epididymitis
8. A patient presents with erectile dysfunction and decreased libido. Laboratory tests reveal low testosterone levels. The most likely cause is
   A. Psychogenic factors
   B. Hypogonadism
   C. Prostatitis
   D. Urethral stricture
9. A 55-year-old male presents with urinary frequency and nocturia. Digital rectal examination reveals a symmetrically enlarged, smooth and firm prostate. The most likely diagnosis is
   A. Prostate cancer
   B. Acute bacterial prostatitis
   C. Chronic bacterial prostatitis
   D. Benign prostatic hyperplasia
10. A patient with a history of intravenous drug use presents with fever, flank pain and costovertebral angle tenderness. Urinalysis is positive for leucocyte esterase and nitrite. The most likely diagnosis is
   A. Acute pyelonephritis
   B. Urolithiasis
   C. Bladder cancer
   D. Glomerulonephritis
11. A 20-year-old male presents with pain and swelling in the scrotum following a sports injury. Ultrasound shows an inhomogeneous testis with areas of increased and decreased echogenicity. The most likely diagnosis is
   A. Testicular torsion
   B. Testicular trauma
   C. Epididymitis
   D. Orchitis
12. A 50-year-old male with a smoking history presents with gross haematuria and irritative voiding symptoms. Cystoscopy reveals a papillary tumour in the bladder. The most likely diagnosis is
   A. Bladder cancer
   B. Acute cystitis
   C. Urolithiasis
   D. Benign prostatic hyperplasia
13. A patient presents with severe loin to groin pain, haematuria and nausea. Noncontrast CT scan shows a 6-mm calculus at the ureterovesical junction. The most likely diagnosis is
   A. Acute pyelonephritis
   B. Renal cell carcinoma
   C. Ureteral stone
   D. Bladder cancer

14. A 60-year-old male presents with a firm, irregular mass on the prostate. Serum PSA is markedly elevated. The most appropriate next step is
    A. Start androgen deprivation therapy.
    B. Perform immediate radical prostatectomy.
    C. Perform transrectal ultrasound-guided biopsy.
    D. Start 5-α reductase inhibitors.
15. A young adult presents with a tender, swollen, red scrotum and fever. Urinalysis is normal. The most likely diagnosis is
    A. Testicular torsion
    B. Orchitis
    C. Epididymitis
    D. Testicular cancer
16. A 45-year-old male presents with a history of recurrent urinary tract infections and a weak urinary stream. Imaging reveals a large bladder diverticulum. The most likely contributing factor is
    A. Bladder cancer
    B. Benign prostatic hyperplasia
    C. Neurogenic bladder
    D. Urethral stricture
17. A patient presents with nocturia, urgency and a sensation of incomplete bladder emptying. Uroflowmetry shows a decreased flow rate. The most likely diagnosis is
    A. Overactive bladder
    B. Urethral stricture
    C. Benign prostatic hyperplasia
    D. Neurogenic bladder
18. A 70-year-old male presents with bone pain and elevated alkaline phosphatase. Digital rectal examination reveals a nodular prostate. The most likely diagnosis is
    A. Prostatitis
    B. Prostate cancer with bone metastases
    C. Benign prostatic hyperplasia
    D. Bladder cancer
19. A 30-year-old male presents with painful urination and a mucopurulent urethral discharge. Gram stain shows gram-negative intracellular diplococci. The most likely diagnosis is
    A. Urethritis caused by *Neisseria gonorrhoeae*
    B. Urethritis caused by *Chlamydia trachomatis*
    C. Nonspecific urethritis
    D. Prostatitis
20. A patient presents with urinary retention and high post-void residual urine volume. The bladder is palpable above the pubic symphysis. The most likely diagnosis is
    A. Acute urinary retention
    B. Chronic urinary retention
    C. Bladder outlet obstruction
    D. Neurogenic bladder

Answers

1. (C); 2. (B); 3. (B); 4. (A); 5. (C); 6. (A); 7. (C); 8. (B); 9. (D); 10. (A); 11. (B); 12. (A); 13. (C); 14. (C); 15. (C); 16. (B); 17. (C); 18. (B); 19. (A); 20. (B)

Self-Assessment Questions

1. A 24-year-old man presented with an exophytic polypoidal growth over the shaft of the penis. Histopathologically, the lesion showed hyperplastic papillary squamous epithelium with koilocytic change. What is your diagnosis? What are the aetiology, recurrence rate and prognosis for this condition?
2. A 75-year-old male patient presented with gross haematuria and loin pain for the past 3 months. On cystoscopy, an exophytic papillary lesion involving the lateral and posterior walls of the bladder was seen. What is your diagnosis? What are the aetiopathogenesis and histological variants of the lesion?
3. A 6-month-old baby boy brought to the outpatient department (OPD) for routine vaccination was incidentally found to have an empty scrotal sac. What is your provisional diagnosis? What are subsequent investigations to be carried out? What are its gross and microscopic features?
4. A 48-year-old male patient presented with an exophytic fungating cauliflower-like mass over the shaft of the penis and glans. He complained of pain over the ulcer and occasional difficulty in passing urine. What is the probable diagnosis? How do you stage this condition?
5. A 35-year-old male patient presented with testicular swelling, which on examination was found to be a bulky, well-circumscribed solid mass measuring approximately 12 × 10 cm. On histopathological examination, the tumour showed poorly demarcated lobules containing sheets of large uniform cells with clear cytoplasm. What is your diagnosis? What are its histological variants? Name a few specific immunohistochemical markers for this tumour.
6. A 40-year-old male patient presented with painless enlargement of the testis, noticed 15 days ago. After a thorough evaluation, provisional diagnosis of testicular tumour was given and radical orchidectomy was performed. Gross examination revealed a solid grey-white tumour with areas of haemorrhage, necrosis, yellowish discoloration and cystic change at foci. What is your diagnosis? What are the possible histopathological components to be expected in such tumours? What is the incidence and diagnostic significance?
7. A 70-year-old male patient presented with difficulty in passing urine and occasional lower abdominal pain for the past few weeks. Per rectal examination showed nodular enlargement of the prostate gland. His PSA levels were 2.4 ng/mL. A biopsy was performed subsequently. What are the expected microscopic findings? What are the aetiopathogenesis and incidence of malignant transformation in this condition?
8. An 80-year-old male patient presented with excruciating pain in the lower spine, along with loss of weight and appetite for the past few weeks. Systematic examination revealed a diffusely enlarged prostate, predominantly the peripheral zone. PSA levels were 32 ng/mL. Radiological assessment showed multiple osteoblastic metabolically active lesions involving the lumbar and thoracic spine. What is your diagnosis? What is the morphological appearance? How will you grade and stage these tumours?
9. A 10-year-old girl was brought to the emergency department with complaints of sudden excruciating pain in the right side of the abdomen, radiating to the groin. A sonogram revealed a 1.2-cm calculus within the right ureter at the level of iliac vessels. What is your diagnosis, and what are the complications associated with this condition?

10. A 30-year-old female patient presented with occasional pain during micturition and lower abdominal pain. Urine examination was normal. On cystoscopy, an exophytic papillary growth, measuring 1 cm in diameter, with a definitive stalk was seen along the lateral wall of the bladder. The adjacent mucosa was unremarkable. The growth was excised and processed for histopathological examination. What is the diagnosis? What are the histopathological findings? What is the overall prognosis for this condition?

Answers

1. Condyloma acuminatum
2. Carcinoma of the urinary bladder
3. Cryptorchidism
4. Carcinoma of the penis
5. Seminoma testis
6. Mixed germ cell tumour of the testis
7. Benign prostatic hyperplasia
8. Prostatic carcinoma
9. Ureteric obstruction due to calculus
10. Urothelial papilloma

Topics for Self-Directed Learning

1. Vesical endometriosis
2. Ormond disease
3. Urachal carcinoma
4. Histopathological variants of prostatic adenocarcinoma
5. Splenogonadal fusion
6. Testicular torsion
7. Role of testicular biopsy in male infertility
8. IgG4-related diseases
9. Phimosis
10. Staging of penile carcinomas

The Female Genital Tract

26

Gayathri Devi Thanigaimani

PA 30.1 Describe the epidemiology, pathogenesis, aetiology, pathology, screening, diagnosis and progression of **carcinoma of the cervix.**

PA 30.2 Describe the pathogenesis, aetiology, pathology, diagnosis, progression and spread of **carcinoma of the endometrium.**

PA 30.3 Describe the pathogenesis, aetiology, pathology, diagnosis, progression and spread of **leiomyomas and leiomyosarcomas.**

PA 30.4 Classify and describe the aetiology, pathogenesis, pathology, morphology, clinical course, spread and complications of **ovarian tumours.**

PA 30.5 Describe the aetiology, pathogenesis, pathology, morphology, clinical course, spread and complications of **gestational trophoblastic neoplasms.**

PA 30.6 Describe the aetiology and morphological features of **cervicitis.**

PA 30.7 Describe the aetiology, hormonal dependence, features and morphology of **endometriosis.**

PA 30.8 Describe the aetiology and morphological features of **adenomyosis.**

PA 30.9 Describe the aetiology, hormonal dependence and morphology of **endometrial hyperplasia.**

CHAPTER OUTLINE

INTRODUCTION

The female genital tract is one of the greatest marvels of nature. It is the only organ in the body capable of forming and nurturing another life to perpetuate and sustain human race on this earth. No blessing comes without a clause, so there are many pathological diseases that may affect the female genital tract and in this chapter we shall see the pathogenesis and morphological changes of a few common conditions.

ANATOMY AND HISTOLOGY

The female genital tract predominantly develops from the Müllerian duct during embryological development. The two ducts on either side fuse in the midline to form the uterovaginal canal, the precursor of the uterine corpus and uterine cervix. This communicates to the exterior through the vagina, the lower part of which develops from an invagination called urogenital sinus. The ovaries develop from the mesothelium of the peritoneum and descend to their location in the pelvis. Let us review the anatomy and histology of the parts of the female genital tract before going on to study their pathology.

Vulva

Anatomy The vulva consists of the whole of the external genitalia including the perineum. The parts include the labia majora, Bartholin gland and labia minora.

Anteriorly, the labia minora enclose the clitoris, which corresponds to the penis in the male. The external urinary meatus lies posterior to the clitoris. The vaginal orifice, covered partially by the hymen, is located posterior to the urinary meatus.

Histology The labia majora and minora are lined by keratinizing stratified squamous epithelium. The majora have skin appendages, whereas the minora are devoid of them. Bartholin glands are composed of acini lined by low columnar epithelium. The ducts are lined by transitional epithelium that becomes squamous near the opening of the duct.

Vagina

Anatomy The vagina is the passage that connects the uterus to the vulval introitus. It is almost flask shaped, with the broad upper part containing the vaginal part of the cervix projecting into it. The vagina is attached to the cervix all circumferentially, with the posterior aspect being the highest, forming a deep posterior fornix.

Histology The vaginal wall is composed of three layers, namely mucosa, muscularis and adventitia. The mucosa is lined by nonkeratinizing stratified squamous epithelium cuboidal cells in the basal layer, prickle cells in the middle and cornified cells superficially. Notably, the subepithelial layer contains erectile tissue and blood vessels.

Cervix

Anatomy The uterus is divided into two portions – the uterine cervix and the uterine corpus. The cervix connects the uterus to the vagina. It is divided into *portio vaginalis* (the part protruding into the vagina) and supravaginal portion (the part above the vagina). The outer exposed surface of the cervix is called the *ectocervix or exocervix*, and the portion in the endocervical canal is called the *endocervix*. The cervix is bound by an *external os* (marking the junction of the ectocervix and the endocervix) and an *internal os* (which is the junction of the endocervix and the endometrium).

Histology The ectocervix is lined by nonkeratinizing squamous epithelium that is continuous with the vagina distally. It is composed of three layers – basal cell, midzone and superficial layer; the morphology of these layers varies with age and hormonal status. The endocervix is lined by a single layer of columnar mucin-secreting cells. The meeting of squamous epithelium with columnar epithelium is called the **squamocolumnar junction** (SCJ) and is located in the ectocervix. Owing to hormonal influence, the lower end of columnar epithelium may partly undergo squamous metaplasia, moving SCJ proximally into the endocervical canal. This zone between the original SCJ and the newly formed SCJ is called the **transformation zone** and is the area of high propensity to undergo malignant transformation due to the susceptibility of these immature squamous cells to human papillomavirus (HPV) infection.

Uterus

Anatomy (Fig. 26.1) The uterus is a pear-shaped organ that measures 7–8 cm along the longitudinal axis. The fallopian tubes enter the uterus on either side. The portion of the uterus above the line joining the fallopian tube orifices is called the *fundus*, the region below it *the body*, and the portion of the uterus at the junction with the cervix is called the *isthmus* or *lower uterine segment*. The wall of the uterus is composed of three layers – the endometrium (which is under hormonal influence), the myometrium (which comprises smooth muscles) and the serosal covering. The hollow cavity of the uterus is shaped like a triangle.

Histology The endometrium of the uterus is composed of stroma and endometrial glands. It is divided into a superficial functional layer and a deep basal layer. The glands and stroma of the functional layer respond to hormonal and ovulatory changes to prepare the endometrium to receive the ovum for implantation, if it has been fertilized. If the ovum is not fertilized, the endometrium is shed off as menstruation and the cycle of changes

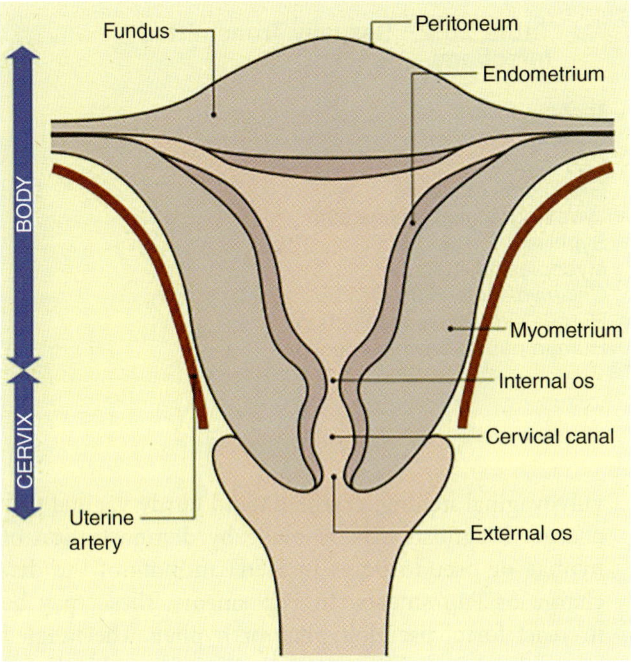

Fig. 26.1 Anatomy of the uterus. (*Source:* From Kamran Abbas, Suna D. Monaghan and Iain Campbell. Uterine physiology. Anaesthesia and Intensive Care Medicine. 2014;15:133-135.)

restarts. The basal layer, however, is made of reserve cells that help in regeneration of the endometrium and do not respond to progesterone levels.

Fallopian Tubes

Anatomy The tubes are about 11–12 cm in length and divided into four segments – the *intramural segment* (within the uterine wall), the *isthmus*, the *ampulla* (dilated portion where fertilisation occurs) and the *infundibulum* (the fimbriated opening into the peritoneal cavity).

Histology The mucosa is lined by ciliated columnar secretory epithelium thrown into folds called plicae. The underlying muscle coat consists of circular and longitudinal layers that help to differentiate the fallopian tubes from the round ligament microscopically.

Ovary

Anatomy The ovaries are paired pelvic organs, measuring about 4 × 2 × 1 cm, located on either side of the uterus. These are attached to the uterus by the ovarian ligament, to the broad ligament through the mesovarium and to the lateral pelvic wall through the infundibulopelvic ligament. These are composed of ovarian follicles that produce oocytes from menarche to menopause. The ovarian follicles may be seen in varying stages such as primordial follicle, maturing follicle, atretic follicle, corpus luteum and corpus albicans. The maturing follicle contains germ cells surrounded by granulosa cells and two layers of theca luteal cells that together produce oestrogen till ovulation. After ovulation, these form the corpus luteum and commence the production of progesterone. If fertilization and implantation do not occur, these cells are phagocytosed by macrophages and replaced by fibroblastic tissue, thereby forming corpus albicans.

Histology The ovary is covered by a single layer of epithelium called surface or *germinal epithelium*. The *stroma* within the ovary is composed of spindle cells resembling fibroblasts arranged in a *storiform* or a whorled pattern. Within the stroma, ovarian follicles in varying stages of development may be seen. Matured and ruptured follicles are represented by the *corpus luteum* and *corpus albicans* (Fig. 26.2).

Placenta

Anatomy The placenta is the organ that enables the survival of the fetus inside the mother's uterus. It serves as an interface between maternal and fetal circulation, enabling diffusion of nutrients, waste and gases. The placenta is made of a network of chorionic villi formed by sprouting

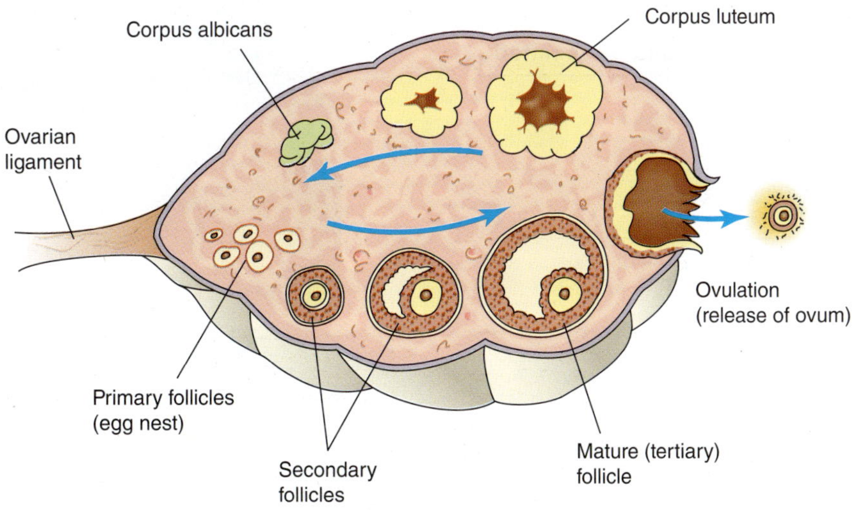

Fig. 26.2 Structure of the ovary.

from the chorion. The maternal blood bathes the outside of the villi. Blood from spiral arteries of the endometrium enters the intervillous space and after the transfer of substances drains into the endometrial veins. On the fetal side, deoxygenated blood enters the placenta through the umbilical arteries, runs through villus vessels and after oxygenation returns back through the umbilical vein.

Histology The cut section of the umbilical cord shows two arteries and one vein. The fetal surface of the placenta is smooth and is covered by membranes, whereas the maternal side is irregular and is divided into cotyledons. Microscopically, numerous villi composed of blood vessels, fibroblasts and macrophages can be seen loosely arranged within a trophoblastic lining. The trophoblasts are of two types – the cytotrophoblasts (which are small round cells with distinct cell membrane, moderate clear to pink cytoplasm and a single vesicular nucleus) and the syncytotrophoblasts (multinucleated large cells with abundant cytoplasm containing vacuoles and a dense nucleus).

INFECTIONS

The female genital tract is a common site of attack for various organisms. Common infections and the organisms associated are shown in Table 26.1.

Although most infections are acquired through sexual transmission and ascending infection (Table 26.2), a few such as mycobacterial infections may be blood-borne.

Infections of the Lower Genital Tract

- **Candidiasis:** Vaginal candidiasis is a condition that reflects the imbalance of vaginal flora and therefore is more common among diabetic patients, pregnant females and those with other conditions of immunosuppression. Affected individuals present with intense vulvovaginal itching, erythema and curdy vaginal discharge. Diagnosis can be made by demonstration of hyphae or pseudospores in KOH mounts of the discharge or Pap smears. In Pap smears, these may be in yeast form, pseudohyphae or hyphae. The tangled pseudohyphae and yeast form give a **'spaghetti and meat ball'** appearance, whereas adherence of squamous cells around pseudohyphae may give a **'shish kebab'** appearance.
- **Trichomoniasis:** It is caused by *Trichomonas vaginalis*, which is a pear-shaped flagellated organism that is sexually transmitted. Patients complain of yellow discharge, dysuria and dyspareunia. In colposcopy, the cervical mucosa appears reddish, with dilated veins giving the appearance of **strawberry cervix** (Fig. 26.3). In the Pap smear, these are seen as pear-shaped organisms with a single flagellum. These are about twice the size of an intermediate cell nucleus, and contain an eccentrically placed nucleus and cytoplasm with red granules.

Table 26.1 Organisms Causing Common Genital Tract Infections

Category	Common Organisms Associated
Organisms causing **lower tract infection**	*Candida* Trichomonas Gardnerella
Organisms that cause **infertility**	*Neisseria gonorrhoeae* Chlamydia
Organisms that cause **preterm delivery**	*Ureaplasma urealyticum* Mycoplasma hominis
Organisms that cause **painful ulcers**	Herpes simplex viruses
Organisms that predispose to **cancer**	Human papillomaviruses

Table 26.2 Sexually Transmitted Infections

Trichomoniasis
Gonorrhoea
Chancroid
Granuloma inguinale
Lymphogranuloma venereum
Syphilis
Mycoplasma infection
Chlamydia infection
Herpes simplex virus infection
Human papillomavirus infection

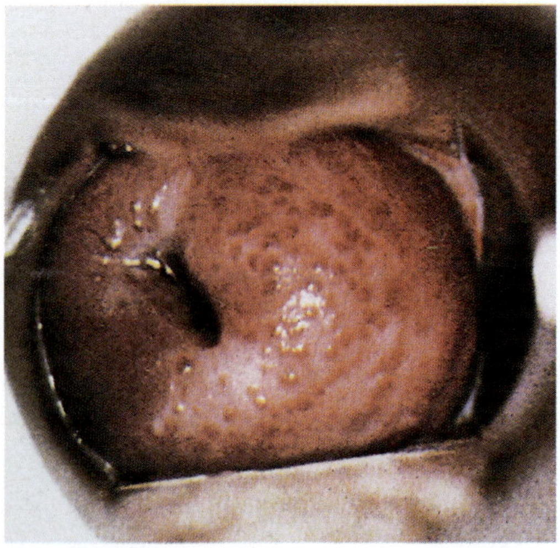

Fig. 26.3 Strawberry cervix – inflamed vaginal mucosa with petechial lesions. (*Source:* From Jane W. Ball, Joyce E. Dains, John A. Flynn, Barry S. Solomon and Rosalyn W. Stewart. Female Genitalia. Seidel's Guide to Physical Examination. 9th edition. Elsevier 2019.)

- **Bacterial vaginosis:** *Gardnerella vaginalis* is a gram-negative bacillus that causes bacterial vaginosis, and the infected patients present with thin, green-grey vaginal discharge with fishy odour. Pap smears show **clue cells** (Fig. 26.4), which are superficial or intermediate squamous cells coated by coccobacilli. Bacterial vaginosis is particularly important in pregnant women because it may cause premature labour.
- **Herpes simplex:** Genital herpes is predominantly caused by herpes simplex virus (HSV) 2 and affects the cervix, vagina and vulva in the decreasing order of frequency. It is acquired by sexual transmission and causes fever, malaise and tender inguinal lymph nodes, followed by genital lesions starting as papule and turning into painful ulcers. Infection of the vagina and cervix may present as vaginal discharge with intense itching, whereas urethral lesions may cause dysuria. The infection may resolve, but the virus remains latent in the lumbosacral ganglia and may get reactivated during stress or in an immunocompromised state. Furthermore, pregnant women with active herpes infection in labour can spread the infection to the newborn during the passage through the birth canal. Prevention of neonatal HSV infection by caesarean section is important in such cases.

Cytopathological studies on the vaginal discharge can identify herpesvirus-infected cells as multinucleated giant cells with ground glass cytoplasm that may contain viral inclusions (Fig. 26.5). Tissue culture can demonstrate the cytopathic effect of the virus. Serology may be helpful in detecting recurrent or latent infection because antibodies are absent in primary infection. Treatment with antiviral agents possibly shortens the course of the disease and reduces its severity.

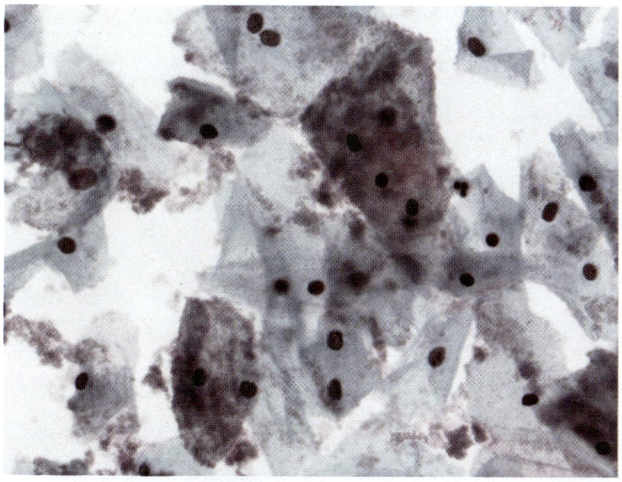

Fig. 26.4 Pap smear showing clue cells, a characteristic feature of *Gardnerella vaginalis* infection. (*Source:* From Sanjiv Manek and Sunanda Dhar. Infections in the gynaecological tract. Diagnostic Histopathology. 2020; 26:575–580.)

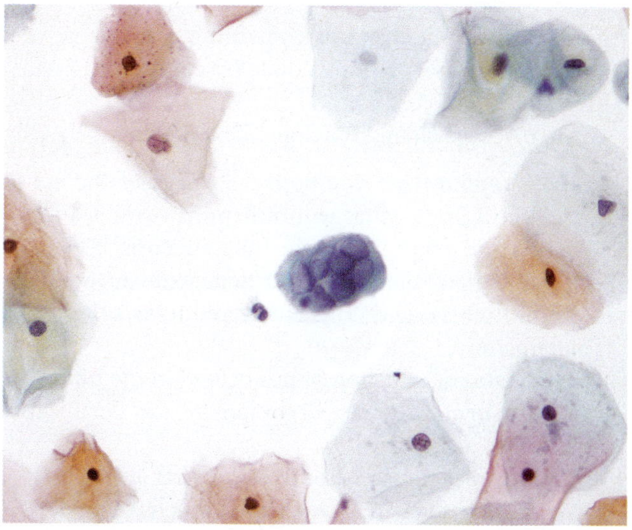

Fig. 26.5 Cervical smear showing HSV infection – multinucleated cell in the centre with ground glass nuclei that contain viral inclusions. (*Source:* From Lora Hedrick Ellenson and Edyta C. Pirog. The Female Genital Tract. Robbins & Cotran Pathologic Basis of Disease. 10th edition. Elsevier 2021.)

Infections of the Upper Genital Tract

Infection of the upper genital tract is referred to as **pelvic inflammatory disease (PID)** and involves infection of most of the structures of the female genital system, causing fever, pelvic pain, adnexal tenderness and vaginal discharge. The common causative agents are *Neisseria gonorrhoeae*, followed by *Chlamydia* and polymicrobia (such as streptococci, staphylococci, *Clostridium perfringens*) causing puerperal infections after events associated with pregnancy and labour.

Gonorrhoea *N. gonorrhoeae* causes ascending infection that may begin in the endocervical mucosa or Bartholin glands and spreads upward, skips the uterus and affects the fallopian tubes, culminating into a tubo-ovarian mass. The complications of PID are enumerated in Table 26.3.

Morphology

Acute inflammatory changes in gonococcal infection involve the mucosa. Inflammatory exudate shows

Table 26.3 Acute and Chronic Complications of Pelvic Inflammatory Disease

Acute Complications	Chronic Complications
Peritonitis	Infertility by tubal obstruction
Septicaemia	Ectopic pregnancy
Endocarditis	Chronic pelvic pain
Meningitis	Adhesions causing intestinal obstruction
Suppurative arthritis	

predominantly neutrophils containing gram-negative diplococci. Confirmation is done by culture or DNA/RNA detection.

Microscopic changes include the following:

- ***Acute suppurative salpingitis:*** Damage of the epithelium lining occurs with inflammatory cell infiltration and exudation in the tubal mucosa.
- Tubal lumen filled with purulent exudate oozing out of fimbrial end: This is referred to as ***salpingo-oophoritis***.
- ***Pyosalpinx:*** Collection of pus occurs in the tubes.
- ***Tubo-ovarian abscess:*** Collection of pus occurs in the tubes and ovary.
- Healing may cause ***chronic salpingitis*** and the reparative changes in the damaged mucosa may lead to narrowing of lumen and infertility.
- Fimbrial end may get obstructed during the healing process, causing ***hydrosalpinx*** good.

Treatment Antibiotics may help to resolve infection in early stages. If the patient develops a tubo-ovarian mass, surgical intervention may be required.

VULVA

BARTHOLIN CYST

Obstruction of the mouth of Bartholin duct by inflammation may cause collection of fluid and cyst formation within the duct. The cysts are usually lined by transitional or squamous epithelium. When the size of cysts increases to about 3–5 cm, the patient may present with discomfort or pain. Treatment includes surgical excision or marsupialization of the cyst. Occasional infection of the gland may lead to Bartholin abscess.

CONDYLOMA ACUMINATUM

Condyloma acuminata are genital warts caused by *HPV 6 and 11.*

Morphology

Condyloma acuminata are usually multifocal and found on the vulva, perineum and perianal region. They may however involve the vagina and cervix also. They are benign and not precancerous.

Microscopy shows that these are papillary exophytic lesions with branching cores of stroma covered by stratified squamous epithelium that may show ***koilocytic changes*** such as perinuclear halo, nuclear enlargement and hyperchromasia.

PAPILLARY HIDRADENOMA

Papillary hidradenoma is a tumour of the vulvar region, which is thought to originate from ectopic mammary tissue because of its close resemblance to intraductal papilloma of the breast. Papillary hidradenomas are mostly benign and present as a well-circumscribed small nodule that may ulcerate.

Morphology

Microscopically, as the name suggests, papillary hidradenomas are composed of a complex branching papillary structure lined by a layer of columnar epithelium with an underlying layer of myoepithelium and may show nuclear pleomorphism and mitotic activity (Fig. 26.6).

EXTRAMAMMARY PAGET DISEASE

Extramammary Paget disease of the vulva is a malignant tumour mostly arising from adnexal stem cells located along the hair follicles and other adnexal structures. Unlike Paget disease of the breast, it is not associated with an underlying malignancy and is mostly confined to the epidermis. Clinically, patients present with an elevated, crusting or scaling erythematous map-like lesion on the vulva.

Morphology

Microscopically, large tumour cells in nests or singles or a continuous layer within the normal epithelial cells can be seen (Fig. 26.7). The cells have clear or pale cytoplasm with nuclear pleomorphism. Tumours cells

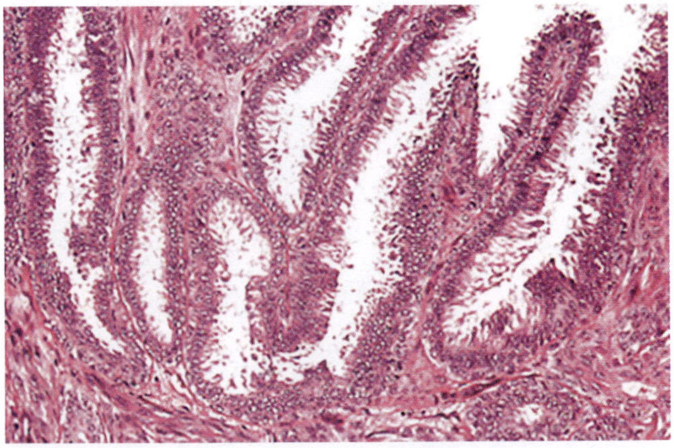

Fig. 26.6 Histology of papillary hidradenoma showing a complex papillary architecture with each papilla lined by double-layered epithelium. (*Source:* From Nooshin K. Brinster, Vincent Liu, A. Hafeez Diwan, Phillip H. McKee. Hidradenoma Papilliferum. In Dermatopathology. Elsevier 2011.)

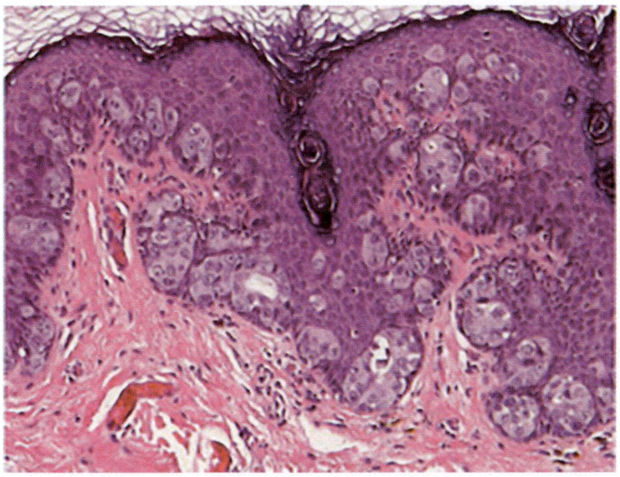

Fig. 26.7 Histology of extramammary Paget disease showing the presence of nests of neoplastic cells within the epithelium. (*Source:* From Renee A. Cowan, Destin R. Black, Lien N. Hoang, Kay J. Park, Robert A. Soslow, Floor J. Backes, Ginger J. Gardner, Nadeem R. Abu-Rustum, Mario M. Leitao, Eric L. Eisenhauer and Dennis S. Chi. A pilot study of topical imiquimod therapy for the treatment of recurrent extramammary Paget's disease. Gynecologic Oncology. 2016;142:139–143.)

contain abundant mucin that can be identified by special stains such as PAS and Alcian blue.

Immunohistochemistry (IHC): Lesions are typically $CK7^+/CK20^-$.

Treatment is by surgical excision. The extent of the disease is microscopically wider than the clinical lesion, and this must be borne in mind because recurrence may occur if incompletely excised. The rare presence of an associated underlying malignancy worsens the prognosis.

VULVAR INTRAEPITHELIAL NEOPLASIA AND CARCINOMA

Vulvar carcinomas are rare lesions contributing to a small (3%) number of female genital tract cancers. These occur in the older age group, older than 50 years, and are often squamous cell carcinomas. Based on their origin and microscopic findings, these are classified into two types as given in Table 26.4.

The risk of malignancy from precursor lesions depends on the duration of the disease and the immune status of the woman. After development of malignancy, prognosis depends on the size of the lesion, depth of invasion and lymph node status. The common nodes involved include the inguinal and pelvic nodes, followed by the iliac and para-aortic nodes. Metastasis to the lung and liver may occur. Treatment is by surgery, vulvectomy with lymph node dissection, but prognosis is poor.

VAGINA

VAGINAL INTRAEPITHELIAL NEOPLASIA AND CARCINOMA

Vaginal carcinomas are squamous cell carcinomas that arise due to spread from cervical squamous carcinoma or as a primary carcinoma of the vagina. In both instances, the predisposing factor is high-risk infection with HPV such as HPV 16 and 18 and the incidence put together constitutes only 1% of female genital tract carcinomas. Primary carcinoma of the vulva may be associated with the precursor lesion, vaginal carcinoma in situ. The most common site of malignancy is the posterior aspect of the upper vagina near the junction with the ectocervix.

Table 26.4 Differences Between Basaloid/Warty Carcinoma and Squamous Cell Carcinoma of the Vulva

Feature	Basaloid and Warty Carcinomas	Keratinizing Squamous Cell Carcinomas
Aetiology	High-risk HPV (HPV 16 & 18)	Not related to HPV infection
Age group	Sixth decade	Eighth decade
Risk factors	Young age at first intercourse, multiple sexual partners, male partner with multiple sexual partners	TP53 mutations
Precursor lesion	Classical VIN including Bowen disease	Differentiated VIN
Microscopy	Classic VIN – increased thickness of epithelium with nuclear pleomorphism, hyperchromasia, lack of differentiation and increased mitosis	Differentiated VIN – atypia of the basal layer with a normal-appearing superficial layer
	Basaloid carcinoma shows nests of basaloid cells that lack differentiation with or without central necrosis; warty carcinoma shows papillary structures and koilocytic changes	Invasive carcinoma shows tongues of malignant squamous epithelium invading the stroma and the presence of abundant keratin pearls

HPV, human papillomavirus; VIN, vulval intraepithelial neoplasia.

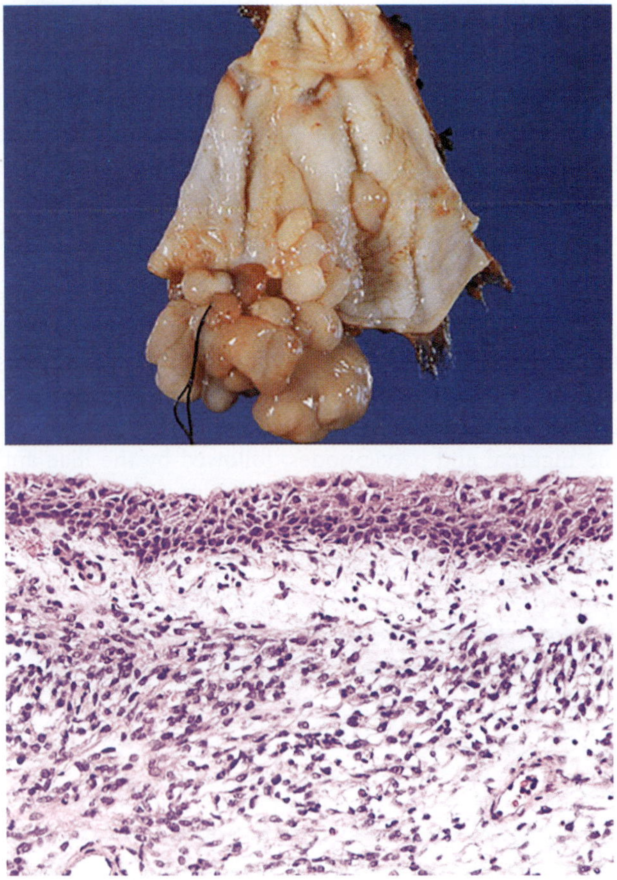

Fig. 26.8 Embryonal rhabdomyosarcoma, gross of excised tumour showing grape-like clusters and microscopy showing the characteristic cambium layer of cells in the submucosa beneath a zone of loose stroma. (*Source:* From Blake Gilks. Vagina. Rosai and Ackerman's Surgical Pathology. 11th edition. Elsevier 2018; Christopher P. Crum, Anna R. Laury, Michelle S. Hirsch, Charles Matthew Quick and William A. Peters. Embryonal Rhabdomyosarcoma. Gynecologic and Obstetric Pathology. Saunders 2016.)

EMBRYONAL RHABDOMYOSARCOMA

Embryonal rhabdomyosarcoma is a rare vaginal tumour that commonly presents in infants and children younger than 5 years as polypoid or round masses protruding from the vagina. These are grape-like in consistency and appearance and hence also called **sarcoma botryoides** (Fig. 26.8).

Morphology

Microscopically, the tumour is composed of **tennis racket–shaped cells** that have oval nuclei and a cytoplasmic protrusion on one end. These cells lie singularly in the loose stroma but tend to crowd around blood vessels and also form a distinct layer beneath the epidermis called **cambium layer**, which is a characteristic feature of this neoplasm.

The tumour may penetrate into the peritoneum by local invasion and cause death. Early diagnosis with surgical treatment and chemotherapy may be helpful.

CERVIX

ACUTE AND CHRONIC CERVICITIS PA 30.6

Inflammation of the cervix is a very common event, as detected in Pap smears and biopsies. Acute and chronic cervicitis is usually asymptomatic and does not have any serious consequence to the individual. However, its knowledge is important because it may sometimes obscure evidence of early precancerous changes.

Protective mechanisms in the cervix: The cervix has protective mechanisms to prevent infection by microorganisms. After menarche, the ovaries start producing oestrogen. This oestrogen stimulates the formation of glycogen within the cervical squamous cells, which appear as empty vacuoles on routine staining. These cells when shed provide the substrate for the growth of aerobic bacteria in the vagina, the most important among them being lactobacilli. The lactobacilli use the glycogen and produce lactic acid that lowers the vaginal pH, making the environment unfavourable for other pathogenic bacteria. Furthermore, the acidic environment enables the lactobacilli to produce hydrogen peroxide, which is a bacteriotoxic agent. Failure of this mechanism results in acute and chronic cervicitis.

Failure of protective mechanisms (Fig. 26.9): The change of cervical and vaginal environment to alkaline pH is associated with an increased risk of infection. This may be due to reduced oestrogen (menopause), alkaline countersecretions (bleeding, sexual intercourse, vaginal douching) or elimination of lactobacilli (antibiotic therapy).

Consequences include the following:

- Asymptomatic inflammation of no clinical relevance

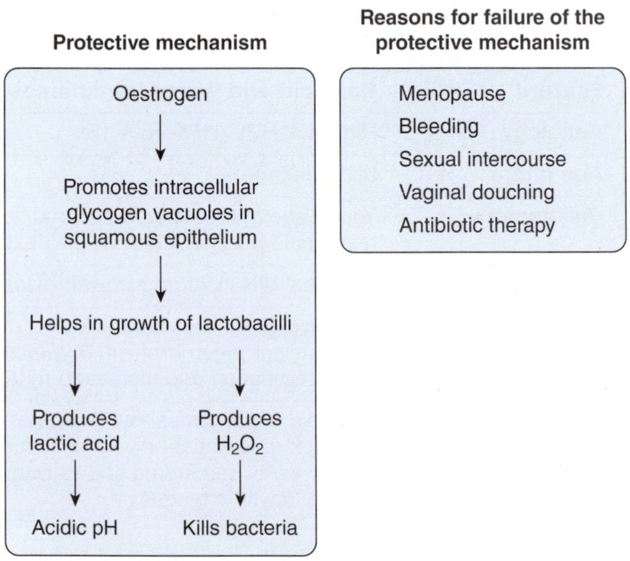

Fig. 26.9 Protective and failure mechanisms for cervicitis.

- Infection by virulent organisms leading to PID
- Reactive changes in epithelial cells leading to misinterpretation of Pap smears

Symptomatic patients may need evaluation with microbiological swabs to determine the nature of infection to check for PID. Pap smears with significant inflammation may be repeated after treating the infection, if any suspicion is raised by the clinician or reporting pathologist.

ENDOCERVICAL POLYPS

Endocervical polyps are benign polypoidal exophytic growths arising from the endocervical lining. These may protrude through the external os as small to large reddish masses and may cause irregular vaginal bleeding, postmenopausal bleeding or postcoital bleeding, thereby mimicking the symptoms of carcinoma. Treatment is by simple excision with or without curettage.

Microscopically, these polyps consist of squamous epithelial lining enclosing a fibromyxomatous stroma containing interspersed dilated endocervical glands.

TUMOURS OF THE CERVIX

Origin, Histology and Prevention of Cancer of the Cervix PA 30.1

Squamous cell carcinoma of the cervix is the most common cancer of this region. The aetiology of this cancer has been shown to have significant association with HPV. Hence, it is important to study about HPV and its role before we venture into studying about cancer of the cervix and its prevention.

Role of HPV in Cervical Neoplastic Changes

HPV is a DNA virus that is typed and named based on its DNA sequence. This virus is classified into high-risk and low-risk types based on its association with malignant transformation. There are 15 high-risk viruses, of which HPV 16 accounts for 60% and HPV 18 for 10% of cervical cancer cases. Apart from cervical cancer, the virus is also associated with squamous cell carcinomas of other sites such as the vagina, vulva, anus, penis, tonsil and other oropharyngeal locations. HPV is a sexually transmitted virus with a higher risk in women with early age of coitus, multiple sexual partners, pregnancy at a younger age (younger than 20 years), coexistent sexually transmitted infections and immunosuppression.

HPV can infect only the basal epithelium and immature epithelium. This makes the transformation zone an easy target to HPV infection, because in the other areas of mature epithelium, there has to be a break in the superficial epithelial cells for HPV to be able to reach the basal layer.

Pathogenesis of HPV Infection Normal RB gene prevents proliferation of cells in the absence of growth signals, and p53 gene stops proliferation of cells with altered or defective DNA. HPV infects immature cells and continues to replicate in maturing cells by the following mechanisms:

- Producing E6 protein that inhibits the p53 gene
- Producing E7 protein that inhibits the Rb gene
- Inhibiting CDK inhibitors p21 and p27
- Dysregulating oncogenes such as MYC due to fusion of viral DNA with host DNA

This results in uncontrolled proliferation of cells that may acquire additional mutations and transform into a neoplasm. However, there has to be additional factors that contribute to this transformation such as cocarcinogens and host immunosuppression. The role of HPV in the development of cervical cancer has been discussed in greater detail in Chapter 7.

Cervical Intraepithelial Neoplasia

The classification of cervical intraepithelial neoplasia (CIN) has changed over the decades from low-grade/high-grade dysplasia to a three-tiered CIN classification to the current two-tiered system that is more relevant from the clinical perspective. The squamous intraepithelial lesions (SILs) are classified into low-grade SILs (LSIL) and high-grade SILs (HSIL). The comparison of terminologies of the three classifications is given in Table 26.5.

LSILs are more common and have a higher replicative rate of virus but have a very low propensity to undergo malignant transformation. These usually regress and are not considered premalignant. HSILs are less common and have a lower replicative rate but cause greater proliferation of epithelial cells and affect their maturation resulting in malignant transformation. About 80% of LSILs and 100% of HSILs are associated with high-risk HPV, the majority being **HPV 16**. HSILs may arise from LSILs or less commonly develop de novo. Their malignant transformation is also influenced by additional factors but takes about a decade.

Table 26.5 Terminologies Used in Cervical Intraepithelial Neoplasia

Dysplasia/Carcinoma In Situ	CIN	SIL, Current Classification
Mild dysplasia	CIN I	LSIL
Moderate dysplasia	CIN II	HSIL
Severe dysplasia	CIN III	HSIL
Carcinoma in situ	CIN III	HSIL

CIN, cervical intraepithelial neoplasia; HSIL, high-grade SIL; LSIL, low-grade SIL; SIL, squamous intraepithelial lesion.

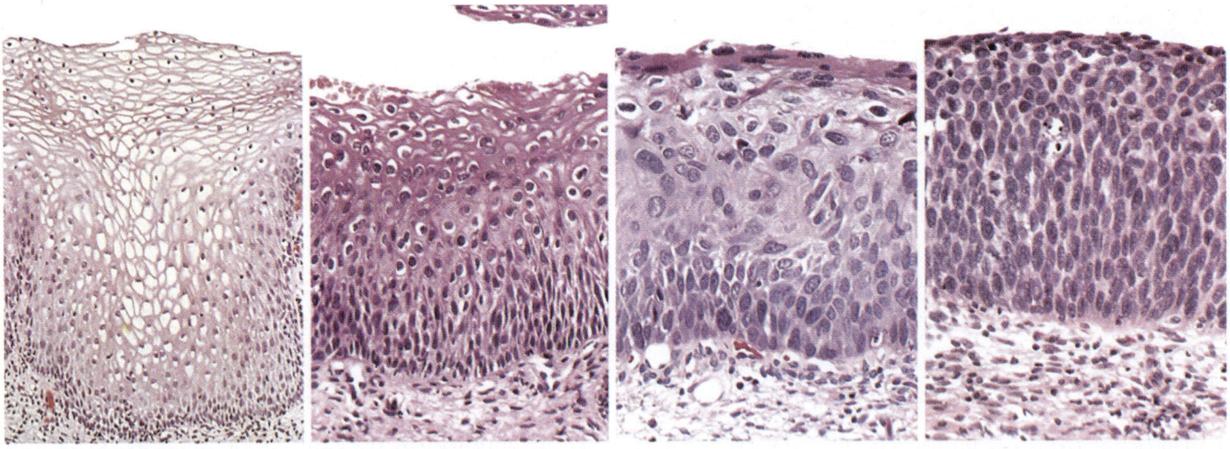

Fig. 26.10 Spectrum of cervical intraepithelial neoplasia: normal squamous epithelium for comparison; low-grade squamous intraepithelial lesion (cervical intraepithelial neoplasia [CIN] I) with koilocytic atypia (vacoulated cytoplasm with prune-like nucleus); high-grade squamous intraepithelial lesion (HSIL) (CIN II) with progressive atypia and expansion of the immature basal cells above the lower third of the epithelial thickness; HSIL (CIN III) with diffuse atypia, loss of maturation and expansion of the immature basal cells to the epithelial surface. (*Source:* From Lora Hedrick Ellenson and Edyta C. Pirog. The Female Genital Tract. Robbins & Cotran Pathologic Basis of Disease. 10th edition. Elsevier 2021.)

Morphology

The histological diagnosis of HPV is based on features collectively called **koilocytic atypia** caused by E4 protein of HPV. It includes the following:

- Perinuclear vacuolation
- Irregularly stained peripheral cytoplasm
- Prune-like nucleus with hyperchromatism and pleomorphism
- Rope-like chromatin
- Multinucleation or binucleation

Based on the extent of epithelium showing these changes, these are classified into high or low grade (Fig. 26.10):

Lower one-third involved: **LSIL**
Upper two-thirds involved: **HSIL**

IHC: **Ki-67** is a proliferative marker that is normally expressed only by the basal layer cells. In HSILs, the cells in the superficial layers also express Ki-67 along with p**16**.

Cervical Carcinoma

Cervical carcinoma has been showing increased incidence across the globe and now ranks as the fourth common cancer in women. It is the second most common cancer in Indian women, next only to breast cancer. Notably, its incidence has been declining in the developing countries due to effective screening programmes and improvement in hygiene and living conditions. However, the incidence in developing and underdeveloped countries is yet to show this trend. Apart from the incidence, the mortality rate of affected patients in the developing countries is also higher than that in developed countries. The average age of cervical carcinoma is about 45 years, which is about a decade or more from the common occurrence of CIN.

The common malignancies of the cervix include the following:

- Squamous carcinoma (80%)
- Adenocarcinoma from adenocarcinoma in situ (precursor lesion) (15%)
- Adenosquamous carcinoma
- Neuroendocrine carcinoma

Aetiology Infection with HPV is an essential event in the development of cervical carcinoma as discussed earlier. However, the progression of HPV infection through the stages of dysplasia, carcinoma in situ to invasive cervical carcinoma is variable in individuals and may be influenced by bacterial factors and host factors.

Bacterial factors: High-risk HPV produce E6 and E7 to inactivate p53 and Rb, respectively.
Host factors: These include immunodeficiency states such as HIV infection, long-term use of oral contraceptives, tobacco smoking, high parity and sexually transmitted infections such as *Chlamydia* infection.

Morphology (Fig. 26.11)

On gross examination, the tumour may be seen as an exophytic growth or may be an infiltrative neoplasm, with the latter more likely to invade surrounding structures.

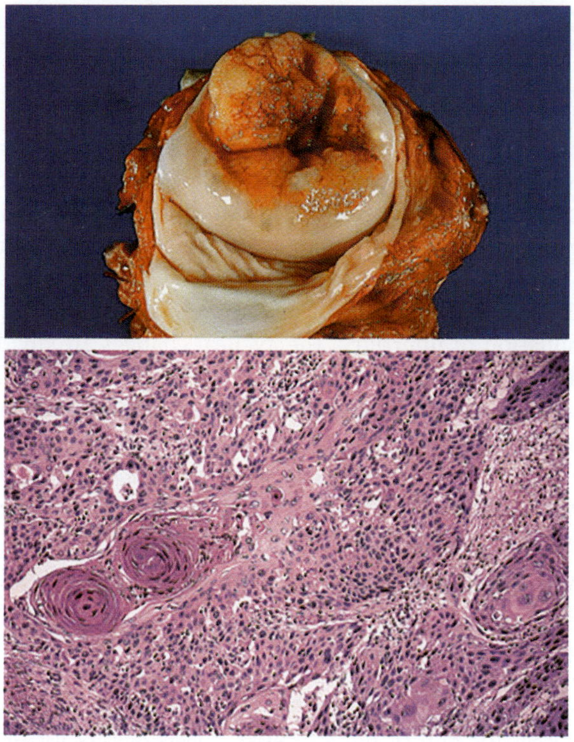

Fig. 26.11 Gross and microscopic images (show nests of neoplastic squamous cells and keratin pearls) of squamous cell carcinoma of the cervix. (*Source:* From Blake Gilks. Uterus: Cervix. Rosai and Ackerman's Surgical Pathology. 11th edition. Elsevier 2018.)

Microscopic examination may show the following features:

Squamous carcinoma: Tongues of malignant squamous cells with a pleomorphic nucleus invading the underlying stroma are present. Keratin pearls may also be seen.
Adenocarcinoma: Proliferating glands with epithelium lining have a hyperchromatic pleomorphic nucleus and lack of mucin in the cytoplasm.
Adenosquamous carcinoma shows a mixture of both components.
Neuroendocrine carcinoma is composed of small round blue cells similar to small cell carcinoma of the lungs.

Clinical Symptoms The common symptoms produced by an exophytic growth include irregular vaginal bleeding and discharge. Involvement of the ureters by lateral growth of the tumour may cause anuria. Involvement of the sciatic plexus in growths infiltrating the parametrium may cause sciatic pain. Involvement of the bladder in anterior spreads may cause urinary symptoms, whereas involvement of the rectum in posterior infiltrating growths may cause bowel symptoms.

The staging system that is used is TNM staging, and the tumour grade (T) in the TNM stage (Table 26.6) is similar to the staging system used earlier called the FIGO (International Federation of Gynaecology and Obstetrics). The

Table 26.6 Staging of Carcinoma of the Cervix

Stage	Description
I	The carcinoma is strictly confined to the cervix (extension to the uterine corpus should be disregarded)
IA	Invasive carcinoma that can be diagnosed only by microscopy, with maximum depth of invasion <5 mm
IB	Invasive carcinoma with measured deepest invasion ≥5 mm (greater than stage IA), lesion to the cervix uteri
II	The carcinoma invades beyond the uterus but has not extended onto the lower third of the vagina or to the pelvic wall
IIA	Involvement limited to the upper two-thirds of the vagina without parametrial involvement
IIB	With parametrial involvement but not up to the pelvic wall
III	Carcinoma involves the lower third of the vagina and/or extends to the pelvic wall and/or causes hydronephrosis or nonfunctioning kidney and/or involves pelvic and/or para-aortic lymph nodes
IV	The carcinoma has extended beyond the true pelvis or has involved (biopsy proven) the mucosa of the bladder or rectum

Source: Reproduced from FIGO staging of cancer of the cervix uteri (2018). https://obgyn.onlinelibrary.wiley.com/journal/18793479.

nodal status and metastases status are mentioned separately as N and M as given in Table 26.7. By combining these three categories (T, N and M), the final staging of the tumour can be obtained in the TNM staging system.

Treatment Microinvasive carcinomas can be treated by conservative surgeries such as cone excision. Invasive carcinomas are treated with more extensive surgery with or without radiotherapy/chemotherapy based on the stage of the tumour. Prognosis of the tumour worsens when it extends beyond the true pelvis, and death is more often due to local extension than due to metastasis.

Table 26.7 Nodal and Metastasis Stages of Cervical Cancer

	Regional lymph nodes (N)
Nx	Regional lymph nodes cannot be assessed
N0	No regional lymph node metastasis
N1	Regional lymph node metastasis (FIGO IIIB)
	Distant metastasis (M)
M0	No distant metastasis
M1	Distant metastasis (including peritoneal spread, involvement of supraclavicular, mediastinal or para-aortic lymph nodes, lung, liver or bone) – FIGO IV B

Screening and Prevention of Cervical Carcinoma

Screening for cervical cancer has markedly reduced the incidence of cervical cancer and related deaths. The ease of the procedure, high sensitivity, cost-effectiveness and time gap between the development of precancerous changes and the development of malignancy have made this possible. The screening methods include the following:

- Pap smear, which is the cytological study of exfoliated cells and scrapings of the cervix
- HPV DNA detection, which has high sensitivity but low specificity

Various screening protocols are followed in different countries. It is generally recommended to start Pap smear screening at 21 years or within 3 years of start of sexual activity (Flowchart 26.1).

- If any abnormality is detected on the Pap smear, a colposcopy is recommended, followed by the acetoacetic acid test in which the abnormal areas appear white and may be biopsied for confirmation. Depending on the severity and the invasion status, ablation or cone excision is performed with careful monitoring and follow-up.
- Currently, vaccines against HPV 16 and 18 are available and are recommended in boys and girls at the age of 11–12 years and also in all men and women until 26 years of age. The vaccine is expected to offer protection for 10 years. Cervical screening should be continued irrespective of vaccine status because vaccine does not offer protection from other high-risk HPV strains.

We shall be discussing more about Pap smear methods and cytological features in chapter 11, 'Basic diagnostic cytology and clinical pathology'.

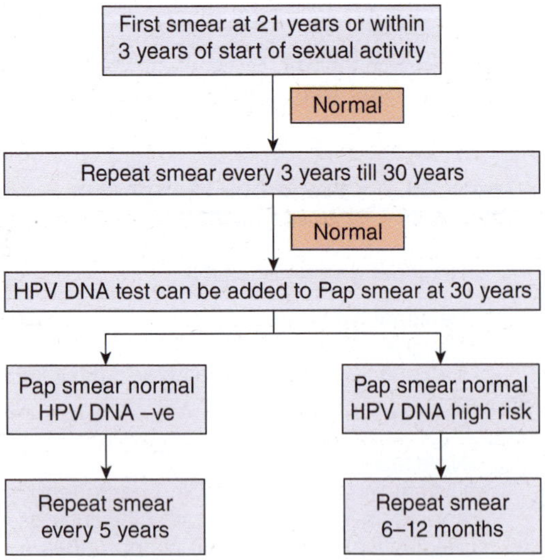

Flowchart 26.1 Protocol for pap smear screening.

ENDOMETRIUM AND BODY OF THE UTERUS

DATING OF ENDOMETRIUM

The uterine endometrium undergoes cyclical changes in response to the hormonal changes of the menstrual cycle, which, in turn, depend on ovulation by the ovary and formation of corpus luteum. Studying the endometrial tissue helps in detecting these cyclic changes and determining the occurrence of ovulation, especially useful in evaluation of infertility. The cyclical changes are divided into proliferative phase and secretory phase and are dominated by oestrogen and progesterone influence, respectively. The presence of secretory changes in the endometrium indicates that ovulation has occurred and progesterone-secreting corpus luteum has been formed. The changes according to the phases are reflected in Table 26.8.

DYSFUNCTIONAL UTERINE BLEEDING

Normal menstruation refers to bleeding in an ovulatory cycle at the end of the secretory phase, lasting for up to 5 days. Any bleeding not fitting into this definition is called **abnormal uterine bleeding**. This is usually associated with lesions such as polyps, endometriosis, submucosal fibroids or cancer. Abnormal uterine bleeding in the absence of any identifiable anatomical cause is called **dysfunctional uterine bleeding (DUB)**. It is attributed to an imbalance or irregularity in the pituitary or ovarian

Table 26.8 Phase-Wise Histological Changes Seen in the Endometrium (Fig. 26.12)

Phase	Histological Features
Menstrual phase	• Endometrial glands and aggregates of stromal cells with necrosis, inflammatory cells and haemorrhage
Proliferative phase	• Glands grow from short to tall and tubular with mitotic figures, lined by columnar epithelium, and later become tortuous with pseudostratification • Stroma goes from dense compact to moderately dense
Ovulation	• Endometrial proliferation stops and differentiation starts
Secretory phase	• Vacuoles filled with secretion begin to appear at the base of the cell, gradually move to the top and discharge the secretions within the lumen of the gland in the late secretory phase • The stroma becomes oedematous and develops spiral arterioles • Towards the end, predecidual changes occur with neutrophilic infiltration

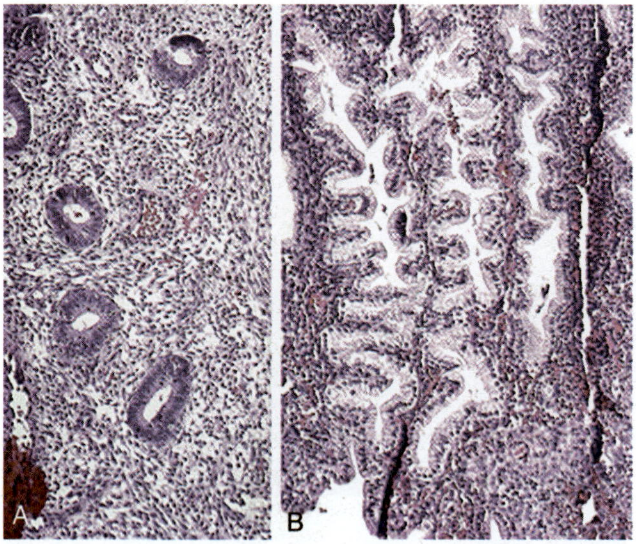

Fig. 26.12 Proliferative phase endometrium (A) showing small round glands in dense stroma and secretory phase endometrium (B) showing convoluted glands lined by columnar cells containing vacuoles in histology. (*Source:* From Blake Gilks. Uterus: Corpus. Rosai and Ackerman's Surgical Pathology. 11th edition. Elsevier 2018.)

hormonal production. The causes of DUB are different in ovulatory and anovulatory cycles.

DUB in the ovulatory group

The causes of DUB in the ovulatory group are as follows:

- Inadequate proliferative phase
- Inadequate secretory phase
- Irregular shedding of endometrium

DUB in the anovulatory group

The cause of DUB in the anovulatory cycle is due to the unopposed action of oestrogen. Ovulation is necessary for transformation of Graafian follicles into progesterone-secreting corpus luteum. In the absence of ovulation, the lack of progesterone predisposes to continuous unrelenting effects of oestrogen on the endometrium. This may cause glandular proliferation, cystic dilation and even endometrial hyperplasia.

The causes of anovulation include the following:

- Endocrine disorders such as thyroid, pituitary and adrenal gland disorders/tumours
- Ovarian hormone–secreting tumours and lesions such as polycystic ovaries
- General metabolic disorders such as malnutrition and obesity.

Role of biopsy in DUB (Fig. 26.13)

Biopsy of the endometrium is performed in cases of irregular menstrual bleeding and menorrhagia in the perimenopausal age group and postmenopausal bleeding. DUB in many cases is a diagnosis of exclusion, so it is necessary to rule out any pathology of the endometrium by performing the biopsy. The presence of proliferative glands with the absence of secretory changes indicates an unopposed action of oestrogen. Atypical

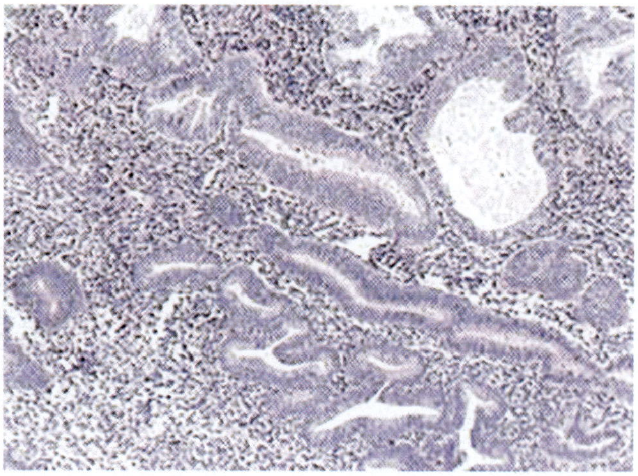

Fig. 26.13 DUB endometrial biopsy showing disorderly proliferative endometrium. (*Source:* From Anne M. Mills and Teri A. Longacre. Endometrial hyperplasia. Seminars in Diagnostic Pathology. 2010;27: 199–214.)

hyperplasia and neoplastic transformation need to be particularly ruled out, and biopsy must be performed before initiating treatment for the patient.

ACUTE AND CHRONIC ENDOMETRITIS

Acute Endometritis

Acute endometritis may occur following childbirth or miscarriage due to the retained placenta or retained products of conception. The common causative organisms are group A β-haemolytic streptococci and staphylococci. Patients are generally treated by removal of the retained products under antibiotic cover.

Chronic Endometritis

The causes of chronic endometritis include the following:

- Chronic pelvic inflammatory disorders such as due to gonorrhoea and *Chlamydia* infection
- Retained products of conception
- Intrauterine contraceptive device
- Blood-borne infections such as tuberculosis

Diagnosis is done by histological examination, which shows **plasma cells in the endometrium**. Swab and culture may be performed to identify the organism but may give false-negative results. Hence, antibiotic treatment may be initiated if clinically indicated to avoid consequences of infection such as salpingitis and infertility.

ENDOMETRIOSIS PA 30.7

Endometriosis refers to the presence of *endometrial tissue at any site other than the uterine lining.* The ectopic tissue may contain glands and stroma, but the presence of stroma is required for the diagnosis. The common sites in the decreasing order of frequency are as follows:

- Ovaries (most common)
- Uterine ligaments
- Rectovaginal septum
- Cul-de-sac
- Pelvic peritoneum
- Large and small bowel and appendix
- Mucosa of the cervix, vagina and fallopian tubes
- Laparotomy scars (least common)

The common theories for the occurrence of ectopic tissue are as follows:

- **Regurgitation theory:** The retrograde flow of menstrual fluid through fallopian tubes into peritoneum
- **Benign metastatic theory:** Migration of endometrial tissue through the lymphovascular route
- **Metaplastic theory:** Development from coelomic epithelium that originally formed the endometrium
- **Extrauterine stem cell theory:** Formation from bone marrow stem cells

The factors that help in the survival of the endometrial tissue in the ectopic site are as follows:

- Release of inflammatory mediators such as prostaglandin E_2, cytokines such as IL-1 and TNF-α, angiogenic factor such as VEGF, proteinases MMP and its inhibitor TIMP
- Presence of enzyme aromatase that produces more oestrogen locally
- Epigenetic alterations that increase its response to oestrogen and decrease its response to progesterone
- Mutations in genes such as PTEN and ARID1A that are shared by ovarian cancers such as endometrioid cancer and clear cell carcinoma in few cases

Clinical Features

Women may present with nonspecific symptoms such as pelvic pain or dysmenorrhoea. Pain during intercourse, micturition (bladder wall involvement) or defecation (rectal wall involvement) may be present, but the problem that brings women to the clinician most often is *infertility*.

Morphology

Gross On laparoscopic examination or during surgery, endometriotic spots appear as bluish red to brown spots on the serosal or mucosal surface. This is due to breakdown of haemoglobin from the cyclical bleeding of the ectopic endometrial tissue in response to oestrogen. The healing process of these foci may lead to the formation of adhesions between various organs. In ovarian endometriosis, blood collects in the form of cyst inside the ovary, forming large, brown, fluid-filled **chocolate cysts** (Fig. 26.14).

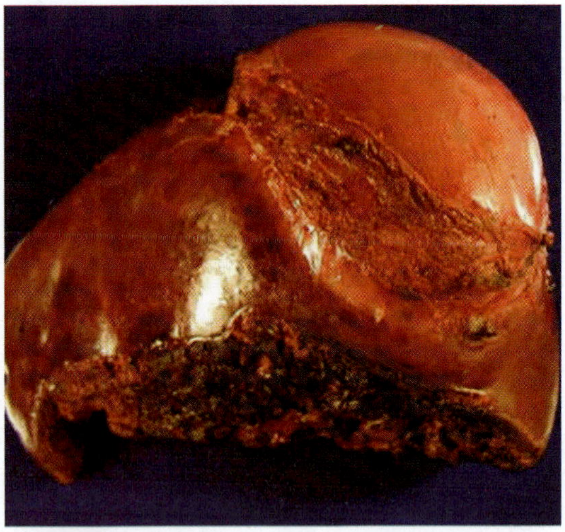

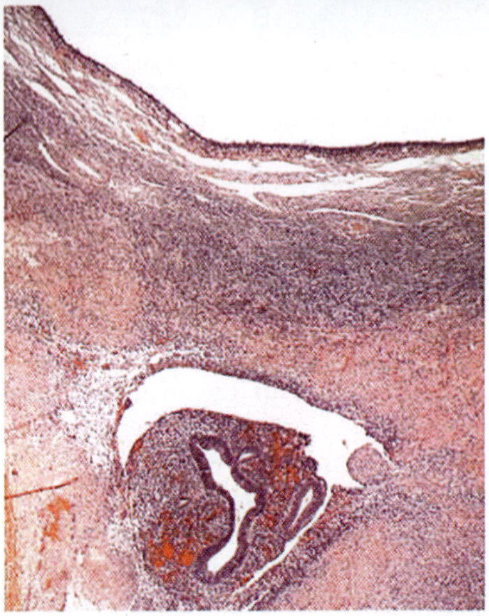

Fig. 26.14 Ovarian chocolate cyst – gross and microscopy showing endometrial glands surrounded by stroma. (*Source:* From Sushilkumar K. Sonavane, Kartikeya P. Kantawala and Christine O. Menias. Beyond the Boundaries—Endometriosis: Typical and Atypical Locations. Current Problems in Diagnostic Radiology. 2011;40:219–232.)

These cysts often form adhesions on the external surface and have a thickened tunica.

Microscopy Microscopic examination shows the presence of endometrial stroma with glands or occasionally only stroma. The presence of only glands is not indicative of endometriosis. Clusters of haemosiderin-containing cyst macrophages may be seen indicative of old bleeding. The presence of atypia in the glandular epithelium or overcrowding of glands similar to endometrial hyperplasia is indicative of **atypical endometriosis** that may progress to become endometrial carcinoma.

Treatment

Treatment of endometriosis depends on the presenting symptoms and the severity of these symptoms. Surgery and hormonal therapy are the two modes of treatment available, with surgery being the first choice in infertility cases because hormonal intervention may affect pregnancy.

ADENOMYOSIS

PA 30.8

Adenomyosis refers to the presence of *endometrial glands and stroma within the myometrium* of the uterus. It differs from endometriosis in location as well as nature. Adenomyosis consists of nonfunctional endometrium basalis, whereas endometriosis contains functional endometrium. It is considered to be due to downward growth of the endometrium and usually regresses postmenopausally. Patients may present with irregular vaginal bleeding, menorrhagia, dysmenorrhoea, dyspareunia or chronic pelvic pain.

Morphology (Fig. 26.15)

Adenomyosis causes irregular, globular enlargement of the uterus due to the associated myometrial hypertrophy surrounding it. The cut surface shows cystic spaces surrounded by hypertrophied muscle and occasional brown spots. Histologically, the glands and stroma should be found at least 2–3 mm away from the basal layer of endometrium to confirm the diagnosis.

Diagnosis is made by ultrasonography and MRI, the latter being superior. Hysterectomy is the treatment of choice in perimenopausal women. Limited resection or hormonal therapy may be tried in women reluctant to undergo hysterectomy, but results vary.

ENDOMETRIAL POLYPS

Endometrial polyps are polypoid exophytic masses that represent localized areas of endometrial hyperplasia. These may be single or multiple and project into the endometrial cavity or even into the endocervical canal when they have a long pedicle. The stroma shows reduced expression of hormonal receptors, and the glands along with the stroma are nonresponsive to progesterone stimulation (Fig. 26.16).

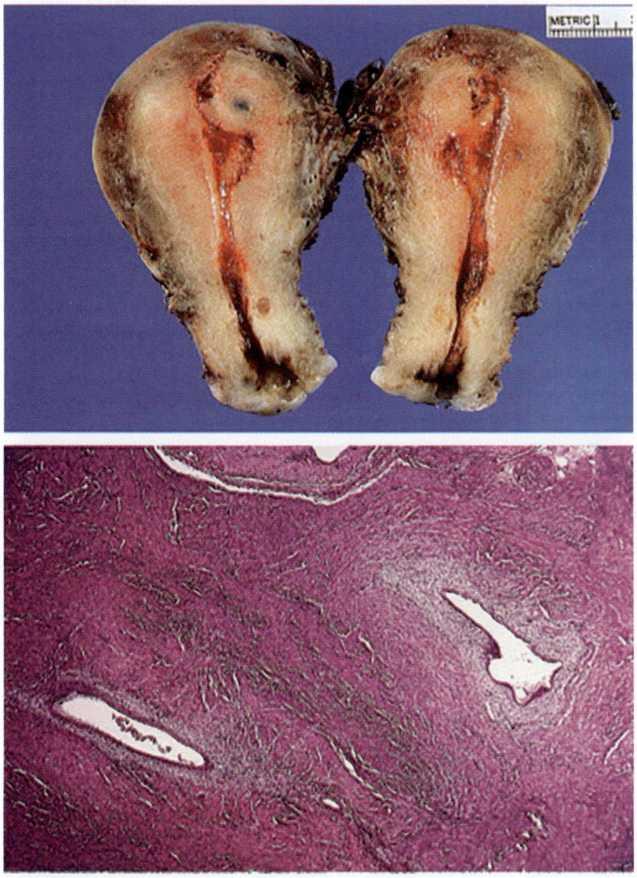

Fig. 26.15 Gross and microscopic appearance of adenomyosis. (*Source:* From Blake Gilks. Uterus: Corpus. Rosai and Ackerman's Surgical Pathology. 11th edition. Elsevier 2018.)

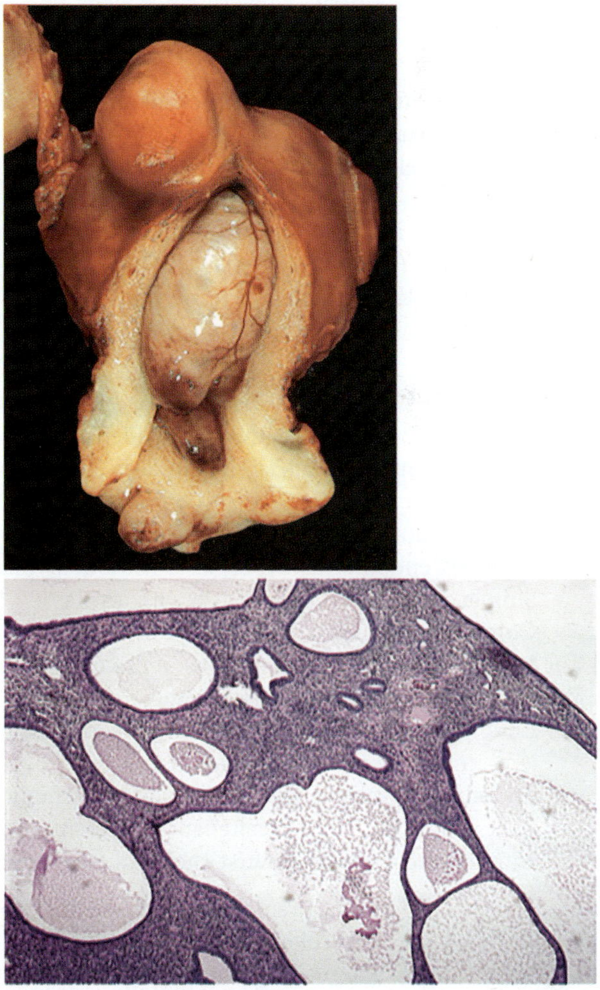

Fig. 26.16 Endometrial polyp: gross and microscopic appearance showing dilated glands. (*Source:* From Blake Gilks. Uterus: Corpus. Rosai and Ackerman's Surgical Pathology. 11th edition. Elsevier 2018.)

Clinically, the polyps may be asymptomatic or present with menorrhagia, intermenstrual bleeding or postmenopausal bleeding. They are composed of glands that show cystic dilation lined by pseudostratified epithelium and thick-walled blood vessels. But the lining epithelium may be flat in postmenopausal women.

Polyps are relatively common in women on tamoxifen therapy for breast cancer because tamoxifen, though anti-oestrogenic to breast tissue, has an oestrogenic effect on endometrium. They may rarely predispose to endometrial carcinoma and are often removed on diagnosis for histological examination.

ENDOMETRIAL HYPERPLASIA PA 30.9

Endometrial hyperplasia refers to excessive proliferation of glands surpassing the stroma, resulting in an *increased gland to stroma ratio*. Risk factors for endometrial hyperplasia include all lesions causing unopposed oestrogen activity. It is important to detect endometrial hyperplasia because it is considered to be a *precursor to endometrial carcinoma*.

Risk Factors

- Obesity (adipose tissue converts androgens to oestrogens)
- Menopause
- Polycystic ovarian syndrome (lack of progesterone due to anovulation)
- Granulosa cell tumours of the ovary (secrete oestrogen)
- Excessive ovarian cortical function (cortical stromal hyperplasia)
- Oestrogen replacement therapy (exogenous oestrogen)

Classification

There have been various classifications for endometrial hyperplasia. The following is the most widely accepted classification for endometrial hyperplasia based on architecture and atypia:

- Simple endometrial hyperplasia without atypia
- Complex endometrial hyperplasia without atypia
- Simple endometrial hyperplasia with atypia
- Complex endometrial hyperplasia with atypia

The above-stated classification was replaced by the WHO classification, which is two tiered:

- Endometrial hyperplasia: Benign, not premalignant, managed with hormonal therapy
- Endometrial intraepithelial neoplasia: Premalignant with a 30% risk of malignant transformation, with hysterectomy as the first choice of treatment

The factors that suggest the premalignant nature of endometrial hyperplasia are as follows:

- Common genetic alterations: PTEN mutations are seen in both endometrial hyperplasia and carcinoma. Cowden syndrome, which is due to a defect in the PTEN gene, is commonly associated with endometrial carcinoma.
- They share the same risk factors with endometrial carcinoma.
- Most cases of carcinoma are preceded by endometrial hyperplasia.
- The severity of hyperplasia and the presence of atypia correlate with the risk of malignant transformation.

Morphology

Endometrial hyperplasia (without atypia) shows an increased gland to stroma ratio. The glands may be irregular with crowding but show the presence of stroma in between (Fig. 26.17). Cystic dilation of glands may also be seen.

Endometrial intraepithelial neoplasia shows complex branching glandular proliferation with intraglandular tufting of cells and minimal scanty stroma (Fig. 26.18).

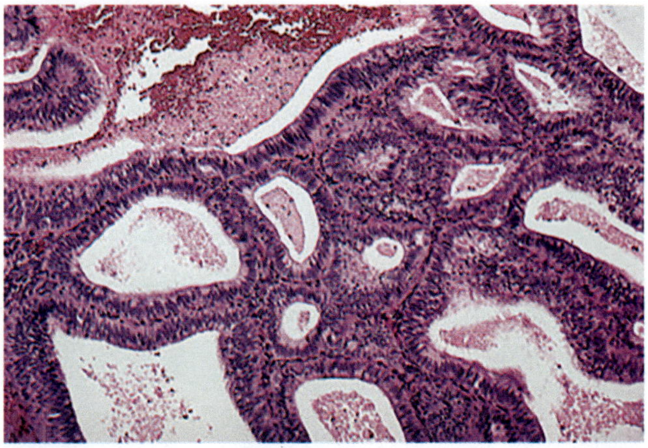

Fig. 26.17 Histology of endometrial hyperplasia without atypia showing crowding of glands and irregularity. (*Source:* From Blake Gilks. Uterus: Corpus. Rosai and Ackerman's Surgical Pathology. 11th edition. Elsevier 2018.)

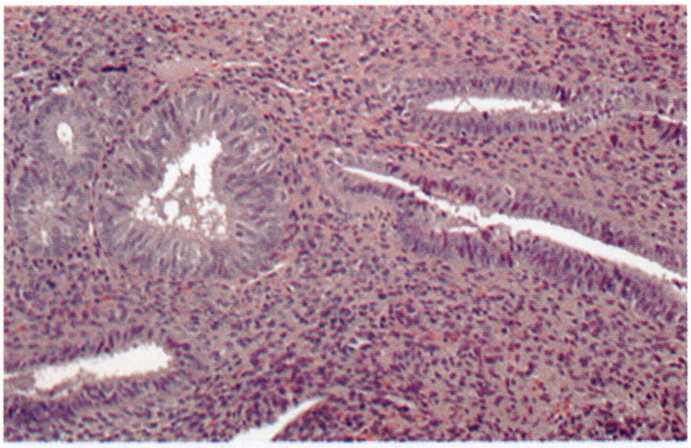

Fig. 26.18 Microscopy of endometrial intraepithelial neoplasia showing back-to-back glands lined by atypical cells. (*Source:* From Blake Gilks. Uterus: Corpus. Rosai and Ackerman's Surgical Pathology. 11th edition. Elsevier 2018.)

The cells lining the glands show nuclear atypia and loss of polarity. The nucleus is vesicular (open chromatin) with prominent nucleoli. This appearance is similar to that of endometrial carcinoma that makes it difficult to confirm the diagnosis on biopsy specimens because subsequent hysterectomy may show an underlying endometrial carcinoma. The presence of metaplasia such as squamous metaplasia may be seen in adjacent areas and does not indicate malignancy.

Management depends on biopsy findings, age of the patient and possibility of adequate follow-up. Surgery is the mainstay in endometrial intraepithelial carcinoma, whereas hormonal therapy and follow-up may be tried in simple endometrial hyperplasia.

MALIGNANT LESIONS OF THE ENDOMETRIUM

Endometrial Carcinoma **PA 30.2**

Endometrial carcinoma is the second most common cancer of the female genital tract, next to cervical carcinoma in India. But it is the most common cancer of the female genital tract in developed countries. It is more common in postmenopausal women but may occur in females of younger age also in whom the tumour is more likely to be well differentiated. Endometrial carcinomas are classified into two types – endometrioid carcinoma and serous endometrial carcinoma.

Type 1 Endometrioid Carcinoma Endometrioid carcinoma accounts for 80% of endometrial carcinomas. These carcinomas resemble proliferating endometrial glands and are due to the action of unopposed oestrogen on the endometrium. The associated premalignant lesion is atypical endometrial hyperplasia. The risk factors associated with endometrioid carcinoma are the same as those of the precursor and include obesity, menopause, polycystic ovarian syndrome, exogenous oestrogens and functional ovarian tumours.

Molecular Basis Endometrioid carcinomas like any other tumours develop due to stepwise acquisition of genetic mutations (Fig. 26.19). The common mutations are listed in Table 26.9.

Morphology

Gross appearance of the tumour may be polypoid or infiltrative (Fig. 26.20). *Invasion of the myometrium and the depth of invasion* are important determinants of the prognosis. The tumour is composed of endometrial glands lined by atypical cells with bridging within the

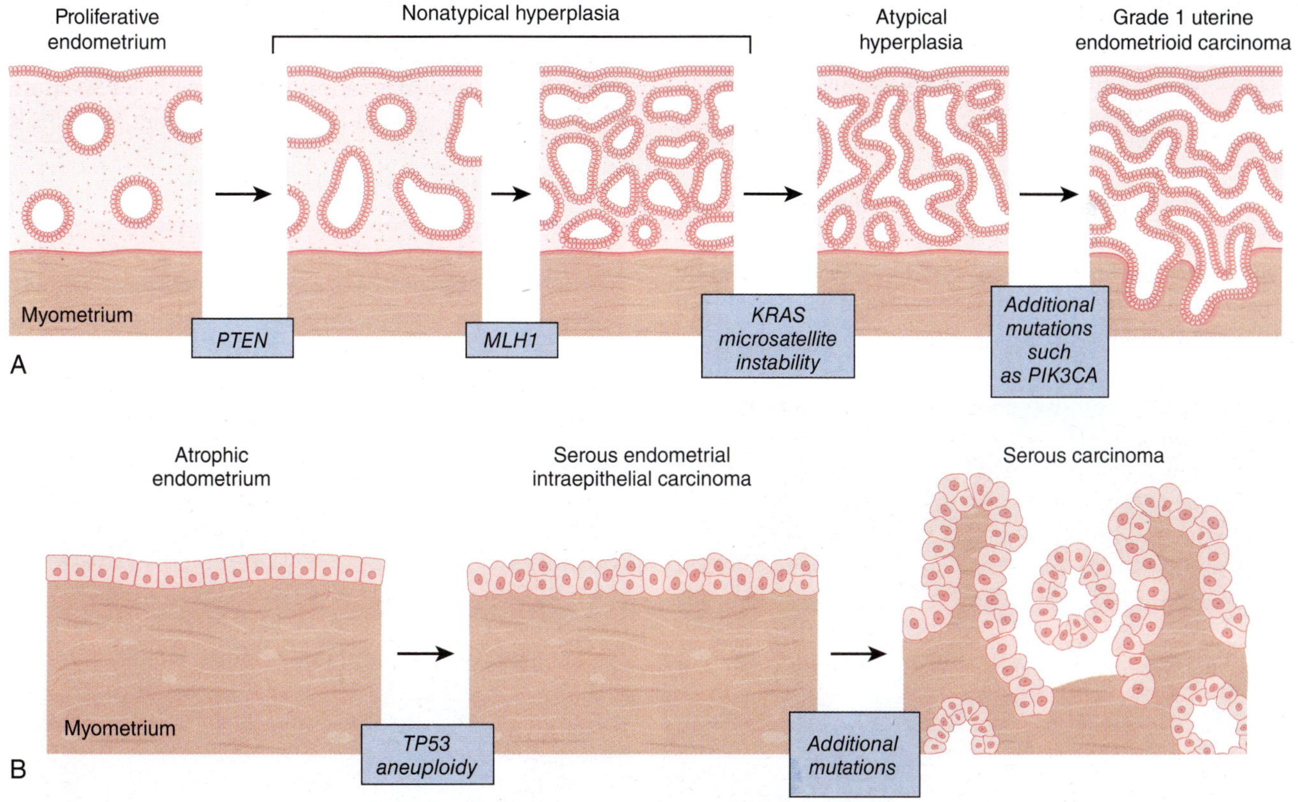

Fig. 26.19 Evolution of (A) endometrioid carcinoma and (B) serous endometrial carcinoma, the sequence. (*Source:* From Lora Hedrick Ellenson and Edyta C. Pirog. The Female Genital Tract. Robbins & Cotran Pathologic Basis of Disease. 10th edition. Elsevier 2021.)

Table 26.9 Early and Late Mutations in Endometrioid Carcinomas

Early Mutations	Late Mutations
Increased PI3K/AKT signals • PTEN mutation • KRAS • ARID1A	Increased PI3K/AKT signals • PIK3CA (aids invasion)
Others • DNA mismatch repair genes	Others • TP53

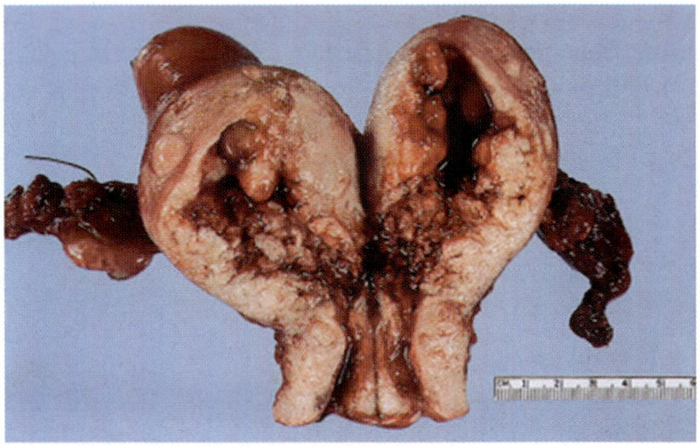

Fig. 26.20 Gross appearance of endometrioid carcinoma showing myometrial extension.

glands (Fig. 26.21). Foci of squamous metaplasia may be present that are predominantly benign appearing. However, tumour grading is based on the appearance of the glandular element only (Table 26.10).

Spread The tumour spreads by invasion into the surrounding structures and organs including the broad ligament. Metastasis to regional lymph nodes and distant organs such as the liver, lung and bones may be seen later in the course of the disease.

Table 26.10 Grading and Staging of Endometrioid Carcinomas

Grading of Tumour
Well differentiated: Composed of only glandular elements Moderately differentiated: Predominantly glands with solid sheets of cells <50% Poorly differentiated: Predominantly solid sheets of cells >50%
Staging of the Tumour
Stage I: Carcinoma is confined to the body of the uterus itself Stage II: Carcinoma involves the uterus and the cervix Stage III: Carcinoma extends outside the uterus but not outside the true pelvis Stage IV: Carcinoma extends outside the true pelvis or involves the mucosa of the bladder or the rectum

Type 2 Serous Carcinoma Serous carcinomas represent about 15% of endometrial carcinomas and typically occur in postmenopausal women and bear a morphological similarity with ovarian serous tumours. The precursor lesion for endometrial serous carcinoma is serous intraepithelial endometrial carcinoma. It originates in atrophic endometrium and differs from endometrial serous carcinoma by the absence of stromal invasion. These tumours are associated with a poorer prognosis because of their nature to exfoliate into the endometrial cavity and spread through the fallopian tube into the peritoneal cavity to form **peritoneal implants**. The common mutation associated with endometrial serous carcinoma is **TP53 mutation** that is often present in the premalignant stage itself.

Morphology

Serous carcinomas of the endometrium develop in the atrophic uterus and have a high propensity to invade deep into the myometrium. These carcinomas show

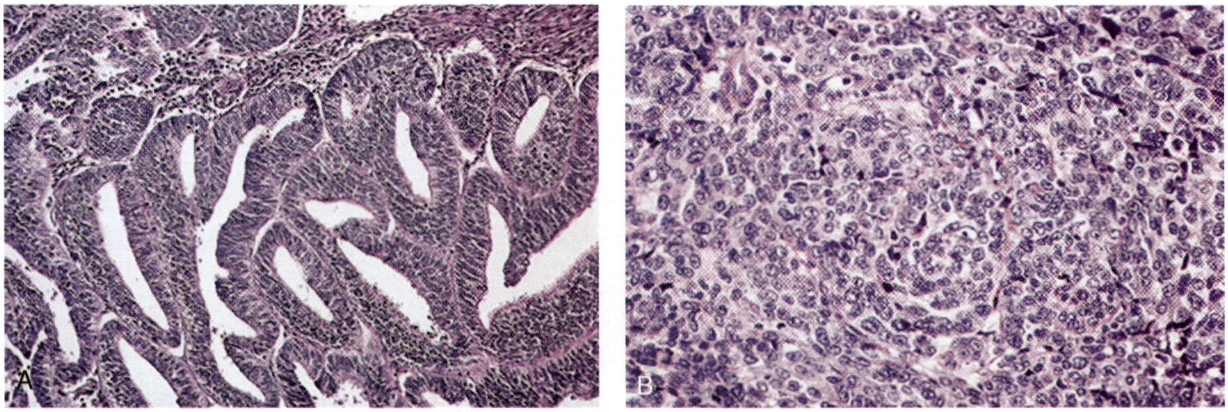

Fig. 26.21 Microscopic appearance of endometrioid carcinoma – well differentiated (A) and poorly differentiated (B). (*Source:* From Blake Gilks. Uterus: Corpus. Rosai and Ackerman's Surgical Pathology. 11th edition. Elsevier 2018.)

significant cytological atypia with marked nuclear pleomorphism and atypical mitosis. Serous intraepithelial endometrial carcinomas show the same changes that are limited to the epithelial surface with no myometrial invasion. Invasive tumours are mostly made of papillary structures and only rarely contain glandular elements (Fig. 26.22).

Grading These tumours are always considered as grade 3 because of their aggressive nature (Table 26.10).

Staging The same staging as in endometrioid carcinoma is used.

Spread These tumours spread superficially through the fallopian tubes or through lymphatics rather than direct invasion.

Recent Updates In the latest WHO classification of uterine tumours, endometrial tumours, irrespective of their histological type, are classified based on POLE gene mutation, mismatch repair gene (MMR) defect and p53 mutation to help in management and determining prognosis. The four categories are as follows:

1. POLE gene mutated (EC-POLE mut)
2. POLE normal, MMR defect (EC-MMRd)
3. POLE and MMR normal, p53 mutated (EC-p53mut)
4. POLE, MMR and p53 normal (EC-NSMP [no specific molecular profile])

Clinical Features Endometrial carcinoma is common in postmenopausal women, peaking between 55 and 65 years of age. The most common presentation is postmenopausal bleeding, which usually makes women seek medical help at an early stage. This helps in better treatment and improves prognosis that depends on the grade and stage of the tumour. Surgery with or without chemotherapy/radiotherapy is used for treating the disease based on the extent of spread. Serous carcinomas have a poorer prognosis, and women are given chemotherapy even in the absence of demonstrable extrauterine disease due to its aggressive nature and chances of silent spread.

Malignant Mixed Müllerian Tumours

Malignant mixed Müllerian tumours (MMMTs) are tumours composed of two components – **epithelial and mesenchymal**. The epithelial component exists in the form of endometrial adenocarcinomas, whereas the mesenchymal component may contain uterine mesenchymal elements such as stromal cells or heterologous malignant cell types like skeletal muscle or cartilage (Fig. 26.23). Evidence shows that most of these tumours are carcinomas that have developed sarcomatous differentiation because mutations found in these tumours are similar to those of endometrioid carcinomas and not to those of sarcomas.

These tumours occur in the older age group and clinically present with postmenopausal bleeding. Prognosis is based on the depth of invasion and staging. The same staging system is used as for endometrioid carcinoma. Biopsy showing heterologous elements is associated with a poor prognosis. Interestingly, metastatic deposits show only the epithelial component.

MYOMETRIAL TUMOURS

Leiomyoma PA 30.3

Leiomyomas are benign tumours of uterine myometrium and are the most common benign tumour in women.

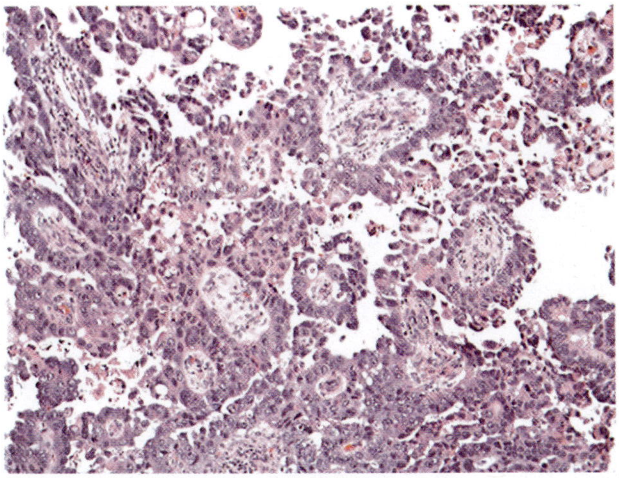

Fig. 26.22 Histopathology of serous endometrial carcinoma with a papillary growth pattern consisting of malignant cells with marked cytological atypia. (*Source:* From Lora Hedrick Ellenson and Edyta C. Pirog. The Female Genital Tract. Robbins & Cotran Pathologic Basis of Disease. 10th edition. Elsevier 2021.)

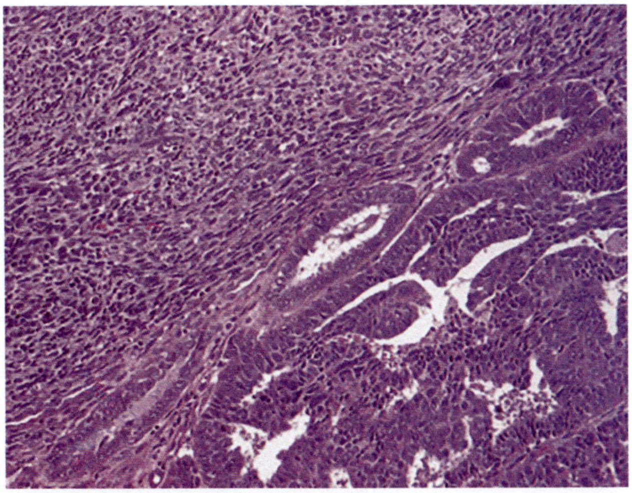

Fig. 26.23 Histopathology of malignant mixed Müllerian tumour showing malignant endometrioid glands and malignant stroma. (*Source:* From Robert A. Soslow, Diagnostic Histopathology, Elsevier 2008.)

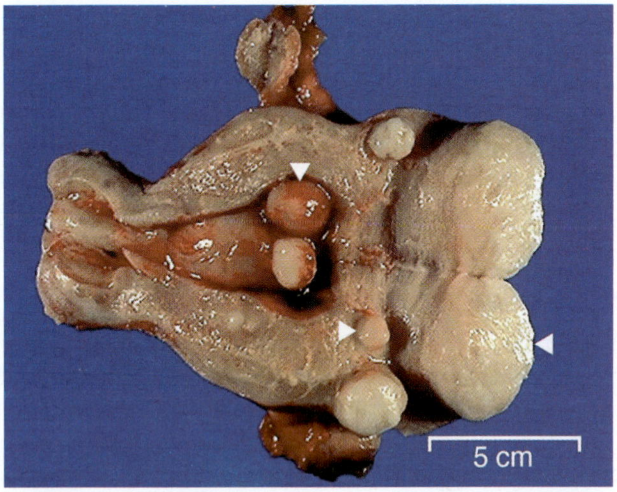

Fig. 26.24 Cut surface of the uterus showing submucosal, intramural and subserosal myoma. (*Source:* From Edward C. Klatt. The Female Genital Tract. Robbins and Cotran Atlas of Pathology. 4th edition. Elsevier 2021.)

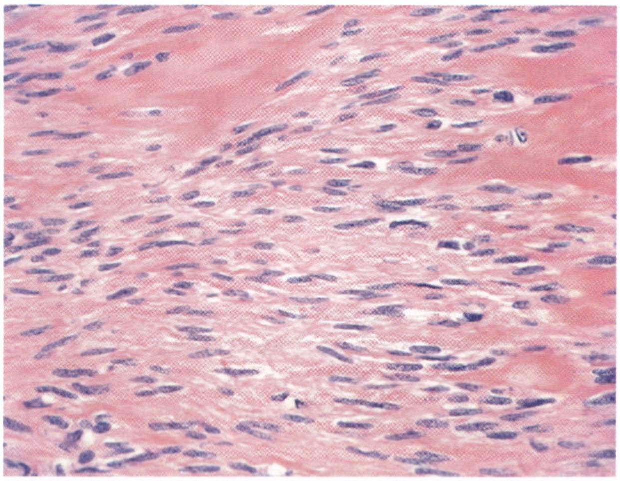

Fig. 26.25 Histology of leiomyoma. (*Source:* From Fibroids (Uterine Myomas). Elsevier Point of Care. 2022.)

These may occur singly or as multiple leiomyomas. About 40% of leiomyomas are associated with chromosomal abnormalities such as HMGIC/HMGIY gene rearrangements or MED12 gene mutations.

Morphology

The uterus appears enlarged and nodular. Leiomyomas may be classified based on the location (Fig. 26.24):

- Within the myometrium (most common) called **intramural**
- Beneath the mucosa called **submucosal**
- Under the serosa on the outer surface called **subserosal**

Irrespective of location, the leiomyomas are well-circumscribed, round, firm, grey-white lesions that vary in size from small to very large tumours. The cut surface shows a whorled appearance and stands out from the surrounding myometrium.

Microscopy shows uniform smooth muscle cells with oval blunt-ended nuclei arranged in whorls (Fig. 26.25). Mitotic figures are rare.

Variants

Occasionally, myomas may show variation in appearance:

- Myomas with necrosis: Red degeneration (Fig. 26.26)
- Myomas with oedema fluid accumulation: Hydropic degeneration
- Myomas with myxoid change: Myxoid leiomyoma
- Myomas with atypical bizarre pleomorphic cells: Symplastic leiomyoma (Fig. 26.27)
- Myomas with increased mitosis: Mitotically active leiomyoma

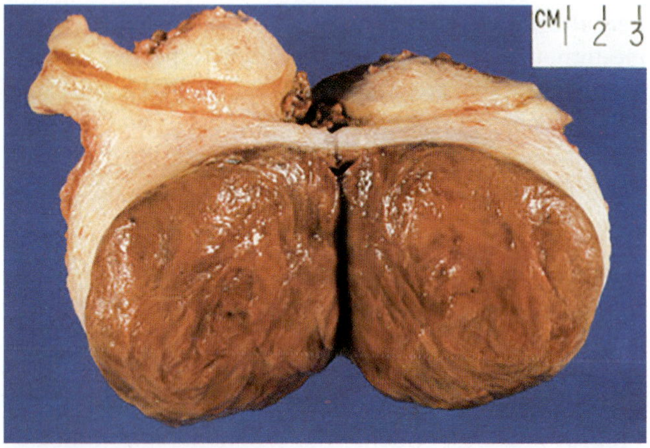

Fig. 26.26 Gross image of myoma with red degeneration. (*Source:* From Blake Gilks. Uterus: Corpus. Rosai and Ackerman's Surgical Pathology. 11th edition. Elsevier 2018.)

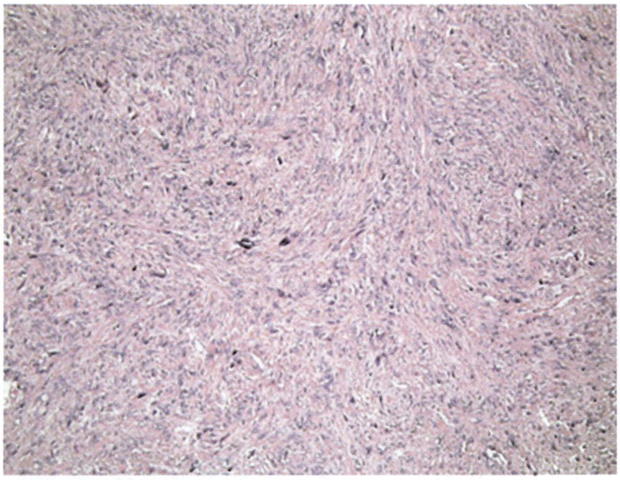

Fig. 26.27 Histology of symplastic leiomyoma composed of cells with atypia. (*Source:* From Christopher P. Crum, Anna R. Laury, Michelle S. Hirsch, Charles Matthew Quick and William A. Peters. Atypical Leiomyoma (Leiomyoma with Bizarre Nuclei). Gynecologic and Obstetric Pathology. Saunders 2016.)

- Myomas that metastasize through blood vessels: Benign metastasizing leiomyoma
- Myomas with multiple peritoneal nodules: Disseminated peritoneal leiomyomatosis
- Myomas with fumarate hydratase deficiency: Are significant because they are part of a syndrome called 'leiomyomatosis/renal cell carcinoma (RCC) syndrome' and the patient needs to be given genetic screening and counselling

Clinical Features Clinically, the size of the leiomyoma does not correlate with clinical symptoms. Women may present with menorrhagia, pelvic pain or urinary symptoms due to pressure on the bladder. Leiomyoma in pregnant women may undergo red degeneration, causing pain, and also affect the fetus, resulting in miscarriage, malpresentation and postpartum haemorrhage. Malignant transformation is extremely rare.

Leiomyosarcoma **PA 30.3**

Leiomyosarcomas are malignant neoplasm of the uterus, originating from the myometrium or endometrial stromal cells. These are associated with genetic mutations such as MED12 as in leiomyoma but do not arise from leiomyomas. The other mutations specific to leiomyosarcoma are TP53 and ATRX. Leiomyosarcomas usually occur in the perimenopausal age group. These are often associated with metastasis to the lung, liver and brain and high chances of recurrence, thereby reducing the 5-year survival rate.

Morphology

Leiomyosarcoma may appear as a polypoid tumour protruding into the uterine lumen or as a fleshy mass within the uterine wall (Fig. 26.28). The features that distinguish it from leiomyoma are *coagulative necrosis, mitotic figures, nuclear pleomorphism and cellularity* in the decreasing order of significance (Fig. 26.29). Sometimes, morphological features of sarcoma may be so subtle that a diagnosis of leiomyosarcoma may seem unjustifiable. This gave way to a separate category of borderline tumours called **soft-tissue neoplasm of uncertain malignant potential (STUMP)**. The following features help us in differentiating leiomyosarcoma from STUMP and some variants of leiomyoma:

- Presence of necrosis with greater than 10 mitoses per 10 high-power fields (HPFs) is generally considered diagnostic of leiomyosarcoma.
- Tumours with only necrosis or only focal increase in mitotic count or only severe atypia are categorized under STUMP.

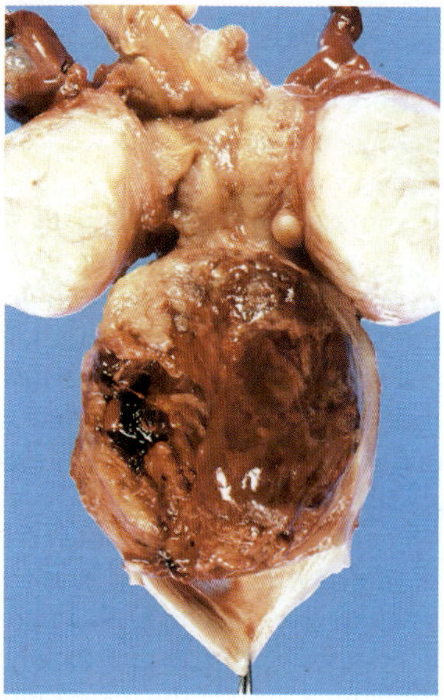

Fig. 26.28 Gross image of leiomyosarcoma exhibiting necrosis and foci of haemorrhage.

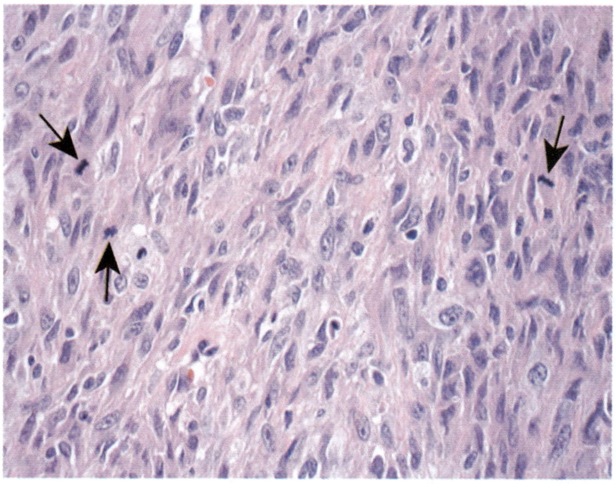

Fig. 26.29 Histology of leiomyosarcoma with nuclear pleomorphism and atypical mitosis. (*Source:* From Lora Hedrick Ellenson and Edyta C. Pirog. The Female Genital Tract. Robbins & Cotran Pathologic Basis of Disease. 10th edition. Elsevier 2021.)

- Tumours without necrosis and only a mild increase in mitotic figures are mitotically active leiomyoma.
- Tumours with only mild to moderate atypia are atypical or symplastic leiomyoma.

Management Uterine leiomyosarcomas tend to spread to the pelvic structures by direct invasion and bloodborne metastasis to the lungs, liver and bones. Spread beyond the uterus and a bigger size of the tumour are associated with a poorer prognosis. Treatment includes hysterectomy with bilateral salpingo-oophorectomy, followed by radiotherapy.

ENDOMETRIAL STROMAL TUMOURS

Endometrial stromal tumours are rare neoplasms made up of proliferating stromal elements with or without benign glands.

Stromal tumours containing malignant stromal component with interspersed benign glands are called **adenosarcomas**. These tumours are sensitive to oestrogen, and treatment by oophorectomy gives good results.

Pure stromal tumours are divided into **benign stromal nodules and stromal sarcomas**. Stromal sarcomas are further divided into low grade and high grade based on their histological appearance. Both have chromosomal translocations forming fusion genes but vary in the fusion gene formed. Low-grade tumours have 50% survival chances after 5 years, whereas high-grade tumours have a much poorer prognosis. This is due to high chances of recurrence, sometimes even at the metastatic sites following treatment at metastatic sites.

FALLOPIAN TUBES

INFLAMMATIONS, CYSTS AND TUMOURS

Inflammation of the fallopian tubes is often due to infections with pyogenic organisms. The common infections include gonorrhoea and *Chlamydia* infection as part of PID discussed earlier. The other infection that is seen in developing countries like India includes tuberculosis, which commonly reaches the tubes by a haematogenous route and presents as infertility or generalized symptoms associated with tuberculosis. The involved tubes show multiple tubercles, which on histological examination reveal caseous necrosis and granulomas.

Common cysts of the fallopian tubes are small cysts lined by flattened serous epithelium thought to arise from Müllerian duct remnants. The small ones along the tubes are called **paratubal cysts**, whereas the larger ones near the fimbriae are called **hydatids of Morgagni**. These are not much of significance except that these may be mistaken occasionally for ovarian cysts during imaging.

Tumours of the tube are rare. These may be benign adenomatoid tumours or malignant adenocarcinoma. The malignant tumours present as a parametrial mass or with bleeding abnormalities. A few may be silent and detected during Pap screening. High-stage tumours are aggressive, causing death in about 40% of women within 5 years of diagnosis.

OVARIES

FOLLICLE CYSTS AND LUTEAL CYSTS

Cysts are often formed in the ovaries from ruptured and unruptured Graafian follicles. These may be multiple and vary in size. It has been proposed that only *cysts larger than 2.5 cm should be called follicular cysts*. These are benign lesions filled with clear serous fluid.

Morphology

Microscopically, these cysts are lined by a granulosa layer surrounded by thecal cells. These grow up to 10 cm in size and may cause pelvic pain or occasionally undergo twisting of the pedicle with haemorrhage. When the cyst lining is of luteinized granulosa cells that appear bright yellow macroscopically, the cysts are called **luteal cysts**.

POLYCYSTIC OVARIES AND STROMAL HYPERTHECOSIS

Polycystic ovarian syndrome or **Stein–Leventhal syndrome** is a complex endocrine disorder seen in up to 10% of women worldwide.

The components include the following:

- Menstrual abnormalities
- Polycystic ovaries
- Chronic anovulation
- Decreased fertility

The associated features are as follows:

- Obesity
- Type 2 diabetes
- Premature atherosclerosis

The metabolic abnormalities that cause these symptoms are as follows:

- Dysregulation of enzymes involved in androgen biosynthesis
- Excessive androgen production
- Insulin resistance
- Altered adipose tissue metabolism

Complications that may occur due to this chronic hormone imbalance are as follows:

- Infertility
- Virilization
- Endometrial hyperplasia
- Endometrial carcinoma

Stromal hyperthecosis is a stromal disorder in which there is hyperplasia of cortical stroma and increased luteinization of stromal cells. This may occur separately or in women with polycystic ovaries.

On gross examination, the ovaries are enlarged and white to tan in colour (Fig. 26.30). In the cut section, these show multiple cysts in the cortex just below the surface with the absence of corpus luteum and corpus albicans, indicating the absence of ovulation. Microscopy shows nests of large vacuolated luteal cells. The cysts show luteinization of the theca interna layer surrounded by a

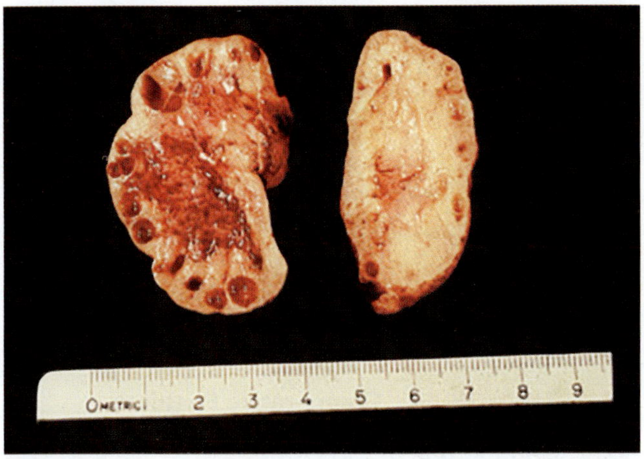

Fig. 26.30 Gross appearance of polycystic ovaries. (*Source:* From Blake Gilks. Ovary. Rosai and Ackerman's Surgical Pathology. 11th edition. Elsevier 2018.)

dense fibrous layer. Patients often present with strong symptoms of virilization.

OVARIAN TUMOURS

PA 30.4

Ovarian tumours contribute up to 3% of tumours in women but are the fifth common cause of cancerous deaths. This is due to the delay in diagnosis of the tumours owing to their asymptomatic nature and late presentation. Benign tumours tend to occur in the reproductive age group, whereas malignant tumours are more common in the older age group. WHO has classified ovarian tumours based on their cell of origin (Table 26.11). The three components of the ovary that give rise to cancer are as follows:

- Surface epithelium
- Germ cells
- Sex cord–stromal cells

Apart from these primary tumours, secondaries may develop in ovaries from primaries of the gastrointestinal (GI) tract, breast and other organs.

The frequency of ovarian tumours is as follows:

- Most common tumours of the ovary are serous tumours.
- Most common benign tumours are benign serous tumours.
- Most common malignant tumours are malignant serous carcinomas, followed by endometrioid carcinomas.
- Most common bilateral tumours are malignant serous carcinomas, followed by metastatic tumours and endometrioid carcinomas.

Table 26.11 Classification of Ovarian Tumours

Surface Epithelial–Stromal Tumours
Serous tumours
Benign (cystadenoma, cystadenofibroma)
Borderline (serous borderline tumour)
Low-grade serous adenocarcinoma
High-grade serous adenocarcinoma
Low-grade serous carcinoma
Mucinous tumours, endocervical-like and intestinal type
Benign (cystadenoma, crytadenofibroma)
Borderline (mucinous borderline tumour)
Malignant (mucinous adenocarcinoma)
Endometrioid tumours
Benign (cystadenoma, cystadenofibroma)
Borderline (endometrioid borderline tumour)
Malignant (endometrioid adenocarcinoma)
Clear cell tumours
Benign
Borderline
Malignant (clear cell adenocarcinoma)
Transitional cell tumours
Benign Brenner tumour
Brenner tumour of borderline malignancy
Malignant Brenner tumour
Epithelial–stromal
Adenosarcoma
Malignant mixed Müllerian tumour
Sex Cord–Stromal Tumours
Granulosa tumours
Fibromas
Fibrothecomas
Thecomas
Sertoli–Leydig cell tumours
Steroid (lipid) cell tumours
Germ Cell Tumours
Teratoma
Immature
Mature
Solid
Cystic (dermoid cyst)
Monodermal (e.g. struma ovarii, carcinoid)
Dysgerminoma
Yolk sac tumour
Choriocarcinoma
Mixed germ cell tumours
Metastatic Cancer From Nonovarian Primary
Colonic, appendiceal
Gastric
Pancreaticobiliary
Breast

SURFACE EPITHELIAL TUMOURS

The surface epithelial tumours develop from ovarian surface epithelium or fallopian tube epithelium. These may be classified based on the following:

- Cell of origin: Serous, mucinous or endometrioid differentiation
- Histological pattern: Cystic, solid or mixed
- Proportion of fibrous tissue: Cystadenoma, cystadenofibroma, adenofibroma in benign tumours
- Atypia and invasion: Benign, borderline and malignant

Surface epithelial tumours are now classified into two types – types 1 and 2 – based on molecular studies (Table 26.12 and Fig. 26.31).

Table 26.12 Features of Type 1 and 2 Surface Epithelial Tumours of the Ovary

Type 1	Type 2
Show progression from benign to borderline to malignant	Are malignant tumours
Are low grade	Are highly aggressive
Develop from borderline tumours of the ovary	Develop from inclusion cysts or fallopian tube epithelium
Include low-grade serous, endometrioid and mucinous tumours	Include high-grade serous carcinomas

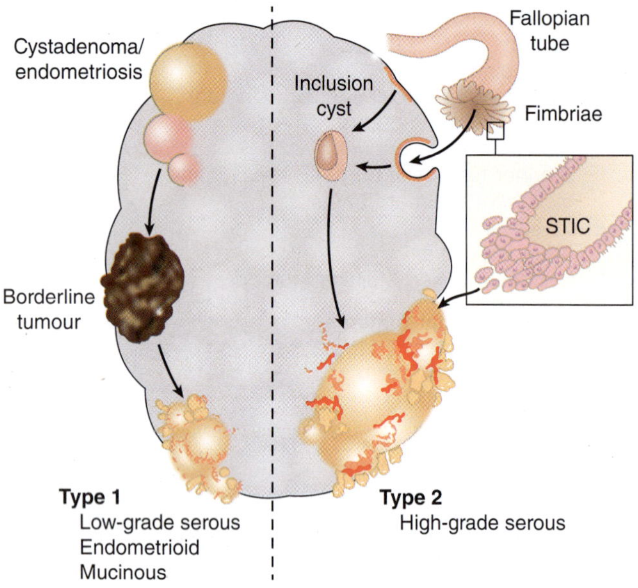

Fig. 26.31 Schematic diagram of the pathogenesis of ovarian epithelial tumours. Type 1 tumours progress from benign tumours through borderline tumours that may give rise to a low-grade carcinoma. Type 2 tumours arise from inclusions cysts/fallopian tube epithelium via intraepithelial precursors that are often not identified. These demonstrate high-grade features. (*Source:* From Lora Hedrick Ellenson and Edyta C. Pirog. The Female Genital Tract. Robbins & Cotran Pathologic Basis of Disease. 10th edition. Elsevier 2021.)

Serous Tumours

Serous tumours constitute 30% of ovarian tumours and 40% of malignant ovarian tumours. Benign and borderline tumours usually present around 20–45 years of age, whereas malignant tumours occur in older women, except familial tumours that may present at a younger age. Risk factors for malignant serous ovarian tumours are listed in Table 26.13.

Based on nuclear atypia, serous carcinomas are classified into low-grade and high-grade carcinomas. This correlates with clinical behaviour of the tumour and prognosis. Recent studies suggest difference in the origin and genetic profile of these carcinomas that are elucidated in Table 26.14.

Table 26.13 Risk Factors and Protective Factors for Malignant Serous Ovarian Tumours

Risk Factors	Protective Factors
Nulliparity Family history Genetic mutations – BRCA1, BRCA2	Oral contraceptives Tubal ligation

Table 26.14 Comparative Features Between Low- and High-Grade Serous Carcinomas of the Ovary

Low-Grade Serous Carcinoma	High-Grade Serous Carcinoma
Arise from borderline serous tumour of the ovary	Arise from serous tubal intraepithelial carcinoma (STIC) of the fallopian tube or serous inclusion cysts of the ovary
Mutations associated are BRAF, KRAS or ERBB2	Mutations associated are TP53, amplification of oncogene PIK3CA, deletion of tumour suppressor Rb gene Familial carcinomas in BRCA1, BRCA2 mutations
Peritoneal spread forms localized noninvasive implants	Peritoneal implants are invasive and widespread
Spread is slow	Wide early metastasis
Better prognosis	Bad prognosis
Survival after 5 years 90%–100%	Survival rate after 5 years 25%, with peritoneal spread to 70% in pure ovarian

Morphology (Table 26.15)

Benign serous tumours may present as cystic masses, with tumour cells lining the cyst wall or embedded on the surface of the ovary (Fig. 26.32). Surface tumours have greater chances of spread to the peritoneum. Histology of benign, borderline (Fig. 26.33) and malignant tumours (Fig. 26.34) is different and helps in making the diagnosis.

IHC: Serous carcinomas of the ovary are $CK7^+/CK20^-$. WT1 positivity helps to differentiate it from mucinous tumours.

Mucinous Tumours

About 20%–25% of ovarian tumours are mucinous tumours. These are common in the reproductive age group and are commonly benign or borderline. Malignant mucinous neoplasms are rare and form only 3% of ovarian

Table 26.15 Morphological Features of Benign, Borderline and Malignant Serous Tumours

	Benign	Borderline	Malignant
Gross	Smooth cyst wall with no epithelial thickening or with small papillary projections	An increased number of papillary projections	Solid or papillary tumour as an irregular mass and fixation or nodularity of the capsule
Bilaterality	20%	30%	66%
Microscopy	Cyst lined by a single layer of columnar epithelium that may have cilia	Complex papillae lined by stratified epithelium and mild nuclear atypia Presence of significant atypia *without stromal invasion* is called micropapillary carcinoma	Complex growth patterns, marked atypia, mitotic figures, ***stromal invasion*** or even frank effacement of the underlying stroma
Psammoma bodies	May be present	May be present	May be present

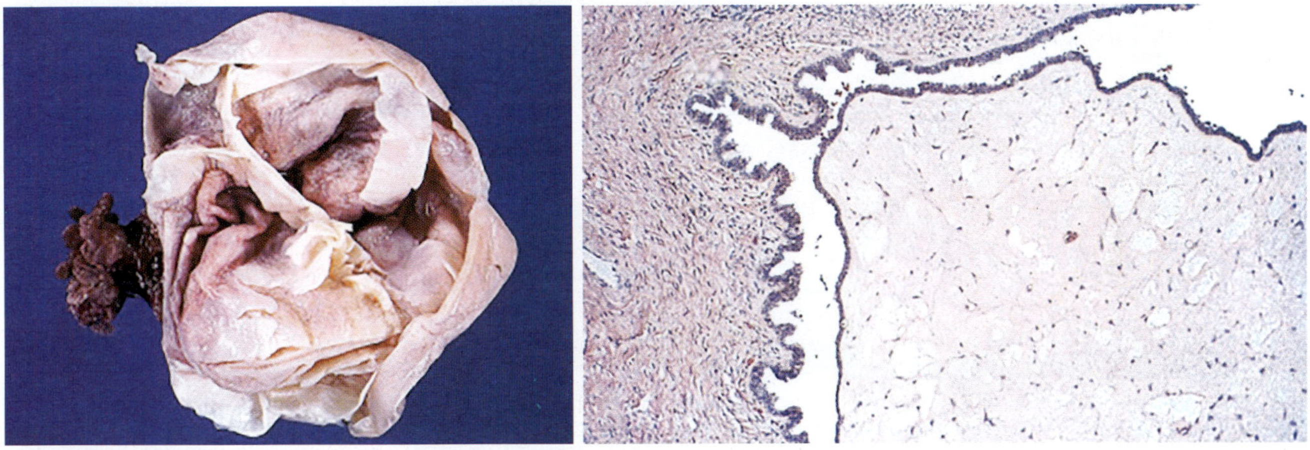

Fig. 26.32 Benign serous tumour – gross image showing a smooth cyst wall and no solid areas, and microscopy showing the cyst wall lined by a single layer of epithelial cells.

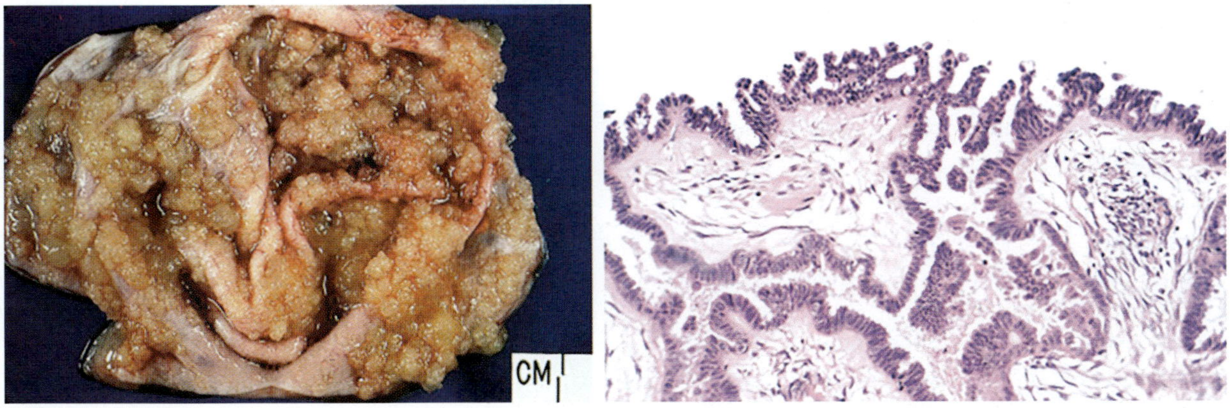

Fig. 26.33 Intermediate serous tumour – gross image showing papillary projections, and microscopy showing complex papillary projections with cells showing atypia but no stromal invasion. (*Source:* From Blake Gilks. Ovary. Rosai and Ackerman's Surgical Pathology. 11th edition. Elsevier 2018; From Lora Hedrick Ellenson and Edyta C. Pirog. The Female Genital Tract. Robbins & Cotran Pathologic Basis of Disease. 10th edition. Elsevier 2021.)

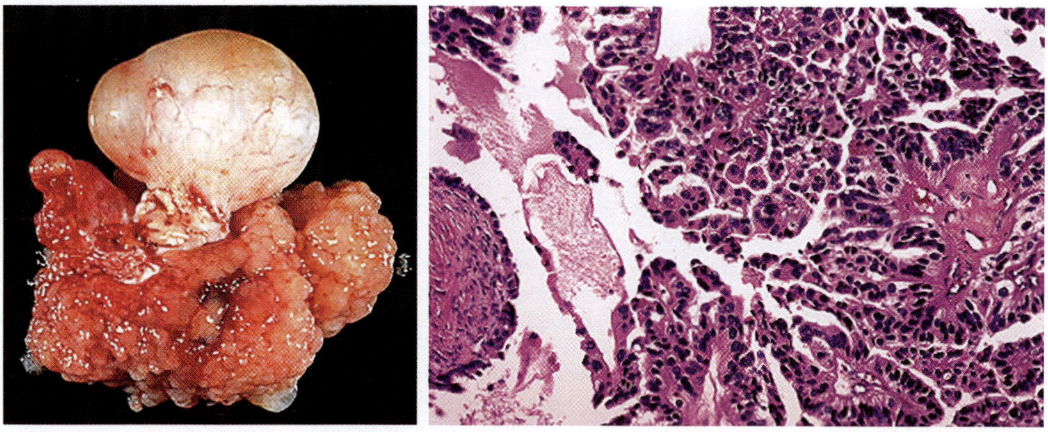

Fig. 26.34 Malignant serous tumour – gross image showing a solid tumour with breach of capsule, and microscopy showing atypical cells invading the stroma. (*Source:* From Blake Gilks. Ovary. Rosai and Ackerman's Surgical Pathology. 11th edition. Elsevier 2018.)

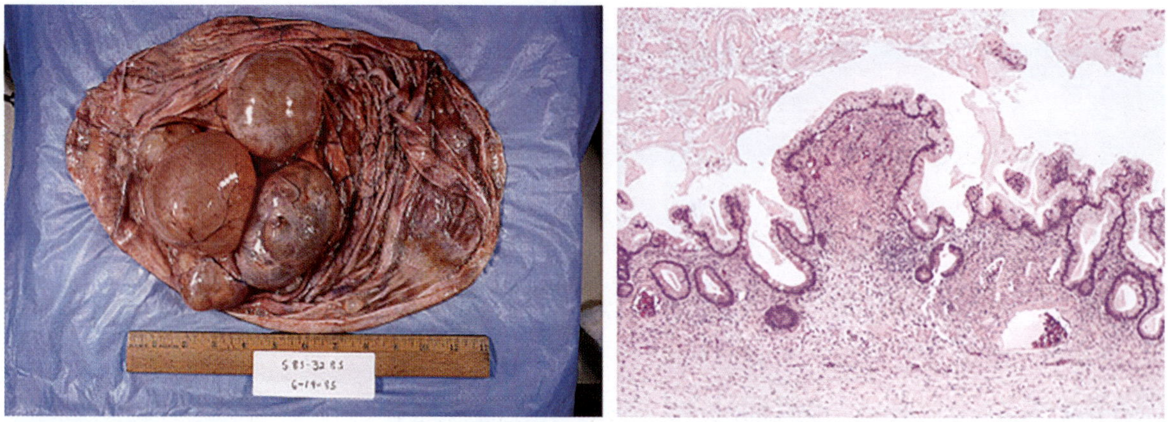

Fig. 26.35 Benign mucinous tumour – gross image showing a multiloculated thin-walled cyst, and microscopy showing the cyst wall lined by a single layer of mucin-containing epithelial cells. (*Source:* From Blake Gilks. Ovary. Rosai and Ackerman's Surgical Pathology. 11th edition. Elsevier 2018; Anne M. Mills and Elisheva D. Shanes. Mucinous Ovarian Tumors. Surgical Pathology Clinics. 2019;12:565–585.)

carcinomas. The common genetic mutations associated with these neoplasms are those of KRAS proto-oncogene, which occur early in the course of development.

Morphology

Mucinous tumours differ from serous tumours as a result of many factors:

- These are less likely to be bilateral (only 5% are bilateral).
- These rarely involve the surface of the ovary.
- These form larger masses.
- These contain mucinous sticky fluid rich in glycoproteins that make them gelatinous.
- Microscopically, the tumours are lined by tall columnar epithelium containing apical mucin and without cilia, resembling gastric, intestinal or endocervical epithelium.

Benign tumours are lined by a single layer (Fig. 26.35), whereas borderline tumours show stratification, tufting or papillary growth without invasion. Mucinous carcinoma shows expansile invasion into the stroma in the form of confluent glands (Fig. 26.36).

IHC: Intestinal-type tumours are CK20 positive, whereas endocervical-type tumours are CA-125 positive. Mucinous tumours have a good prognosis and a 5-year survival rate of about 90%–95% as long as the tumour is confined to the ovaries. Spread of the tumour to the peritoneal surface as implants leads to a condition called ***pseudomyxoma peritonei***. It is charecterised by marked mucinous ascites and adhesions between abdominal and pelvic organs, causing a condition clinically called ***frozen abdomen***.

Endometrioid Carcinoma

Endometrioid tumours are more likely malignant and constitute 10%–15% of ovarian cancers. About 20% of these tumours are associated with ovarian endometriosis and occur about a decade early, whereas 30% coexist with a synchronous (two independent tumours occurring simultaneously) endometrioid carcinoma of

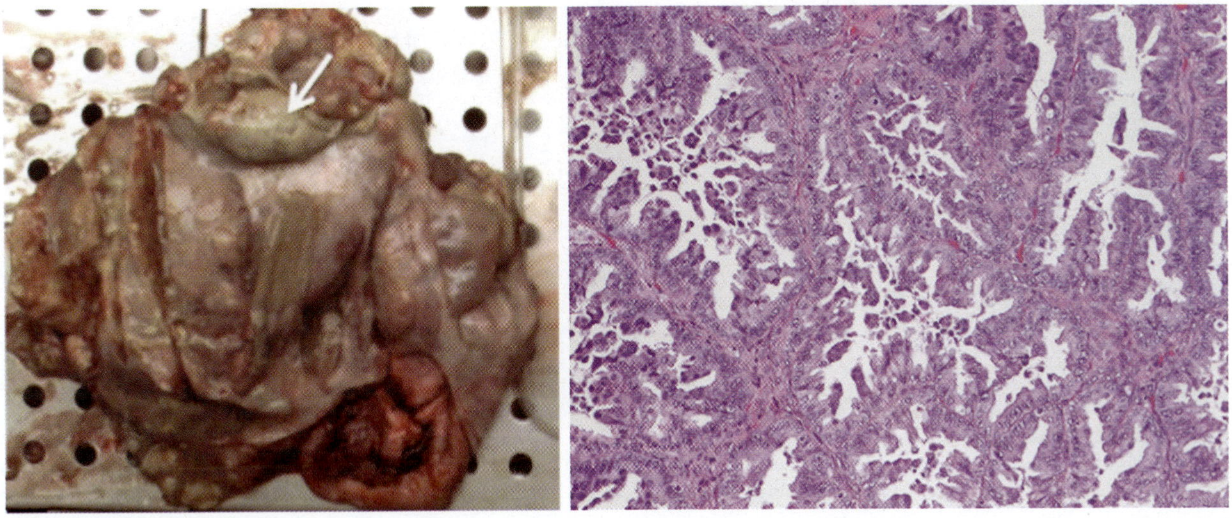

Fig. 26.36 Malignant mucinous tumour – gross image showing a tumour with solid areas (arrow), and microscopy showing a complex papillary structure with stromal invasion of neoplastic cells. (*Source:* From P.-E. Laurent, J. Thomassin-Piana and A. Jalaguier-Coudray. Mucin-producing tumors of the ovary: MR imaging appearance. Diagnostic and Interventional Imaging. 2015;96:1125-1132; Anne M. Mills and Elisheva D. Shanes. Mucinous Ovarian Tumors. Surgical Pathology Clinics. 2019;12:565-585.)

the uterus. These tumours are associated with mutations seen in endometrial carcinomas such as PTEN, KRAS and TP53.

These tumours have a 5-year survival rate of 75% when diagnosed in stage 1.

Morphology

These tumours may be solid or cystic and filled with haemorrhagic fluid (Fig. 26.37). About 40% are bilateral and represent spread of the tumour outside the genital tract. Microscopically, the tumour is composed of glands resembling endometrioid carcinoma occasionally with papillary formation. There may be foci of squamous metaplasia.

IHC: PAX8 positive

Clear Cell Carcinoma

These are rare carcinomas of the ovary composed of a solid sheet of large cells with abundant clear cytoplasm or papillary structures lined by hobnail cells (Fig. 26.38). They sometimes are seen to be associated with **ovarian endometriosis**, or endometrioid carcinoma, and share the same genetic mutations of endometrioid carcinoma. Hence, these are considered as a variant of endometrioid adenocarcinoma. When confined to the ovary, they have a 5-year survival rate of 90%.

Transitional Tumours

These account for 10% of ovarian epithelial tumours and are composed of epithelial cells similar to urothelial transitional epithelium. These tumours are classified into the following types:

- **Benign Brenner tumour:** Usually diagnosed incidentally

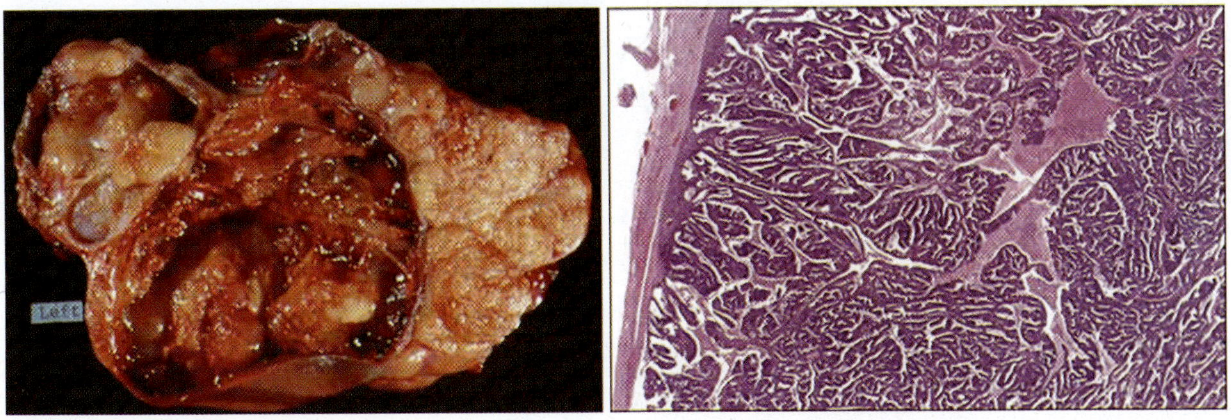

Fig. 26.37 Endometrioid carcinoma – gross image showing a solid cystic tumour filled with haemorrhagic fluid, and microscopy showing a tumour resembling uterine endometrioid tumour. (*Source:* From Jaime Prat. Ovarian Endometrioid, Clear Cell, Transitional, and Mixed Epithelial–Stromal Tumors. Pathology of the Female Reproductive Tract. 3rd edition. Elsevier 2014.)

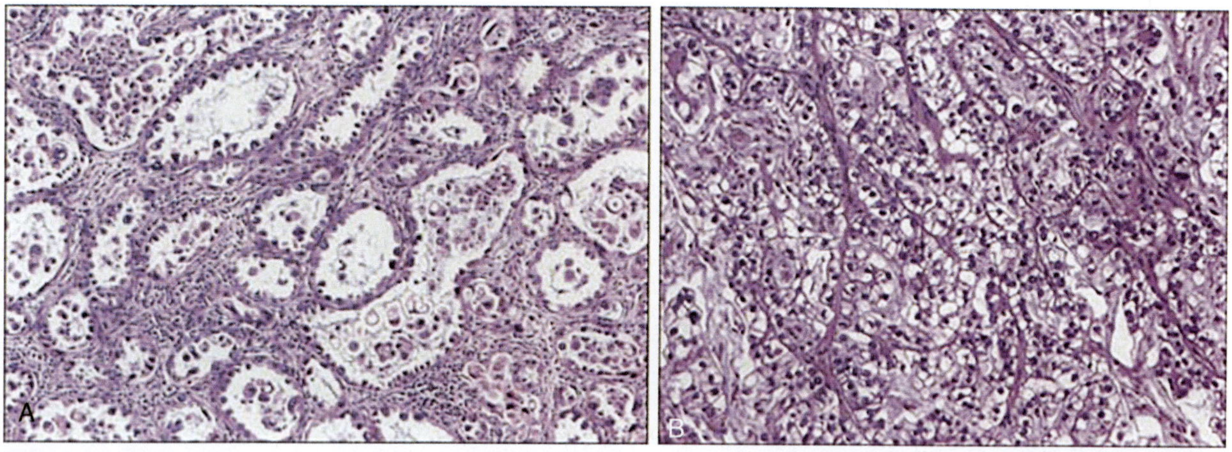

Fig. 26.38 Clear cell carcinoma – microscopy showing hobnail pattern (A) and a clear cell pattern (B). (*Source:* From Jaime Prat. Ovarian Endometrioid, Clear Cell, Transitional, and Mixed Epithelial–Stromal Tumors. Pathology of the Female Reproductive Tract. 3rd edition. Elsevier 2014.)

- **Malignant Brenner tumour:** Considered as grade 1/ low-grade neoplasms
- **Transitional cell carcinoma:** High-grade carcinoma similar to high-grade serous carcinoma

Morphology

These are mostly unilateral, often solid with cystic areas and vary from 1 to 20–30 cm in size. Microscopically, the tumour is composed of fibrous stroma with interspersed nests of transitional epithelium (Fig. 26.39).

Benign Brenner tumour: Benign nests
Malignant Brenner tumour: Benign nests with occasional malignant cells
Transitional cell carcinoma: More than 50% malignant transitional epithelium

Clinical Features of Ovarian Surface Tumours

Ovarian surface epithelial tumours are asymptomatic and present with lower abdominal pain and abdominal mass when the tumours are significantly enlarged. Malignant tumours may be associated with loss of appetite and weight.

Benign tumours can be treated easily with surgical excision, whereas malignant tumours may need postoperative chemotherapy. Malignant tumours often spread into the peritoneal cavity as deposits on the peritoneal surface that may occasionally invade into the underlying tissue. Haematogenous metastasis to the liver, lung and GI tract and lymphatic metastasis to regional lymph nodes may be seen. Measurement of tumour marker CA-125 helps in assessing completeness of treatment, follow-up and recurrence.

Currently, screening of women to identify high-risk mutations such as BRCA1 and BRCA2 and offering prophylactic salpingo-oophorectomy are the only measures available for the prevention of high-grade carcinomas.

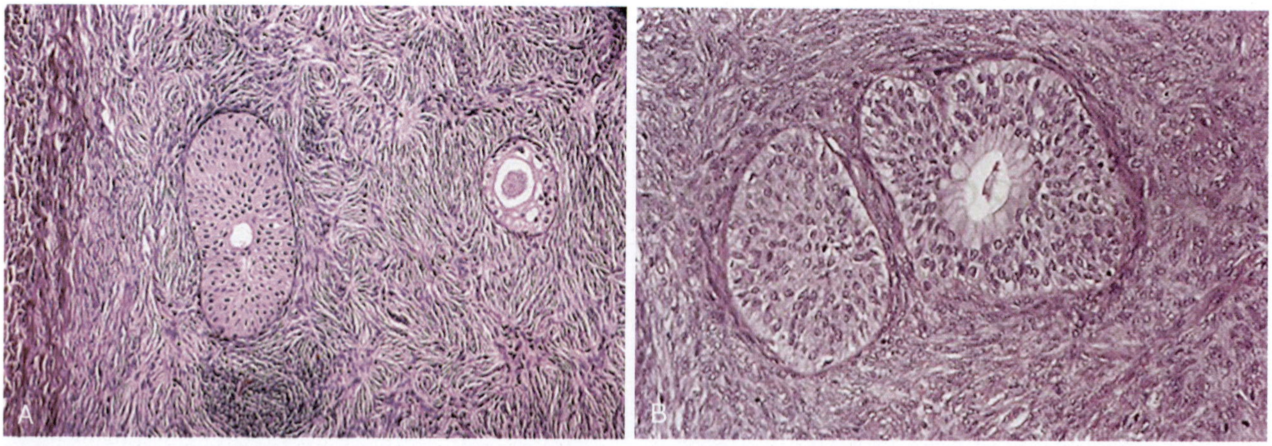

Fig. 26.39 Microscopy of benign Brenner (A) and malignant Brenner (B). (*Source:* A: From Blake Gilks. Ovary. Rosai and Ackerman's Surgical Pathology. 11th edition. B: Diagnostic Pathology: Gynecological, 2nd ed.: Elsevier Inc., 2019; pii:B9780323548151501920/u185-1743-9780323548175.)

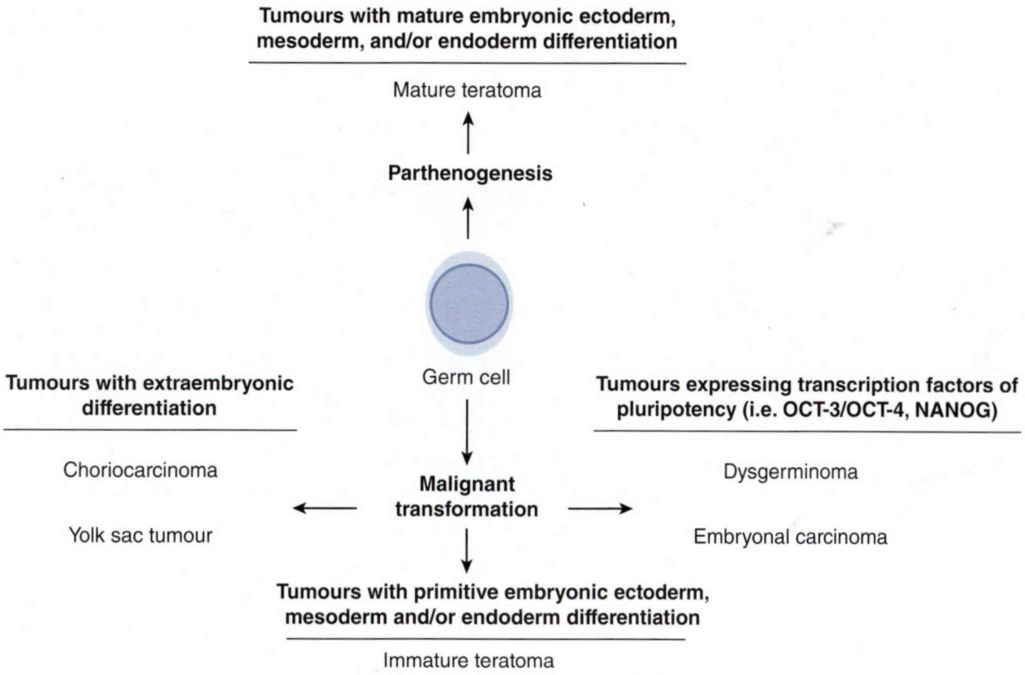

Fig. 26.40 Hypothetical diagram of the origin of germ cell tumours. (*Source:* From Fabiola Medeiros and Kyle C. Strickland. Germ Cell Tumors of the Ovary. Diagnostic Gynecologic and Obstetric Pathology. 3rd edition. Elsevier 2018.)

GERM CELL TUMOURS

Germ cell tumours are more common in the younger age group and constitute about 20% of ovarian tumours. Different types of tumours may develop from the germ cell and have different features and prognosis (Fig. 26.40). Most common among them are benign teratomas.

Teratoma

Teratomas of the ovary are classified into benign mature teratoma (also called dermoid cyst), malignant immature teratoma and monodermal teratoma. Teratomas by definition are composed of tissues originating from more than one germ cell layer or all three germ cell layers – the ectoderm, mesoderm and endoderm.

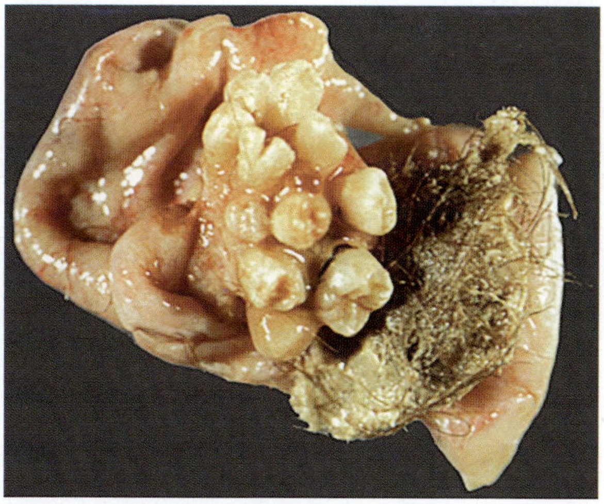

Fig. 26.41 Gross of mature teratoma showing Rokitansky tubercle and hair. (*Source:* From Fabiola Medeiros and Kyle C. Strickland. Germ Cell Tumors of the Ovary. Diagnostic Gynecologic and Obstetric Pathology. 3rd edition. Elsevier 2018.)

Morphology

Benign Mature Teratoma These are cystic structures lined by skin-like epidermis and dermis and hence referred to as **dermoid cyst**. These occur in the reproductive age group and are often incidental findings but occasionally may cause paraneoplastic syndromes such as inflammatory limbic encephalitis that may resolve on surgical excision of the teratoma.

On gross examination, these cysts contain cheesy material, which is the accumulated keratin, and are lined by thin grey glistening epidermis with collection of hair. Areas of calcification and teeth-like protrusions called Rokitansky tubercles may be seen (Fig. 26.41). Microscopic examination shows the lining of the cyst to be keratinizing stratified squamous epithelium with adnexal structures such as sweat glands, sebaceous glands and hair follicles. Foci of thyroid, bone, cartilage or neural tissue may be seen representing other layers. Sometimes, the mature teratoma may be completely solid and difficult to differentiate from immature teratoma. Rarely, any one of the mature components may undergo malignant change – the commonest change being squamous cell carcinoma (Fig. 26.42).

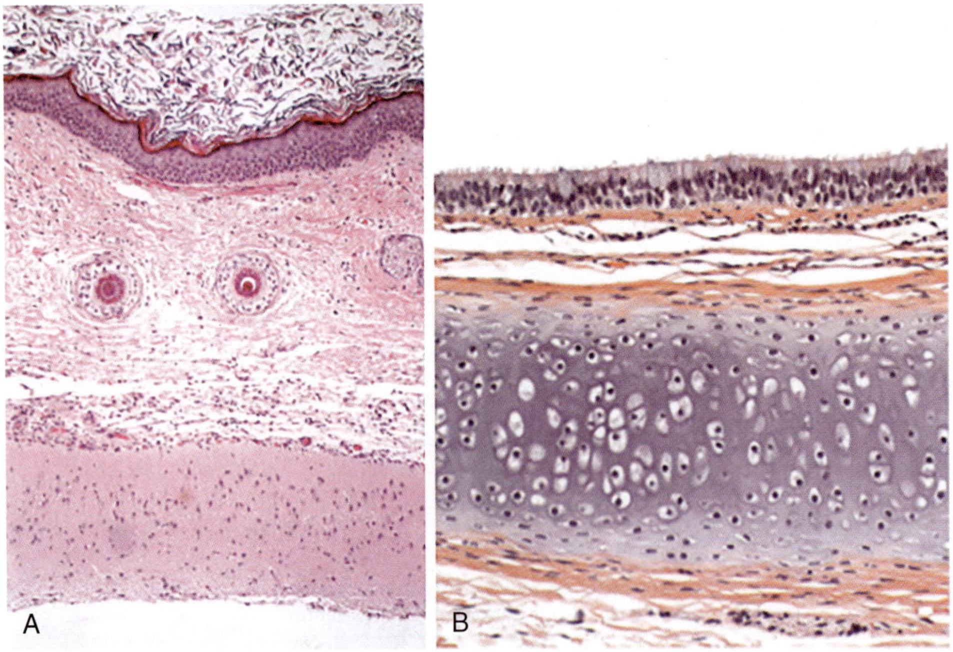

Fig. 26.42 Microscopic images of mature teratoma showing skin with underlying cerebral cortex (A) and respiratory epithelium with underlying cartilage (B). (*Source:* From Fabiola Medeiros and Kyle C. Strickland. Germ Cell Tumors of the Ovary. Diagnostic Gynecologic and Obstetric Pathology. 3rd edition. Elsevier 2018.)

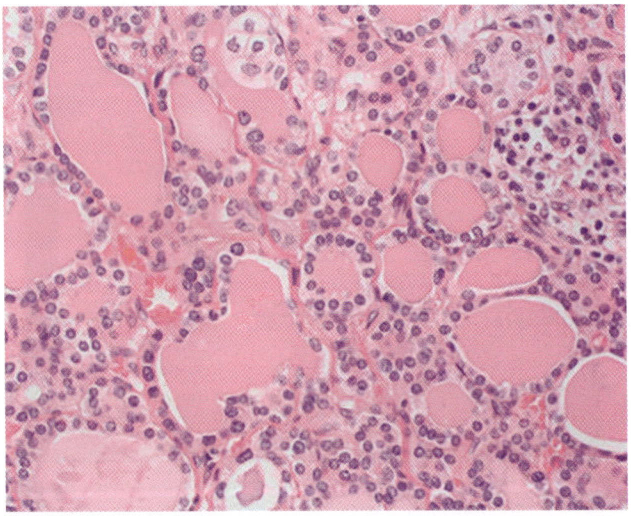

Fig. 26.43 Microscopy of struma ovarii showing benign thyroid follicles.

Monodermal Teratoma These are **specialized teratomas** composed purely of one type of tissue such as thyroid (Fig. 26.43). The most common ones and their presenting features are given in Table 26.16.

Immature Malignant Teratoma These tumours are the most common in teenage and are similar to benign teratomas except for the presence of embryonal and fetal immature tissues.

On gross appearance (Fig. 26.44), these are large solid tumours with smooth external surface. Sectioning shows hair, teeth, cartilage, bone and sebaceous material along with solid areas with haemorrhage and necrosis. Microscopic examination reveals the presence of immature tissue, the most important among them being **immature neuroepithelium**. The proportion of this component is the factor that helps to grade the malignant teratoma, their risk of extraovarian spread and ultimately the prognosis.

Table 26.16 Specialized Teratomas

Tumour	Tissue	Presenting Feature
Struma ovarii	Mature thyroid tissue	Hyperthyroidism
Carcinoid	Neuroendocrine tumour	Carcinoid syndrome in the absence of hepatic metastasis because ovarian veins drain into systemic circulation and not into portal circulation

These tumours are often associated with rapid increase in size, rupture of ovarian capsule and local/distant spread. Stage 1 tumours confined to the ovary have a good prognosis. High-grade tumours even if confined to the ovary require chemotherapy after surgery. If recurrence is not seen within the first 2 years, prognosis is good and chance of cure is high.

Dysgerminoma

These are malignant germ cell tumours constituting 50% of malignant germ cell carcinomas of the ovary. These

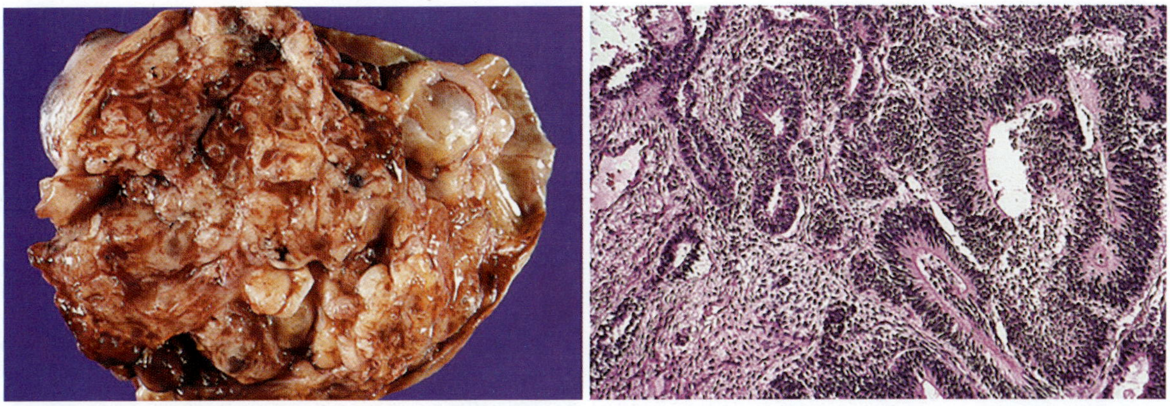

Fig. 26.44 Immature teratoma – gross image showing predominant solid areas, and microscopy showing immature neuroepithelium. (*Source:* From Blake Gilks. Ovary. Rosai and Ackerman's Surgical Pathology. 11th edition. Elsevier 2018.)

represent the ovarian counterpart of seminoma of the testis and present most commonly in the second and third decades of life. **Gonadal dysgenesis** as in the case of pseudohermaphroditism is a risk factor for this tumour.

Molecular profile shows the expression of OCT-3, OCT-4 and NANOG, which are factors maintaining pluripotency as in seminomas and activating mutations of the cKIT gene.

Morphology

Most dysgerminomas are unilateral solid tumours ranging from small to large masses, soft, fleshy, grey-white to pink in appearance on the cut section (Fig. 26.45). Microscopically, these are composed of sheets of large cells with distinct cell margins, clear cytoplasm and a central nucleus. The cells are separated by thin fibrous stroma containing lymphocytic infiltration. High-grade tumours show histological atypia and are aggressive.

IHC: PLAP, cKIT (CD117) positive

Tumour marker: β-Human chorionic gonadotropin (β-hCG), which may be elevated in few cases that show trophoblastic differentiation

For tumours that have not breached the ovarian capsule, salpingo-oophorectomy is curative, whereas for those that have extended beyond the ovary, cure is possible by surgery with chemotherapy.

Yolk Sac Tumour

It is a malignant germ cell tumour arising from cells differentiating to form extraembryonic structure, the yolk sac. It is the second most common germ cell carcinoma usually presenting in children or adolescents with precocious puberty or menorrhagia.

Morphology

These are solid tumours with areas of haemorrhage and necrosis. Microscopy shows a loose network of cells forming the characteristic **Schiller–Duval body** (Fig. 26.46), which is a glomerulus-like structure. It has a central blood vessel surrounded by a layer of cells inside a cystic space lined by similar cells. **Hyaline droplets** may be seen both intracellularly and extracellularly.

IHC: α-Fetoprotein (AFP) positive in hyaline droplets

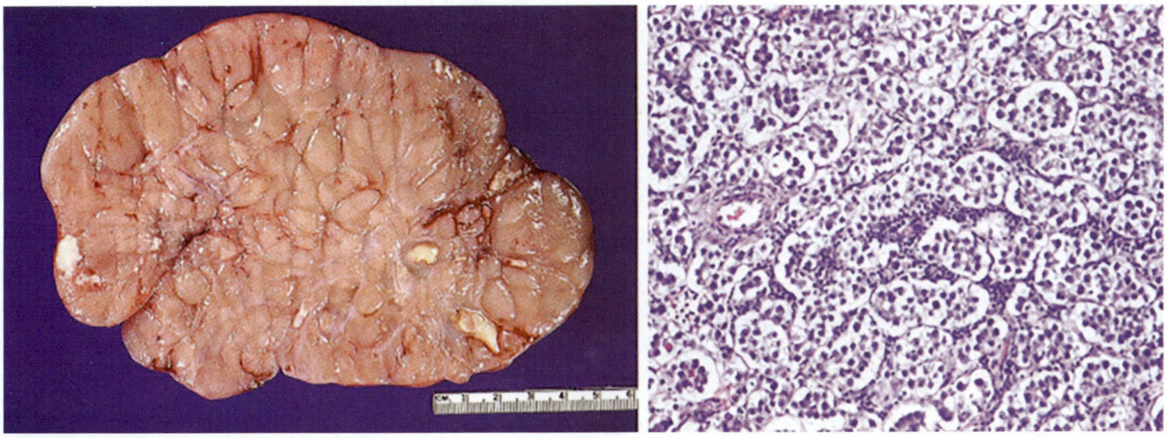

Fig. 26.45 Dysgerminoma – gross image showing a nodular appearance with tan colour, and microscopy showing a nesting pattern.

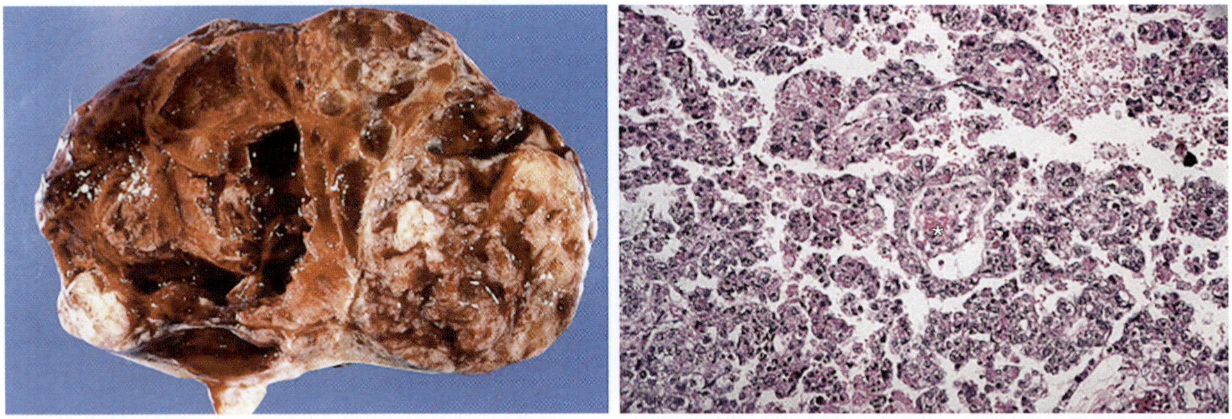

Fig. 26.46 Yolk sac tumour – gross image showing haemorrhage with necrosis and microscopy showing Schiller–Duval bodies (*). (*Source:* From Blake Gilks. Ovary. Rosai and Ackerman's Surgical Pathology. 11th edition. Elsevier 2018.)

Tumour marker: AFP

Combination chemotherapy yields good results.

Choriocarcinoma

These tumours may be of the placental origin or arise from malignant extraembryonic germ cells. Choriocarcinoma of the ovary in postpubertal women is more likely from placental tissue of an ovarian ectopic pregnancy, whereas germ cell origin is the cause in prepubertal girls.

Morphology

Morphology is similar to that of the placental tumour, discussed later, and is composed of cytotrophoblasts, intermediate trophoblasts and syncytiotrophoblasts with abundant mitosis (Fig. 26.47). But the prognosis is worse in an ovarian tumour due to aggressive nature; aggressive metastasis to the lungs, liver and bone; and nonresponsiveness to chemotherapy.

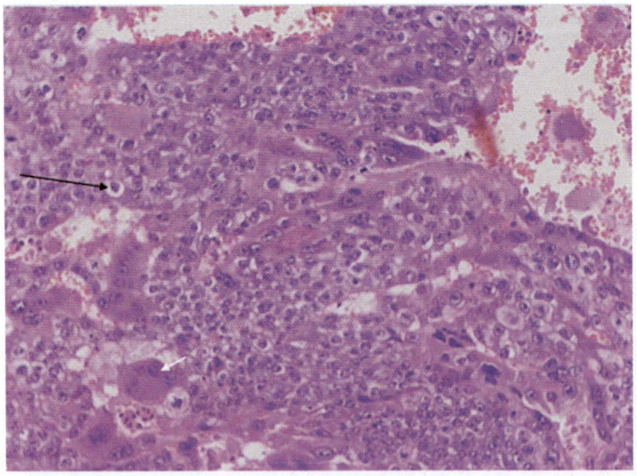

Fig. 26.47 Microscopy of choriocarcinoma showing a tumour composed of cytotrophoblasts (black arrow), intermediate trophoblasts and syncytiotrophoblasts (white arrow) and brisk mitosis of more than 20/HPF. HPF, high-power field. (*Source:* From Mutua Irene et al, Journal of Pediatric Surgery Case Reports, Elsevier 2019.)

Tumour marker: β-hCG

SEX CORD–STROMAL TUMOURS

The undifferentiated mesenchymal cells of ovarian stroma may differentiate into the following:

1. Male-type cells such as Leydig and Sertoli cells that produce androgen and cause virilization
2. Female-type cells such as granulosa and theca cells that produce oestrogen and cause feminization

Granulosa Cell Tumour

These are germ cell tumours that are composed of cells resembling granulosa cells of ovarian follicles. These may occur in any age group but are more common in postmenopausal women. These are classified into the following types:

- **Adult granulosa cell tumours:** More common, occur in older women, present with menorrhagia, proliferative breast lesions, endometrial hyperplasia/carcinoma, associated with FOXL2 gene mutations
- **Juvenile granulosa cell tumours:** Present in the young age with precocious puberty, more aggressive with a greater metastatic potential

Morphology

Granulosa cells in the tumour may be seen to form cords, strands, papillae or sheets. The cells occasionally form small gland-like microfollicles with central acidophilic material called **Call–Exner bodies** (Fig. 26.48). The individual cells are small and polygonal with *nuclear grooves*. Occasional cluster of thecal cells with abundant cytoplasm may be seen.

Granulosa cell tumours elaborate large quantities of oestrogen, producing hyperoestrogenic state in the

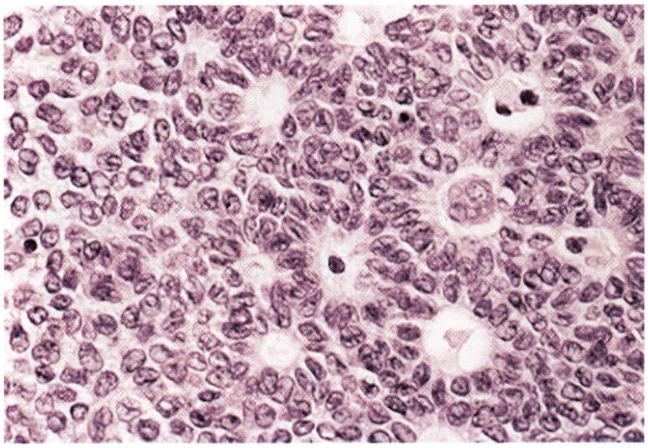

Fig. 26.48 Microscopy of granulosa cell tumour showing Call–Exner bodies and coffee bean nuclei. (*Source:* From Blake Gilks. Ovary. Rosai and Ackerman's Surgical Pathology. 11th edition. Elsevier 2018.)

patients and leading to its related symptoms. They always have malignant potential, but malignant tumours are often low grade and take an indolent course. Surgical management may be followed by recurrences, but such recurrences may also be treated by surgery. Overall, the 10-year survival rate is around 85%.

Fibromas, Thecomas and Fibrothecomas

Tumours of the ovarian stroma may be composed of a varying proportion of fibroblasts and thecal cells. These are mostly benign.

Fibroma: Composed of spindle cells and fibroblasts, and are hormonally inactive
Thecomas: Composed of plump cells with intracellular lipid droplets and elaborate hormones
Fibrothecoma: Mixture of both cells, variable hormonal activity

Morphology

These tumours are mostly unilateral, firm, solid, encapsulated, grey-white mass with a lobulated appearance covered by an intact ovarian serosa (Fig. 26.49). Microscopic examination may show fibroblasts or plump thecal cells or a mixture of both. Rare cases may show marked nuclear atypia and mitotic activity that should be classified as **fibrosarcoma** due to their aggressiveness.

Clinically, the tumour may present as a pelvic mass with associated pelvic pain. Occasionally, tumours larger than 6 cm present with a unique combination of symptoms – ovarian mass with ascites and right-sided pleural effusion – called **Meigs syndrome**. These tumours may be rarely associated with basal cell nevus syndrome.

Sertoli–Leydig Cell Tumours

These are stromal tumours that produce androgens and often cause defeminization and masculinization. The tumour is thus made up of the causative cells, Leydig and Sertoli cells, in various stages of development. These are associated with mutations of the DICER1 gene and commonly occur in young women.

Morphology

Grossly, these are unilateral, solid and grey to brown tumours. Microscopically, these vary in appearance

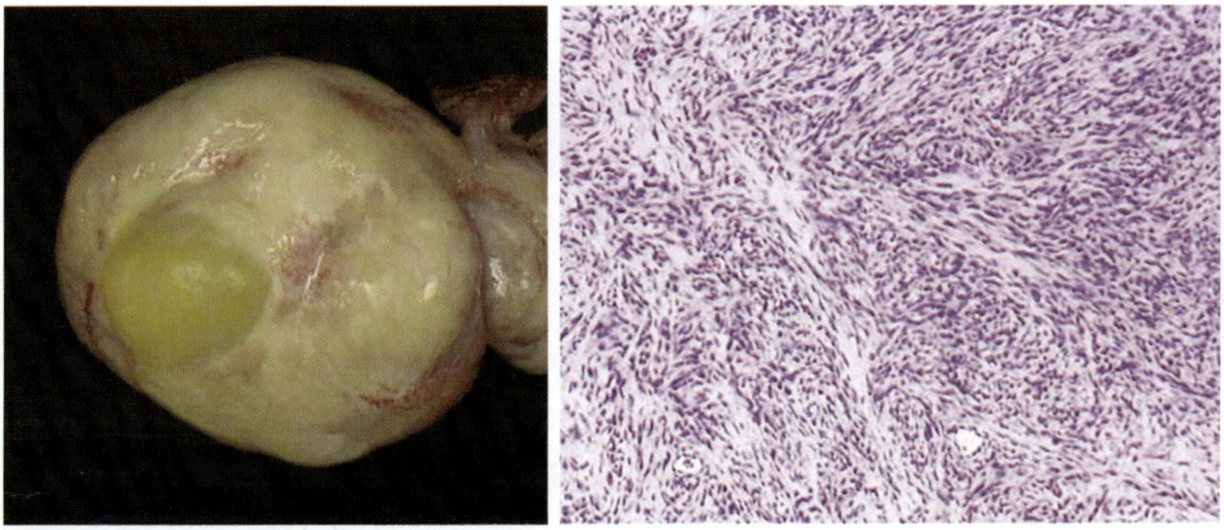

Fig. 26.49 Fibrothecoma – gross image showing a homogeneous grey-white mass, and microscopy showing sheets of spindle cells (fibroblasts). (*Source:* From Christopher P. Crum, Anna R. Laury, Michelle S. Hirsch, Charles Matthew Quick and William A. Peters. Thecoma-Fibroma. Gynecologic and Obstetric Pathology. Saunders 2016; Ming Zhou, George J. Netto and Jonathan I. Epstein. Fibrothecoma. High-Yield Uropathology. Saunders 2012.)

from tubules of Sertoli and Leydig cells in well-differentiated forms to sarcomatous stroma with irregular cords in poorly differentiated tumours. Occasional heterologous components such as bone or cartilage may be seen.

Clinically, these tumours present with defeminization, causing breast atrophy amenorrhoea, loss of hair and sterility. Later on, the women develop hirsutism, voice change and enlargement of the clitoris leading to masculinization.

Metastatic Tumours

Ovarian metastasis may have the following origins:

- From other parts of the female genital tract with Müllerian epithelial origin such as the uterus, contralateral ovary and tubes
- From other organs such as the breast and GI tract

Morphology

Krukenberg tumours are unique tumours that spread to bilateral ovaries by transcoelomic spread from the GI tract, especially the stomach. The ovaries macroscopically appear solid and multinodular. Microscopy shows *signet ring cells* in a background of stromal proliferation in a storiform pattern (Fig. 26.50).

GESTATIONAL TROPHOBLASTIC DISEASES PA 30.5

Gestational trophoblastic disorders constitute a group of disorders that show proliferation of villi or trophoblastic cells. These include hydatidiform mole, choriocarcinoma and placental site trophoblastic tumour (PSTT).

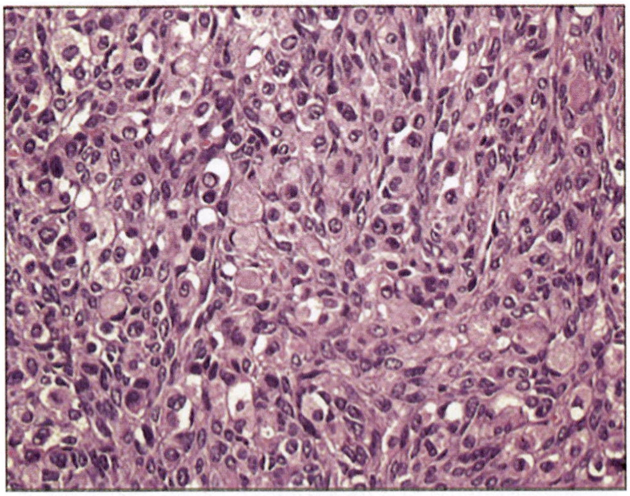

Fig. 26.50 Microscopy of Krukenberg tumour showing signet ring cells. (*Source:* From Emanuela D'Angelo and Jaime Prat. Metastatic Tumors of the Ovary. Pathology of the Female Reproductive Tract. 3rd edition. Elsevier 2014.)

HYDATIDIFORM MOLE

Hydatidiform mole is a placental disorder characterized by oedematous swelling of the villi and proliferation of trophoblasts (Fig. 26.51). The moles are common in the extremes of the reproductive age group, and ultrasonography helps in their diagnosis during early pregnancy. They are associated with an increase in the risk of developing subsequent choriocarcinoma.

The three types of mole are as follows (Table 26.17):

- Partial mole
- Complete mole
- Invasive mole

Clinical Features

Molar pregnancy may present with bleeding in the first trimester or may be identified during routine first trimester scan, which shows snowstorm appearance. Serum hCG levels are elevated more than expected in normal pregnancy. Evacuation of the uterus is performed, and the products appear as translucent grape-like clusters. These women are followed for up to 1 year till serum hCG levels

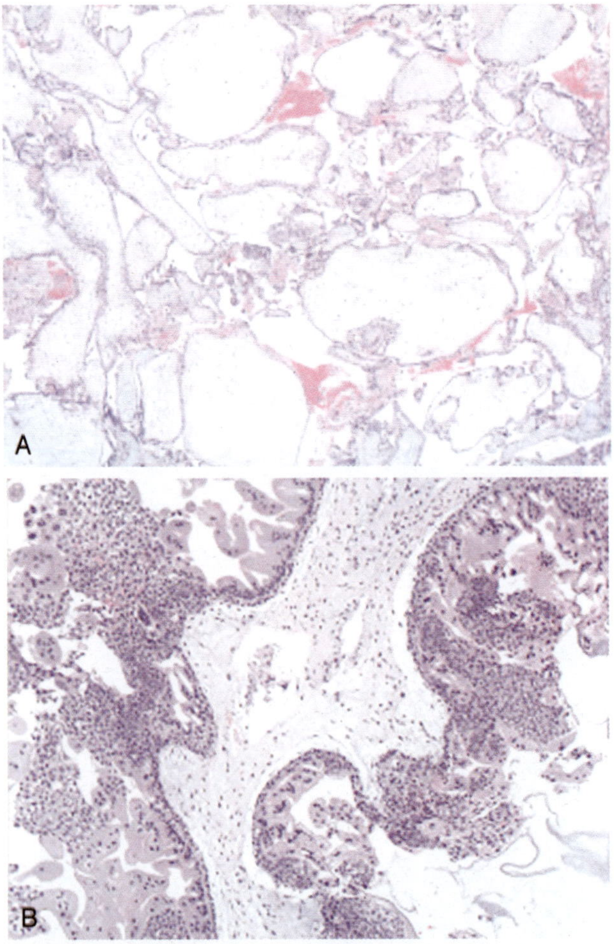

Fig. 26.51 Microscopy of the partial mole showing oedematous villi (A) and the complete mole showing cistern formation and trophoblastic proliferation (B). (*Source:* From Natalia Buza and Pei Hui. Ancillary studies for precision diagnosis of hydatidiform moles. Diagnostic Histopathology. 2017; 23:292–302.)

TABLE 26.17 Comparison of Partial and Complete Moles

Partial Mole	Complete Mole
Fertilization of one egg by two sperms	About 90% formed by duplication of sperm chromosomes inside an empty ovum, whereas 10% from two sperms entering an empty ovum
Maternal chromosomes plus two sets from the paternal side forming 69XXY or 69XXX	No maternal chromosomes, 46XX or 46XY from paternal origin
Fetal tissue present	Embryo dies very early, so no fetal tissue seen
No risk of choriocarcinoma	About 2.5% risk of choriocarcinoma
Microscopy shows partial involvement of villi with focal trophoblastic proliferation	Microscopy shows all villi to be oedematous, swollen with extensive proliferation of trophoblasts

reach the normal value. Persistently elevated hCG in serum is an indication of an invasive mole.

Invasive Mole

Invasion of the myometrium by the atypically proliferating trophoblasts leading to **penetration or perforation of the uterine wall** is called invasive mole. It not only invades adjacent organs such as the parametrium but may also embolize to distant organs such as the lungs. But unlike metastasis, it does not grow there, instead regresses spontaneously. It is diagnosed by a persistent rise in hCG levels and enlargement of the uterus. Treatment is by chemotherapy, but surgery may be needed if perforation of the uterus occurs.

CHORIOCARCINOMA

Choriocarcinoma is a rapidly spreading carcinoma of trophoblastic cells that originated from a previous pregnancy. It occurs in women of the reproductive age group, and it may follow:

- Hydatidiform mole (highest risk)
- Previous abortion
- Normal pregnancy
- Ectopic pregnancy

Morphology

Choriocarcinomas are soft fleshy tumours with marked areas of necrosis and haemorrhage often invading the myometrium even up to serosa or beyond. Microscopically, these are composed of sheets of trophoblasts with atypical mitosis and the *total absence of villi* (Fig. 26.52).

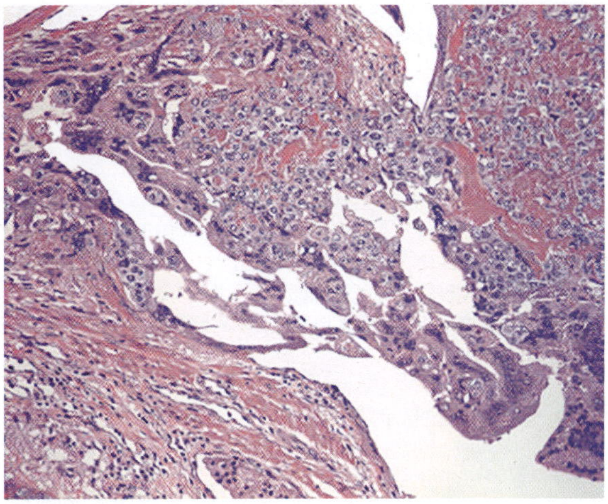

Fig. 26.52 Microscopy of choriocarcinoma admixture of syncytiotrophoblasts and cytotrophoblasts with the absence of villi. (*Source:* From Blake Gilks, Rosai and Ackerman's Surgical Pathology, Elsevier 2018.)

The tumour may occur during the course of normal delivery or up to months following a conception, normal or abnormal. The patient usually presents with bloody or brownish vaginal discharge and blood hCG levels are much elevated. Investigation to check for metastasis is essential due to the nature of the tumour to metastasize early through the haematogenous route to the lungs and vagina. Other sites include the brain, liver, bone and kidney.

Treatment

Treatment is usually by evacuation of the uterus, followed by chemotherapy. This tumour is highly responsive to chemotherapy, and most get cured or achieve 100% remission. Good cure rates and even subsequent normal pregnancies are possible. However, choriocarcinoma that rarely develops from germ cells of the ovary is resistant to chemotherapy and has a bad prognosis.

PLACENTAL SITE TROPHOBLASTIC TUMOUR

PSTT is a placental tumour that occurs following normal pregnancy (75% cases) or hydatidiform mole. It is due to neoplastic proliferation of intermediate trophoblasts that are normally present in extravillous locations such as the implantation area and placental membranes.

Morphology

Gross appearance is that of a well-circumscribed or ill-defined myometrial mass. Necrosis and haemorrhage are inconspicuous. Microscopically, it is composed of large polygonal trophoblastic cells with nuclear pleomorphism invading into the myometrium.

Patients usually present with uterine bleeding or amenorrhoea. β-hCG level is not as elevated as in choriocarcinoma. The tumour is amenable to therapy, but about 15% of patients die due to metastasis.

SELF-ASSESSMENT

Multiple Choice Questions

1. Vaginal tumour presenting as grape-like clusters in young children is
   A. Basaloid vaginal carcinoma
   B. Keratinizing squamous cell carcinoma of the vagina
   C. Sarcoma botryoides
   D. Warty carcinoma
2. The E6 protein produced by HPV leads to cervical carcinoma by
   A. Inhibiting p53 gene
   B. Inhibiting Rb gene
   C. Inhibiting CDK inhibitors
   D. Dysregulating MYC
3. Koilocytic changes in LSIL include all of the following except
   A. Perinuclear vacuolation
   B. Prune-like nucleus
   C. Rope-like chromatin
   D. Irregular nuclear membrane
4. Endometriosis of the ovary leads to the formation of
   A. Chocolate cyst of the ovary
   B. Adenomyosis
   C. Endometrioid carcinoma
   D. Polycystic ovaries
5. Dyspareunia and postcoital bleeding are classical clinical symptoms of
   A. Endometrial polyp
   B. Carcinoma cervix
   C. Adenomyosis
   D. Ectopic pregnancy
6. Which female genital tract malignancy is seen associated with Cowden syndrome?
   A. Carcinoma cervix
   B. Carcinoma endometrium
   C. Serous carcinoma ovary
   D. Mucinous carcinoma ovary
7. The common mutation associated with endometrial serous carcinoma is
   A. TP53
   B. PTEN
   C. KRAS
   D. ARID1A
8. The myomas associated with leiomyomatosis/RCC syndrome are
   A. Benign metastasizing leiomyoma
   B. Disseminated peritoneal leiomyomatosis
   C. Symplastic leiomyoma
   D. Leiomyoma with fumarate hydratase deficiency
9. Most common malignant tumours of the ovary are
   A. Serous tumours
   B. Mucinous tumours
   C. Teratoma
   D. Krukenberg tumour
10. The immunohistochemical marker used to differentiate serous ovarian tumours from mucinous tumours is
    A. CK7
    B. CA125
    C. WT1
    D. TTF
11. The immature tissue used for grading of immature teratoma is
    A. Epidermis
    B. Neuroepithelium
    C. Cartilage
    D. Thyroid
12. Neuroendocrine tissue in specialized teratoma of the ovary presents with
    A. Postmenopausal bleeding
    B. Carcinoid syndrome
    C. Hyperthyroidism
    D. Amenorrhoea
13. Gonadal dysgenesis of the ovary is a risk factor for ovarian
    A. Malignant teratoma
    B. Yolk sac tumour
    C. Choriocarcinoma
    D. Dysgerminoma
14. α-Fetoprotein is a tumour marker for
    A. Yolk sac tumour
    B. Choriocarcinoma
    C. Dysgerminoma
    D. Sertoli–Leydig cell tumour
15. Call–Exner bodies are rosettes of tumour cell arrangements seen in
    A. Yolk sac tumour
    B. Granulosa cell tumour
    C. Yolk sac tumour
    D. Dysgerminoma
16. Meigs syndrome seen in fibroma of the ovary includes all of the following except
    A. Ovarian mass
    B. Ascites
    C. Pleural effusion
    D. Pericardial effusion
17. The mode of spread of Krukenberg tumour to the ovary is
    A. Hematogenous
    B. Lymphatic
    C. Transcoelomic
    D. Direct invasion
18. Absence of maternal chromosomes in the zygote leads to the formation of
    A. Partial mole
    B. Complete mole
    C. Invasive mole
    D. Any of the above
19. The characteristic feature of yolk sac tumour is the presence of
    A. Coffee bean nuclei
    B. Signet ring cells
    C. Hobnail pattern
    D. Schiller–Duval bodies
20. The characteristic feature of choriocarcinoma includes
    A. Focal trophoblastic proliferation
    B. Cistern formation within villi
    C. Complete absence of villi
    D. Penetration of the uterine wall

Answers

1. (C); 2. (A); 3. (C); 4. (A); 5. (B); 6. (B); 7. (A); 8. (D); 9. (A); 10. (C); 11. (B); 12. (B); 13. (D); 14. (A); 15. (B); 16. (D); 17. (C); 18. (B); 19. (D); 20. (C)

Self-Assessment Questions

1. What is the transformation zone in the cervix and what is its significance?
2. A 28-year woman taking oral contraceptives presented to the gynaecology outpatient department (OPD) with vulval itching for the past 5 days and curdy white precipitate. Identify the cause. How will you confirm the diagnosis?
3. A 30-year-old 36-week pregnant woman complains of pain in the vulval area during her antenatal visit. On examination, painful ulcers are seen in the vulva with enlarged tender inguinal lymph nodes. What will you suspect? How will you confirm your diagnosis? What precautions will you advise her?
4. A mother of a 2-year-old girl brings the child to OPD with complaints of passing grape-like masses from the vagina. What is the likely problem?
5. A 32-year-old woman had come to the clinic to discuss her Pap smear report. The report stated that koilocytic changes were seen. What is koilocytic change and what is the cause for it?
6. A 45-year-old woman presented with menorrhagia and irregular vaginal bleeding. Ultrasound scan showed a normal ovary and uterus. What is the likely cause? What is the role of biopsy in this woman?
7. A 45-year-old woman from a village came to the primary health centre (PHC) with postcoital bleeding and irregular spotting. Speculum examination shows a fleshy red growth on the cervix. What is your diagnosis? Write in detail about the pathogenesis, morphology and staging of your diagnosis.
8. What are the risk factors for endometrial hyperplasia? How do you classify it? Explain the morphology findings and their relevance.
9. A 50-year-old woman presented with irregular vaginal bleeding and menorrhagia. Ultrasound scan showed a thickened endometrium. Biopsy was performed that showed glands invading into the myometrium. What is the diagnosis? Explain the pathogenesis and morphology of your diagnosis.
10. Why is serous endometrial carcinoma associated with a poorer outcome than endometrioid?
11. A 35-year-old woman presented with menorrhagia and dysmenorrhoea. On examination, the uterus appeared enlarged. Ultrasound scan showed multiple tumours of varying sizes within the wall of the uterus. What is the likely diagnosis?
12. A 45-year-old woman presented with an enlarged abdomen and loss of appetite and weight. Ultrasound scan showed a large mass in the uterus. Endometrial sampling was normal. Hysterectomy was performed that showed a large mass in the myometrium with necrosis and haemorrhage. What will you suspect?
13. A 26-year-old woman presented to OPD for infertility treatment. She had irregular cycles and on examination had excess facial hair and was obese. What is the cause? How will you evaluate?
14. A 52-year-old woman presented with abdominal distension increasing in size over the past 3 months. Ultrasound scan showed a unilateral enlarged cystic ovary with solid areas filled with clear fluid. What is the possible diagnosis? What is the tumour marker used?
15. A 16-year-old girl presented with acute abdominal pain to the emergency department. Ultrasound scan showed an ovarian cyst that had undergone torsion. She was operated upon, and the cyst sent to pathology showed hair inside it. What is your diagnosis?
16. What is struma ovarii? What complication can it cause?
17. A woman with ovarian tumour had raised α-fetoprotein levels. Histopathology of the tumour mentions about Schiller–Duval bodies. What is the origin of this tumour and what is the prognosis?
18. A 55-year-old woman presented with postmenopausal bleeding. Ultrasound scan showed mildly thickened endometrium and enlarged ovaries, suggesting an ovarian neoplasm. What is your diagnosis? Explain the morphology findings.
19. A known patient with gastric carcinoma developed bilateral enlargement of the ovaries. What are the cause and mechanism?
20. A 23-year-old primigravida woman with 8 weeks' amenorrhoea had complaints of excess vomiting. A few days later, she passed grape-like translucent structures and started bleeding per vaginum. What is the diagnosis? What is the cause for her problem?
21. A 25-year-old woman with a history of complete mole in her previous pregnancy on follow-up showed an increase in β-hCG values. What could be the cause?

Answers

1. Refer text
2. *Candida* infection, refer text
3. Herpes simplex, refer text
4. Embryonal rhabdomyosarcoma
5. HPV induced, refer text
6. Dysfunctional uterine bleeding
7. Cervical carcinoma
8. Refer text
9. Endometrial carcinoma
10. Refer text
11. Multiple leiomyoma
12. Leiomyosarcoma
13. Polycystic ovarian syndrome
14. Ovarian serous tumour, CA125
15. Ovarian teratoma
16. Refer text
17. Yolk sac tumour
18. Granulosa cell tumour
19. Krukenberg tumour
20. Hydatidiform mole (molar pregnancy)
21. Check for development of choriocarcinoma

Topics for Self-Directed Learning

1. Premalignant lesions of the vulva
2. Factors predisposing to pelvic infections
3. Birth anomalies of the uterus
4. Management of abnormal Pap smears
5. Applications of dating of endometrium
6. Follow-up of endometrial hyperplasia
7. Criteria for the classification of myometrial tumours into leiomyoma, STUMP and leiomyosarcoma
8. Stromal tumours of the uterus
9. Lesions of the fallopian tube causing infertility
10. Genetic changes in various ovarian tumours
11. Prevention and screening for surface ovarian tumours
12. Androgenic tumours of the ovary
13. Mixed ovarian tumours
14. Immunohistochemistry profiling of ovarian tumours
15. Placental structural abnormalities
16. Placental changes in preeclampsia and eclampsia
17. Follow-up of molar pregnancy

MIND MAPS

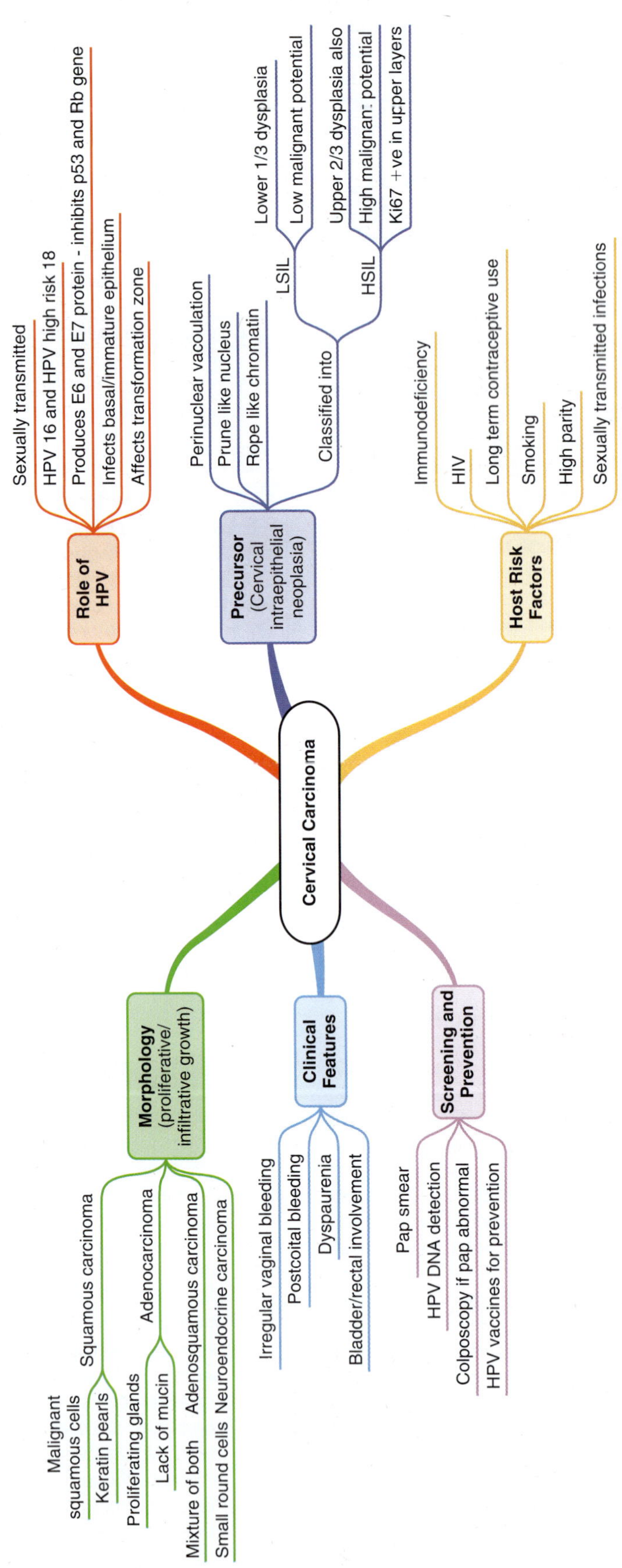

Cervical Carcinoma
Role of HPV
Sexually transmitted
HPV 16 and HPV high risk 18
Produces E6 and E7 protein - inhibits p53 and Rb gene
Infects basal/immature epithelium
Affects transformation zone
Precursor (Cervical intraepithelial neoplasia)
Perinuclear vacoulation
Prune like nucleus
Rope like chromatin
Classified into
LSIL
Lower 1/3 dysplasia
Low malignant potential
HSIL
Upper 2/3 dysplasia also
High malignant potential
Ki67 +ve in upper layers
Host Risk Factors
Immunodeficiency
HIV
Long term contraceptive use
Smoking
High parity
Sexually transmitted infections
Morphology (proliferative/ infiltrative growth)
Squamous carcinoma
Malignant squamous cells
Keratin pearls
Adenocarcinoma
Proliferating glands
Lack of mucin
Adenosquamous carcinoma
Mixture of both
Neuroendocrine carcinoma
Small round cells
Clinical Features
Irregular vaginal bleeding
Postcoital bleeding
Dyspaurenia
Bladder/rectal involvement
Screening and Prevention
Pap smear
HPV DNA detection
Colposcopy if pap abnormal
HPV vaccines for prevention

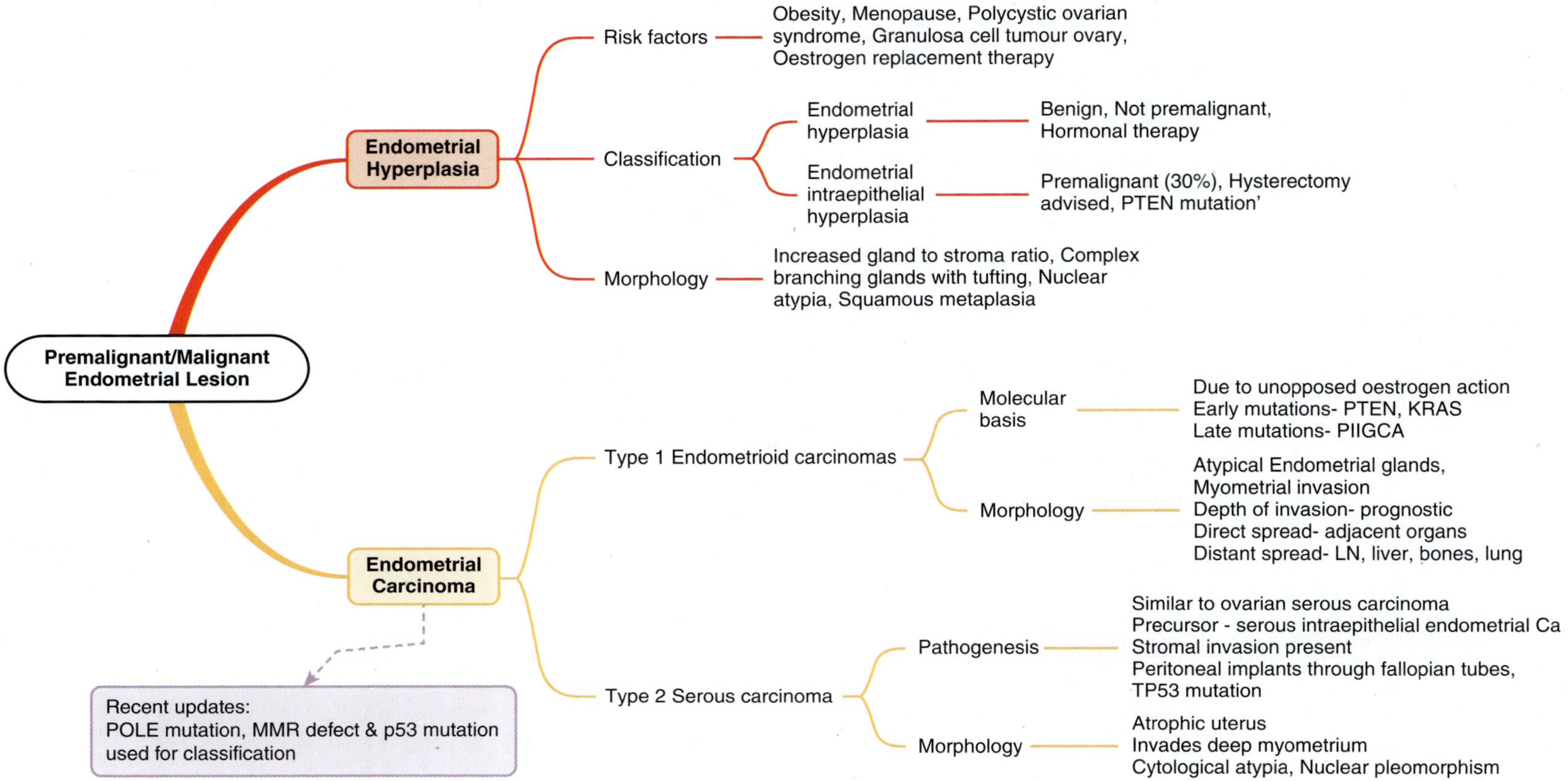
Premalignant/Malignant Endometrial Lesion
Endometrial Hyperplasia
Risk factors
Obesity, Menopause, Polycystic ovarian syndrome, Granulosa cell tumour ovary, Oestrogen replacement therapy
Classification
Endometrial hyperplasia
Benign, Not premalignant, Hormonal therapy
Endometrial intraepithelial hyperplasia
Premalignant (30%), Hysterectomy advised, PTEN mutation'
Morphology
Increased gland to stroma ratio, Complex branching glands with tufting, Nuclear atypia, Squamous metaplasia
Endometrial Carcinoma
Type 1 Endometrioid carcinomas
Molecular basis
Due to unopposed oestrogen action
Early mutations- PTEN, KRAS
Late mutations- PIIGCA
Morphology
Atypical Endometrial glands,
Myometrial invasion
Depth of invasion- prognostic
Direct spread- adjacent organs
Distant spread- LN, liver, bones, lung
Type 2 Serous carcinoma
Pathogenesis
Similar to ovarian serous carcinoma
Precursor - serous intraepithelial endometrial Ca
Stromal invasion present
Peritoneal implants through fallopian tubes,
TP53 mutation
Morphology
Atrophic uterus
Invades deep myometrium
Cytological atypia, Nuclear pleomorphism
Recent updates:
POLE mutation, MMR defect & p53 mutation used for classification

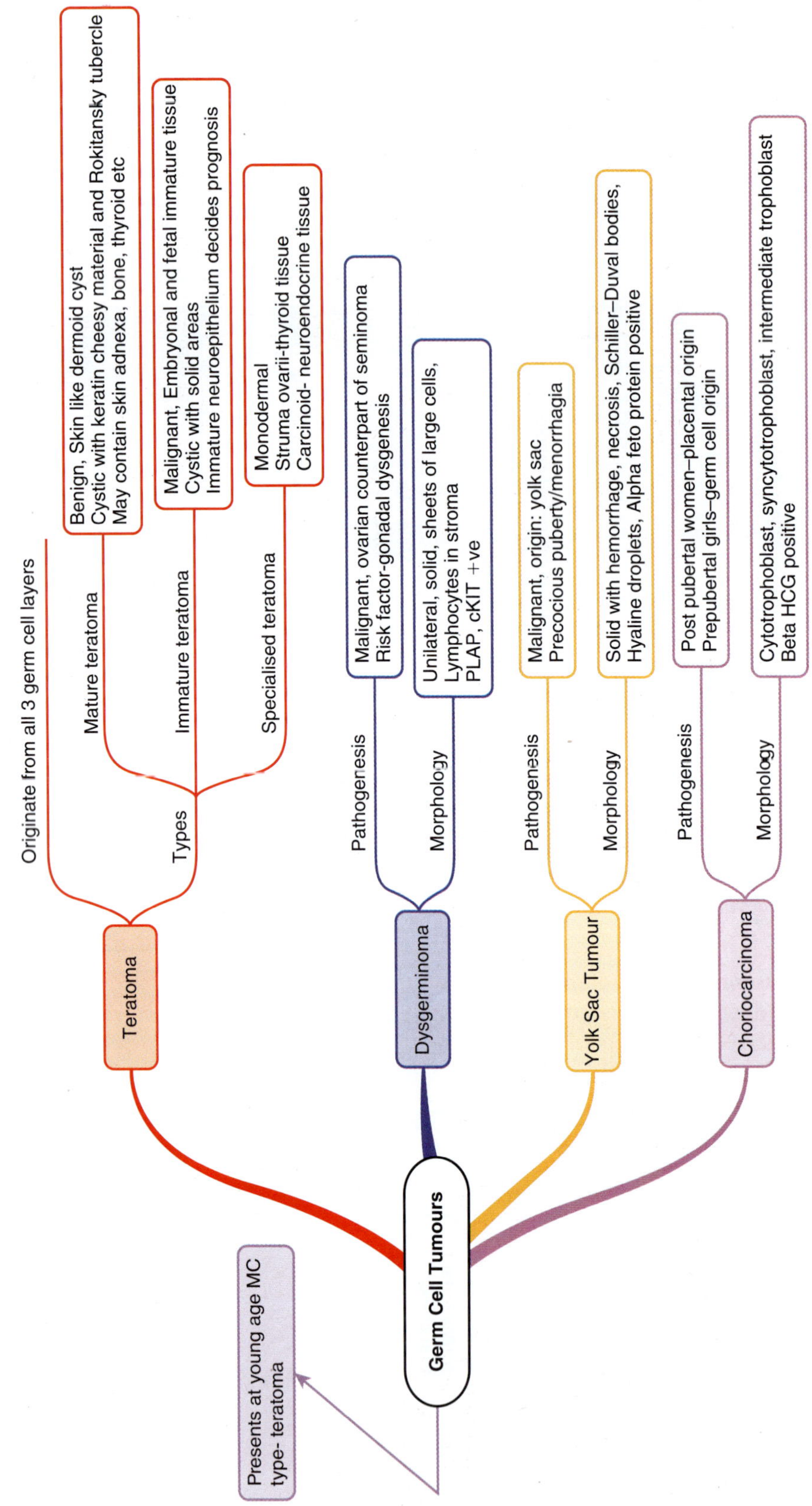
Germ Cell Tumours
Presents at young age MC type- teratoma
Teratoma
Originate from all 3 germ cell layers
Types
Mature teratoma
Benign, Skin like dermoid cyst
Cystic with keratin cheesy material and Rokitansky tubercle
May contain skin adnexa, bone, thyroid etc
Immature teratoma
Malignant, Embryonal and fetal immature tissue
Cystic with solid areas
Immature neuroepithelium decides prognosis
Specialised teratoma
Monodermal
Struma ovarii-thyroid tissue
Carcinoid- neuroendocrine tissue
Dysgerminoma
Pathogenesis
Malignant, ovarian counterpart of seminoma
Risk factor-gonadal dysgenesis
Morphology
Unilateral, solid, sheets of large cells,
Lymphocytes in stroma
PLAP, cKIT +ve
Yolk Sac Tumour
Pathogenesis
Malignant, origin: yolk sac
Precocious puberty/menorrhagia
Morphology
Solid with hemorrhage, necrosis, Schiller–Duval bodies,
Hyaline droplets, Alpha feto protein positive
Choriocarcinoma
Pathogenesis
Post pubertal women–placental origin
Prepubertal girls–germ cell origin
Morphology
Cytotrophoblast, syncytotrophoblast, intermediate trophoblast
Beta HCG positive

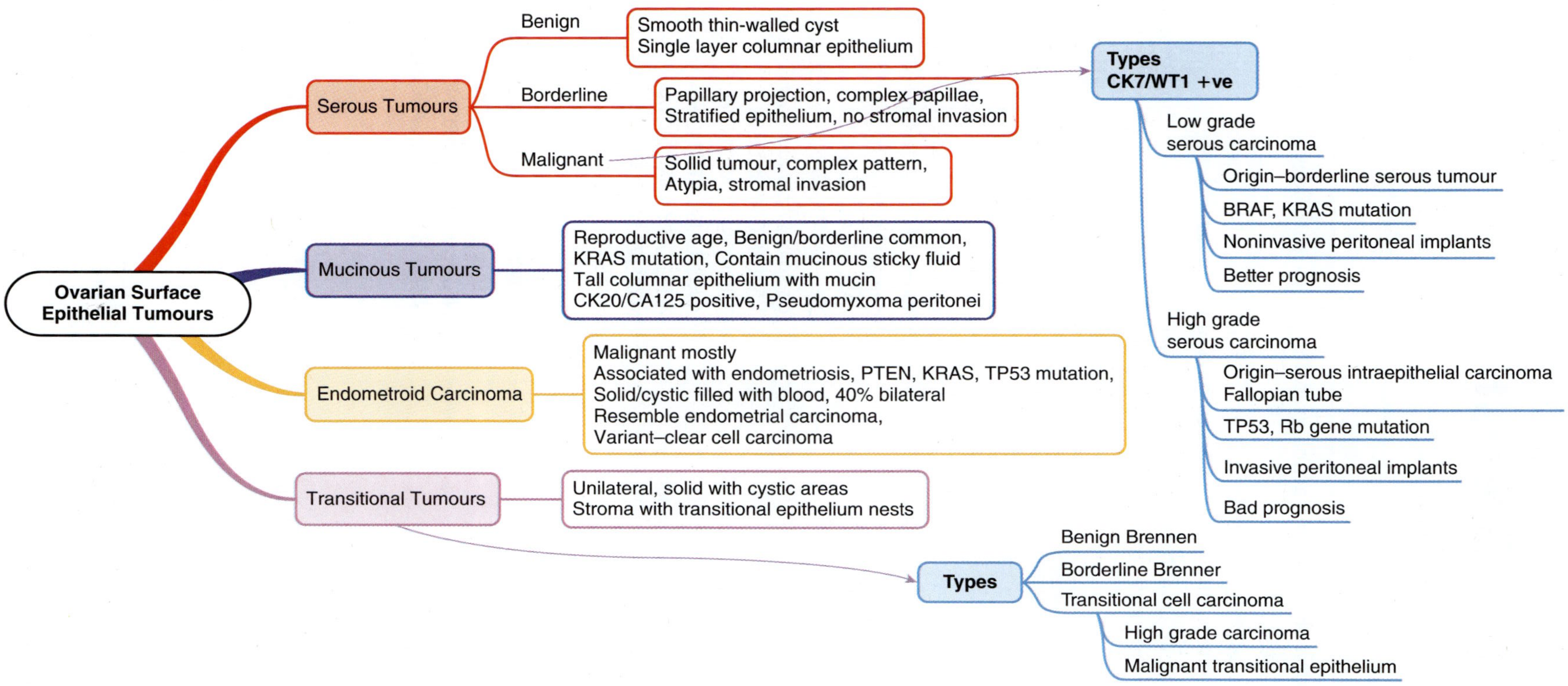
Ovarian Surface Epithelial Tumours
Serous Tumours
Benign
Smooth thin-walled cyst
Single layer columnar epithelium
Borderline
Papillary projection, complex papillae,
Stratified epithelium, no stromal invasion
Malignant
Sollid tumour, complex pattern,
Atypia, stromal invasion
Types
CK7/WT1 +ve
Low grade
serous carcinoma
Origin–borderline serous tumour
BRAF, KRAS mutation
Noninvasive peritoneal implants
Better prognosis
High grade
serous carcinoma
Origin–serous intraepithelial carcinoma
Fallopian tube
TP53, Rb gene mutation
Invasive peritoneal implants
Bad prognosis
Mucinous Tumours
Reproductive age, Benign/borderline common,
KRAS mutation, Contain mucinous sticky fluid
Tall columnar epithelium with mucin
CK20/CA125 positive, Pseudomyxoma peritonei
Endometroid Carcinoma
Malignant mostly
Associated with endometriosis, PTEN, KRAS, TP53 mutation,
Solid/cystic filled with blood, 40% bilateral
Resemble endometrial carcinoma,
Variant–clear cell carcinoma
Transitional Tumours
Unilateral, solid with cystic areas
Stroma with transitional epithelium nests
Types
Benign Brennen
Borderline Brenner
Transitional cell carcinoma
High grade carcinoma
Malignant transitional epithelium

27 The Breast

Rajeswari Kathiah

PA 31.1 Classify and describe the types, aetiology, pathogenesis, pathology and hormonal dependency of **benign breast disease**.

PA 31.2 Classify and describe the epidemiology, pathogenesis, classification, morphology, prognostic factors, hormonal dependency, staging and spread of **carcinoma of the breast**.

PA 31.4 Enumerate and describe the aetiology, hormonal dependency and pathogenesis of **gynaecomastia**.

CHAPTER OUTLINE

INTRODUCTION

Breast, also called mammary gland, is the distinguishing feature of mammals. It is different from all the other organs because of three major reasons:

- Its primary function is to provide nutrition to the young ones.
- It undergoes dynamic changes throughout life.
- It is an organ with social, cultural and personal importance as a symbol of femininity, which has a strong influence on the presentation and management of the diseases arising from it.

Breast diseases are many in number and before discussing the pathology, we briefly review the structural anatomy and physiology of the breast.

ANATOMY (FIG. 27.1)

The breast is an apocrine gland located in the anterior thoracic wall, anterior to the deep fascia and pectoral muscles, separated from them by the retromammary space. Each breast consists of mammary glands surrounded by connective tissue. The mammary glands are modified apocrine sweat glands. These are structurally dynamic, meaning that the anatomical changes depend on the woman's age, phase of the menstrual cycle and reproductive status. Each gland is composed of 15–20 secretory lobes which are separated by fibrous bands called the *suspensory ligaments of the breast (of Cooper)*. Each lobe comprises several lobules, also referred to as the ***terminal duct–lobular unit (TDLU)***, which is the basic functional and histopathological unit of the breast (Fig. 27.2). TDLU consists of a group of 30–50 acini that drain into a terminal duct (intralobular). These terminal ducts drain into larger ducts of the lobes, called the **lactiferous ducts**, and each lactiferous duct dilates to form the **lactiferous sinus** before opening onto the nipple. The nipple is surrounded by a pigmented circular region of skin called the areola, which becomes even more pigmented and prominent during puberty. The areola shows small punctual elevations on its surface, produced by the underlying areolar glands. These are mostly sweat and sebaceous glands, or modified mammary glands called the glands of Montgomery. Their function is to produce secretions with antimicrobial properties to protect the surface of the areola.

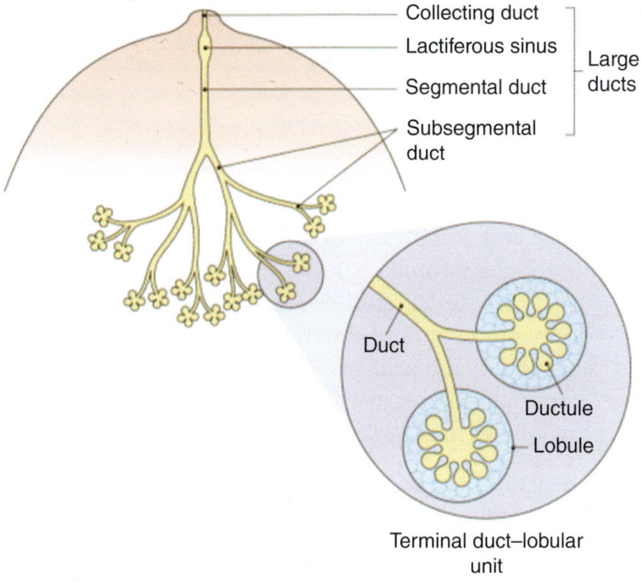

Fig. 27.1 Normal structure of the breast – diagrammatic representation. (*Source:* From Laura C. Collins. Breast. Rosai and Ackerman's Surgical Pathology. 11th edition. Elsevier 2018.)

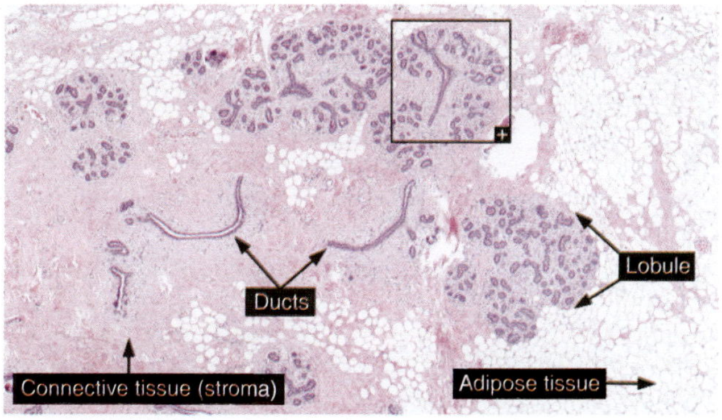

Fig. 27.2 TDLU of breast – microscopy. The breast is divided into 15–25 ***lobules***, each based on a branching ***duct*** system that leads from the collecting ducts to the TDLUs. (*Source:* https://v15.proteinatlas.org/learn/dictionary/normal/breast)

Normal breast – 'rule of two'

- Two types of epithelial cells – luminal cells and myoepithelial cells
- Two types of stroma – interlobular stroma and intralobular stroma
- Two duct structures – large ducts and TDLUs

The ductoalveolar system has dual epithelial lining. The innermost layer (lumen of acini) is made up of luminal ***epithelial cells*** which undergo lactational changes and produce milk. The outer layer is formed by ***myoepithelial cells*** which rest on the basement membrane and form the contractile meshwork to eject milk. Observing the presence of this myoepithelial layer of breast is extremely essential in establishing the benign nature of breast lesions (with very few exceptions), and its absence is a histopathological hallmark of malignancy. The basement membrane is made up of type IV collagen which separates TDLUs from surrounding intralobular stroma. The stroma of the breast is of two types, interlobular and intralobular stroma; the differences between the two are listed in Table 27.1.

PHYSIOLOGY

Hormone Dependency of Benign Breast Diseases PA 31.1

Breast tissue is dependent on hormones for its growth and development. Hormones and growth factors act on stromal and epithelial cells to regulate mammary gland development, maturation and differentiation. Oestrogen

Table 27.1 Differences Between Interlobular and Intralobular Stroma

Interlobular Stroma	Intralobular Stroma
Dense stroma inside each lobe surrounding the lactiferous duct	Loose fibrous stroma surrounding TDLU
Not hormone responsive	Hormone responsive
Rich in fibroblasts	Scattered fibroblasts

TDLU, terminal duct–lobular unit.

mediates development of ductal tissue, progesterone facilitates ductal branching and lobuloalveolar development and prolactin regulates milk protein production. At puberty, oestradiol and progesterone levels increase to initiate breast development. Following this, a complex branching structure results which is composed of 5–10 primary milk ducts originating at the nipple, 20–40 segmental ducts and 10–100 subsegmental ducts ending in glandular units called TDLUs. During the menstrual cycle, the elevations in oestrogen and progesterone levels stimulate cell proliferation during the luteal phase. With this stimulus, breast can increase by as much as 15% in size.

Anatomical and histological structures of the breast undergo substantial changes during the period from early adolescence to menopause under the influence of hormones.

In benign breast disease, the intensity of steroid hormone expression parallels the extent of hyperplasia. Progesterone expression is seen universally in fibroadenomas and benign phyllodes tumours, and approximately 25% of fibroadenomas also express oestrogen receptor (ER).

Oestrogen and progesterone expression is seen in benign breast lesions and in breast carcinoma associated with good prognostic parameters, and it correlates with good response to hormonal therapy (explained later). Hence, assessment of hormone receptor status in patients with breast cancer is routinely practiced nowadays to provide prognostic information and best therapeutic options.

Changes in Breast During Pregnancy and Lactation (Fig. 27.3)

Breast tissue becomes fully mature and functional during pregnancy and lactation.

- Pigmentation of nipple–areolar complex, distension of superficial veins and Montgomery tubercles are more pronounced.
- Enlargement of breast becomes apparent at the fifth month of pregnancy.
- Lactational changes commence approximately day 2–6 postpartum.
- As pregnancy progresses, changes become more pronounced.
- Size and number of lobules increase, epithelial cells enlarge and stroma becomes more vascular with small aggregates of inflammatory cells.
- Epithelial cytoplasm becomes vacuolated, nuclei take on a hobnail appearance (resembles Arias–Stella reaction) and secretions become evident.
- Myoepithelial cells become attenuated in lobules because of enlargement of cells but remain conspicuous in extralobular ducts (second and third trimesters).
- Hormones from corpus luteum and placenta (progesterone, oestrogen, human placental lactogen [hPL]) initially suppress lactation during pregnancy.
- With delivery of the placenta, hPL levels drop precipitously, while prolactin levels remain high and initiate copious milk production.

Changes in Breast After Menopause (Fig. 27.4)

- Reduction of oestrogen and progesterone causes progressive involution and atrophy of TDLUs, reduction in size and complexity of acini and loss of specialized interlobular stroma.
- TDLUs are small, epithelium has less cytoplasm and basement membrane material may appear more prominent and hyalinized.
- As specialized breast stroma also involutes, small atrophic lobules may be seen fully surrounded by fat.

Diseases of the breast, inflammatory, benign and malignant neoplasms, are very common in daily practice,

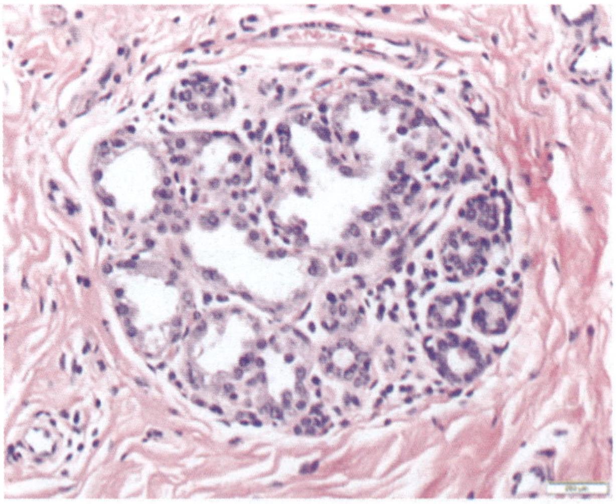

Fig. 27.3 Lactational changes in breast – microscopy. There are numerous round alveoli, with their lumens occupied by the secretory product (milk). (*Source:* From Laura C. Collins. Breast. Rosai and Ackerman's Surgical Pathology. 11th edition. Elsevier 2018.)

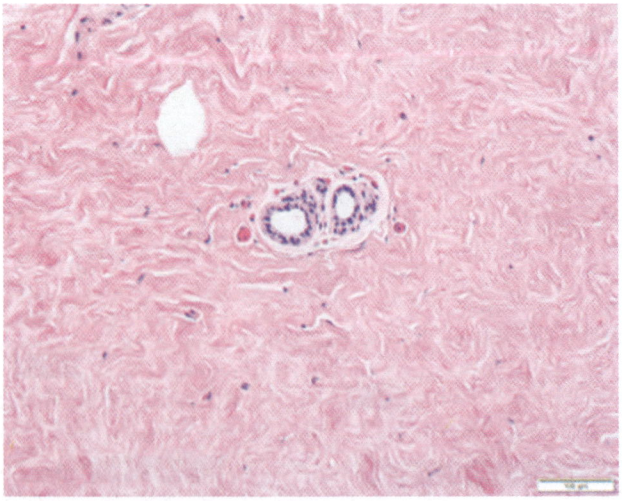

Fig. 27.4 Postmenopausal breast – microscopy. The TDLU undergoes involution leaving few atrophic acini. (*Source:* From Laura C. Collins. Breast. Rosai and Ackerman's Surgical Pathology. 11th edition. Elsevier 2018.)

and the common entities are described in detail after a brief discussion on the presenting clinical features of breast diseases in general.

CLINICAL PRESENTATION OF BREAST DISEASES

The most common clinical presentations in women with breast disease are pain, inflammation, palpable mass, lumpiness without discrete mass and nipple discharge.

1. **Pain – mastalgia or mastodynia**
   Pain is the most common complaint by women with breast disease. Sometimes pain may be associated with menstrual cycle. Most of the painful masses are usually benign, whereas only 10% of breast cancers present with pain. Pain may be cyclical or noncyclical and may be diffuse or localized. Cyclical pain, which is commonly diffuse, occurs in the premenstrual phase and needs just counselling and reassurance, whereas noncyclical and localized pain warrants further workup with radiological and morphological studies along with fine-needle aspiration cytology (FNAC) and biopsy.
2. **Inflammation**
   Inflammation of the breast is a rare symptom and causes erythema and oedema of the entire breast or a portion of it. It is most often caused by infections, which occur commonly during lactation. An important mimic of reactive inflammation is inflammatory breast carcinoma (discussed later).
3. **Palpable mass**
   Palpable mass is the second most common complaint by women with breast disease and is more common in premenopausal women. Most of these are benign and include cysts or fibroadenomas, whereas some may be invasive carcinomas (ICs). Risk of cancer increases with age. Only 10% of breast masses are malignant in women younger than 40 years, whereas 60% of breast masses are malignant in women older than 50 years.
   Most of the malignant lesions become palpable only when they reach a size of around 2 cm and by that time a significant number of them would have metastasized.
4. **Nipple discharge**
   Nipple discharge is the third most common complaint by women with breast disease. Causes of nipple discharge are given in Flowchart 27.1.

INVESTIGATIONS IN BREAST DISEASES

Investigations are to confirm our clinical diagnosis and hence preliminary complete clinical examination is a must.

Mammogram

Mammogram is obtaining X-ray films of breast tissue. It was first introduced in 1980s to detect nonpalpable masses of the breast. It is a safe and noninvasive procedure using very low-voltage, high-amperage X-rays approximately 0.1 cGy. It is used as a screening tool for breast carcinoma in a large population. Best forms of mammogram for breast cancer screening are available today but do not detect all breast cancers. Sensitivity and specificity of the test increase as the age increases.

Possible findings in mammogram

- Calcifications in duct and other tissue
- Mass lesions
- Asymmetric areas
- Dense areas
- New dense area that has appeared since the last mammogram

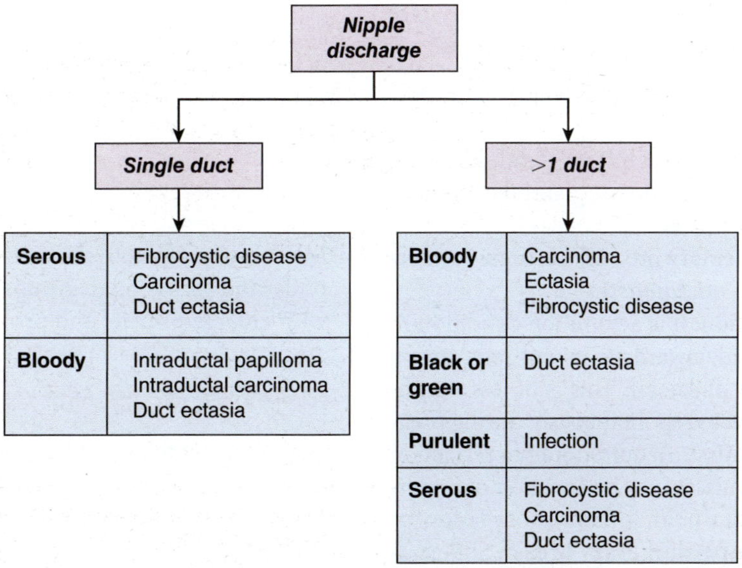

Flowchart 27.1 Causes of nipple discharge.

Principal mammographic signs

- ***Densities:*** Lesion replaces adipose tissue with radiodense tissue forming mammographic densities. Rounded density most commonly represents a benign lesion such as fibrocystic changes or fibroadenomas, whereas an irregular-shaped density raises the suspicion of a malignant lesion. It can identify small, nonpalpable tumours with size less than 1 cm.
- ***Calcifications:*** Calcifications are formed in secretions, necrotic debris or hyalinized stroma. It is usually found in both benign and malignant lesions. In malignant lesions, calcifications are small and numerous and sometimes present in clusters. Ductal carcinoma in situ (DCIS) is most commonly detected as mammographic calcifications.

Limitations of mammography

- Screening mammogram is 5%–15% false-positive and hence requires additional testing such as ultrasonography (USG) or biopsy.
- Mammogram can miss one in five cancers.
- Mammogram in young women is more difficult to interpret because the breast contains more glands and ligaments, resulting in dense breast tissue that can obscure signs of cancers. As age increases, breast tissue becomes fattier and has fewer glands, making it easier to interpret.

Ultrasonography of the Breast

Breast USG is a safe and noninvasive procedure often used as a follow-up test after an abnormal finding on mammogram/MRI. It does not differentiate the mass into benign or malignant in all the cases. It is used to determine the number of lumps or mass, size, shape and location and to differentiate the lumps into fluid-filled cyst or solid mass.

DEVELOPMENTAL DISORDERS

Developmental disorders of the breast are extremely rare except few lesions. Some of them are described here.

Amastia: No glandular tissue (no breast bud), no nipple and no areola

Aplasia: Nipple and areola present but no glandular tissue

Athelia: Very rare, in which the breast glandular tissue is present with no nipple or areola

Hypoplasia: Small rudimentary breasts (i.e. breast underdevelopment), also called ***micromastia***

Congenital nipple inversion: It is a common condition in which the nipple is pulled inward in its entirety during development and may be unilateral. This is of less significance because it gets corrected spontaneously during pregnancy or with simple traction. Acquired nipple retraction has more significance because it may be a marker of underlying infiltrating malignancy or an inflammatory lesion.

Milk line remnants or supernumerary breast: Supernumerary breasts, accessory breast, ectopic breast tissue or polymastia are all synonyms that refer to the presence of breast tissue manifesting as epidermal thickenings anywhere along milk line from axilla to perineum/vulva, arising from probable clusters of primordial breast cells that failed to involute. Though axilla is the most preferred site, other rare sites outside the milk line including the hip, face, foot and shoulder have also been reported.

INFLAMMATORY LESIONS

Inflammation of breast parenchyma is a rare entity and may be because of infectious or noninfectious causes and because of underlying malignancy (inflammatory carcinoma, discussed later).

ACUTE MASTITIS

Acute mastitis is inflammation of the breast tissue which may or may not be associated with bacterial infection. In infective mastitis (acute bacterial mastitis), *Staphylococcus aureus* is the most common pathogen. Less commonly, the pathogen may be a β-haemolytic *Streptococcus* (such as group A or group B *Streptococcus*). Acute bacterial mastitis is most often encountered in lactating mothers, especially in the first month of breastfeeding because of the presence of cracks and fissures in the nipples (often caused by poor feeding technique), and is more common with the first child. The affected breast is erythematous and painful and the patient often has fever. In the beginning, the infection is confined to a single duct system or a portion of the breast, which if not treated spreads to the entire breast with involvement of the draining lymph nodes. Streptococcal infection commonly results in cellulitis, whereas staphylococcal infection often causes single or multiple abscesses. Most cases resolve with antibiotics, and only few cases require surgical draining.

Nonlactational mastitis (less common) can also occur, especially in women with other conditions such as duct ectasia, as periductal mastitis. Tobacco smoking is an important risk factor, causing damage to the subareolar duct walls and predisposing to bacterial infection.

Morphology (Fig. 27.5)

Microscopy of acute mastitis shows abundant neutrophils and occasional groups of reactive ductal cells with enlarged nuclei and prominent nucleoli.

SQUAMOUS METAPLASIA OF LACTIFEROUS DUCTS

Squamous metaplasia of lactiferous ducts is often abbreviated as SMOLD, also referred as ***recurrent subareolar abscess, periductal mastitis and Zuska disease***. It is a change in which the normal double-layer epithelium of the lactiferous ducts is replaced by keratinizing squamous

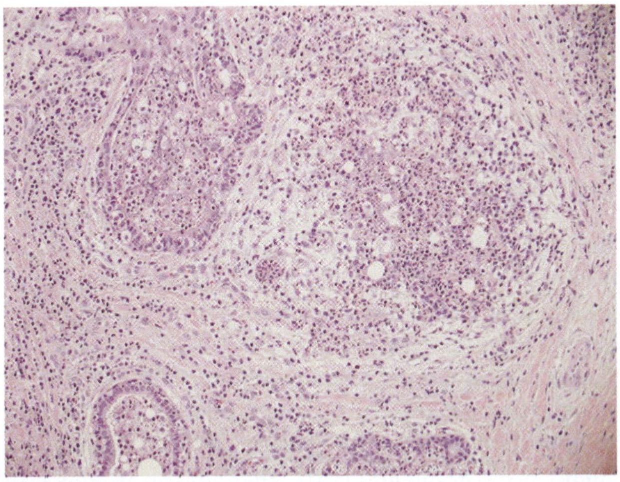

Fig. 27.5 Acute mastitis – microscopy. Note the expanded terminal ductal–lobular unit with infiltration by neutrophils and mononuclear cells. (*Source:* https://www.flickriver.com/photos/jian-hua_qiao_md/8199838977/)

epithelium. It is an uncommon benign change in the breast typically seen in postmenopausal women and has strong association with smoking and tobacco exposure. Decreased level of vitamin A secondary to smoking is attributed to the development of squamous metaplasia. Clinically, affected women present with painful erythematous subareolar mass along with inverted nipple. Single fistulous tract opening at the edge of the areola beneath the smooth muscle of the nipple (the path of least resistance) is a characteristic finding. The lesion may be mistaken for infection.

Pathogenesis

Keratin-producing squamous cells extend abnormally deep into lactiferous sinuses or duct, leading to the formation of keratin plugs which obstruct the duct and cause dilation. At the point when the duct ruptures, it elicits an intense foreign body inflammatory response to the keratin released.

Morphology

Squamous epithelium extending beyond the normal transition point to ductal epithelium (normal transition point is superficial within the duct orifice, at approximately 1–2 mm from the skin surface). Duct spaces filled with keratin debris are seen and may extend into duct spaces lined by normal ductal epithelium. Duct rupture and spillage of keratin debris into the stroma incite an acute and chronic inflammatory response with giant cells surrounding the ducts with squamous metaplasia and keratin debris may be seen to be present within the giant cells in the stroma.

Abscess cavity is drained by a simple incision. Recurrences are common as keratinizing epithelium persists with a simple incision. Hence, en bloc removal of the involved duct and the fistulous tract is done for curative treatment.

Duct Ectasia

Duct ectasia of the breast is the most common cause of greenish discharge from the nipple. The disease is also referred by different terms like, comedomastitis, mastitis obliterans, plasma cell mastitis and periductal mastitis.

Duct ectasia occurs when a milk duct beneath the nipple widens, the duct walls thicken and the duct gets filled with fluid. This is characterized by different degrees of periductal inflammation, periductal fibrosis and duct dilation. It usually occurs in women of perimenopausal and postmenopausal age.

Typically, the age of presentation ranges from 40 to 70 years. Pain, nipple discharge, nipple retraction or a worm-like doughy palpable mass beneath the nipple can be the clinical presentation.

Aetiology is unknown, but some believe that involution seen in postmenopausal women is the primary pathological process of gland atrophy, followed by stasis of secretions leading to leakage of lipid-rich material through the duct wall. This results in periductal inflammation, which is the inciting process that is followed by duct sclerosis, obliteration and ultimately ectasia.

Morphology (Figs 27.6 and 27.7)

Early lesions show dilated ducts that may contain foamy histiocytes, proteinaceous secretions, cholesterol crystals and calcification. The lesion may sometimes be seen as polyps containing histiocytes referred to as ***'lipophagic polyps'***.

Periductal inflammation is characterized by circumferential infiltration of lymphocytes, plasma cells, histiocytes and foreign body giant cells around the duct. It is also called granulomatous *periductal*

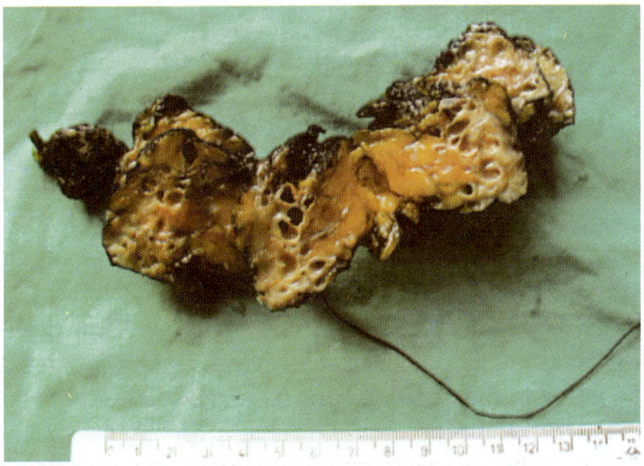

Fig. 27.6 Duct ectasia of the breast – gross. Some of the dilated ducts contain a thick dark material. (*Source:* From Laura C. Collins. Breast. Rosai and Ackerman's Surgical Pathology. 11th edition. Elsevier 2018.)

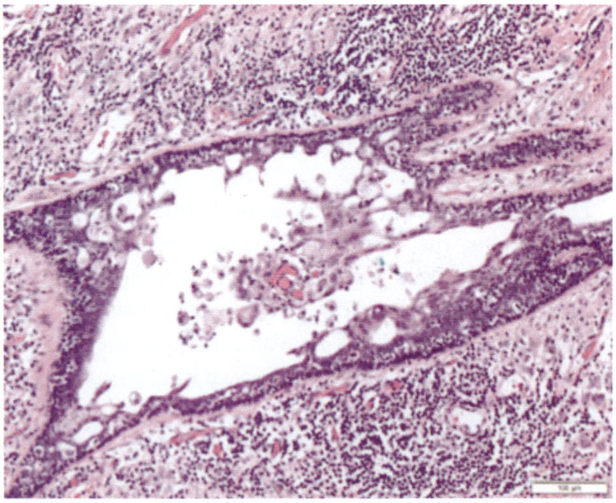

Fig. 27.7 Duct ectasia of the breast – microscopy. There is dilation of a large duct, with accumulation of lipid-rich detritus in the lumen and a florid inflammatory reaction rich in macrophages and plasma cells. (*Source:* From Laura C. Collins. Breast. Rosai and Ackerman's Surgical Pathology. 11th edition. Elsevier 2018.)

mastitis. When plasma cells are more prominent around the duct, then the lesion is termed as ***'plasma cell mastitis'***.

Late lesions present as periductal fibrosis, which is characterized by sclerosis that may lead to duct obliteration, and is called ***'mastitis obliterans'***. The epithelium may be completely destroyed. Sometimes, recanalization around the periphery of ducts by small tubules may be seen which is termed as 'garland pattern'.

Repeated attempts of inflammation and fibrosis can lead to nipple distortion or retraction and, occasionally, patients may present with tender subareolar nodules mimicking invasive malignancies. Hence, careful clinical assessment and biopsy would be required to exclude malignancy in patients with duct ectasia.

Fat Necrosis

Fat necrosis is also known as ***Basler necrosis.*** It is most commonly the result of breast trauma (21%–70%) and the other causes include fine-needle aspiration or biopsy, anticoagulation treatment, radiation therapy and breast infection. Individual patient factors such as smoking, obesity and older age, as well as treatment associated with breast cancer (radiation, chemotherapy and mastectomy), are specifically associated with an increased incidence of breast fat necrosis. Breast fat necrosis may be associated with any breast surgical procedure; however, it becomes the prime concern after mastectomy/reconstruction because fat necrosis can cause breast deformity or may mimic cancer recurrence. It may present as a painless palpable mass, skin thickening, nipple retraction, mammographic densities or calcifications. Its major clinical significance is that it mimics invasive malignancy.

Pathogenesis Fat necrosis is a sterile inflammatory process which results from aseptic saponification of fat by blood and tissue lipase. Lipase is an enzyme that releases fatty acids from triglycerides. These fatty acids form a complex with calcium to undergo saponification. The age of the lesion in fat necrosis dictates its appearance, both grossly and microscopically. Fat necrosis first appears as an area of haemorrhage in fat, which manifests as induration and firmness on gross pathology. Subsequently, saponification occurs, in which the lesion may become yellow, then calcification occurs which presents as a chalky white lesion and lastly when fibrosis occurs, it becomes a yellow–grey mass. In addition, some adipose cells release their contents instead of forming scar as a result of injury, and this results in cystic degeneration. Calcifications frequently develop around the outer lining of the cyst. Fibrosis can surround degenerated fat or oil (***known as 'oil cyst'***), which may persist for months or years.

Morphology (Fig. 27.8)

Fat necrosis is microscopically characterized by mixed inflammatory cell infiltrate composed of histiocytes, lymphocytes, plasma cells and sometimes eosinophils. Lipid-laden foamy histiocytes, multinucleated foreign body-type giant cells formed because of phagocytosis of necrotic adipocytes and haemosiderin deposition, are characteristic findings. Early fibrosis with hypercellular areas of fibroblastic proliferation may be seen. Calcification is seen as amorphous basophilic structures.

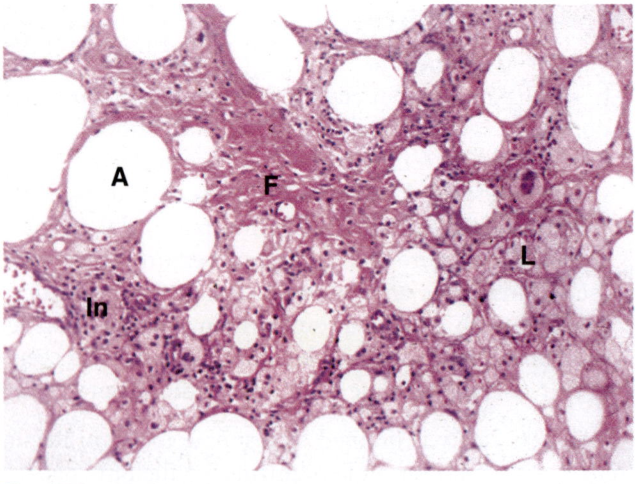

Fig. 27.8 Fat necrosis showing necrotic adipose tissue A, chronic inflammatory cell infiltrate In and lipophages L (macrophages containing lipid, giving their cytoplasm a foamy appearance), fibrosis F and plasma cells.

Lymphocytic Mastopathy

Lymphocytic mastopathy, also named as ***fibrotic mastopathy, diabetic mastopathy or sclerosing lymphocytic lobulitis***, is a benign clinicopathological entity affecting both young and middle-aged women. Its main differential diagnosis is breast carcinoma. It is an uncommon condition often associated with type I/insulin-dependent diabetes or other autoimmune disease but may occur in type II diabetic or nondiabetic patients as well.

It presents as a fibrous breast mass with a prominent lymphocytic infiltrate, most often occurring in patients with long-standing diabetes.

Morphology

Microscopy shows an ill-defined lesion composed of dense intralobular, perilobular and perivascular lymphocytes, lymphoepithelial lesions and lymphoid follicles with germinal centres, along with lobular atrophy and sclerosis. Keloidal ***fibrosis***, histiocytes and fibroblasts are also prominent in late-stage lesions.

Granulomatous Mastitis

Granulomatous mastitis can be divided into granulomatous mastitis and idiopathic granulomatous mastitis.

Granulomatous mastitis occurs as a rare secondary complication of a variety of other conditions such as tuberculosis, fungal infections, sarcoidosis and granulomatosis with polyangiitis. Special forms of granulomatous mastitis occur as a complication of diabetes. Some cases are because of silicone injection or other foreign body reactions.

Idiopathic granulomatous mastitis, also known as ***granular lobular mastitis***, is defined as granulomatous mastitis without any other attributable causes such as those mentioned earlier. It occurs on average 2 years and almost exclusively up to 6 years after pregnancy. The most common clinical presentation is a firm, unilateral, discrete breast mass often associated with an inflammation of the overlying skin. Nipple retraction and even a sinus formation may be present. Because of this, it clinically mimics breast carcinoma.

Morphology

Granulomatous inflammation is usually centred around lobules with lymphocytes, plasma cells, epithelioid histiocytes, multinucleated giant cells and neutrophils. There may be neutrophils forming microabscesses and surrounding empty microcysts, thereby overlapping features with cystic neutrophilic granulomatous mastitis. Usually, necrosis is not seen.

Cystic neutrophilic granulomatous mastitis is due to lipophilic *Corynebacterium*. It occurs in parous women and is similar to idiopathic granulomatous mastitis. Microscopy highlights the presence of granulomas with neutrophils and cystic spaces (hence the name) that contain Gram-positive bacilli.

BENIGN EPITHELIAL LESIONS PA 31.1

NEOPLASMS OF THE BREAST

Neoplasms of the breast can be benign or malignant. Benign breast lesions can be epithelial or stromal, whereas malignant tumours of the breast can be ductal or lobular in simpler terms. Benign epithelial lesions are classified into three categories based on cell proliferation and morphology: nonproliferative, proliferative without atypia and proliferative with atypia.

The vast majority of breast lesions are benign tumours, and we discuss the hormone dependency of breast diseases and benign breast lesions in the subsequent sections.

Nonproliferative Epithelial Breast Diseases

Fibrocystic Disease of Breast Fibrocystic changes of breast comprise a group of diseases with common morphological changes. These are also known as diffuse cystic mastopathy. The term 'fibrocystic change' refers to benign breast changes caused by a hormone-mediated exaggerated breast tissue response. It is most common in premenopausal women in the age group of 30–50 years in whom the presenting symptom is commonly cyclical mastalgia – pain during menstrual cycle. This explains hyperoestrogenism to be a significant aetiological factor. The symptoms have also been observed to subside in the postmenopausal phase when there is a decrease in oestrogen levels. Patients present with painful, tender swellings which are usually bilateral and multifocal.

Morphology

Gross The lesions appear as grey–white fibrous tissue with multiple cysts filled with semitranslucent fluid, giving them the historical name ***blue domed cysts*** because of their blue colour.

Microscopy (Fig. 27.9) Fibrocystic changes of the breast are microscopically characterized by three principal changes – cystic change, which is commonly associated with apocrine change, fibrosis and adenosis.

Cysts: Cystically dilated or ectatic ducts which are lined by metaplastic apocrine ductal cells having abundant eosinophilic granular cytoplasm are seen. The lumen of the cyst shows eosinophilic secretions and foamy macrophages. Calcifications are seen in the lumen of the cyst, which on common mammography

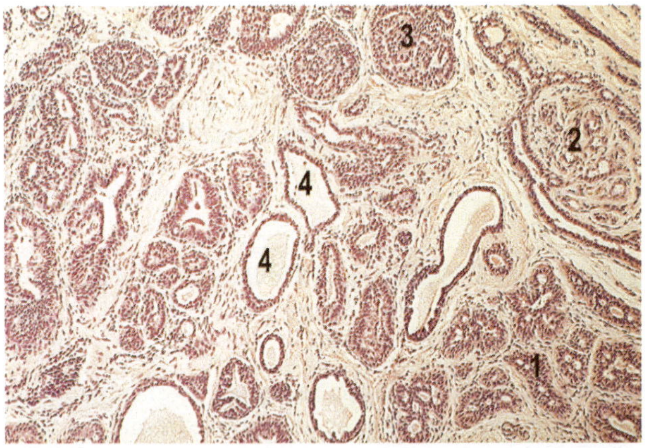

Fig. 27.9 Fibrocystic changes of the breast – microscopy. There is adenosis (1), papilloma formation (2), epithelial hyperplasia (3) and small cysts (4). (*Source:* From J. Louise Jones. Breast. Underwood's Pathology. 7th edition. Elsevier 2019.)

are termed as **'milk of magnesia'**. Cysts disappear following fine-needle aspiration.

Fibrosis: Fibrosis results because of the rupture of cysts leading to release of secretions into the stroma, triggering inflammation causing nodules that can be felt on palpation.

Adenosis: Increase in acini per lobule is defined as adenosis. This is physiological in pregnancy, in which case it is focal. Adenosis by itself is a separate entity and hence discussed elaborately in the next section.

Adenosis Adenosis of the breast is a hyperplastic process primarily involving glands, i.e. an increased number of glandular components. It is a common benign lesion occurring in premenopausal women and is often accompanied by fibrosis.

Types of adenosis

- Apocrine adenosis
- Microglandular adenosis
- Simple adenosis
- Tubular adenosis
- Blunt duct adenosis (now classified as columnar cell change)

Morphology (Fig. 27.10)

Apocrine adenosis: Adenosis with predominant apocrine change.

Microglandular adenosis: Nonlobulocentric proliferation of mammary glands with an infiltrative pattern and lined by a single epithelial layer with a basement membrane.

Simple adenosis: Loosely structured proliferation of acinar or tubular structures, with epithelial and myoepithelial layers, and surrounded by the basement membrane, without distortion of lobular architecture.

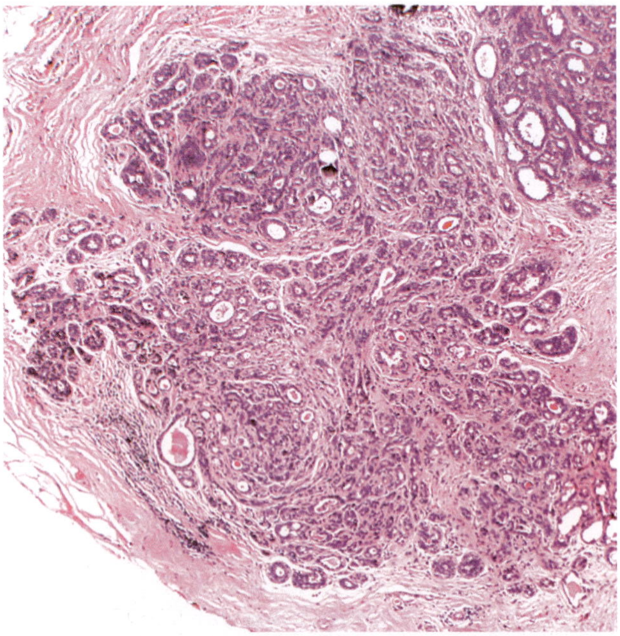

Fig. 27.10 Proliferative breast disease: sclerosing adenosis proliferative breast disease includes lesions that increase the number of epithelial cells, such as this case of sclerosing adenosis. The relative risk (RR) of breast cancer is elevated 1.5–2.0 times, but the great majority of women will not develop cancer.

Tubular adenosis: Haphazard proliferation of branching tubules (two layers).

Few other morphological changes fall under the category of nonproliferative changes. Two such changes are described here:

Lactational adenoma (Fig. 27.11): This lesion is seen in lactating or pregnant women as a palpable

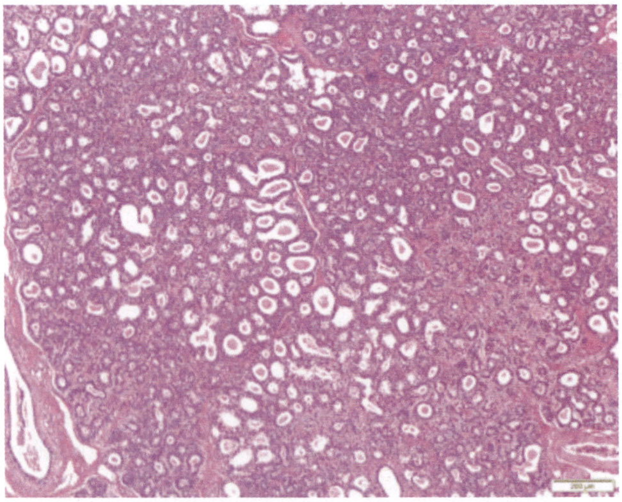

Fig. 27.11 Lactational adenoma – microscopy. The hyperplastic lobules show secretory change. (*Source:* From Laura C. Collins. Breast. Rosai and Ackerman's Surgical Pathology. 11th edition. Elsevier 2018.)

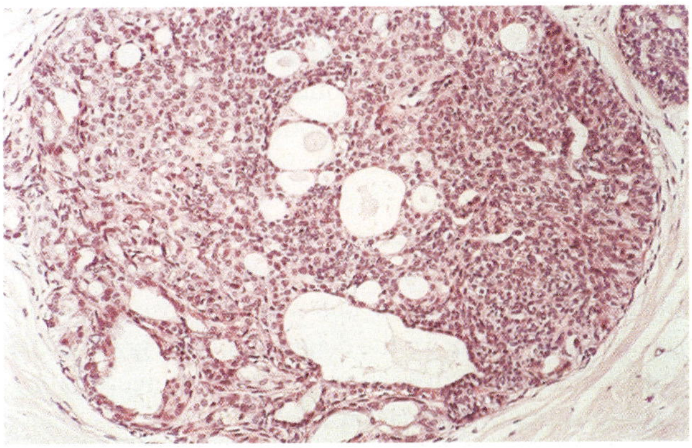

Fig. 27.12 Epithelial hyperplasia – microscopy. The duct lumen is filled by hyperplastic epithelium. (*Source:* From J. Louise Jones. Breast. Underwood's Pathology. 7th edition. Elsevier 2019.)

mass and regress spontaneously after cessation of breastfeeding. Microscopic examination shows normal appearing breast tissue with lactational changes.

Flat epithelial atypia: Flat epithelial atypia is the earliest clonal lesion of the breast that is detectable by microscopy. It is often associated with other lesions of the breast that increase the risk of cancer. It is morphologically characterized by dilated acini and cysts lined by epithelial cells with mild dysplastic changes.

Proliferative Breast Disease Without Atypia

Proliferative breast disease without atypia is defined as an increase in the number of cells and glands with normal morphology. These cells and glands are associated with a minimal increase in the risk of subsequent carcinoma of the breast and are considered as predictors of risk. These are most often detected as mammographic densities, calcifications or incidental findings in biopsies done for other prominent lesions. Uncommonly, these present as a palpable mass. Morphological features of the common lesions are described here.

Morphology

Epithelial cell hyperplasia without atypia (Fig. 27.12): Epithelial hyperplasia is an incidental finding and is morphologically characterized by enlarged TDLUs with dilated acini lined by tightly packed epithelial and myoepithelial cells unlike normal ducts which are lined by a double layer of luminal and myoepithelial cells. Periphery of such lesions shows irregular lumens.

Sclerosing adenosis (Fig. 27.13): Sclerosing adenosis (SA) is a benign proliferative condition characterized by an increased number of acini and their glands. It manifests as multiple small, firm, tender nodules and variable microcysts within the breast. SA commonly affects postmenopausal women but can affect any age group.

SA is a histologically complex entity that consists of enlarged and distorted lobules, containing duplicated and crowded acini, with prominent myoepithelium and stromal fibrosis. It maintains a lobular architecture at low power with rounded and well-defined nodules. Centrally, it is more cellular, with distorted and compressed ductules; peripherally, it has more dilated ductules. Two cell layers are present, but myoepithelial cells may vary from being prominent to indistinct and also intralobular fibrosis, elastosis and apocrine metaplasia may be noted. Florid changes may be seen with pregnancy.

Complex sclerosing lesion (Fig. 27.14): Complex sclerosing lesion is a group of disorders comprising SA,

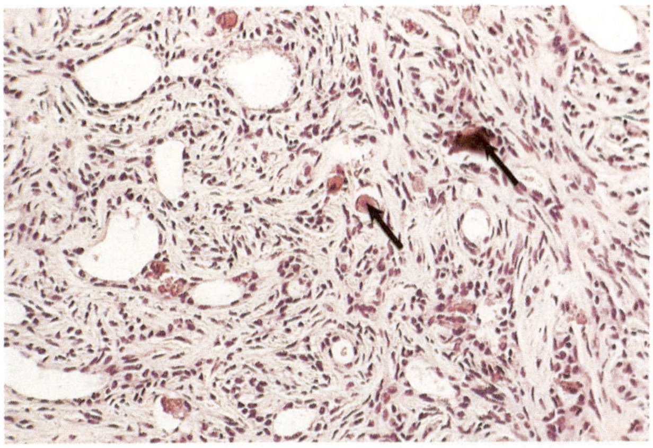

Fig. 27.13 Sclerosing adenosis – microscopy. There are glandular structures with intervening cords of cells in a fibrous stroma. Areas of calcification (arrowed) are also present. (*Source:* From J. Louise Jones. Breast. Underwood's Pathology. 7th edition. Elsevier 2019.)

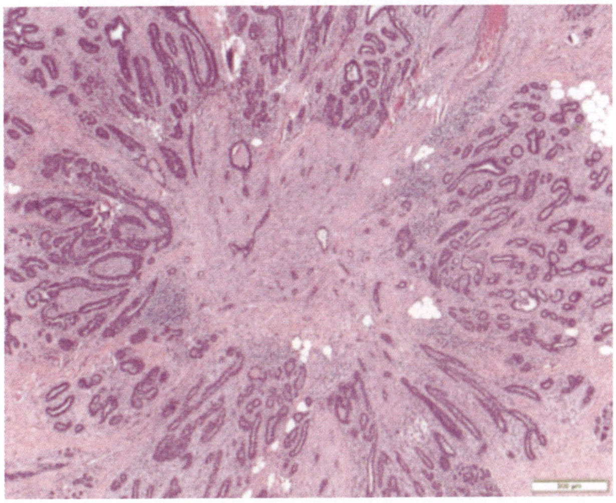

Fig. 27.14 Complex sclerosing lesion/radial scar – microscopy. Typical stellate shape of radial scar as seen on low power. Benign ductular structures are entrapped in the central fibroelastotic stroma. (*Source:* From Laura C. Collins. Breast. Rosai and Ackerman's Surgical Pathology. 11th edition. Elsevier 2018.)

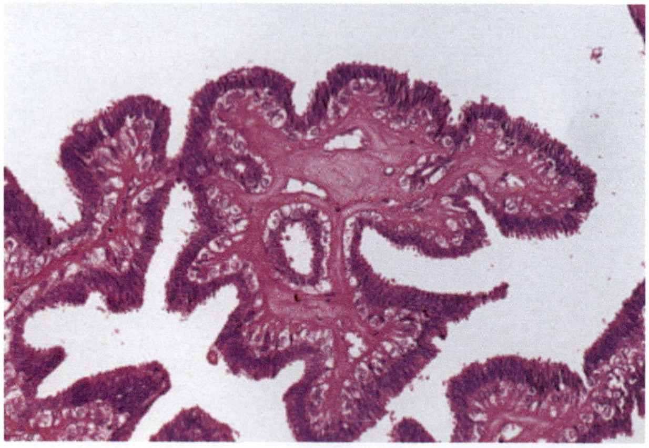

Fig. 27.15 Papilloma – microscopy. Note the complex arborizing architecture and the dual population. (*Source:* From Laura C. Collins. Breast. Rosai and Ackerman's Surgical Pathology. 11th edition. Elsevier 2018.)

papilloma and epithelial hyperplasia. Radial scar is an entity in this group which is characterized by an irregular architecture and hence mimics carcinoma both radiologically and histopathologically. The term 'radial scar' is a misnomer because the lesion is not associated with prior injury or surgery. Microscopy of complex sclerosing lesion reveals a central nidus of entrapped glands in a hyalinized stroma surrounded by radiating projections into the stroma.

Papilloma (Fig. 27.15): Intraductal papillomas are wart-like tumours that grow within the milk ducts of the breast. **Large duct papillomas** (solitary intraductal papillomas) are single tumours that often grow in the large milk ducts near the nipple. The papillomas are a common cause of clear or bloody nipple discharge, especially when it comes from only one breast. These may be felt as a small lump behind or adjacent to the nipple. Sometimes these cause pain. Papillomas may also be found in small ducts in areas of the breast farther from the nipple. Small duct papillomas are often multiple and are less likely to cause nipple discharge. Epithelial hyperplasia and apocrine metaplasia are commonly seen in papillomas.

Nipple adenoma: Nipple adenoma is a benign epithelial proliferation arising near the collecting ducts of the nipple. It presents as an ill-defined nodule, with crusting, erythema and erosion of skin over the nipple.

Microscopically, it is characterized by adenosis or ducts with usual hyperplasia just below the nipple epidermis and is continuous with squamous epithelium of the epidermis, often in a background of fibrosis. Cystic change and keratin cyst may be seen. It may have focal necrosis but without atypia, and the myoepithelial cell layer is retained.

Proliferative Breast Disease With Atypia

Proliferative breast disease with atypia is a group of diseases characterized as an increase in the number of cells and glands with abnormal morphology. There are two types – atypical ductal hyperplasia (ADH), which occurs in the ducts, and atypical lobular hyperplasia (ALH), which occurs in the lobules. Both are associated with a moderately increased risk of carcinoma of the breast.

Atypical Ductal Hyperplasia ADH is characterized by an intraductal clonal epithelial cell proliferation with similar dysplastic features but with the insufficient involvement or volume for the diagnosis of low-grade DCIS. Other names of the disease are B3 lesion (uncertain malignant potential), atypical intraductal hyperplasia, ductal intraepithelial neoplasia and mammary intraepithelial neoplasia. ADH is seen in 5%–17% of specimens from biopsies performed for calcifications.

Morphology (Fig. 27.16)

Microscopy of ADH shows well-defined, evenly spaced monomorphic cells with small rounded nuclei. Variable patterns have been described – solid, cribriform (polarization around lumens), micropapillary (club-shaped). Criteria like size 2 mm or less and space involvement two or fewer spaces or only a portion of the involved space are followed to differentiate ADH from low-grade DCIS.

ADH and ALH express high levels of ER and have a low level of proliferation. These also share chromosomal aberrations with low-grade carcinoma in situ (CIS) and ER^+ invasive breast carcinoma.

Atypical Lobar Hyperplasia ALH is a clonal proliferation of discohesive epithelial cells arising in TDLUs with similar histological features to lobular carcinoma in situ (LCIS) but of insufficient quantity, with distension of less than 50% of the acini.

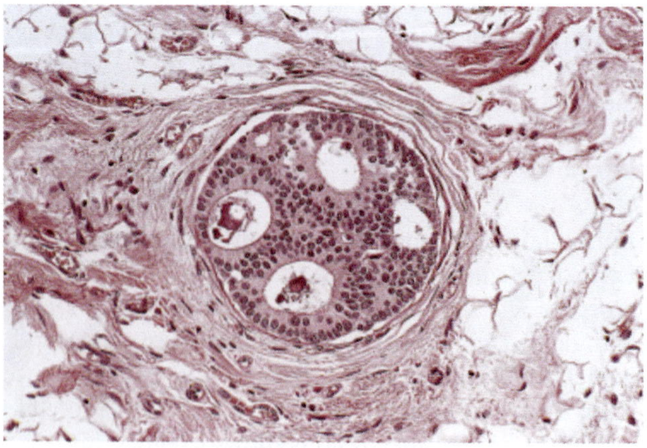

Fig. 27.16 Atypical ductal hyperplasia – microscopy. The small duct space is filled by a relatively uniform single population of epithelial cells that have formed distinctive punched-out luminal spaces. Some polarization of the cells around the luminal spaces is present. (*Source:* From Ian O. Ellis, Andrew H.S. Lee, Sarah E. Pinder and Emad A. Rakha. Tumors of the Breast. Diagnostic Histopathology of Tumors. 5th edition. Elsevier 2021.)

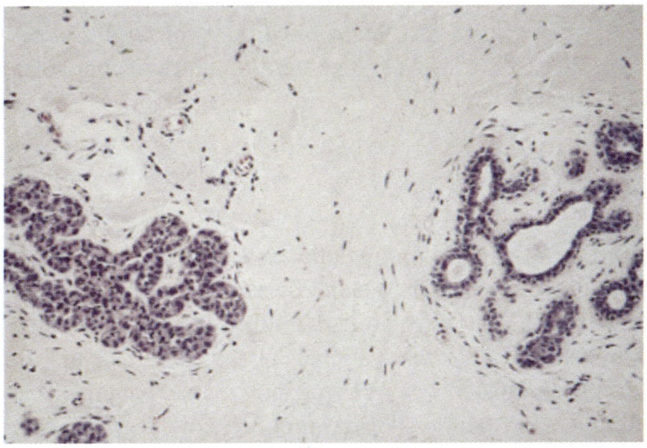

Fig. 27.17 Atypical lobular hyperplasia – microscopy. Two adjacent terminal duct–lobular units. Right, the acini are lined by the normal bilayer of cells; left, a population of cells resembling the normal lining cells is seen, representing mild atypical lobular hyperplasia. (*Source:* From Ian O. Ellis, Andrew H.S. Lee, Sarah E. Pinder and Emad A. Rakha. Tumors of the Breast. Diagnostic Histopathology of Tumors. 5th edition. Elsevier 2021.)

Morphology (Fig. 27.17)

Microscopy of ALH shows a solid, discohesive proliferation of cells that are monomorphic and small, with pale pink cytoplasm and uniform oval nuclei. Some cells have plasmacytoid or signet ring appearance (intracytoplasmic vacuoles).

The usual criteria to differentiate ALH from LCIS are as follows: distension of 50% or more acini within a lobule but not uniformly present throughout the entire lobule or involvement of all acini in a TDLU but does not distend the acini (i.e. calibre of the involved acini is similar to that of uninvolved acini).

ALH is also associated with loss of E-cadherin expression, similar to LCIS.

BENIGN EPITHELIAL CHANGES AND THEIR RELATIVE RISK OF DEVELOPING INVASIVE MALIGNANCY

The relative risk of developing invasive breast carcinoma is different for different groups of benign epithelial changes and is shown in Table 27.2.

Table 27.2 Epithelial Breast Lesions and Their Relative Risk for Breast Carcinoma

Pathological Lesions	Relative Risk
Nonproliferative breast lesions	1.0 (~3%)
Proliferative lesions without atypia	1.5–2 (~5%–7%)
Proliferative lesions without atypia	4–5 (~13%–17%)
Carcinoma in situ	8–10 (~25%–30%)

STROMAL TUMOURS PA 31.1

As already mentioned, stroma of the breast is of two types – intralobular and interlobular, and both give rise to different types of neoplasms. Fibroadenoma and phyllodes tumours arise from intralobular stroma, whereas interlobular stroma gives rise to classical stromal tumours of connective tissue that occur in other sites like lipomas and angiosarcomas and also stromal tumours exclusively seen in the breast such as myofibroblastomas. Here, we restrict our discussion to fibroadenomas and phyllodes tumours because these are most common stromal tumours of the breast. Fibroadenoma and phyllodes tumours are often referred to as 'biphasic tumours' because they also include a variable proportion of non-neoplastic epithelial component along with the neoplastic stromal component. Both the stromal tumours are associated with somatic mutations in the MED12 gene.

FIBROADENOMA

Fibroadenoma is the most common benign tumour of the female breast which is a biphasic tumour composed of a proliferation of both glandular epithelial and stromal components of the TDLU. It almost never turns malignant unless complex features exist.

Morphology

Gross (Fig. 27.18) These tumours are usually less than 3 cm in diameter but may grow to larger sizes. The term 'giant fibroadenomas' is used for tumours that measure more than 5 cm or weigh more than 500 g. These tumours are well-circumscribed, rubbery, greyish white nodules that bulge above the surrounding tissue and often contain slit-like spaces lined by epithelium.

Microscopy (Fig. 27.19) It is a biphasic tumour with a proliferation of both glandular and stromal elements.

There are two growth patterns seen with glandular component:

- **Intracanalicular:** Glands are compressed into linear branching structures by the proliferating stroma.
- **Pericanalicular:** Glands retain open lumens but are separated by the expanded stroma.
  Glandular elements have intact myoepithelial cell layer and are commonly associated with usual type ductal hyperplasia, apocrine metaplasia, cyst formation or squamous metaplasia.
  The stromal component has generally uniform cellularity composed of bland spindle-shaped

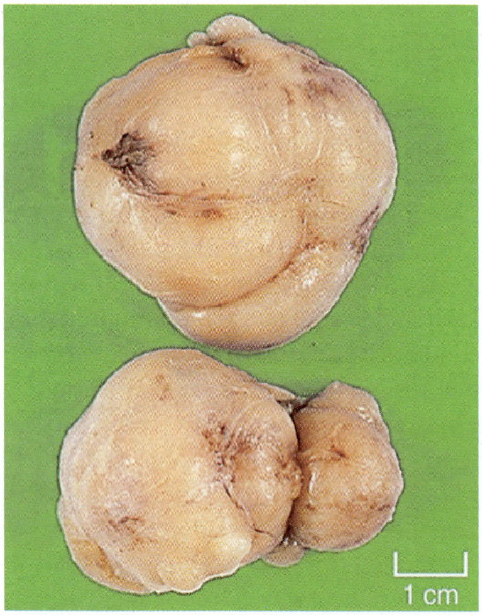

Fig. 27.18 Gross morphology of fibroadenoma. (*Source:* From J. Louise Jones. Breast. Underwood's Pathology. 7th edition. Elsevier 2019.)

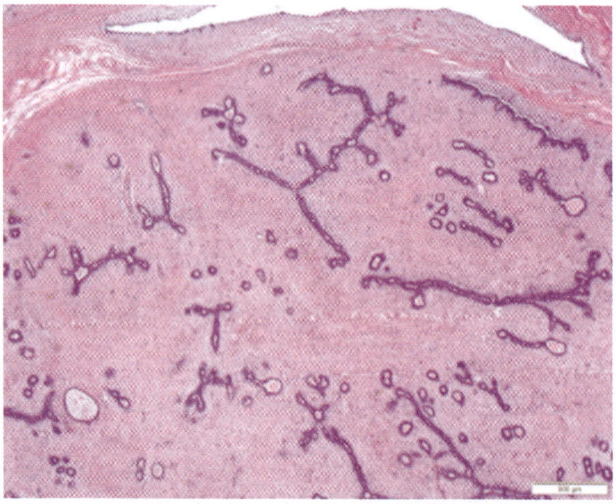

Fig. 27.19 Microscopy of fibroadenoma. Note the circumscribed border, mixed glandular and stromal growth. (*Source:* From Laura C. Collins. Breast. Rosai and Ackerman's Surgical Pathology. 11th edition. Elsevier 2018.)

stromal cells with ovoid or elongated nuclei and no stromal atypia.

Microscopic variants of fibroadenoma

- **Myxoid fibroadenoma:** Fibroadenoma with prominent myxoid stromal change composed of abundant pale, blue–grey extracellular matrix material
- **Complex fibroadenoma:** Fibroadenoma with cysts more than 3 mm in diameter, SA, epithelial microcalcifications or papillary apocrine metaplasia
- **Cellular fibroadenoma:** Fibroadenoma with diffuse stromal hypercellularity
- **Juvenile fibroadenoma:** Fibroadenoma with increased stromal cellularity and increased epithelial hyperplasia with micropapillary projections, a fascicular stromal arrangement and a pericanalicular growth pattern

Clinical Features

Fibroadenoma commonly affects adolescent and young women, with a median age of 25 years, though it can occur at any age. Juvenile fibroadenomas generally occur in younger and adolescent patients younger than 20 years, and complex fibroadenomas are reported in older patients. These present as a painless, firm, mobile, slow-growing mass, which are usually solitary but can be multiple and bilateral.

Fibroadenomas are hormonally responsive and hence grow in size with pregnancy and regress with childbirth. A sudden increase in size during pregnancy and the consequent infarction may clinically mimic malignancy.

PHYLLODES TUMOUR

Phyllodes tumours are benign biphasic tumours resembling fibroadenoma but with their hypercellular mesenchymal component organized in a leaf-like pattern around benign epithelial/myoepithelial lined spaces. These are also called cystosarcoma, which is a misnomer as cystic change is not commonly seen and the tumour is most commonly benign, though intermediate and malignant forms have been reported. Phyllodes means 'leaf' in Greek and the tumour is named so because of its morphological resemblance to a leaf.

Morphology

Gross (Fig. 27.20) Phyllodes tumour is a well-circumscribed, firm, bulging mass. Its cut surface is tan pink to grey. Large lesions have a whorled pattern, with curved clefts resembling leaf buds.

Microscopy (Fig. 27.21) Microscopy of a phyllodes tumour shows circumscribed pushing border and stromal hypercellularity (particularly next to epithelial elements). Benign glandular elements with an intracanalicular pattern with a balanced ratio are noted. Stroma resembles fibroblasts and myofibroblasts. Epithelial component may exhibit hyperplasia and squamous metaplasia. There may be variable areas of haemorrhage, necrosis, fat, bone, cartilage and skeletal muscle. The tumour cells exhibit mild atypia, and the mitotic count is usually less than four mitotic figures/10 HPF (high-power field). Phyllodes tumour can be differentiated from fibroadenoma by the presence of higher cellularity, a higher mitotic count, nuclear pleomorphism, stromal overgrowth and infiltrative borders. Low-grade phyllodes tumours resemble fibroadenomas and high-grade lesions resemble sarcomas.

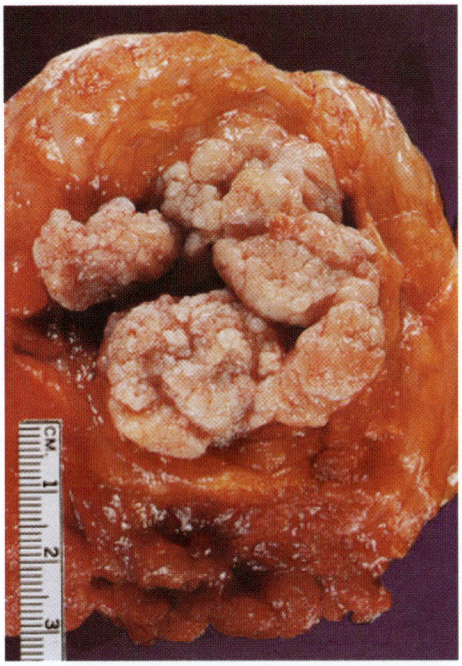

Fig. 27.20 Gross morphology of phyllodes tumour. The cut surface is solid and grey–white and shows the cleft-like spaces. (*Source:* From Laura C. Collins. Breast. Rosai and Ackerman's Surgical Pathology. 11th edition. Elsevier 2018.)

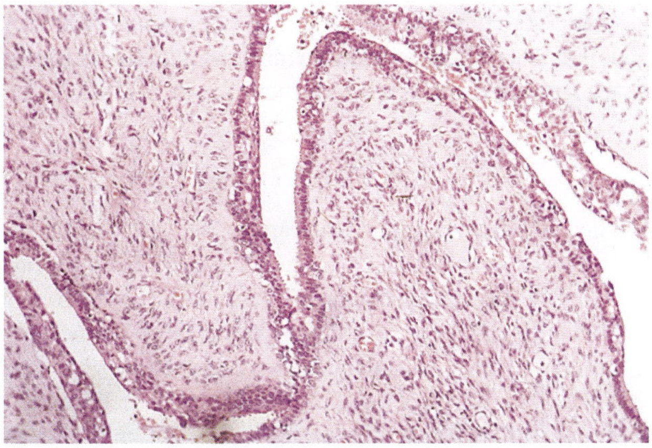

Fig. 27.21 Microscopy of phyllodes tumour. The stroma is cellular and forms club-like fingers covered with epithelium. (*Source:* From J. Louise Jones. Breast. Underwood's Pathology. 7th edition. Elsevier 2019.)

Clinical Features

Phyllodes tumour presents 10–20 years later than the peak age for fibroadenoma and most often present in the sixth decade. Low-grade or benign phyllodes tumours may occasionally recur but never metastasize, whereas borderline and high-grade phyllodes tumours commonly recur unless treated with mastectomy or wide excision. Irrespective of the grade, lymphatic spread is rare and hence lymph node dissection is not indicated. High-grade malignant phyllodes tumours may be associated with distant haematogenous metastases, and only the neoplastic stromal component metastasizes.

GYNAECOMASTIA PA 31.4

Gynaecomastia, the enlargement of breast tissue in males, is a condition that results from an imbalance in the hormonal environment within the body. Specifically, it is characterized by an increase in the ratio of oestrogen (the female hormone) to androgen (the male hormone). This imbalance can lead to the growth of breast glandular tissue. This lesion is typically seen in boys around puberty and adults older than 50 years. It can be unilateral or bilateral and symmetric in puberty and disappears by adulthood. Most cases are idiopathic, and the systemic disorders associated with gynaecomastia are listed in Box 27.1.

The pathogenesis of gynaecomastia involves several key mechanisms and can be influenced by various factors:

Hormonal imbalance

1. Increased oestrogen production:
   This can occur because of increased conversion of androgens to oestrogens by the enzyme aromatase, which is found in adipose (fat) tissue, the skin and other organs.
   Conditions causing hyperoestrogenism, such as liver disease (which impairs the breakdown of oestrogen), or tumours that produce oestrogen, can lead to gynaecomastia.
2. Decreased androgen production or activity:
   Conditions such as hypogonadism (decreased testicular function) can lead to reduced production of testosterone.
   Androgen resistance can also contribute to the development of gynaecomastia.

Physiological gynaecomastia

Neonatal gynaecomastia: Occurs in newborns because of the influence of maternal oestrogens.
Pubertal gynaecomastia: Common in adolescent boys because of transient hormonal fluctuations, where there is a temporary increase in oestrogen relative to androgen.
Senescent gynaecomastia: Seen in older men, partly because of decreased testosterone production and increased body fat (which leads to more oestrogen production through aromatization).

Box 27.1 Causes of Gynaecomastia

- Hyperthyroidism
- Hypogonadism
- Cirrhosis
- Chronic renal failure
- Chronic lung disease
- Hormone use – oestrogen, androgens
- Drugs such as digitalis, cimetidine and spironolactone
- As a paraneoplastic syndrome with bronchogenic carcinoma and germ cell tumours

Pathological gynaecomastia

1. Medication-induced:
   Certain medications can disrupt the balance of oestrogen and androgen. These include antiandrogens, some antibiotics, antiulcer medications, and drugs used in the treatment of cardiovascular diseases and prostate cancer.
   Drugs of abuse like alcohol, heroin, and marijuana can also contribute.
2. Systemic diseases:
   Conditions like liver cirrhosis, kidney failure and hyperthyroidism can alter hormone levels.
   Some tumours, particularly those of the testes, adrenal glands or lungs, can secrete hormones that affect breast tissue.

Morphology

Gross

The lesion is typically a soft, rubbery and firm subareolar mass which is grey–white on the cut surface with ill-defined margins.

Microscopy (Fig. 27.22)

In gynaecomastia, there is proliferation of ductal epithelial and periductal connective tissue in the breast. Early in its development, the condition is characterized by an increase in ductal tissue with periductal oedema and fibroblastic proliferation. As it progresses, there is an increase in fibrous tissue and a reduction in the ductal component.

Diagnosis and Management

Gynaecomastia is diagnosed based on clinical examination and may be confirmed with imaging or tissue biopsy.

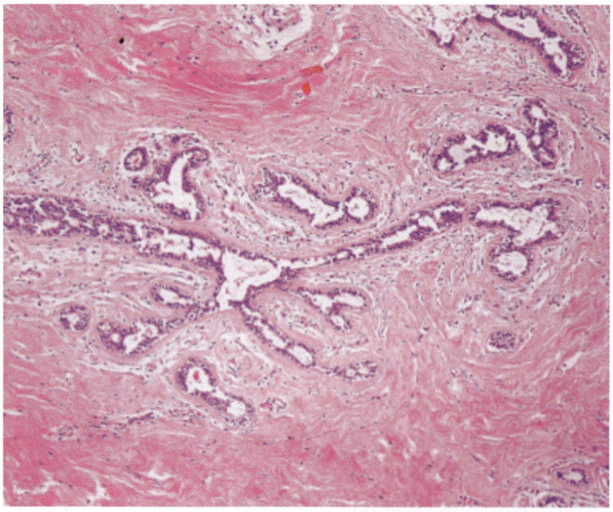

Fig. 27.22 Gynaecomastia – microscopy. Epithelial proliferation surrounded by a hypocellular myxoid halo in gynaecomastia. (*Source:* From Laura C. Collins. Breast. Rosai and Ackerman's Surgical Pathology. 11th edition. Elsevier 2018.)

Management depends on the underlying cause. In many cases, especially if physiological, it may resolve spontaneously. In other cases, treatment of the underlying cause, medication adjustments or surgical intervention may be required.

CARCINOMA OF THE BREAST PA 31.2

Worldwide, breast carcinoma is the most common malignancy affecting women. It is more common in the affluent countries, but breast cancer incidence is steadily rising in the developing countries. Breast carcinoma is a heterogeneous disease morphologically, immunohistochemically as well as at the molecular level, regardless of the race or geographic location. Hence, the prognosis and response to standard treatments can be highly variable from one patient to another. The first step towards customized therapy for breast carcinoma is to understand the heterogeneity of the disease. Pathologists have been aware of breast cancer heterogeneity for a long time and therefore have devised classification systems to stratify them and a grading system to identify tumours with different prognosis. The more recent advances in breast cancer research have increased our understanding of breast cancer and provided us with more refined classification systems. Morphological classification was used widely in the past, but the recent molecular classification is gaining more importance because of its impact on designing personalized treatment protocols.

EPIDEMIOLOGY

For decades together, cervical cancer was the most common cancer in women in India. However, over the last 10 years, breast cancer has been rising steadily and for the first time in 2012, breast cancer was declared as the most common cancer in women in India. Breast cancer has been ranked as the number one cancer among Indian females, with an age-adjusted rate as high as 25.8 per 100,000 women and mortality 12.7 per 100,000 women. The incidence of this disease has been consistently increasing, and it is estimated that it has risen by 50% between 1965 and 1985. The annual percentage change in the incidence ranged from 0.46 to 2.56 for breast cancer. Breast cancer seems to be more common in the younger age group in India, and 52% of all women suffering from breast cancer in India are between 40 and 49 years of age. A significant number of patients are younger than 30 years. The population-based registries show a significant rural–urban division in the breast cancer incidence. However, hospital-based registries may be biased because of varying reference patterns/socioeconomic and other factors. Mortality to incidence ratio was found to be as high as 66 in rural and as low as 8 in urban cases. Breast cancer projection for India during 2020 suggests the number to go high. Better health awareness and availability of breast cancer screening programmes and treatment facilities would cause a favourable and positive clinical picture in the country.

AETIOPATHOGENESIS

Risk Factors

A number of factors have been studied and included in the list of risk factors for the development of breast carcinoma and the leading factor is gender, followed by age, oestrogen exposure, genetic inheritance, environmental and lifestyle changes. All the factors are listed with their relative risk for developing breast carcinoma in Table 27.3.

Pathogenesis and Molecular Classification of Breast Carcinoma

In the beginning of the last century, all the patients with breast malignancy were treated uniformly. But over time, it was observed that patients with the same type of cancer showed varying prognosis and that led to the identification of different morphological variants by pathologists over the last 50 years. Currently, there are 20 major types and 18 minor subtypes of breast cancer that have been defined and included in the recently published WHO classification. However, there are doubts as to whether these variants are biologically significant or not. Now, it is obvious that breast cancer is a heterogeneous disease with different histological and biological properties because of genetic, epigenetic and transcriptome changes, with varying clinical findings, treatment responses and with multiple entities. The basis of all this chaos seems to be based on the absence of specific markers and the inability to understand the epithelial cellular development of breast tissue. But with the advancement of molecular techniques such as gene expression profiling, 'heterogeneity in breast cancer concept' has now become generally accepted. Thus, a new 'taxonomy' was developed for the classification of breast cancer. Pathologists were introduced to the so-called new era 'molecular classification' that has been developed from the traditional, old-fashioned 'morphological' classification. Targeted therapies and, more importantly, individualized treatment programmes have become possible with the implementation of this classification.

Table 27.3 Risk Factors for Developing Breast Cancer

Risk Factors	Relative Risk
Female gender Increasing age Germline mutations of high penetrance Strong family history (more than one first-degree relative, young age, multiple cancers) Personal history of breast cancer High breast density	>4.0
Germline mutations of moderate penetrance High-dose radiation to the chest at a young age Family history (one first-degree relative)	2.1–4.0
Early menarche (age <12 years) Late menopause (age >55 years) Late first pregnancy (age >35 years) Nulliparity Absence of breastfeeding Exogenous hormone therapy Postmenopausal obesity Physical inactivity High alcohol consumption	1.1–2.0

Perou and Sorlie proposed 'molecular classification' terminology in breast cancer for the first time, with a comprehensive study showing the differences in gene expression in 2000. It consisted of four major molecular classes of breast cancer. Molecular subtypes of breast cancer can be classified as follows:

1. **Luminal**
   - Luminal A – $ER^+/PR^+/HER2^-$/low Ki-67
   - Luminal B – $ER^+/PR^+/HER2^-/+$/high Ki-67
2. **HER2 – Overexpression – $ER^-/PR^-/HER2^+$**
3. **Triple-negative breast cancers (TNBCs) – $ER^-/PR^-/HER2^-$**
4. **Basal-like subtype found to be positive for basal marker (CK5/6) expression**

It is simpler to check the expression of proteins by immunohistochemistry (IHC); the molecular classification has become a routine practice in most of the centres across the globe.

Breast cancer develops through many pathways by stepwise accumulation of mutations. A majority of breast cancers are sporadic, and only a minority of them are due to germline mutations. We begin our discussion with the familial breast carcinomas because they have provided good insights into the genetics of breast carcinoma.

Familial Breast Carcinoma

A first-degree relative (mother, daughter, sister) with breast cancer or multiple relatives affected by breast or ovarian cancer (especially before they turned 50 years of age) are considered high-risk factors for developing breast cancer. In some cases, a strong family history of breast cancer is linked to the presence of an abnormal gene associated with a high risk of breast cancer, such as the BRCA1 or BRCA2 gene. In other cases, an abnormal CHEK2 gene may play a role in developing breast cancer.

Genetics: Approximately 5%–10% of breast cancers are thought to be hereditary, caused by abnormal genes passed from parents to their children. Most inherited cases of breast cancer are associated with mutations in two genes:

- ***BRCA1 (BReast CAncer gene 1)***
- ***BRCA2 (BReast CAncer gene 2)***

BRCA1 and BRCA2 are normal genes whose function is to repair cell damage and keep breast, ovarian and other cells growing normally. But when these genes contain mutations that are passed from generation to generation, breast, ovarian and other cancer risks increase. BRCA1 and BRCA2 mutations may account for up to 10% of all breast cancers, or 1 of every 10 cases. Having a BRCA1 or BRCA2 mutation does not mean a person will be diagnosed with breast cancer. Researchers are learning that other single nucleotide polymorphisms (SNPs) may be linked to higher breast cancer risks in women with a BRCA1 mutation as well as women who do not inherit a breast cancer gene mutation.

Women who have a BRCA1 or BRCA2 mutation (or both) can have up to a 72% risk of being diagnosed with breast cancer during their lifetime. Breast cancers associated with a BRCA1 or BRCA2 mutation tend to develop in younger women and occur more often in both breasts than cancers in women without these genetic mutations and also have an increased risk of developing ovarian, colon and pancreatic cancers, as well as melanoma.

BRCA1 and BRCA2 are discussed in Chapter 7. BRCA1- and BRCA2-associated tumours are commonly poorly differentiated. BRCA1-associated tumours are generally triple-negative, whereas BRCA2-related tumours are commonly ER^+.

Other genes: Inherited mutations in other genes are also associated with breast cancer. These abnormal gene changes are much less common than BRCA1 and BRCA2 mutations, which themselves are fairly uncommon. Because of their rarity, they have not been studied as much as the BRCA genes. On the basis of research to date, experts have estimated the levels of breast cancer risk that may be associated with each gene mutation.

Levels of genetic risk are generally defined as high risk, moderate to high risk, moderate risk and uncertain risk.

Most common single-gene mutations associated with inherited susceptibility to breast cancer development are listed in Table 27.4.

Table 27.4 Genes and Their Relative Risk for Development of Breast Carcinoma

Category	Risk %	Genes
High risk	>50%	BRCA1 and BRCA2 TP53 PTEN PALB2
Moderate to high risk	25% >50%	ATM CDH1
Moderate risk	25%–50%	CHEK2 NBN NF-1 STK11
Very low risk	?	BARD1 BRIP1

Sporadic Breast Cancer

Three main pathways have been identified in the evolution of sporadic breast cancer. The initiating mutations dictate the pathways, the biological features, response to treatment, recurrence, metastases and survival. The pathways are discussed briefly (Table 27.5).

1. **Luminal, $ER^+/HER2^-$ tumours:** This group has the widest spectrum of cancers with respect to grades and proliferation rates. Tumours with strong ER^+ are most often PR^+ and are well differentiated with a poor proliferation rate, whereas tumours with low ER^+ and PR^- are poorly differentiated with a high proliferative index. As expected, the most common risk factor for this group is sustained oestrogen exposure. ER^+ precursor lesions are flat epithelial atypia, atypical ductal and lobular hyperplasia. These lesions are the earliest identifiable morphological changes and share the genetic changes seen with invasive lesions like gain of chromosome 1q, losses of chromosome 16q and activating mutations in PIK3CA.
   Luminal tumours are further subclassified into luminal A and luminal B based on their proliferative status.
   Luminal A tumours: Hormonal receptor–positive (ER^+ and PR^+), HER2/neu^- and Ki-67^-. It is the most frequent subtype. It shows a good prognosis and responds well to hormone therapy. Various studies have reported that ER^+ tumours have little response to conventional chemotherapy. Luminal A breast cancers are usually low grade, with slow growth and a better prognosis.
   Luminal B tumours: Hormone receptor–positive (ER^+ and PR^+) with $HER2^+$ or $HER2^-$ and high levels of Ki-67^+. Luminal B cancers generally grow slightly faster than luminal A cancers, and their prognosis is slightly worse than luminal A because they are more aggressive with a high tumour grade.
2. **$HER2^+$ tumours:** These tumours are hormone receptor–negative (ER^- and PR^-) and $HER2^+$. HER2-enriched cancers tend to grow faster than luminal cancers and have a worse prognosis, but these are often successfully treated with targeted therapies aimed at the HER2 protein.
   $HER2^+$ tumours are the result of a pathway associated with amplification of the HER2 gene located on chromosome 17q. This is the most common subtype of breast cancer in patients with germline *TP53* mutations which is referred to as Li–Fraumeni syndrome.
   The HER2 gene encodes a transmembrane tyrosine kinase receptor that binds to its extracellular signals and initiates a signalling cascade, mediating cell proliferation and survival. Approximately 12%–20% of breast cancers either overexpress the HER2 protein or have HER2 gene amplification, resulting in aggressive tumour growth and a poor clinical outcome. Its expression is also

Table 27.5 Features of Molecular Subtypes of Breast Cancer

Feature	Luminal A	Luminal B	$HER2^+$	Triple-Negative Basal Like
Percentage of breast cancers	40%–55%	10%	20%	15%
Most common gene mutations	PIK3CA (45%) TP53 (12%)	PIK3CA (29%) TP53 (29%)	PIK3CA (39%) TP53 (70%–80%)	PIK3CA (9%) TP53 (70%–80%)
Special histological types commonly associated	Tubular Grade 1 or 2 lobular Mucinous Papillary	Grade 3 lobular	Some apocrine, some micropapillary	Medullary features Metaplastic
Patient category	Older women and men	*BRCA2* mutation carriers	Young women, *TP53* mutation carriers	Young women, women of African heritage *BRCA1* mutation carriers
Response to chemotherapy	<10%	10%	ER^+: 15% ER^-: 30%–60%	30%
Relapse pattern	Low rate over many years, long survival possible with bone metastases	Early peak at <10 years, late recurrence possible	Bimodal with early and late (10 years) peaks	Early peak at <8 years, late recurrence rare, survival with metastases rare
Metastatic pattern	Bone (70%), more common than viscera (25%) or brain (<10%)	Bone (80%) more common than viscera (30%) or brain (10%)	Bone (70%), viscera (45%) and brain (30%) all are common	Bone (40%), viscera (35%) and brain (25%) all are common

indicative of a potential response to anti-HER2 therapy but not all $HER2^+$ tumours respond equally well to anti-HER2 therapy. This along with the emergence of resistant clones has led to the trial of many therapeutic agents to overcome this. HER2 can be defined as positive if 10% or more of tumour cells exhibit strong uniform membrane staining.

3. **Basal-like or triple-negative tumours:** $CK5/6^+$ and/or $EGFR^+$, ER^- and PR^- and $HER2^-$. The basal class is so named because of its pattern of expression that is similar to basal epithelial cells and normal myoepithelial cells of mammary tissue. This type of cancer is more common in women with BRCA1 gene mutations. Under normal circumstances, BRCA1 could regularize the proliferation of these cells; low regulation of BRCA1 leads to an abnormal growth of these $CK5/6^+$ cells. These tumours tend to be very aggressive, high grade and are often associated with p53 mutation. Various studies have demonstrated a poor prognosis of this class. It is still not clear if this prognosis is because of a lack of therapeutic options or to an inherent aggressiveness.
4. ***Unclassified (penta*** −ve) tumours: This group of tumours includes ER^- and PR^-, $HER2^-$ and $CK5/6^-$ and $EGFR^-$. Unclassified cases were initially considered to be synonymous with 'normal-like' breast cancers. These tumours cluster with nontumoural breast cells and exhibit overexpression of PIK3R1 and AKR1C1, in addition to other genomic alterations. The current concept states that the 'normal-like' subtype is absolutely different from the unclassified (penta −ve) group. These are very good prognostically and are grouped with the luminal type, as both exhibit low pathological complete remission rates of 6%.

MORPHOLOGICAL TYPES OF IN SITU LESIONS

Most of the breast malignancies are adenocarcinomas, which constitute more than 95% of breast cancers. Invasive ductal carcinoma (IDC) is the most common form of invasive breast cancer. It accounts for 55% of breast cancer cases on diagnosis. Breast carcinomas arise from the same segment of the TDLU. In general, breast carcinoma is divided into CIS and IC. CIS is a noninvasive malignant intraductal or intralobular proliferation of epithelial cells that is confined to the ducts and lobules. Invasive or infiltrative carcinoma refers to a malignant abnormal proliferation of neoplastic cells in the breast tissue which has penetrated through the basement membrane into stroma. IC and CIS are classified as ductal and lobular on the basis of the site from which the tumour originated. Cancers originating from the ducts are known as *ductal carcinomas*, whereas those originating from the lobules are known as *lobular carcinomas*.

Ductal Carcinoma In Situ

DCIS is a neoplastic proliferation of mammary ductal epithelial cells confined to the ductal–lobular system without evidence of invasion through the basement membrane into the surrounding stroma. In total, 3.3%–5.9% of women with DCIS carry a germline mutation in

BRCA1 or *BRCA2* and the prevalence of *BRCA* mutation is significantly greater in women diagnosed with DCIS before the age of 50 years with a personal or family history of breast cancer.

Morphological Types of Ductal Carcinoma In Situ Historically, DCIS has been divided into five architectural subtypes:

a. Comedo
b. Solid
c. Cribriform
d. Papillary
e. Micropapillary

A. ***Comedo*** (Fig. 27.23): The term 'comedo' refers to a yellowish creamy necrotic material that extrudes from the ducts resembling comedones. Histologically, this subtype is characterized by enlarged ducts filled with necrotic debris surrounded by none to a few layers of highly atypical epithelial cells and numerous mitotic figures. Necrosis usually spans more than 90% of the duct cross-section. The abundant necrotic material calcifies and appears as large linear branching calcifications on mammogram. It is categorized as high-grade DCIS.
B. ***Solid:*** 'Solid' cell pattern is the one in which the cancer cells have completely filled the duct. The lumen of ducts or lobules is filled with sheets of cohesive atypical malignant cells which are evenly spaced. It is categorized as low- or intermediate-grade DCIS.
C. ***Cribriform*** (Fig. 27.24): 'Cribriform' pattern refers to the neoplastic cell sheets pierced with numerous small holes with rigid extracellular lumens giving a punched-out appearance similar to the 'holes in Swiss cheese 'or 'ripples'. A cribriform pattern is consistent with a low- or medium-grade DCIS.

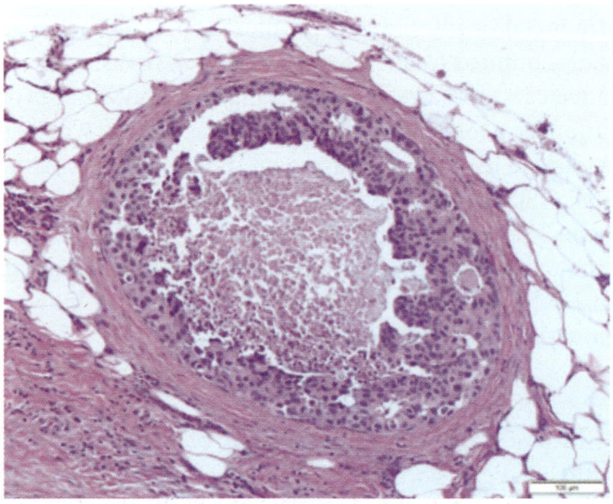

Fig. 27.23 DCIS, comedo – microscopy. (*Source:* From Laura C. Collins. Breast. Rosai and Ackerman's Surgical Pathology. 11th edition. Elsevier 2018.)

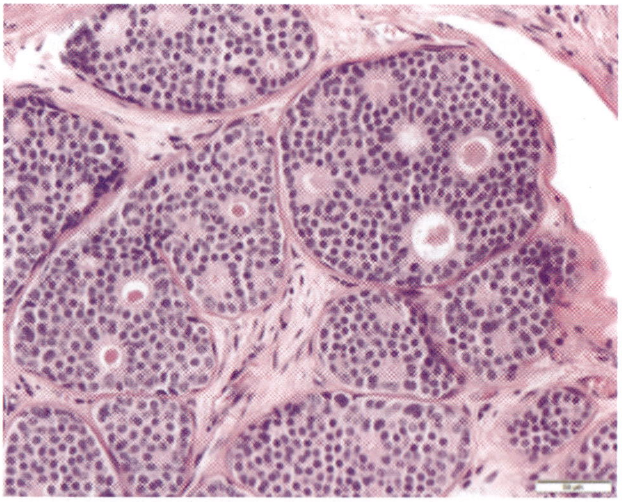

Fig. 27.24 DCIS, cribriform – microscopy. (*Source:* From Laura C. Collins. Breast. Rosai and Ackerman's Surgical Pathology. 11th edition. Elsevier 2018.)

D. ***Papillary:*** A 'papillary' DCIS pattern is the one that is arranged in a 'fern-like' or 'finger-like' pattern within the duct. It contains a prominent fibrovascular septa projecting into duct lumen and the papillary cores generally lack a myoepithelial cell layer.
E. ***Micropapillary:*** It refers to a tumour composed of small clusters of cells within clear stromal spaces resembling dilated vascular channels.

Clinical Features and Management It is very difficult to determine the history and progress of DCIS. Currently, patients with DCIS are managed with excision and radiation therapy. Left untreated, a small low-grade DCIS progresses to invasive malignancy at a rate of 1% per year. When compared with mastectomy, excision has a slightly higher risk of recurrence. The major risk factors for recurrence are high nuclear grade, necrosis, greater extent of the disease and positive surgical margins.

Complete excision of DCIS is not always possible with conservative surgeries because the exact distribution is not reliably revealed by imaging and also because the lesions may not be grossly evident during surgery. Hence, postoperative tamoxifen and radiation are recommended to reduce the recurrence rate.

The invasive malignancy that develops has similar grade, ER and HER2 expression profile like that of the precursor DCIS. As expected, high-grade DCIS has a higher risk of progression to invasive malignancy.

Paget Disease of the Nipple (Fig. 27.25)

Paget disease of the nipple is an uncommon manifestation of breast cancer with an incidence of 1%–4%. It presents as a unilateral erythematous lesion of the nipple with scaling and crusting. Patients complain of intense pruritus and hence the lesion may often be mistaken for eczema. A palpable lump is present in at least half of

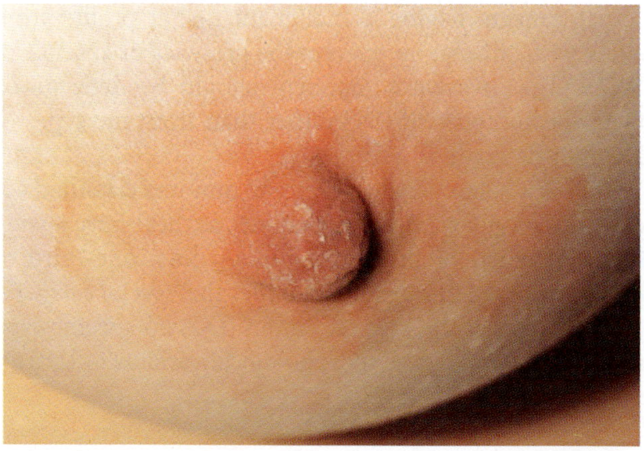

Fig. 27.25 Paget disease of the nipple – clinical picture. Eczematous hyperaemic and eroded clinical appearance. (*Source:* From Laura C. Collins. Breast. Rosai and Ackerman's Surgical Pathology. 11th edition. Elsevier 2018.)

patients with Paget disease of the nipple and a majority of them turn out to be invasive malignancy. Patients without a palpable lump usually have only DCIS.

Morphology (Fig. 27.26)

Microscopically, Paget disease is characterized by the extension of DCIS within the ducts to the nipple skin through lactiferous sinuses without breaching the basement membrane. As the tumour cells disrupt the normal epithelial barrier, the extracellular fluid seeps on to the nipple surface. Paget cells are large with clear cytoplasm and eccentric, hyperchromatic nuclei and are readily detected by nipple biopsy or cytological preparations of the exudate from the nipple.

Invasive malignancies are generally ER^- and $HER2^+$. Prognosis of the underlying malignancy is not influenced by the presence or absence of Paget disease.

Lobular Carcinoma In Situ

LCIS is the lobulocentric proliferation of small uniform cells which fill and distend most of the acini in the involved lobule, in contrast to ALH which only partially involves the lobule by filling up the acini without significant distension. LCIS usually does not show up on mammograms because of lack of desmoplasia and is an incidental microscopic finding with characteristic cellular morphology and multifocal tissue patterns. It is therefore difficult to estimate the actual incidence of LCIS. LCIS is identified in 0.5%–1.5% of benign breast biopsies and in 1.8%–2.5% of all breast biopsies. Age-specific incidence analysis reveals that the magnitude of the incidence is highest among women 50 years or older.

Morphology (Figs 27.27 and 27.28)

Classical LCIS

LCIS is a proliferation cantered in the TDLUs and consists of neoplastic cells that fill and expand most (>50%) of the acini. Pagetoid extension into the terminal ducts with growth of LCIS cells underneath the ductal epithelium is also common. The cross-section of a duct with pagetoid involvement by LCIS has a characteristic 'cloverleaf' pattern. Classical LCIS is a monomorphic, discohesive proliferation of nonpolarized cells of round to oval shape with inconspicuous cytoplasm referred to as 'marbles in a bag'. The nuclei are located in the centre of the cells and are small, round to oval, with a smooth nuclear membrane and inconspicuous nucleoli. Cell borders are indistinct. Intracytoplasmic vacuoles are common, and signet ring cell formation can occur. Mitotic activity is either absent or exceedingly rare. Discohesiveness of the cells is because of loss-of-function mutation of the

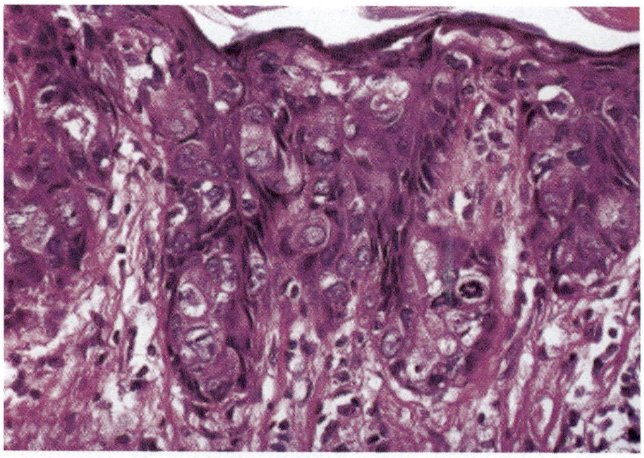

Fig. 27.26 Paget disease nipple – microscopy. Striking cytological atypia in the tumour cells is readily apparent. (*Source:* From Laura C. Collins. Breast. Rosai and Ackerman's Surgical Pathology. 11th edition. Elsevier 2018.)

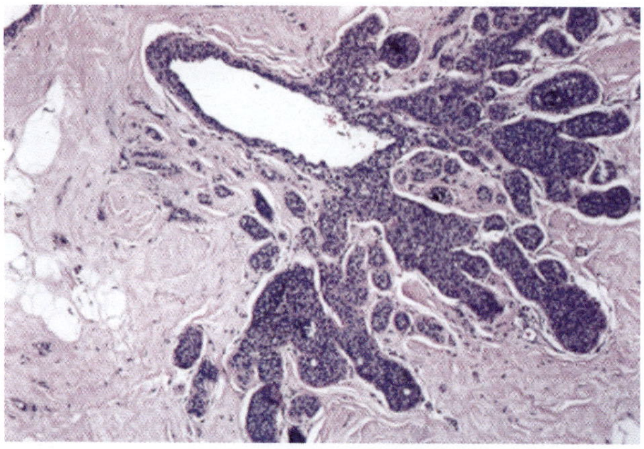

Fig. 27.27 LCIS – microscopy. Typical pattern of involvement of terminal duct–lobular unit by lobular carcinoma in situ. (*Source:* From Laura C. Collins. Breast. Rosai and Ackerman's Surgical Pathology. 11th edition. Elsevier 2018.)

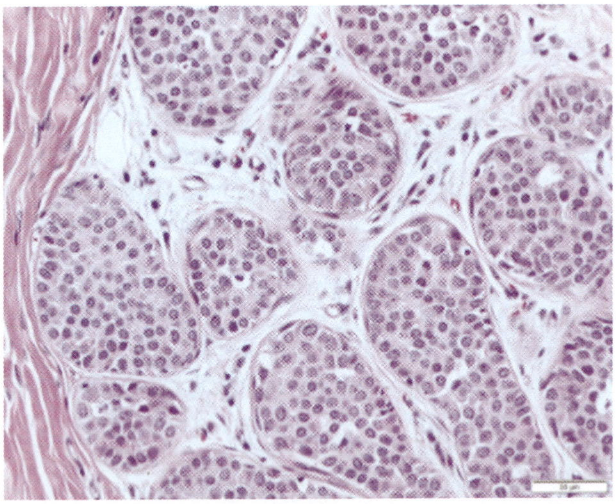

Fig. 27.28 LCIS – microscopy. Marked expansion of a lobular unit by lobular carcinoma in situ. (*Source:* From Laura C. Collins. Breast. Rosai and Ackerman's Surgical Pathology. 11th edition. Elsevier 2018.)

CDH1 gene resulting in the loss of expression of E-cadherin protein similar to lobular carcinoma.

Two types of cells are described:

- **Type A or small cells:** Loosely cohesive cells with uniform small nuclei with homogeneous chromatin and inconspicuous nucleoli
- **Type B or large cells:** Poorly cohesive cells with mild to moderate nuclear variability and prominent nucleoli

The two cell types can coexist in the same patient, in the same breast and even in the same lobule. In the absence of necrosis or marked nuclear pleomorphism, LCIS composed predominantly of large cells is best classified as classical LCIS. Pleomorphic LCIS, P-LCIS, is a variant of LCIS that is characterized by pleomorphic cells, calcifications, architectural distortion and less frequently a mass lesion. Florid LCIS is a newly described variant in which the acini are markedly distended with the absence of intervening stroma.

LCIS cells are most often ER^+, PR^+ and $HER2^-$.

LCIS is a risk factor for the development of invasive lobular carcinoma (ILC) (more commonly than ductal carcinoma), but unlike DCIS there is also an increased risk for the development of carcinoma of the contralateral breast. The incidence of IC is 1% per year. Prophylactic bilateral mastectomy, tamoxifen or more commonly close clinical follow-up and mammographic screening are the management options.

INVASIVE DUCTAL CARCINOMA (IDC)

IDC is the most common form of breast cancer, representing 80% of all breast cancer diagnoses. IDCs are breast cancers having a malignant ductal proliferation along with stromal invasion in the presence or absence of DCIS. The invasive component should be determined from the subtypes of IDC rather than from the types of DCIS or its grade.

IDC is a heterogeneous group of tumours classified according to cytoarchitectural features, as these have a wide scope of morphological variation. At least one-third of breast cancers can be grouped under the '*special category*'. We first discuss the most common IDC, no specific type (NST), followed by the morphological variants of IDC.

Morphology

Classical IDC, NST: IDC, NST, is the most common type of IDC that constitutes approximately 40%–75% of all invasive breast carcinomas. The tumour shows a heterogeneous type of growth, including diffuse sheets, nests, cords or singly distributed cells with a variable amount of ductal differentiation. The amount of ductal differentiation ranges from more than 70% of tumour tissue to complete absence. Tumour cells are pleomorphic, vary in shape and size and usually have prominent nucleoli and numerous mitoses. The areas of necrosis and calcification can be detected in 60% of cases. Foci of squamous metaplasia, apocrine metaplasia or clear cell changes are sometimes present. The amount of stroma is variable, ranging from none to abundant.

Grading of Breast Carcinoma (Fig. 27.29)

Breast carcinoma is graded using the ***Nottingham histological score***, Bloom–Richardson grading system. Three parameters are evaluated for grading – tubule formation, nuclear pleomorphism and mitotic activity.

Grade 1: Well-differentiated carcinomas with predominant tubule formation and small uniform nuclei and a low proliferative rate

Grade 2: Moderately differentiated carcinomas with tubular pattern mixed with a solid or single-cell growth pattern with greater nuclear pleomorphism and a high proliferative rate

Grade 3: Poorly differentiated carcinomas with ragged nests or sheets of cells with enlarged, irregular and pleomorphic nuclei, areas of tumour necrosis and a very high proliferative rate

Clinical Features

Large tumours may invade the dermis causing retraction of the skin or invade the pectoralis muscle and become fixed to the chest wall. Nipple retraction may be seen when the tumour involves the central portion of the breast. Depending on the presenting stage, axillary lymph node metastasis or distant metastases may be present. Rarely, small tumours get obscured by dense breast tissue or lack desmoplastic stromal response and present as

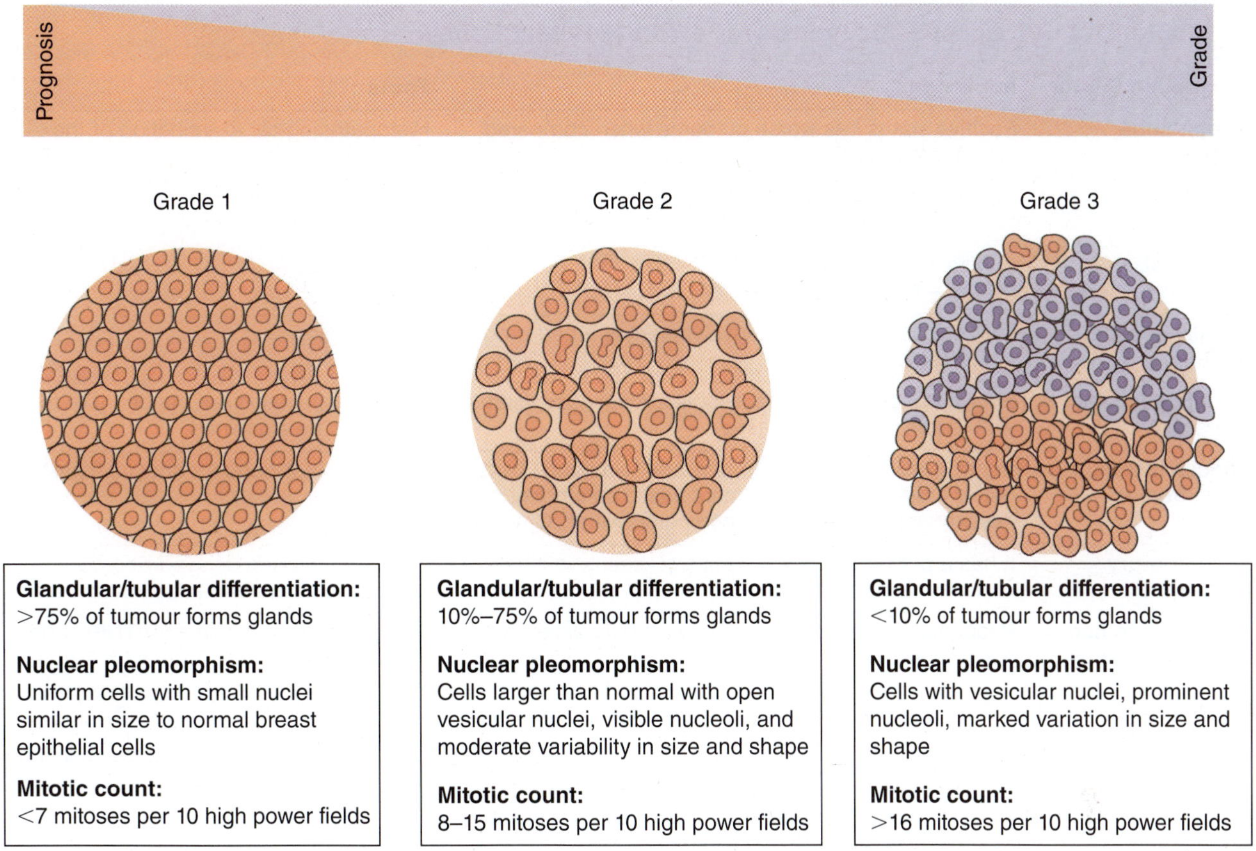

Fig. 27.29 Bloom–Richardson grading for breast carcinoma. (*Source:* https://pathology.jhu.edu/build/assets/breast/_lgImg/breast-cancer-grades-illustration.jpg)

axillary lymph node or distant metastases without a clinically palpable breast lump. Such occult tumours are picked up with imaging techniques.

PROGNOSTIC AND PREDICTIVE FACTORS FOR INVASIVE CARCINOMAS

Biological features of carcinoma and stage of the tumour dictate the prognosis in patients with breast cancer. In general, patients with distant metastases and inflammatory carcinoma have guarded prognosis, whereas for all other tumours the prognosis is best determined by the histopathological evaluation of the primary tumour and the axillary lymph nodes. Two set of factors are important in the evaluation of patients with breast carcinoma – prognostic and predictive factors. Prognostic factors help in assessing the outcome of the disease and designing the treatment protocol, whereas predictive factors enable to predict the likely response of a tumour to a specific form of treatment. Factors associated with tumour extent are prognostic, whereas factors associated with tumour biology are both prognostic and predictive.

Table 27.6 lists the prognostic and predictive factors in breast cancer and the role played by them.

STAGING OF BREAST CARCINOMA

Staging is an important aspect of management of breast cancers, and factors like tumour size, local extension, lymph node status and distant metastases are taken into consideration. There are four types of staging – anatomical, clinical, pathological and postneoadjuvant chemotherapy staging. The latest anatomical staging system widely followed is the American Joint Committee on Cancer (AJCC) 8th edition, anatomical stage (Table 27.7).

Clinical prognostic stage is assigned for all the patients including patients prior to surgery, patients not eligible for surgery and patients who undergo systemic therapy before surgery. Pathological staging is assigned to patients undergoing excision of the tumour before the treatment. Tumour response is assessed histopathologically following administration of neoadjuvant chemotherapy.

MANAGEMENT AND TARGETED THERAPY FOR BREAST CARCINOMA

The aims of treatment in breast cancer are to control local disease and prolong survival of patients by treating known or potential distant metastases and prevent future recurrences. Breast-conserving surgery (and mastectomy when

Table 27.6 Prognostic and Predictive Factors in Breast Cancer

Prognostic Factor	Inference	Facts
Lymph node status	Positive status has worse outcome when compared with negative status	Histopathological examination of the nodes is essential
Distant metastases	Bad prognostic factor	Metastases beyond regional lymph nodes is a crucial factor
Tumour size	<1 cm – good prognosis >4 cm – bad prognosis	Refer staging
Locally advanced tumour	Skin or pectoralis muscle involvement is a bad prognostic factor	Refer staging
Lymphovascular invasion	Poor prognosticator because it is strongly associated with lymph node metastases	Vascular spaces in the periphery of the tumour to be examined
Special histological subtypes	Some special types like tubular, adenoid cystic carry better prognosis, whereas metaplastic carcinoma carries worse prognosis when compared with IDC, NST	Grading is not done for special types
Inflammatory carcinoma	It has a poor prognosis because of extensive invasion of dermal lymphatics	Diagnosis is often delayed because of close resemblance to inflammatory lesion
Response to neoadjuvant therapy	Responsive tumours have a better prognosis than nonresponsive tumours	This is mainly applicable for TNBC and HER2 tumours

IDC, NST, invasive ductal carcinoma, no specific type.

Table 27.7 AJCC 8th Edition, Anatomical Stage

Stage	T – Primary Tumour	N – Lymph Nodes	M – Distant Metastasis	10-Year Survival %
0	Ductal carcinoma in situ	No metastases	Absent	97
I	Invasive carcinoma ≤2 cm	No metastases or only micrometastases	Absent	87
II	Invasive carcinoma >2 cm Invasive carcinoma >5 cm but ≤5 cm	1–3 positive LNs 0–3 positive LNs	Absent	65
III	Invasive carcinoma >5 cm Any size invasive carcinoma Invasive carcinoma with skin or chest wall involvement or inflammatory carcinoma	Negative or positive LNs ≥4 positive LNs Negative or positive LNs	Absent	40
IV	Any size invasive carcinoma	Negative or positive LNs	Present	5

LN, lymph node.

indicated) and radiation therapy provide local control, and systemic therapy in the form of chemotherapy, anti-oestrogen therapy or targeted therapy provides protection against metastasis. The common treatment protocols followed are listed in Table 27.8.

Table 27.8 Treatment Protocols for Systemic Control of Breast Cancers

Breast Cancer – Type	Treatment Option
ER^+ tumours	Hormonal therapy
Highly proliferative tumours	Chemotherapy
$HER2^+$ tumours	HER2 antagonists
Triple-negative tumours	Immunotherapy

ER, oestrogen receptor.

MALE BREAST CANCER

Male breast cancer accounts for only 1% of total breast cancers and has the same risk factors as those in women such as advancing age, first-degree relatives with breast cancer, exposure to oestrogens, ionizing radiation, alcohol consumption, obesity, infertility, prior benign breast disease and Klinefelter syndrome.

The most important factor that plays a role in familial breast cancers is germline mutation of the BRCA2 gene. The other genes that are associated in the genesis of male breast cancer are BRCA1, PTEN, TP53 and PALB2.

Most of the cases in males are of luminal type, and TNBCs and HER2 types are rare. Patients present with a readily palpable subareolar mass as the breast tissue is less and limited to large ducts near the nipple. Hence, the tumours are located close to the skin and thoracic wall and therefore invade these structures earlier, resulting in skin ulceration and chest wall fixation.

Tumours follow the same paths as those in women and involve axillary lymph nodes and in advanced cases present with distant metastases to the lungs, brain, bones and liver.

Men present at a higher stage at a shorter time than women, but when matched stage to stage, prognosis is similar. Cancers are treated with mastectomy and axillary lymph node dissection and radiotherapy with or without systemic therapy when indicated.

OTHER MALIGNANT TUMOURS OF THE BREAST

Other malignant tumours that may occur rarely in the breast are as follows:

- Angiosarcoma
- Non-Hodgkin B-cell lymphoma
- Non-Hodgkin T-cell lymphoma associated with breast implants
- Skin tumours
- Adnexal tumours
- Metastasis from melanoma and ovarian tumours

The morphology of these tumours is exactly the same as how they appear elsewhere and are described in the respective chapters.

LABORATORY APPROACH TO A CASE OF BREAST CARCINOMA

Patients with suspected breast lump initially undergo thorough clinical examination, followed by imaging studies. A tru-cut biopsy or an FNAC is mandatory for the diagnosis of breast carcinoma. Postexcision or postbiopsy pathological investigations are as follows:

- Histopathological examination
- Histopathological grading for IDC, NST
- Assessment of pathological staging
- ER/PR/HER2 by IHC
- CK5/6 if ER/PR$^-$
- HER2 by FISH (fluorescent in situ hybridization)
- Ki-67 to assess proliferative status
- Response to treatment is assessed if neoadjuvant chemotherapy is given before excision
- Genomic profiling wherever possible

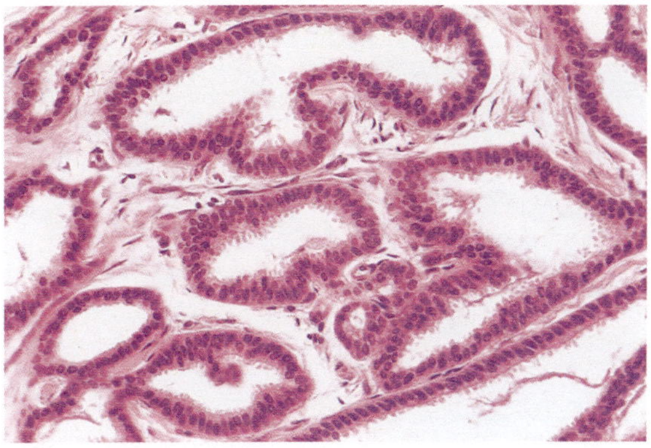

Fig. 27.30 Tubular carcinoma breast – microscopy. Tubular glands lie in a fibrous stroma. (*Source:* From J. Louise Jones. Breast. Underwood's Pathology. 7th edition. Elsevier 2019.)

TUBULAR CARCINOMA (FIG. 27.30)

It is a rare, well-differentiated type of breast carcinoma, constituting approximately 2% of IDCs. It is common in elderly women; it has an excellent prognosis and low likelihood of lymph node metastasis. It is characterized microscopically by the proliferation of angulated, oval or elongated tubules; these cancers typically test positive for oestrogen (ER) and progesterone (PR) receptors, and negative for HER2.

CRIBRIFORM CARCINOMA

It is a rare type with a favourable prognosis, occurring mostly in patients older than 50 years, and accounting for 0.8%–3.5% of breast cancer cases. It exhibits islands of uniform, low-grade tumour cells with a cribriform appearance and clear stromal invasion.

MUCINOUS CARCINOMA (FIG. 27.31)

It is also known as gelatinous or colloid carcinoma, this rare subtype accounts for 2% of breast cancers, primarily affecting women older than 60 years. Tumours are characterized by small clusters of epithelial cells in abundant mucin, usually positive for ER/PR and negative for HER2.

MEDULLARY CARCINOMA (FIG. 27.32)

Previously a special subtype with a favourable prognosis, it is now classified as T-cell–rich IDC. It is common in BRCA1 mutation carriers around 50 years of age; it shows

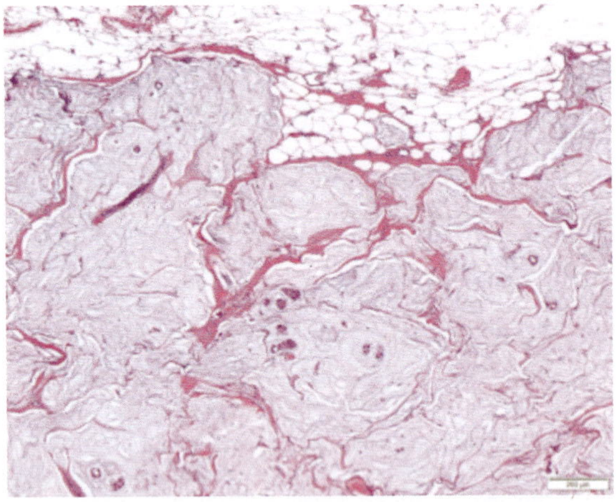

Fig. 27.31 Mucinous carcinoma of the breast – microscopy. Clusters of well-differentiated tumour cells are seen floating in a sea of mucin. (*Source:* From Laura C. Collins. Breast. Rosai and Ackerman's Surgical Pathology. 11th edition. Elsevier 2018.)

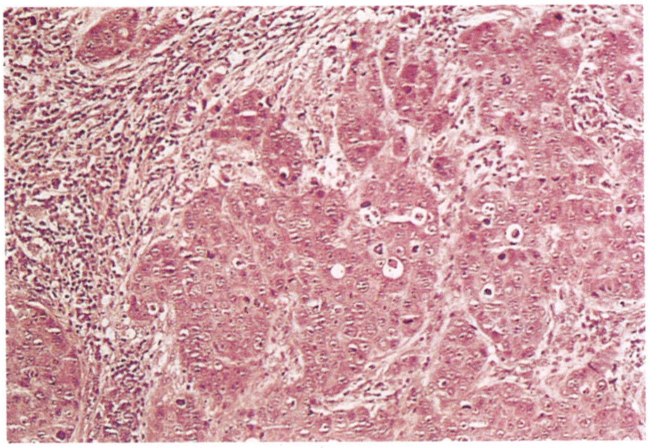

Fig. 27.32 Medullary carcinoma of the breast – microscopy. Large groups of irregularly shaped tumour cells are surrounded by an infiltrate of lymphocytes. (*Source:* From J. Louise Jones. Breast. Underwood's Pathology. 7th edition. Elsevier 2019.)

poorly differentiated cells, diffuse lymphoplasmacytic infiltrate, and frequent 'triple-negative' status (negative for ER, PR, and HER2).

INVASIVE PAPILLARY CARCINOMA

It is a very rare subtype with a better prognosis than classical IDC, affecting mostly postmenopausal women and accounting for less than 2% of invasive breast cancers. It is characterized by papillary structures with malignant cells and a delicate fibrovascular core.

INVASIVE MICROPAPILLARY CARCINOMA (FIG. 27.33)

It represents only 2% of invasive breast cancers, with a poor prognosis because of high incidence of recurrence and lymph node metastasis. It features small epithelial clusters in pseudopapillary structures within clear stromal spaces.

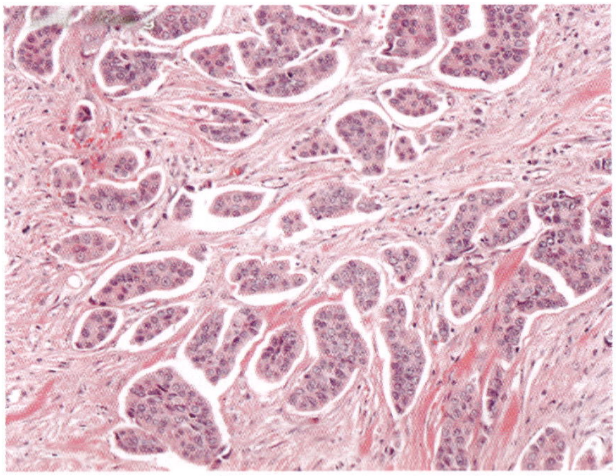

Fig. 27.33 Invasive micropapillary carcinoma of the breast – microscopy. Micropapillary clusters surrounded by lacunar spaces infiltrating through the desmoplastic stroma. (*Source:* https://www.webpathology.com/image.asp?case=293&n=17)

APOCRINE CARCINOMA

It is a rare variant, comprising 1%–4% of breast cancers, with prominent apocrine differentiation. It is characterized by large cells with acidophilic, granular cytoplasm, and often high grade with poor prognosis.

NEUROENDOCRINE TUMOUR

Accounting for approximately 2% of breast carcinomas, these rare tumours resemble neuroendocrine cells and express neuroendocrine markers, common in postmenopausal women.

SECRETORY CARCINOMA

It mimics lactating breast, typically 'triple-negative' but with a good prognosis and rare metastasis.

METAPLASTIC CARCINOMA

It is an aggressive subtype constituting less than 1% of breast cancers, characterized by metaplastic differentiation of various cell types. It affects mainly postmenopausal women around the age of 55 years.

INFLAMMATORY CARCINOMA (FIG. 27.34)

It presents as breast erythema and swelling, often mistaken for an inflammatory lesion. It is IDC with dermal lymphatic invasion and has a poor prognosis.

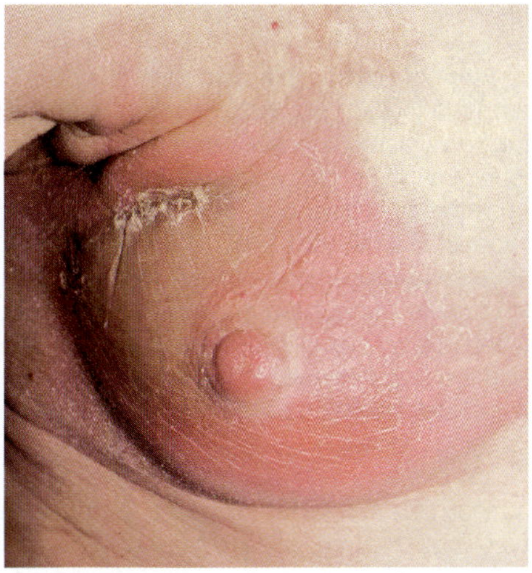

Fig. 27.34 Inflammatory breast carcinoma – cellulitic appearing plaque.

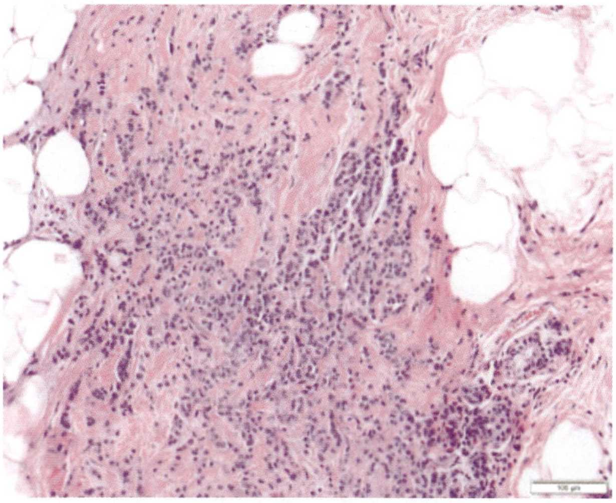

Fig. 27.35 Lobular carcinoma – microscopy, low power. (*Source:* From Laura C. Collins. Breast. Rosai and Ackerman's Surgical Pathology. 11th edition. Elsevier 2018.)

INVASIVE LOBULAR CARCINOMA

It makes up 5%–15% of invasive breast cancers, usually affecting older women. It is characterized by noncohesive, small, round cells with a single-file infiltration pattern. Various histological variants include solid, pleomorphic, tubulolobular, alveolar and mixed types (Figs 27.35 and 27.36).

Each variant has distinct microscopic features and prognostic implications, emphasizing the importance of accurate diagnosis and tailored treatment approaches.

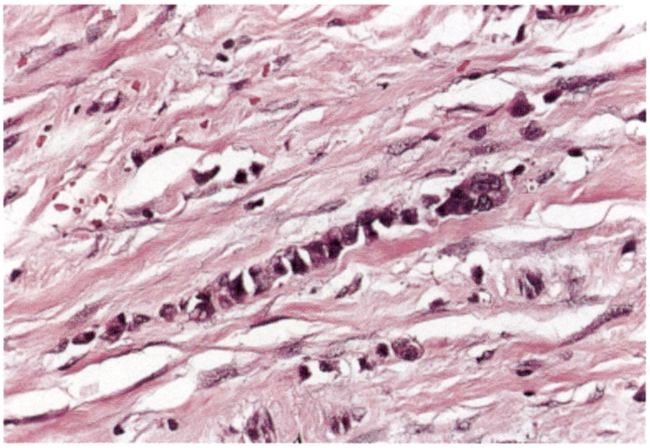

Fig. 27.36 Lobular carcinoma – microscopy, high power. (*Source:* From Laura C. Collins. Breast. Rosai and Ackerman's Surgical Pathology. 11th edition. Elsevier 2018.)

SELF-ASSESSMENT

Multiple Choice Questions

1. A 25-year-old woman presents with a mobile, painless breast lump. Ultrasound suggests a well-circumscribed mass. Which of the following is the most likely diagnosis?
   A. Invasive ductal carcinoma
   B. Fibroadenoma
   C. Phyllodes tumour
   D. Inflammatory breast cancer
2. A 45-year-old patient presents with a rapidly growing breast lump. Biopsy reveals stromal overgrowth. Which of the following is the most likely diagnosis?
   A. Invasive lobular carcinoma
   B. Fibroadenoma
   C. Phyllodes tumour
   D. Invasive ductal carcinoma
3. A patient with a breast mass undergoes a biopsy. The pathology report indicates high levels of ER and PR receptors. This finding is most indicative of:
   A. Triple-negative breast cancer
   B. HER2-enriched breast cancer
   C. Hormone receptor–positive breast cancer
   D. Inflammatory breast cancer
4. In a patient with breast cancer, overexpression of HER2/neu protein is most likely associated with:
   A. Improved prognosis
   B. High grade and aggressiveness
   C. Better response to hormonal therapy
   D. Lower risk of recurrence
5. A 55-year-old woman presents with nipple retraction and Peau d'orange. These clinical features are suggestive of:
   A. Fibrocystic changes
   B. Invasive ductal carcinoma
   C. Ductal carcinoma in situ (DCIS)
   D. Fibroadenoma
6. In a case of nonspecial type (NST) breast cancer, which immunohistochemical marker is typically assessed?
   A. CD10
   B. CK5/6
   C. ER/PR
   D. S100

7. A 40-year-old woman undergoes mammography, revealing a 'spiculated' mass. This finding is most indicative of:
   A. Benign breast lesion
   B. Inflammatory breast cancer
   C. Malignant breast lesion
   D. Fibrocystic changes
8. A breast cancer patient shows lymph node involvement without distant metastasis. According to the TNM staging system, this would be at least stage:
   A. Stage I
   B. Stage IIA
   C. Stage IIB
   D. Stage IIIA
9. A patient's breast tumour biopsy reveals spindle-shaped cells in a leaf-like pattern. Which of the following is the most likely diagnosis?
   A. Fibroadenoma
   B. Phyllodes tumour
   C. Invasive ductal carcinoma
   D. Invasive lobular carcinoma
10. During breast cancer surgery, a 'sentinel lymph node' is identified. The purpose of examining this lymph node is to:
   A. Assess the need for chemotherapy
   B. Determine the extent of breast tissue to remove
   C. Evaluate the spread of cancer
   D. Identify the type of breast cancer
11. A breast cancer patient has a BRCA1 mutation. This mutation most significantly increases the risk for:
   A. HER2-enriched breast cancer
   B. Triple-negative breast cancer
   C. Hormone receptor–positive breast cancer
   D. Phyllodes tumour
12. A mammogram of a 50-year-old woman reveals microcalcifications in a ductal pattern. Which of the following is the most likely diagnosis?
   A. Ductal carcinoma in situ (DCIS)
   B. Invasive ductal carcinoma
   C. Fibroadenoma
   D. Invasive lobular carcinoma
13. In the management of breast cancer, neoadjuvant therapy is primarily used to:
   A. Eradicate distant metastases
   B. Reduce the size of the tumour before surgery
   C. Prevent recurrence after surgery
   D. Treat hormone receptor–positive tumours only
14. A breast lump that fluctuates in size with the menstrual cycle is most characteristic of:
   A. Inflammatory breast cancer
   B. Fibroadenoma
   C. Fibrocystic changes
   D. Invasive ductal carcinoma
15. The presence of orange peel skin and nipple retraction in a patient with breast cancer is most suggestive of:
   A. Early-stage breast cancer
   B. Advanced local disease
   C. Metastatic disease
   D. Benign breast disease

Answers

1. (B); 2. (C); 3. (C); 4. (B); 5. (B); 6. (C); 7. (C); 8. (D); 9. (B); 10. (C); 11. (B); 12. (A); 13. (B); 14. (C); 15. (B)

Scenario-Based Questions

1. A 29-year-old woman presents with a mobile, painless breast lump that she noticed a few months ago. The lump seems to vary slightly in size with her menstrual cycle. Ultrasound imaging shows a well-circumscribed, solid mass. Discuss the likely diagnosis, the differential diagnoses to consider in this patient.
2. A 52-year-old woman undergoes a routine mammogram, which reveals a spiculated mass in the left breast. A subsequent biopsy reveals invasive carcinoma.
   Outline the steps involved in further evaluating this patient, including additional imaging, laboratory tests and the staging process.
3. A patient presents with a large, rapidly growing mass in the breast. Biopsy findings suggest a stromal tumour with areas of cellular atypia and increased mitotic activity.
   Describe the key features and diagnostic criteria of the suspected tumour.
4. A breast cancer patient's pathology report indicates that the tumour is ER-positive and PR-positive.
   Explain the implications of these findings for the patient's treatment plan and prognosis. Discuss the role of hormonal therapy in managing this type of breast cancer.
5. A patient diagnosed with breast cancer is found to have HER2/neu overexpression.
   Discuss the significance of HER2/neu overexpression in breast cancer, including its impact on prognosis. Describe the targeted treatment options available for this type of breast cancer and their mechanisms of action.
6. During a breast cancer surgery, the surgeon identifies and biopsies the sentinel lymph node. The pathology report shows micrometastases.
   Explain the significance of finding micrometastases in the sentinel lymph node in the context of breast cancer treatment and prognosis.
7. A patient undergoing breast cancer screening is found to have clustered microcalcifications on mammogram, which are highly suggestive of malignancy.
   Describe the next steps in the diagnostic process following this radiological finding.
8. A breast cancer patient's biopsy report indicates triple-negative status (ER^-, PR^-, $HER2^-$).
   Discuss the implications of a triple-negative breast cancer diagnosis for treatment and prognosis.
9. A 17-year-old male patient presented with painless diffuse enlargement of both breasts for the past 6 months. What is your diagnosis and how would you approach the case?
10. List the proliferative breast diseases with atypia and describe them.

Topics for Self-Directed Learning

1. Pseudoangiomatous stromal hyperplasia (PASH)
2. FNAC findings in breast lesions
3. Complications of silicone implants in the breast
4. Malignant stromal tumours of the breast
5. Role of frozen section in breast tumours
6. ER, PR, HER2 status assessment in breast cancer
7. Angiosarcoma of breast
8. Postneoadjuvant chemotherapy breast carcinoma, grossing guidelines
9. Postmastectomy lymphangiosarcoma

The Endocrine System

28

Rajeswari Kathiah

PA 32.1 Enumerate, classify and describe the aetiology, pathogenesis, pathology and **iodine dependency of thyroid swellings**.

PA 32.2 Describe the aetiology, cause, iodine dependency, pathogenesis, manifestations, laboratory and imaging features and course of **thyrotoxicosis**.

PA 32.3 Describe the aetiology, pathogenesis, manifestations, laboratory and imaging features and course of **thyrotoxicosis/hypothyroidism**.

PA 32.4 Classify and describe the epidemiology, aetiology, pathogenesis, pathology, clinical and laboratory features, complications and progression of **diabetes mellitus**.

PA 32.5 Describe the aetiology, genetics, pathogenesis, manifestations and laboratory and morphological features of **hyperparathyroidism**.

PA 32.7 Describe the aetiology, pathogenesis, manifestations, laboratory and morphological features and complications of **adrenal insufficiency**.

PA 32.8 Describe the aetiology, pathogenesis, manifestations, laboratory and morphological features and complications of **Cushing syndrome**.

PA 32.9 Describe the aetiology, pathogenesis, manifestations and laboratory and morphological features of **adrenal neoplasms**.

CHAPTER OUTLINE

INTRODUCTION

The endocrine system is a system of ductless internal glands that secrete hormones directly into the blood to act on distant target organs. The function of these glands is controlled by negative feedback from the hormones secreted by them. The major endocrine glands are the thyroid gland and the adrenal glands apart from the other endocrine glands like pituitary, parathyroid, endocrine pancreas, pineal gland, and the gonads. The hypothalamus is the neural control centre for all endocrine systems. The study of the endocrine system and its disorders is known as endocrinology and is an extensive subject. Diseases of some glands are much more prevalent in the population than others and hence, in this chapter, we describe the common diseases of the following glands:

- **Disorders of the thyroid**
- **Disorders of the parathyroid**

- **Disorders of the endocrine pancreas**
- **Disorders of the adrenal gland**

Disorders of the gonads are discussed under the respective chapters.

I. THE THYROID GLAND

ANATOMY, HISTOLOGY AND PHYSIOLOGY PA 32.1

Anatomy

The thyroid gland is the first among the body's endocrine glands to develop as early as the 24th day of gestation. It originates from two main structures: the primitive pharynx and the neural crest. The rudimentary lateral thyroid develops from the neural crest cells, and the median thyroid that forms the bulk of the gland arises from the primitive pharynx.

Initially, it develops as a diverticular outgrowth from the primitive pharynx which is composed of endoderm. It then descends inferiorly to reach its destination in the neck. During its descent, the thyroid connects to the tongue by the thyroglossal duct, which later atrophies and closes off as the foramen caecum before birth. The thyroid is a small endocrine gland with significant effects on the body. It secretes thyroxine and calcitonin which have target effects on multiple organs.

Histology

Microscopically, the thyroid gland is composed of spherical follicles which are the functional units of the gland, lined by follicular epithelial cells that surround a lumen containing colloid (Fig. 28.1). Interspersed between these thyroid follicles or within the wall of the follicles are cells derived from the neural crest called parafollicular C cells. These cells are responsible for secretion of calcitonin.

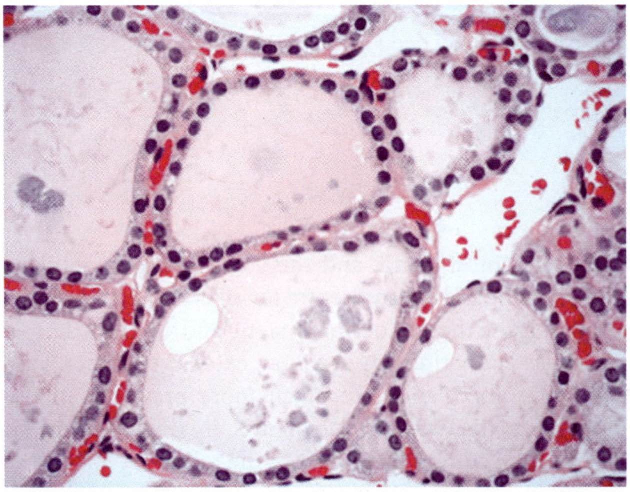

Fig. 28.1 Histology of the thyroid gland containing colloid-filled follicles. (*Source:* From Thyroid Cancer. Elsevier Point of Care. 2022.)

Physiology

The thyroid gland secretes an important hormone called thyroxine, which is regulated by thyroid-stimulating hormone (TSH). TSH is secreted by the pituitary gland, and the whole process is regulated by a negative feedback mechanism. The follicles of the thyroid gland contain colloid composed of thyroxine and several enzymes, importantly thyroid peroxidase, and deiodinase. Iodine is the main nutrient that is needed for synthesis of thyroid hormones. The hormones secreted include triiodothyronine (T_3) and thyroxine (T_4), the former being 10 times more active than the later.

Ingested iodine is transported in the form of iodide and is actively absorbed by the thyroid follicular cells through the transporters present on the cell membrane. Within the follicular cells, iodide is concentrated, oxidized by enzymes such as peroxidase and incorporated into thyroglobulin to form monoiodotyrosine (MIT) and diiodotyrosine (DIT) and later T_3 and T_4. When required, T_3 and T_4 are released into circulation by proteolysis of thyroglobulin and the hormones travel to the target organs bound to specific binding proteins.

The primary functions of the thyroid hormone include the following:

- Maintenance of basal metabolic rate (BMR)
- Heart rate, central nervous system (CNS) activation, gut motility, etc.

Improper levels of secretion of these hormones cause manifestations of several diseases, which can be categorized into the following:

1. **Hypothyroidism**
2. **Hyperthyroidism**
3. **Neoplasms of the thyroid**

The common diseases associated with the categories are discussed in the following sections.

HYPOTHYROIDISM PA 32.3

Hypothyroidism, also called the underactive thyroid or low thyroid, is a disorder caused by functional and structural derangements that interfere with thyroid hormone production. Although it was believed that iodine deficiency is the chief cause of hypothyroidism, population-based studies on the western population have revealed that even with adequate dietary iodine, approximately 0.3%–0.4% of the population had overt hypothyroidism and approximately 4.3%–8.5% had subclinical hypothyroidism. The incidence is much higher in underdeveloped countries. Children with subclinical hypothyroidism often return to normal thyroid function, whereas a small fraction of them develop overt hypothyroidism. Women are more likely to develop hypothyroidism than men. There is a much higher incidence of thyroid diseases, especially hypothyroidism, in persons with Down syndrome and Turner syndrome.

Table 28.1 List of Causes of Hypothyroidism

Mechanism	Causes
Primary Causes	
Iodine deficiency[a]	Dietary deficiency
Autoimmune[a]	Hashimoto thyroiditis
Drugs	Lithium, iodides, etc.
Iatrogenic	Surgery, radioiodine therapy and external irradiation
Congenital	Defects in thyroid development Thyroid hormone resistance syndrome Congenital biosynthetic defect
Secondary Causes	
Pituitary failure	Pituitary tumours Postpartum pituitary necrosis Trauma to pituitary gland
Hypothalamic failure	Trauma to hypothalamus Radiation therapy
Peripheral Causes	
Consumptive hypothyroidism	Increased expression of type 3 deiodinase enzyme by tumour cells
Resistance to thyroid hormone	Tissue-specific hypothyroidism due to decreased sensitivity to thyroid hormone

[a]Most common causes.

Causes of Hypothyroidism

Worldwide, iodine deficiency is the most common cause of hypothyroidism, whereas Hashimoto thyroiditis is the most common cause of hypothyroidism in countries with adequate dietary iodine. The causes of hypothyroidism are broadly divided into two forms, ***primary, central or secondary, and peripheral*** depending on whether the aetiological factor is the thyroid itself or from the higher centres like pituitary and hypothalamus or peripheral tissues (Table 28.1).

All these causes are grouped under three categories – **congenital, iatrogenic and autoimmune** – and are discussed in the subsequent sections.

Manifestations of Hypothyroidism

Individuals with hypothyroidism most often have no symptoms or only minimal symptoms. Numerous signs and symptoms are associated with hypothyroidism, and the common ones are listed in Table 28.2.

Cretinism and myxoedema, two manifestations of severe hypothyroidism, are discussed here.

Cretinism **Cretinism** refers to hypothyroidism that develops in infancy or early childhood and is common in areas with endemic dietary deficiency of iodine. Such conditions are referred to as **endemic cretinism.**

Sporadic cretinism may develop as a result of enzyme defects that interfere with thyroid hormone synthesis.

Clinical features of cretinism (Fig. 28.2)

These include impaired development of the skeletal system and CNS, mental retardation, short stature, coarse facial features, and umbilical hernia, apart from other common signs and symptoms of hypothyroidism.

Myxoedema (Fig. 28.3) **Myxoedema** refers to hypothyroidism in older children and adults, and the term is used synonymously with severe hypothyroidism. However, the term should not be confused with the dermatological change that can occur in Graves disease discussed later.

Clinical Manifestations of Myxoedema Patients present with the usual symptoms of hypothyroidism listed in Table 28.2. In addition, these patients experience slowing down of physical and mental activities along with apathetic intellectual functions. Cardiac output is decreased, and lipid profile is altered with raised low-density lipoprotein (LDL) and cholesterol levels, predisposing to ischaemic changes in the heart. There is also deposition of glycosaminoglycans and hyaluronic acid in various

Table 28.2 Common Signs, Symptoms and Laboratory Investigations of Hypothyroidism

Symptoms	Signs	Laboratory Findings
• Fatigue • Feeling cold • Poor memory and concentration • Constipation • Loss of appetite and weight gain • Breathlessness • Hoarseness of voice • Heavy menstrual bleeding in the beginning, followed by light periods • Poor hearing	• Dry, coarse skin • Cool extremities • Myxoedema • Loss of hair • Bradycardia • Oedema of the limbs • Delayed relaxation of tendon reflexes • Carpal tunnel syndrome • Serous effusions	• TSH elevated • T_4 reduced • Creatinine kinase elevated • Liver enzymes elevated • Cholesterol elevated • Lipoproteins elevated • Antithyroid antibodies positive in autoimmune thyroiditis **Other Tests** Fine-needle aspiration cytology Ultrasonogram Radioactive iodine uptake

T_4, thyroxine; TSH, thyroid-stimulating hormone.

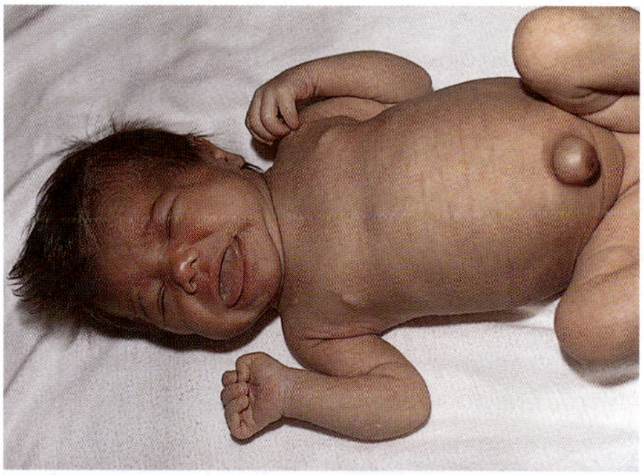

Fig. 28.2 A child with cretinism. Note the coarse facial features, broad nasal bridge, thick lips and umbilical hernia.

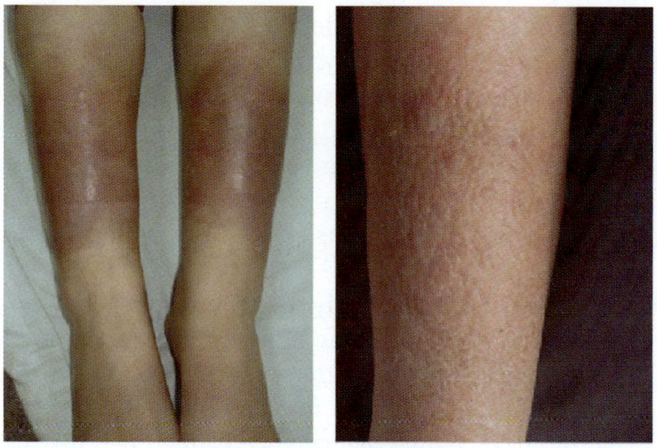

Fig. 28.3 Clinical picture of pretibial myxoedema. (*Source:* https://www.google.com/url?sa=i&url=https%3A%2F%2Fhealthjade.net%2Fpretibial-myxedema%2F&psig=AOvVaw36SXchSSa6lt8wkVqHkJUc&ust=1605694766449000&source=images&cd=vfe&ved=0CAIQjRxqFwoTCLiAkaWtie0CFQAAAAAdAAAAABAD)

tissues, leading to skin changes and voice change (Fig. 28.4). It may also cause broadening and coarsening of facial features and enlargement of the tongue.

Myxoedema coma is a rare state of extreme hypothyroidism. In some cases, it may be the first manifestation of hypothyroidism. Patients with myxoedema coma present with loss of consciousness or confused state of mind, low body temperature without shivering, bradycardia, and reduced breathing effort, apart from other physical findings of hypothyroidism.

Congenital Hypothyroidism

Congenital hypothyroidism is defined as inadequate thyroid hormone production in newborn infants. It can occur because of iodine deficiency, anatomic defect in the gland or inborn error of thyroid metabolism. Congenital hypothyroidism is the most common neonatal endocrine disease, and historically thyroid dysgenesis was thought to be responsible for almost 80% cases. However, recent studies indicate a doubling in the incidence of congenital hypothyroidism in neonates with a normal thyroid which is attributed to lower TSH screening cutoffs, altered ethnicity, and increased multiple and premature births. **Endemic iodine deficiency** is the most common cause associated with congenital hypothyroidism. This is followed by inborn errors of thyroid metabolism, due to blockade of the essential steps in thyroid hormone synthesis. Some neonates diagnosed with primary congenital hypothyroidism may have transient disease and do not develop a permanent state of hypothyroidism.

Iatrogenic Hypothyroidism

Iatrogenic damage to the thyroid gland such as surgical removal of the thyroid gland in toto (total thyroidectomy),

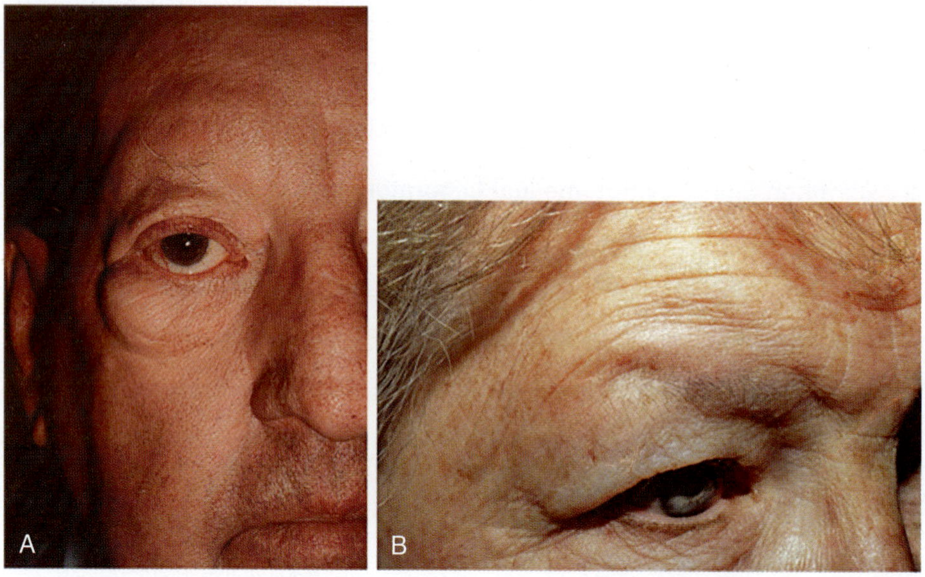

Fig. 28.4 Clinical picture of (A) periorbital infiltration with mucopolysaccharides. (B) Loss of lateral eyebrow in myxoedema. (*Source:* From William D. James, Dirk M. Elston, James R. Treat, Misha A. Rosenbach and Isaac M. Neuhaus. Endocrine Diseases. Andrews' Diseases of the Skin. 13th edition. Elsevier 2020.)

external radiation therapy to the neck and administration of antithyroid drugs can also precipitate hypothyroidism.

Autoimmune Hypothyroidism

As stated earlier, this category is the most common cause of hypothyroidism in iodine sufficient parts of the world. Most of the cases are due to Hashimoto thyroiditis, and the other causes include subacute lymphocytic thyroiditis and granulomatous thyroiditis. Autoimmune destruction of the thyroid gland mediated by autoantibodies and T cells is responsible for the hypothyroid state in patients with these disorders. Autoimmune thyroiditis can be a solitary disease or can occur as a part of autoimmune polyendocrine syndromes.

Clinically, significant causes of autoimmune thyroiditis are as follows:

- **Hashimoto thyroiditis**
- **Subacute lymphocytic thyroiditis**
- **Subacute granulomatous thyroiditis**

Hashimoto Thyroiditis Hashimoto thyroiditis, also known as **chronic lymphocytic thyroiditis** and **Hashimoto disease**, is an autoimmune disease caused by breakdown of self-tolerance to thyroid autoantigens leading to the destruction of thyroid parenchyma by autoantibodies and T cells. This leads to progressive decline in thyroid function and clinical hypothyroidism. The disease is named after the Japanese physician Hakaru Hashimoto, who first described symptoms in persons with *struma lymphomatosa*, an intense infiltration of lymphocytes within the thyroid, in 1912 in a German journal.

Pathogenesis *(Fig. 28.5)* Hashimoto thyroiditis is thought to be due to a combination of genetic and environmental factors. Concordance of disease is seen in 40% monozygotic twins. A variety of circulating autoantibodies are present against thyroid peroxidase, thyroglobulin and TSH receptors, though a minor fraction of people may have no autoantibodies. At the same time, a small percentage of population may also have these autoantibodies without developing Hashimoto thyroiditis.

Hashimoto thyroiditis is associated with polymorphisms in genes regulating T-cell regulation such as *cytotoxic T-lymphocyte–associated antigen-4*, **CTLA4** gene, and *protein tyrosine phosphatase-22*, **PTPN22**. These genes are also associated with the susceptibility to other autoimmune diseases like type 1 diabetes mellitus (T1DM).

As with other diseases due to type 4 hypersensitivity, helper T cells play the key role by activating macrophages, inducing antibodies, and promoting release of cytokines. Self-reactive cytotoxic T cells also contribute by causing destruction of thyrocytes.

All the mediators of autoimmunity, helper T cells, cytotoxic T cells, macrophages, natural killer cells, along with their cytokines, act in coordination to cause destruction of the thyroid follicular epithelial cells.

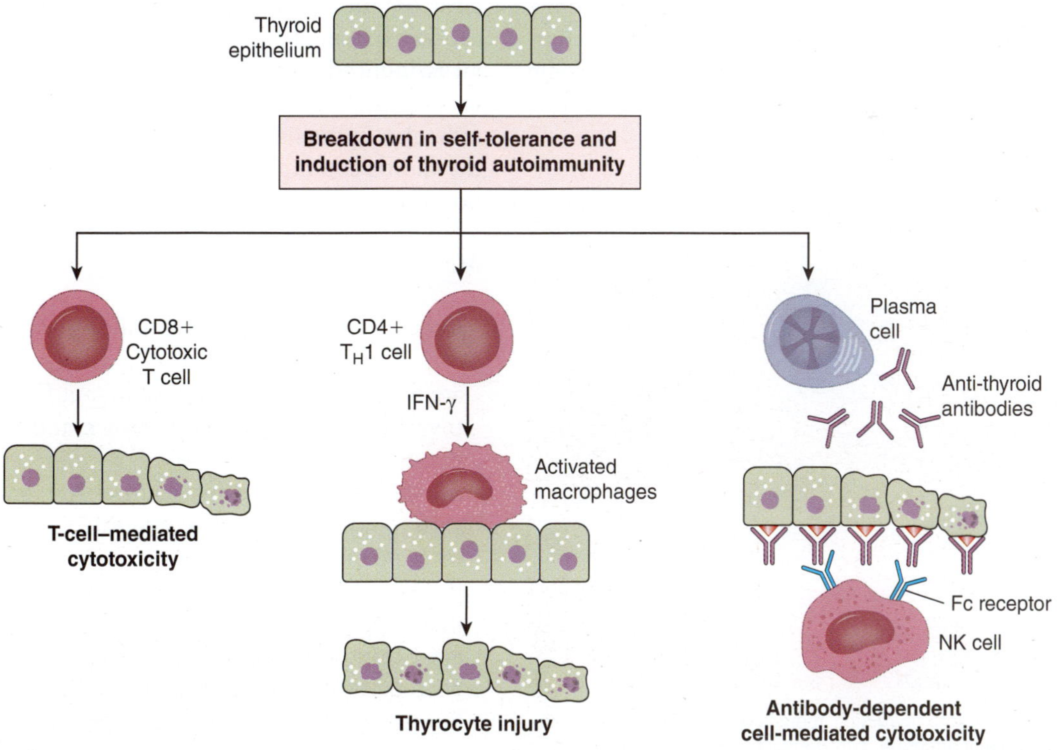

Fig. 28.5 Pathogenesis of Hashimoto thyroiditis. Breakdown of immune tolerance to thyroid autoantigens results in progressive autoimmune destruction of thyrocytes by infiltrating cytotoxic T cells, locally released cytokines or antibody-dependent cytotoxicity. (*Source:* From Vinay Kumar, Abul K. Abbas and Jon C. Aster. Endocrine System. Robbins Basic Pathology. 10th edition. Elsevier 2018.)

Morphology

Gross There is a diffuse and symmetric enlargement of the thyroid gland which is firm and nodular. Thyroid capsule is intact and is well demarcated from surrounding structures. Its cut surface is pale and grey with accentuation of normal lobulation.

Microscopy Prominent feature is the dense infiltration by inflammatory infiltrate consisting of lymphocytes forming lymphoid follicles, and plasma cells, causing destruction of thyroid follicles. There is atrophy of thyroid follicles, with Hürthle cell metaplasia (Fig. 28.6), which is a metaplastic response. The atrophy may be due to interstitial connective tissue, fibrosis.

Hürthle cells are thyroid follicular epithelial cells with abundant eosinophilic, granular cytoplasm. Ultrastructurally, these cells show prominent mitochondria.

Clinical Features Painless enlargement of the thyroid is the usual presentation. The enlargement of the thyroid is mostly symmetric and diffuse, but in some cases, it may present as a nodular lesion mimicking neoplasm. Clinically, patients present with symptoms of hypothyroidism, but in some cases, hypothyroid symptoms are preceded by a phase of thyrotoxicosis termed **hashitoxicosis** caused by the release of thyroxine hormones from the disrupted thyroid follicles. This phase is transient and is soon followed by the progressive hypothyroid state.

Course and Prognosis Patients with Hashimoto thyroiditis is at a high risk for developing other autoimmune disorders. Apart from this, they are also at risk of developing extranodal marginal zone B-cell lymphoma. Some studies suggest that patients with Hashimoto thyroiditis are also at risk of papillary thyroid carcinoma (PTC), hence warranting long-term follow-up.

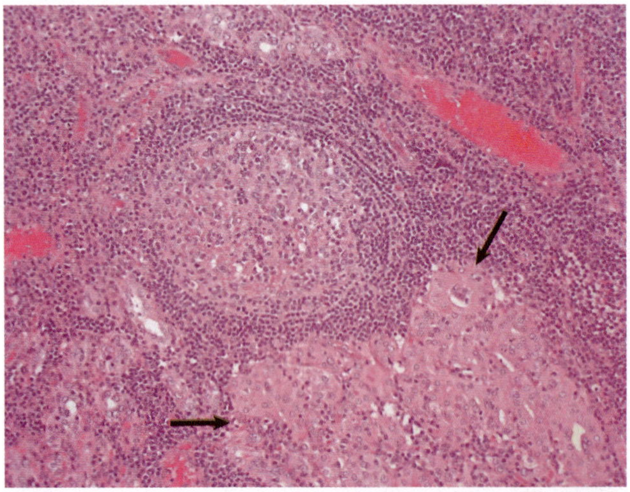

Fig. 28.6 In Hashimoto thyroiditis, there is destruction of follicles by a dense lymphocytic infiltrate with germinal centre formation. Some of the surviving epithelial cells show Hürthle cell change (arrowed). (*Source:* From Timothy J. Stephenson. Endocrine system. Underwood's Pathology. 7th edition. Elsevier 2019.)

Subacute Lymphocytic Thyroiditis Subacute lymphocytic thyroiditis, also referred to as painless thyroiditis, is a form of autoimmune thyroiditis. A variant of subacute lymphocytic thyroiditis that occurs in postpartum females is called **postpartum thyroiditis**. Both entities can be considered as subtypes of Hashimoto thyroiditis and have an autoimmune basis. Antithyroid antibodies are seen as in Hashimoto thyroiditis and the clinical manifestation is also like that of Hashimoto thyroiditis. Microscopic features are also comparable to Hashimoto thyroiditis except for the absence of Hürthle cell metaplastic change and fibrosis.

Subacute Granulomatous Thyroiditis Subacute granulomatous thyroiditis, also referred to as '**de Quervain thyroiditis**', is a self-limited thyroid disorder associated with a triphasic clinical course of hyperthyroidism, hypothyroidism and return to normal euthyroid function.

This is the most common cause of the painful thyroid gland and is also known as '**painful subacute thyroiditis**' and '**migratory thyroiditis**' because of the shifting nature of the pain.

Pathogenesis The most accepted aetiological factor for this entity is a viral illness because episodes often follow upper respiratory tract infections caused by viruses like influenza, adenovirus, mumps and coxsackievirus. The exact pathogenetic mechanism of the disease is still unclear, but the accepted model states that the viral infection causes exposure to a viral or thyroid antigen secondary to virus-induced host tissue damage. This triggers the activity of cytotoxic T lymphocytes that damage the thyroid follicular epithelial cells. Unlike in other autoimmune thyroiditis conditions, the disease is self-limited and does not propagate.

Morphology

Gross The thyroid gland is moderately enlarged and oedematous in de Quervain thyroiditis. Affected areas are firm, yellow–white and stand out from the normal thyroid substance, which is brown and has a rubbery consistency.

Microscopy Microscopic features are patchy. In the early phase, the gland is infiltrated with neutrophils forming **microabscesses**, disrupting the follicles. In the later phase, there is a collection of lymphocytes, macrophages, and plasma cells along with the damaged thyroid follicles. Prominent feature is the presence of **multinucleated giant cells**. At a later stage, fibrosis replaces the foci of inflammatory infiltrate.

Clinical Features Patients present with thyroid pain and symptoms of hyperthyroidism in the beginning, followed by hypothyroid symptoms. The disease is self-limiting, with spontaneous recovery within weeks to months.

HYPERTHYROIDISM

PA 32.2

Hyperthyroidism is characterized by increased hormone synthesis and secretion from the thyroid gland, whereas the term 'thyrotoxicosis' refers to the clinical syndrome of excess circulating thyroid hormones, irrespective of the source. Hyperthyroidism can be due to primary or secondary causes. Primary causes include causes originating from the thyroid, whereas secondary causes include causes originating outside the thyroid, such as TSH-secreting tumours of the pituitary.

Causes of Hyperthyroidism

- Graves disease
- Toxic nodular goitre
- Hyperfunctional thyroid adenoma
- Thyroiditis
- Drug-induced thyroid dysfunction
- Ingestion of excess thyroid hormones as drugs
- TSH-secreting pituitary adenoma

Clinical Course (Table 28.3)

The clinical features of hyperthyroidism are variable and are mainly due to hypermetabolic state induced by excess thyroid hormones and sympathetic overactivity of the nervous system.

Cardiac manifestations are among the earliest and most consistent features of thyrotoxicosis and hence described here. Because of increased peripheral oxygen requirement, cardiac contractility and cardiac output are elevated. Tachycardia and palpitations are common. Cardiomegaly and arrhythmias, especially atrial fibrillation, are common in elderly individuals. Cardiomegaly is a regular finding, and patients may develop congestive cardiac failure. Some patients develop reversible left ventricular dysfunction and low-output heart failure, referred to as '**thyrotoxic or hyperthyroid cardiomyopathy**'.

Microscopic examination of the myocardium reveals focal lymphocytic and eosinophilic infiltration, minimal fibrosis and myofibril fatty changes.

Dermopathy and ophthalmopathy are special features of Graves disease and hence are discussed there.

Table 28.3 Manifestations of Hyperthyroidism

System	Symptoms	Signs
Constitutional	Weight loss Increased appetite Heat intolerance Polydipsia	Weight loss
Cardiovascular	Palpitations	Tachycardia Systolic hypertension Atrial fibrillation
Neuromuscular	Tremor Nervousness Anxiety Fatigue Weakness Sleep disturbances Poor concentration Poor memory	Tremor of the extremities Hyperactivity Hyperreflexia Weakness of pelvic girdle muscles
Gastrointestinal	Hyperdefaecation Nausea Vomiting	Abdominal tenderness
Pulmonary	Dyspnoea	Tachypnoea
Skin	Increased sweating	Warm and moist skin
Reproductive	Menstrual disturbances	
Ocular	Retro-orbital pain Diplopia Irritation	Periorbital oedema Proptosis Ophthalmoplegia
Others		Thyroid acropachy

Management

Laboratory Investigations The most useful screening test for hyperthyroidism is the measurement of **serum TSH levels**, as it is the most sensitive marker, which is decreased in the early phase and even in subclinical phases of the disease. **A combination of low TSH and elevated free T_4** levels confirms the diagnosis of hyperthyroidism.

In some patients, hyperthyroidism is the result of elevated T_3 levels, in which case, T_4 levels may be decreased. In such cases, measurement of serum T_3 is useful. In rare cases of secondary hyperthyroidism caused by lesions in the pituitary, TSH levels are either normal or elevated. In these cases, TSH levels may be checked after TSH stimulation, in which if the normal rise of TSH level is noted, extrinsic or secondary causes of hyperthyroidism can be excluded.

Although measurement of serum TSH levels and free thyroid hormone levels help to confirm hyperthyroidism, radioactive iodine uptake studies of the thyroid gland help in establishing the cause of the hyperthyroidism.

Treatment

Thyrotoxicosis is treated medically by using a combination of drugs: β-blockers to counteract the increased adrenergic tone, thionamide to block the synthesis of new hormones, iodine solution to block the release of thyroid hormones and drugs to inhibit peripheral conversion of T_4 to T_3. Ablation of thyroid function by incorporating radioiodine into the thyroid tissue is also useful in some patients.

Graves disease, the most common cause of thyrotoxicosis, is discussed in detail here.

GRAVES DISEASE

The disease is named after Robert J. Graves, MD, who first described it in a patient in 1835. He described the disorder as 'the disease characterized by violent and long continued palpitations in females'. The disease is also referred to as **Basedow disease**, named after a German physician, Karl Adolph Von Basedow, who described the disease in 1840 without knowing that Graves had described the same disease just a few years ago.

Graves disease, also known as **diffuse toxic goitre**, is an autoimmune disease that affects the thyroid and is also the most common cause of hyperthyroidism. Graves disease is 10 times more common in women than in men and is commonly seen in middle-aged women.

Genetics The exact cause is unclear, and a combination of genetic and environmental factors is implicated. Concordance of disease in seen in monozygotic twins (40%). Genetic susceptibility for Hashimoto and Graves disease is associated with polymorphisms in genes involved in T-cell regulation such as **CTLA4** and **PTPN22**.

It is associated with HLA class II molecule **HLA-DR** (***HLA-DRB1*08*** and ***DRB3*0202).***

Pathogenesis Graves disease is an autoimmune disease characterized by hyperthyroidism due to circulating autoantibodies against many thyroid antigens, most notably against thyrotropin (TSH) receptor. The antibody binds and activates the receptor, leading to increased thyroid hormone synthesis, secretion and growth of the thyroid gland. The most common antibody subtype is called **thyroid-stimulating immunoglobulin (TSI)**. In a minority of patients, TSH receptor blocking antibodies are seen, in whom the presentation is same as that in hypothyroidism. Antibodies to thyroid peroxidase and thyroglobulin are also seen.

Graves disease is characterized by **infiltrative ophthalmopathy**, in which protrusion of eyeballs is a striking feature (Fig. 28.7). Autoimmunity plays a key role in causing ophthalmopathy, and the mechanisms underlying this **exophthalmos** are as follows:

- Mononuclear inflammatory infiltrate in the retro-orbital space
- Oedema of the extraocular muscles
- Deposition of extracellular matrix such as hyaluronic acid and chondroitin
- Increase in the number of adipocytes

The other unique features include pretibial **myxoedema**, which is an infiltrative dermopathy, commonly affecting the skin overlying the tibia, and **acropachy**, which is swelling of extremities with clubbing of fingers and toes due to periosteal new bone formation.

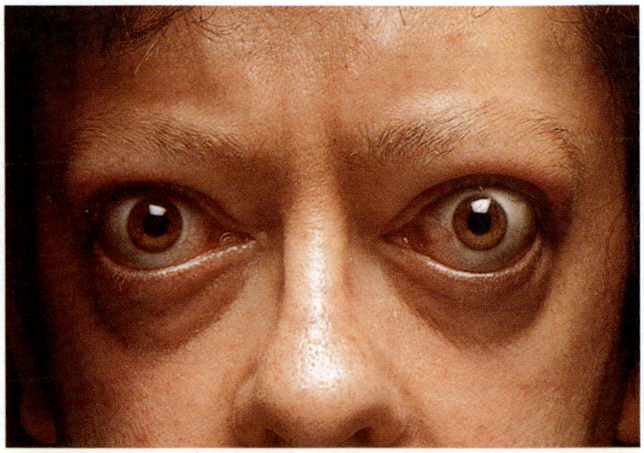

Fig. 28.7 Clinical picture of Graves disease with the classical finding of exophthalmos and lid retraction in Graves disease. (*Source:* From MWJ Strachan and JDC Newell-Price. Endocrinology. Davidson's Principles and Practice of Medicine. 23rd edition. Elsevier 2018.)

Morphology

Gross (Fig. 28.8) The gland is symmetrically enlarged due to diffuse hypertrophy and hyperplasia of thyroid follicular epithelial cells. On the cut section, the thyroid parenchyma appears soft and meaty resembling normal muscle.

Microscopy Microscopically, the follicular epithelial cells show hyperplasia and crowding (Fig. 28.9). This sometimes form small papillae without a fibrovascular core projecting into the lumen of the follicles and encroaching the colloid. The colloid is pale with scalloped margins (Fig. 28.10). Lymphocytes infiltrate the gland along with plasma cells in some areas forming lymphoid aggregates with germinal centre.

Deposition of extracellular matrix and lymphocytic infiltration are seen in the retro-orbital tissues and in the dermis.

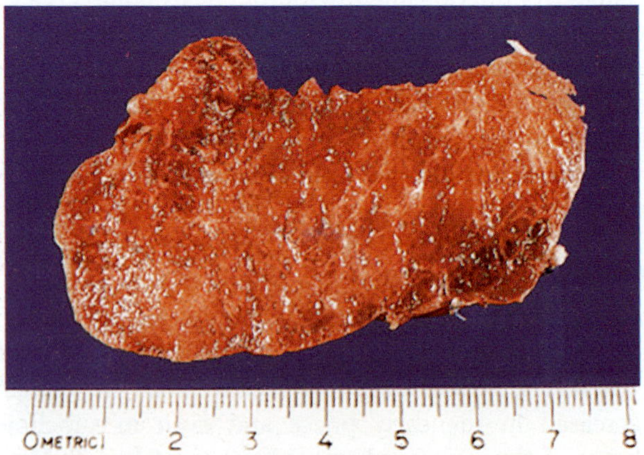

Fig. 28.8 Gross image of Graves disease. A cut surface of the thyroid gland showing diffuse hyperplasia, with a hyperaemic 'juicy' or 'meaty' appearance. (*Source:* From Giovanni Tallini and Thomas J. Giordano. Thyroid Gland. Rosai and Ackerman's Surgical Pathology. 11th edition. Elsevier 2018.)

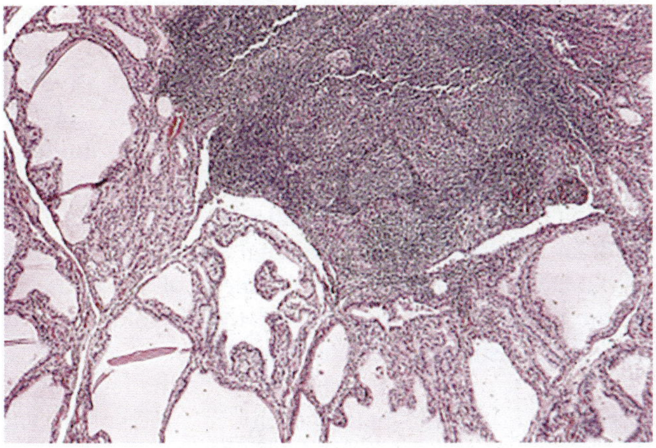

Fig. 28.9 Microscopic picture of Graves disease. Lymphoid follicles with germinal centres and hyperplastic thyroid follicles in diffuse hyperplasia. Note the pale-staining quality of the colloid. (*Source:* From Giovanni Tallini and Thomas J. Giordano. Thyroid Gland. Rosai and Ackerman's Surgical Pathology. 11th edition. Elsevier 2018.)

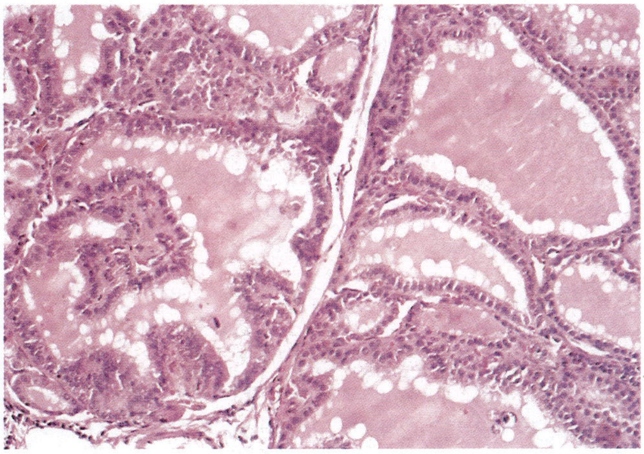

Fig. 28.10 Microscopy of Graves disease. The follicles are lined by tall columnar epithelial cells that are actively resorbing the colloid contained within the follicles, resulting in a 'scalloped' appearance of the colloid. (*Source:* From Vinay Kumar, Abul K. Abbas and Jon C. Aster. Endocrine System. Robbins Basic Pathology. 10th edition. Elsevier 2018.)

Clinical Features Graves disease is characterized by the **triad of hyperthyroidism, infiltrative ophthalmopathy and infiltrative dermopathy**. The presence of thyrotropin receptor antibody in serum and ophthalmopathy on clinical examination distinguish Graves disease from other causes of hyperthyroidism. Patients present with symptoms of hyperthyroidism as mentioned earlier. The degree of each symptom varies from case to case. Retro-orbital changes present as exophthalmos – protrusion of eyeballs. The infiltrative dermopathy or pretibial myxoedema is most seen over the shins as induration and scaly thickening.

Patients may develop congestive cardiac failure, stroke and osteoporosis with muscle weakness. Progression of ophthalmopathy can lead to compromised vision and blindness. Development of thyroid storm in some patients is associated with 20% mortality.

Management Patients are managed with a combination of drugs as mentioned under section Hyperthyroidism. Surgery is indicated only in a minority of patients who present with a large goitre compressing the adjacent structures.

GOITRE

PA 32.1

Goitre is enlargement of the thyroid gland caused by defective synthesis of thyroid hormones due to iodine deficiency. Deficiency of thyroid hormone synthesis leads to a compensatory increase in TSH levels, which, in turn, induces hyperplasia and hypertrophy of thyroid follicular epithelial cells. Most often, such a compensatory increase in the mass of the thyroid gland is sufficient to overcome the hormone deficiency and maintain a euthyroid state. If the underlying pathology is very severe, goitrous hypothyroidism results despite compensatory efforts.

A goitre may present in any of the following ways:

- As an incidental neck swelling
- Symptoms of local compression
- Incidental finding on imaging studies done for related or unrelated medical examinations
- Pain due to inflammation, haemorrhage, necrosis or malignant change
- Signs and symptoms of hypo- or hyperthyroidism

Goitre is of two types:

1. **Diffuse goitre**, also referred to as simple or colloid goitre
2. **Multinodular goitre (MNG)**, in which repeated episodes of hyperplasia and involution result in an irregular enlargement of the thyroid gland

Nontoxic goitre is a term used for goitrous enlargement of the thyroid without any signs and symptoms of hyperthyroidism. Nontoxic goitres can be diffuse or multinodular.

Diffuse Goitre

Diffuse goitre (also called **diffuse nontoxic goitre or simple or colloid goitre**) is an enlargement of the entire thyroid gland without any nodularity. Diffuse goitre is of two types – endemic and sporadic forms.

Endemic Goitre This type of diffuse goitre is the most common type and is seen in areas where soil, water and food supplies have very low levels of iodine. Hence, it is common in hilly and mountainous areas, which are far away from the sea. When more than 10% of the population in a given region have goitre, it is termed endemic goitre. This disorder is a very common, with nearly 200 million people affected, but there has been a decreasing trend because of widespread dietary iodine supplementation programs.

The primary cause is the lack of iodine which impairs the production of thyroid hormones, leading to a compensatory increase in TSH levels. This increase in TSH levels induces hyperplasia and hypertrophy of thyroid follicular epithelial cells, resulting in thyroid gland enlargement.

Apart from the dietary deficiency of iodine, dietary sub stances like goitrogens influence the clinical outcomes. Goitrogens are certain vegetables belonging to the Brassicaceae family such as cauliflower, cabbage, Brussels sprouts, turnips and cassava that on ingestion interfere with the synthesis of thyroid hormones and cause goitre formation.

Sporadic Goitre This type of goitre is less common than endemic goitre and is not restricted to any geographical location. This is very common in females, with a peaking incidence at puberty and in young adult period.

Causes of sporadic goitre

- Idiopathic
- Ingestion of goitrogens
- Dyshormonogenetic goitre

Morphology

In the process of evolution of diffuse goitre, two phases have been identified.

Hyperplastic phase: In this phase, the gland is diffusely and symmetrically enlarged, with the average weight of the gland not exceeding 150 g. The follicles are lined by columnar cells with crowding, which may form projections into the lumen as seen in Graves disease. Colloid accumulation is not uniform as some follicles are highly distended whereas others remain small.

Phase of colloid involution: This phase evolves when the iodine deficiency is corrected with dietary supplements or when the demand for the excessive hormone synthesis ceases. In this phase, the stimulated follicular epithelium involutes to form an enlarged colloid-rich gland, making it brown, glassy and translucent on the cut surface. Microscopically, the follicular epithelial cells are cuboidal and flat with abundant colloid within their lumen.

Clinical Features Most patients with simple goitre remain euthyroid; hence, there are no symptoms of hypo- or hyperthyroidism. Mass effect is usually the reason for which the patients seek medical attention. Children with goitre due to dyshormonogenesis may have features of cretinism.

Laboratory tests show elevated levels of TSH with normal T_3 and T_4.

Multinodular Goitre

MNG is characterized by an irregular enlargement of the gland giving rise to multinodularity of the thyroid gland. It is the result of changes that happen in long-standing simple goitres. Most cases of extreme thyroid enlargement are MNGs. These can arise from both endemic and sporadic goitres and are more common in females but occur at an older age than simple goitre.

Pathogenesis The natural history of MNG is **nodular growth and acquisition of autonomy**. The pathogenesis of MNG consists of diffuse follicular hyperplasia, focal nodular proliferation and eventual acquisition of functional automaticity. The development of MNG is the result of long-term exposure of the thyroid gland to proliferative stimuli as discussed earlier.

Nodule formation is postulated to be the result of inherent and acquired heterogeneity in proliferative and functional upregulation of the follicular epithelial cells.

- Inherent heterogeneity: Thyroid follicular cells are inherently heterogeneous to thyroid hormone production and proliferation in response to TSH stimulation. A subpopulation of follicular cells outgrows other cells and expands to form macroscopic nodules.
- Acquired heterogeneity: On the other hand, follicular cells acquiring activating somatic mutations in the proliferation pathways can expand clonally to form nodules. This mechanism is responsible for nodule formation in 70% of the cases. Somatic mutations resulting in the constitutive activation of TSH receptors are found in 60% of autonomously functioning nodules and are discussed under thyroid adenomas.

The uneven follicular hyperplasia, formation of new follicles and colloid accumulation produce physical stress that leads to rupture of follicles and blood vessels resulting in haemorrhages, scarring and calcification. Scarring leads to nodularity, which is intensified by the preexisting stromal framework of the thyroid gland.

Morphology (Figs 28.11 and 28.12)

Gross The gland is **asymmetrically enlarged with multiple nodules** of varying sizes. However, one nodule may be more prominent and appear as a single large nodule mimicking a solitary adenoma. In contrast to thyroid adenomas, the nodules are unencapsulated. Weight of the thyroid may be increased up to 2 kg, pushing the midline structures laterally. In some cases, the goitre grows downwards behind the sternum and the clavicle to produce intrathoracic or plunging goitre. In some cases, almost the whole lesion hides behind the trachea and the oesophagus. A cut section of the gland shows numerous irregular nodules containing various amounts of colloid. Older lesions have areas of haemorrhages, fibrosis and calcification.

Microscopy Microscopic features include colloid-filled follicles lined by flattened inactive epithelial cells along with areas of follicular epithelial hyperplasia and degenerative changes, as seen in the gross examination.

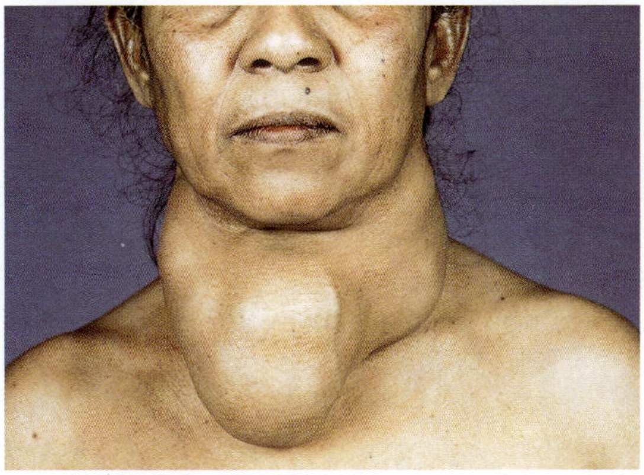

Fig. 28.11 A large multinodular goitre – clinical picture.

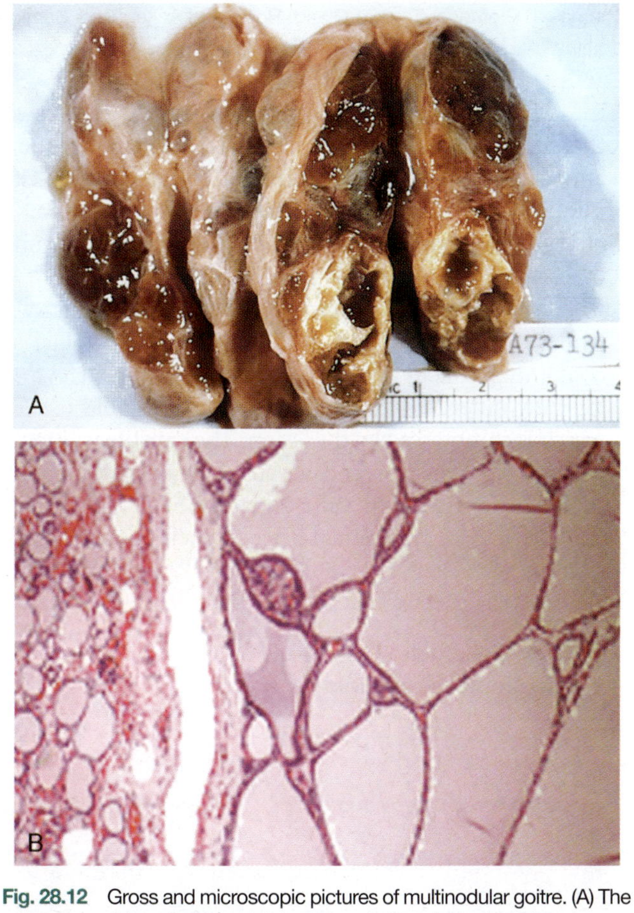

Fig. 28.12 Gross and microscopic pictures of multinodular goitre. (A) The coarsely nodular gland contains areas of fibrosis and cystic change. (B) Hyperplastic nodule with compressed residual thyroid parenchyma on the periphery. The hyperplastic follicles contain abundant pink 'colloid' within their lumina. Note the absence of a prominent capsule, a feature distinguishing such lesions from neoplasms of the thyroid. (*Source:* From Vinay Kumar, Abul K. Abbas and Jon C. Aster. Endocrine System. Robbins Basic Pathology. 10th edition. Elsevier 2018.)

Clinical Features Patients with MNG experience a mass effect, caused by thyroid gland enlargement, as their predominant symptom. Goitre may cause dysphagia or dyspnoea due to airway obstruction. Compression of large vessels in the neck and the upper thorax may result in superior vena cava syndrome.

Most patients remain euthyroid or may have subclinical hyperthyroidism. In a small group of patients, a nodule may become autonomous and precipitate hyperthyroidism because of hyperfunction. This condition of development of toxic MNG is called **Plummer syndrome** and is not associated with other features of Graves disease. Radioiodine uptake studies can be conducted to differentiate a dominant thyroid nodule from thyroid neoplasms.

Though the risk of malignancy is very low (<5%) with MNG, it is not very uncommon. Onset of changes like sudden increase in size and hoarseness of voice should raise the clinical suspicion of malignancy.

SOLITARY THYROID NODULES

Solitary thyroid nodule (STN) is a discrete lesion within the thyroid gland that is clinically or radiologically distinct from the surrounding thyroid parenchyma. Clinical significance of STNs is that up to 5% of them are malignant. The following is a list of thyroid lesions that can present as STN:

- Colloid nodule
- Thyroid cyst
- Thyroiditis
- Thyroid adenoma
- Primary thyroid carcinoma
- Primary lymphoma of thyroid
- Metastatic carcinoma of thyroid

A majority of STNs are benign but need complete evaluation to rule out the possibility of malignancy.

The following features help to categorize STNs:

- Solitary nodules are more likely to be neoplastic than multiple nodules.
- Nodules in men are more likely to be neoplastic than in women.
- Nodules in younger patients are more likely to be neoplastic than those in older individuals.
- Hot nodules are more likely to be benign lesions.
- A history of radiation therapy to the neck is more often associated with malignancy.

These criteria help in stratifying the patients in the beginning of the evaluation. However, a definitive diagnosis can be obtained only by morphological examination by fine-needle aspiration cytology and histopathological examination.

NEOPLASMS OF THE THYROID

Thyroid tumours are relatively common lesions and are the most common endocrine neoplasms. Most of these are benign tumours, but every thyroid tumour should be examined carefully to rule out the possibility of malignancy.

Thyroid adenoma and common thyroid malignancies are discussed in detail here.

Benign Neoplasms: Thyroid Adenoma

Thyroid adenomas originate from follicular epithelial cells of the thyroid and typically present as STNs. Clinically, it is often difficult to distinguish follicular adenomas from dominant nodule of MNG and follicular carcinoma. Though most of the adenomas are nonfunctional without causing hormonal excess, a small subset may be active and produce thyroid hormones causing thyrotoxicosis. In such a scenario, these adenomas are called '**toxic adenomas**'.

Pathogenesis Functioning follicular adenomas occur because of monoclonal expansion of follicular epithelial cells with mutations such as activating mutations in TSH receptor gene and, less frequently, mutations in the adenylate cyclase stimulating G alpha protein gene. These mutations result in increased thyroid hormone secretion independent of TSH. On the other hand, nonfunctioning follicular adenomas, around 20% of them, possess mutations in oncogenes that may predispose them to follicular carcinoma. The mutations that cause this transformation include N-RAS and K-RAS mutations.

Morphology

Gross (Fig. 28.13) Follicular adenomas are **solitary, spherical and well-encapsulated** lesions that are very well demarcated from the surrounding normal thyroid tissue, whereas nodules of MNG are unencapsulated. This finding is very important to differentiate them from MNGs, especially when a dominant nodule of an MNG mimics a solitary nodule clinically. A cut surface of a follicular adenoma shows a soft tumour mass that bulges and compresses the adjacent thyroid tissue, and depending on the amount of colloid present, it may appear grey–white to red–brown. Secondary changes like haemorrhage, fibrosis, calcification and cystic changes are seen as in MNGs.

Microscopy (Figs 28.14 and 28.15) Microscopy of follicular adenoma shows uniform-appearing follicles containing colloid which is architecturally and cytologically different from adjacent normal thyroid tissue which is compressed by the lesion. **The capsule is intact** without any capsular and vascular invasion, which is the hallmark finding to differentiate follicular adenoma from follicular carcinoma. Hence, meticulous examination of the capsule in its entirety is extremely essential. The neoplastic cells may show different patterns:

- Normofollicular (simple)
- Microfollicular (colloid)

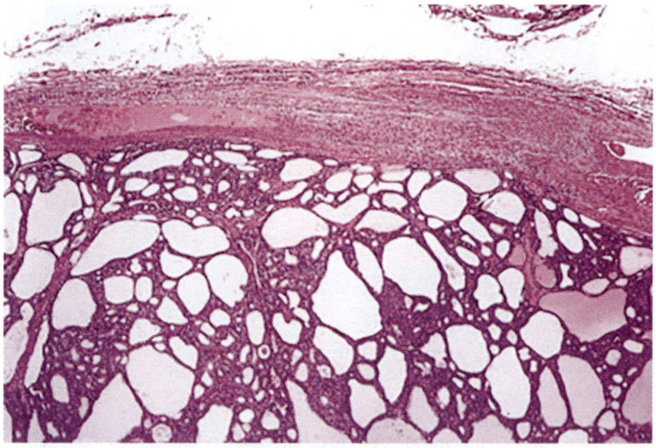

Fig. 28.14 Thyroid adenoma – microscopy. Note the intact fibrous capsule around the tumour. (*Source:* From Giovanni Tallini and Thomas J. Giordano. Thyroid Gland. Rosai and Ackerman's Surgical Pathology. 11th edition. Elsevier 2018.)

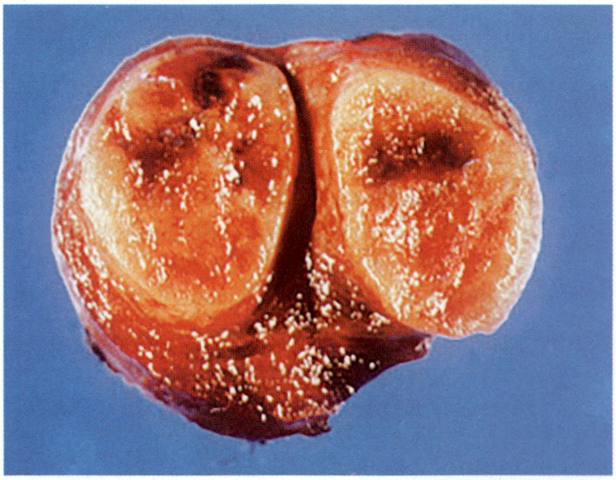

Fig. 28.13 Thyroid adenoma – gross. (*Source:* From Giovanni Tallini and Thomas J. Giordano. Thyroid Gland. Rosai and Ackerman's Surgical Pathology. 11th edition. Elsevier 2018.)

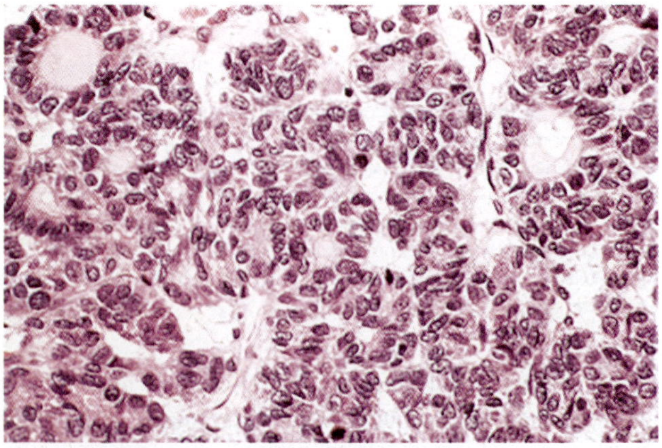

Fig. 28.15 Microscopy of follicular adenoma with a follicular growth pattern. (*Source:* From Giovanni Tallini and Thomas J. Giordano. Thyroid Gland. Rosai and Ackerman's Surgical Pathology. 11th edition. Elsevier 2018.)

- Macrofollicular (fetal)
- Trabecular/solid

There may be a focal papillary pattern as well. Morphologically, the tumour cells are cuboidal to low columnar without much of pleomorphism and mitotic figures are rare. Metaplastic changes like Hürthle cell changes and spindle cell changes may be present.

The term '**atypical adenoma**' is assigned for follicular adenomas exhibiting pleomorphism, cellularity, mitotic figures or necrosis without capsular or vascular invasion.

Clinical Features Most patients with a follicular adenoma present with an STN in an otherwise normal thyroid. Most of these patients are euthyroid and asymptomatic. Patients with larger tumours may present with pressure symptoms like dyspnoea, cough and dysphagia. They may also complain of neck pain caused by a sudden enlargement of the lesion because of haemorrhage and cystic degeneration.

Laboratory Investigations In patients with active adenoma or toxic adenoma, TSH levels are reduced along with elevated levels of T_3 and T_4. An ultrasound examination of the thyroid gland is recommended in all patients with a solitary nodule to help characterize the nodule and to examine the rest of the thyroid gland for other nodules or lesions.

On radionuclide scanning, all inactive adenomas are cold while toxic adenomas are hot. Because 10% of cold nodules can be malignant, such nodules need further evaluation to confirm the benign nature. Though aspiration cytology is widely used to evaluate thyroid lesions, fine-needle aspiration cytology has its limitation in the evaluation of follicular neoplasms. Because capsular integrity must be checked, histopathological examination is the gold standard in the evaluation of follicular neoplasms, which is discussed in detail later.

THYROID MALIGNANCIES (TABLE 28.4)

Thyroid malignancies account for approximately 1%–1.5% of malignancies across the globe. The major thyroid malignancies are as follows:

Papillary carcinoma >85%
Follicular carcinoma >5%–15%
Medullary carcinoma >5%
Anaplastic carcinoma <5%

All carcinomas except medullary carcinoma are derived from follicular epithelial cells of thyroid, whereas medullary carcinoma is the derivative of parafollicular C cells. All these tumours are described separately because of their differences in clinical, pathological, biological and molecular features.

Table 28.4 Summary of Genetic Events in Thyroid Cancers

Tumour	Genetic Alteration
Papillary carcinoma	RET/PTC rearrangement BRAF – gain of function
Follicular carcinoma	RAS – gain of function PIK3CA – gain of function PTEN – loss of function PAX8–PPARG fusion
Anaplastic carcinoma	RAS – rearrangement PIK3CA – rearrangement RET/PTC – rearrangement TP53 – loss of function β-Catenin – gain of function
Medullary carcinoma	RET – gain of function

Papillary Thyroid Carcinoma

PTC is the most common thyroid malignancy that affects individuals between 25 and 50 years of age. It is also the most common thyroid malignancy to develop following exposure to ionizing radiation.

Pathogenesis

Many chromosomal rearrangements have been identified in PTC.

- The first oncogenic events identified in PTC were chromosomal rearrangements involving the RET proto-oncogene, which arises from a paracentric inversion of chromosome 10. RET fusion proteins (the RET/PTC family) play an oncogenic role in approximately 20% of PTCs. More than 15 fusion partners have been studied, but RET/PTC1, RET/PTC2 and RET/PTC3 account for most of the cases. RET/PTC rearrangements produce genes that encode novel fusion proteins with constitutive tyrosine kinase activity inducing autonomous proliferation of follicular epithelial cells.
- NTRK1 and MET proto-oncogenes may be overexpressed or amplified in PTCs.
- Mutation in the BRAF gene leading to BRAF V60E is prominent in PTCs. This mutation is also associated with aggressive clinicopathological characteristics such as extrathyroidal invasion, lymph node metastasis and failure of radioiodine therapy and recurrence of the malignancy.
- In addition to these genetic events, many other mutations in the genes like SFRP1, MMP1, ESM1 and COL13A1 are seen, especially in radiation therapy-associated PTC.

It can also be stressed that RET/PTC, NTRK1 and BRAF mutations are mutually exclusive in most of the cases.

Morphology

Gross (Fig. 28.16) PTC is commonly a **solitary** lesion, but in approximately 20% of cases it may be multifocal. Predominant presentation is a solitary infiltrative solid white tumour with variable cystic changes, fibrosis and calcification. Around 10% of tumours are encapsulated. In some cases, their cut surface shows the presence of **papillary excrescences**, which, if present, is a characteristic finding.

Microscopy (Figs 28.17 and 28.18) The hallmark features of PTC are as follows:

- **Papillary architecture**
  The neoplastic cells in PTC are arranged in the classical complex papillary architecture, with finger-like projections, having a central fibrovascular core and a stalk covered by single to multiple layers of cuboidal epithelial cells. In the well-differentiated forms, neoplastic cells are uniform and cuboidal but in poorly differentiated anaplastic forms, the cells display pleomorphism.
- **Nuclear features**
  Cells of PTC have a classical nuclear morphology and its diagnosis is based on these nuclear features. The features are listed as follows:
  a. **Optically clear nuclei** also referred to as Orphan Annie eye nuclei due to finely dispersed chromatin (Fig. 28.18)
  b. **Intranuclear inclusions** due to invaginations of the cytoplasm (Fig. 28.19)
  c. **Intranuclear grooves** due to the undulating nature of the nuclear membrane

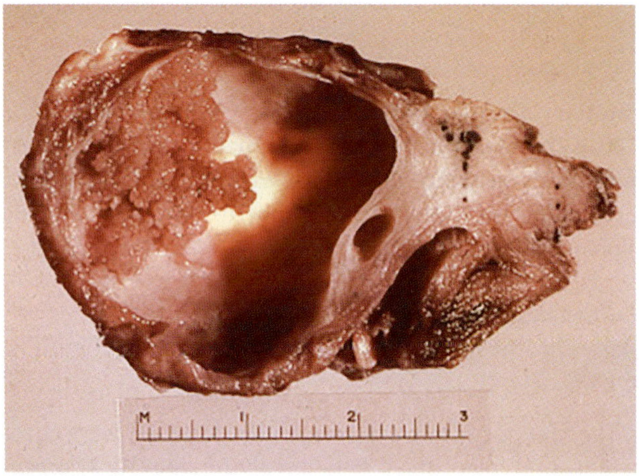

Fig. 28.16 Papillary thyroid carcinoma – gross: predominantly cystic with partly solid and papillary appearance. (*Source:* From Bruce M. Wenig. Neoplasms of the Thyroid Gland. Atlas of Head and Neck Pathology. 3rd edition. Elsevier 2016.)

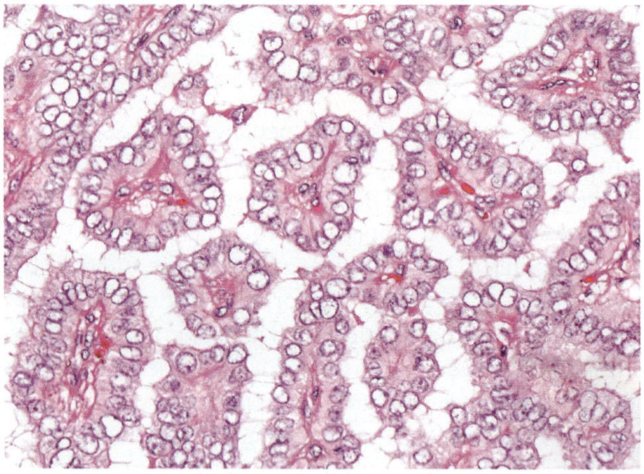

Fig. 28.18 Papillary thyroid carcinoma – microscopy, high power. (*Source:* https://www.google.com/url?sa=i&url=https%3A%2F%2Fwww.pathologyoutlines.com%2Ftopic%2Fthyroidpapillary.html&psig=AOvVaw3QszFd2bJU9ZScJholt-Tu&ust=1605711417134000&source=images&cd=vfe&ved=0CAIQjRxqFwoTCIDW-qjrie0CFQAAAAAdAAAAABAJ)

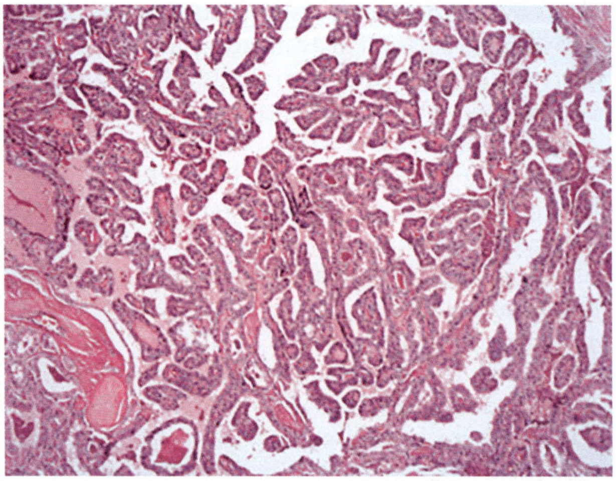

Fig. 28.17 Papillary thyroid carcinoma – microscopy. The scanner view highlights the papillary architecture of the tumour. (*Source:* From Bruce M. Wenig. Neoplasms of the Thyroid Gland. Atlas of Head and Neck Pathology. 3rd edition. Elsevier 2016.)

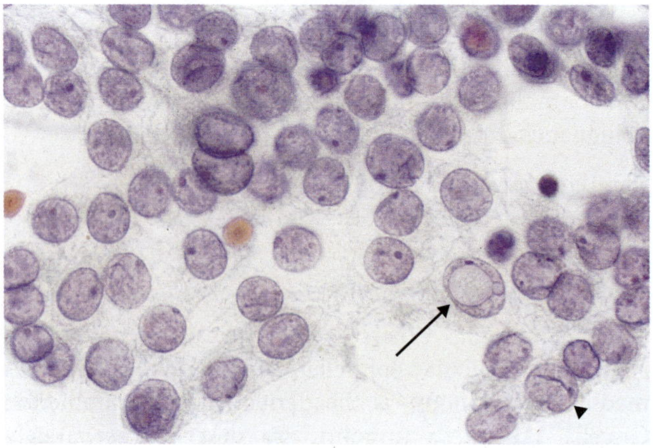

Fig. 28.19 Papillary thyroid carcinoma. Sharply defined intranuclear pseudoinclusion (arrow) and the nuclear groove (arrowhead).

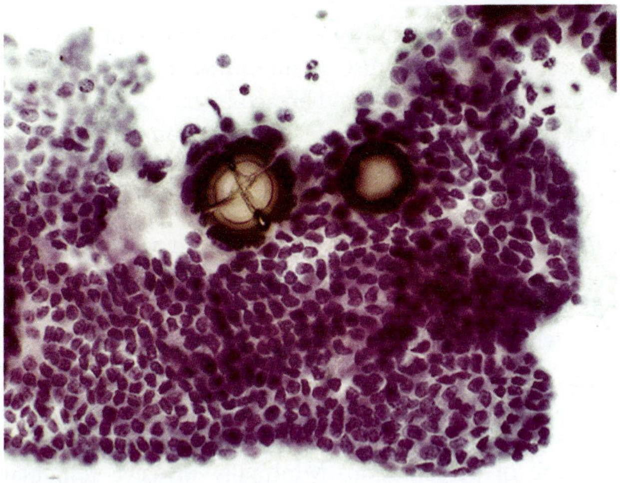

Fig. 28.20 Papillary thyroid carcinoma – cytology. The neoplastic cells are arranged in crowded sheets. Psammoma bodies are present (Papanicolaou stain). (*Source:* From Edmund S. Cibas. Thyroid. Cytology. 5th edition. Elsevier 2021.)

- **Psammoma bodies** (Fig. 28.20)
  Psammoma bodies are concentrically calcified structures seen within the cores of papillae, which, if present, are a specific finding for PTC.
- **Lymphatic invasion and lymph node metastasis** are seen in up to 50% of the cases.

Variants of Papillary Thyroid Carcinoma There are many variants of PTC, with differences in morphology and most importantly in prognosis. The common variants are listed here:

a. **Follicular variant**
b. **Tall cell variant**
c. **Diffuse sclerosing variant**
d. **Cribriform morular variant**
e. **Warthin-like variant**
f. **Solid variant**

Among these variants, the most common is the follicular variant which is described here.

Follicular variant of PTC: This variant of PTC has the nuclear features of papillary carcinoma, but the architecture is completely or predominantly follicular. The tumour can be encapsulated or infiltrative, with the former type being associated with a favourable prognosis. This variant has **RAS** mutations, which are more common than RET/PTC rearrangements.

Papillary microcarcinoma is, in fact, a conventional carcinoma with size **less than 1 cm**. This may be a precursor of typical papillary carcinoma.

Clinical Features In most patients, papillary carcinomas present as incidental thyroid nodules or as cervical lymphadenopathy with occult primary. Thyroid nodules may be indistinguishable from benign and other non-neoplastic lesions of the thyroid. In the advanced stage, hoarseness, dysphagia, cough and dyspnoea may be present. Rarely, blood-borne metastasis to lungs may be present at the time of presentation.

In general, PTCs have an excellent prognosis, with a 10-year survival rate greater than 95%. Patients with advanced stage of the disease have a more guarded prognosis.

Follicular Thyroid Carcinoma

Follicular carcinomas are the second most common thyroid malignancy accounting for 5%–15% of all thyroid malignancies, but in iodine-deficient areas, this account to up to 40% of thyroid cancers. This type of thyroid cancer is more common in women and affects older patients aged 40–60 years when compared with PTC.

Pathogenesis

- Follicular carcinomas are associated with activating mutations of **RAS or the PI-3K/AKT** arm of the receptor tyrosine kinase signalling pathway. RAS mutations can stimulate MAPK and PI3K signalling pathways.
- A fraction of follicular carcinomas is associated with loss-of-function mutation of the **PTEN** gene. These set of mutations are mutually exclusive.
- One-third to one-half of follicular thyroid cancers are associated with a distinctive (2;3) (q13;p25) translocation which creates a fusion gene composed of PAX8 and the peroxisome proliferator activated receptor gene (PPARG). The product of this novel fusion gene has a role in terminal differentiation of cells.

Morphology

Gross (Fig. 28.21) Solitary, well-circumscribed or infiltrative nodule is the classical presentation of follicular carcinoma. With infiltrative borders, the diagnosis is simple whereas the sharply demarcated and encapsulated lesions are difficult to distinguish from follicular adenomas. On the cut surface, the tumour is grey to pink and translucent because of the presence of colloid. Areas of fibrosis and calcification may be seen.

Microscopy Microscopically, the tumour is composed of neoplastic cells arranged in small follicles containing colloid. In poorly differentiated tumours, follicular differentiation is not prominent. **Hürthle cell variant** of follicular carcinoma is characterized by tumour cells with abundant eosinophilic granular cytoplasm. Nuclear features of papillary carcinoma are characteristically absent.

The feature that differentiates follicular adenoma and carcinoma is the presence of **capsular and vascular invasion** (Figs 28.22 and 28.23). This feature can be appreciated only by histopathological examination as, by cytological examination, the capsule cannot be

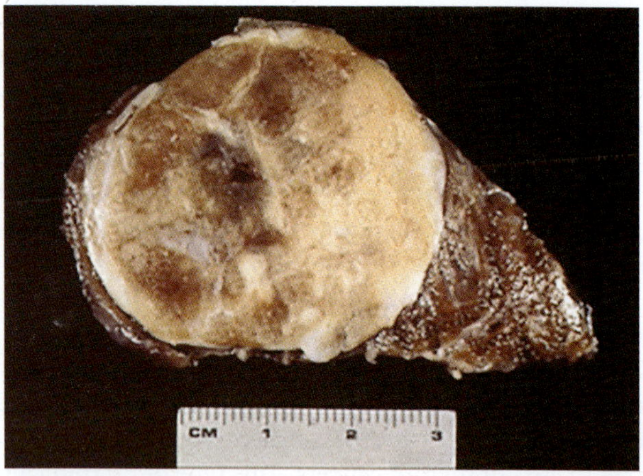

Fig. 28.21 Follicular thyroid carcinoma – gross. The gross appearance of the thyroid tumour is similar to that of follicular adenoma. (*Source:* From Bruce M. Wenig. Neoplasms of the Thyroid Gland. Atlas of Head and Neck Pathology. 3rd edition. Elsevier 2016.)

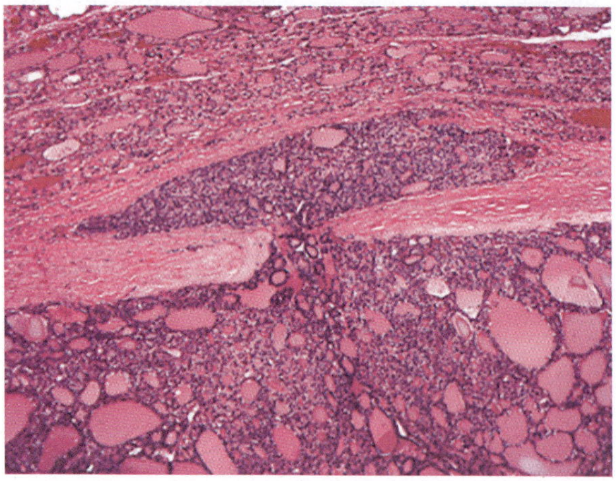

Fig. 28.22 Follicular thyroid carcinoma – microscopy, scanner view. Mushroom-like protrusion of the tumour into the capsule – capsular invasion. (*Source:* From Bruce M. Wenig. Neoplasms of the Thyroid Gland. Atlas of Head and Neck Pathology. 3rd edition. Elsevier 2016.)

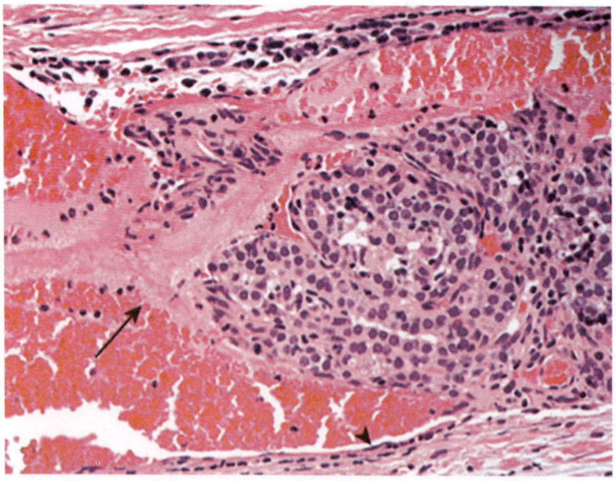

Fig. 28.23 Microscopy of follicular thyroid carcinoma with vascular invasion. Tumour in endothelium-lined vascular spaces *(arrowheads)* with thrombus formation *(arrows)*. (*Source:* From Bruce M. Wenig. Neoplasms of the Thyroid Gland. Atlas of Head and Neck Pathology. 3rd edition. Elsevier 2016.)

inspected. For establishing the diagnosis of malignancy, the capsule must be submitted in entirety and carefully examined for any breach by tumours cells, as well as capsular vessels and vessels beyond the capsule.

Clinical Presentation The most common presentation of follicular carcinomas is the slowly enlarging painless thyroid nodules. Most of them are **cold nodules**. Unlike PTC, which presents with lymphatic invasion in at least half of the cases, follicular carcinoma is associated with vascular invasion and haematogenous metastases. Prognosis is dependent on the extent of invasion and stage at the time of presentation. Minimally invasive follicular thyroid carcinomas have a 10-year survival rate of more than 90%, whereas the prognosis is guarded in widely invasive tumours.

Anaplastic Thyroid Carcinoma

Anaplastic carcinomas of the thyroid are undifferentiated tumours that originate from follicular epithelial cells of the thyroid. These tumours are commonly seen in older individuals, in their seventh decade of life, and are **aggressive** with a high mortality rate of up to 100%. All tumours of this category are of a higher stage. Though this category of thyroid malignancy accounts for less than 5% of thyroid cancers, it accounts for 40% of thyroid cancer-related deaths. At least 25% of patients with anaplastic carcinoma have a history of well-differentiated thyroid carcinoma and another 25% of patients have a simultaneous well-differentiated tumour in the thyroidectomy specimen.

Pathogenesis Anaplastic carcinomas can arise de novo or more commonly from a well-differentiated papillary or follicular carcinoma, as stated earlier. Depending on the well-differentiated component these are associated with, anaplastic carcinomas exhibit the corresponding genetic changes. In addition to these molecular changes, anaplastic carcinomas are associated with **TP53 inactivation or β-catenin activation**, which contribute to its aggressive behaviour.

Morphology

Gross (Fig. 28.24) These tumours are large and solid, with necrosis and haemorrhage. Paucicellular variants have a hard fibrotic mass.

Microscopy Microscopically, these tumours are composed of highly pleomorphic anaplastic cells with a varied morphology. There can be three patterns that occur singly or in combination.

- **Sarcomatoid pattern** is composed of spindle cells.
- **Giant cell pattern** is composed of highly pleomorphic cells and tumour giant cells.

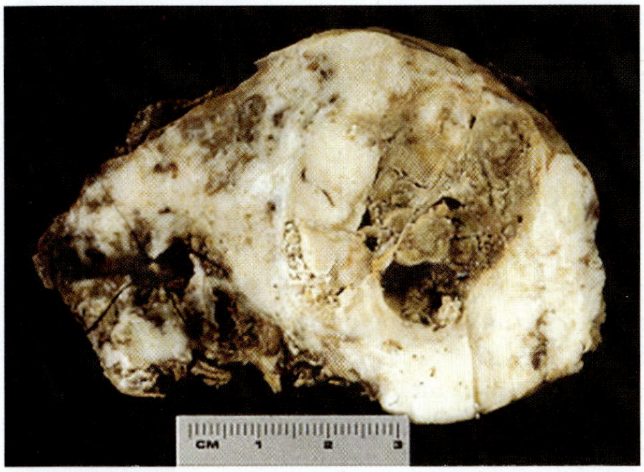

Fig. 28.24 Anaplastic carcinoma – gross. Tan–white tumour with foci of necrosis replacing most of the thyroid gland. The tumour is grossly invading outside the confines of the thyroid gland. (*Source:* From Bruce M. Wenig. Neoplasms of the Thyroid Gland. Atlas of Head and Neck Pathology. 3rd edition. Elsevier 2016.)

- **Epithelial pattern** is composed of squamous or squamoid cells.

There may be foci showing papillary or follicular differentiation, suggesting their origin. Vast areas of necrosis, vascular invasion, increased mitotic figures and areas of heterologous differentiation in the form of bone and cartilage may be seen. The tumour cells are negative for markers of thyroid differentiation such as thyroglobulin.

Clinical Features Patients with anaplastic carcinoma present with a rapidly enlarging neck mass which, in most cases, has spread beyond the thyroid, infiltrating the adjacent neck structures and distant metastasis. Patients may present with symptoms due to compression such as dyspnoea, dysphagia, cough and hoarseness of voice.

Treatment is generally supportive, and the most common causes of death in these patients are local invasion and compression rather than metastasis. The disease is 100% fatal.

Medullary Thyroid Carcinoma

Medullary carcinoma of the thyroid is a neuroendocrine tumour derived from parafollicular C cells which are the derivatives of the neural crest. Like their normal counterparts, tumour cells in medullary thyroid carcinoma secrete **calcitonin**, which also serves as its tumour marker. Some tumours secrete adrenocorticotropic hormone (ACTH) or corticotropin-releasing hormone (CRH). Around 70% of the tumours are sporadic, and the remaining cases are part of **MEN syndrome 2A or 2B or familial medullary thyroid carcinoma**. The usual age group of patients is 40–50 years, but cases occurring as a part of familial syndromes are reported in younger age groups as well.

Pathogenesis Familial medullary thyroid carcinomas occurring in multiple endocrine neoplasia type 2 (MEN2) background are associated with activating mutation of RET proto-oncogene. Of note, **RET mutations** are also associated with 50% of sporadic cases.

Morphology

Gross (Fig. 28.25) Gross presentation is different for sporadic and familial medullary carcinomas. Sporadic tumours present as solitary nodules, whereas familial tumours present commonly as bilateral and multicentric masses. Tumours are commonly located in the mid or upper portion of the gland where the density of C cells is normally high. The tumour is unencapsulated, solid, firm, grey and often with infiltrative borders. Larger tumours have areas of haemorrhage and necrosis. Tumours with size less than 1 cm are called microcarcinomas.

Microscopy (Fig. 28.26) Medullary thyroid carcinomas exhibit a wide variety of morphology and can mimic

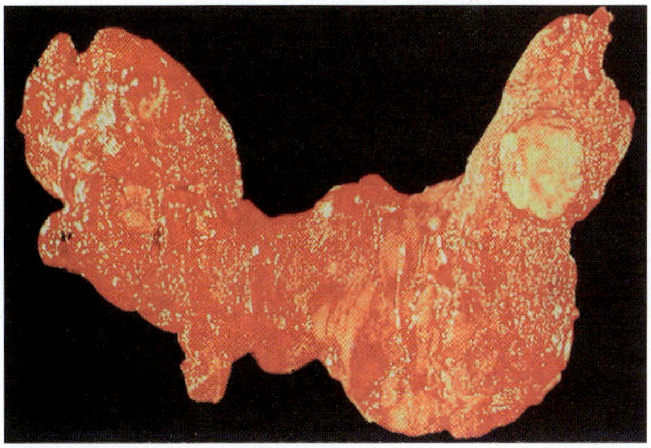

Fig. 28.25 Gross pathology of medullary carcinoma shows a well-defined mass in the thyroid gland.

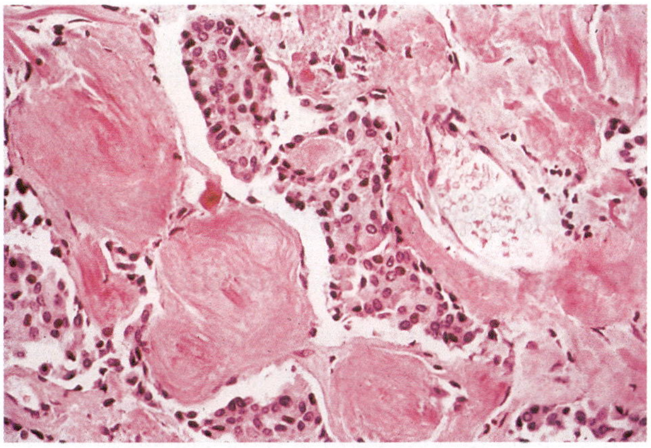

Fig. 28.26 Medullary carcinoma of the thyroid. High-power photomicrograph showing small spherical tumour cells adjacent to masses of amorphous hyaline material; the latter is amyloid.

any other thyroid malignancy. Microscopically, the tumour is composed of polygonal to spindle cells forming nests, trabeculae, follicles or solid sheets often as a mixture of cell types and patterns. Some cases may have more pleomorphic cells.

A striking feature of medullary carcinomas is the presence of **acellular amyloid deposits** in the stroma, which is positive for calcitonin. Surrounding thyroid parenchyma reveals the presence of C cell hyperplasia in familial cases, which is thought to be the precursor lesion. Microcarcinoma has a complex microarchitectural pattern with desmoplastic stroma containing amyloid deposition.

Electron microscopy highlights the presence of dense neurosecretory granules within the cytoplasm of tumour cells. Immunohistochemistry for calcitonin is positive in the tumour cells and amyloid deposits. Amyloid deposits can be highlighted using Congo red stain.

Clinical Features Clinical presentation of sporadic and familial cases differs completely. Sporadic cases present with a painless mass in the neck with or without compression symptoms. In some cases, symptoms due to secretion of hormones like VIP and ACTH cause manifestations like diarrhoea and Cushing syndrome, respectively, and these may the initial manifestations.

Familial cases come to medical attention because of a thyroid mass or symptoms due to endocrine lesions in other organs, as a part of multiple endocrine neoplasia type 2A (MEN2A) or multiple endocrine neoplasia type 2B (MEN2B). In general, medullary carcinomas arising as a part of MEN2B are more aggressive than sporadic cases, MEN2A and familial medullary thyroid carcinoma cases. Hence, prophylactic thyroidectomy is indicated in patients with MEN2 syndrome and RET mutations even in the absence of a thyroid mass.

Apart from calcitonin, the tumour cells also secrete carcinoembryonic antigen, and both of them serve as tumour markers. Unlike other thyroid malignancies, medullary carcinoma is negative for follicular epithelial cell marker such as thyroglobulin.

II. THE PARATHYROID GLAND

ANATOMY, HISTOLOGY AND PHYSIOLOGY

There are four parathyroid glands found near the posterior aspect of the thyroid gland. These are small, bean-shaped organs, weighing 20–40 mg. Parathyroid glands develop from the endoderm of third and fourth pharyngeal pouches and are located along the thyroid gland either in the superior or inferior poles or can be found anywhere along the course taken by the thyroid gland during the developmental process. Parathyroid glands have a distinct, encapsulated smooth surface that is different from that of the thyroid gland which has a more lobular surface. The colour of the gland is typically light brown to tan, which is dependent on its fat content, vascularity and percentage of oxyphil cells in the glands.

Parathyroid glands are made up of chief cells or principal cells and oxyphil cells, which are responsible for secreting parathormone or parathyroid hormone (PTH; Fig. 28.27). PTH is a peptide hormone that is released when blood calcium levels are low. Its main function is to regulate calcium homeostasis. The actions of PTH are listed as follows for a better understanding:

1. PTH secretion induces the release of calcium from the bones by stimulating osteoclasts, which secrete enzymes that degrade bone and release calcium into the interstitial fluid.
2. PTH also inhibits osteoblasts, the cells involved in bone deposition, thereby sparing the blood calcium.
3. PTH causes increased reabsorption of calcium (and magnesium) in the kidney tubules.
4. PTH initiates the production of the steroid hormone calcitriol (also known as 1,25-dihydroxyvitamin D), which is the active form of vitamin D_3, in the kidneys. Calcitriol then stimulates absorption of dietary calcium by the intestines.

The net result of all these actions is elevation of serum free calcium. A negative feedback loop regulates the levels of PTH, with rising blood calcium levels inhibiting further release of PTH.

Diseases of parathyroid glands fall under two categories – hyperfunction and hypofunction of the glands. Tumours are discussed under hyperfunction, as they usually present with features of hyperparathyroidism.

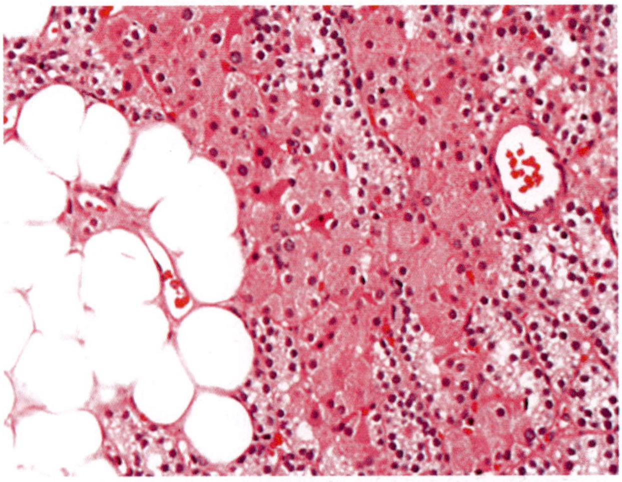

Fig. 28.27 Histology of parathyroid glands. The normal parathyroid gland in adults may include oncocytic cells interspersed with the chief cells as a nodular focus. Note the presence of abundant intraparenchymal mature fat. (*Source:* From Vicky Cheng. Hypoparathyroidism. Elsevier 2022.)

HYPERPARATHYROIDISM

PA 32.5

Hyperparathyroidism is caused by increased levels of PTH and can be classified into three categories:

- Primary hyperparathyroidism
- Secondary hyperparathyroidism
- Tertiary hyperparathyroidism

Primary Hyperparathyroidism

Primary hyperparathyroidism is due to **autonomous production of PTH** by parathyroid glands in the absence of parathyroid stimulation by renal or intestinal diseases. Parathyroid lesions that contribute to this phenomenon are as follows:

- **Adenoma 85%**
- **Hyperplasia 15%**
- **Carcinoma <1%**

Primary hyperparathyroidism usually affects adults older than 50 years and more commonly affects women. Though the disease can have a wide range of clinical presentations, most cases are detected as incidental findings.

As shown in the list, most cases of primary hyperparathyroidism are due to adenoma. Let us discuss the pathology of parathyroid adenoma.

Pathogenesis The cause of increased PTH levels in parathyroid hyperplasia is an increase in the number of cells. But in primary hyperparathyroidism due to adenomas, the normal negative feedback on PTH production by extracellular calcium seems to be lost, resulting in increased parathormone production. There are two genetic changes associated with the development of parathyroid adenomas.

1. **Cyclin D1 activating mutation:** Clonal rearrangements and overexpression of cyclin D1 are associated with more than 50% of cases of parathyroid adenoma.
2. **Multiple endocrine neoplasia type 1 (MEN1) inactivating mutation:** MEN1 gene is inactivated in up to 30% of sporadic and most cases of familial causes of parathyroid adenomas.
   Other causes are as follows:
   - MEN1 syndrome due to mutations in MEN1 and RET
   - Familial hypocalciuric hypercalcemia due to mutations in the parathyroid calcium-sensing receptor (CSAR) gene.

Morphology

Parathyroid adenoma

Parathyroid adenomas are always solitary and look like normal glands and weigh around 0.5–5 g. These are well-circumscribed, encapsulated and soft tan to reddish brown in colour (Fig. 28.28). The glands external to the adenoma are either normal or shrunken because of feedback inhibition caused by hypercalcaemia.

Adenomas are typically made up of uniform polygonal chief cells with some nests of oxyphil cells. In some cases, adenomas can be entirely composed of oxyphil cells, resembling Hürthle cell tumours found in the thyroid, known as oxyphil adenomas. It is important to note that although mitotic figures are uncommon, pleomorphic nuclei may be observed. However, the presence of pleomorphic nuclei should not be considered a sign of malignancy and is referred to as 'endocrine atypia'. In contrast to normal glands, stromal adipocytes are absent in adenomas (Fig. 28.29).

Parathyroid hyperplasia

In parathyroid hyperplasia, classically, all the four glands are involved, but in many cases, there may be asymmetry which may create confusion with adenomas. The total weight of all the glands does not exceed 1 g. Microscopically, the prominent finding is the diffuse or multinodular pattern of chief cell hyperplasia. Like in adenomas, stromal fat is not seen.

Parathyroid carcinoma

These lesions are usually invasive but can also be circumscribed and encapsulated and can be confused with adenomas. The tumour involves only one parathyroid gland and forms a grey–white irregular mass with weight exceeding 10 g, at times. Microscopically, there are nodular or trabecular patterns of uniform chief cells. There is no cytological marker for malignancy, and only invasion and metastasis are the distinguishing features.

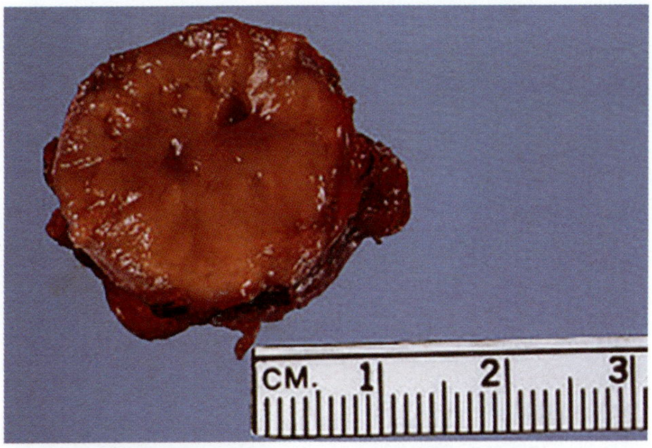

Fig. 28.28 Parathyroid adenoma – gross. Note the circumscription, the homogeneous appearance interrupted by a few foci of fresh haemorrhagic or cystic changes and the brown to yellowish colour. (*Source:* From Thomas J. Giordano. Parathyroid Glands. Rosai and Ackerman's Surgical Pathology. 11th edition. Elsevier 2018.)

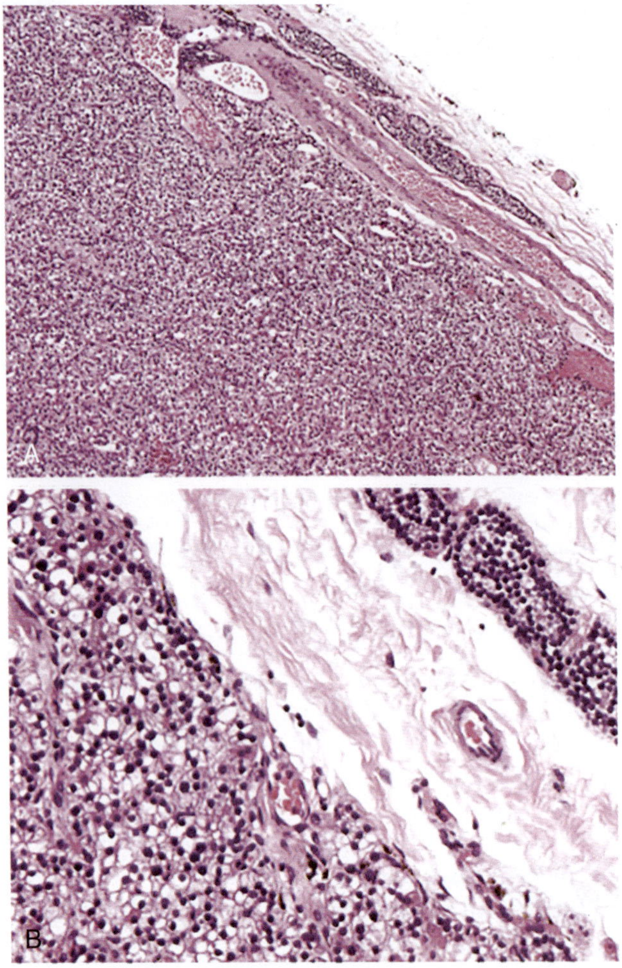

Fig. 28.29 Parathyroid adenoma – microscopy. (A) Note the tumour circumscription and the residual rim of parathyroid tissue in the upper field. (B) Compared with the tumour (left field), the residual parathyroid (right field) shows smaller cells and smaller nuclei. (*Source:* From Christopher D.M. Fletcher. Tumors of the Thyroid and Parathyroid Glands. Diagnostic Histopathology of Tumors. 5th edition. Elsevier 2021.)

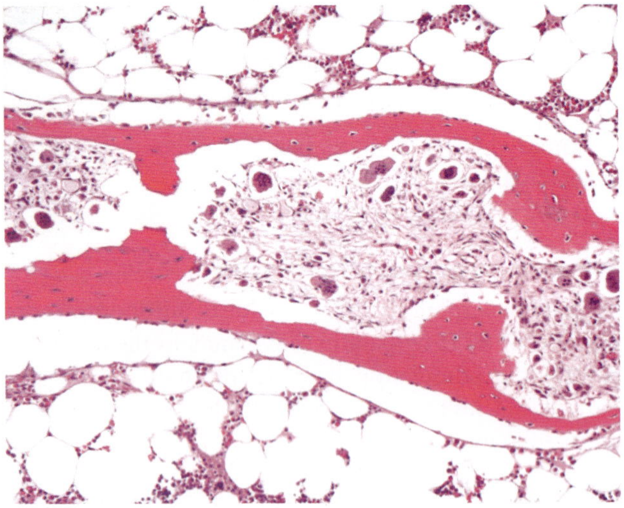

Fig. 28.30 Microscopy of dissecting osteitis seen in hyperparathyroidism – osteoclasts boring into the centre of the trabecula. (*Source:* From Osteomyelitis in Adults. Elsevier Point of Care. 2021.)

Morphological changes can be seen in other organs in primary hyperparathyroidism due to elevated levels of PTH and calcium.

A. **Skeletal system**
Three changes are seen in the skeletal system of patients with symptomatic, untreated, long-term hyperparathyroidism. The changes are due to increased osteoclastic activity induced by hyperparathyroidism.
1. **Osteoporosis:** Common bones affected are cortical bones of phalanges, vertebrae and proximal femur. Predominant changes seen are decreased bone mass and osteoporosis. In the medulla, osteoclasts tunnel into and dissect along the central length of the trabeculae, creating the appearance of railroad track, which is referred to as **dissecting osteitis** (Fig. 28.30). Fibrovascular tissue replaces marrow spaces around the affected surfaces.
2. **Brown tumours** (Fig. 28.31): Osteoporotic changes predispose to microfractures and secondary haemorrhages, followed by infiltration of macrophages and growth of reparative fibrous tissue. These changes create a mass of reactive tissue, referred to as brown tumour. The colour of the lesion is because of vascularity, haemorrhage and deposition of haemosiderin. These lesions commonly undergo secondary cystic changes.
3. **Osteitis fibrosa cystica:** The triad of exaggerated osteoclastic activity, peritrabecular fibrosis and cystic brown tumours is the hallmark feature of severe hyperparathyroidism and is known by the term 'generalized osteitis fibrosa cystica', also called **von Recklinghausen disease of the bone**. This triad is seen only in chronic and severe untreated cases of hyperparathyroidism.

B. **Urinary tract**
Hypercalcaemia induced by hyperparathyroidism precipitates urinary tract stones and nephrocalcinosis, characterized by calcification of renal tubules and interstitium. Renal stones also lead to hypertension, which is an important cause of death.

C. Hypercalcaemia also causes **metastatic calcification** in the sites like gastric mucosa, lungs, myocardium and blood vessels.

Clinical Features Most often patients with hyperparathyroidism are asymptomatic and only a small fraction of patients present with the classical clinical manifestations.

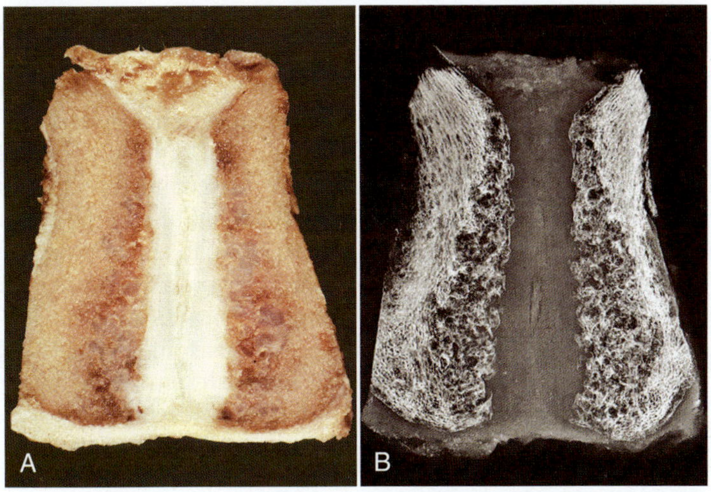

Fig. 28.31 (A) Gross appearance of a symphysis pubis obtained at autopsy from a patient with hyperparathyroidism shows hyperaemia, fibrosis and resorption of the bone on each side of the symphysis. (B) Radiograph of the specimen.

Signs and symptoms are because of PTH elevation and hypercalcaemia. The symptoms are referred to as '**painful bones, renal stones, abdominal groans and psychic moans**'.

Bone pain is because of fractures caused by osteoporosis and osteitis fibrosa cystica.

Renal stones cause renal colic, obstructive uropathy and chronic renal failure.

Gastrointestinal problems like constipation, nausea, peptic ulcers, gallstones and pancreatitis can be present.

CNS symptoms include depression, lethargy and seizures.

Laboratory Findings The most common laboratory finding in patients with hyperparathyroidism is hypercalcaemia.

Hyperparathyroidism is the most common cause of asymptomatic hypercalcaemia, whereas malignancy is the most common cause of symptomatic hypercalcaemia. Yet, malignancy should be ruled out in all cases of hypercalcaemia, be it symptomatic or asymptomatic. In patients with primary hyperparathyroidism, serum PTH levels are inappropriately elevated for the serum calcium levels. In hypercalcaemia induced by nonparathyroid diseases, PTH levels are too low for the serum calcium levels. Apart from hypercalcaemia, other biochemical alterations seen in primary hyperparathyroidism are increased urinary calcium and phosphate levels. Serum phosphate levels may get normalized with phosphate retention caused by secondary renal disease.

Secondary Hyperparathyroidism

Secondary hyperparathyroidism is the **compensatory overproduction of PTH secondary to** hypocalcaemia, typically because of vitamin D deficiency and/or chronic kidney disease. Other causes include inadequate dietary intake of calcium, steatorrhoea. etc.

The mechanism by which chronic renal failure leads to secondary hyperparathyroidism is still not completely understood. Probably, the reduced phosphate excretion by the kidney leads to hyperphosphataemia and hypocalcaemia which, in turn, trigger the parathyroid gland. The other possible mechanism is the decreased availability of 1α-hydroxylase for the synthesis of active form of vitamin D, which leads to reduced intestinal absorption of calcium, resulting in the compensatory overactivity of parathyroid glands.

Morphology

As explained earlier, parathyroid hyperplasia is associated with secondary hyperparathyroidism. Microscopically, the gland shows diffuse or multinodular increase in chief cells with a reduced number of adipocytes in the stroma. Apart from this, metastatic calcification may be seen.

Clinical Features Symptoms of secondary hyperparathyroidism are not so prominent because the symptoms of chronic renal failure dominate the clinical picture. Bony changes are mild and regress with treatment. Metastatic calcification can cause narrowing of the blood vessels, leading to ischaemia in skin, the condition referred to as **calciphylaxis**. Patients generally respond to vitamin D supplements and phosphate binders.

Tertiary Hyperparathyroidism

Tertiary hyperparathyroidism is a state of excessive secretion of PTH following a long period of secondary hyperparathyroidism and resulting in hypercalcaemia. It is due to the development of autonomous parathyroid function following a period of persistent stimulation of parathyroid glands. Surgical removal of three full and one half of the parathyroid glands is the treatment of choice in these cases.

HYPOPARATHYROIDISM

Hypoparathyroidism is characterized by reduced levels of PTH and consequently hypocalcaemia. It can be due to genetic or acquired causes which are described as follows:

- Surgical removal of parathyroid glands in thyroidectomy surgeries
- Autoimmune hypoparathyroidism as a part of autoimmune polyendocrine syndrome due to mutations in the autoimmune regulator gene (AIRE)
- Familial isolated hypoparathyroidism due to mutations in the genes involved in the development of parathyroid glands or in the production of PTH
- As a component of 22q11 deletion syndrome, in which parathyroid glands may be absent.

Clinical Features

The dominant clinical features are because of hypocalcaemia.

The key feature of hypocalcaemia is **tetany** characterized by neuromuscular irritability with symptoms of circumoral numbness, paraesthesia, carpopedal spasm, seizures and laryngospasm leading to choking and death.

Clinical findings include **Chvostek sign**, elicited by tapping the course of the facial nerve and looking for the contractions of the muscles of the eyes, mouth and nose, and **Trousseau sign**, elicited by obstructing the forearm and hand circulation with blood pressure cuff and looking for carpal spasms.

Other clinical features include emotional instability, anxiety, depression, confusion, hallucination and psychosis.

There is also a paradoxical combination of hypocalcaemia with calcification caused by hyperphosphataemia that leads to deposition of phosphate along with the locally available calcium. Such calcification may be seen in basal ganglia and eye lens leading to Parkinson disease–like state and cataract changes.

QT prolongation in the electrocardiogram may occur because of conduction defects induced by hypocalcaemia.

Apart from these, patient may also have dental abnormalities in the form of dental hypoplasia, eruption failures, defective root and enamel formation.

Pseudohypoparathyroidism

Pseudohypoparathyroidism (PHP) is a heterogeneous group of rare endocrine disorders characterized by **resistance to the action of PTH**, manifesting with hypocalcaemia, hyperphosphataemia and increased serum concentration of PTH. Renal function usually is unaffected. There are five variants of PHP.

In 1942, Fuller Albright first introduced the term 'pseudohypoparathyroidism' to describe patients who presented with PTH-resistant hypocalcaemia and hyperphosphataemia along with an unusual combination of developmental and skeletal defects, collectively termed Albright hereditary osteodystrophy. Administration of PTH failed to produce the expected phosphaturia or to stimulate renal production of cAMP in those patients.

The molecular defect lies in the gene ***GNAS1*** encoding the α-subunit of the stimulatory G protein, Gsα, and contributes to at least four different forms of the disease. One subtype is associated with renal resistance to PTH action.

Diagnosis of PHP is defined by the coexistence of hypocalcaemia and hyperphosphataemia with elevated PTH levels in the presence of normal vitamin D values and normal renal function and absence of hypercalciuria.

The goals of treatment are to correct calcium deficiency, prevent complications and reduce morbidity. Intravenous calcium is the initial treatment option for all patients with severe symptomatic hypocalcaemia. Administration of oral calcium and 1α-hydroxylated vitamin D metabolites, such as calcitriol, remains the mainstay of treatment and should be initiated in every patient with a diagnosis of PHP.

III. THE ENDOCRINE PANCREAS

ANATOMY, HISTOLOGY AND PHYSIOLOGY

Anatomy and histology of the pancreas are discussed in Chapter 23. Here, we shall review the physiology of the endocrine pancreas for a better understanding of its diseases.

Physiology of the Pancreas

The pancreas contains around 1 million clusters of cells, the islets of Langerhans, which contain four main types of cells:

- The **alpha (α)-cells** secrete the hormone **glucagon** and make up approximately 20% of each islet. Glucagon plays an important role in blood glucose regulation; low blood glucose levels stimulate its release.
- The **beta (β)-cells** secrete the hormone **insulin** and make up approximately 75% of each islet. Elevated blood glucose levels stimulate the release of insulin.
- The **delta (δ)-cells** account for 4% of the islet cells and secrete the peptide hormone **somatostatin**. Recall that somatostatin is also released by the hypothalamus, stomach and intestines. As an inhibiting hormone, pancreatic somatostatin inhibits the release of both glucagon and insulin.
- The **PP cells** account for approximately 1% of islet cells and secrete the **pancreatic polypeptide hormone**. It is thought to play a role in appetite regulation, as well as in the regulation of pancreatic exocrine and endocrine secretions. Pancreatic polypeptide released following a

meal may reduce further food consumption; however, it is also released in response to fasting.

With this review, we now discuss the pathology of diabetes mellitus (DM) and pancreatic endocrine tumours in the following sections.

DIABETES MELLITUS

PA 32.4

DM is a group of diseases characterized by disturbed carbohydrate metabolism, leading to elevated blood glucose levels (hyperglycaemia) and secretion of glucose in urine (glycosuria) because of insufficient production or functioning of the pancreatic hormone insulin, combined with a few yet undefined predisposing factors.

DM is not a pathogenic entity but a group of aetiologically different metabolic defects. Chronic hyperglycaemia causes long-term secondary damage, dysfunction and failures of various cells, tissues and organs.

History

Clinical features similar to DM were described 3000 years ago by the ancient Egyptians. The term 'diabetes' was first coined by Aretaeus of Cappadocia in CE 81–133. Later, the word 'mellitus' (honey sweet) was added by Thomas Willis (Britain) in 1675, after discovering the sweetness in urine and blood of patients (first noticed by the ancient Indians). It was only in 1776 that Dobson (Britain) confirmed the presence of excess sugar in urine and blood as a cause of the sweetness. In modern time, the history of diabetes coincides with the emergence of experimental medicine. An important milestone in the history of diabetes is the establishment of the role of the liver in glycogenesis and the concept that diabetes is due to excess glucose production by Claude Bernard (France) in 1857. The role of the pancreas in pathogenesis of diabetes was discovered by Mering and Minkowski of Austria in 1889. Later, this discovery constituted the basis for isolation of insulin and clinical use by Banting and Best of Canada in 1921. Trials to prepare an orally administrated hypoglycaemic agent ended successfully by the first marketing of tolbutamide and carbutamide in 1955. History book of diabetes has added many chapters since then and many more are still being added.

Epidemiology

Diabetes is emerging rapidly as one of the most serious health problems of our time. The number of people with diabetes worldwide has more than doubled during the past 20 years, the magnitude which no other disease has ever had. One of the most worrying features of this rapid increase is the emergence of type 2 diabetes in children, adolescents and young adults. Although the role of traditional risk factors for type 2 diabetes, such as genetic, lifestyle and behavioural risk factors, has been given attention, recent research has focussed on identifying the contributions of yet unidentified mechanisms. Most important identified causes include sedentary lifestyle and altered eating habits contributing to obesity and DM. Epidemiological data predict an inexorable and unsustainable increase in global health expenditure attributable to diabetes.

This silent epidemic claims more lives per year than HIV/AIDS and places a severe burden on health care systems and economies worldwide, with the heaviest burden falling on the developing countries. Yet, awareness of the global scale of the diabetes threat remains piteously low. A more recent study provides the following data on diabetes.

Facts and Figures About Diabetes Worldwide

In 2019, approximately 463 million adults (aged 20–79 years) were living with diabetes; by 2045, this figure will rise to 700 million.

The proportion of people with type 2 diabetes is increasing in most countries. Approximately **79%** of adults with diabetes are living in low- and middle-income countries.

One in five people older than 65 years has diabetes.
One in two (232 million) people with diabetes is undiagnosed.
Diabetes has caused 4.2 million deaths.
More than 1.1 million children and adolescents are living with type 1 diabetes.
More than 20 million live births (one in six live births) are affected by diabetes during pregnancy.
Approximately 374 million people are at an increased risk of developing type 2 diabetes.

The present situation of diabetes in developing countries like India is even more worrying because of its rapidly increasing trend not just in incidence but also in the rate of morbidity and mortality associated with it.

Diagnostic Criteria

According to the latest World Health Organization (WHO) and American Diabetes Association (ADA) 2019 guidelines, **one** of the following criteria must be met for a diagnosis of diabetes:

- Fasting plasma glucose (FPG) level 126 mg/dL or more (7.0 mmol/L)
- 2-Hour postprandial glucose level 200 mg/dL or more (11.1 mmol/L) during an oral glucose tolerance test (OGTT)
- HbA_{1c} 6.5% or more (48 mmol/mol)
- Random plasma glucose level 200 mg/dL or more (11.1 mmol/L) in a patient with classic symptoms of hyperglycaemia or hyperglycaemic crisis

  To rule out the possibility of transient hyperglycaemia seen in association with severe infections, burns or trauma, the diagnosis of diabetes requires persistence of hyperglycaemia following recovery from the acute illness.

The WHO criteria for **impaired glucose tolerance** (IGT) are as follows:

- FPG level less than 126 mg/dL (7 mmol/L)
- Plasma glucose level above 140 mg/dL to just below 200 mg/dL (≥7.8 to <11.1 mmol/L) 2 hours after a 75-g glucose load.
- One intervening plasma glucose value at or above 200 mg/dL.

WHO notes that IGT is not a clinical entity but a risk factor for future diabetes and/or adverse outcomes.

These criteria are a better predictor of increased macrovascular risk than the ADA's current intermediate category of impaired fasting glucose (IFG) or prediabetes. Presumably, patients with IFG are at an increased risk for development of DM, but their risk for macrovascular disease does not appear to be as high as for patients with IGT (which is about the same as for patients with frank type 2 diabetes mellitus [T2DM]).

Classification (Table 28.5)

Hyperglycaemia is the defining common feature of all types of diabetes, but aetiology, underlying pathogenic mechanisms, natural history and treatment of the different types of diabetes differ. Ideally, all types of diabetes would be defined by defining features that are specific and exclusive to that type of diabetes. However, some types of diabetes are difficult to classify.

There are many reasons to revisit classification of diabetes. According to the current classification, there are two major types: type 1 and type 2 diabetes. The distinction between the two types has historically been based on the age at onset, degree of loss of β-cell function, degree of insulin resistance, presence of diabetes-associated autoantibodies and requirement of insulin treatment for survival. However, none of these characteristics unequivocally distinguish one type of diabetes from the other, nor account for the entire spectrum of diabetes phenotypes.

Subtyping diabetes is important in clinical care for diagnosis, to guide treatment choices and when making treatment decisions for a person whose glycaemic control is unsatisfactory. An incorrect treatment decision could risk a person developing diabetic ketoacidosis (DKA) or lead to unnecessary insulin therapy in the case of some forms of monogenic diabetes. The phenotype of both T1DM (overweight or obese) and T2DM (younger, normal weight) has changed over time and contributes to clinicians' increasing difficulty in classifying the types of diabetes.

There have been recent calls to review and update the classification system for diabetes. This is because many people with diabetes do not fit into any single category. There have been recent advances in knowledge of pathophysiological pathways and emerging technologies to examine pathology and treatments that act on specific pathways. Finally, there is a trend towards individualized treatment.

- Type 1 and type 2 diabetes are discussed in detail as follows:
- **Monogenic diabetes** can be due to monogenic defects in β-cell function or insulin function, which is a large heterogeneous group of disorders caused by defects in one gene. This group includes all types of MODY – (maturity-onset diabetes of the young).
- **Diseases of the exocrine pancreas** include disorders like fibrocalculous pancreatopathy, pancreatitis, pancreatectomy, trauma, neoplasms, cystic fibrosis and haemochromatosis.
- **Infections** include those caused by cytomegalovirus, congenital rubella, etc.
- **Endocrine disorders** include Cushing syndrome, acromegaly, phaeochromocytoma, hyperthyroidism, glucagonoma, etc.

Before delving into the pathogenesis of diabetes, let us review glucose homeostasis.

Table 28.5 WHO Classification of Diabetes, 2019

Type 1 diabetes
Type 2 diabetes
Hybrid forms of diabetes • Slowly evolving immune-related diabetes of adults • Ketosis-prone type 2 diabetes
Other specific types of diabetes • Monogenic diabetes • Diseases of the exocrine pancreas • Endocrine disorders • Drug or chemical induced • Infections • Uncommon specific forms of immune-mediated diabetes
Unclassified types of diabetes • This category should be used temporarily when there is not a clear diagnostic category, especially close to the time of diagnosis of diabetes
Hyperglycaemia first detected during pregnancy • Diabetes mellitus in pregnancy • Gestational diabetes mellitus

Simpler version of WHO 2019.

Glucose Homeostasis (Fig. 28.32)

Blood glucose level is tightly regulated by three closely related processes:

- Glucose production in the liver
- Uptake and utilization of glucose by peripheral tissues, mainly skeletal muscles
- Actions of insulin and counterregulatory hormones like glucagon on glucose uptake and metabolism

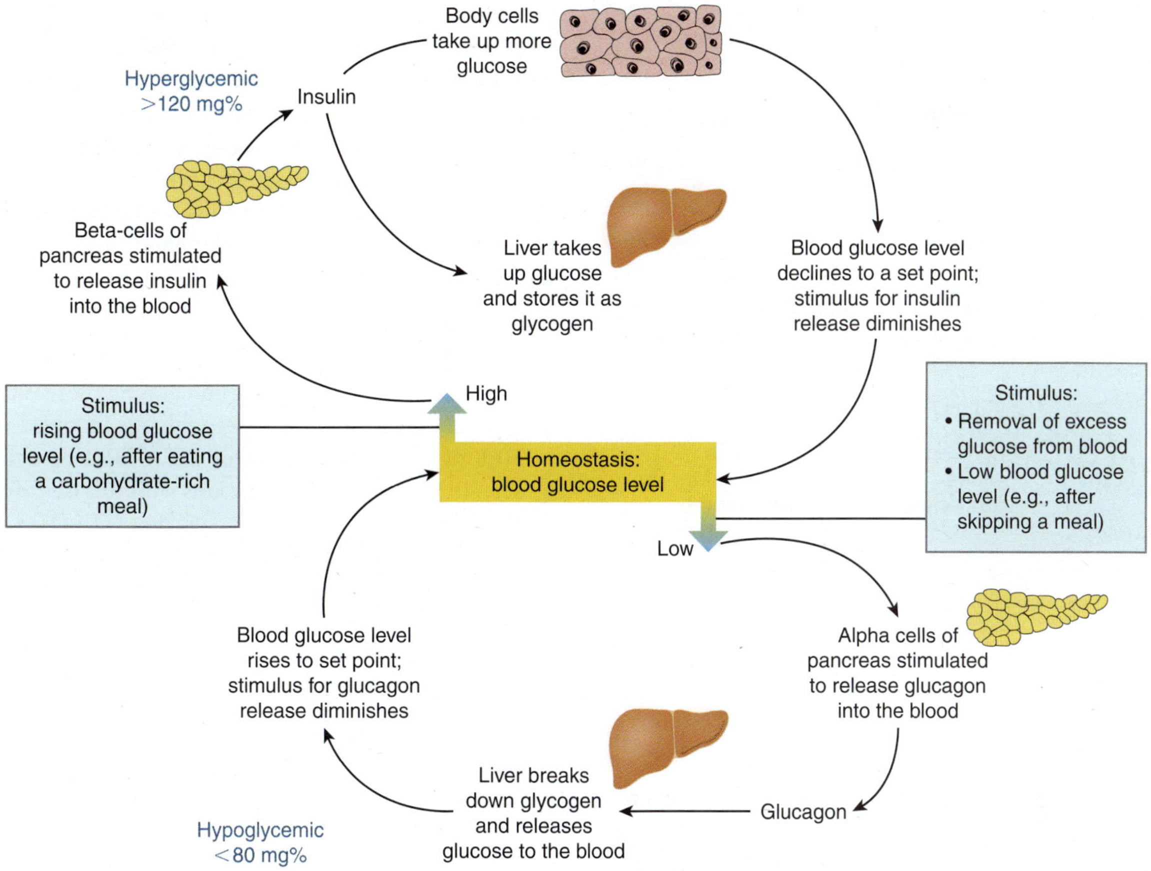

Fig. 28.32 Glucose homeostasis. (*Source:* https://www.google.com/url?sa=i&url=https%3A%2F%2Fwww.researchgate.net%2Ffigure%2FGlucose-homeostasis-in-the-human-body-adapted-from-9_fig1_281056437&psig=AOvVaw3jtaB4-VYDteOxvN3DOMZc&ust=1605786798033000&source=images&cd=vfe&ved=0CAIQjRxqFwoTCKCil5GEjO0CFQAAAAAdAAAAABAD)

Insulin Regulatory Mechanisms

In the insulin synthesis pathway, preproinsulin containing an A-chain, a C-peptide, a B-chain and a signal sequence is translocated into the endoplasmic reticulum of β-cells of the pancreas. The signal sequence is cleaved by a signal peptidase leaving proinsulin. After proinsulin is packaged into vesicles in the Golgi apparatus, the C-peptide is removed, leaving the A-chain and B-chain bound together by disulphide bonds that constitute the insulin molecule.

Glucose-mediated release of insulin: Glucose is the most important stimulus for the synthesis and release of insulin. When there is an increase in blood glucose levels, GLUT-2, a glucose transporter whose function is independent of insulin, facilitates glucose uptake in the pancreatic β-cells, which possess an ATP-sensitive K^+ channel on their membrane. When glucose gets metabolized, ATP molecules are generated, which inhibits the ATP-sensitive K^+ channel, resulting in the membrane depolarization and Ca^{2+} influx. These changes stimulate release of insulin stored within the β-cell granules. This mechanism enables the immediate release of insulin. With the persistence of secretory stimulus, active synthesis of insulin happens.

Incretin-mediated release of insulin: **Incretins** are a group of hormones that act to promote insulin secretion from pancreatic β-cells following food intake. The two incretins are **glucose-dependent insulinotropic polypeptide (GIP)**, secreted by enteroendocrine K cells of the small intestine, and **glucagon-like peptide-1 (GLP-1)**, secreted by L cells in the distal ileum and colon. Elevation of such incretins following food intake is called ***'incretin effect'***. The net result of this incretin effect is insulin release from β-cells coupled with inhibition of glucagon release and delay in gastric emptying. After their release, the incretins are degraded by dipeptidyl peptidases. This incretin effect is blunted in type 2 diabetes. Many researches are currently focussed at increasing the incretin sensitivity and many such drugs are currently in use.

Mechanism of Insulin Action

Insulin has many growth-promoting effects and is the most **anabolic hormone**. The major functions of insulin are as follows (Table 28.6):

- Increase the rate of glucose transport into certain cells like skeletal muscles and adipocytes, thereby increasing the energy level and providing metabolic intermediates required for biosynthetic processes of the cells.
- In muscles, glucose is stored as glycogen or oxidized to ATP, whereas in adipocytes glucose is stored as lipid.

Table 28.6 Metabolic Actions of Insulin

Metabolic Effect	Stimulated by Insulin	Inhibited by Insulin
Carbohydrate metabolism	Glucose transport Glycolysis Glycogen synthesis	Glycogen breakdown Gluconeogenesis
Protein metabolism	Amino acid transport Protein synthesis	Protein breakdown
Lipid metabolism	Triglyceride uptake Lipogenesis	Lipolysis Fatty acid oxidation

- Apart from this lipogenic activity, insulin inhibits lipolysis and proteolysis.
- Insulin has many mitogenic actions, stimulating cell growth and differentiation.

The actions of insulin are summarized in Fig. 28.33.

Insulin receptor is a tetramer with two α- and two β-subunits. Insulin binds to the extracellular domain of the α-subunit following which the β-subunit that possesses tyrosine kinase activity gets activated. This leads to autophosphorylation of the receptor, which, in turn, induces the activation of many intracellular proteins including the insulin receptor substrates (IRSs). This group of substrate proteins activates multiple signalling pathways, promoting metabolic and mitogenic activities. Insulin also promotes the production of GLUT-4, an insulin-sensitive glucose transporter protein which augments glucose intake.

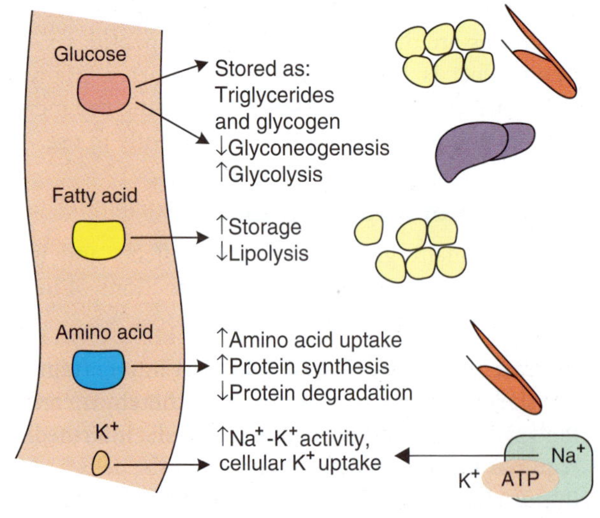

Fig. 28.33 Illustration of insulin actions.

Pathogenesis of Type 1 Diabetes

Autoimmunity is the main aetiology of T1DM. It leads to destruction of islet cells by the immune reactions against β-cells. Type 1 diabetes manifests in the childhood or commonly at puberty and progresses with age. Old terminologies like juvenile diabetes and insulin-dependent DM are now considered imprecise. Both genetic and environmental factors are involved in the evolution of type 1 diabetes.

Genetic susceptibility

More than 30 susceptibility loci have been identified for type 1 diabetes. Most important among these is the HLA gene cluster located on 6p21 which is involved in up to 50% of cases. **HLA-DR2 or HLA-DR4** association is seen in 90%–95% of Caucasians with this disease. When these HLA haplotypes are associated with **DQ8** concurrently, the inherited risk is highest in sibling studies.

Apart from these HLA genes, many non-HLA genes are also involved in the pathogenesis of type 1 diabetes. Few such genes are insulin, polymorphisms of **CTLA4, PTPN22** genes and mutations in the **AIRE** gene.

Environmental factors

Environmental factors play a major role in type 1 diabetes. The most common factor linked is viral infections. The mechanisms by which viral infections precipitate autoimmune reactions are explained in detail in Chapter 6.

Mechanisms of β-cell destruction

Though the autoimmune disease process starts earlier, the disease manifests with its classical features only after 90% of β-cells are destroyed by the autoimmune reaction. The target antigens for autoimmunity are glutamic acid decarboxylase and islet cell autoantigen 512. The mechanisms of cell injury and death caused by autoimmune reactions are explained in Chapter 6. In short, T_H1 helper T cells and cytotoxic T cells mediate β-cell destruction through their cytokines. Autoantibodies are suspected to play a role in the development of type 1 diabetes, but it is still not completely proven.

Pathogenesis of Type 2 Diabetes (Fig. 28.34)

T2DM is a disease with **proinflammatory state**, and its pathogenesis revolves around genetic and environmental factors. The pathogenesis of type 2 diabetes ordinarily begins with the development of insulin resistance and gets compounded later with other factors.

Genetic Factors Concordance rate of greater than 90% is seen in monozygotic twins; with first-degree relatives, the risk of developing this disease is 5- to 10-fold higher. At least 30 genetic loci have been identified, but most of the polymorphisms are associated with insulin secretion.

Environmental Factors **Central obesity** is the most important environmental risk factor for type 2 diabetes

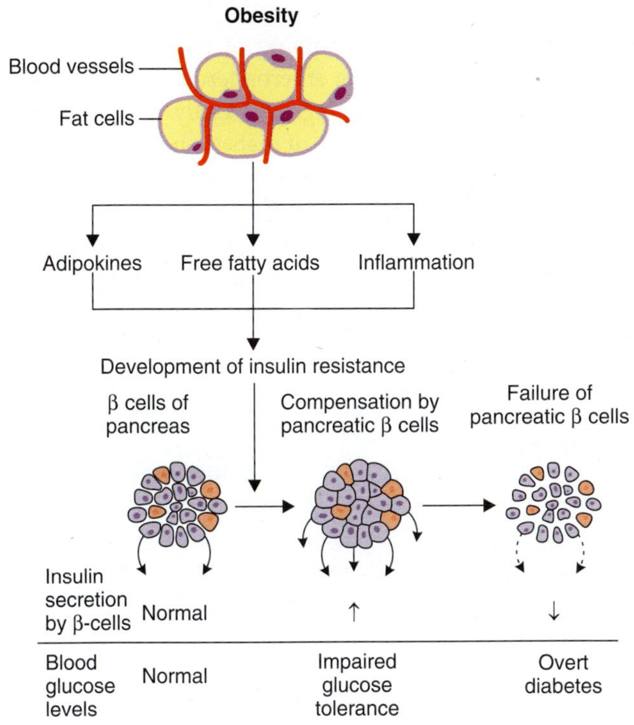

Fig. 28.34 Development of type 2 diabetes.

and is associated with more than 80% of patients. The major mechanism by which obesity contributes to the development of type 2 diabetes is insulin resistance. Apart from obesity, sedentary lifestyle is also a strong risk factor for type 2 diabetes. Hence, weight loss, when coupled with lifestyle modification through exercises, improves insulin sensitivity and benefits patients with type 2 diabetic.

Metabolic Abnormalities in Type 2 Diabetes The two major metabolic defects in type 2 diabetes are as follows:

1. **Insulin resistance**, in which peripheral tissues like skeletal muscles, adipocytes and liver have decreased response to insulin. In the early phase, insulin resistance partners with compensatory β-cell hyperfunction with the resultant hyperinsulinaemia.
2. **β-Cell dysfunction**, due to their failure to adapt to the increased secretion insulin, leads to decreased insulin secretion and contributes to already existing hyperglycaemia in the later phase of the disease.

Both the defects are discussed in detail here.

Insulin Resistance Insulin resistance is seen in the tissues which are normally sensitive to insulin. Insulin resistance leads to the following results:

- Failure to inhibit glycogenolysis
- Failure to promote glucose uptake and glycogenesis in skeletal muscles
- Failure to inhibit lipolysis, resulting in elevated levels of free fatty acids

Role of obesity in insulin resistance As mentioned earlier, obesity is the major contributing factor for insulin resistance and the probable mechanisms are explained as follows:

- **Excess free fatty acids** available in obesity lead to the accumulation of intermediates like diacylglycerol (DAG) which would blunt signalling through insulin receptors.
- **Adipokines** are hormones secreted by adipocytes. In diabetes associated with obesity, the adipokines that encourage hyperglycaemia are elevated and the ones that promote insulin sensitivity such as adiponectin are decreased (Fig. 28.34).
- Elevated levels of free fatty acids and glucose contribute to the **proinflammatory state** seen in diabetes which would ultimately result in insulin resistance and β-cell dysfunction.

β-Cell Dysfunction It is the β-cell dysfunction that results in the development of frank diabetes. Insulin resistance stimulates the β-cells to produce more insulin, and at a point the β-cells are exhausted and no longer able to continue in this altered state. At this point, hyperinsulinaemic state gets replaced by the state of relative insulin deficiency. The factors responsible for β-cell dysfunction are as follows:

- **Lipotoxicity** induced by excess free fatty acids
- **Glucotoxicity** imposed by excess glucose
- **Abnormal incretin effect** inhibiting synthesis of GIP and GLP-1 hormones
- **Amyloid deposition** in the islets seen in almost all patients with long-standing type 2 diabetes

Chronic Complications

The chronic complications of diabetes fall under two categories:

1. **Diabetic macrovascular disease**
   - Atherosclerosis
2. **Diabetic microvascular disease**
   - Retinopathy
   - Nephropathy
   - Neuropathy

Pathogenesis of Chronic Complications Chronic complications stem from hyperglycaemia, insulin resistance and obesity.

Mechanisms Underlying the Development of Complications

1. Formation of advanced glycation end products (AGEs)
2. Activation of protein kinase C
3. Oxidative stress and disturbances in polyol pathways
4. Hexosamine pathways and the formation of fructose-6-phosphate

These mechanisms contribute to end-organ damages associated with diabetes and are discussed briefly here.

1. **Formation of advanced glycation end products**

   AGEs are the products of nonenzymatic reactions that occur between intracellular glucose-derived dicarbonyl precursors and the amino groups of intracellular and extracellular proteins. In the presence of hyperglycaemia, production rate of AGEs is accelerated.

   The receptors for AGEs are RAGE expressed on inflammatory cells, vascular endothelial cells and smooth muscle cells.

   Effects of AGEs are as follows:
   - Deposition of extracellular matrix within walls of blood vessels through release of cytokines and growth factors
   - Enhanced expression of VEGF that plays a dominant role in the development of diabetic retinopathy
   - Cause oxidative stress to the endothelial cells through generation of reactive oxygen species
   - Tilting the endothelium towards procoagulant activity
   - Proliferation of vascular smooth muscle cells and synthesis of extracellular matrix
   - Direct cross-linking of extracellular matrix proteins, leading to loss of vessel wall elasticity, decrease in endothelial cell adhesion, extravasation of fluid and trapping of proteins like LDL, thereby augmenting atherosclerosis and basement membrane thickening, especially in glomeruli. This is the key feature of diabetic nephropathy.
2. **Activation of protein kinase C**

   Hyperglycaemia leads to excessive synthesis of DAG from glycolytic intermediates. These DAG molecules activate intracellular protein kinase C which mediates many downstream events including the production of VEGF, TGF-β and the procoagulant plasminogen activator inhibitor-1.
3. **Oxidative stress and disturbances in polyol pathways** (Fig. 28.35)

   With persistent hyperglycaemia, intracellular glucose levels rise in tissues such as nerves, lens, kidneys and blood vessels that are not dependent on insulin for glucose transport. The excess glucose gets converted to sorbitol by the action of aldose reductase and then to fructose through a reaction that consumes NADPH. This consumption of NADPH in the polyol pathway depletes the reserve of NADPH, affecting the formation of reduced glutathione (synthesis of reduced glutathione needs NADPH). The net result is the reduced availability of the antioxidant and reduced glutathione and the cell suffers oxidative stress.

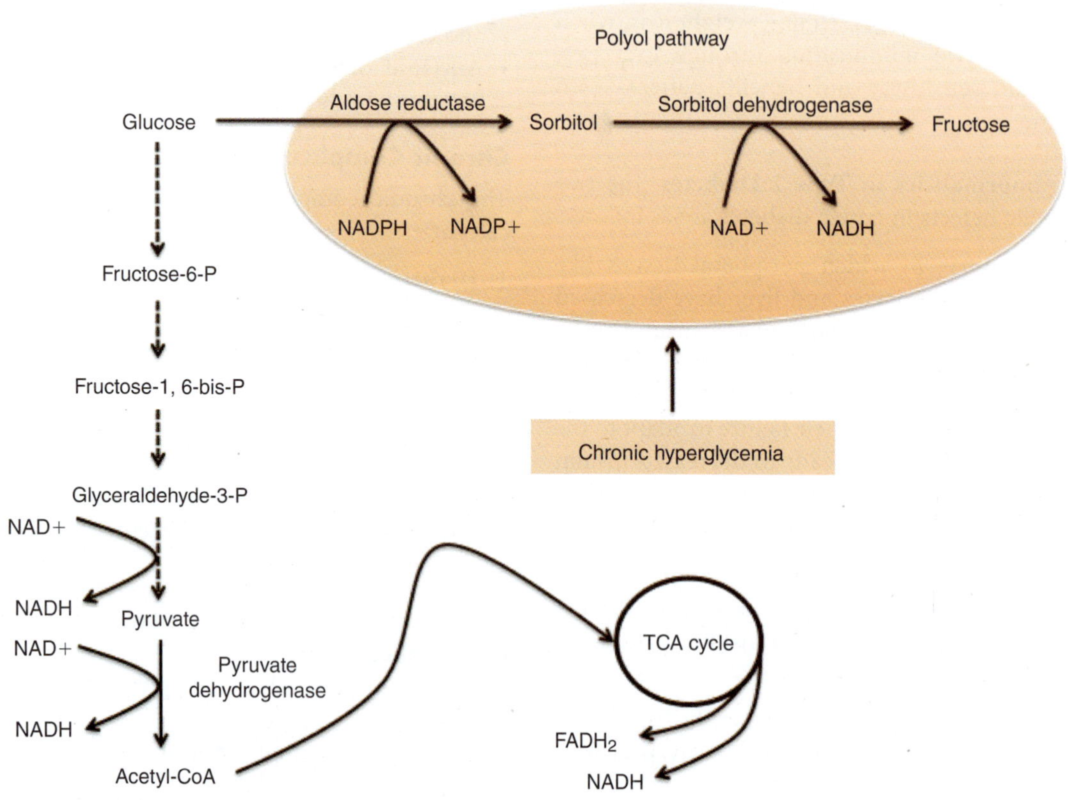

Fig. 28.35 Disturbances in polyol pathways seen in diabetes. Note the depletion of NADPH due to activation of the polyol pathway. (*Source:* Luo X, Wu J, Jing S, Yan LJ. Hyperglycemic Stress and Carbon Stress in Diabetic Glucotoxicity. Aging and Disease. 2016 Jan;7(1):90-110.)

4. **Hexosamine pathways and the formation of fructose-6-phosphate**
   Chronic hyperglycaemia also induces the hexosamine pathways leading to the formation of fructose-6-phosphate which results in the production of excess proteoglycans.

Morphology

Morphology of organs in diabetes is discussed under the following headings: Morphological changes seen in pancreas, diabetic macrovascular disease and microvascular diseases including diabetic nephropathy, retinopathy and neuropathy.

1. **Pancreas**
   Morphological changes in the pancreas are not diagnostic and are not constant findings. These are more often seen in type 1 diabetes rather than type 2 diabetes. The pancreas may show one or more of the following changes in diabetes:
   - Decrease in the number and size of islets
   - Lymphocytic infiltration of the islets
   - Mild reduction in islet cells mass in type 2 diabetes
   - Amyloid deposition within islets in type 2 diabetes
   - Increase in the number and size of the islets induced by maternal hyperglycaemia is a striking feature seen in newborns of diabetic mothers
2. **Macrovascular disease**
   The hallmark feature of diabetic macrovascular changes is **accelerated atherosclerosis** affecting the aorta and other large- and medium-sized blood vessels. Atherosclerosis leads to myocardial infarction and gangrene of the lower extremities, which are extremely common in diabetic patients when compared to nondiabetic patients. Morphology of blood vessels in atherosclerosis is discussed in Chapter 13. Apart from atherosclerosis, hyaline arteriolosclerosis affecting the arterioles also occurs, with a higher incidence in diabetic patients.
3. **Microvascular disease**
   The most characteristic feature of diabetic microangiopathy is diffuse thickening of the basement membrane of the blood vessels of skin, skeletal muscle, retina, renal glomeruli and many nonvascular structures. Despite basement membrane thickening, the blood vessels are leakier in diabetes. This microangiopathy is the basis of diabetic nephropathy, retinopathy and neuropathy. The morphological changes seen in these conditions are described here.
   Diabetic nephropathy
   Diabetic nephropathy is characterized by three major changes in the kidney – **glomerular lesions, vascular lesions and pyelonephritis**.
   A. **Glomerular lesions:** The characteristic glomerular lesions are capillary basement membrane thickening, diffuse mesangial sclerosis and nodular glomerulosclerosis.
      1. **Basement membrane thickening** is not only a universal finding but also the earliest renal finding in diabetes and affects both glomeruli and tubules.
      2. **Diffuse mesangial sclerosis** is due to the increase in mesangial matrix with PAS-positive deposits. Such expansion of the mesangium correlates well with declining renal function and is a marker of disease progression.
      3. **Nodular glomerulosclerosis**, also referred to as **intercapillary glomerulosclerosis** or **Kimmelstiel–Wilson disease**, is due to the deposition of matrix nodules in the periphery of glomerulus. It is a unique feature of diabetes and is pathognomonic of diabetic nephropathy. As the disease progresses, the nodules enlarge and compress the glomerular capillaries. Such nodular lesions are accompanied by the prominent deposition of hyaline material in the capillary loops referred to as '**fibrin caps**' or attached to the Bowman capsule, in which case, they are referred to as '**capsular drops**'.
   B. **Renal vascular changes** are atherosclerosis and arteriolosclerosis, and their morphology is the same as that in other sites.
   C. **Pyelonephritis** is more common in diabetic patients and one special pattern of acute pyelonephritis, **necrotizing papillitis**, is highly prevalent among diabetic patients.
   Diabetic retinopathy
   Eye is one of the commonly affected organs in diabetes. The damages suffered by eyes in diabetes are as follows:
   - Diabetic retinopathy
   - Cataract
   - Glaucoma
   Diabetic neuropathy
   This is seen in almost every patient living with diabetes for more than 15 years and at least half of them present with symptoms. Morphological changes are discussed in Chapter 31.

Clinical Features

Initially, it was thought that type 1 diabetes starts its manifestations in patients younger than 18 years, but now it is understood that it can occur at any age. Though β-cell destruction starts earlier, some acute stress such as infections precipitate the typical manifestations of type 1 diabetes many years after the onset of β-cell dysfunction.

On the other hand, patients of type 2 diabetes are older than 40 years and are obese in most cases. However, this trend is showing a shift towards younger age groups because of the rapid increase in the incidence of childhood and adolescent obesity and changing lifestyles. Most of these patients remain asymptomatic and are diagnosed during routine blood investigations.

The Triad of Diabetes

Onset of type 1 diabetes is characterized by the triad of symptoms due to metabolic derangements – **polyuria, polyphagia and polydipsia** (Fig. 28.36).

Polyuria is the result of osmotic diuresis induced by glycosuria, which occurs when hyperglycaemia exceeds the renal threshold for glucose. Polyuria and the intracellular dehydration caused by hyperosmolarity due to hyperglycaemia are the reasons for polydipsia. The switch in metabolism from the anabolic to catabolic state in the face of insulin deficiency causes a negative energy balance leading to polyphagia.

Despite the increased appetite and catabolic effects, loss of muscle mass and body weight is characteristic of type 1 diabetes.

Complications of Diabetes

Complications seen in diabetic patients are classified into acute metabolic complications and chronic complications. We discuss the complications under these two headings.

Acute Metabolic Complications

1. The most important acute metabolic complication of both types of diabetes is **hypoglycaemia.** This is

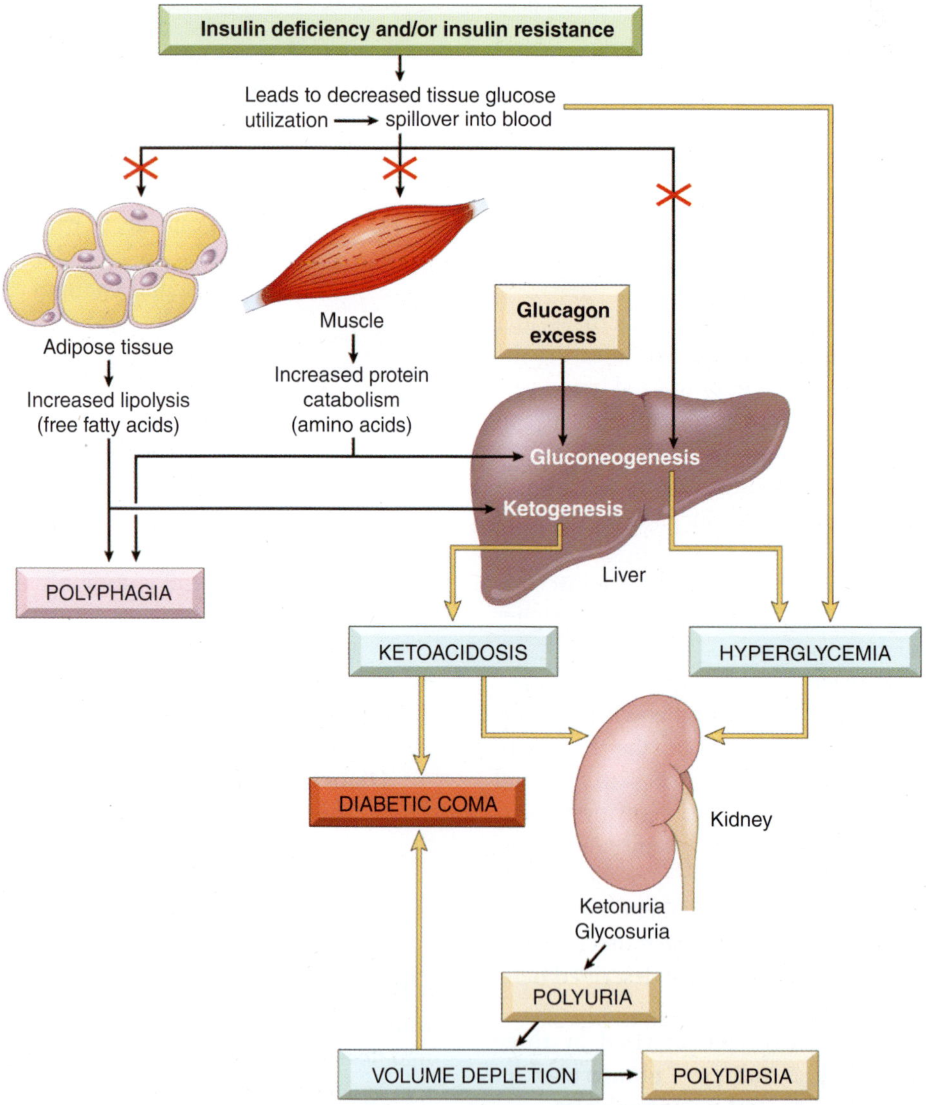

Fig. 28.36 Metabolic derangements as the basis for clinical manifestations in diabetes. Sequence of metabolic derangements seen underlying the clinical manifestations of diabetes. An absolute insulin deficiency leads to a catabolic state, culminating in ketoacidosis and severe volume depletion. These cause sufficient central nervous system compromise that leads to coma and eventual death if left untreated.

usually precipitated by missing a meal, exertion, excess insulin administration or drug overdose. The signs and symptoms include sweating, palpitation, tachycardia, dizziness and confusion. If hypoglycaemia is prolonged and untreated, loss of consciousness occurs, which may later complicate with the development of coma. Oral or intravenous administration of glucose corrects hypoglycaemia.

2. The other most important and dangerous acute metabolic complication of diabetes, especially type 1, is **DKA**. This is the result of insulin deficiency paired with excess glucagon, shifting the metabolism to gluconeogenesis. This leads to exaggerated hyperglycaemia, with osmotic diuresis leading to severe dehydration and ketoacidotic state. In the face of insulin deficiency, ketogenic machinery gets activated. Ketone bodies are the products of oxidation of fatty acyl-CoA molecules, generated by esterification of excess free fatty acids by the action of lipoprotein lipase. This leads to ketonaemia and ketonuria characterized by the presence of ketone bodies in blood and urine, respectively. If dehydration supervenes, urinary excretion of ketone bodies is compromised, resulting in systemic metabolic ketoacidosis, which is a medical emergency. Treatment includes insulin administration with the correction of metabolic acidosis and specific treatment of the precipitating diseases. Ketoacidosis is precipitated in patients because of failure to take insulin or because of other stress such as infections, trauma and drugs. Patients with DKA present with nausea, vomiting, excessive fatigue, acute abdominal pain, a characteristic fruity odour and Kussmaul breathing, a deep laboured breathing. Uncorrected and prolonged state of ketoacidosis leads to CNS depression and eventually coma.
3. Like the high frequency of DKA in type 1 diabetes, type 2 diabetes is associated with **hyperosmolar hyperosmotic syndrome** (HHS). This syndrome typically affects people older than 60 years with polyuria but with no compensatory water intake leading to severe dehydration and hyperosmolarity. In such conditions, the plasma glucose is in the range of 600–1200 mg/dL.

Consequences of Chronic Diabetes

Chronic complications are the major cause of morbidity and mortality in diabetic patients. Such complications take an average 15–20 years to develop and their severity is directly proportional to the degree and duration of diabetes.

Complications stemming from chronic uncontrolled diabetes are as follows:

1. **Macrovascular diseases** leading to myocardial infarction, renal ischaemia and stroke are the most common causes of mortality in diabetic patients.
2. **Diabetic nephropathy** leading to renal failure is one of the leading causes of morbidity and mortality in diabetic patients.
3. **Visual disturbances** and even total blindness are the consequences of diabetic retinopathy.
4. **Distal symmetric polyneuropathy, autonomic neuropathy and diabetic mononeuropathy** are all consequences of diabetic neuropathy.
5. Apart from these, diabetics are vulnerable to many **infections** of the skin, lungs, kidney and other organs. The mechanisms by which their immune response is altered are beyond the scope of this book.

HbA_{1c}

Glycated haemoglobin, also called HbA_{1c} or haemoglobin A_{1c}, is a form of haemoglobin that is chemically linked to a sugar. The formation of sugar–haemoglobin linkage indicates the presence of excess sugar in the bloodstream and is most often indicative of diabetes. HbA_{1c} is of particular interest as it is easy to detect. The process by which glucose attaches to haemoglobin is called glycation and hence the name glycated haemoglobin. HbA_{1c} is a measure of β-*N*-1-deoxy fructosyl component of haemoglobin.

It is measured

- To determine the 3-month average of blood sugar level
- As a diagnostic test for DM
- An assessment for glycaemic control in diabetic patients

The test is limited to 3-month average because of the average life span of red cells which varies around 4 months. Normal levels of blood glucose produce a normal amount of glycated haemoglobin. As the average blood glucose increases, the fraction of glycated haemoglobin increases. In diabetic patients, higher amounts of glycated haemoglobin indicate poor glycaemic control.

The reference range of glycated haemoglobin is as shown as follows:

HbA_{1c}	Diagnosis
<5.7%	Normal
5.7%–6.4%	Prediabetes
>6.5%	Diabetes
>7%	Poor glycaemic control in diabetic patients

PANCREATIC NEUROENDOCRINE TUMOURS

Pancreatic neuroendocrine tumours (PanNETs) are rare tumours of the pancreatic islet cells. These tumours arise from any portion of the pancreas and can be benign or malignant, single or multiple, functional elaborating hormones or nonfunctional. There are no definite morphological criteria for malignancy, and the malignant nature of these tumours is revealed by their metastases, local invasion and vascular invasion. It is observed that 90% of insulin-producing tumours are benign and 60%–90% of all other tumours irrespective of their hormone status are malignant. The genes associated with PanNETs are MEN1,

PTEN, TSC2, alpha-thalassaemia/mental retardation syndrome, X-linked (ATRX), and death-domain associated protein (DAXX).

Here, in this chapter, we discuss the three common clinical syndromes associated with functional pancreatic neoplasms:

- **Hyperinsulinism**
- **Zollinger–Ellison syndrome (ZES)**
- **Multiple endocrine neoplasia (MEN)**

Hyperinsulinism, Insulinoma, β-Cell Tumours

Though rare, these tumours are the most common pancreatic endocrine neoplasms with sufficient production of insulin to cause clinically significant **hyperinsulinaemic hypoglycaemia**. The tumours are seen in older adults, more often in women. A majority of these tumours are benign, with only 5%–10% being malignant.

Morphology

Insulinomas are more common in the head of the pancreas. A majority of the insulinomas are small, and multiple insulinomas are associated with MEN1 syndrome. Its cut surface shows an encapsulated, yellow-tan homogeneous appearance.

Microscopically, the tumour cells resemble giant islets, with cells arranged in trabecular, nested or solid patterns. Individual cells are like any other neuroendocrine tumour cells. Amyloid deposition is characteristically seen in most of the tumours.

Clinical Features Though insulin secretion is seen in 80% of patients, only 20% develop the classical **Whipple triad**, which includes the following:

- Hypoglycaemia symptoms
- Blood glucose levels less than 50 mg/dL
- Symptoms relieved by glucose or symptoms precipitated by fasting or exercise

In other symptomatic cases, hypoglycaemia is mild and the Whipple triad does not manifest. Laboratory investigations confirm the high circulating levels of insulin coupled with a high insulin to glucose ratio. Complete reversal of the symptoms happens with surgical removal of the tumour. Tumour cells are immunohistochemically positive for neuroendocrine markers. Tumours greater than 2 cm are associated with a poorer prognosis.

Zollinger–Ellison Syndrome, Gastrinomas

ZES is caused by a non–β-islet cell, gastrin-secreting tumour of the pancreas that stimulates the acid-secreting cells of the gastric mucosa, with consequent gastrointestinal mucosal ulceration. Cells of origin of these tumours are believed to be the endocrine cells of the gut or the pancreas. **The triad of pancreatic islet cell lesions, hypersecretion of gastric acid and severe peptic ulceration** was first noted by Zollinger and Ellison and hence the name of the tumour.

ZES can occur as sporadic tumours or as part of MEN1 syndrome.

Morphology

The tumours are usually solitary and arise from the so-called **gastrinoma triangle** (Fig. 28.37) formed by the duodenum and peripancreatic soft tissue. In tumours occurring with MEN1 association, these tend to be multifocal. In more than 50% of cases, the tumours are locally invasive and/or metastatic at the time of diagnosis. Tumour cells are bland, and even malignant cells do not express anaplasia. Duodenal and gastric mucosae have multiple peptic ulcers which are resistant to conventional antiulcer treatments. In patients with peptic ulcers in unusual locations like jejunal mucosa, ZES should be suspected and evaluated accordingly.

Clinical Features Apart from the abdominal pain caused by peptic ulcerations, at least half of the patients present with diarrhoea. Management of ZES includes excision of the neoplasm along with use of H^+K^+-ATPase inhibitors for peptic ulcer management. Patients with liver metastases have a guarded prognosis.

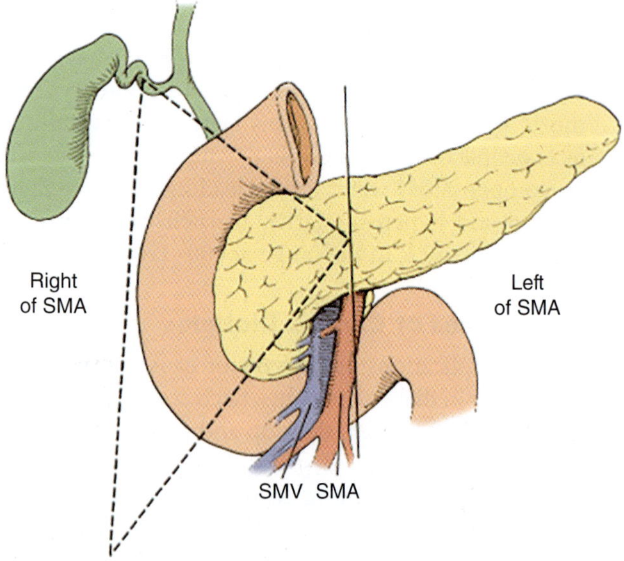

Fig. 28.37 Gastrinoma triangle. Approximately 90% of gastrinomas are thought to arise in this anatomic location. The apex is at the junction of the cystic duct and common bile duct, the inferior aspect lies at the junction of the second and third parts of the duodenum and the medial extent lies at the junction of the head and body of the pancreas. SMA, superior mesenteric artery; SMV, superior mesenteric vein. (*Source:* From Bharti Rathore. Gastrinoma. Elsevier 2022.)

Multiple Endocrine Neoplasia Syndromes

The MEN syndromes are a group of inherited diseases associated with proliferative lesions in multiple endocrine organs. The characteristic features of tumours of the MEN syndrome complex are listed as follows (Fig. 28.38; Table 28.7):

- Tumours affect younger patients.
- Synchronous or metachronous tumours affect multiple endocrine organs.
- Multifocality of tumours can be seen.
- Hyperplastic phase precedes the development of tumour in most lesions.
- The tumours are of aggressive nature with a high rate of recurrence.

There are two types of MEN syndrome, MEN1 and MEN2, which is further subdivided into MEN2A, MEN2B and familial medullary thyroid cancer (FMTC).

MEN1

MEN1 syndrome, also called **Wermer** syndrome, is characterized by diseases of the parathyroid, pancreas and pituitary glands. This syndrome is caused by germline mutation in the MEN1 tumour suppressor gene that normally codes for **menin**. The syndrome is characterized by the following features:

- Parathyroid hyperplasia and adenoma
- Pancreatic endocrine tumours
- Pituitary adenomas most commonly prolactinoma

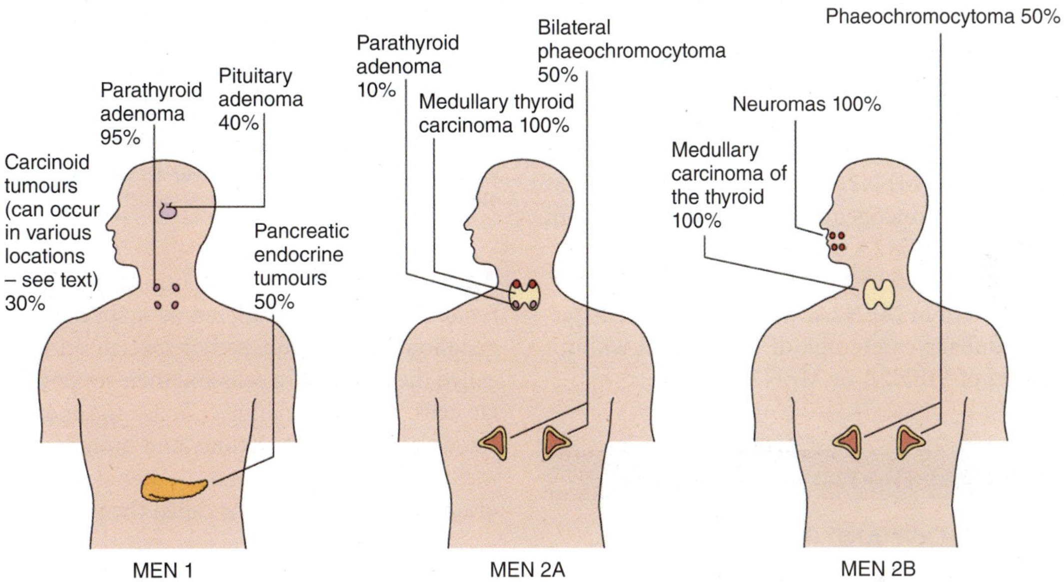

Fig. 28.38 Features of MEN syndromes – illustration. (*Source*: From Harikrashna B. Bhatt, Russell E. Bratman. Multiple Endocrine Neoplasia. Elsevier 2022.)

Table 28.7 Features of MEN Syndromes

Lesion	MEN1 (Wermer)	MEN2A (Sipple)	MEN2B	FMTC
Pituitary adenoma	+			
Parathyroid hyperplasia and adenoma	+	+		
Pancreatic tumours	+			
Medullary thyroid carcinoma		+	+	+
Phaeochromocytoma		+	+	
Paraganglioma				
Insulinoma				
Neuromas and ganglioneuromas of skin and mucosa			+	
Others	Duodenal gastrinoma		Marfanoid habitus	

(*Source:* From Jill P. Crandall and Harry Shamoon. Diabetes Mellitus. Goldman-Cecil Medicine. 26th edition. Elsevier 2020.)

- Along with other tumours such as duodenal gastrinomas, thyroid and adrenocortical adenomas, and lipomas

MEN2

MEN2 syndrome is subclassified into three categories – MEN2A, MEN2B and FMTC.

MEN2A

It is also called **Sipple** syndrome and is characterized by phaeochromocytoma, medullary carcinoma thyroid and parathyroid hyperplasia. MEN2A is due to the germline gain-of-function mutation of **RET** proto-oncogene located on chromosome 10q11.2. If these patients test positive for RET mutation with a family history, prophylactic thyroidectomy is offered to prevent the development of highly aggressive medullary carcinoma thyroid.

MEN2B

Patients with MEN2B syndrome develop medullary thyroid carcinoma and phaeochromocytoma. In addition to these tumours, the syndrome includes neuromas and ganglioneuromas of the skin, mucosa and a marfanoid habitus. MEN2B is due to germline mutation of RET proto-oncogene, which is different from RET mutation of MEN2A.

FMTC

FMTC is a variant of MEN2A, with a strong predisposition to medullary carcinoma of the thyroid without other features of MEN2A or MEN2B.

IV. THE ADRENAL GLAND

ANATOMY, HISTOLOGY AND PHYSIOLOGY

The adrenal gland, also called suprarenal gland, is composed of two embryologically, morphologically and physiologically distinct tissues – the cortex and the medulla. Adrenal cortex is a derivative of the mesoderm which arises from an isolated clump of cells within the urogenital ridge, known as adrenal–gonadal primordium. Adrenal medulla develops from neuroectoderm and is composed of neuroendocrine cells.

The adrenal cortex is the outermost layer of the adrenal gland. The cortex has three distinct layers called 'zones' (Fig. 28.39).

Zona glomerulosa, the outermost layer under the capsule, is the main site for the production of aldosterone, a mineralocorticoid that plays an important role in the regulation of blood pressure.

Zona fasciculata is the middle layer situated between the zona glomerulosa and reticularis. This layer is responsible for the production of glucocorticoids such as cortisol.

Zona reticularis, the innermost layer, produces androgens, mainly dehydroepiandrosterone (DHEA), DHEA sulphate (DHEA-S) and androstenedione, the precursor of testosterone.

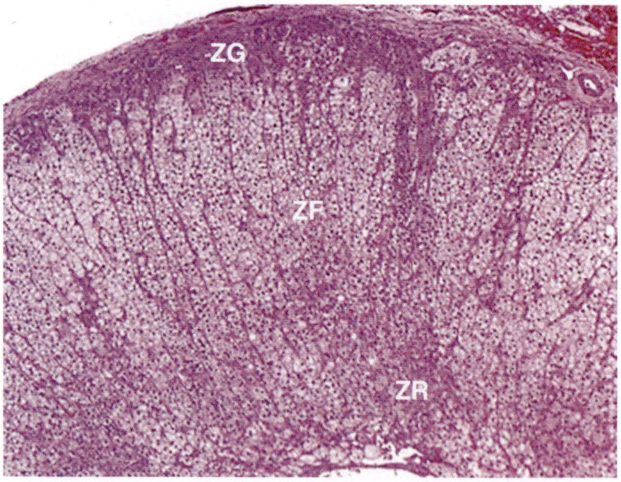

Fig. 28.39 Histology of the adrenal gland – zona glomerulosa (ZG) is at the top of the field beneath the adrenal capsule and forms a thin, discontinuous layer of cells. Most of the cortex is occupied by radial interconnecting cords of zona fasciculata (ZF), which contain cells with pale-staining, lipid-rich cytoplasm. The zona reticularis (ZR) has interconnecting short cords of cells with compact, eosinophilic cytoplasm and congested microvasculature. (*Source:* From Ernest E. Lack and Edina Paal. Adrenal Glands. Urologic Surgical Pathology. 4th edition. Elsevier 2020.)

Adrenal medulla is at the centre of the adrenal gland. Adrenal medulla is considered as a specialized sympathetic ganglion and is composed of specialized neural crest cells called the chromaffin cells and their supporting sustentacular cells. The chromaffin cells are the main source of the catecholamines, adrenaline and noradrenaline. Adrenal medulla along with the extra-adrenal clusters and nodules of neuroendocrine cells is called the paraganglion system.

Diseases of the adrenal cortex and medulla are discussed separately.

DISORDERS OF THE ADRENAL CORTEX

Diseases of the adrenal cortex are divided into hyperfunction, hypofunction and neoplasms.

The diseases of adrenal hyperfunction are due to the hypersecretion of three important hormones of adrenal cortex:

- Cushing syndrome due to excess cortisol
- Hyperaldosteronism due to excess aldosterone
- Adrenogenital or virilizing syndromes due to excess androgens

Cushing Syndrome, Hypercortisolism PA 32.8

Cushing syndrome, also called hypercortisolism, is the collection of signs and symptoms due to prolonged exposure to excessive glucocorticoid hormone. Cushing syndrome can be due to exogenous or endogenous causes (Fig. 28.40). The endogenous causes are divided into ACTH dependent and ACTH independent and are listed in Table 28.8. The most common exogenous cause is the

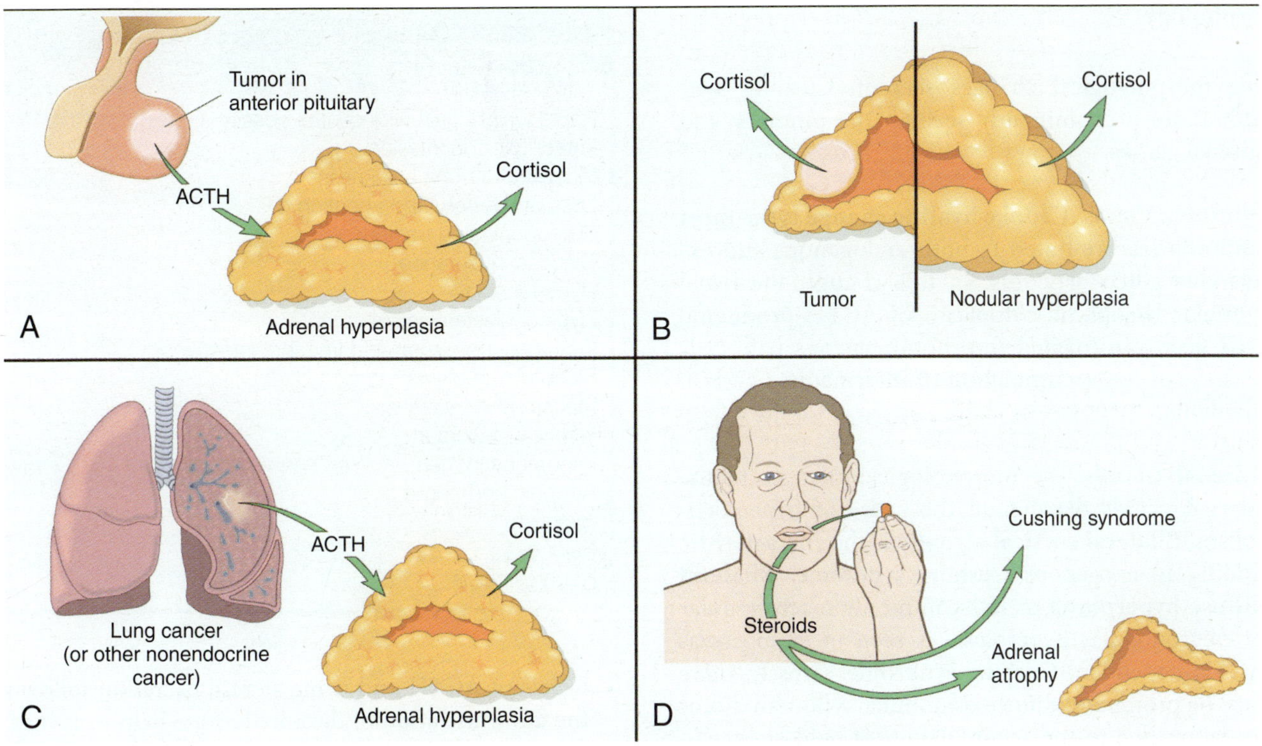

Fig. 28.40 Illustration of various forms of Cushing syndrome. The three endogenous forms and the more common exogenous (iatrogenic) form: (A) pituitary Cushing syndrome; (B) paraneoplastic Cushing syndrome; (C) adrenal Cushing syndrome; and (D) iatrogenic Cushing syndrome. ACTH, adrenocorticotropic hormone.

administration of glucocorticoids, also called iatrogenic Cushing syndrome.

Pathogenesis '**Cushing disease**' is the term used for endogenous hypercortisolism due to ACTH-secreting **pituitary adenomas**. This entity is more common in young women and is characterized by a variable degree of bilateral nodular cortical hyperplasia induced by the elevated levels of ACTH. **Ectopic ACTH** production by tumours like small cell carcinoma of the lung, carcinoids and medullary carcinoma of the thyroid is responsible for approximately 10% of cases of Cushing syndrome and this entity is more common in men older than 40 years. Just like Cushing disease, the adrenal glands show **bilateral cortical hyperplasia**.

ACTH-independent Cushing syndrome is most commonly due to adrenal adenoma and carcinoma and is characterized by highly elevated cortisol levels coupled with low levels of ACTH. In situations with unilateral neoplasm, the uninvolved ipsilateral adrenal cortex and the uninvolved contralateral cortex undergo atrophy because of suppression of ACTH.

Table 28.8 Causes of Cushing Syndrome

Category	Subcategory	Diseases
Endogenous	ACTH dependent	• Cushing disease • ACTH-producing pituitary adenoma[a] • Ectopic corticotropin syndrome
	ACTH independent	• Adrenal adenoma • Adrenal carcinoma • Macronodular hyperplasia • Primary pigmented nodular adrenal disease • McCune–Albright syndrome due to GNAS mutation
Exogenous	Iatrogenic administration of glucocorticoids[b]	

[a]Most common endogenous cause.
[b]Most common cause.

Morphology

The morphological changes seen in Cushing syndrome are predominantly seen in the pituitary and adrenal glands.

Pituitary glands **Crooke hyaline change** is the most common feature noted in both endogenous and exogenous glucocorticoids. In this change, the usual granular basophilic cytoplasm of ACTH-producing cells gets transformed into homogeneous pale cells because of the accumulation of intermediate keratin filaments.

Adrenal Glands The morphological changes in the adrenal glands depend on the cause of hypercortisolism. **Bilateral cortical atrophy** is the characteristic finding in exogenous Cushing syndrome. **Bilateral diffuse hyperplasia** or less commonly macronodular or micronodular hyperplasia is seen in endogenous ACTH-dependent Cushing syndrome. Grossly, there may be prominent diffuse or nodular yellowish discolouration due to the accumulation of lipid-rich cells. Microscopic examination highlights the presence of expanded zona reticularis composed of eosinophilic cells and an outer zone of lipid-rich zona fasciculata in diffuse hyperplasia. In macronodular hyperplasia, there is an admixture of eosinophilic cells and lipid-rich cells. Micronodular hyperplasia is characterized by the presence of tiny pigmented nodules with atrophic intervening areas.

Cushing syndrome due to adrenocortical adenoma shows the presence of encapsulated yellow tumours. Microscopically, the lesions are composed of cells similar to zona fasciculata.

In Cushing syndrome due to adrenocortical carcinomas, unencapsulated tumours larger than adrenal adenomas are seen in the cortex. The tumours display anaplastic features microscopically.

Adjacent adrenal cortex and the contralateral adrenal gland show atrophic features in both benign and malignant functioning tumours.

Clinical Features Symptoms of Cushing syndrome are insidious in onset. Weight gain and hypertension may be the first manifestations. Later, patients develop the more characteristic central pattern of fatty tissue deposition leading to central obesity, moon facies and buffalo hump – the fat deposition in the posterior neck and back. The common clinical features are listed in Box 28.1.

Laboratory Investigations Cushing syndrome is diagnosed on the basis of the following laboratory findings:

- Elevated 24-hour urine free cortisol concentration
- Loss of normal diurnal pattern of cortisol secretion

Box 28.1 Clinical Features of Cushing Syndrome

Rapid weight gain with central obesity
Irritability or depression
Muscle and bone weakness
Loss of memory and attention dysfunction
Osteopenia and fracture
Glucose intolerance
Hypertension
Hypercholesterolaemia
Immunosuppression and frequent infections
Sleep disturbances
Menstrual irregularities
Infertility in women
Impotence in men
Atrophic and fragile skin
Hirsutism
Baldness
Nephrolithiasis

- Levels of ACTH and urine steroid excretion following the administration of dexamethasone help in identifying the cause:
  - Elevated ACTH levels that cannot be supressed by a low-dose dexamethasone but responds to higher doses are seen in pituitary Cushing syndrome. This response is monitored by measuring urinary excretion of 17-hydroxycorticosteroid.
  - Elevated ACTH levels which are completely resistant to low and high doses of dexamethasone are a feature of ectopic ACTH.
  - Low ACTH levels are seen in Cushing syndrome due to adrenal tumour.

Hyperaldosteronism

Hyperaldosteronism, also known as aldosteronism, refers to the chronic excess aldosterone production from the adrenal glands. Hyperaldosteronism may be primary or secondary due to extra-adrenal cause. Primary hyperaldosteronism is due to autonomous overproduction of aldosterone, with resultant suppression of the renin–angiotensin system and reduced plasma renin levels. Secondary hyperaldosteronism is characterized by excess aldosterone release, triggered by the activation of the renin–angiotensin system and also elevated levels of plasma renin.

Primary Hyperaldosteronism Primary hyperaldosteronism, also known as primary aldosteronism, is caused by any one of the following three mechanisms (Fig. 28.41):

- **Bilateral idiopathic hyperaldosteronism** is the most common cause and is characterized by bilateral nodular hyperplasia of adrenal glands.
- **Adrenocortical neoplasms** include adenoma and carcinoma. One-third cases are due to solitary aldosterone-secreting adenoma, an entity referred to as Conn syndrome.

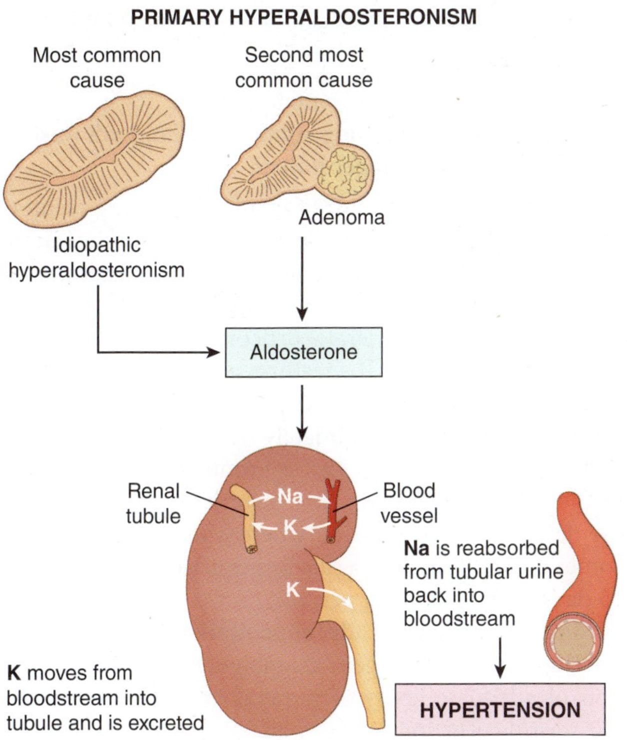

Fig. 28.41 The major causes of primary hyperaldosteronism and its principal effects on the kidney.

- **Glucocorticoid-remediable hyperaldosteronism** is an uncommon cause of primary familial hyperaldosteronism.

Secondary Hyperaldosteronism

Secondary hyperaldosteronism, as stated earlier, is characterized by the elevated plasma renin levels and is caused by any of the following conditions:

- Reduced renal perfusion due to arteriolar nephrosclerosis or renal artery stenosis
- Arterial hypovolaemia and oedema due to congestive cardiac failure, cirrhosis or nephrotic syndrome
- Pregnancy, due to oestrogenic effects on renin

Morphology (Fig. 28.42)

Aldosterone-producing adenomas are solitary, small, well-circumscribed lesions and are more common in women in their fourth decades of life. Their cut surface shows bright yellowish discolouration which on microscopic examination reveals the presence of uniform appearing lipid-rich cortical cells. A hallmark feature is the presence of eosinophilic laminated cytoplasmic inclusions, called **spironolactone bodies**, noted after treatment with the antihypertensive drug spironolactone. Unlike cortical adenomas causing Cushing syndrome, adenomas associated with hyperaldosteronism do not cause atrophy of the adjacent cortex of the ipsilateral and contralateral glands.

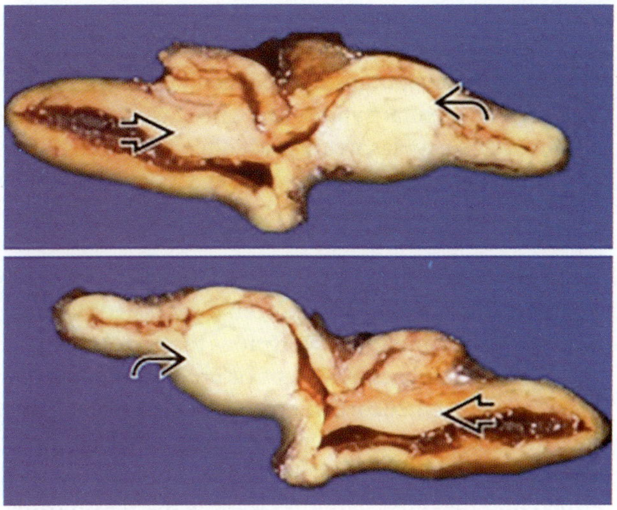

Fig. 28.42 Aldosterone-producing adenoma – gross. (*Source:* Diagnostic Pathology: Endocrine, 2 ed., Vania Nosé, Elsevier Inc., 2018.)

Diffuse and focal hyperplasia of cells resembling zona glomerulosa is the characteristic feature of bilateral idiopathic hyperplasia. As a rule, adrenocortical adenoma must be ruled out as the cause in all cases of hyperaldosteronism.

Clinical Features The most predominant clinical feature of hyperaldosteronism is **hypertension**. Primary aldosteronism is the most common cause of secondary hypertension. Chronic excess of aldosterone levels is associated with cardiovascular compromise due to the expansion of extracellular fluid volume and elevated cardiac output. This may lead to stroke and myocardial infarction. Because of renal salt wasting, **hypokalaemia** is a prominent feature and may lead to muscle weakness, paraesthesias, visual disturbances, etc.

If the plasma aldosterone to renin ratio is elevated in the screening test, aldosterone suppression test must be done to confirm primary hyperaldosteronism.

Patients with primary hyperaldosteronism are treated with aldosterone antagonists, and patients with adenomas are treated with surgical excision.

Adrenogenital Syndromes

Adrenogenital syndromes are primary adrenal or gonadal disorders of sexual differentiation presenting as virilization in females and feminization in males. Here, we discuss the adrenal cause of adrenogenital syndromes.

Adrenal cortex secretes two compounds – **dehydroepiandrosterone and androstenedione**, both of which are converted to testosterone in peripheral tissues. Secretion of these androgens are under the control of ACTH. Hence, adrenogenital syndromes due to excess ACTH can occur as an isolated syndrome or as a part of Cushing disease. The two adrenal causes of adrenogenital syndromes are adrenocortical neoplasms and congenital adrenal hyperplasia. Adrenogenital syndromes with virilization due to adrenocortical neoplasms are most often androgen-secreting carcinomas and are discussed later. Congenital adrenal hyperplasia is discussed here.

Congenital Adrenal Hyperplasia Congenital adrenal hyperplasia is a group of autosomal recessive disorders resulting from mutations of genes that code enzymes mediating the biochemical steps of production of mineralocorticoids, glucocorticoids or sex steroids from cholesterol by the adrenal glands. Any blockage in the process can cause accumulated steroid precursors to be pushed into the other pathways leading to excess production of androgens resulting in virilization, as illustrated in Flowchart 28.1. At the same time, adrenal hyperplasia results because of compensatory increase in secretion of ACTH triggered by the deficiency of cortisol. There may be impairment of aldosterone secretion, leading to salt wasting. Hence, classical congenital adrenal hyperplasia is a syndrome of virilization, salt wasting, elevated ACTH and adrenal hyperplasia.

Enzyme 21-hydroxylase deficiency due to CYP21A2 mutations is the most common cause of congenital adrenal hyperplasia. Flowchart 28.1 illustrates the consequences of 21-hydroxylase deficiency. Clinical symptoms depend on whether the enzyme is partially or completely lost.

The clinical syndromes can be of any of the following categories:

- **Classic salt wasting adrenogenitalism**
- **Simple virilizing adrenogenitalism without salt wasting**
- **Nonclassical adrenogenitalism**

Classic salt wasting adrenogenitalism is the result of total lack of the hydroxylase leading to the blockage in the conversion of progesterone to deoxycorticosterone, as well as of hydroxyprogesterone to deoxycortisol, resulting in the absence of mineralocorticoids and deficiency of cortisols, respectively. The features are salt wasting, hyponatraemia, hyperkalaemia, acidosis, hypotension, cardiovascular collapse and ultimately death. The blockage in cortisol synthesis causes excess production of androgens resulting in virilization. This disorder is picked up on the day of birth in females, whereas in males, it usually comes to attention after a salt-losing crisis, between 5 and 15 days in the postnatal period.

Simple virilizing adrenogenitalism without salt wasting presents with genital ambiguity. There is production of adequate levels of mineralocorticoid to prevent salt wasting. The low levels of glucocorticoids fail to provide feedback inhibition to ACTH. As a result of this, the increased ACTH levels induce excess androgen production leading to virilization.

Nonclassical adrenogenitalism is due to partial deficiency of 21-hydroxylase. Individuals with this syndrome present late during their adulthood with hirsutism, acne or menstrual abnormalities or may be asymptomatic.

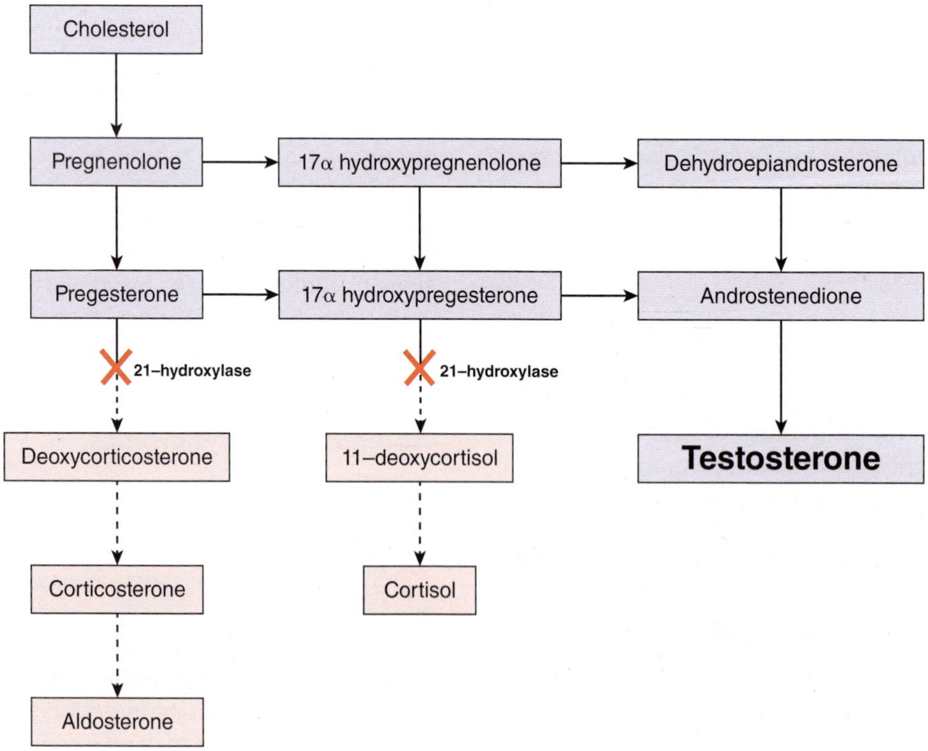

Flowchart 28.1 Consequences of 21-hydroxylase deficiency.

Morphology

Bilateral adrenal glands are hyperplastic, sometimes presenting as a massive enlargement of adrenal glands in all types of congenital adrenal hyperplasia. On the cut section, adrenal glands are thick, nodular and brown in colour because of complete lipid depletion. Microscopically, an admixture of eosinophilic lipid-depleted cells and lipid-laden cells can be observed. In many cases, corticotrophic cell hyperplasia is seen in the anterior pituitary.

Clinical Features Clinical features depend on the enzyme that is deficient and include symptoms due to androgen excess with or without deficiency of aldosterone and glucocorticoid. Because high levels of intra-adrenal glucocorticoids are essential for the synthesis of medullary catecholamines, levels of these hormones are also reduced in these patients. Because of this, these patients are prone to develop hypotension and cardiovascular collapse.

Severe enzyme deficiency is life threatening, with severe vomiting, dehydration and salt wasting.

The onset of symptoms varies from the perinatal period to late adulthood depending on the nature and extent of enzyme deficiency. Prepubertal males present with enlargement of external genitalia, and older males present with oligospermia. Female infants present with features of pseudohermaphroditism, and postpubertal females with acne, hirsutism and acne.

Congenital adrenal hyperplasia should be excluded in any neonate with ambiguous genitalia.

Treatment Patients are treated with exogenous glucocorticoids, which apart from providing the required levels of glucocorticoids also reduce the ACTH levels and thereby suppress the excess formation of steroid hormones. In patients with salt wasting type, mineralocorticoid supplementation is needed.

Adrenocortical Insufficiency PA 32.7

Adrenocortical insufficiency is adrenal hypofunction caused by primary adrenal pathology or ACTH deficiency leading to depressed functioning of adrenal glands (secondary hypoadrenalism). There are three forms of adrenocortical insufficiency:

- **Primary acute adrenocortical insufficiency, adrenal crisis**
- **Primary chronic adrenocortical insufficiency, Addison disease**
- **Secondary adrenocortical insufficiency**

Acute adrenocortical insufficiency occurs because of varied causes as listed in Table 28.9.

In the following sections, Waterhouse–Friderichsen syndrome and Addison disease are discussed.

Table 28.9 Causes of Acute Adrenocortical Insufficiency

Category	Subcategory	Diseases
Primary	Loss of cortical cells	Congenital adrenal hypoplasia Adrenoleucodystrophy Autoimmune adrenal insufficiency Autoimmune polyendocrinopathy syndrome type 1 Autoimmune polyendocrinopathy syndrome type 2 Infections • Tuberculosis • HIV infection • Fungal infections Waterhouse–Friderichsen syndrome Amyloidosis, sarcoidosis Metastatic carcinomatous deposits
	Metabolic failure	Congenital adrenal hyperplasia Drug-induced inhibition of ACTH
Secondary	Hypothalamic pituitary disorder	Inflammation • Tuberculosis • Sarcoidosis • Fungal infection Neoplasm
	Hypothalamic pituitary suppression	Chronic steroid administration Steroid-producing neoplasms

ACTH, adrenocorticotropic hormone.

Waterhouse–Friderichsen Syndrome Waterhouse–Friderichsen syndrome is a rare, yet disastrous and fatal disorder. This disease can occur at any age but is more common in children. The probable explanation for the adrenal haemorrhage is direct bacterial seeding of small blood vessels in the adrenal glands, followed by the development of disseminated intravascular coagulation (DIC) or endothelial dysfunction caused by microbial products and inflammatory mediators.

The characteristic features of this syndrome are as follows:

- Precipitated by bacterial infections by *Neisseria meningitidis*, *Pseudomonas*, pneumococci, *Haemophilus influenzae*, staphylococci, etc.
- Rapidly progressive hypotension leading to shock
- DIC
- Rapidly developing adrenocortical insufficiency due to massive bilateral adrenal haemorrhage

Early recognition and institution of appropriate treatment are the main factors in deciding the prognosis of patients with this disorder, and delayed management is fatal within hours to few days.

Addison Disease Addison disease, also called primary chronic adrenocortical insufficiency and hypocortosolism, is a rare disease due to progressive destruction of the adrenal cortex. Autoimmune destruction of the adrenal cortex caused by an immune reaction against the enzyme 21-hydroxylase is the most common cause of Addison disease, especially in the western world. This may be isolated or in the context of autoimmune polyendocrine syndrome, types 1 and 2, in which other endocrine organs like the thyroid and pancreas may also be affected. The other common causes are tuberculosis (especially in developing and underdeveloped countries), AIDS, metastatic cancers, etc. Genetic causes include congenital hypoplasia and adrenoleucodystrophy.

Morphology

The morphological changes in the adrenal glands are dependent on the aetiology.

The hallmark microscopic features of primary autoimmune adrenalitis include irregularly shrunken glands with only scattered cortical cells in a network of connective tissue. In cases due to tuberculosis and fungal infections, the architecture of adrenal glands is effaced by the granulomatous inflammation. In cases due to metastatic carcinomatous deposits, the architecture is effaced by the infiltrating malignant cells.

Clinical Features In general, clinical manifestations of Addison disease are insidious and do not appear until at least 90% of the adrenal cortex has been destroyed. Early in the disease process, the features are nonspecific, which include progressive weakness, easy fatiguability, anorexia, nausea, vomiting, weight loss and diarrhoea. **Hyperpigmentation** of the sun-exposed areas is a striking feature in patients with primary adrenal disease. This is due to the increased levels of pro-opiomelanocortin (POMC), which is the common precursor of ACTH and melanocyte-stimulating hormone (MSH). Symptoms due to mineralocorticoid deficiency include hyperkalaemia, hyponatraemia, volume depletion and hypotension. **Acute adrenal crisis** is precipitated by stress-like conditions such as infections, surgery and trauma. Features of acute adrenal crisis include severe vomiting, abdominal pain, hypotension, coma and cardiovascular collapse. Early intervention is essential without which the disease can be fatal.

Secondary Adrenocortical Insufficiency Secondary adrenocortical insufficiency is due to disorders of the hypothalamus and pituitary such as infections, infarction, irradiation and tumours. These lesions suppress the release of ACTH and result in hypoadrenalism. In these secondary causes, hyperpigmentation characteristic of primary Addison disease is not seen. Also, in these cases, cortisol and androgen synthesis is suppressed whereas mineralocorticoid synthesis is unaffected. ACTH levels in secondary adrenocortical insufficiency cases are low, and there is a prompt increase in plasma cortisol levels on the administration of exogenous ACTH.

Morphology

Pituitary gland and hypothalamus show the changes according to the underlying disorder. Adrenal glands may be reduced in size with atrophic cortex but medulla is unaffected.

Adrenocortical Neoplasms **PA 32.9**

Adrenocortical adenomas and carcinomas when functional can cause hyperadrenalism. Adults have equal probability of developing adenomas and carcinomas, whereas in children carcinomas are more common than adenomas.

Adenomas are commonly associated with hyperaldosteronism and Cushing syndrome, whereas carcinomas are more often associated with virilizing neoplasm. Not all adrenal neoplasms are functional; a significant percentage of the tumours are nonfunctional.

Morphology

Adrenocortical adenomas

Most of these tumours are incidental findings. Grossly, they appear as well-circumscribed, nodular lesions up to 2.5 cm in size (Fig 28.43). In functional adenomas, the adjacent cortex is atrophic, whereas in nonfunctional adenomas the cortex is normal.

Microscopic features are similar to normal adrenal cortex, though some individual cells may show mild

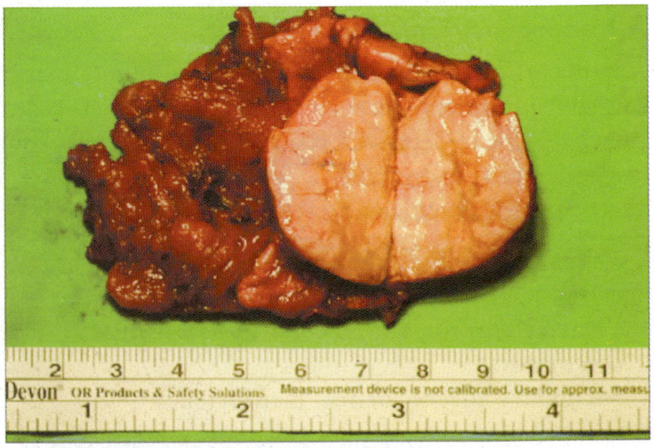

Fig. 28.43 Adrenocortical adenoma – gross. (*Source:* https://www.researchgate.net/publication/221815847/figure/fig3/AS:411267908030467@1475065318811/Gross-appearance-of-adrenal-cortical-adenoma-of-the-differential-diagnosis-of-a-lesion.png)

pleomorphism, which is considered as 'endocrine atypia'. Mitotic figures are not prominent (Fig. 28.44).

Adrenocortical carcinomas

Carcinomas are more often functional than adenomas and are often associated with virilism.

Grossly, these tumours are large lesions exceeding 20 cm in diameter with infiltrating borders Their cut surface is variegated, with many lesions having areas of necrosis, haemorrhage and cystic changes. In most cases, adrenal vein, vena cava and lymphatics are invaded with regional and periaortic nodal involvement.

Microscopically, the tumours may be composed of well-differentiated to highly anaplastic cells admixed with spindle cells.

DISORDERS OF ADRENAL MEDULLA

The two most common neoplasms affecting adrenal medulla are phaeochromocytoma and neuroblastoma. Neuroblastoma is discussed in Chapter 10.

Phaeochromocytoma **PA 32.9**

Phaeochromocytomas are tumours arising from medullary chromaffin cells, which are responsible for the synthesis of catecholamines. The features of phaeochromocytomas are collectively referred to as '**rule of 10s**':

- 10% of phaeochromocytomas are **extra-adrenal**, found in sites such as the organs of Zuckerkandl and carotid body.
- 10% of sporadic adrenal phaeochromocytomas are **bilateral** and close to 50% have familial background.
- 10% of adrenal phaeochromocytomas are **biologically malignant** with the development of metastases.
- 10% of phaeochromocytomas are **not associated with hypertension**. Two-thirds of patients who present with hypertension may have paroxysmal episodes, with highly elevated blood pressure and palpitations which may be fatal if not recognized and treated immediately.

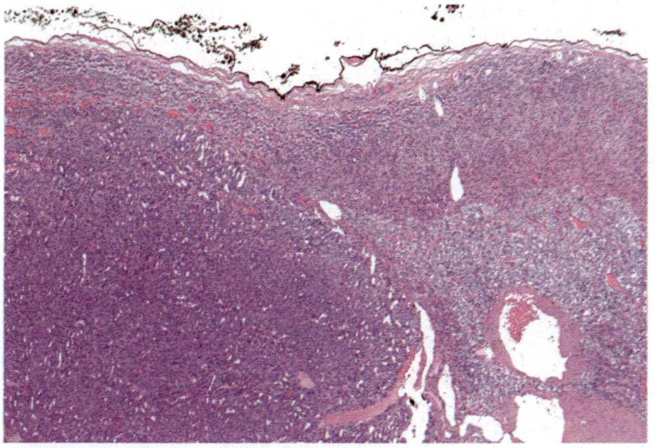

Fig. 28.44 Adrenocortical adenoma – microscopy. (*Source:* https://upload.wikimedia.org/wikipedia/commons/thumb/8/8a/).

Familial cases of phaeochromocytoma are associated with germline mutations involving any of the following genes, RET, NF1 and VHL, as well as the genes encoding components of succinate dehydrogenase complex, SDHB, SDHC and SDHD.

Morphology

Phaeochromocytomas may vary from small, circumscribed, unencapsulated lesions to large haemorrhagic lobulated tumours and weigh from 1 to approximately 4000 g. Remnant adrenal gland can be seen stretched over the surface or attached to one pole. The cut section is yellow–tan, with larger lesions being haemorrhagic, necrotic and cystic (Fig. 28.45). Traditional practice is to incubate fresh tissue of phaeochromocytoma with potassium dichromate solution and to observe the change in colour. The colour changes to dark brown because of oxidation of stored catecholamines and hence the name.

Microscopy of phaeochromocytomas is variable (Fig. 28.46). Classical appearance is the **Zellballen pattern**, in which the tumour cells, also called chief cells, are polygonal to spindle shaped and arranged in small nests, surrounded by supporting sustentacular cells, and the intervening stroma is richly vascular. The nuclei have the characteristic neuroendocrine salt and pepper chromatin. Like any other neuroendocrine tumour, the tumour cells reveal the presence of electron-dense

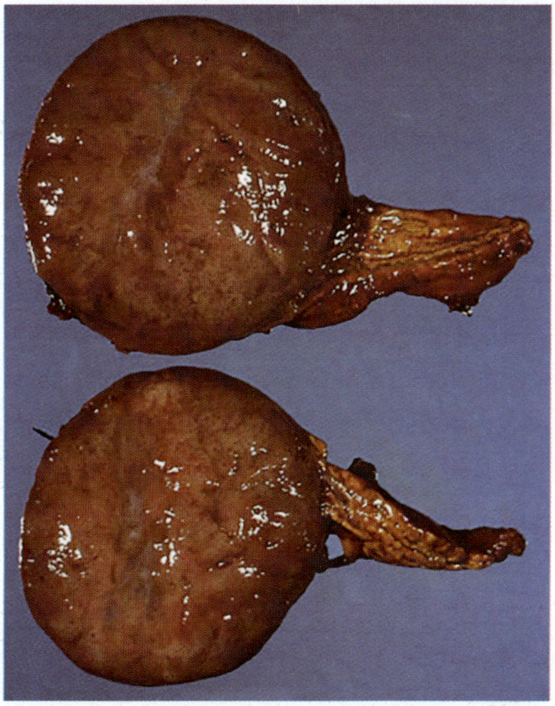

Fig. 28.45 Phaeochromocytoma – gross. The tumour is well demarcated with bulging tan surface on the section with vague lobulation. Residual attached adrenal gland is present. (*Source:* From Ernest E. Lack and Harry P.W. Kozakewich. Tumors of the Adrenal Gland. Diagnostic Histopathology of Tumors. 5th edition. Elsevier 2021.)

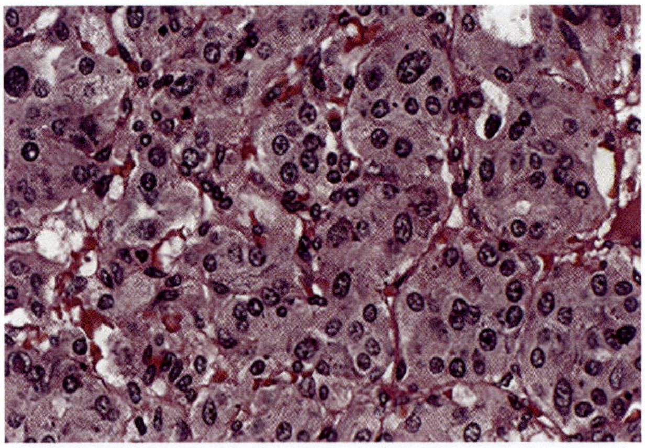

Fig. 28.46 Phaeochromocytoma – microscopy. Note the organoid pattern of arrangement of tumour cells. (*Source:* From Ernest E. Lack and Harry P.W. Kozakewich. Tumors of the Adrenal Gland. Diagnostic Histopathology of Tumors. 5th edition. Elsevier 2021.)

secretory granules by electron microscopy. The chief cells are positive for neuroendocrine markers like chromogranin and synaptophysin, while the peripheral sustentacular cells are S-100 positive.

There are no reliable histological criteria for malignancy, though features like increased mitotic figures, necrosis and spindle cell morphology of tumour cells have been associated with aggressive behaviour of tumours. Capsular and vascular invasion is also not a reliable feature of malignancy. **The criterion for malignancy is the presence of metastases** which may involve lymph nodes, lung, liver or bones.

Clinical Features The prominent clinical feature of phaeochromocytoma is **hypertension** in almost 90% of patients. As mentioned earlier, a significant fraction of patients with phaeochromocytoma may present with **paroxysmal episodes**. Such episodes are associated with headache, tachycardia, palpitations, nausea, vomiting, chest pain, abdominal pain, sweating, tremor and a sense of apprehension. Such episodes may be precipitated by physical exertion, emotional stress, exercise, postural changes or palpation of the tumour. Highly elevated blood pressure leads to congestive cardiac failure, pulmonary oedema, myocardial oedema, ventricular fibrillation and stroke. The cardiac complications of phaeochromocytoma are collectively called '**catecholamine cardiomyopathy**'. It is extremely essential to recognize these tumours because these are rare causes of surgically correctable hypertension.

In few cases, these tumours secrete ACTH or somatostatin and present with features related to these hormones.

Management Laboratory findings of phaeochromocytomas are elevated urine excretion of free catecholamines and their metabolites like vanillylmandelic acid and metanephrines.

Solitary benign tumours are treated with surgical excision with adrenergic blocking drugs during the preoperative and intraoperative periods to prevent hypertensive crisis. Tumours presenting multifocally may require treatment of hypertension over a long period of time.

SELF-ASSESSMENT

Multiple Choice Questions

1. A 35-year-old woman presents with fatigue, weight gain and constipation. Laboratory tests reveal high TSH and low free T_4. What is the most likely diagnosis?
   A. Hyperthyroidism
   B. Hypothyroidism
   C. Graves disease
   D. Thyroiditis
2. A 50-year-old man with a history of renal stones undergoes laboratory tests showing high serum calcium and high PTH. What is the most likely diagnosis?
   A. Primary hyperparathyroidism
   B. Secondary hyperparathyroidism
   C. Tertiary hyperparathyroidism
   D. Hypoparathyroidism
3. A 28-year-old woman presents with palpitations, weight loss and heat intolerance. Physical examination shows a diffusely enlarged thyroid. What is the most likely diagnosis?
   A. Thyroid nodule
   B. Thyroid cancer
   C. Graves disease
   D. Hashimoto thyroiditis
4. A 55-year-old woman with type 2 diabetes has poor glycaemic control despite lifestyle modifications. What is the next best step in management?
   A. Insulin therapy
   B. Oral glucocorticoids
   C. Increase physical activity
   D. Add a sulphonylurea
5. A 45-year-old woman presents with weight gain, hirsutism and hypertension. Laboratory tests show low serum potassium. What is the most likely diagnosis?
   A. Addison disease
   B. Cushing syndrome
   C. Phaeochromocytoma
   D. Hyperthyroidism
6. A 30-year-old man presents with headache, sweating and palpitations. Blood pressure is 180/110 mm Hg. What is the most likely diagnosis?
   A. Hyperthyroidism
   B. Cushing syndrome
   C. Phaeochromocytoma
   D. Hypothyroidism

7. A 60-year-old woman with osteoporosis has a serum calcium of 11.2 mg/dL (normal: 8.5–10.2 mg/dL). What is the most likely cause?
   A. Vitamin D deficiency
   B. Primary hyperparathyroidism
   C. Malignancy
   D. Renal failure
8. A 25-year-old woman presents with amenorrhoea, galactorrhoea and headache. MRI shows a pituitary adenoma. What is the most likely diagnosis?
   A. Cushing disease
   B. Acromegaly
   C. Prolactinoma
   D. Nonfunctioning pituitary adenoma
9. A 40-year-old man presents with increased thirst, urination and unexplained weight loss. Blood tests show high blood glucose. What is the most likely diagnosis?
   A. Type 1 diabetes mellitus
   B. Type 2 diabetes mellitus
   C. Diabetic ketoacidosis
   D. Nondiabetic hyperglycaemia
10. A 70-year-old man has a fasting blood glucose of 126 mg/dL and an HbA_{1c} of 6.5%. What is the most likely diagnosis?
    A. Prediabetes
    B. Type 1 diabetes mellitus
    C. Type 2 diabetes mellitus
    D. Impaired glucose tolerance
11. A 50-year-old woman with a history of thyroidectomy for cancer presents with tingling around her mouth and in her fingertips. What is the most likely cause?
    A. Hypothyroidism
    B. Hypocalcaemia
    C. Hypercalcaemia
    D. Hyperthyroidism
12. A 55-year-old man with a history of hypertension and high cholesterol presents with severe fatigue and weight loss. Laboratory tests reveal hyponatraemia and hyperkalaemia. What is the most likely diagnosis?
    A. Primary hyperaldosteronism
    B. Addison disease
    C. Cushing syndrome
    D. Phaeochromocytoma
13. A 32-year-old woman presents with irregular menstrual periods and difficulty getting pregnant. On examination, she has acne and hirsutism. What is the most likely diagnosis?
    A. Polycystic ovary syndrome (PCOS)
    B. Hyperprolactinaemia
    C. Premature ovarian failure
    D. Hypothyroidism
14. A 45-year-old man presents with severe bone pain and a serum calcium level of 12.4 mg/dL. A bone scan shows multiple lytic lesions. What is the most likely diagnosis?
    A. Osteoporosis
    B. Primary hyperparathyroidism
    C. Metastatic bone disease
    D. Multiple myeloma
15. A 60-year-old woman with a history of thyroid surgery presents with constipation, dry skin and cold intolerance. Laboratory tests reveal a high TSH. What is the most likely diagnosis?
    A. Hyperthyroidism
    B. Hypothyroidism
    C. Thyroid cancer
    D. Nonthyroidal illness
16. A 30-year-old female presents with recurrent kidney stones. Laboratory examination reveals hypercalcaemia and hypophosphataemia. What is the most likely diagnosis?
    A. Primary hyperparathyroidism
    B. Vitamin D intoxication
    C. Sarcoidosis
    D. Renal tubular acidosis
17. A 35-year-old man presents with increased hand size, coarsening facial features and joint pain. What is the most likely diagnosis?
    A. Acromegaly
    B. Cushing syndrome
    C. Hyperthyroidism
    D. Prolactinoma
18. A 55-year-old woman with longstanding rheumatoid arthritis presents with fatigue and joint pain. Laboratory tests show low sodium and high potassium levels. What is the most likely diagnosis?
    A. Addison disease
    B. Cushing syndrome
    C. Secondary hyperparathyroidism
    D. Hypothyroidism
19. A 40-year-old man presents with palpitations, anxiety, tremor and weight loss despite an increased appetite. Laboratory tests show low TSH and high free T_4. What is the most likely diagnosis?
    A. Graves disease
    B. Toxic multinodular goitre
    C. Thyroiditis
    D. Pituitary adenoma
20. A 7-year-old child presents with short stature and delayed bone age. Laboratory tests show low growth hormone levels. What is the most likely diagnosis?
    A. Growth hormone deficiency
    B. Hypothyroidism
    C. Cushing disease
    D. Constitutional growth delay
21. A 50-year-old woman presents with frequent fractures and bone pain. Laboratory tests reveal elevated PTH and serum calcium levels. What is the most likely diagnosis?
    A. Osteoporosis
    B. Primary hyperparathyroidism
    C. Paget disease of bone
    D. Metastatic bone disease
22. A 45-year-old man presents with high blood pressure resistant to treatment. Laboratory tests show low potassium and metabolic alkalosis. What is the most likely diagnosis?
    A. Primary hyperaldosteronism
    B. Cushing syndrome
    C. Phaeochromocytoma
    D. Renal artery stenosis
23. A 30-year-old woman presents with fatigue, weight loss and hypotension. Laboratory tests show low sodium, high potassium and low cortisol levels. What is the most likely diagnosis?
    A. Addison disease
    B. Cushing syndrome
    C. Hyperthyroidism
    D. Hypothyroidism

24. A 65-year-old man presents with an incidentally discovered adrenal mass on imaging. He has no symptoms of hormone excess. What is the most appropriate next step?
    A. Immediate surgery
    B. Hormonal evaluation
    C. Observation and follow-up imaging
    D. Biopsy of the mass
25. A 55-year-old man with diabetes mellitus presents with hypoglycaemia despite reducing insulin dosage. He has no history of kidney or liver disease. What is the most likely cause of his hypoglycaemia?
    A. Insulin overdose
    B. Insulinoma
    C. Noninsulin–mediated hypoglycaemia
    D. Alcohol-induced hypoglycaemia

Answers

1. (B); 2. (A); 3. (C); 4. (D); 5. (B); 6. (C); 7. (B); 8. (C); 9. (B); 10. (C); 11. (B); 12. (A); 13. (A); 14. (D); 15. (B); 16. (A); 17. (A); 18. (A); 19. (A); 20. (A); 21. (B); 22. (A); 23. (A); 24. (C); 25. (B)

Self-Assessment Questions

1. A 30-year-old woman presented with anxiety, sleeplessness, palpitation, heat intolerance, loss of weight and appetite. On examination, it was found that she had diffusely enlarged thyroid, tachycardia, tremors, proptosis and oedema over the shin. What is your provisional diagnosis? Discuss the aetiopathogenesis, morphological features and laboratory findings of the disease.
2. A 30-year-old woman presented with marked thyroid enlargement with no symptoms of hypo- or hyperthyroidism. On examination, the thyroid was found to be enlarged and nodular. What is your provisional diagnosis? Discuss the aetiopathogenesis, morphological features and laboratory findings of the disease.
3. A 32-year-old woman presented with a solitary thyroid nodule. On examination, it was found that the right lobe of the thyroid gland had a solitary nodule which was firm. Ipsilateral cervical node was palpable and firm. What is the probable diagnosis? Discuss the genetics and morphological features of the disease. List down the causes of solitary thyroid nodules.
4. A 35-year-old man presented with thyroid swelling associated with dysphagia and hoarseness. He had a history of illness due to parathyroid hyperplasia. There was also a positive family history of similar thyroid lesions along with adrenal and parathyroid lesions. What is your provisional diagnosis? Discuss the aetiopathogenesis, morphological features and tumour markers for the lesion.
5. A 45-year-old woman was diagnosed with hypercalcaemia when she underwent investigations for preventive health checkup. Following this, her PTH level was checked and was found to be elevated. She did not have any other relevant specific symptoms. What do you think is the cause for asymptomatic hypercalcaemia in this patient? Discuss the types, morphological features and consequences of the disease.
6. A 52-year-old man who was a known case of T2DM and taking oral hypoglycaemic agents for more than 15 years was brought in an unconscious state. There was a history of recent urinary tract infection and skipping of antidiabetic medicines by the patient. His blood sugar was found to be 915 mg/dL. What is your provisional diagnosis? Discuss the pathogenesis and other acute and chronic complications of the disease.
7. A 32-year-old woman presented with recent weight gain and excessive fatigue. There was no history of hypertension or diabetes. On examination, she was found to hypertensive. She also had central obesity, moon facies and hirsutism. Her blood glucose level was elevated. She was also depressed. What is your provisional diagnosis? Discuss the aetiopathogenesis, types and morphological features of the disease.
8. A 45-year-old man who was a known case of tuberculosis and discontinued treatment was brought with complaints of intractable vomiting, abdominal pain and coma. On examination, blood pressure was very low with cold and clammy skin. All these events followed emergency appendicectomy performed on the patient. Laboratory examination results were as follows: hyponatraemia, hyperkalaemia and low cortisol levels. What is your probable diagnosis? Discuss the aetiopathogenesis, morphological features and investigations for the disease.
9. A 40-year-old woman was diagnosed with adrenal mass as an incidental finding while she was being evaluated for an abdominal mass. The lesion was radiologically circumscribed and measured 2.5 cm. The lesion was excised and submitted for histopathological examination. Its cut surface was yellowish, and microscopic examination showed the presence of cells similar to normal adrenal cortex. What is your provisional diagnosis? Discuss the aetiopathogenesis, morphological features, criteria for malignancy and markers for the lesion.
10. A 25-year-old young man was diagnosed with severe hypertension which was found to be resistant to the conventional antihypertensive drugs. He also had paroxysmal episodes of abrupt elevation of blood pressure characterized clinically by chest pain, abdominal pain, nausea, vomiting and a sense of apprehension. On evaluation, he was found to be having an adrenal mass. What is your provisional diagnosis? Discuss the aetiopathogenesis, morphological features, laboratory investigations and markers for the disease.

Answers

1. Graves disease
2. Multinodular goitre
3. Papillary thyroid carcinoma
4. Medullary thyroid carcinoma
5. Primary hyperparathyroidism
6. Hyperosmolar hyperosmotic syndrome
7. Cushing syndrome
8. Acute adrenal insufficiency induced by surgical stress in a known case of tuberculosis
9. Adrenocortical adenoma
10. Phaeochromocytoma

Topics for Self-Directed Learning

1. Pathology of pituitary adenomas
2. Myxoedema coma
3. Drug-induced hypo- and hyperthyroidism
4. Pathogenesis of acropachy of Graves disease
5. Biochemical alterations in different thyroid lesions
6. Radioiodine uptake of different thyroid lesions
7. Radiological findings of different thyroid lesions
8. Immunohistochemistry profile of thyroid carcinomas
9. Familial syndromes associated with phaeochromocytoma
10. Pinealoma
11. Pituitary dwarfism
12. Sheehan syndrome

The Skin 29

A Sathish Selvakumar

PA 34.1 Describe the risk factors, pathogenesis, pathology and natural history of **squamous cell carcinoma of the skin.**

PA 34.2 Describe the risk factors, pathogenesis, pathology and natural history of **basal cell carcinoma of the skin.**

PA 34.3 Describe the distinguishing features between a naevus and melanoma. Describe the aetiology, pathogenesis, risk factors, morphology clinical features and metastases of **melanoma.**

CHAPTER OUTLINE

INTRODUCTION

The skin is the largest organ in the body where varied complicated yet precisely regulated processes at the molecular and cellular level are carried out. It is one of the first line of defences against harmful infectious and physical agents. Apart from these, it also has important sensory functions and endocrine functions such as vitamin D synthesis on exposure to sunlight. The following are some of the important cells and other components that function interdependently and cooperatively.

STRUCTURE OF SKIN

The skin is composed of two major compartments: the epidermis and the dermis. The superficial part of the epidermis, known as the stratum corneum, is composed of dead keratinocytes and acts as a frictional barrier. The epidermis is a dense and poorly vascularized region that is composed of keratinocytes with few melanocytes. The major immune cells in this compartment include Langerhans cells (LCs), dendritic epidermal T cells (DETC; a subset of $\gamma\delta$ T cells) and CD8 T cells. The dermis below is a highly vascularized region, rich in collagen, and elastin fibres, with low cellular density. It is composed of fibroblasts, T cells (CD4 αβ, and γδ), innate lymphoid cells (ILCs), dermal DCs (dDCs), macrophages, mast cells and neutrophils (nonexhaustive list).

The main features of the epidermis, including its cell layers and different cell types are described briefly as follows.

COMPONENTS OF SKIN

Squamous Epithelial Cells (Keratinocytes)

They form a durable physical barrier with the help of tight cell junctions and keratin protein production. They also produce cytokines and defensins involved in cutaneous immune responses.

Melanocytes

Present in the epidermis, they produce melanin pigment that protects against the harmful ultraviolet (UV) radiation in sunlight.

Dendritic Cells

Present in the intraepidermal region, these cells are called LCs. They are involved in the cutaneous immune responses by processing the harmful antigens and also by secreting factors that augment innate immune responses. After migrating to the regional lymph nodes, these cells present the processed antigens to the T lymphocytes and initiate the adaptive arm of the immunity. Dendrocytes are another type of dendritic cell found in the dermis performing similar function.

Lymphocytes

Dendritic cell stimulation causes the T lymphocytes such as the helper ($CD4^+$), cytotoxic ($CD8^+$) and regulatory (Treg) T cells in the regional lymph node to express cutaneous lymphocyte–associated antigen (CLA), an adhesion molecule and chemokine receptors such as CCR4 and CCR10 to home towards the dermis directed by the chemokines secreted by the keratinocytes. These cells express the cytokines that dictate the microscopic patterns and clinical expressions of cutaneous inflammatory and infectious diseases. Few B cells are also found within the dermis and are involved in humoral responses towards antigens.

Like the gut, the skin provides a suitable home for many organisms such as bacteria, fungi, viruses and mites mostly having symbiotic relationships. They prevent colonization by other harmful organisms and also enhances skin immune responses to potential pathogens with much to be explored.

Afferent nerve fibres and neural end organs are responsible for the various types of physical sensations. Autonomic efferent nerve fibres regulate sweat glands and effector pili muscles and also play a role in the innate and adaptive immunity in the dermis.

Merkel cells are located in epithelial basal cell layer and may have neuroendocrine or mechanoreceptor functions.

Adnexal Components

Sweat glands play a pivotal role in body temperature maintenance. Hair follicles manufacture hair shafts and have niches of stem cells that remain dormant and are activated following injury for epithelial cell regeneration. Factors such as prolonged sun light exposure tilts the already delicate homeostasis of the different skin cells leading to deleterious effects such as cutaneous ageing, blunting of immunologic responses to environmental antigens, and favours the development of a variety of premalignant and malignant cutaneous neoplasms. Therapeutic drugs intake and systemic disorders can also have important manifestations in the skin. Skin conditions are very common and as the organ can be visually examined, numerous insights into the functional state of the body can be achieved by careful examination. Critical analysis of the appearance and distribution of skin lesions is essential in formulating diagnoses and in understanding the pathogenesis.

Nomenclature of Common Skin Lesions

Macroscopic Lesions	Description
Macule	A small patch of skin ≤5 mm that is altered in colour, but is not elevated
Patch	A larger area of skin >5 mm that is altered in colour, but is not elevated
Plaque	Elevated, flat-topped lesions >5 mm which may be caused by coalescing papules
Pustule	Pus-filled circumscribed raised lesion
Vesicle and bulla	Fluid-filled raised lesion ≤5 mm is vesicle and similar lesion of larger size is bulla
Excoriation	Loss of portion of epidermis, dermis due to scratching or an exogenous injury
Lichenification	Palpably thickened skin with prominent skin markings
Microscopic Lesions	**Description**
Acanthosis	Diffuse hyperplasia of epidermis
Hypergranulosis	Hyperplasia of stratum granulosum, commonly due to intense rubbing
Spongiosis	Intercellular oedema and rounding of keratinocytes
Parakeratosis	Keratinization with retained nuclei in stratum corneum
Hyperkeratosis	Thickening of stratum corneum
Papillomatosis	Hyperplasia and enlargement of dermal papillae causing undulating surface of epidermis

INFLAMMATORY DERMATOSES

Inflammatory dermatoses are broadly classified into acute and chronic on the basis of their duration. Acute inflammatory dermatoses are of shorter duration and are characterized by inflammatory infiltrate composed of lymphocytes, macrophages, oedema and cell injury, whereas chronic inflammatory dermatoses persist for months to years and are characterized by epithelial atrophy or hyperplasia with or without dermal fibrosis. Common acute and chronic inflammatory dermatoses are discussed here.

ACUTE INFLAMMATORY DERMATOSES

Urticaria

Urticaria (hives) is a common skin disorder, characterized by sudden onset of transient and recurrent wheals which are raised erythematous and oedematous areas of skin associated with pruritis. When the area of involvement is large with the oedema extending into the subcutaneous region, the condition is known as **angioedema**. The lesion can involve any site of the body and angioedema predominantly affects the facial, oropharyngeal and laryngeal regions, hands, feet and genitalia. Acute urticaria lasts up to 24 hours, whereas chronic urticaria can recur over a period of 6–8 weeks. The aetiology is variable and consists of soluble antigens in foods, drugs and insect venom, contact allergens, physical stimuli such as pressure, vibration solar radiation, cold temperature, occult infection, and underlying diseases such as collagen vascular disorders and Hodgkin lymphoma. Hereditary angioedema is a rare condition where recurrent attacks of oedema involves skin, oral cavity, upper respiratory and gastrointestinal tracts, not associated with urticaria. The attacks are often painful and may be stimulated by trauma or emotional stress.

Pathogenesis Urticaria is associated with antigen-induced release of vasoactive mediators from mast cells and eosinophils. The process is an example for localized immediate hypersensitivity (type I) reaction which is mast cell– and IgE-dependent. The exposure to different antigens triggers their binding to IgE antibodies that are attached to mast cells through Fc receptors and results in the histamine release augmented by the complement, especially C5a (the complete process is discussed in Chapter 6). The mechanism can also be mast cell–dependent while IgE-independent which is the result of substances that directly incite the degranulation of mast cells such as opiates, antibiotics, curare and radiographic contrast media. Another form of urticaria which is mast cell– and IgE-independent is triggered by local factors that increase the vascular permeability. A classic example is urticaria caused by exposure to aspirin that inhibits cyclooxygenase and arachidonic acid. Another form known as hereditary angioneurotic oedema is caused by inherited deficiency of C1 inhibitor, resulting in excessive activation of early components of the complement system and production of large number of vasoactive mediators.

Morphology

Gross Macroscopically, the lesions are usually small, pruritic papules to large oedematous plaques. Individual lesions may coalesce to form annular, linear or arciform configurations.

Microscopy Microscopically, the acute lesions show interstitial oedema, dilated venules with endothelial swelling and a paucity of inflammatory cells, whereas the chronic lesions show interstitial oedema along with perivascular and interstitial mixed cell inflammatory infiltrates consisting of mononuclear cells and rare neutrophils and eosinophils. Collagen bundles are more widely spaced with dermal oedema, whereas the epidermis is often unremarkable.

Treatment The main aspect of treatment is to identify the precipitating factors and their elimination and symptomatic relief. Antihistamines are the mainstay of treatment, whereas systemic steroids may be used in severe acute, recalcitrant and urticarial vasculitis. In selected and refractory cases, immunomodulatory drugs and omalizumab (a humanized monoclonal anti-IgE antibody which decreases the circulating level of free IgE) can be used in the treatment of chronic spontaneous urticaria in adults and adolescents (>12 years) not responding to antihistamines.

Acute Eczematous Dermatitis

Eczema, meaning 'to boil over' also referred to as ***spongiotic dermatitis***, has an initiating factor and can be divided into acute, subacute and chronic types. Spongiosis refers to the accumulation of oedematous fluid between the keratinocytes occasionally causing vesicle or bulla formation. Based on the initiating factors, eczematous dermatitis can be subdivided into allergic contact dermatitis, atopic dermatitis, drug-related eczematous dermatitis, photoeczematous dermatitis and primary irritant dermatitis (e.g. because of chemicals).

Pathogenesis The lesion is an example of T-cell–mediated type IV hypersensitivity inflammatory reaction. This reaction consists of an afferent limb, the sensitization or induction phase and an efferent limb, the elicitation limb. The allergens are usually low-molecular-weight proteins (hapten) and are lipid soluble. The allergen with a carrier protein at the site of entry into the skin form neoantigens which are processed by the antigen-presenting cells such as the LCs and they migrate by way of dermal lymphatics to the draining lymph nodes. There they are presented to the naive $CD4^+$ T cells which are then activated and develop into effector and memory cells. If the antigen is re-exposed, then the memory T cells expressing homing molecules (common lymphocyte antigen, lymphocyte function–associated antigen-1, chemokine receptors) migrate to skin sites of antigen localization where they release the cytokines and chemokines and recruit inflammatory cells. This usually occurs within 24–72 hours after exposure and leads to the characteristic lesions. The process is discussed in greater detail in Chapter 6.

Morphology

Gross In acute spongiotic (eczematous) dermatitis, the lesions develop after the exposure to the stimulant and appears as red, erythematous, oedematous, pruritic papulovesicular, oozing, crusted lesions.

Microscopy Microscopically, **spongiosis** is the characteristic histopathological feature and the degree of spongiosis is variable and the keratinocytes may be stellate and surrounded by clear spaces representing the fluid collection with lymphohistiocytic infiltrate (Fig. 29.1). In severe conditions, the oedema seeps into the intercellular spaces of the epidermis, particularly the stratum spinosum that results in intraepidermal vesicles. If the spongiosis is severe, it can lead to **vesicle** formation. If persistent, the lesions develop into raised, scaling plaques because of reactive acanthosis and hyperkeratosis. They are prone to bacterial superinfections, which produce a yellow crusting called **impetiginization**. Drug-induced eczema causes lymphocytic infiltrate, containing eosinophils, around deep as well as superficial dermal vessels, whereas the contact antigens induce mononuclear inflammatory reaction that preferentially affects the superficial dermal layer.

Clinical Features Allergic contact dermatitis is the prototype of acute spongiotic dermatitis secondary to the exposure to poison ivy. Other common causes include nickel, paraphenylenediamine, rubber compounds and cosmetic preservatives. Atopic dermatitis usually involves the younger age group and results because of the complex interaction between genetic, environmental and immunological factors. The lesions commonly affect the face and extensor aspects of infants, whereas these affect the popliteal, antecubital fossa and the sides of the neck in the children and adults. The reaction can occur in relation to an internal circulating antigen that is ingested with food or drug (which is called drug-related eczematous dermatitis). The photoeczematous dermatitis is an increased reactivity to UV and visible light that is brought about by a chemical agent which is a photosensitizing agent, on an immunological basis. Irritants such as alkalis present in soaps, detergents, lye and ammonia-containing compounds cause an inflammatory reaction when it comes into contact with the skin surface in the susceptible individuals.

Treatment Treatment of these conditions mainly involves the search of offending substances and avoiding them. Topical steroids are also useful in their treatment.

Erythema Multiforme/Stevens–Johnson Syndrome/Toxic Epidermal Necrolysis

Historically, the distinction between erythema multiforme (EMF), Stevens–Johnson syndrome (SJS) and toxic epidermal necrolysis (TEN) is blurred. Although EMF and SJS are now considered a separate entity, SJS and TEN are widely regarded as a continuum of hypersensitivity reactions to certain infections and drugs. Any age can be affected and is often associated with infections such as herpes simplex, *Mycoplasma pneumoniae*, histoplasmosis, coccidioidomycosis, typhoid and leprosy. Drugs such as sulphonamides and penicillin are commonly involved. Cancer, lymphomas and collagen vascular diseases are also implicated.

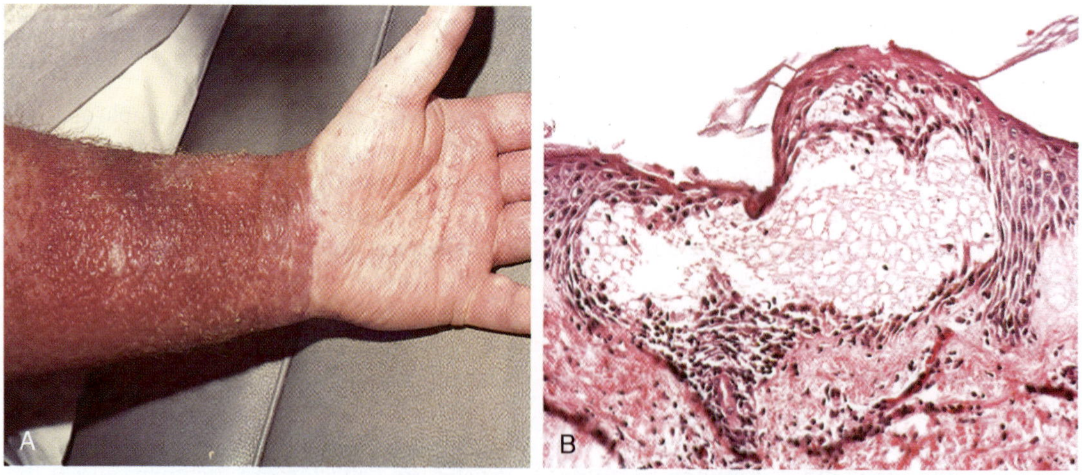

Fig. 29.1 Clinical picture and microscopy of acute eczematous dermatitis. (A) Acute allergic contact dermatitis due to antigen exposure (in this case, laundry detergent in clothing) marked by numerous vesicular lesions on erythematous skin. (B) Oedema within the epidermis creates fluid-filled intraepidermal vesicles. (*Source:* From Alexander J. Lazar. The Skin. Robbins & Cotran Pathologic Basis of Disease. 10th edition. Elsevier 2021.)

Pathogenesis EMF appears to result from a cell-mediated immune reaction. The condition can recur and is most commonly associated with herpes simplex infection and few drugs. Through PCR and in situ hybridization techniques, herpes simplex virus (HSV) DNA can be identified within the lesions. The virus particles remain in the lesions for up to 3 months even after the lesions have healed. Keratinocyte injury is caused by the skin-homing $CD8^+$ cytotoxic T lymphocytes (CTLs) in response to the antigens. $CD8^+$ cytotoxic T cells are more prominent in the central portion of the lesions and the epidermis, whereas the $CD4^+$ helper T cell and LCs are more prevalent in the peripheral portion of the lesions and the dermis. The production of interferon-γ causes an infiltration of leucocytes, monocytes and NK cells. In TEN though the pathogenetic steps remain unclear, majority of the damage is mediated by the cytotoxic T lymphocytes, macrophages, and cytokines such as tumour necrosis factor (TNF)-α.

Morphology

Gross Macroscopically, there is an array of lesions such as macules, papules, vesicles and bullae – 'multiforme' is observed in EMF (Fig. 29.2).

Microscopy EMF is the prototype of the vacuolar form of interface dermatitis which refers to the finding of the presence of inflammatory infiltrates abutting and obscuring the dermoepidermal junction. The common changes include orthokeratosis, necrosis and apoptosis of the individual keratinocytes, vacuolization of the basal cell layer, lymphocytes infiltration along the dermoepidermal junction and the perivascular region. Eosinophils may also be present. Mononuclear cells can be present near the necrotic keratinocytes and are referred to as satellite cell necrosis. With chronicity, there is a moderate infiltrate of lymphohistiocytes at the dermal epidermal region.

In SJS/TEN, the lesions show scattered apoptotic keratinocytes in the epidermis, single-cell necrosis of the keratinocytes to full-thickness epidermal necrosis and subepidermal bulla. The dermal inflammatory infiltration is less when compared with the EMF. In comparison, EMF shows less epidermal necrosis with more of dermal inflammatory infiltration, whereas SJS/TEN shows more epidermal necrosis and less of dermal inflammatory infiltration. However, clinical correlation is essential for a proper diagnosis.

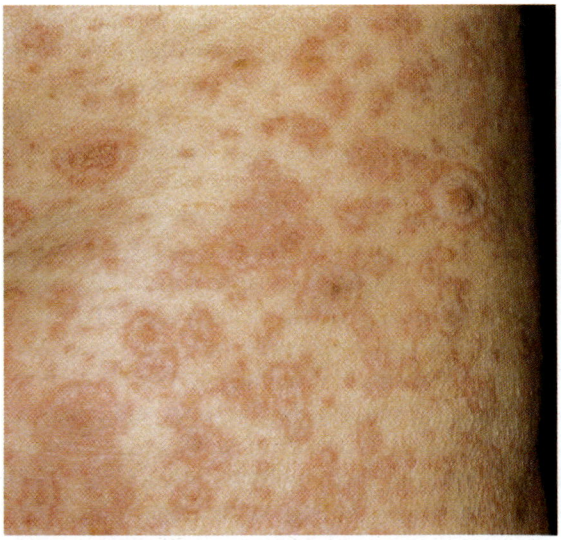

Fig. 29.2 Clinical pictures of EMF/SJS/TEN with typical target lesions that consist of a central blister or zone of epidermal necrosis surrounded by macular erythema. (*Source:* From Erythema Multiforme. Elsevier Point of Care. 2021.)

Erythema Multiforme There is interface change with basal vacuolization, numerous dyskeratotic keratinocytes and a sparse perivascular infiltrate.

Clinical Features EMF is a benign self-limited condition with **symmetric fixed lesions** mainly occurring in the extremities, some of which progress into typical concentric appearing **target-like lesions**. These target-like lesions consist of a pale central blister or zone of epidermal necrosis surrounded by macular erythema. Bullous EMF is a more severe form involving up to 10% body surface area with detachment.

In SJS, the patients present with fever and malaise with cutaneous eruptions consisting of flat atypical targetoid lesions or erythematous or purpuric macules, many with central epidermal necrosis or blister formation involving $<$10% of the body surface. Predominantly, the trunk is affected. The disease is most commonly associated with drugs in adults, whereas it is associated with infections, especially *Mycoplasma pneumoniae* in children, leading to life-threatening sepsis.

TEN, also known as the Lyell syndrome is composed of full-thickness epidermal necrosis involving $>$30% of the body surface area and resembles burns. Clinically, these patients have diffuse erythema, skin tenderness followed by large flaccid bullae and epidermal detachment in sheets. The disease has a high mortality rate because of extensive fluid loss and sepsis. TEN is most commonly associated with drug intake such as NSAIDs, sulphonamides, antibiotics, anticonvulsants, antiretrovirals and allopurinol.

All the three conditions can involve mucosal areas (oral, ocular and/or genital) and cause serious morbidity.

CHRONIC INFLAMMATORY DERMATOSES

Psoriasis

Psoriasis is a common chronic inflammatory dermatosis with an autoimmune basis involving all ages.

Pathogenesis Apart from idiopathic reasons, psoriasis has been proposed to result from complex interactions between altered keratinocyte proliferation and differentiation, genetic, environmental factors, inflammation and immune dysregulation. The autoimmune dysregulation has been linked to genes within the human leuco cyte antigen (HLA) locus with a strong association with HLA-C, particularly with the HLA-Cw*0602 allele. Those individuals who are homozygotes for this allele have a 2.5-fold higher risk for developing psoriasis. Sensitized populations of $CD4^+$ T_H1 and T_H17 cells and activated $CD8^+$ cytotoxic effector T cells enter the skin and accumulate in the epidermis. They secrete an increased amount of cytokines and growth factors that induce keratinocyte proliferation and the characteristic lesions. Interactions between $CD4^+$ T cells, $CD8^+$ T cells, dendritic cells and keratinocytes give rise to a cytokine 'soup'. This mixture contains predominantly the T_H1-type and T_H17-type of cytokines such as interleukin (IL)-12, interferon-γ, TNF and IL-17. Growth factors are also secreted by the lymphocytes that contribute to the epidermal thickening. Psoriatic lesions that can be induced in susceptible individuals by local trauma is known as Koebner phenomenon which can be attributed to the local inflammatory response stimulated by the trauma.

Morphology

Gross The skin of the elbows, knees, scalp, lumbosacral areas, intergluteal cleft and glans penis are the most commonly affected areas. It may cause a total body erythema and scaling, a condition referred to as **erythroderma** (Fig. 29.3). Typical lesions are variable in size and shape, well-demarcated, red to pink to salmon-coloured papules and plaques covered by loosely adherent silvery white scales. As the scales are lifted, multiple, minute, bleeding points can be noted, which is referred to as the **Auspitz sign** and corresponds to the tips of the dermal papillae. Nail changes are seen in 30% of the patients who show yellow-brown discolouration of the nail plates, with pitting, dimpling and separation of the nail plate from the underlying bed (onycholysis), thickening and crumbling.

Microscopy The characteristic findings are seen in the early-scaling papules and near the margins of the advancing plaques. The epidermis shows marked cellular proliferation leading to thickening (acanthosis) with regular downward elongation of rete ridges with thickening in their lower portions (clubbing) often compared to test tubes in a rack. Stratum granulosum layer of the epidermis is thinned or absent and an extensive and confluent overlying parakeratotic scale is seen (Fig. 29.4). Small aggregates of neutrophils collect within the parakeratotic stratum corneum (**Munro microabscesses**) and spongiform pustules. Also, there is thinning of portion of epidermal cell layer that overlies the tips of dermal papillae which are called suprapapillary plates with the occasional presence of small spongiform pustules, and upper epidermal layer pallor are seen. Dilated, tortuous blood vessels within these papillae leads to elongation and oedema. In pustular psoriasis, larger abscess-like accumulations of neutrophils are present directly beneath the stratum corneum. Treatment with TNF blockers has shown good response.

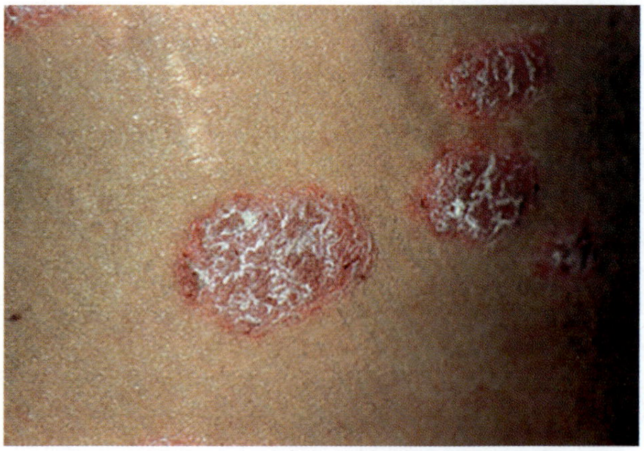

Fig. 29.3 Clinical pictures of psoriasis: Early lesions may be dominated by inflammation. (*Source:* From William D. James, Dirk M. Elston, James R. Treat, Misha A. Rosenbach and Isaac M. Neuhaus. Seborrheic Dermatitis, Psoriasis, Recalcitrant Palmoplantar Eruptions, Pustular Dermatitis, and Erythroderma. Andrews' Diseases of the Skin. 13th edition. Elsevier 2020.)

Clinical Features Apart from the skin lesions, 15% of the patients with psoriasis have associated arthritis. Psoriatic arthritis can be mild or severe with joint deformities, usually involving the terminal interphalangeal joint. A generalized pustular psoriasis is a variant which presents as cutaneous eruption composed of variable numbers of sterile pustules appearing in erythematous and scaly lesions associated with moderate-to-severe constitutional symptoms. This condition is also associated with pregnancy and human immunodeficiency virus (HIV). Clinically, the psoriasis is more severe with acute exacerbations and may be refractory to treatment. Guttate or eruptive psoriasis is observed in young patients and is characterized by an abrupt eruption of small lesions associated with acute group A β-haemolytic streptococcal infection. Psoriasis may also be associated with myopathy, enteropathy and spondylitic joint disease.

Treatment Patient education about the chronic relapsing and remitting nature of the disease, its noncontagiousness,

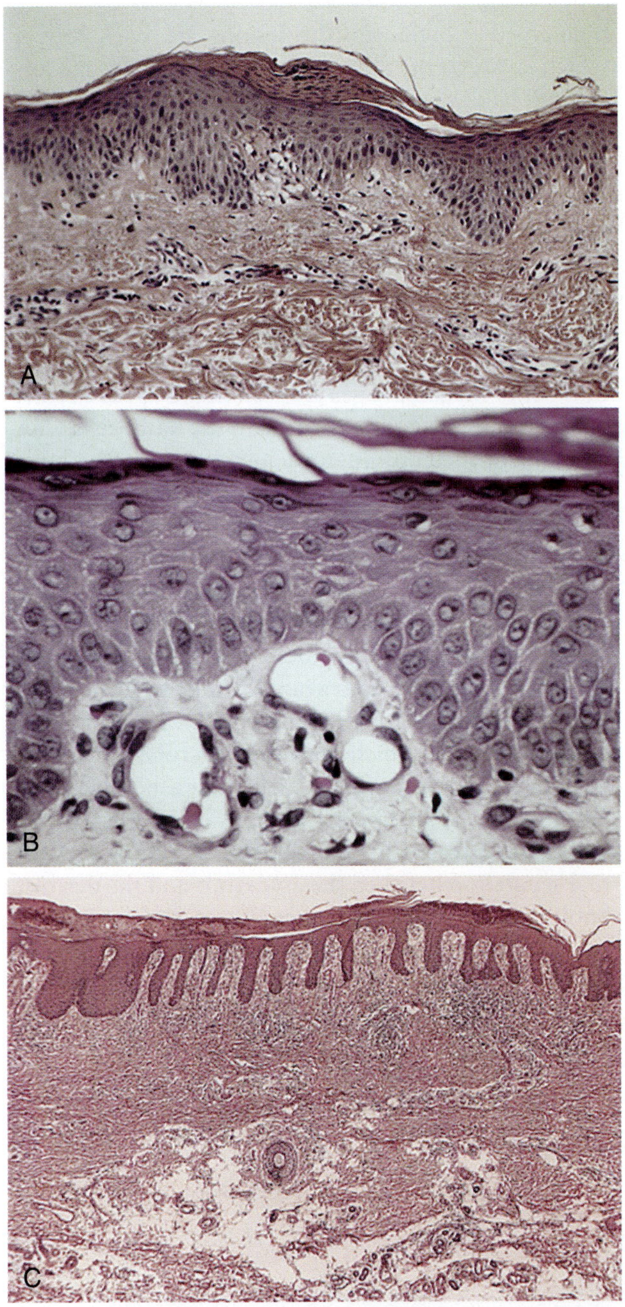

Fig. 29.4 (A) Microscopy of psoriasis showing neutrophils migrating to the summits of the parakeratotic mounds. (B) Dilated vessels are in the papillary dermis (H&E). (C) There is psoriasiform hyperplasia of the epidermis. (*Source:* From James W. Patterson MD, FACP, FAAD. The psoriasiform reaction pattern. Weedon's Skin Pathology. 5th edition. Elsevier 2021.)

drug availability only to control the diseases is the mainstay. In mild diseases, topical therapies with topical corticosteroids are used. Vitamin D analogues and coal tar preparations are also used in mild conditions. Phototherapy is used to treat widespread or refractory disease, and narrow-band ultraviolet B (UVB) is the preferred phototherapy spectrum. Conventional systemic treatment includes vitamin A analogues and methotrexate; cyclosporine particularly acts by modulating the epidermal proliferation and differentiation. Apremilast, which inhibits phosphodiesterase type 4, is recently used in the treatment of severe psoriasis and psoriatic arthropathy. Biologicals such as TNF inhibitors like adalimumab, etanercept and infliximab, IL-12/-23 inhibitors like ustekinumab and IL-17 inhibitor like secukinumab are now used as targeted chemotherapy.

Seborrhoeic Dermatitis

Seborrhoeic dermatitis is a chronic inflammatory dermatosis more common than psoriasis.

Pathogenesis The pathogenesis is unknown. Increased sebum production in response to androgens is believed to be the mechanism involved. In Parkinson disease due to dopamine deficiency, there is an increased sebum production and is associated with an increased incidence of seborrhoeic dermatitis. The lesions are also frequently seen in patients with epilepsy, congestive heart failure, chronic alcoholism, zinc deficiency and HIV infection. Severe form of seborrhoeic dermatitis in HIV-infected individuals is associated with low CD4 counts and the lesions are severe and refractory with atypical distribution. Relationship of the disease occurrence with the colonization of the skin by the fungal genus *Malassezia* is controversial.

Morphology

Gross Macroscopically, the patients develop macules and papules on an erythematous-yellow, greasy base and extensive scaling and crusting are formed on the scalp, ears, eyebrows, nasolabial areas and central chest. Fissures may also be present, particularly behind the ears.

Microscopy The microscopic features are a mixture of those observed in psoriasis and spongiotic dermatitis. The stratum corneum contains focal parakeratosis, with a predilection for the follicular ostia – a finding known as **shoulder parakeratosis**. Occasionally, pyknotic neutrophils are present within the parakeratotic foci (neutrophilic parakeratosis), sometimes with fluid (neutrophilic crust). Mounds of parakeratosis containing neutrophils and serum are present at the ostia of hair follicles, which is called **follicular lipping**. The earlier lesions are spongiotic, whereas the later ones are acanthotic. Superficial perivascular inflammatory infiltrate consists of admixture of lymphocytes and neutrophils. The patients usually have a good response to oral or topical ketoconazole.

Clinical Features In the infants, the scalp ('cradle cap'), face and diaper areas are involved. In the adults, those regions with high density of sebaceous glands such as scalp, forehead (especially the glabella), external auditory canal, retroauricular area, nasolabial folds, presternal area are commonly affected. The lesions are associated with inflammation of epidermis.

Treatment Seborrhoeic dermatitis is usually a self-limiting disease that can be managed by oil massage using mild shampooing that contains antifungal agents. Mild cases can be managed by emollients and mild topical steroids, whereas sever cases require oral antifungals.

Lichen Planus

Lichen planus (LP) is a subacute or chronic dermatosis which is relatively common in general population.

Pathogenesis The disease is idiopathic in origin with the expression of altered antigens in basal epidermal cells or the dermoepidermal junction being given as the explanation for its occurrence. This altered antigenic expression elicits a cell-mediated cytotoxic ($CD8^+$) T-cell response leading to T-lymphocyte infiltration and hyperplasia of LCs.

Morphology

Gross Macroscopically, the lesions are usually small, flat-topped, shiny, polygonal violaceous papules that may coalesce into plaques. The lesions are characteristically described with 'six Ps' namely **pruritic, purple, polygonal, planar, papules or plaques** of LP. These **violaceous lesions** are often highlighted by white dots/lines known as **Wickham striae** that are created by areas of hypergranulosis (Fig. 29.5A). In darkly pigmented individuals, the lesions are dark brown which is due to the release of melanin into dermis following the destruction of the basal cell layer.

Microscopy Microscopically, the lesion shows compact orthokeratosis, wedge-shaped hypergranulosis, irregular acanthosis, vacuolar degeneration of the basal cell layer and a band-like, i.e. a lichenoid dermal lymphocytic, infiltrate in close approximation to the epidermis known as **interface dermatitis** (Fig. 29.5B). Macrophages, few eosinophils and plasma cells are also noticed in the inflammatory infiltrates. Increased number of melanophages are seen in the upper dermis which is because of the damage to the basal cells with subsequent melanin pigment incontinence. The lymphocytes are intimately associated with the basal keratinocytes that show degeneration, necrosis and have resemblance to that of the stratum spinosum cells, an appearance named as **squamatization**. Because of the destructive lymphocytic infiltrate, the dermoepidermal interface takes an angulated zigzag contour causing a **saw-toothed appearance**. Anucleate, necrotic basal layer cells are often incorporated into inflamed papillary dermis, which are termed as colloid, hyaline, cytoid or **Civatte bodies** which have a homogenous eosinophilic appearance. The cells are PAS-positive and diastase resistant. Some lesions may show artefactual separation between the epidermis and the dermis, known as **Max-Joseph spaces**. These spaces develop because of extensive damage to the basal cells. Chronic lesions show features of chronicity such as epidermal hyperplasia, thickening of granular cell layer and stratum corneum.

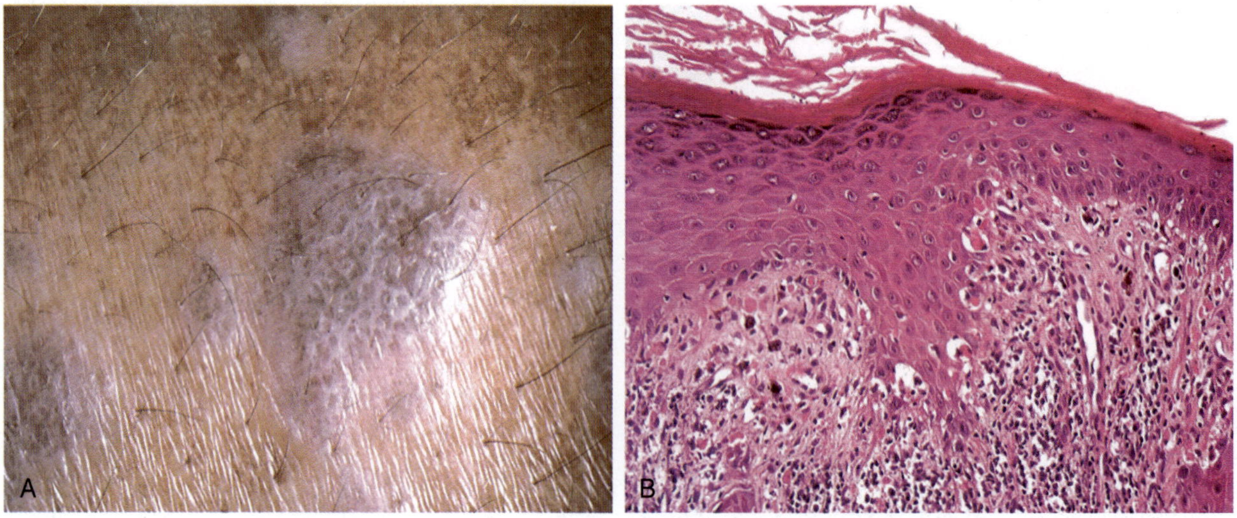

Fig. 29.5 Clinical pictures and microscopy of lichen planus. (A) This flat-topped pink-purple, polygonal papule has a white lace-like pattern of lines that are referred to as Wickham striae. (B) There is a band-like infiltrate of lymphocytes at the dermoepidermal junction, hyperkeratosis and pointed rete ridges (sawtoothing), as a result of chronic basal cell layer injury. (*Source:* From Alexander J. Lazar. The Skin. Robbins & Cotran Pathologic Basis of Disease. 10th edition. Elsevier 2021.)

Clinical Features LP can involve skin, mucous membranes, hair follicles and nails. It most commonly resolves spontaneously within 1–2 years after onset, often leaving a residuum of postinflammatory hyperpigmentation. However, oral lesions may persist for years and usually involve the buccal and glossal mucosa consisting of a lacy reticular network of white coalescent papules. Nails are also involved in 10% of the patients causing roughening, longitudinal ridging and thinning. Squamous cell carcinoma (SCC) has been observed to occur in the site of chronic LP in <1% of cases; an example of carcinogenesis in setting of chronic inflammatory process and Koebner phenomenon is commonly observed in patients with LP. The lesions have a predilection for occurrence over the flexor aspect of the forearms, legs and glans penis.

Treatment The location and severity of the lesion decide the management protocol. Treatment is needed to decrease the associated pruritis, shorten the disease duration and minimize the scarring. Topical corticosteroids, oral histaminics, topical tretinoin, tacrolimus and narrow-band UVB are the preferred drugs for LP management. In sever diseases, systemic corticosteroids, cyclosporine, methotrexate, azathioprine and mycophenolate mofetil have been used.

BLISTERING (BULLOUS) DISEASES

Blistering or bullous disorders frequently involve skin and oral mucosal surfaces. It can occur in unrelated conditions such as herpes virus infection, spongiotic dermatitis, EMF and thermal burns. However, there is a group of bullous disorders where the bullae are the primary occurrence because of acquired or inherited defects of proteins present in the desmosomes and hemidesmosomes. The intercellular adhesion involves the desmosomes, whereas the basal epithelial cells are attached with the basement membrane through hemidesmosomes (Fig. 29.6). These diseases may be life threating because they can lead to dehydration and infections. The level of bulla occurrence has to be assessed properly for diagnosis and better understanding of the pathogenetic mechanisms. The blistering disorders can be divided into those associated with inflammation and those that are not (Flowchart 29.1). Pemphigus, bullous pemphigoid and dermatitis herpetiformis are associated with inflammation, whereas epidermolysis bullosa and porphyria are not associated with inflammation. We will discuss the common blistering disorders.

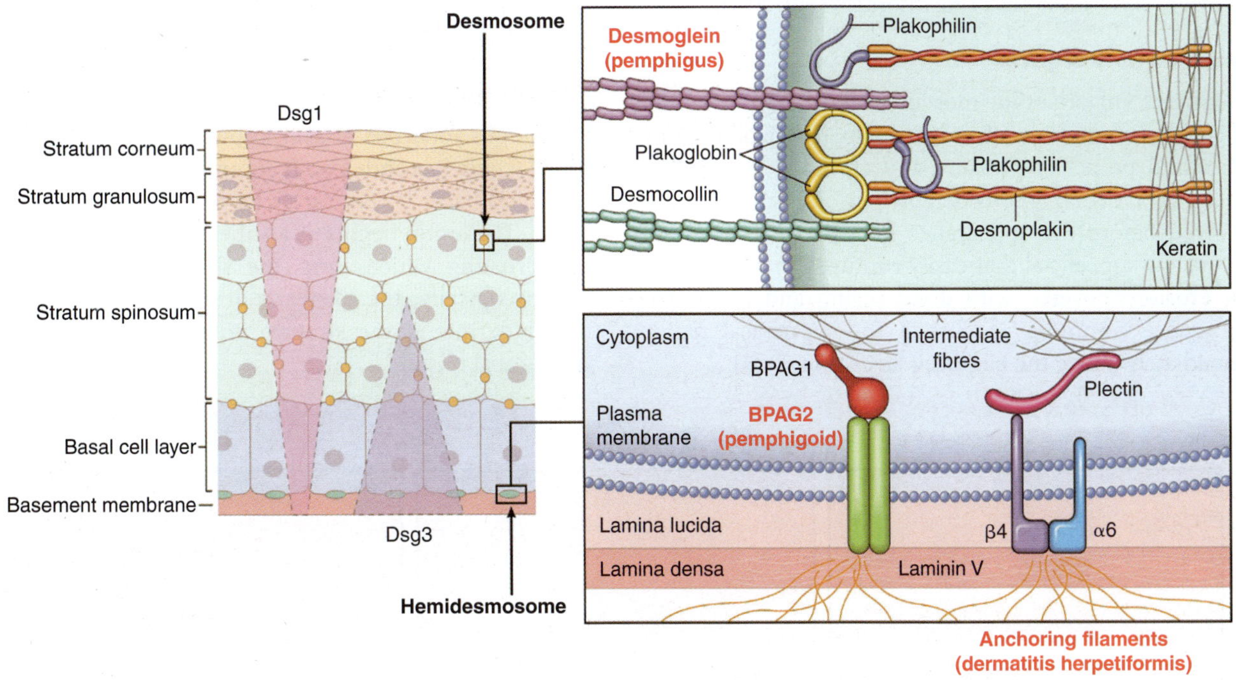

Fig. 29.6 Keratinocyte adhesion molecules and blistering inflammatory disorders. Knowledge of the proteins composing desmosomes and hemidesmosomes is key to understanding blistering disorders. Desmogleins 1 and 3 *(Dsg1, Dsg3)* are functionally interchangeable components of desmosomes but have different distributions within the epidermis *(left panel)*. The major structural proteins of desmosomes and hemidesmosomes are shown in the *right panel*. In pemphigus vulgaris, autoantibodies against Dsg1 and Dsg3 cause blisters in the deep suprabasal epidermis, whereas in pemphigus foliaceus, autoantibodies are against Dsg1 alone, leading to superficial, subcorneal blisters. In bullous pemphigoid, autoantibodies bind BPAG2, a component of the hemidesmosomes, leading to blister formation at the level of the lamina lucida of the basement membrane. Dermatitis herpetiformis is caused by IgA autoantibodies to the fibrils that anchor hemidesmosomes to the dermis. (*Source:* From Alexander J. Lazar. The Skin. Robbins & Cotran Pathologic Basis of Disease. 10th edition. Elsevier 2021.)

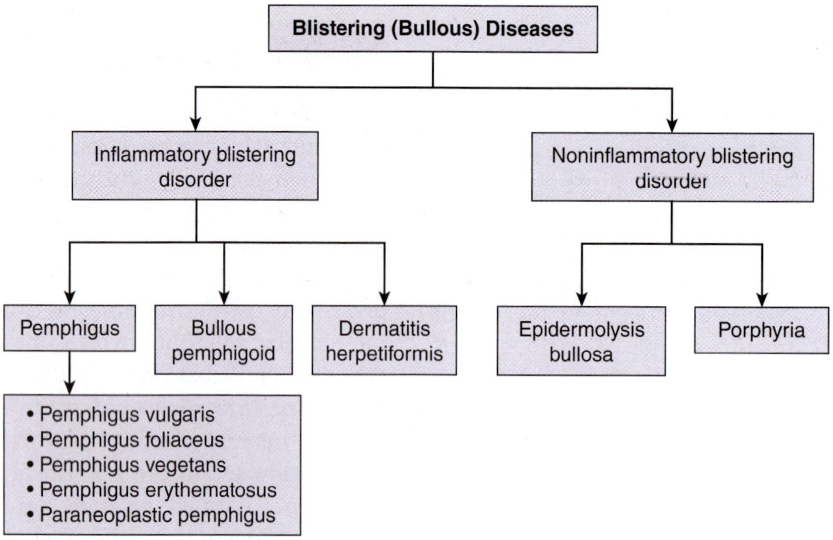

Flowchart 29.1 Classification of bullous disorders.

INFLAMMATORY BLISTERING DISORDERS

Pemphigus is usually a benign blistering disorder caused by the autoantibodies towards the proteins of the desmosomes, which results in the detachment of the intercellular keratinocytic attachments within the epidermis and mucosal epithelium. The level of dehiscence forms the important criteria for the diagnosis of these blistering disorders (Fig. 29.7).

Pemphigus Vulgaris

Pemphigus vulgaris is the most common subtype of pemphigus and commonly affects the scalp, face, axilla, groin, trunk and points of pressure and clinically presents as oral or skin ulcers. A considerable period of time may be involved before the appearance of a bulla. The lesions are usually superficial that easily rupture producing shallow erosions covered with dried serum and crust. The dehiscence commonly occurs at the suprabasal region immediately above the basal cell layer (Fig. 29.8).

Pemphigus Vegetans

Pemphigus vegetans is a rare subtype and clinically the lesions are large, moist, verrucous (wart-like), vegetating plaques and hence the name. The lesions are usually studded with pustules and the groin, axillae and other flexural areas are most commonly affected. The blister is suprabasal in its location, along with overlying epidermal hyperplasia.

Pemphigus Foliaceus

Pemphigus foliaceus is also known as fogo selvagem in Brazil where it is endemic. It commonly affects scalp, face, chest and back. It very rarely involves the mucous membrane. The lesion begins as a superficial area of erythema and crusting which form the sites of blister rupture. Microscopically, the blister is at the superficial part of the epidermis at the stratum granulosum and forms a subcorneal blister.

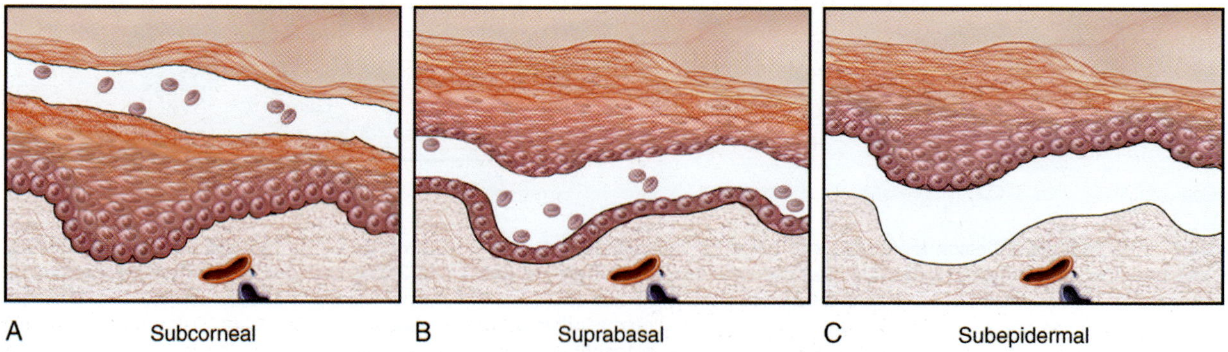

Fig. 29.7 Bulla location in blistering diseases of the skin. Schematic representation of different types of blisters. (A) In subcorneal blisters, the stratum corneum forms the roof of the bulla (as in pemphigus foliaceus). (B) In a suprabasal blister, a portion of the epidermis, including the stratum corneum, forms the roof (as in pemphigus vulgaris). (C) In a subepidermal blister, the entire epidermis separates from the dermis (as in bullous pemphigoid). (*Source:* From Alexander J. Lazar. The Skin. Robbins & Cotran Pathologic Basis of Disease. 10th edition. Elsevier 2021.)

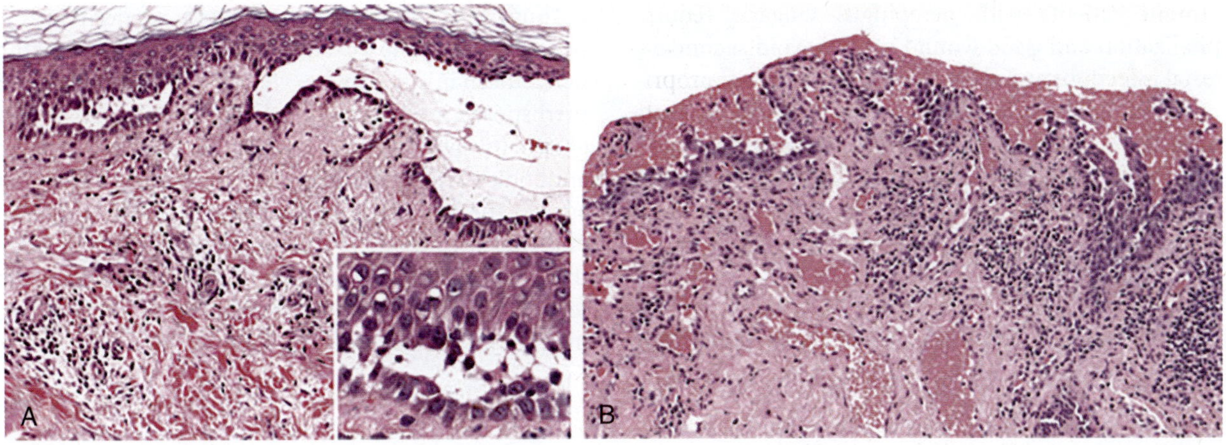

Fig. 29.8 Pemphigus vulgaris – histologic features. (A) Blisters in the skin show suprabasal acantholysis with a few acantholytic cells in the blister cavity (inset). (B) Because blisters in the mouth rarely remain intact, the blister roof is often not seen in oral biopsy specimens. Nonetheless, the diagnosis can be made by the location of the split within the epithelium, the presence of acantholytic cells, and the 'tombstones' appearance of the basal cells. (*Source:* From Masayuki Amagai. Pemphigus. Dermatology. 4th edition. Elsevier 2018.)

Pemphigus Erythematosus

Pemphigus erythematosus is considered to be a localized, less severe form of pemphigus foliaceus. It usually affects the malar area selectively such as in the systemic lupus erythematosus.

Paraneoplastic Pemphigus

Paraneoplastic pemphigus occurs in the setting of a preexisting malignancy which is usually a non-Hodgkin lymphoma.

Pathogenesis All varieties of pemphigus are of autoimmune aetiology where IgG autoantibodies against the desmoglein proteins that form an important component in the intercellular keratinocyte adhesion in the epidermis are found and cause the blister formation. The expression of desmoglein 1 and 3 proteins in the epidermis and the production of autoantibodies to either one or both determines the severity of the blisters. Along with the blister formation, these autoantibodies also stimulate the intercellular proteases. The IgG deposition are seen on direct immunofluorescence method as a characteristic **net-like pattern** of intercellular IgG deposits (Fig. 29.9). These deposits are seen at all the levels of epidermis in pemphigus, whereas only at the superficial layers in pemphigus foliaceus.

Morphology

The common characteristic finding in microscopy in all the subtypes of pemphigus is **acantholysis** which is the dissolution of the intercellular bridges formed by the hemidesmosomes that connect squamous epithelial cells with one another. The acantholytic cells lose their polyhedral shape and become rounded in appearance. In suprabasal blisters seen in pemphigus vulgaris and vegetans, a single layer of intact basal cells forms the blister base and is referred to as a **row of tombstones**. Variable inflammatory infiltrate may be present.

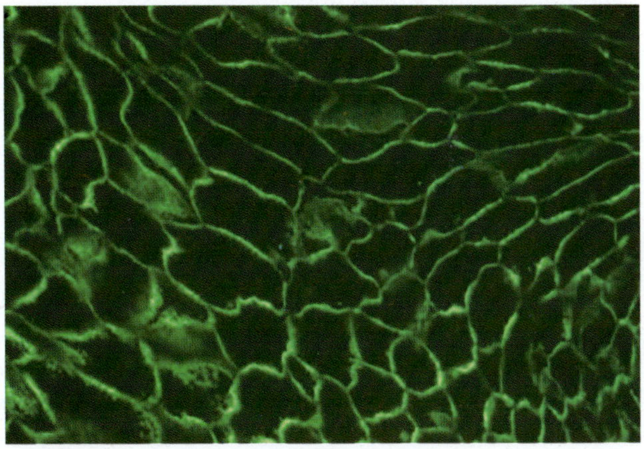

Fig. 29.9 Direct immunofluorescence staining for immunoglobulin of epidermis involved by pemphigus. In pemphigus vulgaris, there is deposition of immunoglobulin along the plasma membranes of keratinocytes in a reticular or fishnet-like pattern accompanied by suprabasal loss of cell-to-cell adhesion (acantholysis). (*Source:* From Kachiu C. Lee. Pemphigus Vulgaris. Elsevier 2022.)

Clinical Features The disease commonly affects patients during the fifth to sixth decade and both the sexes are affected equally.

These lesions are commonly treated with the immunosuppressive agents which help to reduce the titres of the pathogenetic autoantibody levels.

Treatment Patients with pemphigus vulgaris require hospitalization and good wound care to avoid secondary bacterial infections and risk of septicaemia with appropriate antibiotics. Prednisolone and immunosuppressants such as azathioprine, cyclophosphamide and mycophenolate mofetil form the important drugs in the treatment protocol. Anti-CD20 monoclonal antibody rituximab is preferred in patients with recalcitrant disease.

Bullous Pemphigoid

Bullous pemphigoid is also a common skin disorder that presents as bullous lesions of the skin with autoimmune basis.

Morphology

Gross The characteristic lesions are tense bullae containing clear fluid which range from 2 to 8 cm in diameter. These lesions do not rupture easily and heal without scarring, unless infected.
Microscopy Microscopically, the lesions are **subepidermal, nonacantholytic** blisters. Perivascular inflammatory infiltrates composed of lymphocytes, eosinophils, occasional neutrophils, superficial dermal oedema and basal cell vacuolization are noted.

Pathogenesis The autoantibodies are produced against the proteins that are necessary for the adherence of the of basal keratinocytes to the basement membrane. The bullous pemphigoid antigens (**BPAGs**) are the mainstay of the hemidesmosomes and those that are against the BPAG2 frequently result in the blister formation. These autoantibodies stimulate the complement system leading to the recruitment of inflammatory cells such as the neutrophils and eosinophils and result in the bulla formation. In the immunofluorescence study, a continuous linear pattern at the **dermoepidermal junction** is identified.

Clinical Features Bullous pemphigoid commonly affects the inner aspects of the thighs, flexor surfaces of the forearms, axillae, groin and lower abdomen. Oral mucosal lesions can also be found in 10%–15% of the patients after the appearance of the cutaneous lesion. It generally affects the elderly and sometimes presents with urticarial plaques and severe pruritus.

Treatment Oral prednisolone, dapsone, azathioprine, mycophenolate mofetil, cyclophosphamide and tetracycline are used in the treatment of bullous pemphigoid.

Dermatitis Herpetiformis

Dermatitis herpetiformis is a rare disorder with immune basis characterized by urticarial rashes.

Pathogenesis From the association of dermatitis herpetiformis with the intestinal coeliac disease, the pathogenetic mechanism can be viewed where the genetically predisposed individuals develop IgA antibodies to dietary gluten (derived from the wheat protein gliadin). These antibodies cross-react with the anchoring fibrils, mainly against the reticulin that is present in them. These molecules help to attach the epidermal basement membrane to the superficial dermis and therefore a subepidermal blister is produced. A gluten-free diet helps in the improvement of this condition.

Morphology

Gross The lesions occur as bilateral, symmetric, grouped vesicles with urticaria.
Microscopy Microscopically, inflammatory process affects the tips of dermal papillae that are composed of fibrin and neutrophils, forming microabscesses (Fig. 29.10). This causes the dermoepidermal separation at the particular point along with the basal cell layer vacuolization finally resulting in the subepidermal blister formation. A characteristic granular IgA deposit at the tips of the affected dermal papillae is seen in the immunofluorescence study.

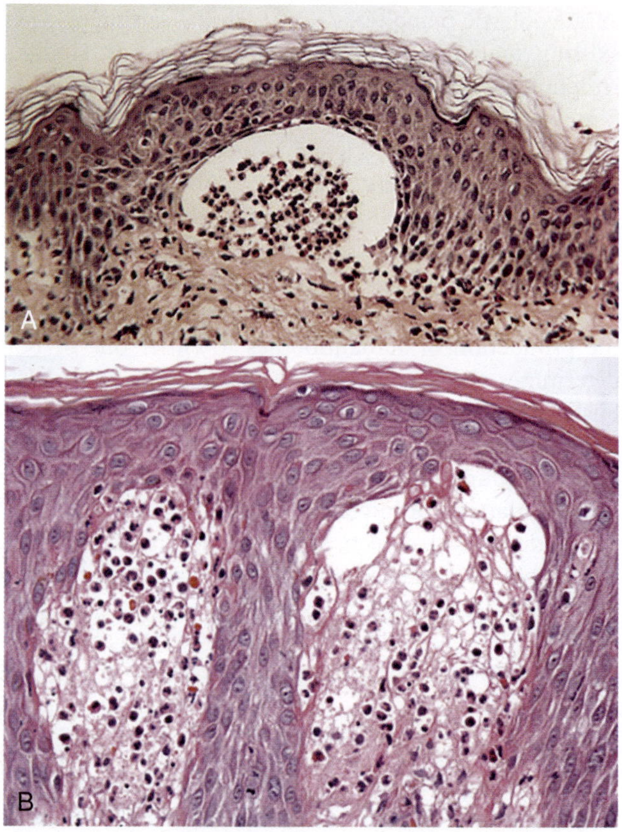

Fig. 29.10 Microscopy of dermatitis herpetiformis. There is a subepidermal blister. (A) A microabscess is present in a dermal papilla. (B) A later lesion with acanthosis and some eosinophils as well as neutrophils in the papillary dermis.

Clinical Features Dermatitis herpetiformis commonly affects the males in the third to fourth decade of life and the lesions commonly occur in the elbows, knees, upper back and buttocks. The disease is associated with the occurrence of intestinal coeliac disease.

Treatment Dapsone is the drug of choice with strict gluten-free diet.

NONINFLAMMATORY BLISTERING DISORDERS

Noninflammatory blistering disorders comprise those disorders with vesicles and bullae that occur because of inherited or acquired defects involving structural proteins of the skin. Epidermolysis bullosa and porphyria are the two important diseases under this category.

Epidermolysis Bullosa

Epidermolysis bullosa is a group of disorders which commonly has inherited defects in the structural proteins such as α6/β4 and α6/β4 integrins which give mechanical support to the skin structure. The lesions commonly occur at the sites of pressure, rubbing or trauma. Different subtypes are present under this entity such as the simplex type, which is most common where there is mutation of genes encoding keratin 14, 15. In the junctional type of epidermolysis bullosa, the dehiscence occurs at the level of lamina lucida and is due to mutations in subunit of laminin or rarely BPAG2 and in the dystrophic type there are mutations in COL7A1 gene encoding type VII collagen where there are subepidermal blister. Mixed type of epidermolysis bullosa shows defects at several levels of basement membrane (Fig. 29.11).

Porphyria

Porphyria is composed of a group of rare, poorly understood inborn or acquired disturbances of porphyrin metabolism. Porphyrins are pigments found in haemoglobin, myoglobin and cytochromes. The disease is classified on the basis of both clinical and biochemical features. Five subtypes are identified, namely congenital erythropoietic porphyria, erythrohepatic protoporphyria, acute intermittent porphyria, porphyria cutanea tarda and mixed porphyria. Clinically, the lesions cause urticaria and are associated with scarring when exposed to sunlight. The location of the vesicles is subepidermal and the dermal blood vessel walls are thickened by glassy deposits of serum proteins, including immunoglobulins.

INFECTIONS

Skin is exposed to frequent trauma and microorganisms making it a vulnerable organ to get frequent infections despite its multilayered protection mechanism as discussed in Chapter 6. Common skin infections in immunocompetent and immunocompromised individuals are discussed in Chapter 8. Here, we discuss the infections that present with skin manifestations primarily.

VERRUCAE

Verrucae or condyloma are contagious squamoproliferative tumours that can occur in skin or mucosal surface and are caused by human papillomavirus (HPV). Classification of warts is based on morphology and anatomic location. Cutaneous warts are traditionally classified as verrucae vulgaris (common warts), verrucae palmares (deep palmar or hand warts), verrucae plantares (deep foot warts, myrmecia), superficial plantar warts (mosaic warts), verrucae planae (plane warts, flat warts), condyloma accuminata (genital warts or venereal warts), condyloma plana (flat cervical condylomas, plane condyloma) and epidermodysplasia verruciformis (EV).

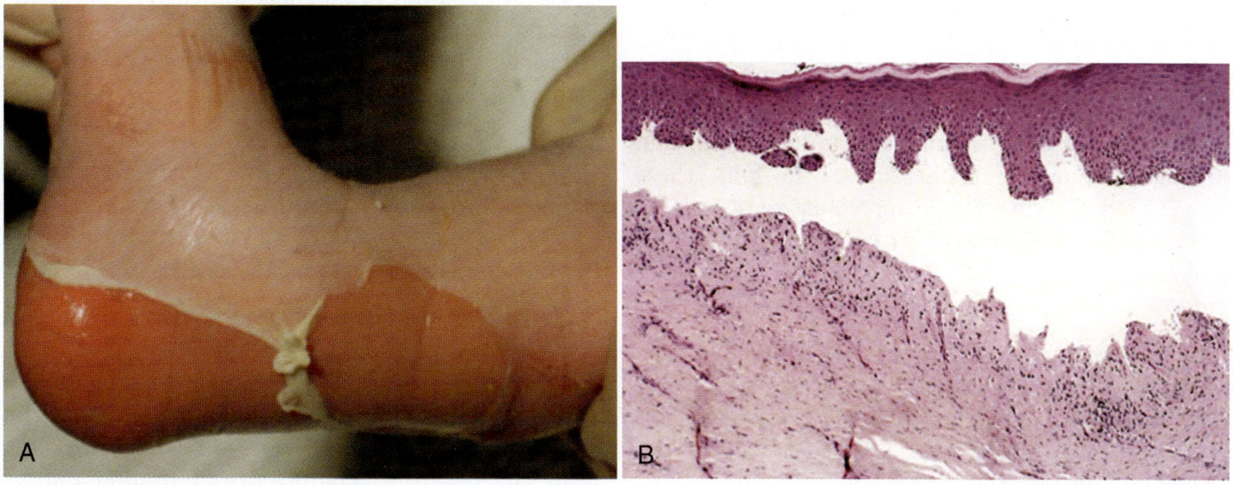

Fig. 29.11 (A) Epidermolysis bullosa – dystrophic type (also known as dystrophic epidermolysis bullosa). (B) There is an infiltrate-poor subepidermal bulla. Scarring is present in the underlying dermis.

The HPVs are DNA viruses which are epitheliotropic and cause many benign and malignant lesions. The lesion occurs equally in both the sexes by direct contact or auto-inoculation and usually spontaneously regresses in 6 months to 2 years.

Benign genital warts are usually caused by HPV-6 and HPV-11. Persistent infection by high risk subtypes HPV-16 and HPV-18 represents the important risk factor for the development of premalignant and malignant lesions. The infection is also aided by suppressed cell-mediated immunity in conditions such as HIV infection, organ transplantation, leukaemia and lymphoma. Viral typing is done by in situ hybridization and polymerase chain reaction. HPVs that produce E6 proteins abolish the p53 function and can have increased risk of oncogenesis. E6 proteins of low-risk HPVs interfere with Notch signalling that is required for the normal maturation of keratinocytes, and may contribute to the formation of warts.

Verruca Vulgaris (Common Wart)

Verruca vulgaris is a benign squamous papillomatous lesion caused by infection with HPV. The lesion commonly occurs in children and adolescents. HPV-2, -1, -4 and -7 are commonly associated with verruca vulgaris.

Morphology

Gross They may be solitary or multiple and found in the exposed parts especially in the fingers and dorsum of the hands and are hard, rough-surfaced papules ranging in diameter from 1.5 to 2 cm. New lesions can also arise in areas of trauma (Koebner phenomenon).
Microscopy Microscopically, the lesions show marked hyperkeratosis, acanthosis, columns of parakeratosis overlying papillomatous projections. **Koilocytes** (large vacuolated cells with pyknotic nuclei) are also seen in the upper part of the epidermis. Dilated blood vessels are seen in the papillomatous projections with variable numbers of lymphocytic infiltration.

Verruca Plantaris (Plantar Wart, Deep Foot Wart, Myrmecia)

Verruca plantaris is a benign, HPV-induced epithelial proliferation occurring on the sole of the foot. These lesions are common in children and young adults.

Morphology

Gross Clinically, they are sharply defined, rounded lesions, with a rough keratotic surface, surrounded by a thickened horn. The surface may have black dots representing thrombosed capillaries. They are divided into superficial warts (mosaic) and deep warts (myrmecia).

Microscopy Microscopically, the mosaic type shows acanthosis, papillomatosis, hyperkeratosis, koilocytes parakeratosis and keratohyalin granules. Myrmecia shows endophytic proliferation of rete ridges covered by thickened keratin and prominent eosinophilic intracytoplasmic inclusions. The regression of the lesions is usually associated with thrombosis of superficial vessels, haemorrhage and necrosis of the epidermis and mixed inflammatory cells.

Verruca Plana (Flat Wart, Verruca Plana Juvenilis)

Verruca planae are benign, HPV-induced slightly elevated flat-topped smooth papules. Children and adolescents are more commonly affected. HPV-3 and HPV-10 are most frequently associated with this lesion. Most of these lesions occur on the back of the hand and fingers, distal forearm, lower leg and face.

Morphology

Gross Clinically, these lesions are small, round-to-oval epidermal papules with a smooth and flat surface, measuring 1–4 mm in diameter.
Microscopy Microscopically, the lesions show hyperkeratosis with basket weave pattern, epidermal hyperplasia with dilatation of the capillaries present in the papillary dermis. Superficial epidermis shows koilocytosis and hypergranulosis.

MOLLUSCUM CONTAGIOSUM

Molluscum contagiosum (MC) is a common self-limited viral disease of the skin and mucosa caused by a DNA poxvirus that only infects humans, called molluscum contagiosum virus (MCV). It is a brick-shaped virus and measures 300 nm in maximal dimension commonly infecting the immunosuppressed individuals. The disease is considered to be transmitted through sexual route, direct skin contact, autoinoculation and fomite transmission.

Morphology

Gross The lesions are usually 2–5 mm dome-shaped pearly or flesh-coloured painless, firm, pruritic papules with central umbilication (Fig. 29.12).

Microscopy Microscopically, the lesions show epidermal lobular acanthosis with inverted epidermal hyperplasia. Prominent granular intracytoplasmic eosinophilic inclusions containing virus particles known as **Henderson–Patterson (molluscum) bodies** are noted in the keratinocytes of stratum spinosum and granulosum (Fig. 29.13).

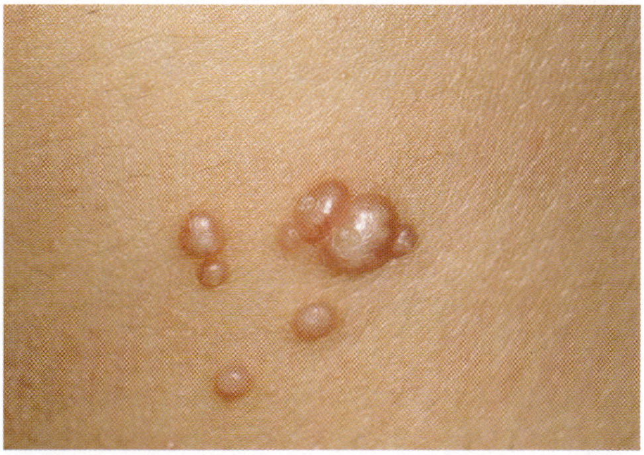

Fig. 29.12 Clinical picture of molluscum contagiosum. Molluscum contagiosum lesions: The lesions, known as mollusca, are small, raised and usually white, pink or flesh-coloured with a dimple or pit in the centre. (*Source:* From Fred F. Ferri. Molluscum Contagiosum. Ferri's Clinical Advisor 2021. Elsevier 2021.)

Clinical Features The lesions can occur anywhere in the body with a predilection for the hair-bearing trunk and the anogenital areas. Frequently, a curd-like material is expressed from the central umbilication that can be smeared and the molluscum bodies can be made more conspicuous with Giemsa or Lendrum's phloxine–tartrazine staining. Rupture of the lesion may incite intense chronic inflammatory cell infiltration.

Treatment The treatment depends on the age of the patient, number and site of the lesions. Children with few lesions are counselled about the spontaneous resolution of the lesions. Treatment is required in patients with numerous, symptomatic, cosmetically concerning lesions that are slow to regress. Mechanical methods of removal by squeezing, applications of irritants and physical destruction by curettage and cryotherapy are used. Immunomodulatory therapies by the usage of topical imiquimod or oral cimetidine are used. Cytotoxic agents such as podophyllotoxin, 5-fluorouracil are also used. Topical 5% cidofovir an antiviral agent is used in HIV patients.

IMPETIGO

Impetigo is the common superficial bacterial infection of skin and is highly contagious. The infection is transmitted through superficial cuts in the skin and can be prevented by proper cleaning and dressing of the wounds. Two forms of impetigo occur, namely impetigo contagiosa (IC) or nonbullous impetigo usually caused by group A β-haemolytic streptococci and bullous impetigo (BI) including the staphylococcal scalded skin syndrome which is caused by *Staphylococcus aureus*. They differ by the size of the pustules.

Impetigo Contagiosa

IC usually occurs in the preschool-aged children and can occur in epidemics. The pathogenesis involves the bacterial species stimulating the innate immune response leading to the destruction of the epidermis and erythematous vesiculopustular lesions externally. The bacteria produce an exfoliative toxin, which is a serine protease enzyme that superficially cleaves desmoglein 1 within or below the stratum granulosum and the dermis is not involved.

Morphology

The lesions often contain numerous neutrophils and very rarely few acantholytic cells at the floor of the vesicopustule beneath the stratum corneum forming a subcorneal pustule. Also, Gram-positive cocci can be

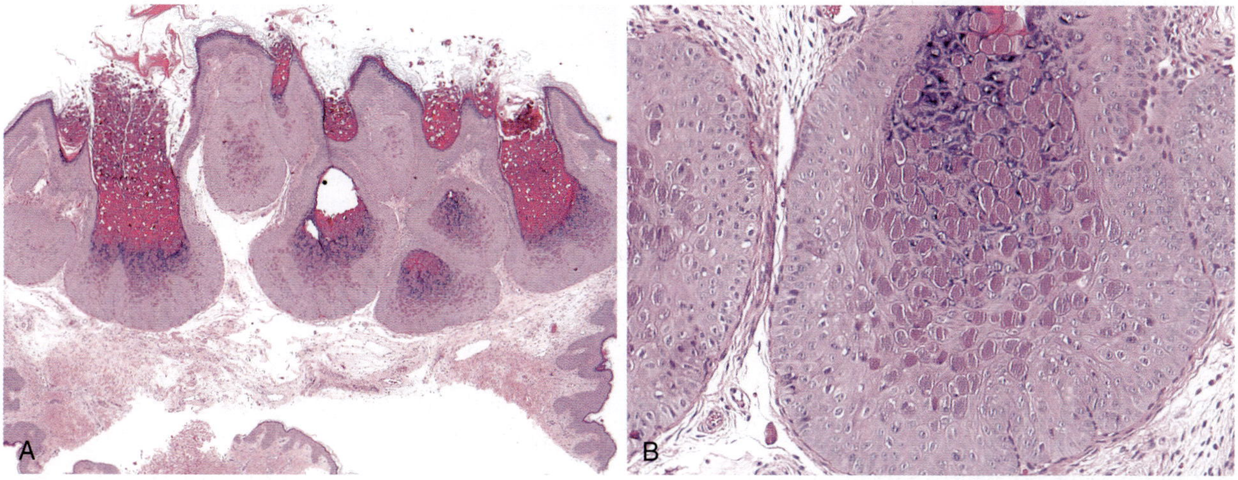

Fig. 29.13 Microscopy of molluscum contagiosum. (A) Biopsy of molluscum contagiosum demonstrates proliferation of characteristic Henderson–Patterson bodies within intraepidermal lobules. (B) High power view showing the intracytoplasmic eosinophilic inclusions. (*Source:* From Wilma F. Bergfeld and Michele Babb Tarbox. Orf Infections and Molluscum Contagiosum. Pathology of Infectious Diseases. Saunders 2015.)

found within the vesicopustule both intra- and extracellularly of the neutrophils. These lesions rupture quickly forming shallow erosions, and are followed by heavy serous exudation with formation of honey-coloured crusts (scabs). The lesions commonly occur on the exposed skin, particularly of the hand and face and are an occasional sequela of acute glomerulonephritis. These lesions should be differentiated from pemphigus foliaceus by presence of more neutrophils, fewer acantholytic cells and presence of Gram-positive cocci in the bulla cavity.

Bullous Impetigo and Staphylococcal Scalded Skin Syndrome

BI predominantly occurs in the newborns, infants, young children and occasionally in adults suffering from suppressed cell-mediated immunity. Phage group II staphylococci produce BI and the staphylococcal scalded skin syndrome. The lesions appear as vesicles that quickly progress to flaccid bullae with little or no surrounding erythema. BI may spread and become generalized and can be very difficult to distinguish from staphylococcal scalded skin syndrome. Staphylococcal scalded skin syndrome, also known as Ritter disease, also occur largely in the newborns and young children.

Morphology

Gross The lesions start abruptly with diffuse erythema and fever. Large, flaccid bullae filled with clear fluid form and they rupture immediately with a loss of large sheets of epidermis. The disease is fatal in <4% of children and >50% in the adults. The disease is transmissible and can lead to the occurrence of epidemics. No phage group II staphylococci can be grown from the bullae of staphylococcal scalded skin syndrome unlike the BI.

Microscopy Histopathological examination shows the lesion to be situated in the uppermost epidermis either below or within the granular layer, and in contrast to IC, there are few or no inflammatory cells seen within the bullous cavity (Fig. 29.14). In BI, the upper dermis may show polymorphous infiltration, whereas in the staphylococcal scalded skin syndrome, the dermis is usually free of any inflammation. The disease can be differentiated from severe EMF where nearly the entire epidermis detaches itself with considerable necrosis of the epidermal cells.

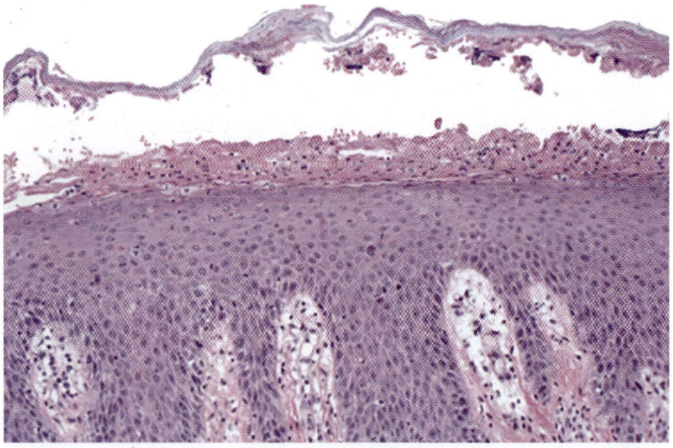

Fig. 29.14 Microscopy of impetigo. Bullous impetigo: There is a subcorneal blister containing inflammatory cells and degenerated keratinocytes. Gram-positive cocci were found (H&E).

SUPERFICIAL FUNGAL INFECTIONS

Superficial fungal infections of the skin correspond to the fungal infection confined to the stratum corneum caused by **dermatophytes**. These organisms can grow in soil and on animals and cause a number of diverse lesions with characteristic distributions, as follows:

Tinea capitis is dermatophytosis of the scalp, which usually occurs in children. It can rarely occur in infants and adults. The lesions are asymptomatic, patchy, with mild erythema, crust formation, scaling and frequent hair loss.
Tinea barbae is a dermatophytosis of the beard area that affects adult men. It is a relatively uncommon infection.
Tinea corporis commonly affects children but can occur in all ages. Excessive heat and humidity, exposure to infected animals are the common predisposing factors. The lesions are expanding, round, slightly erythematous plaque with an elevated scaling border.
Tinea cruris most frequently involves the inguinal areas of obese people during warm weather. The heat, friction and maceration all predispose to its development. The lesions are moist, red patches with raised scaly borders.
Tinea pedis (athlete's foot) occurs as a diffuse erythematous scaling lesion and often localized to the web spaces between the toes. The inflammatory reaction is the result of bacterial superinfection. When the infection spreads to the nails, it is referred to as onychomycosis. The nails are discoloured, thickened with deformed nail plate.
Tinea versicolour usually occurs on the upper trunk and is caused by a yeast named *Malassezia furfur*. The lesions consist of groups of macules of varied size and colour with a fine peripheral scale.

Dandruff is a condition causing flaking of the scalp often leading to lower sociopsychological esteem. Many authors have considered dandruff to be associated with seborrhoeic dermatitis with a role of *Malassezia* yeasts.

Morphology

The microscopic picture varies according to the properties of the organism, the host response and the degree of bacterial superinfection. There may be mild eczematous dermatitis associated with intraepidermal neutrophils. Periodic acid–Schiff stain stains the fungi pink to red because the cell walls contain mucopolysaccharides. They are usually found in the anucleate cornified layer of lesional skin, hair or nails. The organisms can also be cultured for their identification.

Treatment

Topical antifungals in mild cases are used with systemic drugs in severe cases being preferred. Oral antibiotics are used when superadded bacterial infections are noted. Potassium hydroxide (KOH) mounts (wet mount of the clinical specimen) can be used to better visualize the fungal elements.

DISORDERS OF MELANOCYTES

Human melanocytes are distributed in not only the epidermis and in hair follicles but also mucosa, cochlea (ear), iris (eye) and mesencephalon (brain) among other tissues. Melanin is the major colour determinant and is responsible for variations in skin colour. Melanin is contained in special organelles called melanosomes which can be transported to nearby keratinocytes to induce pigmentation. Functionally, melanin serves as protection against UV radiation. Melanocytes also have a role in the immune system.

MELANOCYTIC NAEVUS (PIGMENTED NAEVUS, MOLE)

Melanocytic naevus is a benign, diverse, dynamic and biologically active neoplastic proliferation of the melanocytes. These are the moles that are present in virtually all individuals. This leads to a localized pigmented or nonpigmented lesion that are usually less than 5 mm in diameter.

Pathogenesis

Scientific studies have evidence that naevi have the presence of acquired mutations that lead to constitutive activation of RAS or serine/threonine kinase BRAF which lies in the downstream of RAS. The phenomenon of oncogene-induced senescence reduces the potent transforming activity of RAS signals and prevents many naevi from the progression to melanoma. Oncogene-induced senescence is the permanent growth arrest that follows a brief period of proliferation of melanocytes due to the expression of either activated RAS or BRAF. The growth arrest mediated by the accumulation of p16/INK4a, a potent inhibitor of several cyclin-dependent kinases, including CDK4 and CDK6. This protective response is disrupted in melanoma and in some precursor lesions that give rise to melanoma.

Morphology

Gross The common acquired melanocytic naevi are usually tan to brown to black and are uniformly pigmented. Usually, they are <5 mm across, relatively flat macules or elevated papules with well-defined and rounded borders.

Microscopy Melanocytic naevi are identified by the presence of naevus cells that are different from the ordinary melanocytes by their arrangement in clusters or nests. These cells are relatively rounded and tend to retain their melanin pigment. They undergo a series of morphologic life cycle changes over time, namely the junctional naevus (confined to the epidermis), a compound naevus (has epidermal and dermal extensions) or an intradermal naevus (only intradermal component).

Lentigo simplex is considered to be the early evolving form of melanocytic naevus. These lesions are usually <2 mm and are composed of melanocytes in contiguity with one another near the tips and sides of the rete ridges (Fig. 29.15A).

Junctional naevus is made of well-circumscribed nests of naevus cells lying entirely within the lower epidermis by the tips and the sides of the rete ridges or bulging downwards into the dermis but still in contact with the epidermis (Fig. 29.15B). These cells are regular rounded to cuboidal in appearance with occasional spindled-out forms containing inconspicuous nucleoli, and little or no mitotic activity with varying amounts of melanin pigment.

Compound naevi clinically appear as a pigmented papule or a plaque and histologically they are made up of components of both a junctional and an intradermal naevus (Fig. 29.15C). Naevus cell nests or cords are present in the epidermis and drop off into the dermis region. The naevus cells at the upper part of the dermis are relatively rounder with increased cytoplasm and melanin pigmentation. The deeper naevus cells are much smaller, produce little or no pigment and appear as cords or single spindle-shaped cells, a process termed as **neurotization** or maturation. At the deepest extent of the lesions, these cells often acquire fusiform contours and grow in fascicles resembling neural tissue. This change can be attributed to enzymatic changes, which is the progressive loss of tyrosinase activity and acquisition of cholinesterase activity in deeper regions of lesion extension. These changes are absent in melanomas.

Intradermal naevus shows no junctional activity with nests and cords of naevus cells in the dermis along with few multinucleated naevus cells. In few older involuting lesions, fibrosis, fatty infiltration/metaplasia and neuroid changes can be noted.

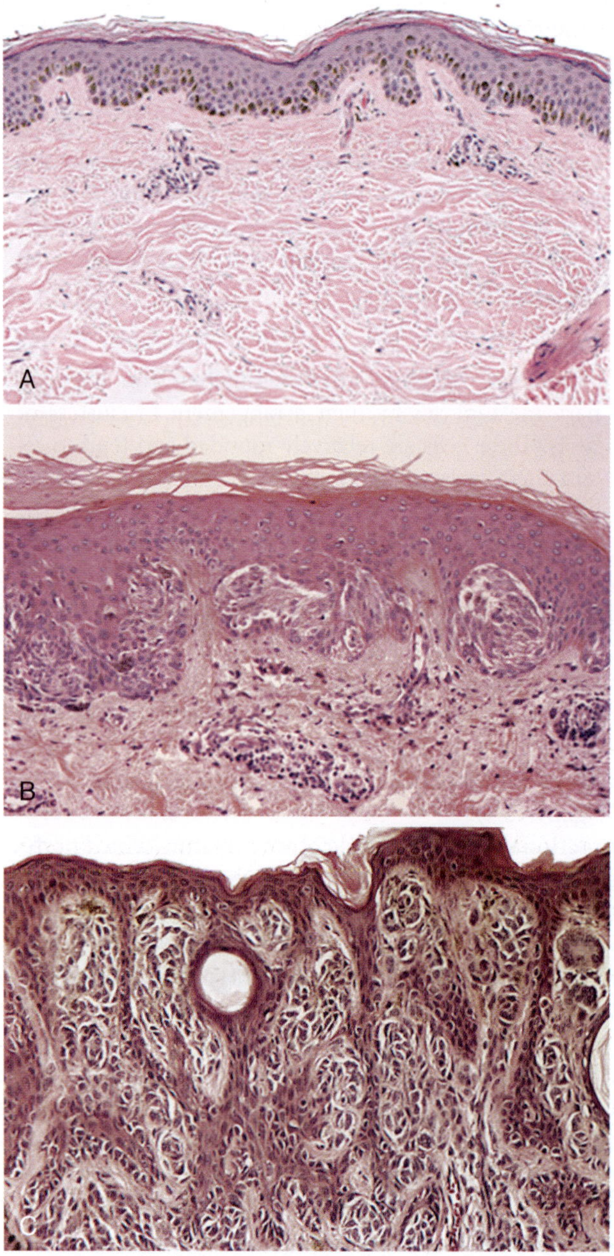

Fig. 29.15 Microscopy of melanocytic naevus. (A) Lentigo simplex. There is mild elongation of pigmented rete ridges. A few scattered lymphocytes and melanophages are present in the papillary dermis (H&E). (B) Junctional naevus. There are discrete nests of naevus cells at the dermoepidermal junction (H&E). (C) Compound naevus. There are both junctional and dermal nests of naevus cells. There is maturation with no cytological atypia (H&E). (*Source:* From Klaus J. Busam. Melanotic Macules. Pathology of Melanocytic Tumours. Elsevier 2019.)

Clinically, compound and intradermal naevi are often more elevated than junctional naevi. Progressive growth of naevus cells from the dermoepidermal junction into the underlying dermis is accompanied by morphologic changes that are taken to be a reflection of oncogene-induced senescence. The clinical and histological diversity of melanocytic naevi necessitates thorough knowledge of their appearance and natural evolution for a proper histopathological diagnosis.

Clinical Features

Clinical appearance such as flat lesions, slightly elevated lesions often with a raised centre and a flat periphery, papillomatous lesions, dome-shaped lesions and pedunculated lesions are noted. Because of hormonal sensitivity, they may become more prominent during pregnancy.

Lesions that are >5 mm in diameter with irregular borders and pigmentation should be considered as a dysplastic naevus (DN). They are rarely present at birth and usually appear in adolescence and early adulthood. They are risk markers, stimulants and potential precursors of melanoma.

They enlarge to a point, stabilize and involute becoming less frequent in the elderly. On the basis of clinical and histological features, melanocytic naevus can be distinguished into two forms: congenital and acquired. The uncommon varieties include blue naevus, spindle and epithelioid cell naevus (Spitz naevus), halo naevus and DN. Acquired melanocytic naevus is the most common type of melanocytic naevi.

DYSPLASTIC NAEVI

DN can occur in sporadic and familial settings as solitary or multiple lesions as many as hundred in number. They may be direct precursors of melanoma and the risk increases with the increase in the number of lesions. Exposure to UVB radiation leading to DNA damage is established as the main cause. In the familial setting, lesions usually appear by puberty and before age 20 and has a high preponderance for progression to malignant melanoma. DN syndrome is an autosomal dominant disorder that has an increased tendency to develop multiple dysplastic naevi and melanoma. By age 60, there is a 50% chance to develop melanoma.

Pathogenesis

Clark and associates described the various stages in the progression of dysplastic naevi to melanoma which is most probably by stepwise acquisition of mutations or epigenetic changes. Frequently these lesions acquire activating mutations in the NRAS and BRAF genes. Patients with DN syndrome often have inherited loss of function mutations in CDKN2A which encodes for several proteins including p16/INK4a, a negative regulator of cyclin-dependent kinase 4 (CDK4) and cyclin-dependent kinase 6 (CDK6). Some affected families have mutations in CDK4 that make the CDK4 protein resistant to inhibition by p16/INK4a. Thus, RAS or BRAF activation and increased CDK4 activity contribute to the development of dysplastic naevi. Increased expression of TERT that encodes the catalytic subunit of telomerase is also implicated in the pathogenesis of DN.

Morphology

Gross DN shows variability in colour, irregular or ill-defined border, background erythema and size usually greater than 4 mm (larger than the acquired naevus), predominantly located on the upper trunk and extremities. These lesions have a pebbly surface with colour variations from tan to dark brown to black. They can also appear as target-like lesions with a darker raised centre and irregular flat periphery. The Dutch working group pronounced the criteria helpful for the clinical diagnosis of DN which included size **≥5 mm in diameter, irregular border, asymmetric shape, irregular pigmentation and red hue**.

Microscopy DN involves both epidermis and dermis with architectural and cytologic atypia. The important microscopic features include size ≥4 mm, junctional component adjacent to a compound naevi component, nested and single melanocytes near the tips and sides of rete ridges, stromal reactions (Fig. 29.16). The cytological atypia includes nuclear enlargement, irregular, angulated, nuclear contours with hyperchromasia and variability in staining and cell size. Naevus cell nests within the epidermis may be enlarged and often fuse or coalescence with adjacent nests. Single naevus cells begin to replace basal cell layer along dermoepidermal junction referred to as **lentiginous hyperplasia**. Superficial dermis shows lymphocytic infiltration, release of melanin from dead naevus cells into the dermis causing melanin incontinence. Linear fibrosis is also seen surrounding the epidermal rete ridges that are involved by the naevus. The risk of melanoma has been associated with the degree of cytological atypia.

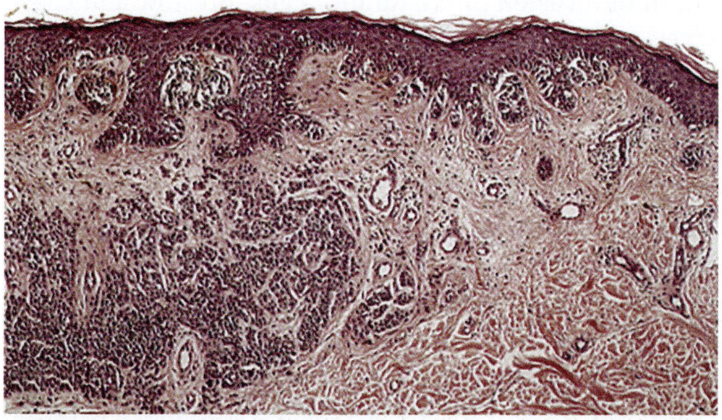

Fig. 29.16 Microscopy of dysplastic naevus. There is a lentiginous proliferation of melanocytes in the basal layer, with some nests of naevomelanocytes in the junctional zone and in the dermis. Only mild cytological atypia is present. (*Source:* From James W. Patterson. Lentigines, nevi, and melanomas. Weedon's Skin Pathology. 5th edition. Elsevier 2021.)

Prognosis and Predictive Factors

In multiple lesions, those lesions that do not demonstrate features different from the predominant type of naevi in the individual should be considered atypical and subjected to biopsy. Regular whole-body photography and melanoma surveillance are useful. The incidence of melanoma in individuals with DN is estimated at 1:3000 and it should be considered as marker for increased risk of melanoma especially in individuals with greater number of lesions.

MELANOMA PA 34.3

Melanoma is a malignant skin tumour of the melanocytes that may arise de novo or within an existing benign or DN frequently occurs because of acquired DNA mutation secondarily after exposure to UV radiation from sunlight. Melanocytes are found in the basal layer of the skin which produces melanin pigment responsible for the skin colouration. The lesion predominantly affects the fair-skinned and light-haired population with the skin, oral, anogenital areas, gastrointestinal tracts, meninges, uvea of eye being some of the most commonly affected sites. The most common skin areas on sun-exposed surfaces that are involved are the upper back in men, back and legs in women. Along with basal cell carcinoma (BCC) and SCC, malignant melanoma forms an important skin tumour which has a high cancer-related mortality rate which can be reduced if detected and treated at an early stage.

Pathogenesis

The pathogenesis of malignant melanoma can be well understood in the light of studying the inherited forms of melanoma which constitutes approximately 10%–15% of melanomas. They are AD, with variable penetrance among the family members. Acquired mutations as already mentioned are strongly associated with **UV radiation-induced DNA damage** and this damage is accentuated in fair-skinned populations where the diminishing melanin production increases the amount of UV DNA damage. The germline mutations frequently affect those genes that regulate cell cycle progression-control genes, progrowth signalling pathways and telomerase functions (Flowchart 29.2).

Mutations That Disrupt Cell Cycle Control Genes

CDKN2A is one of the important genes that is mutated in approximately 40% of the patients with autosomal dominant inherited familial and sporadic melanomas. CDKN2A locus encodes p15, p16 and ARF tumour suppressor genes, of which loss of **p16 and ARF** are clearly implicated in malignant melanoma. p16 helps to reinforce the tumour suppressor ability of RB gene to stop the cells in the G1 phase of the cell cycle by inhibiting CDK4 and CDK6. ARF decreases the degradation of p53 by inhibiting the oncoprotein MDM2 which thereby increases the

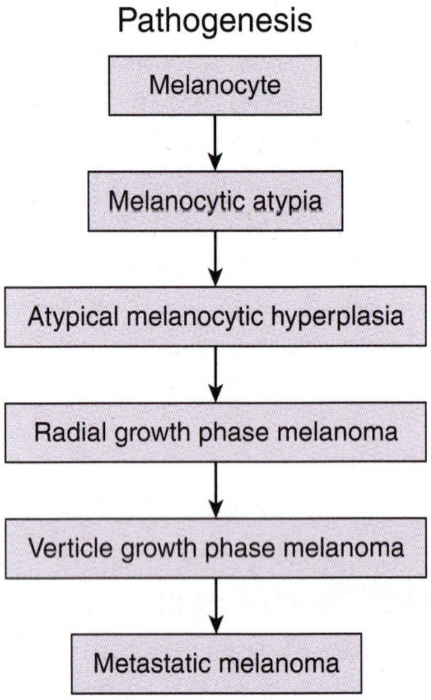

Flowchart 29.2 Pathogenesis of melanoma.

p53 tumour suppressor activity. The overall impact causes the melanocytes to escape the clutches of oncogene-induced senescence and proliferate because of loss of cell cycle control.

Mutations That Activate Progrowth Signalling Pathways The RAS and PI3K/AKT signalling pathways which are involved in the promotion of cell growth and survival are commonly mutated in sporadic melanomas. Activating mutations in BRAF and RAS occur in 40%–50% and 15%–20% of melanomas, respectively. BRAF mutations frequently lead to loss of PTEN tumour suppressor gene that causes an increased activity of PI3K/AKT pathway. However, these mutations are seen in lesser numbers in melanoma lesions that arise in non-sun-exposed regions of the body. Other mutation such as the loss of function mutation of the tumour suppressor gene encoding neurofibromin 1 (NF1) which is a negative regulator of RAS is also noted in melanoma.

Mutations That Activate Telomerase Many cases of sporadic melanomas and rare familial cases have been identified with mutations in the promoter of TERT, the gene that encodes the catalytic subunit of telomerase. This enzyme activity preserves telomeres and protects cells from senescence and is important in the malignant transformation.

Morphology

Gross Macroscopically, melanoma lesion usually presents as an irregularly shaped, asymmetrical lesion with a recent history of change in colour, size, shape or sensation. Ulceration and bleeding portend a poor prognosis. The variations in the colour ranges from shades of black, brown, red, dark blue to grey. The borders of melanomas are frequently irregular and notched up.

Microscopy Microscopical examination of the skin biopsy from the lesional area shows nests of atypical melanocytes usually at the dermoepidermal junction. The individual melanoma cells are larger than the normal melanocytes or cells found in melanocytic naevi which have enlarged nuclei with irregular contours. The nuclear chromatin shows clumping at the periphery of the nuclear membrane, and a prominent red (eosinophilic) nucleolus is the characteristic finding Fig 29.18.

The progression of melanoma can be traced through two phases, namely the radial and vertical growth phases and the morphology of the malignant melanoma cells of both phases is similar.

Radial Growth Phase

This phase corresponds to the horizontal spread of melanoma within the epidermis and/or the superficial dermis. The tumour cells of this phase often lack the capacity to metastasize. The lesions of this phase can be divided into several clinicopathologic classes such as the lentigo maligna which is an indolent lesion, superficial spreading which is the most common type and the acral/mucosal lentiginous which is unrelated to sun exposure.

Vertical Growth Phase

After an unpredictable period of time span, the radial spreading lesions start growing in the vertical direction and invade downward into the deeper dermal layers and clinically present as an expansile mass. These cells of this phase develop the potential to metastasize. Maturation or neurotization that is present in the deeper areas of the benign melanocytic lesions is absent in melanoma. The probability of metastasis strongly correlates with the depth of invasion of the tumour cells. Breslow and Clark levels of system are commonly used for assessing the tumour depth and the Breslow depth assessment method is more specific. The depth corresponds to the distance from the superficial epidermal granular cell layer to the deepest intradermal tumour cells and is known as the **Breslow thickness.** This factor highly correlates with the 10-year survival rate and also helps the surgeon for the margin determination during the surgical resection.

Histopathological features that correlate with the probability of metastatic spread and prognosis are the **tumour depth** (the Breslow thickness) which is considered to be the most important prognostic factor, **number of mitoses, evidence of tumour regression, ulceration, number of tumour-infiltrating lymphocytes and location** (central body or extremity). So, if a tumour has a thinner tumour depth, no or few mitoses ($<1/mm^2$), brisk tumour-infiltrating lymphocyte response, absence of regression and lack of ulceration, then it has a better prognosis.

Sentinel Lymph Node Biopsy

Identification, removal and careful examination of lymph node (or nodes) that is the initial site of drainage (sentinel lymph node) give additional prognostic information about the tumour. Involvement by even a small number of cells called micrometastasis confers a poor prognosis. The degree of involvement and the total number of lymph nodes involved correlate well with overall survival.

Clinical Features

Clinically, the **ABCDE**s, which are the warning features of melanoma should be properly examined and they are **Asymmetry, irregular Borders, variegated Colour, Diameter >6 mm, Evolution** of rapid change in appearance, itching, ulceration, bleeding and pain; presence of these features leads to a poor prognosis (Fig. 29.17). Pain and itching in the lesion are the early signs and most of the lesions are >10 mm and asymptomatic. The most consistent clinical signs include changes in colour, size or shape of a pigmented lesion.

Molecular insights into this tumour have led to success in treating them with drugs that target the RAS and PI3K/AKT pathways and BRAF inhibitors. Antibodies against CTLA4 and PD1 that inhibit immune checkpoint have also tasted some success. Metastatic melanoma is resistant to both chemotherapy and radiotherapy. A small fraction of 'atypical' lesions falls in a histologic grey zone between naevi and melanomas and has been termed melanocytic tumours of uncertain malignant potential. These lesions require complete excision and close clinical follow-up.

BENIGN EPITHELIAL TUMOURS

Benign cutaneous epithelial neoplasms are commonly occurring tumours derived from the keratinizing stratified squamous epithelium of the epidermis and hair follicles and ductular epithelium of cutaneous glands often recapitulating the structures from which they arise. Rarely they are associated with syndromes, e.g. multiple trichilemmomas in Cowden syndrome or multiple sebaceous neoplasms in Muir–Torre syndrome. Few common tumours are discussed here.

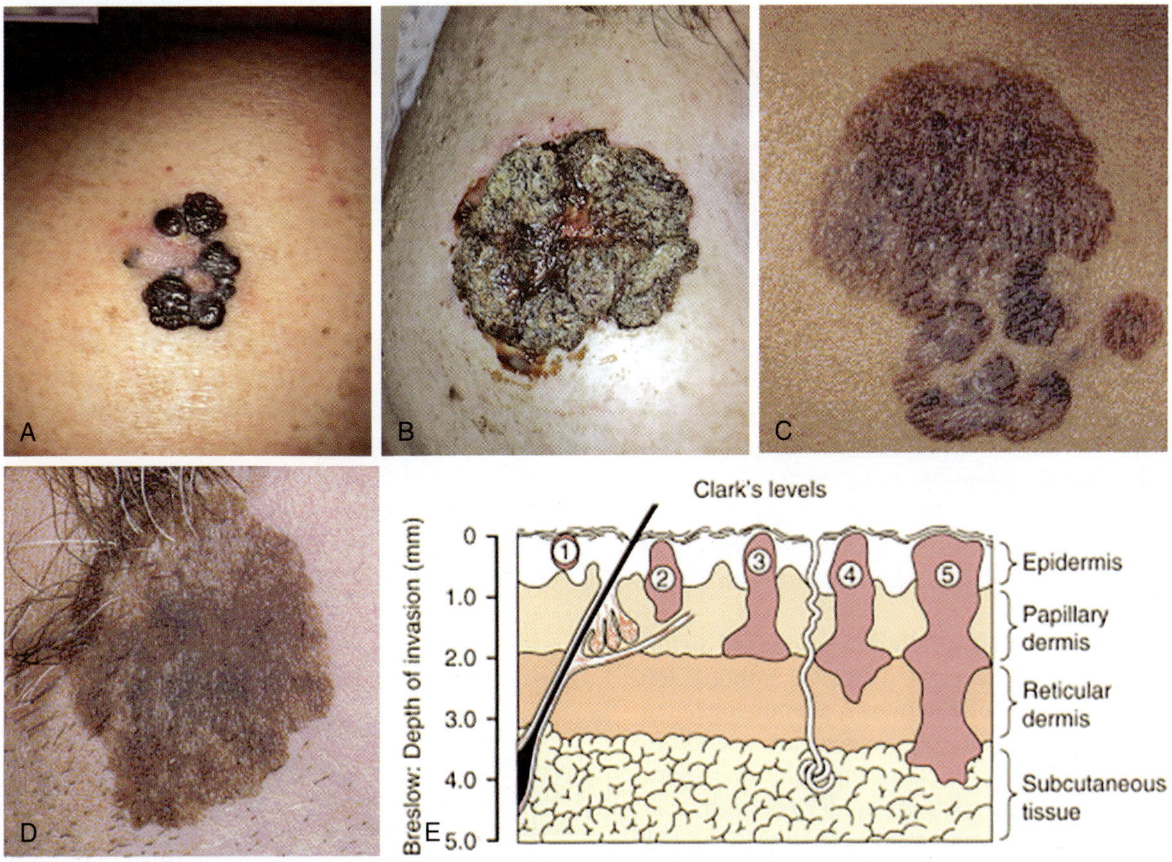

Fig. 29.17 Clinical Pictures of melanoma (Figs A,B,C,D) depicting the ABCDE characteristics of melanoma include Asymmetry, irregular Borders, variegated Colours, large Diameters and Evolution or change over time. (B) Locally advanced melanoma. (E) depicts Clark's levels of invasion: (1) epidermis, (2) extension to papillary dermis, (3) filling the papillary dermis, (4) reticular dermis and (5) subcutaneous fat. *(Source: From Charles W. Kimbrough, Marshall M. Urist, Kelly M. McMasters. Melanoma and Cutaneous Malignant Neoplasms. In Sabiston Textbook of Surgery. Elsevier 2017.)*

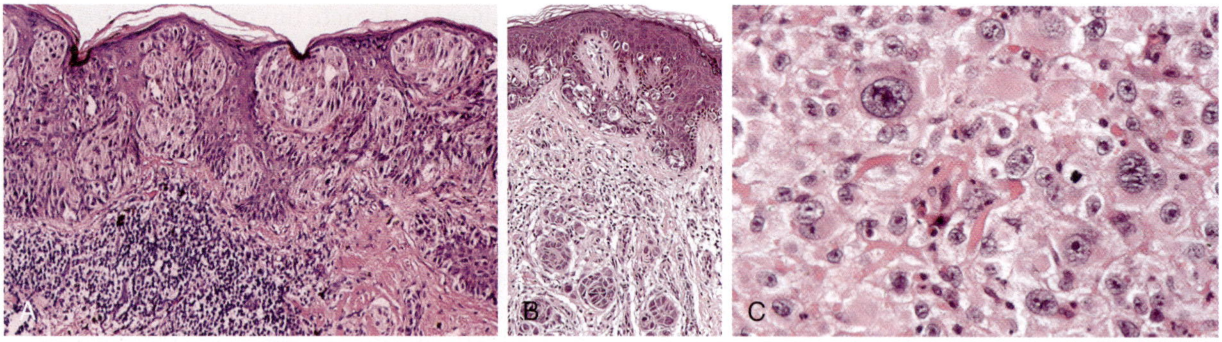

Fig. 29.18 Microscopy of melanoma. (A) Superficial spreading melanoma. The radial growth phase is characterized by the spread of atypical melanocytes along the basilar portion of the epidermis. Also, note the presence of individual melanocytes invading the higher levels of the epithelium. (B) Melanoma: vertical growth phase. In addition to in situ (radial growth phase) tumour, there are multiple nests in the dermis. These are larger than the epidermal ones. (C) Amelanotic melanoma: High power view showing that the tumour cells are very pleomorphic with large vesicular nuclei and prominent nucleoli. (*Source:* A, Brad W. Neville, Douglas D. Damm, Carl M. Allen and Angela C. Chi. Epithelial Pathology. Oral and Maxillofacial Pathology. 4th edition. Elsevier 2016; B, From Jeffrey P. North, Boris C. Bastian and Alexander J. Lazar. Melanoma. McKee's Pathology of the Skin. 5th edition. Elsevier 2020; C, Jeffrey P. North, Boris C. Bastian and Alexander J. Lazar. Melanoma. McKee's Pathology of the Skin. 5th edition. Elsevier 2020.)

SEBORRHOEIC KERATOSIS

Seborrhoeic keratosis is a common epidermal tumour that often occurs as multiple lesions.

Pathogenesis

The growth of seborrhoeic keratosis is derived by the activating mutations in the fibroblast growth factor receptor-3 (FGFR3), a receptor tyrosine kinase. In large numbers, their appearance may form a part of a paraneoplastic syndrome, a sign known as the **Leser–Trélat** sign. This sign is often seen along with the adenocarcinomas of the gastrointestinal tract where the growth of the keratinocytes is stimulated by the transforming growth factor-alpha (TGF-α) produced by tumour cells.

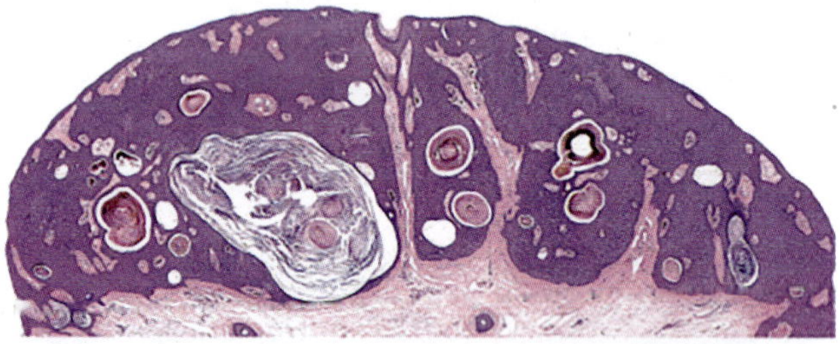

Fig. 29.19 Microscopy of seborrhoeic keratosis (SK). Seborrhoeic keratoses – spectrum of histologic subtypes. Acanthotic type with lobular hyperplasia with prominent horn cysts. (*Source:* From Luis Requena, Celia Requena and Clay J. Cockerell. Benign Epidermal Tumours and Proliferations. Dermatology. 4th edition. Elsevier 2018.)

Morphology

Gross Grossly, seborrhoeic keratosis appears as round, flat, coin-like, sharply demarcated, waxy plaques that vary in diameter and appear to be stuck onto the skin surface. They are tan to dark brown, with a velvety to granular surface. Inspection with a hand lens shows multiple small, round, pore-like ostia impacted with keratin.

Microscopy Microscopically, the lesions are divided into the following varieties, namely acanthotic, irritated, inverted follicular keratosis, adenoid or reticulated, clonal, hyperkeratotic and melanoacanthoma (Fig. 29.19). The lesions are exophytic, sharply demarcated from the adjacent epidermis with a flat base. They show hyperkeratosis, acanthosis and papillomatosis. The acanthotic epidermis is composed of squamous cells and sheets of small cells that resemble the basal cells of the epidermis with variable melanin pigmentation. Exuberant keratin production (hyperkeratosis) is also noted. Small keratin-filled cysts called horn cysts are often noted. If irritated or inflamed, seborrhoeic keratosis develop whirling foci of squamous differentiation resembling eddy currents in a stream. Formation of *in situ* carcinoma within seborrhoeic keratosis called Bowenoid transformation can rarely occur in the lesions of the sun-exposed areas.

Clinical Features

The lesions arise spontaneously mainly on the trunk, extremities, head and neck excluding palm and soles. They commonly occur in the middle-aged or older individuals. In dark-skinned individuals, multiple small lesions on the face termed **dermatosis papulosa nigra occur.** Stucco keratosis are small grey-white seborrhoeic keratosis usually located symmetrically on the distal extremities, especially the ankles. They usually can be scrapped off without any bleeding.

ACANTHOSIS NIGRICANS

Acanthosis nigricans is the thickened hyperpigmented skin with a 'velvet-like' texture. It appears in the flexural areas such as axillae, skinfolds of neck, groin and anogenital regions. Leser–Trélat sign may be the early stage or the incomplete form of the malignant type of acanthosis nigricans. Acanthosis nigricans can be seen under different clinical settings such as malignancy associated, benign, inherited, obesity associated, syndromic, drug induced and mixed.

Benign Type of Acanthosis Nigricans

The lesion usually occurs in the younger age groups with an autosomal dominant type of inheritance associated with obesity, diabetes mellitus, pituitary and pineal tumours.

Malignant Type of Acanthosis Nigricans

The malignant type usually occurs in older individuals with underlying cancers of the gastrointestinal tract, frequently the gastric adenocarcinoma.

Syndromic Acanthosis Nigricans

This type is linked to syndromes associated with insulin resistance such as the HAIRAN syndrome affecting the younger women; there is hyperandrogenaemia (HA), insulin resistance (IR) and acanthosis nigricans (AN). It is also being associated with insulin resistance in obesity, hypothyroidism and congenital generalized lipodystrophy.

Pathogenesis

Increased growth factor receptor signalling in the skin because of activating mutations in FGFR3 leading to epidermal proliferation is commonly pointed out in these lesions. Type 2 diabetes mellitus and hyperinsulinaemia provoke increased stimulation of insulin-like growth factor receptor-1 (IGFR1) and activate FGFR3. Malignant acanthosis nigricans is mediated by the high levels of TGF-α secreted by the malignant cells. The lesion is also associated with skeletal deformities such as achondroplasia and thanatophoric dysplasia.

Morphology

Gross The lesion presents as papillomatous brown patches predominantly in the intertriginous areas. In the extensive cases of the malignant type, mucosal surfaces and the palpebral conjunctiva are also involved.

Microscopy Microscopically, the lesion shows hyperkeratosis, papillomatosis, and slight, irregular acanthosis and usually no hyperpigmentation (Fig. 29.20).

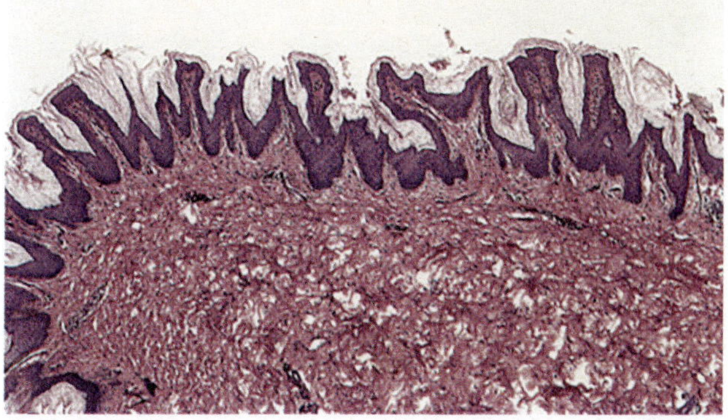

Fig. 29.20 Microscopy of acanthosis nigricans: There is hyperkeratosis and papillomatosis but only mild acanthosis. (*Source:* From James W. Patterson. Miscellaneous conditions. Weedon's Skin Pathology. 5th edition. Elsevier 2021.)

Epidermis and underlying enlarged dermal papillae undulate sharply to form repeating peaks and valleys. Hyperkeratosis imparting the brown colour of the lesions and slight basal cell layer hyperpigmentation are present.

Treatment

Investigations to assess the underlying disorder and its management are essential for the treatment of acanthosis nigricans. Topical keratolytics and depigmenting agents are also helpful in the management.

PREMALIGNANT EPIDERMAL TUMOURS

Premalignant lesions or precancerous conditions are growths that appear on the skin surface that can develop into a skin cancer if left untreated. Actinic keratosis is a precursor lesion of SCC. The majority of these develop out of chronic exposure to sunlight or UV radiation from the sun. Ageing and smoking are other risk factors.

ACTINIC KERATOSIS (SOLAR KERATOSIS)

Actinic keratosis is a precursor lesion of SCC. The word solar refers to *SUN* and the word actinic refers to the various *RAYS* as the causative agent. UVB rays are carcinogenic, whereas the UVA rays can augment the former carcinogenic effects. Usually, they occur as multiple lesions in the sun-damaged skin exhibiting hyperkeratosis, in light-pigmented people of the middle age group. Ionizing radiation, industrial hydrocarbons, arsenicals also can induce such lesions.

Morphology

Gross The lesion is usually <1 cm, tan-brown, red or skin-coloured with rough, **sandpaper-like consistency**

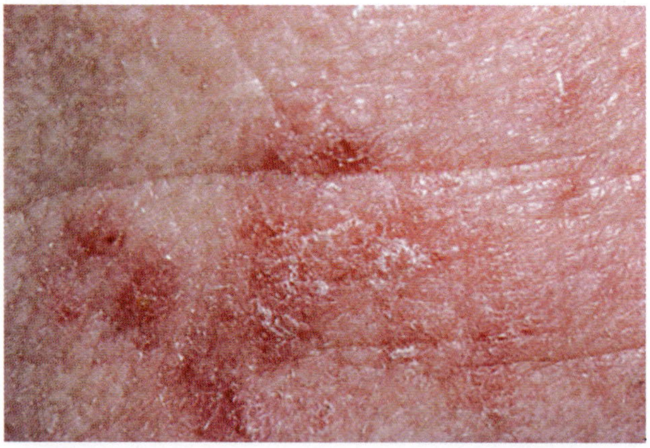

Fig. 29.21 Clinical picture of actinic keratosis: The lesions are flat, red-coloured and covered by an adherent scale with a rough surface. (*Source:* From William D. James, Dirk M. Elston, James R. Treat, Misha A. Rosenbach and Isaac M. Neuhaus. Epidermal Nevi, Neoplasms, and Cysts. Andrews' Diseases of the Skin. 13th edition. Elsevier 2020.)

(Fig. 29.21). Because of the increased keratin production, '**cutaneous horn**' can also be noted. A lesion similar to actinic keratosis can occur in the vermilion border of the lower lip, known as actinic cheilitis.

Microscopy **Microscopically,** actinic keratosis shows keratocytic dysplasias and forms SCCs in situ. Five histological types can be recognized, namely hypertrophic, atrophic, Bowenoid, acantholytic and pigmented and usually occur in different combinations in the same lesion (Fig. 29.22). Stratum corneum is thickened and shows parakeratosis. The **cytologic atypia** is present in the lowermost layers of the epidermis. Atypical basal cells with large, irregular, hyperchromatic nuclei are usually seen. The squamous cells in the mid-epidermis show premature keratinization called **dyskeratosis** with pink or reddish cytoplasm. Superficial dermis contains thickened, blue-grey elastic fibres termed as ***elastosis*** *which can be due to the a*bnormal elastic fibre synthesis by sun-damaged fibroblasts. The upper dermis also consists of chronic inflammatory infiltrates predominantly composed of lymphocytes and plasma cells.

Topical application of imiquimod activates innate immune system through stimulation of Toll-like receptors (TLRs) and is helpful in such lesions.

MALIGNANT EPIDERMAL TUMOURS

Skin tumours develop because of the proliferation of a single or multiple components of the skin such as the keratinocytes, melanocytes, skin appendages and soft tissues. Keratinocytic tumours are derived from epidermal and adnexal keratinocytes. SCC and BCC are the most common malignant epidermal tumours.

SQUAMOUS CELL CARCINOMA PA 34.1

SCC is the second most common primary skin malignancy, exceeded only by BCC. It affects males more than females and less than 5% of these tumours metastasize to regional nodes. They can occur anywhere on the skin and the mucous membrane lined by squamous epithelium. It most commonly arises from sun-damaged skin, and those that arise at the periphery of a chronic ulcer or a scar is termed as **Marjolin ulcer**.

Pathogenesis

DNA damage induced by exposure to UV light from sunlight is considered to be the main cause of cutaneous SCC. Immunosuppression also increases the susceptibility of keratinocytes to infection and transformation by oncogenic viruses such as HPV-5 and HPV-8. It diminishes the immune-mediated elimination of sun-damaged cells. Autosomal recessive disease entity, EV has a high

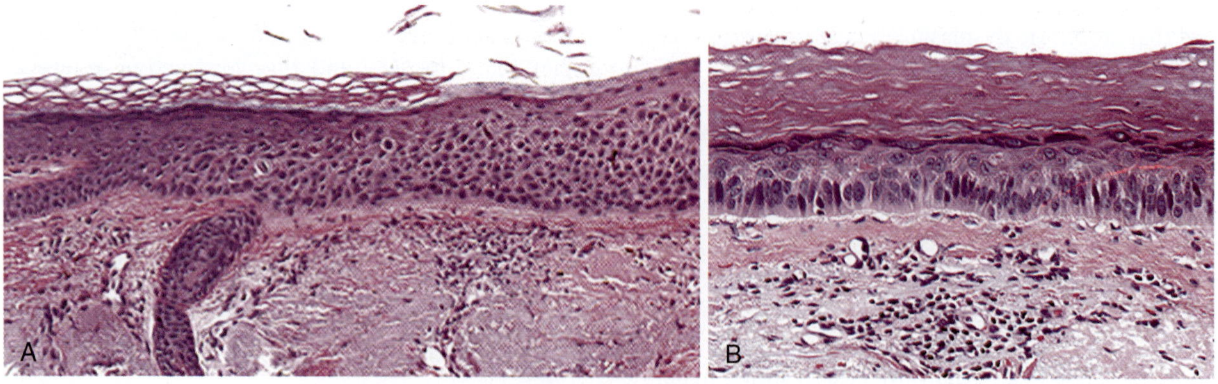

Fig. 29.22 Microscopy of actinic keratosis. (A) Actinic keratosis: Squamous cell atypia and overlying parakeratosis. (B) Actinic keratosis, Bowenoid type: Full-thickness squamous atypia in actinically affected skin. This lesion is also hypertrophic. (*Source:* From Daniel J. Santa Cruz and Alejandro A. Gru. Tumours of the Skin. Diagnostic Histopathology of Tumours. 5th edition. Elsevier 2021.)

susceptibility to cutaneous SCC and oncogenic transformation by the HPV. Tars and oils, chronic ulcers and draining osteomyelitis, ingestion of arsenicals, ionizing radiation, tobacco and betel nut chewing increase the susceptibility to the formation of SCC.

Genetics of Squamous Cell Carcinoma of Skin

TP53 mutations and dysfunction are identified as early events in the development of skin SCC induced by sunlight. The DNA damage by the UV light is efficiently sensed by ataxia-telangiectasia mutated (ATM) and ATM- and Rad3-related (ATR) (checkpoint kinases) and signals are sent out for the upregulation and the stability of p53 which in turn arrests the damaged cells in the G1 phase of the cell cycle and executes the 'high-fidelity' DNA repair or the elimination of the damaged cells by apoptosis (Flowchart 29.3). Because of p53 mutations, these protective functions are disturbed leading to accumulation of further mutations and carcinogenesis. Similar mechanism is also noted in patients with xeroderma pigmentosum, where the inherited mutations in genes in the nucleotide excision repair pathway lead to defective, error-prone repair and accumulation of mutations with increased susceptibility to cutaneous SCC. Multiple driver mutations that increase RAS signalling and that decrease Notch signalling also stem the development of skin SCC along with p53 mutations.

Morphology

Gross SCC of the skin consists of a sharply defined, red, shallow ulcer, covered by a crust, with scaling plaques and surrounded by a wide, elevated and indurated border. SCC that has not invaded through the basement membrane at the dermoepidermal junction is called ***in situ*** SCC (Fig. 29.23). Invasive lesions are nodular with variable keratin production (grossly hyperkeratotic scales) and often show ulceration. Metastasis of the primary tumours is most likely seen in the tumours with a diameter of at least 15 mm and a vertical tumour thickness of 2 mm, decreasing degrees of differentiation, desmoplasia, inflammatory reaction including eosinophils and plasma cells and tumours arising from mucosal surface, inflammatory and degenerative process.

Microscopy The tumour consists of irregular masses of atypical squamous epithelial cells that proliferate downwards breaching the basement membrane into the dermis. The invading tumour front consists of varying proportions of normal and atypical (anaplastic) squamous cells. The atypical squamous cells are enlarged with hyperchromatic nuclei and show great variation in the size and shape of the cells, hyperplasia and hyperchromasia of the nuclei, absence of intercellular bridges, keratinization of the individual cells and presence of atypical mitotic figures. They show variable degrees of differentiation from well-differentiated, moderately differentiated to poorly differentiated tumours with the proportion of the atypical squamous cells higher in the poorly differentiated SCCs. Keratinization takes place in the form of keratin pearls which are composed of concentric layers of squamous cells showing gradually increasing keratinization towards the centre (Fig. 29.24).

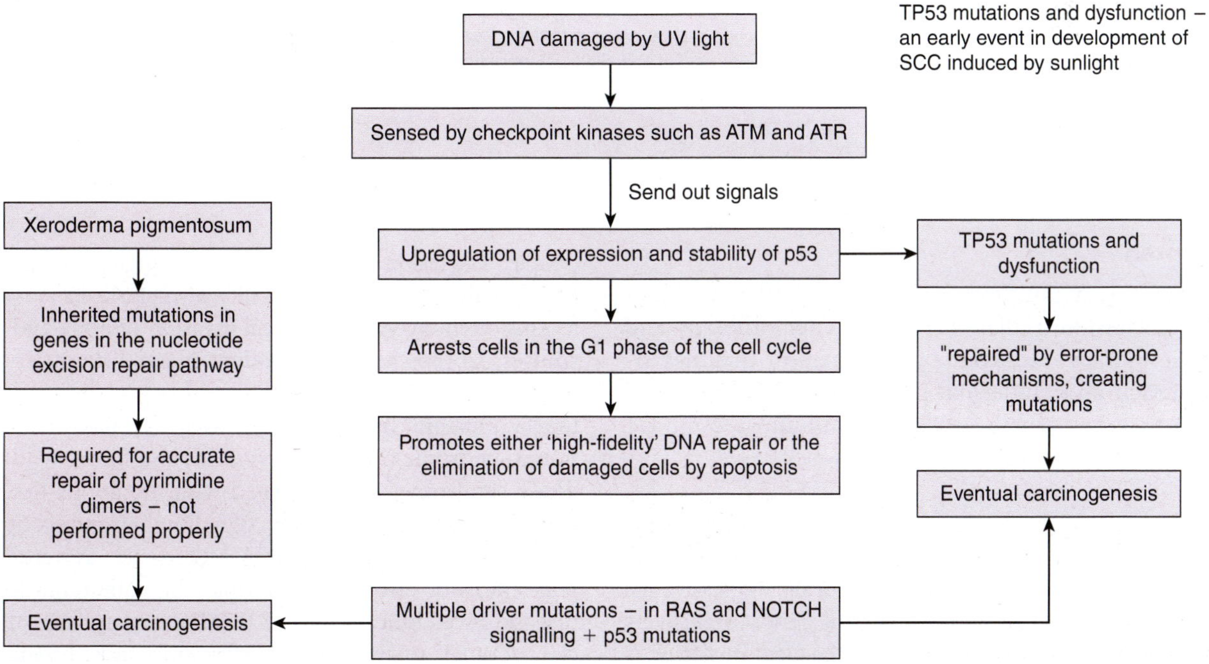

Flowchart 29.3 Genetics of skin squamous cell carcinoma. ATM, ataxia-telangiectasia mutated; ATR, ATM- and Rad3-related).

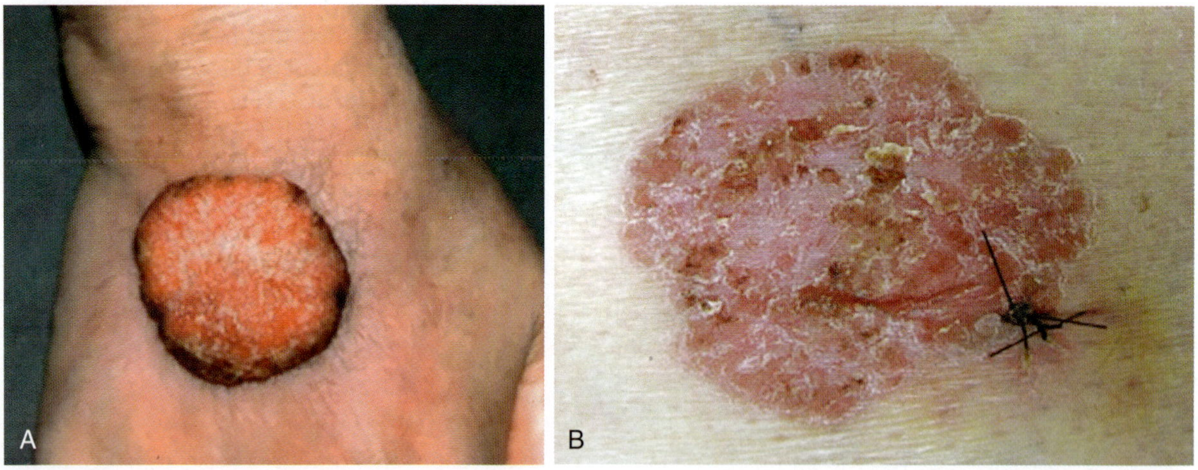

Fig. 29.23 Clinical pictures of squamous cell carcinoma (SCC). (A) Clinical spectrum of cutaneous squamous cell carcinoma – large, fungating nodule on the dorsum of the hand. (B) SCC in situ – a large, discrete, thin, erythematous, scaly plaque on the lower back of a middle-aged man with a fair complexion. (*Source:* From Cutaneous Squamous Cell Carcinoma. Elsevier Point of Care. 2021.)

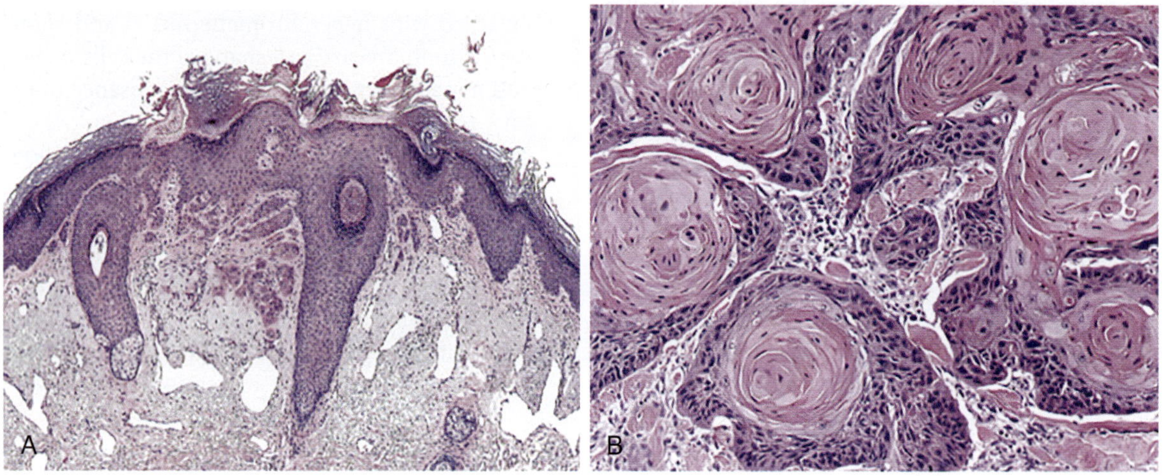

Fig. 29.24 Microscopy of squamous cell carcinoma (SCC). SCC, usual type. Branching lobules extend from an ulcerated surface in this lesion (A). SCC: Range of histopathologic findings. (B) Squamous cell carcinoma lacking pearls. This is an infiltrative squamous carcinoma. (*Source:* A: From Daniel J. Santa Cruz and Alejandro A. Gru. Tumours of the Skin. Diagnostic Histopathology of Tumours. 5th edition. Elsevier 2021; Daniel J. Santa Cruz and Alejandro A. Gru. Tumours of the Skin. Diagnostic Histopathology of Tumours. 5th edition. Elsevier 2021.)

Treatment

Treatment is a multimodality approach that includes surgical excision, radiation therapy, chemotherapy and immunotherapy. Adjuvant chemotherapy includes 5-fluorouracil and epidermal growth factor receptor inhibitors, e.g. cetuximab, a chimeric immunoglobulin G1 monoclonal antibody, is used in high-risk cases.

BASAL CELL CARCINOMA PA 34.2

BCC is the most common distinctive locally aggressive invasive skin cancer of the adults occurring almost exclusively on the hair-bearing skin, especially on the face. The lesion is common in the sun-exposed sites and in lightly pigmented people. The lesion usually occurs as a single, slow-growing lesion with a very rare possibility of metastasis. Advanced lesions often ulcerate with local invasion of bone and facial sinuses, so they are called **rodent ulcers**. There are three rare forms of BCC syndromes with early onset, namely linear unilateral basal cell naevus, nevoid basal cell carcinoma syndrome (NBCCS) (NBCCS) and Bazex syndrome. These syndromes are associated with mutations that activate the Hedgehog pathway signalling. Immunosuppression, inherited defects in DNA repair such as xeroderma pigmentosum also makes the patient vulnerable for the disease. Five clinical types of BCC occur, namely superficial, nodular, micronodular, infiltrating and fibroepithelioma type (Fig. 29.25).

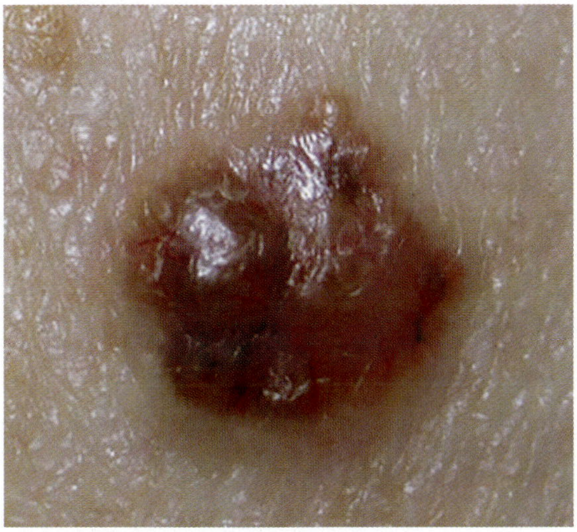

Fig. 29.25 BCC nodular variety – the most common type. (*Source:* From William D. James, Dirk M. Elston, James R. Treat, Misha A. Rosenbach and Isaac M. Neuhaus. Epidermal Nevi, Neoplasms, and Cysts. Andrews' Diseases of the Skin. 13th edition. Elsevier 2020.)

Predisposing Factors

Predisposing factors involve light skin colour with prolonged exposure to strong sunlight. It is more evident in patients with xeroderma pigmentosum. Other predisposing factors include exposure to Roentgen rays and presence of burn scars.

Pathogenesis

Pathogenesis involves mutations that lead to increased Hedgehog signalling; naevoid basal cell carcinoma syndrome (NBCCS; also known as basal cell nevus syndrome or gorlin syndrome); AD disorder characterized by multiple BCCs; age <20 years accompanied by other conditions – medulloblastomas, ovarian fibromas, odontogenic keratocysts, certain developmental abnormalities; gene associated – PTCH, a tumour suppressor gene.

Pathogenesis of NBCCS

NBCCS has the first hit in the form of a germline loss of function mutation in one of the PTCH allele 9q22.3. The second normal allele is inactivated by acquired mutation or because of exposure to mutagens such as the UV light, which forms the second hit in-line with the classical Knudson 'two-hit' hypothesis. PTCH protein is a receptor for sonic Hedgehog (SHH), a component of Hedgehog signalling pathway that determines the polarity during embryonic development and regulates hair follicle formation and hair growth. In the 'off' state, PTCH exists in a complex with another transmembrane protein called SMO (for 'smoothened'). Binding of SHH to PTCH releases SMO, which in turn activates the transcription factor GLI1. In NBCCS there is loss of PTCH function, which results in constitutive activation of SMO and downstream signalling and activation of GLI with translocation of GLI1 into the nucleus turning on the expression of genes that support tumour cell growth and survival. One-third of mutations consist of C→T transitions, which is the hallmark of UV damage.

The lesions occur as small nodules at a much earlier age between puberty and 35 years of age distributed over the face and the body. During the adulthood, the lesions may become neoplastic and become invasive and mutilating leading to death and metastasis.

Morphology

Gross Macroscopically, the lesions may be erythematous, ulcerated, scaly, with pearly border.

Microscopy Microscopically, the tumour cells resemble normal basal cell layer of epidermis with the cells at the periphery of tumour cell islands arranged radially with their long axes in parallel alignment called a peripheral palisading of the lesional cell nuclei. The cells at the centre show haphazard arrangement. In H&E sections, the stroma retracts away from the carcinoma creating clefts/separation artefacts; it assists in differentiating BCC from trichoepithelioma. They arise from the epidermis/follicular epithelium and two patterns are observed, namely the multifocal superficial type and the nodular lesion type (Fig. 29.26). Multifocal growth originates from the epidermis and extends over the skin surface, whereas the nodular lesions grow downward deeply into dermis as cords, islands of variably basophilic cells with hyperchromatic nuclei, embedded in mucinous matrix, surrounded by fibroblasts, lymphocytes.

Treatment

Treatment modalities for BCC include surgical, radiation, medical and other destructive therapies. BCC is usually radiosensitive. In selected cases, imiquimod, topical 5-fluorouracil, interferons and photodynamic therapy are useful.

ADNEXAL TUMOURS

Skin adnexal tumours (SATs) are a large and diverse group of benign and malignant neoplasms. They are uncommon and can be single or multiple, sporadic or familial. Benign adnexal tumours are more common and malignant SATs are rare and are locally aggressive and have the potential for nodal involvement and distant metastasis with a poor clinical outcome.

BENIGN ADNEXAL (APPENDAGE) TUMOURS (SAT)

SATs show morphological differentiation towards one of the four primary adnexal structures present in normal skin: hair follicles, sebaceous glands, apocrine glands and

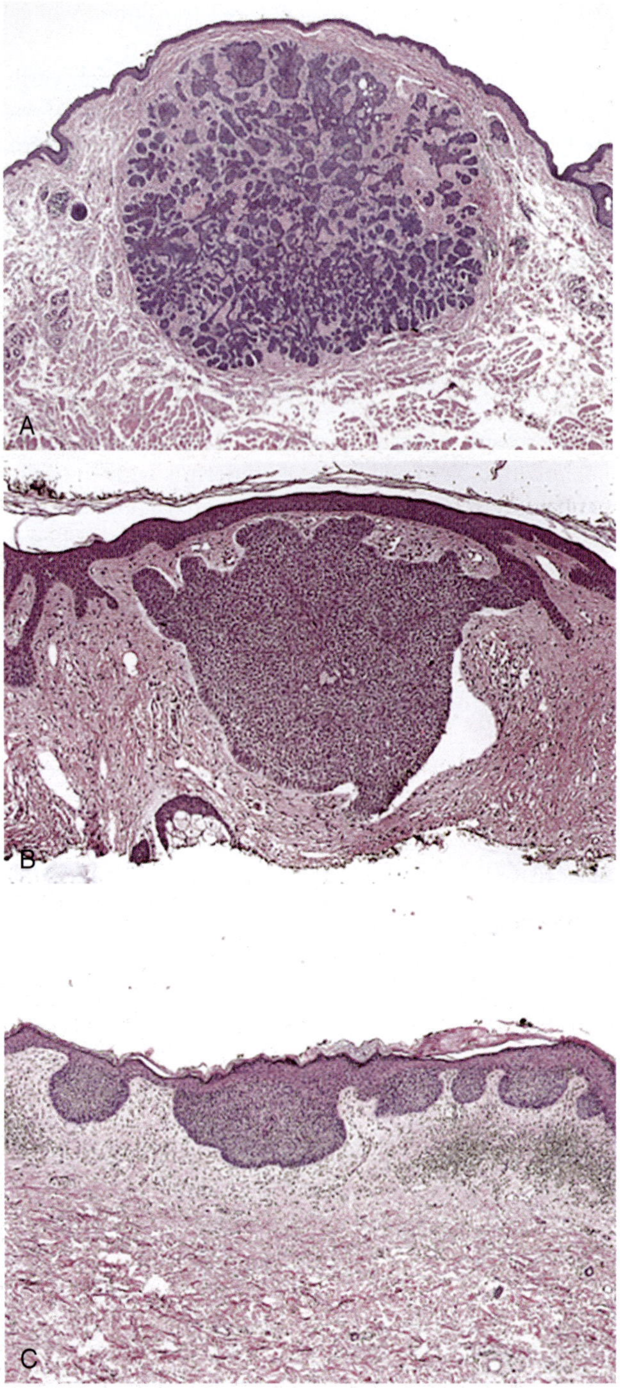

Fig. 29.26 (A) Basal cell carcinoma, common type. There is a nodule composed of insular, basaloid cells. (B) Note the retraction artefact. (C) Basal cell carcinoma, superficial type. Budlike nests of basaloid cells connect to the epidermis across a broad front. (*Source*: From Daniel J. Santa Cruz and Alejandro A. Gru. Tumours of the Skin. Diagnostic Histopathology of Tumours. 5th edition. Elsevier 2021.)

eccrine glands. They also exhibit more than one line of differentiation making their precise diagnosis difficult. Their origin from a pluripotent stem cell is a plausible explanation. Majority of these lesions are benign but their malignant counterpart has also been described. Simple surgical excision is curative; however, they may be a sign of syndromes with internal malignancies, such as trichilemmomas in Cowden disease, a disorder caused by germline mutations in the tumour suppressor gene PTEN that is associated with an increased risk of endometrial cancer and breast cancer and sebaceous tumours in Muir–Torre syndrome. The most common form of presentation of these tumours is as a nondescript, flesh-coloured, solitary or multiple papules and nodules. Some of the important tumours of hair follicles and sebaceous, eccrine and apocrine glands are described here.

Eccrine Poroma

Eccrine poromas are benign adnexal neoplasms with terminal ductal differentiation and can show either eccrine or apocrine differentiation (Fig. 29.27).

Morphology

Gross Lesions predominantly occur on the palms and soles where sweat glands are numerous. It commonly

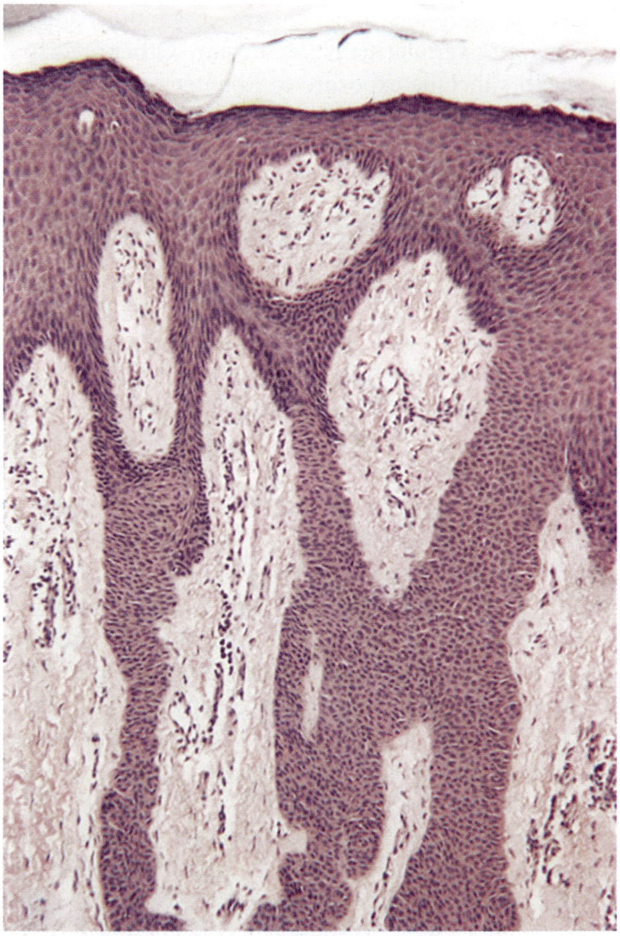

Fig. 29.27 Eccrine poroma. The tumour characteristically grows in the form of anastomosing bands, cords and nests of small tumour cells with multiple connections and attached to the overlying epidermis. (*Source:* From James W. Patterson. Tumours of cutaneous appendages. Weedon's Skin Pathology. 5th edition. Elsevier 2021.)

occurs as dome-shaped papules, nodules or plaques measuring <1 cm in diameter.

Microscopy Microscopically, the lesions are well circumscribed, composed of uniform basaloid and cuboidal cell proliferation with small and irregular nuclei and modest amount of cytoplasm often containing glycogen. These cells extend from the lower part of the epidermis into the dermis as broad columns.

Cylindroma

Cylindroma, is a skin appendageal tumour showing ductal (apocrine or eccrine) differentiation. Inactivating mutations in the tumour suppressor gene CYLD that negatively regulates the oncogenic transcription factor NF-κB are noted. The lesion is also associated with genetic syndromes such as Brooke–Spiegler syndrome (associated with both trichoepithelioma and cylindroma).

Morphology

Gross The lesion commonly occurs on the forehead and scalp. Multiple lesions can coalesce and can produce a hat-like growth, earning the name a turban tumour.

Microscopy Microscopically, the lesion is composed of islands of cells resembling the normal epidermal or adnexal basal cell layer (basaloid cells). These islands of cells are characteristically arranged as pieces of a **jigsaw puzzle,** which fit together within a fibrous dermal matrix (Fig. 29.28).

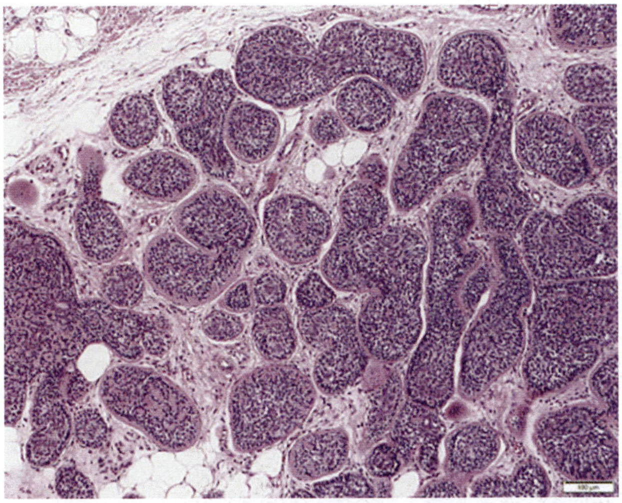

Fig. 29.28 Cylindroma. The basaloid cells are arranged in irregularly shaped islands surrounded by a thin band of hyaline material and containing hyaline droplets. The tumour cells are arranged in jigsaw puzzle–like pattern and hyalinized material within the peripheral islands. (*Source:* From James W. Patterson. Tumours of cutaneous appendages. Weedon's Skin Pathology. 5th edition. Elsevier 2021.)

Syringoma

Syringoma is a benign small skin adnexal lesion with eccrine differentiation.

Morphology

Gross It usually occurs as multiple, small, tan papules in the vicinity of the lower eyelids.

Microscopy Microscopically, the lesions are restricted to the upper reticular dermis. The lesion is composed of nests, cords and tubules of epithelial cells that anastomose and is present within a dense stroma made of collagen bundles and few fibrocytes. The individual cells have eosinophilic to clear cytoplasm and small nuclei with inconspicuous nucleoli (Fig. 29.29).

Pilomatricoma

Pilomatricoma is a relatively common skin adnexal neoplasm showing differentiation towards the matrix and the inner sheath of a normal hair follicle. The lesion is associated with activating mutations in CTNNB1, the gene encoding β-catenin. This pathway is critical for the early hair development, its growth and maintenance. They prefer the hair-bearing region and many occur in the head and neck and the upper extremities.

Morphology

Gross Clinically, the lesions are usually solitary, asymptomatic, slow-growing, firm-to-hard nodules varying in size from 0.5 to 3 cm in diameter. Grossly, the lesion shows lobulation with variable amounts of chalky white or yellowish keratinous material on cut section. Bone formation may also be noted.

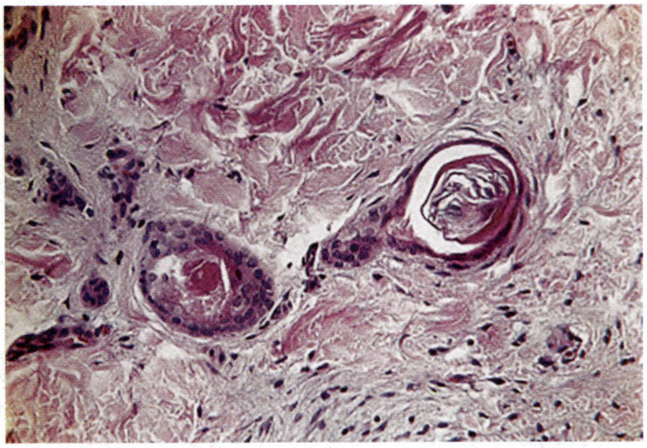

Fig. 29.29 Microscopy of syringoma: Small glandular structures with little 'tails' are typical of this entity. (*Source:* From Steven D. Billings. Tumours and Tumourlike Conditions of the Skin. Rosai and Ackerman's Surgical Pathology. 11th edition. Elsevier 2018.)

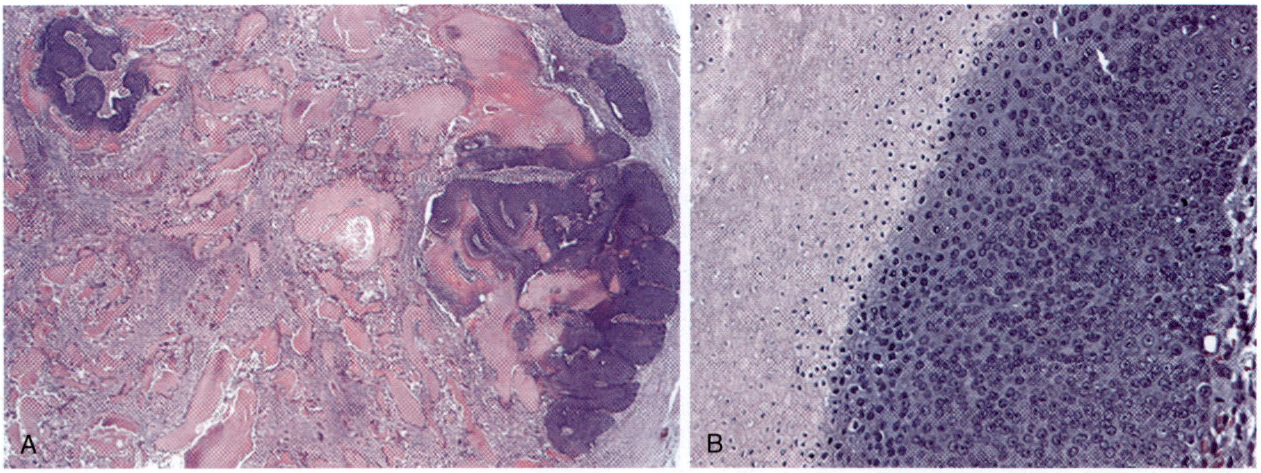

Fig. 29.30 Microscopy of pilomatrixoma. (A) Two cell types present – nests of basaloid cells (dark blue) and shadow cells (pink). (B) Basaloid cells making a transition into shadow cells. (*Source:* A: From Eduardo Calonje, Thomas Brenn, Alexander J. Lazar and Steven D. Billings. Tumours of the hair follicle. McKee's Pathology of the Skin. 5th edition. Elsevier 2020. B: Daniel J. Santa Cruz and Alejandro A. Gru. Tumours of the Skin. Diagnostic Histopathology of Tumours. 5th edition. Elsevier 2021.)

Microscopy Microscopically, the lesion is predominantly located in the dermis region composed of basaloid cells showing trichilemmal or hair-like differentiation similar to the germinal portion of the normal hair bulb. Early and well-developed lesions show small- to large-sized cystic lesions lined focally by aggregations of basaloid cells and filled centrally by large masses of eosinophilic cornified material containing ghost cells and keratin filaments. A transition zone of retained nuclei from basaloid cells to eosinophilic cornified material containing anucleate shadow cells is typically observed. The late regressing tumours are large and cystic with prominent areas of shadow cells and foci of basaloid cells surrounded by inflammatory cells, siderophages, melanophages, giant cells and also foci of metaplastic ossification (Fig. 29.30). Treatment is surgical excision, and malignant transformation may occur rarely.

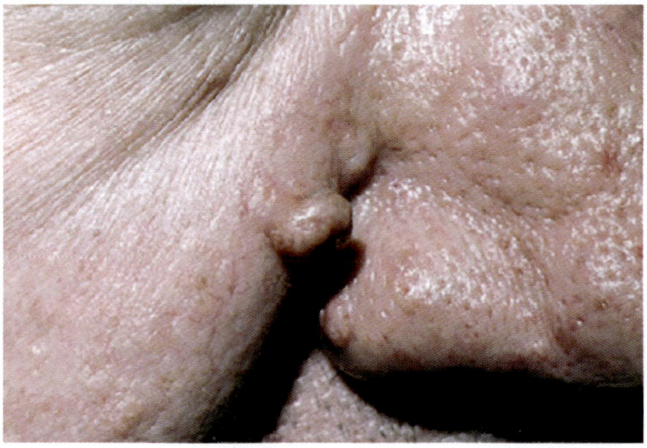

Fig. 29.31 Sebaceous adenomas of Muir–Torre syndrome. (*Source:* From William D. James, Dirk M. Elston, James R. Treat, Misha A. Rosenbach and Isaac M. Neuhaus. Epidermal Nevi, Neoplasms, and Cysts. Andrews' Diseases of the Skin. 13th edition. Elsevier 2020.)

Sebaceous Adenomas

Sebaceous adenoma is a small tumour composed of basaloid cells and fully differentiated sebocytes commonly arising as solitary lesions in the middle age. The lesion can be associated with Muir–Torre syndrome and Lynch syndrome (Fig. 29.31).

Morphology

Macroscopically, these lesions are yellowish covered with scale or crust.

Microscopically, the tumour is well circumscribed, composed of small lobular aggregations of sebocytes with a rim of basaloid cells at the periphery. Mature sebocytes are seen in the central portion of the lesion that have frothy or bubbly cytoplasm because of the presence of lipid vesicles (Fig. 29.32). It has to be differentiated from sebaceous hyperplasia, where the sebaceous lobules are arranged around a centrally placed follicular infundibulum that is connected to the epidermis.

MALIGNANT SKIN ADNEXAL TUMOURS

Although predominantly the skin appendageal tumours are benign, malignant counterparts do exist. Malignant tumours are more common in the apocrine differentiation than the benign forms.

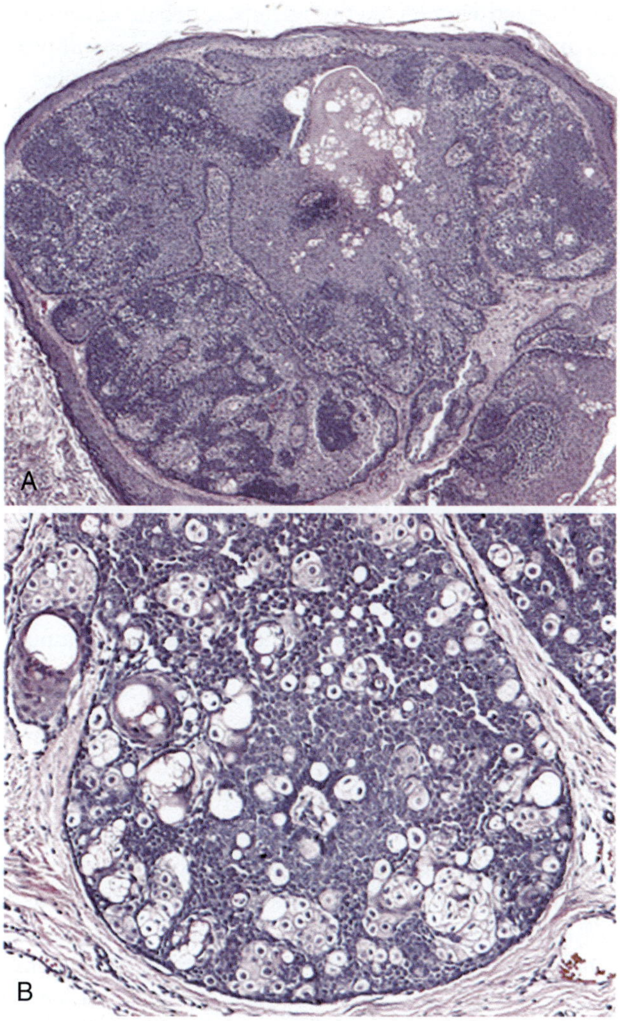

Fig. 29.32 Sebaceous adenoma: Lobules of sebaceous cells with germinal cells. (A) This lesion contains lobules of sebocytes with a modest degree of terminal differentiation. (B) This lesion contains sebocytes with a prominent germinal pattern. (*Source:* From Daniel J. Santa Cruz and Alejandro A. Gru. Tumours of the Skin. Diagnostic Histopathology of Tumours. 5th edition. Elsevier 2021.)

Apocrine Carcinoma

Apocrine carcinoma (AC) is a rare malignant sweat gland neoplasm with apocrine ductal differentiation. Axilla and the anogenital region are most commonly involved by this tumour.

Morphology

Gross Most tumours are solitary, firm or cystic nodules varying in size from 2 to 8 cm in diameter. AC is predominantly a tumour centred in the dermis and tries to reach the subcutaneous region. The tumours are usually poorly circumscribed with infiltrating borders.

Microscopy Microscopically, the tumour growth patterns are highly variable, including tubular, papillary, cystic, cribriform, micronodular and solid formations. The cells have abundant eosinophilic cytoplasm and large, round-to-oval, mostly vesicular nuclei, single prominent eosinophilic nucleolus with characteristic intracytoplasmic PAS-positive diastase-resistant granules. A well-recognized feature of decapitation secretion in the form of apical snouts is usually observed. The surrounding stroma is usually densely fibroblastic or hyaline and may contain prominent lymphoplasmacytic infiltrates.

ACs have the proper adenocarcinoma appearance and should be differentiated from metastatic adenocarcinoma because of their tendency to form gland-like structures. The infiltrative growth pattern is a hint of malignancy in a well-differentiated tumour.

The majority of ACs are slow-growing tumours with prolonged course. The overall mortality is relatively low. Surgical excision is the treatment of choice.

Sebaceous Carcinoma

Sebaceous carcinoma (SC) is a cytologically and/or architecturally malignant neoplasm showing exclusive sebocytic differentiation. Clinically, the lesions present as painless masses and can be multifocal. SCs are slow-growing nodules and can become ulcerated.

Morphology

Gross The common sites include the ocular region from the meibomian gland, trunk, genitals and extremities (Fig. 29.33).

Microscopy Microscopically, the tumour cells show the characteristic sebocytic differentiation consisting of multivesicular and vacuolated clear cytoplasm. The

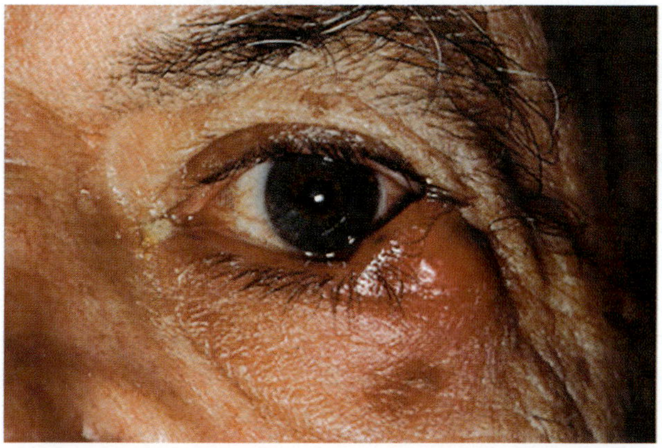

Fig. 29.33 Sebaceous carcinoma in patient with Muir–Torre syndrome. (*Source:* From William D. James, Dirk M. Elston, James R. Treat, Misha A. Rosenbach and Isaac M. Neuhaus. Epidermal Nevi, Neoplasms, and Cysts. Andrews' Diseases of the Skin. 13th edition. Elsevier 2020.)

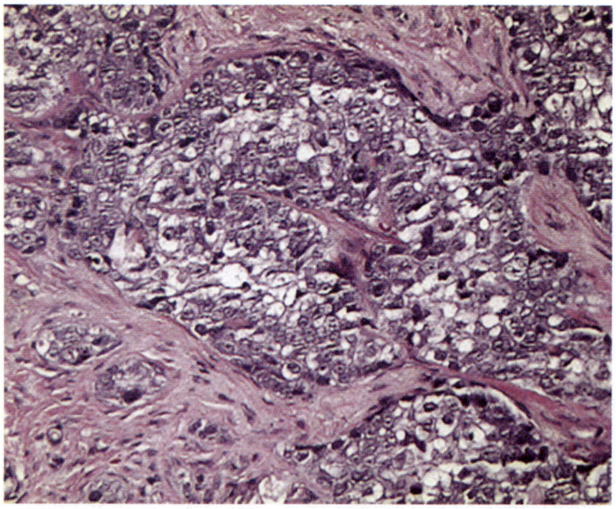

Fig. 29.34 Sebaceous carcinoma with typical cytoplasmic vacuolization. Tumour contains cells with foamy cytoplasm and the cytoplasmic vacuoles are usually small and the nuclei of tumour cells are typically very basophilic and may appear smudged. (*Source:* From Robert Folberg and Amy Lin. Tumours of the Eye and Ocular Adnexa. Diagnostic Histopathology of Tumours. 5th edition. Elsevier 2021.)

tumour mainly occupies the dermal region as lobules of variably atypical polygonal cells, with a fibrovascular stroma that lacks desmoplasia and central areas of comedo-like necrosis may also be seen. The tumour cells show abundant cytoplasm and oval vesicular nuclei with distinct nucleoli with variable mitotic figures (Fig. 29.34). There may be focal squamous differentiation. It may also mimic a variety of cutaneous neoplasms, including BCC.

All SCs have the potential for an association with overlying carcinoma in situ (CIS), or extramammary Paget disease (EPD) of the sebaceous type, or both, in the surface epithelium. The tumour has the capacity for local tumour recurrence, distant metastases, causing tumour-related mortality.

DERMAL TUMOURS

Benign skin tumours need to be differentiated from other more serious conditions to ensure the appropriate treatment. The dermis is composed of connective tissue including collagen and elastic tissue, muscle, vessels, nerves and fat extending from the subcutis. All of these elements may give rise to tumours, either true neoplasms or congenital malformations.

BENIGN FIBROUS HISTIOCYTOMA (BFH) (DERMATOFIBROMA)

The lesion is usually seen in adults as a dermal lesion, occurring on the extremities and trunk of young and middle-aged women. Aetiologically, a debate of whether it is an inflammatory or a neoplastic process is still present but a history of antecedent trauma, insect bites or folliculitis is present in many patients, suggesting an abnormal response to injury and inflammation, although few observations support a clonal origin hinting at a neoplastic process.

Morphology

Gross Grossly, the lesion is ill-defined, single, round, firm-to-hard, tan-to-brown papules or nodules ranging from 1 to 2 cm in diameter. The characteristic 'dimpling' sign, when the lesions are squeezed between the thumb and index finger is frequently noted. Cut section is solid grey-white to yellowish with areas of haemorrhage and lipidization. Multiple dermatofibromas (DFs) sometimes grouped ('agminated') papules are regarded as a marker of immune suppression commonly seen in black females with systemic lupus erythematosus.

Microscopy Microscopy shows an ill-defined non-encapsulated lesion present in the reticular dermis composed of benign, spindle- to round-shaped cells with some of them being fibrocytes or macrophages. Early lesions are rich in macrophages with some forming Touton or foreign body type of giant cells. The spindle-shaped cells are frequently arranged in short fascicles that interweave forming 'storiform pattern' with collagen trapping by lesional cells leading to 'collagen ball formation' at the periphery (Fig. 29.35). Variable number of inflammatory cells, collagen bundles and epidermal, melanocytic and folliculosebaceous hyperplasia are also characteristically present above the lesion.

Immunohistochemical profile: Good reactivity for CD68 and factor XIIIa is observed, especially in the early lesions.

Differential Diagnosis

Dermatofibrosarcoma protuberans (DFSP) (particularly with the cellular variant of DF) and Kaposi sarcoma in the nodular and tumour stage are the important differential diagnosis. DFSP is poorly circumscribed with deeper and irregular infiltration into the subcutis and show CD34-positivity unlike DF. Kaposi sarcoma is characterized by erythrocytes extravasated into slits between interweaving fascicles of spindle-shaped cells and are positive for vascular markers.

Prognosis and predictive factors: Majority of these lesions are benign; incomplete excision may result in recurrence.

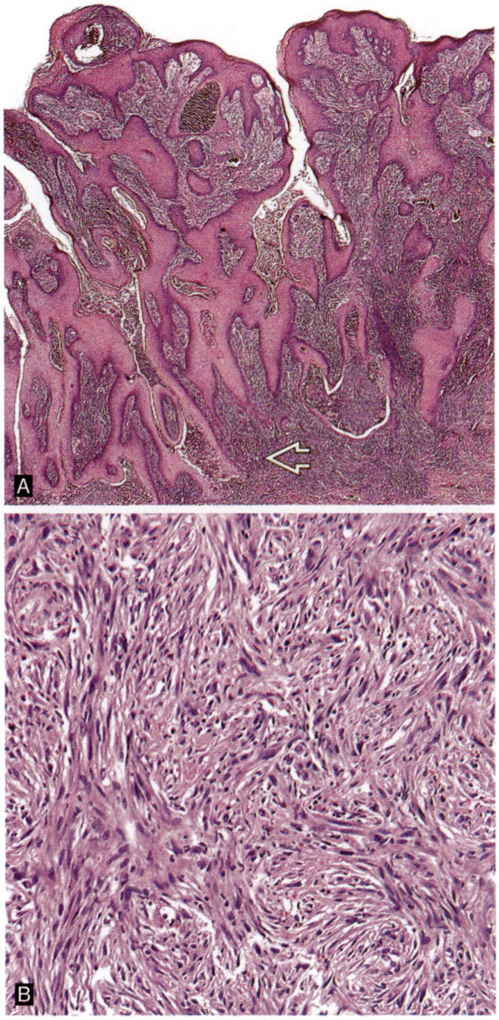

Fig. 29.35 Microscopy of benign fibrous histiocytoma. Dermatofibroma. (A) The epidermis overlying the dermal tumour is acanthotic and papillomatous. (B) The cells have a storiform arrangement. (*Source:* A, Diagnostic Pathology: Genitourinary, 3ed.: Mahul B. Amin, Satish K. Tickoo, Elsevier Inc., 2022. B, Diagnostic Pathology: Head and Neck, 3ed. Lester D.R. Thompson, Brenda L. Nelson, Susan Muller, Elsevier Inc., 2022.)

DERMATOFIBROSARCOMA PROTUBERANS

DFSP is a superficial well-differentiated, low-grade sarcoma occurring in the dermis and subcutis. The lesion is locally aggressive and has a male preponderance occurring in the adulthood mainly involving the chest, back, abdominal wall and the scalp. Clinically, it is a persistent slow-growing cutaneous nodular tumour often with peripheral red or blue discolouration attaining the final protuberant appearance with single or multiple nodularity. Advanced lesions may show superficial ulceration with rare occurrences of metastasis.

Pathogenesis

DFSP is thought to be derived from fibroblast cells that have close linkage to dermal dendrocytes. Balanced translocation between genes encoding collagen 1A1 (COL1A1) and the platelet-derived growth factor-β (PDGFβ) has been identified which leads to overexpression and secretion of PDGFβ that drives the tumour growth.

Morphology

Gross The cut surface of the tumour is grey-white and firm, with occasional areas showing a gelatinous appearance, corresponding to areas of myxoid change, and rarely areas of necrosis are seen.

Microscopy Microscopically, the DFSP diffusely infiltrates the dermis invading into subcutaneous tissue and the fibrous septa of fat. The tumour is typically composed of compact, uniform, slender, mildly atypical, spindle-shaped fibroblasts arranged in a whorled pinwheel (storiform), or cartwheel pattern (Fig. 29.36). Nuclear pleomorphism and mitotic activity are inconspicuous. Overlying epidermis is generally thinned-out with deep extension from the dermis into subcutaneous fat, producing a characteristic 'honeycombing' pattern. Immunohistochemically, DFSP cells label diffusely and strongly with antibodies to CD34 and vimentin. The lesion has to be differentiated from the benign and cellular DF by the absence of epidermal hyperplasia, prominent collagenous stroma and minimal extension into fat lobules in DFSP.

Local wide excision is preferred along with administration of tyrosine kinase inhibitor imatinib mesylate which inhibits the PDGFβ receptor activation and reduces the tumour growth. Incomplete resections may lead to local recurrence of the tumour.

TUMOURS OF MIGRANTS TO SKIN

Lymphocyte migration from the bloodstream into secondary lymphoid organs is essential for maintaining

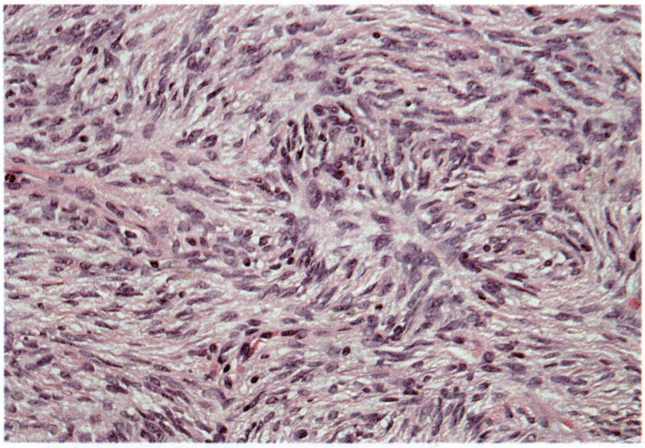

Fig. 29.36 Microscopy of dermatofibrosarcoma protuberans: Storiform or cartwheel pattern of dermatofibrosarcoma protuberans. (*Source:* https://upload.wikimedia.org/wikipedia/commons/3/39/Storiform_pattern_-_very_high_mag.jpg)

homeostasis and for providing efficient defence against pathogens. This migration occurs mostly through high endothelial venules and is partially regulated by signalling cascades involving adhesion and activation. Integrins mediate the firm adhesion of leucocytes to the endothelium that allows for the transmigration of cells into tissue. When lymphomas occur in the skin with no evidence of disease anywhere else at the time of diagnosis, they are called 'primary' cutaneous lymphomas.

MYCOSIS FUNGOIDES (CUTANEOUS T-CELL LYMPHOMA)

Mycosis fungoides (MF) is an idiopathic spectrum of cutaneous T-cell lymphoma (CTCL) with preferential proliferation and homing of neoplastic clonal $CD4^+$ T-helper cells into the skin because of expression of cutaneous lymphocyte antigen (CLA). It is a peripheral, epidermotropic non-Hodgkin T-cell lymphoma of low-grade malignant potential and can occur in any part of the skin tissue.

The disease initially presents in the skin showing clinical progression from patches to plaques and tumours over a period of years with distinct histological, phenotypic and genotypic features.

Morphology

Gross The early patches are circumscribed, scaly, red-brown lesions with discolouration without palpable infiltration of the skin. Plaques evolve out of patches with variable degree of palpable infiltration, whereas the tumours show exophytic growth with ulceration followed by dissemination into the peripheral blood, bone marrow and visceral organs in advanced stages (Fig. 29.37). Development of multiple, large (≥10 cm in diameter), red-brown nodules indicate systemic spread.

Microscopy **Sézary–Lutzner cells:** T-helper cells ($CD4^+$) are the histologic hallmark of MF and form band-like aggregates within the superficial dermis (**epidermotropism**). These cells have infolded nuclear membranes, imparting a hyperconvoluted or cerebriform contour. They invade the epidermis as single cells and small clusters (**Pautrier microabscesses**). Subcorneal, intraepidermal and subepidermal bullous formation may result from confluence of Pautrier microabscesses and the cells also lose the quality of epidermotropism in the advanced nodular lesions and grow deep into the dermis ensuing the systemic spread (Fig. 29.38). The cells are positive for CD2, CD3 and CD4.

Involvement of peripheral blood by malignant T cells with cerebriform nuclei, along with diffuse erythroderma and scaling of entire body is known as the Sézary syndrome having a poor prognosis (Fig. 29.39).

Clinical Features

The disease usually occurs in adults older than 60 years with a male preponderance. Clinically, the patients present with a triad of pruritus, intractable erythroderma and

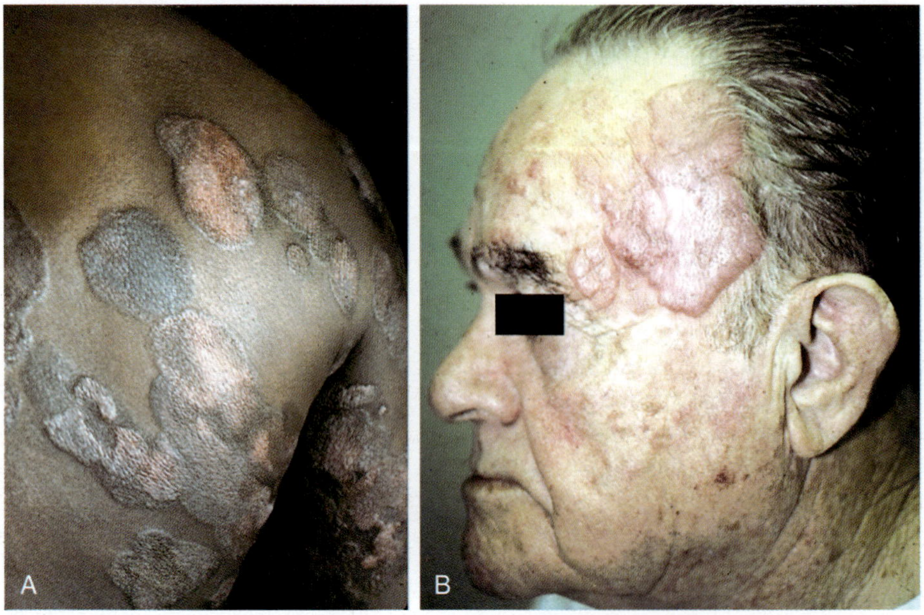

Fig. 29.37 Clinical pictures of mycosis fungoides. (A) Plaques of mycosis fungoides often have a polycyclic appearance. (B) Tumours are more elevated above the skin surface. By the time tumours supervene, sun-exposed skin, such as the face, is often involved. (*Source:* From Jaffe ES et al: Hematopathology, Philadelphia, 2011, WB Saunders.)

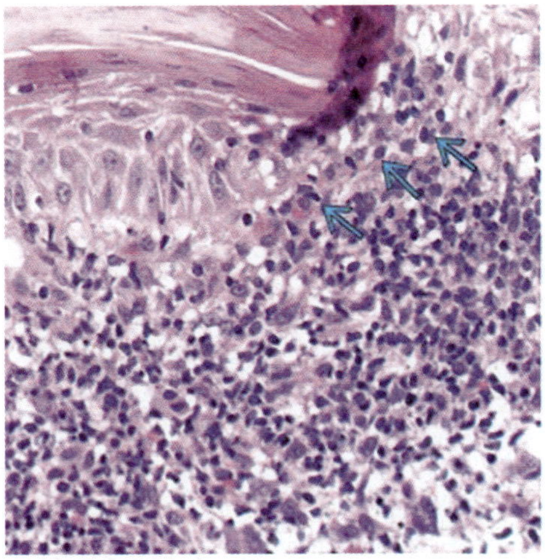

Fig. 29.38 Microscopically, there is infiltration of atypical lymphocytes beneath and also invading the epidermis – epidermotropism. (*Source:* Diagnostic Pathology : Molecular Oncology, 3rd ed.: Mohammad A. Vasef, M. Carmen Frias Kletecka, Aaron Auerbach, et. al., Elsevier Inc., 2024.)

lymphadenopathy. Alopecia, ectropion, nail dystrophy, palmoplantar keratoderma, leonine facies and bacterial skin infection are also the presenting features.

Clinically, MF corresponds to the chronic proliferative process, whereas MF d'emblée presents as an aggressive nodular eruptive variant. The more the percentage of body surface involved with transformation into the plaque

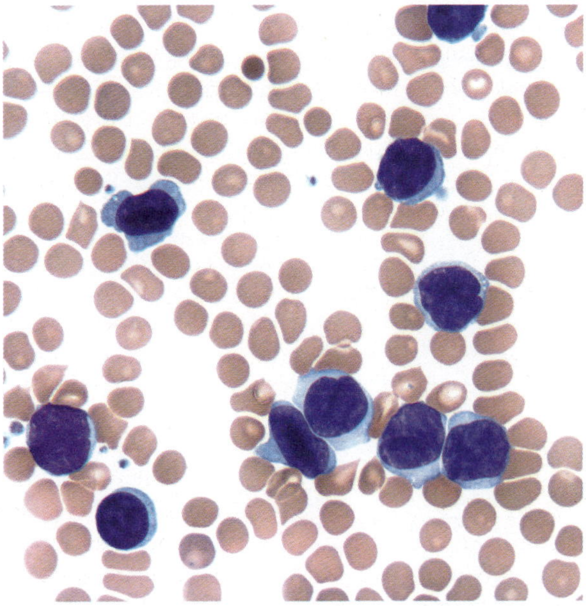

Fig. 29.39 Microscopy of Sézary syndrome. Sézary cells in a peripheral blood smear: Recognition of these cells is no longer critical for the diagnosis because of the advent of clonality studies and flow cytometry. (*Source:* Diagnostic Pathology: Lymph Nodes and Extranodal Lymphomas, 3ed.: L. Jeffrey Medeiros, Roberto N. Miranda, Elsevier Inc., 2023.)

and tumour stage in an elderly patient, the poorer the prognosis. Topical therapy with steroids or UV light is helpful in the early skin lesions, whereas aggressive systemic chemotherapy is suited for the advanced disease.

SELF-ASSESSMENT

Multiple Choice Questions

1. A 65-year-old fair-skinned individual presents with a non-healing ulcer on his face. Biopsy reveals nests of atypical cells with keratin pearls. What is the most likely diagnosis?
   A. Basal cell carcinoma
   B. Squamous cell carcinoma
   C. Melanoma
   D. Naevus
2. A patient with a history of chronic sun exposure presents with a pearly papule with telangiectasias on his nose. Histopathological examination shows basaloid cells with peripheral palisading and clefting. What is the most likely diagnosis?
   A. Basal cell carcinoma
   B. Squamous cell carcinoma
   C. Melanoma
   D. Naevus
3. A suspicious lesion is biopsied and found to have cells with large, irregular nuclei and prominent nucleoli. There is also evidence of keratinization. What is the most likely diagnosis?
   A. Basal cell carcinoma
   B. Squamous cell carcinoma
   C. Melanoma
   D. Naevus
4. A patient presents with a dark, irregularly shaped lesion on her back. Dermoscopy reveals asymmetry, irregular borders and multiple colours. Which of the following features supports a diagnosis of melanoma?
   A. Regular borders
   B. Symmetry
   C. Homogeneous colour
   D. Asymmetry
5. A lesion is excised and histopathological examination reveals a proliferation of melanocytes confined to the epidermis. What is the most likely diagnosis?
   A. Basal cell carcinoma
   B. Squamous cell carcinoma
   C. Melanoma in situ
   D. Naevus
6. A patient presents with a changing mole on his forearm. On examination, you notice asymmetry, irregular borders and variegated colour. What is the most appropriate next step?
   A. Advise the patient to monitor the mole for further changes
   B. Perform a punch biopsy of the lesion
   C. Prescribe topical steroids for the lesion
   D. Reassure the patient that it is likely benign

7. A patient with a history of extensive sun exposure presents with a nodular lesion on her face. Dermoscopy reveals arborizing vessels and ulceration. What is the most likely diagnosis?
   A. Basal cell carcinoma
   B. Squamous cell carcinoma
   C. Melanoma
   D. Naevus
8. A lesion is biopsied and histopathological examination reveals a proliferation of melanocytes with invasion into the dermis. What is the most likely diagnosis?
   A. Basal cell carcinoma
   B. Squamous cell carcinoma
   C. Melanoma
   D. Naevus
9. A patient presents with a dark, irregularly shaped lesion on their leg. Dermoscopy reveals irregular pigmentation and an irregular vascular pattern. What is the most concerning feature for melanoma?
   A. Regular borders
   B. Symmetry
   C. Homogeneous colour
   D. Asymmetry
10. A patient presents with a new pigmented lesion on their back. Dermoscopic examination reveals a regular network of pigmented lines and globules. What is the most likely diagnosis?
   A. Basal cell carcinoma
   B. Squamous cell carcinoma
   C. Melanoma
   D. Naevus

Answers

1. (B); 2. (A); 3. (B); 4. (D); 5. (C); 6. (B); 7. (A); 8. (C); 9. (D); 10. (C)

Self-Assessment Questions

1. A 35-year-old woman presented with complaints of joint pain and plaques of variable sizes with loosely adherent silvery white scales. When the scales are lifted, multiple bleeding points were noted. What is the diagnosis and what is the sign referred to as?
2. A 40-year-old man came with the complaints of flat-topped violaceous papules highlighted by whitish lines (Wickham striae) with pruritis. What is the diagnosis?
3. A 65-year-old man with a history of B-cell lymphoma developed blisters predominantly affecting the oral mucosa. What is the diagnosis?
4. An immunocompromised individual presented with squamoproliferative lesions involving the skin and oral mucosa caused by human papillomavirus. The microscopy showed large vacuolated squamous cells with pyknotic nuclei. What are these cells known as?
5. A 42-year-old woman undergoing chemotherapy for a haematological malignancy developed dome-shaped pearly papule with central umbilication. What are the intracytoplasmic granular inclusions known as?
6. A 50-year-old mason developed an asymmetrical blackish skin lesion with recent history of colour and size. What is the name of the thickness measured from the epidermal granular cell layer to the deepest intradermal tumour cell site?
7. A 45-year-old farmer presented with an ulceroproliferative lesion on the leg in the site of an old scar. Microscopy showed atypical squamous cells with keratin pearl formation. What is the diagnosis?
8. A 58-year-old construction worker with a fair complexion presented with a slow-growing, erythematous, ulcerated lesion with pearly edges on the face for 2 months. Mutation study revealed loss of function mutation in PTCH allele. What is the diagnosis? Describe the microscopy of the lesion.
9. A 15-year-old girl presented with a hard nodule of 2.5 cm in size in the upper arm and the lesion was surgically excised which revealed chalky white material of cut section. What is the diagnosis?
10. A 65-year-old man presented with cervical lymphadenopathy, pruritic skin lesions and erythroderma. The patient also had ectropion and nail dystrophy. What are the characteristic helper T cells of the condition known as?

Answers

1. Psoriasis, Auspitz sign
2. Lichen planus
3. Paraneoplastic pemphigus
4. Koilocytes
5. Henderson–Patterson bodies
6. Breslow thickness
7. Squamous cell carcinoma
8. Basal cell carcinoma; microscopy shows islands of tumour basaloid cells with peripheral palisading along with retraction artefacts
9. Pilomatrixoma
10. Sézary–Lutzner cells

Topics for Self-Directed Learning

1. Role of immunofluorescence in skin lesions
2. Role of immunohistochemistry in malignancies of skin
3. Applications of electron microscopy in skin lesions
4. Skin lesions with syndromic background
5. Cutaneous pseudolymphomas
6. Pathology of cutaneous drug eruptions
7. Autoimmune bullous disorders of skin

Bones, Joints, Soft-Tissue Tumours, Skeletal Muscle and Peripheral Nervous System

30

Vimala Chelladurai, Rajeswari Kathiah, Gayathri Devi Thanigaimani

PA 33.1 Classify and describe the aetiology, pathogenesis, manifestations, radiological and morphological features and complications of **osteomyelitis**.

PA 33.2 Classify and describe the aetiology, pathogenesis, manifestations, radiological and morphological features, complications and metastasis of **bone tumours**.

PA 33.3 Classify and describe the aetiology, pathogenesis, manifestations, radiological and morphological features, complications and metastasis of **soft-tissue tumours**.

PA 33.4 Classify and describe the aetiology, pathogenesis, manifestations, radiological and morphological features and complications of **Paget disease of the bone**.

PA 33.5 Classify and describe the aetiology, immunology, pathogenesis, manifestations, radiological and laboratory features, diagnostic criteria and complications of **rheumatoid arthritis**.

CHAPTER OUTLINE

I. BONES

STRUCTURE AND FUNCTIONS OF BONE

The human skeleton consists of cartilage and bones. There are 206 bones in human body, which constitute to about 12% of the body weight. The bones provide mechanical support, protect the internal organs, take part in mineral homeostasis and also produce niche for blood cell production. Besides the osteoid matrix, bone consists of three main types of cells, namely the osteoblasts, osteoclasts and osteocytes (Fig. 30.1).

CELLS

Osteoblasts are uninucleate cells found on the new bone-forming surfaces. They synthesize and assemble the bone matrix. The osteoblastic activity in the blood can be measured by serum levels of bone-related alkaline phosphatase. Physiological increase in the osteoblastic activity is seen during puberty and pathological increase is seen in conditions such as fracture repair and Paget disease of the bone.

Osteocytes are the osteoblasts which get incorporated into the bone matrix during their synthesis. They occupy a small chamber called lacuna within the bone matrix. The osteocytic lacunae are important to distinguish the woven bone from the lamellar bone.

Osteoclasts which are multinucleated macrophages derived from monocytes help in bone resorption. Their activity in blood is determined by bone-related serum *acid phosphatase.*

MATRIX

Matrix is the extracellular component of bone. It predominantly contains type 1 collagen with a smaller amount of other proteins such as glycosaminoglycans. Bone matrix is composed of 35% of osteoid and 65% of

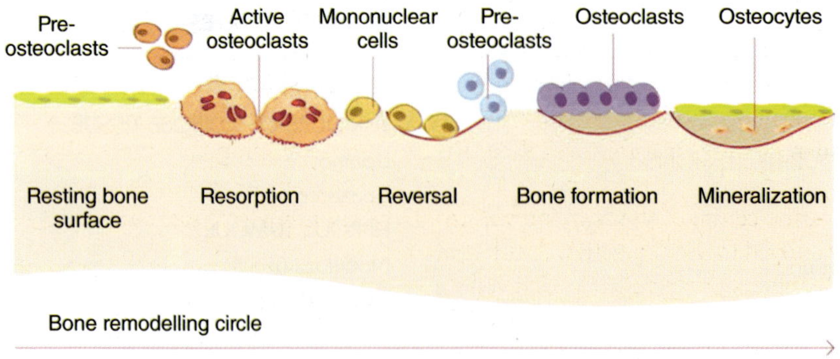

Fig. 30.1 Illustration of active bone formation.

minerals. The hardness of the bone matrix is due to the presence of hydroxyapatite.

Osteoid is composed of many proteins including osteopontin which is synthesized by osteoblasts and is involved in the regulation of bone formation, mineralization and calcium homeostasis. Hence, serum osteopontin level is also a marker of osteoblast activity. Many other factors such as cytokines, growth factors and mechanical forces are involved in the regulation of bone metabolism and maturation.

Bone matrix can be either woven or lamellar.

Woven bone is rapidly produced during fetal development and fracture repair and is composed of haphazardly arranged collagen fibres.

Lamellar bone is slowly produced and is composed of parallelly arranged collagen fibres.

A cross-section of a long bone is composed of the outer cortex and central medulla with bony trabeculae separated by the marrow.

DEVELOPMENT

Bone is a tissue where formation and resorption of the organ takes place regularly over the entire period of growth. *Enchondral ossification* is the process of bone formation from hyaline cartilage during embryogenesis. Majority of the bones are formed by enchondral ossification except for the flat bones such as the skull, mandible and clavicle. These flat bones develop by a process that involves direct conversion of the mesenchymal connective tissue into bone by osteoblastic activity and this process is called *membranous ossification*. In both these ossifications, uncalcified osteoid matrix is formed by osteoblasts which gets mineralized in 2 weeks to form bone.

A long bone is divided into several regions.

Epiphysis: The region between the growth plate and the expanded end of the bone

Metaphysis: The region where the growth plate and the diaphysis meet

Diaphysis: The shaft of the long bones located between the two metaphyses

Enchondral ossification follows the following five steps:

(a) Mesenchymal cells differentiate into chondrocytes.

(b) These chondrocytes secrete the extracellular matrix (ECM) to form the cartilage model of the future bony skeleton and a surrounding membrane called the perichondrium.

(c) The chondrocytes at the centre of the bony model undergo hypertrophy and aid in the deposition of collagen and fibronectin – this altered matric allows calcification. Calcification prevents nutrient supply to the chondrocytes causing them to die by apoptosis. The resultant void in the cartilage template allows capillaries to penetrate, bringing osteogenic cells that activate the conversion of the perichondrium to the periosteum. The proliferating blood vessels and the expanding spaces eventually combine to form the medullary cavity. Osteoblasts further give rise to a thickened area of compact bone at the diaphyseal region of the periosteum referred to as the periosteal collar. This is where the primary ossification centre develops.

(d) The bone is being formed replacing the cartilage in the diaphysis, whereas the cartilage and chondrocytes continue to grow at ends of the bone, contributing to bone length.

(e) After birth, similar ossification centres occur in the epiphysis – secondary ossification centres. Both the primary and the secondary ossification centres fuse during adolescence and early adulthood giving rise to complete bones.

HOMEOSTASIS AND REMODELLING

The bone may look static but undergoes dynamic changes throughout life through a well-regulated physiological process called remodelling. Remodelling of bone takes place at a microscopic locus known as bone multicellular unit (BMU) which consists of coupled osteoblast and osteoclast activity on the bone surface. Osteoclast attachment, resorption, osteoblast attachment and proliferation and, finally, matrix synthesis proceed at BMU and are tightly regulated by cell–cell interactions and cytokines (Fig. 30.2).

The control mechanisms involve several signalling pathways.

1. One such pathway involves three factors:
   (i) RANK receptors expressed on osteoclast precursors
   (ii) RANKL (RANK ligand) which is expressed on osteoblasts and marrow stromal cells
   (iii) Osteoprotegerin (OPG), a secreted decoy receptor that can bind to RANKL, thus blocking the RANK and RANKL interaction
   When stimulated by RANKL, RANK signalling activates the transcription factor NF-κB which helps in generation and survival of osteoclasts
2. Monocyte colony–stimulating factor (M-CSF) produced by osteoblasts: Activation of M-CSF receptor on osteoclast precursor stimulates a tyrosine kinase pathway which also helps in the generation of osteoclasts.
3. WNT/β-catenin pathway – WNT proteins produced by osteoprogenitor cells bind to LRP5 and LRP6 receptors on the osteoblasts and thereby trigger the activation of β-catenin and production of OPG.

Sclerostin which is produced by osteocytes inhibits the WNT/β-catenin pathway.

Germline mutations involving OPG, RANK, RANKL and LRP5 genes cause disturbances of bone metabolism. Hence, the bone formation and bone resorption are

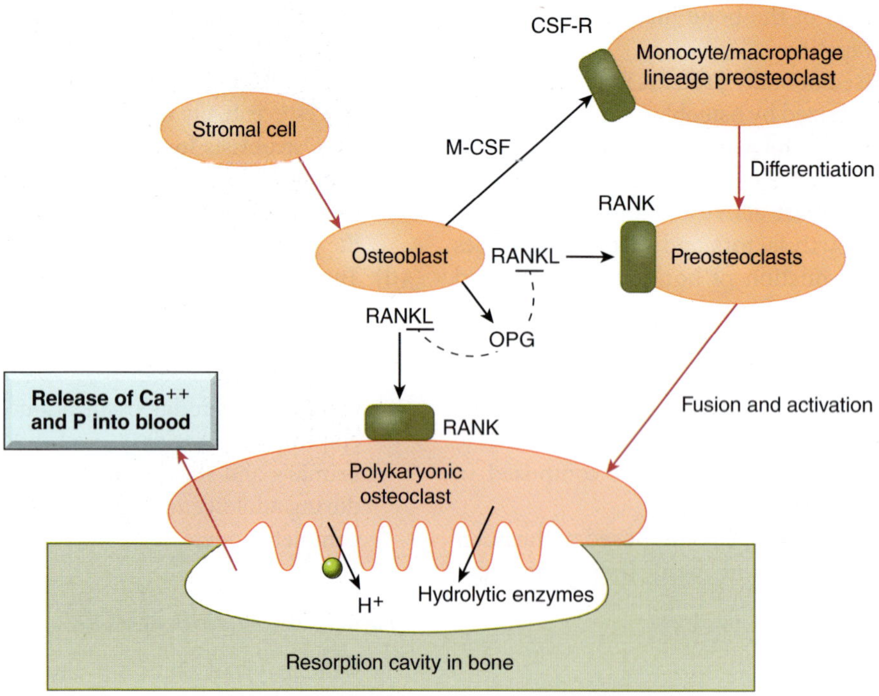

Fig. 30.2 Regulation of osteoclast formation and function.

modulated by the signals that connect to the RANK and WNT signalling pathways.

In the subsequent discussion on the pathologies concerned with bone tissue, we review the clinical features and the imaging findings along with the morphology of the lesion for better understanding and correlation.

DEVELOPMENTAL DISORDERS OF BONE AND CARTILAGE

The developmental disorders of the bone may be inherited or acquired but are most often a result of inherited mutations. They may arise from disorders affecting the ossification locally (dysostosis) or from global disorganization of bone or cartilage (dysplasia).

ACHONDROPLASIA (SIGNAL TRANSDUCTION PROTEIN DEFECT)

Achondroplasia is an autosomal dominant disorder and is the most common cause of dwarfism. About 80% of cases result from new mutations which originate from paternal genes. The remaining cases are inherited from a parent with the disease. The risk of new mutation increases with the age of the father. Children, who inherit both the affected genes because of the presence of the disease in both the parents, typically die intrauterine or in the early infancy period because of respiratory failure caused by the underdeveloped rib cage.

The disease is due to gain-of-function mutations in the FGF receptor 3 gene, FGFR3 gene. This gene contributes to the production of collagen and other structural components of bones and other tissues. In normal development, FGFR3 has a negative regulatory effect on bone growth. The gain-of-function mutation of this gene leads to inhibition of endochondral growth of bones resulting in retarded cartilage growth and shortened proximal extremities with a relatively normal-length trunk, enlarged head, bulging forehead and depression of the root of the nose (Fig. 30.3). The affected individuals usually do not have any change in the longevity of life, IQ or fertility.

The disease is generally diagnosed on the basis of the symptoms but skeletal survey may be helpful and genetic testing is performed in some cases for confirmation. There is no known cure for achondroplasia and some experimental drugs are in trial.

There are two other syndromes with a genetic basis similar to that of achondroplasia: hypochondroplasia and thanatophoric dysplasia.

OSTEOGENESIS IMPERFECTA (COLLAGEN DEFECT)

Osteogenesis imperfecta (OI), also called brittle bone disease, is one of the most common connective tissue matrix diseases caused by defective type 1 collagen synthesis. The disease is heterogenous and is due to mutations in the genes coding for alpha 1 and 2 collagen chains. It is usually autosomal dominant in inheritance. The mutations result in misfolding of collagen polypeptides and defective assembly of higher-order collagen chains. Such defectively assembled mutant collagens also interfere and interrupt the assembly of normal collagen chains, thus exerting a dominant negative effect.

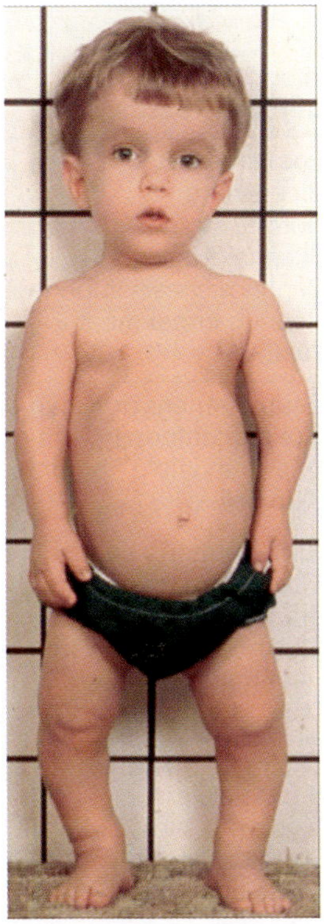

Fig. 30.3 A 3-year-old with achondroplasia with typical features and tibial bowing. (*Source:* From William A Horton Prof, Judith G Hall Prof and Jacqueline T Hecht Prof. Achondroplasia. The Lancet. 2007; 370:162–172.)

Apart from the skeletal system, other collagen-rich tissues such as the joints, skin, ears, eyes and teeth are also affected. The basic abnormalities in OI are marked cortical thinning and attenuation of trabeculae resulting in extreme skeletal fragility and the resultant fractures (Fig. 30.4). The other features of OI are short stature, blue sclera (blue colour is due to visualization of choroid through collagen-deficient translucent sclera), sensorineural hearing loss (due to impeded conductions by the abnormalities of the middle ear and inner ear bones) and dental abnormalities such as small, misshapen, blue-yellow teeth (due to dentin deficiency).

There are four subtypes of OI, of which types I and IV are compatible with survival. Type III is characterized by shortened survival because of progressive deformities, whereas type II is uniformly fatal. The subtypes are listed in Table 30.1.

OSTEOPETROSIS

Osteopetrosis, otherwise known as marble bone disease or Albers-Schönberg disease, is a group of rare genetic disorders in which bone modelling and remodelling are impaired. The disease is characterized by diffuse symmetric skeletal sclerosis due to impaired resorption of bone as a result of defective development and function of osteoclasts. The affected bones are hard but are brittle like a piece of chalk and more prone to fractures.

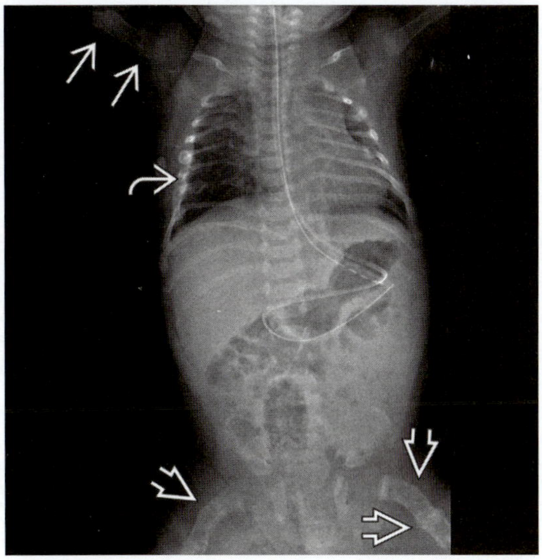

Fig. 30.4 Radiograph of osteogenesis imperfecta. AP radiograph in a 1-month-old patient showing numerous fractures, including the right humerus, multiple ribs and bilateral femurs that show associated bowing (indicated by the arrows). (*Source:* From A. Carlson Merrow and Selena Hariharan. Osteogenesis Imperfecta. Imaging in Pediatrics. Elsevier 2018.)

Osteopetrosis is classified into variants on the basis of both the mode of inheritance and the severity of clinical findings.

Pathogenesis

Osteopetrosis is caused by underlying mutations that interfere with the acidification of the osteoclast resorption pit. Carbonic anhydrase 2 (CA2) is required by the osteoclasts for proton production. Defect in gene for the enzyme CA2 blocks the process of acidification of the resorption pit and prevents the dissolution of calcium hydroxyapatite within the matrix. CA2 also facilitates urinary acidification by renal tubular epithelial cells and so osteopetrosis due to CA2 mutations is accompanied by renal tubular acidosis. Osteopetrosis may also be due to mutation in CLCN7 (chloride channel) that codes for a proton chloride exchanger on the osteoclast surface, required for resorption pit acidification. The classification of osteopetrosis is given in Table 30.2.

Clinical Features

As shown in Table 30.2, clinical features are dependent on the type. The disease is the most severe and fatal in the infantile form because the fetus suffers multiple and fatal intrauterine fractures. Other causes of death include fatal infections as a result of bone marrow failure and congestive cardiac failure due to anaemia.

Radiology

Radiological findings are characteristic and display generalized osteosclerosis. The long bones appear solid with no medullary canal and have bulbous ends, which is referred to as ***Erlenmeyer flask deformity***. The bones may

Table 30.1 Subtypes of Osteogenesis Imperfecta

Type	Mode of Inheritance	Collagen Defect	Clinical Features
I	Autosomal dominant	Decreased synthesis of pro-α1(1) chain Abnormal pro-α1(1) or pro-α2(1) chains	Postnatal fractures Blue sclera Normal stature Skeletal fragility Dentinogenesis imperfecta Hearing impairment Joint laxity
II	Most autosomal recessive Some autosomal dominant New mutations	Abnormally short pro-α1(1) chain Unstable triple helix; abnormal or insufficient pro-α2(1)	Death in utero or within days of birth Skeletal deformity with excessive fragility and multiple fractures Blue sclera
III	Autosomal dominant Autosomal recessive	Altered structure of pro-peptides of pro-α2(1); impaired formation of triple helix	Growth retardation Multiple fractures Progressive kyphoscoliosis Blue sclera at birth that becomes white Hearing impairment Dentinogenesis imperfecta
IV	Autosomal dominant	Short pro-α2(1) chain; unstable triple helix	Postnatal fractures Normal sclerae Moderate skeletal fragility Short stature Sometimes dentinogenesis imperfecta

Table 30.2 Subtypes of Osteopetrosis

Type	Inheritance Pattern	Clinical Features	Bone Marrow Failure	Prognosis
Adult onset	Autosomal dominant	Repeated fractures Asymptomatic Incidental finding	Absent	Good
Infantile	Autosomal recessive	Fractures Anaemia Hydrocephalus Cranial nerve defects Fatal infections	Severe	Poor
Intermediate	Autosomal recessive	Intermediate	None	Poor

be club-like with the appearance of a bone within bone, **endobone**. There may also be evidence of fractures or osteomyelitis. The entire skull is thickened and dense, especially at the base (Fig. 30.5). The neural foramina are small and the exiting nerves may be compressed.

Morphology

Bone biopsy is generally not indicated for the diagnosis because the radiological findings are diagnostic. Histopathological features highlight the failure of the osteoclasts to resorb the skeletal tissue. The bones show decreased or no marrow space because of the persistence of the primary spongiosa in the marrow cavity, beyond the growing phase (Fig. 30.6). Dense irregular bony trabeculae are seen because the deposited bone is not remodelled and the bone is often woven rather than lamellar. The number of osteoclasts varies according to the underlying defect.

Osteopetrosis was the first genetic bone disease treated with haematopoietic stem cell transplantation in which the normal osteoclasts produced from donor stem cells reverse many of the skeletal abnormalities.

METABOLIC DISORDERS OF BONE

Many of the metabolic disorders of bone are acquired and are much more common than genetic disorders of bone. The common disorders are discussed here.

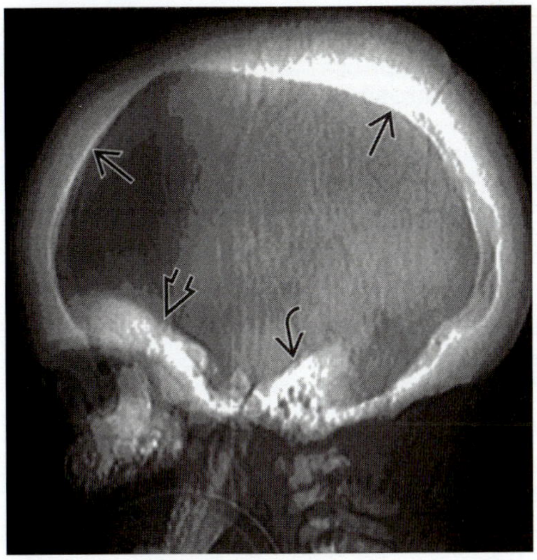

Fig. 30.5 Radiograph of skull in osteopetrosis. Lateral radiograph showing diffuse thickening of the calvarium (indicated by ↪), cranial base (indicated by ⇒) and temporal bone (indicated by →), characteristic of the more severe form of osteopetrosis (autosomal recessive). (*Source:* From Richard K. Gurgel and H. Ric Harnsberger. Skull Base Osteopetrosis. Imaging in Otolaryngology. Elsevier 2018.)

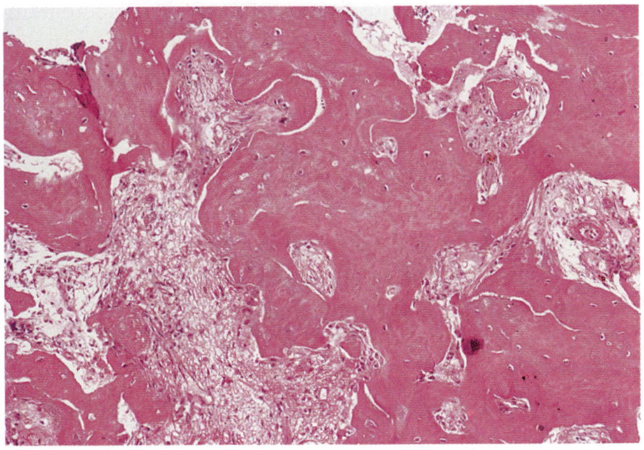

Fig. 30.6 Biopsy of bone in a child with osteopetrosis showing markedly reduced marrow space and numerous osteoclasts in some areas along the endosteal surface. (*Source:* From Daniel A. Arber. Bone Marrow. Rosai and Ackerman's Surgical Pathology. 11th edition. Elsevier 2018.)

OSTEOPENIA AND OSTEOPOROSIS

Decreased bone mass is referred to as **osteopenia**. The severe form of osteopenia that is associated with an increased risk of fractures is called **osteoporosis**. It is a systemic skeletal disease characterized by low bone mass and microarchitectural deterioration of bone tissue. There is a consequent increase in bone fragility leading to fractures. Osteoporosis is the most common metabolic bone disease of the adults globally and it does not become clinically apparent until a fracture occurs.

Aetiology

Bone mineral density (BMD) is an indicator of the bone mass and bone loss. Radiographically, osteopenia is defined as BMD about 1–2.5 standard deviation (SD) below the mean peak bone mass in young adults, whereas a further reduction of BMD below 2.5 SD is called osteoporosis. The disease may be localized to a certain bone or region, such as in disuse osteoporosis of a limb, or may be generalized with the involvement of the entire skeleton as a manifestation of a metabolic bone disease. Generalized osteoporosis may be primary or secondary to a variety of conditions.

The causes of osteoporosis are listed in Box 30.1.

Box 30.1 Causes of Osteoporosis

- **Primary**
  - Idiopathic
  - Postmenopausal
  - Senile
- **Secondary**

  Endocrine disorder
  - Hyperparathyroidism
  - Hyperthyroidism
  - Hypothyroidism
  - Pituitary tumours
  - Neoplasms
    - Multiple myeloma
    - Carcinomatosis
  - Type 1 diabetes
  - Addison disease

  Gastrointestinal
  - Vitamin deficiencies (vitamins C and D)
  - Malabsorption and malnutrition

  Drug induced
  - Alcohol
  - Anticonvulsants
  - Anticoagulants
  - Chemotherapy
  - Corticosteroids

  Others
  - Anaemia
  - Homocystinuria
  - Immobilization
  - Osteogenesis imperfecta
  - Pulmonary disease

Pathogenesis

Peak bone mass is achieved during young adulthood and, as shown in Flowchart 30.1, its extent is determined by hereditary factors, physical activity, diet, muscle strength, hormonal status, etc. After attaining maximal skeletal mass, bone resorption mildly exceeds bone formation, which is the basis for age-related bone loss. The condition averages 0.7% every year. Although both males and females are affected equally, osteoporosis is more commonly seen in elderly postmenopausal women and the process is more rapid in certain populations such as Caucasians.

Risk Factors

Advancing age and postmenopausal state are the two most important causes of osteoporosis. The risk factors

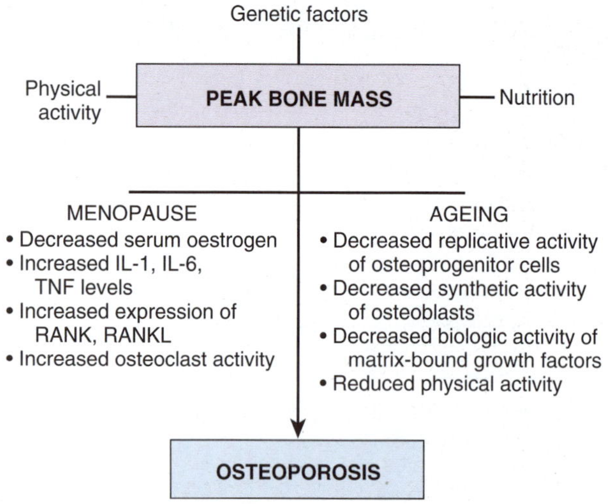

Flowchart 30.1 Pathophysiology of osteoporosis. (*Source:* From Andrew Horvai. Bones, Joints, and Soft Tissue Tumors. Robbins & Cotran Pathologic Basis of Disease. 10th edition. Elsevier 2021.

for osteoporosis are described as follows along with their mechanisms:

- **Ageing:** Osteoblasts in the elderly have a reduced proliferation capacity and biosynthetic potential, thereby reducing their ability to make new bones. This is called senile osteoporosis which is a low turnover variant.
- **Menopause:** Postmenopausal women lose up to 2% of cortical bone and 9% of cancellous bone every year. Oestrogen deficiency in the postmenopausal state is the most common cause of postmenopausal osteoporosis. Oestrogen deficiency leads to increased osteoclast activity and the osteoblasts cannot compensate for the loss.
- **Reduced physical activity:** Mechanical forces are important stimulants for bone remodelling evidenced by higher BMD in athletes. Zero gravity as in astronauts and immobilization reversibly lead to reduction in skeletal mass.
- **Genetic factors:** Variations in vitamin D receptor type account for 75% of variation in maximal peak bone mass. The genes that commonly influence bone mass include RANKL, OPG and RANK (which are key regulators of osteoclast).
- **Nutritional status:** Low calcium level is an important cause of osteoporosis.
- **Hormone deficiency:** Vitamin D deficiency and hyperparathyroidism are also implicated in the development of senile osteoporosis.
- **Other risk factors:** White people and Asians are at a higher risk when compared with Africans. Smoking and alcohol abuse are also implicated in the development of osteoporosis.

Clinical Features

- Although most patients remain asymptomatic for a long time, nonspecific complaints such as bone pain and weakness are quite common. Episode of acute pain may follow a fall or minor trauma. Vertebral fractures are common in thoracic and lumbar vertebrae and cause loss of height leading to 'dowager's hump' with significant deformity (lumbar lordosis and kyphoscoliosis).
- Fractures involving the femoral neck, pelvis or spine can get complicated with the development of pulmonary embolism and pneumonia, which may be fatal in many patients having comorbid conditions.

Table 30.3 Features of Postmenopausal and Senile Osteoporosis

Postmenopausal Osteoporosis (Type I)	Senile Osteoporosis (Type II)
Occurs in 50- to 65-year-old women	Occurs in men and women older than 70 years
Predominant increase in osteoclastic activity	Predominant decrease in osteoblastic activity
Characterized by an accelerated phase of hypo-oestrogenism-related bone loss	Represents bone loss associated with ageing
More significant trabecular bone loss	More significant cortical bone loss
The predominant fractures are vertebral bodies and distal forearm	The predominant fractures are hip, wrist, vertebral

Radiology

Evidence of osteoporosis is detected in radiography only after 30%–40% bone mass is lost. Features evident are flattening of vertebral bodies, and widening and swelling of intervertebral discs with fish mouth appearance. Thoracic and lumbar spines are commonly affected (Table 30.3).

Morphology

The key feature of osteoporosis is bone that is decreased in quantity but normal in histology (Figs 30.7 and 30.8). The entire skeleton is affected but the common sites affected are bones with a high surface area such as the cancellous compartment of the vertebral body. It often results in loss of height in the elderly and may cause microfractures or collapse of vertebrae. **In senile osteoporosis**, the cortex is thinned out by subperiosteal and endosteal resorption and trabecular plates lose their interconnection (Fig. 30.9). In severe cases, the Haversian systems are widened and enlarged, and the cortex mimics cancellous bone.

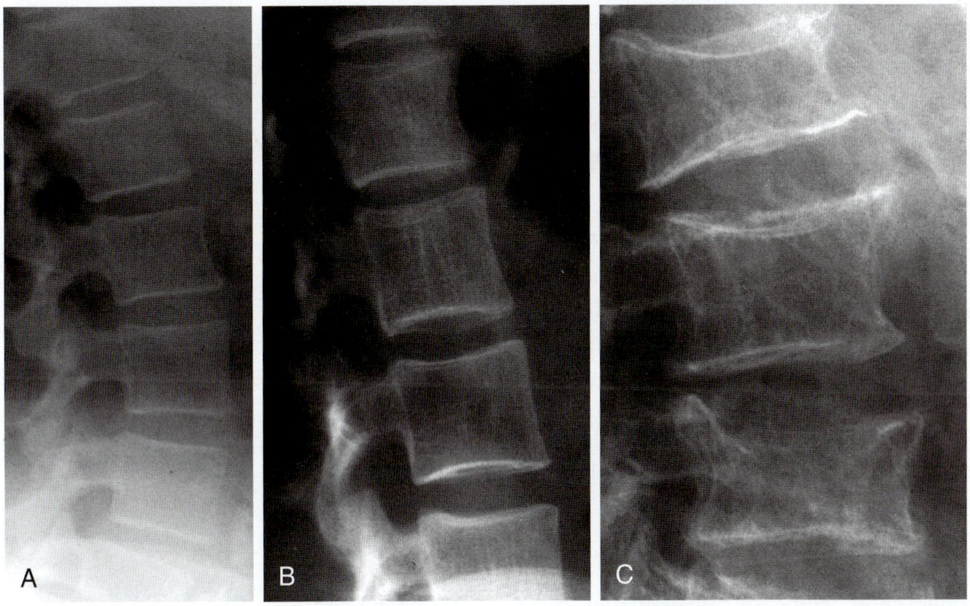

Fig. 30.7 Osteoporosis – radiograph. (A) Lateral lumbar spine radiograph showing normal vertebrae with crisp clear intact endplates. (B) The earliest feature of spinal osteoporosis is prominent vertical striations due to loss of secondary horizontal trabeculae. (C) Multiple vertebral fractures in the lumbar spine of varying types and grades. (*Source:* From Judith E. Adams. Osteoporosis. Musculoskeletal Imaging. 2nd edition. Saunders 2015.)

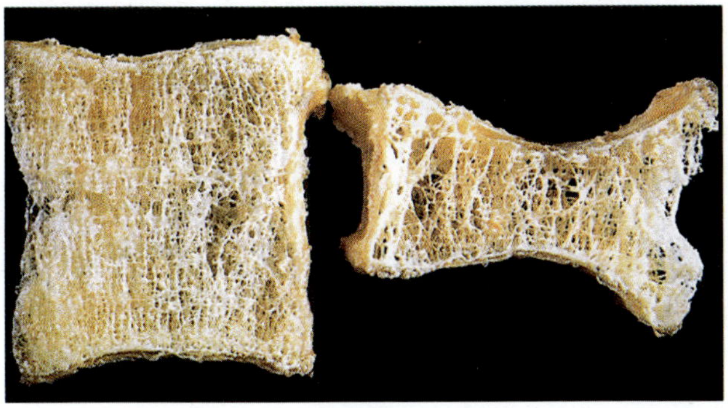

Fig. 30.8 Osteoporotic bone – gross appearance. Osteoporotic vertebral body (right) shortened by compression fractures compared with a normal vertebral body (left). Note that the osteoporotic vertebra has a characteristic loss of horizontal trabeculae and thickened vertical trabeculae. (*Source:* From Andrew Horvai. Bones, Joints, and Soft Tissue Tumors. Robbins & Cotran Pathologic Basis of Disease. 10th edition. Elsevier 2021.)

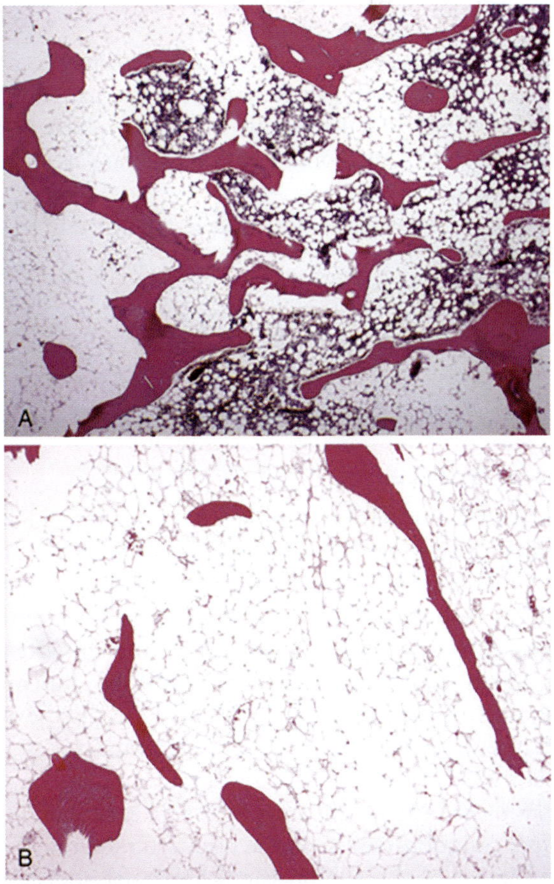

Fig. 30.9 Osteoporosis – microscopy. Scanning magnification of normal bone with broad, anastomosing trabeculae (A) and bone from a patient with osteoporosis (B) showing thin, separated and discontinuous trabeculae. (*Source:* From Andrew E. Horvai and Thomas Link. Osteoporosis. High-Yield Bone and Soft Tissue Pathology. Saunders 2012.)

Management

The investigation of choice to diagnose asymptomatic suspected cases of osteoporosis is specialized radiological imaging techniques that measure BMD, such as quantitative computed tomography and dual-energy X-ray absorptiometry. Serum calcium, phosphorus and alkaline phosphatase levels remain within normal limits.

Osteoporosis is a preventable cause of bone deformities and disabilities. Hence, attention should be focused on prevention of osteoporosis in high-risk patients with exercise, nutritive diet, vitamin D and calcium supplements and drugs such as bisphosphonates to supress osteoclastic activity. Postmenopausal osteoporosis is prevented to some extent by hormone replacement therapy that comes with its own set of complications.

PAGET DISEASE OF BONE (OSTEITIS DEFORMANS) PA 33.4

Paget disease, also referred to as osteitis deformans, is a disorder characterized by increased bone mass but the deposited bone is structurally defective. It is named after English surgeon Sir James Paget, who described it in 1877.

The disease commonly affects older people, and men are more often affected than women. In addition, the disease is most common in Caucasians and is rare in native populations of Scandinavia, China, Japan and Africa. It is the second most common bone disorder in elderly individuals, after osteoporosis.

Pathogenesis

The affected bones show signs of dysregulated bone remodelling at the microscopic level with excess osteoclastic activity followed by a compensatory increase in osteoblastic activity, leading to the formation of disorganized bone. These structural changes cause the bones to weaken resulting in deformities, pain, fracture and arthritis of the associated joints.

The exact cause of the disease is not known and many theories indicate both genetic and acquired causes. Two genes, SQSTM1 and RANK which are involved in the regulation and activation of osteoclasts, are associated with this disease.

Pathogenesis of Paget can be described in four stages (Fig. 13.10):

1. Osteoclastic activity
2. Mixed osteoclastic and osteoblastic activity
3. Osteoblastic activity
4. Malignant degeneration

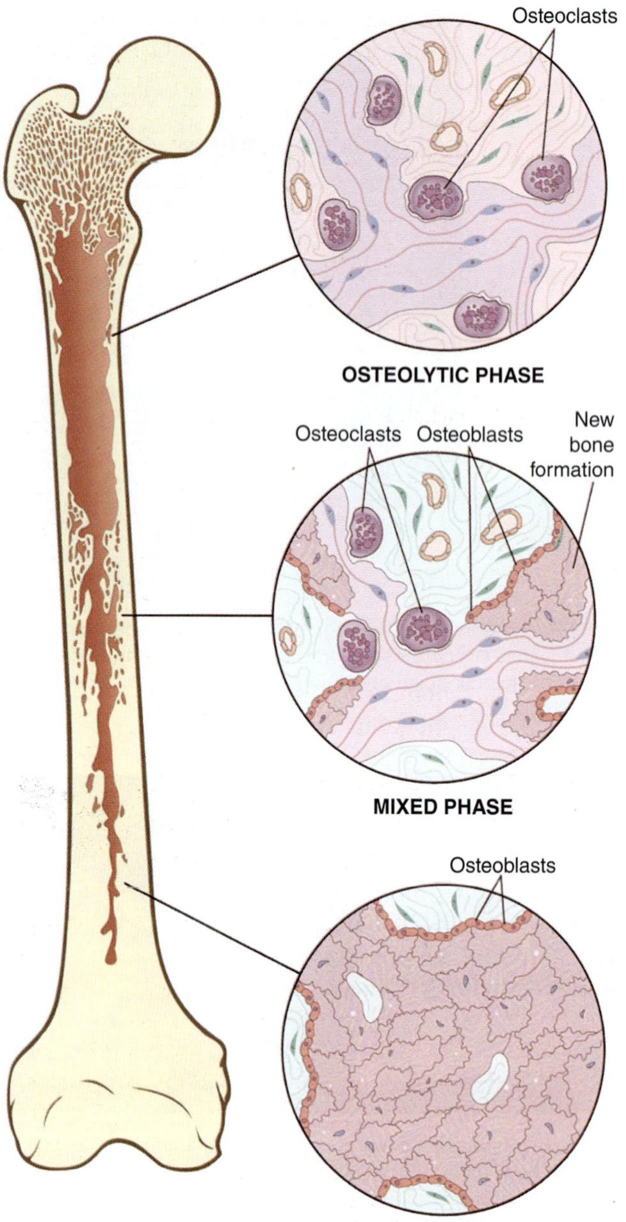

Fig. 30.10 Phases of Paget disease. (*Source:* From Andrew E. Horvai and Thomas Link. Osteoporosis. High-Yield Bone and Soft Tissue Pathology. Saunders 2012.)

Clinical Features

- Patients are usually asymptomatic and identified incidentally. They are often in their late adulthood. Incidence increases with increasing age. Paget disease may affect one bone (monostotic) or multiple bones (polyostotic) with the pelvis, tibia, femur, lumbar vertebrae and skull being most commonly affected, but never involves the entire skeleton. Monostotic disease may involve the pelvis, femur, skull or vertebrae.
- Clinical symptoms are highly variable and are dependent on the extent and stage of the disease. Pain is the most common symptom due to microfractures or due to the new bone compressing the spinal and cranial nerve roots.
- In some patients, there may be enlargement of the craniofacial skeleton that may produce **leontiasis ossea** (lion face) and the cranium may be so heavy that it is difficult for the person to hold the head erect. There may be invagination of the skull base (**platybasia**) and compression of the posterior fossa. Weight bearing leads to anterior bowing of the femurs and tibiae and distortion the femoral heads, resulting in the development of severe secondary osteoarthritis (OA).
- **Chalk stick–type fractures** are common in the weakened bones and usually involve the long bones of the lower extremities. Vertebral compression fractures may lead to spinal cord injury and kyphosis. Rarely, the bones with hypervascularity in severe polyostotic disease can act as an arteriovenous shunt, leading to high-output heart failure or exacerbation of underlying cardiac disease.

- Tumours and tumour-like conditions associated with Paget disease are giant cell tumour, giant cell reparative granuloma, extraosseous masses of haematopoietic tissue and, very rarely, sarcomas.
- The most feared complication of Paget disease is sarcoma (usually an osteosarcoma or fibrosarcoma), which is very rare and occurs in less than 1% of all individuals with Paget disease, and in 5%–10% of those with severe polyostotic disease.

Morphology

There are remarkable variations in the morphology of the affected bones on the basis of the phase in which the bone is examined.

1. The initial **phase of osteoclastic activity** is characterized by an increase in osteoclasts with numerous numbers of resorption pits. The osteoclasts are large with many nuclei (10–12 nuclei), at times even 100 nuclei. These localized areas of pathological destruction of bone tissue are seen radiologically as an advancing lytic wedge in the long bones or skull. In the skull, it is called osteoporosis circumscripta.
2. This phase is soon followed by a **phase of mixed osteoclastic and osteoblastic activity** in which there is an imbalance between osteoblast bone formation and osteoclast resorption. This results in accelerated deposition of newly formed bone that may be woven or lamellar, but eventually it is entirely remodelled into lamellar bone.
3. **Osteosclerotic stage** due to osteoblastic activity is characterized by excessive bone formation that makes the bone compact and dense leading to osteosclerosis. The intense cellular activity produces a chaotic picture of trabecular bone – 'mosaic pattern' – rather than the normal linear lamellar pattern. The mosaic pattern of the lamellar bone, seen in the sclerotic phase, is the hallmark of this disease (Fig. 30.11).
4. In the phase of **malignant degeneration**, the resorbed bone is replaced and the marrow spaces are filled with excess of connective tissue along with increase in vascularity causing the bones to become hypervascular. The bone at this phase is dense and is referred to as 'Pagetic bone'. The newly formed bone is vulnerable to fractures and this stage produces characteristic cotton wool appearance of the bone involved.

Management

Paget disease is diagnosed with its characteristic appearance on X-rays and skeletal survey is indicated in many cases. An elevated level of alkaline phosphatase along with normal levels of serum calcium, phosphate and

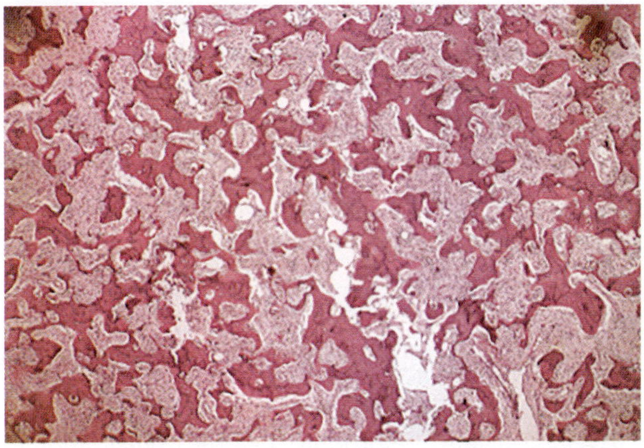

Fig. 30.11 Mosaic pattern of Paget disease – microscopy. (*Source:* From Bruce M. Wenig. Neoplasms of the Thyroid Gland. Atlas of Head and Neck Pathology. 3rd edition. Elsevier 2016.)

aminotransferase in an elderly patient with appropriate clinical and radiological features is highly indicative of the disease. Levels of serum and urine hydroxyproline are also elevated in most patients.

The disease is progressive and slowly worsens with time. There is no specific treatment available for Paget disease and the goal of treatment is to relieve bone pain and prevent the progression of the disease. Bisphosphonates are currently available for the management of Paget disease. Surgery may be required for treatment of fractures and correction of deformities. The patients often need to be under long-term follow-up.

OSTEOMALACIA AND RICKETS

Osteomalacia and rickets are due to defective mineralization of bone matrix. It is different from osteoporosis in which bone mineralization is unaffected but the bone mass is reduced. The disease manifests in the developing skeleton by a set of unique features, a condition known as rickets.

- **Rickets:** It is a disorder in children in which vitamin D deficiency interferes with deposition of bone in the growth plate.
- **Osteomalacia:** Bone formed during remodelling is undermineralized, resulting in weak bones.

Both conditions are due to deficiency of vitamin D or due to its abnormal metabolism and are characterized by weak bones that are prone to fractures.

The diseases are discussed in detail in Chapter 9.

HYPERPARATHYROIDISM

Bone resorption is the key feature of hyperthyroidism and the disease is discussed in detail in Chapter 28. The effects of parathyroid hormone relevant to bone lesions are discussed here.

In hyperparathyroidism, due to oversecretion of parathyroid hormone (PTH), there is an increase in the activity of osteoclasts that leads to bone resorption, which ultimately results in fractures, bony deformities and joint problems.

The effects of PTH are as follows:

- Excess synthesis of active form of vitamin D, $1,25(OH)_2D$, by the kidneys increases release of calcium from bone.
- Osteoclast activation: Elevated levels of PTH cause increased RANKL expression on osteoblasts directly and by the action of activated vitamin D. RANKL stimulates RANK on the osteoclasts activating them.
- Excess calcium resorption by the renal tubules occurs.
- Excess phosphate excretion in the urine occurs.

The net effect of all these events is accelerated bone resorption with the consequent increase in serum calcium levels and weakening of bones. With time, loss of bone mass increases susceptibility to fractures, bone deformation and joint problems.

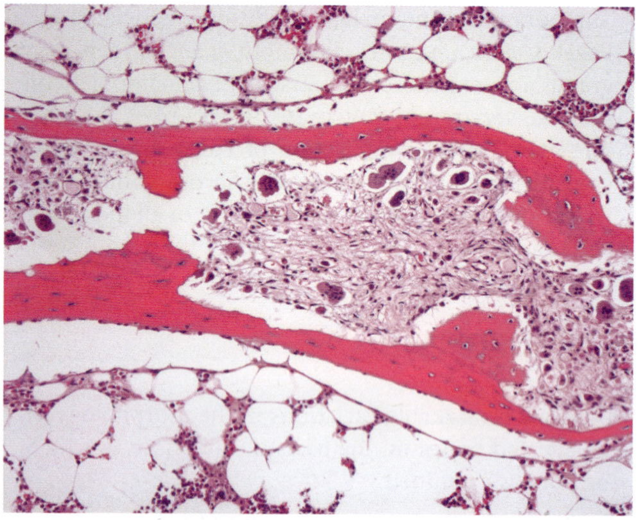

Fig. 30.12 Dissecting osteitis of hyperparathyroidism – osteoclasts boring into the centre of the trabeculum. (*Source:* From Andrew Horvai. Bones, Joints, and Soft Tissue Tumors. Robbins & Cotran Pathologic Basis of Disease. 10th edition. Elsevier 2021.)

Morphology

There are three major changes in the skeletal system if the hyperparathyroidism is symptomatic and untreated – **osteoporosis, brown tumours and osteitis fibrosa cystica**.

- **Osteoporosis:** The osteoporosis in this condition is generalized but is most severe in the phalanges, vertebrae and proximal femur. The increased osteoclast activity affects the cortical bone more than the medullary bone. The osteoclasts tunnel into and dissect the centre of the trabeculum of the cortical bone giving the appearance of a railroad track and this is called dissecting osteitis (Fig. 30.12). The marrow spaces are replaced by fibrosis. Because of decrease in density, the affected bones are more prone to microfractures and haemorrhages.
- **Brown tumour:** The healing process of the above-mentioned fractures and haemorrhages leads to an influx of macrophages and an ingrowth of reparative fibrous tissue leading to the formation of a reactive tissue called **brown tumour**. The lesion is so named because of its colour, which, in turn, is due to the vascularity, haemorrhage and haemosiderin deposition. Brown tumours commonly undergo cystic degeneration.
- **Generalized osteitis fibrosa cystica: Also called** von Recklinghausen disease of bone, it is the term used to denote the combination of increased osteoclastic activity, perivascular fibrosis and cystic brown tumours.

Management

Laboratory tests for primary hyperparathyroidism reveal increase in PTH, hypercalcaemia, hypophosphataemia and hypercalciuria.

Fortunately, osteitis fibrosa cystica is not common nowadays because of early diagnosis of hyperparathyroidism in routine blood investigations and effective control of the disease. Secondary hyperparathyroidism is also associated with similar skeletal changes; the skeletal changes tend to be subtle because the process is generally less severe than primary hyperparathyroidism. In all forms of hyperparathyroidism, control of hyperparathyroidism helps the bone changes to regress or disappear completely.

RENAL OSTEODYSTROPHY

Renal osteodystrophy is a systemic disorder that is usually diagnosed after treatment for end-stage renal disease begins. It represents a constellation of bone abnormalities such as **osteopenia, osteoporosis, hyperparathyroidism and growth retardation**, which occur in patients with chronic renal failure including the changes induced by long-term dialysis. Such changes are more prevalent in the present timeline because of the increase in the incidence of renal failure and the prolongation of survival of such patients with the advancement in the field of medicine. Renal osteodystrophy has been shown to be associated with three types of presentation:

- High-turnover osteodystrophy with increased osteoclastic and osteoblastic activities, with the former predominating
- Low turnover or aplastic with little osteoclastic and osteoblastic activities

- Mixed pattern disease showing a combination of both in different regions

Both high- and low-turnover diseases are associated with an increased risk of skeletal fractures, reduced quality of life and poor clinical outcomes.

Pathogenesis

Renal osteodystrophy has been classically described to be the result of the following mechanisms (Fig. 30.13):

- Hyperparathyroidism secondary to hyperphosphataemia combined
- Hypocalcaemia
  (Both the above-mentioned mechanisms are because of reduced excretion of phosphate by the damaged kidneys.)
- Tubular dysfunction in the kidneys that leads to renal tubular acidosis, which dissolves the hydroxyapatite, resulting in matrix demineralization and osteomalacia
- Reduced renal vitamin D hydroxylation that causes decreased active form of vitamin D, 1,25$(OH)_2$-vitamin D_3, which leads to hypocalcaemia
- Deficiency of BMP-7, which is normally produced by renal tubular cells and is required for osteoblast differentiation and proliferation (this leads to bone weakening)
- Deficiency of FGF-23, which is normally produced by osteocytes, and acts on the kidneys to regulate Klotho-dependent renal phosphate homeostasis and vitamin D hydroxylation (deficiency leads to hyperphosphataemia and hypocalcaemia)

Apart from these mechanisms, dialysis-related metabolic bone disease is due to the use of aluminium-containing dialysate that interferes with calcium deposition on bones causing osteomalacia, secondary hyperparathyroidism and osteitis fibrosa cystica.

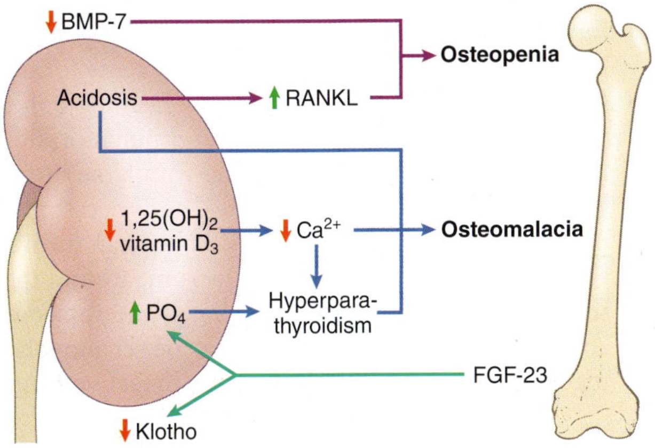

Fig. 30.13 Pathogenesis of renal osteodystrophy. (*Source:* From Andrew Horvai. Bones, Joints, and Soft Tissue Tumors. Robbins & Cotran Pathologic Basis of Disease. 10th edition. Elsevier 2021.)

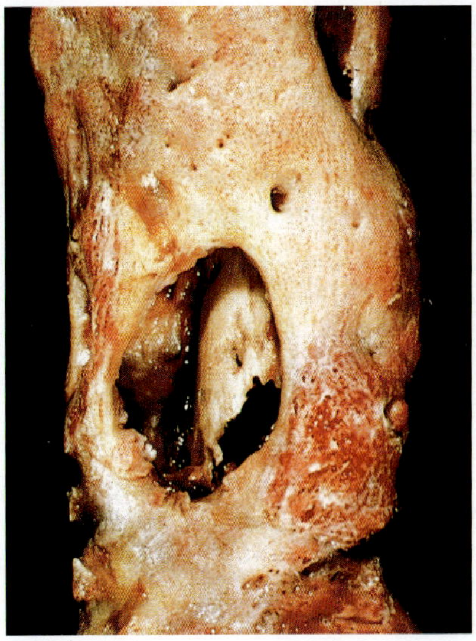

Fig. 30.14 Osteomyelitis – femur. (*Source:* From Osteomyelitis in Adults. Elsevier Point of Care. 2021.)

OSTEOMYELITIS PA 33.1

Osteomyelitis is the inflammation of the bone and bone marrow caused by an infecting organism (Fig. 30.14). The disease commonly manifests as a primary disease of bone, but can also be seen as a complication of any systemic infection.

PATHOGENIES

Osteomyelitis can be caused by bacteria, viruses, parasites and fungi but certain pyogenic bacteria and mycobacteria are the most commonly associated. Although bone is resistant to bacterial colonization, it can get infected in many ways. The organisms may reach the bone through blood or by events such as surgery or trauma, and the process is worsened by the presence of foreign bodies or prostheses that disrupt the integrity of bone. Hence, the major causes of osteomyelitis are classified into two:

- **Primary:** Haematogenous
- **Secondary:** Secondary to trauma, surgery, foreign body, prosthesis or sepsis

Around 20% of adult cases of osteomyelitis are haematogenous, which for unknown reasons are common in males. The overall incidence of osteomyelitis is higher in developing countries because of their poor sanitation and hygiene.

The following are the important factors in the pathogenesis of osteomyelitis:

- Virulence of the infecting organisms
- Underlying illness
- Immune status of the host
- Type, location and vascularity of the bone

Osteomyelitis may be acute or most commonly chronic. Acute osteomyelitis is a surgical and medical emergency that requires immediate antibiotic therapy, surgical drainage and secondary procedure as required. Chronic osteomyelitis is prolonged in its course and can be extremely debilitating with recurrent acute episodes and quiescent periods.

Pyogenic osteomyelitis and mycobacterial osteomyelitis are discussed in detail here.

PYOGENIC (BACTERIAL) OSTEOMYELITIS

Pyogenic osteomyelitis is almost always bacterial in origin and the organisms can reach the bone by blood or direct implantation or by extension from a contiguous site.

Pathogenesis

Almost 50% of the cases are due to unknown bacteria, and *Staphylococcus aureus* is the cause in 80% of cases with known organisms. *S. aureus* expresses receptors to bone matrix components, as collagen, which facilitates its adherence to bone. Sickle cell patients may be infected by *Salmonella* species more commonly than general population. Posttraumatic cases are commonly infected by *Pseudomonas* and mixed bacteria. Other organisms include *E. coli*, *Klebsiella*, *Haemophilus influenzae*, etc.

Common sites affected are areas of rapid growth in children, and distal and proximal femur, proximal tibia, humerus and distal radius, which are at an increased risk of trauma. The vertebral column is also a common site for osteomyelitis in adults. The location of infection in the bones is influenced by the osseous blood circulation, which is different for different age groups:

- In neonates: Metaphysis and epiphysis
- In older children: Metaphysis
- In adults: Epiphyses and subchondral regions

In children, the initiating bacteraemia is caused by simple mucosal injuries or from minor skin infections. In adults, it is often a complication of open fractures, surgical procedures and infection of foot ulcers in immunocompromised and diabetic patients.

Osteomyelitis affecting infants is dangerous because the epiphyseal infection can spread to the adjacent joint that may be affected badly by the development of suppurative arthritis, articular cartilage destruction and permanent disability.

Clinical Features

The common presentation is in the form of a nonspecific systemic illness with fever with chills, tiredness and throbbing pain over the involved bone. Occasionally, adults may present with only localized pain. Blood count tests may indicate pyogenic infection by neutrophilic leucocytosis. X-ray shows a lytic focus surrounded by sclerosis representing dead bone surrounded by reactive new bone. Identification of pathogen is by bone and tissue biopsy. Treatment is with surgical curettage under antibiotic cover.

Radiology

X-ray examination of the suspicious limb may show displacement of deep muscle planes in the early stages, which may be confirmed by comparison with X-ray of the opposite limb. Apart from the soft-tissue changes, the development of lytic changes in the bone may take up to 2–3 weeks. Hence, MRI is a more sensitive imaging modality for the diagnosis. Subperiosteal abscess and collection of purulent debris within the bone marrow may be identified by MRI, and osteomyelitis can be easily differentiated from soft-tissue lesions.

Morphology

Osteomyelitis is designated as acute, subacute or chronic, on the basis of the clinical duration of the disease.

- **Acute osteomyelitis** presents with acute inflammatory cells, vascular congestion, oedema, small-vessel thrombosis and bone necrosis. Necrotic bone on bone biopsy appears whiter than living bone because of the loss of blood supply, and in microscopy shows extensive resorption and inflammatory exudates. Spread of infection to the cortex lifts the periosteum from the cortex, especially in children, in whom it is loosely attached. This may lead to the formation of subperiosteal abscess, compromising subperiosteal blood supply. This disruption in medullary and periosteal blood supply causes extension of the necrotic process producing large areas of dead bone (Fig. 30.15). The subperiosteal abscess may rupture on the surface, forming discharging sinuses. The dead bone, known as sequestrum, may crumble, releasing fragments through the sinus tract.
- **Subacute osteomyelitis** differs from acute form in the type of inflammatory infiltrate. It shows more lymphocytes and plasma cells than the acute form.
- **Chronic osteomyelitis** lesions show necrotic bone, formation of reactive new bone and polymorphonuclear leucocyte exudation along with large numbers of lymphocytes, histiocytes and occasional plasma cells. The newly developed bone can form a shell of living tissue, called involucrum, around the segment of the infected bone. Small intraosseous abscesses called Brodie abscess may be seen involving the cortex surrounded by sclerotic reactive bone.

Failure of treatment may occur in 5%–25% of cases, especially in cases with delayed diagnosis, inadequate treatment, extensive necrosis of bone or immunosuppression.

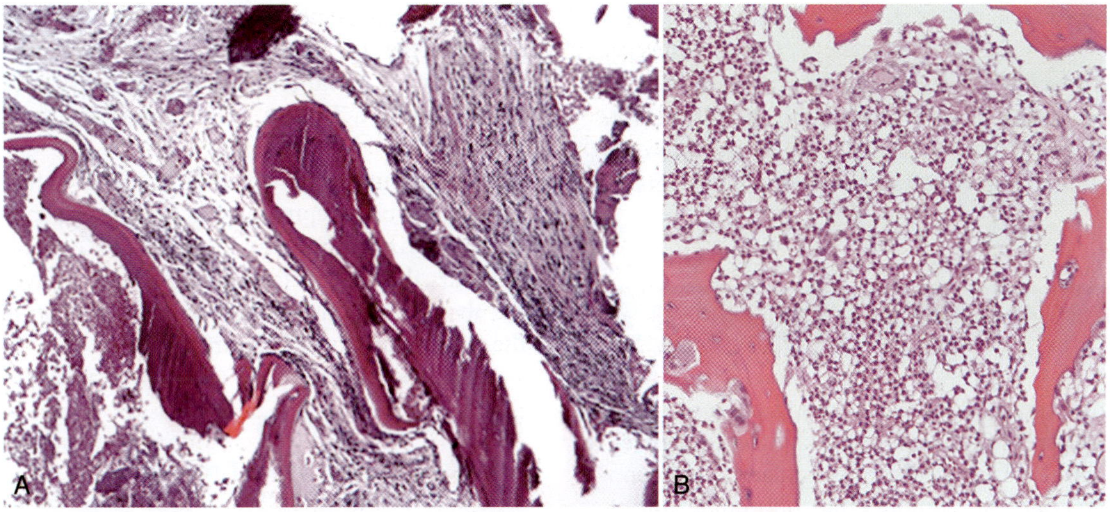

Fig. 30.15 Osteomyelitis – microscopy showing bone and fibrous tissue with inflamed marrow (A) and neutrophilic microabscess (B) that is uninterrupted sheet of neutrophils filling at least one intertrabecular space. (*Source:* From Meenakshi Bindal and Brian Krabak. Acute Bacterial Sacroiliitis in an Adult: A Case Report and Review of the Literature. Archives of Physical Medicine and Rehabilitation. 2007;88: 1357–1359.)

Such cases develop chronic osteomyelitis whose complications include pathological fracture, secondary amyloidosis, endocarditis and sepsis.

MYCOBACTERIAL OSTEOMYELITIS

About 1%–3% of patients with tuberculosis have bone infection, usually from focus of acute visceral disease, direct extension or lymphatics. Advanced cases are associated with cutaneous sinuses, which cause secondary bacterial infections. The common sites are the vertebrae, hip, knee, ankle, elbow and wrist and involve synovium, epiphysis or metaphysis.

Morphology

Caseous necrosis and granuloma with central necrosis, epithelioid cells and giant cells of Langhans type are characteristic, similar to other sites. Tuberculosis spondylitis (Pott disease) commonly involves the spine, causing destruction of the discs and vertebrae resulting in permanent compression fractures (Fig. 30.16). It produces scoliosis or kyphosis and neurological deficits because of spinal cord and nerve root compression.

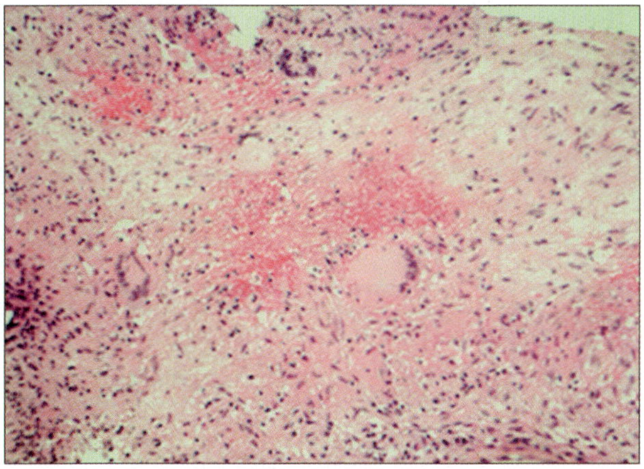

Fig. 30.16 Tuberculous osteomyelitis – microscopy showing necrotizing granulomatous inflammatory infiltrate. (*Source:* From Dan Lebowitz, Line Wolter, Christiane Zenklusen, Amine Chouiter and Raffaele Malinverni. TB Determined: Tuberculous Osteomyelitis. The American Journal of Medicine. 2014;127:198-201.)

SKELETAL SYPHILIS

Treponema pallidum and *Treponema pertenue* rarely involve bones because the infection caused by these is diagnosed and treated before bone involvement occurs. In congenital syphilis, bone involvement starts from the fifth month of gestation and is fully developed at birth, whereas patients with acquired syphilis produce bone lesions in the tertiary stage (2–5 years) after exposure of the organism.

Morphology

The spirochaetes localize in the areas of active enchondral ossification (osteochondritis) and the periosteum (periostitis) and produce massive reactive periosteal bone deposition on the medial and anterior surfaces of the tibia called saber shin. In acquired syphilis, the bone is involved in the tertiary stage (after 2–5 years of the initial infection), and the commonly involved bones include the nasal bone, palate, skull and long tubular bones such as tibia.

Microscopy

Syphilis involving bone is characterized by oedematous granulation tissue with plasma cells and necrotic bone. Silver histochemical stain can be used to demonstrate the spirochaetes within the inflammatory tissue.

TUMOURS AND TUMOUR-LIKE LESIONS PA 33.2

Bone tumours are a very challenging diagnosis for the treating surgeons because of the disfiguring surgeries required for their management. Secondary bone deposits and haematopoietic tumours far outnumber primary bone neoplasms. However, these tumours are a significant number that affect the survival and quality of life of the population. The most common primary bone malignancies are osteosarcoma, chondrosarcoma and Ewing sarcoma.

Benign tumours are often an incidental diagnosis but sometimes cause pain. Malignant tumours are mostly diagnosed in advanced stages. The presenting age and the location of the tumour along with the radiographic findings help to identify the type of tumour. But a biopsy is required for the definitive diagnosis.

The tumours are classified on the basis of the lineage of cell that has been represented in the tumour or on the basis of the matrix produced by the neoplastic cells (Table 30.4). Tumours that do not fall into any category on the basis of the above-mentioned criteria are classified on the basis of the clinicopathological features.

TUMOUR-LIKE LESIONS

Fibrous Cortical Defect and Nonossifying Fibroma

Fibrous cortical defect and nonossifying fibroma

Also called metaphyseal fibrous defect, fibrous cortical defect is a benign abnormality common in children younger than 2 years. It involves the metaphysis of the distal femur and proximal tibia. Often less than 0.5 cm, it can also be more than 5 cm in size and it is described by the term nonossifying fibroma. Though

Table 30.4 Classification of Bone Tumours

Origin	Nature	Tumour	Age (Years)	Bones More Commonly Affected (in Order of Frequency)	Usual Location Within Long Bone
Bone forming	Benign	Osteoma	40–50	Skull, facial bone	–
		Osteoid osteoma	10–30	Femur, tibia, humerus	Metaphysis
		Osteoblastoma	10–30	Vertebrae, tibia, femur	Metaphysis
	Malignant	Osteosarcoma	10–25	Femur, tibia, humerus	Metaphysis
Cartilage forming	Benign	Chondroma	10–40	Hands and feet, ribs, femur	Diaphysis
		Osteochondroma	10–30	Femur, tibia, humerus	Metaphysis
		Chondroblastoma	10–25	Femur, tibia, humerus	Epiphysis
		Chondromyxoid fibroma	10–25	Tibia, femur, feet	Metaphysis
	Malignant	Chondrosarcoma	30–60	Pelvis, ribs, femur	Diaphysis (central), metaphysis (peripheral)
Unknown aetiology	Benign	Giant cell tumour	20–40	Femur, tibia, radius	Epiphysis, metaphysis
		Aneurysmal bone cyst	10–20	Vertebrae, flat bones, femur	Metaphysis
	Malignant	Ewing sarcoma/PNET	5–20	Femur, pelvis, tibia	Diaphysis, metaphysis
Notochordal	Malignant	Chordoma	40–60	Sacrococcygeal, spheno-occipital, cervical vertebrae	–
Hematopoietic	Malignant	Plasma cell myeloma	40–60	Vertebrae, pelvis, ribs	Diaphysis, metaphysis, epiphysis
		Malignant lymphoma, large cell and mixed cell types	30–60	Femur, pelvis, vertebrae	Diaphysis, metaphysis
Histiocytic	Benign	Langerhans cell histiocytosis	5–15	Skull, jaw, humerus	Metaphysis, diaphysis

differing by size, histologically both the lesions are identical.

X-ray

Sharply demarcated radiolucency surrounded by thin zone of sclerosis

Morphology

The lesions are grey to yellow-brown, granular and well circumscribed, which on histology show storiform pattern of arrangement of fibroblasts along with macrophages and multinucleated giant cells. Haemosiderin is usually present.

Fibrous dysplasia

Fibrous dysplasia is a benign fibro-osseous lesion that may involve one (monostotic) or multiple (polyostotic) bones affecting mostly children and young adults. It is a developmental disorder of bone resulting in the failure to form mature lamellar bone. It consists of mass forming developmental defect composed of woven bone and fibroblast-like spindle cells. Chromosomal abnormality arises because of somatic gain-of-function mutation during development in GNAS1, which leads to elevated intracellular cyclic adenosine monophosphate (cAMP) that interrupts the normal osteoblast differentiation from precursors, and it has been described in many patients.

Monostotic forms are common than polyostotic. Monostotic form is seen in the femur, tibia, ribs, jawbones, humerus and calvarium.

X-ray shows ground-glass appearance and well-defined margination (Fig. 30.17).

Polyostotic form involves multiple bones and it frequently affects the lower extremities and pelvis. It involves the femur, skull, tibia, humerus, ribs, fibula, radius, ulna, mandible and vertebrae. It is associated with spontaneous fractures and skeletal deformities. A rare complication is malignant transformation into sarcoma.

Mazabraud syndrome: There occurs fibrous dysplasias with soft-tissue myxomas

McCune–Albright syndrome: Polyostotic disease with café-au-lait skin pigmentations and endocrine abnormalities. It is characterized by polyostotic bone lesions, skin pigmentations and precocious puberty.

Morphology

Gross: The lesions are well circumscribed, intramedullary in origin, varying in size, tan white and gritty. Areas of cyst formation or haemorrhage may be identified.

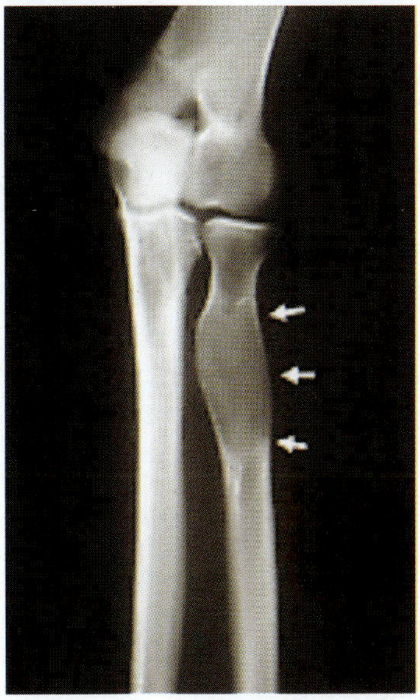

Fig. 30.17 Fibrous dysplasia – anteroposterior radiograph of the forearm reveals a well-circumscribed intramedullary lesion within the proximal radius with the so-called ground-glass appearance (white arrows). (*Source:* From Fibrous Dysplasia and McCune-Albright Syndrome. Elsevier Point of Care. 2021.)

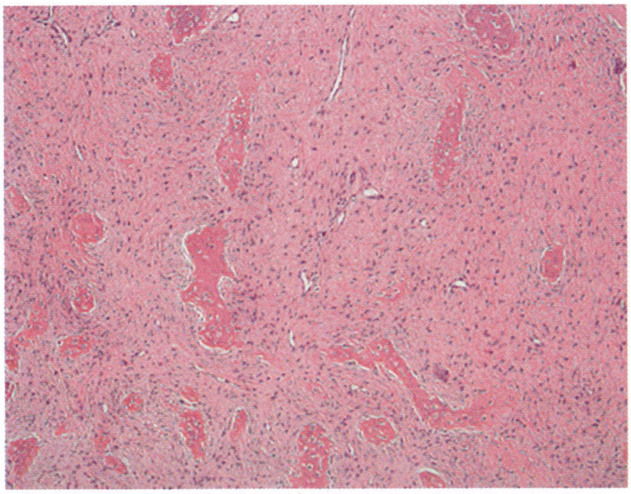

Fig. 30.18 Biopsy of fibrous dysplasia lesion showing irregularly shaped woven bone spicules surrounded by fibrous stroma. The surfaces of the trabeculae are devoid of osteoblasts. (*Source:* From John D. Reith. Bone and Joints. Rosai and Ackerman's Surgical Pathology. 11th edition. Elsevier 2018.)

Microscopy: Tumour is composed of branching and anastomosing irregular trabeculae of woven bone surrounded by benign-looking fibroblasts (Fig. 30.18). These spicules of woven bones in curvilinear shapes resemble Chinese letters likened as 'Chinese letter pattern'.

Secondary aneurysmal bone cyst (ABC)–like changes may also be seen.

BONE-FORMING TUMOURS

Tumours that form unmineralized osteoid or mineralized woven bone fall under this category. They may be benign or malignant. The benign tumours include osteoma, osteoid osteoma and osteoblastoma, whereas osteosarcoma is the malignant counterpart.

Osteoma

Osteoma is a benign bone-forming tumour composed of compact or mature trabecular bone, limited almost exclusively to flat bone of the skull and face, especially the nose and paranasal sinuses.

Morphology

Gross: The tumour is sessile, polypoid in shape with bosselated smooth surface.
Microscopy shows dense compact trabecular bone. The outer surface is sharply demarcated and lined by respiratory epithelium in nasal and sinus tumours.

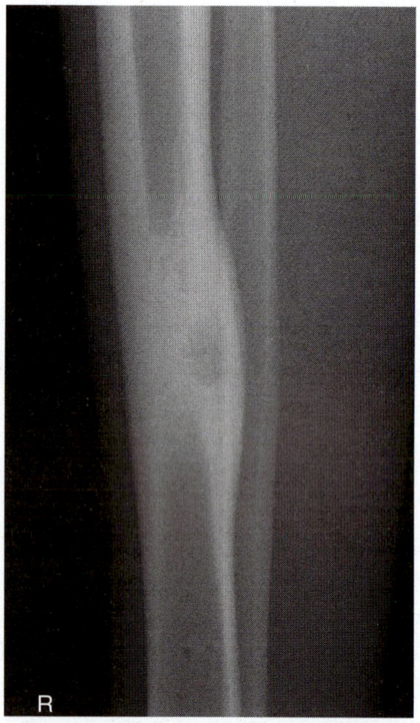

Fig. 30.19 Osteoid osteoma of tibia – radiology showing a radiolucent central nidus surrounded by dense, reactive bone. (*Source:* From John D. Reith. Bone and Joints. Rosai and Ackerman's Surgical Pathology. 11th edition. Elsevier 2018.)

Osteoid Osteoma

Osteoid osteomas are small, benign, bone-forming tumours associated with pain and limited growth potential. They are commonly seen in young individuals (younger than 20 years) in the appendicular skeleton, especially in long bones such as the femur and tibia (50%). Pain occurs because of production of prostaglandin E_2 in the reactive zone. Clinically, patients present with intense localized pain, nocturnal in nature relieved by nonsteroidal anti-inflammatory drug (NSAIDs) or aspirin. Radiographically, a central nidus surrounded by sclerotic bone is seen (Fig. 30.19).

Morphology

The tumours are well circumscribed, round-to-oval mass, haemorrhagic and gritty tan with size less than 2 cm. Microscopy of the tumour shows a circumscribed neoplasm with a central nidus composed of randomly interconnecting trabeculae of woven bone that are rimmed by single layer of osteoblasts (Fig. 30.20). The stroma surrounding the tumour bone consists of loose connective tissue with many dilated and congested capillaries.

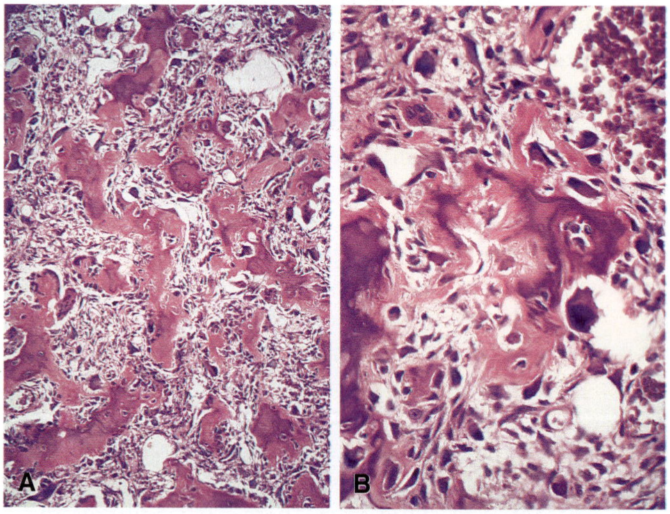

Fig. 30.20 Osteoid osteoma – microscopy showing (A) woven bone surrounded by plump osteoblasts. (B) The stroma is cellular and well vascularized. (*Source:* From John D. Reith. Bone and Joints. Rosai and Ackerman's Surgical Pathology. 11th edition. Elsevier 2018.)

Osteoblastoma

Osteoblastoma is a benign bone-forming tumour composed of anastomosing trabeculae of osteoid and woven bone lined by osteoblasts. It is also known as giant osteoid osteoma because of the histological similarity. The only feature that morphologically differentiates the two lesions is the size. Affected patients complain of nocturnal pain that is less likely relieved by NSAIDs, unlike in osteoid osteoma.

Wide skeletal distribution frequently arises within the posterior elements of the vertebral column and long tubular bones. When the tumour involves the spine, patients may present with neurological symptoms due to spinal cord or nerve root compression.

Morphology

Grossly, the tumour is larger than 2 cm, involving the metaphysis. A curetted tumour appears as gritty haemorrhagic mass, whereas intact tumours are well demarcated with scalloped edges. Microscopy of the lesion shows anastomosing trabeculae of osteoid with woven bone rimmed by a layer of benign activated osteoblasts surrounded by numerous osteoclasts (Fig. 30.21). The stroma contains dilated capillaries and areas of large, dilated, blood-filled sinusoids. Loose connective tissue may be seen between intertrabecular spaces. Rarely, the tumours may show cartilaginous matrix and degenerative atypia. Mitotic rate is minimal.

Osteosarcoma

Osteosarcoma is the most common malignant high-grade bone tumour in which the tumour cells produce osteoid (bone). It most commonly presents in young individuals younger than 20 years – but about 25% of them may present in older age, making the presentation bimodal. Men may show a slightly increased tendency than women. The risk factors that predispose to this tumour in adults include radiation exposure, Paget disease and bone infarcts. The most common location is in the metaphysis of long bones, especially around the knee joint with the involvement of the lower end of the femur or upper end of the tibia or proximal humerus.

Pathogenesis As noted earlier, these tumours are often seen in adolescents near the growth plate of long bones. This can be explained by the fact that this is a common location for increased cell proliferation during the pubertal growth spurt of individuals. Rapid proliferation of cells forms a fertile ground for new mutations that predispose to malignant transformation. About 70% of osteosarcomas are associated with mutations of tumour suppressor genes. The common mutations include:

- Mutation in RB gene is present in 70% of sporadic cases (a patient with hereditary retinoblastoma has a high risk of developing osteosarcoma).
- p53 mutations may also be associated with osteosarcoma as evident in its increased incidence in patients with Li–Fraumeni syndrome.
- MDM2 and CDK4 are overexpressed in many low-grade osteosarcomas.
- INK4A is inactivated in many osteosarcomas, which encodes tumour suppressor gene p14 and p16.
- FGFR1 gene amplification may also be present.

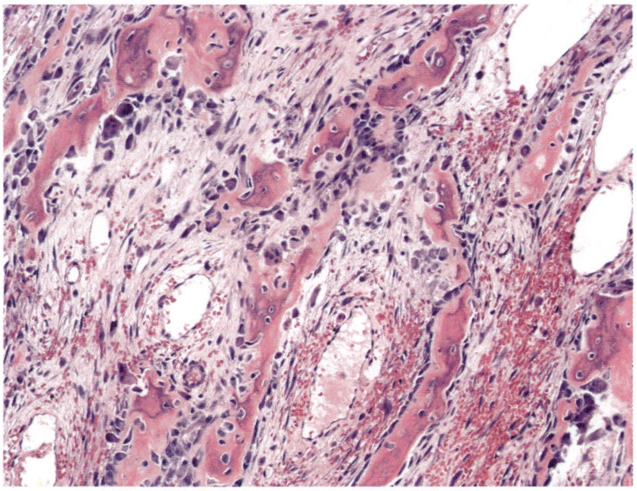

Fig. 30.21 Osteoblastoma – microscopy showing woven bone with prominent osteoblasts, fibrovascular stroma and blood vessels. (*Source:* From John D. Reith. Bone and Joints. Rosai and Ackerman's Surgical Pathology. 11th edition. Elsevier 2018.)

Classification Osteosarcomas may be classified on the basis of various factors:

- On the basis of the anatomical site, they may be classified into intramedullary, surface or extraskeletal osteosarcomas. Intramedullary osteosarcomas are the most common type and are commonly referred to as conventional osteosarcomas. The surface osteosarcomas may be intracortical, periosteal or parosteal in location.
- On the basis of the histological grading, the tumours may be classified into low grade and high grade that may reflect in the prognosis of the tumour.
- On the basis of origin of the tumour, they may be called primary in the absence of predisposing factors or secondary when the predisposing conditions such as Paget disease, bone infarcts, previous radiation or OI are present.
- On the basis of the histological features, osteosarcomas may be osteoblastic, chondroblastic or fibroblastic. But this distinction does not affect the prognosis or treatment of the patient. Some of the special variants that warrant mentioning are the telangiectatic, small cell and giant cell types.

Clinical Features Symptoms of osteosarcoma may be present for weeks or months before patients are diagnosed. The most common presenting symptom is pain, particularly pain with activity. Pathological fractures are not particularly common with or without rise in serum alkaline phosphatase. The patients may present with metastasis at the time of presentation itself, which makes the prognosis poor.

Radiographic Findings Large destructive, mixed lytic and blastic mass with infiltrative margins may be seen on X-ray.

Elevation of the periosteum occurs because of reactive bone formation as a result of irritation of the periosteum by the tumour when it penetrates the cortex. This gives

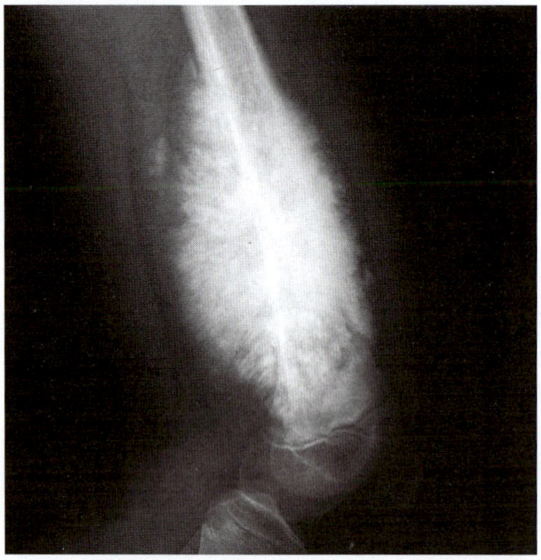

Fig. 30.22 Radiograph of distal femur, osteosarcoma showing sunburst appearance due to brisk periosteal new bone formation. (*Source:* From A. Carlson Merrow and Selena Hariharan. Approach to Pediatric Musculoskeletal System. Imaging in Pediatrics. Elsevier 2018.)

the characteristic Codman triangle and the so-called sunray appearance (Fig. 30.22). The bone under the periosteum in the Codman triangle is not the tumour but is composed of the reactive bone only.

Morphology

Gross The tumour appears bulky with the cut surface being gritty and grey white showing areas of haemorrhage and necrosis (Fig. 30.23). Osteosarcoma may destroy the cortex and produce soft-tissue mass. It may also penetrate the epiphyseal plate or enter the joints, but these are infrequent.

Microscopy The neoplasm is composed of tumour cells of varying size and shape with intermingled large bizarre multinucleated cells and cells with atypical mitosis. The formation of neoplastic osteoid bone by tumour cells is diagnostic. The neoplastic bone usually has a fine, lace-like architecture (Fig. 30.24). In some cases, the tumour cells may produce cartilage or fibrous tissue also. Vascular invasion and extensive necrosis are also common.

Occasionally, tumour foci may be seen at other areas of the same bone discontinuous with the primary lesion. When it is within the reactive region of the primary lesion, it is called satellite lesion, and when it occurs outside the reactive area in the normal bone, it is called skip metastasis. The presence of any of these worsens the prognosis. The common site of metastasis is to the lung by blood dissemination followed by other bones, pleura and visceral organs. Lymphatic spread is very uncommon in this tumour.

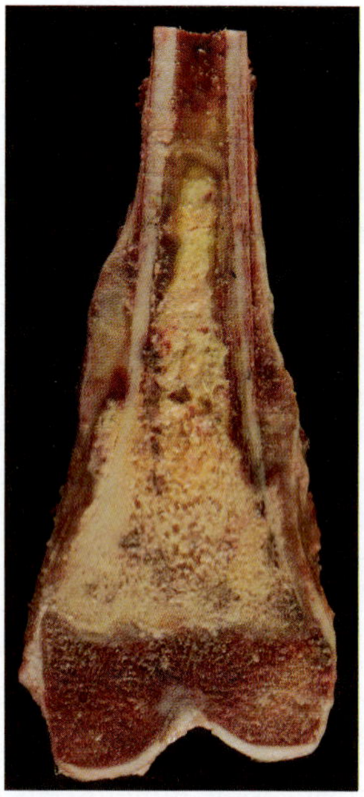

Fig. 30.23 Osteosarcoma – gross image of distal femur. (*Source:* From John D. Reith. Bone and Joints. Rosai and Ackerman's Surgical Pathology. 11th edition. Elsevier 2018.)

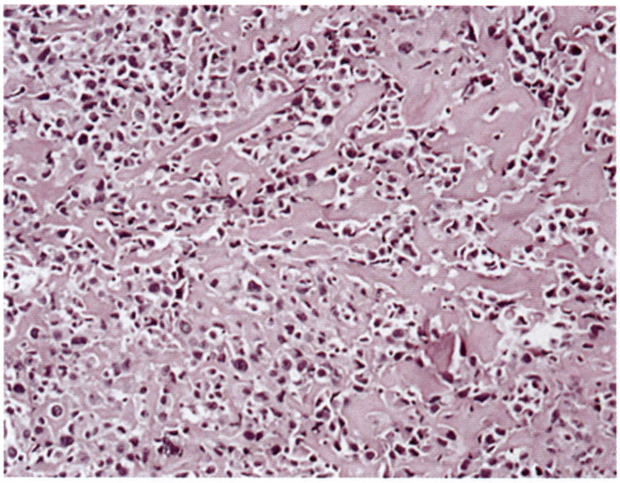

Fig. 30.24 Osteosarcoma – microscopy showing filigree pattern – (thin, randomly arborizing osteoid intercalating between neoplastic cells that show marked nuclear atypia). (*Source:* From Andrew E. Horvai and Thomas Link. Conventional Osteosarcoma. High-Yield Bone and Soft Tissue Pathology. Saunders 2012.)

CARTILAGE-FORMING TUMOURS

Cartilage-forming tumours are tumours that form cartilaginous material, especially hyaline or myxoid cartilage. Fibrous and elastic cartilage are only rarely produced. Most of the common benign and malignant primary bone tumours come under this category. Cartilaginous tumours are more commonly benign than malignant.

Osteochondroma

Osteochondromas are the most common bone tumours accounting for 20%–50% of all benign osseous tumours.

They are surface bone lesions composed of both medullary and cortical bone with hyaline cartilage caps. They are more common in men than in women, and often present in late adolescence or early adulthood. Multiple osteochondromas are seen in multiple hereditary exostosis (autosomal dominant hereditary disease) associated with loss-of-function mutation in EXT gene (EXT1 or EXT2) and often present earlier during childhood.

These lesions are seen only in bones showing endochondral ossification. The most common site is the metaphysis of long bones: femur > humerus > tibia. Involvement of flat bones (scapula and ilium) may occur.

Clinical Features Osteochondromas are often asymptomatic. Symptoms, if present, may be secondary to fracture, malignant transformation, compression of adjacent neurovascular structures, bursal formation or bursitis or palpable mass. Patients with multiple hereditary exostosis are generally more severely affected and present at a younger age with multiple osseous deformities such as bowing of the extremities, short limbs and short stature.

Radiology The lesions are often found around the knee joint localized to the surface of the bone. They present as perpendicular outgrowths with medullary and cortical continuity in the region of the metaphysis of the long bones. The lesions may be sessile or pedunculated and contain thin, lobulated cartilaginous cap, which may be calcified.

Morphology

Grossly, they are sessile or pedunculated mass measuring about 1–20 cm in size with hyaline cartilage cap. Microscopy shows a cap composed of hyaline cartilage of varying thickness, covered peripherally by perichondrium (Fig. 30.25). The cartilage exhibits enchondral ossification with newly formed bone lining the inner side in the stalk and the head. The cortex of the stalk appears to merge with the cortex of the host bone. Marrow elements may be present within the bony stalk and head and they are contiguous with those of the native bone.

Osteochondromas usually stop growing following closure of growth plate in early adulthood. They require removal only if symptomatic or for cosmetic reasons. Transformation into secondary chondrosarcoma is very rare.

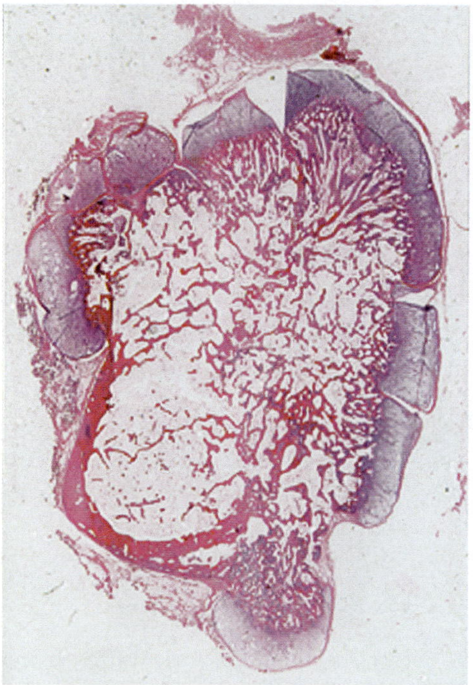

Fig. 30.25 Osteochondroma – microscopy showing mature bone covered by a well-differentiated cartilaginous cap. (*Source:* From John D. Reith, Rosai and Ackerman's Surgical Pathology, Elsevier 2018.)

Chondroma

Chondromas are benign tumours composed of mature hyaline cartilage. They generally have a limited growth potential and are not locally aggressive. These tumours are called enchondromas when they occur in the medullary canal of the bone and juxtacortical chondromas when they occur on the surface of the bone. They may be solitary or multiple. Ollier disease and Maffucci syndrome are nonhereditary disorders characterized by multiple enchondromas. Chondromas possess associations with somatic mutations in isocitrate dehydrogenase 1 (IDH1) and 2 (IDH2) genes. The mutations are rare and often sporadic.

Clinical Features Enchondromas are asymptomatic lesions usually identified incidentally in radiographs performed for other reasons. The symptoms if present are often found as a result of a pathological fracture as pain. Enchondromas may present at any age, although the classic presentation is in the second decade of life. Enchondromatosis syndromes present typically before age 10 years. Majority of these lesions occur in the small bones of the hands and feet. The next most common sites are the long tubular bones. Of the long bones, the femur is the most commonly involved site.

Radiology Chondromas are seen as circumscribed lucencies with central irregular calcifications, a sclerotic rim and an intact cortex (Fig. 30.26).

Morphology

These lesions are mostly smaller than 3 cm, well circumscribed, pale blue and solid, resembling cartilage

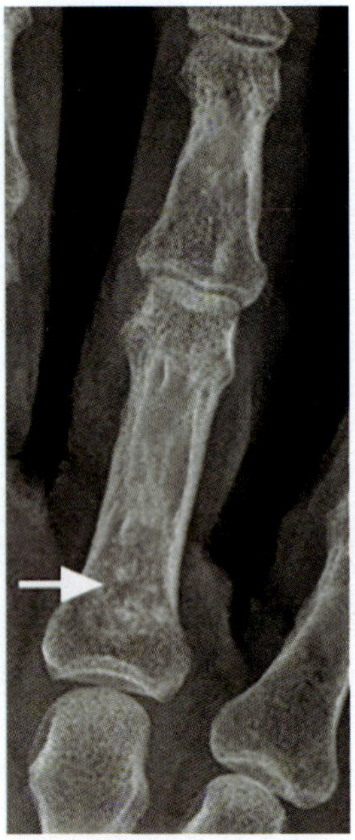

Fig. 30.26 Enchondroma – radiograph showing enchondroma of the third finger located in the proximal phalanx (arrow). (*Source:* From A. Larbi, P. Viala, P. Omoumi, F. Lecouvet, J. Malghem, C. Cyteval and B. Vande Berg. Cartilaginous tumours and calcified lesions of the hand: A pictorial review. Diagnostic and Interventional Imaging. 2013;94:395-409.)

but without myxoid changes. If they are calcified, they appear ivory white on cutting.

Microscopically, the lesions consist of well-circumscribed nodules of mature hyaline cartilage with varying cellularity. Normal marrow separates the cartilaginous lobules, which may be partially enclosed in mature lamellar bone. Within the lesion, areas of myxoid change or focal necrosis with foci of fine or coarse calcifications may be seen. Cellular tumours are often seen in Maffucci and Ollier syndromes containing chondrocytes with atypical nuclei mimicking chondrosarcoma.

Chondromas have a limited growth and treatment may vary from simple observation to surgical curettage. Malignant transformation to chondrosarcoma may be seen in multiple enchondromatosis. People with Maffucci syndrome, apart from multiple chondroma, may develop spindle cell haemangiomas and other malignancies such as brain gliomas.

Chondroblastoma

Chondroblastoma is a rare primary bone tumour of young age, which typically arises in the ends of the long bones. It is often painful and causes joint effusions with restriction of joint mobility. About 95% of cases involve mutations in either H3F3A or H3F3B gene.

Radiology It is characterized by a well-defined osteolytic lesion involving an epiphysis or secondary ossification centre with 50% of cases showing internal calcifications within the lesion.

Morphology

The curettings of the tumour are soft, friable, red to grey, or brown resembling granulation tissue. There may be flecks of gritty, calcific material in the curettings.

Microscopically, chondroblastoma is composed of sheets of neoplastic mononuclear chondroblasts with abundant pink cytoplasm and hyperlobulated nuclei with grooves. Interspersed among the mononuclear cells are osteoclast-like giant cells. Chondroid differentiation is almost always present (pink vs. blue matrix). The unique feature is the presence of pericellular fine calcification called chicken-wire calcification (Fig. 30.27).

Chondrosarcoma

Chondrosarcomas are malignant cartilaginous neoplasms with diverse morphological features and clinical behaviour. About 20% of all primary malignant tumours of the bone are chondrosarcomas. The majority of chondrosarcomas are sporadic, but they may develop from the malignant transformation of osteochondromas and enchondromas.

Chondrosarcomas arising in multiple osteochondroma syndrome exhibit mutations in EXT gene, whereas both chondromatosis-related and sporadic chondrosarcomas may have IDH1 and IDH2 mutations. Chondrosarcoma is a tumour of adulthood and older age. The majority of patients are older than 50 years at diagnosis, with a male predominance. Chondrosarcoma usually presents as painful, progressively enlarging mass. The commonest locations involved in chondrosarcoma are the bones of the axial skeleton (pelvis, scapula, sternum and ribs) followed by the proximal femur and proximal humerus.

Different types of chondrosarcoma have been described, which include:

- Conventional chondrosarcoma, which accounts for nearly 90% of all chondrosarcomas
- Dedifferentiated chondrosarcoma
- Clear-cell chondrosarcoma
- Mesenchymal chondrosarcoma
- Juxtacortical chondrosarcoma
- Secondary chondrosarcoma

Secondary chondrosarcomas are those that occur on a preexisting benign cartilaginous lesion.

Radiology Chondrosarcomas are usually greater than 5 cm in size. The bony contour appears thinned and

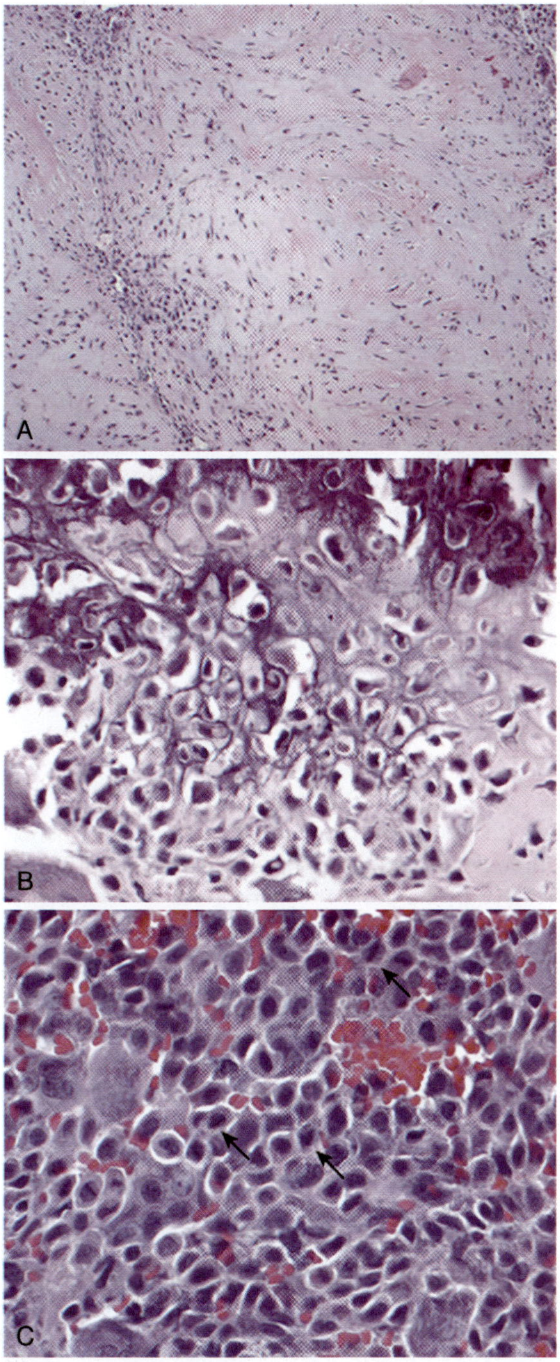

Fig. 30.27 Chondroblastoma – microscopy. The classic triad of histological findings in chondroblastoma includes fibrochondroid matrix (A), chicken-wire calcifications (B) and mononuclear cells with nuclear grooves (arrows) (C). (*Source:* From Andrew E. Horvai and Thomas Link. Chondroblastoma. High-Yield Bone and Soft Tissue Pathology. Saunders 2012.)

expanded, and multiple surface erosions (endosteal scalloping) are seen. The extent of bone destruction depends on the histological grade of the tumour. The periosteum overlying the lesion may be elevated. This leads to new bone formation that results in hazy cortical irregularity and fuzziness or parallel periosteal new bone formation. This is in contrast with osteosarcomas, which results in

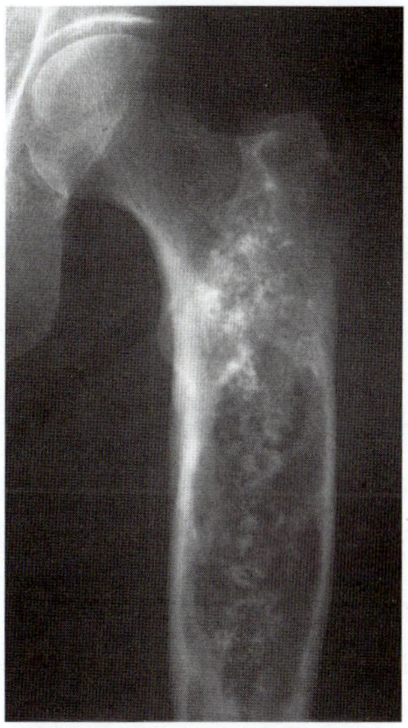

Fig. 30.28 Chondrosarcoma – radiograph of the femur showing an extensive central chondrosarcoma with typical chondroid matrix, cortical expansion and thickening with endosteal scalloping. (*Source:* From Lee Alexander Grant and Nyree Griffin. Malignant Bone Tumours. Grainger & Allison's Diagnostic Radiology Essentials. 2nd edition. Elsevier 2019.)

perpendicular periosteal new bone formation giving a sunburst appearance. The characteristic finding which aids the diagnosis is the typical 'ring-and-arc' chondroid matrix mineralization (Fig. 30.28).

Morphology

Grossly, the tumours are large bulky masses with nodules of glistening grey-white, translucent cartilage often gelatinous or myxoid. Focal calcifications and areas of necrosis are present.

Microscopy of the lesion shows chondroid matrix with increased cellularity, and binucleate cells.

These tumours can be classified into the following three histological grades, depending on findings of cellularity, atypia and pleomorphism:

i. **Grade I** (low grade): It is cytologically similar to enchondroma; cellularity is higher, with occasional plump nuclei having open chromatin structure.
ii. **Grade II** (intermediate grade): It is characterized by a definite and increased cellularity; distinct nucleoli are present in most cells, and foci of myxoid change may be seen.
iii. **Grade III** (high grade): It is characterized by high cellularity, prominent nuclear atypia and the presence of mitosis.

Variants of Chondrosarcoma Dedifferentiated chondrosarcomas: These are low-grade chondrosarcomas with a second high-grade component that does not produce cartilage.

Clear-cell chondrosarcomas: They are tumours composed of malignant chondrocytes in sheets that have abundant clear cytoplasm, numerous osteoclast-type giant cells and reactive bone formation.
Mesenchymal chondrosarcomas: These tumours are composed of islands of well-differentiated hyaline cartilage surrounded by small round cells in sheets.

TUMOURS OF UNKNOWN ORIGIN

This category includes primary tumours of the bone that do not arise from bone cells or cartilage cells.

Ewing Sarcoma

Ewing sarcoma is an aggressive tumour of adolescents and young adults, which constitutes 10%–15% of all bone sarcomas. It is the second common sarcoma of bone only next to osteosarcoma. It shows slight predilection to men than to women. It is a primitive round cell malignant tumour that lacks differentiation.

Pathogenesis Ewing sarcoma and the peripheral primitive neuroectodermal tumour are found to contain the reciprocal translocation between chromosomes 11 and 22, t(11;22). In affected individuals, t(11;22)(q24;q12) fuses one of the exons from EWS and FLI1 to form the fusion message. The most common combination is EWS exon 7 fused to FLI1 exon 6 (type 1 translocation) that occurs in approximately 50%–64% of tumours of Ewing sarcomas.

Clinical Features Ewing sarcoma usually affects the diaphysis of long bone and the commonest sites are the lower extremity followed by the pelvis, upper extremity, axial skeleton and ribs. The femur is the most frequently affected bone, with the tumour usually arising in the midshaft. Presenting symptoms include localized pain and a palpable tender mass mimicking an infectious aetiology. Back pain may indicate a paraspinal, retroperitoneal or deep pelvic tumour. Systemic symptoms of fever and weight loss often indicate metastatic disease.

Morphology

The tumour is ill defined, soft, tan-white with areas of haemorrhage and necrosis involving the medulla and cortex with periosteal elevation.

Microscopy of the tumour shows small round cells with uniform round nuclei containing finely dispersed chromatin and inconspicuous nucleoli, and a narrow rim of clear or vacuolated cytoplasm due to the presence of glycogen (PAS - granular positive) (Fig. 30.29). Either Homer Wright rosettes (round groupings of cells with a central fibrillary core) or Flexner–Wintersteiner rosette (central lumens) may be seen.

Ewing sarcoma is an aggressive tumour, but if managed with neoadjuvant chemotherapy, surgery and follow-up chemotherapy, 5-year survival of about 75% may be achieved. The presence of necrosis in excision specimen indicates good response to chemotherapy.

Osteoclastoma/Giant Cell Tumour

Osteoclastoma is a benign and locally aggressive primary bone neoplasm composed of mononuclear round to spindle cells with numerous evenly dispersed osteoclast-like giant cells. It usually arises in individuals in their 20s to 40s.

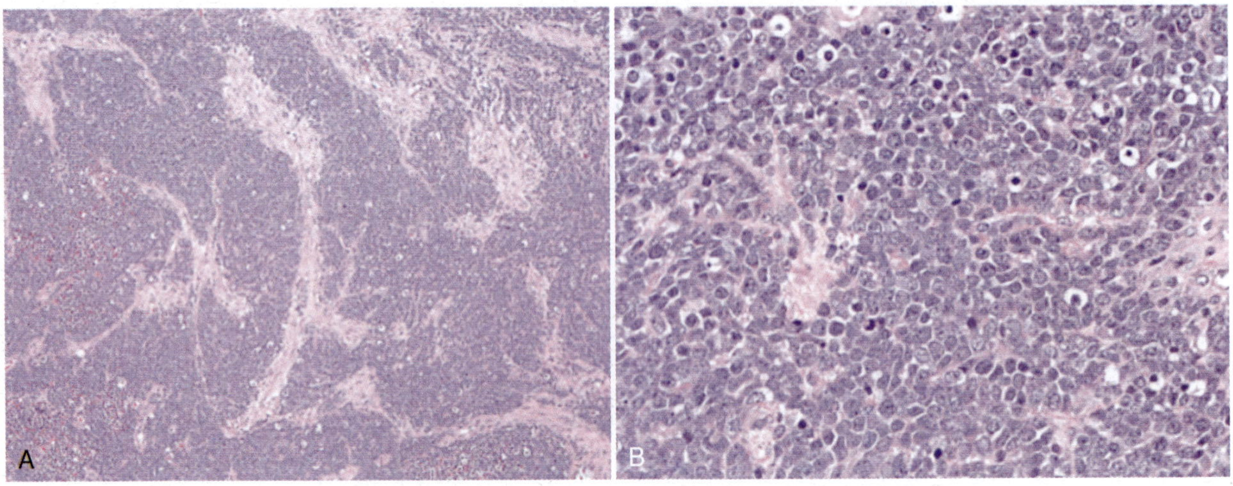

Fig. 30.29 Ewing sarcoma – (A and B) microscopy showing sheets of small blue round cells separated by fibrous septa. (*Source:* From John D. Reith. Bone and Joints. Rosai and Ackerman's Surgical Pathology. 11th edition. Elsevier 2018.)

Pathogenesis RANKL on neoplastic preosteoblasts binds to RANK (receptor activator of nuclear factor κB) on non-neoplastic macrophage-like osteoclast precursors. In the presence of M-CSF, this promotes osteoclast differentiation and giant cell formation. H3F3A genetic alterations have been detected in 95% of GCT. The lack of communication that normally exists between osteoblasts and osteoclasts is responsible for the lytic nature of the tumour.

Clinical Features Pain is the most common presenting symptom. Swelling and deformity are associated with larger lesions. Soft-tissue extension is common. The incidence of pathological fracture at presentation is 11%–37%. The common site is in the epiphysis and adjacent metaphysis of long bones (distal radius, proximal humerus, distal femur, proximal tibia). Other bones (proximal sacrum, vertebrae, skull base) may also be involved.

Radiography Expansive lytic lesion without any sclerosis or periosteal reaction, often destroying the overlying cortex and producing a bulging soft-tissue mass, is noted (Fig. 30.30). Hence, the radiological appearance is often described as soap bubble appearance.

Morphology

The tumour appears as a large, red-brown mass that usually undergoes cystic degeneration, with areas of haemorrhage and necrosis (Fig. 30.31). Microscopy of the tumour shows numerous osteoclast-like giant cells uniformly distributed throughout the tumour (Fig. 30.32). Most of the giant cells are larger than normal osteoclasts with numerous (>50) nuclei. The nuclei of the giant cells and the mononuclear cells are similar with prominent nucleoli. Necrosis/mitotic activity may be present.

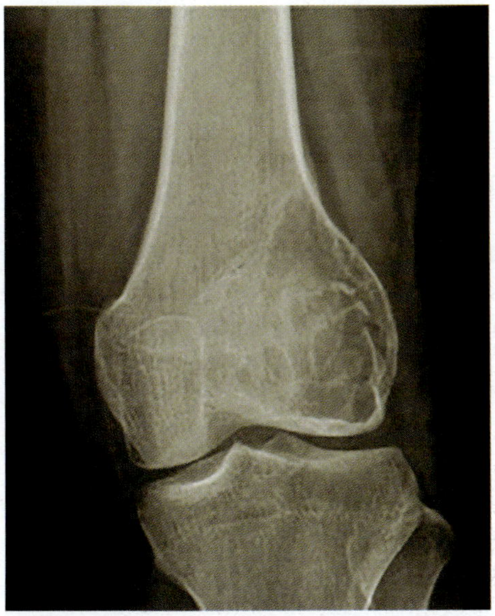

Fig. 30.30 Osteoclastoma – radiograph of the left knee showing a well-defined, osteolytic lesion at the lateral femoral condyle with an ill-defined sclerotic rim and extension to subchondral portion. (*Source:* From Byeong-Joo and Yong-Koo Park. Giant cell tumor of bone: updated molecular pathogenesis and tumor biology. Human Pathology. 2018;81:1-8.)

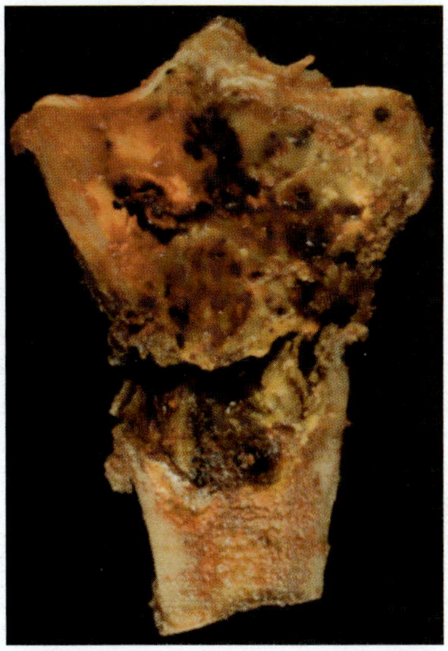

Fig. 30.31 Osteoclastoma – gross. Note the presence of a red brown haemorrhagic tumour in proximal tibia. (*Source:* From John D. Reith. Bone and Joints. Rosai and Ackerman's Surgical Pathology. 11th edition. Elsevier 2018.)

Osteoclastoma are usually benign tumours and do not metastasize. However, around half of the patients develop local recurrence and about 4%–5% of them develop metastatic lesions in the lung that are not fatal mostly.

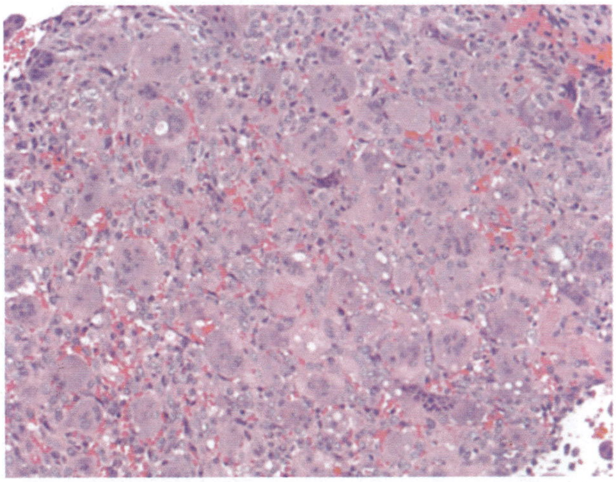

Fig. 30.32 Osteoclastoma – microscopy showing tumour composed of multinucleated giant cells and stromal cells. (*Source:* From John D. Reith. Bone and Joints. Rosai and Ackerman's Surgical Pathology. 11th edition. Elsevier 2018.)

The newer drug, RANKL inhibitor denosumab shows some promise in the treatment of this tumour.

Aneurysmal Bone Cyst

ABC is a benign tumour characterized by multiloculated blood-filled cystic spaces that are locally destructive and weaken bones to the point of pathological fracture. They are most common in the femur, tibia and vertebrae. The vast majority of ABCs present in the metaphysis of long bones. The majority of primary ABC lesions demonstrate rearrangements of chromosome 17p13 that upregulates the TRE17/USP6 oncogene, which halts osteoblastic maturation.

Radiography Cystic or osteolytic lesions with thin 'egg-shell' sclerotic well-defined borders are a characteristic feature of ABC (Fig. 30.33). The enclosed cavity contains fluid-filled levels separated by internal septa. The surrounding bone may be pushed outwards because of expansive nature of the lesion.

Morphology

Grossly, the tumour is a spongy, multiloculated, haemorrhagic lesion. A thin subperiosteal shell of new bone surrounds the structure and contains cystic blood-filled cavities (Fig. 30.34).

Microscopically, the blood-filled cystic spaces are separated by cellular septa containing fibroblasts, giant cells and reactive woven bone (Fig. 30.35).

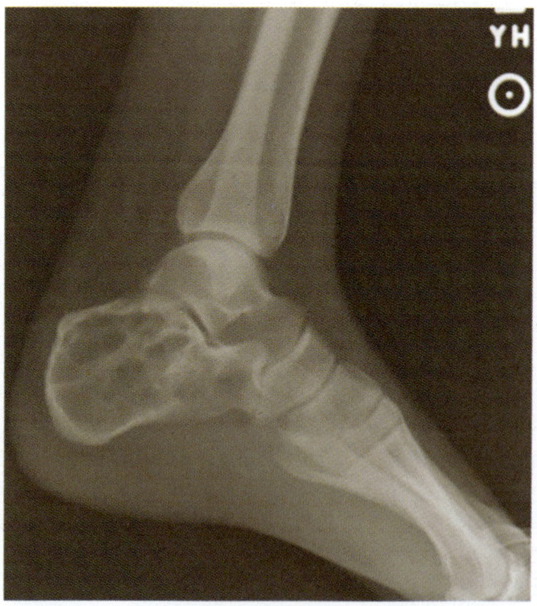

Fig. 30.33 Aneurysmal bone cyst – radiograph showing an aneurysmal bone cyst with a multicystic appearance. (*Source:* From John D. Reith. Bone and Joints. Rosai and Ackerman's Surgical Pathology. 11th edition. Elsevier 2018.)

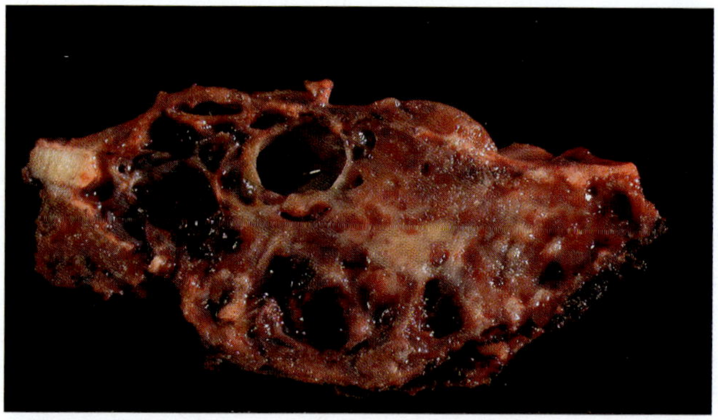

Fig. 30.34 Aneurysmal bone cyst – gross; contains multiple blood-filled cystic spaces. (*Source:* From John D. Reith. Bone and Joints. Rosai and Ackerman's Surgical Pathology. 11th edition. Elsevier 2018.)

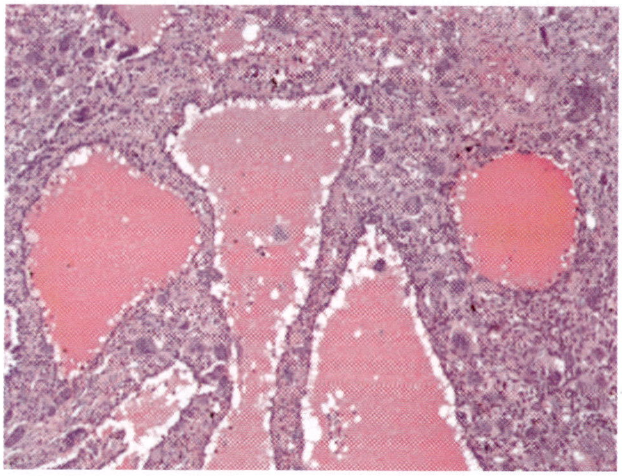

Fig. 30.35 Aneurysmal bone cyst – microscopy showing multiple blood lakes surrounded by a giant cell–rich fibroblastic proliferation. (*Source:* From John D. Reith. Bone and Joints. Rosai and Ackerman's Surgical Pathology. 11th edition. Elsevier 2018.)

METASTATIC TUMOURS OF BONE

Metastatic tumours of the bone are the most common skeletal malignancies. The common pathways of spread include direct spread, lymphatic or haematogenous spread and intraspinal seeding. In adults, 75% of the bone metastasis occurs from cancer of the prostate, breast, kidney and lung (Fig. 30.36). In children, the most common primary tumours with secondaries to bone are neuroblastoma, Ewing sarcoma, rhabdomyosarcoma and Wilms tumour. Most of the metastatic tumours are multifocal. They usually involve the haematopoietic marrow of the axial skeleton (vertebral column, pelvis, ribs, skull and sternum).

X-rays of these lesions show an entirely lytic or entirely blastic or mixed lytic and blastic picture. Pure osteoblastic secondaries are from prostatic adenocarcinoma. Pure lytic tumours are from carcinomas of the kidney, lung, gastrointestinal tract and malignant melanoma (Fig. 30.37).

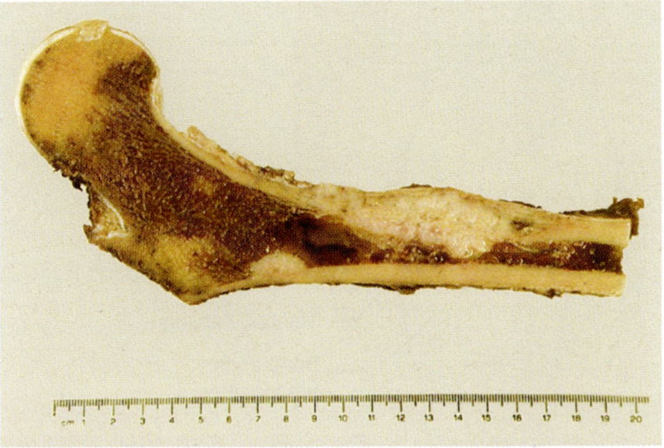

Fig. 30.36 Bone metastases – gross; shows metastatic deposits. (*Source:* From Alexandra K. Freeman, Vaiyapuri P. Sumathi and Lee Jeys. Metastatic tumours of bone. Surgery. 2018;36:35–40.)

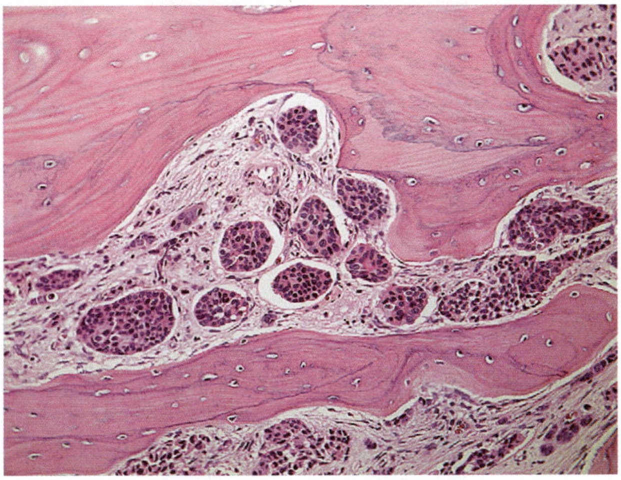

Fig. 30.37 Bone metastases – microscopy showing metastatic breast carcinoma. (*Source:* From Alexandra K. Freeman, Vaiyapuri P. Sumathi and Lee Jeys. Metastatic tumours of bone. Surgery. 2018;36:35–40.)

II. JOINTS

Joints are the point of contact between two or more bones that function to enable mechanical movement. They are of two types:

- Solid (nonsynovial) joints: They lack joint space and have minimal movement. They serve to provide mechanical stability. They may be:
  a. Fibrous synarthroses – joined by fibrous tissue, e.g. cranial sutures
  b. Cartilaginous synchondroses – joined by cartilage, e.g. manubrium sterni and pubis
- Cavitated (synovial) joints: They have a joint space lined by synovium that contains synovial fluid. They permit a wide range of movement.

The synovium is lined by two types of cells – type A synoviocytes (similar to macrophages) and type B synoviocytes (similar to fibroblasts) – and lacks a basement membrane. The type B cells produce hyaluronic acid and other proteins required by the joint. The synovial fluid is a hyaluronic acid–rich filtrate of plasma that helps in lubrication of the joints.

Another important component of the joint is the articular hyaline cartilage. It is an effective shock absorber and acts as a water-resistant surface, thereby providing resistance to stress and vertical load transmission. The production and degradation of the components of the cartilage is by the chondrocytes. They produce the degradative enzymes in the inactive stage, and also keep these enzymes this way by producing inhibitors of these enzymes. Hence, degradation of the cartilage happens only when the inhibitor levels decrease and the degrading enzyme gets activated. This is mediated by inflammatory cytokines such as interleukin (IL)-1 and tumour necrosis factor (TNF)-β produced by the indigenous cells such as chondrocytes, fibroblasts and synoviocytes and by external inflammatory cells entering the joint during inflammation. Excessive release of these inflammatory mediators is the major cause of articular destructive diseases.

OSTEOARTHRITIS

AETIOLOGY

Osteoarthrosis or OA is the commonest degenerative joint disease that results in structural and functional failure of synovial joints due to degeneration of the cartilage. It can be classified into two categories – primary OA and secondary OA. **Primary OA** is diagnosed in the absence of a predisposing trauma or disease. **Secondary OA** presents following preexisting joint abnormality, fracture, diabetes, obesity, ochronosis or haemochromatosis. Women are more commonly affected, especially in the knee joint and joints of the hand.

Pathogenesis

Risk factors for developing OA include age, female gender, obesity, anatomical factors, muscle weakness and joint injury. OA is a disease of the entire joint sparing no tissues. Inflammation occurs as cytokines and metalloproteinases are released into the joint. These agents are involved in the excessive matrix degradation over the productive capacity that results in cartilage degeneration. Inflammatory molecules that have been associated with OA include IL-17, 15-hydroxyeicosatetraenoic acid, prostaglandin E_2, IL-1β, TNF-α, IL-1 receptor antagonist and uric acid.

In early OA, swelling of the cartilage usually occurs because of the increased secretion of inflammatory mediators, synthesis of collagens, proteoglycans and protease; this reflects an effort by the chondrocytes to repair

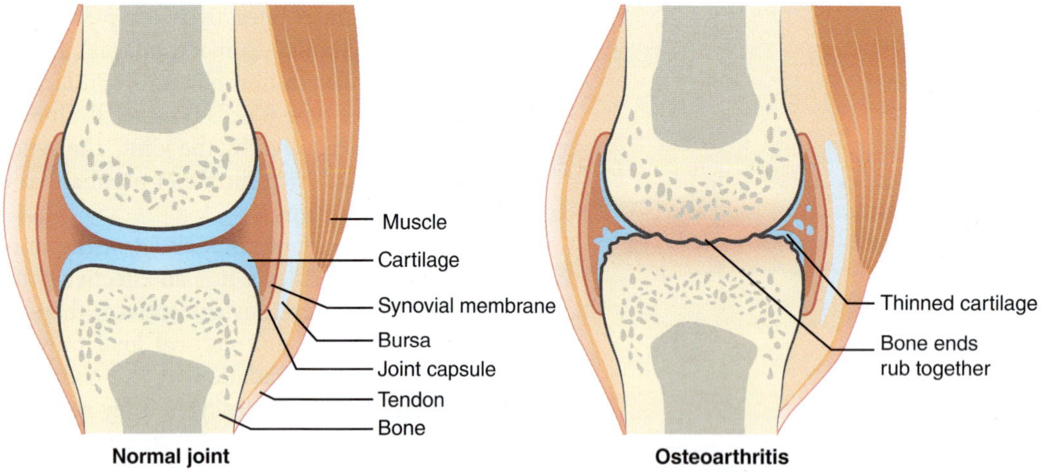

Fig. 30.38 Schematic representation of normal joint versus osteoarthritic joint.

the cartilage damage. However, proinflammatory cytokines result in deterioration of chondrocyte metabolism (Fig. 30.38). This stage may last for years or decades that act to remodel the cartilaginous matrix.

As OA progresses, there is loss of chondrocytes and the level of proteoglycans eventually drops very low, causing loss of cartilage, thereby markedly deteriorating joint surface integrity.

Clinical Features

Individuals are mostly asymptomatic until their 50s. **The presenting symptoms include** deep aching joint movements that worsen with activity, limitation in range of movements and crepitus. The common sites involved are the hips, knees, lumbar and cervical vertebrae, and proximal and distal interphalangeal joints. Later, the patients develop muscle spasm and atrophy and neurological deficits because of the newly formed reactive bones (osteophytes) causing nerve root compression. The other clinical features include **Heberden nodes** in distal interphalangeal joints (F > M) and **loose bodies within the joint space** when a portion of articular cartilage breaks off and continues to grow.

RADIOLOGY

The findings on imaging include deformity of joint with loss of bone substance and cartilage, loss of joint space, migration of joint, osteophyte formation, sclerosis of subchondral bone and subchondral bone cysts (Fig. 30.39). It is important to remember that the degree of damage noted radiographically does not correlate with the severity of the clinical symptoms.

Morphology

Morphological changes seen in OA include loss of cartilage (polished appearance) – eburnation, osteophyte formation and subchondral cysts with mucoid fluid surrounded by sclerotic bone. Owing to the weakening of the affected bone, small fractures through the articulating bone are a common finding. Loose bodies formed from the dislodged pieces of cartilage and subchondral bone are a common finding, which are referred to as joint mice.

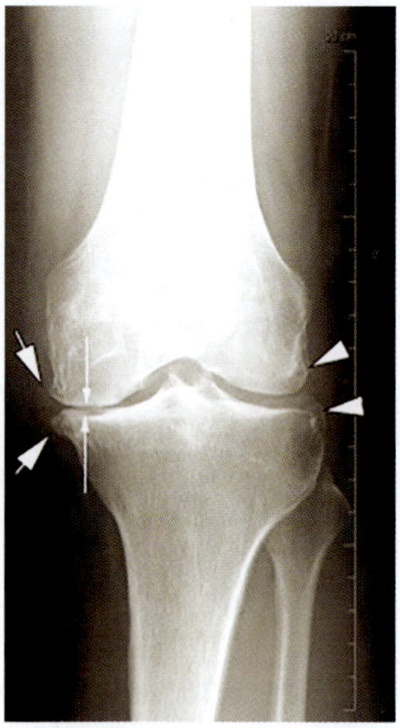

Fig. 30.39 X-ray of knee joint showing large marginal osteophytes at the medial joint space (large arrows) and smaller osteophytes at the lateral femur and tibia (arrowheads). In addition, there is definite medial narrowing of joint space (thin, long arrows).

MANAGEMENT

The objective of OA treatment includes alleviation of pain and improvement of functional status because none of the available treatment modalities can stop the degeneration of the cartilage. Comprehensive management of the disease involves both nonpharmacological and pharmacological therapies. Nonpharmacological interventions include patient education, heat and cold therapy, weight loss, exercise and physiotherapy.

Pharmacotherapy of OA involves oral, topical and/or intra-articular injections. Acetaminophen and oral NSAIDs are the most popular options for OA and are usually the initial choice of pharmacological treatment. Topical NSAIDs are less efficacious than their oral counterparts. Intra-articular steroid injections can also be a treatment option for OA, especially in a setting of acute pain.

RHEUMATOID ARTHRITIS PA 33.5

Rheumatoid arthritis (RA) is a chronic systemic autoimmune disease characterized by inflammatory arthritis and extra-articular involvement. The arthritis is nonsuppurative and proliferative in nature. The extra-articular manifestations may involve the heart, blood vessels, skin and lungs and may resemble other autoimmune disorders such as SLE and systemic sclerosis. Women are predominantly involved than men, with a ratio of 3:1, and presentation may be as early as second decade up to fourth decade.

AETIOLOGY

Several genetic, environmental, hormonal, immunological and infectious factors may play significant roles. The risk of developing RA has been associated with HLA-DRB1 alleles: HLA-DRB1*04, HLA-DRB1*01 and HLA-DRB1*10. It involves small bones of the hands first and later the wrist, elbow and knee.

Pathogenesis

RA is predominantly a type IV hypersensitivity reaction mediated by $CD4^+$ helper T cells. The additional components are mediated by the self-directed antibodies. As a result of this combination, the synovium in RA is infiltrated by innate immune cells (monocytes, dendritic cells, mast cells) and adaptive immune cells - $CD4^+$ T helper 1, T-helper 17, B cells and plasma cells. These cells, especially the T_h1 cells, produce cytokines and chemokines such as TNF, IL-6 and granulocyte-monocyte colony-stimulating factors that activate the endothelial cells and cause further increase in immune cells within the synovial compartment. Fibroblast and inflammatory cells lead to osteoclast generation resulting in bone erosion. The role of the various cytokines in the pathogenesis is elucidated in Table 30.5.

Patients with RA contain antibodies to citrullinated proteins. The antibodies to citrulline are called anticitrullinated protein antibodies (ACPA). They can be of IgG, IgM or IgA isotypes. ACPA can bind citrullinated residues on self-proteins such as vimentin, fibronectin, fibrinogen, histones and type 2 collagen, which leads to complement activation. Apart from ACPA, these individuals may also have IgA and IgM antibodies directed against Fc portion of IgG that get deposited within the joints eliciting an immune response. They are called the rheumatoid factor. Although they may be present in 80% of patients, they are not specific to RA. However, the presence of antibodies in RA is associated with increased morbidity and mortality.

Table 30.5 Role of Cytokines in Rheumatoid Arthritis

Cytokine	Produced By	Effect
INF-γ	Th cells	Activates macrophages and synovial cells
RANKL	Expressed on activated T cells	Stimulates bone resorption by osteoclasts
IL-17	T_h17 cells	Recruits neutrophils and monocytes
IL-1 and TNF	Macrophages	Stimulates synovial cells to produce proteases that degrade the cartilage

IL, interleukin; TNF, tumour necrosis factor.

Clinical Features

General malaise, fatigue and musculoskeletal pain (due to IL-1 and TNF) are the common presenting symptoms. The small joints (metacarpophalangeal and proximal interphalangeal) of the hands and feet are commonly affected. The classical feature noted is the stiffness of the joints in the morning or following inactivity.

COMPLICATIONS

Destruction of tendons, ligaments and joint capsules produces swan neck deformity, radial deviation of the wrist, ulnar deviation and flexion–hyperextension of the fingers. Joints are unstable with minimal range of motion and nearly 50% of the patients have spinal involvement.

EXTRA-ARTICULAR LESIONS

The **skin** shows subcutaneous rheumatoid nodules that are firm, nontender and round to oval and commonly seen in the ulnar aspect of the forearm, elbows, occiput and lumbosacral areas. **Blood vessels** exhibit acute necrotizing vasculitis involving small and large arteries. Eye manifestations include uveitis and keratoconjunctivitis. Peripheral neuropathy may be present. Long-term complications include systemic amyloidosis.

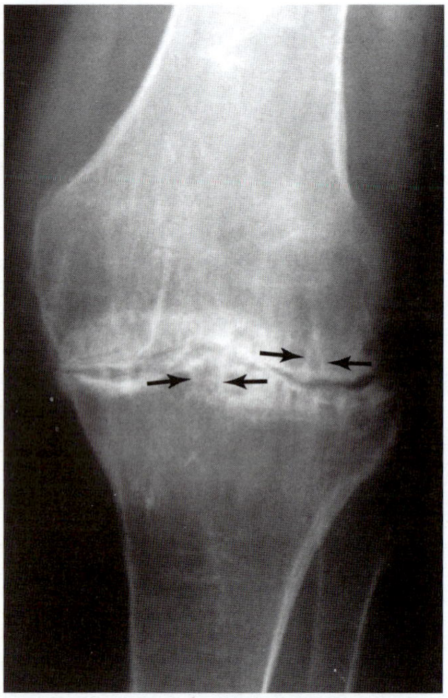

Fig. 30.40 Rheumatoid arthritis imaging showing diffuse joint space narrowing with subchondral cyst formation present (arrows). Absence of spurs/osteophytes helps to differentiate from osteoarthritis. (*Source:* From Fred A. Mettler. Skeletal System. Essentials of Radiology. 4th edition. Elsevier 2019.)

RADIOLOGY

Early stages of the disease or the X-ray may show osteopenia near the joint with soft-tissue swelling, and a smaller than normal joint space (Fig. 30.40). As the disease progresses, bony erosions and subluxation may be present even in the absence of pain.

LABORATORY INVESTIGATIONS

The laboratory investigations include the inflammatory markers CRP and ESR, which tend to be elevated; the antibody serology to detect rheumatoid factor and ACPA; and the investigations that are performed to determine the presence of systemic involvement of other organs, such as blood count tests and renal and liver function tests.

DIAGNOSTIC CRITERIA

In 2010, the American College of Rheumatology and European League Against Rheumatism laid down the criteria for diagnosis of new patients and also gave the criteria of who needed to be screened for this disorder. The criteria are given in Box 30.2.

Box 30.2 The 2010 American College of Rheumatology/European League Against Rheumatism Classification Criteria for RA

	Score
Target population (who should be tested?): 1) Patients who have at least one joint with definite clinical synovitis (swelling) 2) Patients with the synovitis not better explained by another disease Classification criteria for RA (score-based algorithm: add score of categories A–D; a score of ≥6 out of 10 is needed for classification of a patient as having definite RA)	
A. Joint involvement	
One large joint	0
Two to 10 large joints	1
One to three small joints (with or without involvement of large joints)	2
Four to 10 small joints (with or without involvement of large joints)	3
>10 joints (at least one small joint)	5
B. Serology (at least one test result is needed for classification)	
Negative RF *and* negative ACPA	0
Low positive RF *or* low positive ACPA	2
High positive RF *or* high positive ACPA	3
C. Acute phase reactants (at least one test result is needed for classification)	
Normal CRP and normal ESR	0
Abnormal CRP or normal ESR	1
D. Duration of symptoms	
<6 weeks	0
≥6 weeks	1

ACPA, anticitrullinated protein antibodies; RA, rheumatoid arthritis.

Morphology

Gross Joints have oedematous, thick, hyperplastic synovium, covered by delicate and bulbous fronds.

Microscopy **The destruction of the joints may occur in three stages – inflammation, pannus formation and ankylosing fibrosis. In the first stage, the microscopic features include:**

- **Synovial hyperplasia** and proliferation (Fig. 30.41A)
- **Dense inflammatory cell infiltrate** composed of CD4 T cells, B cells (forming lymphoid follicles), plasma cells and macrophages (Fig. 30.41B)
- Increased vascularity (with haemosiderin deposition) due to neoangiogenesis
- Osteoclastic activity in underlying bone making way for the inflamed synovium to penetrate the bone
- Fibrinopurulent exudate on the synovial and joint surfaces

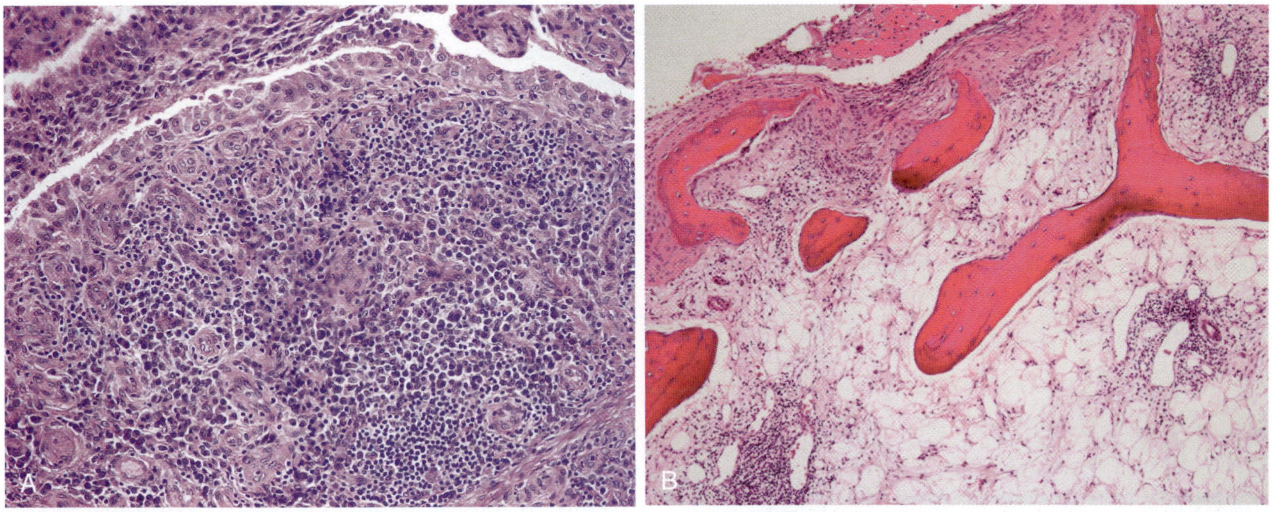

Fig. 30.41 Rheumatoid arthritis – biopsy shows synovial hyperplasia and lymphoplasmacytic infiltration in early stages (A) and destruction of the articular surface by pannus, as well as lymphoid aggregates in the subchondral bone in later stages (B). (*Source:* From John D. Reith. Bone and Joints. Rosai and Ackerman's Surgical Pathology. 11th edition. Elsevier 2018.)

In the next stage, the joint surface is covered by the pannus that is composed of oedematous synovium, inflammatory cells, granulation tissue and fibroblasts. It causes destruction and erosion of the joint cartilage. In later stages, there is periosteal erosion, subchondral cyst formation, inflammation and fibrinoid deposits leading to complete destruction of the articular cartilage and fusion of the opposing bone by fibrosis called fibrous ankylosis that may get ossified to form bony ankylosis.

There is no complete cure for RA, but treatments can improve symptoms and slow the progression of the disease. Disease-modifying antirheumatic drugs (DMARDs) are initiated as soon as the diagnosis of RA is made. NSAIDs and immunosuppressive drugs may be added for improvement of treatment effectiveness and relief of symptoms. Surgical intervention may include synovectomy, tenosynovectomy, arthroplasty and tendon realignment when indicated.

SERONEGATIVE SPONDYLOARTHROPATHIES

Seronegative spondyloarthropathies (SpA) (Table 30.6) are a family of rheumatological disorders that include:

- Ankylosing spondylitis
- Psoriatic arthritis
- Enteropathic arthritis
- Reactive arthritis (formerly Reiter syndrome)

Pathogenesis

The spondyloarthropathies are chronic inflammatory diseases that most commonly involve the sacroiliac joints and the axial skeleton, with hip and shoulder joints less frequently affected. The primary pathology is in the ligamentous attachments that exhibit chronic inflammation by inflammatory cells such as $CD4^+$ and $CD8^+$ T lymphocytes and macrophages. Cytokines such as TNF-α and transforming growth factor-β (TGF-β) are also a part of the inflammatory process leading to fibrosis and ossification at the sites.

Table 30.6 Seronegative Spondyloarthropathies

Types	Features	Site	HLA-B27 Association
Ankylosing spondylitis	Causes destruction of articular cartilage and bony ankylosis	Sacroiliac joints and apophyseal joints (between tuberosities and processes)	Yes
Reactive arthritis	Triad – arthritis, conjunctivitis and gonococcal urethritis or cervicitis	Knee, ankle and feet	Yes
Enteropathic arthritis	Owing to gastrointestinal tract infection (e.g. *Yersinia, Shigella, Campylobacter*) and also associated with inflammatory bowel disease including Crohn disease and ulcerative colitis	Knee and ankle; at times, wrist, fingers and toes	–
Psoriatic arthritis	Chronic inflammatory arthropathy associated with psoriasis	Peripheral joints of hands and feet as well as axial joints	Yes

Table 30.7 Types of Infectious Arthritis

Types	Features	Site	Organism
Suppurative arthritis	Direct infection of joint space by bacterial organisms	Knee, hip and shoulder	*H. influenzae*, *S. aureus* and *Salmonella*
Mycobacterial arthritis	Chronic progressive monoarticular infection	Hip, knee and ankle	*Mycobacterium tuberculosis*
Lyme arthritis	Dissemination of infection from skin to joints	Knees, shoulder, elbow and ankle	*Borrelia burgdorferi* (transmitted by deer ticks)
Viral arthritis			HIV, alphavirus, parvovirus B19, rubella virus, Epstein–Barr virus and hepatitis B and C virus

INFECTIOUS ARTHRITIS

Infectious arthritis, also known as joint infection or septic arthritis, is the invasion of a joint by an infectious agent resulting in joint inflammation. It can be infected by direct spread or from a site of soft-tissue abscess and focus of osteomyelitis. Types of infectious arthritis are given in Table 30.7.

CRYSTAL-INDUCED ARTHRITIS

It refers to a joint disorder (called *arthropathy*) that is characterized by accumulation of small *crystals* in one or more *joints*. Endogenous crystals involve monosodium urate (gout), calcium pyrophosphate dehydrate (pseudogout) and calcium phosphate. Exogenous crystals involve corticosteroid ester crystals and talcum.

GOUT

It refers to general inflammatory response triggered because of the precipitation of urate crystals in and around joints. Disease is characterized by hyperuricaemia with plasma urate level more than 6.8 mg/dL. Monosodium urate (MSU) crystals can be deposited in all tissues mainly in and around the joints forming tophi. The first metatarsophalangeal joint is the commonly affected joint followed by the ankles and knees. Gout causes 2%–5% of chronic joint diseases.

Types

Primary (90% of cases): Cause is unknown with gout as the major manifestation of the disease.
Secondary (10% of cases): Owing to a known underlying disease, plasma urate levels are increased.

Pathogenesis

Hyperuricaemia → precipitation of urate crystals in joints → (also stimulates production of IL-1) interaction of MSU crystals with mononuclear phagocytes and neutrophils → lysis of neutrophils releases lysosomal enzymes and free radicals → tissue injury and inflammation.

Clinical Features

Repeated attacks of acute arthritis lead to chronic tophaceous arthritis with tophi formation in the inflamed synovial membrane and periarticular tissue eventually causing loss of joint function. The gold standard of diagnosis is identification of MSU crystals in the synovial fluid using polarized light microscopy.

Morphology

Acute arthritis commonly affects the first toe. The diagnostic MSU crystals are seen as long, needle-shaped, slender, negative birefringent crystals under polarized light, in the aspirated synovial fluid, also containing scattered lymphocytes, plasma cells and macrophages (Fig. 30.42). Most crystals can be identified within the cytoplasm of the neutrophils.

Chronic gout evolves because of multiple episodes of acute attacks causing precipitation of urate crystals with characteristic presence of tophi. Tophi represent deposition of MSU crystals in tissues in and around the affected joints. The synovium appears hyperplastic, fibrotic and thickened because of inflammatory cells. The renal complications caused by MSU crystals are called gouty nephropathy leading to uric acid nephrolithiasis and pyelonephritis.

Medications such as NSAIDs, colchicine and corticosteroids can be used to treat acute attacks and prevent future attacks. They can also reduce the risk of development of tophi from urate crystal deposits.

PSEUDOGOUT/CHONDROCALCINOSIS

Pseudogout or chodrocalcinosis refers to general inflammatory response triggered by the precipitation of calcium

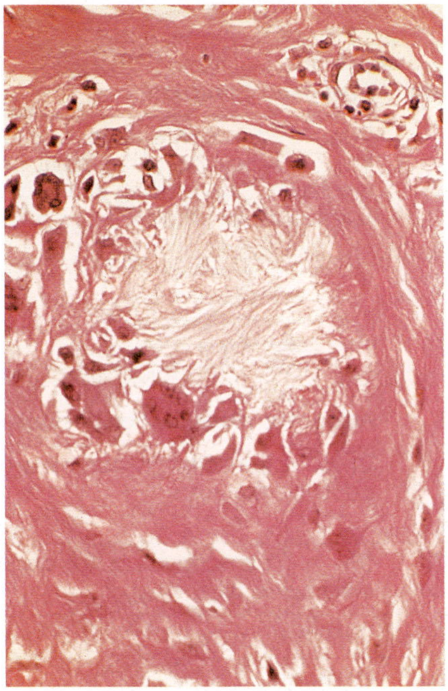

Fig. 30.42 Gout – a lesion of periarticular gout showing a foreign body-type giant cell reaction to the deposited crystals. (*Source:* From John D. Reith. Bone and Joints. Rosai and Ackerman's Surgical Pathology. 11th edition. Elsevier 2018.)

pyrophosphate in patients older than 80 years. Calcium pyrophosphate crystal deposition disease (CPPD) is divided into hereditary, sporadic and secondary (with prior joint damage). The knees and wrist are the most commonly affected. Generally, the affected patients are asymptomatic and the symptomatic patients can be treated symptomatically with NSAIDs.

Pathophysiology

It develops first in menisci and intervertebral discs, and may seed the joints and produce a neutrophilic response. Fifty percent of the affected individuals get significant joint damage.

Morphology

Gross: Chalky white friable deposits are seen.
Microscopy: Rhomboid or coffin-shaped crystals of 0.5–5 μm, which are weak positively birefringent, are seen.

III. SOFT TISSUES

TUMOURS PA 33.3

Soft tissue is the supportive tissue of various organs and the nonepithelial, extraskeletal structures excluding lymphohaematopoietic tissues. The term soft tissue includes fibrous tissue, adipose tissue, synovial tissue, blood vessels, muscle, lymphatics and peripheral nervous system, embryologically derived from mesoderm, except peripheral nerves that are derived from ectoderm. Tumours of soft tissue are a heterogenous group of neoplasms that have been classified according to their histogenetic features. Benign tumours are more common than malignant. Malignant soft-tissue tumours commonly metastasize through blood to the lungs, liver, bones and brain unlike epithelial tumours that commonly metastasize through lymphatics.

Pathogenesis

Majority of soft-tissue tumours are sporadic and a minor fraction of the tumours is associated with genetic syndromes such as neurofibromatosis type 1 (NF1), Li–Fraumeni syndrome and Osler–Weber–Rendu syndrome. Environmental factors such as radiation and certain toxins are also implicated in the genesis of soft-tissue sarcomas. The genetics of sarcomas is heterogenous with 20% of tumours having simple karyotype, and around 80% of chromosomal abnormalities and mutations in genes are detected by molecular and cytogenetic studies of these tumours and are routinely used to complement traditional morphological studies. Chromosomal abnormalities commonly seen with soft-tissue tumours are listed in Table 30.8.

CLASSIFICATION

Soft-tissue tumours are classified on the basis of their clinical features and pathology.

Clinical classification includes the following categories:

- **Benign** – cured by completed excision, no recurrence, e.g. lipoma
- **Intermediate, locally aggressive** – locally infiltrative and destructive; no metastasizing; e.g. desmoid tumour
- **Intermediate, rarely metastasizing** – locally infiltrative, destructive and recurrent; 2% metastasize; e.g. dermatofibrosarcoma protuberance
- **Malignant** – locally infiltrative, destructive and recurrent; rate of metastasis high; e.g. rhabdomyosarcoma

Pathological classification of soft-tissue tumours is based on cellular differentiation, immunohistochemistry and molecular diagnostics. Important prognostic indicators are stage (size and depth) and grade (degree of differentiation).

TUMOURS OF ADIPOSE TISSUE

LIPOMA

Lipoma is a benign soft-tissue tumour composed of mature adipocytes with uniform nuclei resembling normal

Table 30.8 Chromosomal Abnormalities

Tumours	Cytogenetic Abnormality	Gene Fusion	Proposed Function
Ewing sarcoma	t(11;22)(q24;q12) t(21;22)(q22;q12)	EWS-FLI1 EWS-ERG	Disordered protein with multiple functions, including aberrant transcription, cell cycle regulation, RNA splicing and telomerase
Clear-cell sarcoma	t(12;22)(q13;q12)	EWS-ATF1	
Desmoplastic small round cell tumour	t(11;22)(p13;q12)	EWS-WT1	
Extraskeletal myxoid chondrosarcoma	t(9;22)(q22;q12)	EWS-CHN	
Myxoid liposarcoma	t(12;16)(q13;p11)	FUS-DDIT3	Adipocytic differentiation is arrested
Synovial sarcoma	t(x;18)(p11;q11)	SS18-SSX1 SS18-SSX2 SS18-SSX4	Chimeric transcription factor interrupts cell cycle control
Rhabdomyosarcoma – alveolar	t(2;13)(q35;q14)	PAX3-FOXO1 PAX7-FOXO1	Chimeric transcription factor, disrupt skeletal muscle differentiation
Alveolar soft part sarcoma	t(x;17)(p11;.2;q25)	TFE3-ASPL	Unknown
Nodular fasciitis	t(22;17)	MYN9-USP6	Unknown

fat. It is the most common mesenchymal and soft-tissue tumour of adulthood. Lipoma is subclassified into conventional lipoma, fibrolipoma, angiolipoma, spindle cell lipoma and myelolipoma. It is usually subcutaneous in location with the common sites being the trunk, back, shoulder, neck and proximal extremities.

Morphology

Gross: Lipoma appears as bright yellow homogeneous mass with thin fibrous capsule (only in superficial lesions) and trabeculae with greasy cut surface.
Microscopy: Encapsulated tumour with lobules of mature adipocytes separated by delicate fibrous septa is present.

LIPOSARCOMA

It is the most common sarcoma of adulthood. Malignant tumour is composed of adipocytes. Common incidence is fifth to seventh decade. Unlike lipoma that arises from the mature adipose tissue, liposarcoma arises from lipoblasts that are primitive mesenchymal cells and are deep seated. It is commonly seen in retroperitoneum and popliteal fossa.

Morphology

Gross: Circumscribed, infiltrative and nodular mass, 5 cm or more in diameter, is seen. The cut surface is grey-white to yellow, myxoid and gelatinous with areas of haemorrhage (Fig. 30.43).

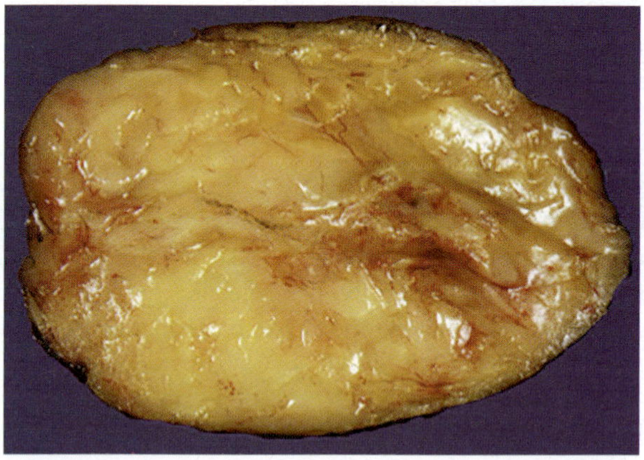

Fig. 30.43 Lipoma – gross. Note the circumscribed homogenous mass with greasy appearance and the presence of delicate capsule on the surface. (*Source:* From Andrew E. Horvai and Thomas Link. Lipoma and Lipomatosis. High-Yield Bone and Soft Tissue Pathology. Saunders 2012.)

Microscopy: Hallmark of diagnosis is the presence of univacuolated or multivacuolated lipoblasts. The vacuoles are due to the fat in the cytoplasm (Fig. 30.44).

Variants of Liposarcoma

Well-differentiated liposarcoma – varying adipocyte size, fibrous septations, atypical, hyperchromatic nuclei in adipocytes or stromal cells (lipoblasts may be present but are not required for the diagnosis) (Fig. 30.45A)
Myxoid liposarcoma – abundant basophilic ECM, scattered lipoblasts, delicate 'chicken-wire' or 'crow's feet' vasculature (Fig. 30.45B)

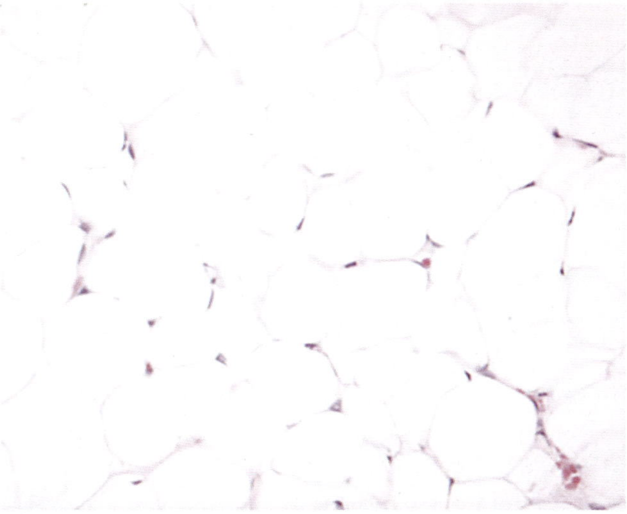

Fig. 30.44 Microscopy of lipoma – note the presence of uniform population of adipocytes with small eccentric nuclei. (*Source:* From Andrew E. Horvai and Thomas Link. Lipoma and Lipomatosis. High-Yield Bone and Soft Tissue Pathology. Saunders 2012.)

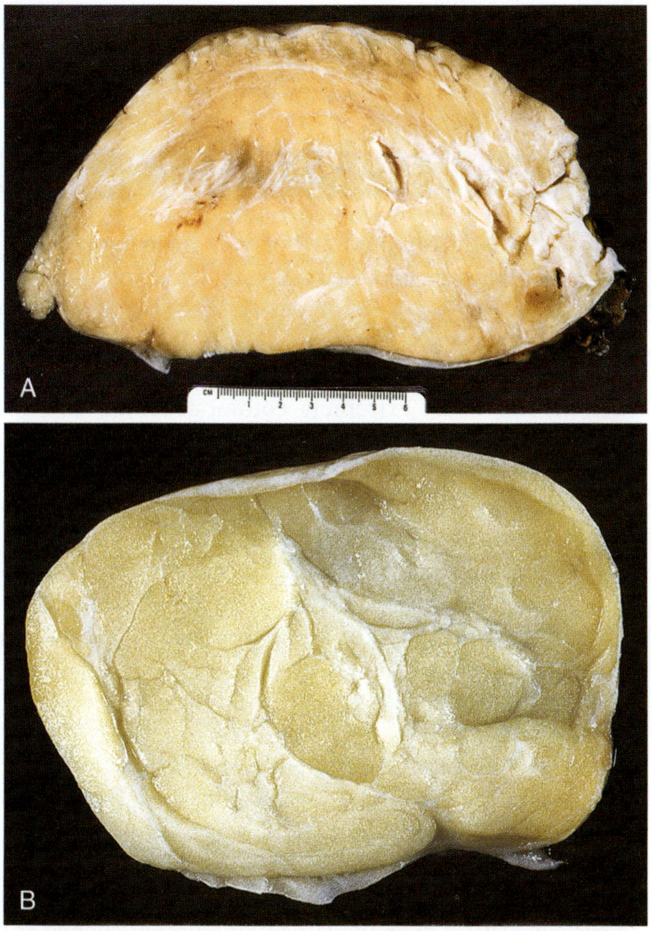

Fig. 30.45 Liposarcoma – gross. (A) Well-differentiated liposarcoma resembles lipoma and (B) myxoid liposarcoma. Note the gelatinous appearance. (*Source:* From John R. Goldblum, Andrew L. Folpe and Sharon W. Weiss. Liposarcoma. Enzinger and Weiss's Soft Tissue Tumors. 7th edition. Elsevier 2020.)

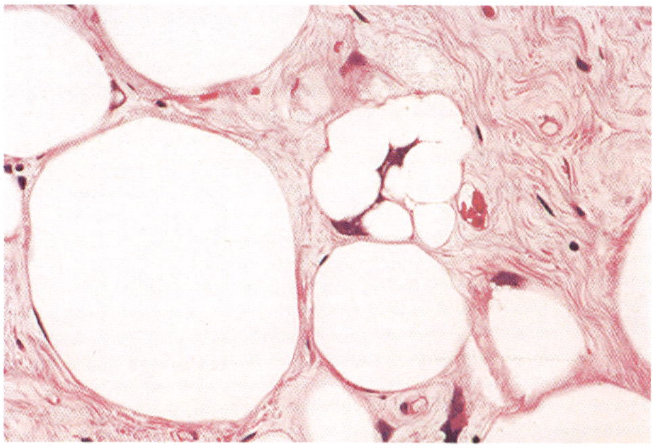

Fig. 30.46 Microscopy of liposarcoma – note the presence of multivacuolated lipoblast. (*Source:* From John R. Goldblum, Andrew L. Folpe and Sharon W. Weiss. Liposarcoma. Enzinger and Weiss's Soft Tissue Tumors. 7th edition. Elsevier 2020.)

Pleomorphic liposarcoma – sheets of anaplastic cells with bizarre nucleus and variable amounts of lipoblasts that are typically large and multivacuolated (Fig. 30.46)

FIBROUS TUMOURS

NODULAR FASCIITIS

Nodular fasciitis is a benign, self-limited proliferating lesion common among young adults in the upper extremity with 25% of cases having a previous history of trauma. It is a self-limited clonal neoplastic process that presents as a subcutaneous 'growth' over few weeks that eventually regresses. It shows fibroblastic and myofibroblastic proliferation. Nodular fasciitis spontaneously regresses or if excised, it rarely recurs.

Cytogenetics: MYH9-USP6 is the most common fusion product resultant of t(17;22) translocation.

Morphology

Gross: It is a solitary lesion seated in the deep dermis, subcutis or muscle. It is circumscribed, rarely infiltrative, with size of 5 cm or less in diameter.

Microscopy shows a vast array of pattern histologically and composed of uniform, plump, immature, spindled fibroblasts and myofibroblasts in fascicles (Fig. 30.47). A gradient of maturation (zonation) effect with peripheral hypercellular and central hypocellular is typical. Many times, it is seen with mucoid/myxoid pools (microcysts). Mitotic activity is abundant. Scattered lymphocytes, histiocytes and osteoclast-type giant cells might be present. Areas of extravasated erythrocytes are often present.

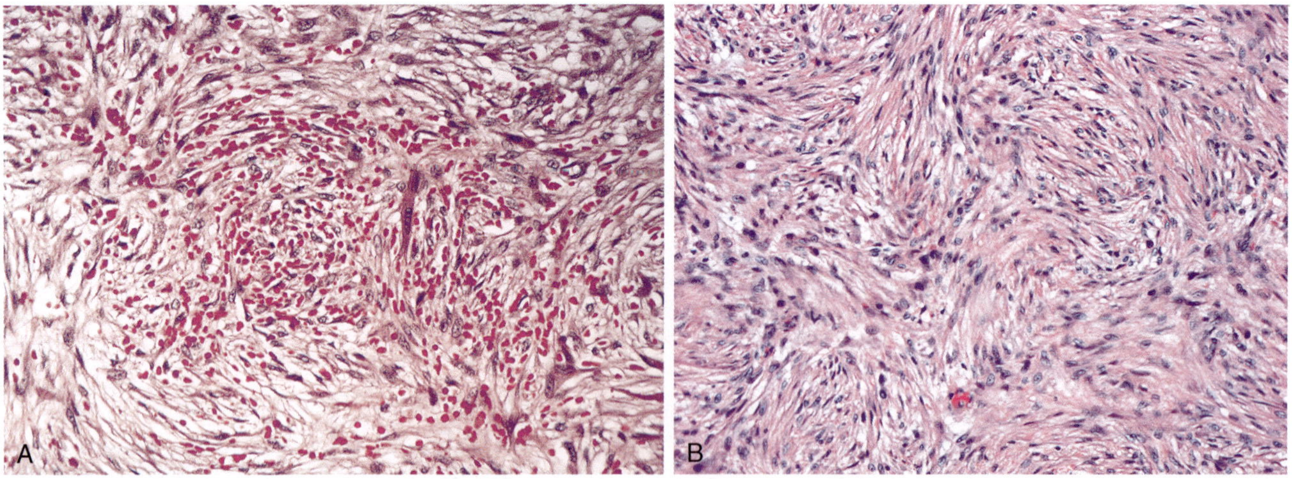

Fig. 30.47 Microscopy of nodular fasciitis. (A) Microhaemorrhages between bundles of fibroblasts and (B) storiform growth pattern in nodular fasciitis. (*Source:* From John R. Goldblum, Andrew L. Folpe and Sharon W. Weiss. Benign Fibroblastic/Myofibroblastic Proliferations, Including Superficial Fibromatoses. In Enzinger and Weiss's Soft Tissue Tumors. 7th edition. Elsevier 2020.)

FIBROMATOSIS

Fibromatosis can be superficial or deep depending on the plane of involvement.

Superficial fibromatosis is infiltrative fibroblastic proliferation causing local deformity. It is subclassified into palmar, plantar and penile clinically on the basis of the location. **Palmar (Dupuytren contracture)** is the most common subtype. Nodular proliferation of palmar aponeurosis either unilaterally or bilaterally leads to puckering and dimpling of the overlying skin over a period of time. This leads to flexion contractures affecting the fourth and fifth fingers of the hand. **Plantar** form is usually unilateral without contractures. **Penile (Peyronie disease)** is common in the dorsolateral aspect of the penis causing curvature towards the side of contractures (penile strabismus) or constriction of the urethra.

Deep fibromatosis, **also called desmoid tumour**, is a locally aggressive tumour that does not metastasize. It is more common among women aged 20–30 years. This is usually seen in the abdominal region (abdominal fibromatosis) and also seen in extra-abdominal sites such as the shoulder girdle or the mesentery. Mutations of APC or CTNNB1 (β-catenin) genes are common.

Morphology

Gross: It is typically 1–15 cm, and may be poorly defined or well circumscribed, grey-white and firm mass. The cut surface is gritty and coarsely trabeculated.
Microscopy: Long sweeping fascicles of bland fibroblasts set in a collagenous stroma are seen. Histology resembles a scar.

Fibromatosis is a benign tumour that may cause local deformity with a bland course (superficial fibromatosis) or with infiltrative borders and a propensity for local recurrence (deep fibromatosis). Although half of palmar and plantar fibromatoses progress, others do not. Recurrence is common even after excision. According to the World Health Organization, it is classified as an intermediate soft-tissue tumour related to the sarcoma family.

SMOOTH MUSCLE TUMOURS

Smooth muscle tumours are of two main types – the benign leiomyoma and the malignant leiomyosarcoma.

LEIOMYOMA

Leiomyoma is an extremely common benign smooth muscle tumour, which is also referred to as fibroid, myoma and leiomyofibroma. Leiomyoma mostly arises from the uterus and is also the most common neoplasm in women during reproductive years. Myomas that arise from the erector pili muscles are called pilar leiomyoma, which is seen in the skin, nipples, scrotum, etc. These tumours have been dealt with in detail in Chapter 26.

Leiomyosarcoma

Leiomyosarcoma is a malignant smooth muscle tumour that is common among adults, predominantly affecting women. It contributes to 10% of adult soft-tissue sarcomas. Most common uterine sarcoma often arises from the retroperitoneum and superficial or deep soft tissues. It is also seen arising from the large blood vessels such as the inferior vena cava. Its morphology has been dealt with in Chapter 26.

Leiomyosarcomas often present as painless firm tumours. Small, superficial or cutaneous tumours have a good prognosis. Retroperitoneal tumours are large, unresectable and fatal. For resectable tumours, treatment is excision with a clear margin. Death is often due to local recurrences and metastasis.

TUMOURS OF UNCERTAIN ORIGIN

A significant percentage of soft-tissue tumours lack obvious differentiation towards a defined mesenchymal tissue type. They are referred to as tumours of uncertain origin, after extensive workup.

SYNOVIAL SARCOMA

Synovial sarcoma is a malignant soft-tissue sarcoma with variable differentiation. The name is a misnomer because these tumours arise from places that lack synovium, and their morphological features are inconsistent with an origin from synoviocytes. Synovial sarcomas typically present as deep-seated masses close to the large joints, tendon sheaths, bursae and joint capsules. Common chromosomal translocation associated with this tumour is t(x;18)(p11;q11) involving genes SS18 and SSX1, SSX2 or SSX4. The most common locations are the lower extremities.

Morphology

Gross The size of the tumour varies depending on the growth rate. It grossly appears as grey white, round to multilobulated and encapsulated with the cut surface showing areas of haemorrhage, necrosis, foci of calcification and cystic spaces.

Microscopy Morphological types of synovial sarcoma include monophasic or biphasic:

Monophasic: Monotonous cells with scant cytoplasm, vesicular nucleus, dense chromatin and inconspicuous nucleoli growing in tightly packed fascicles are present.
Biphasic: Along with the above-mentioned features, it has additional gland-like structures composed of cuboidal to columnar epithelial cells. Myxoid matrix, calcification and hyalinization are also seen. In IHC, both variants of tumour cells are positive for cytokeratin (Fig. 30.48).
Poorly differentiated: Highly cellular round cells with hyperchromatic nuclei and frequent mitotic activity and necrosis are present.

Synovial sarcomas are aggressively treated with limb-sparing surgery and chemotherapy. In general, synovial sarcomas have high recurrence rates.

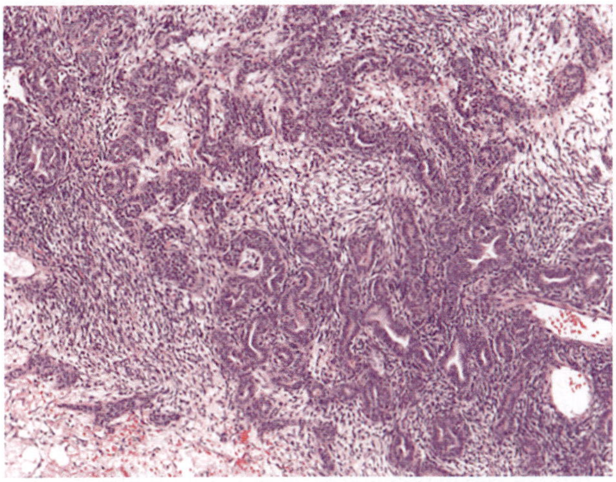

Fig. 30.48 Microscopy of synovial sarcoma with biphasic appearance. Note the close apposition of epithelial structures with malignant spindle cells. (*Source:* From John R. Goldblum, Andrew L. Folpe and Sharon W. Weiss. Other Malignant Soft Tissue Tumors, Including Those of Uncertain Type. In Enzinger and Weiss's Soft Tissue Tumors. 7th edition. Elsevier 2020.)

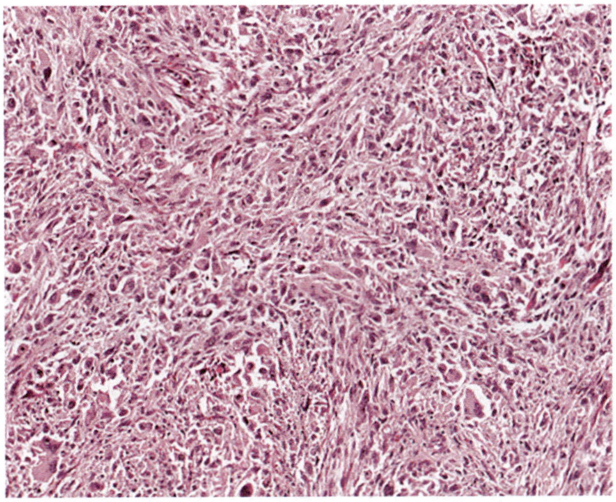

Fig. 30.49 Microscopy of undifferentiated pleomorphic sarcoma showing obvious pleomorphic cells arranged in vague storiform pattern. (*Source:* From John R. Goldblum, Andrew L. Folpe and Sharon W. Weiss. Undifferentiated Pleomorphic Sarcoma. In Enzinger and Weiss's Soft Tissue Tumors. 7th edition. Elsevier 2020.)

UNDIFFERENTIATED PLEOMORPHIC SARCOMA

Undifferentiated pleomorphic sarcoma (UPS) is a diagnosis of exclusion. It is a high-grade malignant mesenchymal tumour that cannot be categorized into another category with histomorphology, immunophenotyping or molecular genetics. Thorough search should be made to look for the presence of other components to rule out dedifferentiated sarcoma. Microscopically, the tumour is composed of fibroblasts, myofibroblasts and histiocyte-like cells (Fig. 30.49). UPSs are aggressive tumours that are treated aggressively.

IV. SKELETAL MUSCLES

The skeletal muscle is one of the three significant muscle tissues in the human body and has unique structural, cellular and molecular characteristics. It also possesses unique patterns of injury and repair. Skeletal muscle forms by fusion of mononucleated myoblasts to form multinucleated myotubes. Furthermore, they mature into myofibres of varying length that contain thousands of nuclei. Each skeletal muscle consists of thousands of myofibres wrapped together by connective tissue sheaths forming fascicles. Each fascicle contains a tiny pool of stem cells referred to as satellite cells that contribute to muscle regeneration after injury. The individual bundles of muscle fibres in a skeletal muscle are known as fasciculi. The outer connective tissue sheath surrounding the entire muscle is known as epimysium. The connective tissue sheath covering each fasciculus is known as perimysium, and the innermost sheath surrounding individual muscle fibre is known as endomysium. Each muscle fibre is composed of a number of myofibrils containing a number of myofilaments. When bundled together, all the myofibrils get arranged in a unique striated pattern forming sarcomeres that are the fundamental contractile unit of a skeletal muscle. The two most significant myofilaments are actin and myosin filaments that are arranged distinctively to form various bands on the skeletal muscle.

INHERITED DISEASES

Inherited diseases of skeletal muscle, also referred to as hereditary myopathies, are a heterogeneous group of inherited disorders characterized by progressive weakness and degeneration of skeletal muscles. This group of disorders is caused by mutations in different genes that encode for proteins that play major roles in muscle structure and function. Hence, muscle weakness and hypotonia are typical clinical manifestations in most of the hereditary myopathies. Histopathological features of many inherited myopathies may overlap and historically inherited myopathies are subdivided on the basis of inheritance pattern, pattern of muscle involvement, age of onset, clinical course and pathogenesis.

CONGENITAL MYOPATHIES

Congenital myopathies are a group of genetic muscle disorders characterized clinically by hypotonia and weakness. The disorder is usually present from birth, with a static or slowly progressive clinical course and, in some cases, delayed motor development later in childhood.

The three most common types of congenital myopathies are as follows:

- Central core and multiminicore myopathies (core myopathies) – autosomal dominant
- Centronuclear myopathy
- Nemaline myopathy

They are distinguished by their histological features, symptoms and prognosis.

The diagnosis of congenital myopathy is indicated by characteristic clinical findings and is confirmed by MRI of muscles and muscle biopsy. Recently, the genetic basis of many of the different forms of congenital myopathy has been identified and DNA testing is sometimes performed depending on the results of clinical evaluation and other tests.

Central Core Myopathy and Multiminicore Myopathy (Core Myopathies)

Central core myopathy and multiminicore myopathy (core myopathies) are the most common forms of congenital myopathy and are commonly associated with RYR1 (ryanodine receptor 1) 19q13.1 mutation. The mode of inheritance is autosomal dominant. Core myopathies are characterized by cytoplasmic cores on muscle biopsy in which oxidative enzyme staining is absent; regions may be peripheral or central, focal, multiple or extensive. Most affected patients develop hypotonia and muscle weakness. This may present as 'floppy infant' in neonates, but sometimes symptoms of core myopathy do not manifest until adulthood. Many infants also elicit facial weakness. Weakness is nonprogressive, and life expectancy is normal, but some patients are severely affected and may become wheelchair-bound. A fraction of patients has a high risk of developing malignant hyperthermia.

Centronuclear Myopathy

Centronuclear myopathy is characterized by the centralization of nuclei on muscle biopsy. This myopathy may be X-linked, autosomal dominant or autosomal recessive but most genes implicated encode membrane-trafficking proteins.

X-linked forms are the most common and most severe, and most affected children have weakness; some have more severe weakness and hypotonia at birth and do not survive beyond 1 year of life.

Autosomal dominant forms typically manifest in adolescence or adulthood with exercise-induced myalgia, bifacial weakness, ptosis and external ophthalmoplegia.

Centronuclear myopathy is characterized by many fibres containing nuclei in the geometric centre of the myofibres.

Nemaline Myopathy

Nemaline myopathy is one of the common congenital myopathies that can be autosomal dominant or recessive. Causative mutations have been identified in 10 genes and all are related to the production of thin-filament proteins.

Clinical features of nemaline myopathy may be severe, moderate or mild. Severely affected patients may have weakness of respiratory muscles and respiratory failure. Moderate disease causes progressive weakness in muscles of the face, neck, trunk and feet, but life expectancy may be near normal. Mild disease is nonprogressive and life expectancy is normal.

Treatment of congenital myopathy is supportive and includes physical therapy, which may help in preserving the function.

MUSCULAR DYSTROPHIES

Muscular dystrophies are a group of inherited, progressive muscle disorders resulting from defects in one or more genes needed for normal muscle structure and function, which typically manifest between childhood and adulthood.

Duchenne dystrophy is the most common form of muscular dystrophy, followed by Becker dystrophy and facioscapulohumeral dystrophy. Duchenne dystrophy is a more severe form, whereas Becker dystrophy has a later onset with milder symptoms. Common types with better understood pathogenesis are discussed here.

Duchenne Muscular Dystrophy and Becker Muscular Dystrophy

Duchenne muscular dystrophy follows the classical X-linked recessive inheritance pattern caused by mutations of the dystrophin gene, the largest known human gene, at the Xp21.2 loci. Majority of Duchenne dystrophies are caused by a single or multiexon deletion or duplication. In Becker dystrophy, majority of the patients have a deletion.

Pathogenesis Duchenne and Becker muscular dystrophies are caused by the loss-of-function mutations in the dystrophin gene located on the X chromosome, a 427-kDa protein found on the cytoplasmic surface of the plasma membrane of muscle fibres (the sarcolemma) in skeletal and cardiac muscles. These disorders are referred to as dystrophinopathies.

Dystrophin provides mechanical stability to the sarcolemma and is likely involved in force transmission between the intracellular contractile apparatus and ECM, which envelops the fibre and is connected to the tendon (Fig. 30.50). In the absence of dystrophin, the sarcolemma becomes fragile and is unable to withstand the stress of normal muscle contractions. This leads to increased intracellular Ca^{2+}, which activates proteases that result in muscle death or necrosis. Necrotic fibres become replaced by fat, which can be an apparent 'pseudohypertrophy', especially in the muscles of the lower leg associated with weakness (Fig. 30.51). Dystrophin is also seen in cardiac muscle and in the central nervous system; hence, both are affected.

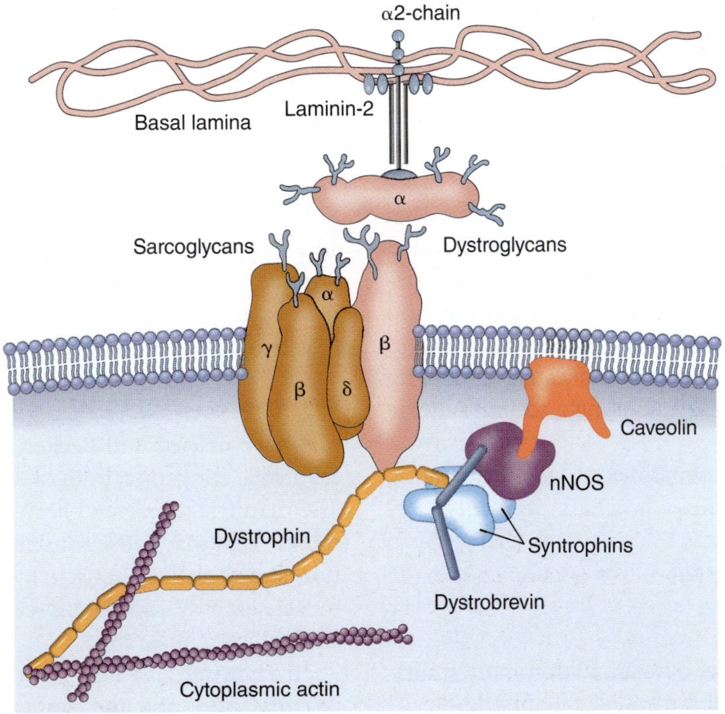

Fig. 30.50 Relationship between the cell membrane (sarcolemma) and the sarcolemma-associated proteins. (*Source:* From Peter Pytel and Douglas C. Anthony. Peripheral Nerves and Skeletal Muscles. Robbins & Cotran Pathologic Basis of Disease. 10th edition. Elsevier 2021.)

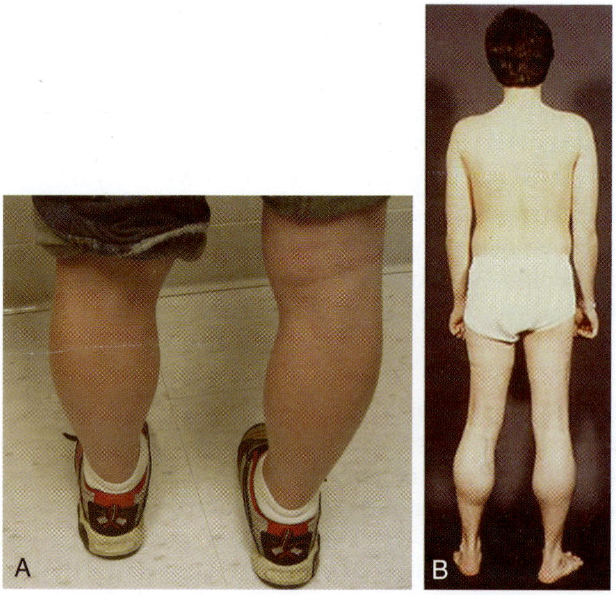

Fig. 30.51 (A) Calf pseudohypertrophy in an 8-year-old boy with Duchenne muscular dystrophy and (B) Becker muscular dystrophy in a 24-year-old man. Dystrophy of the shoulder girdle and calf pseudohypertrophy are evident. (*Source:* From William J. Groh, Gordon F. Tomaselli and Douglas P. Zipes. Neurologic Disorders and Cardiovascular Disease. Braunwald's Heart Disease: A Textbook of Cardiovascular Medicine. 11th edition. Elsevier 2019.)

Morphology

Morphological changes include marked variation in myofibre size with segmental myofibre degeneration and regeneration associated with small, atrophic fibres. Increased endomysial fibrosis and fatty replacement of muscle is a characteristic feature of disease progression. IHC shows complete absence of membrane-associated dystrophin.

As the disease is X-linked, females are carriers of the mutation and are asymptomatic or may be mildly affected when there is unfavourable lyonization. Diagnosis is suspected by characteristic clinical findings, age at onset and family history suggestive of X-linked inheritance. Serum creatinine kinase is elevated 100 times because of ongoing muscle damage. Genetic studies will help to find out the dystrophin mutation.

Treatment of dystrophinopathies is still challenging and supportive care remains the main modality. Researches are ongoing towards offering gene therapy as a successful plan of management.

Myotonic Dystrophy

Myotonic dystrophy is a rare autosomal dominant multisystem disorder associated with skeletal muscle weakness. The disease affects both voluntary and involuntary muscles.

The disease is characterized by myotonia – delayed relaxation after muscle contraction, weakness and wasting of distal limb muscles (especially in the hand) and facial muscles (ptosis is especially common) and cardiomyopathy. Cataracts and endocrinopathy can also occur. Two types are recognized, with different genetic loci. DM 1 involves a mutation of the DMPK (myotonic dystrophy protein kinase) gene located on chromosome 19. DM 2 is a milder form that involves mutation of ZNF9 gene located on chromosome 3.

Emery–Dreifuss Dystrophy

Emery–Dreifuss dystrophy (EMD) is a disease with multiple modes of inheritance. Muscle weakness and wasting can begin any time before age 20 years and commonly affect the biceps and triceps. Genes associated with EMD encode nuclear lamina proteins, and it is caused by mutations in the gene encoding lamin A/C (autosomal) and emerin (X-linked).

Early contractures are characteristic of the disease. Cardiomyopathies associated with conduction abnormalities are associated with a high likelihood of sudden death.

Facioscapulohumeral Muscular Dystrophy

Facioscapulohumeral muscular dystrophy (FSHD) is characterized by weakness of facial muscle and shoulder girdle. It is an autosomal dominant disorder. FSHD is caused by abnormal expression of the DUX4 gene, which is located on the long arm of chromosome 4.

Limb-Girdle Muscular Dystrophy

Limb-girdle muscular dystrophy is a group of heterogeneous disorders that includes autosomal dominant and autosomal recessive disorders. The disease often begins in childhood and is slowly progressive, impacting the proximal muscles. Several chromosomal loci have been identified for autosomal dominant (5q) and recessive (2q, 4q [beta-sarcoglycan], 13q [gamma-sarcoglycan], 15q [calpain, a calcium-activated protease] and 17q [alpha-sarcoglycan or adhalin]) forms. Structural (e.g. dystrophin-associated glycoproteins) or nonstructural (e.g. proteases) proteins can be affected.

Myotonia Congenita

Thomsen disease and Becker disease are the two forms of myotonia congenita, both of which involve the same gene. The manifestations are because of delay in contraction of muscle that may cause muscle stiffness. Clinical examination shows skeletal muscle hypertrophy due to sustained muscle activity and the increased muscle bulk gives them an 'athletic' appearance.

In Thomsen disease, the onset is in the first year of life or early childhood and starts in the upper limbs and face, whereas in Becker disease, it begins later in childhood in the lower limbs, and has muscle hypertrophy.

INFLAMMATORY MYOPATHIES

Inflammatory disorders of skeletal muscle include polymyositis, dermatomyositis and inclusion body myositis (IBM). Dermatomyositis occurs in children and adults, whereas all the other forms of myositis develop mostly in middle-aged individuals. The diagnosis is challenging and usually requires testing of autoantibodies, skeletal muscle biopsy, histological evaluation, MRI and Electromyography (EMG).

Dermatomyositis

Dermatomyositis is a multisystem autoimmune disease that affects children and adults, characterized clinically by progressive symmetrical proximal muscle weakness and specific skin manifestations, including Gottron papules (scaling erythematous eruptions or dusky red patches over the knees, knuckles, elbows), heliotrope rash (lilac-coloured lesions over the upper eyelids) and macular erythema (Fig. 30.52). The disease primarily affects small blood vessels, which is the basis of muscular damage and also leads to changes that can be seen, which are telangiectasias in the nail folds, eyelids and gums.

Pathogenesis Dermatomyositis is associated with antibodies, especially antinuclear antibodies (ANA). Majority of people with dermatomyositis test positive for ANA and lesser population of people has myositis-specific autoantibodies that include anti-Mi2 antibodies (directed against a helicase involved in nucleosome remodelling), anti-Jo1 antibodies (directed against the enzyme histidyl t-RNA synthetase) and anti-P155/P140 antibodies (directed against many transcriptional regulators).

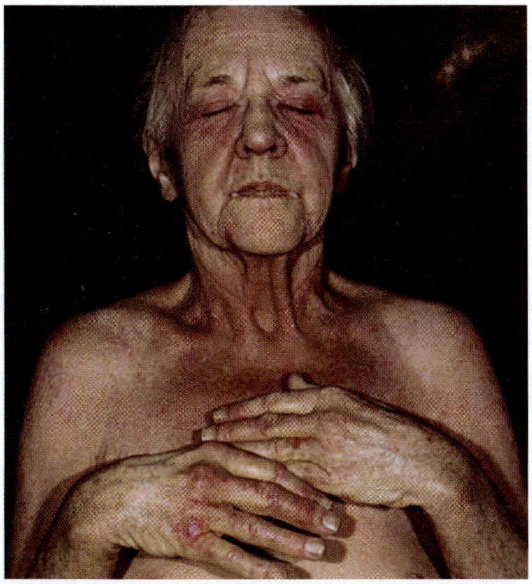

Fig. 30.52 Dermatomyositis – Gottron papules on finger joints and periorbital heliotrope rash in dermatomyositis. (*Source:* From James G.H. Dinulos. Connective Tissue Diseases. Habif's Clinical Dermatology. 7th edition. Elsevier 2021.)

Morphology

Muscle biopsy shows the presence of mononuclear inflammatory infiltrate, especially in the perimysial connective tissue and around blood vessels. Perifascicular atrophy is the distinct feature of dermatomyositis (Fig. 30.53). Segmental fibre necrosis and regeneration are also noted. The endothelial cells become swollen and necrotic, and develop tubuloreticular inclusions and microvacuoles that are linked to a type 1 interferon response, seen with an electron microscope.

The disease may affect adults or children and the patients experience slow-onset muscle weakness and myalgia. One-third of patients develop dysphagia because of the involvement of oesophageal and oropharyngeal muscles. Cardiac involvement is commonly seen, whereas cardiac failure is rare.

Polymyositis

Polymyositis is an adult-onset inflammatory myopathy related to dermatomyositis and IBM. Patients typically present with weakness and/or loss of muscle mass in the proximal musculature and there may be inflammatory involvement of the heart and the lungs.

Pathogenesis Polymyositis is characterized by T-cell-mediated injury. Infiltrating $CD8^+$ and $CD4^+$ T cells are prominent in affected muscles.

Morphology

The inflammatory infiltrate in polymyositis is found in the endomysium (Fig. 30.54). Degenerating necrotic, regenerating and atrophic myofibres are found in random or patchy distribution. Perifascicular atrophy and perivasculitis are absent unlike in dermatomyositis.

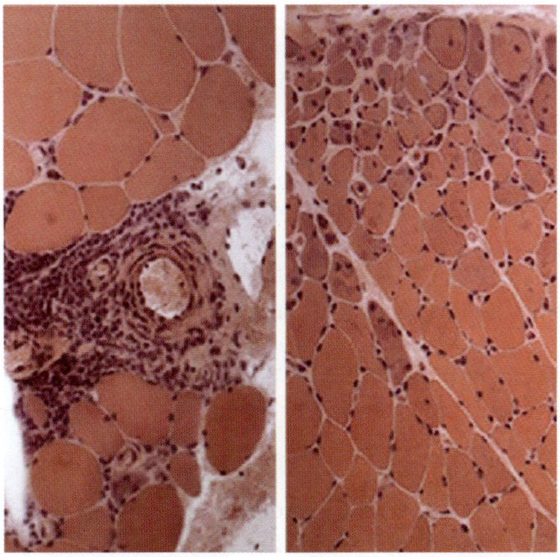

Fig. 30.53 Microscopy of dermatomyositis with dense inflammatory infiltrate at perivascular site and prominent perifascicular atrophy.

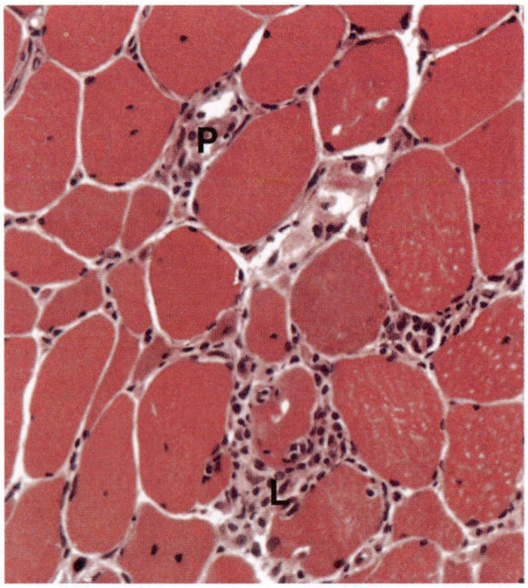

Fig. 30.54 Microscopy of polymyositis with the characteristic appearance of necrosis of individual muscle fibres, a lymphoid infiltrate (L) and phagocytosis (P) of muscle fibre debris. (*Source:* From Geraldine O'Dowd, Sarah Bell and Sylvia Wright. Nervous system. In Wheater's Pathology: A Text, Atlas, and Review of Histopathology. 6th edition. Elsevier 2020.)

Inclusion Body Myositis

IBM is an autoimmune chronic progressive myopathy seen in patients older than 50 years. It is also the most common myopathy seen in individuals older than 65 years. Severe weakness in quadriceps more than in hip flexors and a weakness of finger flexors more than of shoulder abductors are observed.

Pathogenesis Activation of T cells is central to the disease and is likely an antigen-driven response, which is suggested by the presence of abundant antigen-presenting cells in the muscle fibres. Antibody to cN1A (cytosolic 5′-nucleotidase) has also been recently described in the pathogenesis of IBM.

Morphology

Inflammatory cell infiltrate rich in cytotoxic $CD8^+$ T cells with macrophages invading and the $CD4^+$ T cells and macrophages surrounding the non-necrotic muscle fibres is a prominent feature. 'Rimmed vacuoles' (abnormal cytoplasmic inclusions) are seen with Gomori trichrome stain (Fig. 30.55). Tubulofilamentous inclusions are seen in myofibres by electron microscopy. In chronic cases, endomysial fibrosis and fatty replacement are seen.

Patients with inflammatory myopathies are treated with immunosuppressants that improve the prognosis of dermatomyositis and polymyositis, whereas IBM responds poorly.

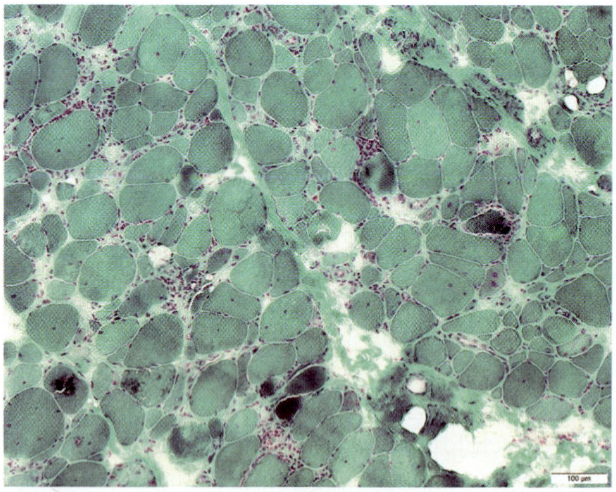

Fig. 30.55 Microscopy of inclusion body myositis showing inflammation, aggregates and vacuoles (Gomori trichrome stain).

TOXIC MYOPATHIES

Toxic myopathy is a diverse group of disorders affecting skeletal muscles caused by a variety of medications and toxins. Many substances including commonly prescribed medications can produce adverse effects on muscle, causing toxic myopathies. Cholesterol-lowering medications such as statins have been the most widely prescribed drugs that have been described to cause a myopathy. Long-term administration of chloroquine or hydroxychloroquine for treatment of systemic autoimmune disorders causes progressive muscle weakness in a significant number of patients. Alcohol can cause necrotizing myopathy leading to rhabdomyolysis, myoglobinuria and renal failure. Clinical features range from mild muscle pain and cramps to severe weakness with rhabdomyolysis, renal failure and even death. Hypothyroidism, hyperthyroidism (thyrotoxic myopathy) and hyperparathyroidism are common causes of elevated CK and muscle weakness with external ophthalmoplegia and always should be considered when toxic myopathy is suspected.

A past and present medication history is important, because withdrawing the offending agent usually leads to improvement of myopathy because the muscle cells have the capacity to regenerate.

SKELETAL MUSCLE TUMOURS

TUMOURS

Rhabdomyoma and rhabdomyosarcoma are the tumours of striated muscles. Most often, they are malignant.

RHABDOMYOMA

Rhabdomyoma is a rare benign tumour with mature skeletal muscle differentiation. The most common locations are the upper neck, tongue, larynx and pharynx. This tumour is frequently associated with individuals with tuberous sclerosis.

MORPHOLOGY

Gross

Tumours range in size from 1 to 3 cm and are soft, circumscribed with tan-red-brown colour. They may have a nodular or lobulated appearance.

Microscopy

Rhabdomyomas are circumscribed but unencapsulated. The tumour cells are large, round to oval with eosinophilic cytoplasm, often vacuolated containing glycogen. The cells with vacuolated appearance are referred to as spider cells because of the appearance similar to spider webs. Special stain used is phosphotungstic acid–haematoxylin (PTAH) to demonstrate cross-striations. No mitotic activity or atypia is seen unlike in rhabdomyosarcoma.

The tumour cells are positive for PAS because of their glycogen content and are also positive for skeletal muscle markers such as muscle-specific actin, desmin and myoglobin by IHC.

Excision of the tumour is generally curative, but may recur if incompletely excised.

RHABDOMYOSARCOMA (RMS)

Rhabdomyosarcoma is a malignant soft-tissue tumour with skeletal muscle phenotype. There are four subtypes of the tumour, although mixtures are common:

- Embryonal (most common in childhood/adolescence)
- Alveolar
- Pleomorphic (predominant in adults)
- Spindle cell or sclerosing

Most of the lesions in children are seen in the head and neck, and genitourinary tract. Among adolescents, the common sites are the paratesticular, trunk and abdominal regions.

There is also site predilection for the variants of the tumour. Head and neck tumours are more often embryonal types. Extremity tumours are more often have alveolar histological type and 80% of genitourinary RMS are embryonal type.

Alveolar rhabdomyosarcomas possess fusion of FOXO1 gene with PAX3 or PAX7 because of t(2;13) or t(1,13). PAX3 is a transcription factor that plays a role in skeletal muscle differentiation and the fusion protein interferes with differentiation process. The other subtypes of rhabdomyosarcoma are genetically varied.

MORPHOLOGY

Embryonal rhabdomyosarcoma usually appears before 20 years and is the most common subtype seen in childhood and adolescence. The malignant cells resemble skeletal muscle of various stages of embryogenesis containing sheets of round and spindle cells in a myxoid matrix. Cells with visible cross-striations (rhabdomyoblast/strap cells) are present. When they develop along the walls of the hollow, mucosa-lined structures (bladder, vagina, nasopharynx), they are called 'sarcoma botryoides' because of their appearance being similar to a bunch of grapes. The botryoid variant frequently shows a 'cambium layer', which is a hypercellular area due to tumour cell condensation just beneath the epithelial layer. It has a better prognosis.

Alveolar rhabdomyosarcoma usually occurs before 20 years of age. Tumour is composed of nests of malignant cells arranged in alveolar spaces adhering peripherally (hobnail/tombstone appearance). The neoplastic cells are uniform, round with little cytoplasm. Occasional strap cells are present.

Pleomorphic rhabdomyosarcoma is a high-grade sarcoma containing undifferentiated cells. Cross-striations are rarely seen. Tumours may express myogenin, desmin and myosin; the demonstration becomes essential to establish the skeletal muscle origin. This type carries a poor prognosis.

Spindle cell or sclerosing rhabdomyosarcomas are characterized by the fascicular or storiform arrangement of spindle-shaped cells with or without the presence of rhabdomyoblasts.

Rhabdomyosarcomas are aggressive tumours and are treated with surgical excision and chemotherapy with or without radiotherapy. Prognosis is also influenced by the type and site of the tumour.

V. PERIPHERAL NERVE SHEATH TUMOURS

TUMOURS

Majority of peripheral nerve sheath tumours show Schwann cell differentiation. They can be both benign and malignant. These tumours can be located within the dura or in the periphery, along the course of the nerves.

Three common types are schwannoma, neurofibroma and malignant peripheral nerve sheath tumour (MPNST).

The special features of peripheral nerve sheath tumours are as follows:

- Malignant transformation of a preexisting benign tumour is rare.
- Peripheral nerve sheath tumours have a common association with familial tumour syndromes such as NF1, NF2 and schwannomatosis.

- Malignant transformation of preexisting benign plexiform neurofibroma is a common event in the context of NF1.

SCHWANNOMA

Schwannoma is a benign, encapsulated tumour of the nerve sheath with Schwann cell differentiation.

PATHOGENESIS

Schwannomas may occur spontaneously or may be associated with familial tumour syndromes like NF2, schwannomatosis or Carney syndrome. NF2 may be due to a loss-of-function mutation in the protein merlin. The NF2 gene on chromosome 22, the merlin gene (also called schwannomin), encodes for the merlin protein. Specific gene mutations in the NF2 gene cause the inactivation of the gene, thus preventing the formation of the merlin protein.

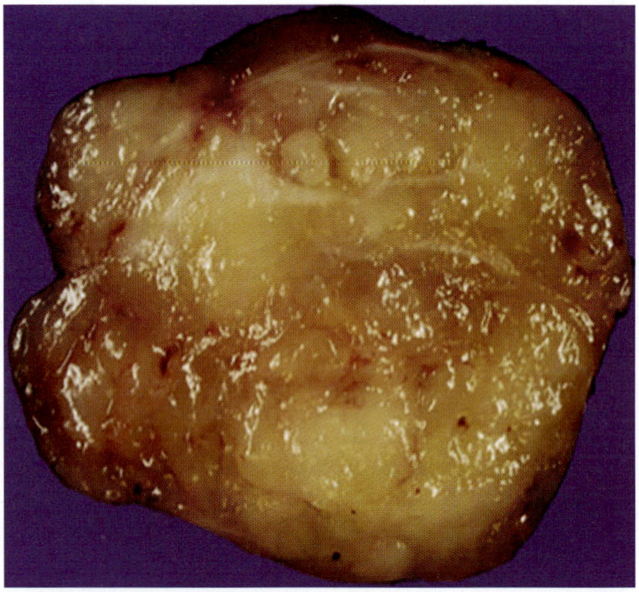

Fig. 30.56 Schwannoma – gross. The cut surface showing the typical yellow-tan, solid, somewhat lobulated appearance. (*Source:* From Andrew E. Horvai and Thomas Link. Schwannoma. High-Yield Bone and Soft Tissue Pathology. Saunders 2012.)

CLINICAL FEATURES

It is more common in the upper limbs, followed by the head and neck area. Pain and neurological symptoms are uncommon unless the tumour is large and there is compression to the involved nerve or adjacent structures. Lesions in proximal nerves may cause distal symptoms. If these masses occur in well-defined compartments (e.g. wrist or ankle), they can present as either carpal tunnel or tarsal tunnel syndrome. Similarly, involvement of the vestibular branch of the eighth nerve can cause tinnitus and hearing loss. Deep-seated tumours are mainly in the posterior mediastinum and retroperitoneum.

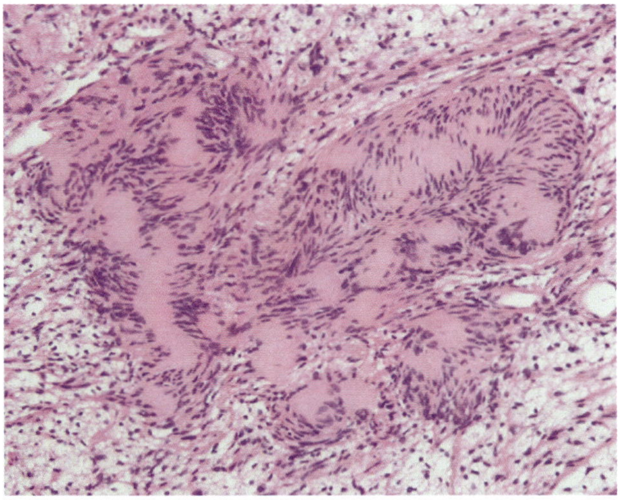

Fig. 30.57 Schwannoma – microscopy showing Antoni A, B areas and nuclear palisading. (*Source:* Chen S., Badve S. (2018) Schwannoma, Mediastinal. In: Allen T.C., Suster S. (eds) Pathology of the Pleura and Mediastinum. Encyclopedia of Pathology. Springer, Cham.)

MORPHOLOGY

Gross

Tumour is usually solitary, firm, glistening and grey mass (Fig. 30.56). Capsule is derived from the perineurium and the nerve of origin may be present at the periphery. Large tumours may be cystic.

Microscopy

Schwannomas are well-circumscribed, encapsulated tumours with biphasic pattern composed of dense and loose areas. **Antoni A areas** are dense cellular regions with predominantly benign spindle cells in many intersecting fascicles; they may palisade around eosinophilic regions and a nuclear-free zone. Nuclear palisading around fibrillary processes called Verocay bodies is often seen in cellular areas that are positive for S100 staining. In **Antoni B areas**, cells are loose and less cellular and have a background of loose connective tissue that is myxomatous in appearance (Fig. 30.57). Large tumours may be cystic and areas of haemorrhage may also be seen. IHC is positive for S100.

NEUROFIBROMA

Neurofibroma is the most common benign nerve sheath tumour composed of Schwann cells admixed with perineurial-like cells, fibroblasts, mast cells and $CD34^+$ spindle cells. Neurofibromas are either sporadic or inherited which are NF1 associated and are caused by a biallelic inactivation of the tumour suppressor gene NF1 that is located on 17q11.2.

There are three main types of neurofibromas – superficial, diffuse and plexiform.

Superficial neurofibromas are pedunculated well-circumscribed nodules in the dermis or subcutaneous tissue; they are solitary in case of sporadic and multiple in NF1 associated.

Diffuse neurofibromas are poorly defined tumours with expansile proliferation around adnexal structures, extending into the subcutaneous tissue and adipose tissue; they present as elevated lesions on the skin.

Plexiform neurofibroma is pathognomonic for NF1 with an increased risk of malignant transformation.

PATHOGENESIS

Neurofibromas are caused by a biallelic inactivation of the tumour suppressor gene NF1 that is located on 17q11.2. As explained in Chapter 7, neurofibromin inhibits RAS activity by stimulating the activity of GTPase. Decreased production of neurofibromin protein, which is a tumour suppressor, results in various clinical features.

MORPHOLOGY

Grossly, neurofibromas are tan white with a glistening cut surface (Fig. 30.58).

Microscopy

Superficial Cutaneous Tumour Superficial cutaneous neurofibromas are small unencapsulated tumours containing cellular elements such as neoplastic Schwann cells, axons admixed with perineurial-like cells, fibroblasts, $CD34^+$ spindle cells and mast cells with mucinous stroma and collagen (Fig. 30.59).

Diffuse Neurofibroma These are morphologically similar to superficial cutaneous neurofibromas, but these are poorly circumscribed and spread laterally along the tissue planes diffusely infiltrating the dermis and subcutaneous connective tissue. They frequently show **organoid structures resembling Meissner corpuscles.**

Plexiform Neurofibroma This variant consists of **thickened nerve fascicles** that appear **tortuous** (entrapping associated axons) because they are sectioned in various planes. At times, these are referred to as 'bag of worm' because of their appearance. There is an increased amount of myxoid matrix in the endoneurium. Lesions with increased cellularity and nuclear atypia are more prone to malignant transformation.

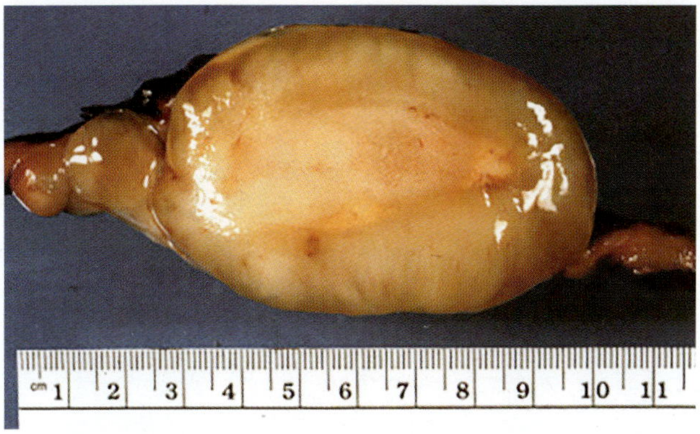

Fig. 30.58 Neurofibroma – gross. Note the fusiform expansion of the nerve involved. (*Source:* From John R. Goldblum, Andrew L. Folpe and Sharon W. Weiss. Benign Tumors of Peripheral Nerves. Enzinger and Weiss's Soft Tissue Tumors. 7th edition. Elsevier 2020.)

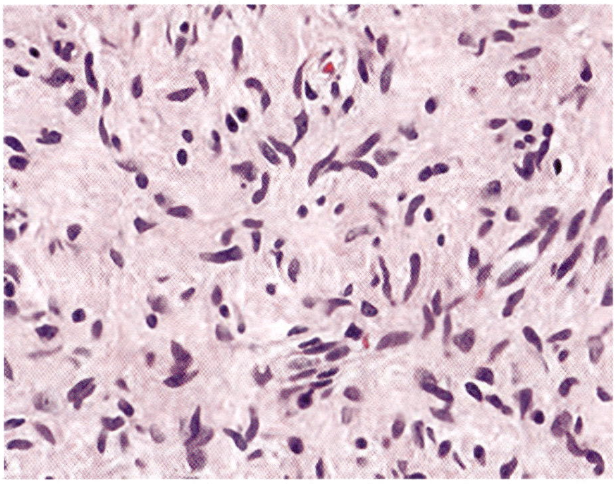

Fig. 30.59 Neurofibroma – microscopy showing spindle cells with wavy nuclei without pleomorphism, arranged in fascicles and intermixed with (wire-like) collagen.

Schwann cells in neurofibromas are strongly positive for S100.

Plexiform neurofibromas when multiple and deep seated have a high risk of transforming into a malignant nerve sheath tumour in a subset of patients with NF1 and hence need surgical excision and close follow-up.

NEUROFIBROMATOSIS TYPE 1 AND TYPE 2

Neurofibromatosis Type 1

NF1 is an autosomal dominant disorder belonging to a group of inherited cancer predisposition syndromes caused by germline mutations in the genes of RAS/mitogen-activated protein kinase (MAPK pathway) (Fig. 30.60). It is caused by genetic defect in the tumour suppressor gene NF1 located on chromosome 17q11, which encodes neurofibromin.

Clinical Features Diagnostic criteria of NF1 are met if two or more of the following are present:

- $\geq$6 café-au-lait patches $>$0.5 cm in prepubertal individuals or $>$1.5 cm in postpubertal individuals

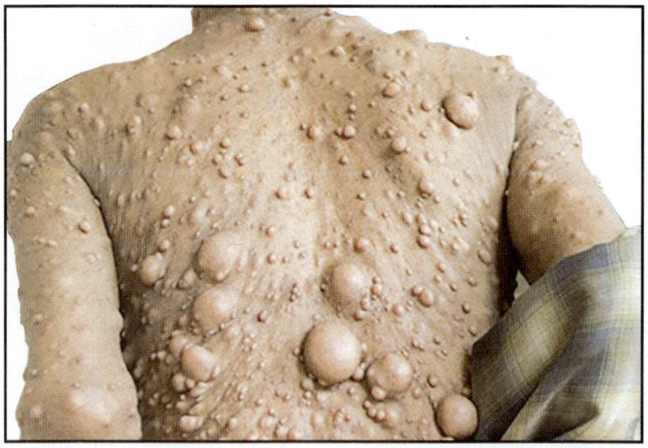

Fig. 30.60 Neurofibromatosis type 1 with multiple cutaneous neurofibromas.

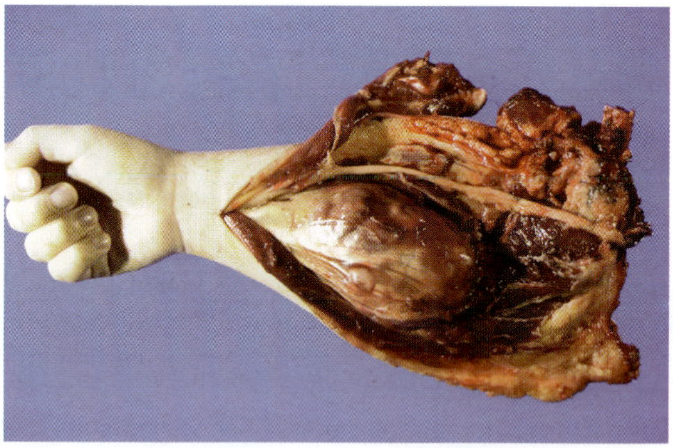

Fig. 30.61 Amputated specimen showing MPNST arising from a forearm nerve. (*Source:* Image courtesy of drbloodmoney on Flickr. CC BY SA 2.0.)

- ≥2 neurofibromas of any type or 1 plexiform neurofibroma
- Axillary or inguinal freckling
- ≥2 Lisch nodules (pigmented nodules of the iris)
- Optic glioma
- Sphenoid dysplasia or thinning of long bone cortex with or without pseudoarthrosis
- First-degree relative diagnosed with NF1

Other features include mental retardation, seizures, skeletal defects, Gastrointestinal stromal tumor (GIST), gynaecomastia and non-neural tumours such as pheochromocytoma.

Different forms include segmental NF, gastrointestinal NF, familial spinal and familial café-au-lait spots.

Neurofibromatosis Type 2

It is also an autosomal dominant disorder, affecting 1 in 40,000 individuals. It occurs because of the inactivating germline mutation in NF2 located in chromosome 22q12.2. This locus codes for the protein merlin also called schwannomin, which is involved in the formation and movement of cells. The severity is based on the type of mutation. Nonsense and frameshift mutations cause more severe phenotypes.

Clinical Features The hallmark feature of NF2 is bilateral vestibular schwannoma (diagnostic feature of this syndrome), causing tinnitus and hearing loss. Other manifestations include cutaneous schwannoma, meningioma, ependymoma, neurofibroma and glioma. Tumours of NF2 located in the brain or in the spinal cord may cause morbidity and reduced life span.

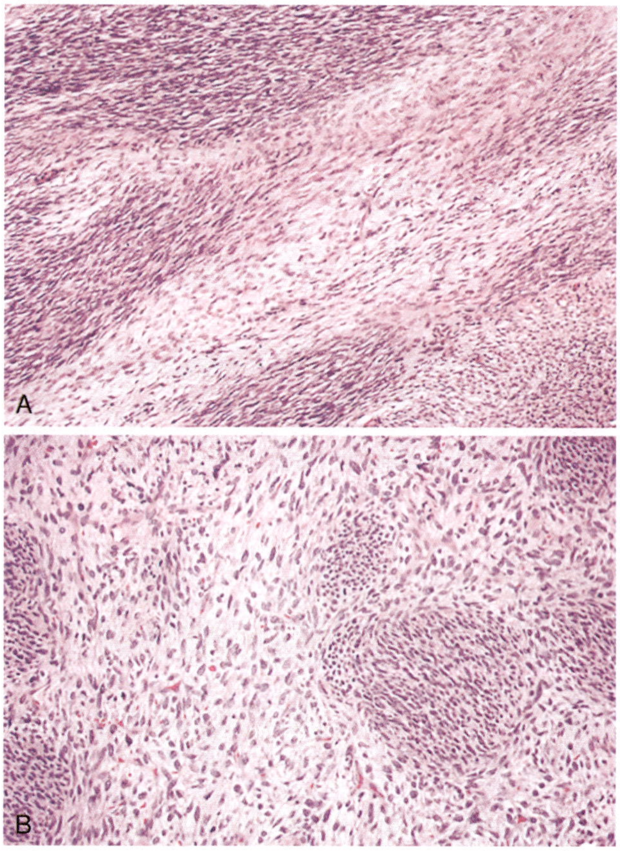

Fig. 30.62 MPNST – microscopy. (A and B) Typical appearance of MPNST with densely cellular areas alternating with less cellular areas, creating a marbleized appearance. (*Source:* From John R. Goldblum, Andrew L. Folpe and Sharon W. Weiss. Malignant Peripheral Nerve Sheath Tumors. Enzinger and Weiss's Soft Tissue Tumors. 7th edition. Elsevier 2020.)

MALIGNANT PERIPHERAL NERVE SHEATH TUMOUR

MPNST are high-grade neoplasms arising from the peripheral nerves. These tumours arise from a preexisting nerve sheath tumour in NF1 that is due to a genetic mutation on the 17th chromosome, which causes tumours along the nervous system or in the setting of prior radiation therapy. At least half of the cases can be sporadic with no association with NF1 and prior radiation. Although the tumours can arise from any anatomic location, the most common sites are the trunk and extremities, followed by that head and neck.

MORPHOLOGY

Gross

Tumours are larger than 5 cm, fusiform to globoid, large, fleshy and pseudoencapsulated with areas of haemorrhage and necrosis (Fig. 30.61).

Microscopy

There is marbling appearance under low power because of the presence of hyper- and hypocellular areas with perivascular accentuation. Individual tumour cells have anaplastic nuclear features, whorled structures and epithelioid appearance of perivascular tumour cells noted with areas of mitosis and necrosis (Fig. 30.62). Heterologous differentiation in the form of skeletal muscle or other elements is seen in 10%–15% of cases.

IHC is positive for S100 (only in 50% of cases); nestin and SOX10 favour a diagnosis of MPNST.

MPNSTs have generally aggressive behaviour with frequent metastatic disease and local recurrence.

SELF-ASSESSMENT

Self-Assessment Questions

1. A 62-year-old postmenopausal woman came with complaints of severe low back pain following minor injury. Radiological examination revealed fracture of L4–L5 vertebrae with shortening and flattening. What is the most probable diagnosis? Discuss the aetiopathogenesis, morphology and diagnostic workup of the disease.
2. A 65-year-old male patient was brought with features of quadriparesis. On examination and investigations, he was found to have kyphosis and spinal cord compression. He also had enlargement of the skull, breathlessness, pedal oedema and other features of cardiac failure. What is your probable diagnosis? Discuss the pathogenesis and morphological features of the disease.
3. A 12-year-old male child was brought with complaints of fever, fatigue, loss of weight and intense pain over the shin. Blood investigations revealed neutrophilia with toxic changes. What is your probable diagnosis? Discuss the aetiopathogenesis and morphological features of the disease.
4. A 16-year-old male patient was brought with complaints of breathlessness. There was also history of easy fatiguability and loss of appetite and weight. On examination, it was found that he had a mass around the knee that was found to be destructive with infiltrative margins. What is your probable diagnosis? Discuss the aetiopathogenesis, morphological features and investigations performed for the disease.
5. A 35-year-old man presented with pathological fracture of the proximal humerus. Radiological examination revealed the presence of lytic lesion. The lesion was excised, which appeared as honeycomb on gross examination. What is your probable diagnosis? Discuss the aetiopathogenesis and morphological features of the disease.
6. A 52-year-old woman presented with pathological fracture of the pelvis. Radiological examination revealed the presence of lytic lesion in the pelvic bone. PET scan revealed the presence of multiple bony lesions along with increased uptake in the left breast. What is your probable diagnosis? Discuss the aetiopathogenesis and morphological features of the disease.
7. A 33-year-old woman came with complaints of knee joint pain and early morning stiffness that is progressive in nature. On examination, she also had multiple subcutaneous nodules, purpuric spots and photophobia. What is your probable diagnosis? Discuss the aetiopathogenesis, morphological features and the investigations performed for the disease.
8. A 48-year-old woman presented with large thigh mass that recently increased in size. On examination, it was found that the mass was 14 × 12 × 7 cm on the anterior aspect of the right thigh with firm-to-hard consistency and irregular margins. What is the differential diagnosis in this case? How would you like to investigate further?

Answers

1. Osteoporosis
2. Paget disease
3. Osteomyelitis
4. Osteosarcoma
5. Osteoclastoma
6. Skeletal metastases from breast cancer
7. Rheumatoid arthritis
8. Soft-tissue sarcoma – liposarcoma, MPNST, etc.

Topics for Self-Directed Learning

1. Lytic lesions of bone
2. Sclerotic lesions of bone
3. Retroperitoneal tumours
4. Role of IHC markers in the evaluation of bone tumours
5. Evaluation of bone metastasis
6. Role of IHC in the evaluation of soft-tissue tumours
7. Pathology of Guillain–Barré syndrome
8. Toxic neuropathies
9. Pathology of myasthenia gravis
10. Patterns of peripheral nerve damage
11. Mitochondrial myopathies

MIND MAPS

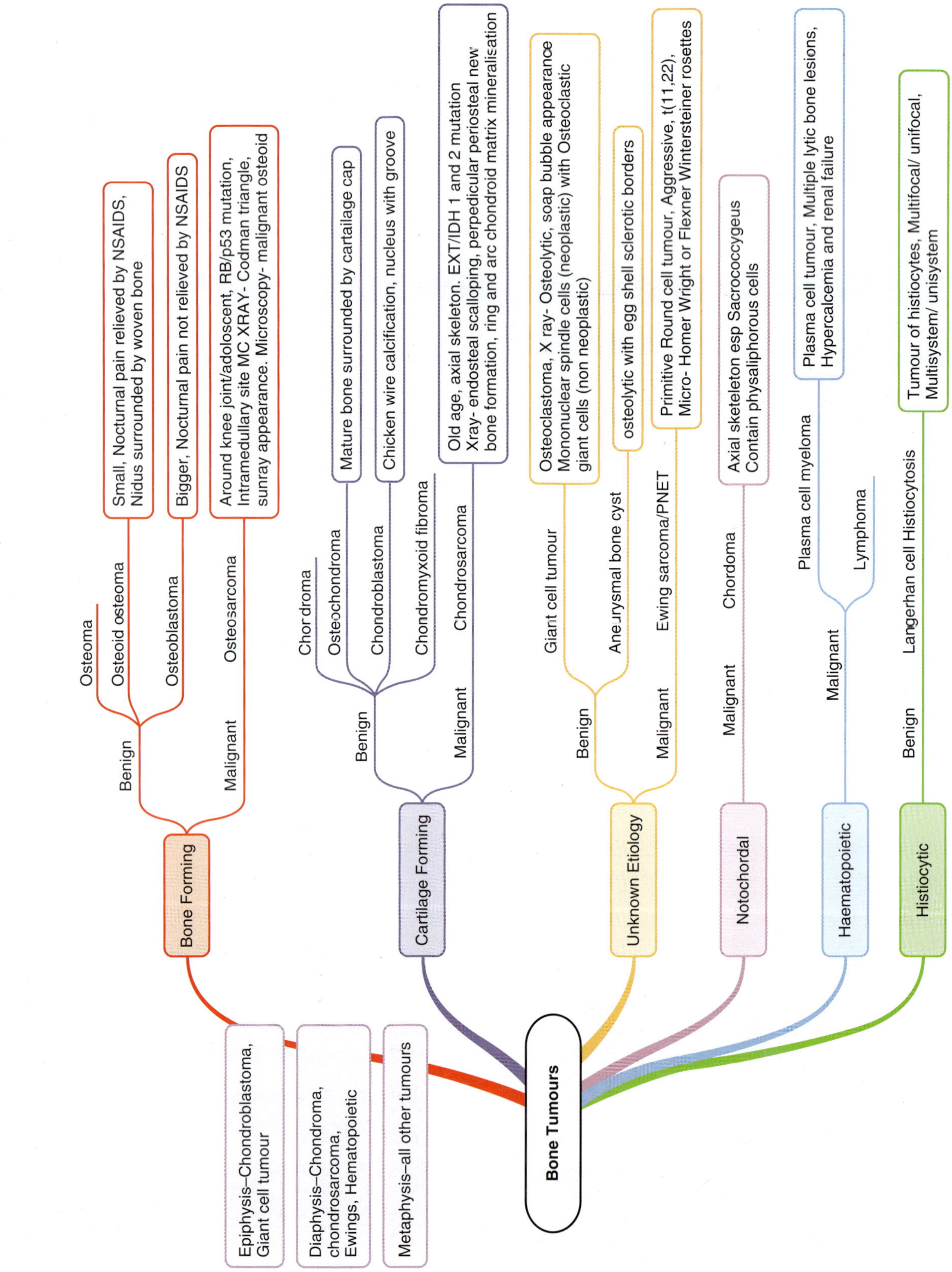
Bone Tumours
Epiphysis–Chondroblastoma, Giant cell tumour
Diaphysis–Chondroma, chondrosarcoma, Ewings, Hematopoietic
Metaphysis–all other tumours
Bone Forming
Benign
Osteoma
Osteoid osteoma
Small, Nocturnal pain relieved by NSAIDS, Nidus surrounded by woven bone
Osteoblastoma
Bigger, Nocturnal pain not relieved by NSAIDS
Malignant
Osteosarcoma
Around knee joint/adoloscent, RB/p53 mutation, Intramedullary site MC XRAY- Codman triangle, sunray appearance. Microscopy- malignant osteoid
Cartilage Forming
Benign
Chondroma
Osteochondroma
Mature bone surrounded by cartilage cap
Chondroblastoma
Chicken wire calcification, nucleus with groove
Chondromyxoid fibroma
Malignant
Chondrosarcoma
Old age, axial skeleton. EXT/IDH 1 and 2 mutation Xray- endosteal scalloping, perpedicular periosteal new bone formation, ring and arc chondroid matrix mineralisation
Unknown Etiology
Benign
Giant cell tumour
Osteoclastoma, X ray- Osteolytic, soap bubble appearance Mononuclear spindle cells (neoplastic) with Osteoclastic giant cells (non neoplastic)
Aneurysmal bone cyst
osteolytic with egg shell sclerotic borders
Malignant
Ewing sarcoma/PNET
Primitive Round cell tumour, Aggressive, t(11,22), Micro- Homer Wright or Flexner Wintersteiner rosettes
Notochordal
Malignant
Chordoma
Axial sketeleton esp Sacrococcygeus Contain physaliphorous cells
Haematopoietic
Malignant
Plasma cell myeloma
Plasma cell tumour, Multiple lytic bone lesions, Hypercalcemia and renal failure
Lymphoma
Histiocytic
Benign
Langerhan cell Histiocytosis
Tumour of histiocytes, Multifocal/ unifocal, Multisystem/ unisystem

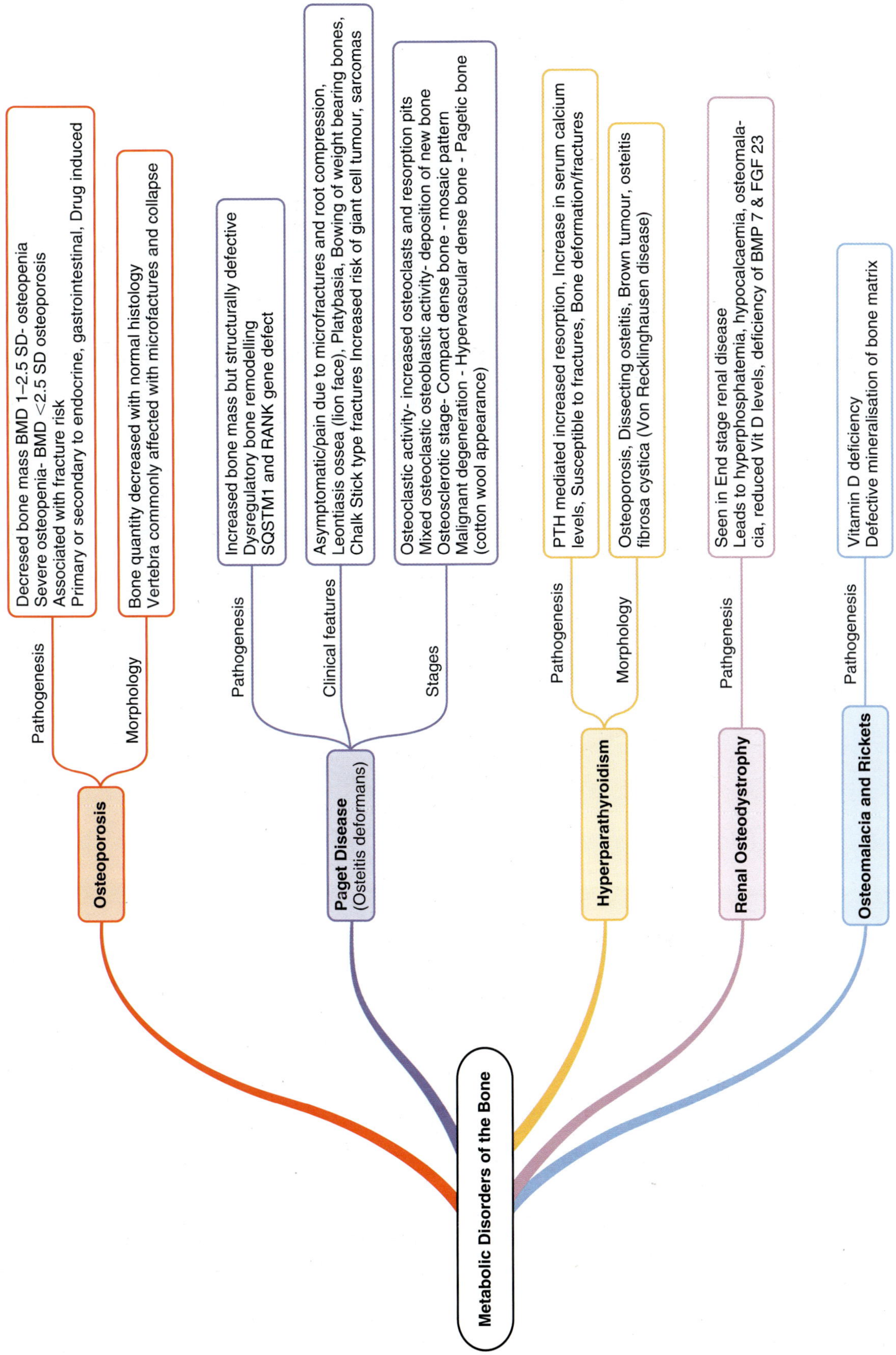
Metabolic Disorders of the Bone
Osteoporosis
Pathogenesis
Decresed bone mass BMD 1–2.5 SD- osteopenia
Severe osteopenia- BMD <2.5 SD osteoporosis
Associated with fracture risk
Primary or secondary to endocrine, gastrointestinal, Drug induced
Morphology
Bone quantity decreased with normal histology
Vertebra commonly affected with microfactures and collapse
Paget Disease
(Osteitis deformans)
Pathogenesis
Increased bone mass but structurally defective
Dysregulatory bone remodelling
SQSTM1 and RANK gene defect
Clinical features
Asymptomatic/pain due to microfractures and root compression,
Leontiasis ossea (lion face), Platybasia, Bowing of weight bearing bones,
Chalk Stick type fractures Increased risk of giant cell tumour, sarcomas
Stages
Osteoclastic activity- increased osteoclasts and resorption pits
Mixed osteoclastic osteoblastic activity- deposition of new bone
Osteosclerotic stage- Compact dense bone - mosaic pattern
Malignant degeneration - Hypervascular dense bone - Pagetic bone
(cotton wool appearance)
Hyperparathyroidism
Pathogenesis
PTH mediated increased resorption, Increase in serum calcium
levels, Susceptible to fractures, Bone deformation/fractures
Morphology
Osteoporosis, Dissecting osteitis, Brown tumour, osteitis
fibrosa cystica (Von Recklinghausen disease)
Renal Osteodystrophy
Pathgenesis
Seen in End stage renal disease
Leads to hyperphosphatemia, hypocalcaemia, osteomala-
cia, reduced Vit D levels, deficiency of BMP 7 & FGF 23
Osteomalacia and Rickets
Pathogenesis
Vitamin D deficiency
Defective mineralisation of bone matrix

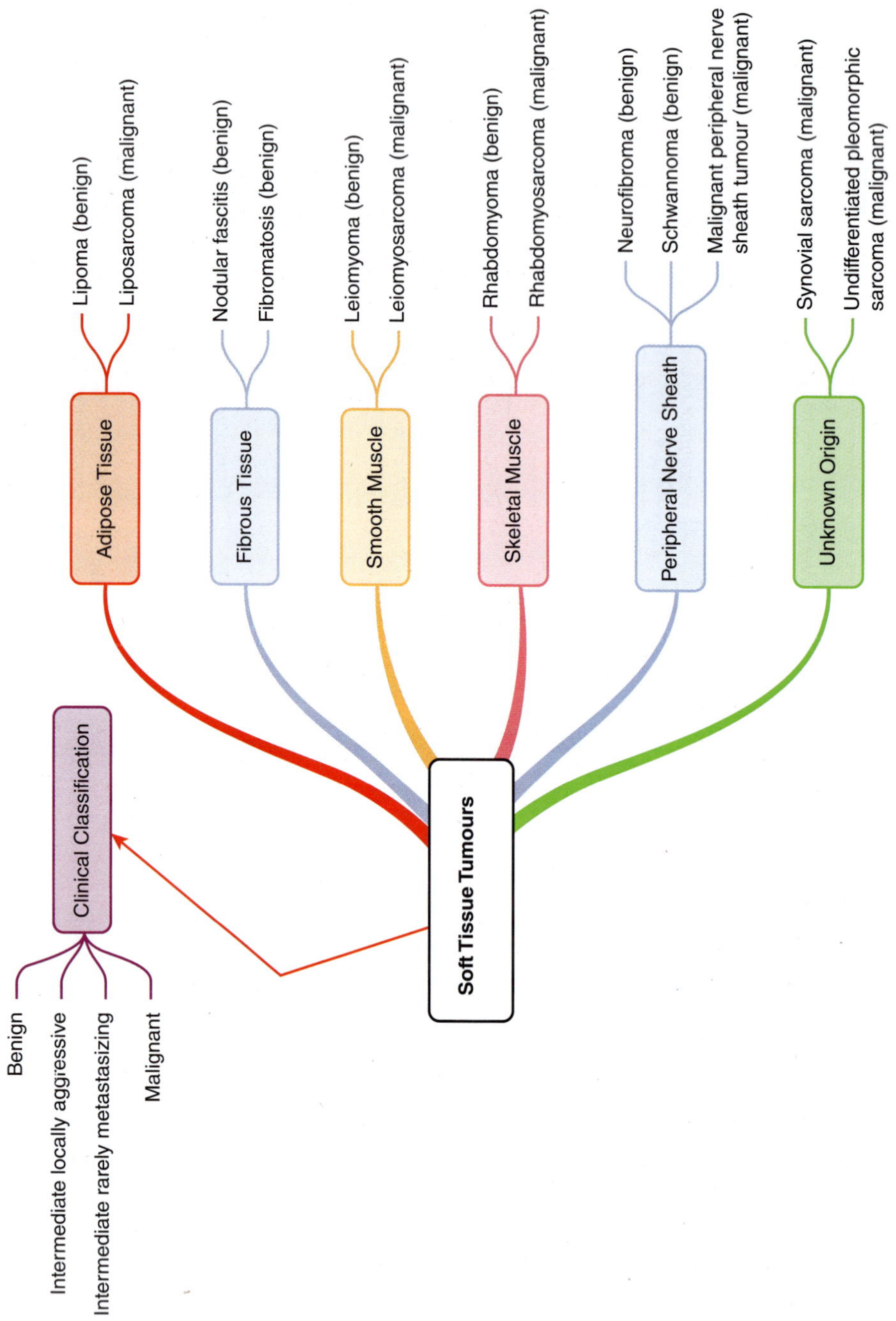

Soft Tissue Tumours
Clinical Classification
Benign
Intermediate locally aggressive
Intermediate rarely metastasizing
Malignant
Adipose Tissue
Lipoma (benign)
Liposarcoma (malignant)
Fibrous Tissue
Nodular fascitis (benign)
Fibromatosis (benign)
Smooth Muscle
Leiomyoma (benign)
Leiomyosarcoma (malignant)
Skeletal Muscle
Rhabdomyoma (benign)
Rhabdomyosarcoma (malignant)
Peripheral Nerve Sheath
Neurofibroma (benign)
Schwannoma (benign)
Malignant peripheral nerve sheath tumour (malignant)
Unknown Origin
Synovial sarcoma (malignant)
Undifferentiated pleomorphic sarcoma (malignant)

Central Nervous System and Eye

31

G Anushuya

PA 35.1 Describe the aetiology, types and pathogenesis, differentiating factors and CSF findings in **meningitis**.

PA 35.2 Classify and describe the aetiology, genetics, pathogenesis, pathology, presentation, sequelae and complications of **CNS tumours**.

PA 36.1 Describe the aetiology, genetics, pathogenesis, pathology, presentation, sequelae and complications of **retinoblastoma**.

CHAPTER OUTLINE

ANATOMY AND HISTOLOGY

ANATOMY

The nervous system consists of two parts – **the central nervous system** (CNS) that includes the brain and the spinal cord, and the **peripheral nervous system** that connects CNS to the rest of the body. The brain and spinal cord serve as the main centres that correlate and integrate neural information. The brain is divided into three different parts – the forebrain, the midbrain and the hindbrain. It lies in the cranial cavity and is continuous with the spinal cord through the foramen magnum. It is surrounded by three meninges – the dura mater, the arachnoid mater and the pia mater; these are continuous with the corresponding meninges of the spinal cord. The cerebrospinal fluid (CSF) is contained in the subarachnoid space and surrounds the brain and spinal cord. It also circulates in the ventricular system consisting of the third ventricle, lateral ventricles and fourth ventricle. The fourth ventricle is connected by the cerebral aqueduct to the third ventricle, superiorly, and continues as the central canal of the spinal cord, inferiorly. The foramen of Luschka and Magendie help in communication with the subarachnoid space, thus bathing the entire nervous system inside out.

Glial tissue has glial cells and neurons. **Neurons** are the functional units of CNS. *Glial cells* are the supporting cells such as the *astrocytes* and *oligodendrocytes*. Neurons are **terminally differentiated** cells that have lost the dividing property. They have distinctive property depending on their locations. Let us see the histology of the cerebral cortex.

HISTOLOGY

The cerebral cortex contains **outer grey matter** composed of nerve cell bodies and **inner white matter** composed of nerve fibres. The outer grey matter lies beneath the pia–arachnoid meninges and is called the neocortex. It is made of the following six layers that merge with each other:

- Plexiform layer containing horizontally arranged nerve cells
- Outer granular layer containing small pyramidal neurons
- Outer pyramidal layer containing medium-sized pyramidal neurons
- Inner granular layer containing large pyramidal neurons
- Inner pyramidal or Purkinje layer containing larger pyramidal neurons
- Polymorphous layer that lacks pyramidal cells

The cerebellar cortex also contains outer grey matter and inner white matter. The grey matter is composed of three layers – molecular layer, Purkinje layer and granular layer.

Certain areas of this chapter that are not included in competencies are dealt with briefly to help the readers focus on the important topics but also be aware of the plethora of the conditions that may affect CNS.

Injury to CNS shows pattern of clinical signs and symptoms depending on the region of the brain involved. However, neurons *respond in some identifiable ways* to any incited insults. The next section discusses the reactions of the cells of CNS to injury.

REACTION OF CELLS OF CENTRAL NERVOUS SYSTEM TO INJURY

The cells of CNS undergo a spectrum of functional and morphological changes in response to injury. Recognizing these patterns helps in understanding the mechanism of cellular injury and the type of disease (Flowchart 31.1).

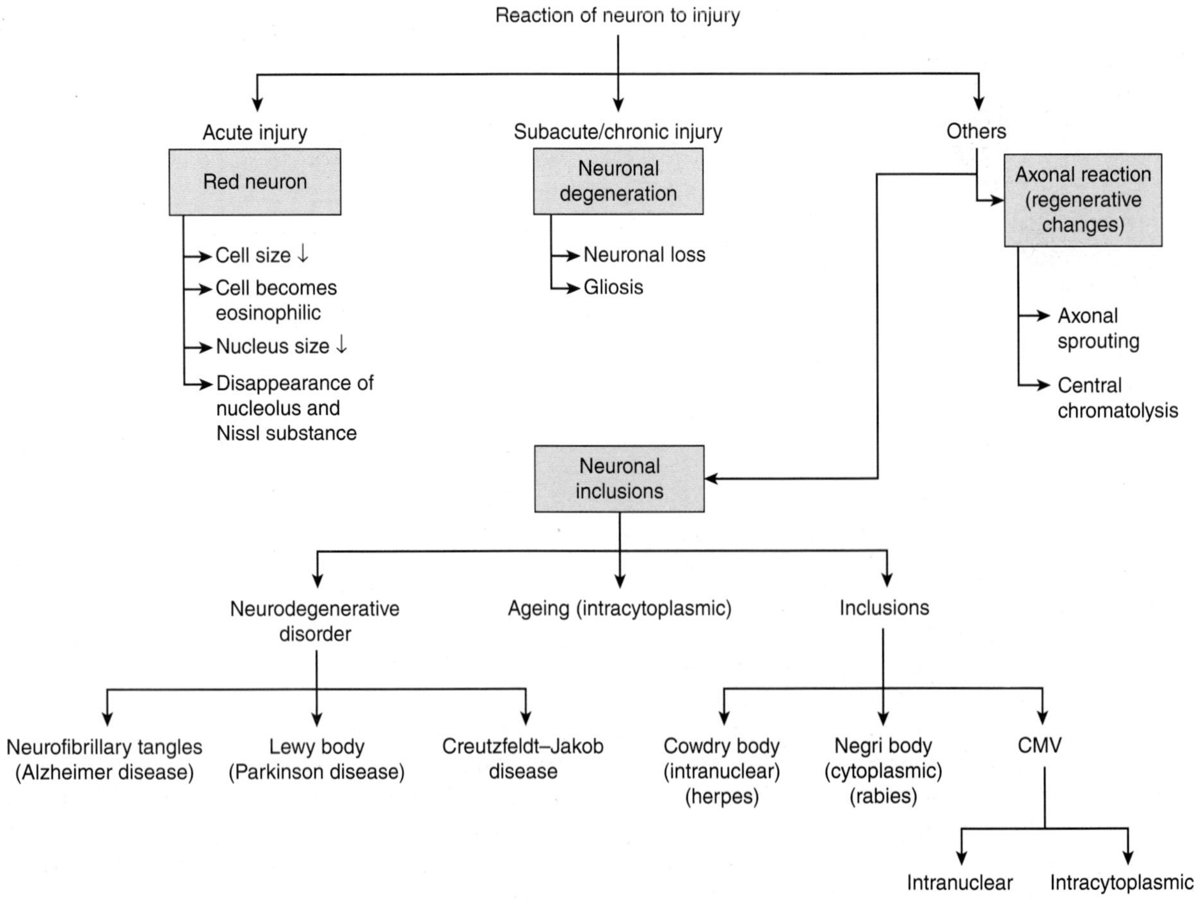

Flowchart 31.1 Summary of reactions of neurons to injury.

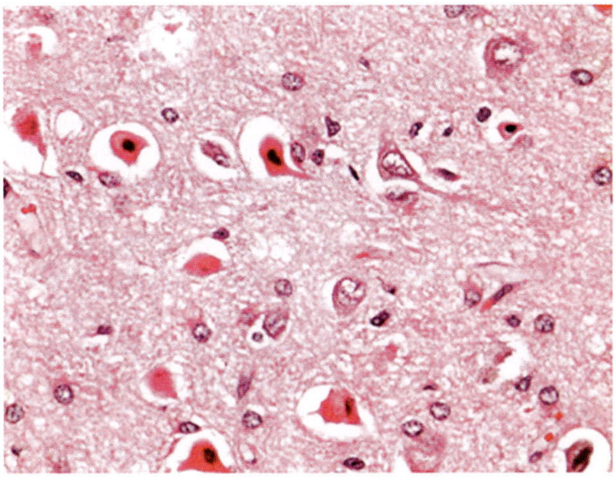

Fig. 31.1 Acute hypoxic-ischaemic injury in the cerebral cortex. The cell bodies are shrunken and eosinophilic ('red neurons'), and the nuclei are pyknotic. (*Source:* Vinay Kumar, Abul K. Abbas and Jon C. Aster, Central Nervous System, in Robbins Basic Pathology, 10th Edition, © 2018 by Elsevier Inc.)

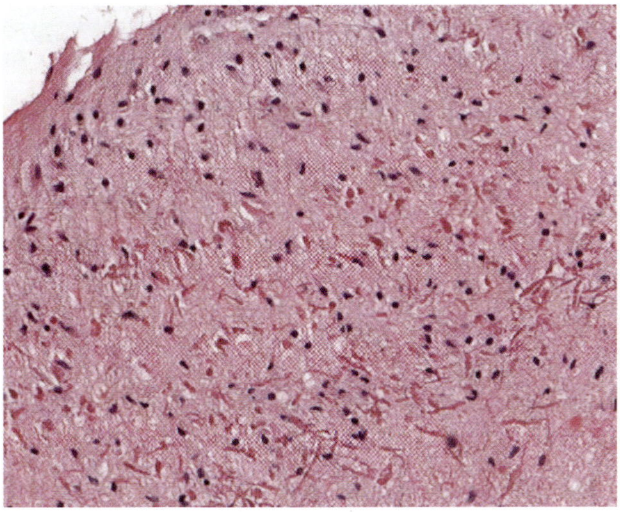

Fig. 31.2 Rosenthal fibres that appear as brightly eosinophilic, rounded, elongated or carrot-shaped structures in haematoxylin and eosin–stained sections. (*Source:* David Ellison, Pathologic reactions in the CNS, in Neuropathology, 3rd Edition, © 2013, Elsevier Limited.)

Reactions of neurons to injury: Neurons exhibit changes such as formation of 'red' neurons, (Fig. 31.1) neuronal degeneration, axonal degeneration and formation of inclusions such as Cowdry bodies in herpes and Negri bodies in rabies.

Reactions of astrocytes to injury: The changes include gliosis and formation of gemistocytic astrocytes, Rosenthal fibres (Fig. 31.2), corpora amylacea and Lafora bodies.

Reactions of microglia to injury: These cells respond to injury by proliferating and forming rod cells, microglial nodules and by neuronophagia.

Reactions of other cells: Oligodendroglial cells respond by undergoing apoptosis or by formation of inclusions and ependymal cells respond by forming granulations

CEREBROVASCULAR DISEASE

Cerebrovascular disease is resultant of injury to the brain as a consequence of ischaemia and haemorrhage. Stroke includes all these conditions occurring within a short span of time. Cerebrovascular disease can be grouped into two processes.

HYPOXIA, ISCHAEMIA AND INFARCTION

The brain is a very sensitive organ. Cerebral blood flow is maintained constant despite the fluctuation in blood pressure and intracranial pressure by an intact autoregulation mechanism. In case of ischaemia, the anatomic site and the size of the lesion determine the clinical deficit. Irrespective of the cause, the survival of the penumbra (region between the normal brain and the necrotic tissue) depends on the duration of hypoxia, the rapidity of the reduction of flow and the collateral circulation. Apart from the cellular injury changes occurring elsewhere, **inappropriate release of excitatory neurotransmitters also contributes to the** injury of the brain. **Neurons** are the **most sensitive** to ischaemic injury followed by oligodendrocytes and astrocytes. Ischaemia may be global or focal.

- **Global cerebral ischaemia**
  Global ischaemia is caused by incidents such as shock, cardiac arrest and severe hypotension. Severe global cerebral ischaemia causes widespread neuronal death leading to persistent vegetative state if the person survives and may culminate in 'brain death', evidenced by absent reflexes and respiratory drive.
- **Focal cerebral ischaemia**
  Focal cerebral ischaemia is caused by **arterial occlusion** or hypoperfusion causing localized reduction of blood supply to a part of the brain that may be due to emboli, in situ thrombi or vasculitis. Ischaemia, if prolonged, leads to infarction. The duration of ischaemia and the presence of collateral flow (as established by the circle of Willis) determine the size of the infarct and the extent of tissue damage.

HYPERTENSIVE CEREBROVASCULAR DISEASE

Uncontrolled hypertension can cause cerebrovascular diseases such as lacunar infarcts, slit haemorrhages, hypertensive encephalopathy and massive hypertensive intracerebral haemorrhage, warranting aggressive management.

Lacunar infarcts: These are single or multiple tiny, cavitary infarcts caused due to occlusion of deep penetrating arteries and arterioles in individuals with hypertension.
Slit haemorrhages: Rupture of the small, penetrating vessels in the brain often leads to tiny haemorrhage that resolves eventually leaving a slit-like cavity surrounded by brownish discoloration.

Hypertensive encephalopathy: It occurs in patients with malignant hypertension, and is characterized by headache, vomiting, confusion and convulsions with cerebral dysfunction culminating in coma. Accompanying elevated intracranial pressure requires rapid therapeutic intervention because spontaneous remission is unlikely. An oedematous brain with or without tonsillar or transtentorial herniation is seen during autopsy.

INTRACRANIAL HAEMORRHAGE

Haemorrhages can be intraparenchymal or within the cranium but outside the brain (subarachnoid haemorrhage).

Intraparenchymal haemorrhage is caused by rupture of tiny vessels within the brain that leads to stroke. They are nontraumatic haemorrhages in old age caused by hypertension, cerebral amyloid angiopathy, coagulation disorders, vasculitis, neoplasms, aneurysms and vascular malformations. Hypertension is the most common risk factor causing deep brain parenchymal haemorrhage. Charcot–Bouchard microaneurysms is the term used for minute aneurysms seen in chronic hypertension that are often the sites of rupture.

Subarachnoid haemorrhage is often caused due to cerebral artery saccular (*'berry'*) aneurysm (Fig. 31.3) rupture. The other causes include traumatic haematoma extension, vascular malformation, tumours and haematological disturbances. The most common intracranial aneurysm type is saccular aneurysm. Other aneurysm types include fusiform (due to atherosclerosis involving the basilar artery), traumatic, mycotic and dissecting. The latter three variants along with saccular aneurysm involve the anterior circulation, yet cause cerebral infarction and not subarachnoid haemorrhage.

Saccular aneurysms – formerly known as berry aneurysms – are thin-walled outpouchings usually located at the arterial branch point. They may range from few millimetres to 3 cm in size. They are often seen in the anterior circulation in the circle of Willis, the most common site being the junction of the anterior communicating artery with the anterior cerebral artery. The aetiopathogenesis of aneurysm has been dealt with in detail, which the students are encouraged to refer for better understanding. Rupture of aneurysm can occur anytime but occurs at an increased rate with acute increase in intracranial pressure such as in straining while passing stool or sexual orgasm. Sudden rupture causes blood to be forced into the subarachnoid space leading to excruciating headache with loss of consciousness. Death occurs in 25%–50% of patients during the first rupture. However, subsequent unpredictable bleeding occurs in survivors and prognosis worsens with each episode of bleeding. Subarachnoid haemorrhage on healing may cause meningeal fibrosis with scarring, causing obstruction to the CSF flow along with disruption of normal CSF resorption.

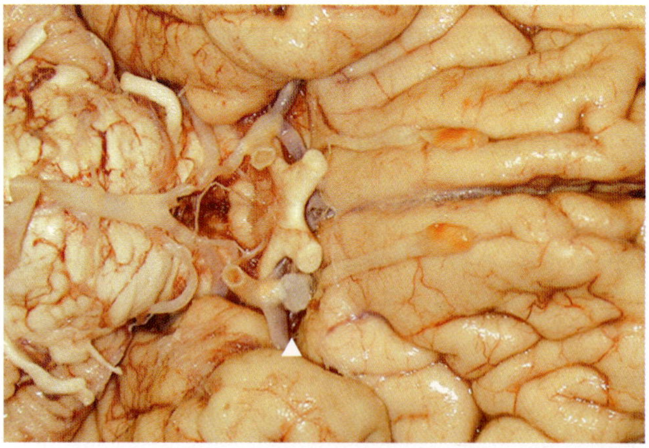

Fig. 31.3 Berry aneurysm. A nonruptured saccular (berry) aneurysm (▲) is seen at the bifurcation of the left middle cerebral and anterior communicating arteries of the circle of Willis at the base of the brain. (*Source:* Edward C. Klatt, The Central Nervous System, in Robbins and Cotran Atlas of Pathology, 4th Edition, © 2021 by Elsevier, Inc.)

INFECTIONS

Infections are an important cause of damage to the nervous system either directly by the causative agent injuring the neurons or glia, or indirectly by producing microbial toxins. This gets worsened with superadded destructive effects of the inflammatory response, or other immune-mediated mechanisms.

ROUTES OF ENTRY

The routes by which microbial organisms enter CNS are as follows:

- **Haematogenous spread** is the most common. Organisms enter CNS through the arterial circulation or by retrograde venous spread via anastomoses with facial veins.
- **Direct implantation of microorganisms** may be due to trauma or congenital malformations such as meningomyelocele, in which case organisms have direct access.
- **Direct extension** occurs from infected adjacent structures such as teeth, skull, air sinuses or vertebrae.
- Viruses may travel **along the peripheral nerves** such as in herpes zoster virus and rabies.

MECHANISM OF INJURY

ACUTE FOCAL SUPPURATIVE INFECTIONS

Brain Abscess

Brain abscess is an isolated focus of necrosis of the brain with associated inflammation, frequently caused by bacterial infection. It may be due to direct implantation of the organism; by local extension from adjoining foci such as mastoiditis/paranasal sinusitis; by haematogenous spread with the primary site being the heart, lungs or long bones of the extremities; or by spread following tooth extraction.

Predisposing factors include:

- Acute bacterial endocarditis, which causes multiple brain abscesses
- Congenital heart disease with right-to-left shunt in which the pulmonary filtration of organisms does not occur
- Chronic pulmonary sepsis such as bronchiectasis
- Systemic disease with immunosuppression

The most common offending organisms are streptococci and staphylococci in nonimmunosuppressed patients.

Morphology

Abscesses are distinct lesions with liquefactive necrosis in the centre. The lesion is surrounded by exuberant granulation tissue along with neovascularization that is leaky causing vasogenic oedema (Fig. 31.4). Also seen in the surrounding region is a zone of reactive gliosis showing many gemistocytic astrocytes.

Clinical Features Abscesses in the brain are destructive lesions leading to **focal progressive neurological deficits** along with signs and symptoms of increased intracranial pressure. CSF shows elevated white cell count and increased protein concentration with normal glucose content level. The source of infection can be apparent or may be traced to an asymptomatic small distant focus. **Complications** of brain abscess include fatal herniation due to increased intracranial pressure, abscess rupture leading to ventriculitis or meningitis and also venous sinus thrombosis. High mortality rate may be reduced to less than 10% with surgery and antibiotic treatment.

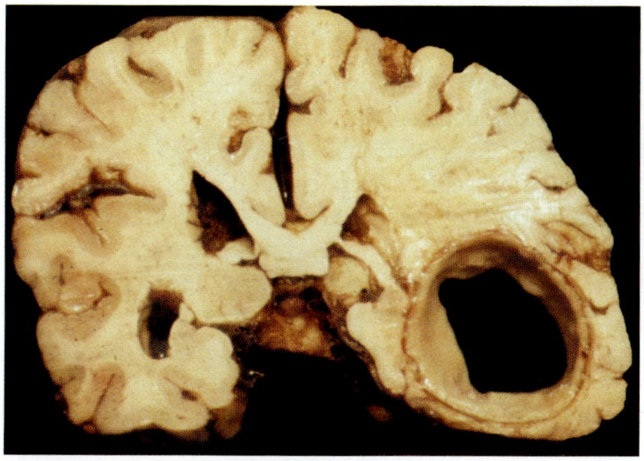

Fig. 31.4 Gross – brain abscess. Coronal section of the brain demonstrates an abscess cavity in the right temporal lobe. Note the fibrous capsule that separates the abscess from the surrounding brain parenchyma. The pus has drained out of the cavity. (*Source:* Sandra Camelo-Piragua and E. Tessa Hedley-Whyte, Infections of the Nervous System, in Diagnostic Pathology of Infectious Disease, 2nd Edition, © 2018 by Elsevier, Inc.)

Subdural Empyema

Bacteria and a few fungi infecting the skull bones or the sinuses may spread to the subdural space causing subdural empyema. This condition leaves the arachnoid and the underlying subarachnoid space unaffected. However, a large subdural empyema can produce mass effect or thrombophlebitis of the veins situated in the subdural space, leading to venous occlusion and infarction of the brain. Most patients present with fever, headache and neck stiffness along with symptoms due to the source of infection. The CSF profile is similar as in brain abscess. Without treatment, the patients develop focal neurological deficits, lethargy and coma. With prompt surgical drainage, resolution and complete recovery are possible, with the only residuum being a thickened dura.

Extradural Abscess

Extradural abscess is usually associated with osteomyelitis, often arising from an adjoining focus of infection such as sinusitis or following a surgical procedure. If the process involves the spinal epidural space, it may lead to spinal cord compression which is a neurosurgical emergency.

MENINGITIS PA 35.1

Meningitis is the inflammation of **leptomeninges and CSF in the subarachnoid space** usually due to infection, whereas meningoencephalitis is the term used to refer to the inflammation of the brain parenchyma along with meninges. Infections are the most common causes of meningoencephalitis and meningitis, but they may also occur in response to certain chemical irritants introduced into the subarachnoid space such as in **chemical meningitis**.

Acute meningitis is broadly **classified on the basis of** aetiology and evolution as:

- Acute pyogenic meningitis (bacterial)
- Aseptic meningitis (acute/subacute viral)

Acute Pyogenic (Bacterial) Meningitis

Successful vaccination has markedly reduced the prevalence of acute bacterial meningitis and the epidemiology of the causative organisms has changed because of the same. Affected individuals typically show **signs of meningeal irritation** such as neck stiffness, photophobia, headache, clouding of consciousness and irritability, in addition to **systemic signs** such as fever. If left untreated, it may be fatal.

The aetiological agent shows variation on the basis of the age:

- In neonates: Group B streptococci and *E. coli*
- In adults and elderly: *S. pneumoniae* and *L. monocytogenes*, which are the most common
- In adolescents and young adults: *N. meningitidis*

H. influenzae–induced meningitis has markedly reduced following vaccination.

In **Waterhouse–Friderichsen syndrome**, meningococcal and pneumococcal meningitis cause haemorrhagic infarction of the adrenal glands with septicaemia and cutaneous petechiae.

In immunosuppressed individuals, purulent meningitis is caused by *Klebsiella* or anaerobic organisms that present with atypical signs and uncharacteristic CSF findings, making the diagnosis difficult.

CSF findings:

1. Increased CSF pressure is present.
2. CSF is frankly purulent or cloudy.
3. Neutrophils are >90,000/mm^3 in CSF.
4. Protein concentration is increased.
5. Glucose content is reduced.
6. Bacteria may be demonstrated by smear or can be cultured even before the appearance of neutrophils.

Acute Aseptic (Viral) Meningitis

It is an acute-onset meningitis causing signs of meningeal irritation, fever and altered sensorium but is microbial culture negative. It is usually due to viral aetiology but can be caused by rickettsial, bacterial or autoimmune causes also. The condition is treated symptomatically and is **self-limiting**. Isolation of the organism by molecular methods is possible in only minority of cases. Enteroviruses are the most common (80%) aetiology. Other causes include arboviruses such as Eastern and Western equine encephalitis virus, mumps, herpes family viruses, lymphocytic choriomeningitis virus, adenovirus, measles and HIV, and nonviral causes such as tuberculosis.

There is seasonal and geographical variation in the organism. It has a less severe clinical course.

CSF findings:

- Lymphocytic pleocytosis
- Protein elevation: Moderate
- Glucose content: Nearly normal

Rupture of an epidermoid cyst into the subarachnoid space causes an **aseptic meningitis**–like picture because of introduction of a chemical irritant, an example of chemical meningitis. CSF in these cases is sterile with neutrophilic pleocytosis, increased protein concentration and normal sugar content.

Morphology of Acute Meningitis

Gross The exudate covers the surface of the brain and is seen within the leptomeninges with engorged meningeal vessels. A difference in anatomic distribution of the exudate has been observed depending on the causative organism:

1. *H. influenzae* meningitis: Exudate in the skull base
2. Pneumococcal meningitis: Exudate over cerebral convexities, adjoining the sagittal sinus (pus in the exudate tracks along blood vessels on the surface of the brain; fulminant meningitis produces **ventriculitis** [the inflammation of the ventricles])

Microscopy Microscopy shows that neutrophils fill the subarachnoid space in severely affected areas, whereas they are seen around the leptomeningeal blood vessels in less severe cases. Bacteria can be demonstrated by Gram stain in untreated meningitis. Fulminant meningitis shows the inflammatory cell infiltrate on the walls of leptomeningeal veins causing venous thrombosis, haemorrhagic infarctions in the brain and focal inflammation in the brain parenchyma (**cerebritis**). Leptomeningeal fibrosis is a sequela of pyogenic meningitis leading to **hydrocephalus**. Pneumococcal meningitis produces large amounts of gelatinous exudate due to the capsular polysaccharide produced by the organism that promotes arachnoid fibrosis termed **chronic adhesive arachnoiditis**.

CHRONIC BACTERIAL MENINGOENCEPHALITIS

Mycobacterium tuberculosis, *Borrelia* and *Treponema pallidum* species may cause chronic bacterial infection of the brain and meninges.

Tuberculosis

Tuberculosis of CNS involves the meninges or the brain; it may be a part of active disease elsewhere in the body or may be an isolated lesion subsequent to seeding from a silent lesion elsewhere, usually the lungs. The pathogenesis of tuberculosis has already been described earlier in Chapters 8 and 19.

Clinical Features The patient presents with malaise, mental confusion, headache and vomiting.

CSF findings:

- CSF shows pleocytosis, consisting of mononuclear cells with neutrophils.
- Protein concentration is elevated.
- Glucose level is moderately reduced or normal.

Complications of chronic tubercular meningitis:

- Hydrocephalus due to arachnoid fibrosis
- Infarction of the underlying brain due to obliterative endarteritis causing arterial occlusion
- Dissemination of infection through CSF, can involve the spinal cord, subarachnoid space affecting the nerve roots, choroid plexus and ependyma
- **Tuberculomas** – space-occupying lesions in the brain mimicking CNS tumours

CNS tuberculosis in patients with acquired immunodeficiency syndrome (AIDS) is similar but with less host reaction. HIV-positive individuals are also at the risk of developing disseminated *Mycobacterium avium-intracellulare* infection. This lesion is identified by the

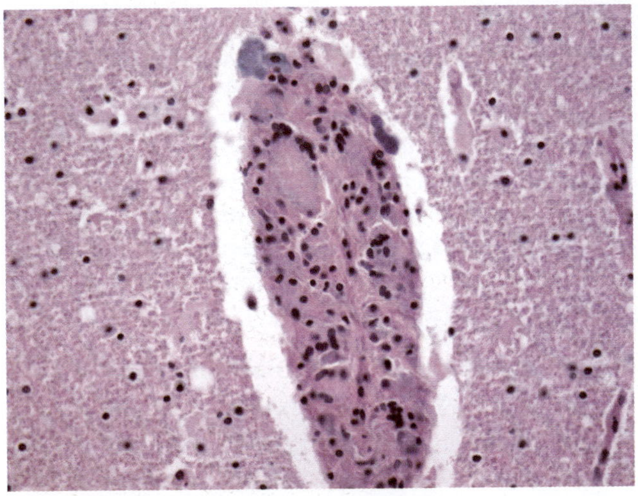

Fig. 31.5 Microscopy of a tuberculoma showing a rounded collection of epithelioid macrophages with a multinucleated giant cell. (*Source:* Sandra Camelo-Piragua and E. Tessa Hedley-Whyte, Infections of the Nervous System, in Diagnostic Pathology of Infectious Disease, 2nd Edition, © 2018 by Elsevier, Inc.)

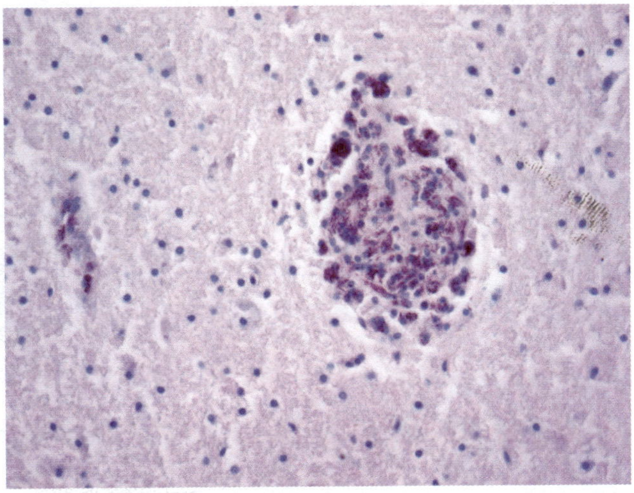

Fig. 31.6 Microscopy of tuberculosis – acid-fast stain (AFB) demonstrates numerous mycobacteria. Numerous organisms are more likely to be seen in infections with atypical mycobacteria in immunosuppressed hosts. (*Source:* Sandra Camelo-Piragua, E. Tessa Hedley-Whyte (2018). Diagnostic Pathology of Infectious Disease (2nd ed.). St Louis, MO: Elsevier.)

confluent sheets of macrophages containing the organisms. The granulomas are few or none.

Morphology

Tuberculosis of CNS presents as diffuse meningoencephalitis with the following findings:

1. A gelatinous or fibrinous exudate in the subarachnoid space of the base of the brain is seen surrounding the cranial nerves and obscuring the cisterns.
2. Discrete white areas of inflammation may be seen over the leptomeninges.
3. Tuberculoma is a well-circumscribed intraparenchymal mass of about few centimetres in diameter, causing mass effect. Active lesions have caseous necrosis in the centre surrounded by granulomas, whereas inactive lesions show calcification.

Microscopy shows the following findings:

- Mixed inflammatory cells consisting of lymphocytes, macrophages and plasma cells
- Well-formed caseating granulomas with Langhans giant cells seen in florid cases (Fig. 31.5)
- Obliterative endarteritis with intimal thickening seen involving the arteries running in the subarachnoid space
- Tuberculous bacilli, which are demonstrated with the help of acid-fast stains (Fig. 31.6)

Neurosyphilis

The **tertiary stage** of syphilis may manifest as neurosyphilis in about 10% of untreated patients. HIV-infected patients are at an increased risk of developing neurosyphilis, especially acute syphilitic meningitis or meningovascular disease, due to impaired cell-mediated immunity. The pathogenesis of syphilis is discussed in detail in Chapter 8.

Morphology

Syphilis can lead to meningovascular neurosyphilis, paretic neurosyphilis and tabes dorsalis in CNS. It presents as a mixed pattern and the commonly observed combination is tabes dorsalis and paretic disease (taboparesis).

- **Meningovascular neurosyphilis** presents as chronic meningitis affecting the cerebri basalis with variable involvement of the cerebral convexities. The spinal leptomeninges may be involved. **Heubner arteritis** – an obliterative endarteritis, which is characterized by perivascular inflammatory infiltrate composed of plasma cells and lymphocytes – can be seen (Fig. 31.7). **Cerebral gummas** are plasma cell–rich mass involving the meninges extending into the parenchyma.
- **Paretic neurosyphilis** presents insidiously as progressive cognitive impairment (delusions of grandeur) terminating in severe dementia (general paresis of the insane). It is caused by invasion of the brain by *T. pallidum* damaging the parenchyma of the frontal lobe, cortex and other areas of the isocortex. These foci show neuronal loss, gliosis, proliferation of microglia (rod cells) and iron deposits (demonstrated by Prussian blue stain). Iron deposits in the perivascular region are presumably due to damage of the microcirculation causing haemorrhage. The spirochaetes may be rarely demonstrated in tissue sections.

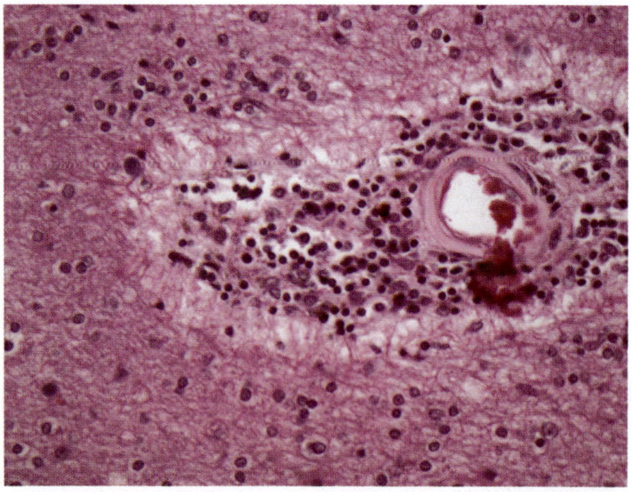

Fig. 31.7 Microscopy of Heubner arteritis of brain showing perivascular lymphoplasmacytic inflammation in a case of syphilis. (*Source:* Sandra Camelo-Piragua and E. Tessa Hedley-Whyte, Infections of the Nervous System, in Diagnostic Pathology of Infectious Disease, 2nd Edition, © 2018 by Elsevier, Inc.)

- **Tabes dorsalis** is due to sensory axonal damage in the dorsal roots. This causes ataxia (locomotor ataxia), impaired joint position sense and loss of pain sensation, leading to damage of the skin and joint (**Charcot joints**). Other sensory disturbances include loss of deep tendon reflexes and 'lightning pains'. Microscopy of the spinal cord shows pallor and atrophy in the dorsal column due to loss of both myelin and axons. Organisms cannot be demonstrated in the cord lesions.

Neuroborreliosis (Lyme Disease)

Neuroborreliosis is a CNS disease caused by spirochaete *Borrelia burgdorferi* and is transmitted by *Ixodes* tick, a vector. It has varying clinical presentations such as facial nerve palsy, aseptic meningitis, polyneuropathies and encephalopathy. Microscopy shows focal microglial proliferation in the brain with extracellular organisms.

VIRAL MENINGOENCEPHALITIS

Some viruses infect the nervous system specifically (**neurotropism**). Some infect specific cells of CNS (e.g. oligodendrocytes), whereas others have a predilection for particular areas of the brain (the limbic system or medial temporal lobes). The following manifestations of CNS can be caused by viral infection:

- CNS involvement can be confined to cerebral parenchyma – **encephalitis** or associated with meningeal involvement (**meningoencephalitis**). It may simultaneously involve the spinal cord (**encephalomyelitis**).
- **Latency** is characteristic of viral infections of CNS (progressive multifocal leucoencephalopathy [PML], herpes zoster). The influenza pandemic in 1918 led to **postencephalitic parkinsonism**, a slowly progressive degenerative syndrome after many years of the viral illness.
- Even in the absence of direct viral penetration into CNS, systemic viral infections may cause **immune-mediated damage**, such as perivenous demyelination.
- In utero infection with rubella causes **congenital malformations.**

Arthropod-Borne Viral Encephalitis

Arboviruses cause epidemic encephalitis in tropical regions. They cause high mortality and severe morbidity. The pathogenic arboviruses are Japanese B (Far East), tick-borne (Russia and Eastern Europe) and Murray Valley (Australia and New Guinea) that are prevalent all over the world. In the Western hemisphere, the most important ones are West Nile, Eastern and Western equine, Venezuelan, La Crosse and St. Louis. These viruses have animal hosts and arthropod vectors. Clinically, the patients develop focal signs such as ocular palsies and reflex asymmetry. Generalized neurological deficits such as confusion, seizures, delirium or coma may be seen also. West Nile encephalitis presents as polio-like syndrome with paralysis due to involvement of the spinal cord.

CSF findings:

- CSF pressure is elevated mildly.
- It appears colourless.
- Protein level is elevated.
- Glucose level is normal.
- Initially, neutrophilic pleocytosis is seen followed by lymphocytosis.

Morphology

The following microscopic findings may be seen:

- Perivascular lymphocytic and sometimes neutrophilic infiltration are seen.
- Multiple foci of grey and white matter necrosis are found.
- **Neuronophagia** – evidence of neuronal necrosis involving single cell, with phagocytosis of the debris – may be particularly seen.
- Microglial nodules – small aggregates of microglial cells – are seen around necrotic foci.
- Necrotizing vasculitis with associated focal haemorrhages is seen in severe cases.
- Intracellular inclusion bodies are seen in certain viral infections.
- The causative virus is identified by a combination of molecular, ultrastructural and immunohistochemical methods.

Herpes Simplex Virus Type 1

Children and young adults are most commonly affected by herpes simplex virus type 1 (HSV-1) encephalitis. Only 10% of the patients have a history of herpetic infection. The clinical features include alterations in mood, behaviour and memory. Virus detection in CSF samples is done with ease by polymerase chain reaction (PCR)–based methods and this method helps in recognition of patients with less severe disease. Successful antiviral therapy has significantly reduced the mortality rate. HSV-1 encephalitis, in some patients, has a subacute course with weakness, lethargy, ataxia and seizures as the clinical manifestations, which evolves over a protracted period of 4–6 weeks.

Morphology

The medial and inferior regions of the temporal lobes, and the orbital gyri of the frontal lobes are involved in HSV encephalitis and are severely affected. Microscopy shows haemorrhagic necrosis in the severely affected areas and intranuclear viral inclusion bodies – **Cowdry type A** in infected neurons and glia (Fig. 31.8).

Herpes Simplex Virus Type 2

Herpes simplex virus type 2 (HSV-2) can infect the nervous system. It causes meningitis in adults. Severe encephalitis is seen in 50% of neonates born by vaginal delivery to mothers with active HSV genital infections. Coexisting HIV infection with HSV-2 may cause acute haemorrhagic and necrotizing encephalitis.

Varicella Zoster Virus (Herpes Zoster)

Primary infection with varicella causes chickenpox, one of the childhood exanthems without neurological involvement. Severe CNS involvement by herpes zoster is rare. Herpes zoster may cause granulomatous arteritis. In immunocompromised individuals, herpes zoster may cause **acute encephalitis** characterized by numerous well-circumscribed demyelinating lesions that undergo subsequent necrosis.

Cytomegalovirus

CNS involvement due to CMV infection is seen in immunosuppressed individuals (patients with AIDS) and fetus of an infected mother. In utero infection causes periventricular necrosis with severe brain destruction leading to periventricular calcification and microcephaly. The pathogenesis of CMV is discussed in detail in Chapter 8.

Morphology

It can infect all the cells of CNS including neuronal, ependymal, glial or endothelial cells. Subacute encephalitis with CMV inclusion–bearing cells is seen in immunocompromised individuals (Fig. 31.9). Paraventricular subependymal area of the brain is predominantly affected where it causes choroid plexitis and severe haemorrhagic necrotizing ventriculo-encephalitis.

Painful radiculoneuritis can be seen due to involvement of the lower spinal cord and its roots. Enlarged cells with **intracytoplasmic and intranuclear inclusions** may be seen readily by light microscopy. CMV infection is confirmed by immunohistochemistry.

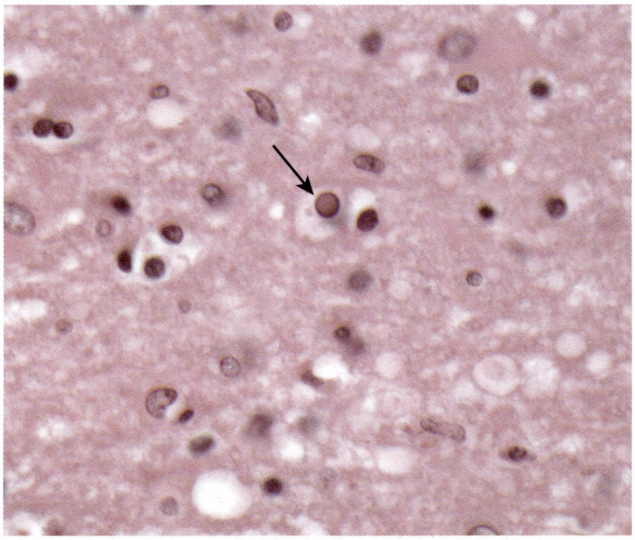

Fig. 31.8 Microscopy of herpes simplex virus type 1 – Cowdry type A – brain parenchyma showing intranuclear viral inclusion *(arrow)* with glassy chromatin. (*Source:* Sandra Camelo-Piragua and E. Tessa Hedley-Whyte, Infections of the Nervous System, in Diagnostic Pathology of Infectious Disease, 2nd Edition, © 2018 by Elsevier, Inc.)

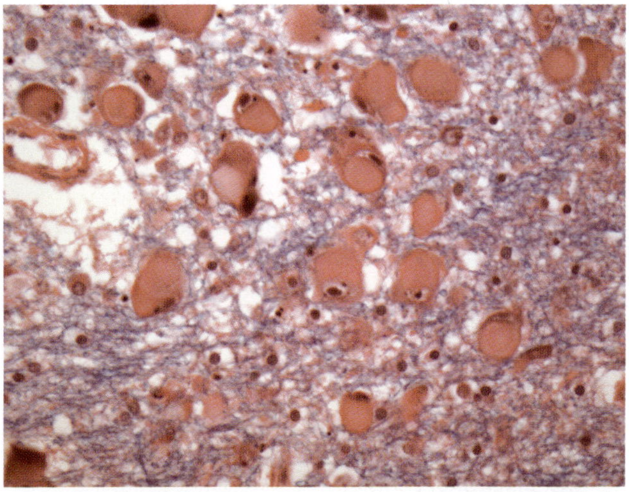

Fig. 31.9 Microscopy of cytomegalovirus – inclusions. Note the large size of the inclusion-bearing cells compared with the normal oligodendrocytes and astrocytes in the background. (*Source:* Sandra Camelo-Piragua and E. Tessa Hedley-Whyte, Infections of the Nervous System, in Diagnostic Pathology of Infectious Disease, 2nd Edition, © 2018 by Elsevier, Inc.)

Poliomyelitis

Paralytic poliomyelitis has been successfully eradicated by vaccination; however, it poses a serious health problem in few countries. Poliovirus infection in unimmunized individuals causes mild subclinical gastroenteritis, similar to the other picornavirus group of enteroviruses. In a subset of the susceptible population, the virus invades the nervous system.

Morphology

The motor neurons in the anterior horn of the spinal cord, in acute cases, show perivascular mononuclear cell cuffs and neuronophagia. The inflammatory reaction confines itself to the anterior horns but may extend to the posterior horns. When severe, the damage may cause cavitation. Poliovirus RNA can be isolated in anterior horn cell motor neurons. The virus can sometimes involve the cranial motor nuclei.

Autopsy findings in patients with symptomatic poliomyelitis show neuronal loss with gliosis and atrophy in the involved anterior horns of the spinal cord, and mild inflammatory infiltrate with denervation atrophy of the affected muscle.

Clinical Features CNS infection manifests as signs of meningeal irritation and CSF examination shows features of **aseptic meningitis**. The disease may or may not progress to involve the spinal cord. Spinal cord involvement produces permanent neurological residue of flaccid paralysis with muscle wasting and hyporeflexia of the involved segment. Motor neuron destruction may cause paresis or paralysis. Involvement of the diaphragm and intercostal muscles compromises respiration causing death. One of the complications of acute infection is myocarditis. After 25–35 years of initial illness, some patients develop post-polio syndrome characterized by progressive weakness with muscle atrophy and pain.

Rabies

It causes **severe encephalitis** and is transmitted by the bite of a rabid dog or rarely by other wild mammals that are reservoirs. Certain species of bats may transmit the disease even without a bite.

Morphology

- Gross examination of the brain shows oedema with vascular congestion.

Microscopy shows degeneration of neurons with inflammatory reaction that is widespread but most severe in the brainstem. It may also involve the basal ganglia, dorsal root ganglia and spinal cord. The

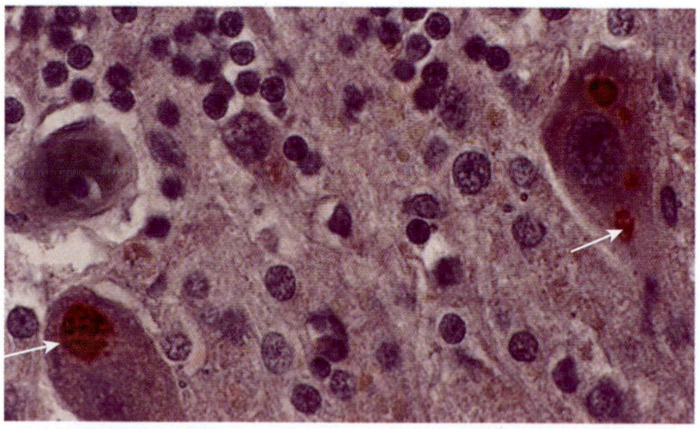

Fig. 31.10 Microscopy of rabies – Purkinje cells show well-circumscribed, eosinophilic intracytoplasmic inclusions (Negri bodies) *(arrow)*. (*Source:* David Ellison, Acute viral infections, in Neuropathology, 3rd Edition, © 2013, Elsevier Limited.)

pathognomonic microscopic finding is the **Negri bodies** that are round to oval, eosinophilic intracytoplasmic inclusions, in the sites devoid of inflammation such as pyramidal neurons of the hippocampus and Purkinje cells of the cerebellum (Fig. 31.10). Rabies virus can be demonstrated ultrastructurally within Negri bodies and by immunohistochemistry.

Clinical Features The virus travels along the peripheral nerves from the wound site to enter CNS. The incubation period varies between 1 and 3 months, depending on the distance between the brain and the wound. The disease begins with a prodrome of fever, malaise and headache besides local paraesthesia around the wound that is diagnostic. On progression, the patients exhibit CNS sensitivity. The touch is perceived as pain with violent motor response. The patients may have convulsions and signs of meningeal irritation. They have hydrophobia (aversion to water) seen as foaming in the mouth due to contracture of the pharyngeal muscles on swallowing. As the disease progresses, flaccid paralysis ensues. Periods of mania alternate with stupor. The disease finally progresses to coma eventually leading to death due to respiratory failure.

Human Immunodeficiency Virus

In times prior to antiretroviral therapy, neuropathological changes were demonstrated in as much as 80%–90% of cases with AIDS, during postmortem examination. Damage to the nervous system may be directly by the virus, by opportunistic infections or by primary CNS lymphomas (Epstein–Barr virus [EBV]-positive B-cell tumours). The multidrug antiretroviral therapy has dramatically reduced these complications. In 10% of patients, within 1–2 weeks of seroconversion, HIV produces aseptic meningitis. The virus can be isolated from CSF and antibodies to HIV can be demonstrated. Acute phase of HIV invasion of CNS on microscopy shows mild lymphocytic meningitis and perivascular inflammation with myelin loss. **Microglia** is the only cell in CNS to express the chemokine receptors

(CCR5 or CXCR4) and the CD4 coreceptor, both of which are required for infection by HIV. HIV encephalitis is seen on autopsy in individuals during the chronic phase. An interesting phenomenon called **'immune reconstitution inflammatory syndrome' (IRIS)** is seen in patients with AIDS after successful therapy. This syndrome presents as clinical deterioration after initiating therapy. It is an exuberant inflammatory response that is 'reconstituted' during antiretroviral therapy. Paradoxically, IRIS in CNS causes exacerbation of opportunistic infections. There is intense inflammation due to influx of $CD8^+$ lymphocytes. HIV-associated dementia causing severe cognitive changes may develop in spite of effective therapy. This disorder is due to inflammatory activation of microglial cells. Neuronal dysfunction in this setting is due to a cascade of toxic effects of HIV-derived proteins and inflammatory cytokines.

Progressive Multifocal Leucoencephalopathy

PML is **JC polyomavirus–induced encephalitis**. The virus has a predilection to infect **oligodendrocytes** producing demyelination as the principal pathological effect. It exclusively infects **immunocompromised** individuals. Primary infection is **asymptomatic** in spite of the fact that most people are exposed to JC virus by 14 years of age. PML occurs because of **reactivation of virus** in immunosuppressed patients such as those with chronic myeloproliferative or lymphoproliferative disease, patients on monoclonal antibody therapy targeting integrins and patients with AIDS who are immunosuppressed.

Subacute Sclerosing Panencephalitis

Subacute sclerosing panencephalitis (SSPE) is a rare entity affecting **children or young adults** characterized by progressive cognitive decline, spasticity of limbs and seizures. Acute infection with **measles**, after a long latent period of months or years, causes SSPE in children or young adults. Nonproductive, persistent infection of CNS by an altered measles virus, formed by several changes in the viral genes, attributes to this disease.

It is characterized by **widespread gliosis and myelin degeneration**. **Viral inclusions** are seen largely within the nuclei of oligodendrocytes and neurons with variable inflammation of white and grey matter besides neurofibrillary tangles. Ultrastructural study shows that the inclusions contain nucleocapsids characteristic of measles and immunohistochemistry for measles virus antigen is positive. The incidence of the disease has fallen sharply because of vaccination programmes, but it persists in nonimmunized populations.

FUNGAL MENINGOENCEPHALITIS

Fungal meningoencephalitis primarily affects **immunocompromised** individuals. The widespread **haematogenous dissemination** in these patients leads to infection affecting the brain. Haematogenous dissemination is the most common route to infect the brain; however, **direct extension**, such as in **mucormycosis**, can occur in the setting of diabetes mellitus. The most frequent causative organisms include *Aspergillus fumigatus*, *Candida albicans* and *Mucor* species, whereas *Cryptococcus neoformans*, *Histoplasma capsulatum*, *Coccidioides immitis* and *Blastomyces dermatitidis* may involve CNS following primary pulmonary or cutaneous infection in a clinical setting of immunosuppression. These infections occur in endemic regions. Fungal infection of CNS causes three major forms of injury – vasculitis, parenchymal invasion and chronic meningitis. **Vasculitis** is a feature of mucormycosis and aspergillosis that are vasoinvasive. It is seen occasionally with other infections such as candidiasis. Vasculitis is followed by vascular thrombosis causing haemorrhagic infarction that is subsequently invaded by the causative organism. **Parenchymal infection** by the fungus causes the formation of abscesses or granulomas and it coexists with meningitis. Parenchymal involvement is most commonly seen with *Candida* and *Cryptococcus*. *Candida* produces numerous microabscesses, with or without granuloma. A common opportunistic infection in patients with AIDS, cryptococcosis, can be indolent, evolving over months to years or have a fatal, fulminant course within 2 weeks. CSF has a high concentration of protein and is paucicellular. Cryptococcal **meningitis** can be demonstrated in CSF, as mucoid encapsulated yeasts, visualized with special stains or detected indirectly with assays for cryptococcal antigens.

Morphology

Cryptococcal infection causes chronic meningitis involving the basal leptomeninges, which appears thickened and opaque because of reactive connective tissue. Hydrocephalus may be seen because of obstruction to the flow of CSF through the foramen of Luschka and Magendie. Sections of the brain, especially in the distribution of the lenticulostriate arteries of the basal ganglia, show a gelatinous material in the subarachnoid space and small cysts reminiscent of 'soap bubbles' (Fig. 31.11). Perivascular (Virchow–Robin) spaces are expanded consisting of aggregates of organisms with little or no inflammation and gliosis. Meninges show infiltrates consisting of chronic inflammatory cells and fibroblasts with cryptococci (Table 31.1).

OTHER INFECTIONS OF CNS

CNS can be involved by other infectious disease such as:

- Protozoal infections such as malaria, toxoplasmosis, amebiasis and trypanosomiasis
- Metazoal infections such as cysticercosis and echinococcosis

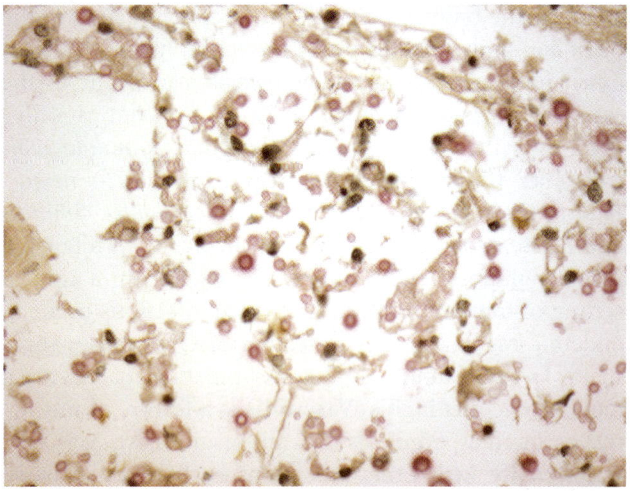

Fig. 31.11 Microscopy of cryptococcal meningitis. Mucicarmine staining highlights the polysaccharide capsule around the yeasts in the subarachnoid space. (*Source:* Sandra Camelo-Piragua and E. Tessa Hedley-Whyte, Infections of the Nervous System, in Diagnostic Pathology of Infectious Disease, 2nd Edition, © 2018 by Elsevier, Inc.)

- Rickettsial infections such as typhus and Rocky Mountain spotted fever

The pathogeneses of all infections mentioned next are discussed in detail in Chapter 8, and hence we will be describing the features relevant to CNS here.

Cerebral Malaria

Cerebral malaria, a **rapidly progressive encephalitis**, is a complication of ***Plasmodium falciparum*** infection associated with a high mortality. Cerebral involvement by malaria produces vascular dysfunction resulting in reduced cerebral blood flow. An acute phase characterized by ataxia, seizures and coma is followed by long-term cognitive deficits, which is seen in 20% of children following cerebral malaria.

Cerebral Amoebiasis

Naegleria species is known to cause fatal, rapidly progressing necrotizing encephalitis, whereas infection with *Acanthamoeba* produces chronic granulomatous meningoencephalitis. Amoebae may be morphologically similar to activated macrophages. Definitive identification relies on immunofluorescence studies, molecular methods and culture. **Methenamine silver or PAS stain** helps visualize the organisms.

Cerebral Toxoplasmosis

It is seen in a setting of **HIV-associated immunosuppression**. ***Toxoplasma gondii*** causes subacute infection of the brain that lasts over a 1- to 2-week period and it may be focal or diffuse. **Multiple ring-enhancing lesions** as seen in tuberculosis, CNS lymphoma and fungal infections are seen on imaging studies. Maternal infection during **early pregnancy** affects the brain of the developing fetus causing multifocal necrotizing and calcifying lesions.

Morphology

It causes brain abscess involving the grey–white junction of the cerebral cortex and deep grey nuclei, and less commonly in the brainstem and cerebellum. It rarely involves the spinal cord. Acute lesions show a necrotic centre, petechial haemorrhage surrounded by inflammatory infiltrate consisting of acute and chronic inflammatory cells, macrophages and proliferating blood vessels. The periphery of the necrotic foci shows **free tachyzoites** as well as **encysted bradyzoites**. The organisms can be identified by **Giemsa stains** or routine haematoxylin and eosin **(H&E)** staining but are clearly demonstrated by **immunohistochemistry**.

Table 31.1 Differences Between Various Types of Meningitis

Characteristics	Bacterial Meningitis	Aseptic (Viral) Meningitis	Fungal Meningitis	Tuberculosis
Appearance	Clear, cloudy or purulent	Clear	Clear or cloudy	Clear or opaque (cobweb appearance)
Opening pressure	Elevated (>25 cm H_2O)	Normal or elevated	Elevated	Elevated
WBC count	>100 cells/μL (>90% neutrophils); partially treated cases may have as low as 1 WBC/μL	10–1000 cells/μL (lymph but PMN early)	10–500 cells/μL	50–500 cells/μL (early PMN, then lymph)
Glucose level	Low (<40% of serum glucose)	>60% serum glucose (may be low in HSV infection)	Low	Low
Protein level	Elevated (>50 mg/dL)	Elevated (>50 mg/dL)	Elevated	Elevated

HSV, herpes simplex virus.

The blood vessels surrounding the lesion have prominent **intimal proliferation**, which sometimes show **frank vasculitis with fibrinoid necrosis and thrombosis.** Chronic lesions show small cystic areas with scattered lipid and haemosiderin-laden macrophages and surrounded by gliosis. Organisms are difficult to be identified in chronic lesions.

PRION DISEASES

A rapidly progressive neurodegenerative disorder caused by '***contagious***' pathogenic misfolded protein having the characteristics of an infectious organism constitutes prion disease. These abnormal misfolded prion proteins (PrP) cause '**spongiform change**' in the neurons and glia. It encompasses the following diseases in humans: Creutzfeldt–Jakob disease (CJD), fatal familial insomnia (FFI), Gerstmann–Sträussler–Scheinker syndrome and kuru.

PATHOGENESIS AND MOLECULAR GENETICS

The characteristic features with respect to pathogenesis of prion disease are given next.

Normal neurons contain a 30-kDa cytoplasmic protein PrP that exists as an α-helix isoform (PrPc). A conformational change leads to the formation of abnormal β-pleated sheet isoform (PrPsc) that resists proteinase K–mediated digestion, leading to its accumulation in the neural tissue causing prion disease. PrPsc protein has a property of inducing a self-propagating process that facilitates further conversion of PrPc molecules to PrPsc molecules, progressing the disease, and this unique feature explains transmission of prion diseases. PrPsc protein also causes cytoplasmic vacuoles and cell death by an unknown mechanism. PRNP gene encoding the PrP protein is a highly conserved gene. Familial variants of prion diseases can be due to a lot of mutations of PRNP gene. Such mutations lead to a faster conversion of PrPc protein to PrPsc protein leading to familial CJD.

CREUTZFELDT–JAKOB DISEASE

CJD, though rare, is the **most common prion disease** manifesting clinically as a rapidly progressive dementia. The sporadic form of CJD has an annual incidence of approximately 1 per 1,000,000 people. Familial forms are caused by mutations in PRNP gene. Peak incidence is noted in the **seventh decade** of life. Iatrogenic transmission has been observed following deep implantation of electrode in the brain, corneal transplantation and contaminated human growth hormone supplementation. Clinical signs of the disease are noted as subtle behavioural changes and changes in memory, which subsequently are followed by rapid downgrade. This disease is invariably fatal. Patients on an average survive for 7 months after initial symptoms. Extensive atrophy of the involved grey matter is seen in long-term survivors.

Variant Creutzfeldt–Jakob Disease

The United Kingdom, in 1995, reported cases of CJD-like illness affecting young adults. This variant CJD (vCJD) lacked the classical presenting features of CJD such as early prominent behavioural changes, and had a slower disease progression than in individuals with CJD. Pathological features and molecular findings were however similar to those of CJD. vCJD was linked to **bovine spongiform encephalopathy** exposure. It was transmitted by food contaminated with bovine spongiform encephalopathy agent as well as by blood transfusion. PRNP gene has no alterations and the disease seems to be due to codon 129 Met/Met homozygosity.

DEMYELINATING DISEASES

Demyelinating disease encompasses a group of acquired disorders of CNS, characterized by selective damage to myelin (which overwhelms the regenerative capacity) with relative initial sparing of axons that are damaged later on with disease progression. This loss of myelin causes disturbances in the transmission of electrical impulses through axons. Myelin loss can be due to the following reasons: immune-mediated injury of myelin (multiple sclerosis [MS]) and infections (JC virus infection of oligodendrocytes in PML). Leucodystrophies comprise inherited disorders that affect synthesis/turnover of myelin and are categorized as metabolic disorders.

MULTIPLE SCLEROSIS

MS is the most common **demyelinating disorder** of autoimmune aetiology. It forms discrete white matter lesions, delineated in space causing neurological deficits. Its prevalence is approximately 1 per 1000 persons in most of Europe and the United States. The disease clinically presents at any age. However, it is relatively rare in childhood or after 50 years. It affects women twice as often as men. A **relapsing and remitting** course of neurological defects of variable duration followed by partial recovery of neurological function is the characteristic presentation of MS. Frequency of relapse decreases over time with neurological deterioration.

Pathogenesis

Autoimmune injury of myelin sheath components is the main event. Genetic as well as environmental factors are involved in its pathogenesis. **DR2 extended haplotype** of the major histocompatibility complex has a strong effect. Genome-wide association studies (GWAS) initially identified association of the disease with IL-2 and IL-7 receptor genes and genes encoding proteins such as cytokines and their receptors and cytoplasmic signalling molecules. Immune mechanisms of myelin damage include T_H1 cell–secreted cytokines such as IFN-γ that activates macrophages and T_H17 cell–promoted recruitment of leucocytes along with a small role of humoral immunity. Hence, treatment with immunomodulators and agents that deplete B cells has shown to be beneficial. A probable role by viral infection such as EBV has also been implicated.

Morphology

MS is a **white matter disease** of the brain and spinal cord but may extend into the deep grey matter.

Gross Morphology shows well-circumscribed, slightly depressed, grey-tan, glassy, irregularly shaped **plaques** that are firmer than the surrounding white matter because of sclerosis. Plaques are observed adjoining the lateral ventricles, frequently involving the optic nerves with optic chiasma, ascending as well as descending fibre tracts, brainstem, cerebellum and spinal cord.

Microscopy Microscopy depends on the nature of the lesion. **Active plaque** is a lesion that has abundant lipid-rich macrophages containing PAS-positive debris with relative preservation of axons and reduced oligodendrocytes. Perivascular cuffs of lymphocytes and monocytes are present centred around small veins at the outer edge of the lesion. In time, reactive changes of astrocytes are seen. As lesions become quiescent, the inflammatory cells slowly disappear.

These plaques range from microscopic areas to confluent large lesions of the deep white matter. Demyelination can be demonstrated by using stains for myelin. In **inactive plaques**, myelin can be little to none, with reduced oligodendrocyte, prominent astrocytic proliferation and gliosis. Old gliotic plaques show few axons with severe demyelination. Abnormally thinned-out myelin sheaths that are considered to be the evidence of incomplete, partial remyelination can be demonstrated at the outer edge (Fig. 31.12).

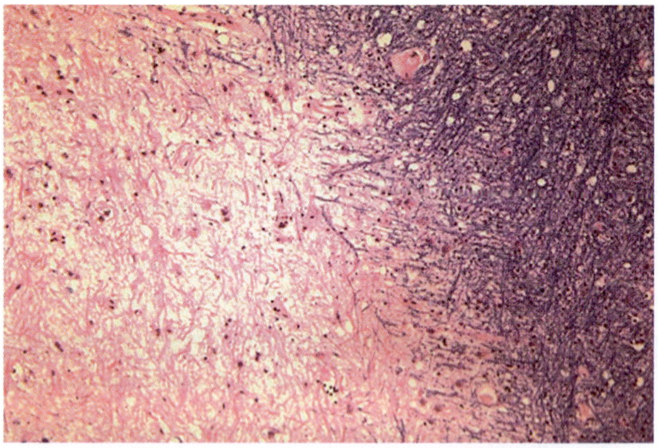

Fig. 31.12 Microscopy of multiple sclerosis. This Luxol fast blue stain for myelin shows lack of staining with demyelination on the left in a sharply demarcated MS plaque, with residual blue staining myelinated white matter at the right. (*Source:* Edward C. Klatt, The Central Nervous System, in Robbins and Cotran Atlas of Pathology, 4th Edition, © 2021 by Elsevier, Inc.)

Clinical Features

The entire CNS may be involved. Optic neuritis and retrobulbar neuritis presenting as unilateral visual impairment are frequent initial manifestations of MS. But only 10%–50% of individuals presenting with optic neuritis develop MS. Brainstem involvement produces ataxia, nystagmus, cranial nerve signs and internuclear ophthalmoplegia due to interruption of the medial longitudinal fasciculus fibres. Spinal cord lesions cause motor and sensory impairment of the limbs and trunk, spasticity and difficulties with the voluntary control of bladder function. CSF examination shows a mild elevation of protein level with **oligoclonal IgG bands** and moderate pleocytosis. IgG elevation indicates the presence of a small clone of self-reactive, activated B cells in CNS.

NEURODEGENERATIVE DISEASES

Neurodegenerative diseases include entities characterized by the progressive loss of functionally related group of neurons. Current classification is postulated on the basis of recent genetic and molecular studies because these disorders have many shared features. Neurodegenerative diseases have a predilection for certain anatomic locations and cause specific cellular abnormalities (e.g. tangles, plaques and Lewy bodies).

PATHOGENESIS

These disorders are collectively referred to as '**proteinopathies**' because of the common pathogenesis of accumulation of protein aggregates. Protein aggregates are formed because of accumulation of abnormally configured proteins that are resistant to clearance or because of defective clearance of normal proteins. Variable factors such as genetic, environmental or stochastic allow gradual accumulation of these proteins. These protein aggregates cause stress response along with direct toxicity to neurons. They may affect the normal adjoining cells by promoting protein aggregation in the latter, and may spread from one site in the brain to another. But only prions of prion disease are transmissible, whereas proteins in Alzheimer disease (AD) and Parkinson disease (PD) are not. These aggregates are seen histologically as **inclusions** – a diagnostic hallmark of the disease.

ALZHEIMER DISEASE

AD is the most common cause of dementia in older adults. Patients become symptomatic after 50 years of age and present with insidious impairment of higher cognitive function. The disease incidence increases with age. Later, disturbances of visuospatial orientation, memory, judgement, language and personality emerge. The affected individual, over a period of 5–10 years, becomes mute, profoundly disabled and immobile. Both sporadic form and familial form (5%–10%) exist, the former being more common. A combination of clinical assessment with radiology allows an accurate diagnosis in 80%–90% of cases. However, histopathological examination is necessary for a definitive diagnosis.

Molecular Genetics and Pathogenesis

Excessive production and defective removal lead to **accumulation of two proteins** (Aβ peptides in the neuropil and microtubule binding protein tau) in specific areas of the brain. The two pathological hallmarks of AD (evident in end stage) are **plaques and tangles**, which develop intracellularly but later are seen extracellularly after neuronal death causing neuronal dysfunction. Plaques represent aggregated Aβ protein, whereas tangles are aggregates of the protein tau. Pathogenesis of AD involves primarily **Aβ and tau**, apart from several other genetic and host factors. Aβ protein generation appears to be the crucial initiating event, whereas tau deposits are important in pathogenesis of progressive supranuclear palsy, frontotemporal lobar degenerations and corticobasal degeneration. The following genetic mutations are responsible for the familial form of AD:

- Mutations in APP gene encoding for Aβ protein cause familial AD.
- Increased copy number of chromosome 21 that contains the APP gene (trisomy 21) cause familial AD.
- Point mutations in protease complexes that produce Aβ from APP cause familial AD.
- Mutations in the gene for tau do not initiate AD but rather cause frontotemporal lobar degenerations.

Morphology

Gross Gross examination reveals the following: The brain shows varying cortical atrophy with widening of the cerebral sulci that is most pronounced in the frontal, temporal and parietal lobes. Medial temporal lobe structures such as the hippocampus and amygdala are usually involved in the earlier course of the disease and are severely atrophied with disease progression. Compensatory ventricular enlargement termed **hydrocephalus ex vacuo** occurs secondary to the reduced brain volume, caused by atrophy.

Microscopy Microscopy shows **neuritic (senile) plaques, neurofibrillary tangles** with concurrent neuronal loss and reactive gliosis (Fig. 31.13). The plaques are frequently observed in the hippocampus, amygdala and neocortex, whereas they relatively spare primary motor and sensory cortices. Neuritic plaques contain both Aβ40 and Aβ42 peptides. Neuritic plaques are localized spherical collections (20–200 μm) of dystrophic neurites surrounding the central amyloid core with a clear halo. The amyloid core demonstrated by Congo red contains several abnormal proteins like Aβ.

Microglial cells and reactive astrocytes are seen at their periphery. **Diffuse plaques** are formed by amyloid-like Aβ peptide deposition without surrounding

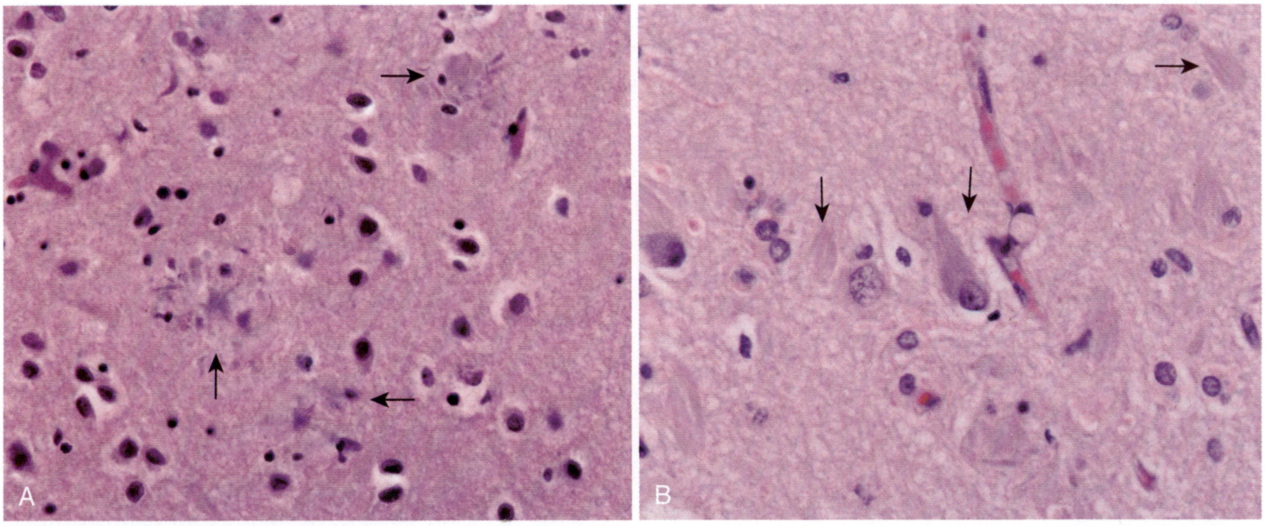

Fig. 31.13 Microscopy of Alzheimer disease. (A) Plaques with dystrophic neurites surrounding amyloid cores are visible *(arrows)*. (B) Neurofibrillary tangle is present within one neuron, and several extracellular tangles are also present *(arrows)*. (*Source:* Marta Margeta and Arie Perry, The Central Nervous System, in Robbins & Cotran Pathologic Basis of Disease, 10th Edition, © 2021 by Elsevier, Inc.)

neuritic process. They represent the early stage of plaque seen in the superficial parts of the cerebral cortex, basal ganglia as well as cerebellar cortex. Diffuse plaques are made up of Aβ42. **Neurofibrillary tangles** are tau-containing filaments in neuronal cytoplasm that displace or encircle the nucleus.

'Globose' tangles are elongated 'flame'-shaped structures in round cells with basket weave–like fibres around the nucleus in the pyramidal neurons. Microscopically, they are identified as basophilic fibrillary structures with H&E staining. Neurofibrillary tangles resist clearance because they are insoluble and may be seen as **'ghost' or 'tombstone' tangles** even after neuronal death in tissue sections. They can be demonstrated clearly by silver staining such as Bielschowsky stain and by immunohistochemistry directed against tau.

Sites showing these neurofibrillary tangles are cortical neurons, entorhinal cortex, the amygdala, pyramidal cells of the hippocampus, the raphe nuclei as well as the basal forebrain. Tangles are not specific to AD, being found in other diseases also.

Clinical Features AD is a slowly progressive disease that takes over a period of 10 years to develop. Initially, it presents as forgetfulness with memory disturbances, followed later by loss of mathematical skills, language deficits and learned motor skills. In the advanced stage, the person becomes mute, incontinent and unable to walk.

Treatment initiated in preclinical stages is aimed at clearing Aβ from the brain by immunological approaches, interrupting generation of Aβ by drugs that targets BACE (β-secretase 1) or γ-secretase and drugs preventing alterations in tau.

PARKINSON DISEASE

PD is a hypokinetic movement disorder due to **loss of dopaminergic neurons** in the substantia nigra. The clinical signs include masked facies (diminished facial expression), slow voluntary movements, rigidity, a 'pill-rolling' tremor and stooped posture with festinant gait (short accelerated steps). PD is caused by reduction in the striatal dopamine content due to destruction of dopaminergic neurons of the substantia nigra that release dopamine into the striatum. The severity of the motor syndrome is proportionate to the dopamine deficiency and replacement of dopamine is the mainstay of treatment. This is not an exclusive disease of dopaminergic neurons but begins in the brainstem, involves substantia nigra and eventually affects the cerebral cortex, causing cognitive impairment. Several other neurodegenerative disorders, dopaminergic antagonists and toxins can produce symptoms of parkinsonism. Parkinsonism is diagnosed by a triad of **rigidity, tremor and bradykinesia** – after ruling out other causes. Pesticide exposure is a risk factor for PD, but caffeine and nicotine seem to be protective.

Molecular Genetics and Pathogenesis

Protein accumulation and mitochondrial abnormalities with neuronal loss in the substantia nigra and elsewhere in the brain lead to PD. PD can be sporadic (mostly) or genetic.

- **α-Synuclein gene** encoding a lipid-binding protein associated with synapses is identified as the cause of autosomal dominant PD. α-Synuclein is the major component of **Lewy body** – the diagnostic hallmark of PD. Mutations in α-synuclein, though rare, may be due to point mutations/amplifications of the site on chromosome 4q21 that contains the gene. Polymorphisms in α-synuclein promoter sequence can alter its expression, influencing the risk of PD. α-Synuclein forms aggregates as well as small oligomers that seem to be the most toxic to neurons. Prion-like pattern of spread of these aggregates from cell to cell is seen even in PD. α-Synuclein-containing Lewy bodies and Lewy neurites appear initially in the medulla and then ascend the brainstem, extending into limbic structures and finally the neocortex.
- **Mitochondrial dysfunction** is a feature of autosomal recessive form of PD caused by mutation in genes encoding proteins PINK1, DJ-1 and parkin. DJ-1 acts as a transcriptional regulator, but during oxidative stress, it relocates into mitochondria and is responsible for the cytoprotective effects. PINK1, a kinase, during mitochondrial dysfunction, recruits parkin that is an E3 ubiquitin ligase. Normally, PINK1 and parkin combination promotes mitophagy – a process of clearance of dysfunctional mitochondria. Patients with sporadic PD have reduced mitochondrial complex I in the brain. It is a component of oxidative phosphorylation cascade.
- Autosomal dominant PD is more commonly caused by mutation in gene encoding LRRK2 (leucine-rich repeat kinase 2) and such mutation can also be seen in sporadic cases. LRRK2, a cytoplasmic kinase, can cause PD by gain-of-function mutation by hyperphosphorylation of normal targets.

Morphology

Gross Gross finding in PD shows pallor of the substantia nigra and locus coeruleus due to loss of the pigmented catecholaminergic neurons (Fig. 31.14).
Microscopy Lewy bodies are eosinophilic, round to oblong inclusions with a dense core bounded by a pale halo seen singly or multiply in the cytoplasm of the remaining neurons. They are seen in cholinergic cells of the basal nucleus of Meynert (with neuronal loss), brainstem nuclei, locus coeruleus and dorsal motor nucleus of the vagus. Neuronal loss is associated with

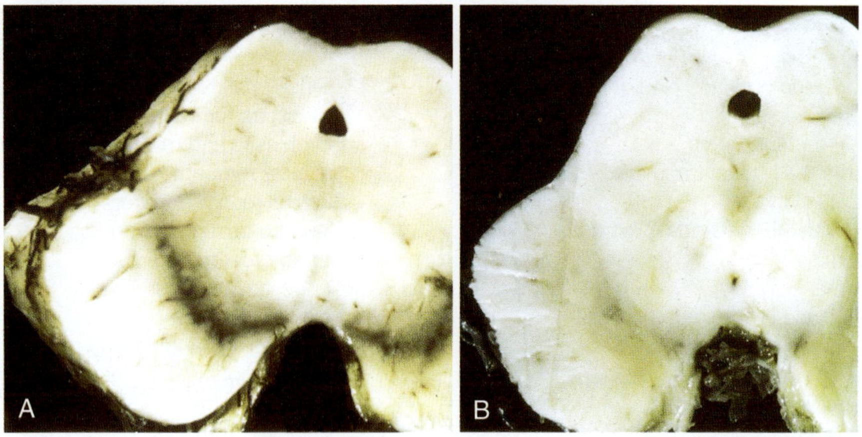

Fig. 31.14 Gross and microscopy of Parkinson disease. (A) Normal substantia nigra. (B) Depigmented substantia nigra in idiopathic Parkinson disease. (*Source:* Marta Margeta and Arie Perry, The Central Nervous System, in Robbins & Cotran Pathologic Basis of Disease, 10th Edition, © 2021 by Elsevier, Inc.)

gliosis. Dystrophic processes containing α-synuclein are Lewy neurites. Ultrastructurally, Lewy bodies show fine filaments of α-synuclein that are densely packed in the core and loose at the edge.

Dementia with Lewy bodies: With advancing age, 10%–15% of patients with PD develop dementia. This disorder characteristically has a fluctuating course with hallucinations and signs of frontal lobe involvement.

Atypical parkinsonism syndromes: 'Atypical parkinsonism syndromes' have clinical features of parkinsonism such as bradykinesia and rigidity, along with the presence of additional signs and symptoms. They are minimally responsive to treatment with levodopa and are also known as 'Parkinson plus syndrome'. They include conditions such as tauopathies that consist of progressive supranuclear palsy, corticobasal degeneration and synucleinopathy like multisystem atrophy.

Management: There is no definitive lab or imaging test recommended for PD. **DaTscan** is a technique that allows doctors to visualize the brain's dopamine system. Treatment includes supportive therapy such as physiotherapy and drugs such as levodopa. Initially, there is prompt response to levodopa replacement therapy but treatment cannot reverse morphological changes or stop the disease progression and drug therapy seems to be less effective when the symptoms worsen. Deep brain stimulation is used as a therapy for the motor symptoms. Early therapeutic trials with neural transplantation and gene therapy are recent ventures in treating PD.

TUMOURS OF THE BRAIN PA 35.2

The annual incidence of the CNS tumours is variable for intracranial and intraspinal tumours. The former has an incidence of 10–17 per 100,000 persons, whereas the incidence of the latter is 1–2 per 100,000 persons. Majority of the tumours are primary, whereas one-fourth to one-half are due to metastasis. CNS tumours account for approximately 20% of all childhood cancers. About 70% of childhood CNS tumours involve the posterior fossa, whereas tumours in adults occur to the same percentage in the supratentorial cerebrum. The clinical course of these patients is strongly dependent on the location and patterns of growth. Even a benign meningioma can cause cardiorespiratory arrest if it compresses vital centres in the medulla.

The **World Health Organization (WHO) classification** categorizes tumours from grade I to IV and also uses molecular genetics for diagnosis, which can be met with only by large centres. Thus, for the classification system to be followed universally, the surrogate immunohistochemical methods are made available, and this facilitates molecular genetics to be incorporated in the diagnosis. Treatment protocols are hence based on the current WHO classification.

Even the most malignant gliomas rarely metastasize outside CNS. '**Drop metastasis**' is the term used for tumours that encroach the subarachnoid space and tend to spread through CSF, hence causing an implantation along the brain or spinal cord at a distance from the original tumour site. Tumour recurrence represents clonal evolution of the same tumour, hence occurs with upgradation to a higher histological grade and designation.

A simplied version of the WHO classification of CNS tumours 2021 is given in Box 31.1. This section enlightens about the few common CNS tumours and meningeal tumours along with familial tumour syndromes.

GLIOMAS

The term gliomas include astrocytomas, oligodendrogliomas and ependymomas. They are the most common primary brain tumours. These tumours arise from a common

Box 31.1 The 2021 WHO Classification of Tumours of the Central Nervous System (Simplified)

1. Gliomas, Glioneuronal tumours and Neuronal tumours
   - Adult-Type Diffuse Gliomas
     Astrocytoma, IDH-mutant
     Oligodendroglioma, IDH-mutant and 1p/19q-codeleted
     Glioblastoma, IDH-wildtype
   - Paediatric-Type Diffuse Low-Grade Gliomas
     Diffuse astrocytoma
     Angiocentric glioma
   - Paediatric-Type Diffuse High-Grade Gliomas
     Diffuse midline glioma,
     Diffuse hemispheric glioma,
   - Circumscribed Astrocytic Gliomas
     Pilocytic astrocytoma
     Pleomorphic xanthoastrocytoma
   - Glioneuronal and Neuronal Tumours
   - Ependymal Tumours
2. Choroid Plexus Tumours
   - Choroid plexus papilloma
   - Choroid plexus carcinoma
3. Embryonal Tumours
   - Medulloblastomas
   - Other CNS embryonal tumours
     Atypical teratoid/rhabdoid tumour
     CNS neuroblastoma
4. Pineal Tumours
   - Pineocytoma
   - Pineoblastoma
5. Cranial and Paraspinal Nerve Tumours
   - Schwannoma
   - Neurofibroma
   - Perineurioma
   - Malignant peripheral nerve sheath tumour
6. Meningioma
7. Mesenchymal, Non-meningothelial Tumour Involving CNS
   - Soft tissue tumours
     Fibroblastic and myofibroblastic tumours
     Vascular tumours
     Skeletal muscle tumours
   - Chondro osseous tumours
   - Notochordal tumours
8. Melanocytic Tumours
   - Meningeal melanocytoma
   - Meningeal melanoma
9. Haematolymphoid Tumours Involving CNS
   - CNS lymphomas
   - Histiocytic Tumours
10. Germ Cell Tumours
    - Teratoma
    - Germinoma
    - Embryonal carcinoma
    - Yolk sac tumour
    - Choriocarcinoma
    - Mixed germ cell tumour
11. Tumours of the Sellar Region
    - Craniopharyngioma
    - Pituicytoma
    - Pituitary adenoma/pituitary neuroendocrine tumour
12. Metastatic tumours
13. Genetic Tumour Syndromes involving CNS
    - Neurofibromatosis type 1
    - Neurofibromatosis type 2
    - Tuberous Sclerosis
    - von Hippel Lindau Syndrome
    - Li-Fraumani syndrome
    - Cowden syndrome
    - Naevoid Basal Cell Carcinoma Syndrome

(*Source: Neuro-Oncology*, Volume 23, Issue 8, August 2021, Table 1, Pages 1231–1251.)

progenitor cell that differentiates along one of the cellular lineages of mature cell types (astrocytes, oligodendrocytes and ependymal). There is certain anatomic predilection with specific age distribution for some tumours in the brain. The current WHO classification divides the gliomas as diffuse adult-type glioma, low-grade paediatric glioma, high-grade paediatric glioma and circumscribed glioma as tabulated earlier. We will discuss, subsequently, about each subtype that is in line with the curriculum and within the scope of this textbook.

Astrocytoma: IDH Mutant

The patients with astrocytomas – IDH-mutant, CNS WHO grade 2 or 3 tumours – present in their thirties or forties (median age, 38 years) with a slight male predominance, whereas patients with CNS WHO grade 4 tumours tend to be seen in slightly older individuals. *IDH-mutant astrocytoma rarely affects adolescents and is uncommon in patients older than 55 years.*

Astrocytomas with IDH1/IDH2 mutation arise in any region of CNS usually centred near or within the frontal lobes yet most commonly involving the supratentorial compartment besides affecting the brainstem and spinal cord.

Molecular Genetics and Aetiopathogenesis *Most IDH-mutant astrocytomas are sporadic. GWAS* demonstrate *a link between IDH-mutant gliomas and low-frequency SNP at 8q24.21.*

Glioma with IDH1 and IDH2 mutations causes a gain-of-function state of the metabolic enzymes IDH1 and IDH2, which increases production of oncometabolite 2-hydroxyglutarate. In addition, IDH-mutant astrocytomas harbour loss-of-function mutations in TP53, ATRX and combined whole-arm deletions of 1p and 19q. Homozygous deletion of CDKN2A ± CDKN2B is associated with CNS WHO grade 4.

Morphology

Gross Diffuse astrocytomas may range in size from few centimetres to those that replace an entire hemisphere.

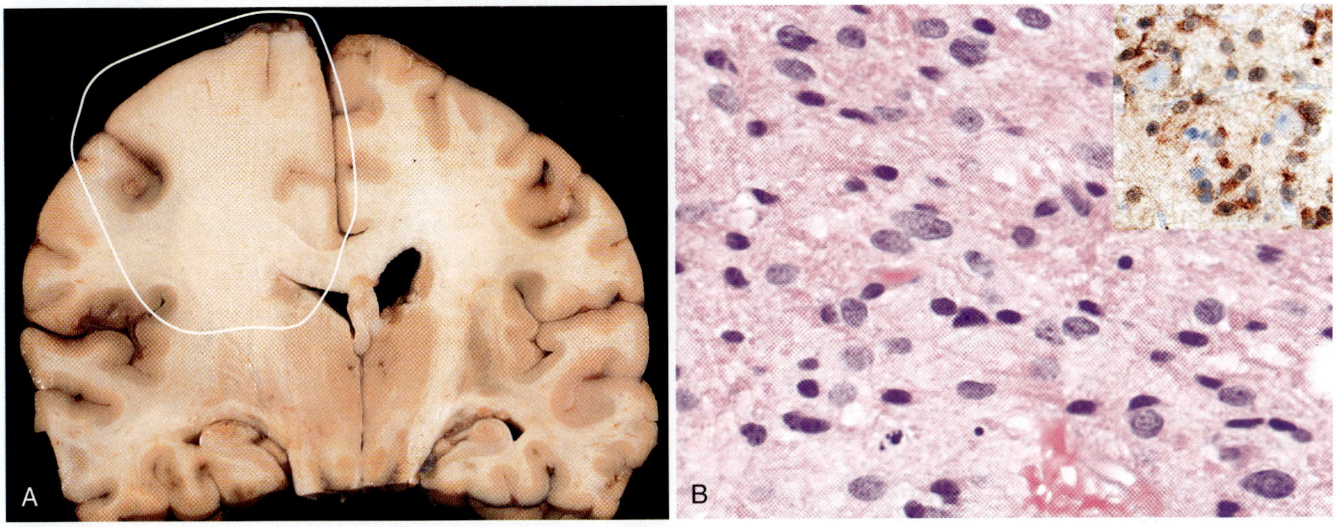

Fig. 31.15 Astrocytoma – IDH mutant. (A) Gross examination at autopsy shows the expanded left frontal white matter with blurring of the corticomedullary junction due to infiltrative tumour *(circled region).* (B) Microscopy of white matter shows enlarged, irregular, hyperchromatic nuclei that appear embedded within the native fibrillary matrix of the brain; the smaller round and oval nuclei are native oligodendrocytes and reactive astrocytes, respectively. (Inset) An immunostain for IDH1 R132H is positive for mutant protein in tumour cells, some of which surround the larger immunonegative cortical neurons ('perineuronal satellitosis'). (*Source:* Marta Margeta and Arie Perry, The Central Nervous System, in Robbins & Cotran Pathologic Basis of Disease, 10th Edition, © 2021 by Elsevier, Inc.)

They are grey, ill-defined, infiltrative and expansile tumours that distort the brain. The cut surface may be soft and gelatinous or firm, with cystic degeneration (Fig. 31.15A). Higher-grade examples may show similar features, but large coalescent zones of yellowish discolouration due to necrosis and/or haemorrhage may also be present.

Microscopy

Grade	Criteria
Astrocytoma IDH mutant, grade 2 (Figs 31.15B and 31.16)	Well-differentiated, diffusely infiltrative astrocytic lesion with an IDH1/IDH2 mutation lacking features of anaplasia • Mitotic activity is not detected • Absence of microvascular proliferation, necrosis, along with homozygous deletions of CDKN2A ± CDKN2B
Astrocytoma IDH mutant, grade 3	IDH1 or IDH2 mutation–positive, diffusely infiltrative astrocytic glioma with anaplasia and increased mitotic activity • Absence of microvascular proliferation, necrosis, along with homozygous deletions of CDKN2A ± CDKN2B
Astrocytoma IDH mutant, grade 4	IDH1 or IDH2–mutation positive, diffusely infiltrative astrocytic glioma with any of the microvascular proliferation necrosis homozygous deletions of CDKN2A and/or CDKN2B

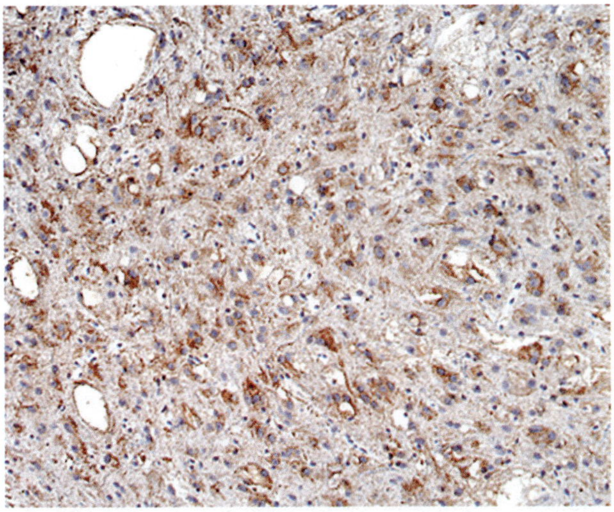

Fig. 31.16 Microscopy of astrocytoma – IDH mutant. GFAP stain shows positivity and highlights irregular clusters of neoplastic cells with variable quantities of cytoplasm and few coarse processes. (*Source:* Daniel J. Brat and Arie Perry, Astrocytic and Oligodendroglial Tumors, in Practical Surgical Neuropathology: A Diagnostic Approach, 2nd Edition, © 2018 by Elsevier, Inc.)

Immunohistochemistry:

Immunohistochemical assays used as surrogates for genetic alterations (IDH1 p.R132H positivity, p53 strong nuclear expression of p53 in >10% of tumour cells, loss of nuclear ATRX expression)

Glioblastoma, IDH-Wildtype Previously called glioblastoma multiforme, abbreviated as GBM, they are the most common malignant brain tumour in adults. Glioblastoma accounts for 15% of all intracranial neoplasms and 45%–50% of all primary malignant brain tumour. Glioblastoma, IDH-wildtype, is a diffuse, astrocytic glioma that has IDH-wildtype with H3-wildtype along with one or more of the histological/genetic features given next besides astrocytic differentiation: diffuse growth pattern showing nuclear atypia, marked cellular pleomorphism and mitotic activity, microvascular proliferation, necrosis, TERT promoter mutation, EGFR gene amplification and +7/−10 chromosome copy-number changes.

It commonly affect individuals of age between 55 and 85 years. It is more common in men. Glioblastoma, IDH-wildtype, is positioned in cerebral hemispheres along the subcortical white matter and deeper grey matter. Tumour infiltration extends through the corpus callosum into the contralateral side also. Glioblastoma, IDH-wildtype, also affects the brainstem, cerebellum and spinal cord.

Molecular Genetics and Aetiopathogenesis Irradiation of the head and neck region is one of the most important risk factors for the development of glioblastoma. Tumour-associated macrophages (TAMs) are attracted to and reprogrammed by gliomatous cells by secretion of chemokines and other soluble factors to promote gliomagenesis by enhancing invasion, angiogenesis and immunosuppression. Trisomy 7 and monosomy 10 are the most frequent chromosomal alterations in glioblastoma

Morphology

Gross Glioblastoma was the name given because of gross morphology of these tumours that had variegated appearance within the same tumour. The tumour has firm to soft areas, white to yellow necrotic area admixed with areas showing cystic degeneration and haemorrhage.

Microscopy Glioblastoma, IDH-wildtype, is a highly cellular, diffusely infiltrating glioma composed of poorly differentiated astrocytic tumour cells showing nuclear atypia and marked pleomorphism. Mitotic activity is readily identifiable and brisk. Microvascular proliferation along with necrosis, which may or may not be associated with perinecrotic palisading, is the characteristic diagnostic feature (Fig. 31.17). In IDH- and H3-wildtype diffuse glioma, at least one of the above-mentioned features (microvascular proliferation or necrosis) would suffice for the diagnosis of glioblastoma. Subtypes of glioblastoma, to name a few, would be giant cell glioblastoma, small cell glioblastoma, epithelioid glioblastoma, heavily lipidized glioblastoma, glioblastoma with epithelial and mesenchymal metaplasia, and gliosarcoma.

Microscopy is similar to that of anaplastic astrocytoma with few additional features that include serpentine pattern of necrosis in hypercellular areas (Fig. 31.17).

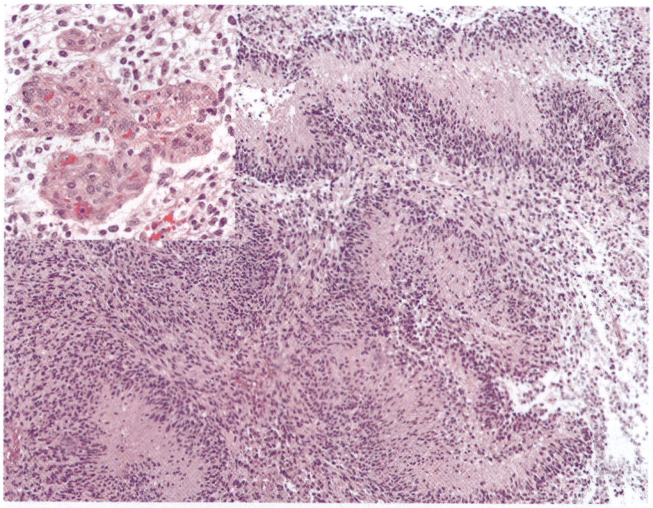

Fig. 31.17 Microscopy of glioblastoma – serpiginous foci of palisading necrosis (tumour nuclei lined up around the red anucleate zones of necrosis). (Inset) Microvascular proliferation. (*Source:* Marta Margeta and Arie Perry, The Central Nervous System, in Robbins & Cotran Pathologic Basis of Disease, 10th Edition, © 2021 by Elsevier, Inc.)

Tumour cells border the necrotic areas, producing a pattern referred to as **pseudopalisading**. Vascular/endothelial cell proliferation occurs because of VEGF produced by the malignant astrocytes in response to hypoxia and this vascular cell proliferation causes tuft of cells to bulge into the lumen of the vessel (the minimal criterion being double-layered endothelial cells).

IHC: GFAP and nuclear positivity of OLIG2 are reliable markers along with Ki-67 index, which will be high corresponding to high proliferative index.

Clinical Features of Astrocytoma The symptoms of diffuse astrocytoma are variable according to its location and growth rate. Diffuse astrocytoma remains stable over a number of years, progressing slowly; the mean survival is more than 5 years. Clinical deterioration follows because of progression to a higher histological grade that grows rapidly. Neuroimaging shows the tumour mass with surrounding oedema in the brain. High-grade astrocytomas have contrast enhancement on imaging studies because of abnormal 'leaky' vessels causing a permeable blood–brain barrier.

Glioblastoma has a very poor prognosis. Most patients with glioblastoma die within 15–18 months after chemoradiation. Some patients with glioblastomas benefit with maximal safe surgery, radiation, bevacizumab (where approved) and alkylating chemotherapy, as well as immunological interventions. This marked heterogeneity observed in treatment response reflects the biological heterogeneity of the disease.

Pilocytic Astrocytoma (WHO Grade I)

Pilocytic astrocytoma is a circumscribed astrocytic neoplasm with pilocytic (bipolar hair-like) cells, compact yet myxoid regions with Rosenthal fibres and eosinophilic granular bodies. It is characterized by MAPK pathway gene alterations. Pilocytic astrocytoma is the most common glioma in children and young adults. Common sites are the cerebellum, the other sites being floor and walls of the third ventricle, the optic nerves and cerebral hemispheres. Pilocytic astrocytoma is a slow-growing tumour. Sporadic pilocytic astrocytoma is also the principal CNS tumour type in a group of neurodevelopmental diseases associated with germline mutations in MAPK pathway genes. This includes neurofibromatosis type 1 (NF1), Noonan syndrome and encephalocraniocutaneous lipomatosis. NF1 is caused by NF1 germline mutation, whereas Noonan syndrome is due to mutations in PTPN11 or RAF1 and encephalocraniocutaneous lipomatosis is caused by FGFR1 germline mutations.

Morphology

Pilocytic astrocytoma is usually cystic but can be a solid, well-circumscribed and, rarely, infiltrative lesion. Tumours are biphasic, with 'microcystic' and fibrillary areas.

Pilocytic astrocytomas are low to moderately cellular neoplasm. Neoplastic cells have a varied morphology with piloid and oligodendrocyte-like cells (Fig. 31.18). Nuclei are round to oval. Giant cells with nuclear clusters in horseshoe shape (pennies-on-a-plate pattern) are seen. Hyperchromasia and nuclear pleomorphism may be obvious in some cases but mitotic figures are rarely seen. Cases that have a brisk mitotic activity imply an aggressive behaviour. Rosenthal fibres and eosinophilic granular bodies are seen in varying proportion. Stroma may be myxoid with microcystic change apart from degenerative changes like hyalinized vessels, calcifications and haemorrhages. Histological patterns that can be seen in pilocytic astrocytoma are the following:

(1) a biphasic pattern, compact areas with bipolar cells and Rosenthal fibres alternating with loose, microcystic regions having oligodendrocyte-like cells
(2) Compact, piloid pattern, with lots of Rosenthal fibres
(3) Dispersed pattern

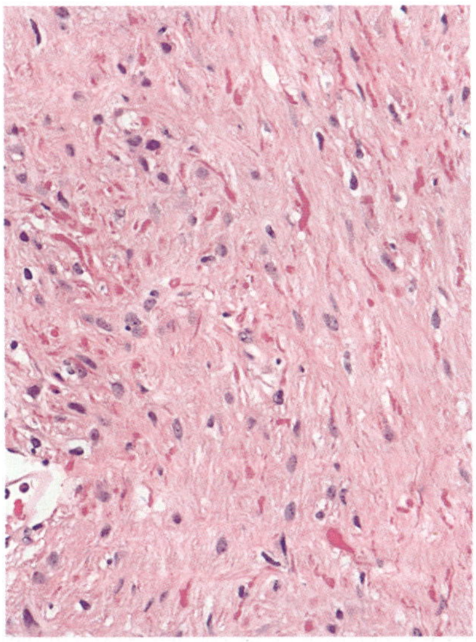

Fig. 31.18 Pilocytic astrocytoma. Higher magnification reveals oval to irregular tumour nuclei resembling those of diffuse astrocytoma, but with numerous Rosenthal fibres (brightly eosinophilic corkscrew-shaped inclusions) in the background. (*Source:* Marta Margeta and Arie Perry, The Central Nervous System, in Robbins & Cotran Pathologic Basis of Disease, 10th Edition, © 2021 by Elsevier, Inc.)

Tumours from the optic tract extending into the hypothalamic region have an ominous clinical course because of their location.

Oligodendroglioma

Oligodendroglioma, IDH-mutant and 1p/19q-codeleted, is a diffusely infiltrating glioma with IDH1 or IDH2 mutation and codeletion of chromosome arms 1p and 19q (CNS WHO grade 2 or 3). It occurs most commonly between 35 and 44 years of age with a slight male predominance. Patients present with neurological complaints, especially seizures. The lesions occur in the white matter of the cerebral hemispheres, usually the frontal lobe.

Molecular Genetics The most common genetic aberrations in oligodendrogliomas are IDH1 and IDH2 mutations, seen in up to 90% of oligodendrogliomas, and foretell a better prognosis. Codeletion of chromosomes 1p and 19q occurs in approximately 80% of cases. Codeletion of 1p/19q has a good response to treatment with chemoradiotherapy, whereas the tumours without codeletion 1p/19q are resistant to chemotherapy. The defining alteration in oligodendrogliomas is missense mutation affecting IDH1 codon 132/IDH2 codon 172 apart from whole-arm deletions of 1p and 19q. TERT promoter hotspot mutations can also be seen in cases with IDH1/IDH2 mutation and codeletion of 1p/19q.

Morphology

Gross examination shows well-circumscribed, grey gelatinous mass with cysts and focal haemorrhage and calcification. Calcification may impart a gritty texture while grossing and may be seen as intratumoural stones.

Classic oligodendroglioma cells have slightly larger round nuclei than normal oligodendrocytes with increased chromatin density or stippled salt-and-pepper pattern with a distinct nuclear membrane (Fig. 31.19). After routine processing, the tumour cells appear rounded with a crisp cell membrane and clear cytoplasm around a centrally placed nucleus giving a fried-egg appearance, which is a helpful diagnostic feature due to artefact. This artefact is not seen in frozen sections, smear preparations and rapidly fixed tissue. The

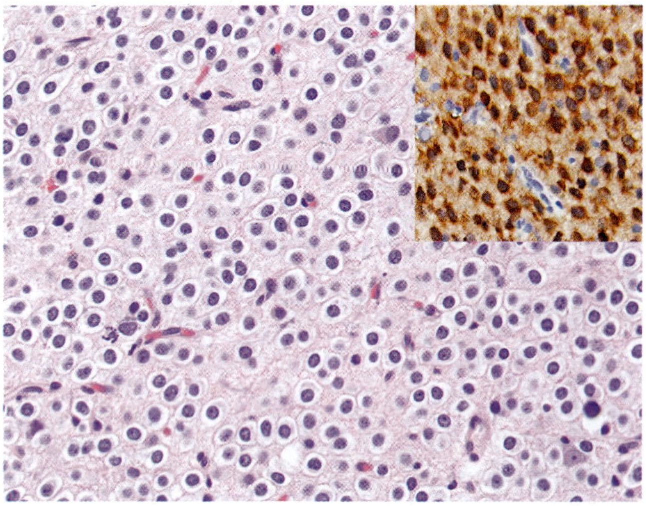

Fig. 31.19 Microscopy of oligodendroglioma. Tumour nuclei are round, with cleared cytoplasm forming 'halos' and vasculature composed of thin-walled capillaries. Tumour cells are usually positive for IDH1 R132H–mutant protein *(inset)*. *(Source:* Marta Margeta and Arie Perry, The Central Nervous System, in Robbins & Cotran Pathologic Basis of Disease, 10th Edition, © 2021 by Elsevier, Inc.)

tumour has a delicate network of anastomosing capillaries exhibiting the characteristic **chicken-wire pattern**. Reactive astrocytes are prominent at the tumour borders. GFAP-positive 'minigemistocytes' or 'microgemistocytes' can be seen.

Immunohistochemistry Most oligodendrogliomas are immunopositive for antibody against IDH1 p.R132H, which helps in differentiating it from other clear cell tumours, and non-neoplastic and reactive lesions. IDH-mutant with 1p/19q-codeleted oligodendrogliomas show nuclear expression of ATRX and lack widespread nuclear p53 staining.

Treatment Factors associated with favourable outcomes are younger patient age at diagnosis, frontal lobe involvement, presenting with seizures and high postoperative Karnofsky score, apart from macroscopic complete surgical removal. Adequate surgical resection has been associated with a longer overall survival (OS). Radiotherapy, chemotherapy and postsurgical resection are often deferred until tumour progression to deter possible therapy-associated neurotoxicity.

Ependymoma

Ependymomas originate from the ependymal lining of the ventricular system of the brain and the obliterated part in the spinal cord. The fourth ventricle is the common site in children while the spinal cord is the common site in adults especially adults with neurofibromatosis type 2.

Pathogenesis The supratentorial ependymomas are associated with ZFTA or YAP1 fusion and infratentorial tumours are classified as PFA or PFB based on their unique molecular alterations while spinal tumours are defined by the presence of MYCN amplification. Tumours in the above locations but lacking these molocular features are called Ependymoma- Not otherwise specified.

Morphology

The most common site of supratentorial ependymomas are the cerebral hemispheres with or without connection to the ventricular system. They occur in children and adults with incidence decreasing with age coinciding with increase in frequency in spinal tract. Posterior fossa ependymomas occur in the roof (common in PFA variant), lateral wall and floor of fourth ventricle (common in PFB variant). They may be found herniating into the spinal canal thorough the foramen magnum enveloping the cranial nerves and vessels. Spinal tumours are commonly located in the cervical or cervicothoracic region of spinal cord.

These tumours are well circumscribed with soft spongy consistency and tan colour. Calcification if present ay give a gritty texture to the tumour.

Microscopically these tumours are composed of small regular round to oval cells with round nuclei and indistinct cytoplasmic borders. They show presence of **pseudorosettes** composed of cells arranged around vessels with a nuclei free zone surrounding the blood vessel composed of fibrillary processes and **true ependymal rosettes** which are cells arranged around gland like spaces (Fig. 31.20). The supratentorial ones show a unique branching vascular pattern not seen in other variants. Nuclear pleomorphism and mitotic activity may be seen and are more common in posterior fossa tumours. Spinal ependymomas may mimick pilocytic astrocytomas by the presence of spindle shaped cells with bipolar processes.

The unique variant myxopapillary ependymoma is usually composed of elongated tumour cells arranged around hyalinized blood vessels with an intervening accumulation of myxoid material which is PAS positive. They are Grade 1 and are the most common tumours of the filum terminale and conus medullaris of the spinal cord and have a relatively better prognosis.

Clinical features The patient may present with focal neurological deficits depending on the location of the tumour or symptoms of increased intracranial tension.

Immunohistochemistry done shows positivity for GFAP and S100 around blood vessels and in perivascular pseudorosettes. Most but not all tumours also show positivity for EMA. Diagnosis of the tumour is complete only after molecular typing is done for categorization of the lesion as the prognosis depends on the molecular characteristics of the tumour.

Prognosis The prognosis depends of the completeness of surgical resection of the tumour. Overall supratentorial

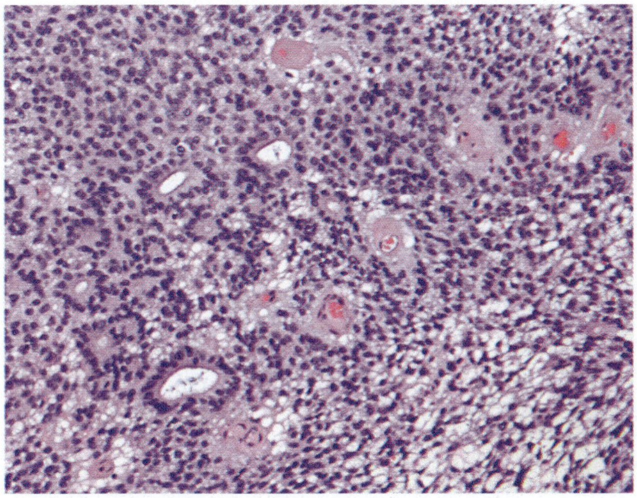

Fig. 31.20 Microscopy of ependymoma. The microscopic appearance includes both true rosettes (with a gland-like central lumen) and perivascular pseudorosettes (nuclear-free zone composed of fibrillary processes radiating towards a central blood vessel). (*Source:* Marta Margeta and Arie Perry, The Central Nervous System, in Robbins & Cotran Pathologic Basis of Disease, 10th Edition, © 2021 by Elsevier, Inc.)

tumours have poorer prognosis than infratentorial ones in adults. Complete resection followed with radiotherapy helps to reduce recurrence and gives good prognosis in tumours that have not metastatized. Invasion into surrounding brain parenchyma, inability to resect completely and metastasis are indicators of poor prognosis. Drop metastasis through CSF is seen in as many as 15% of cases especially ones with higher histological grades.

Medulloblastoma

The most common embryonal tumour is medulloblastoma. This malignant embryonal tumour accounts for 20% of brain tumours in children involving the cerebellum. These largely undifferentiated WHO grade IV tumours express neuronal as well as glial markers. Medulloblastoma is classified taking into account the molecular and histopathological features. Consensus that was based on available datasets established four principal molecular groups – WNT-activated, sonic hedgehog (SHH)–activated, group 3 and group 4. Tumours in the WNT and SHH groups show activation of their respective cell signalling pathways. Non-WNT/non-SHH medulloblastomas comprise group 3 and group 4 tumours.

We will be confining the discussion of this tumour to its prototype, i.e., medulloblastoma histologically defined.

Medulloblastomas, Histologically Defined Medulloblastoma, an embryonal neuroepithelial tumour located in the posterior fossa, shows on histology small, poorly differentiated cells with high N:C ratio, high mitosis and apoptosis.

Sites involved are the following:

Classic medulloblastomas: Cerebellar midline is in the fourth ventricle. Classic medulloblastoma, WNT- or SHH-activated, involves the cerebellar peduncle and hemisphere laterally.

Desmoplastic/nodular (D/N) medulloblastomas involve the cerebellar hemisphere and the vermis. They usually involve the cerebellar hemispheres in adults.

Medulloblastomas with extensive nodularity (MBENs) involve the vermis, along with the adjoining hemispheres.

Large cell/anaplastic (LC/A) medulloblastomas have a predilection for the cerebellar midline, fourth ventricle and adjacent brainstem and cerebellar structures. SHH activation type of LC/A medulloblastomas has lateral localization with extracerebellar extension.

Imaging On MRI, classic medulloblastomas are identified as homogeneous, hyperintense, contrast-enhancing mass in the midline.

Epidemiology Classic medulloblastomas account for 70%–80% of all medulloblastomas. They have a predilection for any age while being common in childhood (60%–70%). Classic morphology is seen across all four genetically defined medulloblastoma types but more so in WNT-activated and non-WNT/non-SHH medulloblastomas.

Aetiopathogenesis Classic medulloblastomas, in rare cases, demonstrate mismatch repair deficiency syndrome, germline APC, BRCA2 or PALB2 mutation, or Rubinstein–Taybi syndrome.

D/N medulloblastoma or MBEN can occur in naevoid basal cell carcinoma syndrome (NBCCS). D/N medulloblastomas arise from granule cell progenitors that form the external granule cell layer during cerebellar development. These progenitors depend on the mitogen, SHH – produced by Purkinje cells. MBENs arise from cerebellar fetal granular layer or cerebellar velum.

Majority of LC/A medulloblastomas are sporadic. SHH-activated, TP53-mutant medulloblastoma is diagnosed in the setting of Li–Fraumeni syndrome.

Non-WNT/non-SHH group 3 LC/A medulloblastomas seem to arise from a stem cell–like population present in the early developing cerebellum.

Morphology

Macroscopic Appearance Classic medulloblastomas appear as friable pink masses, occasionally with macroscopic foci of necrosis (Fig. 31.21A).

D/N medulloblastomas tend to be firm and circumscribed, reflecting intratumoural desmoplasia.

MBENs tend to be firm, grape-like and well circumscribed.

LC/A medulloblastomas appear as friable, greyish-pink masses, occasionally with macroscopic foci of necrosis. At surgery, LC/A medulloblastomas often show cerebellar and brainstem invasion.

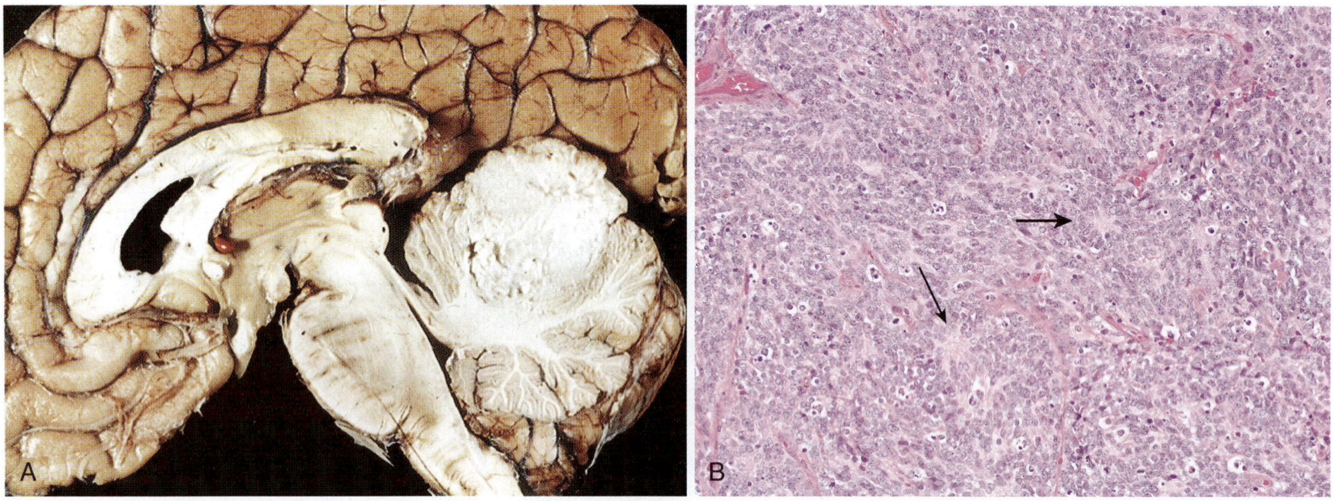

Fig. 31.21 Classic variant medulloblastoma. (A) Sagittal section of brain showing medulloblastoma replacing part of the superior cerebellar vermis. (B) The microscopic appearance of classic medulloblastoma includes primitive-appearing 'small blue cells' that form sheets and Homer Wright (neuroblastic) rosettes with central neuropil *(arrows)*. (*Source:* Marta Margeta and Arie Perry, The Central Nervous System, in Robbins & Cotran Pathologic Basis of Disease, 10th Edition, © 2021 by Elsevier, Inc.)

Classic Medulloblastoma Classic medulloblastoma is the archetype of CNS small blue round cell tumour. It consists of poorly differentiated embryonal cells that are tightly packed, with hyperchromatic nuclei of various shapes. Homer Wright rosettes can be seen in classic medulloblastomas (Fig. 31.21B). Mitosis is high and apoptotic bodies are found. Classic medulloblastomas express specific neural markers like CD56 (NCAM1), MAP2 and NSE.

Desmoplastic/Nodular Medulloblastoma D/N medulloblastoma is characterized by tightly packed, poorly differentiated cells with pleomorphic hyperchromatic nuclei producing extensive intercellular reticulin fibres surrounding reticulin-free zones (pale islands).

Medulloblastoma With Extensive Nodularity MBEN is large lobular with reticulin-free zones and has a rich neuropil-like matrix. These zones have small cells with round nuclei in a streaming pattern, with variable neurocytic differentiation.

Large Cell/Anaplastic Medulloblastoma As the name implies, these tumours have large cell and anaplastic features. Anaplasia is seen as marked nuclear pleomorphism with high mitosis and apoptotic bodies. Cytoplasmic pseudoinclusions, nuclear moulding and cell wrapping are the typical features.

Clinical Features Most patients present with symptoms and signs of raised intracranial pressure from noncommunicating hydrocephalus due to occlusion of the fourth ventricle. Medulloblastoma causes nausea, vomiting, headache, dizziness, tiredness, poor coordination, double vision and unsteady gait. These symptoms may be due to the tumour per se or as a result of raised intracranial pressure.

At diagnosis, classic medulloblastoma has disseminated to the leptomeninges in as many as 40% of cases. They are highly malignant but the tumour is radiosensitive. The prognosis of the patient depends on the variant and the treatment. While aggressive subtypes have only 20% to 30%, 5-year survival the better ones like WNT- activated medulloblastoma have 100%, 5-year survival.

MENINGIOMAS

Meningioma is a family of neoplasms derived from the meningothelial cells of the arachnoid mater attached to the dura (CNS WHO grades 1, 2 or 3). In the United States, meningioma occurs at an average annual age-adjusted rate of 8.58 cases per 100,000 population, and accounts for 37.6% of CNS tumours. It may be found on external surfaces of the brain as well as inside the ventricular system, in which case it arises from stromal arachnoid cells of the choroid plexus. A known risk factor for meningioma development is a past history of radiotherapy for the head and neck.

Molecular Genetics

The most common genetic abnormality observed in meningioma is loss of chromosome 22(22q). Meningiomas are common in the setting of neurofibromatosis type 2 (NF2) because of deletion of the region 22q12 that represents NF2 gene encoding the protein merlin. NF2 gene mutation is observed in 50%–60% of sporadic meningiomas also, leading to the absence of merlin protein in many cases. NF2 mutations are more often associated with high-grade meningiomas because of chromosomal instability (additional chromosomal aberrations are seen with chromosome 22 loss). Apart from NF2 mutations, the other most common mutation is TNF-receptor-associated factor 7 (TRAF7) mutation, which constitutes a subset of meningioma with a lower histological grade because of greater chromosomal stability. Meningiomas express progesterone receptors and tend to grow rapidly during pregnancy.

Morphology

Gross Meningiomas are well-defined dura-based mass extending onto the overlying bone. They are found compressing the brain at the site of the lesion and still can be easily separated. Grossly, they appear as bosselated encapsulated masses. Meningioma rarely may grow en plaque, in which the tumour forms a sheet-like covering along the dural surface. This type is associated with hyperostotic reactive change of the adjoining bone. The cut surface of the tumour is firm, fibrous to finely gritty and sometimes contains calcified psammoma bodies. Evidence of necrosis and frank haemorrhage is absent on gross examination (Fig. 31.22A).

Microscopy Microscopy may show various histological patterns but is unrelated to prognosis. Meningiomas constitute WHO grade I lesions unless mentioned otherwise and include the following:

- **Meningothelial ('syncytial') meningioma:** The meningothelial subtype of meningioma has epithelioid cells forming syncytia-like lobules, demarcated by fine collagen septa. The cells are monomorphic, with few nuclei demonstrating nuclear holes and pseudoinclusions, with abundant eosinophilic cytoplasm (Fig. 31.22B). Meningothelial meningiomas have AKT1 p.E17K mutations, apart from TRAF7 mutations, or SMO and PIK3CA mutations.
- **Fibroblastic meningioma:** The fibrous subtype of meningioma have spindle cells arranged in fascicles, interlacing bundles and storiform pattern in a collagen-rich matrix (Fig. 31.22C). EMA expression may be weak or absent, whereas S100 staining is strong. Fibrous meningiomas show 22q deletion and mutation of the retained NF2 allele, akin to transitional and psammomatous meningiomas. They seem to arise more commonly involving the skull base.
- **Transitional meningioma:** The transitional subtype shows admixture of lobular (meningothelial) and

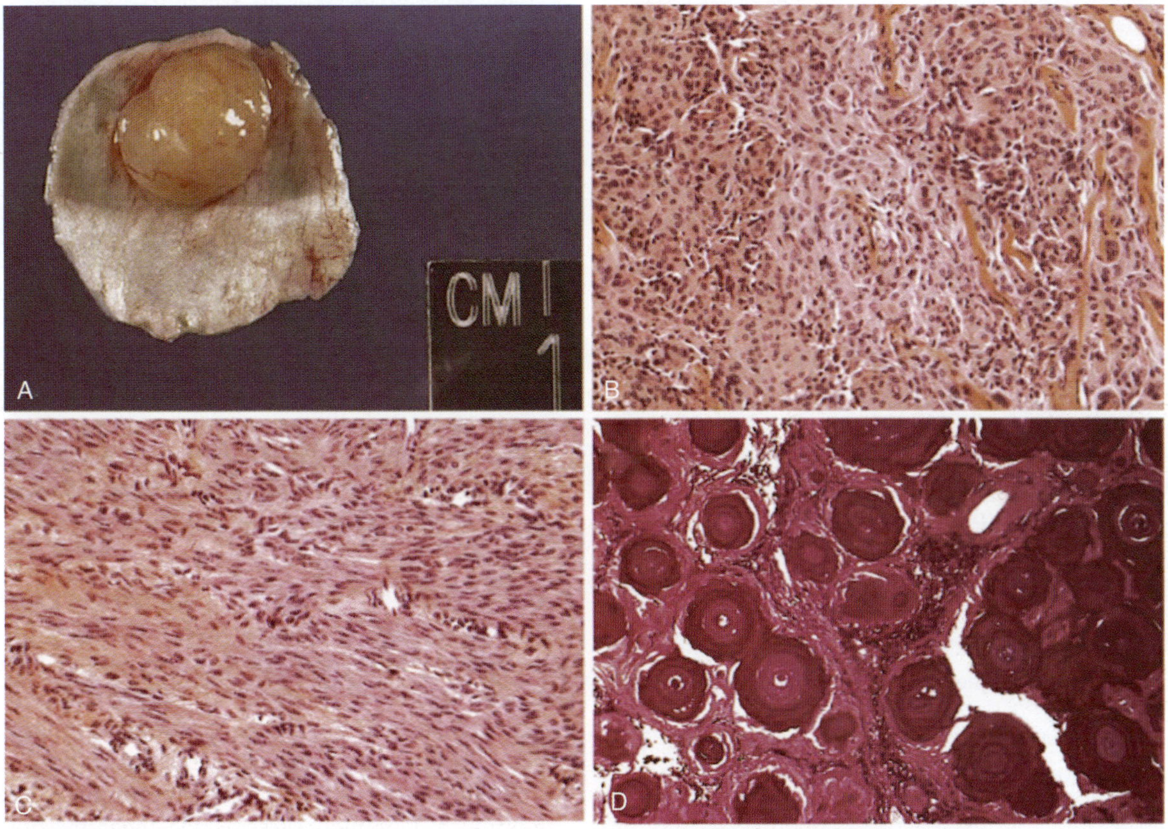

Fig. 31.22 Meningioma. (A) Gross appearance of a typical meningioma showing a well-circumscribed, tan-yellow mass attached to the dura. (B) Syncytial meningioma (WHO grade I) marked by lobules of cells separated by fibrovascular septa. Whorling of cells in the lobules is common. (C) Fibroblastic meningioma (WHO grade I) characterized by a proliferation of monomorphic spindled cells. (D) Numerous laminated calcified structures mark a psammomatous meningioma (WHO grade I). (*Source:* Marta Margeta, Arie Perry (2021). Robbins & Cotran Pathologic Basis of Disease (10th ed.). St Louis, MO: Elsevier.)

fascicular (fibrous) patterns as well as transitional features, which seem to be between the two prototypes that are admixed in this tumour. Psammoma bodies and whorl formation are frequent in this subtype. They often arise from the convexity. Just like fibrous and psammomatous meningiomas, transitional meningiomas also show 22q deletions and NF2 mutations.

- **Psammomatous meningioma:** Psammoma bodies predominate in this variant more than the viable tumour cells. They are seen as large, confluent, calcified mass (Fig. 31.22, CS). Meningioma cells may be rare to virtually absent, but can be demonstrated by immunohistochemistry with EMA or SSTR2A. Noncalcified foci show features of fibrous or transitional subtypes. This subtype commonly occurs in the thoracic spine region of middle-aged or elderly women. Like fibrous and transitional meningiomas, psammomatous meningiomas demonstrate 22q deletions and NF2 mutations.
- **Angiomatous Meningioma:** Numerous thin- or thick-walled hyalinized small blood vessels are seen admixed with meningioma cells that may be hard to find and identify as meningioma cells. Angiomatous areas can also be seen admixed with microcystic or metaplastic areas, and cells may show degenerative nuclear atypia. Angiomatous, microcystic and metaplastic meningiomas have high-frequency gain of chromosome 5.
- **Microcystic Meningioma:** Microcysts formed by cells having thin, elongated processes are seen creating a cobweb-like background. These cysts can be identified macroscopically or radiologically. Degenerative nuclear atypia can raise the suspicion of a higher grade, yet these are typically benign. Gain of chromosome 5 is common. Cerebral oedema is frequent, as in angiomatous and secretory meningiomas.
- **Secretory Meningioma:** It is characterized by focal gland-like epithelial differentiation having PAS-positive eosinophilic secretions with or without KLF4 and TRAF7 mutations.
  These eosinophilic secretions called pseudopsammoma bodies are positive for carcinoembryonic antigen (CEA) apart from epithelial and secretory markers. The tumour cells can be positive for CEA and cytokeratins. Peritumoural oedema is common. KLF4 p.K409Q and TRAF7 mutations characterize this subtype.
- **Lymphoplasmacyte-Rich Meningioma:** Lymphoplasmacyte-rich meningioma, a rare subtype, shows features of extensive chronic inflammatory infiltrates over the meningothelial component. Plasma cells are scant, and macrophages often predominate. Caution needs to be exercised to distinguish this subtype from inflammatory disorders with focal meningothelial hyperplasia.
- **Metaplastic Meningioma:** The metaplastic subtype of meningioma has mesenchymal components – osseous, myxoid, cartilaginous, lipomatous and xanthomatous tissues, focally or extensively.
  The morphology of metaplastic meningioma may be that of angiomatous and microcystic meningiomas, and chromosome 5 gain is a frequent alteration in all three subtypes.
- **Atypical Meningioma:** It is an intermediate-grade meningioma with features of at least three of the following: high cellularity, sheeting (uninterrupted patternless or sheet-like growth), small cells with a high N:C ratio, prominent nucleoli, foci of noniatrogenic necrosis and/or increased mitosis, and invasion of adjacent brain parenchyma.
  Increased mitotic activity is defined as ≥2.5 mitoses/mm^2 (i.e. ≥4 mitoses per/10 HPF). The risk factors for atypical meningioma includes male gender, non-skull base location and prior surgery. It is associated with a high recurrence rate despite adequate resection, and bone involvement seems to be an important factor that increases recurrence risk. Brain invasion by meningioma is identified by tongue-like, irregular protrusions of tumour cells into GFAP-positive parenchyma, without leptomeninges in between. Genetic changes like homozygous CDKN2A and/or CDKN2B deletion or TERT promoter mutation are suggestive of CNS WHO grade 3 meningioma and are found to be clinically aggressive.
- **Anaplastic (Malignant) Meningioma:** Anaplastic meningiomas account for 1%–3% of meningiomas. This high-grade meningioma may (1) resemble carcinoma, melanoma or high-grade sarcoma; (2) have markedly elevated mitotic activity; (3) harbour TERT promoter mutation; and/or (4) have homozygous CDKN2A and/or CDKN2B deletion. It has mitotic count of ≥20 mitoses/10 HPF. Extensive necrosis and brain parenchymal invasion are often seen in these tumours. The presence of TERT promoter mutation, homozygous deletion of CDKN2A and/or CDKN2B *and* loss of H3 p.K28me3 (K27me3) are associated with a poor prognosis.
  Certain other subtypes of meningioma are clear cell meningioma, chordoid meningioma, papillary meningioma and rhabdoid meningioma

Clinical Features Meningiomas have neither a significant risk of recurrence nor an aggressive course. They are rare in children and have a female predominance (3:2). It has been observed that the ratio alters to 10:1 (F:M) in case of spinal meningiomas, which are of psammomatous morphology. These slow-growing tumours present with nonlocalizing symptoms or with signs due to compression of the brain underneath. Common sites include the convexity of the brain along the parasagittal region, dura along the lateral convexity, sphenoid wing, sella turcica, olfactory groove and foramen magnum. Tumours are frequently solitary; however, multiple lesions should raise the suspicion of NF2 when associated with glial tumours or acoustic neuromas. They are treated by combined radiation therapy and surgery. The first treatment for a malignant meningioma is surgery, if possible. Other tumours that present as dura-based masses are solitary fibrous tumours, metastases and poorly differentiated sarcomas.

Primary Diffuse Large B-Cell Lymphoma of CNS It was earlier referred to as primary CNS lymphoma, which is now renamed diffuse large B-cell lymphoma of CNS (CNS-DLBCL). The cytological and most of its molecular features correspond to those of its systemic counterpart. Primary CNS-DLBCLs are predominantly solitary brain lesions (65% of cases), with the rest being multifocal lesions. Tumour location in descending order of frequency will be the cerebral hemisphere (38%), thalamus with the basal ganglia (16%), corpus callosum (14%), periventricular region (12%) or cerebellum (9%). The leptomeninges may be involved. Presenting complaints are psychomotor slowing, cognitive dysfunction and focal neurological symptoms besides less common findings like headache, seizures and cranial nerve palsies. Eye floaters and blurred vision are symptoms of ocular involvement. Tumour cells are the mature, late germinal-centre exit B cells arising from self/polyreactive precursor cells, which escaped elimination, due to early acquisition of MYD88 mutations. Due to dysregulated germinal-centre reaction, the tumour cells have increased self/polyreactivity, causing the tumour B-cell receptor to bind to various CNS antigens, which explains, in part, the affinity and confinement of this lymphoma to the CNS microenvironment. Tumour cells have rearranged and somatically mutated Ig genes with ongoing somatic hypermutation. They also show persistent BCL6 activity.

Morphology

Gross CNS-DLBCLs may be single or multiple mass in the brain parenchyma, usually in the cerebral hemisphere. Often, they are adjacent to the ventricular system. The tumour may be greyish tan or yellow, with central necrosis with firm, friable, granular or haemorrhagic areas. Demarcation from adjacent parenchyma is variable.
Microscopy These are cellular patternless diffuse tumours. They show extensive necrosis with interspersed islands of lymphoma cells (large cells with pleomorphic nuclei and ldistinct nucleoli) and angiocentric distribution of similar cells that then invade into the surrounding parenchyma. Mitotic activity is brisk. Tumour cells are admixed with reactive inflammatory cells consisting of mature, small T and B lymphocytes (Fig. 31.23).
Immunophenotype The tumour cells are mature B cells that are positive for PAX5, CD19, CD20, CD22 and CD79a. Tumours show surface expression of IgM and IgD, with either kappa or lambda light chain restriction. Most cells express BCL6 (60%–80%) and MUM1 (IRF4) (90%), whereas plasma cell markers (CD38 and CD138) are negative. CD10-positive CNS lymphoma with DLBCL morphology should prompt an investigation for systemic DLBCL that could have spread to CNS.

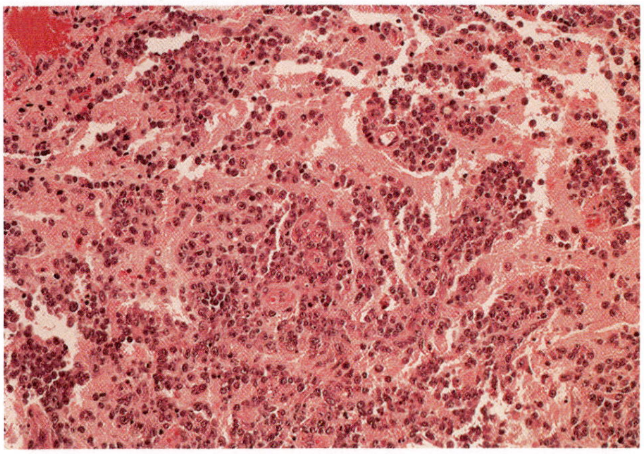

Fig. 31.23 Microscopy of primary DLBCL – CNS-DLBCL. Angiocentric arrangement of tumour cells. (*Source:* Richard A. Prayson, Non-Glial Tumors, in Neuropathology, 2nd Edition, © 2012, 2005 by Saunders, an imprint of Elsevier Inc.)

CNS-DLBCL has a poor outcome than systemic DLBCL. A minority of younger patients can be cured. Old age, especially more than 65 years, is a major negative prognostic factor because it is associated with reduced survival apart from an increased risk of neurotoxicity. High-dose methotrexate-based polychemotherapy is the induction therapy of choice. Consolidative whole-brain irradiation may improve progression-free survival, but not OS; however, it can increase the risk of neurotoxicity causing cognitive dysfunction, if patients are older than 60 years.

Germ Cell Tumours

These primary CNS tumours are commonly seen along the midline, especially involving the pineal and suprasellar regions. They account for 0.2%–1% of brain tumours in Europe, whereas their incidence is higher at around 10% in Japan. They are most common in the first two decades of life. Of the germ cell tumours, **teratomas** are found to be more common type of the congenital tumours. Pineal region germ cell tumours have a strong male predominance, whereas it is not so in the case of suprasellar lesions. The source of germ cells in CNS, though unclear, has been postulated to arise from **'rests'** remaining in CNS per se or migrating from elsewhere at a later stage of development. Gonadal germ cell tumour metastasis to CNS is common, so a diagnosis of primary germ cell tumour of CNS must be made after excluding the possibility of a non-CNS primary tumour. Classification of germ cell tumours of the brain is the same as that of the testis, yet a seminomatous histology in the testis is named germinoma in CNS. Their response to chemoradiotherapy is similar to that of germ cell tumours in other sites. Tumour marker level such as α-fetoprotein and β-human chorionic gonadotropin may be measured in CSF for diagnosing and gauging response to therapy.

METASTATIC TUMOURS

Intracranial tumours due to carcinomatous metastatic deposits account for as high as one-quarter to one-half of intracranial tumours in hospitalized patients. Most common primary tumours that metastasize to the brain (up to 80%) are the **lung**, **breast**, kidney, skin (melanoma) and gastrointestinal tract. Other rare tumours such as choriocarcinoma also metastasize to the brain, whereas tumours such as prostatic adenocarcinoma almost never metastasize. Metastatic disease frequently involves the meninges also. Metastatic tumours can be the initial manifestation of a cancer presenting clinically as a mass lesion. Metastases may require emergency intervention when they involve the subdural or epidural space leading to spinal cord compression.

Morphology

Parenchymal lesions are discrete mass, frequently at the grey and white matter junction surrounded by a zone of oedema. Microscopically, the tumour brain interface is well defined with the exception of melanoma. In melanoma, the individual cells invade the surrounding brain. In melanoma, nodules of tumour cells have central necrosis that are surrounded by reactive gliosis. Meningeal carcinomatosis presents as nodules studded on the surface of the brain, spinal cord and intradural nerve roots and is frequently associated with lung and breast carcinoma.

Clinical Features

Headache and seizure constitute the two most common presenting symptoms.

Cognitive dysfunction and motor dysfunction are the other important signs. The most definitive therapy is selected on the basis of the number, size and location of brain metastasis apart from the primary tumour type, its extent, control of the systemic disease and the patient's performance status. Therapy for brain metastasis includes treatment directed against the tumour itself along with supportive treatment including glucocorticoids, antiepileptic drugs and anticoagulants.

FAMILIAL TUMOUR SYNDROMES

Numerous familial syndromes are known to cause tumours of the nervous system as follows:

- **Cowden syndrome:** It is an autosomal dominant disorder caused mainly by germline pathogenic variants of PTEN (*affecting* the PI3K/AKT signalling pathway activity), and is identified by multiple hamartomas involving tissues arising from all three germ cell layers along with a high risk of thyroid, breast, endometrial, renal and colon cancers. In CNS, adult-onset dysplastic cerebellar gangliocytoma (Lhermitte–Duclos disease) is considered to be pathognomonic.
- **Li–Fraumeni syndrome:** It is an autosomal dominant disorder caused by pathogenic sequence variants of the tumour suppressor gene TP53 on chromosome 17p13.1. It is characterized by multiple primary neoplasms in both children and adults, especially osteosarcomas, soft-tissue sarcomas, breast cancer, adrenocortical carcinoma and brain tumours – medulloblastomas.
- **NBCCS – Gorlin syndrome:** It is an autosomal dominant disease caused by germline pathogenic variants of genes encoding those involved in hedgehog signalling pathway, like PTCH1, SUFU and rarely GPR161. Patients present with developmental disorders and are predisposed to benign as well as malignant tumours like palmar/plantar dyskeratotic pits, odontogenic keratocysts, intracranial calcifications, intratarsal keratinous eyelid cysts, cutaneous basal cell carcinomas, macrocephaly and medulloblastomas (D/N subtypes). In the next section, the familial syndromes known to cause CNS tumours are elaborated in detail.

Tuberous Sclerosis Complex

It is a group of autosomal dominant disorders caused by pathogenic variants of TSC1 on 9q or TSC2 on 16p. It is characterized by hamartomas, benign neoplastic lesions that affect CNS and various non-neural tissues. The incidence is approximately 1 in 6000 births. TS is due to mutation involving chromosome 9q34 (TSC1 locus) encoding for a protein called hamartin. A more common mutation involving chromosome 16p13.3 (TSC2 locus) encodes tuberin. These two proteins together form a complex that inhibits kinase mTOR, a key protein synthesis regulator, which is involved in anabolic metabolism. This syndrome presents with seizures, autism, mental retardation along with hamartomas and benign neoplasms of the brain.

Diagnostic criteria for TS (2012) are as follows:

Genetic diagnostic criteria

Identification of TSC1 or TSC2 pathogenic mutation in DNA from normal tissue is sufficient to make a diagnosis of tuberous sclerosis.

Clinical diagnostic criteria

Major features

1. Hypomelanotic macules (≥3, at least 5 mm in diameter)
2. Angiofibromas (≥3) or fibrous cephalic plaque
3. Ungual fibromas (≥2)
4. Shagreen patch

5. Multiple retinal hamartomas
6. Cortical dysplasias (including tubers and cerebral white matter migration lines)
7. Subependymal nodules
8. Subependymal giant cell astrocytoma
9. Cardiac rhabdomyoma
10. Lymphangioleiomyomatosis[a]
11. Angiomyolipomas (≥2)[a]

Minor features

1. Confetti-like skin lesions
2. Dental enamel pits (≥3)
3. Intraoral fibromas (≥2)
4. Retinal achromic patch
5. Multiple renal cysts
6. Nonrenal hamartomas

Definite diagnosis: Two major features[a] **OR** one major feature with at least two minor features

[a]Combination of these two major features does not meet the diagnostic criteria

Von Hippel–Lindau Disease

It is an autosomal dominant disorder caused by pathogenic germline variants of the VHL tumour suppressor gene (chromosome 3p25.3). It is characterized by haemangioblastoma of CNS or retina, phaeochromocytoma, clear cell renal cell carcinoma (RCC), pancreatic neuroendocrine tumours and endolymphatic sac tumours (ELSTs). The disease has an annual incidence rate of 2.8 cases per 100,000 population. VHL type 1 is characterized by RCCs (phaeochromocytomas are rare or absent) and haemangioblastomas and it is caused by deletions, truncations and missense mutations *of VHL*. Type 2A is characterized by phaeochromocytomas (RCCs are rare) and haemangioblastomas, caused by missense mutations. Type 2B is characterized by a high frequency of haemangioblastomas, phaeochromocytomas and RCCs. It is also caused by missense mutations. Type 2C is characterized by only phaeochromocytomas (haemangioblastomas and RCCs are absent), and it is also caused by missense mutations. In CNS, haemangioblastoma involving the cerebellum and retina has been observed, but may involve other sites in CNS also. Haemangioblastomas are highly vascular neoplasms. VHL gene is a tumour suppressor gene. It encodes for a protein (VHL) that is located on chromosome 3p25.3. The VHL protein has various functions, and is involved in protein degradation. VHL protein is a component of ubiquitin ligase complex that downregulates a transcription factor named hypoxia-induced factor 1 (HIF-1). HIF-1 regulates the expression of erythropoietin, vascular endothelial growth factor and other growth factors. It also regulates the genes that control cell growth and cellular metabolism that are likely to contribute towards tumour formation. The erythropoietin dysregulation seems to be responsible for polycythaemia associated with haemangioblastomas seen in approximately 10% of cases.

Morphology

Grossly, haemangioblastomas show large fluid-filled cysts with mural nodule. Numerous capillary-sized vessels along with thin-walled larger vessels are seen with stromal cells that contain lightly PAS-positive, vacuolated, lipid-rich cytoplasm. The stromal cells are of uncertain histogenesis expressing inhibin that can be demonstrated by immunohistochemistry and are considered as the neoplastic elements in haemangioblastoma.

Cerebellar haemangioblastomas when symptomatic are treated by resection, whereas laser therapy is a treatment modality used for retinal haemangioblastomas.

Neurofibromatosis

Neurofibromatosis is a familial tumour syndrome presenting with tumours of PNS and CNS. It can be due to two autosomal dominant disorders, namely NF1 and NF2. NF1 is more common and has a frequency of 1 in 3000. It has features of cutaneous hyperpigmented macules (café au lait spots), gliomas of the optic nerve, neurofibromas of the peripheral nerve and pigmented nodules of the iris (Lisch nodules). On the contrary, NF2 has a frequency of 1 in 40,000–50,000. It commonly shows features of bilateral vestibulocochlear nerve schwannomas along with multiple meningiomas and spinal cord ependymoma. The pathogenesis of this condition is explained in detail in Chapter 7 and its morphology in Chapter 30.

PARANEOPLASTIC SYNDROMES

Paraneoplastic syndrome may also involve CNS and/or peripheral nervous system and on occasions be the first sign of an underlying malignant neoplasm. Paraneoplastic syndromes are explained in detail in Chapter 7.

Pathogenesis

Molecular mimicry seems to be the underlying mechanism of paraneoplastic syndrome, in which the immune response developed against tumour antigens cross-reacts with antigens found in CNS or peripheral nervous system.

Few classic examples are as follows:

- Patients with uterine, ovarian or breast carcinoma have circulating **PCA-1 antibody (anti-Yo)** causing cross-reactions with Purkinje cells leading to **subacute cerebellar degeneration**.
- Circulating **ANNA-1 antibody (anti-Hu)** that recognizes neuronal nuclei in CNS and peripheral nervous system is associated with small-cell carcinoma of the lung. It produces **limbic encephalitis**–like presentation involving the brainstem alone or with limbic system involvement.
- **Opsoclonus** (an eye movement disorder) with myoclonus is most commonly associated in children with neuroblastoma.

The peripheral nervous system can also be affected as follows:

- **Lambert—Eaton myasthenic syndrome** is due to antibodies towards voltage-gated calcium channel found in the presynaptic portion of the neuromuscular junction.
- Circulating VGKC-complex antibody causes peripheral neuropathy because it cross-reacts with voltage-gated potassium channel.

Paraneoplastic syndromes can be treated by immunotherapy that involves removal of circulating antibodies along with immunosuppression. This treatment modality proves effective in those syndromes that have plasma membrane–reactive antibodies such as VGKC and NMDAR. Tumour removal also results in improvement in other cases.

EYE

NORMAL STRUCTURE OF THE EYE

The main function of the eye is to aid vision. It in turn depends on a transparent focusing system consisting of the cornea and lens, transparent media composed of aqueous humour and vitreous humour, and a normal retina with the neural conduction system. The eyelids are covered externally by the skin and internally by the conjunctiva, which in turn is reflected over the eyeball. The lacrimal gland is a compound racemose gland situated at the upper outer angle of the orbit.

The globe of the eye consists of three layers – the cornea– sclera, choroid–iris and retina. The cornea has a layer of stratified epithelium externally, which is a continuation of the conjunctiva lying over the cornea. The subepithelial stroma is a fibrous connective tissue coated on its interior by the posterior endothelium-lined elastic membrane named Descemet's membrane. The sclera consists of dense fibrous tissue, which is the thickest posteriorly. The choroid is a vascular membrane associated with the sclera. The choroid is thicker anteriorly forming ciliary processes and ciliary body containing ciliary muscle. It continues anteriorly as the iris that is found anterior to the lens. It has similar structure like that of the choroid but contains pigmented cells. The uveal tract is composed of three parts – the iris anteriorly and the choroid with the ciliary body posteriorly.

The retina lines the choroid internally. It has multiple layers of cells and their synapses, which are of three types – the rods and the cones that are the external photoreceptor cells, the intermediate relay layer of bipolar cells and the innermost layer of ganglion cells with their axons continuing as the optic nerve starting at the optic disc. The central fovea is a specialized area in the retina consisting of only photosensitive cones, devoid of photoreceptor rods and blood vessels.

The lens is a biconvex structure formed by laminated transparent tissue covered by an elastic capsule. The anterior chamber is filled with the aqueous humour, and is bound by the cornea anteriorly and the iris posteriorly, with the anterior aspect of the lens exposed in the pupil. The anterior chamber containing aqueous humour is a triangular space extending from the posterior aspect of the iris, the anterior surface of the lens and the ciliary body forming the apex at the pupillary margin. The posterior chamber is the large space posterior to the lens containing gelatinous vitreous humour. The cornea and lens receive their nutrients from the aqueous humour produced by the ciliary process.

The intraocular pressure is maintained normally at 15–20 mm Hg that depends on the rate of aqueous production and the resistance in the outflow system.

Having discussed the normal structure of the eye, the subsequent section discusses in detail the retinoblastoma.

Retinoblastoma PA 36.1

Retinoblastoma is a malignant neoplasm derived from the retina that usually arises in early childhood. It is a tumour of neurosensory retina involving on progression the vitreous cavity, optic nerve, ocular coats and periocular tissues. A white pupillary reflex – leucocoria, due to the retinal tumour – is the hallmark clinical feature of retinoblastoma observed in 63% of cases. The second most common presenting sign is strabismus (10% of cases); however, the combination of leucocoria with strabismus is seen less frequently (4% of cases). Diagnosis of retinoblastoma may be confirmed in the clinic with dilated eye examination. A noninvasive diagnostic imaging modality – ocular ultrasound – can also help detect the mass and characteristic dystrophic calcifications within the tumour.

The most common age of presentation is 6 months to 2 years.

Aetiopathogenesis Retinoblastoma originates from developing retinal cells, especially the cone progenitors. In >98% of RB1−/− tumours, carcinogenesis inactivation of the RB1 tumour suppressor gene initiates the tumorigenesis. Heritable retinoblastoma is due to constitutional mutation (first hit) and subsequently a somatic alteration (second hit). Nonheritable retinoblastoma, on the other hand, is initiated when the somatic mutation arises in the same vulnerable cell.

Retinoblastomas that occur because of germline mutations are frequently bilateral and can be accompanied by pinealoblastoma, in which case they are termed **'trilateral'** retinoblastoma.

Morphology

Gross Macroscopically, the tumour has a white encephaloid appearance that contains white flecks of calcification. Various growth patterns are recognized. **Endophytic retinoblastomas** arise from the retina, remaining attached to it, and invade the vitreous. **Exophytic retinoblastomas** arises from the outer layers of the retina causing retinal detachment, which is high and bullous leading to anterior displacement of the lens, iris and secondary angle closure. (Figs 31.24 and 31.25).

Microscopy Retinoblastoma shows poorly differentiated neuroblastic (retinoblasts) cells with scant cytoplasm and hyperchromatic nuclei giving an intense basophilic appearance, giving its name small blue round call tumour. Mitotic figures and apoptotic bodies are common. The tumour can outgrow its blood supply causing necrosis with foci of dystrophic calcification, which is a helpful diagnostic feature.

Rosettes with central tangle of neurofilamentary neuropil surrounded by nuclei may be seen and are called Homer Wright rosettes. They represent neuroblastic differentiation and are a typical finding in neuroblastoma, apart from other neuroendocrine tumours. Flexner–Wintersteiner rosette represents early retinal differentiation (Fig. 31.26). It has a central lumen filled with mucopolysaccharide corresponding to the subretinal space that is surrounded by the tumour cells. Retinoblastoma becomes less well differentiated with increasing age. Rarely, retinoblastomas can undergo true spontaneous regression. This phenomenon occurs as a result of vascular occlusion secondary to severe neovascular glaucoma. Histopathological features associated with high-risk of metastasis include extraocular extension, massive posterior uveal invasion which is greater than 3 mm in diameter and/or full-thickness choroidal involvement, and retrolaminar optic nerve invasion.

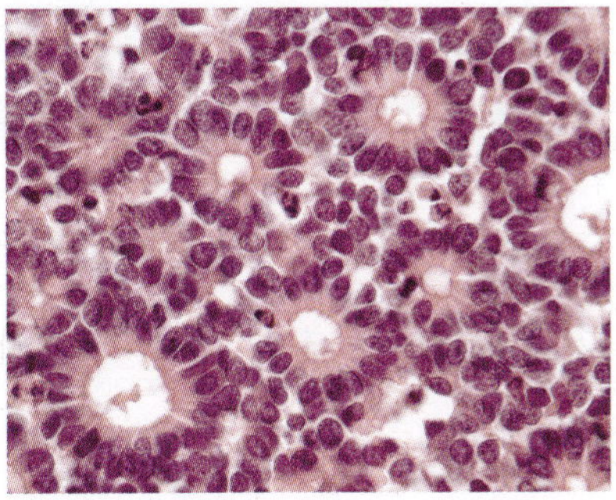

Fig. 31.26 Flexner–Wintersteiner rosettes. (*Source:* Ralph C. Eagle, Ocular Tumors, Ophthalmology Secrets in Color, 4th Edition. © 2016 by Elsevier, Inc.)

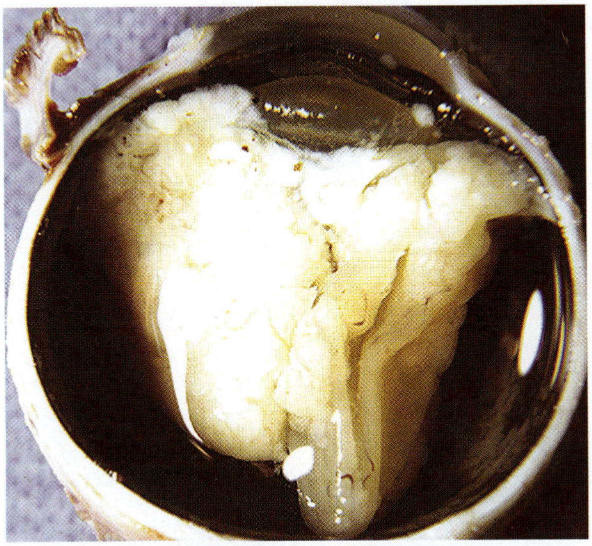

Fig. 31.24 Gross picture of retinoblastoma – endophytic retinoblastoma. Retinoblastoma grows inward from neural retina and fills vitreous compartment of eye. (*Source:* Myron Yanoff and Joseph W. Sassani, Retinoblastoma and Simulating Lesions, in Ocular Pathology, 8th Edition, © 2020, Elsevier Inc.)

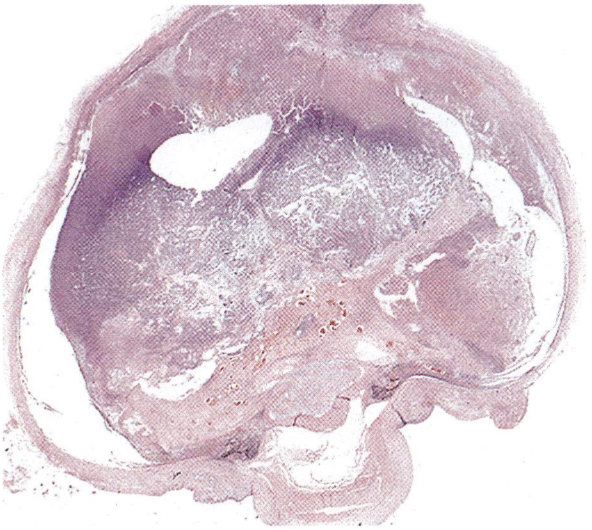

Fig. 31.25 Whole mount image of removed eyeball shows complete retinal detachment with partially necrotic tumour collapsing the anterior chamber. (*Source:* Myron Yanoff and Joseph W. Sassani, Ocular Pathology, 8th Edition, © 2020, Elsevier Inc.)

Treatment decision for retinoblastoma in order of priority is the following: life of the child, second vision and third globe salvage. The natural history of retinoblastoma without therapy is 100% mortality. Recently, therapy to salvage an eye is being optimized to achieve 98% survival. Enucleation is preferred for patients with high-risk features such as optic nerve enlargement or enhancement on MRI scanning.

Retinoblastoma metastasizes to the brain and bone marrow, whereas it spreads seldom to the lungs. Prognosis is poor whenever there is invasion of the optic nerve, extraocular extension or choroidal invasion.

SELF-ASSESSMENT

Scenario-Based MCQs

Scenario I

A 25-year-old female college student presents to the clinic with complaints of fever, severe headache and confusion. She mentions attending a crowded music festival 2 days ago. On examination, neck stiffness and photophobia are noted.

1. Given the patient's recent exposure history, which pathogen is the most likely cause of her symptoms?
   A. *Streptococcus pneumoniae*
   B. Haemophilus influenzae
   C. *Neisseria meningitidis*
   D. *Listeria monocytogenes*
2. What diagnostic test is essential for confirming the diagnosis of meningitis in this patient?
   A. Blood culture
   B. Chest X-ray
   C. Lumbar puncture
   D. CT scan of the head
3. Which physical examination finding supports the diagnosis of meningitis and suggests meningeal irritation?
   A. Positive Babinski reflex
   B. Positive Romberg sign
   C. Positive Brudzinski sign
   D. Presence of nystagmus

Scenario II

A 60-year-old male presents to his primary care physician with complaints of progressive weakness in his left arm and leg, along with frequent headaches. Neurological examination reveals decreased sensation and strength on the left side of the body.

4. On the basis of the patient's symptoms, which region of CNS is the most likely affected?
   A. Brainstem
   B. Spinal cord
   C. Cerebellum
   D. Frontal lobe
5. What imaging modality is the most appropriate initial investigation for confirming the presence of a CNS tumour in this patient?
   A. MRI of the brain and spine
   B. CT scan of the head
   C. PET scan
   D. EEG
6. Which of the following is a potential complication of CNS tumours in this patient?
   A. Pulmonary embolism
   B. Brain herniation
   C. Osteoporosis
   D. Myocardial infarction

Scenario III

A 4-year-old child is brought to the paediatrician's office by his parents due to concerns about a white pupil in the left eye. On examination, leucocoria is observed.

7. What is the most likely diagnosis on the basis of the patient's clinical presentation?
   A. Cataract
   B. Retinoblastoma
   C. Glaucoma
   D. Macular degeneration
8. Which genetic mutation is commonly associated with the development of retinoblastoma?
   A. APC gene mutation
   B. RB1 gene mutation
   C. BRCA1 gene mutation
   D. TP53 gene mutation
9. What is a potential sequela of retinoblastoma if not treated promptly?
   A. Sensorineural hearing loss
   B. Osteosarcoma
   C. Brain haemorrhage
   D. Orbital cellulitis

Scenario IV

A 55-year-old woman presents with a history of progressive headaches, visual disturbances and difficulty with balance. MRI reveals a well-circumscribed, enhancing mass lesion in the cerebellum.

10. What is the most common primary brain tumour in adults?
    A. Glioblastoma
    B. Medulloblastoma
    C. Meningioma
    D. Astrocytoma
11. What histopathological feature is characteristic of the glioblastoma?
    A. Rosettes
    B. Psammoma bodies
    C. Pseudopalisading necrosis
    D. Homer Wright rosettes
12. What genetic alteration is commonly associated with the development of glioblastoma?
    A. EGFR amplification
    B. BRCA1 mutation
    C. APC gene mutation
    D. RB1 gene mutation
13. Which type of brain tumour is most commonly associated with neurofibromatosis type 1 (NF1)?
    A. Glioblastoma multiforme
    B. Medulloblastoma
    C. Meningioma
    D. Schwannoma
14. What is the primary cell of origin for medulloblastoma?
    A. Oligodendrocytes
    B. Astrocytes
    C. Neurons
    D. Granule cell precursors
15. Which histopathological feature is characteristic of a meningioma?
    A. Pseudopalisading necrosis
    B. Psammoma bodies
    C. Rosettes
    D. Homer Wright rosettes

Answers

1. (C); 2. (C); 3. (C); 4. (D); 5. (A); 6. (B); 7. (B); 8. (B); 9. (D); 10. (C); 11. (C); 12. (A); 13. (D); 14. (D); 15. (B)

Self-Assessment Questions

1) A 40-year-old man presented in casualty with altered sensorium and seizure. On examination, it was found that he had neck rigidity. A CSF examination revealed a cloudy fluid with the following findings: elevated polymorphonuclear leucocytes (PNLs), increased protein levels and decreased glucose levels. What is the diagnosis? Describe the aetiology, types and pathogenesis, and differentiating features in CSF of this condition.
2) A 19-year-old, married, Asian woman, with a strong history of tuberculous contact, presented in a clinical set-up with a headache, backache and mild lower limb weakness for 4 months. Initial CSF report showed lymphocyte predominance, high protein, low glucose and positive mycobacterial culture on BACTEC medium. What is the diagnosis? Describe the aetiology, types and pathogenesis, and differentiating features in CSF of this condition.
3) An 18-year-old woman presented with fever, headache, photophobia and neck stiffness. CSF findings showed lymphocytic pleocytosis, moderate protein elevation and nearly normal glucose content. What is the diagnosis? Describe the aetiology, types and pathogenesis, and differentiating features in CSF of this condition.
4) A 12-year-old boy presented with headaches that are worse in the morning, nausea, vomiting, seizures and changes in mood. MRI showed a large cystic component with a brightly enhancing mural nodule in the posterior fossa. What is the diagnosis? Classify and describe the aetiology, genetics, pathogenesis, pathology and complications of this condition.
5) A 57-year-old man presented in casualty with seizures and three episodes of incoherent speech for several hours within 1 month prior to hospitalization. A contrast-enhanced T1-weighted MRI showed a left temporal tumour surrounded by massive oedema. What is the diagnosis? Classify and describe the aetiology, genetics, pathogenesis, pathology and complications of this condition.
6) A 58-year-old woman presented in OPD with severe giddiness not responding to treatment. A parasagittal noncontrast T1-weighted MRI showed isointense mass lesion attached to the dura. What is the diagnosis? Discuss in detail about the aetiopathogenesis and morphology of this condition.
7) A 2-year-old male child presented with leucocoria with exophthalmos of the left eye. A positive family history was elicited. What is the diagnosis? Describe the aetiology, genetics, pathogenesis, pathology and presentation of the condition.

Answers

1. Pyogenic meningitis – *Streptococcus pneumoniae*
2. Tubercular meningitis
3. Aseptic viral meningitis
4. Pilocytic astrocytoma
5. Glioblastoma
6. Meningioma
7. Retinoblastoma

Topics for Self-Directed Learning

1. Malformations and developmental disorders
2. Traumatic lesion of the central nervous system
3. Central pontine myelinolysis
4. Huntington disease
5. Amyotrophic lateral sclerosis (ALS)
6. Neuronal storage diseases
7. Leucodystrophies
8. Mitochondrial encephalomyopathies
9. Tumours of CNS

Appendix: Histopathology, Cytopathology and Haematology Diagrams

HISTOPATHOLOGY

FATTY LIVER

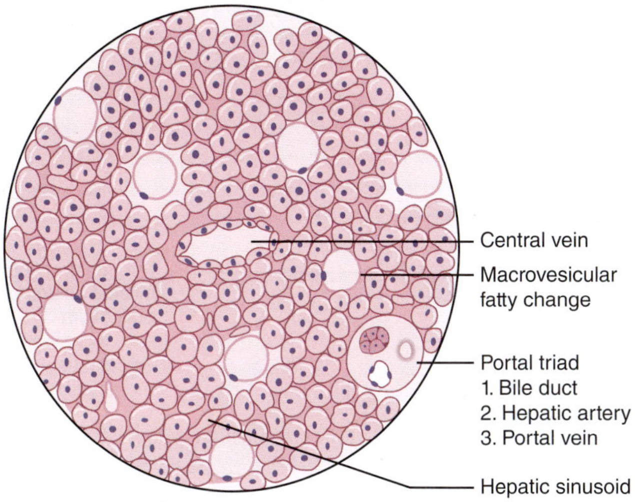

MONCKEBERG'S CALCIFIC SCLEROSIS

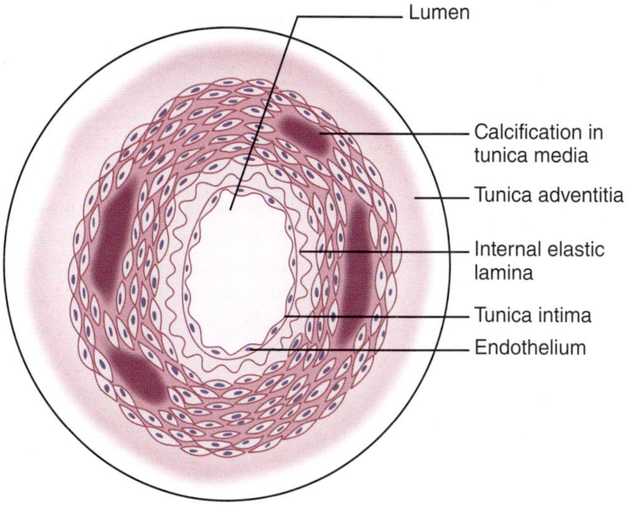

ACUTE APPENDICITIS

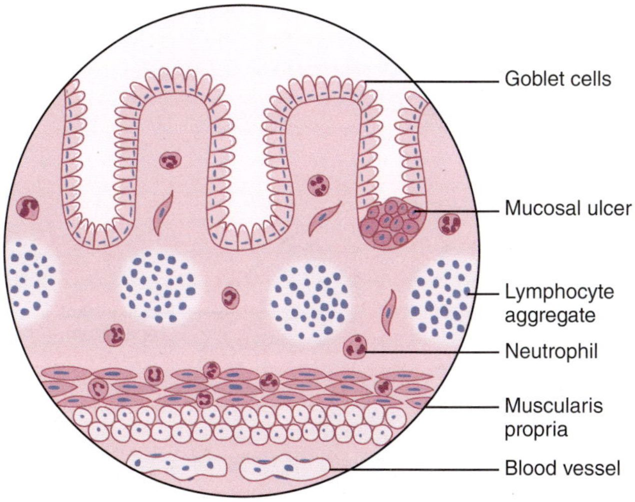

GRANULATION TISSUE

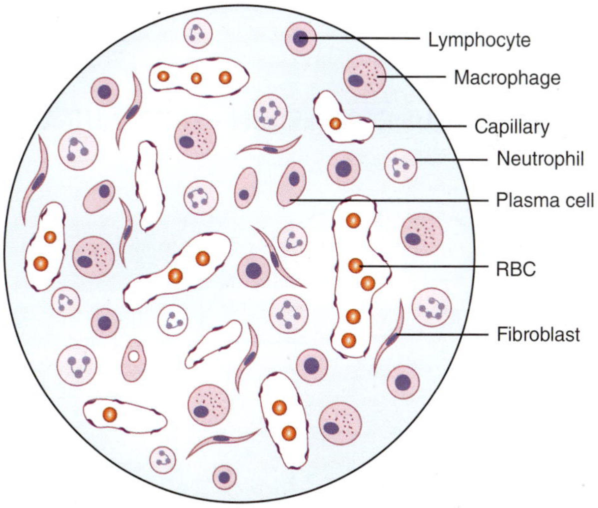

THROMBUS – VESSEL

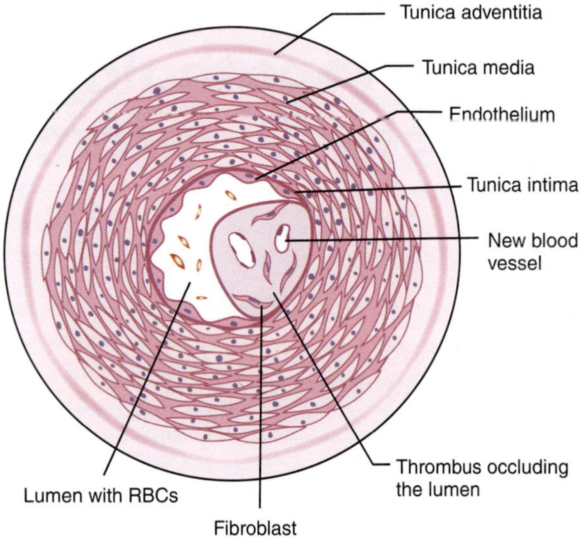

CHRONIC VENOUS CONGESTION – LUNG

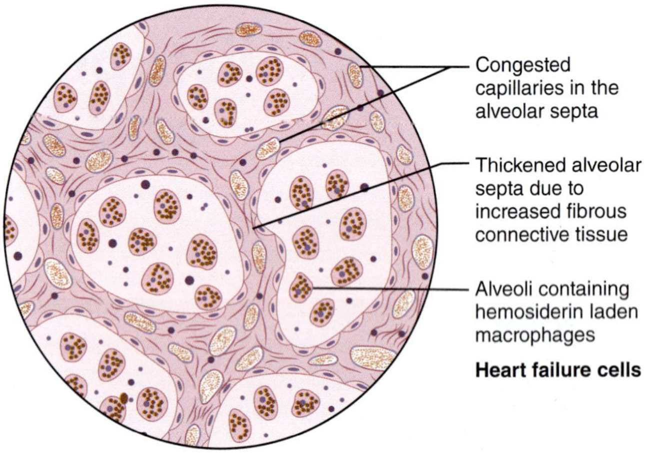

INFARCT – SPLEEN

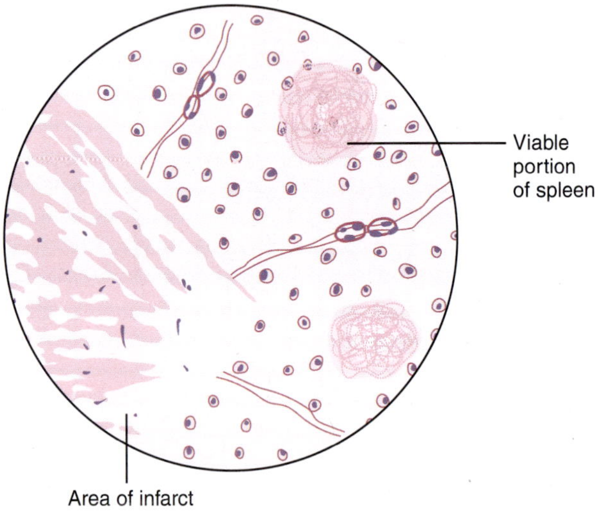

RHINOSPORIDIOSIS

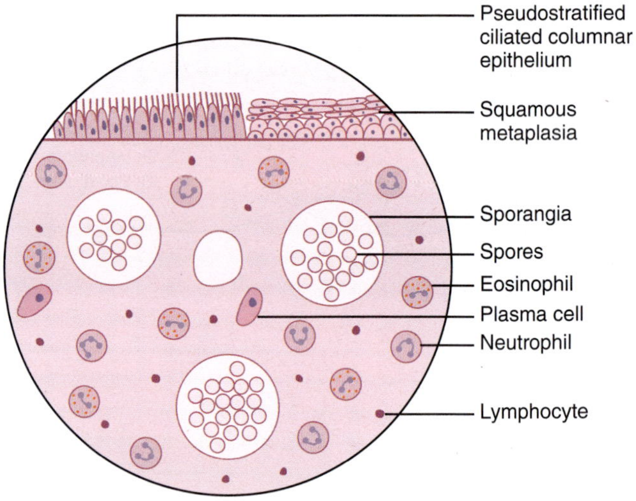

CHRONIC VENOUS CONGESTION – LIVER (NUTMEG LIVER)

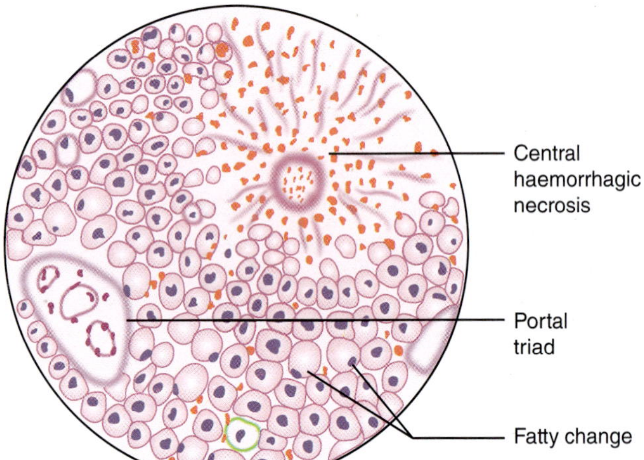

ACTINOMYCOSIS

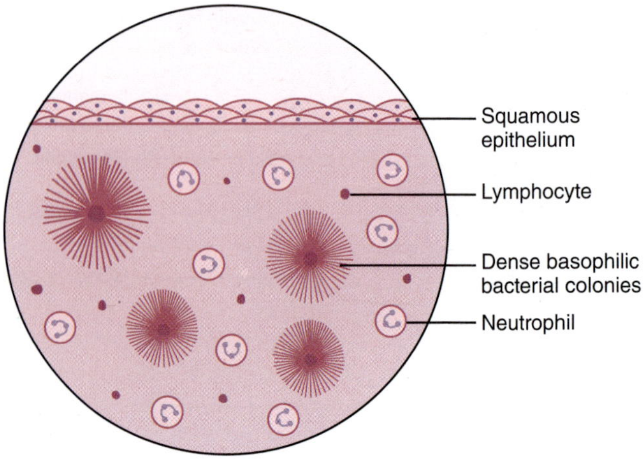

CASEATING TUBERCULOUS LYMPHADENITIS

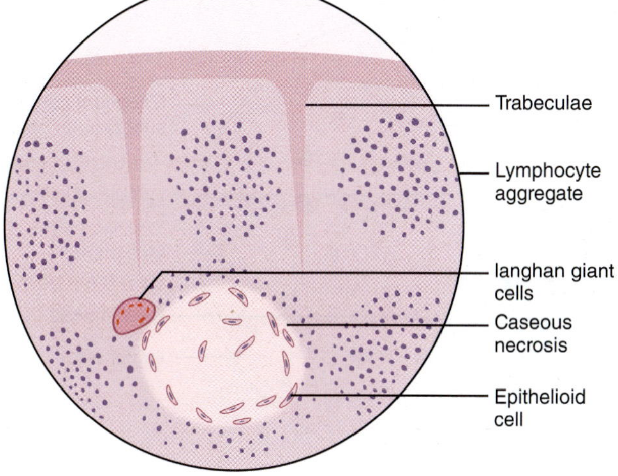

CAPILLARY HAEMANGIOMA

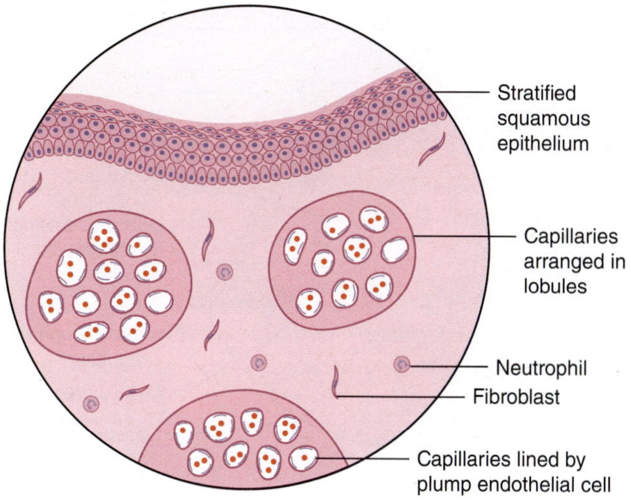

HYDATID CYST

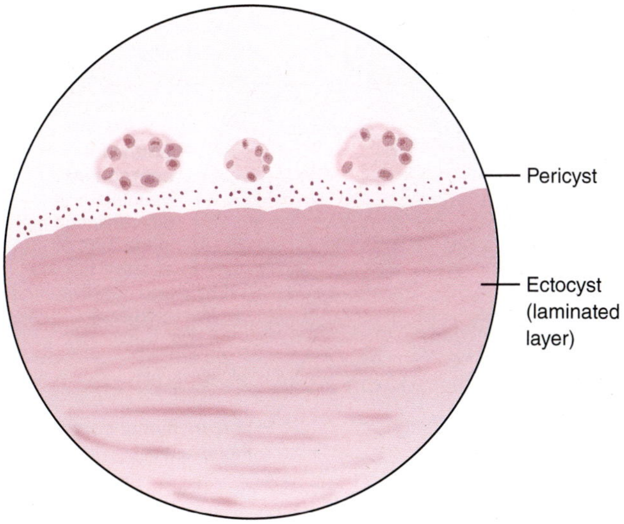

SQUAMOUS PAPILLOMA

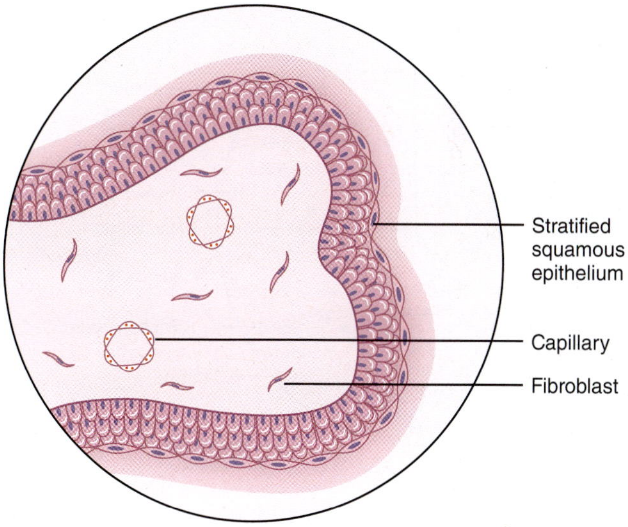

CAVERNOUS HAEMANGIOMA

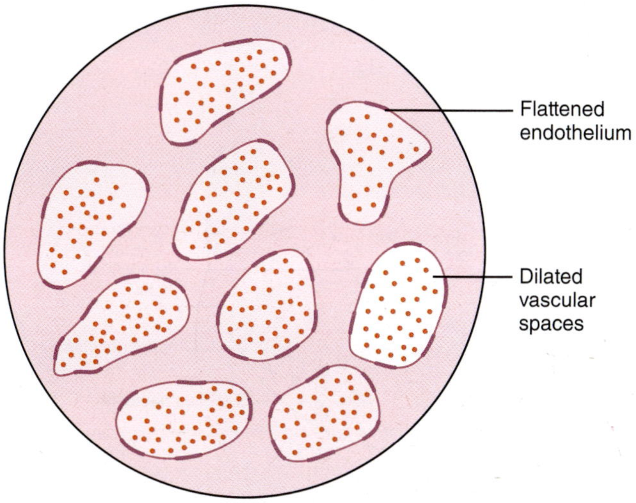

LIPOMA

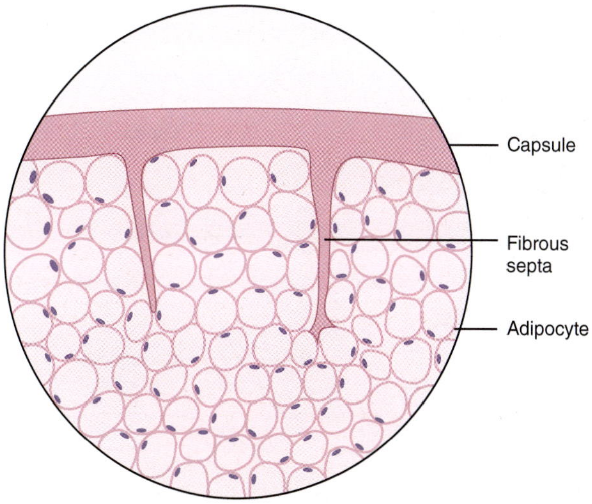

PLEOMORPHIC ADENOMA

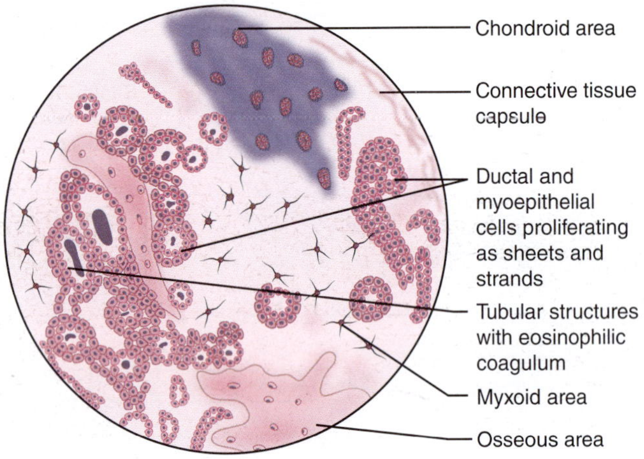

SQUAMOUS CELL CARCINOMA, SECONDARIES IN LYMPH NODE

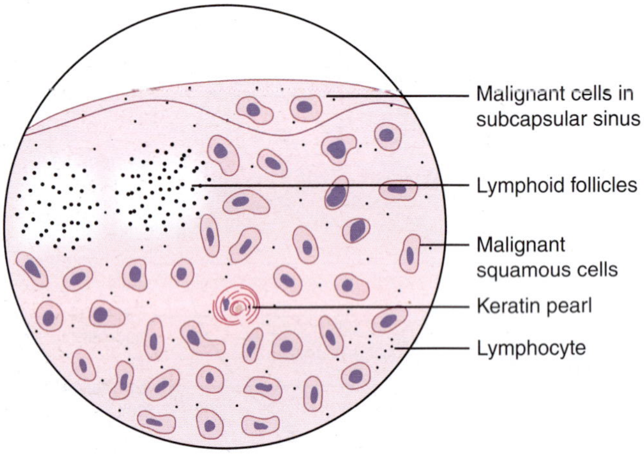

TERATOMA

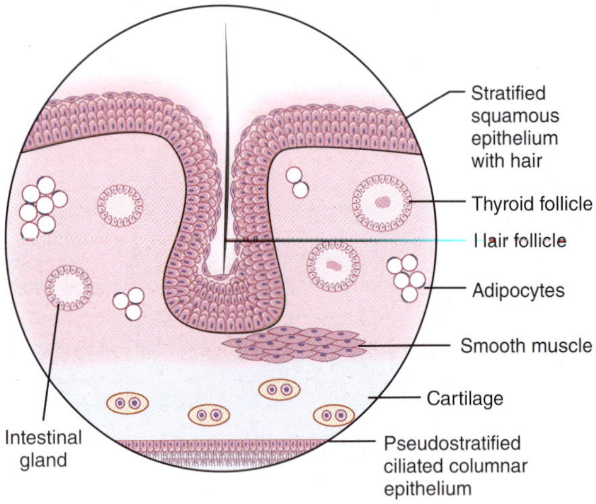

WILMS TUMOUR (NEPHROBLASTOMA)

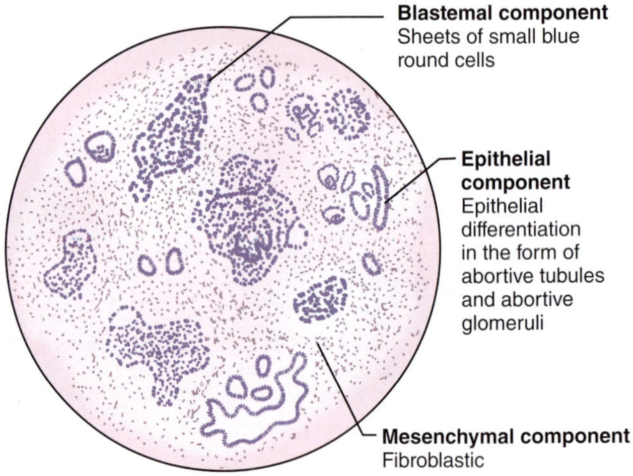

CHONDROMA

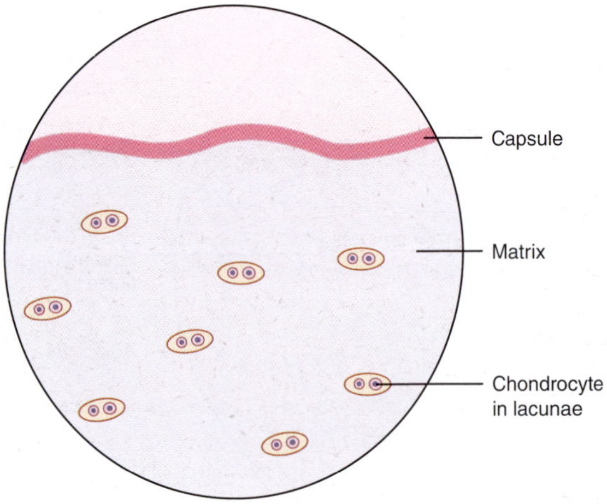

TUBERCULOSIS – LUNG

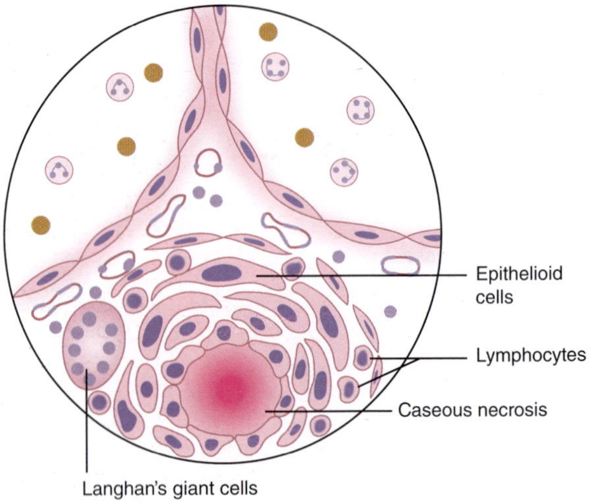

ADENOCARCINOMA COLON

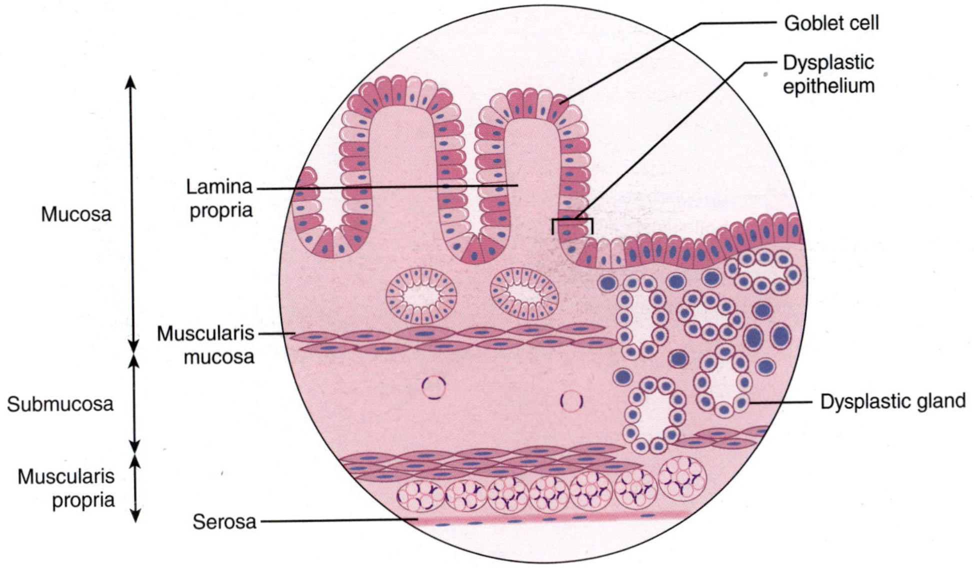

GASTRIC CARCINOMA

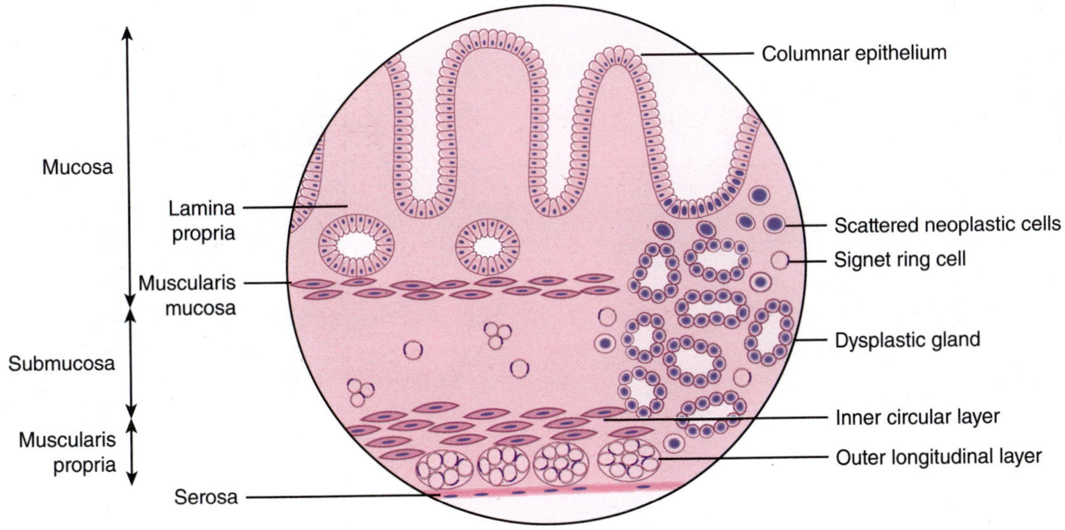

GASTRIC ULCER

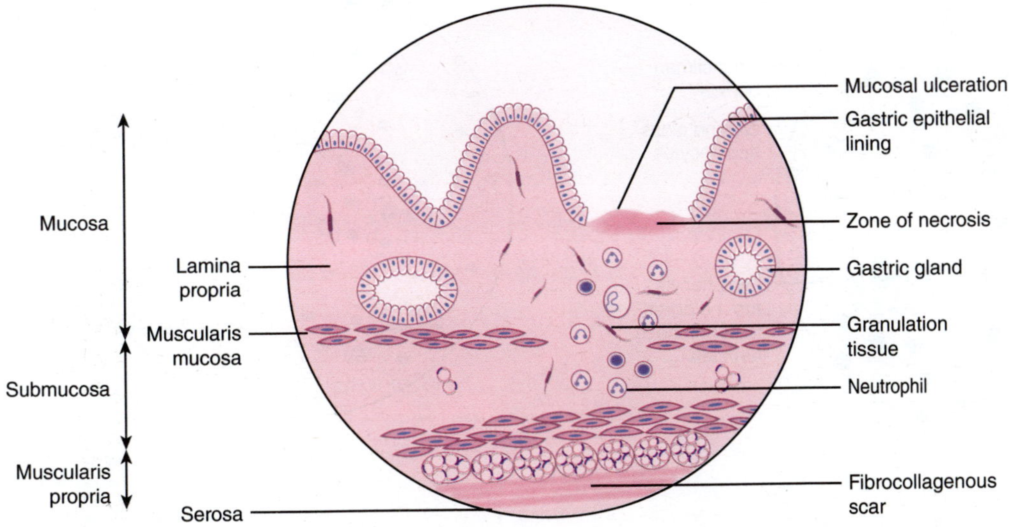

TUBERCULOSIS – INTESTINE

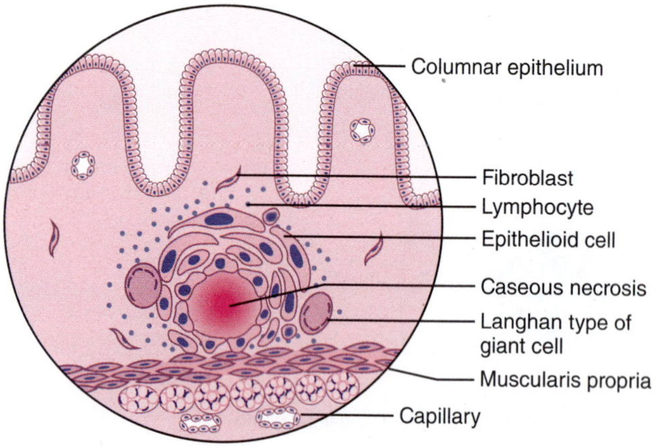

CHRONIC HEPATITIS C

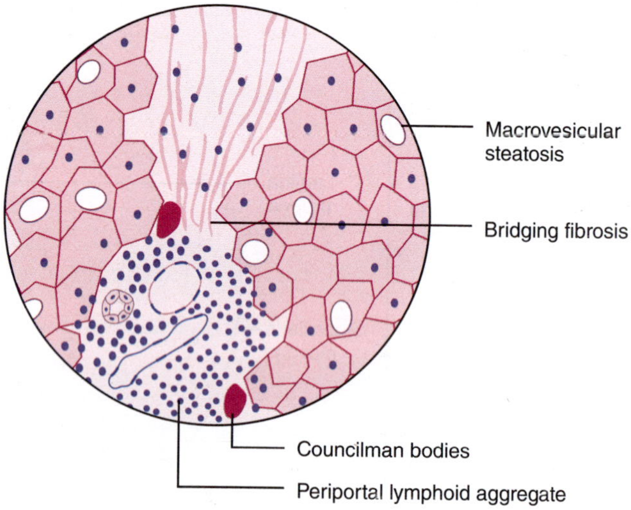

EMPHYSEMA – LUNG

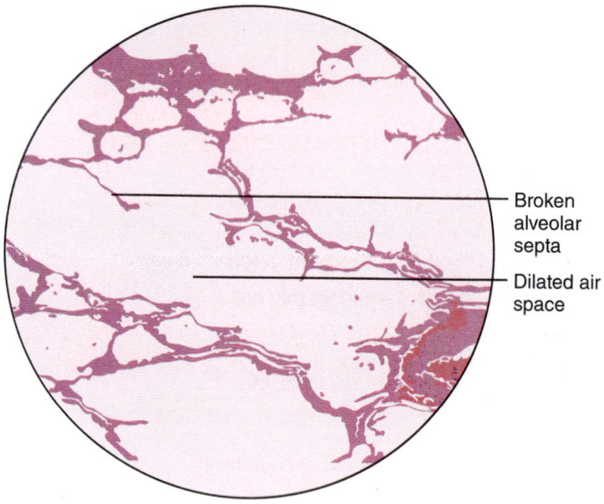

CIRRHOSIS – LIVER

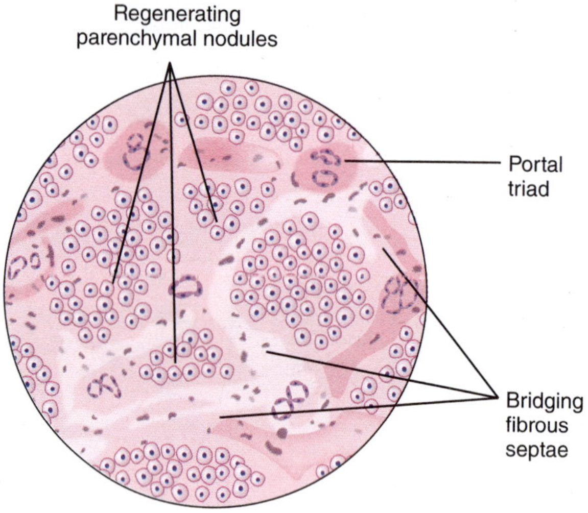

HEPATITIS B

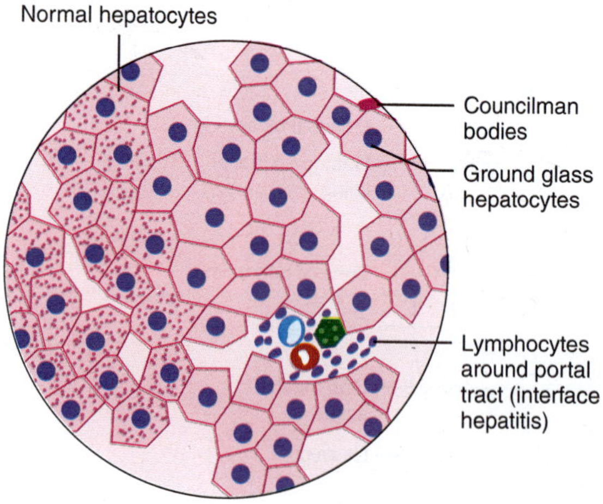

HEPATOCELLULAR CARCINOMA

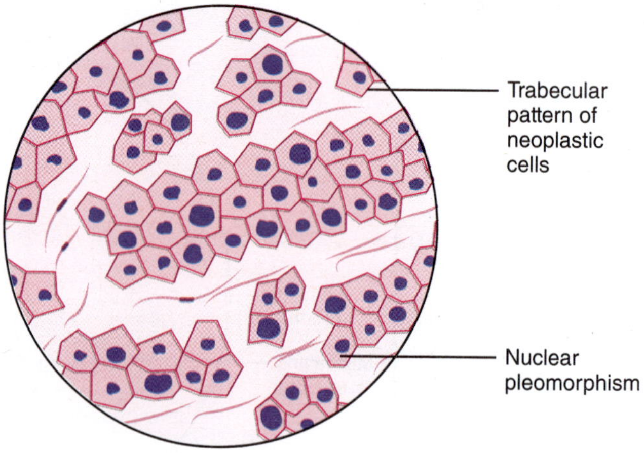

CHRONIC PYELONEPHRITIS

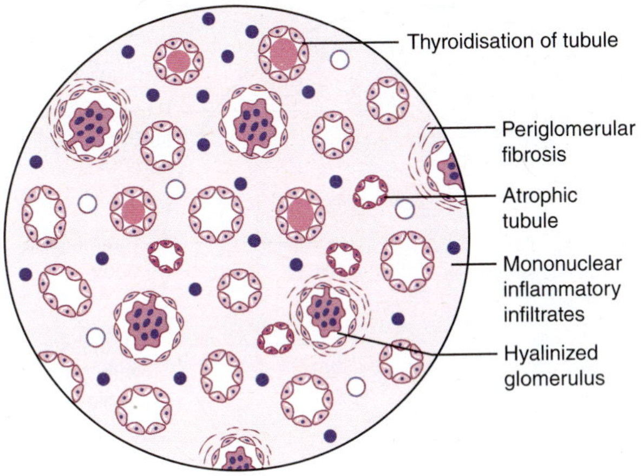

INFILTRATING DUCTAL CARCINOMA – BREAST

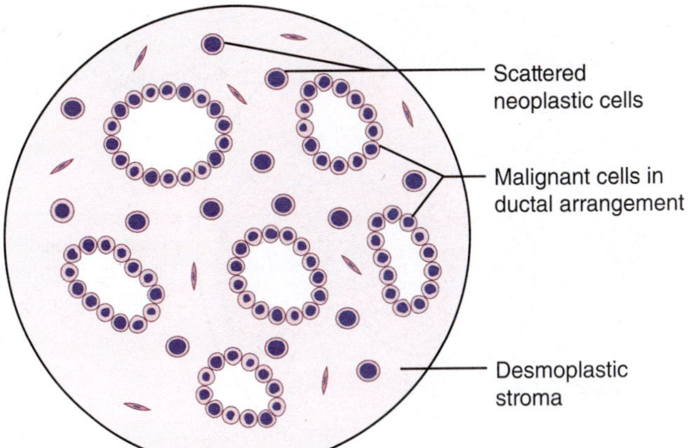

RENAL CELL CARCINOMA (CLEAR CELL TYPE)

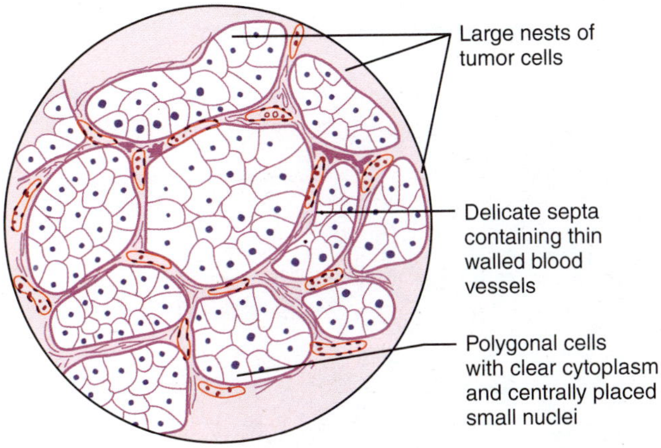

SEMINOMA

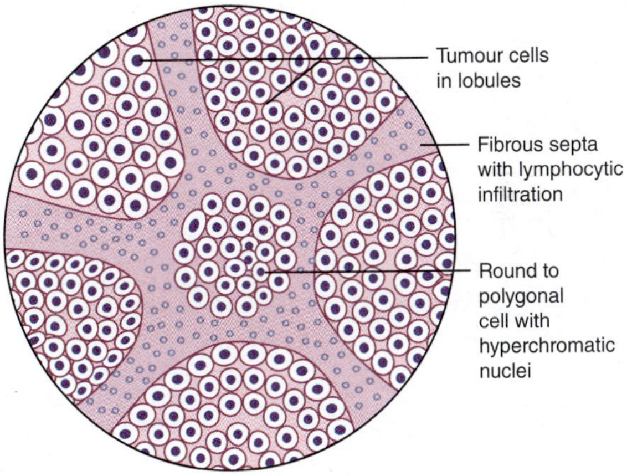

FIBROADENOMA – BREAST

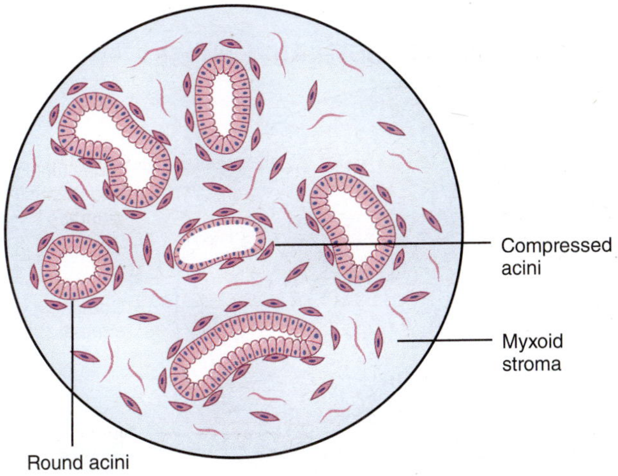

COLLOID GOITRE

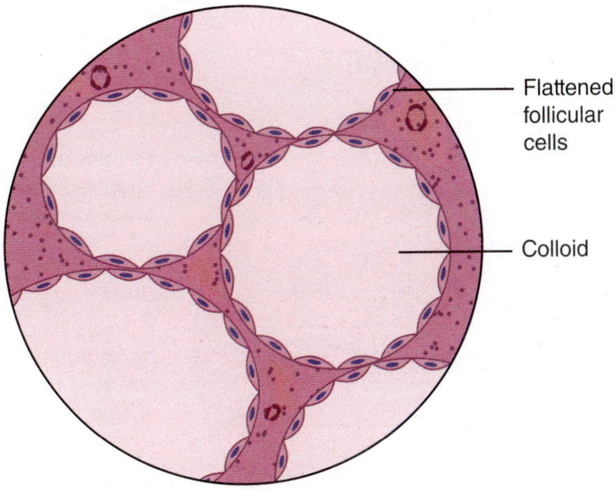

MULTINODULAR GOITRE

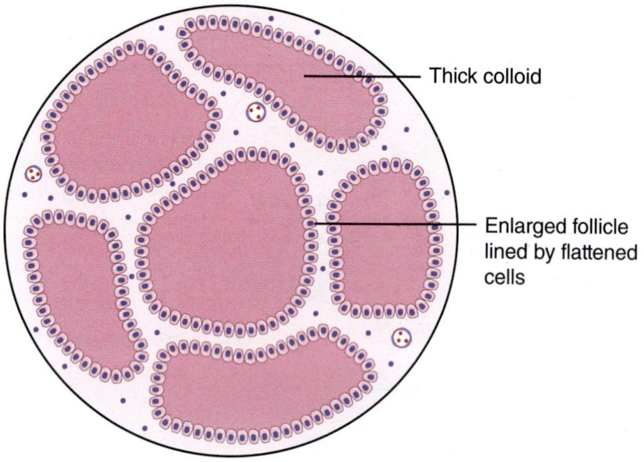

PAPILLARY CARCINOMA – THYROID

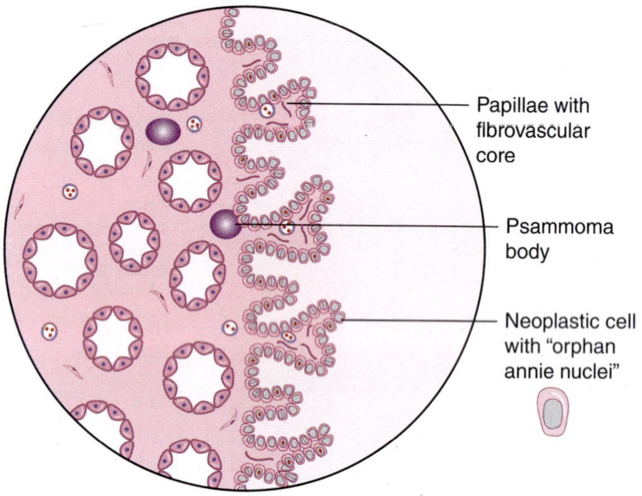

TOXIC GOITRE

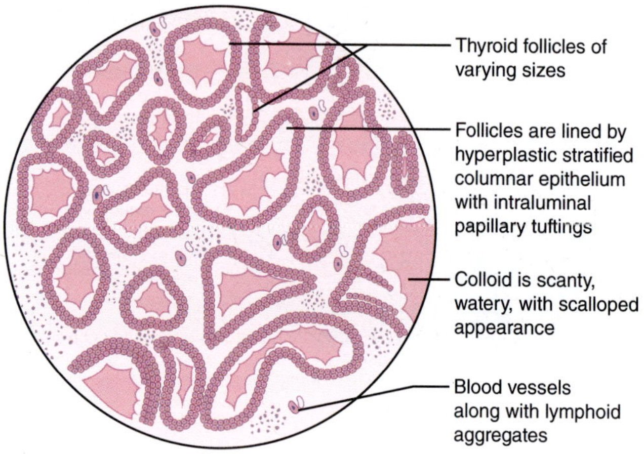

FOLLICULAR CARCINOMA - THYROID

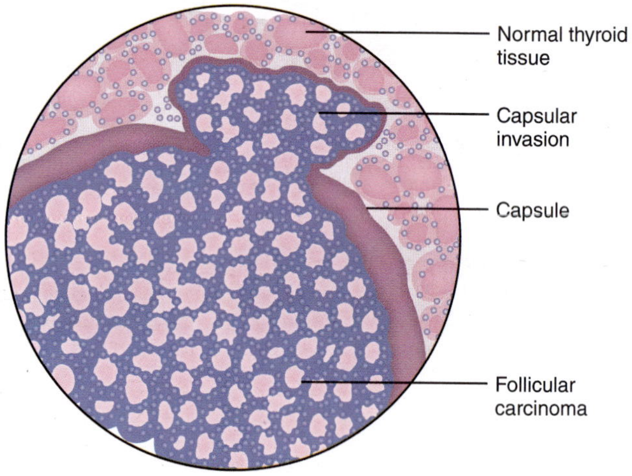

HASHIMOTO'S THYROIDITIS

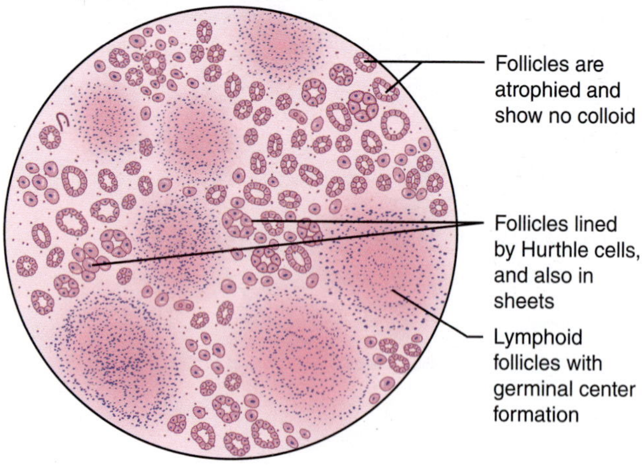

ENDOMETRIUM – PROLIFERATIVE PHASE

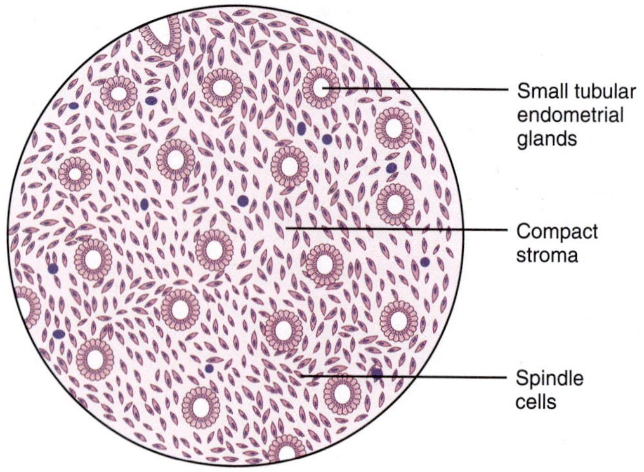

ENDOMETRIUM – SECRETORY PHASE

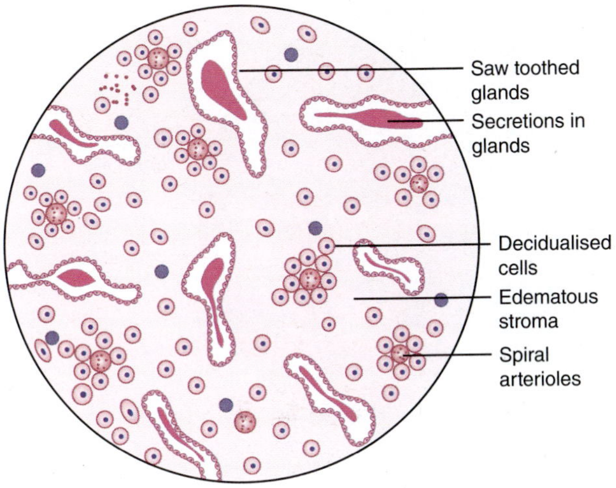

WELL DIFFERENTIATED ENDOMETRIAL ADENOCARCINOMA

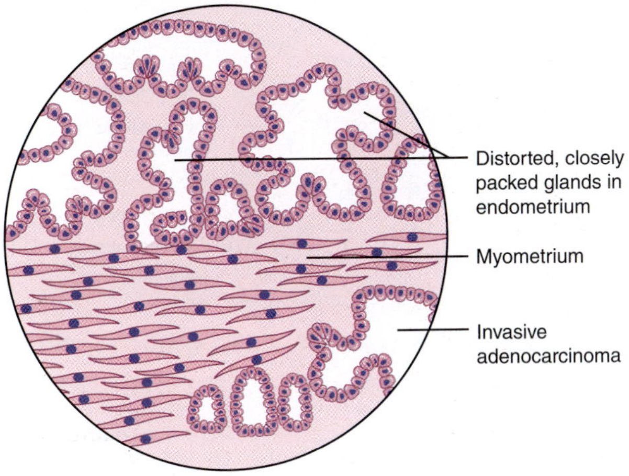

LEIOMYOMA

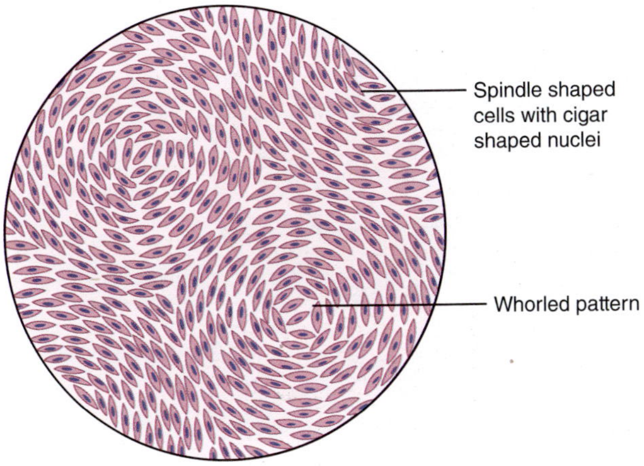

BENIGN PROSTATIC HYPERPLASIA

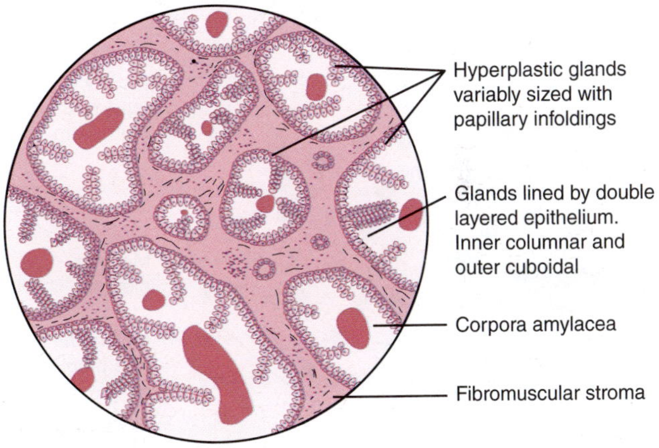

HYDATIDIFORM MOLE

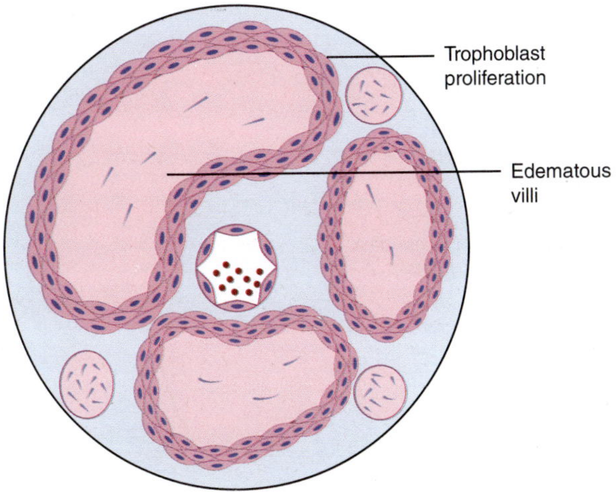

BASAL CELL CARCINOMA

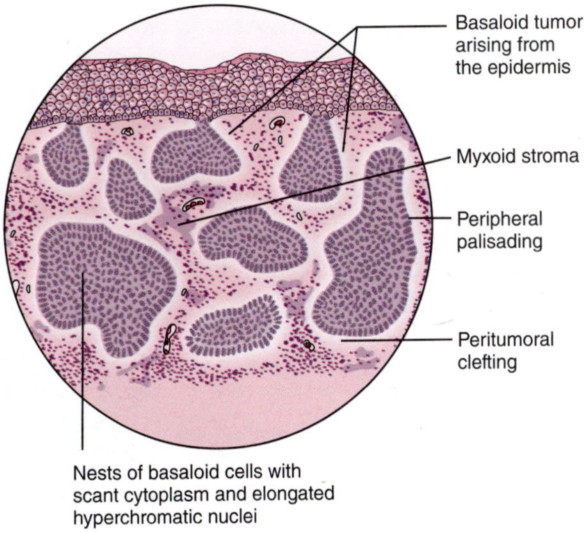

SQUAMOUS CELL CARCINOMA

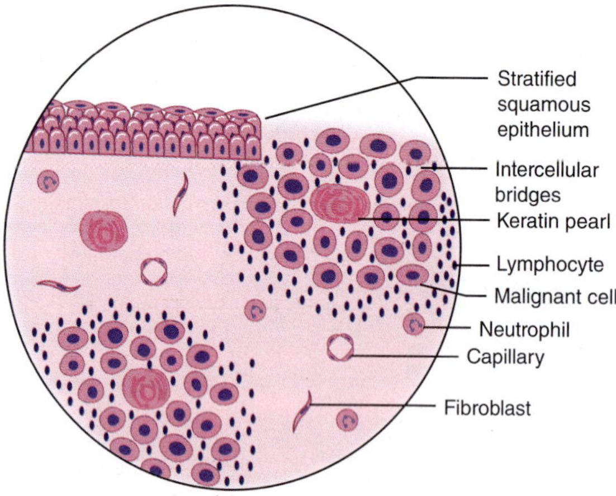

GIANT CELL TUMOUR (OSTEOCLASTOMA)

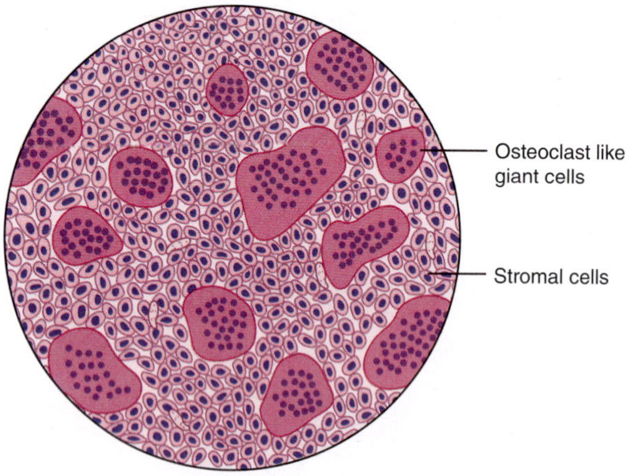

MALIGNANT MELANOMA

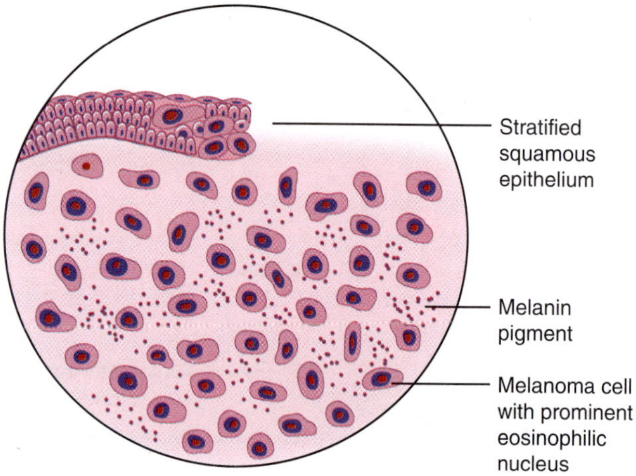

OSTEOSARCOMA

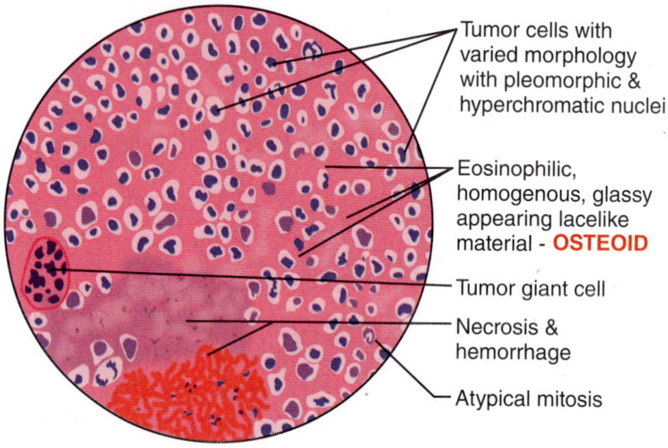

MENINGIOMA

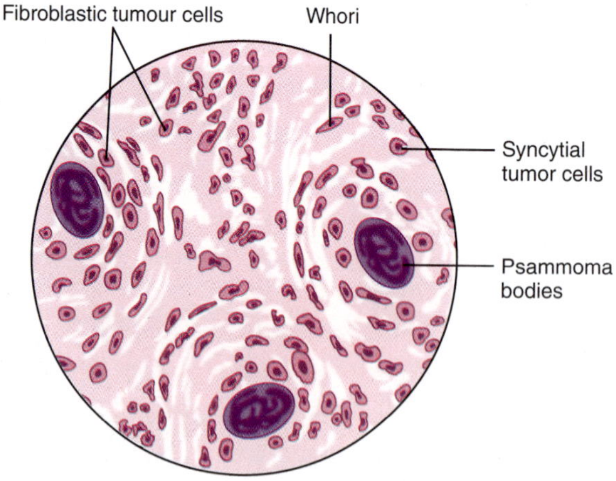

CYTOLOGY

TUBERCULOUS LYMPH NODE

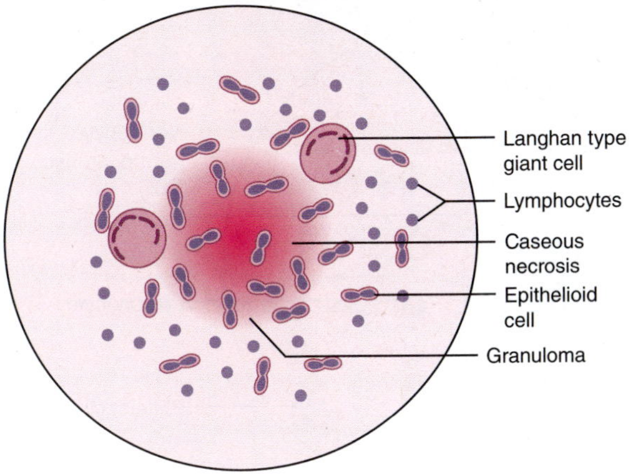

ASCITIC FLUID – POSITIVE FOR MALIGNANCY

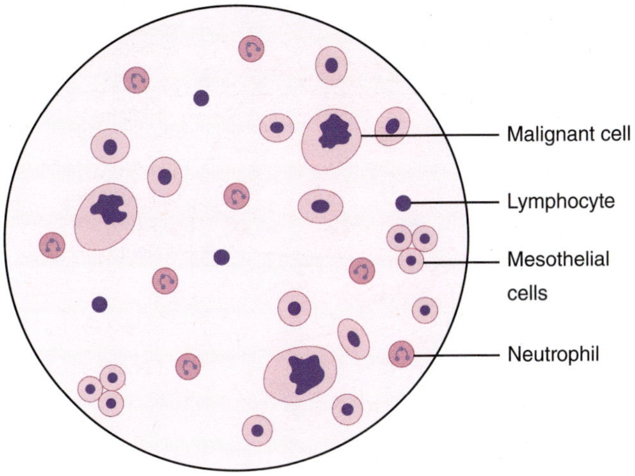

FIBROADENOMA BREAST

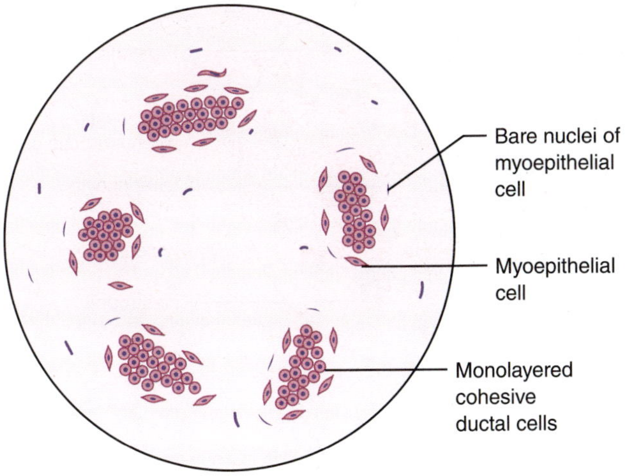

PAP SMEAR (ESTROGENIC PHASE)

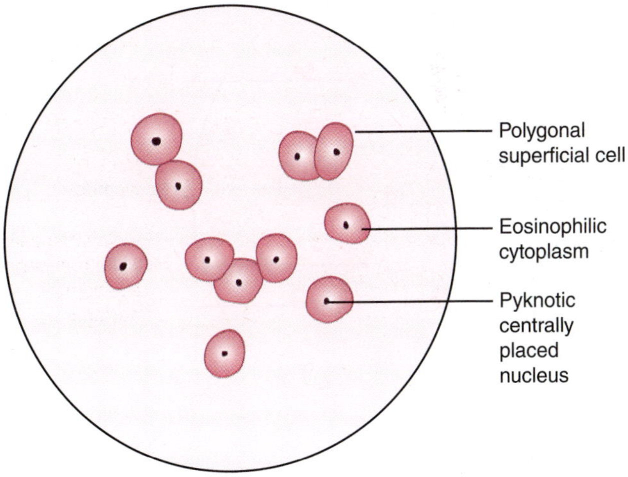

CARCINOMA BREAST

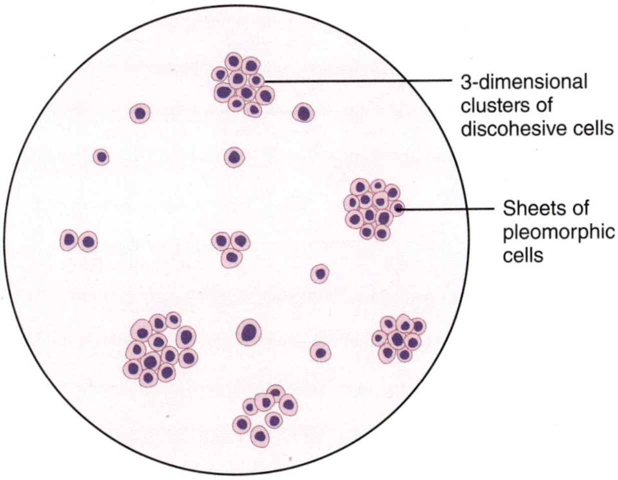

PAP SMEAR (PROGESTOGENIC PHASE)

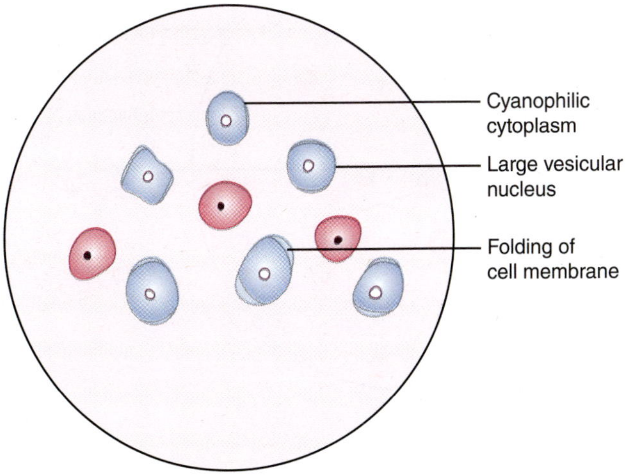

HEMATOLOGY

MICROCYTIC HYPOCHROMIC ANEMIA

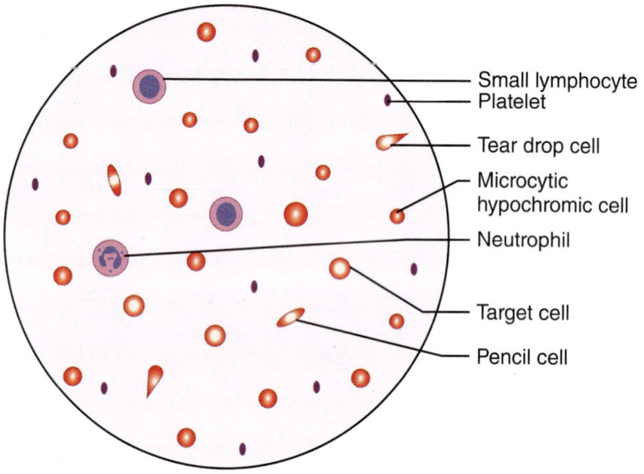

THROMBOCYTOSIS

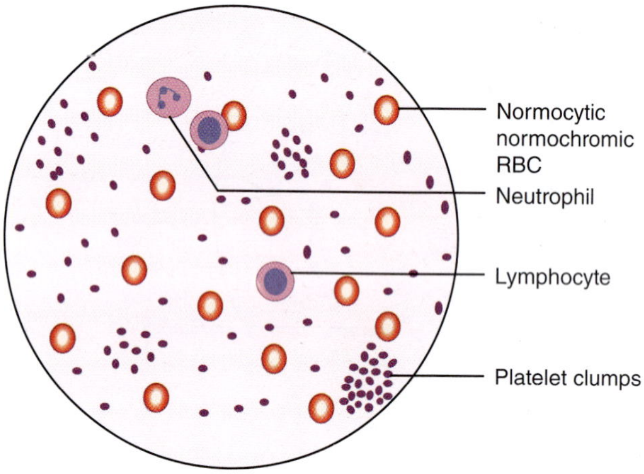

NEUTROPHILIA

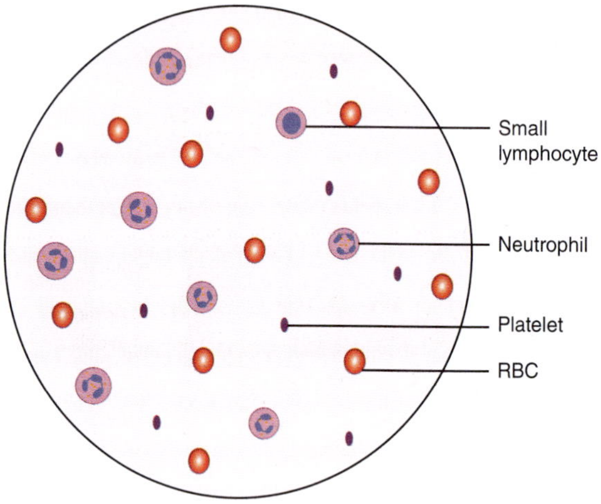

THROMBOCYTOPENIA

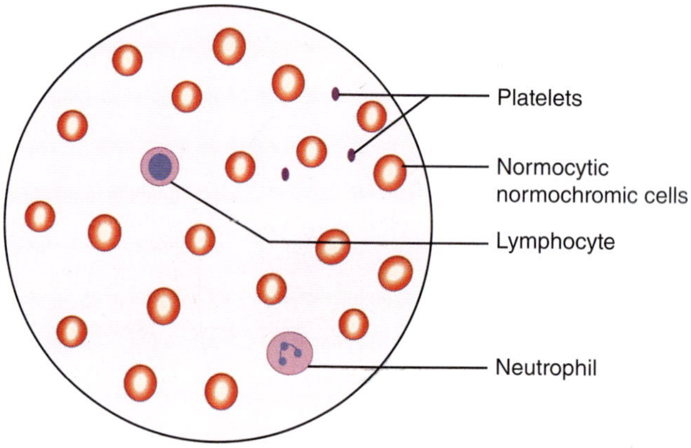

EOSINOPHILIA

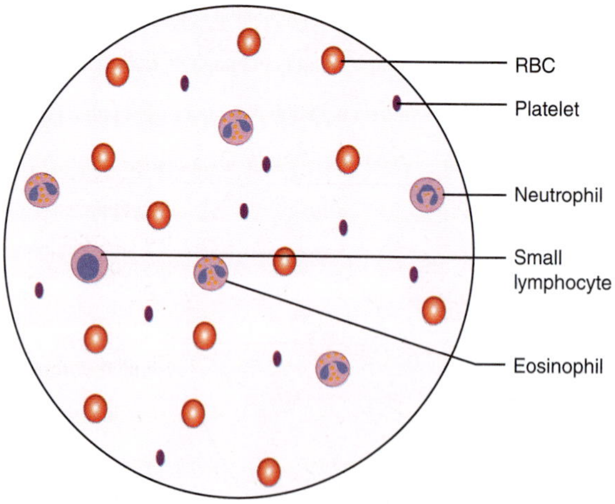

HEMATOLOGY –THALASSEMIA

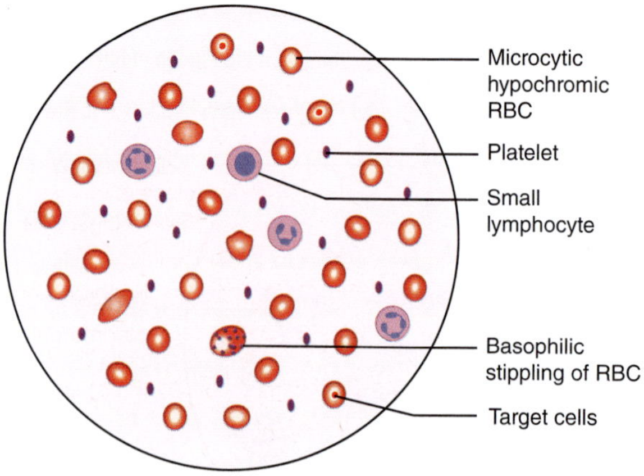

MEGALOBLASTIC ANEMIA

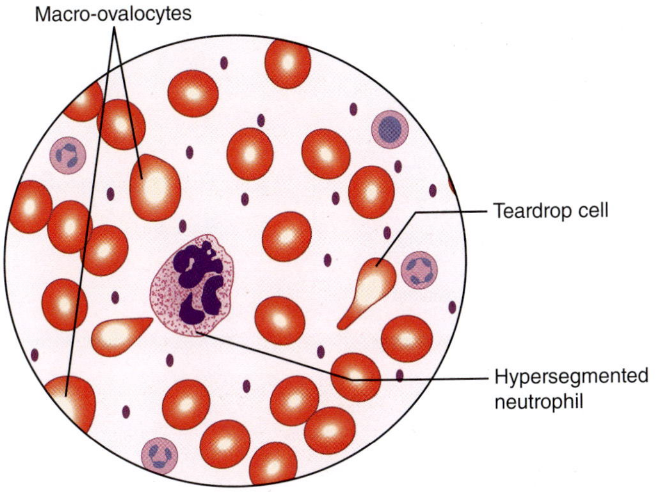

SICKLE CELL ANEMIA

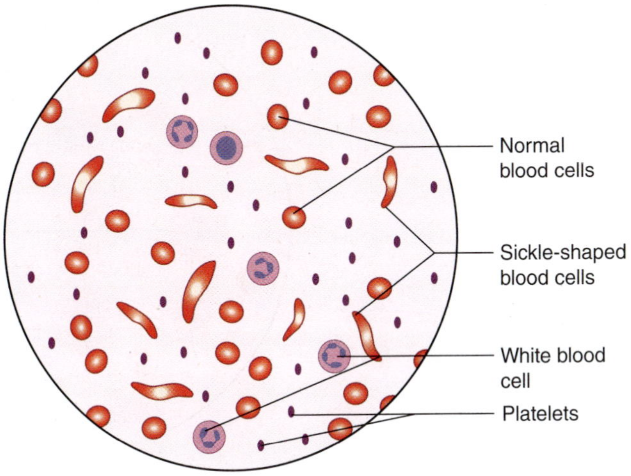

MALARIAL PARASITE POSITIVE – PLASMODIUM VIVAX

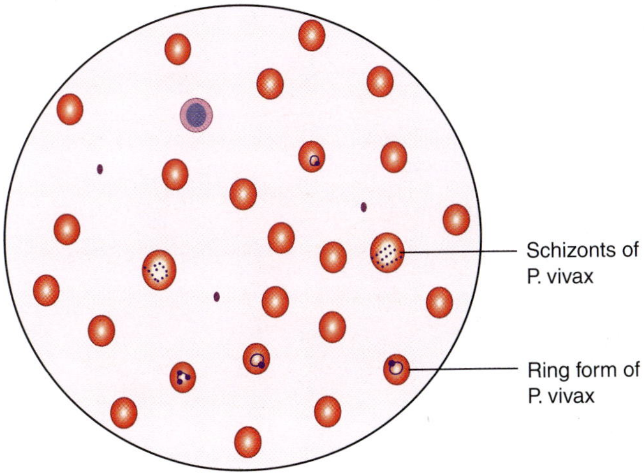

ACUTE MYELOID LEUKEMIA

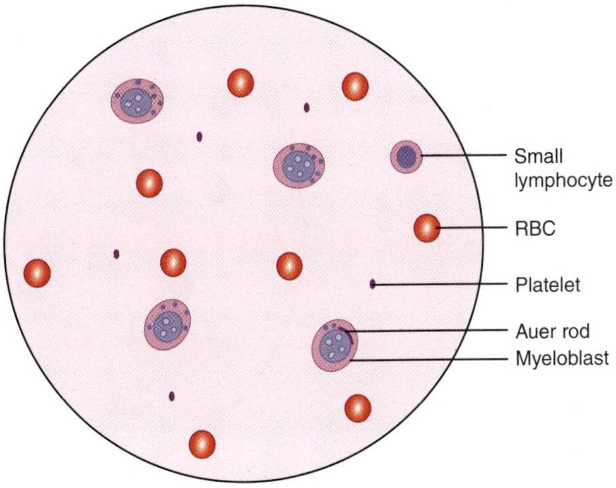

IDIOPATHIC THROMBOCYTOPENIA – BONE MARROW ASPIRATE

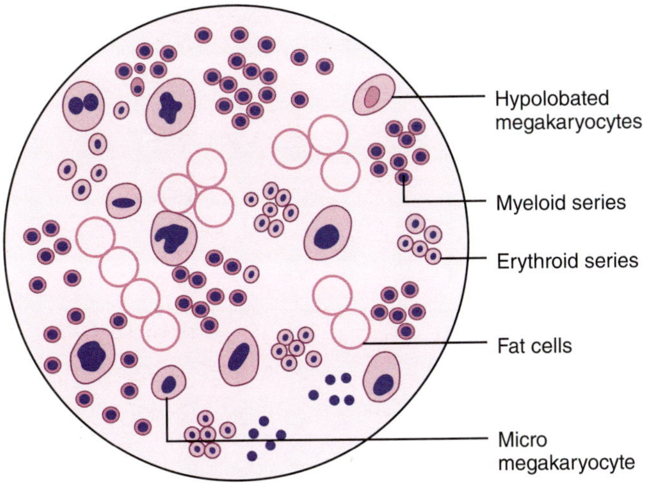

ACUTE LYMPHOBLASTIC LEUKEMIA

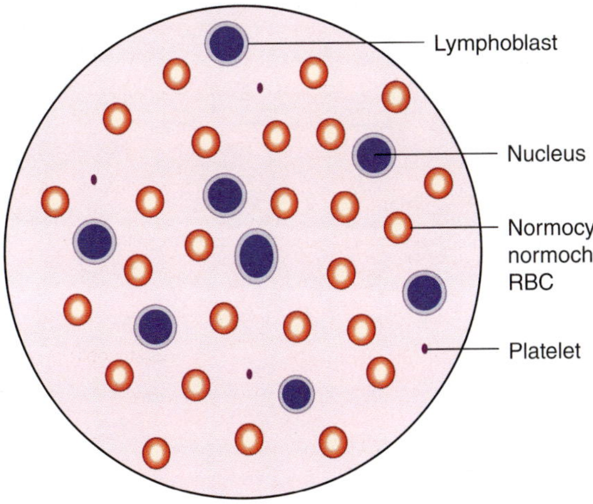

CHRONIC MYELOID LEUKEMIA

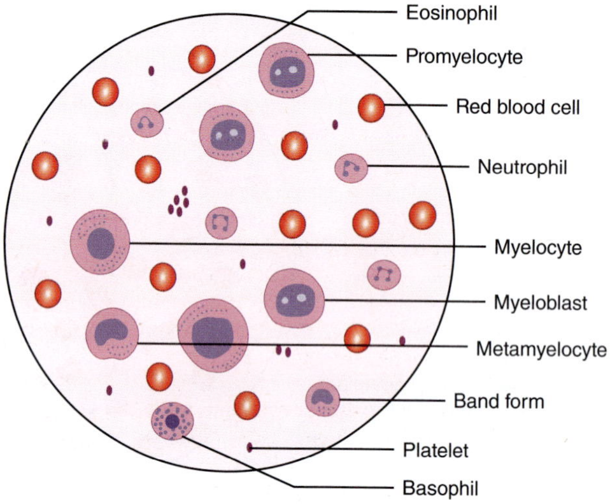

CHRONIC LYMPHOCYTIC LEUKEMIA

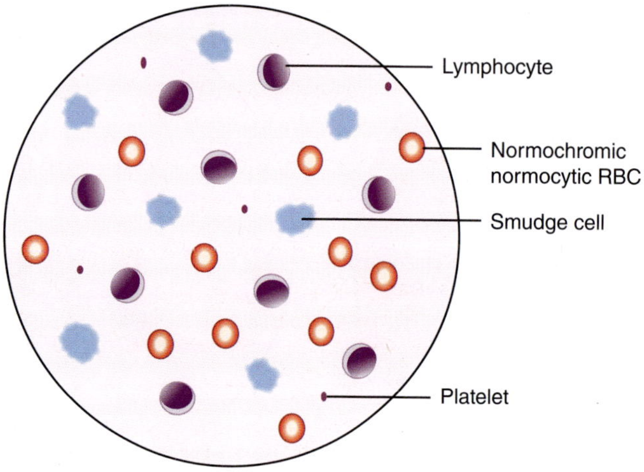

Index

A

B

D

E

F

G

L

M

N

Q

R

S

T